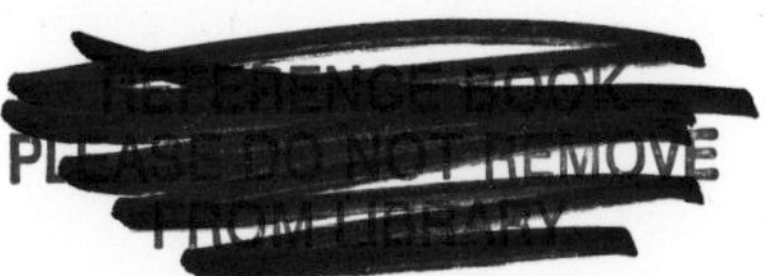

OPERATIVE TECHNIQUES IN FOOT AND ANKLE SURGERY

ALSO AVAILABLE IN THIS SERIES

OPERATIVE TECHNIQUES IN FOOT AND ANKLE SURGERY

Editor: Mark E. Easley
Editor-In-Chief Sam W. Wiesel

OPERATIVE TECHNIQUES IN ORTHOPAEDIC PEDIATRIC SURGERY

Editor: John M. Flynn
Editor-in-Chief Sam W. Wiesel

OPERATIVE TECHNIQUES IN ORTHOPAEDIC TRAUMA SURGERY

Editors: Paul Tornetta III
Gerald R. Williams
Matthew L. Ramsey
Thomas R. Hunt III
Editor-in-Chief Sam W. Wiesel

OPERATIVE TECHNIQUES IN SHOULDER AND ELBOW SURGERY

Editors: Gerald R. Williams & Matthew L. Ramsey
Editor-in-Chief Sam W. Wiesel

OPERATIVE TECHNIQUES IN SPORTS MEDICINE SURGERY

Editor: Mark D. Miller
Editor-in-Chief Sam W. Wiesel

OPERATIVE TECHNIQUES IN ADULT RECONSTRUCTION SURGERY

Editors: Jarvad Parvizi & Richard H. Rothman
Editor-in-Chief Sam W. Wiesel

OPERATIVE TECHNIQUES IN HAND, WRIST, AND FOREARM SURGERY

Editors: Thomas R. Hunt III
John M. Flynn
Editor-in-Chief Sam W. Wiesel

OPERATIVE TECHNIQUES IN FOOT AND ANKLE SURGERY

Mark E. Easley, MD
EDITOR

Associate Professor of Orthopaedic Surgery
Co-Director, Foot and Ankle Fellowship
Duke University Medical Center
Durham, North Carolina

Sam W. Wiesel, MD
EDITOR-IN-CHIEF

Professor and Chair
Department of Orthopaedic Surgery
Georgetown University Medical School
Washington, DC

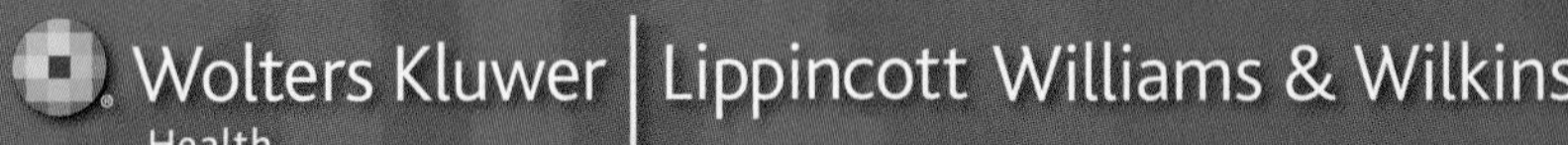
Wolters Kluwer | Lippincott Williams & Wilkins
Health
Philadelphia • Baltimore • New York • London
Buenos Aires • Hong Kong • Sydney • Tokyo

Acquisitions Editor: Robert A. Hurley
Developmental Editor: Grace Caputo, Dovetail Content Solutions
Product Manager: Dave Murphy
Manufacturing Manager: Ben Rivera
Design Manager: Doug Smock
Compositor: Maryland Composition/ASI
Copyright 2011

Two Commerce Square
2001 Market Street
Philadelphia, PA 19103

Printed in China

Library of Congress Cataloging-in-Publication Data

Operative techniques in foot and ankle surgery / Sam W. Wiesel, editor-in chief ; Mark E. Easley, editor.
p. ; cm.
Chapters derived from Operative techniques in orthopaedic surgery / editor-in-chief, Sam Wiesel. c2010.
Includes bibliographical references and index.
Summary: "Operative Techniques in Foot and Ankle Surgery provides full-color, step-by-step explanations of all operative procedures in podiatry. It contains the chapters on the foot and ankle from Sam W. Wiesel's Operative Techniques in Orthopaedic Surgery. Written by experts from leading institutions around the world, this superbly illustrated volume focuses on mastery of operative techniques and also provides a thorough understanding of how to select the best procedure, how to avoid complications, and what outcomes to expect. The user-friendly format is ideal for quick preoperative review of the steps of a procedure. Each procedure is broken down step by step, with full-color intraoperative photographs and drawings that demonstrate how to perform each technique.
Extensive use of bulleted points and tables allows quick and easy reference. Each clinical problem is discussed in the same format:
definition, anatomy, physical exams, pathogenesis, natural history, physical findings, imaging and diagnostic studies, differential diagnosis, non-operative management, surgical management, pearls and pitfalls, postoperative care, outcomes, and complications. To ensure that the material fully meets residents' needs, the text was reviewed by a Residency Advisory Board"—Provided by publisher.
ISBN 978-1-60831-904-6 (hardback)
1. Foot—Surgery. 2. Ankle—Surgery. I. Wiesel, Sam W. II. Easley, Mark E. III. Operative techniques in orthopaedic surgery.
[DNLM: 1. Foot—surgery. 2. Ankle—surgery. 3. Orthopedic Procedures. WE 880 O6153 2011]
RD563.O655 2011
617.5'85—dc22

2010018356

Care has been taken to confirm the accuracy of the information presented and to describe generally accepted practices. However, the authors, editors, and publisher are not responsible for errors or omissions or for any consequences from application of the information in this book and make no warranty, expressed or implied, with respect to the currency, completeness, or accuracy of the contents of the publication. Application of the information in a particular situation remains the professional responsibility of the practitioner.

The authors, editors, and publisher have exerted every effort to ensure that drug selection and dosage set forth in this text are in accordance with current recommendations and practice at the time of publication. However, in view of ongoing research, changes in government regulations, and the constant flow of information relating to drug therapy and drug reactions, the reader is urged to check the package insert for each drug for any change in indications and dosage and for added warnings and precautions. This is particularly important when the recommended agent is a new or infrequently employed drug.

Some drugs and medical devices presented in the publication have Food and Drug Administration (FDA) clearance for limited use in restricted research settings. It is the responsibility of the health care provider to ascertain the FDA status of each drug or device planned for use in their clinical practice.

To purchase additional copies of this book, call our customer service department at (800) 638-3030 or fax orders to (301) 223-2320. International customers should call (301) 223-2300.

Visit Lippincott Williams & Wilkins on the Internet at LWW.com. Lippincott Williams & Wilkins customer service representatives are available from 8:30 am to 6 pm, EST.

CCS0311

10 9 8 7 6 5 4 3 2

Dedication

To my wife, Mary Lynne, and my children, Ford, Benson, and Charlotte, for patiently tolerating the time I spent away from them while I pursued this academic endeavor, and to my parents, Barbara and Dennis Easley, whose guidance and support prepared me for a career in academic medicine. —MEE

CONTENTS

SECTION V SPORTS-RELATED PROCEDURES FOR ANKLE AND HINDFOOT

CONTRIBUTORS

Jorge I. Acevedo, MD
Associate Clinical Faculty
Department of Orthopedic Surgery
University of Miami
Wellington Regional Medical Center
Royal Palm Beach, Florida

Samuel B. Adams, Jr., MD
Resident
Department of Orthopaedic Surgery
Duke University Medical Center
Durham, North Carolina

Robert S. Adelaar, MD
Medical College of Virginia
Richmond, Virginia

Oladapo Alade, MD
Private Practice
Houston, Texas

Richard Alvarez, MD
Southern Orthopedic Foot Center
Chattanooga, Tennessee

Annunziato Amendola, MD
Professor and Callaghan Chair
Department of Orthopaedic Surgery
University of Iowa
Iowa City, Iowa

John G. Anderson, MD
Associate Professor
Michigan State University College of Human Medicine
Co-Director
Grand Rapids Orthopaedic Foot and Ankle Fellowship
Assistant Program Director
Grand Rapids Orthopaedic Residency Program
Orthopaedic Associates of Michigan
Grand Rapids, Michigan

Robert B. Anderson, MD
Chief, Foot and Ankle Service
Department of Orthopaedic Surgery
Carolinas Medical Center, OrthoCarolina
Charlotte, North Carolina

Michael S. Aronow, MD
Associate Professor
Department of Orthopaedic Surgery
University of Connecticut Health Center
Farmington, Connecticut

Mathieu Assal, MD
Orthopaedic Surgery Service
Geneva University Hospital
Geneva, Switzerland

Vikrant Azad, MD
Research Fellow
Department of Orthopaedics
University of Medicine and Dentistry of New Jersey
NJ Medical School
Newark, New Jersey

Alexej Barg, MD
Orthopaedic Clinic
Kantonsspital
Lirstal, Switzerland

Michael Barnett, MD
Assistant Professor of Orthopaedic Surgery
Director of Undergraduate Orthopaedic Education
Wright State University Boonshoft School of Medicine
Dayton, Ohio

Heather Barske, MD
Department of Orthopaedic Surgery
University of Manitoba
Winnipeg, Manitoba, Canada

Douglas N. Beaman, MD
Clinical Assistant Professor
Department of Orthopaedic Surgery
Oregon Health Sciences University
Summit Orthopaedics
Portland, Oregon

Christoph Becher, MD
Department of Orthopaedic Surgery
Hannover Medical School
Hannover, Germany

Karl Bergmann, MD
Department of Orthopaedics
University of Medicine and Dentistry of New Jersey
NJ Medical School
Newark, New Jersey

Gregory C. Berlet, MD, FRCS(C)
Chief, Foot and Ankle
Department of Orthopedics
Orthopedic Foot and Ankle Center
Ohio State University
Westerville, Ohio

James L. Beskin, MD
Clinical Assistant Professor
Department of Orthopedics
Tulane University
Director, Foot & Ankle Section
Orthopedic Residency Program
Atlanta Medical Center
Atlanta, Georgia

Eric M. Bluman, MD, PhD
Assistant Professor
Department of Orthopaedic Surgery
Harvard University
Brigham and Women's Hospital
Boston, Massachusetts

Donald R. Bohay, MD
Associate Professor
Department of Orthopaedic Surgery
Michigan State University
Orthopaedic Associates of Michigan
Grand Rapids, Michigan

Michel Bonnin, MD
Department of Orthopaedic Surgery
Centre Orthopédique Santy
Lyon, France

Michael E. Brage, MD
Assistant Professor of Clinical Orthopedics
Director, Foot and Ankle Services
Department of Orthopaedic Surgery
University of California, San Diego
South County Orthopaedic Specialists
Laguna Woods, California

Lloyd C. Briggs, Jr., MD
Associate Clinical Professor
Department of Orthopaedic Surgery
Orthopaedic Institute of Ohio
Lima, Ohio

Matteo Cadossi, MD
PhD Student
Department of Human Anatomy and Pathophysiology of Musculoskeletal System
2nd Orthopaedic Department
Istituto Orthopedico Rizzoli
University of Bologna
Bologna, Italy

John T. Campbell, MD
Institute for Foot and Ankle Reconstruction at Mercy
Mercy Medical Center
Baltimore, Maryland

Fabio Catani, MD
Professor of Orthopaedics
Department of Orthopaedic Surgery
Istituto Orthopedico Rizzoli
University of Bologna
Bologna, Italy

Wen Chao, MD
Department of Orthopaedic Surgery
PennCare—Pennsylvania Orthopaedic Foot and Ankle Surgeons
Philadelphia, Pennsylvania

Timothy Charlton, MD
Assistant Professor of Clinical Orthopaedics
Keck School of Medicine
University of Southern California
USC Orthopaedic Surgery Associates
Los Angeles, California

Christopher P. Chiodo, MD
Brigham Foot and Ankle Center at Faulkner Hospital
Boston, Massachusetts

Thomas O. Clanton, MD
Professor of Orthopaedic Surgery
The University of Texas Medical School at Houston
Director, Foot and Ankle Sports Medicine
The Steadman Clinic
Vail, Colorado

Michael P. Clare, MD
Director of Fellowship Education, Foot & Ankle Fellowship
Florida Orthopaedic Institute
Tampa, Florida

J. Chris Coetzee, MD, FRSCS
Minnesota Orthopedic Sports Medicine Institute
Eden Prairie, Minnesota

Bruce Cohen, MD
Department of Orthopedic Surgery
Carolina Medical Center
Charlotte, North Carolina

Jean-Alain Colombier, MD
Department of Orthopaedic Surgery
Clinique de L'Union
Saint Jean, France

Michael J. Coughlin, MD
Chief of Orthopaedics
St. Alphonsus Regional Medical Center
Clinical Professor of Surgery
Department of Orthopaedics
Oregon Health Sciences University
Boise, Idaho

Justin S. Cummins, MD, MS
Department of Orthopedic Surgery
SMDC Health System
Duluth, Minnesota

Richard J. deAsla, MD
Co-Director, Foot and Ankle Unit
Instructor
Department of Orthopaedic Surgery
Harvard Medical School
Boston, Massachusetts

Bryan D. Den Hartog, MD
Assistant Clinical Professor
Department of Orthopaedics
Sanford School of Medicine
Rapid City, South Dakota

Jonathan T. Deland, MD
Chief, Foot and Ankle Service
Associate Attending Orthopaedic Surgeon
Hospital for Special Surgery
Associate Professor
Department of Orthopaedic Surgery
Weill Cornell Medical College
New York, New York

James K. DeOrio, MD
Associate Professor
Division of Orthopedic Surgery
Department of Surgery
Duke University
Durham, North Carolina

Matthew J. DeOrio, MD
The Orthopedic Center
Huntsville, Alabama

Benedict F. DiGiovanni, MD
Associate Professor of Orthopaedics
University of Rochester Medical Center
Rochester, New York

Christopher W. DiGiovanni, MD
Director and Professor
Brown University Orthopaedic Residency Program
Chief, Foot and Ankle Service
Department of Orthopaedic Surgery
The Warren Alpert School of Medicine
Brown University
Rhode Island Hospital
Providence, Rhode Island

Brian Donley, MD
Director, Center for Foot and Ankle
Department of Orthopaedic Surgery
Cleveland Clinic
Cleveland, Ohio

Thomas Dreher, MD
Orthopaedic Department
University of Heidelberg
Heidelberg, Germany

Brad Dresher, MD
Department of Orthopaedics
Penrose St. Francis Medical Center
Colorado Springs, Colorado

Mark E. Easley, MD
Associate Professor of Orthopaedic Surgery
Co-Director, Foot and Ankle Fellowship
Duke University Medical Center
Durham, North Carolina

Patrick Ebeling, MD
Associate Clinical Instructor
Department of Orthopaedic Surgery
University of Minnesota
Burnsville, Minnesota

Andrew J. Elliott, MD
Assistant Professor
Department of Orthopaedic Surgery
Hospital for Special Surgery
New York, New York

Cesare Faldini, MD
Professor of Orthopaedics
Department of Human Anatomy and Pathophysiology of Musculoskeletal System
2nd Orthopaedic Department
Istituto Orthopedico Rizzoli
University of Bologna
Bologna, Italy

Nicholas A. Ferran, MBBS, MRCSEd
Specialist Registrar
Department of Trauma and Orthopaedics
Lincoln County Hospital
Lincolnshire, United Kingdom

Lamar L. Fleming, MD
Professor and Chairman
Department of Orthopaedics
Emory University School of Medicine
Atlanta, Georgia

Adolph S. Flemister, Jr., MD
Associate Professor
Department of Orthopaedics
University of Rochester
Rochester, New York

Austin T. Fragomen, MD
Limb Lengthening Specialist
Fellowship Director, Director of Education, and Director of Limb Lengthening and Deformity Service
Hospital for Special Surgery
New York, New York

Carol Frey, MD
Assistant Clinical Professor of Orthopedic Surgery (Volunteer)
University of California, Los Angeles
Manhattan Beach, California

Delan Gaines, MD
Department of Sports Medicine
Southeastern Orthopedic Center
Savannah, Georgia

Richard E. Gellman, MD
Clinical Assistant Professor
Department of Orthopaedic Surgery
Oregon Health Sciences University
Summit Orthopaedics
Portland, Oregon

Sandro Giannini, MD
Professor of Orthopaedics
Department of Human Anatomy and Pathophysiology of Musculoskeletal System
2nd Orthopaedic Department
Istituto Orthopedico Rizzoli
University of Bologna
Bologna, Italy

Brian D. Giordano, MD
Department of Orthopaedics
University of Rochester
Rochester, New York

Jason P. Glover, DPM
Department of Foot and Ankle Surgery
Rutherford Hospital
Rutherfordton, North Carolina

John S. Gould, MD
Professor of Surgery/Orthopaedics
University of Alabama at Birmingham
Birmingham, Alabama

Gregory P. Guyton, MD
Department of Orthopedic Surgery
Union Memorial Hospital
Baltimore, Maryland

Steven L. Haddad, MD
Associate Professor of Clinical Orthopaedic Surgery
University of Chicago Pritzker School of Medicine
Section Head, Foot and Ankle Surgery
NorthShore University HealthCare Systems
Illinois Bone and Joint Institute, LLC
Glenview, Illinois

Sigvard T. Hansen, Jr., MD
Professor
Director, Sigvard T. Hansen, Jr., MD Foot and Ankle Institute
Department of Orthopaedics and Sports Medicine
University of Washington
Seattle, Washington

Paul Hamilton, BMedSci, FRCS(Tr&Orth)
Senior Clinical Fellow
Department of Orthopaedics
Guy's and St. Thomas' NHS Foundation Trust
London, England

William G. Hamilton, MD
Clinical Professor
Department of Orthopedic Surgery
Columbia University College of Physicians and Surgeons
New York, New York

Thomas G. Harris, MD
Assistant Professor
Department of Orthopaedics
UCLA-Harbor Medical Center
Torrance, California

Paul J. Hecht, MD
Associate Professor
Department of Orthopaedic Surgery
Dartmouth Hitchcock Medical Center
Lebanon, New Hampshire

W. Bryce Henderson, BSc, MD, FRCSC
Chief of Orthopedics
Department of Orthopedic Surgery
Red Deer Hospital, Central Alberta
Alberta, Canada

John E. Herzenberg, MD, FRCSC
Director, International Center for Limb Lengthening
Rubin Institute for Advanced Orthopedics
Sinai Hospital of Baltimore
Baltimore, Maryland

Beat Hintermann, MD
Associate Professor of Medicine
Orthopaedic Clinic
University of Basel
Liestal, Switzerland

Stefan G. Hofstaetter, MD
Orthopaedic Senior Resident
Department of Orthopaedics
Klinikum Wels-Grieskirchen
Wels, Austria

George B. Holmes, Jr., MD
Assistant Professor
Director, Section of Foot and Ankle
Rush University Medical Center
Westchester, Illinois

Jason M. Hurst, MD
Associate Partner
Joint Implant Surgeons
New Albany, Ohio

James J. Hutson, Jr., MD
Associate Clinical Professor
Department of Orthopedic Surgery
Miller School of Medicine
University of Miami
Miami, Florida

Christopher F. Hyer, DPM, FACFAS
Co-Director, Foot and Ankle Fellowship
Orthopedic Foot & Ankle Center
Westerville, Ohio

Clifford L. Jeng, MD
Institute for Foot and Ankle Reconstruction
Mercy Medical Center
Baltimore, Maryland

Shine John, DPM, AACFAS
Private Practitioner
Foot Specialists
Georgetown, Texas

Catherine E. Johnson, MD
Department of Orthopaedic Surgery
Massachusetts General Hospital
Watertown, Massachusetts

Jeffrey E. Johnson, MD
Associate Professor
Chief, Foot and Ankle Service
Department of Orthopaedic Surgery
Barnes-Jewish Hospital at Washington University Medical Center
St. Louis, Missouri

Thierry Judet, MD
Chief
Department of Orthopedics
Hopital Raymond Poincare
Garches, France

Kevin L. Kirk, DO
Chief
Orthopedic Surgery Service
San Antonio Military Medical Center
Houston, Texas

Alex J. Kline, MD
Department of Orthopaedic Surgery
University of Pittsburgh Medical Center
Pittsburgh, Pennsylvania

Markus Knupp, MD
Department of Orthopaedics
Kantonsspital Liestal
Liestal, Switzerland

Sameh A. Labib, MD
Assistant Professor of Orthopedic Surgery
Director of Foot and Ankle Service
Emory University
Atlanta, Georgia

Bradley M. Lamm, DPM, FACFAS
Head, Foot and Ankle Surgery
International Center for Limb Lengthening
Rubin Institute for Advanced Orthopedics
Sinai Hospital of Baltimore
Baltimore, Maryland

Geoffrey S. Landis, DO
Tucson Orthopaedic Institute Oro Valley
Oro Valley, Arizona

Johnny T. C. Lau, MD, MSc, FRCSC
Assistant Professor of Surgery
University Health Network – Toronto Western Division
Toronto, Ontario, Canada

Ian L. D. Le, MD
Department of Orthopaedic Surgery
Duke University Medical Center
Durham, North Carolina

Alberto Leardini, DPhil
Movement Analysis Laboratory
Istituto Orthopedico Rizzoli
Bologna, Italy

Simon Lee, MD
Assistant Professor
Department of Orthopaedic Surgery
Rush University Medical Center
Westchester, Illinois

Johnny Lin, MD
Assistant Professor
Department of Orthopaedic Surgery
Rush University Medical Center
Westchester, Illinois

Sheldon Lin, MD
Associate Professor
Department of Orthopaedics
University of Medicine and Dentistry of New Jersey
NJ Medical School
Newark, New Jersey

Umile Giuseppe Longo, MD
Consultant
Department of Orthopaedic and Trauma Surgery
Campus Biomedico University
Rome, Italy

Deianira Luciani, MD
PhD Student
Department of Human Anatomy and Pathophysiology of Musculoskeletal System
2nd Orthopaedic Department
Istituto Orthopedico Rizzoli
University of Bologna
Bologna, Italy

Nicola Maffulli, MD, MS, PhD, FRCS(Orth.)
Professor of Orthopaedic and Trauma Surgery
Centre for Sports and Exercise Medicine
Barts and The London School of Medicine and Dentistry
London, England

Ansar Mahmood, MD
Department of Trauma and Orthopaedic Surgery
Keele University School of Medicine
Stoke on Trent, Staffordshire, United Kingdom

Peter Mangone, MD
Department of Orthopaedic Surgery
Mission Hospitals Health System
Asheville, North Carolina
Margaret R. Pardee Hospital
Hendersonville, North Carolina

Jeffrey A. Mann, MD
Private Practice
Oakland, California

Roger A. Mann, MD
Department of Orthopaedic Surgery
Oakland Bone and Joint Specialists
Oakland, California

Arthur Manoli, MD
Department of Orthopedic Surgery
Michigan International Foot & Ankle Center
Pontiac, Michigan

Javier Maquirriain, MD, PhD
Director, Orthopaedic Department
Director, Sports Medicine Research Department
Centro Nacional de Alto Rendimiento Deportivo
Buenos Aires, Argentina

Richard M. Marks, MD, FACS
Assistant Professor
Department of Orthopaedic Surgery
Medical College of Wisconsin
Milwaukee, Wisconsin

William C. McGarvey, MD
Associate Professor
Residency Program Director
Department of Orthopaedic Surgery
University of Texas Medical School at Houston
Houston, Texas

Angus M. McBryde, MD
Director
Ankle and Foot Fellowship
American Sports Medicine Institute
St. Vincent's – Birmingham
Birmingham, Alabama

Ronan McKeown, MB, BCh, BAO, MD, FRCSI(T&O)
Craigavon Area Hospital
Portadown
Co. Armagh, Ireland

Siddhant Mehta
Research Fellow
Department of Orthopaedics
University of Medicine and Dentistry of New Jersey
NJ Medical School
Newark, New Jersey

Marc Merian-Genast, MD
Clinical Assistant Professor
Department of Orthopedics
University of Saskatoon
Regina, Saskatchewan, Canada

Stuart D. Miller, MD
Attending
Department of Orthopaedic Surgery
Union Memorial Hospital
Baltimore, Maryland

Andrew P. Molloy, FRCS(Tr & Orth), MR
Department of Trauma and Orthopaedics
University Hospital Aintree
Liverpool, England

Mark S. Myerson, MD
Institute for Foot and Ankle Reconstruction at Mercy
Mercy Medical Centre
Baltimore, Maryland

Caio Nery, MD
Professor of Medicine
Department of Orthopaedics and Traumatology
Federal University of São Paulo, Brazil
São Paulo, Brazil

Christopher W. Nicholson, MD
Department of Orthopedics
The Doctors Hospital of Tatnall
Savannah, Georgia

Florian Nickisch, MD
Assistant Professor of Orthopaedic Surgery
Department of Orthopaedics
University of Utah
Salt Lake City, Utah

James A. Nunley II, MD
Chairman and Professor
Department of Orthopaedic Surgery
Duke University
Durham, North Carolina

Tahir Ögüt, MD
Associate Professor of Medicine
Department of Orthopaedics and Traumatology
Istanbul University Cerrahpasa Medical Faculty
Istanbul, Turkey

Blake L. Ohlson, MD
Fellow
Department of Orthopaedics
Union Memorial Hospital
Baltimore, Maryland

Martin J. O'Malley, MD
Associate Professor of Orthopaedics
Hospital for Special Surgery
New York, New York

Enyi Okereke, MD[†]
Associate Professor of Orthopedic Surgery
University of Pennsylvania School of Medicine
Chief, Division of Foot and Ankle Surgery
University of Pennsylvania Health Systems
Philadelphia, Pennsylvania

Justin Orr, MD
Division of Orthopaedic Surgery
Department of Surgery
William Beaumont Army Medical Center
El Paso, Texas

Fred W. Ortmann, MD
Greensboro Orthopaedics
Greensboro, North Carolina

Thomas G. Padanilam, MD
Clinical Assistant Professor
Department of Orthopaedic Surgery
University of Toledo
Toledo, Ohio

Geert I. Pagenstert, MD
Assistant Professor
Department of Orthopaedic Surgery
University Hospital Basel
Basel, Switzerland

Dror Paley, MD, FRCSC
Director, Paley Advanced Limb Lengthening Institute
St. Mary's Hospital
West Palm Beach, Florida

Selene G. Parekh, MD, MBA
Associate Professor
Division of Orthopaedics
Department of Surgery
Duke University
Durham, North Carolina

Terrence M. Philbin, DO
Clinical Assistant Professor
Department of Orthopaedic Surgery
The Ohio State University College of Medicine and Public Health
Orthopedic Foot and Ankle Center
Weiterville, Ohio

Phinit Phisitkul, MD
Clinical Assistant Professor
Department of Orthopaedics
University of Iowa
Iowa City, Iowa

Michael S. Pinzur, MD
Professor
Department of Orthopaedic Surgery and Rehabilitation
Loyola University Medical Center
Maywood, Illinois

Gregory C. Pomeroy, MD
New England Foot and Ankle Specialists
Portland, Maine

George E. Quill, Jr., MD
Clinical Instructor of Orthopaedics
University of Louisville School of Medicine
Director of Foot and Ankle Services
Louisville Orthopaedic Clinic
Louisville, Kentucky

Steven M. Raikin, MD
Associate Professor
Director, Foot and Ankle Service
Department of Orthopaedic Surgery
Rothman Institute at Thomas Jefferson University Hospital
Philadelphia, Pennsylvania

Keri A. Reese, MD
South Bay Orthopaedic Specialists
Clinical Instructor, Volunteer
Department of Orthopaedic Surgery
University of California, Irvine, School of Medicine
Torrance, California

David R. Richardson, MD
Assistant Professor
Resident Program Director
Department of Orthopaedic Surgery
University of Tennessee—Campbell Clinic
Memphis, Tennessee

Mark A. Reiley, MD
Department of Orthopaedic Surgery
Berkeley Orthopaedic Medical Group, Inc.
Berkeley, California

Pascal Rippstein, MD
Department for Foot and Ankle Surgery
Schulthess Clinic
Zurich, Switzerland

Mark Ritter, MD
Department of Orthopedic Surgery
Methodist Sports Medicine Center
Indianapolis, Indiana

Venus R. Rivera, MD
Foot and Ankle Fellow
Department of Orthopaedic Surgery
Union Memorial Hospital
Baltimore, Maryland

Robert Rochman, MD
Private Practice
Royal Palm Beach, Florida

Matteo Romagnoli, MD
2nd Clinic of Orthopaedic Surgery
Istituto Orthopedico Rizzoli
Bologna, Italy

Michael M. Romash, MD
Orthopedic Surgeon
Orthopedic Foot and Ankle Center of Hampton Roads
Sports Medicine and Orthopedic Center
Chesapeake, Virginia

S. Robert Rozbruch, MD
Institute for Limb Lengthening and Complex Reconstruction
Hospital for Special Surgery
Weill Cornell Medical College
New York, New York

S. Robert Rozbruch, MD
Institute for Limb Lengthening and Complex Reconstruction
Hospital for Special Surgery
Weill Cornell Medical College
New York, New York

G. James Sammarco, MD, FACS
Professor
Department of Orthopaedic Surgery
Tulane University School of Medicine
Clinical Professor
Department of Orthopaedic Surgery
University of Cincinnati Medical Center
Cincinnati, Ohio

Vincent James Sammarco, MD
Department of Orthopedic Surgery
Cincinnati Sports Medicine and Orthopaedic Center
Cincinnati, Ohio

Thomas P. San Giovanni, MD
Department of Orthopedic Surgery
UHZ Sports Medicine Institute
Coral Gables, Florida

Amy Sanders, RN, BSN/PAC
Physician's Assistant
Columbia Orthopaedic Group
Columbia, Missouri

Roy W. Sanders, MD
Clinical Professor of Orthopaedics
University of South Florida
Chief, Department of Orthopaedics
Tampa General Hospital
Director, Orthopaedic Trauma Services
Florida Orthopaedic Institute
Tampa, Florida

Bruce J. Sangeorzan, MD
Professor of Orthopedics and Sports Medicine
University of Washington/Harborview Medical Center
Seattle, Washington

James Santangelo, MD
Staff Orthopaedic Surgeon
Womack Army Medical Center
Fort Bragg, North Carolina

Michael Scherb, MD
Fellow
Department of Orthopaedics
Union Memorial Hospital
Baltimore, Maryland

Aaron T. Scott, MD
Assistant Professor
Department of Orthopaedic Surgery
Wake Forest University Baptist Medical Center
Winston-Salem, North Carolina

Steven L. Shapiro, MD
Savannah, Georgia

Scott B. Shawen, MD
Assistant Professor
Department of Surgery
Uniformed Services University of Health Sciences
Bethesda, Maryland

Paul S. Shurnas, MD
Director, Foot and Ankle
Columbia Orthopaedic Group
Columbia, Missouri

Sam Singh, MD
Director, CathLab and Continuing Medical Education
San Joaquin Community Hospital
Bakersfield, California

Bertil W. Smith, MD
Department of Orthopaedic Surgery
University of California at San Diego
San Diego, California

Ronald W. Smith, MD
Associate Clinical Professor
Department of Orthopaedic Surgery
University of California at Los Angeles
Balance Orthopaedic Foot and Ankle Center
Long Beach, California

Emmanouil D. Stamatis, Lt Colonel MD, FHCOS, FACS, PhD
Orthopaedic Department
General Army Hospital
Athens, Greece

Michael M. Stephens, MSc(Bioeng.), FRCSI
Associate Professor
Department of Orthopaedic Surgery
Cappagh National Orthopaedic Hospital
Dublin, Ireland

Karen M. Sutton, MD
Assistant Professor
Department of Orthopaedic Surgery
Yale University
New Haven, Connecticut

Yoshinori Takakura, MD
Department of Orthopaedic Surgery
Nara Medical University
Nara, Japan

Virak Tan, MD
Associate Professor
Department of Orthopaedics
University of Medicine and Dentistry of New Jersey
NJ Medical School
Newark, New Jersey

Yasuhito Tanaka, MD
Department of Orthopaedic Surgery
Nara Medical University
Nara, Japan

James P. Tasto, MD
Clinical Professor
Department of Orthopaedic Surgery
University of California at San Diego
Founder, San Diego Sports Medicine & Orthopaedic Center
San Diego, California

Dean C. Taylor, MD
Professor of Orthopaedic Surgery
Co-Director, Sports Medicine Fellowship
Duke University Medical Center
Durham, North Carolina

Ahmed M. Thabet, MD, PhD
Lecturer of Orthopaedic Surgery
Benha University
Benha, Egypt

Hajo Thermann, MD, PhD
Professor
Center for Knee and Foot Surgery/Sports Trauma
ATOS Clinic Center
Heidelberg, Germany

Sandra L. Tomak, MD
Department of Orthopedic Surgery
Center for Orthopaedics
New Haven, Connecticut

Brian C. Toolan, MD
Associate Professor of Surgery, Foot and Ankle
Director, Residency Program of Orthopaedic Surgery
The University of Chicago Hospitals
Chicago, Illinois

Hans-Joerg Trnka, Univ. Doz. Dr.
Foot and Ankle Center
Vienna, Austria

H. Robert Tuten, MD
Associate Clinical Professor
Department of Orthopedic Surgery
Medical College of Virginia
Richmond, Virginia

Victor Valderrabano, MD, PhD
Professor and Chairman
Orthopaedic Department
University Hospital Basel
Basel, Switzerland

C. Niek van Dijk, MD, PhD
Professor of Medicine
Department of Orthopaedic Surgery
Academic Medical Center
University of Amsterdam
Amsterdam, The Netherlands

Francesca Vannini, MD, PhD
2nd Orthopaedic Department
Istituto Orthopedico Rizzoli
Bologna, Italy

Emilio Wagner, MD
Associate Professor
Department of Orthopedic and Trauma Surgery
Universidad del Desarrollo/Clinica Allemana
Santiago, Chile

Markus Walther, MD, PhD
Professor of Orthopaedic Surgery
Orthopaedic Hospital Munich-Harlaching
Munich, Germany

Keith L. Wapner, MD
Clinical Professor
Department of Orthopedic Surgery
Pennsylvania Hospital
University of Pennsylvania
Philadelphia, Pennsylvania

Anthony Watson, MD
Assistant Professor
Department of Orthopaedic Surgery
Drexel University College of Medicine
Philadelphia, Pennsylvania

Troy Watson, MD
Director, Foot and Ankle Institute
Department of Orthopaedic Surgery
Institute of Orthopaedic Surgery
Las Vegas, Nevada

Wolfram Wenz, MD
Head of Unit for Pediatric Orthopaedics and Foot Surgery
Department of Orthopaedics
University of Heidelberg
Heidelberg, Germany

Michael G. Wilson, MD
Assistant Professor
Department of Orthopaedic Surgery
Harvard Medical School
Brigham and Women's Hospital
Boston, Massachusetts

Dane K. Wukich, MD
Assistant Professor
Department of Orthopaedic Surgery
UPMC Cancer Center Physicians
Pittsburgh, Pennsylvania

Gilbert Yee, MD, Med, MBA, FRCSC
Department of Surgery
The Scarborough Hospital
Toronto, Ontario, Canada

Alastair Younger, MD, ChB, MSc, ChM, FRCS(C)
Ambulatory Care Physician Leader
Providence Health Care
Director, BC Foot and Ankle Clinic
Vancouver, British Columbia, Canada

PREFACE

I am honored to serve as foot and ankle section editor of *Operative Techniques in Orthopaedic Surgery*. I must admit that it was a daunting task to start a textbook from scratch. This process quickly revealed two truths: (1) this endeavor cannot be done without the unselfish contributions of this collection of outstanding foot and ankle educators and (2) such a project is never complete. I am fortunate to have so many foot and ankle experts share their techniques to make this textbook state-of-the-art. I am also fortunate to be charged with this assignment in a modern era when topics or newer techniques not included in this first edition may still be added as periodic web-based updates. I have benefitted immensely from this experience and trust that this textbook allows healthcare providers to optimize patient care.

Mark E. Easley

FOREWORD

Dr. Easley and his contributors can feel extremely satisfied with the educational product which comprises this text. This foot and ankle section of *Operative Techniques in Orthopaedic Surgery* is the most comprehensive and yet user friendly technique-based text available today. It is a must for those surgeons practicing in the subspecialty, as well as for the generalist with an occasion interest. The information provided will save many surgeons the stress that can be involved with preoperative decision making and procedural specifics.

Dr. Easley is an internationally recognized leader in the field of foot and ankle surgery and his vast professional and personal associations provided the foundation for this project, one that undoubtedly required countless hours of hard work. Dr. Easley successfully assembled a collection of renowned and world-class experts to write on subjects and techniques of which they have personal interest and vast experience. The format of these individual chapters allows for extensive exposure to the topic at hand, and yet in a manner that is easy to follow; filled with teaching pearls and potential perils. The inclusion of intraoperative color photos and illustrations rounds out the point-by-point explanation of the technique presented. The reader will find easy reference for all aspects of the entity presented, and will be quite happy to find the authors' suggestion on postoperative management as well.

As one reviews the table of contents, he/she will be amazed at the spectrum of subjects highlighted in a very organized fashion. I truly commend and thank Dr. Easley for his dedication to this project as he has provided our specialty with a state-of-the-art "go-to" instructional text. It is without a doubt the best of its class and will be a must for any foot and ankle surgeon's library. Congratulations Mark!

—Robert Anderson

My reaction to reading the table of contents was wow! This is incredibly complete and comprehensive. Indeed this text is an excellent compendium of thought from foot and ankle surgeons around the world which has been carefully assembled to give various view points, opinions ideas and alternative techniques. This has been so well put together by Mark Easley, and so very different from traditional text books on similar topics. What is going to be incredibly helpful to the reader is that this includes alternative approaches by leaders in the field covering different variations of pathology and deformity. It is an exciting and innovative textbook.

—Mark Myerson

I am deeply honored to have been selected to provide a foreword for this outstanding text, which is actually a comprehensive master piece of foot surgery, that has been edited by my friend, my colleague, and my partner, Mark Easley. Mark has accomplished in this textbook what many others have attempted to do, but have failed. The text is concise, it is up-to-date, it is beautifully illustrated, and it provides a ready guide for virtually every currently performed procedure in the foot and ankle arena. For most people a text like this would be a lifetime accomplishment. Mark Easley has been able to edit and direct this book in a very short period of time, and he has been able to have most of the chapters written by *the authoritative source*. I can only marvel at the amount of work and effort that went into such a comprehensive text.

—James A. Nunley

ACKNOWLEDGMENTS

I acknowledge my mentors and colleagues, Mark Myerson, Lew Schon, Robert Anderson, Hodges Davis, Jim Nunley, and Jim DeOrio, whose tireless commitment to academic orthopaedic surgery continues to inspire me, and the tremendous contributions of the authors who shared their expertise to make this textbook possible.

—MEE

RESIDENCY ADVISORY BOARD

The editors and the publisher would like to thank the resident reviewers who participated in the reviews of the manuscript and page proofs. Their detailed review and analysis was invaluable in helping to make certain this text meets the needs of residents today and in the future.

Daniel Galat, MD
Dr. Galat is a graduate of Ohio State University College of Medicine and the Mayo Clinic Department of Orthopedic Surgery residency program.
He is currently serving at Tenwek Hospital in Kenya as an orthopedic surgeon.

Lawrence V. Gulotta, MD
Fellow in Sports Medicine/Shoulder Surgery
Hospital for Special Surgery
New York, New York

Dara Chafik, MD, PhD
Southwest Shoulder, Elbow and Hand Center PC
Tuscon, Arizona

GautamYagnik, MD
Attending Physician
Orthopaedic Surgery
DRMC Sports Medicine
Dubois, Pennsylvania

Gregg T. Nicandri, M.D.
Assistant Professor
Department of Orthopaedics (SMD)
University of Rochester
School of Medicine and Dentistry
Rochester, New York

Catherine M. Robertson, MD
Assistant Clinical Professor
UCSD Orthopaedic Surgery—Sports Medicine
San Diego, California

Jonathan Schoenecker, MD
Assistant Professor
Departments of Orthopaedics, Pharmacology and Pediatrics
Vanderbilt University
Nashville, Tennessee

Chapter 1 Distal Chevron Osteotomy: Perspective 1

Hans-Joerg Trnka and Stefan G. Hofstaetter

DEFINITION

- The first reports of a distal metatarsal osteotomy date back to Reverdin, who described in 1881 a subcapital closing-wedge osteotomy for the correction of hallux valgus deformity.
- The chevron osteotomy has become widely accepted for correction of mild and moderate hallux valgus deformities. In the initial reports by Austin and Leventen[1] and Miller and Croce,[13] no fixation was mentioned. They suggested that the shape of the osteotomy and impaction of the cancellous capital fragment upon the shaft of the first metatarsal provided sufficient stability to forego fixation.
- To increase the indication for this technically simple osteotomy, internal fixation and a lateral soft tissue release have been added.

ANATOMY

- The special situation distinguishing the first metatarsophalangeal (MTP) joint from the lesser MTP joints is the sesamoid mechanism.
  - On the plantar surface of the metatarsal head are two longitudinal cartilage-covered grooves separated by a rounded ridge. The sesamoids run in these grooves.
  - The sesamoid bone is contained in each tendon of the flexor hallucis brevis; they are distally attached by the fibrous plantar plate to the base of the proximal phalanx.
- The head of the first metatarsal is rounded and cartilage-covered and articulates with the smaller concave elliptic base of the proximal phalanx.
- Fan-shaped ligamentous bands originate from the medial and lateral condyles of the metatarsal head and run to the base of the proximal phalanx and the margins of the sesamoids and the plantar plate.
- Tendons and muscles that move the great toe are arranged in four groups:
  - Long and short extensor tendons
  - Long and short flexor tendons
  - Abductor hallucis
  - Adductor hallucis
- Blood supply to the metatarsal head
  - First dorsal metatarsal artery
  - Branches from the first plantar metatarsal artery

PATHOGENESIS

- Extrinsic causes
  - Hallux valgus occurs predominantly in shoe-wearing populations and only occasionally in the unshod individual.
  - Although shoes are an essential factor in the cause of hallux valgus, not all individuals wearing fashionable shoes develop this deformity.
- Intrinsic causes
  - Hardy and Clapham found in a series of 91 patients a positive family history in 63%.
  - Coughlin[2] reported that a bunion was identified in 94% of 31 mothers whose children inherited a hallux valgus deformity.
  - Association of pes planus with the development of a hallux valgus deformity has been controversial.
  - Hohmann was the most definitive that hallux valgus is always combined with pes planus.
  - Coughlin[2] and Kilmartin[7] noted no incidence of pes planus in the juvenile patient.
  - Pronation of the foot imposes a longitudinal rotation of the first ray, which places the axis of the MTP joint in an oblique plane relative to the floor. In this position the foot appears to be less able to withstand the deformity pressures exerted on it by either shoes or weight bearing.
  - The simultaneous occurrence of hallux valgus and metatarsus primus varus has been frequently described. The question of cause and effect continues to be debated.

PATIENT HISTORY AND PHYSICAL FINDINGS

- Patient history often includes:
  - Pain in narrow shoes
  - Symptomatic intractable keratoses beneath the second metatarsal head (in 40% of patients)
  - Lateral deviation of the great toe
  - Pronation of the great toe
  - Keratosis medial plantar underneath the interphalangeal joint
  - Bursitis over the medial aspect of the medial condyle of the first metatarsal head
  - Hypermobility of the first metatarso-cuneiform joint
- Physical examination for hallux valgus deformity includes the following:
  - Hallux valgus angle: Normal is 15 degrees or less.
  - Intermetatarsal angle: Normal is 9 degrees or less.
  - Measurement of the position of the medial sesamoid relative to a longitudinal line bisecting the first metatarsal shaft
    - Grade 0: no displacement of sesamoid relative to the reference line
    - Grade I: overlap of less than 50% of sesamoid relative to the reference line
    - Grade II: overlap of greater than 50% of sesamoid relative to the reference line
    - Grade III: sesamoid completely displaced beyond the reference line
  - Joint congruency: measuring the lateral displacement of the articular surface of the proximal phalanx with respect to the corresponding articular surface of the metatarsal head, as seen on a dorsoplantar roentgenogram

IMAGING AND OTHER DIAGNOSTIC STUDIES

- Radiographs of the foot should always be obtained with the patient in the weight-bearing position with AP, lateral, and oblique views. The following criteria are examined:
  - Hallux valgus angle
  - Intermetatarsal angle
  - Sesamoid position
  - Joint congruency
  - Distal metatarsal articular angle: the relationship between the articular surface of the first metatarsal head and a line bisecting the first metatarsal shaft (normal is 10 degrees or less)
  - Arthrosis of the first MTP joint

DIFFERENTIAL DIAGNOSIS

- Ganglion
- Hallux rigidus

NONOPERATIVE MANAGEMENT

- Comfortable wider shoes
- Orthotics?
- Spiral dynamics physiotherapy in adolescents

SURGICAL MANAGEMENT

Indications

- Symptomatic hallux valgus deformity with a first intermetatarsal angle of up to 16 degrees
- Stable first metatarso-cuneiform joint

Contraindications

- Narrow metatarsal head so that adequate translation is not possible
- Intermetatarsal angle of more than 16 degrees
- Impaired vascular status
- Skeletally immature patient
- Severe osteoarthritic changes

Preoperative Planning

- Standard weight-bearing AP and lateral radiographs are mandatory.
- The hallux valgus and intermetatarsal angles and tibial sesamoid position are measured.
- A preoperative drawing is helpful.
- Clinical examination includes measurement of active and passive range of motion of the first MTP joint as well as inspection of the foot for plantar callus formation indicative of transfer metatarsalgia and stability of the first tarsometatarsal joint.

Positioning

- The foot is prepared in the standard manner.
- The patient is positioned supine.
- An ankle tourniquet is optional.

Approach

- The lateral soft tissue release is performed through a dorsal approach.
- The chevron osteotomy is performed through a straight midline incision.

TECHNIQUES

LATERAL SOFT TISSUE RELEASE

- The procedure is typically performed under a peripheral nerve block.
- Make a dorsal 3-cm longitudinal incision over the first web space (TECH FIG 1A).
- Continue deep dissection bluntly.
- Insert a lamina spreader and a Langenbeck retractor to expose the first web space.
- Divide the lateral joint capsule (metatarso-sesamoid

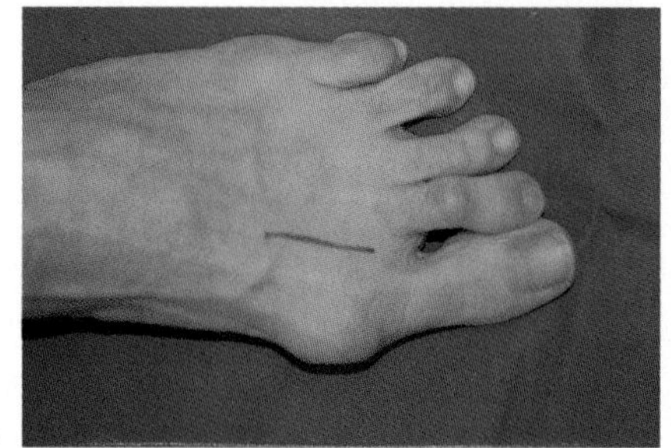

A

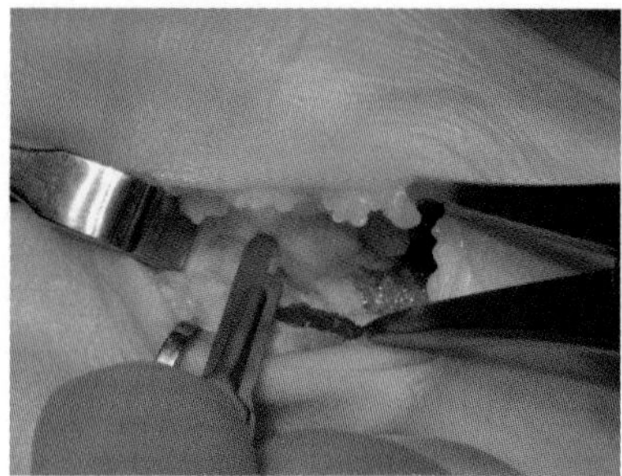

B

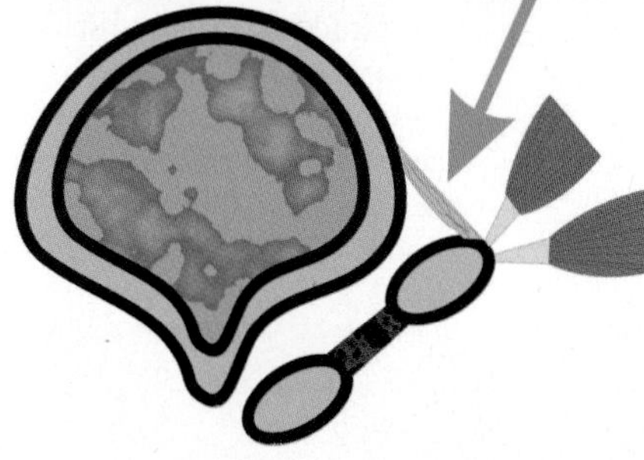

C

TECH FIG 1 • **A.** Skin incision over the first web space. **B, C.** Release of the metatarso-sesamoidal ligament. *(continued)*

ligament) immediately superior to the lateral sesamoid. Fenestrate the lateral capsule at the first MTP joint (**TECH FIG 1B,C**). Apply a varus stress to the hallux to complete the lateral release (**TECH FIG 1D**).

- Place one or two sutures between the lateral capsule of the first MTP joint and the periosteum of the second metatarsal.

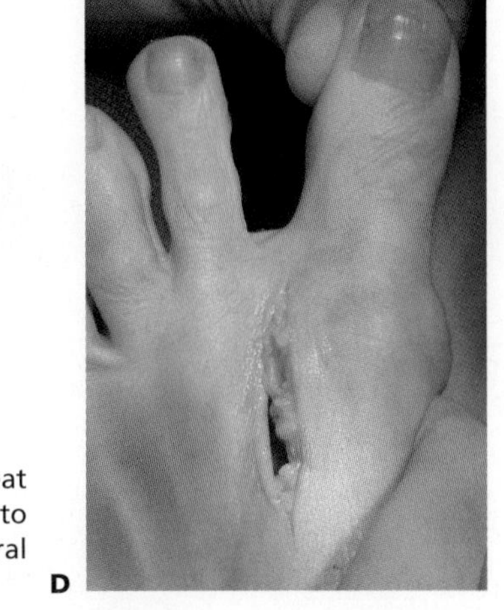

TECH FIG 1 • *(continued)* **D.** The great toe is brought into 20 degrees varus to demonstrate the release of the lateral structures.

CHEVRON OSTEOTOMY

- Externally rotate the leg. Make a second skin incision at the medial aspect of the first MTP joint (**TECH FIG 2A**).
- Perform careful dissection to avoid any damage to the dorsomedial nerve. Open the medial MTP joint capsule with an inverted L-type incision (**TECH FIG 2B,C**). Inspect the joint for degenerative changes.
- Expose the metatarsal head and place Hohmann retractors dorsal and plantar just extra-articular of the first MTP joint. The plantar Hohmann retractor protects the plantar artery to the metatarsal head, and the dorsal retractor protects the dorsal intra-articular blood supply originating from the capsule.
- Minimally shave the medial eminence to achieve a plane surface but also to preserve as much metatarsal head width as possible (**TECH FIG 2D**). This is one of the most important principles if a chevron osteotomy is carried out in a moderate to severe deformity.

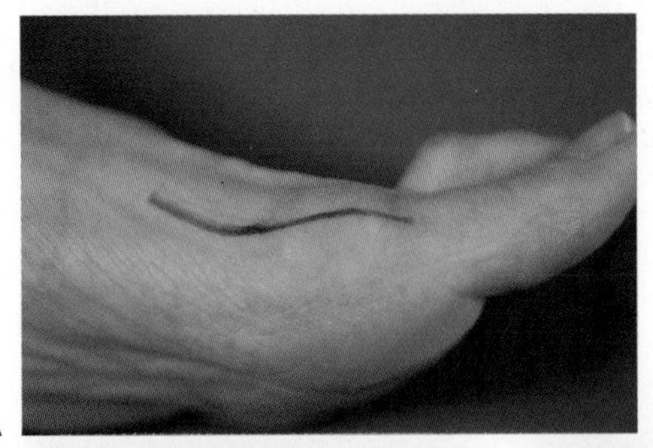

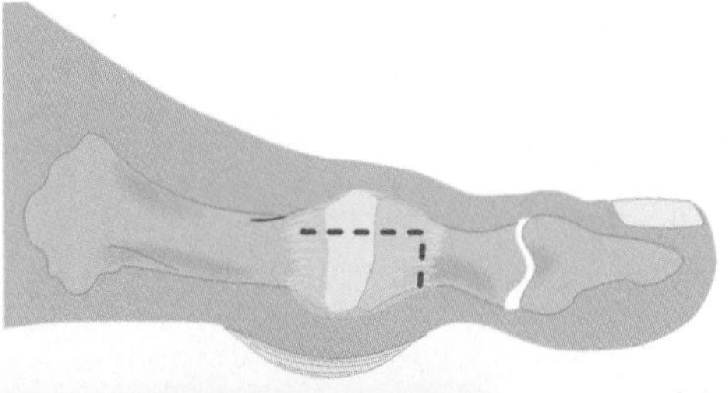

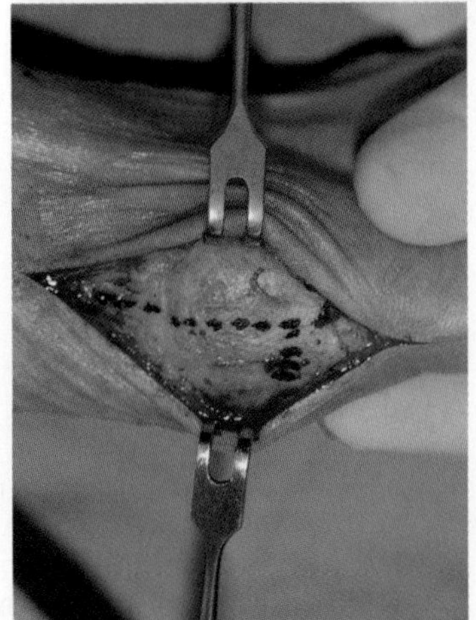

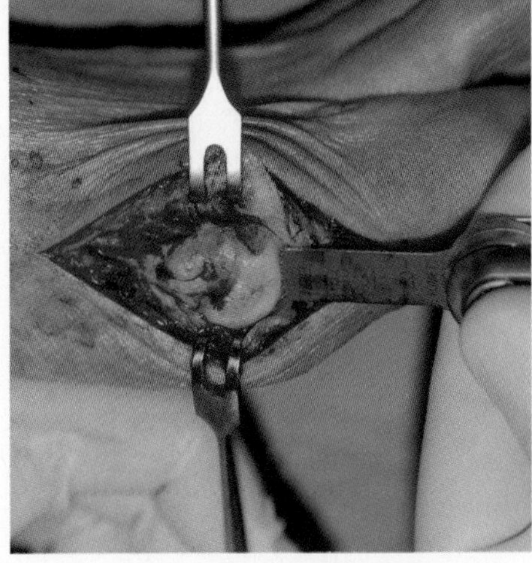

TECH FIG 2 • **A.** Medial skin incision for the osteotomy. **B, C.** Inverted L-type capsular incision. **D.** The medial eminence is minimally resected.

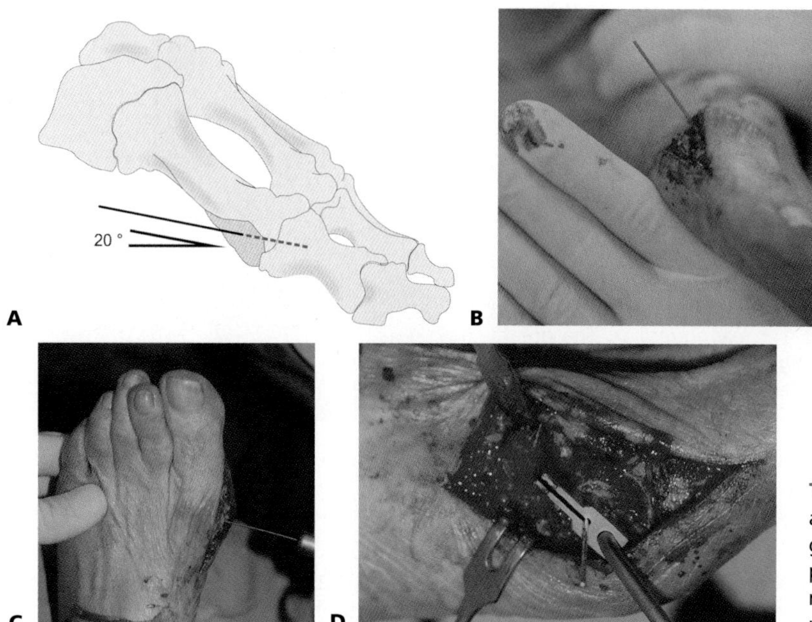

TECH FIG 3 • A–C. A guidewire marks the apex of the osteotomy. It should be 10 degrees inclined from medial to lateral, and pointing at the head of the fourth metatarsal. **D.** The osteotomy is performed using an osteotomy guide.

- Drill a 1.0-mm Kirschner wire slightly dorsal to the center of the exposed medial eminence. This wire is generally inclined 20 degrees from medial to lateral, aiming at the head of the fourth metatarsal (**TECH FIG 3A–C**). In the situation of an elevated position of the first metatarsal, the inclination may be increased. If shortening or lengthening of the first metatarsal is needed, the wire may be aimed to the fifth or third metatarsal head.
- Using a saw guide (**TECH FIG 3D**), make two cuts with an oscillating power saw so that they form an angle of 60 degrees proximal to the drill hole.
- Once the capital fragment is freely mobile, pull the metatarsal shaft medially by using a towel clip while pushing the metatarsal head laterally with the help of the thumb of the other hand (**TECH FIG 4A,B**).
- If the distal metatarsal articular angle is increased, a wedge from the distal dorsal cut may be excised to place the metatarsal head in a more varus position. If there is only a minor increase of the distal metatarsal articular angle, this may also be achieved by impacting the metatarsal head onto the shaft.
- Insert a guidewire for a cannulated Charlotte multiuse compression screw (Wright Medical Technology) from the distal dorsal metatarsal shaft obliquely to lateral plantar of the metatarsal head (**TECH FIG 4C,D**).

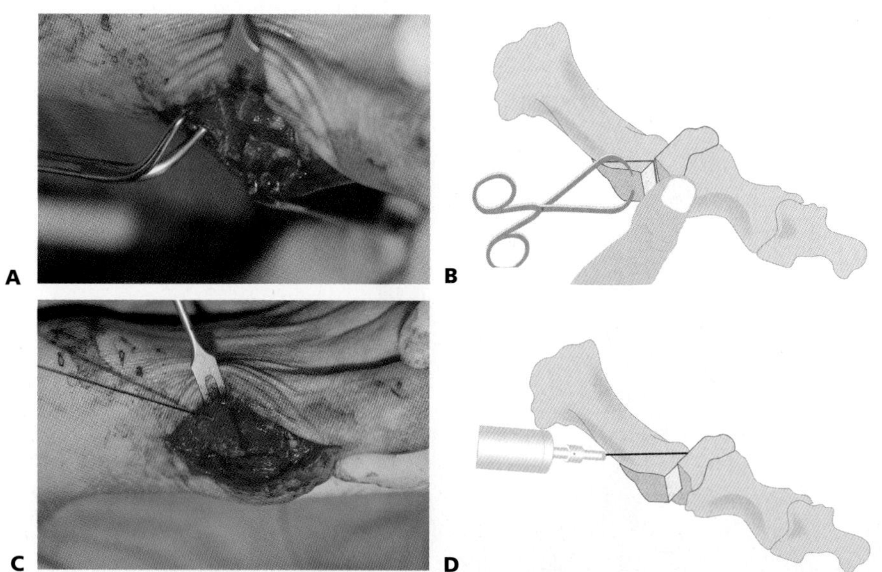

TECH FIG 4 • A, B. The metatarsal head is pushed laterally while the metatarsal shaft is pulled medially. **C, D.** A guidewire for the 3.0 Charlotte multiuse compression screw (Wright Medical Technology) is placed.

- Check the position of the osteotomy and the guidewire with a C-arm or a FluoroScan.
- Measure the length of the screw with the cannulated depth gauge (**TECH FIG 5A**). The multiuse compression screws are designed to be totally self-tapping and self-drilling. However, to avoid dislocation of the head, use the cannulated drill (**TECH FIG 5B**) and cannulated head drill (**TECH FIG 5C**).
- Insert the screw (**TECH FIG 5D**).
- Excise the medial eminence in line with the metatarsal shaft, taking care not to excise too much bone off the metatarsal head (**TECH FIG 5E**).
- While an assistant holds the great toe in a slightly overcorrected position, repair the medial joint capsule with U-type sutures, and tighten the first web space sutures (**TECH FIG 5F**).

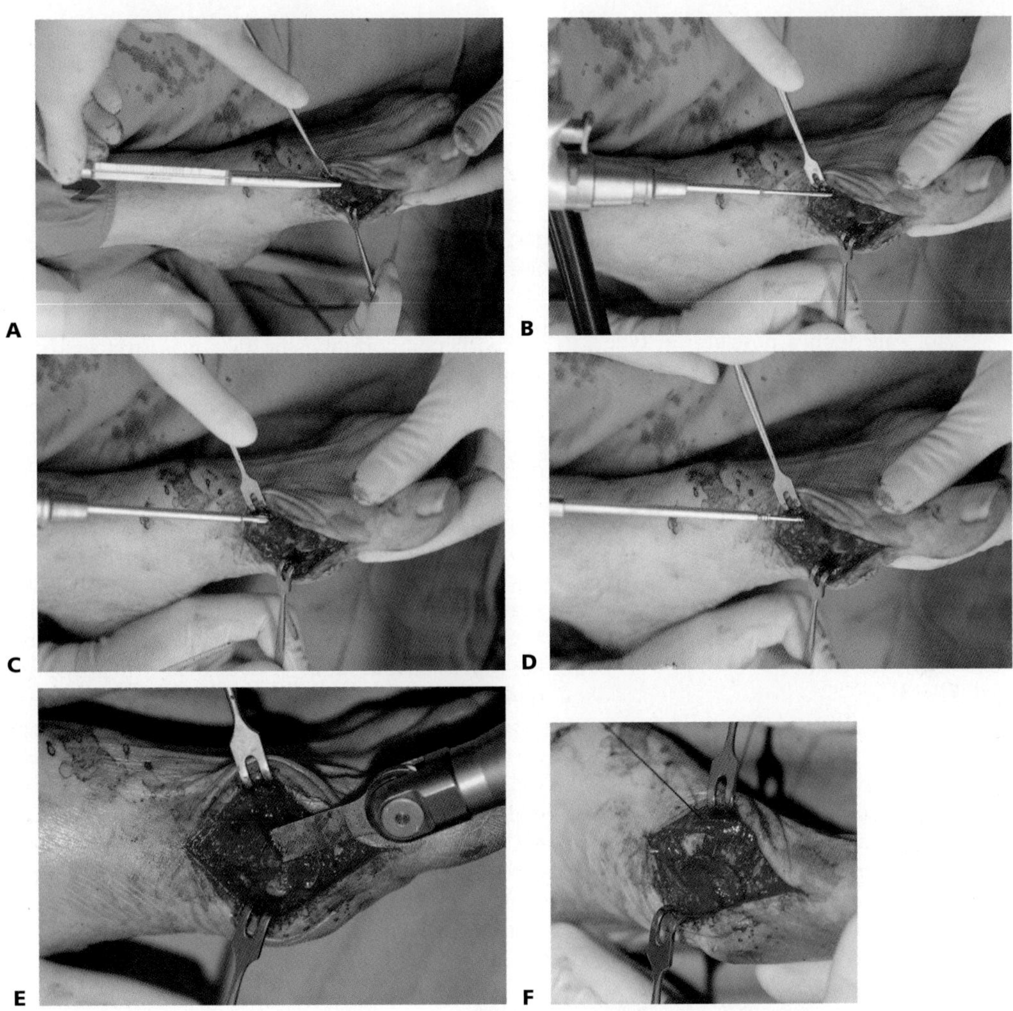

TECH FIG 5 • **A.** Length determination using the depth gauge. **B.** Predrilling with the Charlotte cannulated drill. **C.** Preparing a countersunk area with the Charlotte cannulated head drill. **D.** The screw is inserted until the head is completely countersunk within the bone. **E.** The medial eminence is resected. **F.** Closing of the medial capsule with U-type sutures.

PEARLS AND PITFALLS

Lateral tilt of the metatarsal head	■ Lateral release to avoid lateral tilting of the head, intraoperative FluoroScan control
Avascular necrosis	■ Careful soft tissue dissection
Intraoperative fracture of the metatarsal head	■ A guidewire at the apex of the osteotomy will prevent overpenetration of the distal fragment with the saw blade.

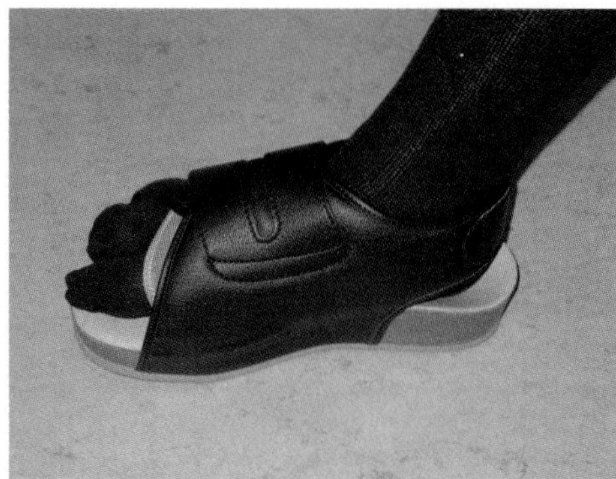

FIG 1 • Rathgeber postoperative shoe (OFA Rathgeber, Germany).

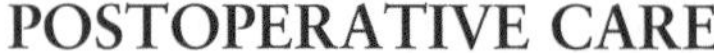

POSTOPERATIVE CARE

- Starting immediately postoperatively, ice application to the foot is helpful to reduce swelling.
- Provided that the bone quality was intraoperatively sufficient, patients are allowed to walk with a postsurgical type shoe (OFA Rathgeber) (**FIG 1**) on the same day (limited for 4 weeks).
- Weekly changes of the tape dressing are necessary.
- An alternative to weekly dressing changes is the postoperative hallux valgus sock, which also reduces postoperative edema (**FIG 2**).
- Radiographs are taken intraoperatively and at 4 weeks of follow-up.
- After radiographic union is achieved, normal dress shoes with a more rigid sole are allowed.
- After 4 weeks physiotherapy to achieve normal forefoot function is recommended (**FIG 3**).

OUTCOMES

- In the early years of this technique it was limited to patients 50 years and younger. This was represented by the study of Johnson et al,[5] which established a contraindication for using a chevron osteotomy in patients older than 50 years. However, Trnka[21–23] and Schneider[19] have proven that age is not a limiting factor for the chevron osteotomy.

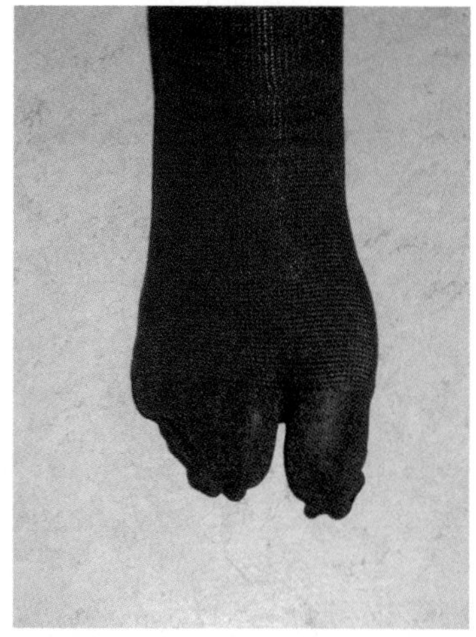

FIG 2 • Postoperative hallux valgus compression stocking for use after suture removal.

- Another important issue that was stretched out over the years was the combination of a lateral soft tissue release and a distal chevron osteotomy. Earlier reports have expressed concern about an increased risk of avascular necrosis if a lateral release is performed in addition to a chevron osteotomy. Jahss,[6] Mann,[9–11] and Meier and Kenzora[12] have all suggested that avascular necrosis frequently accompanies distal Chevron with lateral soft tissue release, citing an incidence of up to 40%. Pochatko[16] and Trnka[21–23] could not support this in their publications and found no increased risk of avascular necrosis.
- Chevron osteotomy was for many years limited to mild hallux valgus deformities.[18,20] Designed primarily without fixation, the concern was stability and loss of fixation. As it became more obvious that a lateral soft tissue release is important for correction of more severe deformities, this concern gained weight. According to papers by Harper[4] and Sarrafian,[18] lateral displacement is limited up to 50% of metatarsal width.
- Over a period of 14 years we have modified and developed the chevron osteotomy. By reviewing each step of the development with clinical studies, we now perform a chevron osteotomy with lateral soft tissue release and single screw fixation.

A 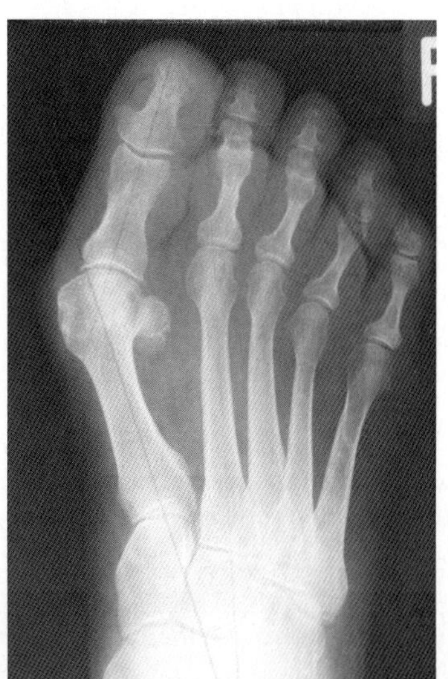

B 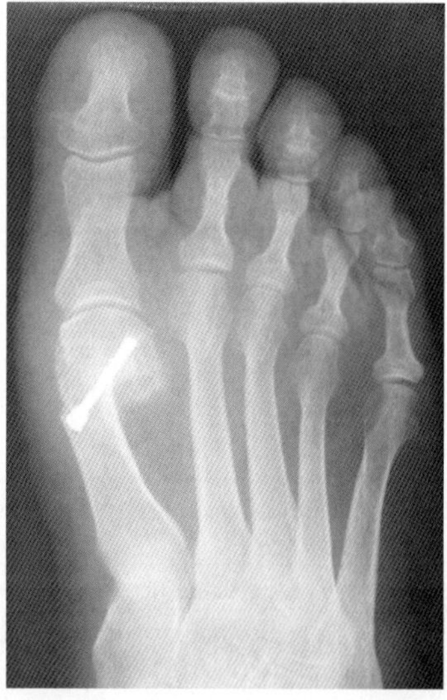

FIG 3 • A 72-year-old woman before surgery (**A**) and after surgery (**B**).

- Trnka et al[22] reported in 2000 a series of 43 patients (57 feet) with 2-year and 5-year follow-up. Radiographic evaluation revealed a preoperative average hallux valgus angle of 29 degrees and a preoperative average intermetatarsal angle of 13 degrees. At the 2-year follow-up, those angles averaged 15 and 8 degrees, respectively, and at the 5-year follow-up, they averaged 16 and 9 degrees. The results at these two follow-up periods proved that the chevron osteotomy is a reliable procedure for mild and moderate hallux valgus deformity and that there are no differences in outcome based on age.
- Schneider et al[19] reported in 2004 a series of 112 feet (73 patients) with a minimum follow-up of 10 years. For 47 feet (30 patients), the results were compared with those from an interim follow-up of 5.6 years. The AOFAS score improved from a preoperative mean of 46.5 points to a mean of 88.8 points after a mean of 12.7 years. The first MTP angle showed a mean preoperative value of 27.6 degrees and was improved to 14.0 degrees. The first intermetatarsal angle improved from a preoperative mean of 13.8 degrees to 8.7 degrees. The mean preoperative grade of sesamoid subluxation was 1.7 on a scale of 0 to 3 and improved to 1.2. Measured on a scale of 0 to 3, arthritis of the first MTP joint progressed from a mean of 0.8 to 1.7. The progression of arthritis of the first MTP joint between 5.6 and 12.7 years postoperatively was statistically significant. Excellent clinical results after chevron osteotomy not only proved to be consistent but also showed further improvement over a longer follow-up period. The mean radiographic angles were constant, without recurrence of the deformity. So far, the statistically significant progression of first MTP joint arthritis has not affected the clinical result, but this needs further observation.
- Sanhudo[17] retrospectively reviewed 50 feet with moderate to severe hallux valgus deformity in 34 patients with a mean follow-up of 30 months. There was a mean AOFAS score improvement of 39.6 (44.5 to 84.1) points. The hallux valgus angle and intermetatarsal angle improved a mean of 22.7 degrees and 10.4 degrees, respectively. He concluded that the chevron osteotomy is also indicated for moderate to severe hallux valgus deformity.

COMPLICATIONS

- Avascular necrosis of the metatarsal head
  - A lateral release does not increase the incidence.[16]
- Hallux varus
- Malpositioning
- Loss of fixation

REFERENCES

1. Austin DW, Leventen EO. A new osteotomy for hallux valgus: a horizontally directed "V" displacement osteotomy of the metatarsal head for hallux valgus and primus varus. Clin Orthop Relat Res 1981;157: 25–30.
2. Coughlin MJ. Roger A. Mann Award. Juvenile hallux valgus: etiology and treatment. Foot Ankle Int 1995;16:682–697.
3. Hardy RH, Clapham JC. Observations on hallux valgus based on a controlled series. J Bone Joint Surg-Br 1951;33:376–391.
4. Harper MC. Correction of metatarsus primus varus with the chevron metatarsal osteotomy. An analysis of corrective factors. Clin Orthop Relat Res 1989;253:180–198.
5. Johnson JE, Clanton TO, Baxter D, et al. Comparison of chevron osteotomy and modified bunionectomy for correction of mild to moderate hallux valgus deformity. Foot & Ankle 1991;12:61–68.
6. Jahhs MH. Hallux valgus: further considerations—the first metatarsal head. Foot & Ankle 1981;2:1–4.
7. Kilmartin TE, Wallace WA. The significance of pes planus in juvenile hallux valgus. Foot Ankle 1992;13:53–56.
8. Kuhn MA, Lippert FG III, Phipps MJ, et al. Blood flow to the metatarsal head after chevron bunionectomy. Foot Ankle Int 2005;26:526–529.
9. Mann RA. Bunion surgery: decision making. Orthopedics 1990;13: 951–957.
10. Mann RA, Coughlin MJ. Adult hallux valgus. In: Coughlin MJ, Mann RA, eds. Surgery of the Foot and Ankle. St. Louis, MO: Mosby, 1999: 150–269.
11. Mann RA, Donatto KC. The chevron osteotomy: a clinical and radiographic analysis. Foot Ankle Int 1997;18:255–261.
12. Meier PJ, Kenzora JE. The risks and benefits of distal metatarsal osteotomies. Foot & Ankle 1985;6:7–17.
13. Miller S, Croce WA. The Austin procedure for surgical correction of hallux abductor valgus deformity. J Am Pod Ass 1979;69: 110–118.
14. Muhlbauer M, Zembsch A, Trnka HJ. Short-term results of modified chevron osteotomy with soft tissue technique and guide wire fixation: a prospective study [in German]. Z Orthop Ihre Grenzgeb 2001;139: 435–439.
15. Myerson MS. Hallux valgus. In: Myerson MS, ed. Foot and Ankle Disorders. Philadelphia: WB Saunders, 2000:213–288.
16. Pochatko DJ, Schlehr FJ, Murphey MD, et al. Distal chevron osteotomy with lateral release for treatment of hallux valgus deformity. Foot Ankle Int 1994;15:457–461.
17. Sanhudo JA. Correction of moderate to severe hallux valgus deformity by a modified chevron shaft osteotomy. Foot Ankle Int 2006;27: 581–585.
18. Sarrafian SK. A method of predicting the degree of functional correction of the metatarsus primus varus with a distal lateral displacement osteotomy in hallux valgus. Foot Ankle 1985;5:322–326.
19. Schneider W, Aigner N, Pinggera O, et al. Chevron osteotomy in hallux valgus: ten-year results of 112 cases. J Bone Joint Surg Br 2004; 86B:1016–1020.
20. Shereff MJ, Yang QM, Kummer FJ. Extraosseous and intraosseous arterial supply to the first metatarsal and metatarsophalangeal joint. Foot Ankle 1987;8:81–93.
21. Trnka HJ, Hofmann S, Salzer M, et al. Clinical and radiological results after Austin bunionectomy for treatment of hallux valgus. Arch Orthop Trauma Surg 1996;115:171–175.
22. Trnka HJ, Zembsch A, Easley ME, et al. The chevron osteotomy for correction of hallux valgus: comparison of findings after two and five years of follow-up. J Bone Joint Surg Am 2000;82A: 1373–1378.
23. Trnka HJ, Zembsch A, Wiesauer H, et al. Modified Austin procedure for correction of hallux valgus. Foot Ankle Int 1997;18:119–127.

Chapter **2**

Distal Chevron Osteotomy: Perspective 2

Paul Hamilton, Sam Singh, and Michael G. Wilson

SURGICAL MANAGEMENT

- The primary indication for a chevron osteotomy is symptomatic hallux valgus deformity with a moderate deformity with an intermetatarsal angle of less than 15 degrees. The first metatarsocuneiform joint should be stable. The osteotomy can also be used to correct an abnormal distal metatarsal articular angle. It is used as a sole procedure in those presenting with minimal transfer symptoms.

Preoperative Planning

- AP and lateral weight-bearing radiographs of the foot are evaluated for metatarsal length, intermetatarsal angle, hallux valgus angle, distal metatarsal articular angle, and interphalangeal angle for cases that may require a proximal phalangeal osteotomy to obtain complete correction. Congruency of the joint, presence of osteophytes, the size of the bony medial eminence, and the position and condition of the sesamoids are noted.

Positioning

- Surgery is performed on an outpatient basis.
- Prophylactic antibiotics are administered.
- A thigh tourniquet is applied.
- The patient is positioned supine with a sandbag under the ipsilateral buttock so the big toe points to the ceiling.

TECHNIQUES

CHEVRON OSTEOTOMY

- Perform the distal soft tissue release through a first web space incision. Take care to avoid stripping the lateral metatarsal head soft tissues. We then perform the osteotomy in a step manner as described below.
- Approach the metatarsal through a medial longitudinal incision extending from a point 1 cm proximal to the medial eminence to the medial flare of the proximal phalanx. This can be extended distally if a phalangeal osteotomy is required. Identify the dorsal medial cutaneous nerve and incise the medial capsule sharply in a single longitudinal direction (**TECH FIG 1A**). Expose the medial eminence and resect it 1 mm medial to the sagittal sulcus (**TECH FIG 1B**). The most important part of the exposure is the identification of the plantar vascular supply (**TECH FIG 1C**). The osteotomy must be extracapsular. This plantar vascular supply must remain attached to the capital fragment to minimize any risk of avascular necrosis (AVN).
- The apex of the osteotomy is defined as the center of an imaginary ellipse or circle started by the articular surface of the metatarsal. Mark the apex with ink (**TECH FIG 2A**).
- Create the transverse limb of the osteotomy from the apex to the plantar surface of the metatarsal. The obliquity of this cut varies, the most important factor being that the osteotomy must remain extra-articular and the plantar vascular supply must be maintained to the metatarsal head (**TECH FIG 2B**). Complete the osteotomy through to the lateral side.
- Perform the vertical osteotomy by measuring a 90-degree angle to the plantar cut and then angling the saw blade to reduce this angle by 10 to 20 degrees. The exact angle is not crucial; we find aiming for the angle to be between 60 and 80 degrees produces a stable osteotomy (**TECH FIG 2C**). Complete this osteotomy to the lateral side to allow displacement of the head fragment. Take care to protect the extensor hallucis longus tendon while performing the vertical osteotomy.
- Use a sharp towel clip to grasp the proximal fragment and use the thumb to apply lateral displacement to the capital fragment (**TECH FIG 3A**). We allow a maximum of 50% displacement. A McDonald dissector can be used to tease the capital fragment over if required.

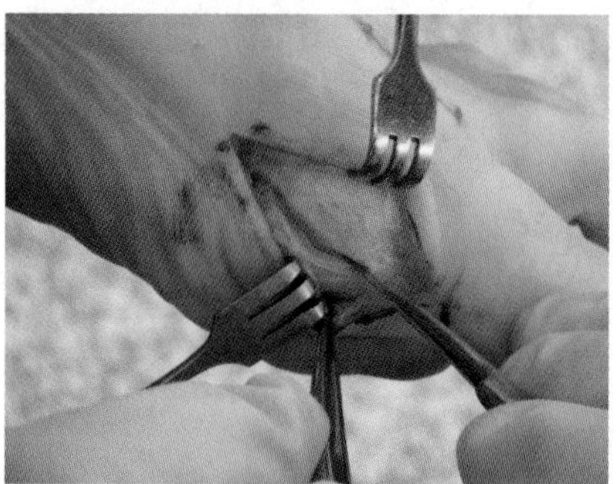
A

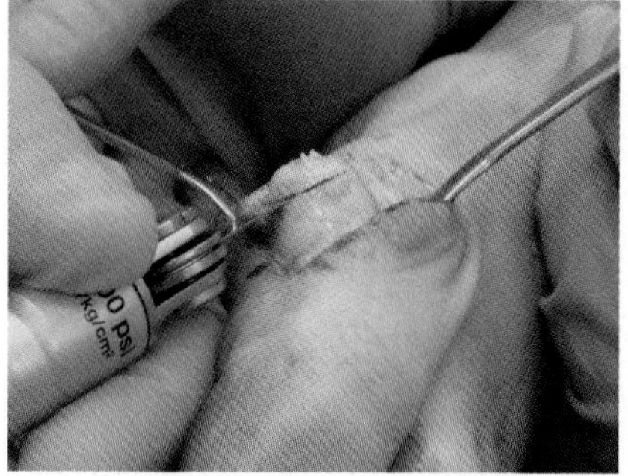
B

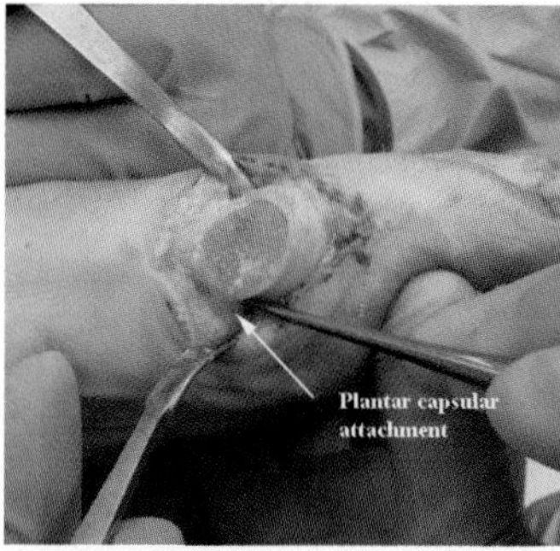

C

TECH FIG 1 • **A.** After the skin is incised and the dorsomedial nerve is protected, the capsule is incised in a longitudinal fashion. **B.** The medial eminence is resected. **C.** Exposure and preservation of the plantar capsular attachment.

- Use in-line force to compress the head fragment onto the shaft, allowing cancellous impaction (**TECH FIG 3B**). This aids in the immediate stability of the osteotomy while fixation is achieved.
- We prefer fixation using a 1.6-mm Kirschner wire, although a compression screw can also be used. We pass the Kirschner wire in a retrograde fashion under direct vision from the plantar head obliquely across to the proximal fragment and through an appropriately placed small skin incision (**TECH FIG 3C**). Back the wire out to leave it a few millimeters deep to cartilage, thus maintaining excellent fixation without penetrating the joint. Shave the redundant neck cortex, approximating to 50% of the protruding portion.
- Imbricate the medial capsule with a strong absorbable suture while holding the hallux in a neutral or slightly abducted position with the aid of a swab.
- Confirm the reduction in the intermetatarsal angle, screws, and relocation of the sesamoids with image intensification with the foot flat on the image intensifier. Assess the need for a proximal phalangeal osteotomy.
- Close the wound in layers with continuous Monocryl to the skin and apply a forefoot bandage to maintain the correction.

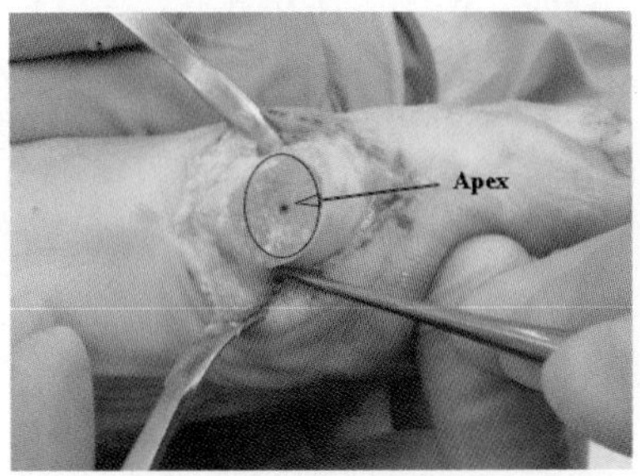

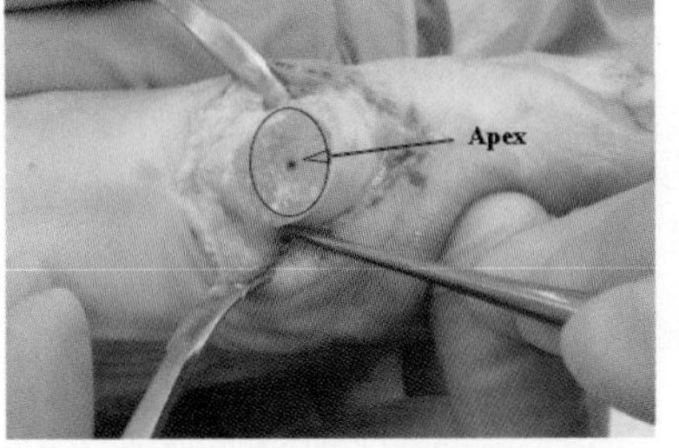

A

B

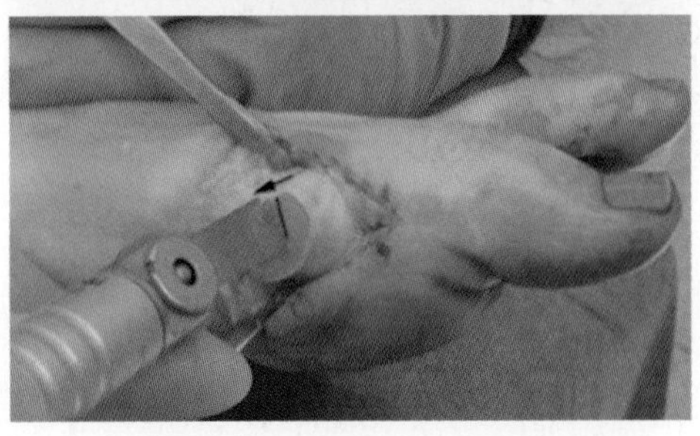

C

TECH FIG 2 • **A.** An imaginary ellipse based on the articular surface is made and the center is marked with ink. This is used as the apex of the osteotomy. **B.** The longitudinal cut is performed, ensuring that the proximal limb is extra-articular and the vascular bundle is maintained to the head. **C.** The saw blade is placed at 90 degrees to the longitudinal cut and then angled to produce a chevron osteotomy of between 60 and 80 degrees.

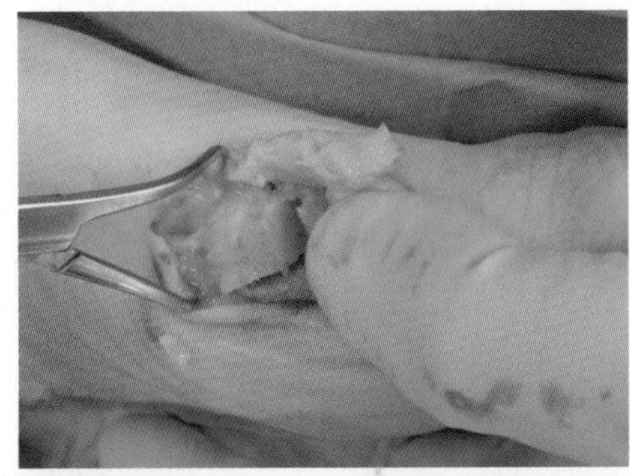

A

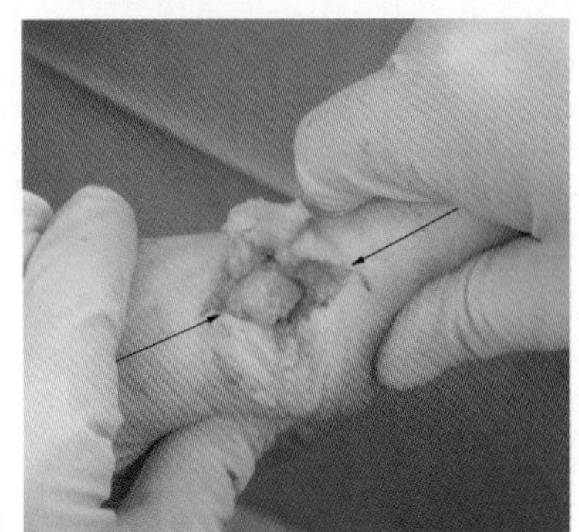

B

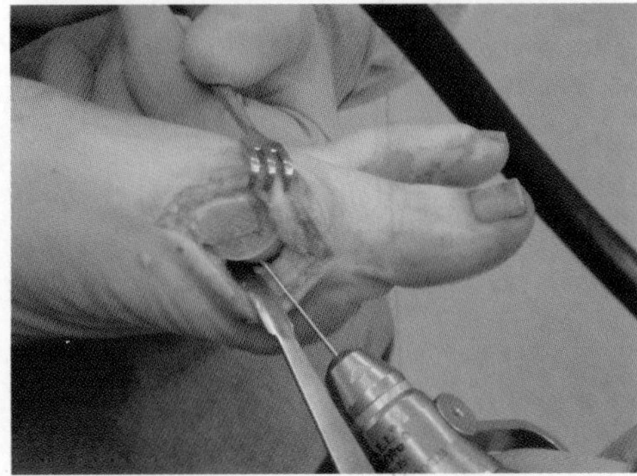

C

TECH FIG 3 • **A.** The osteotomy is displaced and held with a clip. **B.** In-line compression is performed to impact the cancellous fragments together to increase stability. **C.** A 1.6-mm Kirschner wire is passed in a retrograde fashion across the osteotomy site.

PEARLS AND PITFALLS

Exposure	■ The most important part of the exposure is that of the plantar vascular bundle. Failure to do so may compromise the blood supply to the metatarsal head.
Osteotomy	■ If displacement of the osteotomy is difficult, check that all cuts have been completed. A limited lateral capsulotomy may be performed if needed, restricting the knife cuts to the lateral soft tissues distal to the metatarsal head.
Distal metatarsal articular angle correction	■ To correct an abnormal distal metatarsal articular angle, a small medial wedge from the vertical limb of the osteotomy can be performed. This will make the osteotomy more unstable, and care must be taken to achieve good fixation.

POSTOPERATIVE CARE

- If safe, patients are discharged home on the day of surgery with strict advice to elevate the foot whenever resting for the first 2 weeks.
- In most cases they are allowed to bear weight on their heel and lateral forefoot in a hard-soled postoperative shoe.
- Cast immobilization is not required.
- The wound is inspected at 2 weeks, at which time the hallux is restrapped and patients are taught simple passive and active toe flexion–extension exercises.
- At 4 weeks postoperatively the osteotomy is assessed. The Kirschner wire is removed in the outpatient setting.
- At 6 weeks the osteotomy is checked radiologically, and if there is consolidation at the line of the osteotomy, the patient is instructed to wear a wide shoe or sneaker and to progress to full weight bearing as tolerated. Strapping of the hallux is discontinued at this time.

OUTCOMES

- The chevron osteotomy is the most commonly performed distal chevron osteotomy for mild hallux valgus in the United States,[4] and outcomes are excellent.[2,5,9]
- AVN with the use of a lateral release remains a concern. Recent reports suggest very low rates of AVN when correcting moderate deformities with the chevron osteotomy with a lateral release.[1,3,5,7] The improved correction that we see with a lateral release means that we perform it in every case.
- Evidence also now suggests that concern that the osteotomy should be reserved for patients under 50 years old may not be true, with equivalent results in differing age groups.[6,8]

COMPLICATIONS

- Complications include AVN, stiffness, wound problems, infection, undercorrection, overcorrection, fractures, chronic regional pain disorder, and deep vein thrombosis. Delayed union and nonunion are rare complications with the use of fixation.

REFERENCES

1. Kuhn MA, Lippert FG III, Phipps MJ, et al. Blood flow to the metatarsal head after chevron bunionectomy. Foot Ankle Int 2005; 26:526–529.
2. Nery C, Barroco R, Réssio C. Biplanar chevron osteotomy. Foot Ankle Int 2002;23:792–798.
3. Peterson DA, Zilberfarb JL, Greene MA, et al. Avascular necrosis of the first metatarsal head: incidence in distal osteotomy combined with lateral soft tissue release. Foot Ankle Int 1994;15:59–63.
4. Pinney S, Song K, Chou L. Surgical treatment of mild hallux valgus deformity: the state of practice among academic foot and ankle surgeons. Foot Ankle Int 2006;27:970–973.
5. Potenza V, Caterini R, Farsetti P, et al. Chevron osteotomy with lateral release and adductor tenotomy for hallux valgus. Foot Ankle Int 2009;30:512–516.
6. Schneider W, Aigner N, Pinggera O, et al. Chevron osteotomy in hallux valgus: ten-year results of 112 cases. J Bone Joint Surg Br 2004; 86B:1016–1020.
7. Singh SK, Jayasakera N, Nazir S, et al. Use of a polydioxone (PDS) suture to stabilize the chevron osteotomy: a review of 30 cases. J Foot Ankle Surg 2004;43:306–310.
8. Trnka HJ, Zembsch A, Easley ME, et al. The chevron osteotomy for correction of hallux valgus: comparison of findings after two and five years of follow-up. J Bone Joint Surg Am 2000;82A:1373–1378.
9. Trnka HJ, Zembsch A, Weisauer H, et al. Modified Austin procedure for correction of hallux valgus. Foot Ankle Int 1997;18:119–127.

Chapter 3 Biplanar Distal Chevron Osteotomy

Caio Nery

DEFINITION

- Hallux valgus is a common condition that can affect both adults and adolescents.[2,4] Patients complain of pain and restriction with activities of daily living because of the lateral deviation of the great toe, the medial deviation of the first metatarsal, and the onset of inflammation at the progressively worsening medial eminence of the first metatarsal head.

ANATOMY

- The first metatarsophalangeal (MTP) joint's complex anatomy is directly related to its complex physiology. The concave articular surface of the great toe's proximal phalanx articulates with the convex first metatarsal head. Its physiologic relationship is maintained by the surrounding articular capsule and collateral ligaments.[4] At the plantar aspect of the first MTP joint, the sesamoid complex acts as a rail on which the first metatarsal head glides congruently with the intrinsic and extrinsic tendons, providing power and stability to the joint.[10]

PATHOGENESIS

- Congruent first MTP joint (physiologic distal metatarsal articular angle [DMAA])
  - The literature suggests that that lateral deviation of the great toe is the primary event leading to hallux valgus deformity. This primary deforming force has a reciprocal relationship with metatarsus primus varus; the first and second intermetatarsal angle (IMA) worsens with an increase in the hallux valgus angle (HVA), and vice versa.[10,16] The valgus of the proximal phalanx produces forces whose vectors determine the lateral deviation of the head of the first metatarsal.[6,7,10,12]
- Congruent first MTP joint (increased DMAA)
  - With an increased DMAA, hallux valgus is present despite congruency of the first MTP joint. The articular surface of the first metatarsal head is in a valgus position relative to the first metatarsal shaft axis; therefore, hallux valgus is present even without an imbalance of the muscle forces on the first MTP joint.[12] However, this imbalance leads to a worsening of the deformity. Hallux valgus with an increased DMAA is less common than the incongruent type and typically occurs in men and younger patients (juvenile hallux valgus).[4,6,7]

NATURAL HISTORY

- Shoe wear may contribute to the development of hallux valgus deformity.[2,10,13] A narrow and triangular toe box combined with high heels may force lateral deviation of the great toe, leading to a mechanical disadvantage of the abductor hallucis muscle.
- Persistence of these deforming forces may create a relative lateral displacement of the extensor hallucis longus and flexor hallucis longus tendons, which in turn may increase valgus deviation of the great toe. Eventually, the first MTP joint's medial capsule and collateral ligament become attenuated, while its lateral soft tissues become contracted.
- The laterally deviated hallux proximal phalanx exerts a varus-producing force to the first metatarsal head, thereby worsening the metatarsus primus varus deformity.[16] Since the sesamoid complex is attached to the proximal phalanx, the sesamoid position typically remains anatomic as the first metatarsal head subluxates medially. Progression of this displacement often produces the functional deficits and pronation of the great toe.[10]
- Because the first MTP joint is stable and congruent but malaligned with respect to the first metatarsal axis (increased DMAA), juvenile and adolescent hallux valgus deformity should prompt evaluation for potential associated pathology, such as metatarsus adductus, hypermobility, or ligamentous laxity.

PATIENT HISTORY AND PHYSICAL FINDINGS

- Patients typically complain of pain over the first metatarsal head's medial eminence, especially while standing and walking in a narrow toe box shoe. Occasionally, patients develop a symptomatic bursitis over the medial eminence.
- Pain plantar to the first metatarsal head suggests a symptomatic and incongruent articulation of the sesamoids with the first metatarsal head. Compensation for this discomfort may lead to transfer metatarsalgia.
- An imbalance of forefoot pressures created by the malalignment of the first ray secondary to hallux valgus may also lead to transfer metatarsalgia.
- We routinely review the patient's general health, activity level, and family history of hallux valgus. We always check for comorbidities that may have a direct impact on the success of corrective bunion surgery, particularly diabetes, arthritis, and neurovascular diseases.[2,10]
- To fully appreciate the degree of hallux valgus deformity, the involved foot must be examined with the patient standing.
- We evaluate the range of motion and alignment of the ankle, hindfoot, midfoot, and forefoot with the patient standing and walking.
- Pronation of the hallux is also best assessed with the patient standing.
- The lesser toes are carefully examined for deformities, which can be rigid or supple, requiring different types of treatment.[14]
- Pronation of the great toe must be assessed as well as the presence of callosities under the toes and forefoot associated with metatarsalgia.[1,10]
- Passive correction of hallux valgus is attempted. With the patient standing, pressure is applied over the lateral face of the great toe, trying to correct its valgus deviation. Patients with passive correctable lateral deviation of the great toe will need less invasive or hazardous procedures for the treatment of their hallux valgus deformity, particularly the adductor hallucis release.

- Hypermobility of the first ray can have an influence on the onset of the hallux valgus deformity as well as on its treatment.
- It is easy to differentiate the flexible and rigid forms of hammer or claw toes by applying thumb pressure in the forefoot sole and elevating the metatarsal heads; in the flexible forms, the deformities reduces or disappears completely; in the rigid forms, the maneuver does not change the hammer or claw toes.
- A positive MTP joint drawer sign indicates the presence of a capsulitis and instability of the joint due to the lesion of the plantar capsule or collateral ligaments, more commonly the lateral portion of the plantar plate.

IMAGING AND OTHER DIAGNOSTIC STUDIES

- Hallux valgus must be assessed with a minimum of AP and lateral weight-bearing radiographs of the foot.
- The HVA is determined by the intersection of the diaphyseal axes of the first metatarsal and the proximal phalanx. Arbitrarily, a normal HVA does not exceed 15 degrees (**FIG 1A**).
- The IMA is the angle between the diaphyseal axes of the first and second metatarsals. Arbitrarily, a normal IMA does not exceed 9 degrees (**FIG 1B**).
- The sesamoid position is determined by its relationship with the first metatarsal diaphyseal axis. Typically the sesamoids remain in their anatomic position; with progressive hallux valgus deformity, the first metatarsal head progressively subluxates medially in relation to the sesamoids.
  - Normal (grade 0) sesamoid position: The tibial and fibular sesamoids are equidistant from the bisecting line of the first metatarsal.
  - Sesamoid position grades 1 to 3: Grades 1 through 3 signify an increasingly greater lateral position of the tibial sesamoid relative to the bisecting line of the tibial shaft axis, with grade 3 indicating that the tibial sesamoid is positioned completely lateral to the reference line (**FIGS 1C AND 2**).
  - The interphalangeal angle (IPA) is measured between the axis of both the proximal and distal phalanx of the great toe; arbitrarily, its normal value is up to 10 degrees.
  - The DMAA is obtained by the intersection of the line that connects the articular edges of the head and the line bisecting the first metatarsal shaft. The DMAA normal value is up to 8 degrees (**FIG 3**).[13,15] Inter-and intra-observer reliability for measuring the DMAA is poor.
  - The proximal phalanx articular angle is measured between the tangent to the proximal articular surface of the proximal phalanx of the great toe and the line bisecting the diaphyseal axis of the same phalanx. It is considered normal up to 10 degrees.

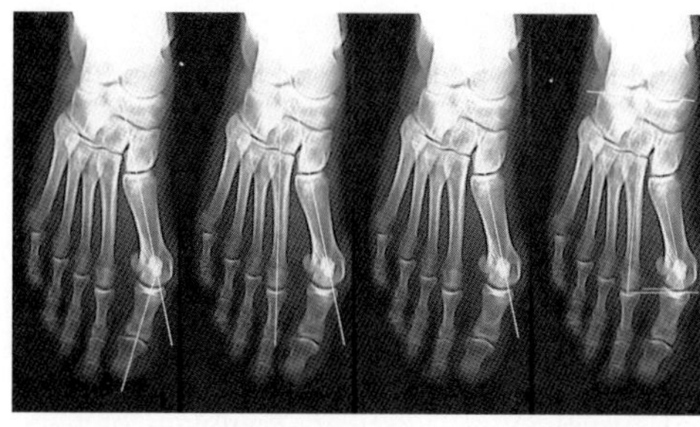

FIG 1 • AP radiograph of a patient with hallux valgus. *Left,* Hallux valgus angle (*HVA;* up to 15 degrees). *Second from left,* First intermetatarsal angle (*IMA;* up to 9 degrees). *Second from right,* Sesamoid position. In this patient, the tibial sesamoid is divided into two halves by the diaphyseal axis of the first metatarsal, which means the beginning of a grade 2 sesamoid subluxation (normal is grade 0). *Right,* Relative length of the first and second metatarsals; normal is up to 5 mm.

  - Relative length of the first and second rays is measured pre- and postoperatively. Most osteotomies lead to shortening of the first metatarsal. In our experience, greater than 5 mm of first metatarsal shortening of the first metatarsal frequently results in transfer metatarsalgia (**FIG 1D**).

DIFFERENTIAL DIAGNOSIS

- Hallux valgus interphalangeus
- Hallux rigidus
- Sesamoiditis

NONOPERATIVE MANAGEMENT

- Patient education
  - While there is no concrete evidence that shoe wear causes hallux valgus, we believe that wearing shoes with tight toe boxes and high heels contributes to the worsening of deformity.
  - Patients with intrinsic factors contributing to hallux valgus, such as an increased DMAA, should be educated that they are particularly prone to external forces worsening their hallux valgus deformity.[4]
- Orthotic devices and insoles may relieve symptoms but generally do not correct deformity. Moreover, patients already in need of wider toe boxes may need to find shoes with extra depth to accommodate both their foot deformity and the orthotic device. In juvenile hallux valgus (skeletally immature patients), the use of a custom-made night splint could limit the progression but cannot reverse the deformity.[11]

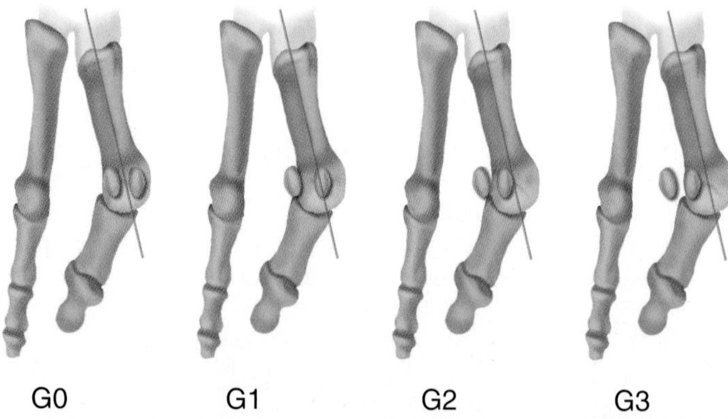

FIG 2 • Evaluation of hallucal sesamoid position. Grade 0, no displacement of sesamoids relative to the middle diaphyseal axis of the first metatarsal (normal). Grade 1, overlap of less than 50% of the tibial (medial) sesamoid to the reference line. Grade 2, overlap of more than 50% of the tibial sesamoid to the reference line. Grade 3, tibial sesamoid completely displaced beyond the reference line.

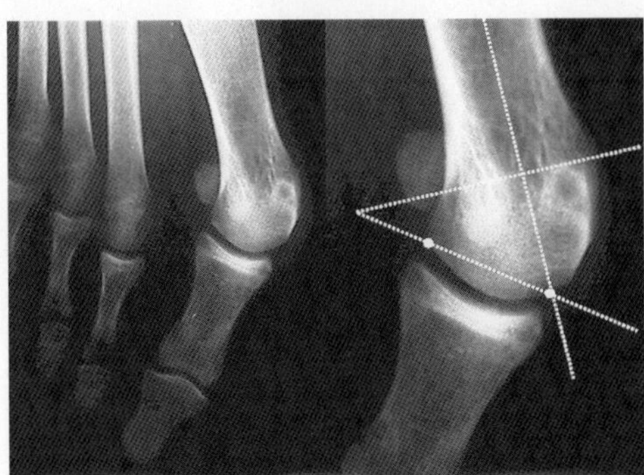

A

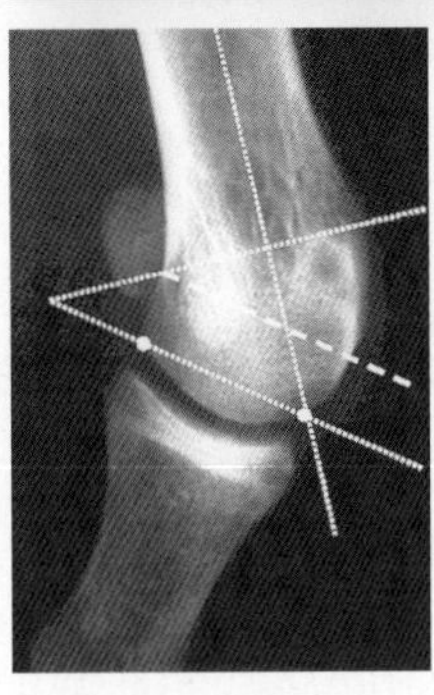

B

FIG 3 • **A.** AP radiograph from a patient with juvenile hallux valgus in which the absolute congruence of the metatarsophalangeal joint can be noted. The misalignment of the distal articular surface of the metatarsal determines the hallux valgus deformity. **B.** Both edges of the metatarsal head articular surface are marked. The distal metatarsal articular angle is measured between the line that connects the articular edges and the perpendicular to the diaphyseal axis of the first metatarsal. The normal value is up to 8 degrees.

- In skeletally mature patients, intermittent use of a corrective splint does not adequately counterbalance many hours of shoe wear with a narrow toe box and a high heel.

SURGICAL MANAGEMENT

- The primary indication for the biplanar distal chevron osteotomy is moderate hallux valgus deformity with a 1–2 IMA of 14 degrees or less associated with a DMAA greater than 8 degrees.[15]
- Reports of the traditional distal chevron technique over the past two decades suggest that comparable outcomes are achieved for younger and older patients.[9]
- In our hands, contraindications to any distal first metatarsal osteotomy for hallux valgus correction include asymptomatic deformity; a 1–2 IMA exceeding 15 degrees; first MTP joint stiffness or degenerative arthritis; and osteoporosis or osteopenia.

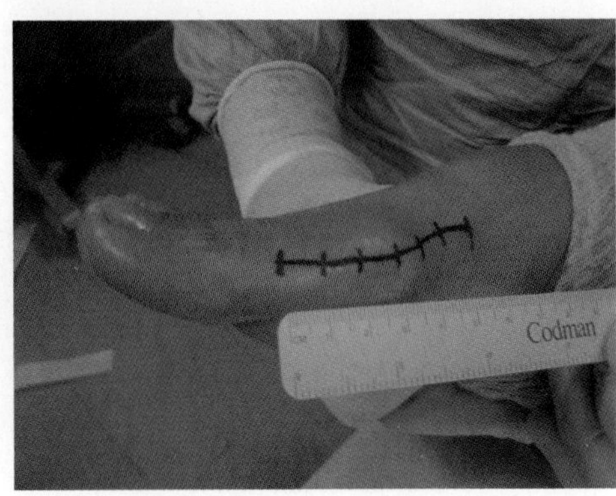

FIG 4 • The skin incision is centered over the medial eminence.

Preoperative Planning

- Satisfactory neurovascular status
- Is the hallux valgus passively correctible? The surgeon should assess associated lesser toes deformities, including fixed versus flexible deformity, impingement or overlap on the first toe, and presence of plantar calluses.
- Using radiographic measurements from preoperative weight-bearing radiographs of the foot, we always have a preoperative estimation of the required lateral translation of the first metatarsal head and wedge resection to correct the increased DMAA.

Positioning

- The patient is positioned supine, with the plantar aspect of the operated foot in line with the end of the operating table.
- We stand on the side of the table immediately adjacent to the operated foot; our assistant stands at the end of the table.
- We routinely use a tourniquet.

Approach

- A 5-cm longitudinal midaxial medial incision is made, centered over the medial eminence (**FIG 4**).
- Careful subcutaneous dissection is performed to protect the dorsal and plantar medial sensory nerves to the hallux.
- While the distal metatarsal metaphysis must be exposed, periosteal stripping is kept to a minimum and the lateral vascular supply to the first metatarsal head remains protected.
- In our experience, with the proper indications outlined above, we rarely need to perform a risky lateral dissection of the adductor hallucis tendon at the joint line.
  - A routine portion of the exposure, lateral dislocation of the metatarsal head, serves as a physiologic release of the adductor hallucis by bringing its phalangeal insertion closer to its origin.[9,10,15]

CAPSULOTOMY

- I use a Y-shaped incision over the medial face of the MTP joint capsule, creating three distinct flaps that I reapproximate at the completion of the procedure to achieve optimal tensioning (**TECH FIG 1A,B**).
- A short V capsular flap attached to the base of the hallux proximal phalanx may be used as an anchor to correct the deformity. I always preserve the relatively thin dorsal capsular flap continuous with the lateral capsule to maintain the blood supply to the first metatarsal head. The stout plantar capsular flap attached to the sesamoids serves to re-establish the optimal first metatarsal head–sesamoid position when tensioned after completion of the osteotomy.

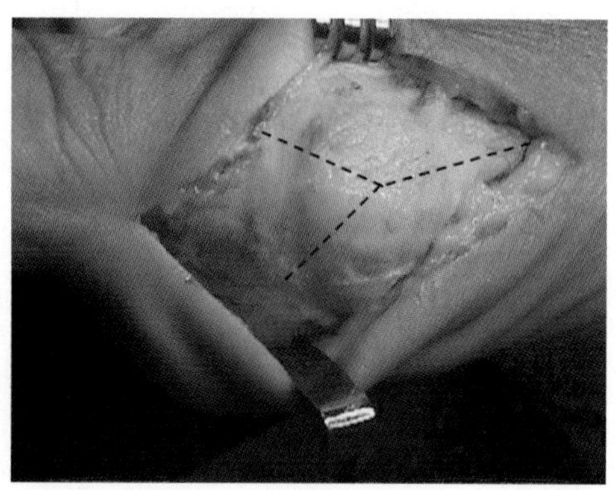

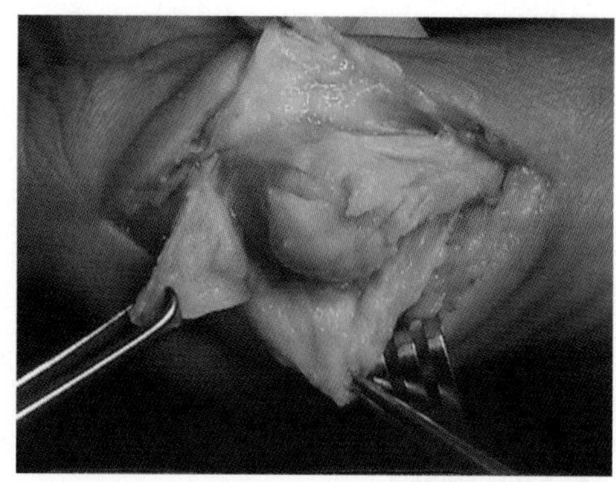

TECH FIG 1 • **A.** The Y figure over the medial face of the metatarsophalangeal joint demarcating the capsular flaps. **B.** Following the Y figure, the articular capsule is divided to create the three flaps: a V flap attached to the base of the proximal phalanx, a thin dorsal flap, and a strong plantar flap.

MEDIAL AND DORSAL METATARSAL HEAD EXPOSURE

- After capsulotomy the first metatarsal head's medial eminence and sagittal groove are exposed.
- Starting at the medial aspect of the sagittal groove, I resect the medial eminence with a small oscillating saw from dorsal to plantar, in line with the medial edge of the foot (**TECH FIG 2A,B**).
  - I make sure to preserve the integrity of the metatarsal head and medial cortex of the metatarsal shaft (**TECH FIG 2C,D**).
- Occasionally, a "dorsal bunion" is present in the absence of degenerative change. I routinely resect this dorsal eminence in line with the dorsal cortex of the metatarsal shaft to eliminate any chance for impingement and potentially improve cosmesis (**TECH FIG 2E**).

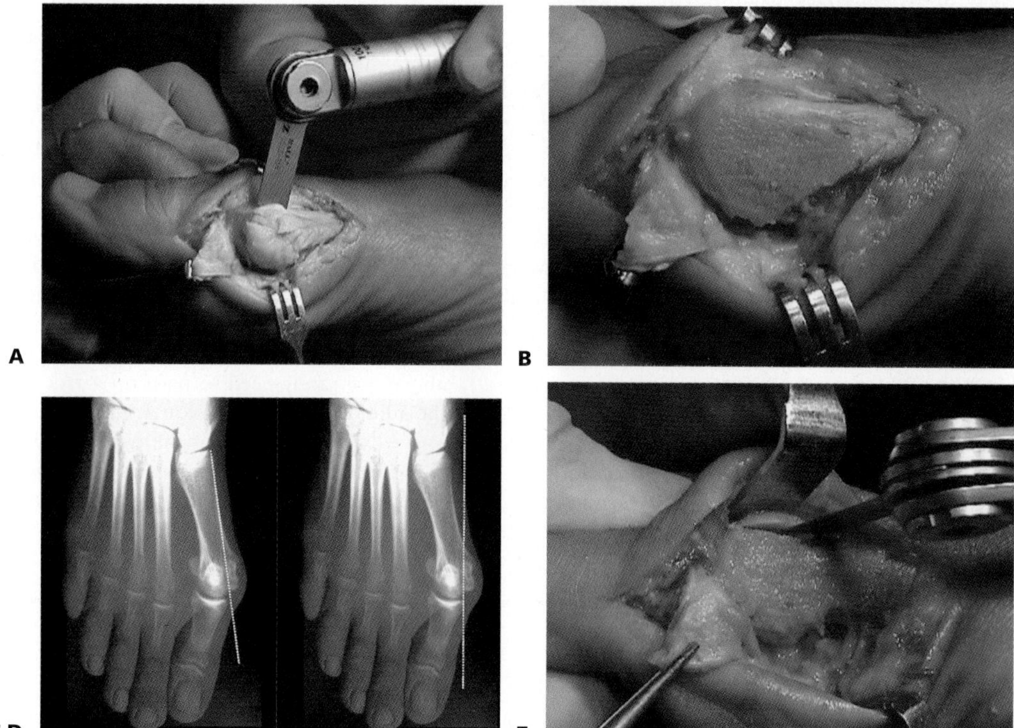

TECH FIG 2 • **A, B.** The beginning of the medial prominence removal. With the sagittal groove used as a guide, the saw is oriented in a dorsoplantar direction. **C.** The medial osteotomy must follow the medial border of the foot to preserve the integrity of the metatarsal head and diaphysis. The wrong way to do this is shown. **D.** The right way to proceed to the prominence resection is shown. **E.** The dorsal prominence of the metatarsal head is resected in line with the dorsal diaphyseal cortex.

OSTEOTOMY

- As a point of reference, I mark the geometric center of the first metatarsal head with a sharp instrument on the prepared medial surface (**TECH FIG 3A**). From this point I draw the segments (arms) of the planned osteotomy.
- I cut the plantar arm of the osteotomy parallel to the inferior surface of the foot (**TECH FIG 3B**), thereby creating a broad and stable surface area to promote healing between the two osteotomy fragments.
- According to the preoperative radiographic DMAA estimate, I plan a medially based wedge resection as part of the dorsal limb osteotomy to rotate the capital fragment into a more physiologic relationship with the first metatarsal shaft. Three methods exist to determine the correct size for the medial wedge to be removed[15]:
  - A trigonometric formula (wedge width = tan DMAA × first metatarsal head width [in millimeters])
  - Drawing the wedge corresponding to the measured DMAA over the AP radiographic image of the first metatarsal
  - By direct vision during the operation, make the distal cut parallel to the distal metatarsal articular surface and the proximal cut perpendicular to the long axis of the first metatarsal (**TECH FIG 3C–E**).
- The saw blade must not violate the inferior portion of the metatarsal head fragment.
- In my experience, each millimeter of lateral metatarsal head translation corresponds to one degree of 1–2 IMA correction. Using average physiologic dimensions, the metatarsal head may be translated laterally up to 6 mm to create a 9-degree 1–2 IMA without forfeiting osteotomy stability.
- After dorsal wedge resection and simultaneous to lateral translation, rotate the metatarsal head to create a physiologic DMAA and achieve optimal bony apposition at the dorsal aspect of the osteotomy.[9,12]
- Gentle longitudinal traction on the hallux and concomitant pressure with the thumb over the medial capital fragment facilitates lateral displacement (**TECH FIG 3F**).
- By driving the great toe as a joystick, the capital fragment is rotated under direct vision to correct the DMAA.

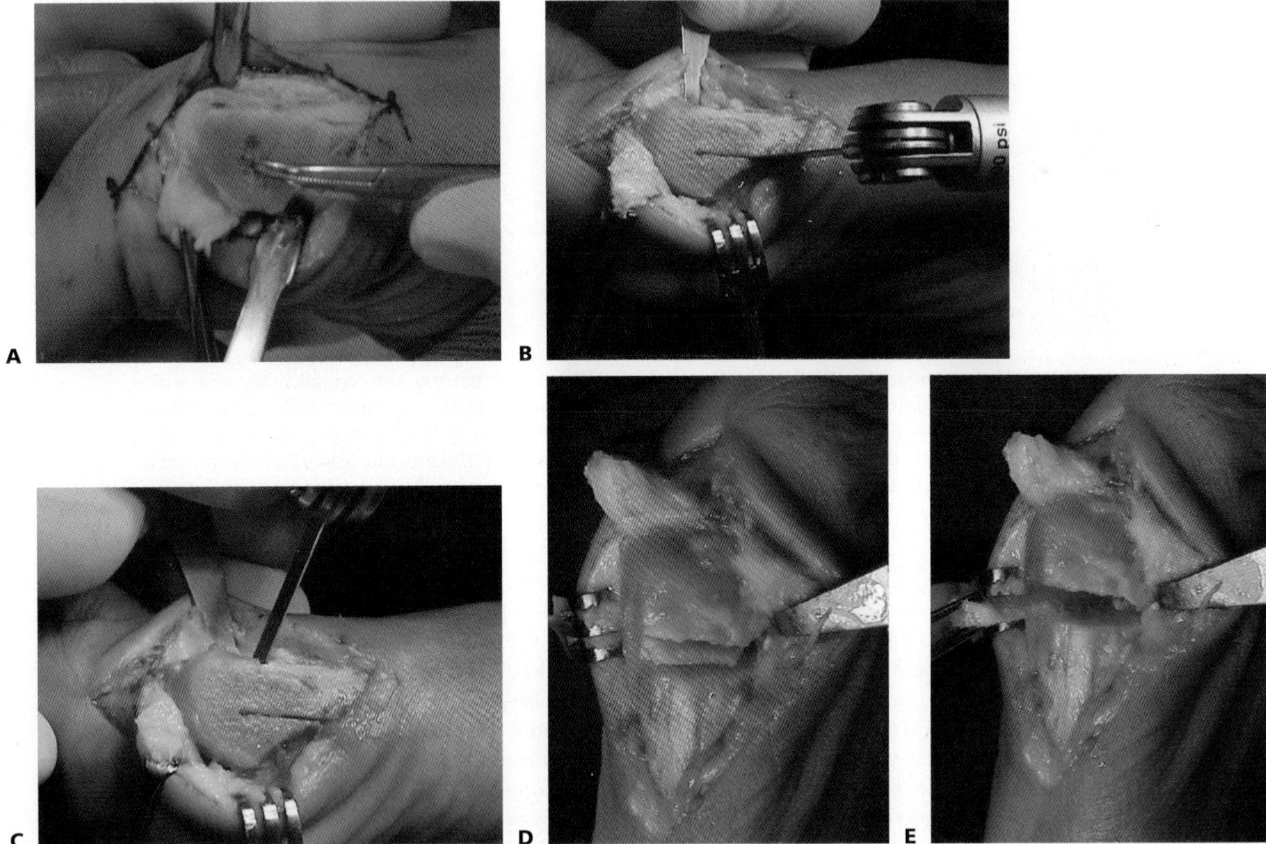

TECH FIG 3 • **A.** Marking the geometric center of the metatarsal head. **B.** The plantar arm of the osteotomy, parallel to the plantar surface of the foot. **C.** The positioning of the saw during the planning of the dorsal arm of the osteotomy. There is a posterior inclination of 10 to 15 degrees to create an acute vertex for the osteotomy. **D.** The dorsal segment of the osteotomy is made using two cuts. The distal one is parallel to the distal articular surface, and the proximal cut is perpendicular to the metatarsal diaphyseal axis so that a medially based wedge is produced. **E.** The metaphyseal bone wedge is removed. *(continued)*

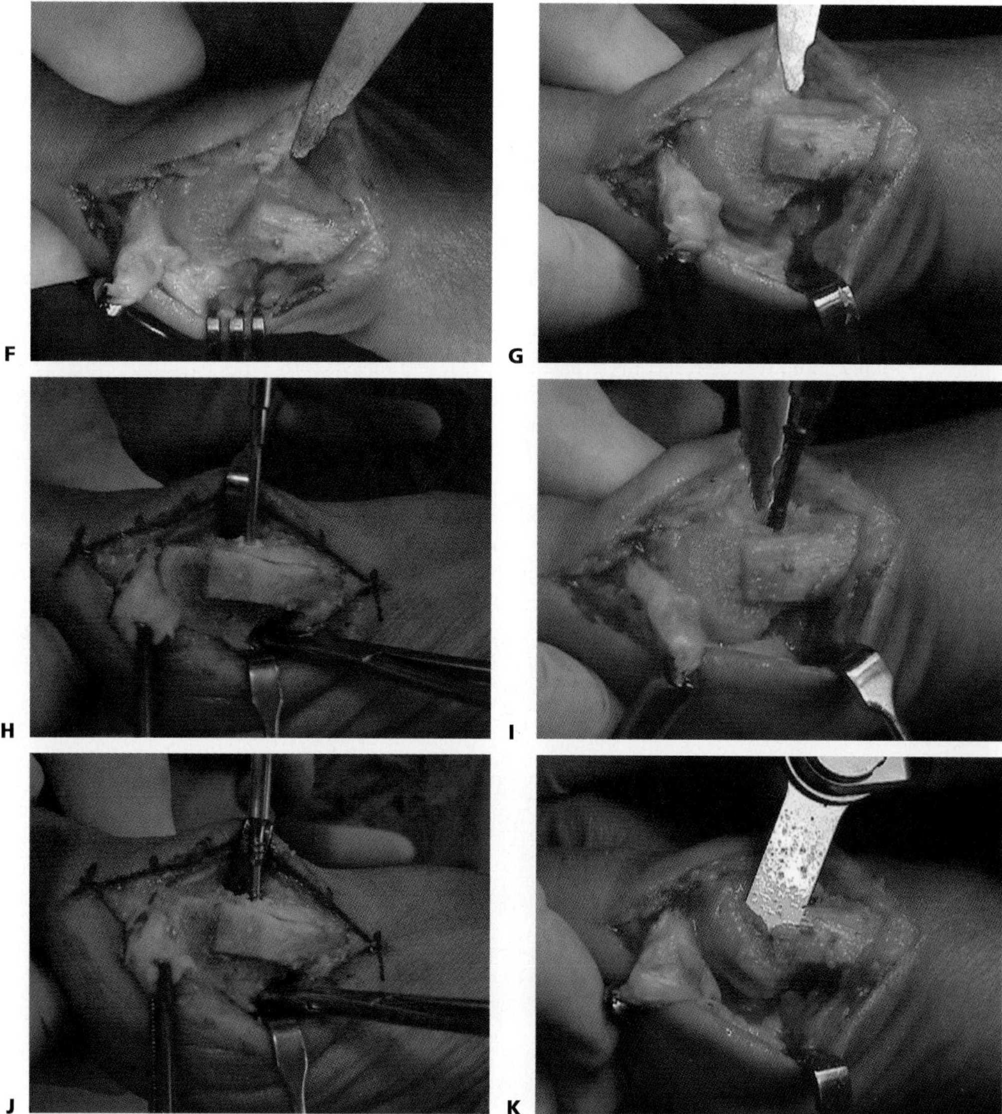

TECH FIG 3 • *(continued)* **F.** With light distraction applied on the great toe, the cephalic fragment is laterally dislocated and internally rotated to reduce both the intermetatarsal angle and the distal metatarsal articular angle. **G.** Gentle pressure is applied on the great toe to coapt the osteotomy site. **H.** Making a drill hole at the dorsal aspect of the metaphysis of the metatarsal. **I.** The introduction of a 2.7-mm screw to achieve the bone fixation. **J.** Bone fixation with a Herbert-type screw. **K.** The metaphyseal remaining portion must be removed from dorsal to plantar to clear the medial border of the metatarsal.

- Once the proper positioning of the fragments is obtained, apply gentle pressure on the great toe to coapt the osteotomy site (TECH FIG 3G).
- In our experience, it is not necessary to check the position of the fragments and the amount of correction with fluoroscopy but, for those who think that it is advisable, this is the right moment to do that. You can use a 1.2-mm Kirschner wire to maintain the fragments temporarily during the fluoroscopic checking.
- I routinely secure the osteotomy with a single screw, either a solid screw placed in lag fashion or a headless cannulated or noncannulated dual-pitch compression screw, while maintaining manual reduction of the osteotomy.
  - Screw position: 5 mm proximal to the dorsal arm of the biplanar chevron osteotomy, on the first metatarsal shaft (TECH FIG 3H)
  - Screw trajectory: I aim the screw 10 degrees distally and 15 degrees laterally to target the optimal portion of the laterally translated distal fragment, compress the fragments, and limit the risk of penetrating the plantar articular surface.[9]
- Using a 2.7-mm solid screw
  - Initial 2.0-mm drill hole, followed by overdrill of the near cortex with a 2.7-mm drill to create a lag effect
  - Because of the screw trajectory and relatively thin overlying capsule and skin, consider using a countersink.
  - Insertion of the 2.7-mm screw to carefully compress the osteotomy and maintain reduction (TECH FIG 3I)
- Using a headless cannulated or noncannulated dual-pitch screw
  - Guide pin (if cannulated)

- Dual-diameter drill corresponding to the particular screw system
- Insertion of the screw after proper screw length has been determined, with compression of the fragments and stability created at the osteotomy (**TECH FIG 3J**)
- Carefully resect the residual medial prominence of the proximal fragment with an oscillating saw, directing the saw blade from dorsal to plantar while avoiding any violation of the first metatarsal diaphysis (**TECH FIG 3K**).

- I routinely irrigate the first MTP joint with saline solution to remove undesirable detritus.

CAPSULORRHAPHY

- I judiciously resect redundant medial capsule. Holding the proximal phalanx in optimal alignment relative to the long axis of the first metatarsal in both the sagittal and transverse planes facilitates determining the overlap of residual medial capsule.
  - In anticipation of some tendency toward recurrence of deformity, I typically hold the hallux in a slight varus and plantarflexion position.
  - In my experience, this optimal position is best maintained by the assistant holding the first metatarsal, the MTP joint, and hallux between the thumb and the second finger of the assistant's hand so that the hallux rests in the space between the assistant's first and second metacarpals (**TECH FIG 4A,B**).
- With the assistant maintaining the optimal position, I resect the redundant capsular flaps.
- Next, I check the relationship of the medial sesamoid and first metatarsal head, applying greater tension to the plantar flap to reduce the head on the sesamoids if necessary. I place a 2-0 nonabsorbable buried suture at the central corners of both the dorsal and plantar capsular flaps and systematically close the capsulotomy from distal to proximal (**TECH FIG 4C**).
- Appose the residual V-shaped flap attached to the medial aspect of the proximal phalanx to the previously sutured dorsal and plantar flaps.
- In my experience, removing greater capsular redundancy from the dorsal portion of the phalangeal flap facilitates correction of hallux pronation (**TECH FIG 4D–F**).
- I use a single suture, which is placed at the center of the Y, where the capsular flaps meet (**TECH FIG 4G**).
  - Once the medial capsulorrhaphy is complete, the assistant releases the toe. Ideally, the hallux should maintain its corrected alignment without external support.
  - Occasionally I augment the capsulorrhaphy with complementary tensioning sutures to obtain the desired position. Again the hallux must be held in the corrected position, or even slight varus as noted above (**TECH FIG 4H**).

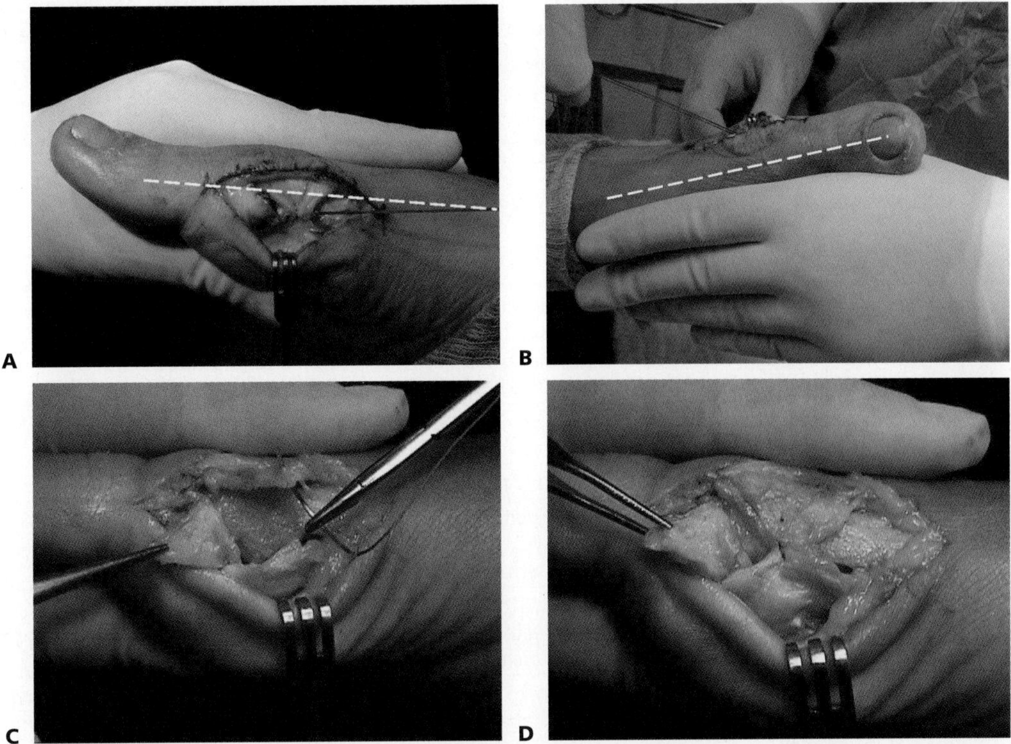

TECH FIG 4 • **A, B.** The best way to keep the hallux in the right position during the capsulorrhaphy. The great toe must be aligned with the first metatarsal in the sagittal and transverse planes. **C.** After resecting the excess, the dorsal flap is sutured to the plantar capsular flap. **D.** The V-shaped flap attached to the proximal phalanx is apposed to the dorsal and plantar flaps. *(continued)*

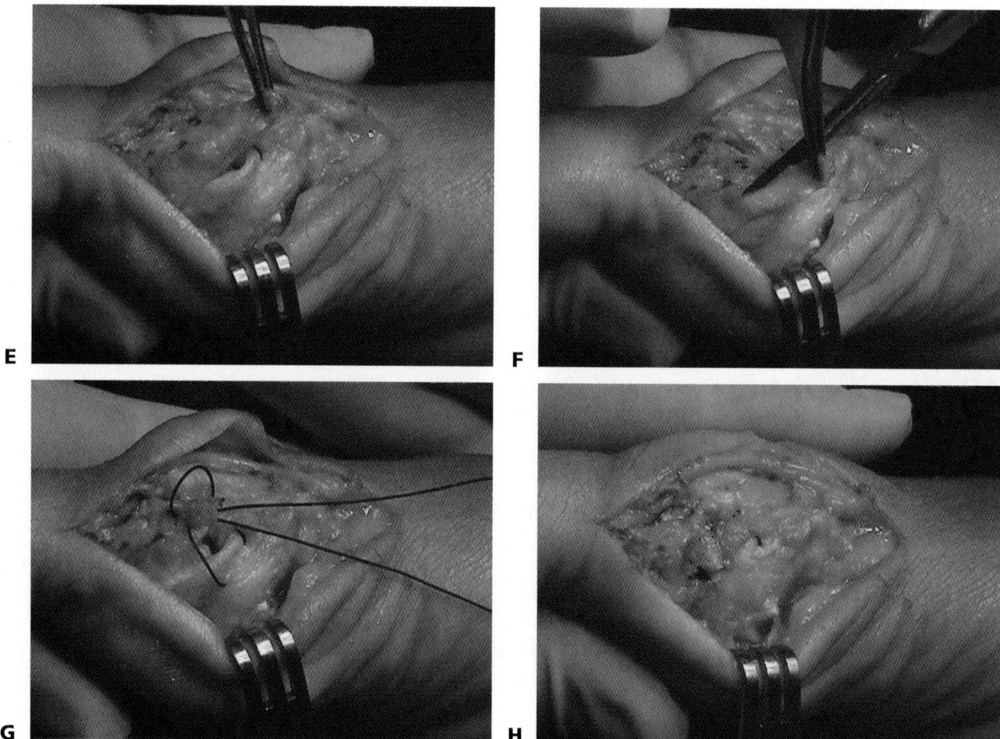

TECH FIG 4 • *(continued)* **E, F.** The excess of the V flap is determined and resected. **G.** A single suture is placed in the vertex of the V-shaped flap. After the toe is released, its adequate position is checked. **H.** While the great toe is kept at the right position, the capsular suture is finished.

- Close the subcutaneous tissue with interrupted absorbable sutures.
- I favor using absorbable subcuticular sutures and interrupted fine nylon suture in young patients (more favorable skin) and older patients (less favorable skin), respectively. I routinely use a bunion dressing, or H dressing, in the first web space to relieve tension on the medial capsulorrhaphy. I wrap the forefoot with a sterile cotton bandage followed by an adhesive bandage that maintains slight compression on the first metatarsal.

PEARLS AND PITFALLS

Indications	■ I favor a proximal first metatarsal osteotomy with a 1–2 IMA greater than 15 degrees. ■ In my experience, the power of 1–2 IMA correction is limited by the width of the metatarsal head. ■ In general, 1 mm of lateral translation equals 1 degree of 1–2 IMA correction. ■ A biplanar osteotomy is not required unless the DMAA exceeds 8 degrees.
Approach	■ I routinely perform the skin incision 2 mm dorsal to the medial midaxial line to identify and protect the dorsomedial sensory nerve to the hallux.
Capsular flaps	■ Develop the capsular flaps carefully to allow optimal soft tissue balancing during capsulorrhaphy.
Medial eminence resection	■ Perform the medial eminence resection in line with the medial foot, not the medial aspect of the first metatarsal. ■ Less resection is better (limits potential for varus)!
Osteotomy	■ The plantar arm should be parallel to the plantar plane of the foot. ■ The apex of the wedge to be resected dorsally should coincide with the lateral cortex of the head to avoid shortening of the metatarsal.
Screw fixation	■ Direct the drill and screw laterally to capture the plantar "tongue" of the distal fragment. ■ Avoid placing a screw that penetrates the plantar cortex at the metatarsal head–sesamoid complex. ■ Remember to countersink the dorsal metaphyseal cortex when using a 2.7-mm screw.
Capsulorrhaphy	■ Be sure that your assistant maintains the great toe at the right position during capsulorrhaphy.
Dressing	■ Should maintain the great toe in the optimal position for 3 weeks.

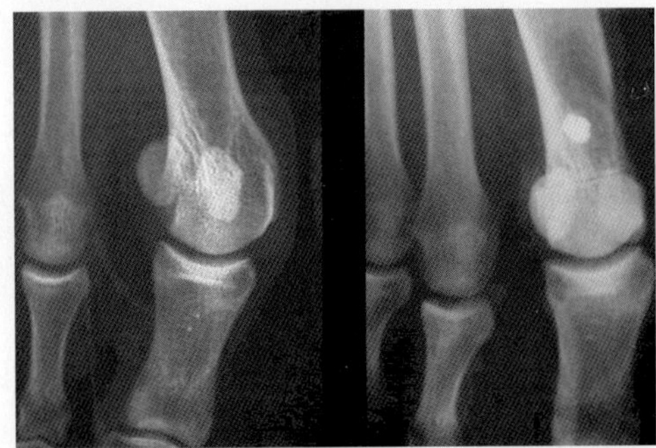
A

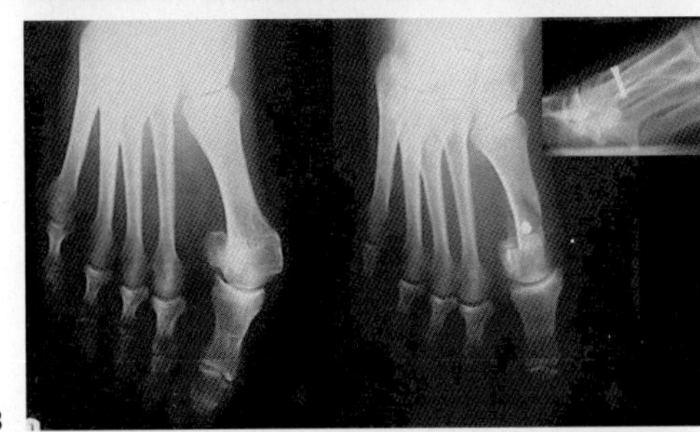
B

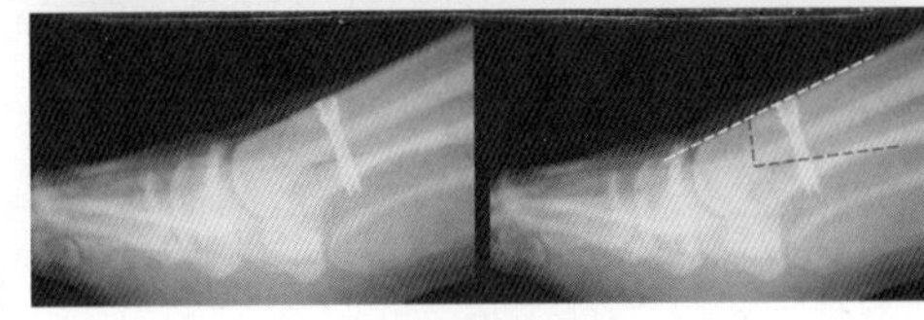
C

FIG 5 • **A.** Preoperative and postoperative radiographic images of a right foot with hallux valgus with increased distal metatarsal articular angle (DMAA), treated by the biplanar chevron osteotomy. The correction of the DMAA and the sesamoid position is easy to see. The valgus of the great toe was also satisfactorily corrected. **B.** In these images, we can see the correction obtained with the biplanar distal chevron osteotomy. The cephalic fragment was 6 mm laterally dislocated to correct the intermetatarsal angle (IMA) and the sesamoid position. The DMAA and hallux valgus angle (HVA) were corrected to normal values. In the lateral view, we can see the size and position of the screw used in the fragment fixation. **C.** Lateral views of a patient treated by the biplanar distal chevron osteotomy, where we can see both the plantar and dorsal arms of the osteotomy, the position of the screw used in its fixation, and the alignment of the cephalic fragment with the metatarsal diaphysis resulting from the dorsal fragment resection.

POSTOPERATIVE CARE

- Anticipated dried blood may harden the bandage and create pressure-related symptoms postoperatively. This occurs often enough that we routinely change the patient's bandage on postoperative day 3 or 4.[10]
- We allow my patients to bear weight in a Barouk postoperative shoe after the first dressing change. This orthosis concentrates the patient's weight on the rear of the foot while protecting the forefoot. Our patients do not routinely require crutches or assistive devices, but the occasional elderly patient with comorbidities may benefit from temporary use of a walker.
- We routinely change the bandage for my bunion patients at 10-day intervals to confirm that proper great toe alignment is maintained. To confirm that the alignment and reduction are maintained, we obtain a radiograph of the operated foot at 3 weeks after surgery. In our experience, at 1 month postoperatively patients may transfer to a pair of soft and wide lace-up shoes and initiate hallux range-of-motion exercises.
- In our practice, it takes an average of 3 to 4 months for patients to reach the maximum range of motion and return to regular shoe wear and full activity.

OUTCOMES

- Patient satisfaction rates after distal biplanar chevron osteotomy for moderate hallux valgus deformity approach 90%, depending on appropriate patient expectations and selection.[15]
- In our experience, the procedure reliably and reproducibly corrects the 1–2 IMA, HVA, and increased DMAA (**FIG 5**).

COMPLICATIONS

- Complications are similar to other distal first metatarsal osteotomies for correction of hallux valgus.
- Recurrence or undercorrection
  - Inappropriate preoperative planning
    - Stretching the indications
  - Usually due to inadequate:
    - Lateral translation
    - Rotation of the first metatarsal head
    - Soft tissue balancing during the capsulorrhaphy
  - Lack of proper postoperative bunion dressing
- Avascular necrosis of the head of the first metatarsal
  - Overzealous lateral soft tissue stripping
  - Overpenetration of the saw blade into the lateral capsule
  - Although radiographic first metatarsal head changes are frequently observed after distal metatarsal osteotomies, they rarely progress to symptomatic necrosis and collapse of the metatarsal head.[8]
- First MTP joint stiffness
  - In our experience, joint stiffness responds to physical therapy and advancing the weight-bearing status. We maintain that slight overcorrection and some MTP joint stiffness is preferable to undercorrection and full MTP joint motion.
- Hallux varus
  - Overresection of the medial capsule
  - Unnecessary overrelease of the lateral capsule and adductor hallucis tendon

REFERENCES

1. Alexander IJ. Disorders of the first MTP joint. In: The Foot: Examination and Diagnosis, ed 2. New York: Churchill Livingstone, 1997:69–82.
2. Campbell JT. Hallux valgus: adult and juvenile. In: Richardson EG. OKU: Foot and Ankle 3. Rosemont, IL: American Academy of Orthopaedic Surgery, 2004:3–15.
3. Coughlin MJ. Metatarsophalangeal joint instability in the athlete. Foot Ankle 1993;14:309–319.
4. Coughlin MJ. Roger A. Mann Award: Juvenile hallux valgus: etiology and treatment. Foot Ankle Int 1995;16:682–697.
5. Coughlin MJ. Forefoot disorders. In: Baxter DE, ed. The Foot and Ankle in Sport. St Louis: Mosby, 1994:221–244.
6. Coughlin MJ, Carlson RE. Treatment of hallux valgus with an increased distal metatarsal articular angle: evaluation of double and triple first ray osteotomies. Foot Ankle Int 1999;20:762–770.
7. Coughlin MJ: Hallux valgus with increased DMAA. In: Nunley JA, Pfeffer GB, Sanders RW, et al, eds. Advanced Reconstruction Foot and Ankle. Rosemont, IL: American Academy of Orthopaedic Surgery, 2004:3–18.
8. Easley ME, Kelly IP. Avascular necrosis of the hallux metatarsal head. Foot Ankle Clin 2000;5:591–608.

9. Johnson KA. Chevron osteotomy. In: Master Techniques in Orthopaedic Surgery: The Foot and Ankle. New York: Raven, 1994: 31–48.
10. Myerson MS. Hallux valgus. In: Foot and Ankle Disorders. Philadelphia: WB Saunders, 2000:213–288.
11. Nery C, Mizusaki J, Magalhães AAC, et al. Tratamiento conservador del hallux valgus juvenil mediante ortesis nocturnas. Rev Española Cir Osteo 1997;187:32–37.
12. Nery C, Barrôco R, Maradei S, et al. Osteotomia em chevron biplana: apresentação de técnica. Acta Ortop Brasil 1999;7:47–52.
13. Nery C, Réssio C, Netto AA, et al. Avalição radiológica do hálux valgo: estudo populacional de novos parâmetros angulares. Acta Ortop Brasil 2001;9:41–48.
14. Nery C. Tornozelo e pé. In: Barros TEP, Lech O, eds. Exame Físico em Ortopedia, Sarvier. São Paulo, 2001:267–300.
15. Nery C, Barroco R, Réssio C. Biplanar chevron osteotomy. Foot Ankle Int 2002;23:792–798.
16. Piggot H. The natural history of hallux valgus in adolescence and early adult life. J Bone Joint Surg Br 1960;42B:749–754.

Chapter 4 Extending the Indications for the Distal Chevron Osteotomy

James L. Beskin

DEFINITION

- The distal chevron osteotomy has proven to be a reliable, reproducible method of bunion repair for mild to moderate deformity. By altering the location and displacement of the osteotomy, the indications can be expanded to more complex deformities while preserving the straightforward surgical exercise.
- The apex of the chevron osteotomy can be modified to a more proximal location along with a reduced angle to provide a stable healing surface that facilitates maximal lateral translation.
- The proximal location of the osteotomy also reduces the risk of avascular necrosis and permits safe lateral capsule release needed for larger corrections.
- This technique facilitates treatment for moderate to severe bunion deformity with a straightforward surgical method using limited, readily available internal fixation.

ANATOMY

- Factors contributing to a bunion deformity vary among individuals. The diverse anatomic features require scrutiny during surgical planning.
- Pertinent to the corrective factors of a translational osteotomy is the width of the distal metatarsal. The amount of correction may be limited in a small, narrow, or "hourglass" shaped bone.
- The distal metatarsal articular angle (DMAA) may be altered by varus or valgus rotation during a distal osteotomy. This additional corrective factor should be addressed during the surgical planning.
- The position of the sesamoids needs to be assessed for optimal correction. Station III subluxation usually requires a lateral capsule release to restore normal joint mechanics.
- Hypermobility of the first ray should be evaluated. Correction by lateral translation of the distal metatarsal may be compromised if the cuneiform–metatarsal joint is unstable.

IMAGING AND DIAGNOSTIC STUDIES

- Weight-bearing AP and lateral radiographs are used to determine bone morphology, associated disease, and deformity parameters used in decision making.
- The ideal correction is based on a line drawn along the first metatarsal that is parallel to the second metatarsal shaft and touches the medial base of the first metatarsal or cuneiform. This line crosses the first metatarsal shaft bisector near the ideal location for a corrective osteotomy. It also estimates the amount of translational correction needed (**FIG 1**).
- The grade of sesamoid subluxation is evaluated to determine whether a lateral capsular release is indicated. The DMAA is assessed to determine any varus or valgus rotational correction needed at the time of the osteotomy.

SURGICAL MANAGEMENT

Positioning

- The patient is positioned supine. When regional ankle block anesthesia is used, an ankle tourniquet is applied. Otherwise, a thigh tourniquet can be used for general or spinal anesthesia.

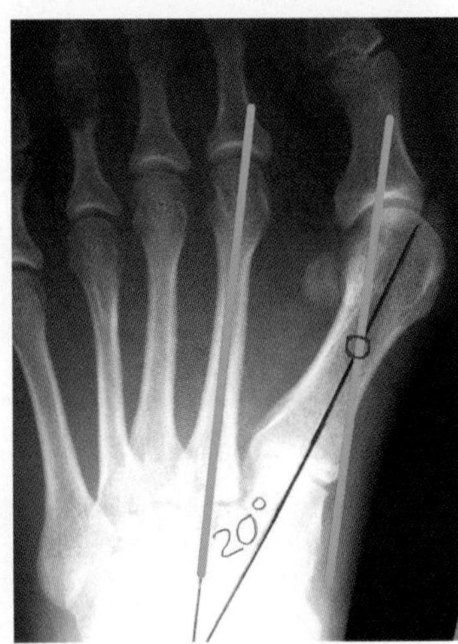

FIG 1 • The "ideal correction" is found by drawing a line parallel to the second metatarsal bisector that touches the base of the first metatarsal. The position where this line crosses the first metatarsal bisector helps determine the location and degree of translation needed for the first metatarsal osteotomy.

SOFT TISSUE PREPARATION

- When significant sesamoid subluxation is present (grade II or III), use a dorsal first web incision to expose the lateral capsule.
- A Freer elevator is helpful to probe and identify the dorsal margin of the subluxed lateral sesamoid. Then incise the capsule longitudinally from the phalanx to well proximal to the lateral sesamoid. The adductor tendon is plantar to this incision and is preserved. Leave the intermetatarsal ligament intact. The purpose of this longitudinal cut is to allow medialization of the plantar sesamoid complex at the time of capsule repair from the medial side.
- Expose the joint through a medial longitudinal incision. Identify and protect the superficial peroneal nerve. Mobilize the tissues to expose the capsule from the medial sesamoid inferiorly to the extensor hallucis longus tendon superiorly. The medial plantar digital nerve is also at risk and needs to be protected as the dissection nears the medial sesamoid.

- Cut the capsule longitudinally and slightly plantar to the center of the metatarsal. Reflect the capsule to expose the medial metatarsal eminence and the joint, but preserve it on the dorsal or plantar aspect to minimize risk of vascular insult.

BONE PREPARATION

- Remove the medial eminence with a power saw. The amount of bone is based on radiographic interpretation. Avoid excessive removal to prevent hallux varus. Usually the cut is 1 to 2 mm medial to the articular margin or the sagittal groove.
- Determine the apex of the osteotomy and mark it with a surgical pen (**TECH FIG 1**). It is typically 15 to 20 mm from the articular surface. Outline the proximal limbs at an angle of about 35 to 45 degrees. If the limbs are too short, there may be instability; if they are too long, there may be difficulty translating or rotating the distal head portion.

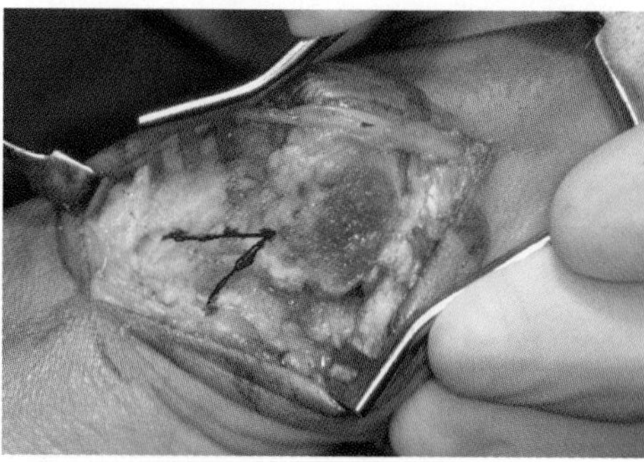

TECH FIG 1 • Usual location for the osteotomy.

- Next, use a Freer elevator to gently strip the periosteum and soft tissue over the area where the osteotomy is anticipated to cut the dorsal and plantar aspects of the metatarsal. Again, leave the tissues distal to the bone cut in place to minimize vascular compromise.
- The osteotomy can be affected by saw position with a dorsal, plantar, proximal, or distal angulation. Generally, a straight or neutral cut is best.
- After completing the osteotomy, the distal head fragment should be readily mobilized. Translation is facilitated by applying traction to the toe with one hand and using the other hand to pull with a towel clip on the apex of the proximal metatarsal. Thumb pressure against the head while maintaining traction will allow repositioning of the metatarsal with minimum force (**TECH FIG 2A**). If the head fragment is not readily mobilized, the osteotomy needs to be rechecked and cut.
- Since the osteotomy is usually proximal to the metaphyseal bone, the lateral cortex often appears as a spike. The distal head is then perched on this lateral process to maintain length (**TECH FIG 2B**). Up to 90% translation is possible and satisfactorily stabilized with Kirschner wires. Slight varus or valgus tilt can be applied as indicated by the DMAA.
- Using 0.054 smooth Kirschner wires, direct a pin from the proximal third of the metatarsal, medially exiting the lateral cortex and then entering the distal head fragment. These three points of fixation help maximize stability

A

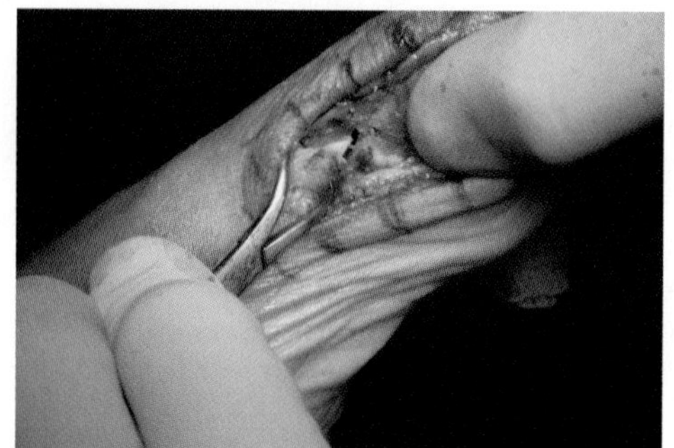

B

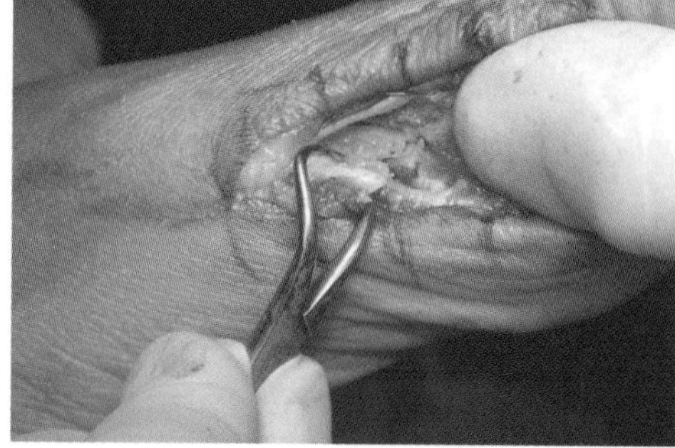

C

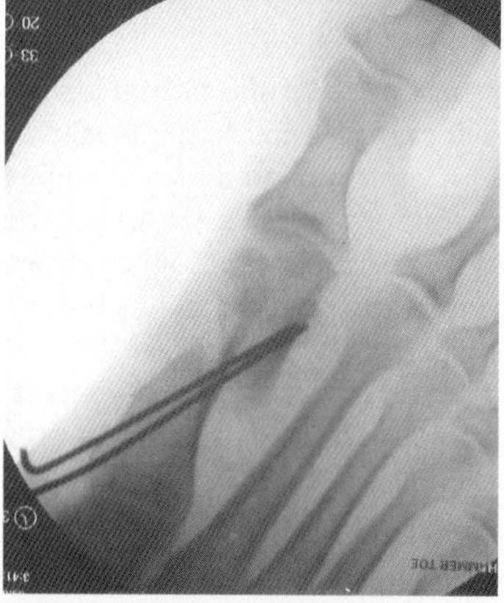

TECH FIG 2 • **A.** The osteotomy is translated laterally with traction and thumb pressure on the distal end while counterpressure is applied with a towel clip to the medial spike of the proximal end. **B.** The lateral cortex of the proximal metatarsal provides a stable spike to perch the distal head fragment.

with large corrections (TECH FIG 3). Place a second similar pin and check the position with radiographic control. Pins are typically bent and left out percutaneously but can be cut adjacent to the bone and removed electively.

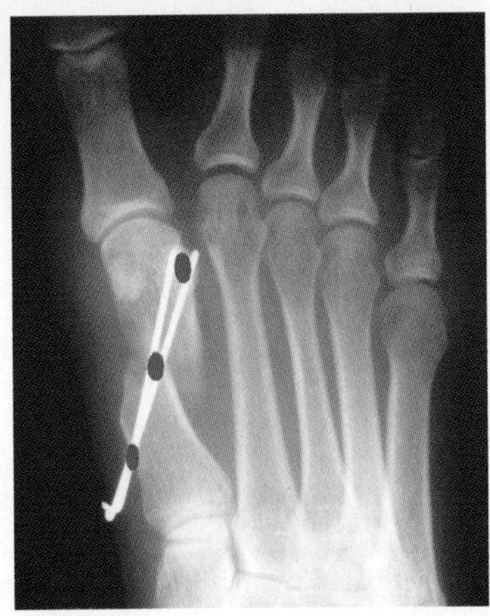

TECH FIG 3 • Optimal pin placement. Note contact with the medial and lateral aspect of the proximal metatarsal before entering the distal head fragment.

- Cut the large prominence of bone from the proximal, medial metatarsal and contour it in line with the distal head's medial margin. It is important to cut this back proximal enough to avoid a residual bump at the mid-metatarsal area (TECH FIG 4).

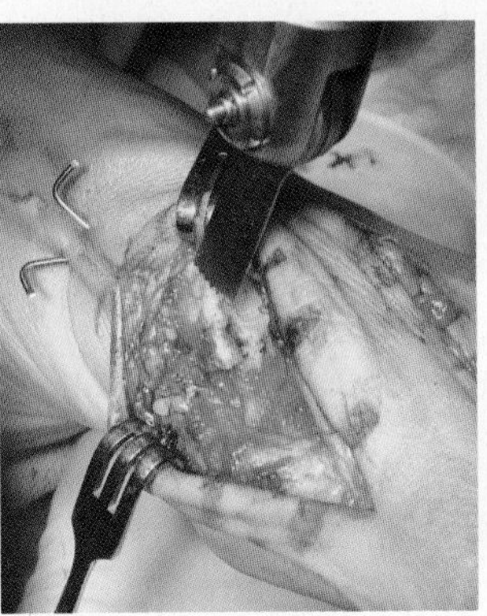

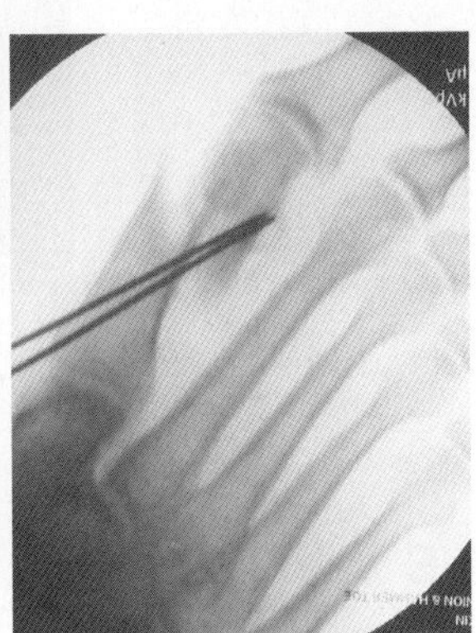

TECH FIG 4 • The saw is used to remove the remaining medial "bump" of the first metatarsal. This needs to be contoured in line with the medial metatarsal head to avoid symptoms at this area postoperatively.

SOFT TISSUE CLOSURE

- Tighten the medial capsule by removing a U-shaped wedge of tissue from the plantar aspect near the medial sesamoid. The amount of tissue removed is judged to allow adequate correction of the hallux valgus. Next, repair the capsule defect in the plantar limb. Then perform a "pants-over-vest" closure between the plantar and dorsal capsule to improve sesamoid position. The goal is to bring the medial sesamoid to the medial margin of the metatarsal head (TECH FIG 5). Skin closure and bunion dressings are then applied.

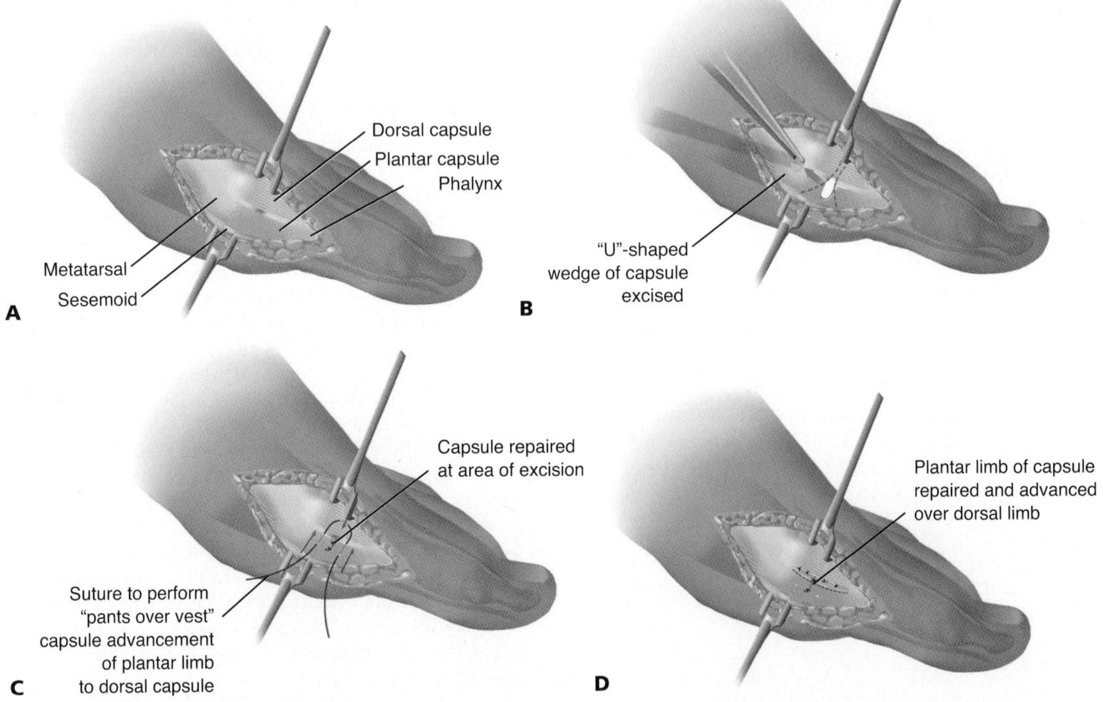

TECH FIG 5 • **A.** The longitudinal capsule incision. **B.** A U-shaped wedge of capsule is removed and sutured to tighten the plantar limb of the capsule and correct the hallux valgus. **C.** Suture is placed in a "pants-over-vest" technique to advance the plantar limb of the capsule medial and dorsal. **D.** The remaining capsule is closed.

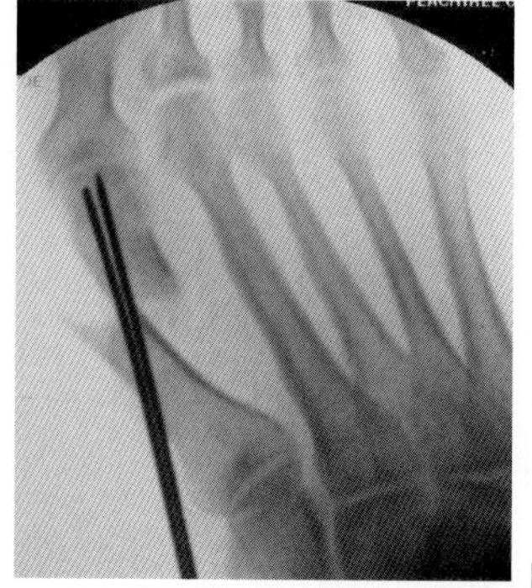
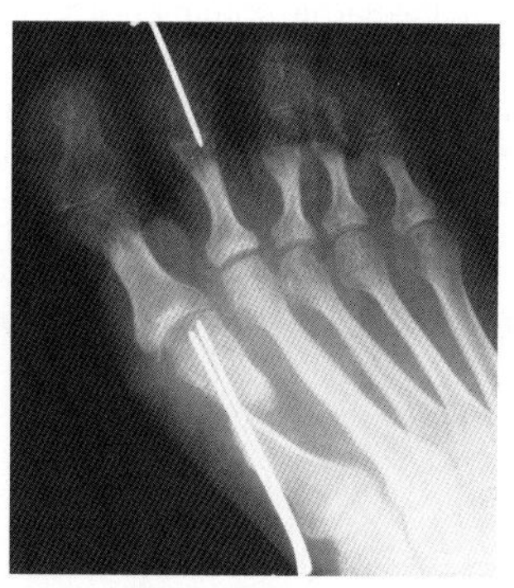
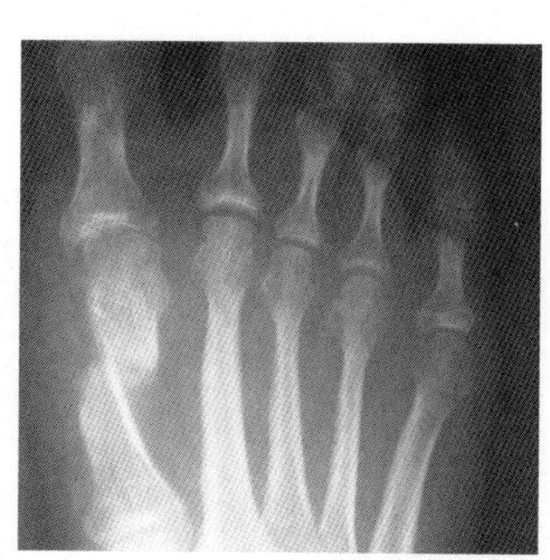
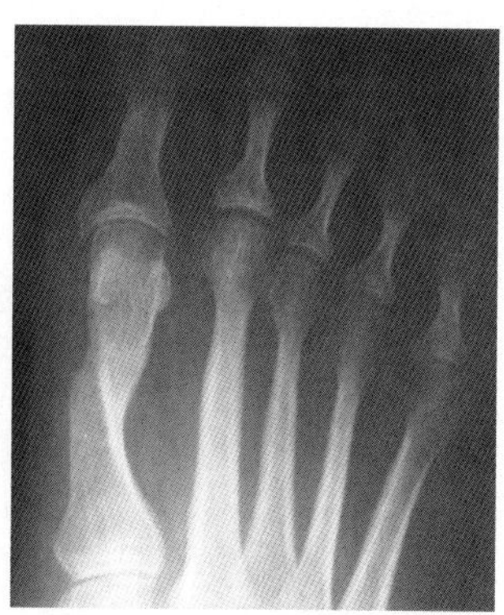

FIG 2 • **A.** Intraoperative radiographic appearance of the osteotomy. The "medial bump" still needs removal from the metatarsal. Office radiographs at 2 weeks (**B**), 8 weeks (**C**), and 12 months (**D**).

PEARLS AND PITFALLS

- Avoid routine lateral adductor release to reduce the risk of hallux varus unless specifically indicated by the clinical situation. The increased lateral translation of the osteotomy usually decompresses the lateral structures. The main focus is to realign the sesamoids under the metatarsal head.
- An aggressive contouring of the proximal portion of the metatarsal is necessary to reduce the risk of a residual bony bump near the osteotomy site. This often goes into the medullary canal. The Kirschner wires need to be placed proximal enough to avoid being cut out during this maneuver.
- Two Kirschner wires are recommended to reduce the risk of head migration until healing callus has developed.

POSTOPERATIVE CARE

- Patients are instructed to keep the limb elevated the majority of the first 2 weeks postoperatively. They are allowed to "heel walk" in a postoperative shoe with crutches provided for longer distance or pain management.
- At 2 weeks, sutures are removed and another bunion dressing is applied. The patient is instructed to passively dorsiflex and plantarflex the toe.
- At 5 weeks the pins are removed and the patient is taught to use a compression wrap and toe spacer. Aggressive range-of-motion exercises are initiated.
- Patients are followed on a 3- to 4-week basis to monitor healing and alignment (**FIG 2**).
- With larger osteotomy translation and correction, radiographic healing can take 3 months or more. However, the osteotomy is usually stable for activities of daily living within 2 months. Sports and strenuous activities may require 3 to 5 months of healing.

OUTCOMES

- We assessed 72 procedures in 62 patients operated on between Jan. 1, 2002, and Dec. 30, 2003. AOFAS scores and radiographic assessments were obtained from 39 at an average of 27.6 months after surgery.[5]
- AOFAS scores averaged 93.3, with complete radiographic healing in all patients.
- Hallux valgus angle correction averaged 22.3 degrees and intermetatarsal angle correction averaged 7.7 degrees.

COMPLICATIONS

- Complications included three symptomatic hallux varus deformities that were felt to be due to routine adductor release. This has been revised to a limited lateral capsule release as described here with preservation of the adductor tendon in most cases.
- There were three symptomatic medial diaphyseal "bumps" due to inadequate resection of the medial metatarsal after translation. This is now being addressed with more aggressive medial contouring.
- There was one symptomatic dorsal malunion and one case of surgical neuritis of the peroneal nerve branches.
- Only three cases of new or increased transfer lesions were identified.
- No cases of avascular necrosis were identified.

REFERENCES

1. Antonio J, Sanhudo V. Correction of moderate to severe hallux valgus deformity by a modified chevron shaft osteotomy. Foot Ankle Int 2006;27:581–585.
2. Austin DW, Leventen EO. A new osteotomy for hallux valgus. Clin Orthop Relat Res 1981;157:25–30.
3. Harper MC. Correction of metarsus primus varus with the chevron metatarsal osteotomy. Clin Orthop Relat Res 1989;243:180–183.
4. Johnson KA, Cofield RH, Morrey BF. Chevron osteotomy for hallux valgus. Clin Orthop Relat Res 1979;142:44–47.
5. Murawski D, Beskin JL. Increased displacement maximizes the utility of the distal chevron osteotomy for hallux vagus deformity correction. Foor Ankle Int 2008;29:155–163.
6. Oh I, Kim MK, Lee SH. New modified technique of osteotomy for hallux valgus. J Orthop Surg 2004;12:235–238.
7. Sanhudo JA. Extending the indications for distal chevron osteotomy. Foot Ankle Int 2000;21:522–523.
8. Sarrafian SK. A method of predicting the degree of functional correction of the metatarsus primus varus with a distal lateral displacement osteotomy in hallux valgus. Foot Ankle Int 1985;5:322–326.
9. Schneider W, Aigner N, Pinggera O, et al. Chevron osteotomy in hallux valgus: ten-year result of 112 cases. J Bone Joint Surg Br 2004; 86B:1016–1020.
10. Stienstra JJ, Lee JA, Nakadate DT. Large displacement distal chevron osteotomy for the correction of hallux valgus deformity. J Foot Ankle Surg 2002;41:213–220.
11. Thordarson D, Ebramzadeh E, Moorthy M, et al. Correlation of hallux valgus surgical outcome with AOFAS forefoot score and radiological parameters. Foot Ankle Int 2005;26:122–127.

Chapter 5 The Minimally Invasive Hallux Valgus Correction (SERI)

Sandro Giannini, Cesare Faldini, Francesca Vannini, Matteo Cadossi, and Deianira Luciani

DEFINITION

- Hallux valgus is a deformity of the forefoot characterized by progressive lateral subluxation of the proximal phalanx of the first toe on the first metatarsal head. It is considered pathologic when the patient experiences symptoms associated with a valgus deviation (hallux valgus angle [HVA]) greater than 15 degrees (**FIG 1**).[7,8]
- Hallux valgus is more common in adult women. It is often bilateral, and in many cases it is associated with other foot deformities, such as lesser toe or hindfoot or midfoot deformities that may exacerbate the pathology.[14]
- Hallux valgus is often a progressive disease that compromises the physiologic function of the first metatarsophalangeal (MTP) joint and potentially the entire forefoot.

ANATOMY

- The first metatarsal is the broadest and shortest of the five metatarsals, and the distal condyle of the first metatarsal head articulates with the proximal phalanx of the great toe. In addition, the plantar aspect of the first metatarsal head articulates with the sesamoids, which are contained in the flexor brevis hallucis tendon.
- The relationship of the medial and lateral sesamoids is maintained by the intersesamoid ligament. In association with the ligaments of and muscle balance about the first MTP joint, the sesamoid complex contributes to stabilizing the first MTP joint.
- When functioning properly, the first MTP joint optimizes push-off of the hallux during gait.[4]
- While physiologically the first MTP joint has a wide motion arc in the sagittal plane, it exhibits very little flexibility in the coronal plane. Hallux valgus occurs with greater than physiologic coronal plane motion of the first MTP joint.
- The first metatarsal head receives its main dorsal blood supply from the first dorsal metatarsal artery, a major contributor to an extracapsular anastomosis at the first MTP joint. On the plantar aspect of the first metatarsal head, the blood supply is from a combination of capsular arteries, branches of the first plantar metatarsal artery, and the first dorsal metatarsal artery.[15,17]

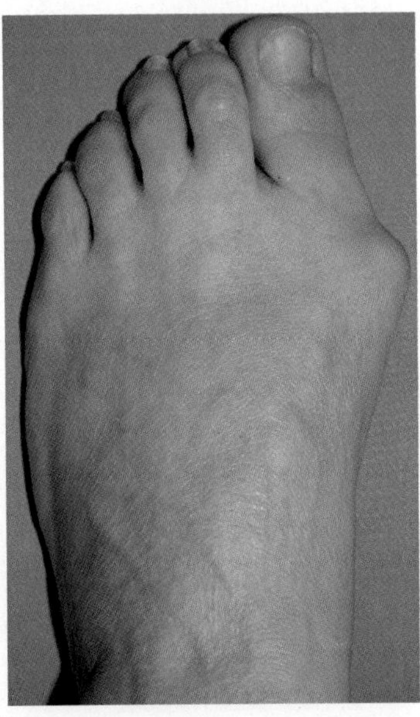

FIG 1 • Hallux valgus deformity in a female patient 50 years old.

PATHOGENESIS

- The pathogenesis of hallux valgus is not fully understood.
- In some patients, hallux valgus deformity may be due to congenital malalignment, neurologic conditions, systemic disease (such as rheumatoid arthritis), connective tissue disorders (with greater than physiologic ligamentous laxity), valgus deviation of the lesser toes, or trauma.[3,4,12,13]
- Several factors that may compromise the normal biomechanics of the foot have been implicated in the development of hallux valgus, including hereditary factors, shape of the first MTP joint, shoe wear, pes planus, and metatarsus adductus.[1–3,10,18,19]
- Controversy remains over the greatest primary cause leading to hallux valgus: valgus deviation of the hallux or metatarsus primus varus.[5,7–11]

PATIENT HISTORY AND PHYSICAL FINDINGS

- With loss of the physiologic balance of the first MTP joint, dynamic muscle function leads to progression of hallux valgus deformity in the majority of cases.
- Progressive hallux valgus may create other forefoot problems, including bursitis of the first MTP joint (**FIG 2**), callosities, and onychocryptosis (between the first and the second toe).
- Advanced hallux valgus may diminish first MTP joint function to the point that it leads to lesser toe deformity (claw and hammer toes) and associated transfer metatarsalgia (**FIG 3**).
- For ideal decision making in the management of hallux valgus, the following factors must be considered: pain, mobility and stability of the first MTP joint, and associated deformity.
- The site of the pain should be evaluated. The pain is often localized at the prominent medial eminence. At times, an inflamed

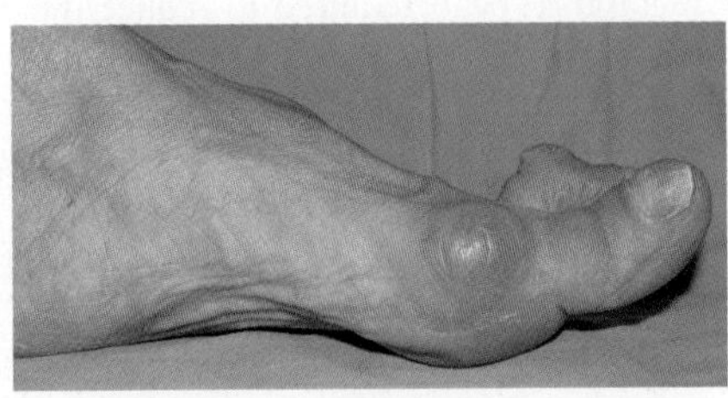

FIG 2 • Inflamed bursitis in a female patient 63 years old.

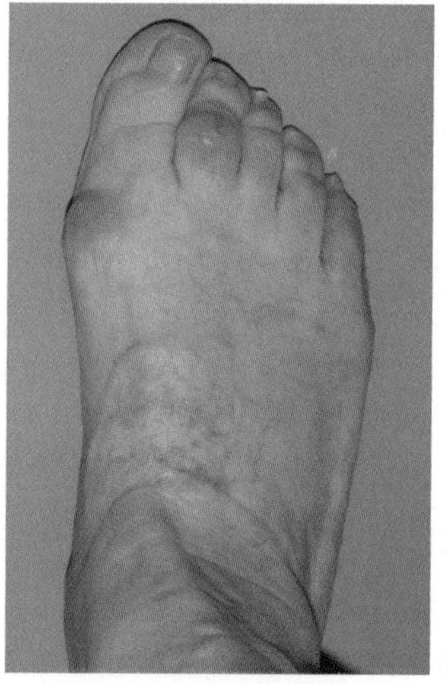

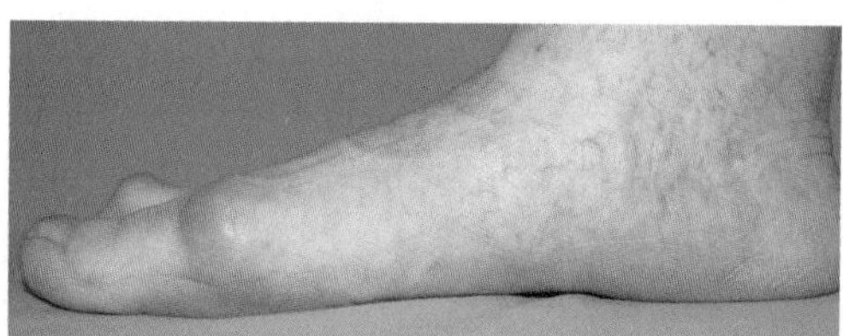

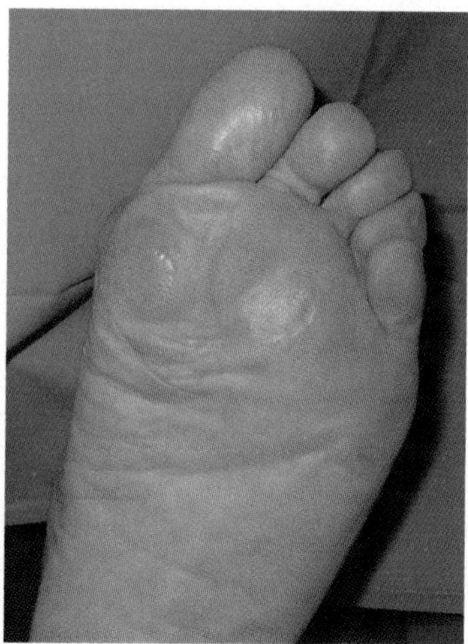

FIG 3 • **A,B.** Dorsoplantar and lateral view of a case of hallux valgus associated with a lesser toes deformity in a female patient 58 years old. **C.** Plantar view of a case of hallux valgus associated with metatarsalgia and plantar callosity in a female patient 55 years old.

bursa, a site of tenderness, overlies the prominent medial eminence. In advanced hallux valgus the pain should be referred to the lateral metatarsal head.

- Hallux mobility at the first MTP joint should be evaluated. Range of motion of the first MTP joint should be checked both in its resting valgus position and its correct neutral position. Any limitation may be a sign of first MTP joint incongruency or arthritis and should be evaluated radiographically.
- Stability of the first MTP joint should be assessed. Severe instability of the first MTP is a contraindication for use of the SERI technique.
- Associated lesser toe deformities, such as clawtoes, result in metatarsal overload and callus formation, often creating symptoms that exceed those directly related to the hallux.

IMAGING AND OTHER DIAGNOSTIC STUDIES

- A standard radiographic examination, including AP and lateral weight-bearing views of the forefoot, allows the assessment of arthritis and congruency of the joint; measurement of the HVA, intermetatarsal angle (IMA), and distal metatarsal articular angle (DMAA); and calculation of the metatarsal formula,[16,20,21] especially the relation between the length of the first and the second metatarsal.
- Preoperative planning is performed using the preoperative weight-bearing radiographs of the foot. In particular, we assess the radiographs to determine the desired obliquity of the bone cut and the amount of mediolateral and dorsoplantar shift of the metatarsal head required to reduce the metatarsal head over the sesamoid complex and correct an increased DMAA (**FIG 4**).

NONOPERATIVE MANAGEMENT

- Comfortable shoes with a wide toe box and sole may reduce the pressure on the first metatarsal head's medial prominence. In severe deformity, custom-made shoes or insoles with a metatarsal support may relieve symptoms attributable to transfer metatarsalgia and associated plantar callus formation.
- Nonoperative treatment of hallux fails to correct the deformity; it only accommodates to it. Given that hallux valgus deformity tends to progressively worsen, probably due to muscle imbalance about the first MTP joint, symptoms may abate only with surgical correction when conservative treatment proves inadequate.

SURGICAL MANAGEMENT

Indications for SERI Technique

- In our experience, the SERI ("simple, effective, rapid, inexpensive") technique is effective in correcting mild to moderate hallux valgus, with HVA and IMA not exceeding 40 degrees and 20 degrees, respectively.
- The SERI technique may be applied to congruent and incongruent hallux valgus deformity. The operation is indicated in case of hallux valgus presenting with any degree of DMAA and a mild degenerative arthritis of the first MTP joint.
- Specific contraindications to the SERI technique are severe degenerative arthritis, stiffness, or severe instability of the first MTP joint.

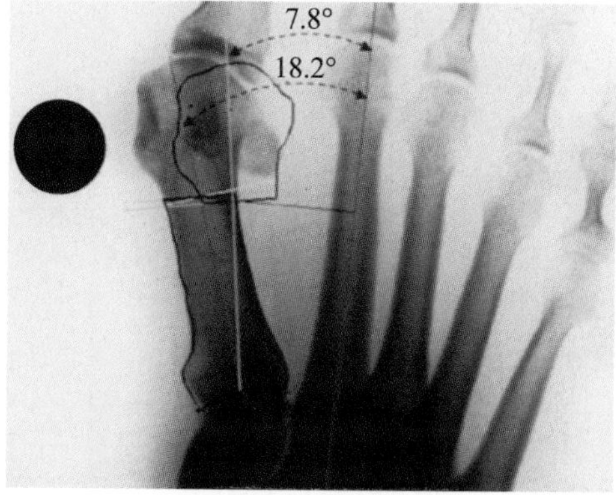

FIG 4 • Preoperative planning for hallux valgus correction by the SERI osteotomy.

- Before surgery, the patient's foot or feet (simultaneous bilateral procedures) are scrubbed using disinfectant soap solution.
- Several anesthetic techniques can be used. We usually prefer a sciatic nerve block using ropivacaine hydrochlorate monohydrate 7.5 mg/mL.
- The patient is placed in a supine position, with the lower extremity externally rotated with the foot's lateral border contacting the operating table.
- After the foot is exsanguinated, an Esmarch elastic bandage is used as an ankle tourniquet with adequate padding.
- The SERI technique does not require a lateral soft tissue release, particularly with a flexible hallux valgus deformity, because the lateral soft tissues relax with lateral translation of the first metatarsal head. Even with slight stiffness of the first MTP joint we do not perform a lateral release, instead applying an intraoperative manual stretch to the adductor hallucis by forcing the hallux in a varus position.
- Make a 1-cm medial longitudinal incision midaxially just proximal to the medial eminence through the skin and subcutaneous tissue, directly to the medial aspect of the first metatarsal (**TECH FIG 1A**). The capsule of the joint is spared.
- Retract the soft tissues dorsally and plantarly using two 5-mm retractors (**TECH FIG 1B**).
- If performed as described, the medial aspect of the first metatarsal neck will be adequately exposed.
- Perform a complete osteotomy using a standard pneumatic saw with a 9.5 × 25 × 0.4-mm blade (Hall Surgical, Linvatec Corp., Largo, FL) (**TECH FIG 1C**). In the sagittal plane, the osteotomy is performed with 15 degrees of inclination from dorsal to plantar and distal to proximal. The inclination of the osteotomy in the mediolateral direction is perpendicular to the foot axis (ie, to the long axis of the second metatarsal bone) if the length of the first metatarsal bone must be maintained. If shortening of the metatarsal bone or decompression of the MTP joint is necessary, as in the case of mild arthritis, the osteotomy is inclined in a distal to proximal direction up to 25 degrees. More rarely, if a lengthening of the first metatarsal bone is necessary (ie, if the first metatarsal bone is shorter than the second or if laxity of the MTP joint is present), the osteotomy is inclined in a proximal to distal direction as much as 15 degrees.
- With a small osteotome, mobilize the head.
- Using a standard wire driver, insert a single-tipped 2.0-mm Kirschner wire retrograde through the incision into the soft tissue immediately adjacent to the proximal and distal phalanges of the hallux, in the longitudinal axis of the great toe (**TECH FIG 1D**).
- The Kirschner wire exits at the medial tip of the toe close to the toenail. Regrasp it with the wire driver (**TECH FIG 1E**) and retract it so that its proximal tip rests at the level of the osteotomy (**TECH FIG 1F**).
- Using a small grooved lever to prize the osteotomy (**TECH FIG 1G**), obtain the correction by moving the metatarsal head depending on the pathoanatomy of the deformity (**TECH FIG 1H,I**).
- If pronation of the first metatarsal bone is present, obtain the correction with a derotation of the hallux at the osteotomy up to the neutral position of the first metatarsal head.
- After correcting the HVA, IMA, DMAA, and pronation, advance the Kirschner wire antegrade into the diaphysis of the first MTP joint so that its proximal tip reaches the metatarsal base (**TECH FIG 1J**).
- Expose the medial prominence at the osteotomy site on the distal aspect of the metatarsal shaft by two retractors and remove it using a pneumatic saw or a rongeur (**TECH FIG 1K**).
- The wound requires only a single 3-0 absorbable suture to reapproximate the skin.
- Bend and cut the segment of the Kirschner wire that is protruding from the tip of the toe in routine fashion.
- In our experience, the SERI technique may be performed as simultaneous bilateral procedures or combined with concomitant correction of associated foot deformities.

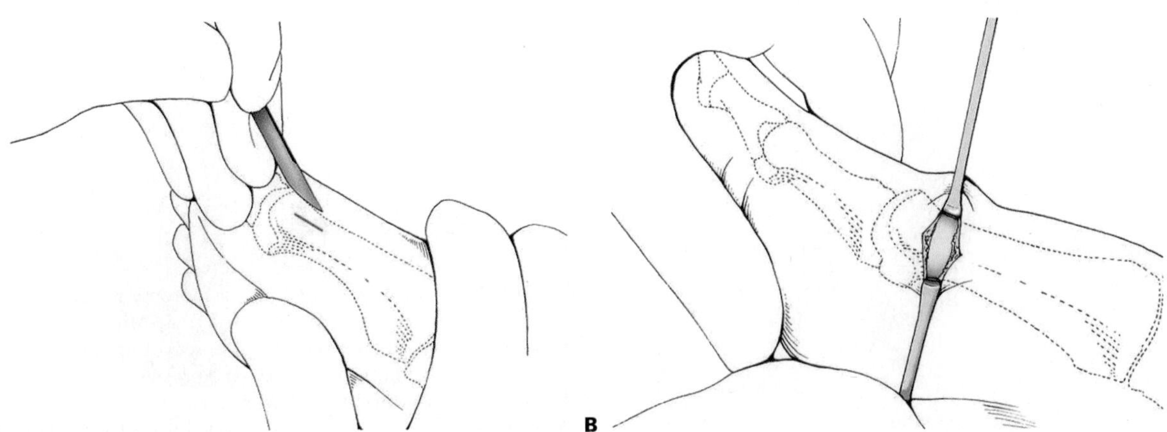

TECH FIG 1 • **A.** Surgical field showing the 1-cm medial incision. **B.** Retracting the soft tissues. *(continued)*

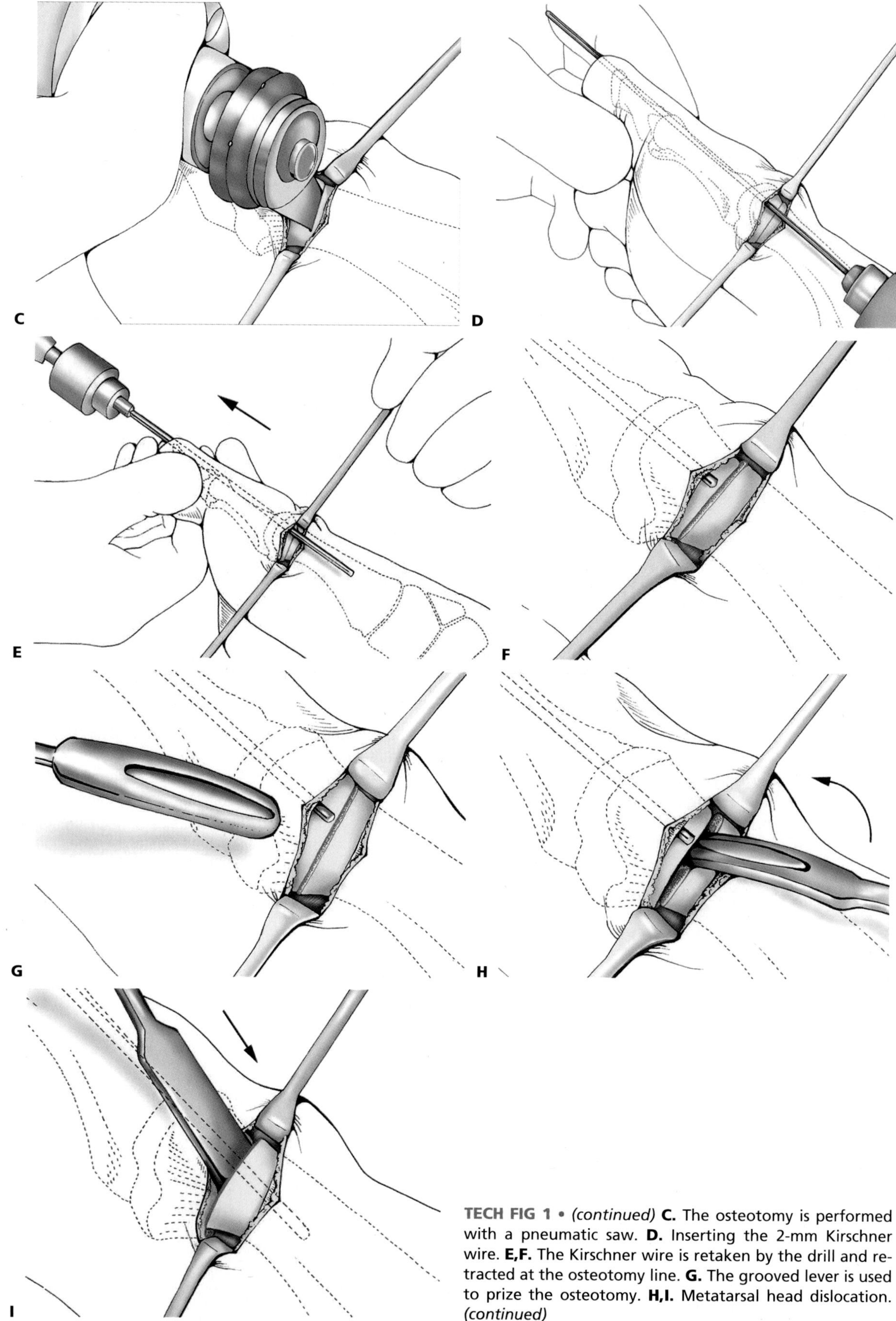

TECH FIG 1 • *(continued)* **C.** The osteotomy is performed with a pneumatic saw. **D.** Inserting the 2-mm Kirschner wire. **E,F.** The Kirschner wire is retaken by the drill and retracted at the osteotomy line. **G.** The grooved lever is used to prize the osteotomy. **H,I.** Metatarsal head dislocation. *(continued)*

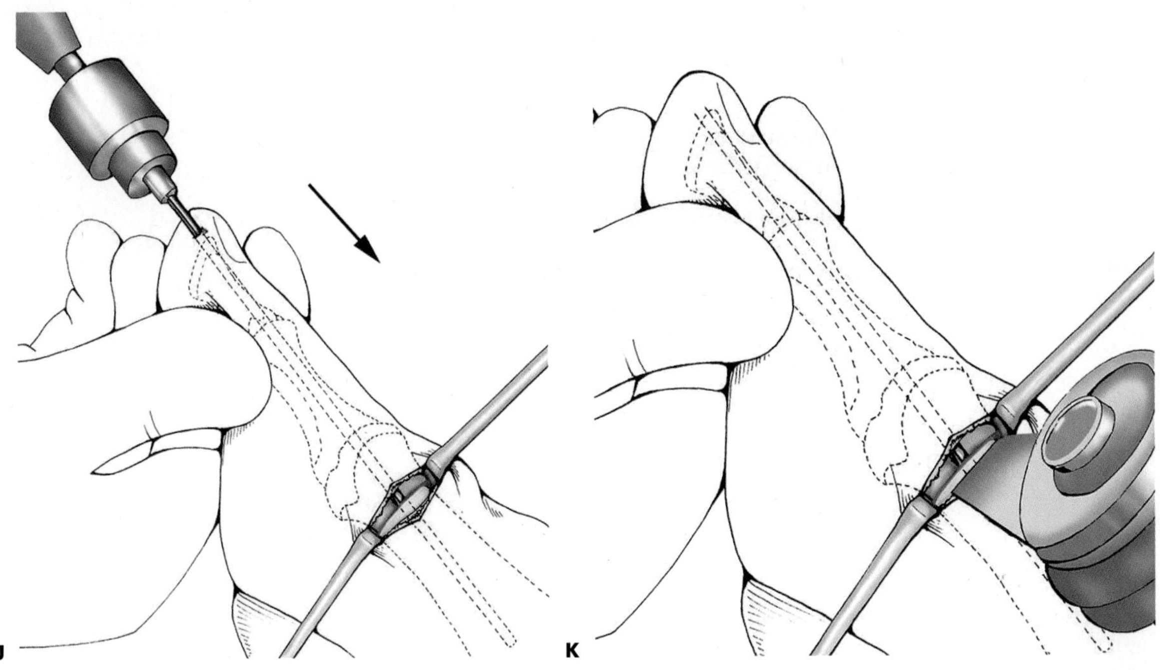

TECH FIG 1 • *(continued)* **J.** The Kirschner wire is inserted in the diaphyseal channel. **K.** Proximal stump regularization.

PEARLS AND PITFALLS

- A 15-degree inclination in the osteotomy from dorsal to plantar and distal to proximal affords stability to the osteotomy to limit dorsal displacement of the metatarsal head with weight bearing.
- If shortening of the metatarsal or decompression of the MTP joint is necessary, the osteotomy should be inclined in a distal–proximal direction up to 25 degrees. More rarely, if lengthening of the metatarsal is necessary, the osteotomy should be inclined in a proximal–distal direction up to 15 degrees (**FIG 5**).
- An adjustment of the final intraoperative correction of the first metatarsal head in the mediolateral dislocation plane of the metatarsal head is dictated by the position of the K-wire in the metatarsal diaphysis. Greater correction warrants a more lateral placement of the wire within the metatarsal shaft. Greater plantar displacement of the metatarsal head necessitates placing the K-wire more dorsally into the soft tissue immediately adjacent the metatarsal head (**FIG 6**).

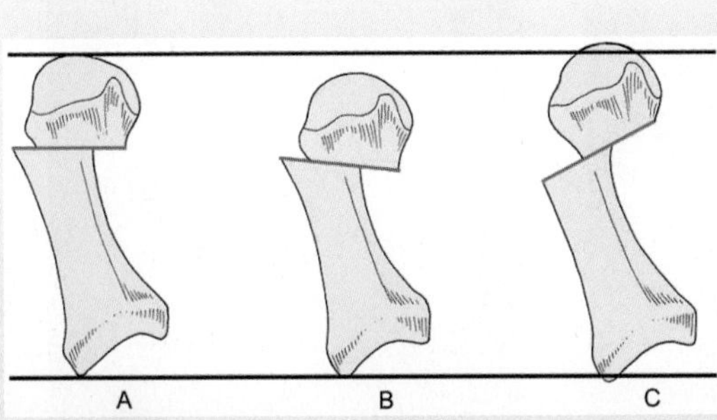

FIG 5 • Possibilities of metatarsal lengthening or shortening by using different SERI osteotomy inclinations.

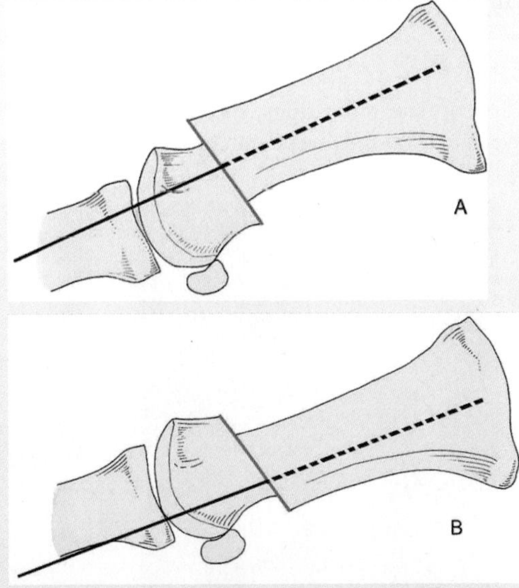

FIG 6 • Possibility of plantar or dorsal dislocation of the metatarsal head.

- To correct the DMAA, the Kirschner wire must be introduced obliquely into the medial soft tissues in a mediolateral direction (**FIG 7**). Then, manual adduction of the hallux must be performed to rotate the metatarsal head, correcting the DMAA.
- In our experience, an osteotomy performed proximal to the recommended position increases the risk of first metatarsal malunion and nonunion.
- If the Kirschner wire is inserted into the phalanx rather than immediately adjacent to the phalanx, it has been our experience that the DMAA cannot be properly corrected.
- Excessive shortening of the first metatarsal may lead to overload of the lesser toes.
- Like most other corrective procedures for hallux valgus, the SERI technique is not indicated for hallux valgus associated with moderate to severe hallux rigidus.

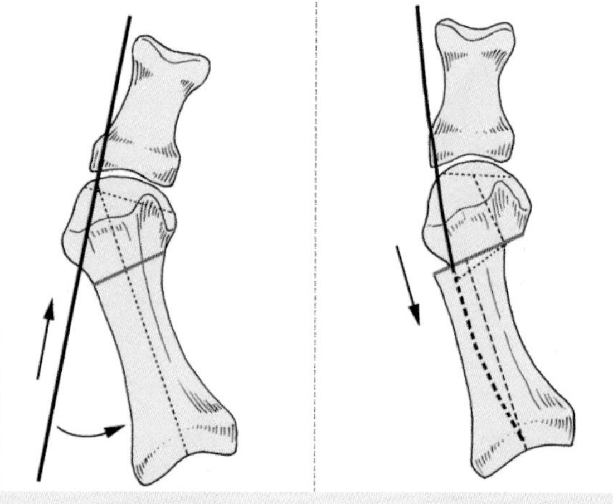

FIG 7 • Correction of distal metatarsal articular angle.

POSTOPERATIVE CARE

- After the completion of the surgery, a mildly compressive gauze dressing is applied to the wound and forefoot (**FIG 8**) and AP and oblique radiographs are obtained to confirm the placement of the osteotomy and the correction of any characteristics of the deformity.
- Ambulation is allowed immediately using "talus" shoes. These shoes maintain the foot in the talus position of the ankle, allowing weight bearing on the hindfoot and discharging weight from the forefoot. Foot elevation is advised when the patient is at rest in the immediate postoperative period.
- Kirschner wire fixation due to wire bending upon insertion produces a very stable and elastic stabilization, maintaining the same position obtained during surgery and favoring early healing of the osteotomy combined with early weight bearing.
- After 1 month, the dressing, suture, and Kirschner wire are removed. Passive and active exercises with cycling and swimming are advised and comfortable normal shoes are worn, gradually returning to standard footwear.
- As a rule, significant postoperative swelling does not last for more than 1 month.

OUTCOMES

- With appropriate indications, the SERI technique of minimally invasive distal metatarsal osteotomy is simple, effective, rapid, and inexpensive, giving satisfactory results in more than 90% of cases.
- This technique is easily repeated, without removal of the eminence and without open lateral release. It is minimally invasive but performed under direct line of vision and without radiations.
- Normally, the osteotomies heal well, with callus evident after an average of 3 months.
- The radiographic evaluation showed significant correction of the parameters over time (**FIG 9**).
- No severe complications, such as avascular necrosis of the metatarsal head, nonunion of the osteotomy, or hallux varus, were observed.
- All the metatarsal bones remodeled themselves over time, even in cases with significant offset at the osteotomy (few millimeters of bony contact). In our experience, the healing of the osteotomy and the remodeling capability of the metatarsal bone are not related to the offset at the osteotomy, but it is necessary to obtain a bony contact.

COMPLICATIONS

- There was a 1.9% rate of delayed union of the osteotomy (over 4 months). In our experience, delayed union is not related to the amount of displacement or correction at the osteotomy.
- There was a 2.1% rate of skin irritation or erythema about the Kirschner wire at the tip of the great toe.

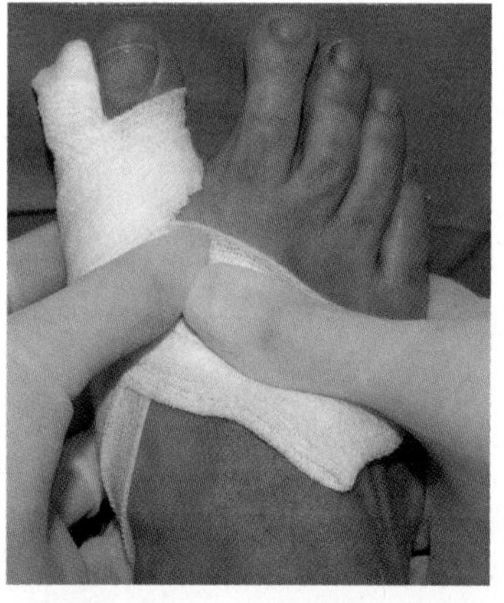

A

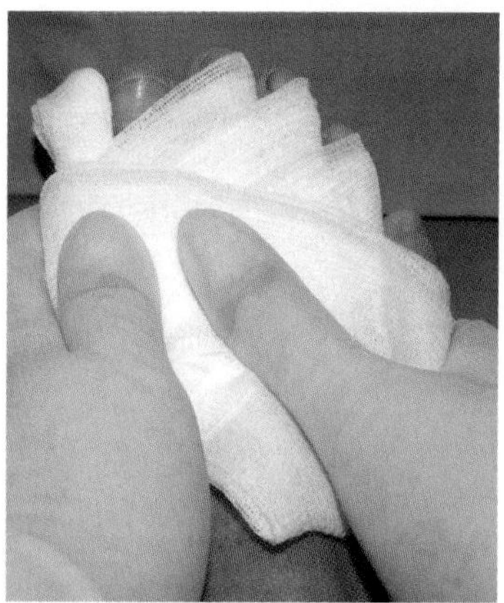

B

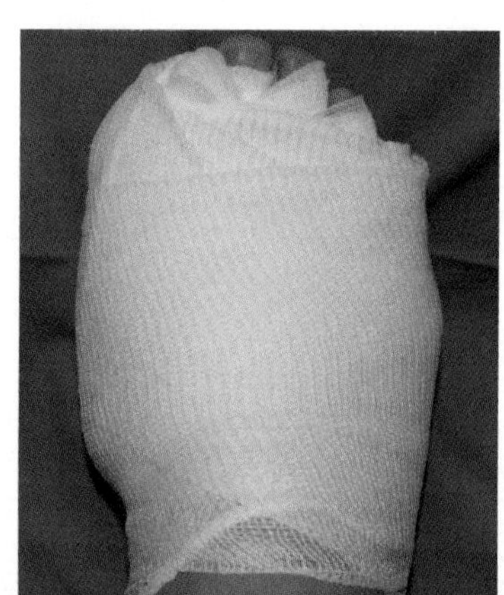

C

FIG 8 • Step-by-step application of the gauze compression dressing.

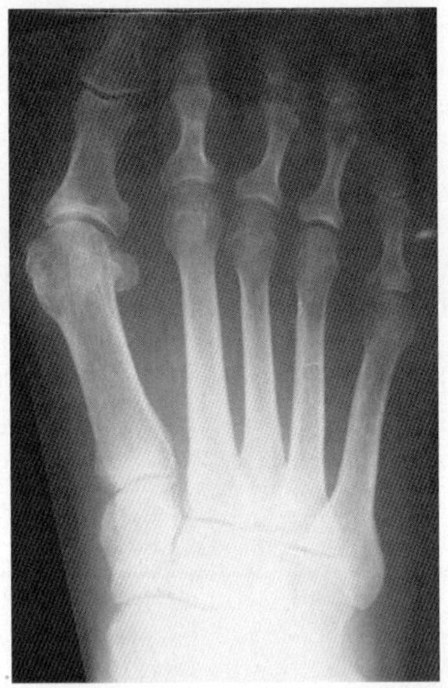
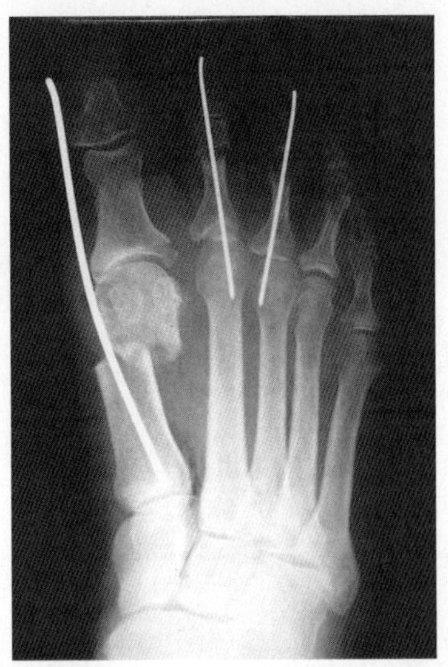
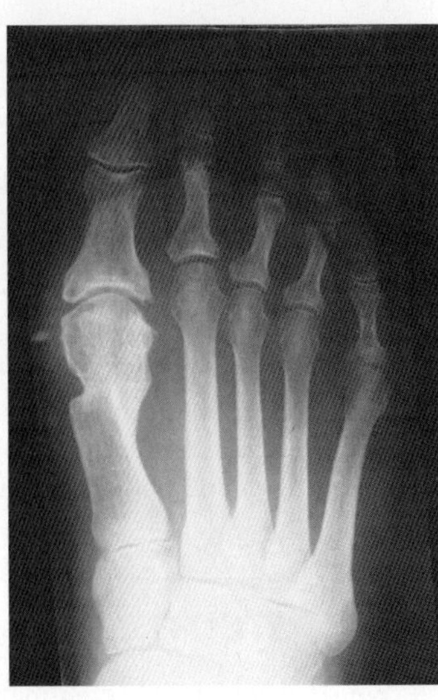

FIG 9 • **A.** Dorsoplantar radiographs showing a hallux valgus deformity in a female patient 50 years old. **B.** Postoperative radiograph. **C.** Radiographs at 3 years of follow-up.

- There was a 12% rate of transfer metatarsalgia with plantar callosities under the second and third metatarsal heads, resolving by the use of insoles with metatarsal support.
- There was a 0.5% rate of deep vein thrombosis.

REFERENCES

1. Coughlin MJ. Juvenile hallux valgus: etiology and treatment. Foot Ankle Int 1995;16:682.
2. Coughlin MJ. Hallux valgus. J Bone Joint Surg Am 1996;78A:932.
3. Coughlin MJ, Jones CP. Hallux valgus: demographics, etiology, and radiographic assessment. Foot Ankle Int 2007;28:759–777.
4. Dragonetti L. Inquadramento eziopatogenetico e clinico dell'alluce abdotto-valgo. In: Malerba F, Dragonetti L, Giannini S. Progressi in Medicina e Chirurgia del Piede; 6, L'alluce valgo. Bologna, Italy: Aulo Gaggi, 1997.
5. Fritz GR, Prieskorn D. First metatarsocuneiform motion; a radiographic and statistical analysis. Foot Ankle Int 1995;16:117.
6. Giannini S, Ceccarelli F, Mosca M, et al. Algoritmo nel trattamento chirurgico dell'alluce valgo. In: Malerba F, Dragonetti L, Giannini S, eds. Progressi in Medicina e Chirurgia del Piede; 6, L'alluce valgo. Bologna, Italy: Aulo Gaggi, 1997:155–165.
7. Hardy RH, Clapham JCR. Observations on hallux valgus: based on a controlled series. J Bone Joint Surg Br 1951;33B:376.
8. Hardy RH, Clapham JCR. Hallux valgus. Lancet 1952;1:1180–1183.
9. Klaue K. Hallux valgus and hypermobility of the first ray: causal treatment using tarso-metatarsal reorientation arthrodesis. Ther Umsch 1991;48:817.
10. Klaue K, Hansen ST, Masquelet AC. Clinical, quantitative assessment of tarsometatarsal mobility in the sagittal plane and its relation to hallux valgus deformity. Foot Ankle Int 1994;15:9.
11. Lapidus PW. Operative correction of the metatarsus varus primus in hallux valgus. Surg Gynecol Obstet 1934;58:183.
12. Mann RA, Coughlin MJ. Hallux valgus: etiology, anatomy, treatment and surgical considerations. Clin Orthop Relat Res 1981;157: 31–41.
13. Mann RA, Coughlin MJ. Adult hallux valgus. In: Coughlin MJ, Mann RA. Surgery of the Foot and Ankle. St. Louis: Mosby, 1999: 150–269.
14. Piqué-Vidal C, Solé MT, Antich J. Hallux valgus inheritance: pedigree research in 350 patients with bunion deformity. J Foot Ankle Surg 2007;46:149–154.
15. Sarrafian SK, ed. Anatomy of the Foot and Ankle: Descriptive, Topographic, Functional. Philadelphia: JB Lippincott, 1983.
16. Shereff MJ, Yang QM, Kummer FJ. Extraosseous and intraosseous arterial supply to the first metatarsal and the first metatarsophalangeal joint. Foot Ankle 1987;8:81.
17. Shereff MJ, DiGiovanni L, Bejjani FJ, et al. A comparison of non-weight-bearing and weight-bearing radiographs of the foot. Foot Ankle 1990;10:306.
18. Shrine IB. Incidence of hallux valgus in a partially shoe-wearing community. Br Med J 1965;1:1648.
19. Sim-Fook L, Hodgson AR. A comparison of foot forms among the non-shoe and shoe-wearing Chinese population. J Bone Joint Surg Am 1958;40A:1058.
20. Suzuki J, Tanaka Y, Takaoka T, et al. Axial radiographic evaluation in hallux valgus: evaluation of the transverse arch in the forefoot. J Orthop Sci 2004;9:446–451.
21. Tanaka Y, Takakura Y, Kumai T, et al. Radiographic analysis of hallux valgus: a two-dimensional coordinate system. J Bone Joint Surg Am 1995;77A:205.

Chapter 6 Akin Osteotomy

Paul Hamilton and Sam Singh

SURGICAL MANAGEMENT

- The primary indication for an Akin osteotomy is hallux valgus interphalangeus or in cases where residual hallux valgus causes pressure on the second toe on the load stimulation test. It is most commonly used to accompany a scarf or chevron osteotomy. An isolated Akin is contraindicated in the treatment of hallux valgus. We use a proximal medial closing wedge osteotomy that is fixed by a varisation screw (Depuy, Warsaw, IN).
- The osteotomy is fashioned within metaphyseal cancellous bone, ensuring excellent cancellous healing. The osteotomy, by being close to the apex of the deformity at the interphalangeal joint, allows for more powerful correction.

TECHNIQUES

AKIN OSTEOTOMY

- We describe an eight-step method for performing the Akin osteotomy.
- The exposure is performed usually as an extension to the midline longitudinal incision from the metatarsal osteotomy. If performed as an isolated procedure, the exposure must allow visualization of the metatarsophalangeal joint proximally and the shaft of the proximal phalanx distally. The exposure of the shaft of the phalanx may require excision of overlying fatty tissue.
- After dissecting directly onto bone, complete the exposure by periosteal elevation above and below the phalanx. Place two small pointed retractors above and below the phalanx to protect the extensor and flexor tendons (**TECH FIG 1A**).
- Position a 1-mm Kirschner wire in the midportion of the phalanx in the sagittal plane approximately 3 mm distal to the phalangeal flare (**TECH FIG 1B**).
- Traction on the big toe allows us to visualize the joint to ensure the wire is not intra-articular (**TECH FIG 2A**).
- Remove the Kirschner wire and mark the hole (**TECH FIG 2B**).

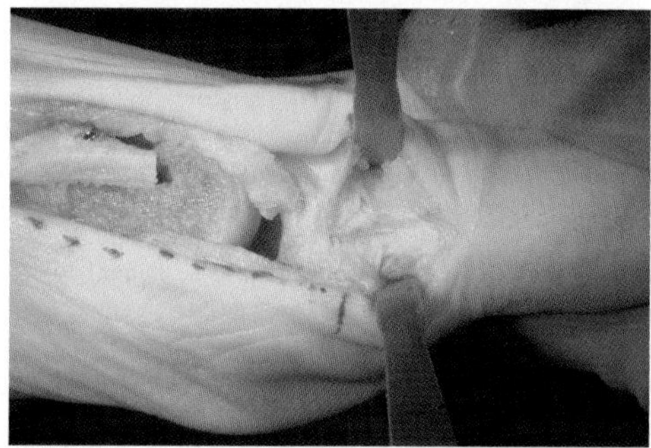
A

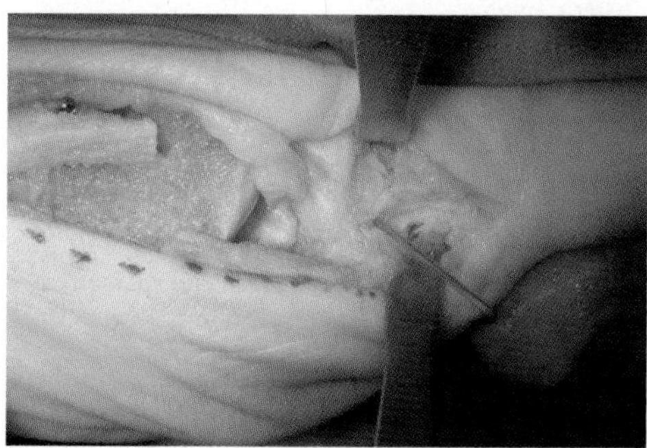
B

TECH FIG 1 • A. Incision is made directly to bone with subperiosteal dissection above and below the proximal phalanx. **B.** Kirschner wire position on proximal phalanx parallel to phalangeal base.

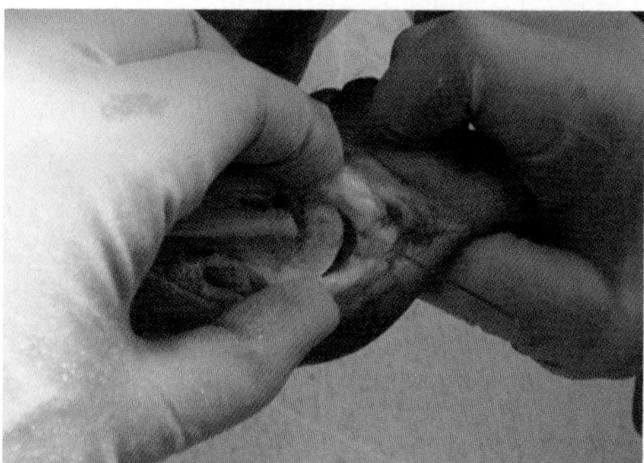
A

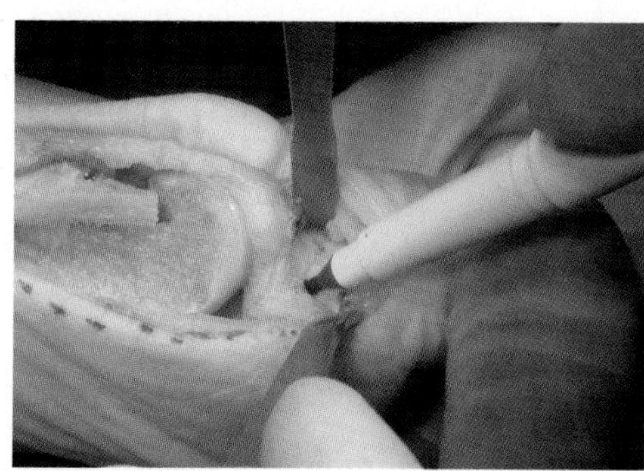
B

TECH FIG 2 • A. The joint is checked to confirm the Kirschner wire has not penetrated the articular surface. **B.** The Kirschner wire position is marked.

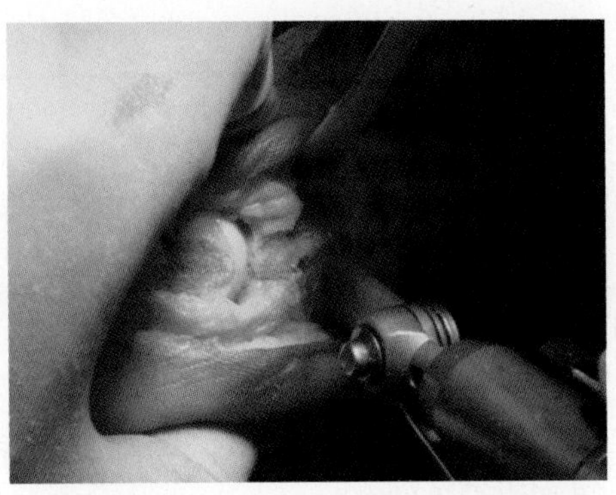

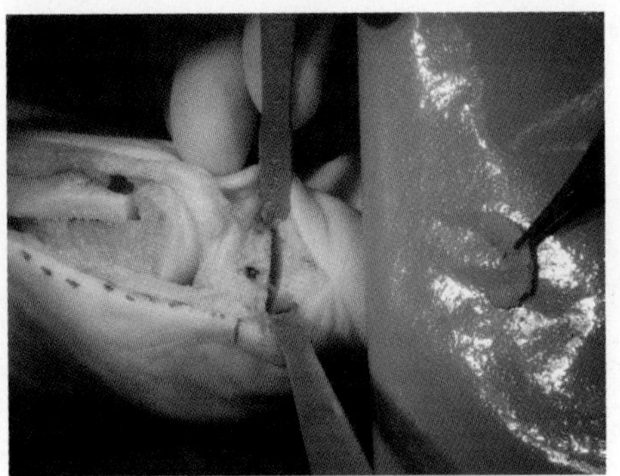

TECH FIG 3 • **A.** The osteotomy is performed parallel to the phalangeal base. **B.** The second cut is performed to produce a small sliver of bone.

- Make the proximal cut parallel to the phalangeal base (**TECH FIG 3A**). To maintain control of the osteotomy, score the lateral cortex but do not penetrate it with the saw blade, thus allowing it to act as a hinge. Perform the second osteotomy to produce a wafer of bone with the apex laterally (**TECH FIG 3B**). When removed it should look like a fine slice of lemon. Use direct pressure to close the wedge. This "greensticks" the intact but weakened lateral cortex.

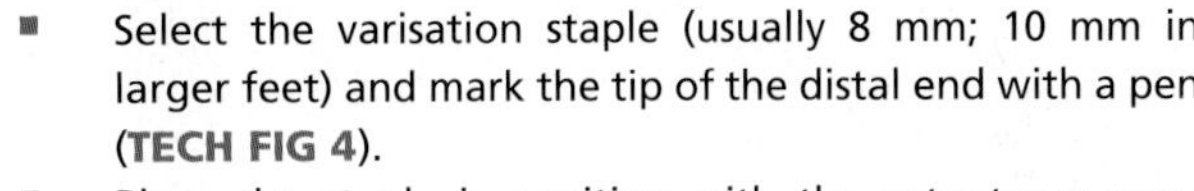

- Select the varisation staple (usually 8 mm; 10 mm in larger feet) and mark the tip of the distal end with a pen (**TECH FIG 4**).
- Place the staple in position with the osteotomy compressed. Check that it is on the midportion of the phalanx in the sagittal plane (**TECH FIG 5A**). The distal staple leaves an ink mark; drill this mark with a 1-mm Kirschner wire (**TECH FIG 5B**) and then mark the hole. The position for the staple can then be identified by the two bone marks.
- While maintaining compression, insert the staple in the predrilled holes. Check for stability of the fixation (**TECH FIG 5C**), and again axial traction confirms the staple is not in the joint.
- Close the wound in layers with continuous Monocryl to skin, and apply a forefoot bandage to maintain the correction.

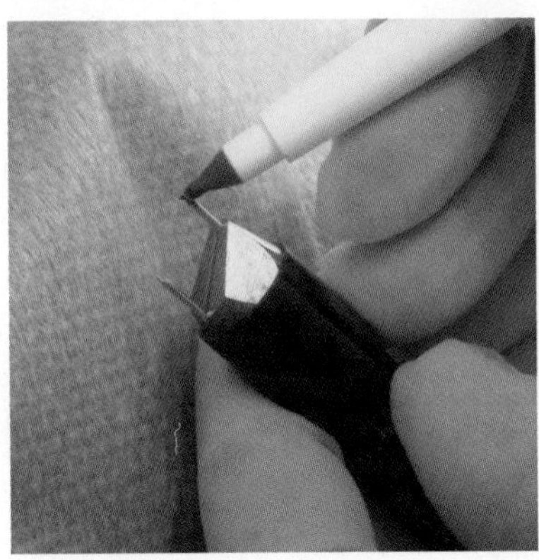

TECH FIG 4 • The staple is marked with a pen.

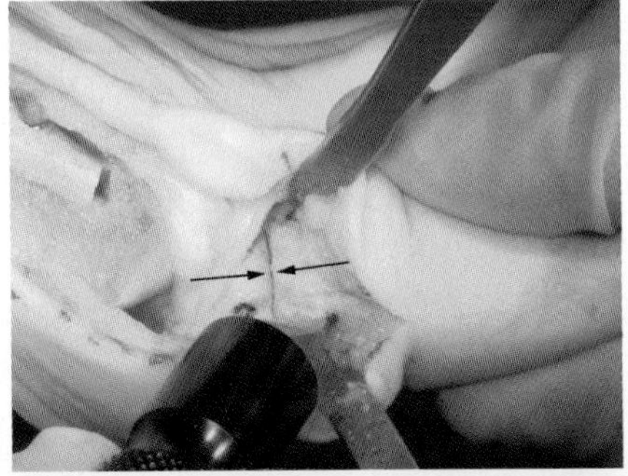

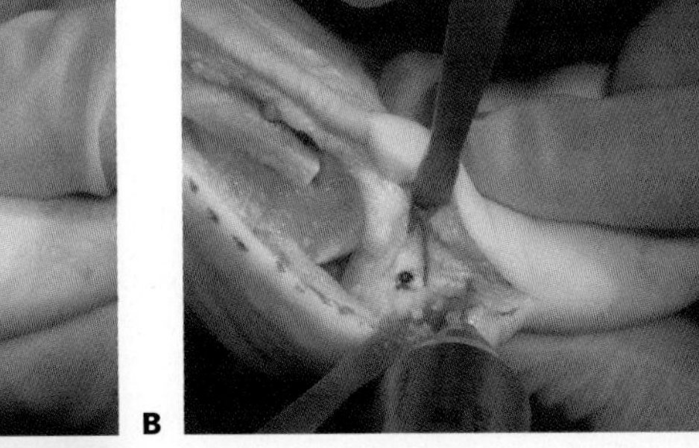

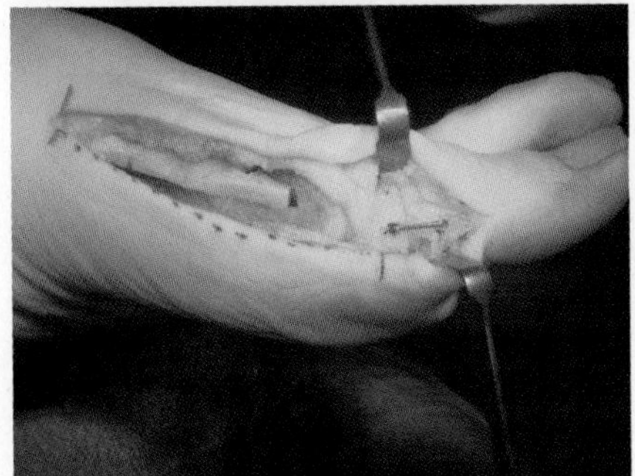

TECH FIG 5 • **A.** The osteotomy is compressed and the marked staple is placed in the correct position. **B.** The distal mark is then drilled with a Kirschner wire. **C.** The staple is inserted with the osteotomy compressed.

PEARLS AND PITFALLS

Exposure	▪ The orientation of the osteotomy can be difficult if performed in the absence of a metatarsal osteotomy. Avoid the temptation to use a small incision, instead taking care to expose the metatarsophalangeal joint and the shaft of the phalanx.
Staple insertion	▪ Resistance may be encountered when inserting the staple due to the hard subchondral bone. Avoid using excess force when inserting the staple, as this may fracture the lateral "greensticked" cortex. Either repeat the Kirschner wire drilling or accept the staple 2 to 3 mm proud if a good hold is achieved.
Inadvertent lateral cortex fracture	▪ If the lateral cortex if fractured, then a compression screw is inserted from medial to lateral spanning the osteotomy.
Overcorrection	▪ The osteotomy is very powerful as it is at the apex of the deformity. Aim for a very fine segment of bone; it can be cut again if required.
Unable to greenstick the lateral cortex	▪ Often a rectangle of bone as opposed to a wedge has been removed. Forcing it to close will crack the lateral cortex. Instead use a gentle to-and-fro motion with the running saw while applying gentle compressive force. This thins the lateral cortex until the osteotomy closes without "bouncing back" once pressure is removed.

POSTOPERATIVE CARE

- See Chapter FA-7 on scarf osteotomy.

OUTCOMES

- The most common indication for an Akin osteotomy is in combination with a metatarsal osteotomy for hallux valgus. Outcomes are therefore reported together with satisfaction rates at between 85% and 95%.[1,2,4] Very few studies have concentrated solely on the Akin.

COMPLICATIONS

- Complications of this osteotomy are rare[3] but can include nonunion, nerve damage, infection, displacement of the osteotomy, and overcorrection or undercorrection. Failure to recognize propagation of the lateral cortex may increase the risk of subsequent displacement.

REFERENCES

1. Frey C, Jahss M, Kummer FJ. The Akin procedure: an analysis of results. Foot Ankle 1991;12:1–6.
2. Garrido IM, Rubio ER, Bosch MN, et al. Scarf and Akin osteotomies for moderate and severe hallux valgus: clinical and radiographic results. Foot Ankle Surg 2008;14:194–203.
3. Hammel E, Abi Chala ML, Wagner T. Complications of first ray osteotomies: a consecutive series of 475 feet with first metatarsal Scarf osteotomy and first phalanx osteotomy. Rev Chir Orthop Reparatrice Appar Mot 2007;93:710–719.
4. Mitchell LA, Baxter DE. A Chevron-Akin double osteotomy for correction of hallux valgus. Foot Ankle 1991;12:7–14.

Chapter 7 Scarf Osteotomy

Paul Hamilton and Sam Singh

SURGICAL MANAGEMENT

- The primary indication for a Scarf osteotomy is symptomatic hallux valgus deformity with an intermetatarsal angle of less than 20 degrees. The first metatarsocuneiform joint should be stable. It is a versatile osteotomy that can allow shortening, lengthening, rotation, displacement, or plantarization of the first metatarsal head. Thus, indications include symptomatic hallux valgus with or without mild transfer symptoms, juvenile hallux valgus with an abnormal distal metatarsal articular angle, arthritic hallux valgus not severe enough for a fusion, and revision surgery in suitable cases.

Preoperative Planning

- AP and lateral weight-bearing radiographs of the foot are evaluated for metatarsal length, intermetatarsal angle, hallux valgus angle, distal metatarsal articular angle, and interphalangeal angle for cases that may require a proximal phalangeal osteotomy to obtain complete correction. Congruency of the joint, presence of osteophytes, the size of the bony medial eminence, and position and condition of the sesamoids are noted.

Positioning

- Surgery is performed on an outpatient basis.
- Prophylactic antibiotics are administered.
- A thigh tourniquet is applied.
- The patient is positioned supine with a sandbag under the ipsilateral buttock so the big toe points to the ceiling.

SOFT TISSUE RELEASE AND BUNIONECTOMY

- Approach the metatarsal through a medial longitudinal incision extending from the first tarsometatarsal joint to the medial flare of the proximal phalanx (**TECH FIG 1A**). This can be extended distally if a phalangeal osteotomy is required. Identify the dorsal medial cutaneous nerve and incise the medial capsule sharply in a single longitudinal direction. Expose the medial eminence and resect it 1 mm medial to the sagittal sulcus (**TECH FIG 1B**). Overresection can lead to a postoperative varus deformity. Expose the metatarsal shaft using subperiosteal sharp dissection, taking care to protect the plantar neck vascular bundle to the metatarsal head (**TECH FIG 1C**). The proximal plantar exposure can be performed safely without any disruption to the plantar blood supply. Use a large Langenbeck retractor to protect and retract the plantar flap. The tarsometatarsal joint is identified but does not need to be exposed.
- Perform a lateral release of the first metatarsophalangeal joint by exposing the first web space with aid of a lamina spreader as an "over the top" technique. This does not compromise the plantar blood supply. Use a banana blade to perform the sharp dissection (**TECH FIG 1D**). Release the tendinous insertion of the adductor hallucis muscle onto the fibula sesamoid and proximal phalanx. Release the suspensory metatarsal–sesamoid ligaments and make multiple sharp perforations in the lateral capsule at the joint line if required. Apply a varus force to the hallux, completing the capsular release (**TECH FIG 1E**).
- This release can also be performed through a separate first web space incision if preferred.

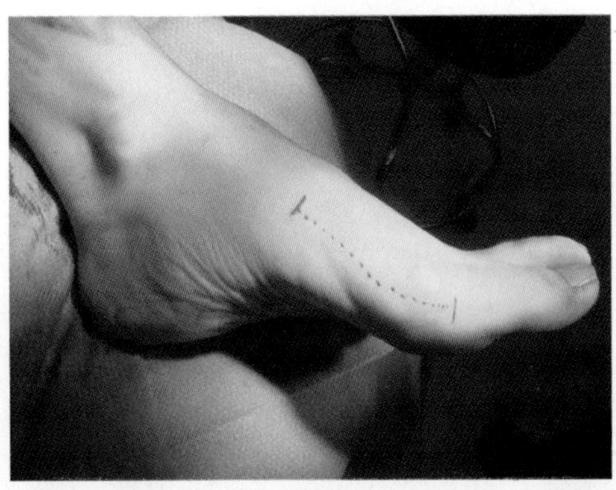

A

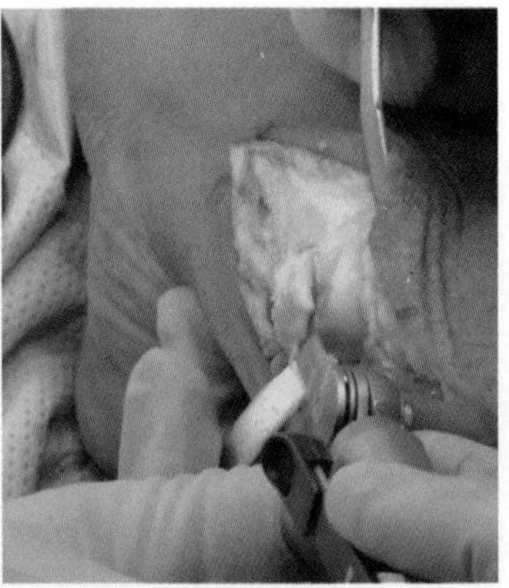

B

TECH FIG 1 • **A.** The incision is made from the tarsometatarsal joint to the base of the phalanx. **B.** Resection of the medial eminence. *(continued)*

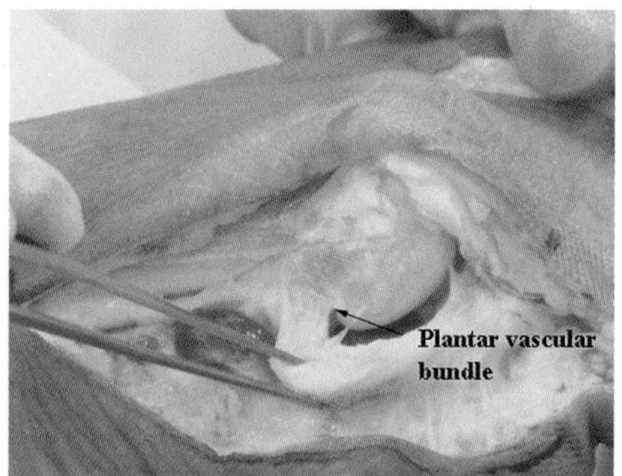

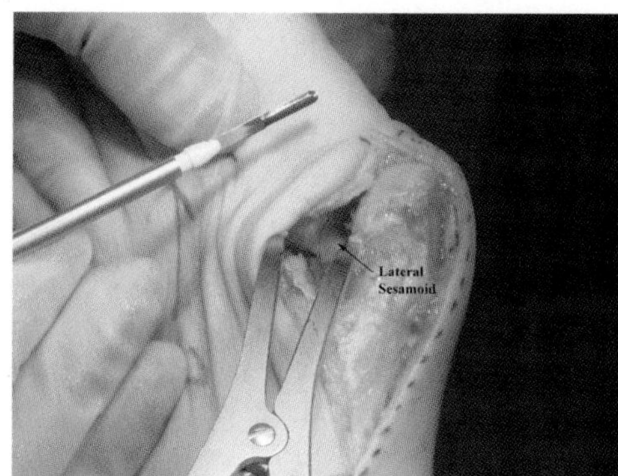

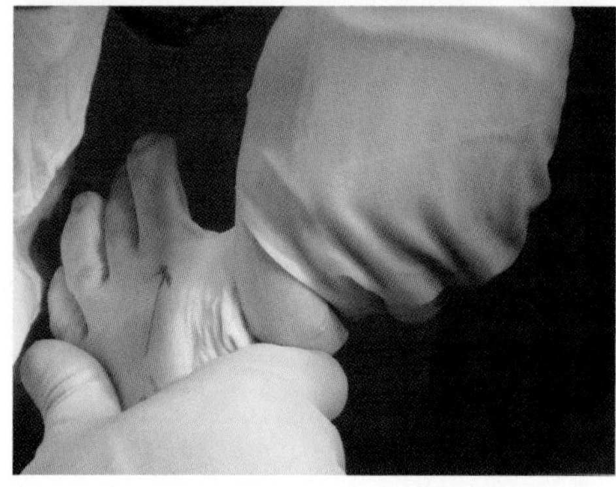

TECH FIG 1 • *(continued)* **C.** Plantar exposure protecting vascular supply to metatarsal head. **D.** First web space exposure and adductor release using a Banana blade. **E.** Varus force is applied to complete lateral release.

SCARF OSTEOTOMY

- Make the cut starting with the medial longitudinal cut. This is begun distally 5 mm from the articular surface and 2 to 3 mm from the dorsal surface of the metatarsal and finished 5 mm from the tarsometatarsal joint, 2 to 3 mm from the proximal plantar surface of the metatarsal (**TECH FIG 2A**). Make the longitudinal cut in the same plane as the plantar orientation of the metatarsal (**TECH FIG 2B**). This allows a degree of plantarization of the metatarsal head. Using a large Langenbeck retractor helps to visualize the plantar metatarsal surface. Perform the transverse cuts at 60 degrees to the longitudinal cut as a chevron. Both cuts are directed proximally, avoiding convergence laterally, which would hinder translation (**TECH FIG 2C**). When performing the distal cut, elevate the hand to complete the lateral cut (**TECH FIG 2D**). Separate the two fragments, taking care not to lever the fragments. These steps may need to be repeated if there has been failure to complete all the cuts, but take care to avoid double cutting. Release of the capsule from the lateral side may be needed if it is preventing displacement (**TECH FIG 2E**).

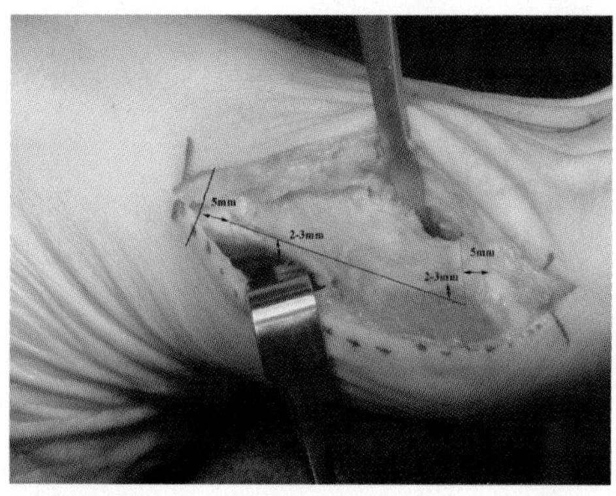

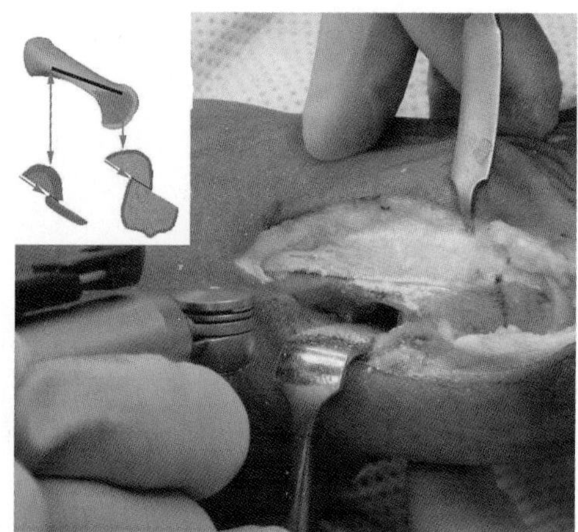

TECH FIG 2 • **A.** Position of the osteotomy. **B.** Longitudinal cut in the same plane as the plantar metatarsal surface. *(continued)*

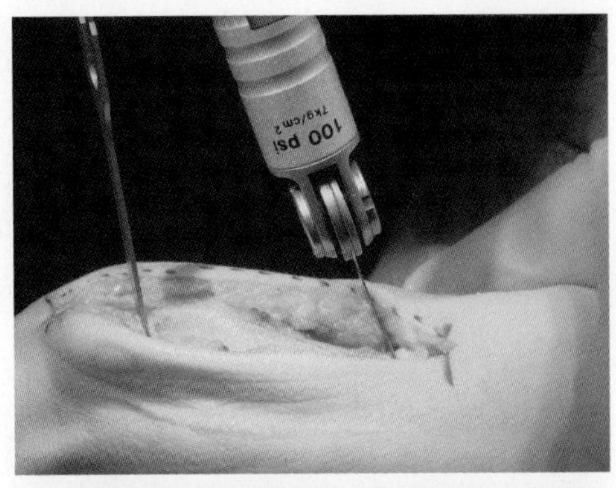

C

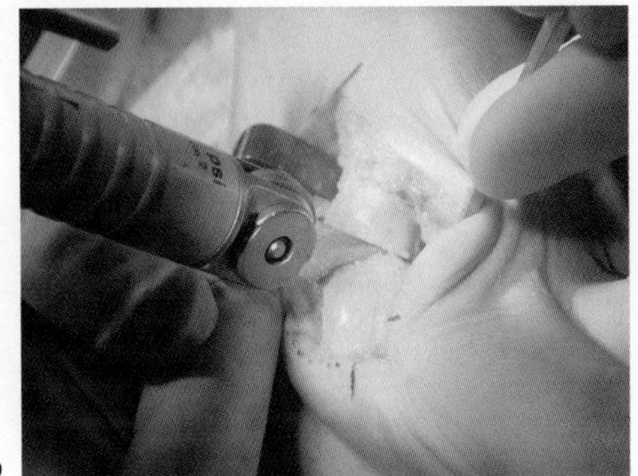

D

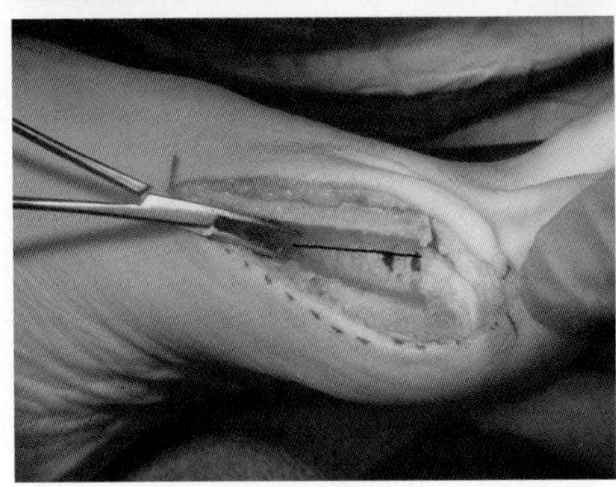

E

TECH FIG 2 • *(continued)* **C.** Transverse cuts, avoiding convergence. **D.** The hand is elevated to complete the distal transverse cut. **E.** Release of the capsule from the proximal end.

- Perform displacement or rotation with guidance from preoperative radiographs by using a clamp on the distal lateral cortex (**TECH FIG 3A**). Use a compression clamp to hold the displacement (**TECH FIG 3B**). Up to two thirds of lateral displacement can be obtained while maintaining a strong lateral strut and good bone apposition.
- Obtain screw fixation using Barouk screws (Depuy, Warsaw, IN). These are cannulated, self-tapping screws with a long distal thread and a threaded head to allow compression and burial of the head. Place the distal screw first. Pass the guidewire from the proximal fragment obliquely into the head (**TECH FIG 4A**). Directly visualize the guidewire in the joint, and withdraw it to be flush with the articular surface so that it can be measured (**TECH FIG 4B**). A screw at least 4 mm less than the measured amount is used to avoid intra-articular penetration. During the drilling over the guidewire, ensure that the drill countersink is seated fully to avoid inadvertent fracture of screw placement (**TECH FIG 4C**). Directly inspect the joint. Compress the osteotomy further with the clamp. Place the second guidewire for the proximal screw in the midline in an oblique direction to reach the plantar cortex of the distal fragment (**TECH FIG 4D**). Measure it by withdrawing the guidewire so as to be flush with the cortex. Retraction of the plantar tissue protects and allows direct visualization of the wire and the drill. This screw length equals the measurement from the wire. Directly visualize the screw to confirm compression and length (**TECH FIG 4E**).

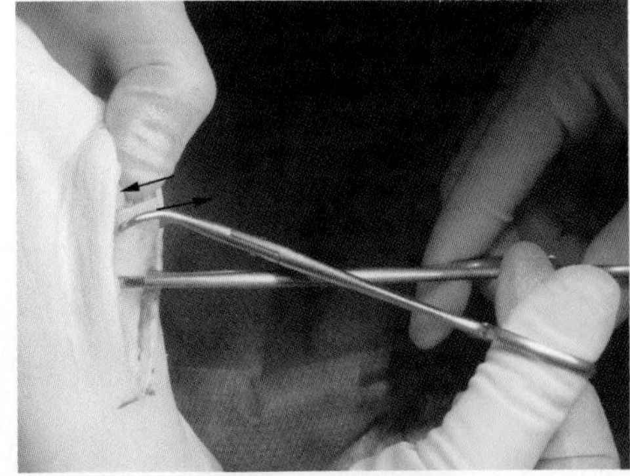

A

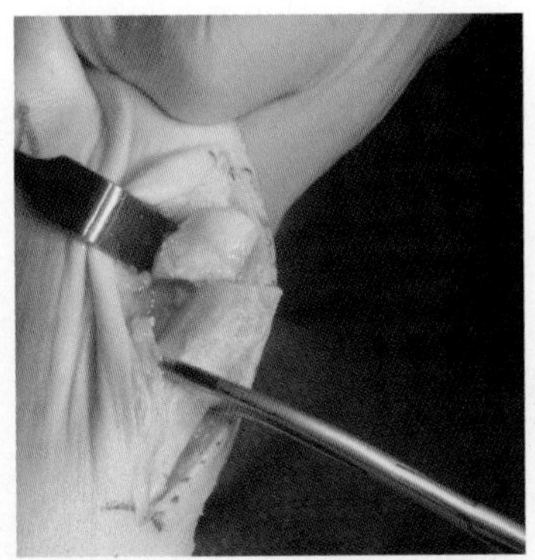

B

TECH FIG 3 • **A.** Method of displacement of the fragment. **B.** Compression clamp applied after displacement.

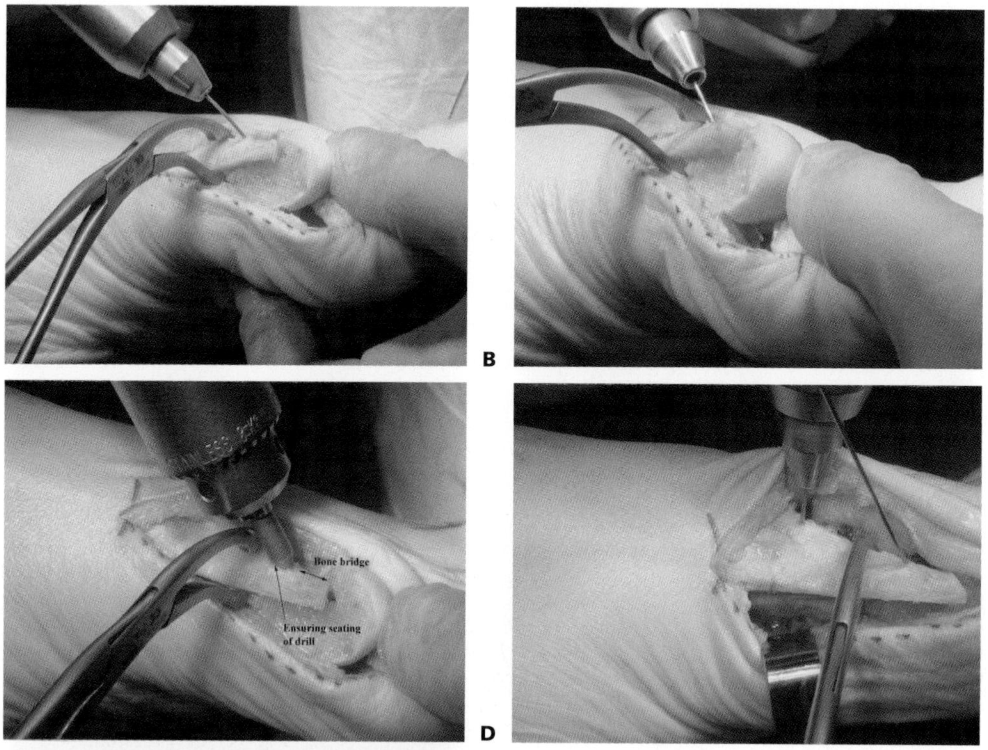

TECH FIG 4 • **A.** Distal wire placement. **B.** Distal wire position in metatarsal head. **C.** Seating of distal drill over wire. **D.** Proximal wire placement. **E.** Screw length and compression checked.

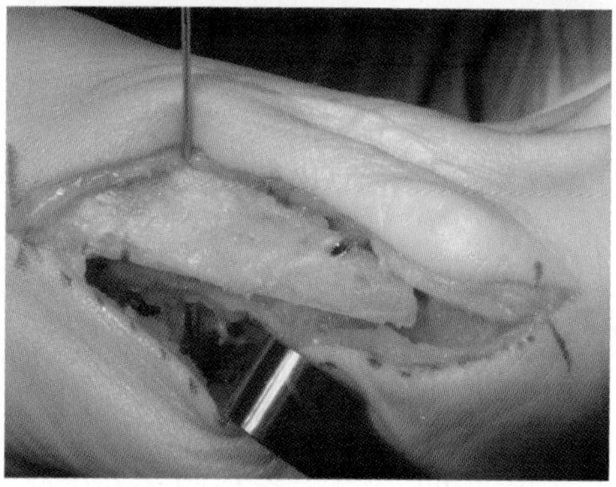

- Resect the medial distal aspect of the dorsal fragment (TECH FIG 5) and check the osteotomy for stability.
- Imbricate the medial capsule with a strong absorbable suture while holding the hallux in a neutral or slightly abducted position with the aid of a swab (TECH FIG 6).
- Confirm the reduction in the intermetatarsal angle, screws, and relocation of the sesamoids with image intensification with the foot flat on the image intensifier (TECH FIG 7). Assess the need for a proximal phalangeal osteotomy.
- Close the wound in layers with continuous Monocryl to skin and apply a forefoot bandage to maintain the correction.

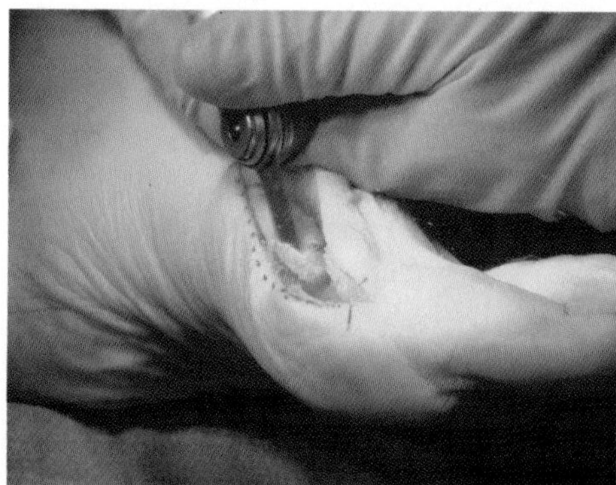

TECH FIG 5 • Residual medial bony protuberance excised.

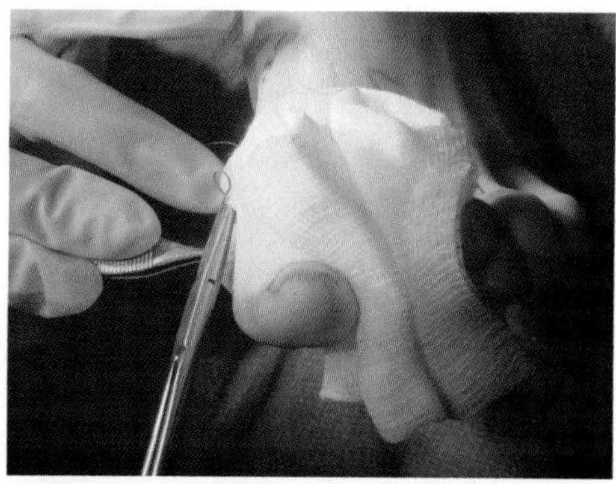

TECH FIG 6 • Capsule sutured in slightly abducted position.

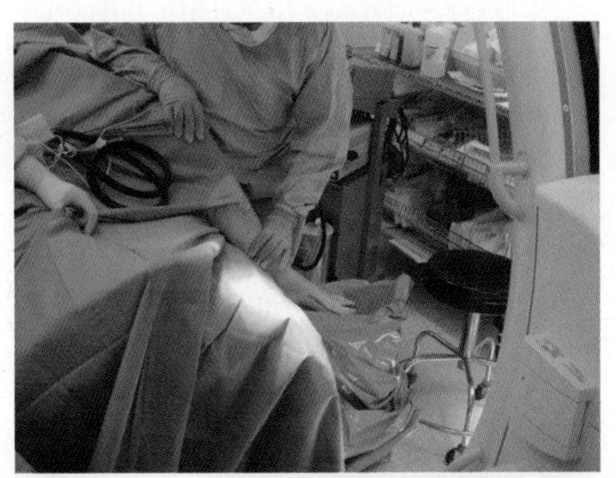

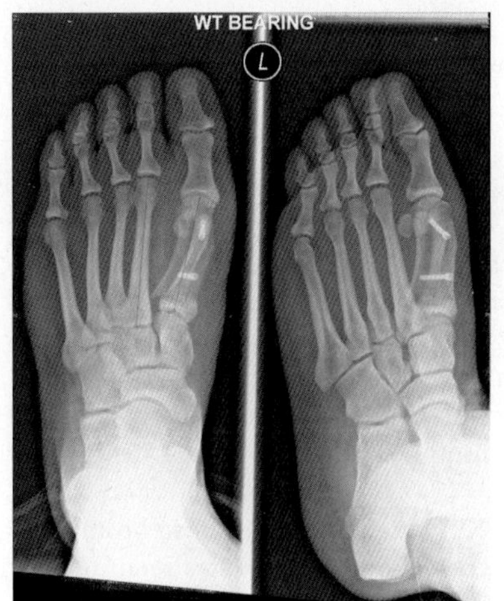

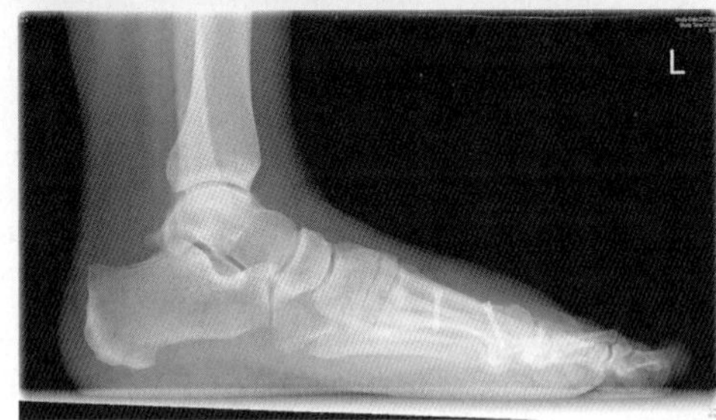

TECH FIG 7 • **A.** Image intensifier radiographs taken on table with foot "weight-bearing" image intensifier plate. **B, C.** AP, oblique, and lateral radiographs of a scarf osteotomy.

PEARLS AND PITFALLS

Ensure adequate soft tissue release on the dorsal fragment.	▪ After completing the cuts successfully, if displacement is still difficult, then check that the periosteum is not tethering the distal lateral corner of the proximal fragment.
Divergent transverse cuts	▪ Avoid convergent transverse cuts, as this will make displacement difficult.
Rotational osteotomy to correct distal metatarsal articular angle	▪ If using the Scarf osteotomy to correct the distal metatarsal articular angle, then excise a wedge of bone from the proximal, lateral, plantar fragment to allow for displacement and to avoid impingement onto the second metatarsal. A shorter Scarf can also be used.
Longitudinal cut	▪ The direction of the longitudinal cut can depress the metatarsal head, depending on the requirement.
Transverse cut	▪ Double cutting the transverse cuts can shorten the osteotomy in cases where the joint is very stiff or there is very severe hallux valgus deformity.
Screws	▪ Direct visualization of the metatarsophalangeal joint is made to avoid joint penetration. Take care to avoid seating the proximal screw too deep into the very thin dorsal cortex, as this may reduce screw hold.
Proximal plantar exposure	▪ This is a safe exposure and does not compromise the blood supply to the metatarsal. It is a vital step: once completed, it allows orientation of the longitudinal cut parallel to the plantar surface; identification of the flare of the first tarsometatarsal joint ensures the transverse cut is not intra-articular; and a clear view of the lateral plantar surface allows the surgeon to pass the guidewire under direct vision and check the screw length.

POSTOPERATIVE CARE

- If safe, patients are discharged home on the day of surgery with strict advice to elevate the foot whenever resting for the first 2 weeks.
- In most cases they are allowed to bear weight on their heel and lateral forefoot in a hard-soled postoperative shoe.
- Cast immobilization is not required.
- The wound is inspected at 2 weeks, at which time the hallux is restrapped and patients are taught simple passive and active toe flexion–extension exercises.
- At 5 weeks postoperatively the osteotomy is assessed with radiographs. If there is some consolidation at the line of the osteotomy the patient is instructed to wear a wide shoe or sneaker and to progress to full weight bearing as tolerated.

Strapping of the hallux is discontinued at this time. Delayed union or nonunion is rare with this osteotomy.

OUTCOMES

- The Scarf osteotomy is now a widely used method of correction for hallux valgus; it is particularly popular in Europe. Satisfaction rates range from 88% to 92%,[2,3,8,9] equivalent to those of the chevron osteotomy,[4,5] including patients defined as having severe hallux valgus. In a review of five recent publications[4,6,8–10] the hallux valgus angle was improved on average by 16 degrees (range 11 to 21), the intermetatarsal angle by 6.4 (range 3 to 10), and the AOFAS score by 45 (range 37 to 55).
- A learning curve for performing the Scarf osteotomy has also been noted, with higher complication rates seen in early series.[1]

COMPLICATIONS

- The main complication seen is stiffness, which occurs in up to 5% of cases.[7] Other complications include wound problems, infection, undercorrection, overcorrection, fractures, chronic regional pain disorder, and deep vein thrombosis. Delayed union and osteonecrosis are rare complications. Fracture risk can be reduced by preserving the lateral strut when placing the proximal screw and by using a long longitudinal cut.

REFERENCES

1. Barouk LS, Barouk P. The Scarf first metatarsal osteotomy in the correction of hallux valgus deformity. Interact Surg 2007;2:2–11.
2. Berg RP, Olsthoorn PG, Pöll RG. Scarf osteotomy in hallux valgus: a review of 72 cases. Acta Orthop Belg 2007;73:219–223.
3. Crevoisier X, Mouhsine E, Ortolano V, et al. The Scarf osteotomy for the treatment of hallux valgus deformity: a review of 84 cases. Foot Ankle Int 2001;22:970–976.
4. Deenik AR, Pilot P, Brandt SE, et al. Scarf versus chevron osteotomy in hallux valgus: a randomized controlled trial in 96 patients. Foot Ankle Int 2007;28:537–541.
5. Deenik A, van Mameren H, de Visser E, et al. Equivalent correction in Scarf and chevron osteotomy in moderate and severe hallux valgus: a randomized controlled trial. Foot Ankle Int 2008;29:1209–1215.
6. Garrido IM, Rubio ER, Bosch MN, et al. Scarf and Akin osteotomies for moderate and severe hallux valgus: clinical and radiographic results. Foot Ankle Surg 2008;14:194–203.
7. Hammel E, Abi Chala ML, Wagner T. Complications of first ray osteotomies: a consecutive series of 475 feet with first metatarsal Scarf osteotomy and first phalanx osteotomy. Rev Chir Orthop Reparatrice Appar Mot 2007;93:710–719.
8. Jones S, Al Hussainy HA, Ali F, et al. Scarf osteotomy for hallux valgus: a prospective clinical and pedobarographic study. J Bone Joint Surg Br 2004;86B:830–836.
9. Lipscombe S, Molly A, Sirikonda S, et al. Scarf osteotomy for the correction of hallux valgus: midterm clinical outcome. J Foot Ankle Surg 2008;47:273–277.
10. Perugia D, Basile A, Gensini A, et al. The scarf osteotomy for severe hallux valgus. Int Orthop 2003;27:103–106.

Chapter **8**

Proximal Crescentic Osteotomy

Roger A. Mann and Jeffrey A. Mann

SURGICAL MANAGEMENT

- The distal soft tissue procedure and proximal metatarsal osteotomy has been widely used for bunion corrections for more than 30 years. It is a reliable, reproducible procedure that can be used to treat a wide range of bunion deformities.
- The procedure is indicated for a hallux valgus deformity with an incongruent metatarsophalangeal joint, an intermetatarsal angle of more than 10 to 12 degrees, and a distal metatarsal articular angle of less than 10 degrees.
- It is carried out in three main steps:
  - Release of the contracted lateral capsular structures: the adductor hallucis tendon, the transverse metatarsal ligament, and the lateral joint capsule
    - By freeing up these three structures the sesamoid sling can be replaced beneath the first metatarsal head.
  - Preparation of the medial joint structures
    - Exposure and plication of the medial joint capsule
    - Excision of the medial eminence
  - Exposure of the base of the first metatarsal and proximal crescentic metatarsal osteotomy

TECHNIQUES

RELEASE OF THE LATERAL JOINT STRUCTURES

- Make a 2.5-cm incision on the dorsal aspect of the first web space between the first and second metatarsal heads.
  - Deepen this incision through the subcutaneous tissue.
- Place a Weitlander retractor to expose the web space.
  - On the floor of the web space lies the adductor hallucis, which passes obliquely to insert into the lateral sesamoid and the base of the proximal phalanx (**TECH FIGS 1 AND 2**).
- Identify the capsule between the subluxated fibular sesamoid and the lateral base of the first metatarsal head.
- Use a scalpel to release the capsule. By extending the incision distally in this interval, detach the adductor hallucis tendon from its insertion into the base of the proximal phalanx.
- Detach the adductor tendon from the lateral aspect of the fibular sesamoid, dissecting proximally until the flexor hallucis brevis muscle tissue is noted (**TECH FIG 3**).
- Place a Weitlander retractor between the first and second metatarsal heads, placing the transverse metatarsal ligament under tension (**TECH FIGS 2 AND 4**).
- Transect this ligament.
  - While carrying out this step, it is important that only ligamentous tissue is cut because directly beneath the

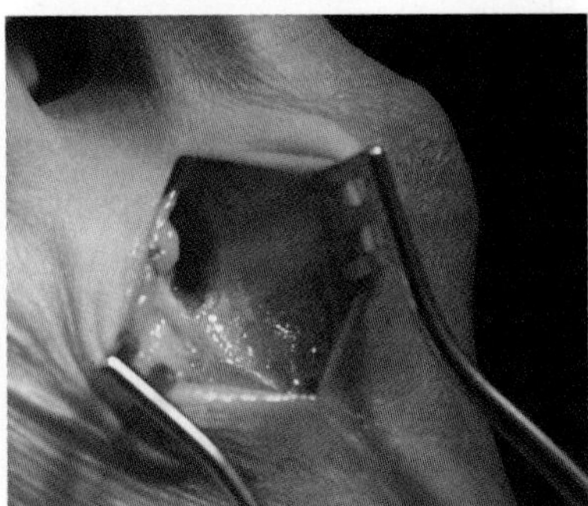

TECH FIG 1 • Dissection of the first web space, showing the adductor hallucis tendon.

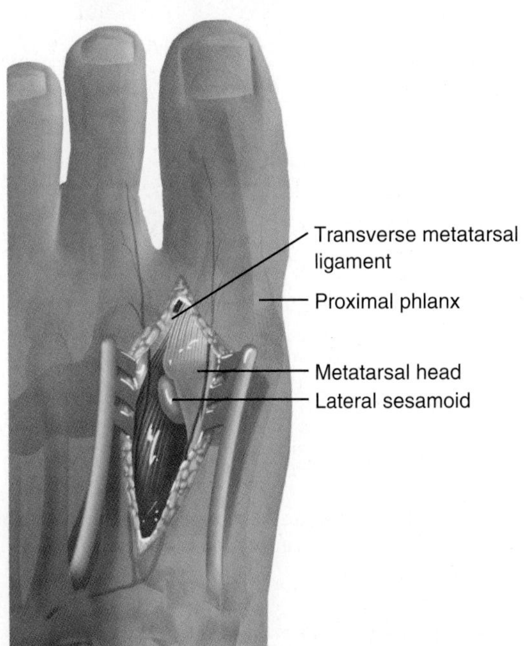

TECH FIG 2 • Diagram of Techniques Figure 1, illustrating the insertion of the adductor hallucis tendon into the base of the proximal phalanx and lateral sesamoid. Note the position of the transverse metatarsal ligament.

ligament lies the common nerve to the first web space and the accompanying vessels.

- Release the lateral joint capsule.
  - Make an incision through the dorsal aspect of the joint capsule at the level of the joint line, and pass the knife blade to the plantar aspect of the metatarsal (**TECH FIGS 5 AND 6**).
  - With the blade well seated against the bone, pass the scalpel proximally, stripping the origin of the capsule off the metatarsal head over a distance of about 1.5 cm.
  - This creates a flap of the lateral joint capsule to be used later in the repair (**TECH FIG 7**).
- Bring the hallux into about 25 degrees of varus, which ensures that no lateral contracture remains.

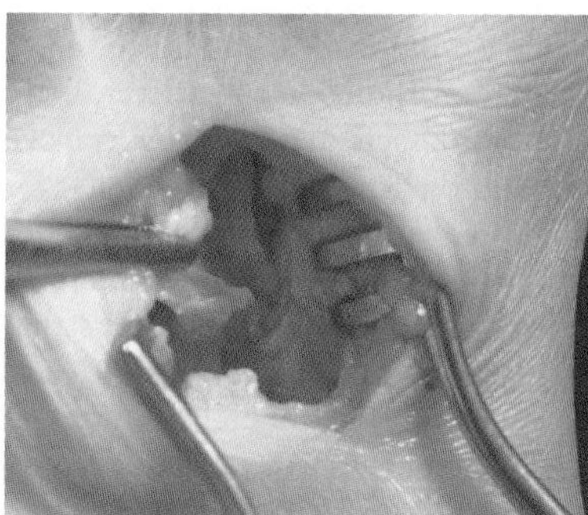

TECH FIG 3 • The adductor tendon has been detached from the lateral aspect of the fibular sesamoid and is being held in the forceps.

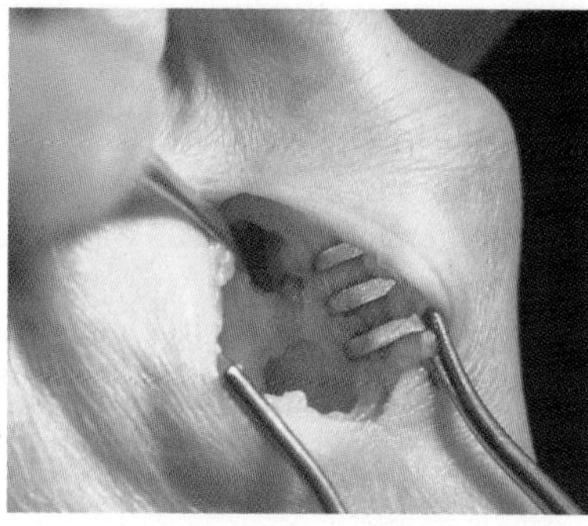

TECH FIG 4 • The transverse metatarsal ligament is placed under tension using a Weitlander retractor.

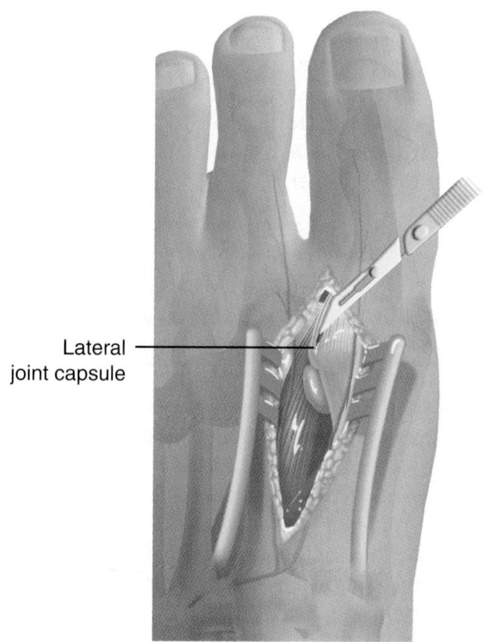

TECH FIG 6 • Diagram of Techniques Figure 5, illustrating the lateral joint capsule of the first metatarsophalangeal joint.

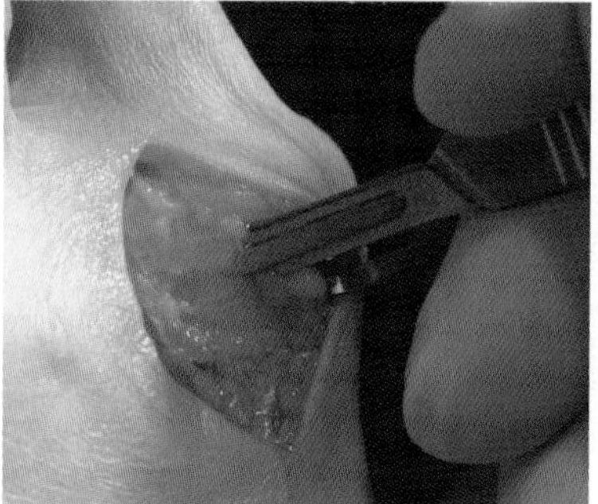

TECH FIG 5 • The scalpel has been placed through the dorsal aspect of the lateral joint capsule of the first metatarsophalangeal joint.

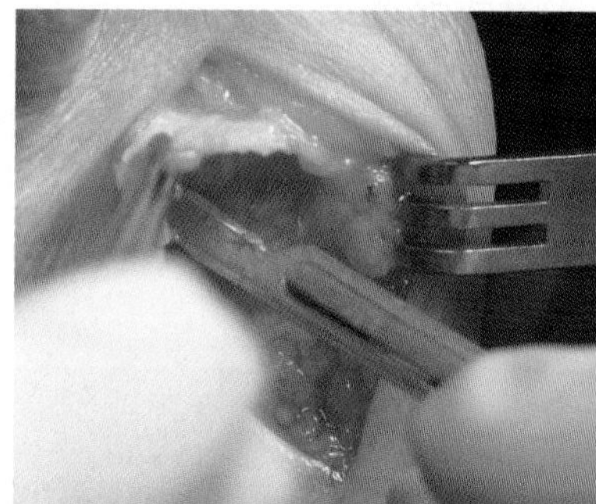

TECH FIG 7 • The origin if the lateral joint capsule has been stripped off the metatarsal head, creating the flap of tissue held in the forceps.

PREPARATION OF THE MEDIAL JOINT CAPSULE

- Approach the medial joint capsule through a longitudinal incision in the midline starting at the middle of the proximal phalanx and proceeding proximally just past the medial eminence.
- Identify the plane between the subcutaneous tissue and the joint capsule; take care to work along this plane.
  - Dissecting dorsally at first, pull the skin flap away from the capsule to expose the dorsal medial cutaneous nerve, which is then carefully retracted.

- Next, dissect the skin flap off the plantar half of the capsule until the abductor hallucis muscle and tendon are identified.
  - Take care in this area, because the plantar medial cutaneous nerve lies just plantar to the abductor tendon.
- The capsulotomy that we prefer starts with a vertical cut in the medial joint capsule, made 2 to 3 mm proximal to the base of the proximal phalanx.
- Make a second, parallel cut 3 to 8 mm proximal to the first cut, depending on the severity of the hallux valgus deformity. A more severe deformity requires more resection of tissue from the medial joint capsule (**TECH FIG 8**).
- Bring together these two parallel capsular cuts dorsally through an inverted V-shaped incision.
- On the plantar side, make an upright V-shaped incision through the abductor hallucis tendon that ends at the tibial sesamoid (**TECH FIG 9**).
- Remove this capsular tissue (**TECH FIG 10**).
- While making the cut through the abductor hallucis tendon, keep the tip of the knife blade inside the joint to avoid damaging the plantar medial cutaneous nerve.
- Make an incision through the joint capsule on the dorsal aspect of the medial eminence.
- Peel the capsular flap proximally and plantarward until the medial eminence is completely exposed (**TECH FIGS 11, 12, AND 13**).

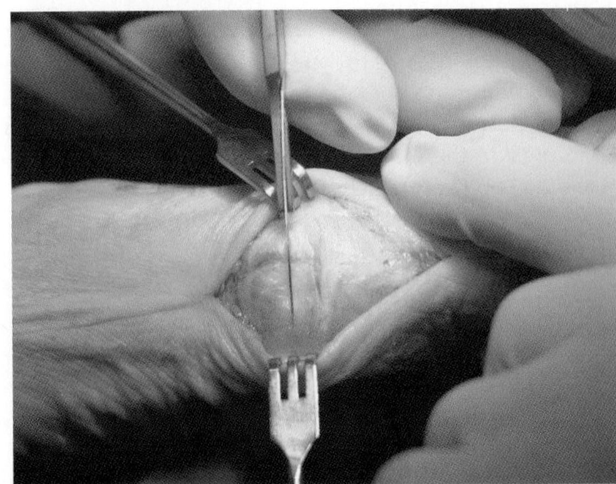

TECH FIG 8 • Exposure of the medial joint capsule, showing the parallel cuts that represent the vertical limbs of the capsulotomy.

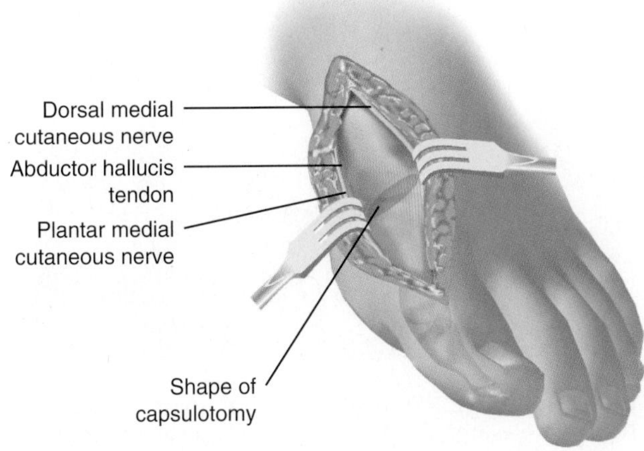

TECH FIG 9 • Diagram of Techniques Figure 8, demonstrating the shape of the medial joint capsulotomy.

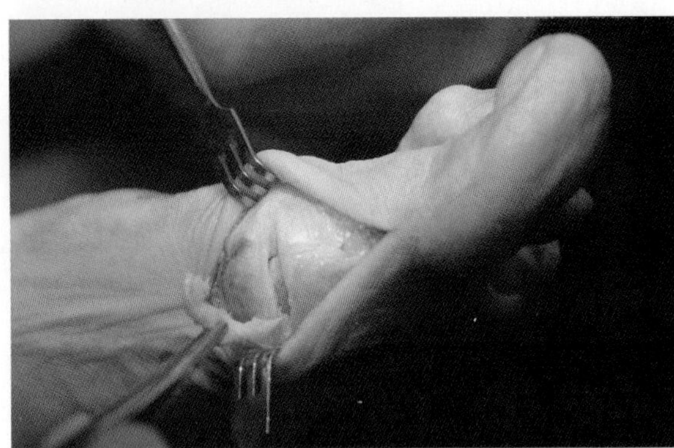

TECH FIG 10 • Removing the medial joint capsular tissue.

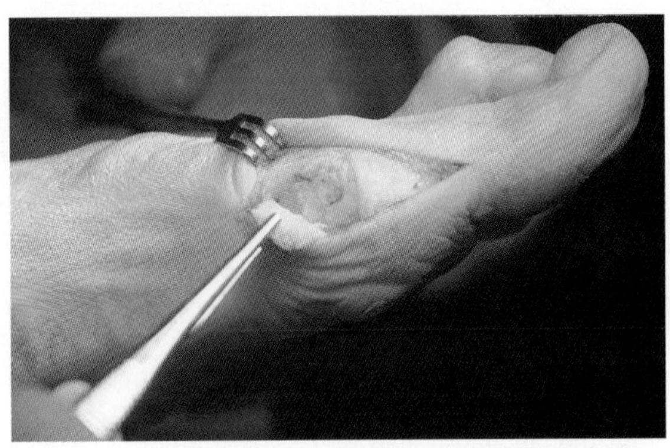

TECH FIG 11 • A dorsal incision is made and the capsular flap is peeled proximally and plantarward.

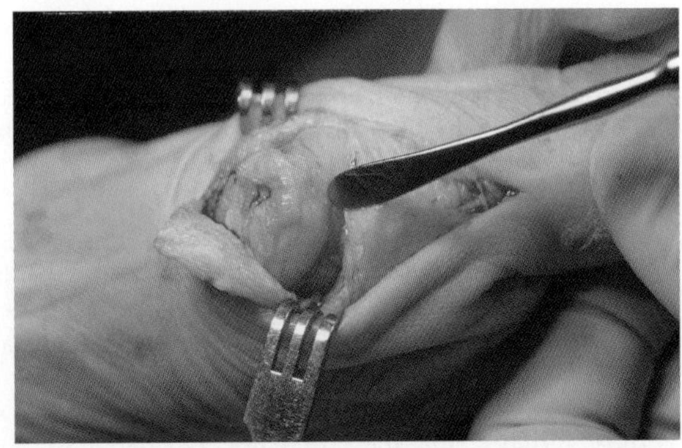

TECH FIG 12 • The medial eminence has been completely exposed. The sagittal sulcus is demonstrated by the Freer elevator.

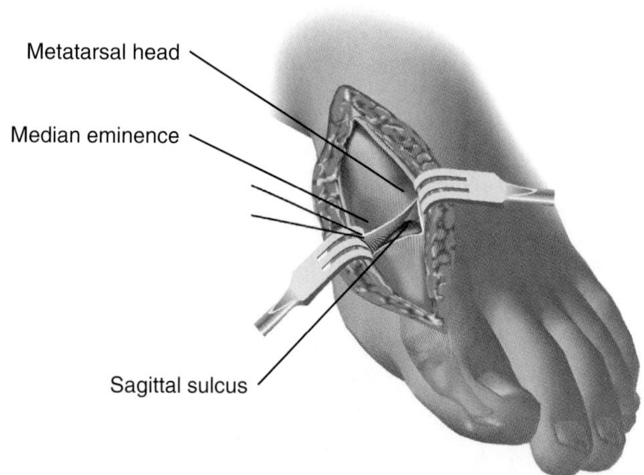

TECH FIG 13 • Diagram of the medial eminence after the capsular flap has been retracted. Note the sagittal sulcus.

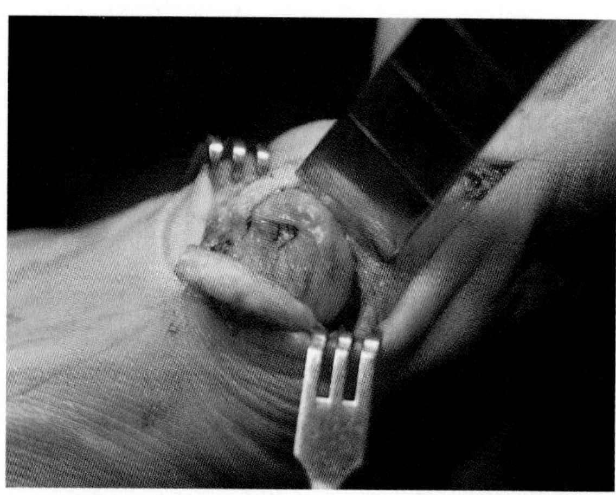

TECH FIG 14 • The osteotomy to remove the medial eminence is started 1 to 2 mm medial to the sagittal sulcus and is performed in line with the medial aspect of the metatarsal shaft.

- Perform an osteotomy to remove the medial eminence.
  - Start the osteotomy 1 to 2 mm medial to the sagittal sulcus; the osteotomy is in line with the medial aspect of the metatarsal shaft (**TECH FIG 14**).
  - The medial eminence can be removed with a 16-mm osteotome or with a saw blade. This is strictly the choice of the operating surgeon.
- After performing the osteotomy, inspect the metatarsal to be sure there are no rough edges of bone. Rongeur off any bony prominence.

APPROACH TO THE PROXIMAL CRESCENTIC OSTEOTOMY

- Make an incision directly over the extensor hallucis longus tendon, from just proximal to the metatarsal cuneiform joint distally about 2.5 to 3 cm.
  - Usually a large vessel crosses this plane; cut or cauterize it when the approach is made.
- Mobilize the extensor tendon and retract it either medially or laterally to expose the metatarsal shaft.
- As the metatarsal shaft is exposed, it is not necessary to be subperiosteal.
  - Working just above the periosteal plane allows the tissues to move easily.
- Identify the metatarsal cuneiform joint.
  - Make a mark on the metatarsal 1 cm distal to the joint; this is where the crescentic osteotomy will be created.
  - Make a second mark on the metatarsal 1 cm distal to the osteotomy site; this is where the screw will be placed that stabilizes the osteotomy (**TECH FIGS 15 AND 16**).
  - To confirm that the osteotomy site is correct, note the flare on the lateral aspect of the metatarsal that marks the junction of the diaphyseal and metaphyseal bone.
    - This is located about 1 cm distal to the metatarsal cuneiform joint.
- Advance a guide pin for the 4.0-mm cannulated screw a short distance into the metatarsal, beginning at the marked site.
  - The pin should be angled at about 50 degrees to the long axis of the metatarsal in the sagittal plane (**TECH FIG 16**). At this angle the pin and subsequent screw will pass into the plantar aspect of the proximal metatarsal fragment and will not violate the joint.
- Carry out the osteotomy using a crescent-shaped saw blade.
  - This blade comes in two lengths. It is easier to start with a shorter blade and then use the longer blade if necessary to complete the osteotomy (**TECH FIGS 16 AND 17**).

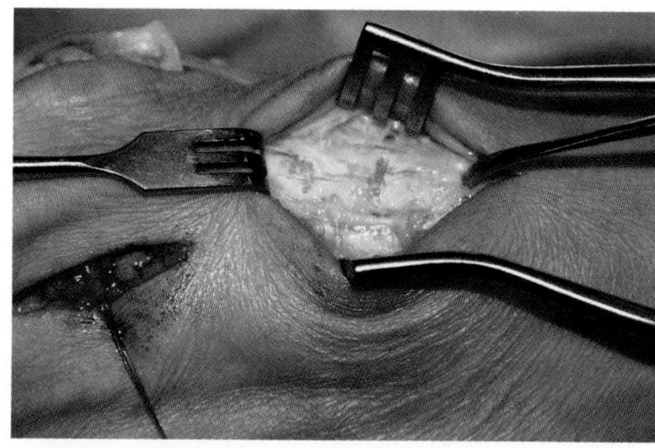

TECH FIG 15 • The first metatarsal shaft is exposed. The Freer elevator points to the metatarsocuneiform joint. One centimeter distal to the joint marks the site of the osteotomy, and 1 cm more distally marks the screw insertion site.

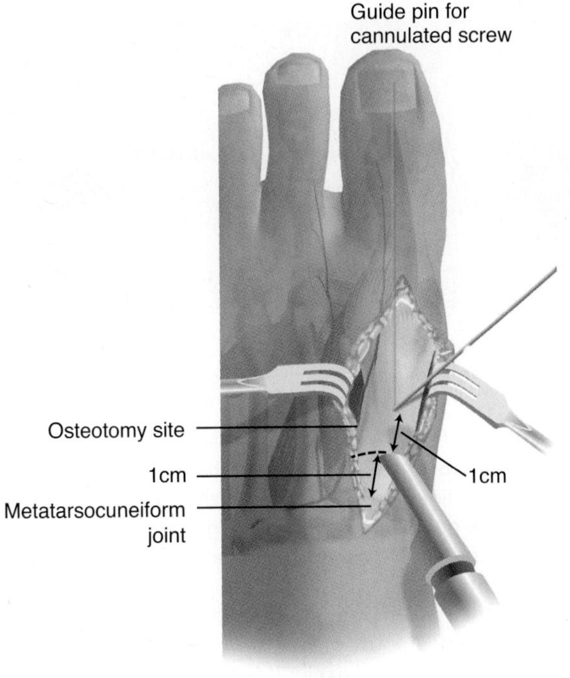

TECH FIG 16 • Diagram of the first metatarsal shaft demonstrating the metatarsocuneiform joint. Note the osteotomy site and angle of the saw blade. Also note the screw insertion site.

- Positioning of the foot in preparation for the osteotomy is a critical part of this procedure.
  - Sit at the side of the table holding the foot in one hand.
  - Hold the foot in a neutral position in regard to dorsiflexion–plantarflexion and inversion–eversion.
  - Place the saw with the concavity facing proximally, toward the heel.
  - The angle of the saw blade should be neither perpendicular to the bottom of the foot nor perpendicular to the metatarsal, but about halfway between those positions (**TECH FIG 16**).

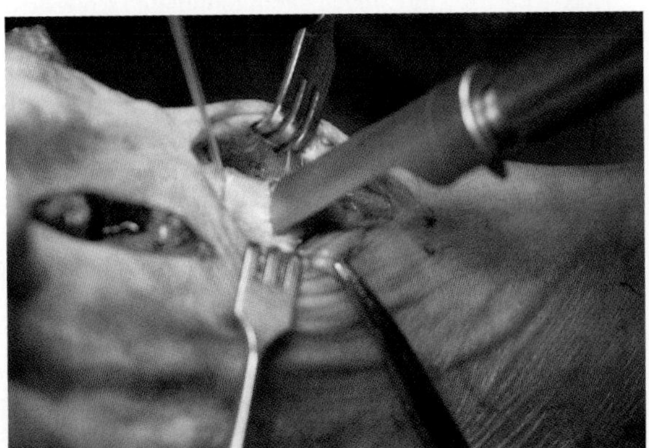

TECH FIG 17 • The osteotomy is performed with a crescent-shaped saw blade.

- Start the osteotomy cut by applying firm pressure to the blade.
  - After making the initial cut into the bone, carefully evaluate the position of the saw blade to be sure that it will cut through the lateral cortex of the metatarsal shaft.
  - Sometimes in a wide metatarsal the blade will not penetrate both cortices.
    - If the medial cortex is not completely cut, it is safe and simple to complete the osteotomy in this area.
    - However, it is difficult and potentially dangerous to complete an osteotomy laterally, as there is a major artery in the space between the first and second metatarsals that could be harmed.
- Make the cut by moving the saw in a medial–lateral direction along the arc of the saw blade.
  - While cutting, apply a little bit of pressure to the blade toward the heel, as this helps to stabilize the blade in the plane of its cut.
  - Once the cut is established, moving the saw blade back and forth without a lot of pressure plantarward will produce a nice smooth cut.
- It is important that the cut passes all the way through the metatarsal so that the distal portion of the bone is totally free and has no bony attachments to the proximal fragment.
- If a medial piece of bone is still present, use a 4- to 6-mm osteotome to cut through the bone.
- Pass a knife blade along the medial side of the cut to be sure that the cut is completely free of any bony or periosteal attachment.
- Return your attention to the first web space.
  - Place a figure 8 suture of 2-0 chromic into the cut end of the adductor hallucis tendon. It is easier to place this stitch before the osteotomy site has been reduced.

CORRECTION OF THE OSTEOTOMY

- Correcting the osteotomy is the most technically demanding part of the bunion procedure.
  - The objective is to stabilize the base of the metatarsal while rotating the distal portion of the metatarsal around the osteotomy site.
- The first step is to push the proximal portion of the cut metatarsal in a medial direction so that it is at the medial excursion of the metatarsal cuneiform joint.
  - This can be accomplished with a Freer elevator (**TECH FIGS 18 AND 19**).

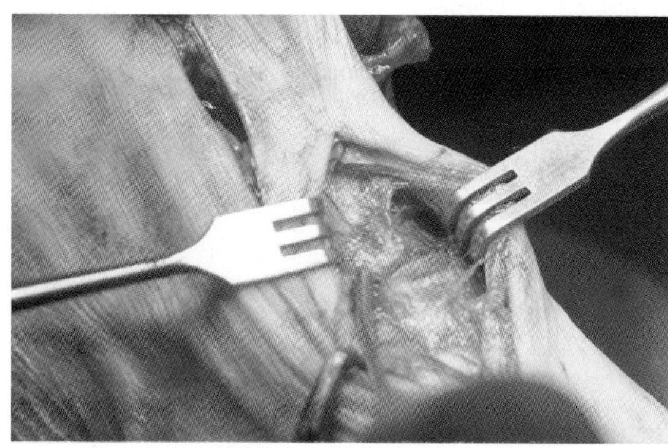

TECH FIG 18 • The osteotomy is corrected by pushing the proximal portion of the cut metatarsal in a medial direction (note the Freer elevator) while rotating the distal aspect of the metatarsal in a lateral direction around the osteotomy site.

- Grasp the metatarsal head firmly with your other hand and rotate the distal aspect of the metatarsal in a lateral direction around the osteotomy site.
  - Examining the osteotomy site demonstrates that the distal fragment rotates no more than 2 to 3 mm around the "crescent" (Tech Figs 18 and 19).
- Hold the osteotomy site in this alignment and drill the previously placed guide pin across the osteotomy site until the plantar cortex is engaged.
  - Once this occurs, the osteotomy site is reasonably stable.
- Measure the guide pin to determine the screw length, which is usually 28 to 30 mm.

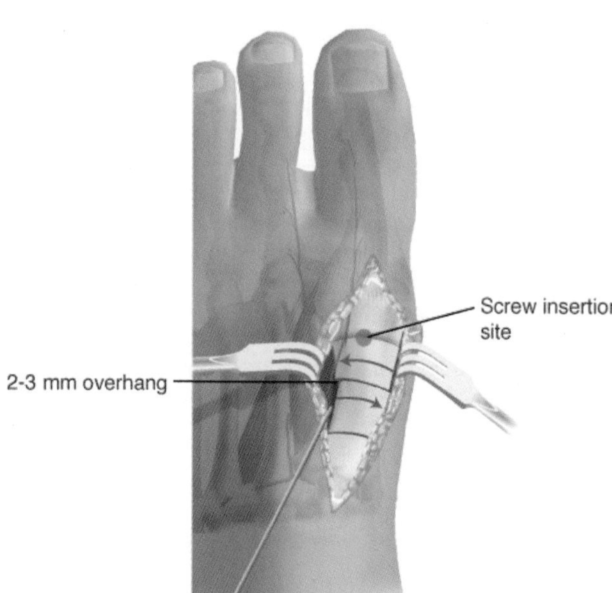

TECH FIG 19 • Diagram of the osteotomy site. The surgeon's hand is pushing the metatarsal shaft in a lateral direction. The Freer elevator is pushing the metatarsal base in a medial direction. Note the 2- to 3-mm overhang on the lateral aspect of the osteotomy site.

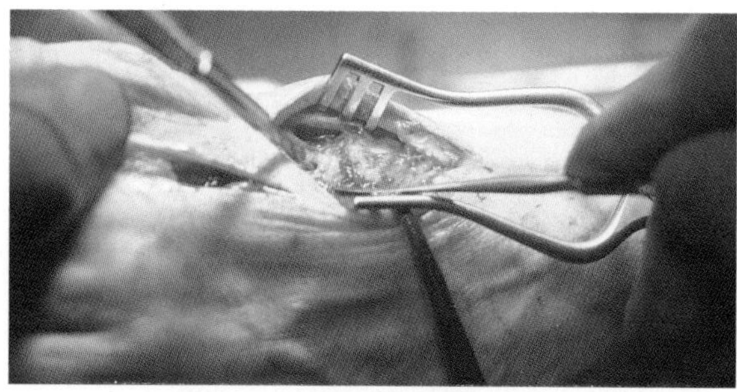

TECH FIG 20 • The osteotomy site is being held while the cannulated drill is advanced over the guide pin.

- When learning to perform this procedure, or if there is a question as to the alignment of the osteotomy, at this point obtaining a radiograph is warranted.
  - If the guide pin is not providing adequate stability, a second pin or Kirschner wire can be used for supplemental fixation while evaluating the radiograph.
  - If the radiograph shows that the intermetatarsal angle is not sufficiently closed down, remove the guide pin and remanipulate the osteotomy site until the intermetatarsal angle is adequately corrected.
- While holding the osteotomy site corrected, overdrill the guide pin with the appropriate-sized drill for the cannulated screw set (TECH FIG 20).
  - Usually it is adequate to advance the drill to a position just past the osteotomy site, so that the guide pin does not back out when the drill is removed.
- Use a countersink, mainly on the distal side of the screw hole, to make the screw head less prominent. However, excessive countersinking can cause the screw head to be pulled through the screw hole site and produce instability of the osteotomy site.
- Place a partially threaded 4.0-mm cannulated screw across the osteotomy site and carefully tighten it (TECH FIG 21).
  - Be cautious as the screw is tightened because the island of bone is only about 5 or 6 mm and can be cracked if the screw is tightened too firmly.
- Check the stability of the osteotomy site by moving the distal fragment in the sagittal plane, looking for any motion at the osteotomy site.
  - Mild instability of the osteotomy can be addressed by carefully tightening the screw or by adding a small-diameter Kirschner wire for supplemental fixation.
  - Occasionally a small plate may need to be added to the first metatarsal to secure the osteotomy if there is gross instability.

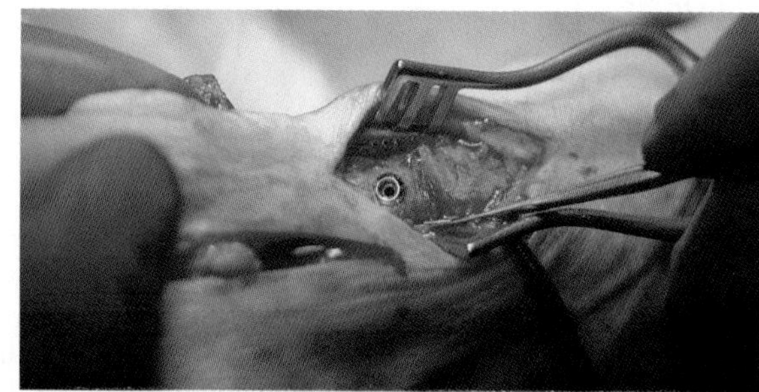

TECH FIG 21 • The cannulated screw has been placed to stabilize the osteotomy site.

RECONSTRUCTION OF THE MEDIAL JOINT CAPSULE

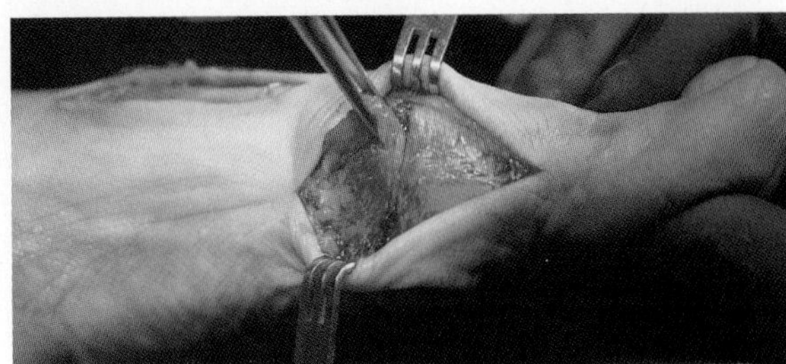

TECH FIG 22 • With the toe held in neutral position, the medial capsular flaps are checked for proper alignment.

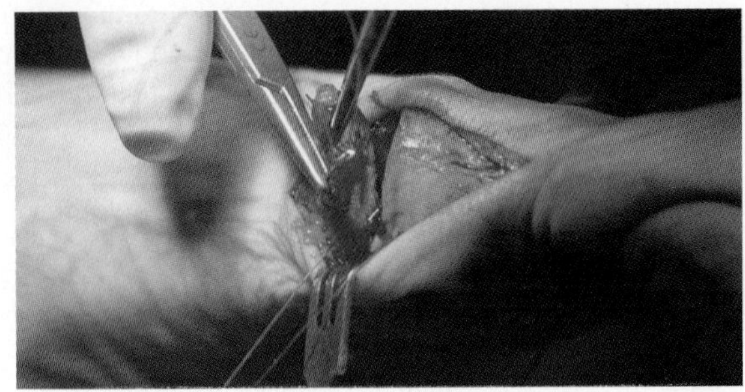

TECH FIG 23 • The first suture for repairing the medial joint capsule is placed as plantar as possible; it incorporates the abductor hallucis tendon.

- The first step in reconstructing the medial joint capsule is to hold the great toe in correct alignment:
  - Neutral dorsiflexion–plantarflexion
  - 0 to 5 degrees of varus
- Rotate the toe to correct pronation, which brings the sesamoids back underneath the metatarsal head.
  - Reduction of the sesamoids has been achieved if they are visible along the plantar aspect of the medial eminence.
- Pull the proximal joint capsule distally to see whether the proximal and distal flaps of the capsule juxtapose one another (TECH FIG 22).
- If they do, then the capsular flaps are approximated.
- If insufficient capsule has been removed, then more capsular tissue needs to be removed before it is plicated.
  - The capsular flaps should not be overlapped in a "pants over vest" fashion, as this creates too much bulk over the medial eminence.
- To repair the medial capsule, place four to six sutures of 2-0 chromic into the joint capsule with the toe held in correct alignment.
- The first suture is placed as plantar as possible and incorporates the abductor hallucis tendon (TECH FIG 23).
  - The suture line progresses dorsally (TECH FIG 24).
- Once the sutures are placed and tied, check the alignment of the toe.
  - The toe should be in neutral position as far as varus and valgus is concerned, or possibly in a little bit of varus.
  - In general, if the final alignment of the toe is in more than 5 degrees of valgus, extra capsular tissue should be removed.
- Return your attention to the first web space.
  - Sew the adductor hallucis tendon (already tagged with a suture) to the flap of capsule that was stripped off the metatarsal head.
  - If the toe had been positioned in a little too much varus when plicating the medial capsule, tension can be placed on this web space repair to prevent a hallux varus from occurring.
- Thoroughly irrigate the wounds with antibiotic solution and then close them with interrupted silk.
- Apply a sterile compression dressing and then release the tourniquet.

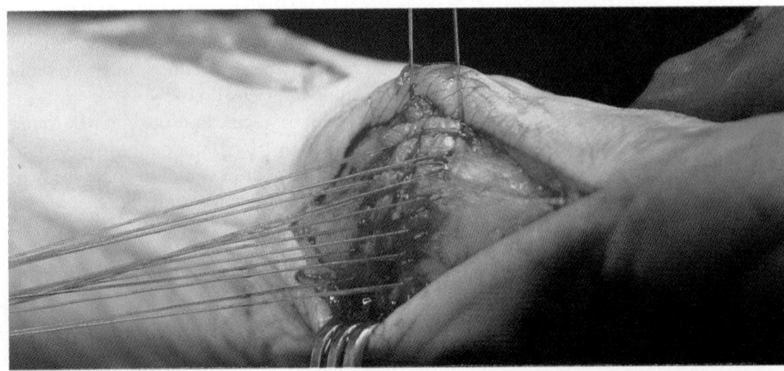

TECH FIG 24 • A total of four to six sutures are used to repair the medial joint capsule.

PEARLS AND PITFALLS

Indications	▪ Incongruent metatarsophalangeal joint ▪ Intermetatarsal angle of more than 10 to 12 degrees ▪ Distal metatarsal articular angle of less than 10 degrees
First web space dissection	▪ Release the entire adductor hallucis tendon off its insertion in the sesamoid and proximal phalanx. ▪ Check adequate release of lateral structures by pulling the toe into maximum varus. ▪ Do not dissect plantar to the transverse metatarsal ligament.
Medial capsulotomy	▪ Start with a 3-mm medial capsulotomy for a milder bunion deformity and a larger medial capsulotomy for a more advanced bunion deformity. ▪ Avoid the dorsal and plantar medial cutaneous nerves. ▪ When plicating the medial capsule, do not overlap the capsular flaps in a "pants over vest" fashion, as this creates too much bulk over the medial eminence.
Medial eminence osteotomy	▪ The median eminence osteotomy is started 1 to 2 mm medial to the sagittal sulcus and is performed in line with the medial aspect of the metatarsal shaft.
Crescentic metatarsal osteotomy	▪ The crescentic osteotomy is performed 1 cm distal to the metatarsocuneiform joint, at the flare of the base of the proximal phalanx. ▪ The angle of the saw blade for the osteotomy cut should be neither perpendicular to the bottom of the foot nor perpendicular to the metatarsal, but about halfway between those positions.
Fixation of metatarsal osteotomy	▪ The guide pin for the cannulated screw should be angled at about 50 degrees to the long axis of the metatarsal. ▪ Leave adequate bone bridge (1 cm) between the cannulated screw and the metatarsal osteotomy. ▪ Avoid penetrating the metatarsal cuneiform joint with the screw fixating the osteotomy site.
Correcting metatarsal osteotomy	▪ Avoid overcorrection or undercorrection of the metatarsal osteotomy. Check the alignment with a fluoroscan if there is any doubt as to the degree of correction.

POSTOPERATIVE CARE

- The initial postoperative dressing is changed 1 to 2 days after surgery.
  - A dressing incorporating firm gauze and adhesive tape is used to hold the toe in correct alignment.
  - The patient is permitted to ambulate in a postoperative shoe.
- The patient is seen about 8 to 10 days after surgery, at which point the sutures are removed and a radiograph is obtained.
- Based on the alignment of the toe in this radiograph, it is determined how the toe is dressed—namely, into a little more varus or valgus, or held in a neutral position.
- The dressings are changed on a weekly basis to ensure that the alignment of the toe remains correct.
- At 3 to 5 weeks after surgery another radiograph is obtained to confirm the alignment of the toe.
  - If the alignment is not correct, it can still be corrected by pulling the toe into more varus or valgus, depending on what the radiograph dictates.
- After 8 weeks the dressings are removed and the patient is started on range-of-motion exercises.

OUTCOMES

- Proximal metatarsal osteotomy and distal soft tissue release decreases the bunion deformity to an average of 10 degrees and decreases the intermetatarsal angle to an average of 5 degrees.
- A 90% to 95% rate of patient satisfaction has been reported, as well as improvements in pain level and improvements in overall function.

COMPLICATIONS

- Recurrence of hallux valgus deformity
- Hallux varus
- Dorsiflexion of metatarsal osteotomy
- Nonunion of osteotomy site
- Delayed union of osteotomy site

REFERENCES

1. Dreeban S, Mann RA. Advanced hallux valgus deformity: long-term results utilizing the distal soft tissue procedure and proximal metatarsal osteotomy. Foot Ankle Int 1996;17:142–144.
2. Mann RA, Coughlin MJ. Adult hallux valgus. In: Coughlin MJ, Mann RA, eds. Surgery of the Foot and Ankle, 7th ed. St. Louis: Mosby, 1999.
3. Thordarson DB, Rudicel SA, Ebramzadeh E, et al. Outcome study of hallux valgus surgery—an AOFAS multi-center study. Foot Ankle Int 2001;22:956–959.

Chapter 9 Ludloff Osteotomy

Hans-Joerg Trnka and Stefan G. Hofstaetter

DEFINITION

- Symptomatic hallux valgus associated with a first intermetatarsal angle greater than 15 degrees is typically corrected with a proximal first metatarsal osteotomy and distal soft tissue procedure when nonoperative treatment fails.
- Multiple techniques for the hallux valgus deformity correction have been decribed.[5]
- In 1918 Ludloff[4] described an oblique osteotomy from the dorsal–proximal to distal–plantar aspects of the first metatarsal, and the procedure was performed without internal fixation.
- The procedure recently gained renewed attention when Myerson[1,6] recommended adding internal fixation and modified several parts of the technique.
- The modified Ludloff osteotomy has been extensively studied with biomechanical and mathematical investigations.

ANATOMY

- The special situation distinguishing the first metatarsophalangeal (MTP) joint from the lesser MTP joints is the sesamoid mechanism.
  - On the plantar surface of the metatarsal head are two longitudinal cartilage-covered grooves separated by a rounded ridge. The sesamoids run in these grooves.
  - The sesamoid bone is contained in each tendon of the flexor hallucis brevis; they are distally attached by the fibrous plantar plate to the base of the proximal phalanx.
- The head of the first metatarsal is rounded and cartilage-covered and articulates with the smaller concave elliptical base of the proximal phalanx.
- Fan-shaped ligamentous bands originate from the medial and lateral condyles of the metatarsal head and run to the base of the proximal phalanx and the margins of the sesamoids and the plantar plate.
- Tendons and muscles that move the great toe are arranged in four groups:
  - Long and short extensor tendons
  - Long and short flexor tendons
  - Abductor hallucis
  - Adductor hallucis
- Blood supply to the metatarsal head
  - First dorsal metatarsal artery
  - Branches from the first plantar metatarsal artery

PATHOGENESIS

- Extrinsic causes
  - Hallux valgus occurs almost exclusively in shoe-wearing populations, but only occasionally in the unshod individual.
  - Although shoes are an essential factor in the cause of hallux valgus, not all individuals wearing fashionable shoes develop this deformity.
- Intrinsic causes
  - Hardy and Clapham[2] found, in a series of 91 patients, a positive family history in 63%.
  - Coughlin[5] reported that a bunion was identified in 94% of 31 mothers whose children inherited a hallux valgus deformity.
  - The association of pes planus with the development of a hallux valgus deformity has been controversial.
  - Hohmann was the most definitive proponent that hallux valgus is always combined with pes planus.
    - Coughlin[5] and Kilmartin noted no incidence of pes planus in the juvenile patient.
    - Pronation of the foot imposes a longitudinal rotation of the first ray that places the axis of the MTP joint in an oblique plane relative to the floor. In this position the foot appears to be less able to withstand the deformity pressures exerted on it by either shoes or weight bearing.[11]
    - The simultaneous occurrence of hallux valgus and metatarsus primus varus has been frequently described. The question of cause and effect continues to be debated.

PATIENT HISTORY AND PHYSICAL FINDINGS

- Physical findings associated with hallux valgus deformity include the following:
  - Pain in narrow shoes
  - Symptomatic intractable keratoses beneath the second metatarsal head (in 40% of patients)
  - Lateral deviation of the great toe
  - Pronation of the great toe
  - Keratosis medial plantar underneath the interphalangeal joint
  - Bursitis over the medial aspect of the medial condyle of the first metatarsal head
  - Hypermobility of the first metatarsocuneiform joint
- Physical examination for hallux valgus deformity should include the following:
  - Hallux valgus angle measurement: Normal is 15 degrees or less.
  - Intermetatarsal angle measurement: Normal is 9 degrees or less.
  - Sesamoid position measurements
  - Joint congruency

IMAGING AND OTHER DIAGNOSTIC STUDIES

- Radiographs of the foot should always be obtained with the patient in the weight-bearing position, with AP, lateral, and oblique views. The following criteria are examined:
  - Hallux valgus angle
  - Intermetatarsal angle
  - Sesamoid position
  - Joint congruency
  - Distal metatarsal articular angle: the relationship between the articular surface of the first metatarsal head and a line bisecting the first metatarsal shaft (normal is 10 degrees or less)
  - Arthrosis of the first MTP joint

DIFFERENTIAL DIAGNOSIS

- Ganglion
- Hallux rigidus

NONOPERATIVE MANAGEMENT

- Comfortable wider shoes
  - Orthotics?
  - Spiral dynamics physiotherapy in adolescents

SURGICAL MANAGEMENT

- Indications
  - Symptomatic hallux valgus deformity with a first intermetatarsal angle of more than 15 degrees
  - Stable first metatarsal-cuneiform joint
- Contraindications
  - Narrow metatarsal so that adequate rotation of the dorsal fragment is not possible
  - Severe osteoporosis
  - Skeletally immature patient
  - Severe osteoarthritic changes

Preoperative Planning

- Standard weight-bearing AP and lateral radiographs are mandatory.
- The hallux valgus and intermetatarsal angles and tibial sesamoid position are measured.
- A preoperative drawing is helpful.
- Clinical examination includes measurement of active and passive range of motion of the first MTP joint as well as inspection of the foot for plantar callus formation indicative of transfer metatarsalgia and stability of the first tarsometatarsal joint.

Positioning

- The foot is prepared in the standard manner.
- The patient is positioned supine.
- An ankle tourniquet is optional.

Approach

- The lateral soft tissue release is performed through a dorsal approach.
- The Ludloff osteotomy is performed through a straight midline incision.

TECHNIQUES

LATERAL SOFT TISSUE RELEASE

- The procedure is typically performed under the peripheral nerve.
- Make a dorsal 3-cm longitudinal incision over the first web space (**TECH FIG 1A,B**).
- Continue deep dissection bluntly.
- Insert a lamina spreader and a Langenbeck retractor to expose the first web space.
- Divide the lateral joint capsule (metatarsal-sesamoid ligament) immediately superior to the lateral sesamoid. Fenestrate the lateral capsule at the first MTP joint (**TECH FIG 1C,D**).
- Apply a varus stress to the hallux to complete the lateral release (**TECH FIG 1E**).
- Place one or two sutures between the lateral capsule of the first MTP joint and the periosteum of the second metatarsal.

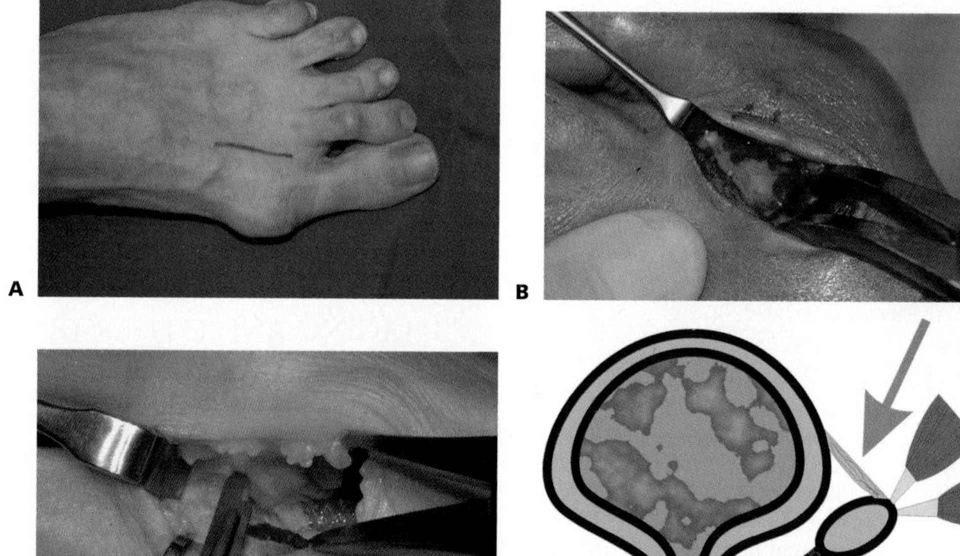

TECH FIG 1 • **A.** A dorsal 3-cm longitudinal incision is made over the first web space. **B.** A lamina spreader and a Langenbeck retractor are inserted to expose the first web space. **C, D.** Release of the metatarsal-sesamoid ligament. *(continued)*

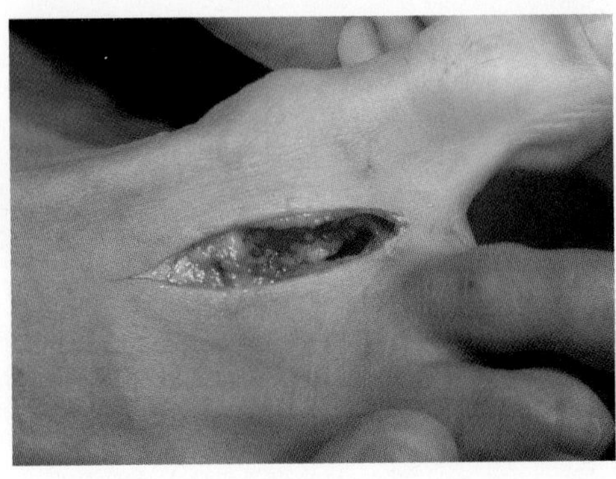

TECH FIG 1 • *(continued)* **E.** The great toe is brought into 20 degrees varus to demonstrate the release of the lateral structures.

LUDLOFF OSTEOTOMY

Incision and Exposure

- Make a midaxial skin incision over the medial first MTP joint, extending to the first tarsometatarsal joint (**TECH FIG 2A,B**).
- After careful subcutaneous dissection to avoid damage to the dorsomedial nerve bundle, expose the periosteum of the first metatarsal and insert dorsal–proximal and distal–plantar Hohmann retractors (**TECH FIG 2C**).
- Perform an L-shaped medial capsulotomy and split the periosteum up to the first tarsometatarsal joint level. Minimize periosteal dissection (**TECH FIG 2D,E**).

Beginning the Osteotomy

- Plan an oblique first metatarsal osteotomy from the dorsal–proximal first metatarsal (immediately distal to the first tarsometatarsal joint) to the plantar–distal first metatarsal (immediately proximal to the sesamoid complex). First mark the osteotomy with the electrocautery (**TECH FIG 3A**).
- The osteotomy is inclined from medial to lateral plantar at an angle of 10 degrees (**TECH FIG 3B**).
- Perform only the dorsal two thirds of the osteotomy initially to guarantee a stable situation (**TECH FIG 3C,D**).

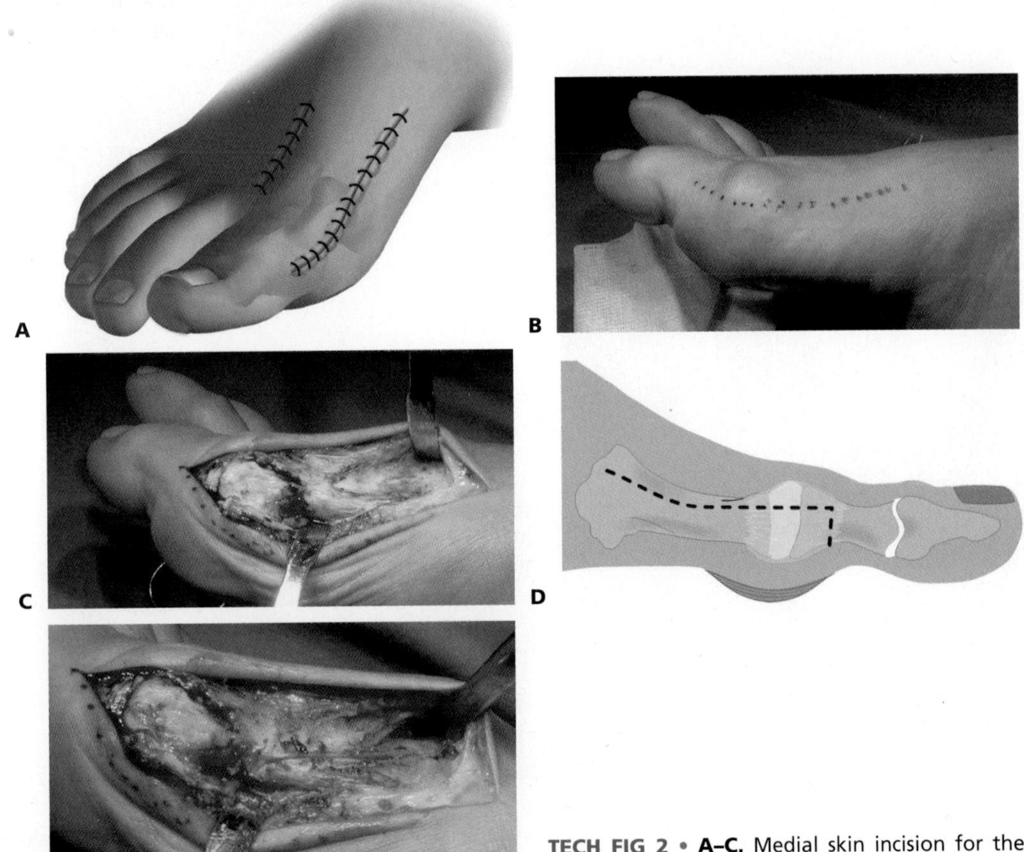

TECH FIG 2 • **A–C.** Medial skin incision for the osteotomy. **D, E.** Exposure of the metatarsal.

TECHNIQUES

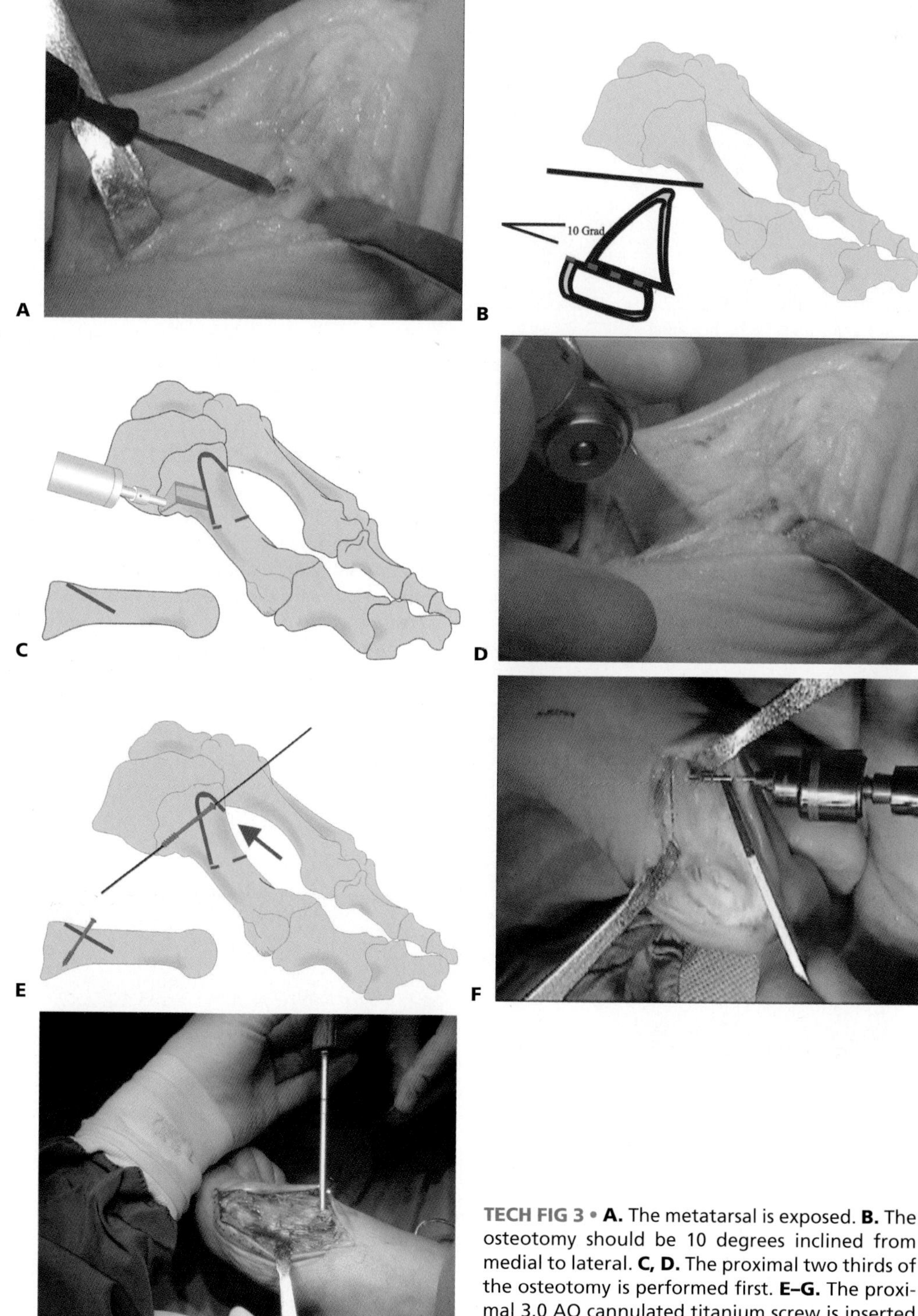

TECH FIG 3 • **A.** The metatarsal is exposed. **B.** The osteotomy should be 10 degrees inclined from medial to lateral. **C, D.** The proximal two thirds of the osteotomy is performed first. **E–G.** The proximal 3.0 AO cannulated titanium screw is inserted but not tightened.

- Insert a guidewire for a 3.0-mm or 4.0-mm cannulated screw (Synthes, Paoli, PA) or a Charlotte multiuse compression screw (Wright Medical Technology) in the proximal aspect of the dorsal fragment perpendicular to the osteotomy (**TECH FIG 3E,F**).
- Insert the first screw without full compression and complete the osteotomy (**TECH FIG 3G**).

Osteotomy Completion and Internal Fixation

- Complete the plantar third of the osteotomy (**TECH FIG 4A,B**).
- Using a towel clip, gently pull the plantar fragment medially, and rotate the dorsal fragment laterally with

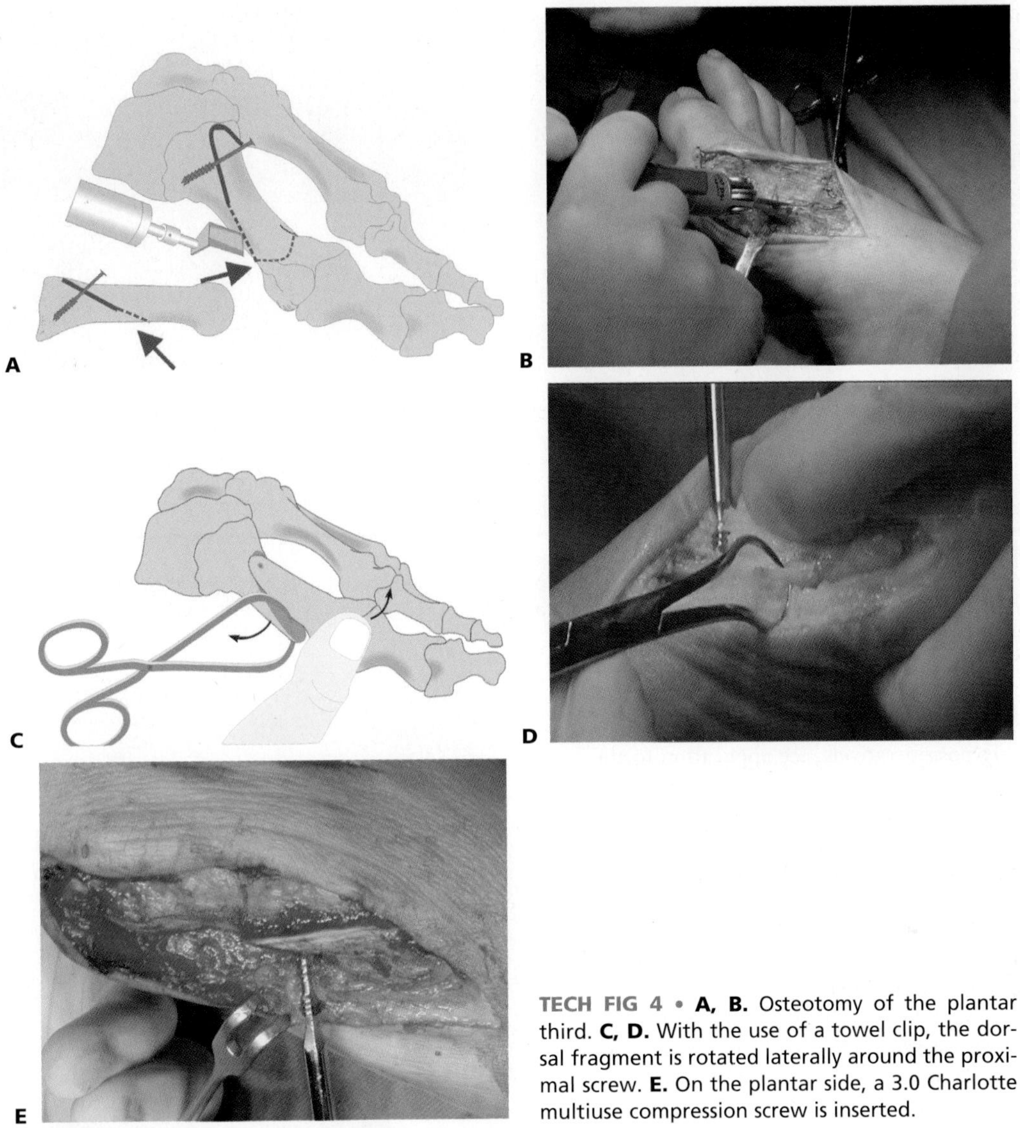

TECH FIG 4 • **A, B.** Osteotomy of the plantar third. **C, D.** With the use of a towel clip, the dorsal fragment is rotated laterally around the proximal screw. **E.** On the plantar side, a 3.0 Charlotte multiuse compression screw is inserted.

gentle thumb pressure on the first metatarsal head's medial aspect (TECH FIG 4C,D).

- After confirming the desired correction fluoroscopically, tighten the first screw to secure the osteotomy.
- Insert a second Charlotte multiuse compression screw from plantar to dorsal across the distal aspect of the osteotomy (TECH FIG 4E).

Completion and Closure

- Resect the medial eminence (TECH FIG 5A). This is not done before the osteotomy because otherwise too much of the metatarsal head might be resected.
- Shave the slight medial bone prominence at the osteotomy smooth with the edge of the saw blade (TECH FIG 5B).

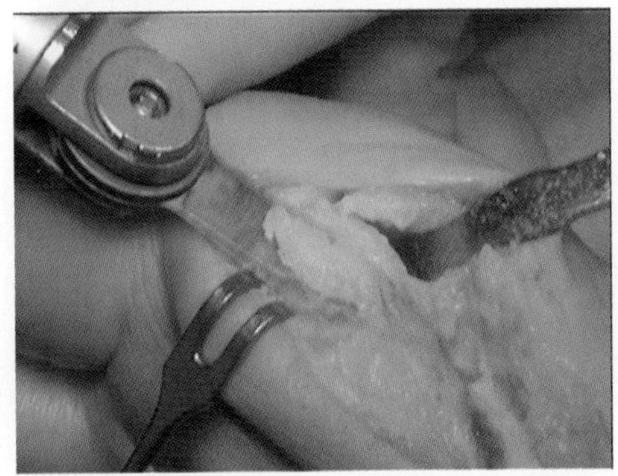

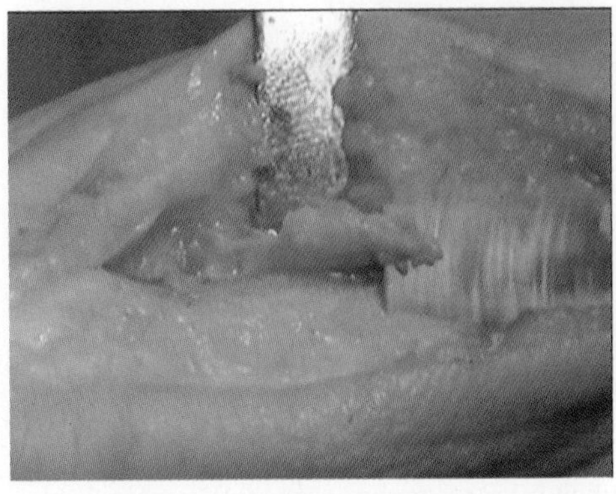

TECH FIG 5 • **A, B.** The medial eminence is resected. *(continued)*

- While an assistant holds the great toe in a slightly overcorrected position, repair the medial joint capsule with U-type sutures, and tighten the first web space sutures (**TECH FIG 5C**).
- Wrap the foot in a traditional, mildly compressive wet-and-dry bunion dressing.

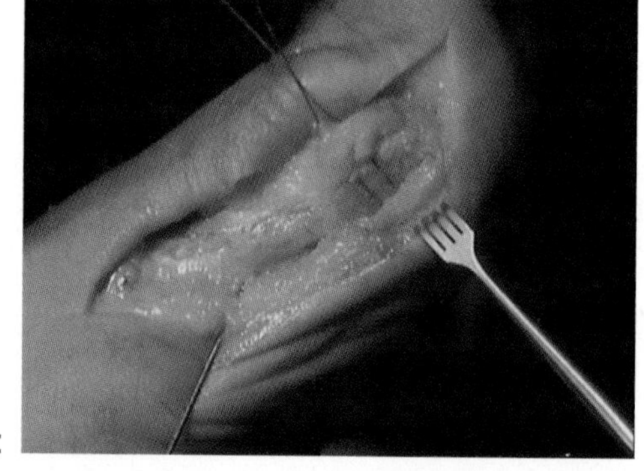

TECH FIG 5 • *(continued)* **C.** Closing the medial capsule with U-type sutures.

PEARLS AND PITFALLS

- Avoid short osteotomy because it would create too small of a contact area.
- There should be a long enough distance between the two screws; otherwise, the rotational control is not guaranteed.
- When the screws do not have enough bite, use a cast for postoperative treatment.

POSTOPERATIVE CARE

- Starting immediately postoperatively, ice application to the foot is helpful to reduce swelling.
- Provided that the bone quality was intraoperatively sufficient, patients are allowed to walk with a postsurgical cork-soled shoe (OFA Rathgeber Health Shoes) or an OrthoWedge-type shoe (Darco) on the same day.
- If the bone quality was not sufficient, the patient is put in a walker boot or a short-leg cast.
- Weekly changes of the tape dressing are necessary.
- An alternative to weekly dressing changes is the postoperative hallux valgus compression stocking, which also reduces postoperative edema (**FIG 1**).
- Radiographs are taken intraoperatively and at 6 weeks of follow-up.
- After radiographic union is achieved, normal dress shoes with a more rigid sole are allowed.
- After 6 weeks, physiotherapy to achieve normal forefoot function is recommended (**FIG 2**).

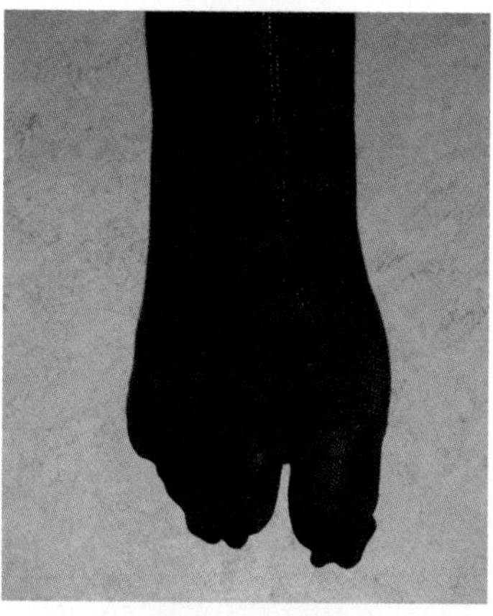

FIG 1 • Postoperative hallux valgus compression stocking, for use after suture removal.

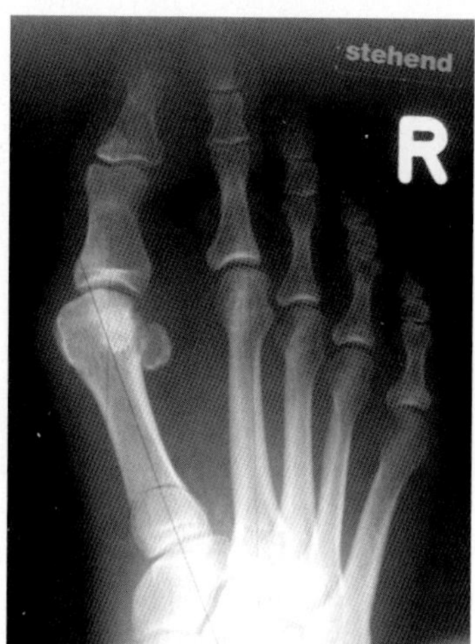

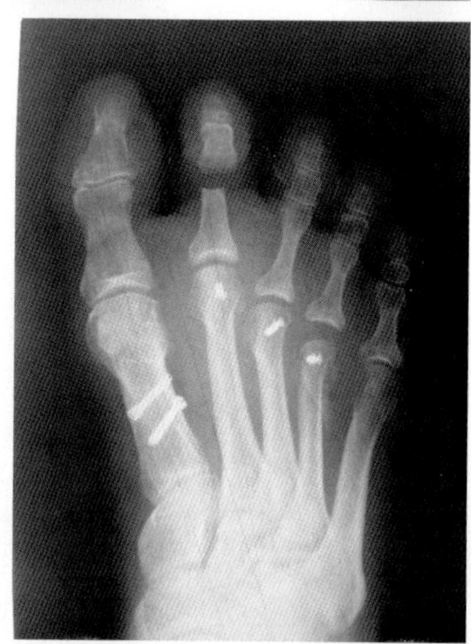

FIG 2 • 50-year-old woman (**A**) before surgery and (**B**) 2 years after the Ludloff osteotomy and Weil osteotomy 2 to 4.

OUTCOMES

- Chiodo et al[1] presented their results on 82 consecutive Ludloff cases. Follow-up was possible in 70 cases (85%) at an average of 30 months (range 18 to 42 months). In their series, no symptomatic transfer lesions were found on the second metatarsal. The mean AOFAS forefoot score improved from 54 to 91 points. The mean hallux valgus and first intermetatarsal angles before surgery were 31 degrees and 16 degrees, respectively; postoperatively they averaged 11 degrees and 7 degrees. Complications included prominent hardware requiring removal (7%, 5/70), hallux varus deformity (6%, 4/70), delayed union (4%, 3/70), superficial infection (4%, 3/70), and neuralgia (4%, 3/70). The average patient age was not mentioned in the study.
- Saxena and McCammon[9] reported the results of 14 procedures in 12 patients with the original technique. The mean hallux valgus angle was corrected from 30.1 to 13.4 degrees and the intermetatarsal angle from 15.9 to 10.8 degrees.
- Weinfeld[14] reported in 2001 a series of 31 patients. The mean hallux valgus angle was corrected from 36.7 to 10.8 degrees and the mean first intermetatarsal angle from 14.8 to 3.9 degrees.
- Trnka et al[12] reviewed the results of 99 patients (111 feet), with an average age of 56 years (range 20 to 78 years), in a multicenter study. The average AOFAS score improved significantly from 46 ± 11 points before surgery to 88 ± 13 points at follow-up. Patients under 60 years of age had a significantly higher AOFAS score (90 ± 12 points) than patients over 60 years of age (82 ± 17). The average preoperative hallux valgus angle of 35 ± 7 degrees decreased significantly to 8 ± 9 degrees, and the average intermetatarsal angle decreased significantly from 17 ± 2 degrees to 8 ± 3 degrees. All osteotomies united without dorsiflexion malunion. In the early postoperative period, 17% (18/111) had bony callus formation at the osteotomy site.

COMPLICATIONS

- Potential complications are similar to other proximal osteotomies.
- Hallux varus in 8% and 6%
- Delayed union
- Loss of fixation
- Iatrogenic fracture

REFERENCES

1. Chiodo CP, Schon LC, Myerson, MS. Clinical results with the Ludloff osteotomy for correction of adult hallux valgus. Foot Ankle Int 2004;25:532–536.
2. Hardy R, Clapham J. Observations on hallux valgus. J Bone Joint Surg Br 1951;33B:376–391.
3. Hofstaetter SG, Gruber F, Ritschl P, et al. [The modified Ludloff osteotomy for correction of severe metatarsus primus varus with hallux valgus deformity.] Z Orthop Ihre Grenzgeb 2006;144:141–147.
4. Ludloff K. Die Beseitigung des Hallux valgus durch die schräge planta-dorsale Osteotomie des Metatarsus I. Arch Klin Chir 1918; 110:364–387.
5. Mann RA, Coughlin MJ. Adult hallux valgus. In: Coughlin MJ, Mann RA, eds. Surgery of the Foot and Ankle. St. Louis, MO: Mosby, 1999:150–269.
6. Myerson MS. Hallux valgus. In: Myerson MS, ed. Foot and Ankle Disorders. Philadelphia: WB Saunders, 2000:213–288.
7. Nyska M, Trnka HJ, Parks BG, et al. Proximal metatarsal osteotomies: a comparative geometric analysis conducted on sawbone models. Foot Ankle Int 2002;23:938–945.
8. Nyska M, Trnka HJ, Parks BG, et al. The Ludloff metatarsal osteotomy: guidelines for optimal correction based on a geometric analysis conducted on a sawbone model. Foot Ankle Int 2003; 24:34–39.
9. Saxena A, McCammon D. The Ludloff osteotomy: a critical analysis. J Foot Ankle Surg 1997;36:100–105.
10. Shereff MJ, Yang QM, Kummer FJ. Extraosseous and intraosseous arterial supply to the first metatarsal and metatarsophalangeal joint. Foot Ankle 1987;8:81–93.
11. Trnka HJ, Hofstaetter SG. The Ludloff osteotomy. Techniques Foot Ankle Surg 2005;4:263–268.
12. Trnka HJ, Hofstaetter SG, Hofstaetter JG, et al. Intermediate-term results of the Ludloff osteotomy in 111 feet. J Bone Joint Surg Am 2008;90A:531–539. Erratum in: J Bone Joint Surg Am 2008;90A:1337.
13. Trnka HJ, Parks BG, Ivanic G, et al. Six first metatarsal shaft osteotomies: mechanical and immobilization comparisons. Clin Orthop Relat Res 2000;381:256–265.
14. Weinfeld SB. The Ludloff osteotomy for correction of hallux valgus: results of 31 cases by one surgeon. Presented at the 31st Annual Meeting of the American Orthopaedic Foot and Ankle Society, San Francisco, CA, March 3, 2001.

Chapter 10 Mau Osteotomy

Jason P. Glover, Christopher F. Hyer, and Gregory C. Berlet

DEFINITION

- Hallux valgus is a static subluxation of the first metatarsophalangeal (MTP) joint with medial deviation of the first metatarsal and lateral or valgus rotation of the hallux. A medial or dorsomedial prominence is present and usually called a bunion.
- The development of hallux valgus is debated but occurs almost exclusively in shod populations.[11,15,18] Other causes that may contribute to a hallux valgus deformity include heredity,[4,6,14,25] pes planus,[9,10,12,19,21] metatarsus primus varus,[10,23] systemic arthritis,[16,20,24] neuromuscular disorders, excessive roundness of the metatarsal head,[2] and abnormal obliquity of the first metacarpal joint.[13] Hypermobility may also be another causative factor in the formation of a bunion, and a first metatarsal–cuneiform joint fusion may be an appropriate alternative procedure.
- Hallux valgus can lead to painful motion of the joint or difficulty with footwear.
- Surgical correction of bunion deformity is a common procedure. For larger deformities a proximal osteotomy of the first metatarsal is required. The Mau proximal osteotomy technique is an accepted and proven technique. This osteotomy has the advantage over other proximal osteotomies of being inherently stable, having a reproducible surgical technique, and minimizing the common complications of other proximal osteotomies.

ANATOMY

- The first MTP joint is two joints with a ball-and-socket type of joint between the first metatarsal and proximal phalanx. The second portion is a groove on the plantar first metatarsal that articulates with the dorsal surface of two sesamoids. These joints share a common capsule and interrelated muscles.
- Collateral ligaments are fan-shaped ligaments that originate from the medial and lateral epicondyles of the first metatarsal head. These ligaments run vertical, horizontal, and oblique from the first metatarsal head, proximal phalanx, and sesamoids.
- The sesamoids (medial and lateral) are separated by a rounded ridge (crista) and are connected by the intersesamoidal ligament. The lateral sesamoid is also connected to the plantar plate of the second metatarsal head by the transverse intermetatarsal ligament. In addition to collateral ligament attachments, each sesamoid is contained by a separated tendon of the flexor hallucis brevis muscle.
- Intrinsic muscles that insert on the proximal phalanx are the abductor hallucis (plantar medial) and the oblique–transverse head of the adductor hallucis (plantar lateral phalanx). Both of these tendons also blend in with the flexor hallucis brevis to invest each corresponding sesamoid. These intrinsic muscles act to maintain alignment of the hallux and balance the forces of each other.
- Extrinsic muscles include the flexor hallucis longus (FHL) and extensor hallucis longus (EHL). The FHL lies within a groove plantar to the intersesamoidal ligament. It proceeds distally to insert into the base of the distal phalanx. The EHL runs over the dorsal surface of the proximal phalanx and inserts into the base of the distal phalanx. Over the first MTP the EHL is anchored to the sesamoids by the extensor sling.

PATHOGENESIS

- The development of hallux valgus varies depending on the causative factor.
- The function of the abductor hallucis muscle is to plantarflex, adduct, and invert the proximal phalanx. The reverse is true for the adductor hallucis muscle. When these muscles act together, a straight plantarflexion force is produced and the transverse–frontal plane forces are neutralized.
- When the adductor hallucis muscle gains the mechanical advantage, such as in removing the tibial sesamoid or pronation, a hallux valgus deformity may ensue. The sesamoids are pulled laterally, thus eroding the crista. The metatarsal head is pushed medially, stretching the medial ligaments, and the abductor hallucis slides beneath the metatarsal head, pronating the hallux.
- As the deformity progresses, the EHL and FHL have been shown to become a dynamic deforming force.

NATURAL HISTORY

- The progression of a hallux valgus deformity is usually gradual, but when multiple causative factors are present, progression can be more rapid. As the deformity progresses, the hallux drifts laterally and either over or under a stable second digit. Over time the second MTP joint can dislocate. As the hallux drifts laterally, it assumes less weight bearing and a diffuse callus may occur underneath the second metatarsal head.

PATIENT HISTORY AND PHYSICAL FINDINGS

- The chief compliant of a bunion deformity is usually pain. Pain can be located over several areas in a bunion deformity: median eminence, dorsal first MTP joint, medial or lateral sesamoids, or impingement on the second digit.
- A thorough general medical history may include gout, osteoarthritis, rheumatoid arthritis, diabetes, or peripheral vascular disease.
- Other important factors include style of shoes and if any shoe gear modification has been attempted, physical activity of the patient, and occupational demands.
- Patient expectations are also very important. Goals of surgery should include increasing activity and decreasing pain. Forewarning the patient of limitations after surgery is necessary, such as the possibility of not returning to tight fashionable shoes.
- The physical examination should start with the patient weight bearing to assess the bunion and lesser toe deformities and compare them to the other foot.

- Evaluation of the vascular status is important. The perfusion is determined by palpating the posterior tibial and dorsal pedis arteries. Perfusion of a digit can be assessed by the capillary refill. Appropriate vascular studies such as transcutaneous oxygen, ankle–brachial index, digital pressures, and segmental pressures are useful when perfusion to the foot is in doubt.
- The first MTP joint range of motion is assessed for crepitus, pain, or impingement if a dorsal spur is present. Motion is also assessed with the hallux in a corrected position to determine the degree of associated contracture of the soft tissues. Normal range of motion is 70 to 90 degrees of dorsiflexion. Joint range of motion is compared to that of the opposite foot.
- Transverse plane mobility is assessed by distracting the hallux while the metatarsal head is pushed laterally to see clinical reduction of the intermetatarsal angle.
- The median eminence is assessed for its prominence and underlying bursa. Neuritic pain can be elicited from the nearby dorsal or plantar cutaneous nerves.
- The tibial and fibular sesamoids are directly palpated while putting the joint through a range of motion to indicate intra-articular derangement.
- The first tarsometatarsal joint excursion is assessed by grasping proximal to this joint and moving the first metatarsal and comparing it to the opposite foot. Normal range of motion is 10 mm of excursion. A hypermobile first ray is more than 15 mm of excursion.
- Range of motion of the hallux interphalangeal joint is evaluated in the transverse and sagittal plane, as well as joint quality.
- Pain may also occur from lesser toe deformities or transfer lesions that may accompany the bunion deformity. A symptomatic intractable plantar keratoma beneath the second metatarsal head is present in the majority of patients.[17] Other associated problems include neuromas, corns, and tailor's bunion.

IMAGING AND OTHER DIAGNOSTIC STUDIES

- The radiologic examination should include weight-bearing lateral, AP, and oblique views.
- Several measurements are obtained using these radiographs to determine the severity of the bunion deformity, including the intermetatarsal 1–2 angle (IM1–2), hallux valgus angle (HVA), tibial sesamoid position, distal metatarsal articular angle (DMAA), and congruency of the first MTP joint.
  - The IM1–2 angle is determined by measuring the angle subtended by the lines bisecting the longitudinal axis of the first and second metatarsals.
    - Normal is less than 9 degrees (**FIG 1**).
  - The HVA is determined by measuring the angle subtended by the lines bisecting the first metatarsal and proximal phalanx of the hallux.
    - Normal is 15 degrees or less (**FIG 2**).
  - Tibial sesamoid position describes the relationship of the tibial sesamoid to the bisection of the first metatarsal.
    - The position of the sesamoid is determined by a numerical sequence of one to seven with increasing deformity.
    - Normal is a position of 1 to 3 (**FIG 3**).
  - The DMAA is the angle subtended by a line representing the articular cartilage of the first metatarsal head and a perpendicular line to the bisection of the shaft of the first metatarsal.
    - Normal measures less than 8 degrees (**FIG 4**).

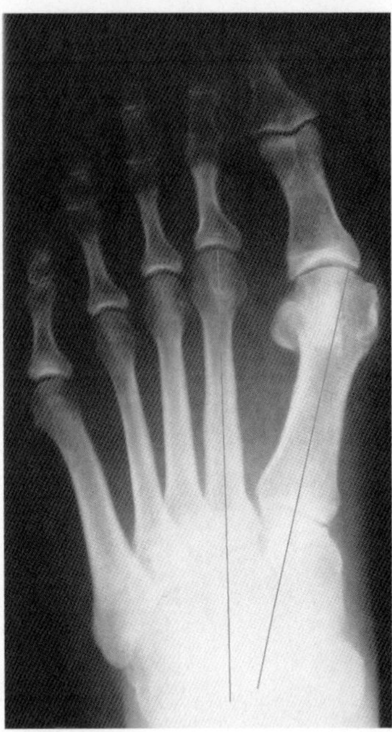

FIG 1 • The intermetatarsal (IM) angle measures the splay between the first and second metatarsals.

    - An increase in the DMAA may demonstrate a structural deformity in the head of the metatarsal.
  - The first MTP joint may be described as congruent, deviated, or subluxed.
    - A congruent joint is one in which the cartilage surfaces of the first metatarsal head and proximal phalanx are parallel.
    - A deviated joint is one in which the cartilage lines intersect at a point outside of the joint.

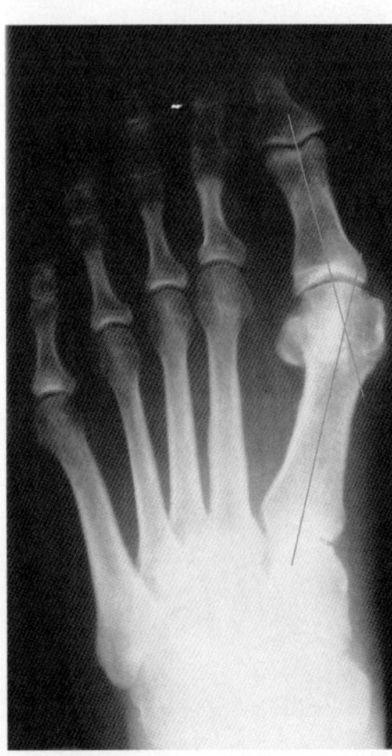

FIG 2 • The hallux valgus angle (HVA) measures the angle formed between the proximal phalanx and first metatarsal.

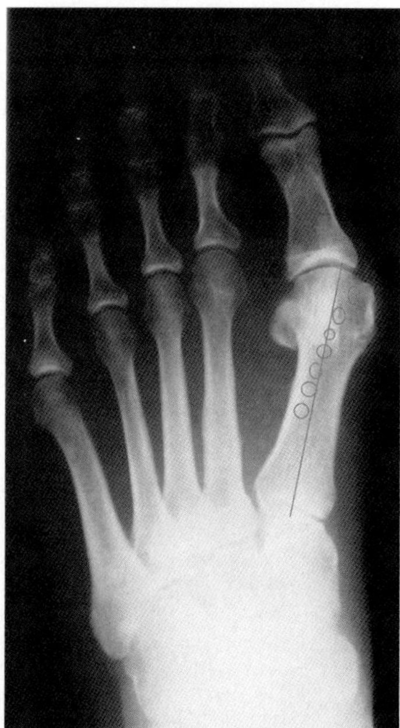

FIG 3 • The tibial sesamoid position describes the position of the tibial sesamoid relative to the bisection of the first metatarsal.

- In a subluxed joint, the cartilage lines intersect within the joint (**FIG 5**).
- Degenerative arthritis at the first MTP joint can be evaluated on each weight-bearing radiograph.

DIFFERENTIAL DIAGNOSIS

- Metatarsus primus varus
- Hallux varus
- Gout
- Hallux rigidus

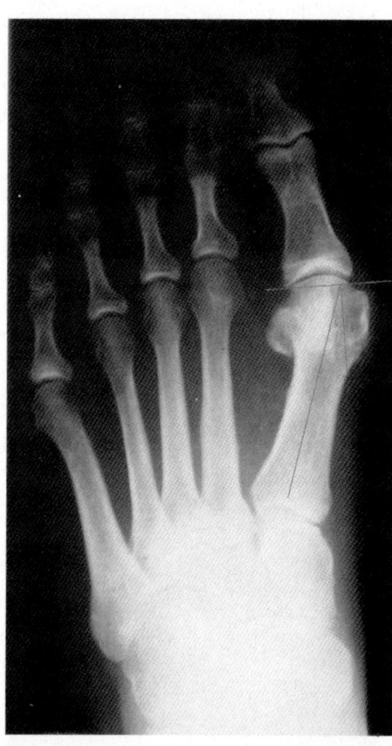

FIG 4 • The distal metatarsal articular angle (DMAA) measures the relationship of the articular surface of the first metatarsal head to the bisection of the first metatarsal.

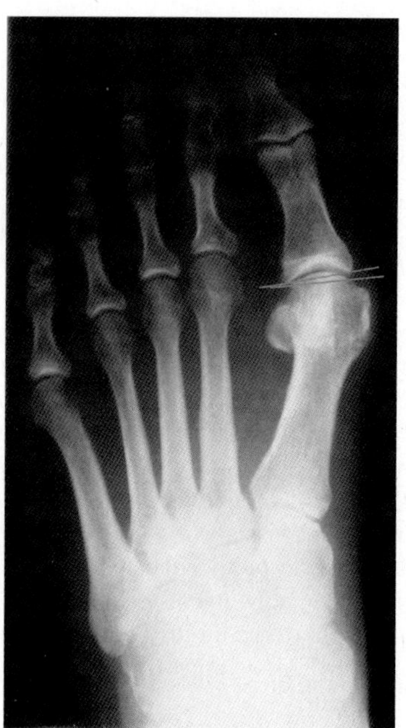

FIG 5 • A deviated joint in which the articular surfaces are not parallel with each other.

NONOPERATIVE MANAGEMENT

- Conservative treatment options for hallux valgus deformities are limited.
- Shoe wear modifications such as an extra-wide and deep toebox can help accommodate the deformity. Also a soft upper leather can be stretched over the bunion to provide accommodation.
- Custom-made shoes may help individuals reluctant or unable to undergo a surgical procedure.
- Bunion pads, night splints, and toe spacers tend to be of little use.
- A custom-made orthosis may be beneficial if an associated flatfoot deformity is present. The use of an orthosis has not been demonstrated to prevent a hallux valgus deformity or slow its progression. Others have proposed using orthoses postoperatively to prevent recurrence.

SURGICAL MANAGEMENT

- Bunions can be classified by their severity. This classification is used to facilitate the decision-making process of how to treat the deformity.
  - Mild bunion: HVA less than 20 degrees, congruent joint, IM angle less than 11 degrees. Pain is usually due to a medial eminence.
  - Moderate bunion: HVA 20 to 40 degrees, incongruent joint, IM angle 11 to 18 degrees. The hallux is usually pronated and presses against the second digit.
  - Severe bunion: HVA more than 40 degrees, subluxed joint, IM angle more than 18 degrees. Hallux is often overriding or underlapping the second digit; painful transfer lesion underneath the second metatarsal head; possible arthritic changes to the first MTP joint.
- The indications for hallux valgus surgery using the Mau osteotomy include:
  - Painful moderate to severe bunion deformity
  - Deformity unresponsive to conservative treatment

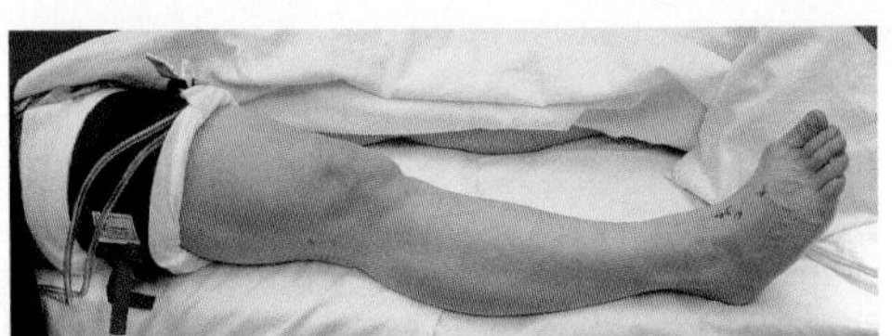

FIG 6 • A well-padded thigh tourniquet set to 300 mm Hg.

Preoperative Planning

- Routine preoperative clearance is obtained via history and physical. This may include an electrocardiogram, chest radiograph, and laboratory workup.
- A prophylactic antibiotic of choice is given 30 minutes before the procedure. Also, one tablet of 200 mg celecoxib (Celebrex) is given.

Positioning

- The patient is placed supine on the operating table with a bump placed under the contralateral hip.
- A well-padded pneumatic thigh tourniquet is used and set to 300 mm Hg (**FIG 6**).

Approach

- Typically two incisions are used to provide adequate exposure.
  - The first incision is placed over the first web space and the second is placed on the medial aspect of the first metatarsal.
  - The second incision starts at the first tarsometatarsal joint and courses distal and medially over the first MTP joint for the distal soft tissue procedure (**FIGS 7 AND 8**).

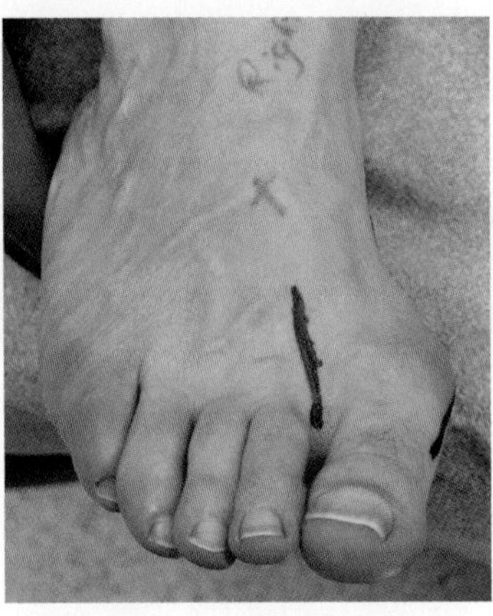

FIG 7 • Incision placed over the first web space for lateral joint release.

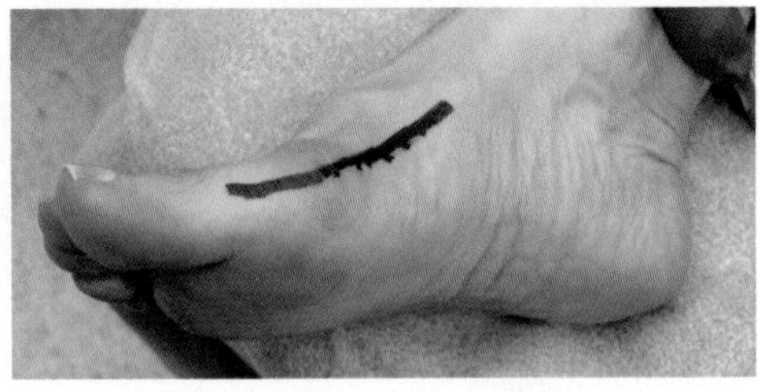

FIG 8 • Medial incision starts at the first tarsometatarsal joint and courses distal and medially for the distal soft tissue procedure.

LATERAL RELEASE OF THE FIRST METATARSOPHALANGEAL JOINT

- Using an incision in the first web space (**TECH FIG 1**), perform the lateral release first. Carry dissection through the subcutaneous layer.
- Typically the first structure incised is the superficial portion of the transverse ligament.
- Use blunt dissection to view the lateral first MTP joint and fibular sesamoid.
- Release the adductor tendon from the plantar–lateral base of the proximal phalanx and fibular sesamoid (**TECH FIG 2**).
- Incise the deep portion of the transverse ligament. The lateral capsule of the first MTP joint is "pie crusted" and a varus stress is placed on the joint.

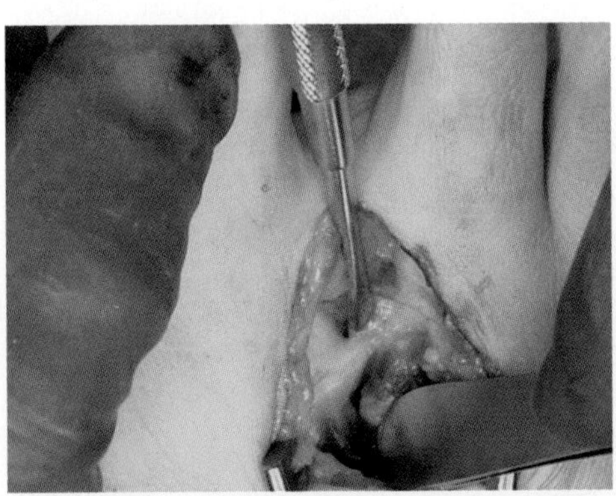

TECH FIG 1 • The first structure identified in a lateral release is the superficial portion of the deep transverse metatarsal ligament.

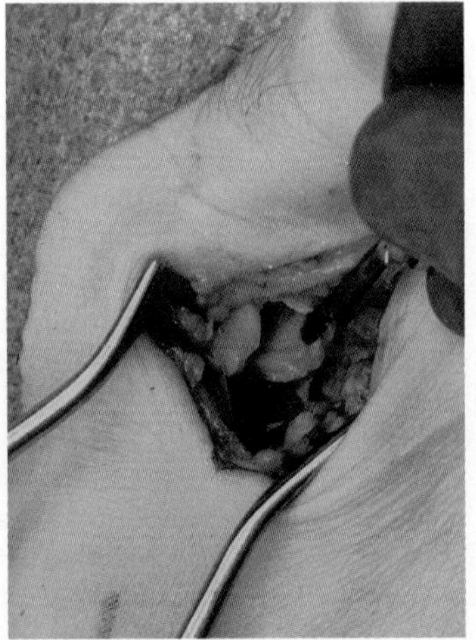

TECH FIG 2 • Blunt dissection is carried deep to identify and release the adductor hallucis tendon.

MEDIAL CAPSULORRHAPHY

- Using a standard medial approach, perform an inverted-L capsulotomy. The alternative dorsal–medial skin incision, which is placed over the first dorsal metatarsal artery and nerve, can cause nerve irritation and entrapment.
- This allows exposure of the enlarged medial eminence and release of the stretched medial sesamoid suspensory ligament (**TECH FIG 3**). Remove the periosteum from the metatarsal head medially and dorsally but keep it intact at the neck plantarly to preserve the nutrient artery.
- Resect the medial eminence using a sagittal saw (**TECH FIG 4**).
  - Take the eminence from dorsolateral to plantar–medial. Remove the eminence in this orientation to prevent staking of the metatarsal head and loss of the sagittal groove, which can lead to medial subluxation of the tibial sesamoid and promote hallux varus.

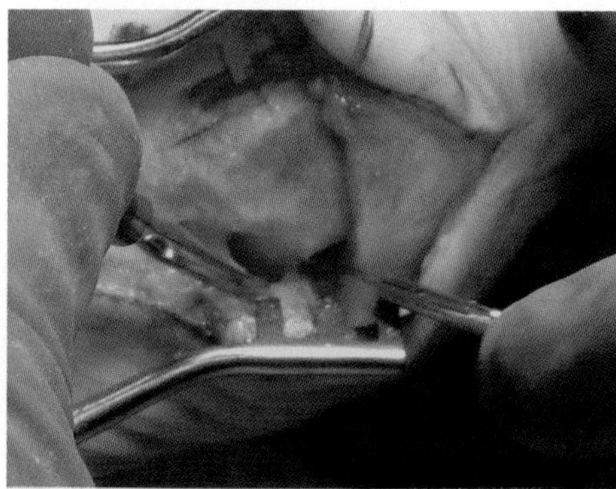

TECH FIG 3 • Release of the stretched medial sesamoid suspensory ligament.

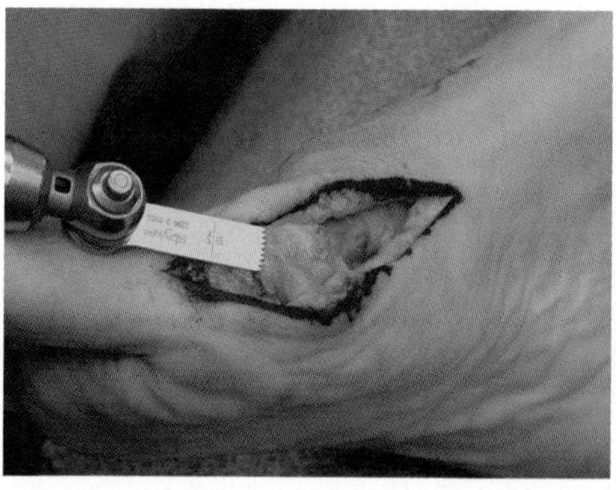

TECH FIG 4 • Minimal exostectomy of the medial eminence.

MAU OSTEOTOMY

- Carry the dissection deep to the first metatarsal shaft. The skin incision can be placed slightly plantar to the first metatarsal to avoid surrounding neurovascular structures such as the first dorsal metatarsal artery and nerve. With this incision, a potentially nonpainful scar results as the incision is not placed directly over bone. The extensor hallucis longus tendon is not encountered with this incision and is retracted safely.
- Identify the first tarsometatarsal joint but do not disturb the capsule. An 18-gauge needle can be placed in the joint for reference.
- Starting 1 cm from the first tarsometatarsal joint, reflect the periosteum plantar-proximal to dorsal-distal only in line with the osteotomy, thereby preserving the rest of the periosteum (**TECH FIG 5**). Much of the periosteum is retained to promote adequate bone healing.
- The osteotomy does not incorporate the entire metatarsal shaft as does the traditional Mau osteotomy. The osteotomy ends in the midshaft of the first metatarsal.
- Complete the osteotomy with a sagittal saw parallel to the weight-bearing surface to prevent unwanted dorsal angulation of the first metatarsal. The Mau is started proximal-plantar and ends distal-dorsal (**TECH FIG 6**). A self-retaining retractor is useful to protect the surrounding neurovascular and tendinous structures. Using the straight medial incision avoids tendinous structures and allows excellent visualization of the medial metatarsal shaft to complete the osteotomy. To maintain complete control while completing the osteotomy, a smooth guide pin for the selected cannulated screw can be placed perpendicular across the completed proximal portion of the osteotomy. Then the osteotomy can be completed without fear of losing the orientation.
- After completing the osteotomy, rotate the distal fragment. Optimal rotation of the osteotomy may be facilitated by placing a large reduction bone clamp on the first metatarsal head and neck of the second metatarsal to help reduce the IM1–2 angle (**TECH FIG 7**).

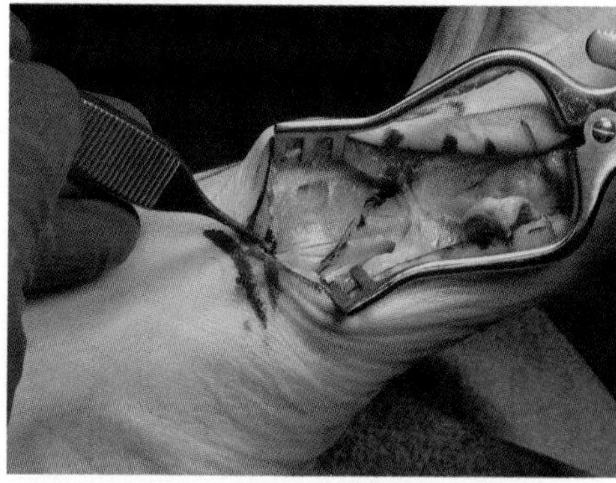

TECH FIG 5 • Identification of the first tarsometatarsal joint (pick-ups) and line of the osteotomy 1 cm distal to the joint.

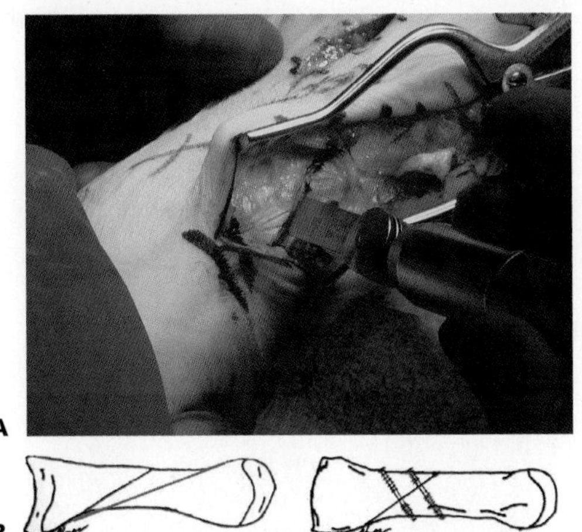

TECH FIG 6 • A. Sagittal saw is placed parallel to the weight-bearing surface of the foot and the osteotomy is completed from proximal-plantar to distal-dorsal. **B.** The traditional Mau osteotomy (*red line*) and the slight modification (*black line*). The modified Mau does not incorporate the entire metatarsal shaft as does the traditional Mau osteotomy. The modified Mau osteotomy with two-screw fixation.

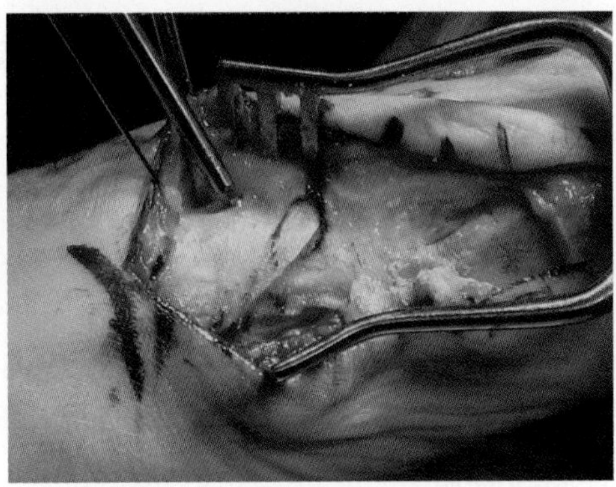

TECH FIG 8 • Temporary fixation of the osteotomy with two parallel Kirschner wires from dorsal to plantar.

- Place two temporary Kirschner wires (0.025 inch) from dorsal to plantar perpendicular to the osteotomy site (TECH FIG 8).
- Reduction of the IM1–2 angle is mostly obtained by rotation of the distal fragment. It is acceptable to allow slight lateral translation of the distal fragment relative to the proximal fragment to further correct the IM angle.
- We recommend using intraoperative fluoroscopy to confirm proper position of the first metatarsal head over the tibial sesamoids, congruent joint alignment, and satisfactory orientation of the osteotomy. We use a towel clip to provisionally advance the capsule into the desired position to assess sesamoid alignment (TECH FIG 9). Redundant capsular tissue is excised and optimal correction is obtained with a tibial sesamoid position less than 2 and an IM1–2 angle less than 9 degrees. About 4 mm of redundant capsule is removed from the inverted-L portion of the capsulotomy to help reduce and advance the sesamoids upon closure. With larger deformities, more capsule may need to be removed to reduce the tibial sesamoid position adequately. To correct pronation of the hallux, the towel clip can be rotated to correct the deformity, and a double simple suture is placed to maintain the correction.
- We use two 2.5- or 3.0-mm headless cannulated screws for final fixation.

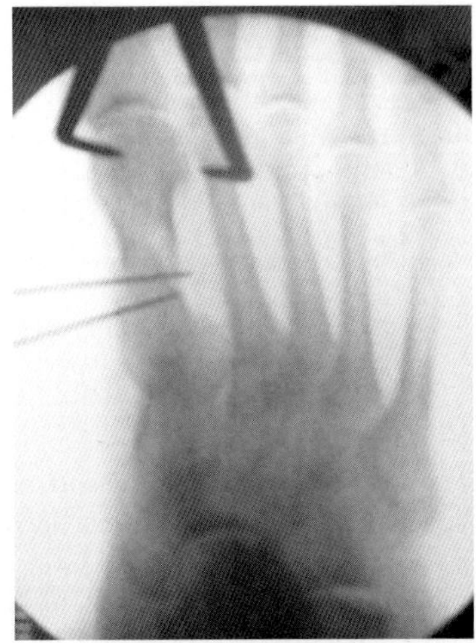

TECH FIG 7 • Operative and fluoroscopy images showing reduction of IM1–2 angle with large reduction bone clamps. The clamp is placed medially at the first metatarsal head and laterally around the second metatarsal head.

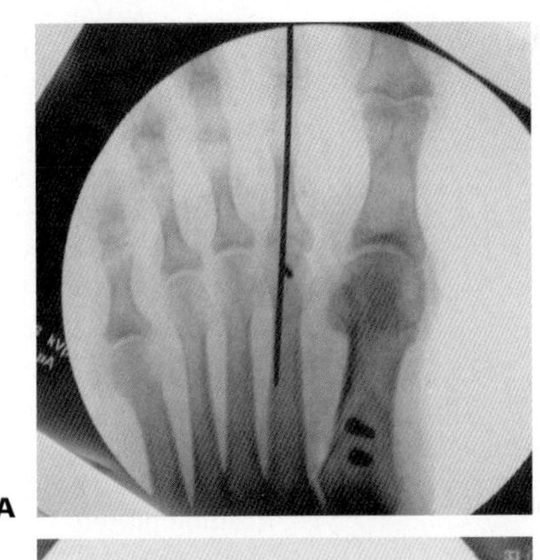

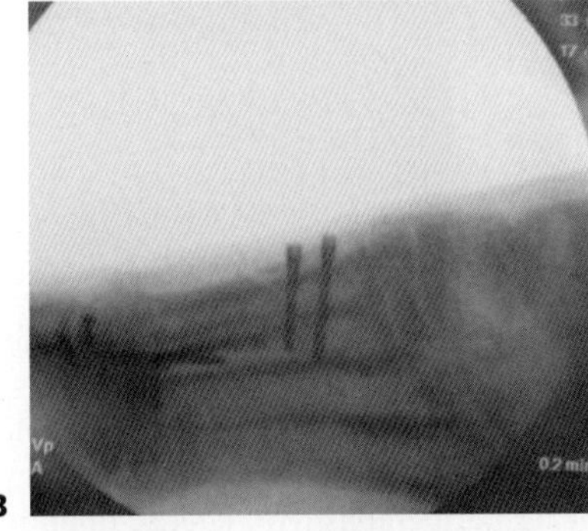

TECH FIG 9 • Intraoperative fluoroscopy of AP and lateral foot, showing final fixation and excellent reduction of the IM1–2 angle.

TECHNIQUES

CLOSURE

- To complete the medial capsulorrhaphy, close the capsule using a double simple suture technique with 0-0 absorbable suture (**TECH FIG 10**).
  - Placing a sponge in the first interspace while closing the capsule will splint the toe in the corrected position.
- Close the subcutaneous layer with 2-0 absorbable suture. The skin is closed based on the surgeon's preference, with either a running subcuticular closure with 5-0 absorbable suture or simple interrupted sutures with 3-0 nylon.
- Place a soft toe spica dressing by dividing a sponge in thirds and wrapping lateral to medial around the hallux to maintain correction. Use caution to prevent aggressive splinting, which can cause overcorrection and potential hallux varus.

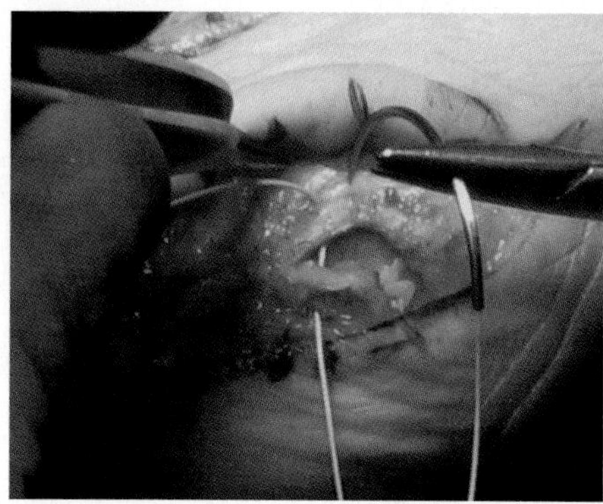

TECH FIG 10 • Completion of the medial capsulorrhaphy with capsule repaired in a double simple suture technique with 0-0 absorbable suture.

PEARLS AND PITFALLS

Incision	▪ Incision is placed medial to the first metatarsal and slightly plantar to avoid the surrounding neurovascular structures. This allows fast deep dissection.
Medial capsulorrhaphy	▪ Placing a varus stress on the hallux will expose redundant capsular tissue that can be incorporated within the L portion of the capsulotomy and can be adequately removed.
Osteotomy	▪ The periosteum is elevated only in line with the osteotomy. The proximal portion of the osteotomy should be at least 1 cm distal from the first tarsometatarsal joint. This will also prevent placement of the osteotomy within the first tarsometatarsal joint. ▪ The saw blade is kept parallel to the weight-bearing surface of the foot to prevent unwanted dorsal angulation of the first metatarsal head after completion of the osteotomy. ▪ To maintain complete control of the osteotomy, a guidewire for the cannulated screw can be placed perpendicular in the completed proximal portion of the osteotomy. The osteotomy can be completed dorsal-distally without fear of losing the orientation.
IM1–2 reduction	▪ Reduction can be achieved with large reduction clamps or by using a Freer elevator on the lateral portion of the proximal fragment and placing counterpressure on the first metatarsal head. Intraoperative fluoroscopy is recommended after placing temporary fixation to achieve an IM angle less than 9 degrees.
Screw placement	▪ Placing a screw too distal may cause fracture of the dorsal portion of the osteotomy site. Allow adequate space between the screws and the distal aspect of the osteotomy to prevent fracture.
Unrecognized hypermobility of the first tarsometatarsal joint	▪ This may result in the inability to effectively reduce the IM1–2 angle after temporary fixation. If encountered, the fist tarsometatarsal joint may be temporarily pinned and permanent fixation placed. The pin across the first tarsometatarsal joint can be removed 4 to 6 weeks postoperatively.

POSTOPERATIVE CARE

- The patient is placed in a soft toe spica dressing after surgery and instructed to remain partially weight bearing on the heel in a surgical shoe.
- Two weeks after surgery the sutures are removed and the patient is fully weight bearing in a surgical shoe.
- Three weight-bearing radiographs (AP, lateral, oblique) are obtained at each visit until bony healing of the osteotomy site is seen.

OUTCOMES

- After a proximal osteotomy and distal soft tissue release, 90% to 95% patient satisfaction rates have been reported.[3,5,17]
- One study reviewed retrospective results of the Mau osteotomy and found excellent correction of a moderate to severe bunion deformity in 24 patients.[8]
- Biomechanical studies using sawbones and fresh frozen cadaver models showed superior stability with the Mau

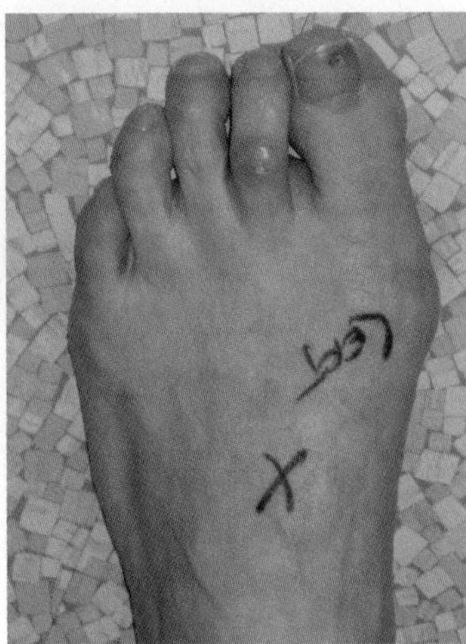

FIG 9 • Preoperative weight-bearing appearance of the bunion deformity.

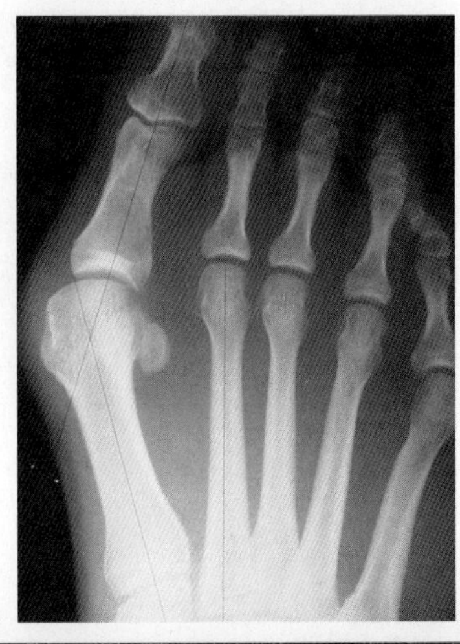

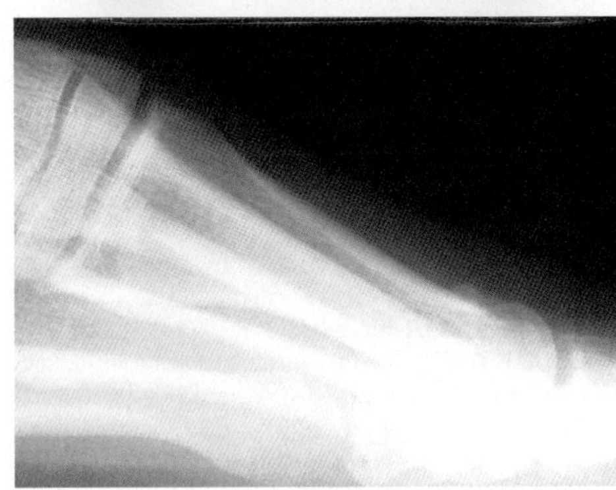

FIG 11 • Preoperative weight-bearing AP and lateral foot radiographs.

osteotomy in terms of fatigue, strength, and stiffness compared to other proximal osteotomies.[1,22] The Mau osteotomy is an inherently stable osteotomy that allows early postoperative weight bearing without the need for cast immobilization as required for other proximal osteotomies due to complications such as dorsal malunion and nonunion. The Mau is a stable osteotomy due to the dorsal shelf to help reduce dorsal displacement forces and broad bony apposition to facilitate two-screw fixation.

- The authors performed a follow-up study comparing the Mau and crescentic osteotomies. Both osteotomies showed comparable correction of the moderate to severe bunion deformity, but significantly more complications were associated with the crescentic osteotomy. Complications included dorsal malunion, placement of screws within the tarsometatarsal joint, and nonunion.[7]
- The Mau osteotomy is technically easier to perform than other proximal osteotomies with fewer complications, as seen in two studies, and excellent correction of a bunion deformity (**FIGS 9–12**).

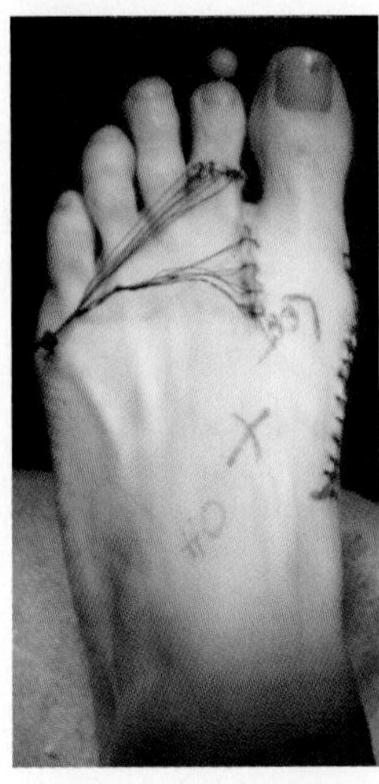

FIG 10 • Final postoperative appearance and closure with 3-0 suture.

COMPLICATIONS

- One of the most common complications after bunion surgery is recurrence. This may be due to selection of the inappropriate procedure to correct the moderate to severe bunion deformity or intraoperative failure to obtain an adequate alignment to correct the deformity.
- Hallux varus is a complication that occurs less often than recurrence. It occurs as a result of overcorrection of the deformity and is much more difficult to correct.
- Other complications include shortening, dorsal malunion, and transfer lesions, which can occur with all proximal osteotomies.

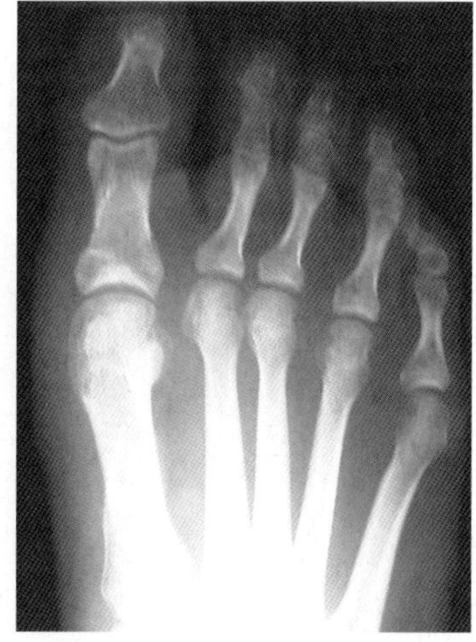

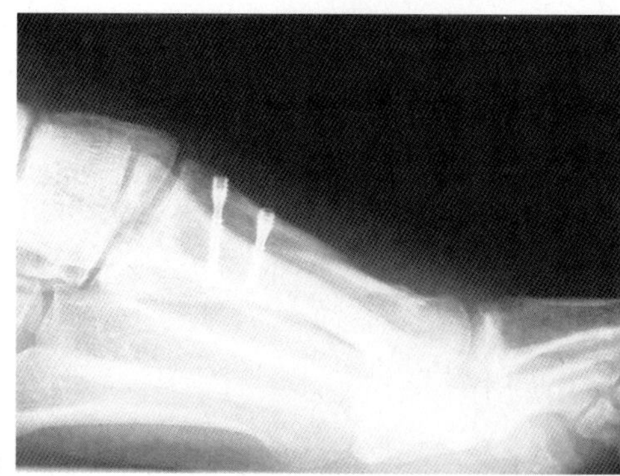

FIG 12 • Postoperative weight-bearing AP and lateral foot radiographs showing excellent reduction of the IM1–2 angle.

REFERENCES

1. Acevedo JI, Sammarco VJ, Boucher HR, et al. Mechanical comparison of cyclic loading in five different first metatarsal shaft osteotomies. Foot Ankle Int 2002;23:711–716.
2. Brahm SM. Shape of the first metatarsal head in hallux rigidus and hallux valgus. J Am Podiatr Med Assoc 1988;78:300.
3. Chiodo C, Schon L, Myerson MS, et al. Clinical results with the Ludloff osteotomy for correction of adult hallux valgus. Foot Ankle Int 2004;25:532–536.
4. Coughlin MJ. Juvenile hallux valgus: etiology and treatment. Foot Ankle Int 1995;16:682–697.
5. Easley ME, Kiebzak GM, Davis WH, et al. Prospective, randomized comparison of proximal crescentic and proximal chevron osteotomies for correction of hallux valgus deformity. Foot Ankle Int 1996;17:307–316.
6. Ellis VH. A method of correcting metatarsus primus varus. J Bone Joint Surg Br 1951;33B:415.
7. Glover JP, Hyer CF, Berlet GC, et al. A comparison of crescentic and Mau osteotomies for correction of hallux valgus. J Foot Ankle Surg 2008;47:103–111.
8. Glover JP, Hyer CF, Berlet GC, et al. Early results of the Mau osteotomy for correction of moderate to severe hallux valgus. J Foot Ankle Surg 2008;47:237–242.
9. Greenburg GS. Relationship of hallux abductus angle and first metatarsal angle to severity of pronation. J Am Podiatr Assoc 1979;69:29.
10. Hardy RH, Clapham JR. Observations on hallux valgus. J Bone Joint Surg Br 1951;33B:376.
11. Hoffman P. Conclusions drawn from a comparative study of the feet of barefooted and shoe-wearing peoples. Am J Orthop Surg 1905;3:105.
12. Hohmann G. Der hallux valgus und die uebrigen Zchenverkruemmungen. Ergeb Chir Orthop 1925;18:308–348.
13. Hyer CF, Philbin TM. The obliquity of the first metatarsal base. Foot Ankle Int 2004;25:728–732.
14. Johnston O. Further studies of the inheritance of hand and foot anomalies. Clin Orthop 1956;8:146.
15. Kato T, Watanabe S. The etiology of hallux valgus in Japan. Clin Orthop Relat Res 1981;157:78.
16. Kirkup JR, Vidigal E, Jacoby RK, et al. The hallux and rheumatoid arthritis. Acta Orthop Scand 1977;48:527.
17. Mann RA, Rudicel S, Graves SC, et al. Hallux valgus repair utilizing a distal soft tissue procedure and proximal metatarsal osteotomy: a long-term follow-up. J Bone Joint Surg Am 1992;74A:124–129.
18. Meyer M. A comparison of hallux abducto valgus in two ancient populations. J Am Podiatr Assoc 1979;69:65.
19. Ross FD. The relationship of abnormal foot pronation to hallux abducto valgus, a pilot study. Prosthet Orthotics Int 1986;10:72.
20. Rubin LM. Rheumatoid arthritis with hallux valgus. J Am Podiatr Assoc 1968;58:481.
21. Stevenson MR. A study of the correlation between neutral calcaneal stance position and relaxed calcaneal stance position in the development of hallux abducto valgus. Master's thesis, 1991.
22. Trnka HJ, Parks BG, Ivanic G, et al. Six first metatarsal shaft osteotomies: mechanical and immobilization comparisons. Clin Orthop Relat Res 2000;381:256–265.
23. Truslow W. Metatarsus primus varus or hallux valgus? J Bone Joint Surg Am 1925;7A:98.
24. Vidigal EC, Kirkup JR, Jacoby RK, et al. The rheumatoid foot: pathomechanics of hallux deformities. Rev Assoc Med Bras 1980;26:23.
25. Wallace WA. Predicting hallux abducto valgus. J Am Podiatr Med Assoc 1990;80:509.

Chapter 11

Proximal Chevron Osteotomy With Plate Fixation

Matthew J. DeOrio and James K. DeOrio

DEFINITION

- Correction of major bunion deformities through the proximal portion of the first metatarsal is widely recognized as the established method of reducing the angle between the first and second metatarsal.[1–4]
- More than 138 techniques have been described for bunion correction, with widely varied methods of fixation of these osteotomies including pins or screws.
  - Pins provide little inherent stability and have been associated with postoperative infections.
  - Getting excellent fixation of screws can be a problem in cases in which there is poor bone quality.
- Plates, although widely used in all other osteotomies, have not been employed in bunion surgery because of the fear of prominence and irritation of the patient's foot.
- Recently, the use of locking plates and locking screws has been increasing in the orthopaedic world. The locking plates provide a fixed-angle device, which allows for a potentially stronger method of fixation.[2]
- The advantages of plate fixation for the patient include no external pins, potentially no second procedure to remove hardware, less pain because the osteotomy is stable, and early full or at least partial weight bearing.
- Advantages for the surgeon are that it is possible to do any osteotomy for the first metatarsal and that excellent and secure fixation is obtained.
- Although many different configurations of the osteotomy can be used, the proximal chevron osteotomy permits a greater degree of correction compared with distal osteotomies. It does this through both an angular and translational displacement of the distal portion of the first metatarsal.[2]

SURGICAL MANAGEMENT

Approach

- The procedure is performed through a single midmedial approach to the first metatarsal with the use of an Esmarch tourniquet (**FIG 1**).

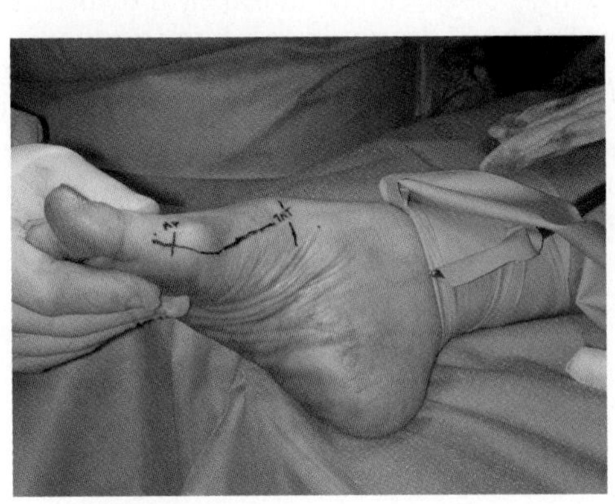

A

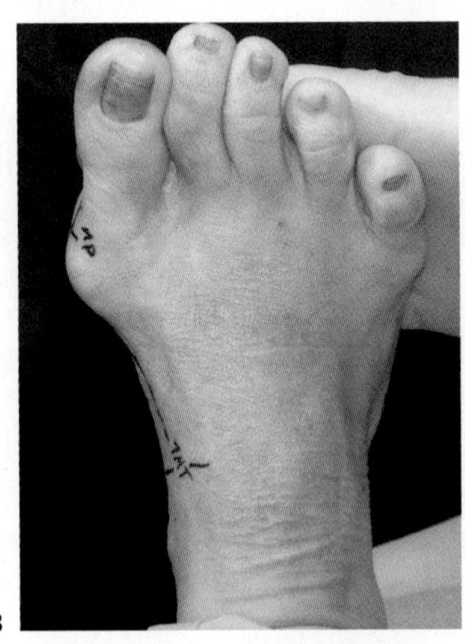

B

FIG 1 • **A.** Simulated weight-bearing view of foot. **B.** A mid-medial approach to the first metatarsal is used. The first metatarsophalangeal and first tarsometatarsal joints are identified.

SKIN AND CAPSULAR INCISION

- The skin and subcutaneous tissues are incised sharply to expose the first metatarsophalangeal (MTP) joint capsule. Care is taken to protect the medial dorsal and plantar cutaneous nerves.
- A vertical capsular resection is performed to remove about 3 to 5 mm of capsule just proximal to the base of the proximal phalanx (**TECH FIG 1**).
- A dorsomedial incision is made in the capsule parallel to the first metatarsal, creating a plantarly based capsular flap with exposure of the medial eminence.

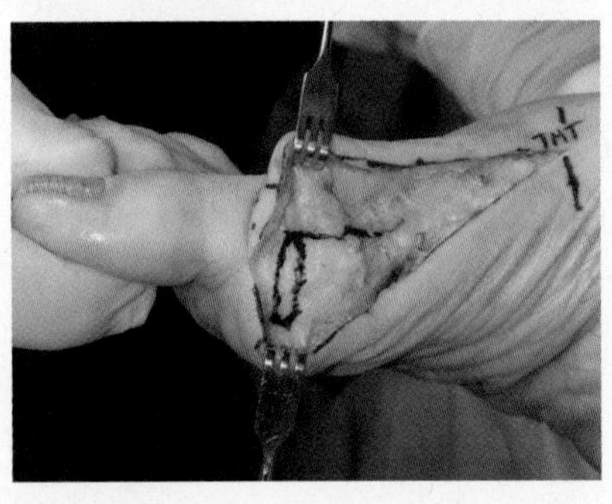

TECH FIG 1 • Thick skin flaps are preserved, and a vertical segment of redundant capsule is excised.

RELEASE OF LATERAL JOINT STRUCTURES

- The lateral soft tissues are released from within the metatarsophalangeal joint after distraction of the sesamoids from the first metatarsal with a lamina spreader. First use a blunt Freer elevator to develop some room and then cut the capsular tissue with a sharp no. 15 blade (**TECH FIG 2**).
- Complete release can be confirmed when the toe can be brought into about 15 degrees of varus through the MTP joint.
- The proximal first metatarsal is subsequently exposed both dorsally and plantarly.

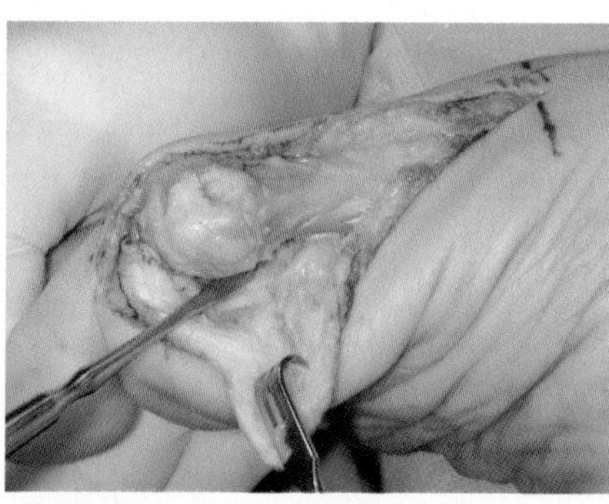

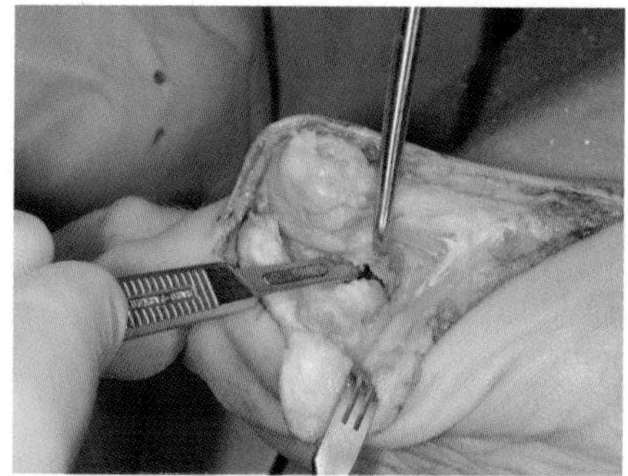

TECH FIG 2 • A. A plantar and proximally based capsular flap is created, and the capsule is released with a Freer elevator. **B.** A no. 15 blade is used to complete the release of the lateral capsular attachment to the lateral sesamoid.

METATARSAL OSTEOTOMY

- The location of the tarsometatarsal (TMT) joint is confirmed, and a point is marked about 20 mm distally from the first TMT joint for the apex of the osteotomy and at the midpoint in the dorsal plantar direction.
- A proximally based chevron osteotomy is created at an angle of about 60 degrees using a microsagittal saw.
- Complete release, both plantarly and dorsally, is confirmed, and care is taken not to fracture either limb of the chevron osteotomy (**TECH FIG 3**).
- The proximal fragment is grasped with a towel clamp, and the distal fragment angulated laterally.
  - It also is translated 3 to 5 mm laterally and plantarly enough to coapt the superior portion of the chevron, leaving an opening in the plantar portion of the osteotomy (**TECH FIG 4**).

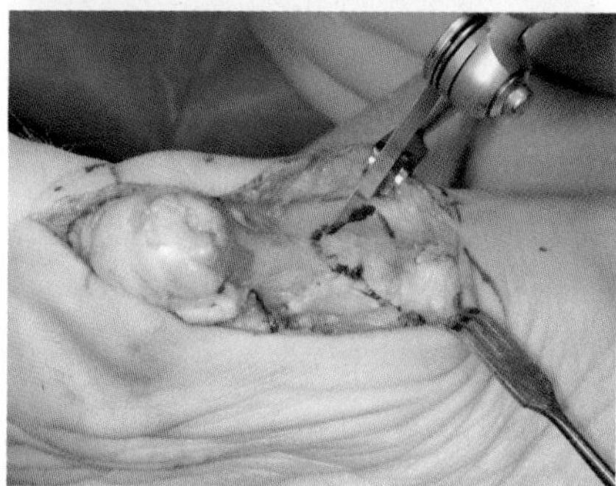

TECH FIG 3 • A microsagittal saw is used to create a 60-degree chevron osteotomy with the apex 20 mm from the tarsometatarsal joint.

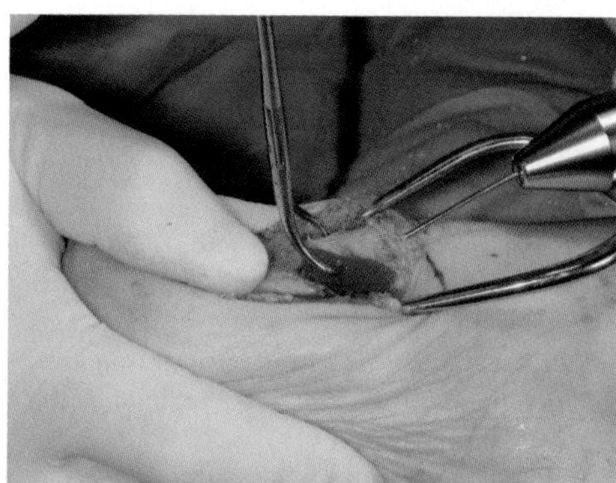

TECH FIG 4 • A pointed towel clip is used to hold the proximal metatarsal while the shaft is angulated and translated laterally to decrease the 1–2 intermetatarsal angle and narrow the foot. A K-wire is advanced from the TMT joint into the shaft to hold the correction temporarily.

OSTEOTOMY FIXATION

- The translated position is secured temporarily with a 0.062-inch K-wire.
- The prominent proximal fragment is cleaned of periosteum and removed flush with the distal fragment.
- The largest removed portion is then placed as bone graft between the fragments at the opening created in the chevron osteotomy from the plantar translation (TECH FIG 5A,B).
- A four-hole hole locking plate is used to bridge the osteotomy medially (TECH FIG 5C).
  - Care is exercised to avoid penetrating the TMT articulation with screws.
- The medial eminence is removed 1 mm medial to the sagittal sulcus (TECH FIG 5D).
- The K-wire is removed, stability is confirmed, and correction and alignment are confirmed with fluoroscopy (TECH FIG 6).

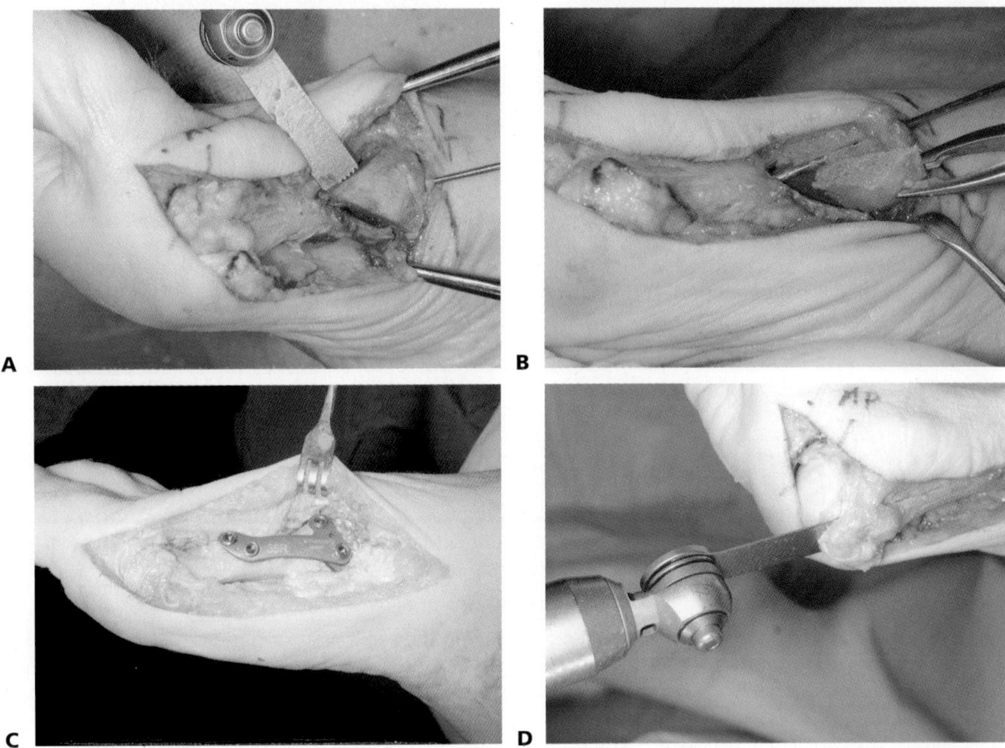

TECH FIG 5 • **A,B.** The prominent proximal bone is removed with a saw. The opening created by plantar flexing the metatarsal creates a gap into which the removed bone may be impacted. **C.** A four-hole locking plate is applied at the osteotomy site. **D.** The prominent medial eminence is removed 1 mm medial to the sagittal sulcus.

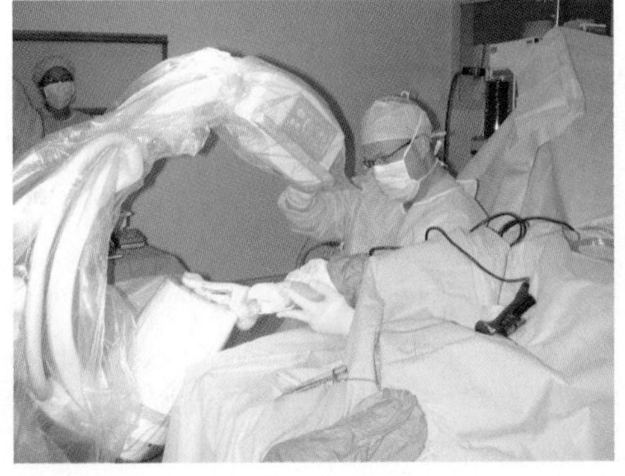

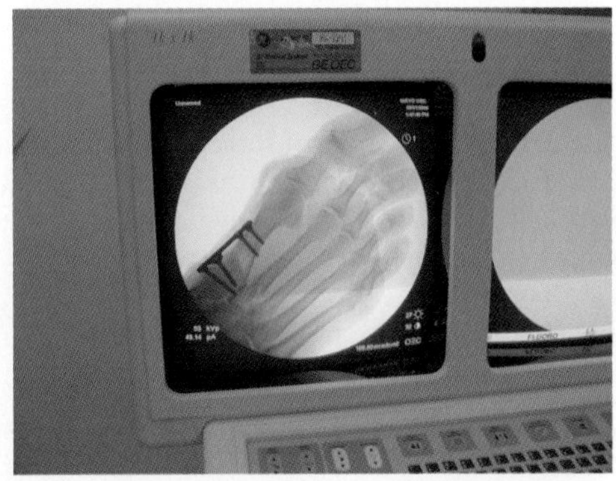

TECH FIG 6 • **A,B.** Correction of the hallux valgus angle and the 1–2 intermetatarsal angle is confirmed with fluoroscopy.

TECHNIQUES

CAPSULE AND SOFT TISSUE CLOSURE

- Meticulous capsular closure is performed with 2-0 Vicryl sutures holding the toe in slight varus and supination (**TECH FIG 7**).
- The deep tissues also are closed over the plate to avoid later plate removal.
- The skin is closed with interrupted vertical mattress 4-0 nylon sutures and a compressive dressing (**TECH FIG 8**).

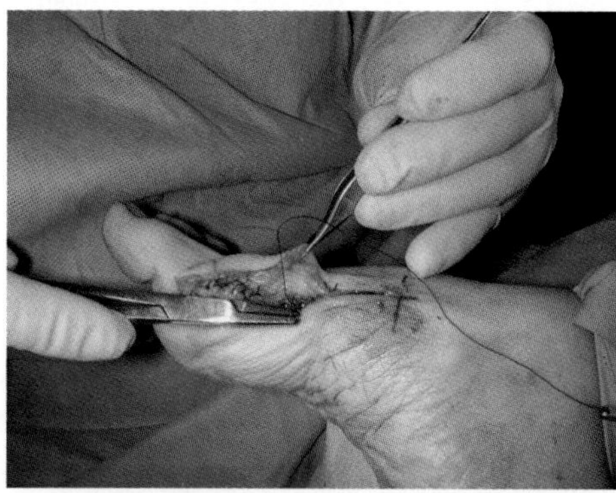

TECH FIG 7 • The capsular flaps are closed with 2-0 interrupted Vicryl sutures with the hallux held in good position. Soft tissue coverage of the plate also is obtained.

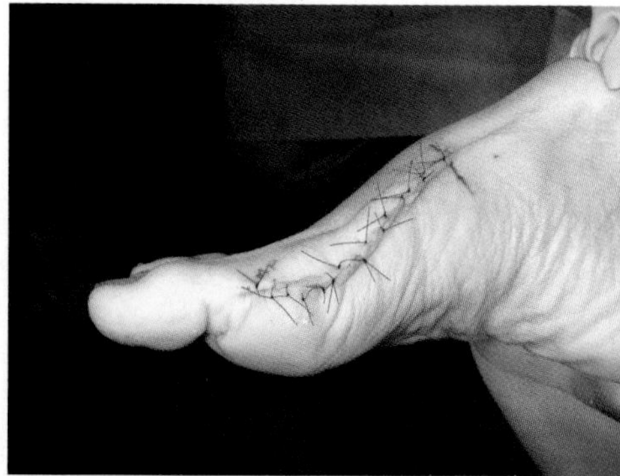

TECH FIG 8 • The skin is closed with interrupted 4-0 nylon vertical mattress sutures.

PEARLS AND PITFALLS

Indications	■ Large symptomatic hallux valgus deformity with minimal degenerative change and a 1–2 intermetatarsal angle greater than 15 degrees.
Exposure	■ During the approach, dissect thick tissue flaps to allow for improved wound healing.
Metatarsal osteotomy	■ Pay particular attention to keeping the saw in the same plane while performing the proximal chevron osteotomy to ensure good bony apposition at the site of fixation. Do not overcorrect the 1–2 metatarsal angle; a negative angle will cause hallux varus.
Locking plate fixation	■ If the plate requires contouring, do not bend the plate through the locking holes or the screws will not seat properly in the plate.
Capsular closure	■ By removing redundant medial capsule during the approach, the capsule repair can be accomplished more efficiently at the conclusion of the procedure. The great toe should be positioned in slight varus, about 2 degrees, to allow healing of the capsular tissues in a good position. These tissues will stretch over time. Do not overtighten the capsule, because this will overcorrect the toe position and result in varus malalignment. Capsular imbrication also can be used to correct pronation deformity of the hallux.

POSTOPERATIVE CARE

- Bunion dressings are applied at the time of surgery, and sutures are removed 2 to 3 weeks from the date of surgery.
- Heel weight bearing can be allowed immediately postoperatively, with advancement to weight bearing as tolerated in a regular shoe at 6 weeks postoperatively.
- Radiographs are obtained at 6 weeks and 3 months.

REFERENCES

1. Easley ME, Kiebzak GM, Davis WH, et al. Prospective, randomized comparison of proximal crescentic and proximal chevron osteotomies for correction of hallux valgus deformity. Foot Ankle Int 1996;17:307–316.
2. Gallentine JW, DeOrio JK, DeOrio MJ. Bunion surgery using locking-plate fixation of proximal metatarsal chevron osteotomies. Foot Ankle Int 2007;28(3):361–368.
3. McCluskey LC, Johnson JE, Wynarsky GT, et al. Comparison of stability of proximal crescentic metatarsal osteotomy and proximal horizontal "V" osteotomy. Foot Ankle Int 1994;15:263–270.
4. Sammarco GJ, Russo-Alesi FG. Bunion correction using proximal chevron osteotomy: A single-incision technique. Foot Ankle Int 1998;19:430–437.

Chapter 12

Closing Wedge Proximal Osteotomy

Sam Singh and Michael G. Wilson

SURGICAL MANAGEMENT

- The primary indication for a proximal closing wedge osteotomy is a symptomatic hallux valgus deformity with a first intermetatarsal angle (IMA) of 14 degrees or greater.
- The first metatarsocuneiform (MC) joint should be stable. We evaluate stability of this joint both by physical examination and radiographs. On physical examination, the cuneiform is stabilized in one hand while the first metatarsal is translated superiorly and inferiorly with the other hand. On weight-bearing radiographs, the MC joint is inspected for incongruency on the AP view and plantar widening on the lateral view. We favor a Lapidus-type procedure for hallux valgus associated with first MC joint instability.
- Relative contraindications to this osteotomy include mild osteoarthritic changes in the first metatarsophalangeal (MTP) joint and the presence of an inflammatory arthropathy. In the presence of mild osteoarthritic changes, an active individual who understands the possible future need for a fusion may remain a candidate for a corrective osteotomy. Similarly, given the improved medical management of inflammatory arthropathy, an informed patient with well-managed rheumatoid arthritis may also be a candidate for reconstructive hallux valgus surgery rather than fusion.
- Absolute contraindications to this osteotomy are advanced osteoarthritis of the first MTP joint or the skeletally immature patient, in whom the very proximal nature of this osteotomy can jeopardize the growth plate.

Preoperative Planning

- AP and lateral weight-bearing radiographs of the foot are evaluated for metatarsal length, IMA, and hallux valgus angle. Congruency of the joint, the size of the bony medial eminence, and the position of the sesamoids are noted. We routinely mark the proposed osteotomy on the radiograph (**FIG 1**).

Positioning

- We perform this procedure on an outpatient basis. Prophylactic antibiotics are administered. A thigh tourniquet is applied. The patient is positioned supine with a small sandbag placed under the ipsilateral buttock to ensure the foot points up, allowing for easier osteotomy orientation.

Approach

- We perform the proximal closing wedge osteotomy with a distal soft tissue procedure through two incisions. The first is a dorsal first web space incision extended proximally in a lazy-S curve to the dorsal first MC joint. This incision allows access for lateral release and proximal osteotomy. The second medial midaxial incision over the first MTP joint is the traditional approach for medial capsulotomy, medial eminence resection, and medial capsular plication.

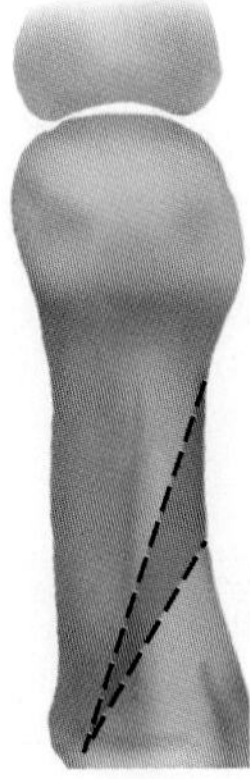

FIG 1 • Line diagram showing the closing wedge osteotomy.

SOFT TISSUE RELEASE AND BUNIONECTOMY

- Perform a standard lateral release of the first MTP joint through a dorsal incision centered over the first web space.
- After incising the skin, continue deep dissection bluntly.
- Using sharp dissection, release the tendinous insertion of the adductor hallucis muscle onto the fibular sesamoid and proximal phalanx; we have not found it necessary to reattach this structure proximally (**TECH FIG 1A**).
- Release the suspensory metatarsal–sesamoid ligaments and make multiple sharp perforations in the lateral capsule at the joint line. Apply a varus force to the hallux, completing the capsular release.
- Approach the medial eminence through a midline longitudinal incision extending from just proximal to the medial eminence to the base of the proximal phalanx. Identify the dorsal medial cutaneous nerve and incise the medial capsule sharply in a longitudinal direction (**TECH FIG 1B**). Expose the medial eminence and resect it 1 mm medial to the sagittal sulcus. Overresection can lead to a postoperative varus deformity.

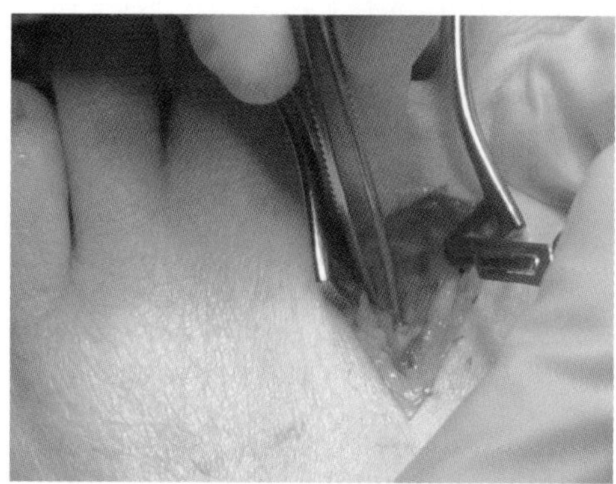

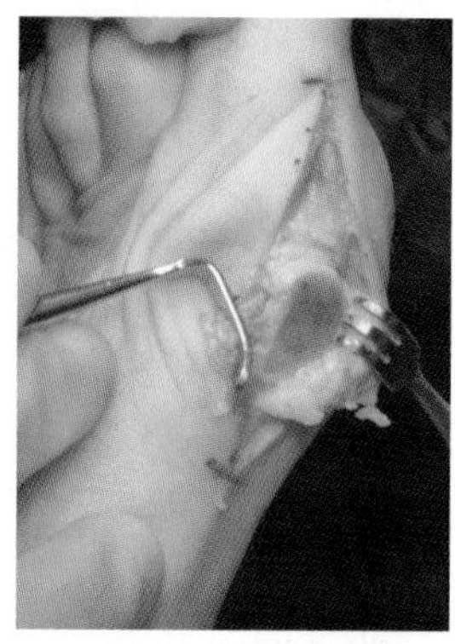

TECH FIG 1 • **A.** The adductor hallucis tendon is released off the proximal phalanx and fibula sesamoid. The suspensory ligaments of the fibula sesamoid are released. **B.** Medial capsulotomy and exostectomy.

CLOSING WEDGE OSTEOTOMY

- Extend the first web space incision in an S shape to the first MC joint (TECH FIG 2A). Approach the dorsal metatarsal shaft through the interval between the extensor hallucis brevis and extensor hallucis longus. Retraction with two small pointed retractors facilitates exposure of the metatarsal base.
- The proposed wedge for resection has its apex on the medial cortex about 3 mm from the MC joint. The proposed long oblique osteotomy should leave a large residual proximal fragment for maximal contact area and solid fixation. The first cut, the proximal of the two, is perpendicular to the weight-bearing axis of the foot. This is demonstrated during surgery by the simulated weight-bearing test. To maintain control of the osteotomy, the medial cortex is scored but not penetrated with the saw blade (TECH FIG 2B).
- After making the second distal cut, excise a lateral wedge-shaped wafer of bone; this leaves a defect, which is compressed with a towel clip. This "greensticks" the intact but weakened medial cortex and the IMA is reduced (TECH FIG 2C–E).
- Insert two 2.7-mm cortical screws (Synthes, Paoli, PA) from the lateral to medial cortex in a lag screw fashion (TECH FIG 3AB). The small size of the proximal fragment

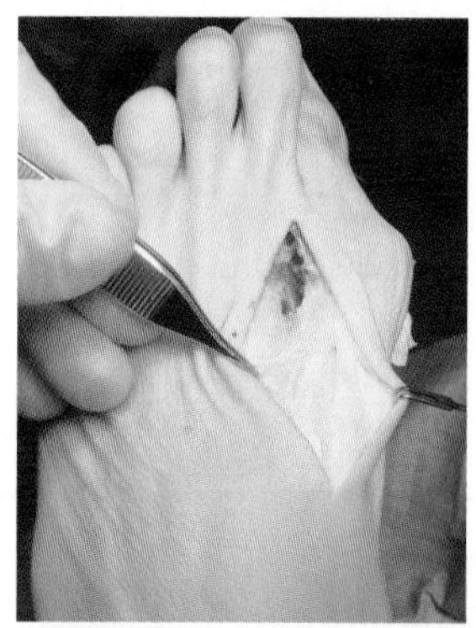

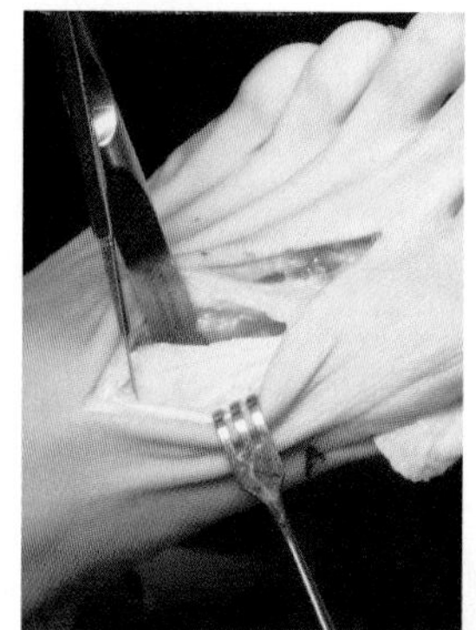

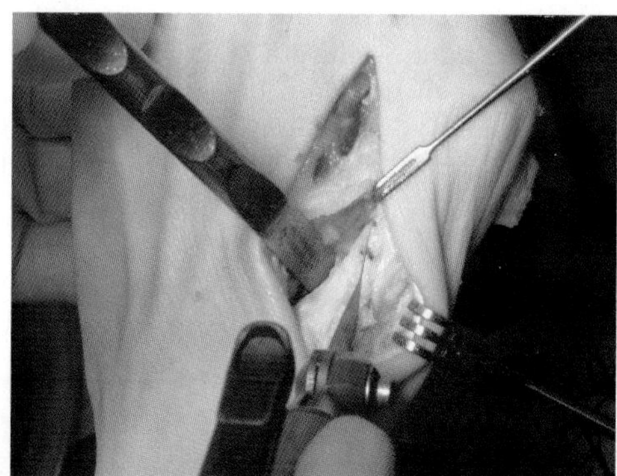

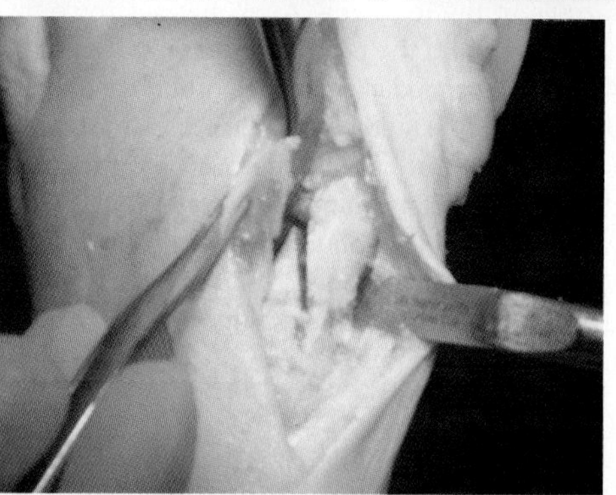

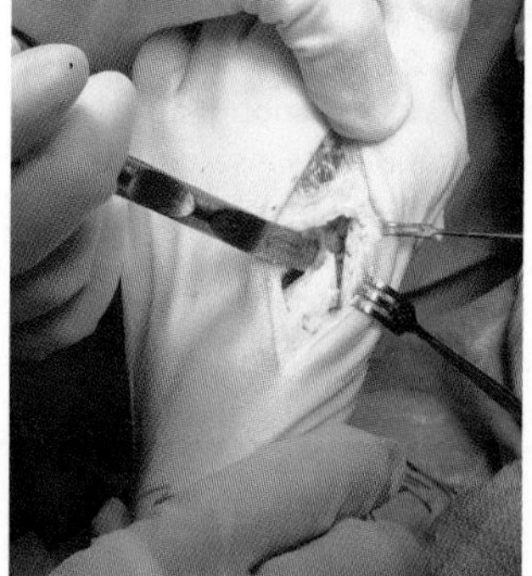

TECH FIG 2 • **A.** The web space incision is extended proximally in a lazy-S shape toward the base of the first metatarsal. The extensor hallucis brevis is identified and protected. **B.** The first tarsometatarsal joint is localized to define the limit of the cut. **C–E.** The two osteotomies leave a wedge-shaped segment of bone, which is removed.

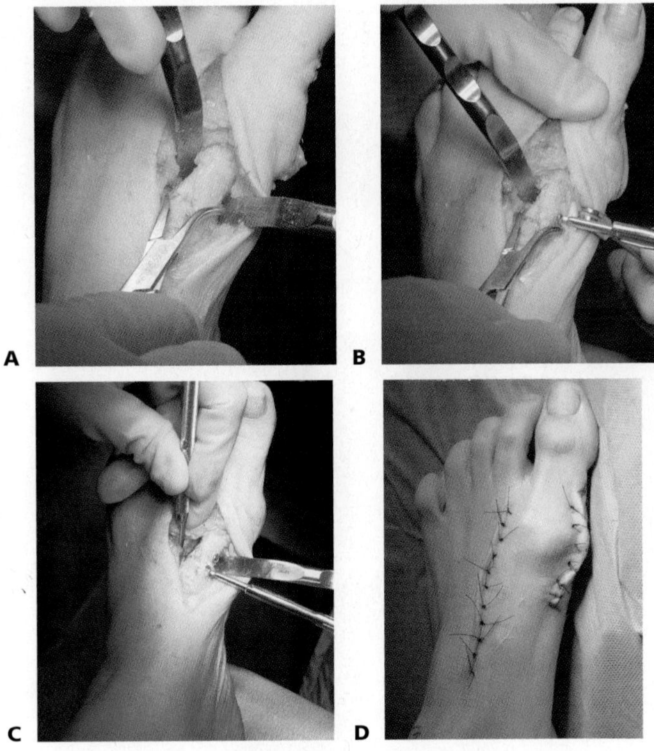

TECH FIG 3 • A. Compression with the clamp "greensticks" the medial cortex. **B, C.** Two screws are inserted in a lag screw fashion. **D.** The capsule is repaired. The skin is closed.

does not allow both screws to be parallel to the osteotomy, but this is not vital, as compression has already been obtained with the reduction forcep.

- Confirm the reduction in the IMA, screws, and relocation of the sesamoids with image intensification.
- Imbricate the medial capsule with a strong absorbable suture while holding the hallux in a neutral or slightly abducted position (TECH FIG 3C).
- Close the wounds in layers with interrupted nylon sutures to the skin and apply a forefoot bandage to maintain the correction (TECH FIG 3D).

PEARLS AND PITFALLS

Keep the center of correction proximal.	▪ The apex of the deformity is the MC joint. To maximize the power of the osteotomy, the center of correction should be as close to the joint as possible, leaving a safe bridge of medial cortex.
Beware the short osteotomy!	▪ If the osteotomy is too short it will exit the lateral cortex too proximally, leaving a small proximal fragment. This compromises the contact area and stability of the osteotomy, precludes adequate fixation, and decreases the corrective power of the osteotomy.
Maintain continuous control of the osteotomy.	▪ By only scoring the medial cortex, complete control of the osteotomy segments is maintained at all times.
Avoid early full weight bearing.	▪ The excessive sagittal loading can lead to a dorsiflexion malunion.

POSTOPERATIVE CARE

- If safe, patients are discharged home on the day of surgery with strict advice to elevate the foot whenever resting for the first 2 weeks.
- In most cases patients are allowed to bear weight on their heel and lateral forefoot in a hard-soled postoperative shoe.
- In noncompliant patients or those with poor bone quality and fixation, we do not hesitate to use cast immobilization from the outset.
- The wound is inspected and sutures are removed at 2 weeks, at which time the hallux is restrapped and patients are taught simple passive and active toe flexion–extension exercises.

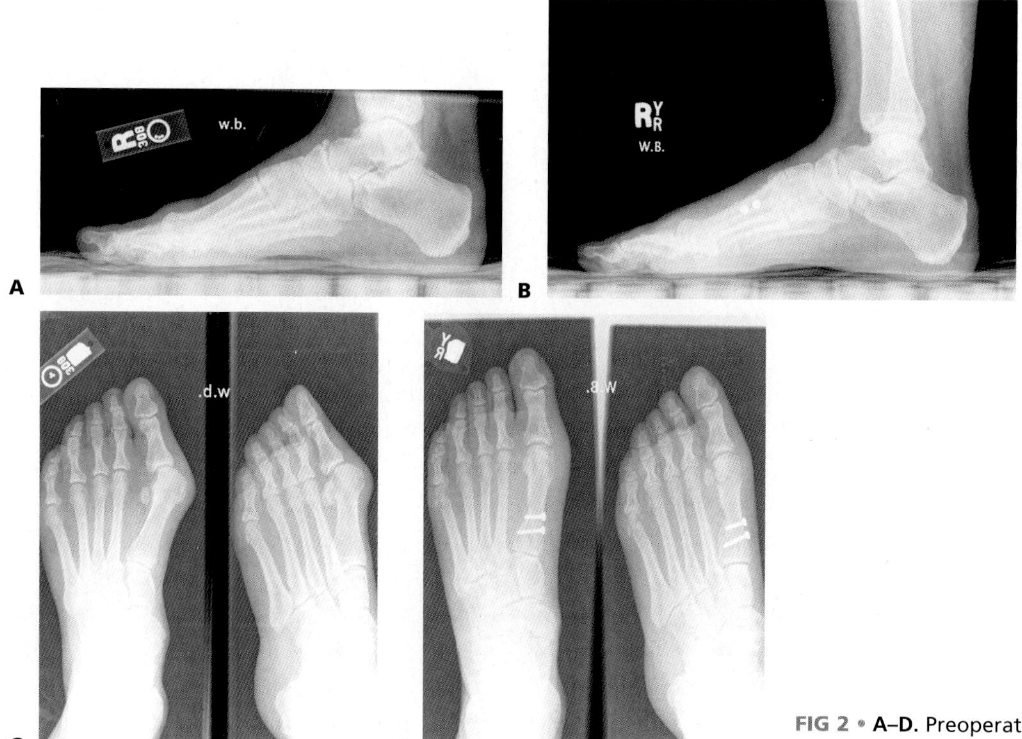

FIG 2 • **A–D.** Preoperative and postoperative radiographs.

- At 6 weeks postoperatively the osteotomy is assessed with radiographs (**FIG 2A–D**). If there is some consolidation at the line of the osteotomy, the patient is instructed to wear a wide shoe or sneaker and to progress weight bearing as tolerated. Strapping of the hallux is discontinued at this time. If there is evidence of a delayed union, the patient is kept non–weight-bearing in a hard-soled postoperative shoe.

OUTCOMES

- A review of our first 40 cases with an average age at surgery of 51 years identified one case of transfer metatarsalgia in a patient who had not had it before surgery, one malunion due to loss of fixation, one delayed union requiring prolonged immobilization, and one asymptomatic nonunion. Shortening of the first metatarsal was minimal with this technique, with an average of 0.98 mm (−1 to 3 mm). In the subset of 11 patients with a severe deformity and an IMA exceeding 18 degrees (range 18 to 22 degrees) the average postoperative IMA was 7.8 degrees, with an average 1.8 mm of shortening.
- Some studies have reported more shortening (average of 5 mm) with similar osteotomies, but this may be due to two factors: (1) a transverse rather than long oblique closing wedge osteotomy and (2) dorsiflexion malunion (which may make the metatarsal appear shorter on radiographic evaluation).
- The stability of this osteotomy is not compromised even when correcting hallux valgus with a large intermetatarsal deformity. This is in contrast to the Scarf, Ludloff, or proximal crescentic osteotomies, where bone contact area is substantially reduced.

COMPLICATIONS

- Those of any hallux valgus surgery: iatrogenic fracture, injury to the dorsal medial cutaneous nerve, superficial infection, loss of fixation, and delayed union
- The risk of iatrogenic fracture can be minimized by using appropriate-diameter screws, leaving a bridge of at least 3 mm between screws, and both drilling and tapping the near cortex (even when using a self-tapping screw).

REFERENCES

1. Mann RA, Rudicel S, Graves SC. Repair of hallux valgus with a distal soft-tissue procedure and proximal metatarsal osteotomy: a long-term follow-up. J Bone Joint Surg Am 1992;74A:124–129.
2. Trnka HJ, Muhlbauer M, Zembsch A, et al. Basal closing wedge osteotomy for correction of hallux valgus and metatarsus primus varus: 10- to 22-year follow-up. Foot Ankle Int 1999;20:171–177.
3. Trnka H-J, Parks BG, Ivanic G, et al. Six first metatarsal shaft osteotomies: mechanical and immobilization comparisons. Clin Orthop Relat Res 2000;381:256–265.
4. Ruch JA, Banks AS. Proximal osteotomies of the first metatarsal in the correction of hallux abducto valgus. In: McGlamry ED, Banes AS, Downey MS, eds. Comprehensive Textbook of Foot Surgery. Baltimore: Williams & Wilkins, 1987:195–211.

Chapter 13

Proximal Metatarsal Opening Wedge Osteotomy

Paul S. Shurnas, Mark E. Easley, Troy Watson, and Amy Sanders

DEFINITION

- Symptomatic hallux valgus, or bunion deformity, is a common problem seen in foot and ankle and general practice clinics.
  - Historically, it is seen almost exclusively in persons who wear shoes.
  - It is characterized by a painful prominence at the medial aspect of the great toe.
- The deformity is exemplified by lateral deviation (valgus) of the great toe proximal phalanx and medial (varus) deviation of the first metatarsal.
- Juvenile hallux valgus deformity usually is a combination of valgus inclination of the metatarsal articular surface (i.e., increased distal metatarsal articular angle [DMAA]) and varus deformity of the first metatarsal.
- Deformity may be classified as mild, moderate, or severe, evaluated on weight-bearing radiographs of the foot and based on the following criteria:
  - The degree of valgus at the metatarsophalangeal (MTP) joint or hallux valgus angle (HVA)
  - The degree of varus deformity of the first metatarsal or 1–2 intermetatarsal angle (IMA)
- Advanced deformity is more complex, and the hallux exhibits the following:
  - Toe pronation noted clinically by medial rotation of the toenail
  - Sesamoid subluxation noted on the anteroposterior (AP) radiograph and sesamoid view
  - Medial capsular laxity and lateral capsular contracture

ANATOMY

- The great toe MTP joint is unique when compared to the lesser MTP joints because of the sesamoid complex, unique tendon insertions, and ligamentous support about the joint (**FIG 1**).
  - The sesamoid ligaments mesh with the collateral ligaments both medially and laterally.
- The tendons of the flexor hallucis brevis, abductor and adductor hallucis, plantar aponeurosis, and joint capsule coalesce to form the plantar plate, surrounding and stabilizing the first metatarsal head (**FIG 2**).
  - Because there are no true tendon insertions on the first metatarsal head, it is vulnerable to varus deviation.
  - An intermetatarsal facet occasionally is present between the first and second metatarsal bases, sometimes creating a rigid metatarsus primus varus.
- The first metatarsal blood supply is derived from arterial supply primarily through the lateral midshaft, and its flow is distal.
  - Intraosseous flow is variable with respect to proximal and distal branches.
  - The primary arterial sources are the first dorsal and plantar metatarsal arteries and the superficial branch of the medial plantar artery.[8]
- The DMAA is defined by the relationship between the metatarsal long axis and the distal metatarsal articular surface lateral inclination (**FIG 3**).

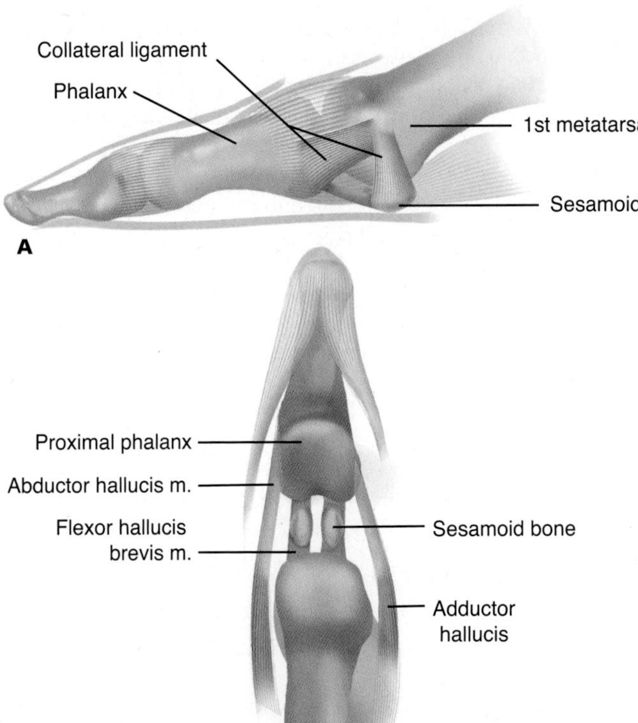

FIG 1 • Collateral ligaments and sesamoid tendon relations. **A.** Collateral S mesh with sesamoid complex. **B.** Sesamoid and tendon relations about the metatarsophalangeal (MTP) joint.

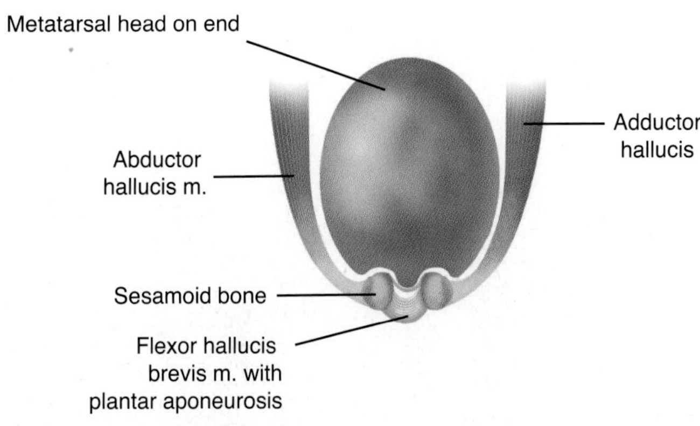

FIG 2 • Plantar plate contributions.

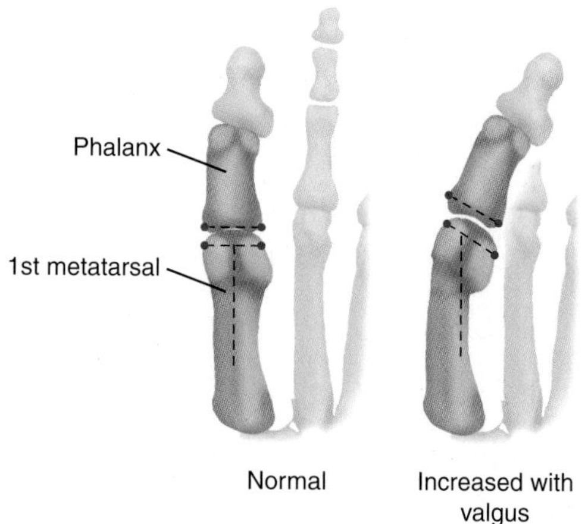

FIG 3 • Distal metatarsal angle (DMAA).

PATHOGENESIS

- The concept of a hallux valgus deformity with a congruent or subluxated MTP joint is important (**FIG 4**).
  - Whereas hallux valgus with a subluxated joint usually is progressive, congruent joints tend to be static deformities.
  - Congruent joint hallux valgus deformity is associated with an increased DMAA and juvenile hallux valgus.
- A flat metatarsal head, with little convexity, is associated with hallux rigidus.[3]
- A rounded metatarsal head is associated with greater MTP instability and hallux valgus. As the proximal phalanx deforms laterally, the metatarsal head shifts medially, increasing both the HVA and 1–2 IMA.[6]
- The inciting event leading to hallux valgus is poorly understood. Typically, with longstanding subluxated hallux valgus deformity, the medial capsule attenuates and the lateral capsule contracts.
  - The sesamoid complex remains in its physiologic position as the metatarsal head shifts medially. The weak link is thought to be the medial capsule immediately superior to the insertion of the abductor hallucis.[6]
  - Ultimately, the abductor hallucis slides plantar to the metatarsal head, leading to a lack of intrinsic muscle stability to the first MTP joint, with resultant pronation of the phalanx (**FIG 5**).

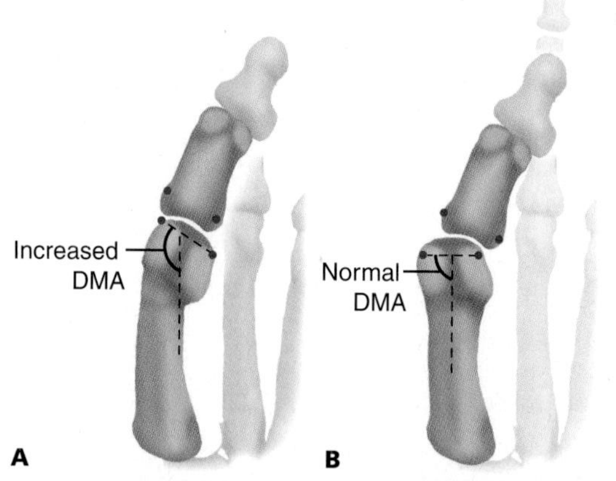

FIG 4 • Congruent versus subluxed joint. **A.** A congruent joint may be associated with hallux valgus when the DMAA is increased, as seen in juvenile hallux valgus. **B.** Joint in subluxed position.

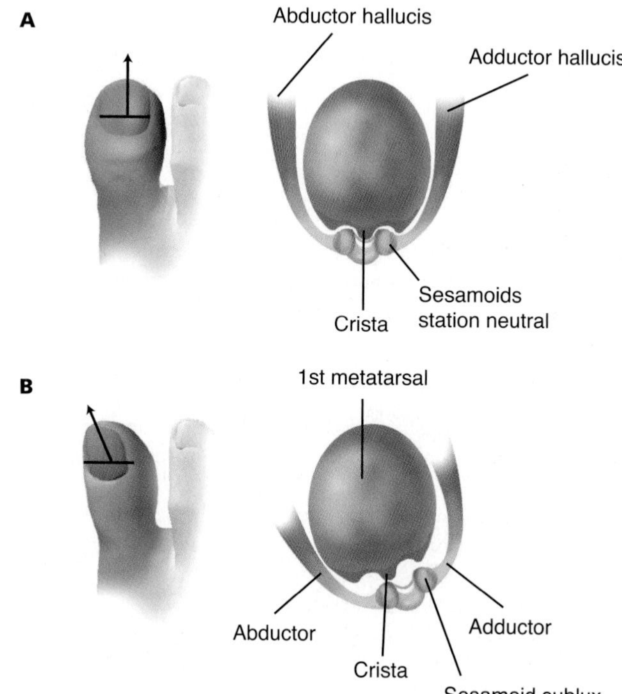

FIG 5 • The abductor hallucis slides under the metatarsal head, contributing to pronation of the toe. **A.** End-on view of toe and nail (normal). **B.** End-on view with pronation.

- With deformity progression, callus may develop along the plantar, medial interphalangeal (IP) joint. A lateral weight shift away from the hallux to the lesser MTP joints may occur, creating lesser MTP joint instability and further callus formation.

NATURAL HISTORY

- Hallux valgus with a subluxated joint usually is progressive, and the pathogenesis described in previous sections commonly is observed over time.
- Hallux valgus associated with a congruent joint tends to be more static in terms of deformity.
- Subluxated and congruent deformities may become symptomatic over time due to shoe pressure, cutaneous nerve irritation, bursitis, callus formation and a painful medial eminence.
- With progressive or painful deformities, other lesions may develop, such as associated lesser toe deformities, Morton's neuroma, lesser MTP joint capsular instability, stress fractures, skin ulceration, and hallux or lesser MTP joint dislocation.

PHYSICAL FINDINGS

- A reddened prominence over the medial aspect of the great toe MTP joint, or "bunion," often develops with pressure from shoe wear (Table 1).
- Many patients exhibit callus formation under the second or third metatarsal heads because the displaced first metatarsal is not bearing weight in a balanced manner with the lesser metatarsal heads.
- On palpation of the foot, most patients are tender over the medial eminence or show irritability in the cutaneous nerve.
- A large dorsal metatarsal prominence is more commonly associated with hallux rigidus and is not typical of symptomatic hallux valgus.

Table 1 Key History and Physical Findings of Hallux Valgus

Chief Complaint	Painful cherry-red prominence over medial aspect of MTP joint: atypical pain is plantar MTP joint (sesamoiditis)
Duration	Worsening pain and deformity the last 6 months to 1 year
Inspection	Swollen, reddened medial eminence with lateral deviation of the toe, often pronated with severe deformity
Palpation	Slight crepitus, bursitis, tender to touch over prominence, slight warmth, smooth and nearly full range of motion without pain
Deformity	Valgus (lateral) toe deviation varus metatarsal deviation and with severe deformity: pronation of the toe (the nail is rotated medially)
Key Differential	Rigidus; extreme pain, swelling (boggy) and warmth with gout or inflammatory condition
Aggravating Factors	Constrictive or unsupportive shoe wear worsens the pain, activity related pain is common when in shoes

- Joint range of motion in hallux valgus, even with severe deformity, usually is well preserved, without crepitance, and with minimal pain.
  - Range of motion also is checked while gently reducing the deformity out of valgus.
- Chronic deformities or congruent joints with increased DMAA may exhibit less dorsiflexion at the MTP joint.
- Palpation of the first metatarsal cuneiform (MTC) joint is performed.
  - Prominence, swelling, and pain with cantilever stress of the first MTC joint, if present, should be noted.
  - Mobility of the first MTC joint and gastrocnemius tightness are assessed.
- Other painful areas are sought out, including those with callus formation, the lesser MTP joints, intermetatarsal spaces, bunionette deformities, and hammer toes.
- We routinely also analyze the patient's gait, with particular attention focused on the stance phase and evaluation of hindfoot position and status of the longitudinal arch.
- Hindfoot joints are examined, tendon strength is checked, and general alignment about the foot and ankle are noted. In select patients, correction of concomitant pes planovalgus deformity, either simultaneously or in a staged fashion, may be warranted, because a valgus hindfoot may predispose to progression or recurrence of hallux valgus.
- Pulses are palpated, sensation is assessed, and the skin is inspected. Poor circulation should prompt a vascular evaluation, and loss of protective sensation may indicate neuropathy and may be a contraindication to corrective hallux valgus surgery. Previous forefoot incisions should be noted and considered in preoperative planning.

IMAGING AND DIAGNOSTIC STUDIES

- Weight-bearing AP and lateral radiographs are routinely obtained.
  - MRI, CT, and bone scans are rarely indicated. The reported normal radiographic values of the hallux MTP joint are a hallux valgus angle (HVA) no greater than 15 degrees, a 1–2 IMA of no more than 9 degrees, and an IP angle of less than 10 degrees.[5,6]
  - Standardized mid-diaphyseal reference points are used to measure the HVA and IMA.
  - The IP angle is measured by a line bisecting the base of the proximal phalanx and the long axis of the phalanx.
- Although precise measurement of the DMAA has been controversial, it is critical that it be considered, because subtotal correction and persistent deformity will result if it is not addressed at the time of surgery.
  - A DMAA of more than 15 degrees is considered increased.[1,2] It is measured based on the AP weight-bearing radiograph (Fig. 3).
- Hallux valgus interphalangeus (HVI) is measured by the IP angle. HVI has been associated primarily with hallux rigidus,[3] but occasionally it occurs with hallux valgus.
  - Proximal first metatarsal osteotomies and distal soft tissue procedures do not correct an increased HVI; phalangeal osteotomies are required to correct HVI.
  - MTC instability may be indicated by a first MTC angle of more than 10 degrees or excess joint obliquity on the weight-bearing AP radiograph, plantar gapping of more than 2 mm on the lateral weight-bearing view, or an intermetatarsal os.
  - Although first ray hypermobility is controversial, in select patients, an increased 1–2 angle may be best corrected with a first MTC arthrodesis in lieu of a proximal first metatarsal osteotomy.
- An intermetatarsal facet at the base of the first and second metatarsals may directly impede correction of the 1–2 IMA.
- Hallux valgus associated with advanced arthrosis of the first MTP joint may preclude joint-preserving operations, and typically is best managed with a first MTP joint arthrodesis.

DIFFERENTIAL DIAGNOSIS

- Inflammatory arthritis of many varieties can result in hallux valgus.
- Traumatic hallux valgus or hallux varus can occur.
- Adult or congenital flatfoot, posterior tibial tendon deficiency, generalized hyperlaxity, and first MTC instability can exacerbate hallux valgus.
- Tarsal coalition or symptomatic accessory navicular with associated hallux valgus may occur.
- Neuromuscular disorders are associated with hallux valgus.

NONOPERATIVE MANAGEMENT

- Shoe wear modification, the mainstay of nonoperative management, includes shoe stretching, wider toe box shoes, and, occasionally, accommodative orthotics.
- Toe spacers, night splints, bunion pads or posts, and other inventive devices may help reduce symptoms.

SURGICAL MANAGEMENT

- More than 120 procedures have been described to surgically correct hallux valgus, including a variety of proximal first metatarsal base, shaft, and distal osteotomies.
- The goals of an ideal proximal base osteotomy are reliable, powerful, predictable correction with stable fixation to allow for early weight bearing.
  - Proximal metatarsal opening wedge osteotomy (PMOW) with a newer low-profile plate fixation system (Arthrex, Inc., Naples, FL) is, in our opinion, nearly ideal for addressing those goals.

PROXIMAL METATARSAL OPENING WEDGE OSTEOTOMY

- PMOW combined with a distal soft tissue procedure (ie, lateral capsular release and medial capsular placation) is considered for moderate to severe hallux valgus, hallux valgus associated with a short first ray, a 1–2 IMA of more than 12 degrees, and recurrent hallux valgus, either after a distal procedure alone or as an adjunct to a distal procedure if subtotal correction is achieved.
- Two or three 3-cm incisions are used, depending on which distal procedure is being performed.
  - The first longitudinal incision is centered over the medial eminence, and a simple bunionectomy is performed in a routine fashion.
  - We prefer to use an inverted L-shaped capsulotomy and save bone resected from the medial eminence to use as autograft in the PMOW.
  - Alternatively, cancellous graft may be harvested from the lateral calcaneus through a 1- to 2-cm lateral heel incision.
  - We make the longitudinal incision for the PMOW dorsomedially, beginning just distal to the first MTC joint.
- The superficial peroneal nerve branch to the hallux and the extensor hallucis longus tendon must be identified and protected.
- The osteotomy is initiated medially about 1.5 cm distal to the joint, slightly oblique (about 20–30 degrees) toward the lateral aspect of the first metatarsal base, without violating the lateral cortex (**TECH FIG 1A**). Minimal periosteal stripping is required.
- The osteotomy is gently opened with three successive osteotomes (largest blade first) from the PMOW set, and care is take to preserve the lateral hinge of bone and soft tissue, if possible. "Stacking" osteotomes diminishes the risk of breaking the lateral cortex, which is more likely to occur when a single osteotome is used to lever the osteotomy open.
  - Once the osteotomy is opened, manual pressure over the medial eminence and a mini lamina spreader (supplied in the set) are used to obtain the desired correction and verified fluoroscopically.
  - Alternatively, a measuring wedge (also provided in the set) may be utilized.
  - If the lateral cortical hinge should fail, the mini lamina spreader is quite useful.
- The osteotomy site is held open and the plate applied as described, which typically reduces the lateral cortex.
- To gain further support to the lateral cortex, one of the proximal screws may be placed not only through the plate but also across the osteotomy to capture the distal lateral cortex. Alternatively, an additional oblique screw may be added outside the plate.
- About 5% of our cases have resulted in lateral cortex fracture with no delay in healing or modification in the postoperative protocol.

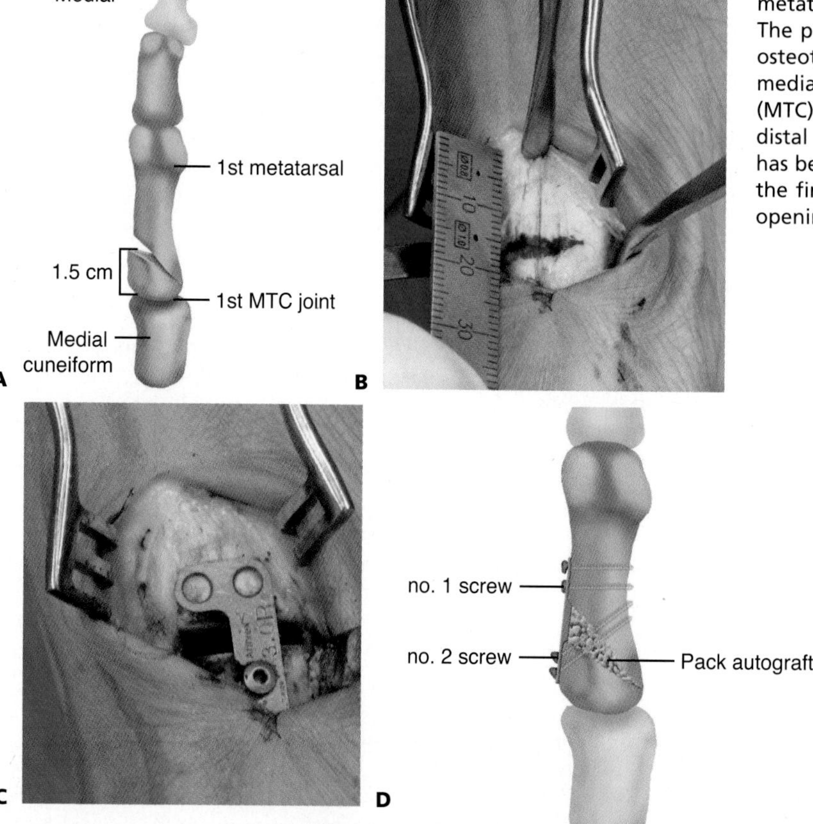

TECH FIG 1 • A. Site and position of first metatarsal opening wedge osteotomy. The proximal metatarsal opening wedge osteotomy is initiated about 1.5 cm distal medial to the first metatarsal cuneiform (MTC) joint. **B.** Site of osteotomy 1.5 cm distal to the first MTC joint. **C.** The plate has been set into position by insertion of the first screw. **D.** Screw placement with opening wedge plate.

- *Based on the authors' clinical data utilizing the oblique osteotomy, a general rule for preoperative planning is approximately 3 degrees of correction per millimeter of opening wedge.*
- The desired wedge is selected and the first screw is placed in the distal hole closest to the osteotomy to set the plate (**TECH FIG 1B,C**).
- The next screw placed is in one of the proximal holes. We prefer to place both of these screws obliquely across the apex of the osteotomy (**TECH FIG 1D**).
  - If there is any concern about stability, an additional screw can be placed obliquely outside the plate to enhance the construct.
- The final screw is placed distally.
- With the plate securely fixed, fluoroscopy is used with the foot flat on the table to verify a congruent joint and increased DMAA or to determine whether any further correction is required.
- With subluxated deformities, the PMWO is combined with a modified McBride bunionectomy using two or three incisions.
  - The third incision, if used, is for the first web space. However, with this technique an aggressive lateral release typically is not required.
- If the joint is congruent with an increased DMAA or if still more correction is desired, a biplanar chevron incision with a long dorsal limb is used (**TECH FIG 2A–C**).
- Any IP deformity or residual pronation can be treated with an Akin osteotomy.
- The capsule is repaired through a drill hole at the metadiaphyseal junction or with mattress suture technique proximally if the tissue quality is satisfactory. The soft tissues over the osteotomy site are closed in a layered fashion, after autologous graft is impacted.
- Nylon sutures are used for the skin.

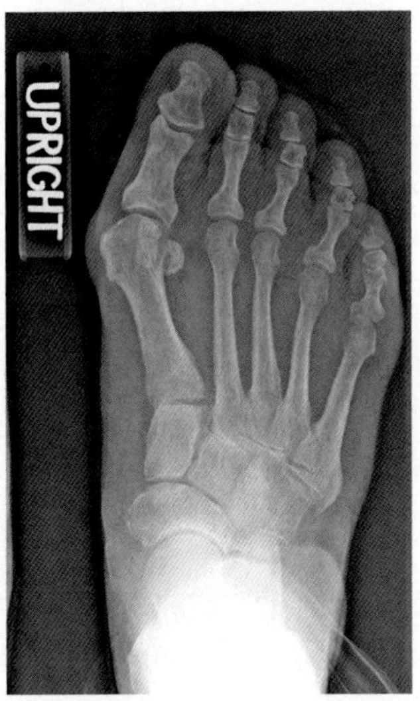

A

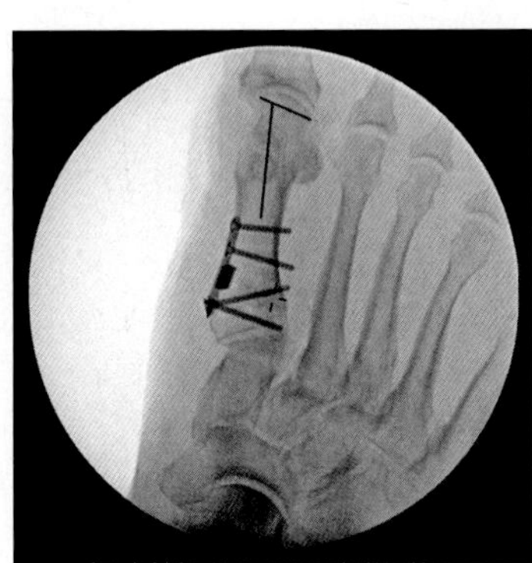

B

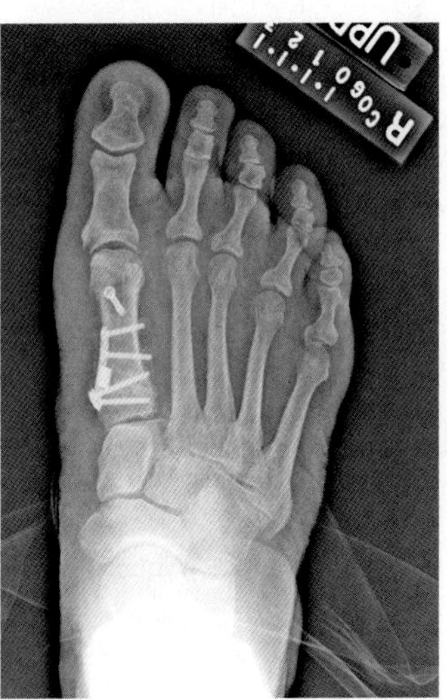

C

TECH FIG 2 • **A.** Preoperative weight-bearing AP radiograph shows a severe hallux valgus deformity with a bipartite tibial sesamoid and mild degenerative changes. **B.** Intraoperative radiograph shows good correction of the 1–2 IMA to less than 9 degrees but an increased DMAA of 25 degrees. **C.** Six week postoperative weight-bearing AP radiograph shows good alignment post-PMOW first metatarsal and distal biplanar chevron bunionectomy.

PEARLS AND PITFALLS

- Start slightly oblique (10–15 degrees) osteotomy at least 1.5 cm distal to the first tarsometatarsal joint.
- A small lamina spreader is useful to obtain desired correction.
- The opposite side plate may fit better on the base of the first metatarsal in some people.
- Avoid an aggressive lateral release; pie-crusting release through the joint is usually enough.
- Distal biplanar chevron osteotomy or similar correction for the DMAA is often needed.
- Careful not to enter the joint with the oblique osteotomy; verify cut with radiology.
- Lateral cortex disruption can occur; temporary Kirschner wire fixation will stabilize.
- Plate removal is lower in clinical studies.[7]
- Varus overcorrection is reduced.[10]
- Although the DMAA is not increased because of PMOW, it becomes more easily recognized and should be treated to optimize the results.

POSTOPERATIVE CARE

- We prefer to use a carefully wrapped Coban dressing with a figure 8 toe cradle in the operating room and for the first 3 weeks postoperatively.
- A soft Velcro bunion splint is used thereafter for 6 weeks.
  - The last 2 weeks are nighttime use only.
- Patients are seen 5 days after surgery and every 10 to 14 days, depending on the amount of swelling they experience.
- Sutures are removed 2 to 3 weeks postoperatively.
- We routinely place the patient's operated foot in a short controlled ankle motion (CAM) walker immediately after surgery and allow heel weight bearing in the boot as tolerated.
  - Patients are allowed full weight bearing on the foot at 6 weeks, first in the boot and then with a relatively rapid transition out of the boot into a comfortable shoe.
- Range of motion is initiated to the MTP joint 10 to 14 days postoperatively.
- Our routine is to assess healing with weight-bearing radiographs at 3, 6, and 14 weeks postoperatively.

OUTCOMES

- Wukich et al[11] reported on 14 patients using PMOW with modified McBride bunionectomy for moderate and severe deformities during 1 year of follow-up. They found no instances of malunion or nonunion, and experienced excellent and reliable correction with complete patient satisfaction.
- Cooper et al[4] reported on 25 patients using the same technique during their first year of experience and noted excellent correction and healing and no adverse outcomes with complete patient satisfaction.
  - The authors reported about 2 degrees correction of 1–2 IMA per mm of opening wedge using a flat cut at the base of the metatarsal.
- Sargas[7] reported greater than 90% good and excellent results in a retrospective review of patients treated by proximal opening wedge osteotomy of the first metatarsal and distal procedure with a low incidence of complications and plate and screw removal.
  - The opposite side plate was used with excellent correction and minimal or no need for removal.
- Shurnas[9] reported cadaveric biomechanical results comparing proximal chevron osteotomy and PMOW, finding no difference in load to failure, ultimate strength, or stiffness.
- Shurnas[9] also reported the initial experience on 50 patients: 25 with at least 1 year of follow-up and 25 with 6 months to 1 year of follow-up.
  - The author reported about 3 degrees correction of 1–2 IMA per mm of opening wedge using an oblique osteotomy.
  - The mean postoperative IMA and HVA were 3 degrees and 11 degrees, respectively, with a mean change in IMA and HVA of 12 degrees and 20 degrees, respectively.
  - Mean time to radiographic and clinical healing was 5.8 weeks, with no instances of nonunion, malunion, or delayed union.
  - All patients were satisfied with their outcome, and mean range of motion was not significantly different comparing preoperative and postoperative values.
  - There was an insignificant increase in the mean first metatarsal protrusion distance of 1.9 mm but no instances of shortening, elevatus, or hardware failure.
- A prospective study of patients who have undergone PMOW and various distal procedures for subluxed, congruent, and juvenile deformities is ongoing.
- Shurnas[9] reported on a retrospective review of more than 90 patients with moderate and severe hallux valgus treated by proximal opening wedge osteotomy and distal procedure with a minimum of 2 years follow-up.
  - The authors reported better than 90% good and excellent results.
  - Plate and screw removal was required in about 15%.
  - There were two varus deformities that required arthrodesis.
  - There was one nonunion in a patient with true metal allergy.

COMPLICATIONS

- Five screws broken during insertion that were stabilized with an additional screw outside the plate without requiring healing delay or regimen change
- Five hardware removals for symptomatic hardware
- The primary author had five varus overcorrections:
  - Four of less than 8 degrees; the patients are completely satisfied and asymptomatic.
  - One of 15 degrees varus, which has been revised with follow-up pending.
- The primary author had two cases of recurrence
  - One due to capsule repair laxity, but the patient is satisfied with a 15-degree HVA.
  - The other recurrence was due to technical error. The first MTC joint was penetrated, leading to instability that required a Lapidus procedure.

REFERENCES

1. Coughlin MJ. Juvenile hallux valgus. In: Coughlin MJ, Mann RA, eds. Surgery of the Foot and Ankle, ed 7. St. Louis, MO: CV Mosby, 1999:270–319.
2. Coughlin MJ, Carlson RE. Treatment of hallux valgus with an increased distal metatarsal articular angle: Evaluation of double and triple first ray osteotomies. Foot Ankle Int 1999;20:762–770.
3. Coughlin MJ, Shurnas PS. Hallux rigidus: Demographics, etiology, and radiographic assessment. Foot Ankle Int 2003;24:731–743.
4. Cooper MT, Berlet GC, Shurnas PS, et al. Proximal opening-wedge osteotomy of the first metatarsal for correction of hallux valgus. Surg Technol Int 2007;16:215–219.
5. Hardy RH, Clapham JCR. Observations on hallux valgus. J Bone Joint Surg 1951;33:376.
6. Mann RA, Coughlin MJ. Adult hallux valgus. In: Coughlin MJ, Mann RA, eds. Surgery of the Foot and Ankle, ed 7. St. Louis, MO: CV Mosby, 1999:150–269.
7. Sargas NP. Proximal opening wedge osteotomy of the first metatarsal for hallux valgus using a low profile plate. Foot Ankle Int 2009;30:976–980.
8. Shereff MJ, Yang QM, Kummer FJ. Extraosseous and intraosseous arterial supply to the first metatarsal and metatarsophalangeal joint. Foot Ankle Int 1987;8:81–93.
9. Shurnas PS. Proximal opening wedge osteotomy of the 1st metatarsal: biomechanical and clinical evaluation. Proceedings of the AAOS Annual Meeting, Chicago, March 22–26, 2006.
10. Shurnas PS, Watson TS, Crislip TW. Proximal first metatarsal opening wedge osteotomy with a low profile plate. Foot Ankle Int 2009;30:865–872.
11. Wukich DK, Roussel AJ, Dial D. Opening wedge osteotomy of the first metatarsal base: A technique for correction of metatarsus primus varus using a new titanium opening wedge plate. Oper Tech Orthop 2006;16:76–81.

Chapter 14 Lapidus Procedure

Ian L. D. Le and Sigvard T. Hansen, Jr.

DEFINITION

- Paul W. Lapidus originally described a procedure for the correction of hallux valgus in 1934.
- This procedure was founded on the premise that hallux valgus was a secondary phenomenon to metatarsus primus varus arising from first tarsometatarsal (TMT) hypermobility and a medially oriented first TMT joint.
- The original Lapidus procedure entailed excision of the lateral aspect of the medial cuneiform and first TMT arthrodesis coupled with a distal first metatarsophalangeal (MTP) capsulorrhaphy.
- Many modifications of the original Lapidus procedure have been made, primarily advocating rigid internal fixation as a means for maintenance of reduction, lower nonunion rates, and earlier healing and mobilization.

ANATOMY

- The goal of foot surgery is to obtain a plantigrade position with normal underlying mechanical alignment to allow for weight bearing, shock absorption, accommodation, and power for efficient painless gait.
- Weight should be evenly distributed across the six weight-bearing surfaces, consisting of the paired sesamoids underlying the first metatarsal head, the lesser metatarsals, and the calcaneus.
- The lateral column of the foot is designed for mobility to accommodate to uneven surfaces while the medial column, including the first TMT joint, is more rigid to allow efficient power for push-off.
- The first TMT joint is typically 30 mm deep.

PATHOGENESIS

- Equinus is often an underlying pathologic feature predisposing the midfoot to increased repetitive tension and subsequent longitudinal collapse and instability.
- In particular, patients develop first TMT hypermobility potentially in both the axial and sagittal planes.
- Axial instability presents as metatarsus primus varus and resultant hallux valgus.
- Sagittal instability presents as a dorsiflexed first metatarsal with predisposition to dorsolateral peritalar subluxation.
- Furthermore, many patients have a medially oriented first TMT joint and tendency toward metatarsus primus varus.

NATURAL HISTORY

- Symptomatic hallux valgus associated with metatarsus primus varus with underlying first TMT hypermobility and equinus presents with progressive deformity and pain.
- In the face of underlying pathologic first TMT hypermobility or equinus, the hallux valgus deformity will inevitably progress over time in both symptomatology and degree of deformity.
- Consequently, it is imperative to treat any underlying pathology concomitantly with treatment of the hallux valgus deformity.

PATIENT HISTORY AND PHYSICAL FINDINGS

- Physical examination methods include:
  - First TMT hypermobility. The examiner rests the index and middle finger of one hand over the dorsal aspect of the first TMT joint to monitor motion. The thumb of that hand rests under the lesser metatarsals. The other hand grasps the first metatarsal between the thumb and fingers and moves it up and down and side to side. Minimal motion should be palpated at this joint. Excessive motion or translation is pathologic and indicative of first TMT hypermobility and instability. Occasionally intercuneiform instability is noted.
  - Equinus/Silfverskiöld test. The examiner corrects the hindfoot to neutral subtalar position and checks dorsiflexion range of motion both with the knee in straight extension and flexed 30 degrees. The forefoot appears wide and splayed with a narrow hindfoot. An inability to obtain neutral dorsiflexion with the knee in straight extension that corrects with flexion is indicative of isolated gastrocnemius equinus. An inability to obtain neutral dorsiflexion in both knee extension and flexion is indicative of soleus and gastrocnemius equinus.
  - First MTP range of motion. The examiner assesses flexion and extension of the first MTP and repeats the test with the first metatarsal held in a corrected position out of varus. Loss of significant range of motion in a corrected position is indicative of loss of congruency at the MTP joint. Consideration may be needed for additional distal metatarsal osteotomy.
  - Lesser metatarsalgia. With hypermobility of the first TMT joint, the first metatarsal is relatively elevated compared to the adjacent lesser metatarsals, resulting in pain and callosities. Callosities are seen beneath the lesser metatarsals, and the skin under the first metatarsal head is often soft from lack of weight bearing. Claw toes and extensor recruitment can result in distal migration of the plantar forefoot fat pad, exacerbating lesser metatarsalgia.

IMAGING AND OTHER DIAGNOSTIC STUDIES

- Plain weight-bearing radiographs including AP, lateral, and oblique views of the foot should be obtained. Every effort should be made to obtain a true lateral radiograph with talar dome overlap.
- Features of first TMT hypermobility
  - Signs of second and third metatarsal overload (hypertrophied cortical thickening, stress fracture)
  - Dorsal translation or dorsiflexion of first metatarsal
  - Plantar widening at the first TMT joint

- First, second, third TMT arthrosis
- First MTP dorsal osteophytes
- Occasionally plain radiographs of the ankle are needed to rule out adjacent involvement.
- Axial sesamoid view can be helpful to assess the extent of metatarsosesamoid arthrosis and degree of sesamoid subluxation.
- Full-length hip-to-ankle radiographs are obtained if there is suspicion of an underlying lower extremity malalignment.
- Seldom is a CT scan, MRI, or other imaging modality needed.

DIFFERENTIAL DIAGNOSIS

- Hallux rigidus
- Metatarsosesamoid arthrosis
- Lesser metatarsalgia
- Interdigital neuroma
- Gout or other inflammatory arthropathy

NONOPERATIVE MANAGEMENT

- Many patients with hallux valgus and hypermobility of the first TMT joint are asymptomatic.
- However, once symptoms develop, progression is inevitable, in particular in patients with underlying equinus contractures.
- Initially management can be directed at resolving local symptoms, including nonsteroidal anti-inflammatories, activity modification, rest, weight loss, shoe modifications, and orthotics.
- In patients with equinus, a well-directed physiotherapy stretching protocol can be helpful.

SURGICAL MANAGEMENT

- Indications
  - Hallux valgus with associated metatarsus primus varus and first TMT hypermobility
  - Hallux valgus with first TMT arthrosis
  - Revision of failed hallux valgus surgery
- Contraindication
  - Open physeal growth plates

Preoperative Planning

- AP foot plain radiographs are reviewed for:
  - Hallux valgus angle (normal less than 15 degrees)
  - Intermetatarsal angle (normal less than 9 degrees)
  - Angle of first TMT joint
  - Proximal phalangeal articular angle (normal less than 10 degrees)
  - Degree of sesamoid subluxation
  - Relative lengths of metatarsal heads
- Lateral foot plain radiographs are reviewed for:
  - Talar first metatarsal angle
- Based on the above, the surgeon formulates an operative plan, including:
  - Degree of correction
  - Need to excise lateral wedge from medial cuneiform
  - Need for concomitant second or third metatarsal shortening
- Intraoperatively the surgeon assesses for equinus and the need for percutaneous Achilles tendon lengthening or gastrocnemius slide.

Positioning

- The patient is placed supine on a radiolucent table with a padded wedge or bump under the ipsilateral hip to correct external rotation.
- The arm is placed across the chest and the ulnar nerve is padded.
- A tourniquet is applied to the thigh proximal enough to allow access to the proximal tibia for possible bone graft.
- Once the limb is prepared and draped, a towel bump is placed beneath the knee to allow access to the dorsum of the foot.

TECHNIQUES

CORRECTION OF METATARSUS PRIMUS VARUS AND PREPARATION OF FIRST TARSOMETATARSAL JOINT

- Make an incision about 8 cm long between the extensor hallucis longus and brevis, roughly in line with the lateral aspect of the first metatarsal and medial cuneiform (**TECH FIG 1A, B**).
- Protect the deep peroneal nerve, dorsalis pedis artery, and dorsal cutaneous nerves.
- Identify the first TMT joint by moving the first metatarsal, and reflect the capsule sharply off bone using the Henry angle of dissection.
- Using a quarter-inch osteotome, remove the dorsal osteophytes over the first TMT joint and save them for bone graft.
- At this point, the joint is prepared in one of two ways:
  - If there is a need to correct a medially angled first TMT joint, use an oscillating saw. First insert an elevator to determine the slope of the joint. Resect a lateral wedge of bone from the medial cuneiform. Remove the piece and check it to ensure that adequate plantar bone was removed. Resect a minimal amount of bone from the first metatarsal base, again ensuring that enough plantar bone is removed. Avoid excessive metatarsal shortening.
  - If there is no medially angled first TMT joint or if there is an excessively short first metatarsal, then prepare the joint using a series of curved osteotomes and curettes. This will give two congruent opposing surfaces for arthrodesis.
- Use an oblong curette to ensure there is no residual plantar lip resulting in excessive dorsiflexion. The first TMT joint is 28 to 30 mm deep.
- Drill each side of the joint with a 2.0-mm drill (**TECH FIG 1C**).
- This should leave a lateral gap in the first TMT joint.

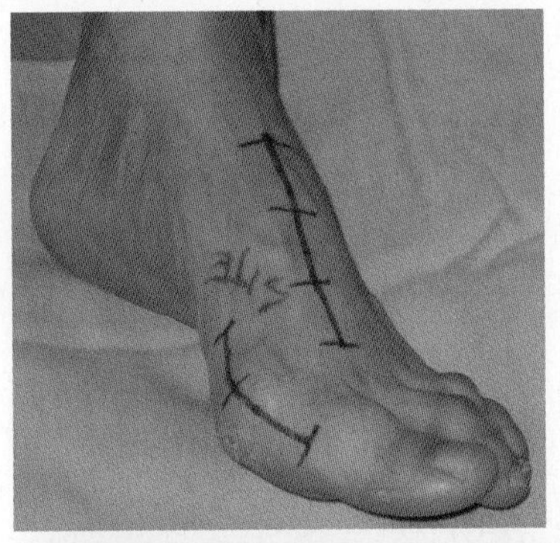

A

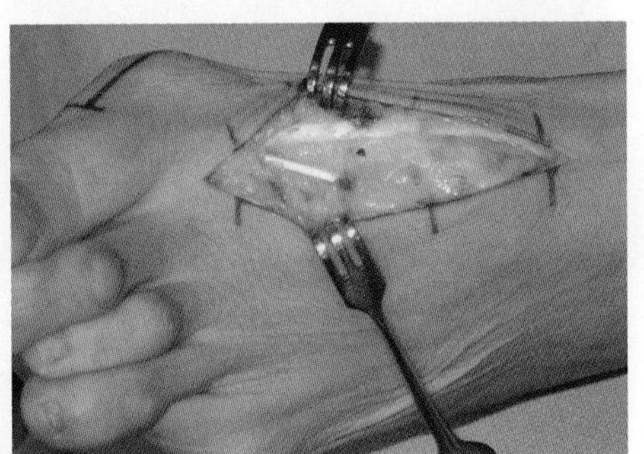

B

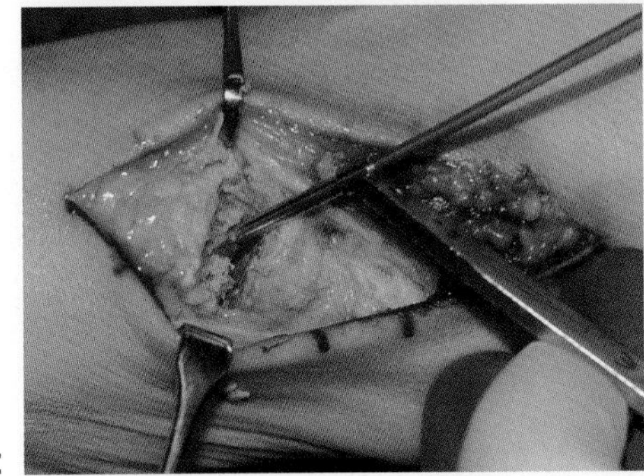

C

TECH FIG 1 • **A.** Planned incisions. **B.** Step 1, incision between extensor hallucis longus and extensor hallucis brevis. **C.** Step 1, joint preparation.

DISTAL SOFT TISSUE PROCEDURE

- Extend the dorsal incision down to the first web space, taking care to avoid the digital nerves.
- Deep to the attenuated intermetatarsal ligament is the fibular sesamoid and adductor hallucis tendon; leave it intact.
- Protect the fibular sesamoid, identify the first MTP capsule, and incise it longitudinally (TECH FIG 2).
- Make a separate medial incision over the first MTP joint, again watching for the crossing dorsal cutaneous nerves.
- Develop a flap superficial to the first MTP capsule, taking care to avoid thinning the capsule itself.
- Sharply incise the capsule full thickness longitudinally and reflect it plantar and dorsal.
- Tease back the capsular reflections to the first metatarsal head proximally to release the scarred synechiae and allow the sesamoid to move independently.
- Grasp the plantar capsule with a Kocher. With gentle pressure, the metatarsal head should be easily reducible over the sesamoids while simultaneously correcting the intermetatarsal angle and closing the gap at the first TMT joint.
- Resect a minimal amount of medial eminence with a rongeur to allow shaping of the medial metatarsal head into a rounded surface.

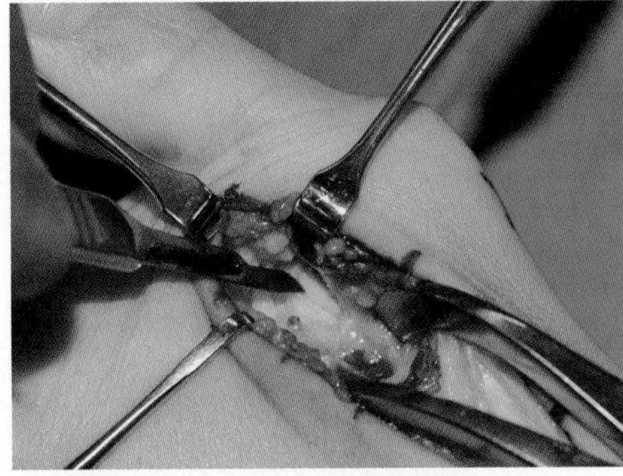

TECH FIG 2 • Step 2, distal soft tissue release.

STABILIZATION

- Before stabilization, hold the foot in a reduced position and palpate the forefoot to ensure it is plantigrade.
- Temporary Kirschner wires may be helpful if assistance is unavailable.
- Burr a bone trough in the mid-dorsal aspect of the first metatarsal about 2 cm away from the joint and tapering out distally.
- Place a 4.0-mm screw after drilling in a lag screw fashion with a 4.0-mm and then a 2.9-mm drill (TECH FIG 3).
- Place a second 4.0-mm lag screw from the dorsal medial cuneiform to the plantar aspect of the first metatarsal base.
- Stabilize this construct by placing a last 4.0-mm screw from the first metatarsal into the base of the second metatarsal.
- Drill this last screw in a lag manner but avoid excessive tightening to prevent overcorrection of the intermetatarsal angle.

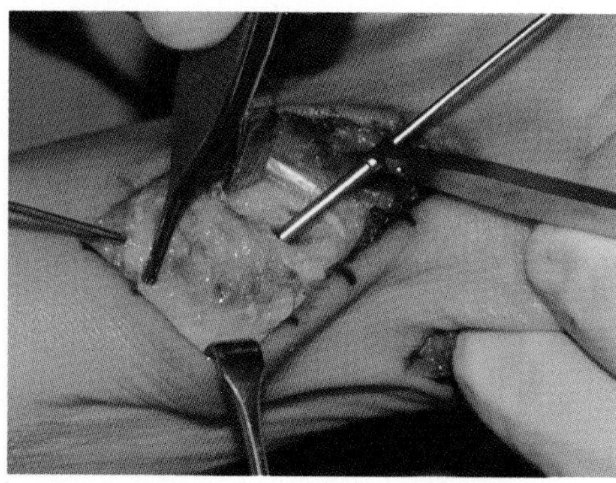

TECH FIG 3 • Step 3, fixation.

BONE GRAFTING

- Use a 5.0-mm burr to create two small troughs on the dorsomedial and dorsolateral aspects of the first TMT joint to serve as sites for shear-strain-relieving bone graft (**TECH FIG 4A, B**).
- Also place bone graft in any gaps at the arthrodesis site.
- Bone graft is obtained from the local procedure or proximal tibial bone graft.

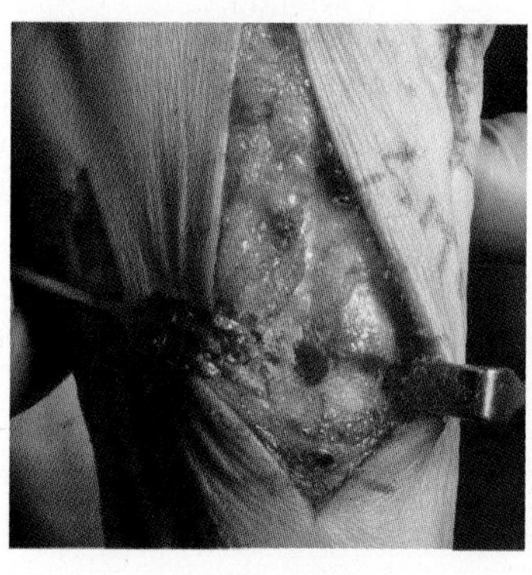

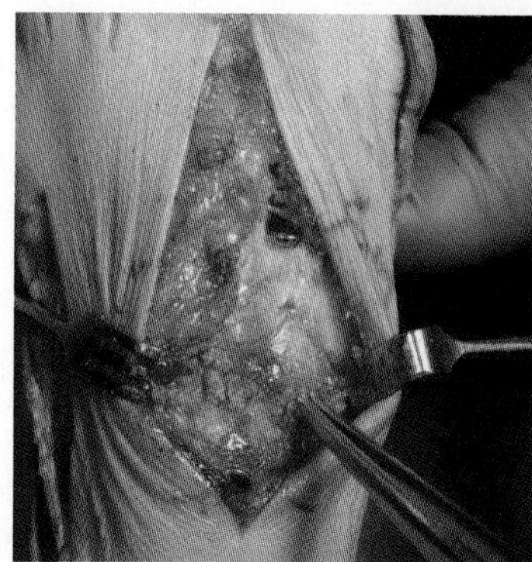

TECH FIG 4 • **A.** Step 4, bone graft trough. **B.** Step 4, shear strain relieving bone graft.

INTRAOPERATIVE RADIOGRAPHS

- Obtain AP, lateral, and oblique films to ensure appropriate positioning and correction, which is often not seen in detail under C-arm fluoroscopy (**TECH FIG 5A, B**).

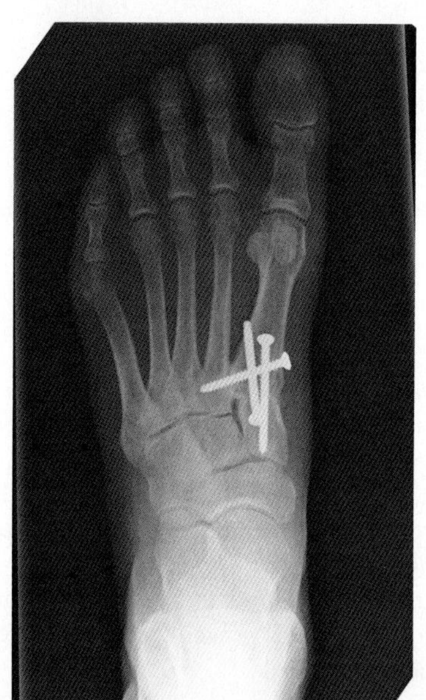

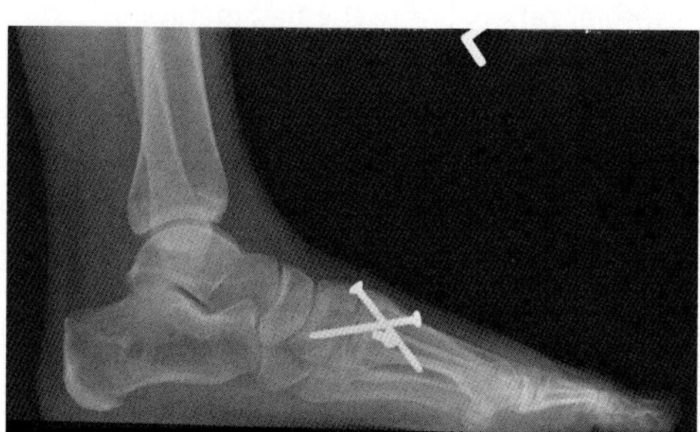

TECH FIG 5 • **A.** Final AP radiograph. **B.** Final lateral radiograph.

TECHNIQUES

WOUND CLOSURE

- Plicate the medial first MTP capsule. Excessive capsule may be excised if redundant.
- It should not be necessary to overtighten the capsule to correct the hallux valgus.
- Close the remaining incisions in layers.

ADDITIONAL PROCEDURES TO CONSIDER

- Gastrocnemius slide or percutaneous Achilles tendon lengthening
  - Persistent equinus and forefoot overload
- Akin osteotomy
  - Presence of associated hallux valgus interphalangeus
- Second or third metatarsal shortening
  - Loss of metatarsal head parabola
  - Particularly problematic in patients wearing high-heeled shoes

PEARLS AND PITFALLS

Persistent dorsiflexed first metatarsal or lesser metatarsalgia	▪ Failure to resect plantar aspect of the first TMT joint
Nonunion	▪ Inadequate joint preparation or inadequate fixation, lack of bone graft
Hallux varus	▪ Overcorrection of intermetatarsal angle ▪ Release of adductor hallucis tendon

POSTOPERATIVE CARE

- A well-molded below-knee plaster cast is applied with a single anterior univalve to accommodate postoperative swelling.
- The cast is overwrapped with fiberglass before discharge.
- Analgesia is best managed with a popliteal peripheral nerve catheter.
- Six weeks of heel weight bearing in static stance phase only is prescribed.
- The patient is mobilized on a knee scooter.
- Progressive weight bearing is allowed between 6 to 12 weeks in a removable boot.
- The patient is weaned out of the removable boot into standard shoes at 12 weeks.

OUTCOMES

- With appropriate surgical indications, surgical technique, and patient compliance, the patient satisfaction rate is greater than 90%.
- Recurrence of hallux valgus is rare.

COMPLICATIONS

- See the Pitfalls section.

REFERENCES

1. Bendnarz PA, Manoli A. Modifed Lapidus procedure for the treatment of hypermobile hallux valgus. Foot Ankle Int 2000;21:816–821.
2. Coetzee JC, Wickum D. The Lapidus procedure: a prospective cohort outcome. Foot Ankle Int 2004;25:526–531.
3. Hansen ST. Hallux valgus surgery: Morton and Lapidus were right. Clin Podiatr Med Surg 1996;13:347–354.
4. Lapidus PW. The author's bunion operation from 1931 to 1959. Clin Orthop 1960;12:119–135.
5. Morton DJ. The Human Foot. Morningside Heights, NY: Columbia University Press.
6. Morton DJ. Evolution of the longitudinal arch of the human foot. J Bone Joint Surg 1924;22:56–90.
7. Sangeorzan BJ, Hansen ST Jr. Modified Lapidus procedure for hallux valgus. Foot Ankle Int 1989;9:262–266.

Chapter 15

Revision Hallux Valgus Correction

J. Chris Coetzee, Patrick Ebeling, and Mark E. Easley

DEFINITION

- Recurrent hallux valgus is a partial or complete return of valgus deformity at the first metatarsophalangeal (MTP) joint after surgical correction.
- Metatarsus primus varus is an increase in the first–second intermetatarsal angle due to obliquity or hypermobility of the first tarsometatarsal joint.

ANATOMY

- The first tarsometatarsal joint is 27 to 30 mm deep and irregularly shaped (**FIG 1**).
- The dorsalis pedis artery and deep peroneal nerve are just lateral to the extensor hallucis longus tendon (**FIG 2**).
- The two heads of the adductor hallucis muscle converge to a single tendon and insert on the lateral sesamoid at the first MTP joint.
- The sesamoids are contained in the capsuloligamentous complex of the MTP joint.
- The dorsal medial cutaneous branch of the superficial peroneal nerve runs along the dorsal medial aspect of the first MTP joint.
- The plantar medial cutaneous branches of the medial plantar nerve run along the plantar aspect of the first MTP joint near the articulations of the sesamoids.

PATHOGENESIS

- Recurrence of hallux valgus is most often due to an improperly chosen initial procedure or improper surgical technique.
- Less frequently, factors such as poor bone or tissue quality, infection, patient noncompliance, and instrumentation failure can lead to recurrent hallux valgus.
- A major cause of recurrent hallux valgus is unrecognized metatarsus primus varus.
- If uncorrected, metatarsus primus varus creates a valgus moment at the first MTP joint.
- An intact adductor hallucis or a tight lateral joint capsule will exacerbate the valgus moment.

NATURAL HISTORY

- Some partial recurrences of hallux valgus may be tolerable with nonoperative treatment.
- If there is an uncorrected metatarsus primus varus, the deformity will most likely progress over time.
- The medial prominence can result in pain, tenderness, and an overlying bursitis.
- Progressive deformity often leads to second toe overload and, ultimately, to arthritis at both the first and second tarsometatarsal joints.
- Lesser metatarsal overload, whether due to shortening of the first metatarsal or subluxation of the sesamoids, is a common reason for secondary surgery.
- Arthritis can develop at the sesamoid–first metatarsal articulations.
- Prolonged hallux valgus, especially with an incongruent joint, can lead to degenerative changes at the first MTP joint.

PATIENT HISTORY AND PHYSICAL FINDINGS

- Patients report valgus deformity at the first MTP joint that either is recurrent or was never fully corrected (**FIG 3**).
- The examiner should evaluate for symptoms associated with metatarsus primus varus:
  - Hypermobility of the first tarsometatarsal joint
    - Mobility of the first tarsometatarsal joint is tested by holding the lesser metatarsal heads stable with one hand while passively dorsiflexing the first metatarsal head.

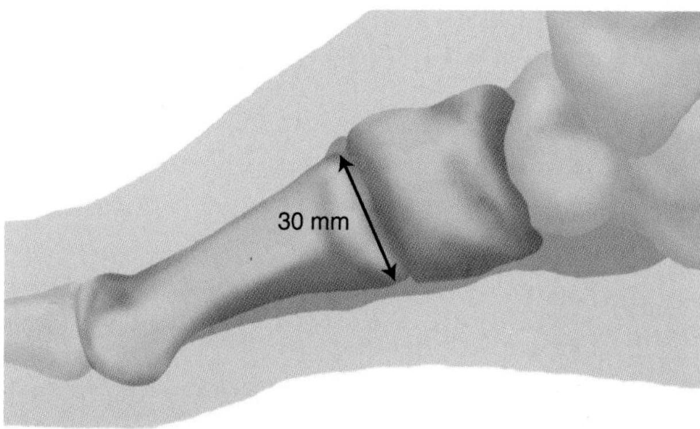

FIG 1 • Lateral view of the first tarsometatarsal joint. The joint is an average of 30 mm deep.

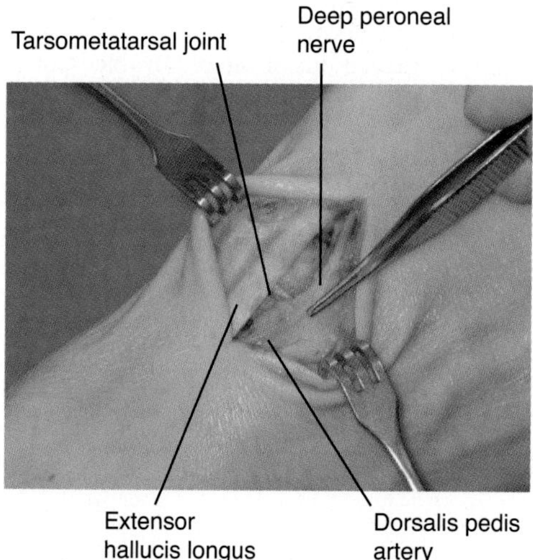

FIG 2 • The extensor hallucis longus over the tarsometatarsal joint. The dorsalis pedis and deep peroneal nerve are just lateral to the tendon.

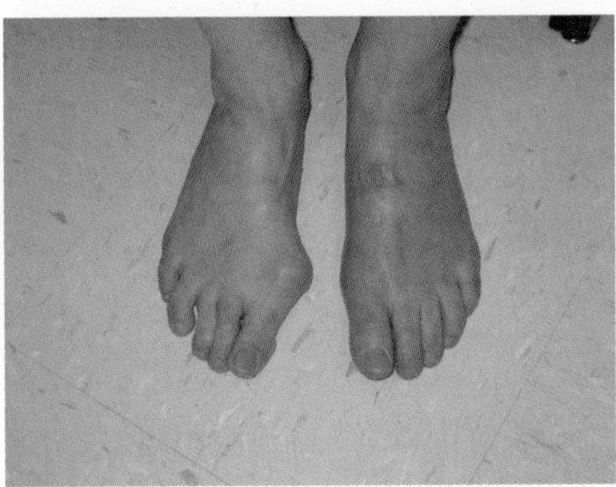

FIG 3 • Picture after previous bilateral distal bunion procedures. The left side is 6 months after revision with a Lapidus procedure and the right side is preoperative.

- Hypermobility has been defined as elevation of the first metatarsal head more than 5 to 8 mm above the level of the second metatarsal head (**FIG 4**).
- Hypermobility at the tarsometatarsal joint creates a valgus moment at the MTP joint, which may contribute to failure of distal hallux valgus correction.
- Degenerative changes at the first tarsometatarsal joint
  - Tenderness at the joint line
  - Osteophytes at the dorsal aspect of the joint
- Second metatarsal overload
  - Patients may report feeling as if there is a rock in their shoe.
  - Tenderness under the second MTP joint

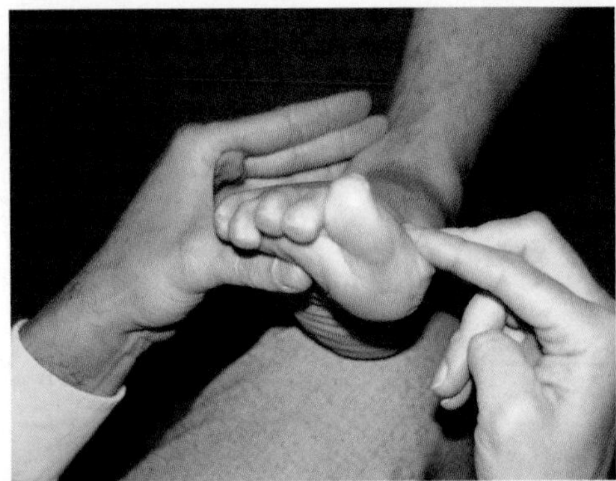

A

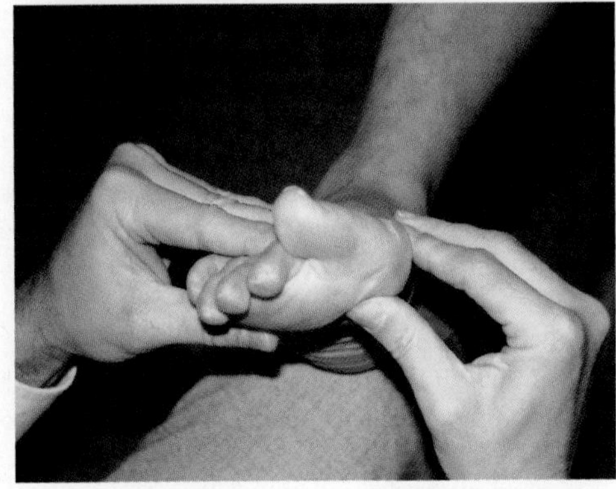

B

FIG 4 • First tarsometatarsal hypermobility.

  - Callosity or ulceration under the second MTP joint
  - Claw toe deformity[3] (**FIG 5**)
- Passive correction of the metatarsus primus varus may reduce the hallux valgus deformity.
- The examiner should check for lesser toe overload.
  - The medial lesser toes should be inspected for claw toe or hammer toe deformity, overlap, large plantar callus, or plantar ulcers. The plantar surface of the MTP joints is palpated for tenderness. The proximal phalanx is translated to evaluate for instability of the MTP joint.
  - Lesser toe overload is often associated with hypermobility of the first tarsometatarsal joint or a dorsiflexion deformity of the first ray.
- Range of motion of the first MTP joint with the hallux valgus deformity corrected is an indication of expected motion after surgical correction. Severely limited motion may be an indication for a fusion of the MTP joint.
- In general, the more severe the deformity, the greater the pronation of first MTP joint on weight bearing.[5]
- Patients are evaluated for other potential causes of the recurrent deformity:
  - Infection
  - Failure of fixation
  - Generalized ligamentous laxity
  - Osteoporosis

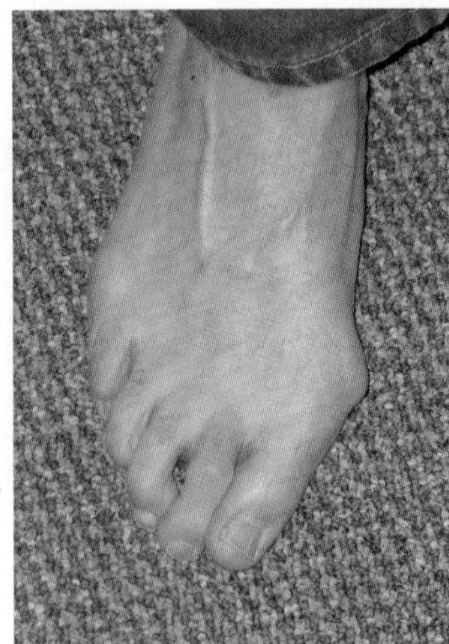

A

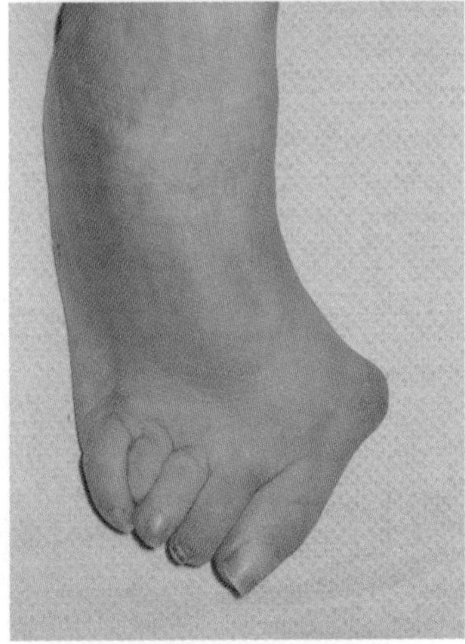

B

FIG 5 • Claw toe deformity.

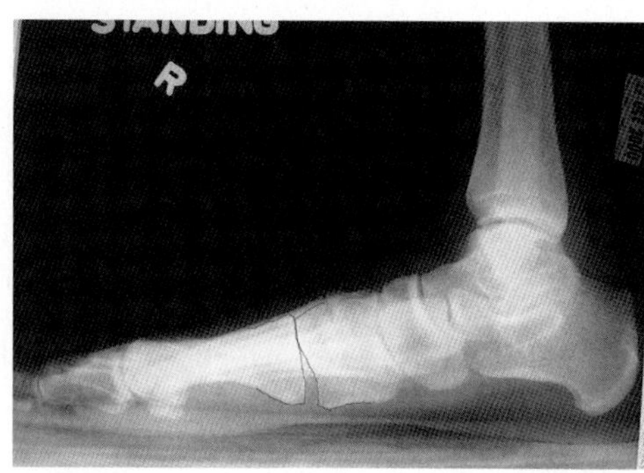

FIG 6 • Plantar gapping of the first tarsometatarsal joint as well as dorsal translation of the first metatarsal on weight-bearing radiographs.

IMAGING AND OTHER DIAGNOSTIC STUDIES

- AP, lateral, and oblique weight-bearing radiographs of the foot should be obtained and evaluated for the following:
  - Surgical changes from the initial surgery, including any retained instrumentation
  - Congruency of first MTP joint
  - Plantarflexion of the first ray
  - Hallux valgus angle
    - Angle between long axes of first metatarsal and proximal phalanx
    - Normal is less than 15 degrees
  - First–second intermetatarsal angle
    - Angle between long axes of first and second metatarsals
    - Normal angle is less than 9 degrees.
  - Distal metatarsal articular angle
    - Angle between long axis of metatarsal shaft and base of distal metatarsal joint surface
    - Normal is less than 15 degrees.
  - Radiologic signs of metatarsus primus varus
    - Increased first–second intermetatarsal angle
    - Plantar gap at first tarsometatarsal joint on weight-bearing lateral image (**FIG 6**).
    - Claw toe deformity

DIFFERENTIAL DIAGNOSIS

- Loss of fixation
- Generalized tissue laxity
- Infection

NONOPERATIVE MANAGEMENT

- Shoe wear modification
  - Wide toe box
  - Low heels
- Orthotics
  - Medial arch support for associated pes planus
  - Metatarsal pad for associated second toe overload
- Activity modification

SURGICAL MANAGEMENT

- It is important to determine what the previous procedure entailed.
- Seldom can a failed distal or shaft procedure be revised with another such procedure.
- Most salvage procedures rely on stabilizing the base of the first metatarsal. It is also possible to get more angular correction at the base of the metatarsal.

Preoperative Planning

- Retained instrumentation may need to be removed.
- The age and position of previous incisions must be taken into account.
- The surgeon must take into account the need for shortening of the lesser metatarsals, correction of claw toes, and the addition of an Akin phalangeal osteotomy to correct concurrent deformities.

Positioning

- The patient is positioned supine.
- A tourniquet is placed on the proximal thigh.
- The foot should be positioned to allow access for intraoperative imaging.

Approach

- The approach depends on the procedure to be performed.

TECHNIQUES

EXAMPLE CASE (Courtesy of Mark E. Easley, MD)

Background

- Thirty-three year old woman post distal bunion correction (details unknown).
  - Persistent symptomatic hallux valgus deformity (**TECH FIG 1A**)
  - Has failed nonoperative management of this problem
  - Motion well preserved in first MTP joint
  - Overload phenomenon second metatarsal head but no deformity in second toe
- Radiographs (**TECH FIG 1B,C**)
  - Prior distal procedure to first metatarsal head
  - Increased 1–2 intermetatarsal angle
  - Increased hallux valgus angle
  - Questionnable increase in the distal metatarsal articular angle
  - Relatively short first metatarsal compared to second metatarsal
  - No obvious second toe deformity

Distal Soft Tissue Procedure

- Dorsomedial approach, because that is what was used previously, but extended more proximally to perform the proximal osteotomy.
- Lateral release also performed through a separate first webspace incision
  - This puts the blood supply to the metatarsal head at risk if a simultaneous distal osteotomy is performed
    - Medial and lateral soft tissues released
    - Complete disruption of the intraosseous blood supply to the head

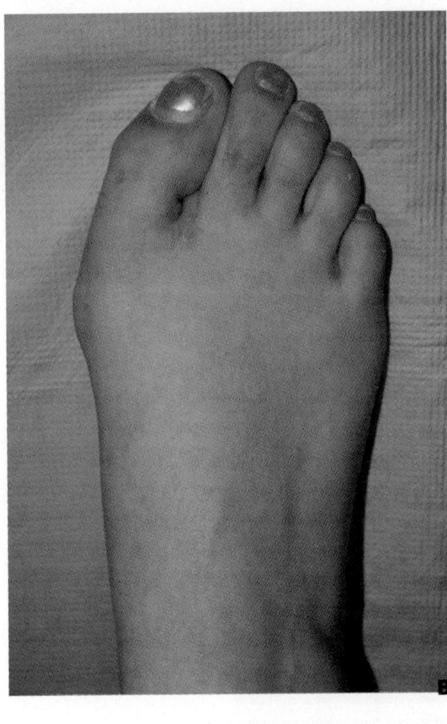

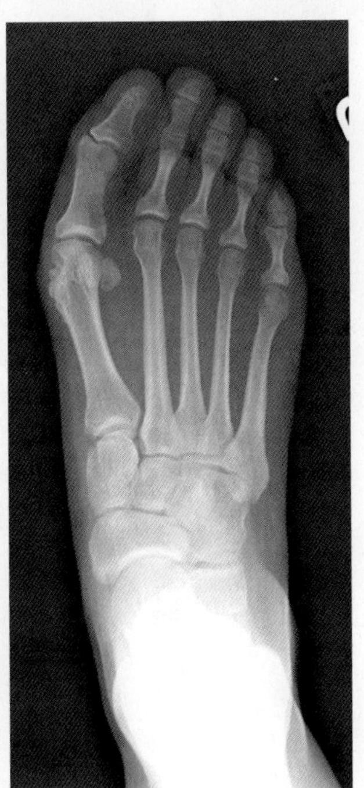

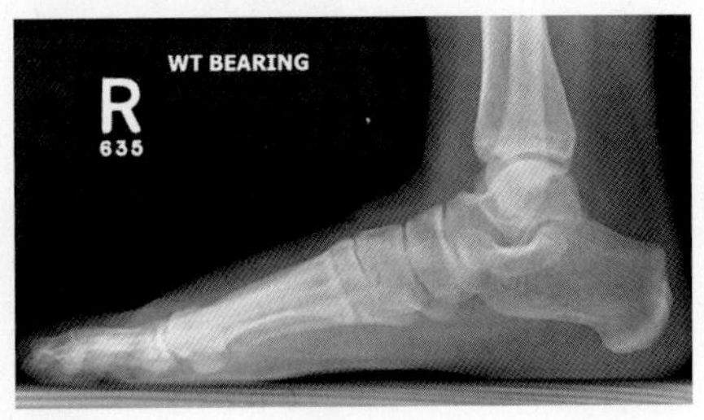

TECH FIG 1 • Preoperative evaluation of 33-year-old woman with failed prior bunion correction. **A.** Clinical view. **B.** AP weight-bearing radiograph. **C.** Lateral weight-bearing foot x-ray.

- Therefore, lateral release must be performed judiciously
  - Distal to the lateral capsule that contains vessels to the metatarsal head
- With the exposure, the actual (not radiographic) distal metatarsal articular angle (DMAA) can be evaluated (**TECH FIG 2**)

Proximal Osteotomy

- In this case, a proximal medial opening wedge osteotomy was performed
  - It may not lengthen the first metatarsal but the risk of shortening is diminished
  - All traditional osteotomies, when they heal, shorten slightly; however, an opening wedged osteotomy may not have that tendency.
  - The goal was to preserve length given that the patient was experiencing a second metatarsal head overload.

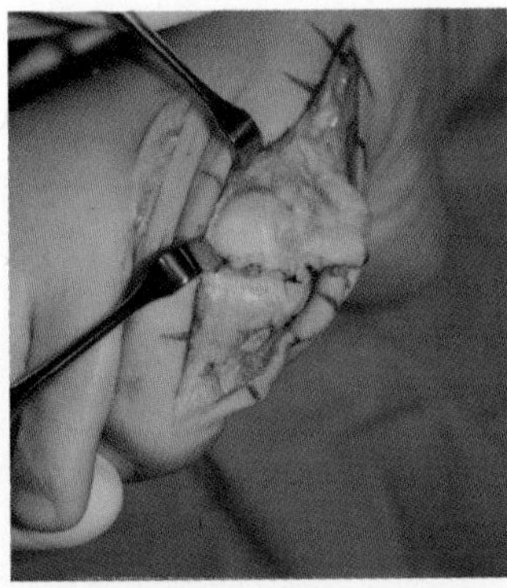

TECH FIG 2 • Suggestion of increased DMAA (metatarsal head oriented laterally relative to first metatarsal shaft). Note lateral release performed through a separate dorsal first webspace incision.

  - Given the the osteotomy is performed from the medial side and the lateral cortex is left intact, it also has less of a tendency to develop a dorsiflexion malunion.
- Fluoroscopy is used to determine the trajectory of the osteotomy and the depth of the saw cut (**TECH FIG 3A**)
- We make the osteotomy in the oblique plane to increase the surface area and target the more proximal aspect of the lateral metatarsal base where the cortex is wider and the soft tissue support is greater (**TECH FIG 3B**)
- The saw cut approaches the lateral cortex without violating it
- The osteotomy is gently opened with a three osteotome technique (**TECH FIG 3C–E**)
- The medial plate with spacer is placed and secured with screws. (**TECH FIG 3F**)
  - One of the proximal screws may be placed across the osteotomy to lend further support to the construct (**TECH FIG 3G**)
- We typically bone graft the osteotomy with bone graft harvested from the lateral calcaneus

Distal Biplanar Chevron Osteotomy

- The proximal osteotomy increases the already greater-than-physiologic DMAA.
- Furthermore, greater correction is warranted in this revision case with considerable hallux valgus deformity
- We check a pin under fluoroscopic guidance to determine the orientation of the osteotomy. (see Tech Fig 3G)
- A distal biplanar chevron osteotomy (Reverdin-Green osteotomy) affords greater correction, satisfactory stability, and a simple means of correcting the increased DMAA (**TECH FIG 4A**).

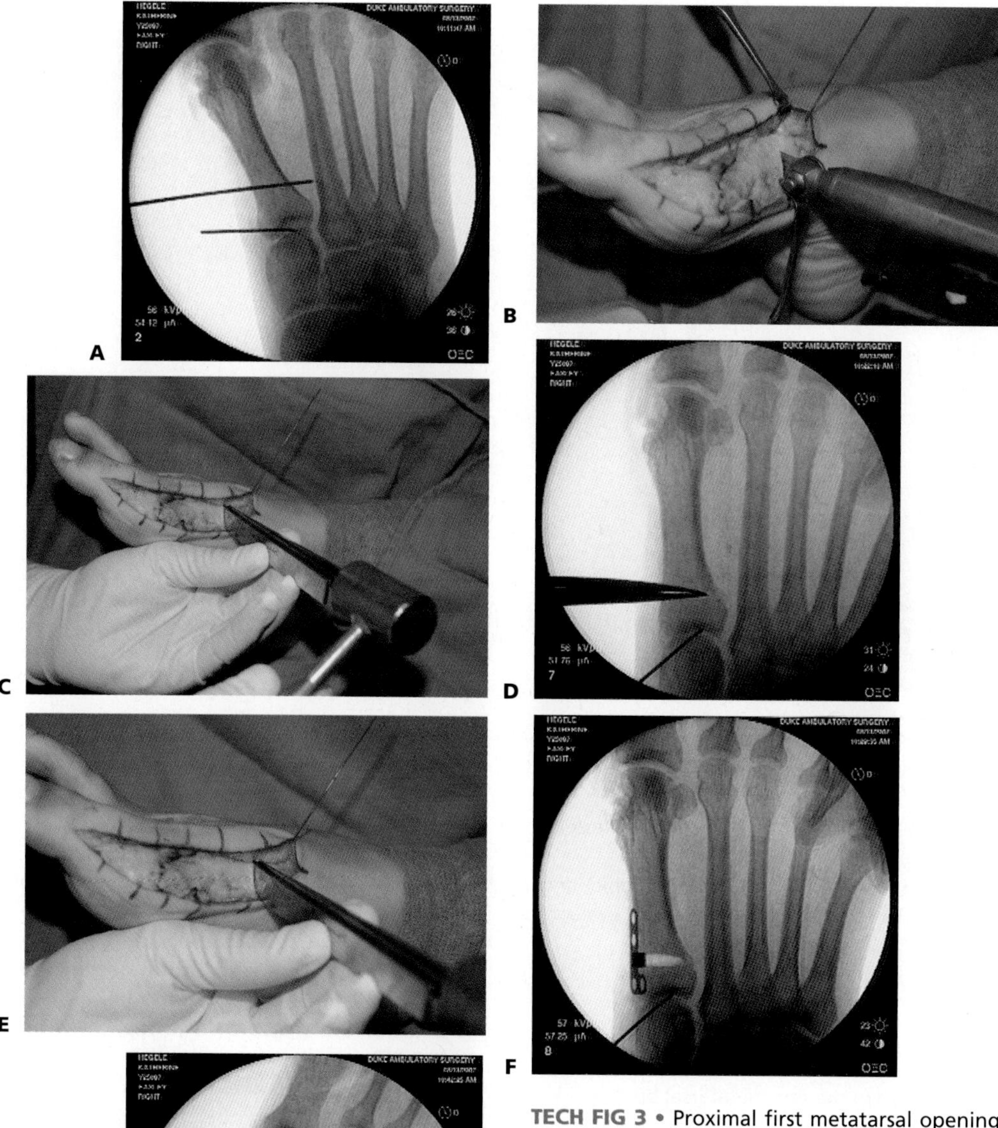

TECH FIG 3 • Proximal first metatarsal opening wedge osteotomy. **A.** Fluoroscopic view of reference pin to guide saw blade trajectory. **B.** Microsagittal saw for osteotomy (note saw blade is perpendicular to metatarsal shaft). **C.** Triple osteotome technique for opening the osteotomy. **D.** Fluoroscopic view of triple osteotomy technique. (Note lateral cortex intact). **E.** Close up of triple osteotome technique. **F.** Initial positioning of medial opening wedge plate. **G.** Reference pin to orient osteotomy. (Note final fixation of proximal osteotomy.)

  - The osteotomy has a long plantar limb the provides large surface area for healing and excellent contact for screw placement (TECH FIG 4B)
  - The short dorsal limb may be modified with a medial closing wedge osteotomy that allows correction of the increased DMAA. (TECH FIG 4C–G)
- We routinely secure this osteotomy with a single screw placed in lag fashion (TECH FIG 4H)
- The medial prominence is resected (TECH FIG 4I)

Akin Osteotomy

- We typically employ an oblique Akin osteotomy (TECH FIG 5A–H)
  - Abundant surface area for healing
  - Screw can be placed from proximal to distal perpendicular to the osteotomy
- Some rotation is still possible to correct the pronation deformity

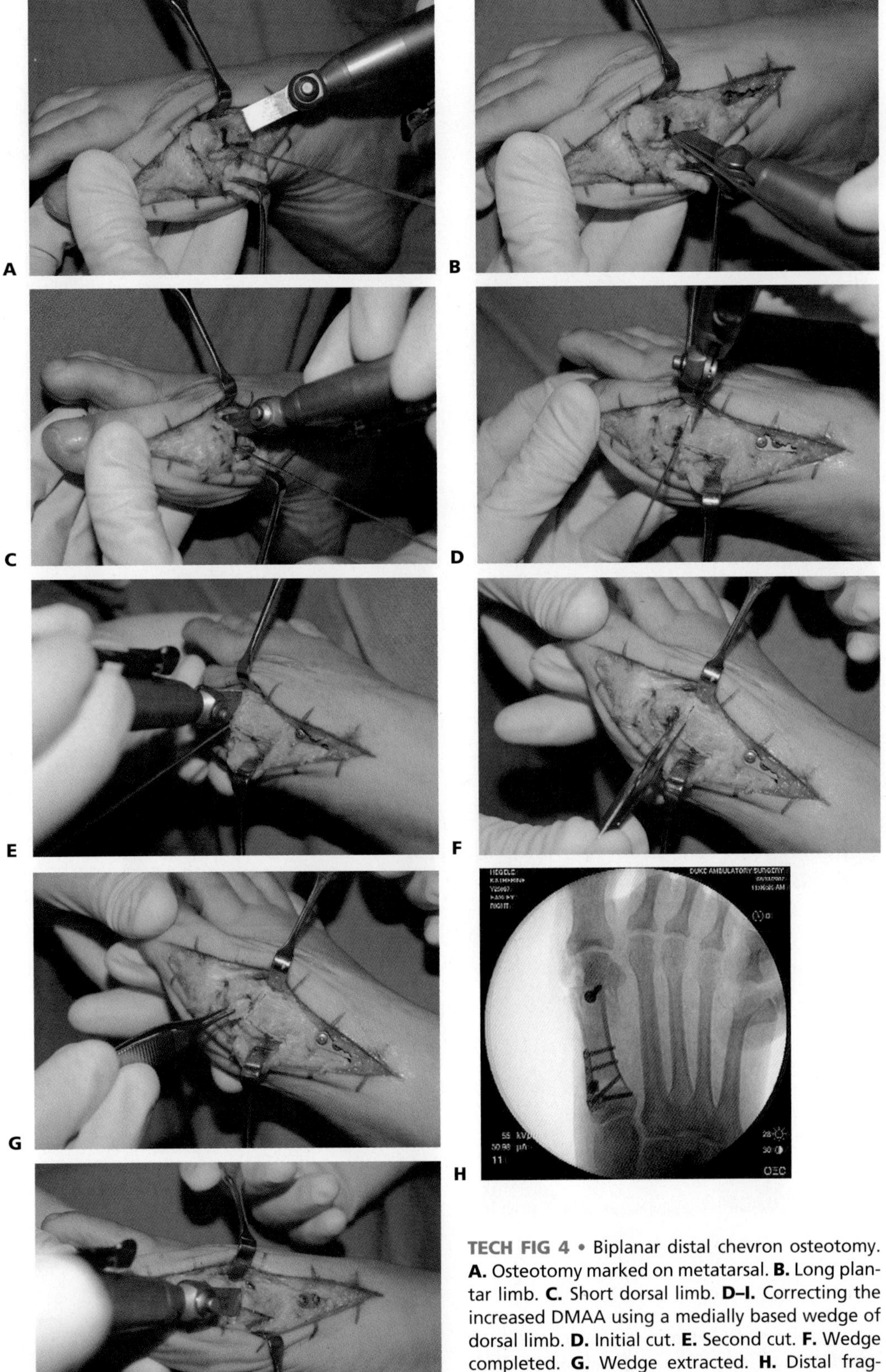

TECH FIG 4 • Biplanar distal chevron osteotomy. **A.** Osteotomy marked on metatarsal. **B.** Long plantar limb. **C.** Short dorsal limb. **D–I.** Correcting the increased DMAA using a medially based wedge of dorsal limb. **D.** Initial cut. **E.** Second cut. **F.** Wedge completed. **G.** Wedge extracted. **H.** Distal fragment translated laterally, oriented properly, and secured with a screw to the proximal fragment. **I.** Medial prominence resected.

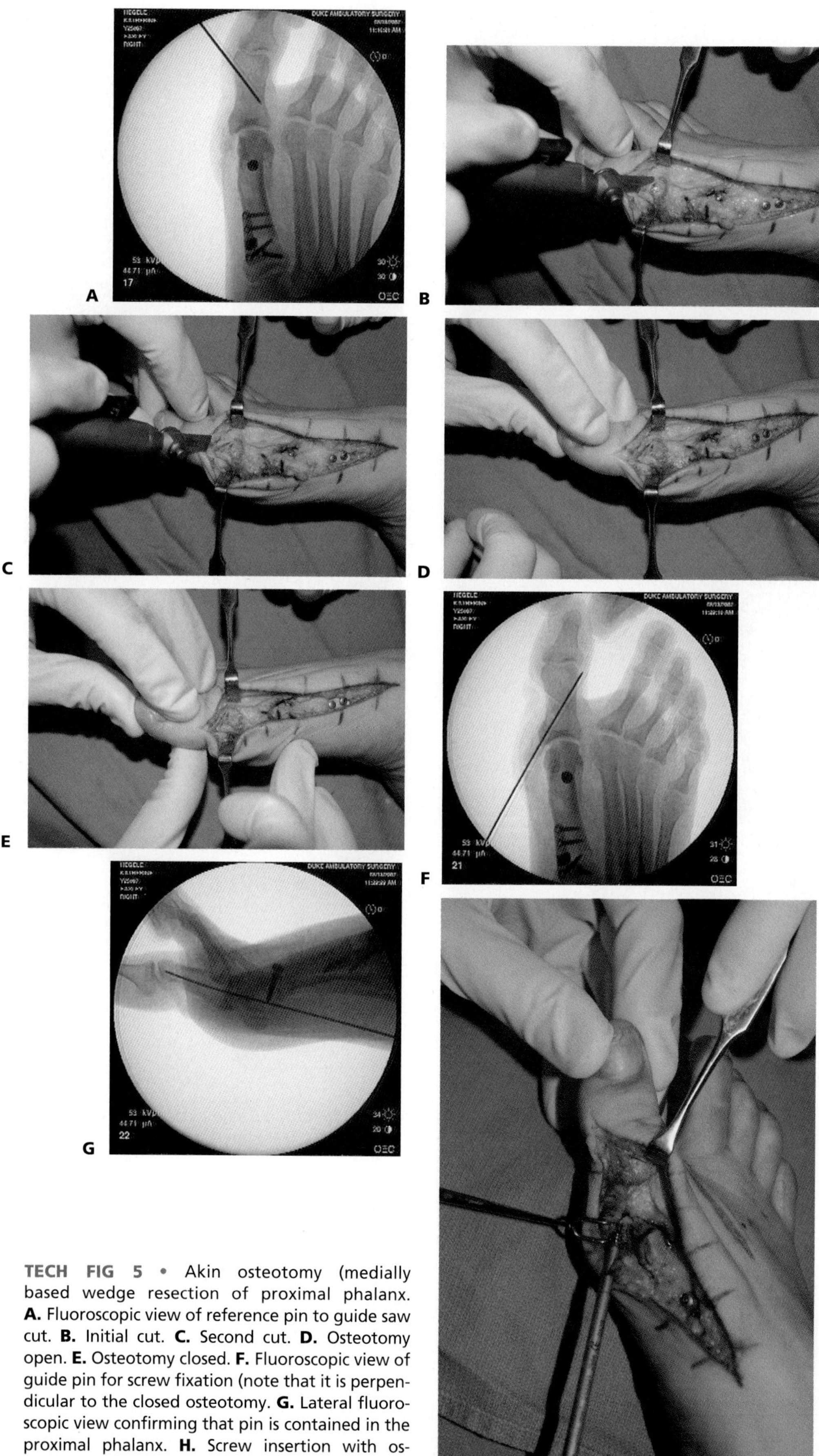

TECH FIG 5 • Akin osteotomy (medially based wedge resection of proximal phalanx. **A.** Fluoroscopic view of reference pin to guide saw cut. **B.** Initial cut. **C.** Second cut. **D.** Osteotomy open. **E.** Osteotomy closed. **F.** Fluoroscopic view of guide pin for screw fixation (note that it is perpendicular to the closed osteotomy. **G.** Lateral fluoroscopic view confirming that pin is contained in the proximal phalanx. **H.** Screw insertion with osteotomy reduced.

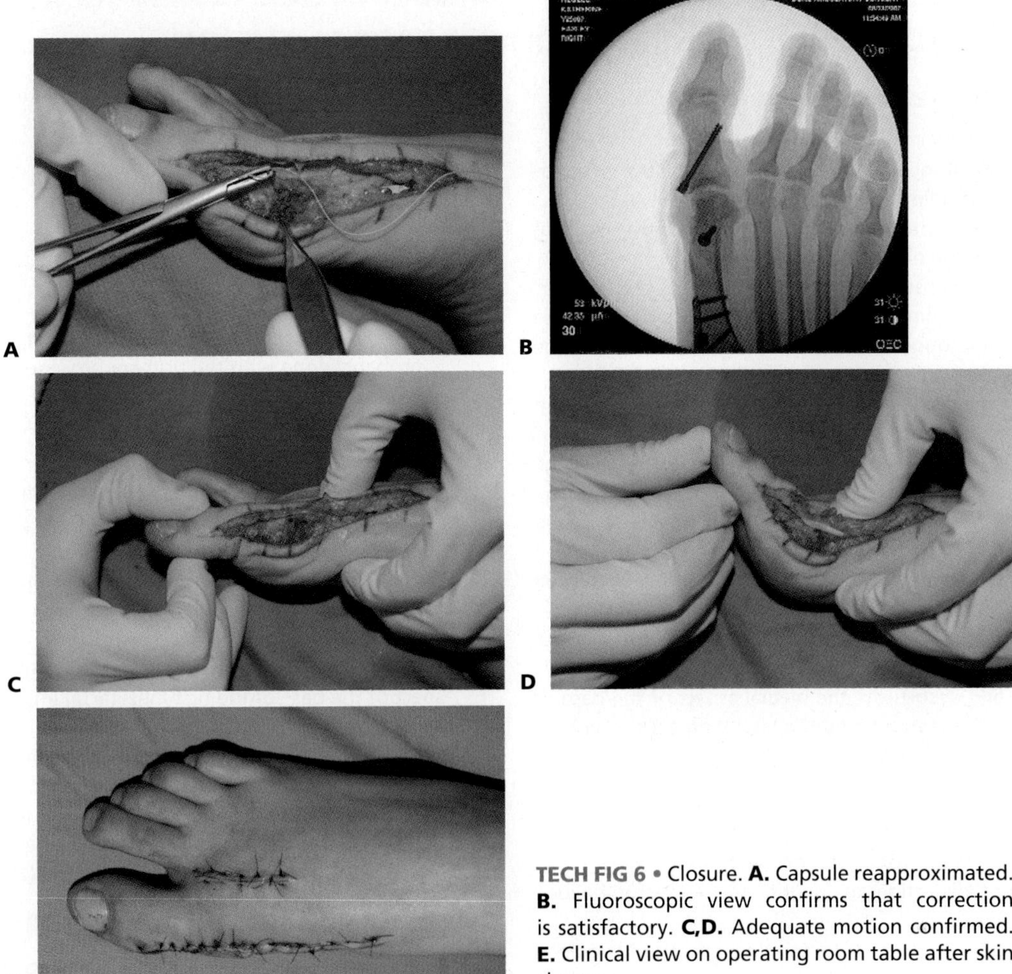

TECH FIG 6 • Closure. **A.** Capsule reapproximated. **B.** Fluoroscopic view confirms that correction is satisfactory. **C,D.** Adequate motion confirmed. **E.** Clinical view on operating room table after skin closure.

Closure

- The capsule is reapproximated (TECH FIG 6A)
- The correction of the axial deformity is achieved with the bony realignment, not the capsular closure (TECH FIG 6B)
  - However, we attempt to correct pronation by suturing the distal plantar capsule to proximal dorsal capsule.
- Motion should be maintained after the capsule is closed (TECH FIG 6C,D).
- Final fluoroscopic images to confirm alignment is appropriate (see Tech Fig 6B)
  - We strive for a slight overcorrection since the tendency is for recurrence, particularly in a revision procedure (TECH FIG 6E; see Tech Fig 6B).
- Postoperative management is the same as for other bunion procedures (TECH FIG 7A–D).

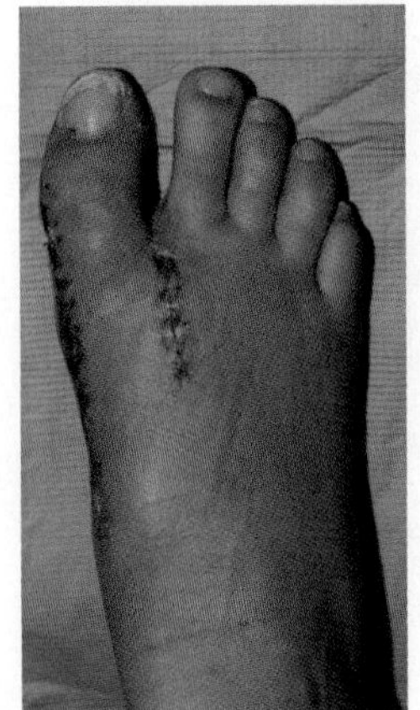

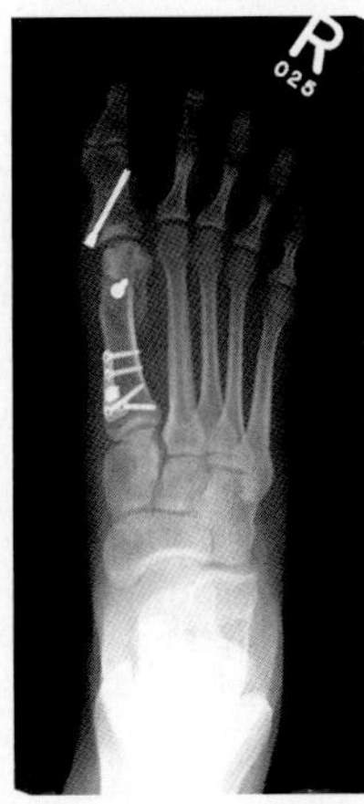

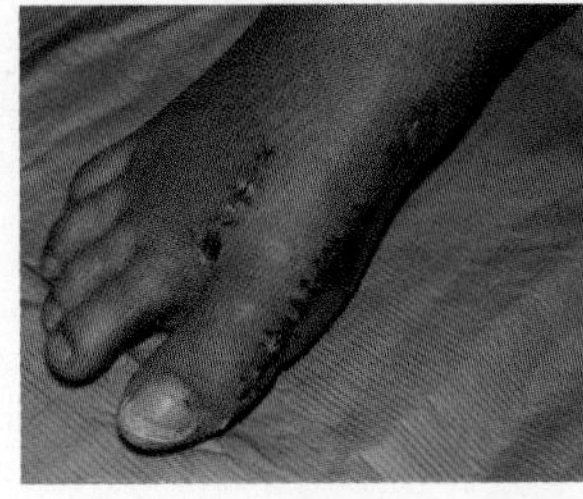

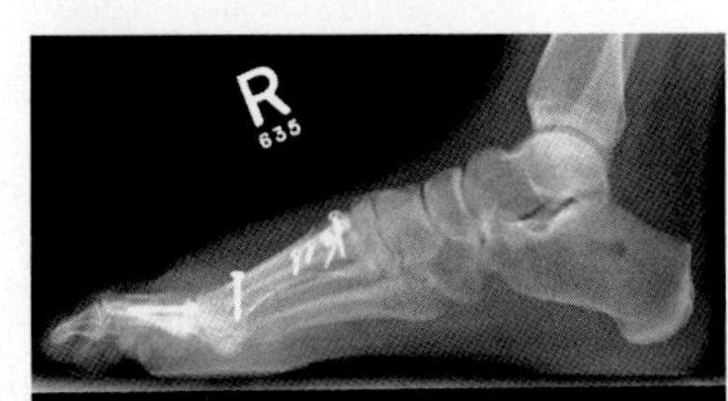

TECH FIG 7 • **A.** Early follow-up clinical view. **B.** Weight-bearing AP foot radiograph. **C.** Another clinical perspective at early follow-up. **D.** Lateral foot radiograph.

LAPIDUS PROCEDURE (FIRST TARSOMETATARSAL FUSION)

First Tarsometatarsal Joint Preparation

- Make a 6-cm incision over the dorsum of the first tarsometatarsal joint.
- Identify the interval between the extensor hallucis longus and the extensor hallucis brevis.
- Incise the capsule over the first and second tarsometatarsal joints and expose the joints. Release the capsule all around the medial and lateral borders of the joint to allow adequate exposure (**TECH FIG 8A,B**).
- Remove the cartilage from the first tarsometatarsal joint using small osteotomes and small curettes.
  - If the first metatarsal is shortened, only cartilage should be removed.
  - If the first metatarsal is long, a small laterally based wedge can be removed from the medial cuneiform.
  - A small plantarly based osteotomy can be performed to plantarflex the first metatarsal if necessary.
- Use a 2.0-mm drill to perforate the subchondral surfaces of the joint.
- Expose and decorticate the medial aspect of the base of the second metatarsal and the lateral aspect of the base of the first metatarsal (**TECH FIG 8C**).

Lateral Soft Tissue Release

- Make a 2-cm incision in the first web space.
- Use blunt dissection to identify the adductor hallucis tendon.
  - Identify and protect the terminal branch of the deep peroneal nerve.
- Incise the adductor hallucis tendon at the lateral aspect of the fibular sesamoid.
- Incise the lateral capsule longitudinally to allow reduction of the sesamoids.
- Force the MTP joint into varus to complete the lateral release.

Medial Exostectomy

- Make a direct medial incision over the first MTP joint.
- Incise the capsule in line with the incision.
  - A wedge of capsule can be removed to facilitate reduction of the sesamoids.
  - Remove any residual prominence. Most of this was probably done with the primary procedure.

Fixation of the First Tarsometatarsal Joint

- Reduce the first metatarsal parallel to the second.
  - Confirm that the first metatarsal is parallel and properly rotated.
- Place a 3.5-mm cortical screw across the first tarsometatarsal joint from proximal to distal using a compression technique.
- Place a second 3.5-mm cortical screw from the medial aspect of the base of the first metatarsal into the base of the second metatarsal.
- Bone graft obtained from removal of the medial prominence can be placed in the first–second intermetatarsal space to augment the fusion.
- Use intraoperative imaging to confirm the position of the screws and reduction of the deformity (**TECH FIG 9**)

Capsular Repair and Wound Closure

- Repair the medial capsulectomy with absorbable suture.
- It should not be necessary to overtighten the capsule to maintain the alignment of the MTP joint.
- Close the wounds in layers.

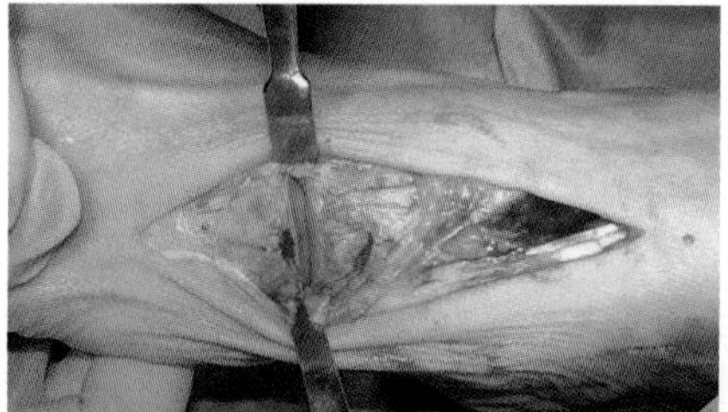

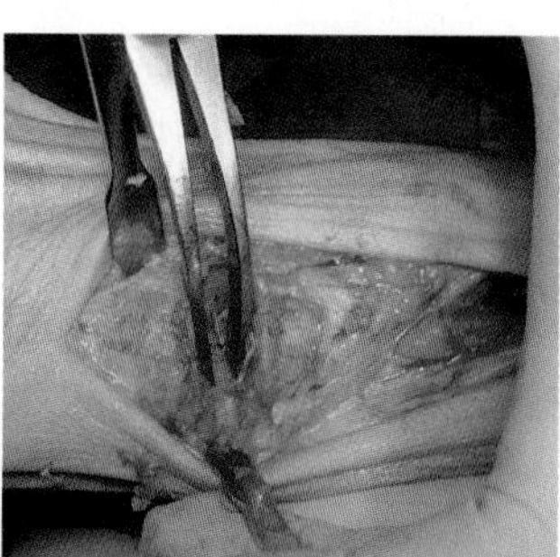

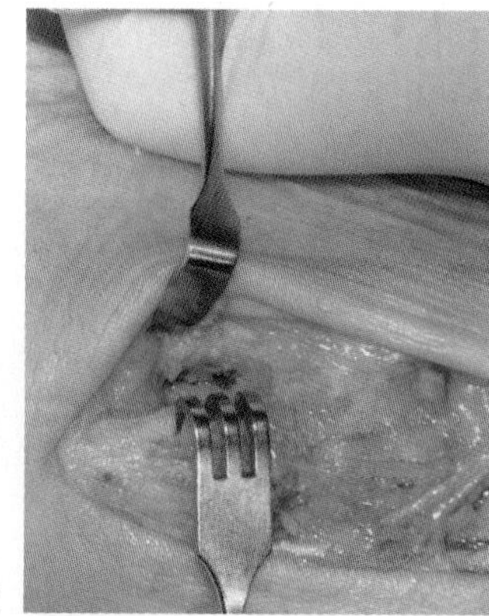

TECH FIG 8 • A,B. With the initial exposure, only the dorsal 10 to 15 mm of the tarsometatarsal joint is visualized. A small lamina spreader or distractor is required to expose the plantar half of the joint. This is a requirement of the procedure to avoid fusing the joint in dorsiflexion. With the distractor in place, the medial aspect of the base of the second metatarsal can be denuded of soft tissue to prepare for intermetatarsal fusion. **C.** Decortication of the lateral aspect of the base of the first metatarsal and the medial aspect of the second metatarsal to allow fusion.

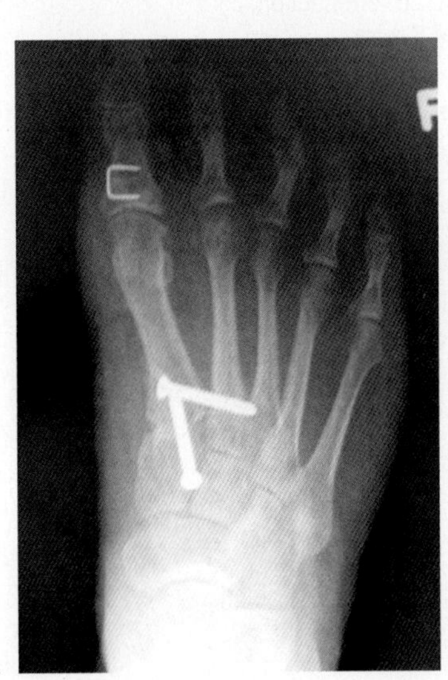

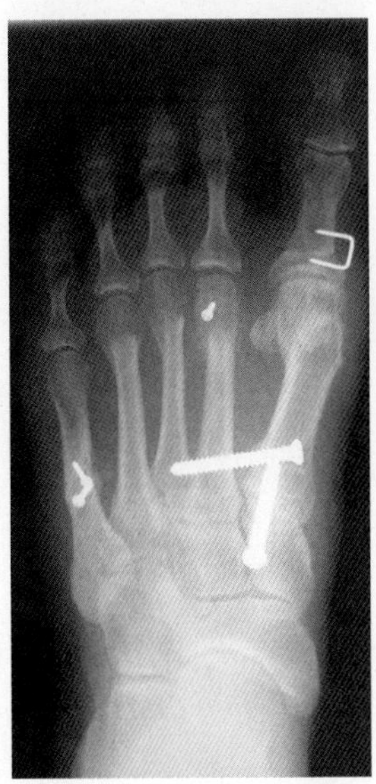

TECH FIG 9 • Screw placement for a salvage of a failed distal procedure. **A.** The first metatarsal length was well preserved with the initial procedure. **B.** The first metatarsal length was such that a second metatarsal shortening was indicated to limit second metatarsal overload.

LUDLOFF METATARSAL OSTEOTOMY

- This procedure could be used instead of a Lapidus procedure (TECH FIG 10).

Indications

- Smokers or patients with other medical issues that would delay a tarsometatarsal fusion
- Patients unable to be non–weight-bearing for an extended period (eg, obesity, rheumatoid arthritis, contralateral joint problems, shoulder problems)
- Patients with less severe deformities: correction achieved will be 8 to 16 degrees

Technique[1,6]

- Make an incision over the medial aspect of the first metatarsal.
- The optimal osteotomy starts on the dorsum, 1 cm from the tarsometatarsal joint, and extends distal and plantar to a point just proximal to the sesamoid articulation.
- The osteotomy should be angled 10 degrees plantarly in the coronal plane.
- The axis of rotation should be within 5 mm from the proximal end of the osteotomy.
- Insert the proximal screw first. It is usually done from dorsal to plantar. This serves as the axis of rotation of the distal (capital fragment).
- Once the desired reduction is obtained, a second screw is inserted (TECH FIG 11).

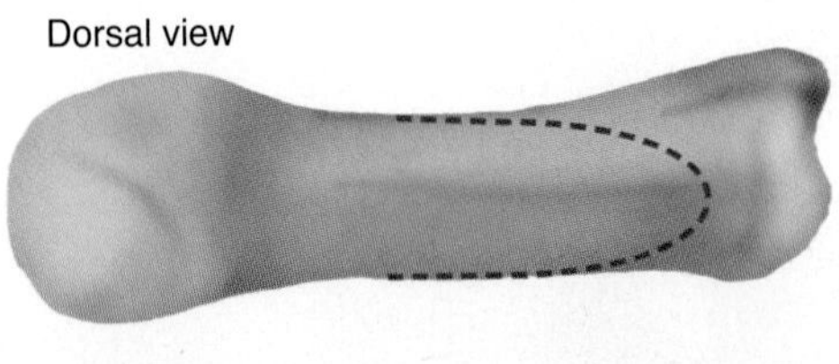

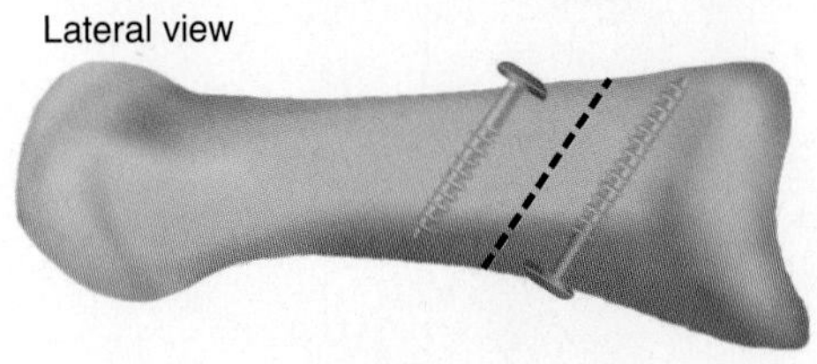

TECH FIG 10 • Ludloff osteotomy: long oblique from dorsal–proximal to plantar–distal.

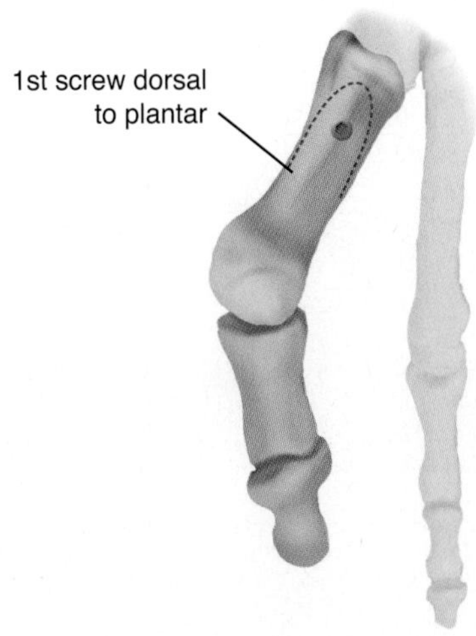

TECH FIG 11 • Ludloff osteotomy. The proximal screw is placed first, from dorsal to plantar. The distal (capital) portion of the metatarsal is now rotated laterally to correct the intermetatarsal angle. This is followed by the second screw, usually from plantar to dorsal. *(continued)*

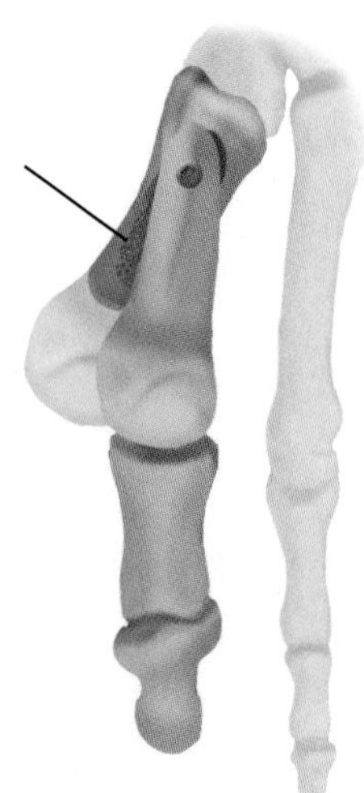

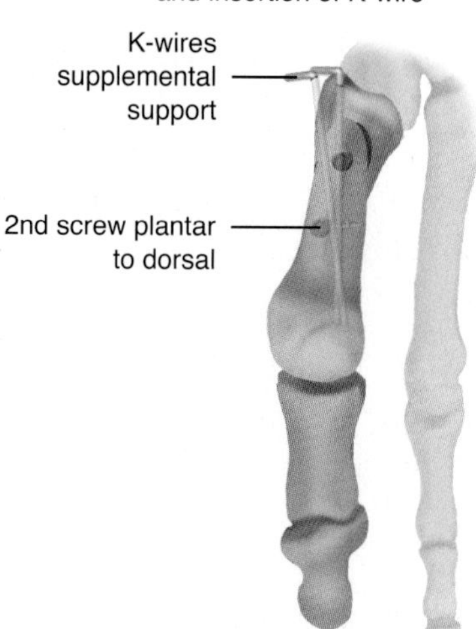

B C

TECH FIG 11 • *(continued)*

DORSAL OPENING-WEDGE OSTEOTOMY

Indications

- Dorsal malunion of a proximal metatarsal osteotomy
- Dorsal malunion or nonunion of a Lapidus procedure (**TECH FIG 12A**)

Technique

- Make a 6-cm incision over the dorsum of the first metatarsal base.
- Identify the interval between the extensor hallucis longus and the extensor hallucis brevis.
- Perform an osteotomy 1.5 cm distal to the first tarsometatarsal joint, leaving the plantar cortex intact.
- For a failed Lapidus procedure, the osteotomy is done through the previous fusion site.
- Place a triangular, tricortical bone graft with the wide surface placed dorsally to plantarflex the first metatarsal.
  - Either an allograft or an iliac crest autograft can be used.
  - A small distractor is helpful in distracting and keeping the osteotomy open.
- Fix the osteotomy with a small fragment screw from distal to proximal across the bone graft or with a dorsal plate that spans the bone graft (**TECH FIG 12B**).

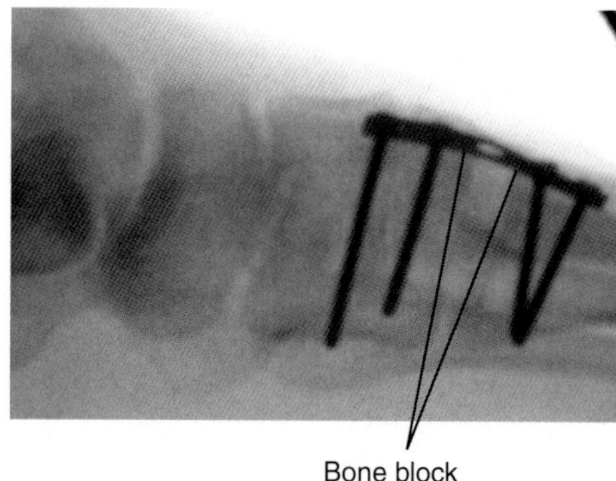

A

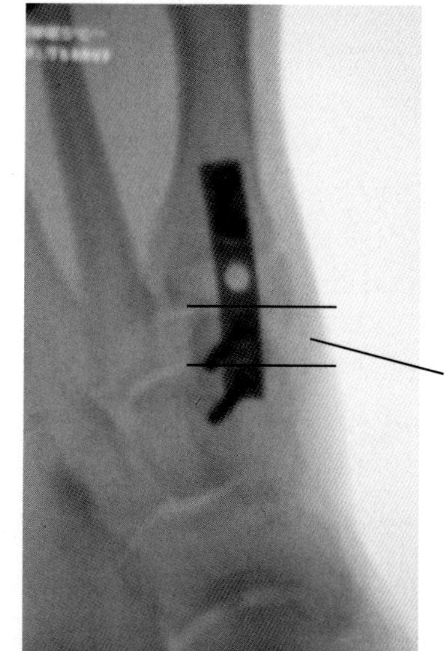

B

TECH FIG 12 • A. Dorsiflexion malunion of a proximal metatarsal osteotomy. **B.** Dorsal open-wedge osteotomy and bone grafting of a malunion of a Lapidus procedure.

Wound Closure and Postoperative Care

- Close the wound in layers.
- Apply a well-padded short-leg cast in the operating room.
- The patient may be partial weight bearing on the heel only for 6 to 8 weeks.
- At 2 weeks the cast is removed to allow suture removal and a wound check.
- A new short-leg cast or a cast boot is applied for another 4 to 6 weeks until bony healing is seen on radiographs.

GREAT TOE FUSION

Indications

- Severe degenerative changes of the first MTP joint secondary to previous bunion surgery
- Avascular necrosis of the metatarsal head
- Severe recurrence of a hallux valgus in a rheumatoid patient

PEARLS AND PITFALLS

Lapidus procedure: Indications	▪ Depending on the pathology, there are simpler treatment options for primary bunion surgery. ▪ A modified Lapidus procedure is not indicated in the absence of metatarsus primus varus or first ray hypermobility. ▪ The modified Lapidus procedure does not correct an increased distal metatarsal articular angle. If there is a significant increase in the distal metatarsal articular angle, a distal medial closing-wedge osteotomy or an Akin procedure is also required. ▪ If there is a dorsiflexion malunion from a previous proximal osteotomy, a corrective osteotomy may be necessary instead of a Lapidus procedure.
First tarsometatarsal joint preparation	▪ Take care not to inadvertently shorten the first metatarsal. Use a saw very sparingly, if ever. ▪ The first tarsometatarsal joint is about 25 to 30 mm deep, and take care to expose and prepare the entire joint surface to avoid fusing the joint in dorsiflexion. ▪ A small Inge retractor or a smooth lamina spreader is invaluable in exposing the joint.
Lateral soft tissue release	▪ The terminal branch of the deep peroneal nerve is vulnerable to injury in the first web space. ▪ Excessive lateral release can lead to a hallux varus deformity.
Medial exostectomy Fixation of the first tarsometatarsal joint	▪ Only a minimal medial exostectomy may be needed. ▪ Avoid dorsiflexion and pronation of the first metatarsal. ▪ Failure to appropriately expose and denude the plantar aspect of the joint can lead to a dorsiflexion malunion. ▪ To ensure appropriate position, it is helpful to hold the metatarsals in one hand while the screws are placed. ▪ Careful preparation of the first–second intermetatarsal joint is mandatory to minimize the incidence of nonunion.
Shortening of the first metatarsal	▪ It is not uncommon to find the first metatarsal shortened with the initial bunion procedure. ▪ If that is the case, and if there are signs of significant second metatarsal overload, a second and sometimes third metatarsal shortening osteotomy should be done.

POSTOPERATIVE CARE

- The wounds are dressed.
- A slipper great toe spica fiberglass cast is placed in the operating room.
- At 2 weeks, the cast is removed to allow wound check and suture removal.
- A new slipper cast or a postoperative bunion shoe is applied for an additional 4 weeks.
- Patients are non–weight-bearing on the operative foot for 6 weeks.
- If there is radiographic and clinical evidence of fusion at 6 weeks, then the cast is removed and physical therapy is begun.
- At 8 weeks, patients can often return to swimming and biking.
- More vigorous physical activity is delayed until 3 months after surgery.

OUTCOMES

- In appropriately chosen patients, the Lapidus procedure is a reliable option for recurrent hallux valgus.
- A prospective cohort study reported an 80% satisfaction rate after the Lapidus procedure for recurrent hallux valgus in carefully selected patients.
- The same prospective cohort study suggested an increased risk of nonunion in smokers.[2]

COMPLICATIONS

- Nonunion of the first tarsometatarsal fusion is the most common complication (6% to 10%).
- Transfer metatarsalgia due to dorsiflexion malunion of the first metatarsal or lesser metatarsal length discrepancy
- Failure to reduce the sesamoids due to rotational malunion of the first metatarsal or inadequate lateral release
- Hallux varus due to excessive lateral release
- Painful instrumentation
- Nerve injury
- Infection

REFERENCES

1. Beischer AD, Ammon P, Corniou A, et al. Three-dimensional computer analysis of the modified Ludloff osteotomy. Foot Ankle Int 2005;26:627–632.
2. Coetzee JC, Resig SG, Kuskowski M, et al. The Lapidus procedure as salvage after failed surgical treatment of hallux valgus: a prospective cohort study. J Bone Joint Surg Am 2003;85A:60–65.
3. King DM, Toolan BC. Associated deformities and hypermobility in hallux vlgus: an investigation with weightbearing radiographs. Foot Ankle Int 2004;25:251–253.
4. Klaue K, Hansen ST, Masquelet AC. Clinical, quantitive assessment of first tarsometatarsal mobility in the sagittal plane and its relation to hallux valgus deformity. Foot Ankle Int 1994;15:9–13.
5. Mann R. Disorders of the first metatarsophalangeal joint. J Am Acad Orthop Surg 1995;3:34–43.
6. Nyska M, Trnka HJ, Parks BG, et al. The Ludloff metatarsal osteotomy: guidelines for optimal correction based on a geometric analysis conduction on a sawbone model. Foot Ankle Int 2003;24:34–39.

Chapter 16 Metatarsal Lengthening in Revision Hallux Valgus Surgery

James A. Nunley II and Jason M. Hurst

DEFINITION

- Shortening of the first metatarsal may occur after first metatarsal osteotomies for hallux valgus correction.
- If the first metatarsal is considerably shortened, the patient may develop painful transfer metatarsalgia of the lesser toes.

ANATOMY

- The physiologically normal first metatarsal is generally of similar length to or slightly shorter than the neighboring second metatarsal.
- This length relationship between the first metatarsal and the lesser metatarsals allows for a smooth, progressive weight transfer and optimizes the windlass mechanism during gait.
- The relative plantar position of the first metatarsal head (and sesamoids) also makes the windlass mechanism more effective in transferring weight to the lesser toes and may compensate for a physiologically shorter first metatarsal.

PATHOGENESIS

- Some metatarsal shortening occurs with the majority of all first metatarsal osteotomies performed during hallux valgus correction.
- An iatrogenically shortened first metatarsal can disrupt the normal forefoot weight transfer mechanism and cause a pathologic overload of the adjacent metatarsals.
- Relative dorsiflexion of the metatarsal head can also occur after hallux valgus correction with metatarsal osteotomy, exacerbating the mechanical disadvantage of the shortened metatarsal and further contributing to transfer metatarsalgia.

NATURAL HISTORY

- Transfer metatarsalgia generally does not resolve spontaneously, particularly if coupled with a concomitant forefoot fat-pad atrophy.
- Mild transfer metatarsalgia is generally well tolerated as the patient is able to modify gait, stance, and activity to compensate.
- However, the problem may progress, with painful callus formation developing under the lesser metatarsal heads. Severe, recalcitrant transfer metatarsalgia may cause debilitating forefoot pain that often persists until normal forefoot biomechanics are restored or reasonable footwear accommodation is used.

PATIENT HISTORY AND PHYSICAL FINDINGS

- The great toe usually but not always appears shorter than the adjacent metatarsal, especially when compared to the contralateral foot (**FIG 1**).
- The plantar surface of the forefoot usually but not always has calluses under the lesser metatarsal heads.
- The lesser metatarsal heads are tender.
- When examined simultaneously, the first metatarsal head (and sesamoids) may appear elevated and more proximal relative to the second metatarsal head, particularly when compared to the contralateral foot.
- The medial forefoot incisions from prior forefoot surgery must be noted in anticipation of potential revision surgery.
- Hallux metatarsophalangeal (MTP) joint alignment must be examined. A recurrence of hallux valgus deformity after prior surgery will need to be corrected in conjunction with metatarsal lengthening.
- Hallux MTP joint motion must be determined. Stiffness and crepitance may suggest arthrosis that may favor first MTP joint arthrodesis over first metatarsal lengthening (**FIG 2**).

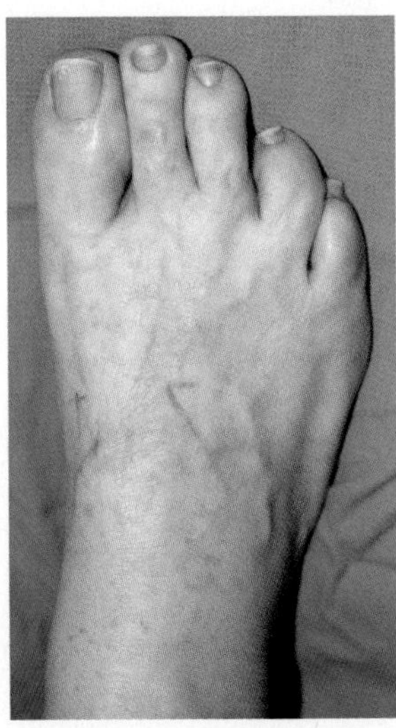

FIG 1 • Foot with relatively short first metatarsal after distal first metatarsal osteotomy.

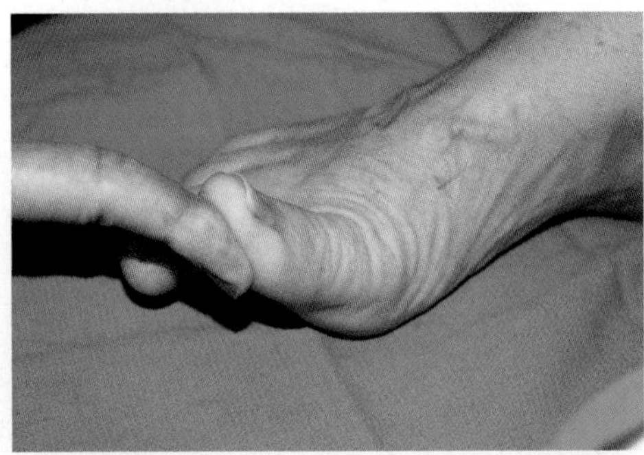

FIG 2 • Assessing range of motion of hallux metatarsophalangeal joint before metatarsal lengthening.

IMAGING AND OTHER DIAGNOSTIC STUDIES

- Weight-bearing plain radiographs are mandatory; we recommend bilateral radiographs to include the contralateral foot for comparison.
- AP radiographs of the symptomatic foot indicate the amount of first metatarsal shortening, the presence of residual deformity (particularly the first metatarsal head–sesamoid relationship), the nature of the prior hallux valgus surgery, and the integrity of the first MTP joint (**FIG 3A**).
- Lateral radiographs suggest the degree of concomitant elevation of the first metatarsal.
- Contralateral foot radiographs provide some indication of the required lengthening, which is useful in surgical planning (**FIG 3B**).

DIFFERENTIAL DIAGNOSIS

- Recurrence of hallux valgus
- First metatarsal head avascular necrosis
- Dorsiflexed malunion of first metatarsal

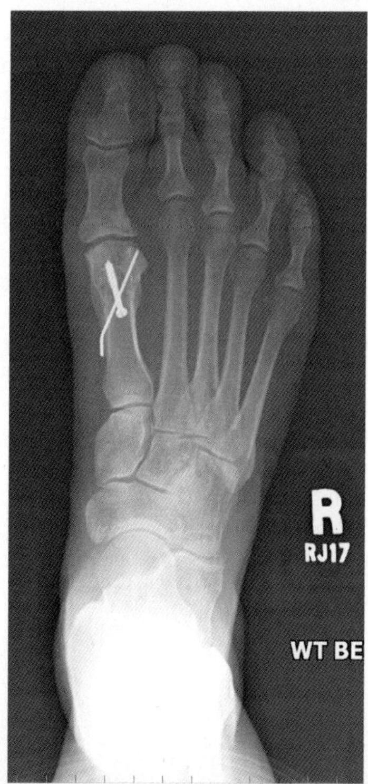

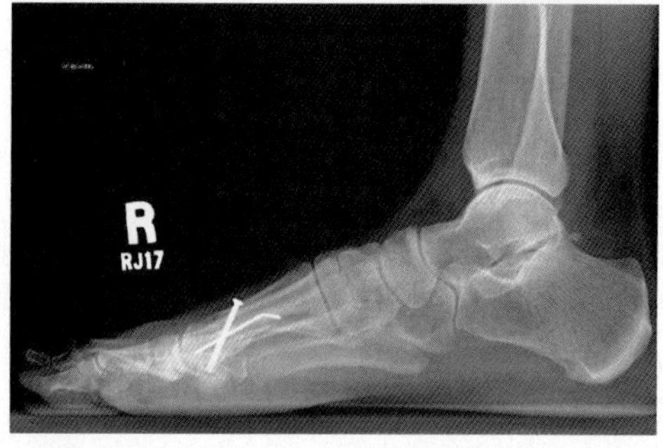

FIG 3 • Preoperative radiographs of foot before hardware removal, application of external fixator, and metatarsal corticotomy. **A.** AP view. **B.** Lateral view.

NONOPERATIVE MANAGEMENT

- Oral anti-inflammatory medication
- Shoe wear modification (ie, greater stiffness in combination with a rocker sole to unload the forefoot)
- Orthotics with medial posting for the first metatarsal and metatarsal support for the lesser metatarsals

SURGICAL MANAGEMENT

- Surgical management is indicated when nonoperative treatments have failed and other causes are not responsible for the forefoot pain and transfer metatarsalgia.
- Two broad categories may be considered in the surgical management of transfer metatarsalgia secondary to a short first metatarsal: (a) shortening of the lesser metatarsals and (b) lengthening of the first metatarsal. With severe first metatarsal shortening, a combination of these two approaches may need to be considered. First metatarsal lengthening affords the advantage of correcting the problem at its source in lieu of performing surgery on lesser metatarsals that are physiologically normal but subject to an overload phenomenon.

Preoperative Planning

- Weight-bearing plain radiographs are essential to plan the desired lengthening and potential realignment of the metatarsal and MTP joint, determine the need for hardware removal from previous surgery, and identify potential arthritis in the MTP joint (Fig 3). The contralateral first metatarsal, if not previously operated, serves as an ideal template to determine how a more physiologic first metatarsal anatomy may be restored. To account for magnification, relative lengths of the first and second metatarsals may be used as a reference.
- Once the patient is deemed appropriate for metatarsal lengthening, the appropriate position for the external fixator half-pins and corticotomy should be planned radiographically.

Positioning

- The patient should be placed in the supine position on the operating table.
- A bump should not be placed under the ipsilateral hip to allow external rotation of the leg and better access to the medial side of the foot.

Approach

- A four-pin single-plane external fixator will be placed along the medial border of the first metatarsal and a short, longitudinal dorsal approach to the metatarsal is needed to perform the metatarsal osteotomy (**FIGS 4, 5**). The incision may need to incorporate or be within previous surgical scars to minimize the risk of soft tissue complications.
- The four drill holes for the external fixator pins are created percutaneously, under fluoroscopic guidance, using a 1.5-mm Kirschner wire or the small-diameter drill corresponding to the particular external fixator set.
- After percutaneous placement of the four external fixator pins, a longitudinal dorsal approach to the metatarsal is used to perform the metatarsal corticotomy.
- Occasionally, a distal soft tissue procedure is necessary and surgical incisions must be planned carefully. In our experience, this procedure is most effective for a shortened first metatarsal and satisfactory alignment of the first MTP joint.

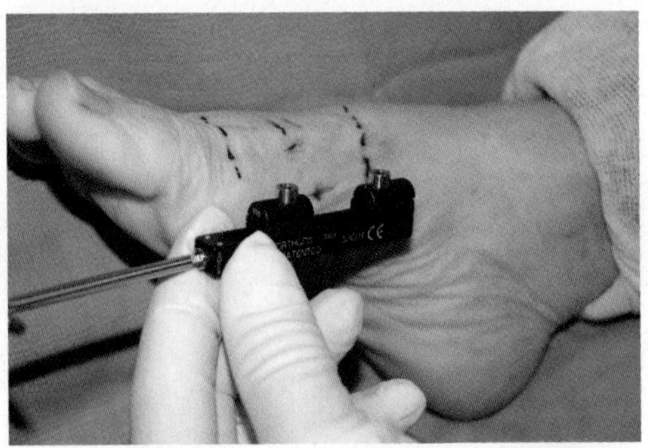

FIG 4 • External fixator is held against metatarsal to determine appropriate adjustment of fixator.

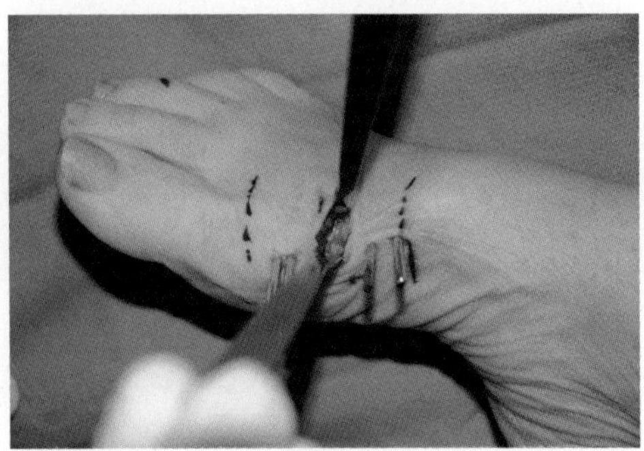

FIG 5 • Minimally invasive incision for metatarsal corticotomy with minimal periosteal stripping.

PLACEMENT OF THE EXTERNAL FIXATOR PINS

- Using a surgical marker, plan the incision for the corticotomy by drawing a 2-cm line along the middle third of the dorsal border of the first metatarsal (Fig 4).
- Using the closed external fixator as a drill guide, create four drill holes (two proximal and two distal) percutaneously along the medial side of the metatarsal using a 1.5-mm Kirschner wire. The external fixator must not be fully distracted when using it as a drill guide; however, it should be slightly distracted in order to apply initial compression after performing the corticotomy.
- With respect to sequence of drill holes, we recommend creating the most distal drill hole first and the most proximal one second, after which these half-pins are secured and the external fixator is attached. This sequence ensures that a monorail external fixator is parallel to the first metatarsal. Alternatively, a hinged external fixator may be employed that can be adjusted to accommodate the pins while still creating longitudinal distraction (**TECH FIGS 1–4**). Place all four pins into the drill holes in a similar percutaneous fashion, and check their position using fluoroscopy (**TECH FIG 5**).
- Some external fixator half-pins are tapered (eg, 2.5-mm tapered threads with 3.0-mm shafts) and thus should not be advanced beyond the lateral cortex of the first metatarsal and then reversed, as they will then lose their stability.

A

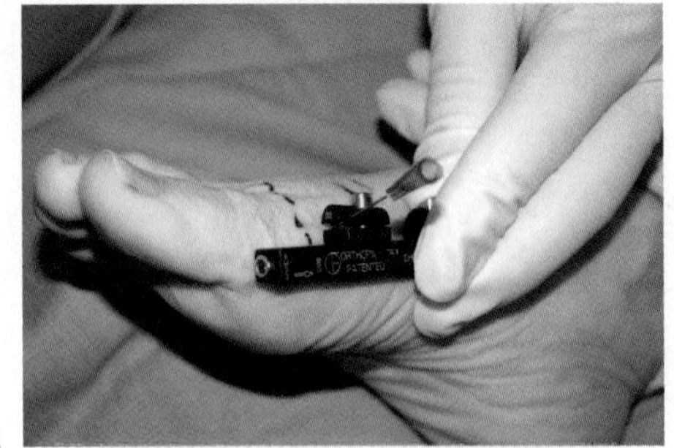

B

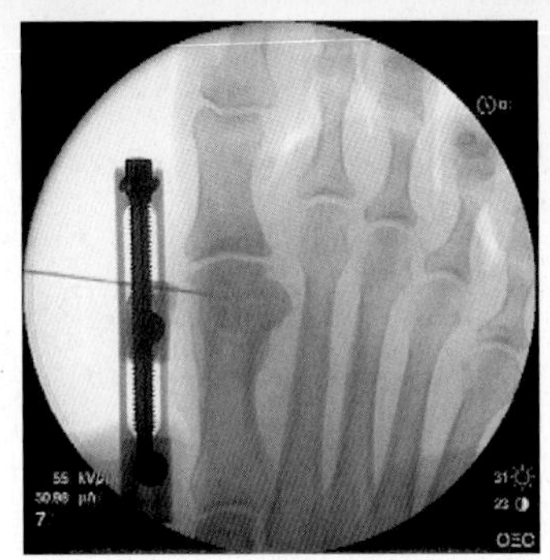

TECH FIG 1 • Determining proper location for external fixator, using a needle as a reference. **A.** Clinical view. **B.** Fluoroscopic view.

A

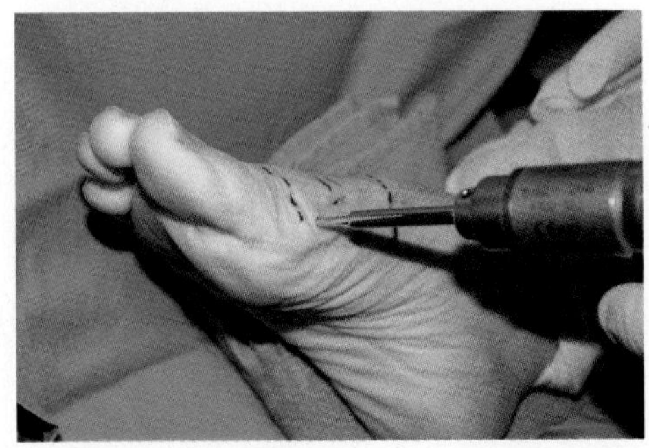

B

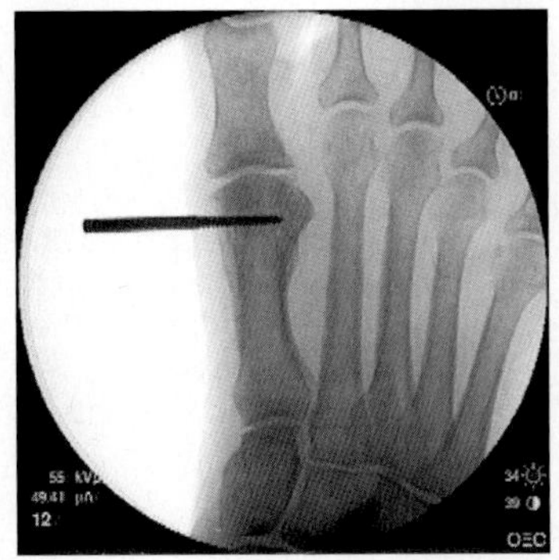

C

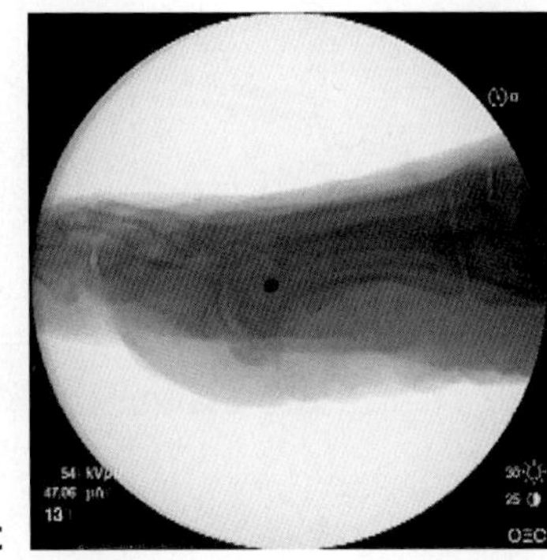

TECH FIG 2 • First pin placed in distal first metatarsal. **A.** Clinical view. **B.** AP fluoroscopic view. **C.** Lateral fluoroscopic view.

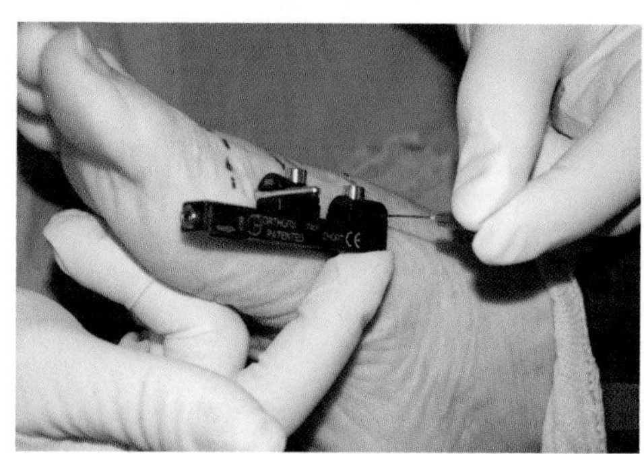
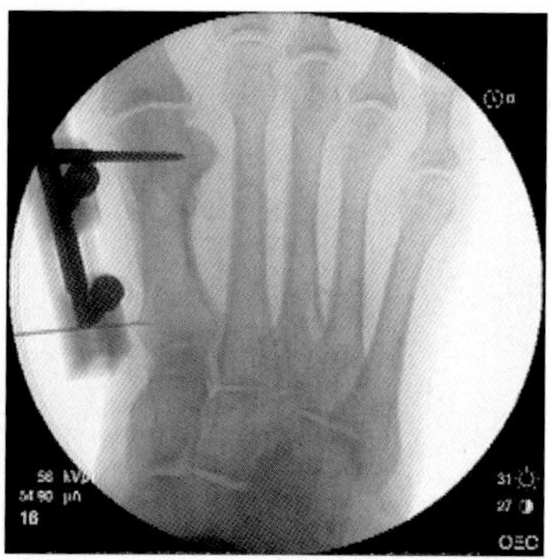

TECH FIG 3 • Determining optimal proximal pin position. **A.** Clinical view. **B.** Fluoroscopic view.

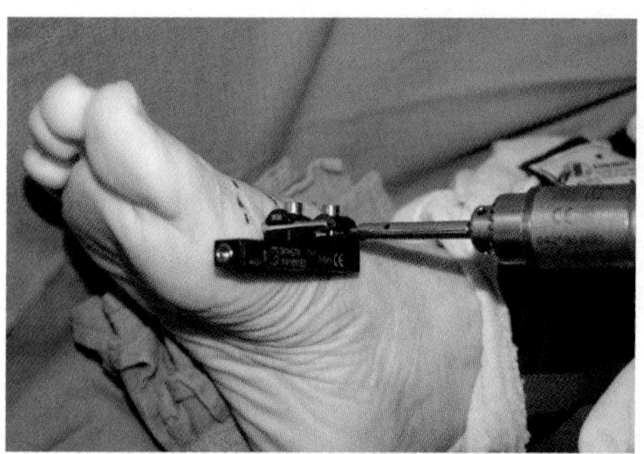
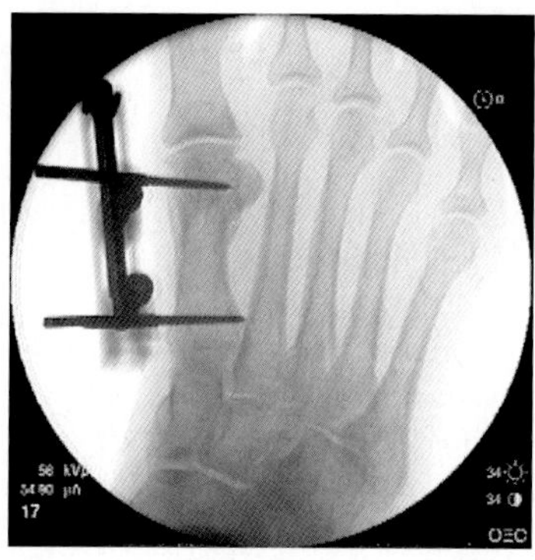
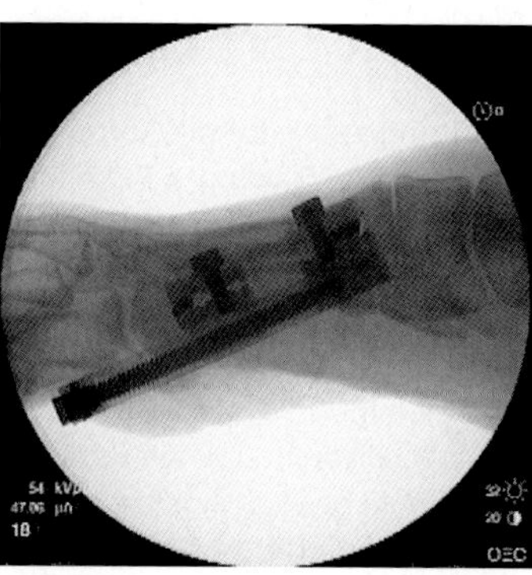

TECH FIG 4 • Placing second pin in proximal first metatarsal. **A.** Clinical view. **B.** AP fluoroscopic view. **C.** Lateral fluoroscopic view.

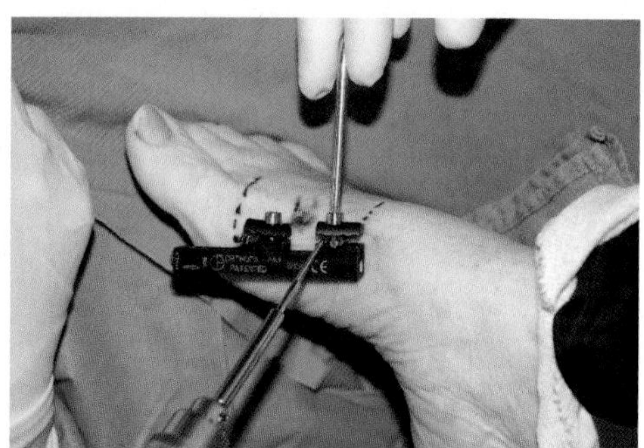
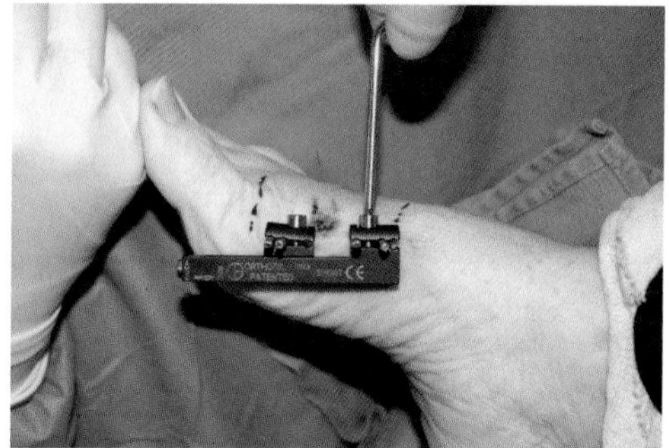
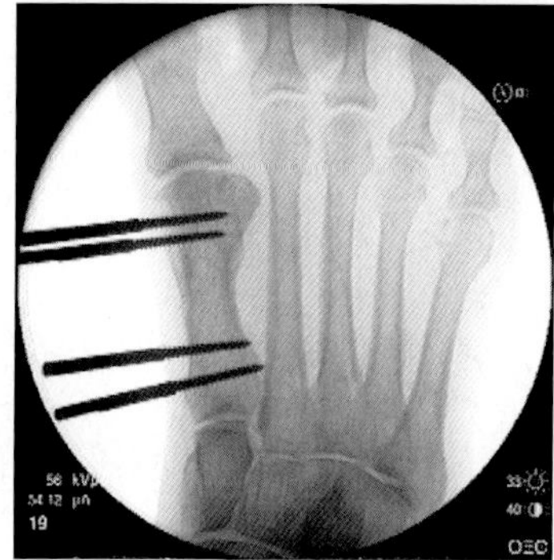

TECH FIG 5 • Final two pins placed. **A.** Second most proximal pin being placed. **B.** External fixator tightened. **C.** Fluoroscopic view of all four pins secured. (Note that external fixator was removed; no further adjustments are made, so that the external fixator may be repositioned on the pins so that the metatarsal maintains its anatomic alignment.)

CREATING THE CORTICOTOMY

- Make a 2-cm incision along the dorsal border of the metatarsal between the central two fixator pins (Fig 5).
- Dissect sharply to bone and incise the periosteum transversely at the site of the planned corticotomy. Avoid unnecessary periosteal stripping; the periosteum only needs to be elevated directly at the corticotomy site.
- Make a transverse osteotomy using a mini-sagittal saw while simultaneously cooling the blade with iced saline irrigation (**TECH FIG 6**).

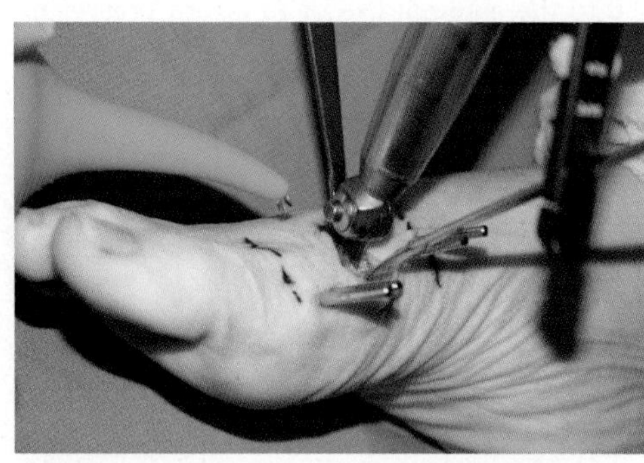

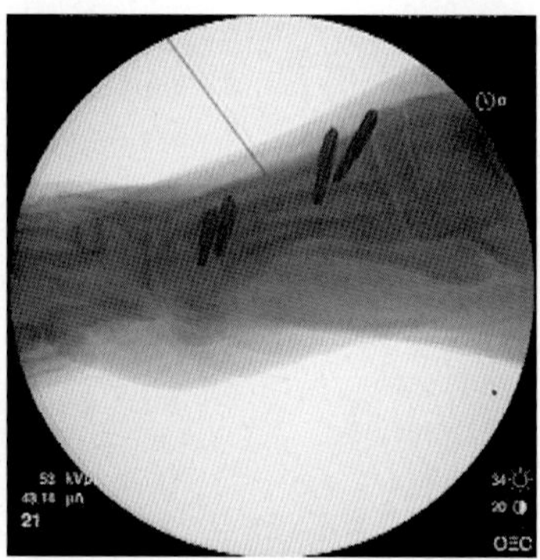

TECH FIG 6 • A. Corticotomy being performed (irrigation is being performed to diminish the risk of bone necrosis from the saw). **B.** Before making the corticotomy, the ideal location is confirmed fluoroscopically (the external fixator has been removed to allow for better access during corticotomy).

APPLYING THE EXTERNAL FIXATOR

- After creating the corticotomy, confirm adequacy and distractibility of the distal and proximal first metatarsal segments with careful distraction through the external fixator and fluoroscopic confirmation (**TECH FIG 7**).
- Compress the corticotomy using the external fixator; little compression is required—essentially the width of the saw blade. Using fluoroscopic imaging, verify adequate bone-on-bone contact of the two first metatarsal segments and secure the fixator set screws (**TECH FIGS 8, 9**). Occasionally, there is slight subluxation of the two first metatarsal segments, and this should be adjusted so that the bony apposition is anatomic.

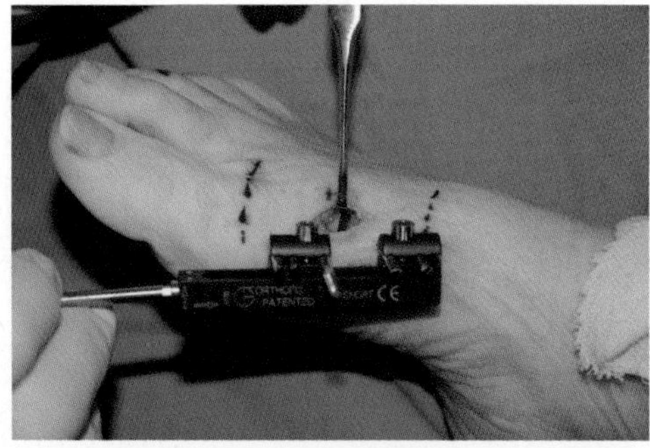

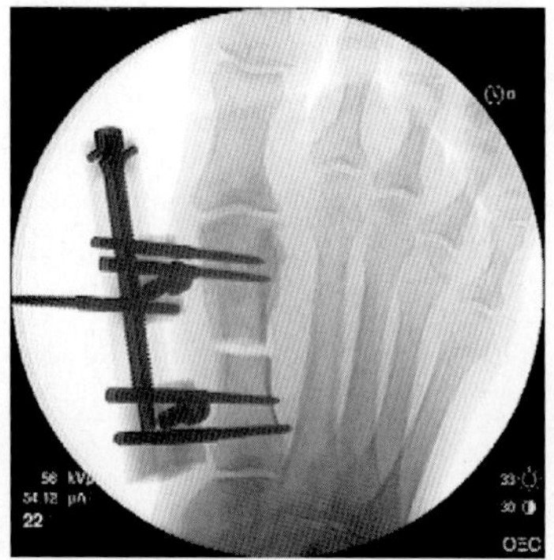

TECH FIG 7 • The external fixator is replaced with the metatarsal in its preoperative position and the corticotomy is distracted to confirm that it is complete.

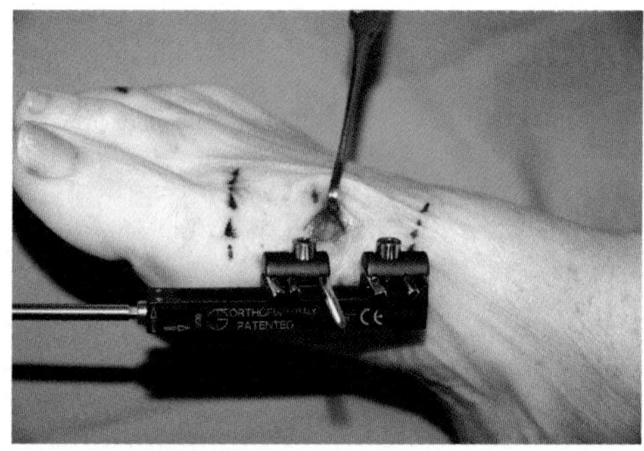

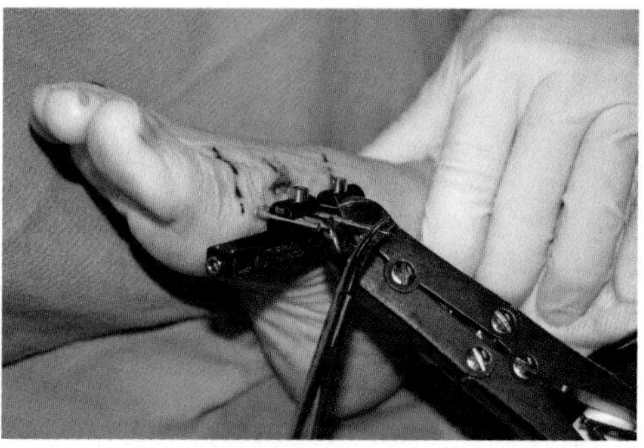

TECH FIG 8 • Additional "dummy" pins are added to the external fixator to afford greater fixator stability. **A.** Adding the pin. **B.** Trimming the pin.

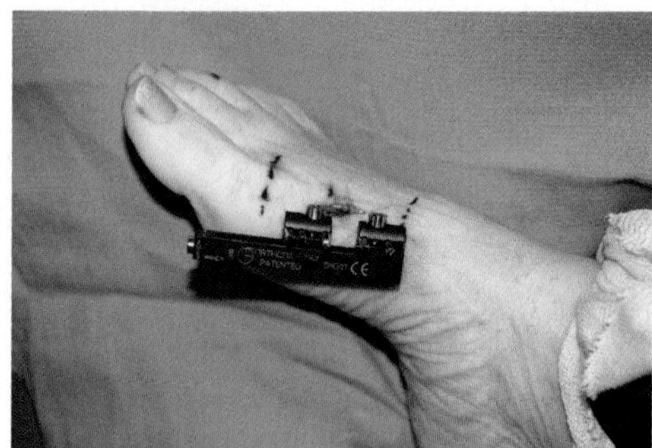

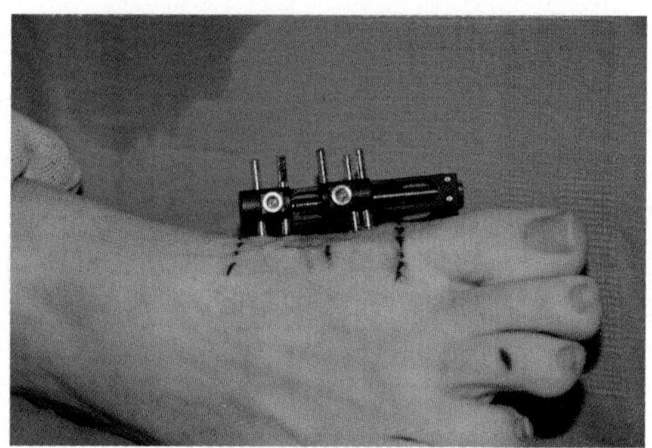

TECH FIG 9 • The corticotomy is compressed to its anatomic, preoperative position, and the external fixator is tightened.

WOUND CLOSURE

- We approximate the periosteum with 4–0 absorbable polyglactin suture and close the skin with 4-0 nylon suture.
- Apply a soft dressing. The patient can be discharged to home non–weight-bearing the same day of the procedure.

PEARLS AND PITFALLS

Placement of the external fixator pins	■ Use the external fixator as a drill guide. ■ Be sure to place the distal two pins in the plantar half of the distal fragment. This helps impart relative plantarflexion of the distal fragment and metatarsal head, thus limiting the potential for first metatarsal elevation.
Creating the corticotomy	■ Cool the saw blade to limit thermal necrosis of the bone edges.
Applying the external fixator	■ The wound may be reapproximated before placing the fixator, but be sure to verify good bony contact clinically and using fluoroscopic imaging.
Sequence of external fixator pins	■ Placing the distal- and proximal-most pins first ensures that the external fixator is parallel to the first metatarsal and that no pin will violate the MTP or tarsometatarsal joints.
Stiffness of the first MTP joint	■ In our experience, with gradual distraction, preoperative motion of the first MTP joint is not compromised.
Formation of bone ("regenerate")	■ Bone or callus does not form immediately with distraction at the corticotomy site; it may lag several weeks behind.
Failure of the regenerate to form	■ Occasionally, the regenerate will not form despite appropriate distraction technique. Once the full desired distraction has been achieved, alternating quarter-turn distraction and compression may stimulate formation of the regenerate. Use of an external bone stimulator may be considered. As a last resort, the intercalary segment may be bone grafted and internal fixation may be substituted for the external fixator, albeit only with a history of clean and healthy pin sites (the risk of infection with internal fixation is increased after previous external fixation in close proximity).
Duration of the external fixator	■ Generally, the regenerate becomes adequately stable for external fixator removal by 8 to 10 weeks, but occasionally 12 to 14 weeks is required. We routinely remove the external fixator in the office setting.

POSTOPERATIVE CARE

- The patient is kept non–weight-bearing. The first metatarsal needs to be protected until the regenerate has formed at the lengthening site. Weight bearing may compromise the stability of the corticotomy and the external fixator; moreover, weight bearing is not axial at the corticotomy site.
- We routinely see the patient in the clinic about 7 days postoperatively for wound inspection, patient education on distraction, and initiation of first metatarsal lengthening.
- We typically set the distraction rate for 1 mm per day (a quarter-turn of the external fixator every 6 hours).
- The patient should be given instructions in pin care and the number of days to distract the device to yield the desired length.
- We encourage daily first MTP joint range of motion to prevent joint contracture.
- The patient should return to the clinic regularly for radiographs to verify adequate distraction, appropriate position of the distal segment, and passive range of motion of the first MTP joint (**FIG 6**).
- The lengthening phase is complete once the first metatarsal has reached the desired length, typically the physiologic length based on the first–second metatarsal length ratio from the physiologically normal contralateral foot.
- Partial weight bearing is allowed when there is radiographic evidence of consolidation within the distracted segment, so long as it does not impinge on the external fixator. Boot or brace modifications typically allow for weight bearing even with the external fixator in place (**FIG 7**).
- The fixator is removed once there is satisfactory radiographic consolidation of the regenerate. The patient can resume full weight bearing once the fixator is removed, but we recommend several weeks of protected weight bearing in a surgical shoe or boot to avoid fracture through the half-pin holes, which are potential stress risers (**FIG 8**).

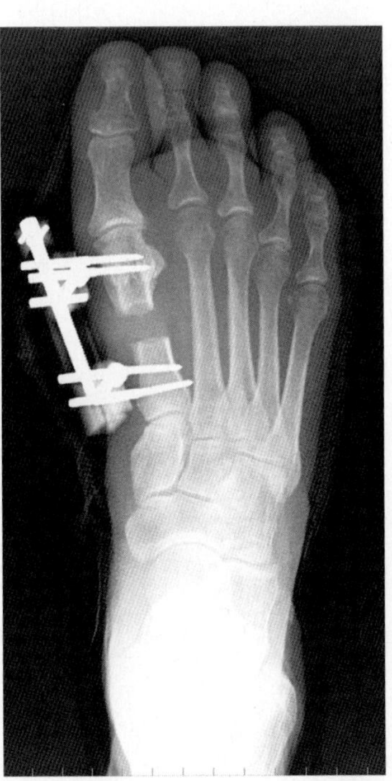

FIG 6 • Distraction at 3 weeks (regenerate is not yet evident).

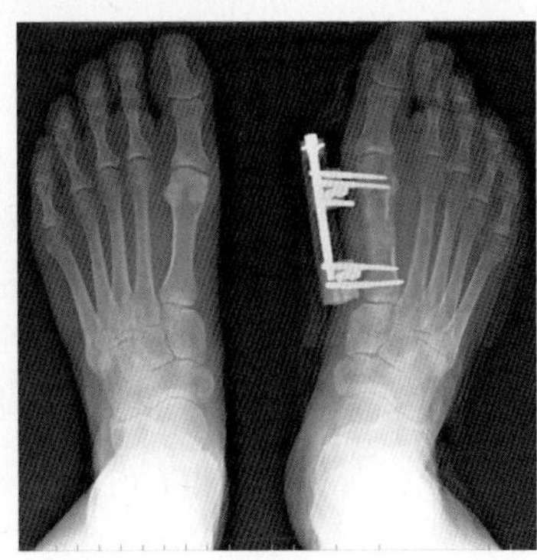

FIG 7 • Distraction at 10 weeks, regenerate present, but not mature.

- Figure 3 shows the radiographic clinical progression throughout the lengthening treatment.

OUTCOMES

- See the 2007 study by Hurst and Nunley.[2]

COMPLICATIONS

- Pin tract infection (inadequate pin care)
- First MTP joint stiffness (failure to perform intermittent first MTP joint range of motion)
- Early consolidation of distracted segment (distraction schedule too slow)
- Loss of hallux valgus correction (rare, with routine distraction schedule)
- Dorsiflexion of the metatarsal head (poor pin placement or premature removal of external fixator)
- Nonunion (poor fixation or stability of external fixator or premature removal of external fixator)

A

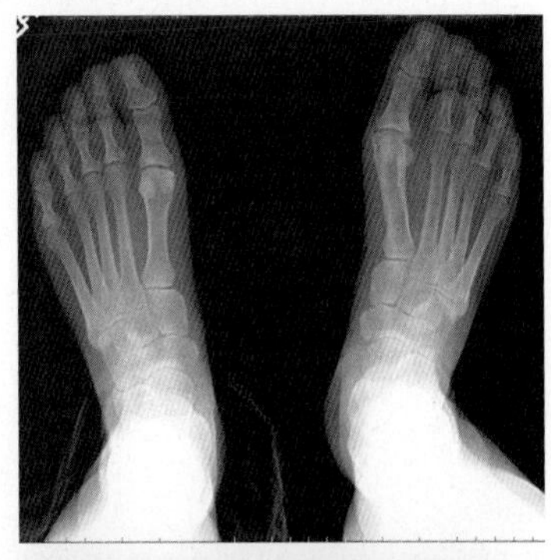

B

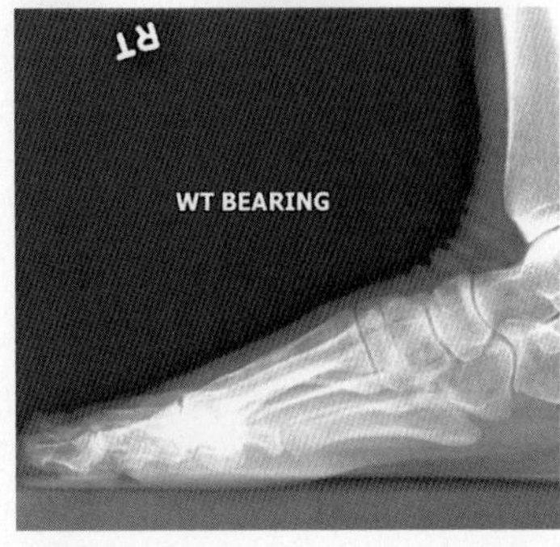

FIG 8 • Radiographic appearance at final 12-month follow-up. First metatarsal consolidation is complete and adequate lengthening has been obtained.

REFERENCES

1. Holden D, Siff S, Butler J, et al. Shortening of the first metatarsal as a complication of metatarsal osteotomies. J Bone Joint Surg Am 1984;66A:582–588.
2. Hurst JM, Nunley JA II. Distraction osteogenesis for the shortened metatarsal after hallux valgus surgery. Foot Ankle Int 2007;28: 194–198.
3. Jones RO, Harkless LB, Baer MS, et al. Retrospective statistical analysis of factors influencing the formation of long-term complications following hallux abducto valgus surgery. J Foot Surg 1991;30: 344–349.
4. Mather R, Hurst J, Easley M, et al. First metatarsal lengthening. Tech Foot Ankle Surg 2008;7:25–30.
5. Nunley JA. The short first metatarsal after hallux valgus surgery. In Nunley JA, Pfeffer GB, Sanders RW, et al, eds. Advanced Reconstruction: Foot and Ankle. Rosemont, IL: American Academy of Orthopaedic Surgeons, 2004:31–33.
6. Nyska M, Trnka H, Parks BG, et al. Proximal metatarsal osteotomies: a comparative geometric analysis conducted on sawbone models. Foot Ankle Int 2002;23:938–945.
7. Sammarco GJ, Idusuyi OB. Complications after surgery of the hallux. Clin Orthop Relat Res 2001;391:59–71.
8. Saxby T, Nunley JA. Metatarsal lengthening by distraction osteogenesis: a report of two cases. Foot Ankle 1992;13:536–539.
9. Urbaniak JR, Richardson WJ. Diaphyseal lengthening for shortness of the toe. Foot Ankle 1985;5:251–256.

Chapter **17** # Moberg Osteotomy

Thomas G. Harris and Ronald W. Smith

DEFINITION

- Hallux rigidus is a degenerative condition of the first metatarsophalangeal (MTP) joint.
- This leads to a functional limitation of motion of this joint, especially with respect to dorsiflexion.
- Other terms, such as hallux limitus and dorsal bunion, have also been used to describe this condition.
- Hallux rigidus affects about 3% of the adult population.[5]
- This chapter pertains to the surgical procedure of a dorsal closing wedge osteotomy of the proximal phalanx, popularized by Moberg. Although it was initially recommended for young patients (under 18 years of age), Moberg extended the indications to include adults.[8]
- It is usually performed in conjunction with a cheilectomy.

ANATOMY

- Usually dorsiflexion is blocked by a dorsal osteophyte on the metatarsal head. In some cases there is an osteophyte or ossicle on the dorsum of the base of the proximal phalanx. Dorsiflexion is also limited by contracture of the plantar portion of the MTP joint capsule.
- Articular erosion is characteristically seen on the dorsum of the articular surface of the first metatarsal head and, to a lesser extent, on the dorsum of the base of the proximal phalanx.
- The medial and plantar aspect of the MTP joint is usually spared until later in the disease process (**FIG 1**).

PATHOGENESIS

- The primary etiology of the hallux rigidus is not known.
- A common cause is trauma, and hallux rigidus may occur after a fracture, sprain, or crush injury. Furthermore, it is thought that microtrauma may injure the articular cartilage over time, leading to degeneration.[4]

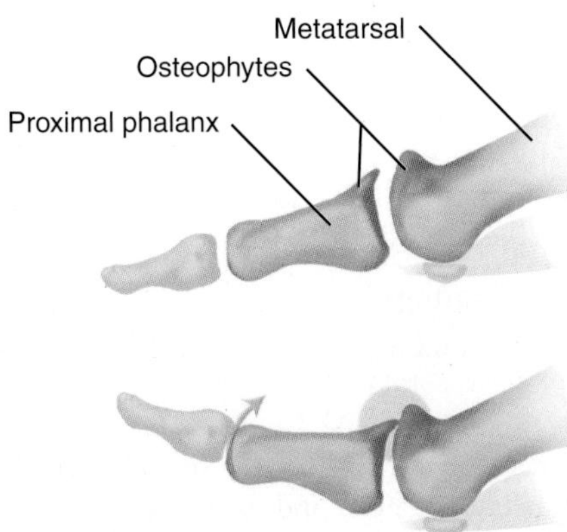

FIG 1 • Hallux rigidus: dorsiflexion of proximal phalanx produces painful impingement at the metatarsophalangeal joint.

- Systemic conditions such as gout and rheumatoid arthritis can also cause degeneration of the first MTP joint, simulating the idiopathic form.

NATURAL HISTORY

- Hallux rigidus is more common in adults than adolescents.
- Generalized degenerative changes tend to progress with increasing age, but this has not been linked with symptoms.[9]
- Women are affected more often than men and boys, and the condition is often bilateral.

PATIENT HISTORY AND PHYSICAL FINDINGS

- Patients usually describe an insidious onset of activity-related pain at the first MTP joint.
- Swelling and stiffness are common complaints.
- On physical examination in the characteristic case, dorsiflexion motion is measurably limited and plantarflexion motion with force is painful. In some cases, forceful dorsiflexion is also painful, but not as painful as forceful plantarflexion.
- Limitation of dorsiflexion usually leads to problems with running, walking on inclines, and wearing high-heeled shoes.
- The increasing dorsal prominence can lead to problems with shoe wear.
- Paresthesias may rarely occur distal to the MTP joint with the compression of the dorsal cutaneous nerves by the dorsal osteophyte and tight-fitting shoes.
- Adaptive gait measures such as a supinated forefoot to unload the painful medial forefoot may lead to lateral foot pain and calluses.[6]
- There is usually generalized enlargement of the joint due to a combination of osteophytes and soft tissue swelling.
- In severe cases with full loss of cartilage and motion, there is sometimes no irritability even with forced flexion. These patients often just have pain because of the osteophytic enlargement causing impingement in the shoe. In these cases, a simple cheilectomy with limited dissection often leads to satisfactory results. These are patients often in their 70s and 80s.
- Interphalangeal joint hyperextension may develop to compensate for restricted MTP joint dorsiflexion, but this is very uncommon.[2]
- Axial loading of the great toe is usually not painful unless severe degeneration or a large osteochondral defect is present.
- Passive plantarflexion of the hallux can also produce pain, as this is thought to bring the inflamed synovium and MTP capsule over the dorsal osteophyte.

IMAGING AND OTHER DIAGNOSTIC STUDIES

- Three weight-bearing views (AP, lateral, and oblique) of the foot are usually sufficient.

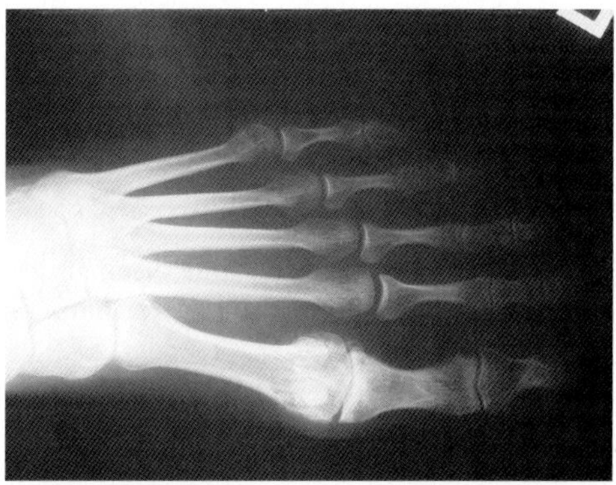

FIG 2 • AP weight-bearing view of foot showing decreased metatarsophalangeal joint space. The surgeon must be wary not to overestimate joint space loss on the AP view alone because overhanging osteophytes may cause joint space to appear obliterated.

- Weight-bearing views are important, because non–weight-bearing views often obscure the dorsal first metatarsal osteophyte. In the non–weight-bearing views, the toes are usually in passive extension, and this may obscure the dorsal osteophyte.
- The AP view is important to assess the amount of medial or lateral joint narrowing.
- The AP view can overestimate the amount of degenerative change as osteophytes may overlie the joint, creating the impression that the joint space is abnormally decreased. Also, a non–weight-bearing AP view can exaggerate the narrowing of the MTP joint space because of the passive extension posturing of the toes at the MTP joint.
- Lateral osteophytes are common and are often early indicators of hallux rigidus. They are also notable at the base of the proximal phalanx. Occasionally, these osteophytes seen on the AP view at the MTP joint are medial.
- Occasionally, a CT scan is useful for detecting osteochondral injuries. MRI can be useful as well for detecting chondral damage (**FIGS 2 AND 3**).

DIFFERENTIAL DIAGNOSIS

- MTP synovitis
- Hallux valgus
- Sesamoiditis or sesamoid fracture

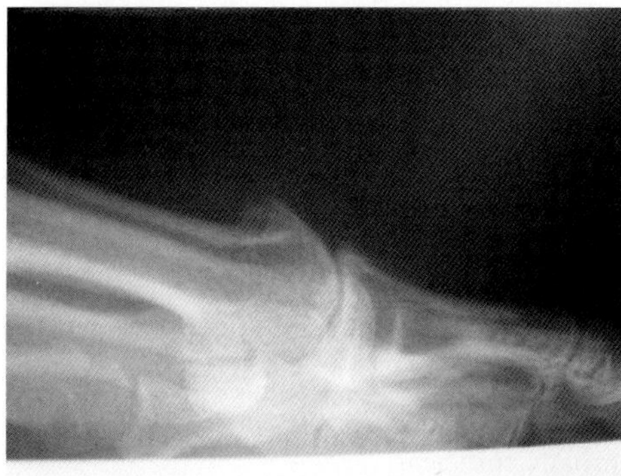

FIG 3 • Lateral weight-bearing view of foot showing dorsal osteophytes of metatarsal head and proximal phalanx.

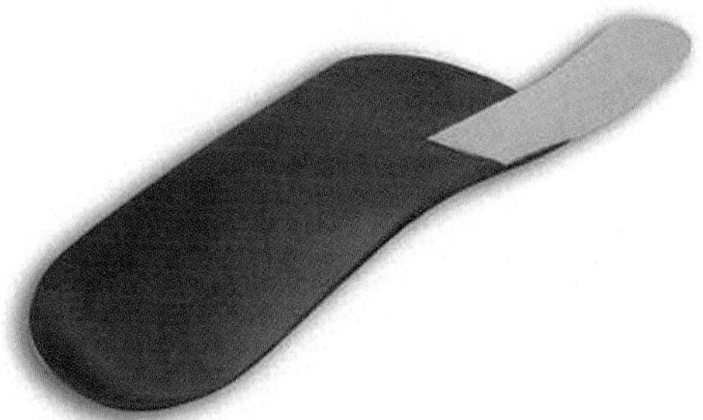

FIG 4 • Typical Morton type of extension to an orthotic. This is thought to decrease dorsiflexion at the metatarsophalangeal joint.

NONOPERATIVE MANAGEMENT

- The decision to pursue nonoperative treatment depends on the patient's symptoms and the extent of the degenerative changes. Patients with mild synovitis and minimal complaints can be treated with rest and anti-inflammatory medications.
- The hallux can be taped or braced to limit dorsiflexion, thus resting the joint.
- There are many devices available to increase the rigidity of the medial forefoot. This limits the motion of the MTP joint, thus minimizing the dorsiflexion impingement pain.
  - A Morton extension is an example (**FIG 4**).
- Steroid injections can be given in the MTP joint. This will help with pain relief but does not slow the degenerative process.
- Standard shoes with a high toe box are helpful for cases of hallux rigidus. This increases the space for the dorsal osteophytes and reduces pressure on the irritable joint.
- A shoe with a stiff-soled rocker bottom is also helpful and helps with gait smoothness.
- These shoe-wear modifications can be effective, but patient compliance and acceptance vary from case to case.
- A study by the senior author with a minimum follow-up of 14 years showed that the pain associated with hallux rigidus remained the same in 22 of 24 feet.[9]

SURGICAL MANAGEMENT

- We routinely perform a cheilectomy with a proximal phalanx osteotomy. The osteotomy is not a stand-alone procedure but is used to augment the effect of the cheilectomy.[10]
- If the osteotomy is to be combined with a cheilectomy, stable internal fixation is important to secure the osteotomy so that early motion of the MTP joint can be started within 1 to 2 weeks after the surgery.

Preoperative Planning

- All radiographs and other imaging studies should be closely reviewed.
  - Special attention should be directed to the lateral radiograph. This study will show the dorsal osteophytes from the distal metatarsal head and proximal phalanx.
- No specific physical examinations need to be done under anesthesia, but it is important to document the passive range of motion (both dorsiflexion and plantarflexion) before the onset of the procedure.
  - The surgeon should alert the patient that we are "stealing" motion from plantarflexion and giving it to dorsiflexion.

Positioning

- The patient is placed supine on the operating table. A Martin-type tourniquet in applied to the supramalleolar region of the ankle.
- The procedure is usually done under ankle block anesthesia.
- A mini C-arm is also used during the procedure and should be available.
- Antibiotics are given before the procedure.
- Positioning is not as important for this procedure as for other operations (**FIGS 5 AND 6**).

Approach

- Usually a dorsomedial approach is used and the extensor hallucis longus (EHL) is retracted laterally. This will provide good access to both the medial and lateral sides of the MTP joint.
- A directly medial approach to the first MTP joint can be used as well, but this approach can limit access to the lateral side of the joint.

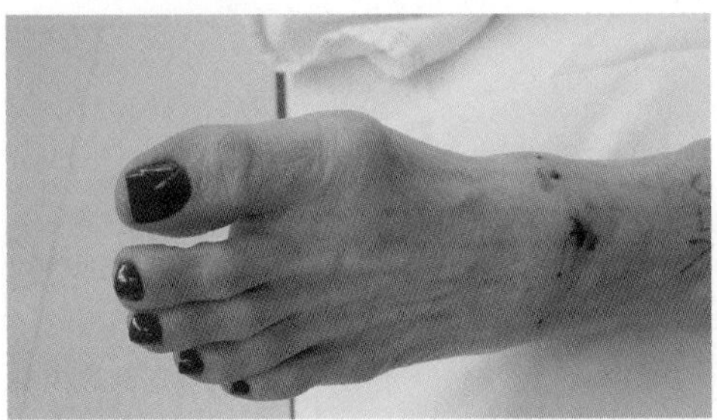

FIG 5 • Operative photograph of foot; note dorsal prominence at metatarsophalangeal joint. Small areas of hemorrhage are from prior ankle block.

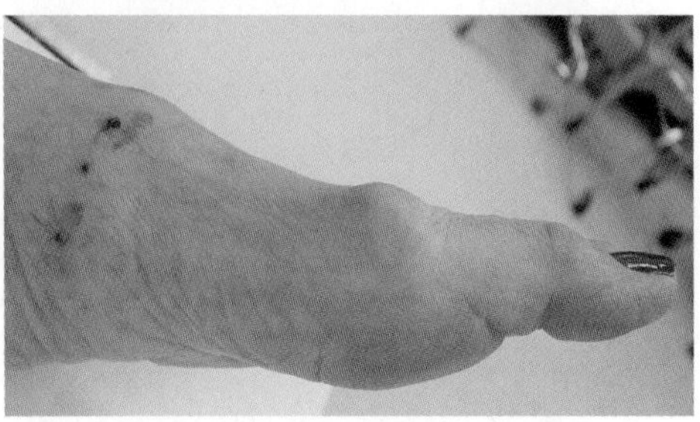

FIG 6 • Lateral operative photograph of foot; note dorsal prominence at metatarsophalangeal joint. Small areas of hemorrhage are from prior ankle block.

APPROACH AND CHEILECTOMY

- Make a dorsomedial incision, taking care to identify and protect the dorsomedial cutaneous nerve.
- Retract the EHL laterally.
- Make the MTP capsulotomy in line with the skin incision; the capsule edges can be tagged with a 2-0 Vicryl suture for ease of identification later.
  - If they are not tagged, carefully identify the dorsal capsule during closure.
  - Retract the capsular edges both plantarly and dorsally.
- Inspect the MTP joint closely.
  - Examine the joint surfaces for osteochondral defects or chondral flaps, as well as overall degeneration within the MTP joint.
- Use a reciprocating saw to remove 1 to 2 mm of the medial eminence.
  - This is done to promote healing of the capsule to the bone.
- Perform a dorsal cheilectomy of the metatarsal head, as described elsewhere. Bone is removed flush with the surface of the dorsum of the metatarsal neck.
  - We try to limit our resection to only the degenerated area of the metatarsal head.
- It is important to gain access to and inspect the lateral side of the MTP joint.
  - Increase the lateral exposure as needed.
  - Osteophytes, which can be hard to detect on radiographs, are often evident on the lateral side of the joint. If present, these osteophytes are removed.
- If present, remove osteophytes or ossicles from the proximal phalanx with a rongeur (**TECH FIGS 1–4**).

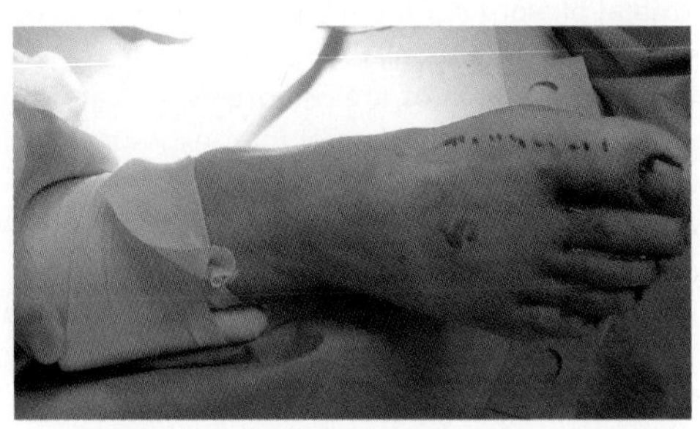

TECH FIG 1 • Operative photograph showing typical line of incision; note tourniquet at supramalleolar region.

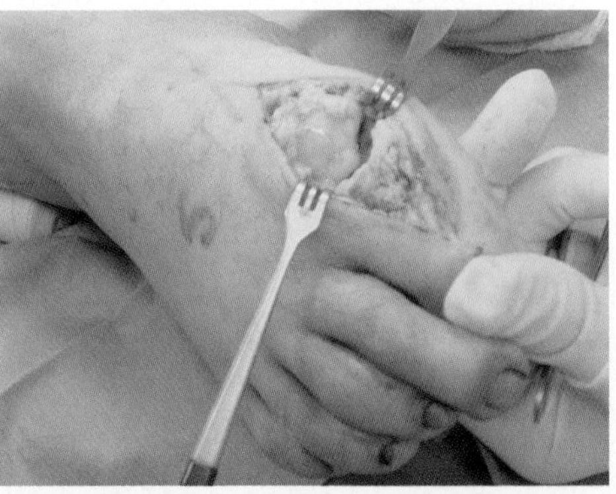

TECH FIG 2 • Operative photograph showing the metatarsophalangeal joint widely exposed. The extensor hallucis longus tendon is retracted laterally. Note exuberant osteophytes on metatarsal head and also osteophytes overhanging from proximal phalanx.

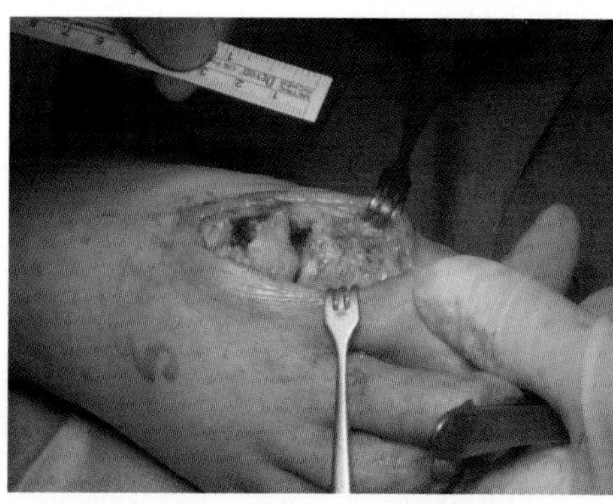

TECH FIG 3 • Operative photograph showing metatarsophalangeal joint after cheilectomy and medial eminence resection. Soft tissue around area of future proximal phalanx osteotomy has been removed.

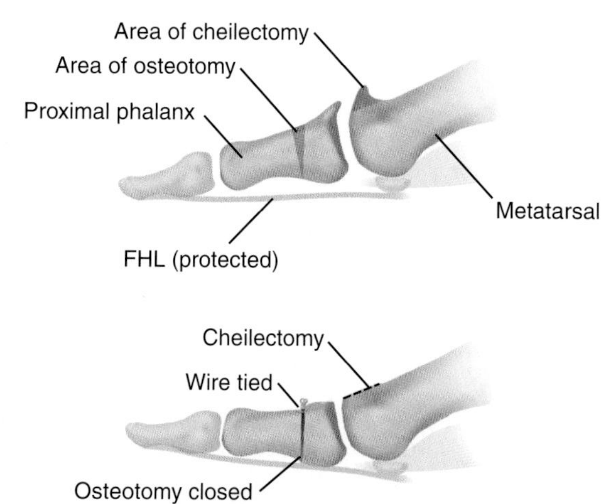

TECH FIG 4 • Schematic of cheilectomy and proximal phalanx osteotomy. Shaded areas will be removed. Protection of the flexor hallucis longus is paramount.

PROXIMAL PHALANX OSTEOTOMY

- We now shift our attention to the proximal phalanx. For the plantar osteotomy, expose the plantar aspect of the proximal phalanx sufficiently to protect the flexor hallucis longus (FHL) tendon.
- During the creation of the osteotomy, be careful to ensure you have enough lateral joint exposure to protect the EHL tendon.
- Place a 0.062-inch smooth Kirschner wire transversely from medial to lateral as a guidewire.
  - It is placed parallel and as close to the articular surface of the proximal phalanx as possible without entering the joint.
  - Use a mini C-arm to verify the proper extra-articular placement of the Kirschner wire. Place the guidewire such that the osteotomy is made just distal to the guide pin.
  - Once the placement of the Kirschner wire has been verified, the osteotomy can begin.
- To maximize the amount of dorsiflexion of the tip of the toe, make the osteotomy as close to the articular surface as feasible. However, if the proximal fragment is too small, sometimes it will fragment postoperatively.
- Use an oscillating saw with a 0.5-cm blade width to make the first cut in the phalanx just distal to the surface of the Kirschner wire.
  - The initial cut is incomplete, leaving the plantar cortex intact.
  - This protects the FHL and maintains stability in the phalanx in preparation for the second cut.
- Make a second, oblique cut measured 5 mm distal to the first cut.
  - In very mild cases of hallux rigidus, a 3–4 mm wedge is used.
  - Keep this cut as parallel as possible to the first cut, looking at the dorsal surface.
    - This width is measured with a sterile ruler.
    - If the two cuts are not parallel, an angular deformity (hallux valgus or varus) can ensue.
  - If there is significant preoperative abductus (lateral angulation), it may help the appearance of the toe to make the medial part of the wedge bigger than the lateral side.
  - As with the first cut, it is important not to finish the osteotomy completely.
- Weaken the remaining plantar cortex with multiple 1.5-mm drill holes. The osteotomy is then completed or "greensticked" (dorsiflexion) manually (**TECH FIGS 5–7**).

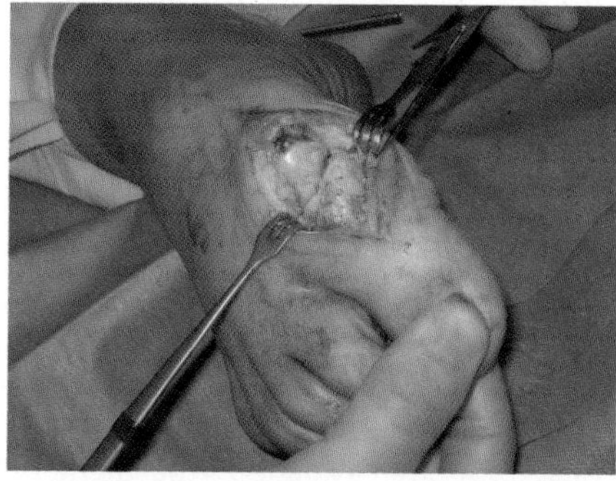

TECH FIG 5 • Operative photograph demonstrating placement of Kirschner wire from medial to lateral to ensure extra-articular placement of osteotomy.

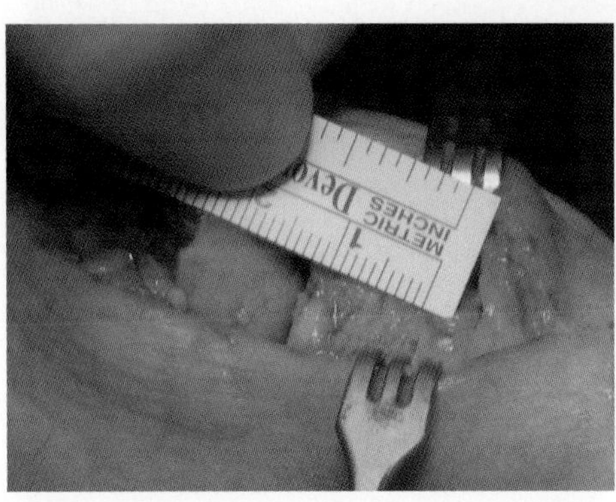

TECH FIG 6 • Operative photograph showing sterile ruler to measure exact dimension of osteotomy.

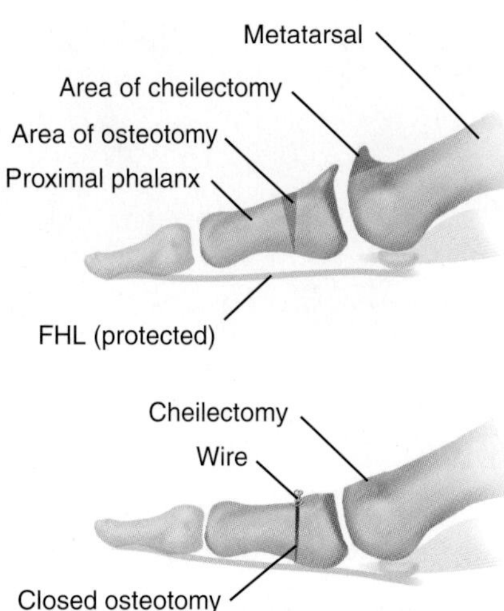

TECH FIG 7 • Schematic showing placement of Kirschner wire to ensure extra-articular placement of Kirschner wire.

FIXATION OF THE OSTEOTOMY AND CLOSURE

- Fix the osteotomy with 28-gauge wire.
- The wire is placed through 1.5-mm drill holes.
- Make one drill hole at the proximal dorsomedial aspect of the basal fragment.
    - Start this hole just adjacent to the articular cartilage at the base of the proximal phalanx and angle it about 45 degrees toward the intramedullary cavity.
    - This starting point is about 4 mm from the osteotomy and helps to avoid breakage of a rather fragile tunnel.
    - It is helpful to pass the wire from proximal to distal; this places most of the tension on the distal side of the osteotomy when the wire is pulled through the distal segment.
- Start the distal drill hole 3 to 4 mm from the osteotomy and angle it about 45 degrees to the plane of the proximal phalanx.
- A wire pass instrument can be used to retrieve the 28-gauge wire passed through the proximal aspect of the osteotomy.
    - As an alternative, a wire passer can be fashioned from the terminal 6 inches of the 28-gauge fixation wire.
- The other 28-gauge wire is modified in the following ways:
    - A 6-inch piece of 28-gauge wire is folded onto itself to form a small loop.
    - The loop is compressed with a small hemostat to fit through the 1.5-mm hole. We usually fold the wire onto itself and form a small loop with the aid of a small hemostat, or mosquito.
    - This loop is then passed into the distal drill hole and into the osteotomy site.
    - Once located within the osteotomy, usually with the assistance of a small hemostat, the created loop is expanded and made larger.
    - This loop is made large enough so the wire from the proximal osteotomy site can be placed through it.
- Once the proximal wire is placed through the loop, the wire with the loop is pulled distally, pulling the proximal wire with it.
- The assistant places dorsiflexion pressure on the plantar tip of the hallux, closing the wedge osteotomy site as the wire is tightened and twisted.
    - While the surgeon applies finger tension on the wire, maintaining a closed osteotomy, the wire is twisted about five revolutions.
    - The wire is cut, leaving about 5 mm of residual wire to be bent and placed against the bone.
- Close the capsule with nonabsorbable suture, usually 2-0 in diameter.
    - Try to completely cover the osteotomy site with soft tissue. Sometimes this is not possible, given the limited amount of distal capsule and thin periosteum.
- Close the skin with nylon type suture in an interrupted fashion.
- Apply a soft dressing consisting of a nonadherent dressing, 4 × 4 gauze, and 4-inch Kling.
- Apply a 2- or 3-inch elastic bandage over this, and the patient is placed in a hard-soled postoperative shoe (**TECH FIGS 8–15**).
- Alternatively, 0.045-inch K-wires or mini fragment screw fixation may be used to secure the osteotomy site.

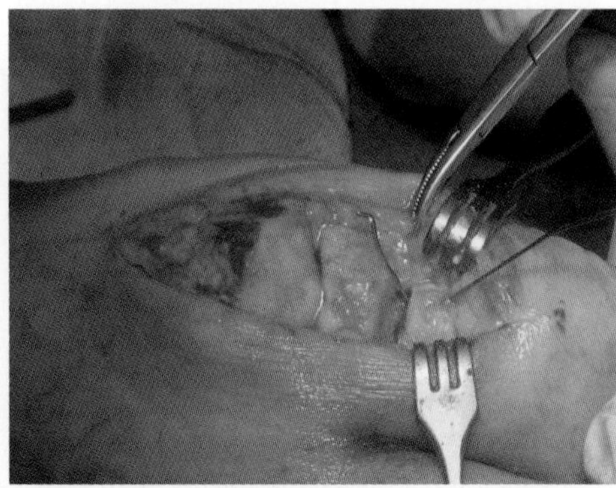

TECH FIG 8 • Operative photograph of 28-gauge wire loop going into distal aspect of osteotomy.

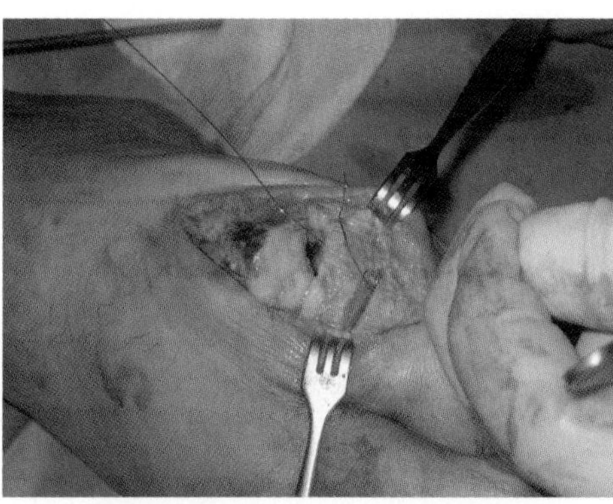

TECH FIG 9 • Operative photograph of 28-gauge wire going into wire loop from proximal to distal.

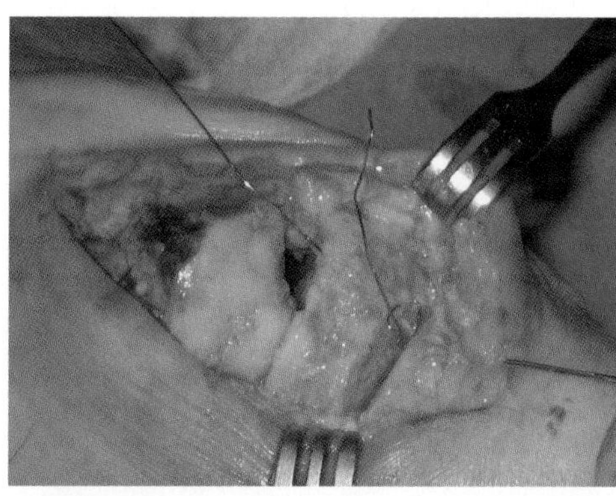

TECH FIG 10 • Operative photograph showing close-up of wire going into loop.

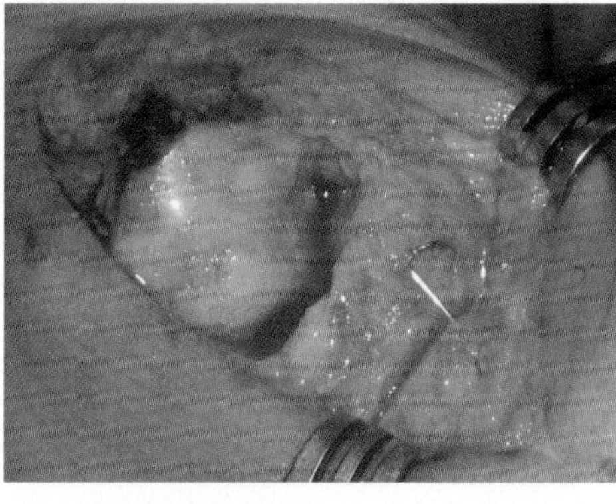

TECH FIG 11 • Operative photograph of wire tied and placed into soft tissue over osteotomy.

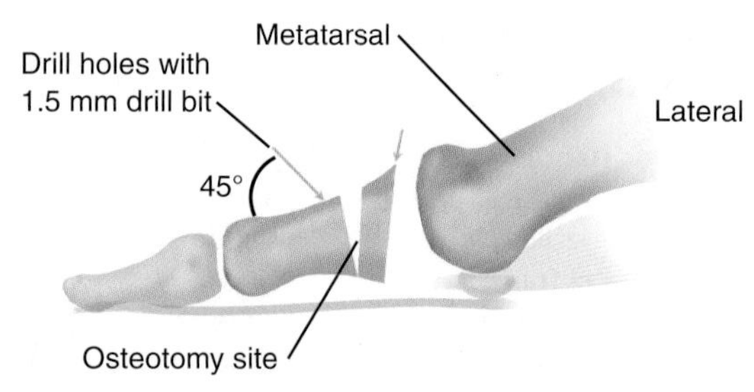

TECH FIG 12 • Creation of proximal and distal drill holes with 1.5-mm drill. Note that the plantar cortex is intact.

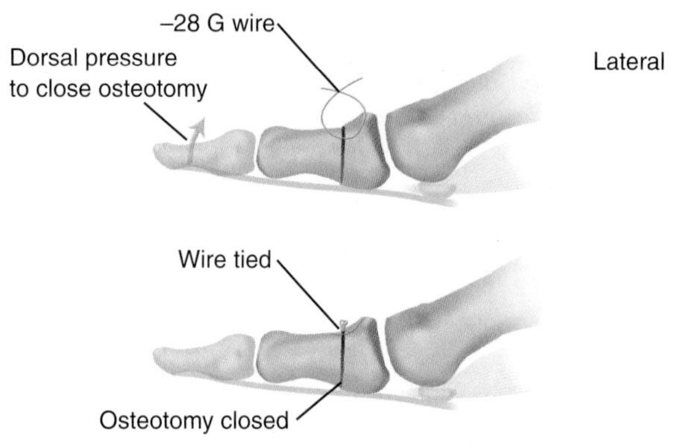

TECH FIG 13 • Dorsal pressure is used to close the osteotomy; the wire is tied; the osteotomy is closed.

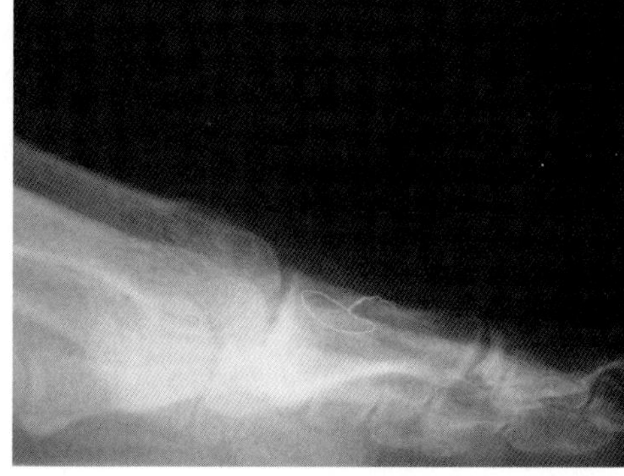

TECH FIG 14 • Lateral radiograph showing healed osteotomy and area of resection from cheilectomy.

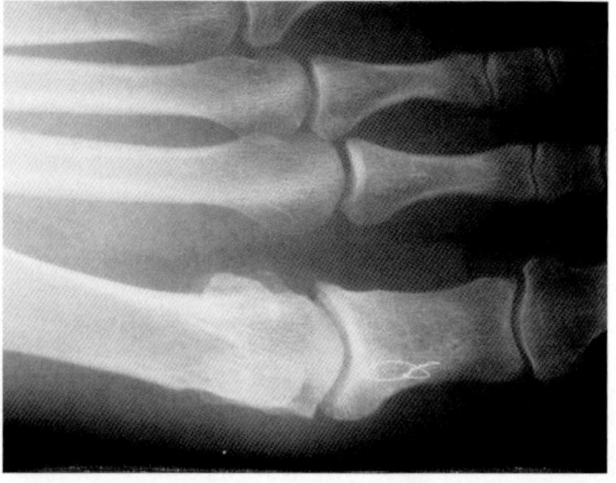

TECH FIG 15 • AP radiographs displaying healed osteotomy of proximal phalanx.

PEARLS AND PITFALLS

Indications	▪ If the MTP joint has end-stage degeneration, the patient may have residual postoperative pain and be better served with an arthrodesis.
Intra-articular osteotomy	▪ Use of Kirschner wire and a mini C-arm can decrease the incidence of an intra-articular placement of the proximal limb of the osteotomy.
Angular deformity after surgery	▪ Extreme care should be taken to make the second cut of the osteotomy as parallel as possible to the first. "Parallel" is from the perspective of looking at the dorsal surface of the proximal phalanx. ▪ It is important to visualize the medial and lateral aspect of the joint and the proximal phalanx.
FHL injury	▪ Careful exposure of the proximal phalanx is essential. ▪ Incomplete plantar osteotomy and "greensticking" the osteotomy after multiple drill holes
Nonunion	▪ Rare, but bony apposition is important, as is solid fixation with the wire technique described ▪ Greensticking of the plantar cortex is also helpful.
Proximal fragment fracture	▪ Creation of 1.5-mm drill hole as close to the proximal articular cartilage as possible ▪ Avoid making the osteotomy too close to the articular surface, let alone cutting into the articular surface. ▪ Pull wire from proximal to distal.

POSTOPERATIVE CARE

- Postoperatively, patients are placed in a hard-soled shoe for 6 weeks.
- Weight bearing as tolerated is allowed the day after surgery when blood coagulation is complete.
- Patients are initially seen 7 to 10 days after surgery. The patient is instructed to massage the operative site to desensitize the wound beginning 1 week postoperatively.
- Passive dorsiflexion exercises of the MTP joint are begun 2 weeks after surgery.
- Plantarflexion-type exercises are not started until 4 weeks postoperatively to avoid early tension on the wire fixation of the osteotomy site.
- Less emphasis is placed on plantarflexion unless the resting posture of the hallux is above ground.

OUTCOMES

- The use of a dorsal closing wedge osteotomy increases the space at the dorsal MTP joint. In effect, the osteotomy draws the dorsal aspect of the phalanx away from the dorsal aspect of the first metatarsal head. The osteotomy may reduce the joint compression force on the dorsum of the first MTP joint during the toe-off phase of gait.
- In one long-term study, eight women who had 10 toes treated for hallux rigidus by dorsal wedge osteotomy of the proximal phalanx were reviewed after an average follow-up of 22 years (no cheilectomies were done in this study).[1] Five toes were symptom-free, four others did not restrict walking, and only one had required metatarsophalangeal fusion. The authors concluded that dorsal wedge osteotomy afforded long-lasting benefits for hallux rigidus.

COMPLICATIONS

- Intra-articular osteotomy
- FHL injury and laceration
- Angular deformity after surgery
- Fragmentation of the proximal fragment of the proximal phalanx
- Nonunion[3]
- Malunion, including rotational malunion[1]
- Failure to improve
- EHL injury and laceration

REFERENCES

1. Citron N, Neil M. Dorsal wedge osteotomy of the proximal phalanx for hallux rigidus: long-term results. J Bone Joint Surg Br 1987; 69B:835–837.
2. Feldman R, Hutter J, Lapow L, et al. Cheilectomy and hallux rigidus. J Foot Surg 1983;22:170–174.
3. Frey CC, Jahss MJ, Kummer FJ. The Akin procedure: an analysis of results. Foot Ankle Int 1991;12:1–6.
4. Giannestras NJ. Foot Disorders: Medical and Surgical Management, 2nd ed. Philadelphia: Lea & Febiger, 1973:400.
5. Gould N, Schneider W, Ashikaga T. Epidemiological survey of foot problems in the continental United States: 1978–1979. Foot Ankle Int 1980;1:8–10.
6. Mann RA, Clanton TO. Hallux rigidus: treatment by cheilectomy. J Bone Joint Surg Am 1988;70A:400–406.
7. McMaster MJ. The pathogenesis of hallux rigidus. J Bone Joint Surg Br 1978;60B:82–87.
8. Moberg E. A simple procedure for hallux rigidus. Clin Orthop Relat Res 1979;142:55–56.
9. Smith RW, Katchis SD, Ayson LC. Outcomes in hallux rigidus patients treated nonoperatively: a long-term follow-up study. Foot Ankle Int 2001;22:462–470.
10. Thomas PJ, Smith RW. Proximal phalanx osteotomy for the surgical treatment of hallux rigidus. Foot Ankle Int 1999;20:3–12.

Chapter 18 Dorsal Cheilectomy for Hallux Rigidus

Richard M. Marks

DEFINITION

- Hallux rigidus refers to limited dorsiflexion of the first metatarsophalangeal (MTP) joint as a result of dorsal osteophyte impingement.
- Plantarflexion is typically not limited, but may be restricted if a large dorsal osteophyte is present.
- In advanced stages, global arthrosis of the first MTP joint is present.

ANATOMY

- The first MTP joint is supported medially and laterally by collateral ligaments that provide medial–lateral stability (**FIG 1**).
- The plantar aspect of the joint consists of (1) the sesamoid complex, including attachments of two slips of the flexor hallucis brevis, which invest the sesamoids (**FIG 2**), and (2) the plantar plate, a thick fibrous band of tissue that additionally invests and supports the sesamoids. The flexor hallucis longus runs between the sesamoids (**FIG 3**).
- The dorsal aspect of the joint includes the capsule, the attachment of the extensor hallucis brevis to the base of the proximal phalanx, and the extensor hallucis longus within the extensor hood.

PATHOGENESIS

- Congenital hallux rigidus (tends to be bilateral)
- Concomitant hallux interphalangus
- A flat, or chevron-shaped MTP joint. This tends to concentrate stresses more centrally.
- Abnormal joint biomechanics
- Trauma to the dorsal articular cartilage, either by a direct blow, or repetitive microtrauma
- Cartilage damage secondary to inflammatory reactions from gout or inflammatory arthritis

NATURAL HISTORY

- Abnormal stresses across the MTP joint—through alterations of biomechanics, increased concentration of dorsal cartilage stresses and wear, inflammatory reaction, or direct cartilage injury—result in reactive dorsal osteophyte and marginal osteophytes. If those stresses are not alleviated or corrected, more global arthritic changes may evolve.

PATIENT HISTORY AND PHYSICAL FINDINGS

- Sagittal range of motion is assessed (**FIG 4**). Pain is typically elicited with extremes of motion, secondary to dorsal impingement, and with plantar motion traction on the dorsal osteophyte.
- A postive grind test indicates more global arthritis, a relative contraindication for cheilectomy.
- Note presence or absence of tenderness with the sesamoid complex exam.

IMAGING AND OTHER DIAGNOSTIC STUDIES

- Standing anteroposterior (AP), lateral, and oblique radiographs are required (**FIG 5**).
  - The joint space may be obliterated by osteophytes on the AP radiograph, so the oblique radiograph may provide a better view of the retained joint surface.
  - The AP radiograph is useful to evaluate medial and lateral osteophytes, and the lateral radiograph will reveal the

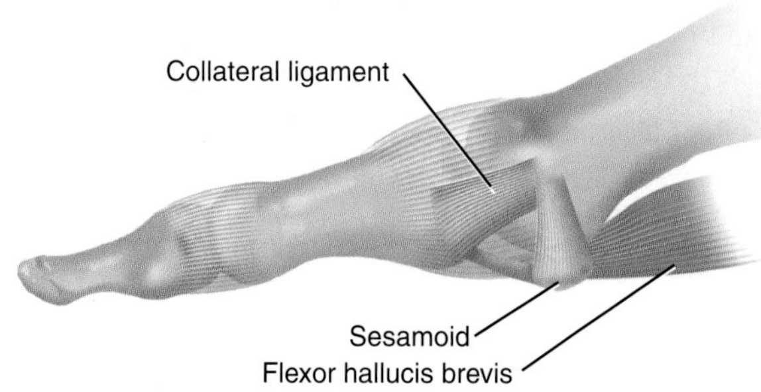

FIG 1 • Medial aspect of first MTP joint anatomy. Collateral ligaments afford medial-lateral stability.

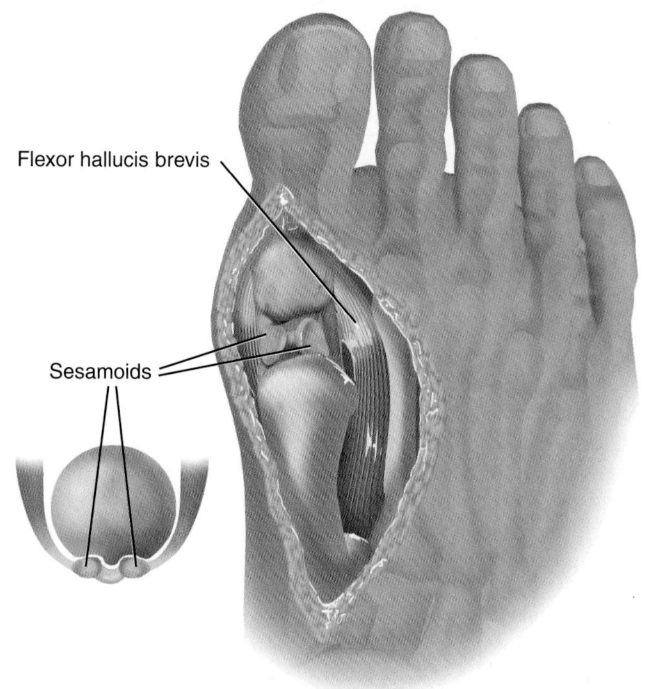

FIG 2 • Dorsal aspect of first MTP joint anatomy.

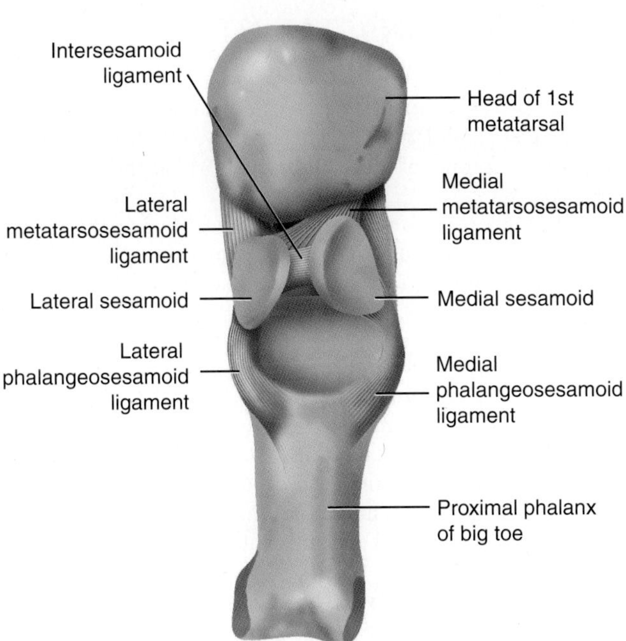

FIG 3 • Detail of first MTP joint anatomy with detail of sesamoid complex.

presence of metatarsus elevatus, and the extent of the dorsal osteophyte.

- Axial sesamoid view will provide additional information about the sesamoid complex.
- Magnetic resonance imaging is helpful if osteochondral defect of the metatarsal head is suspected (**FIG 6**).

DIFFERENTIAL DIAGNOSIS

- Arthrosis (advanced hallux rigidus)
- Osteochondral defect
- "Turf toe," sesamoid complex injury
- Gout

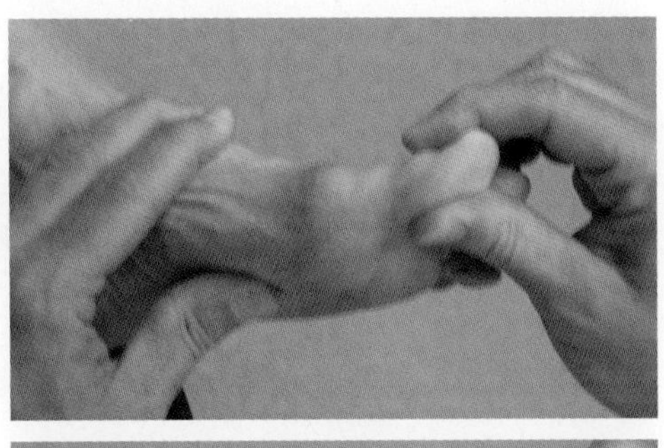

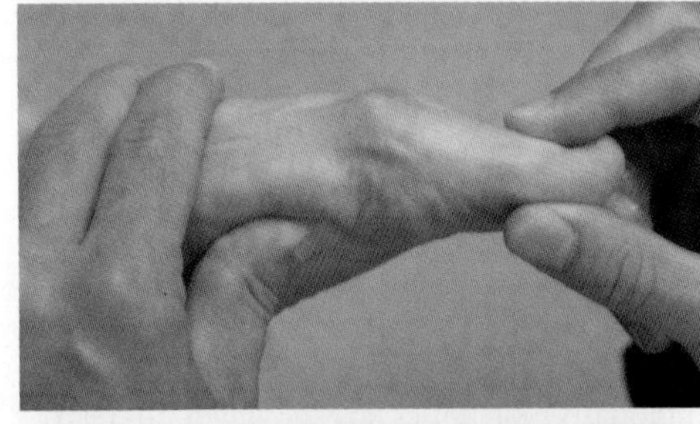

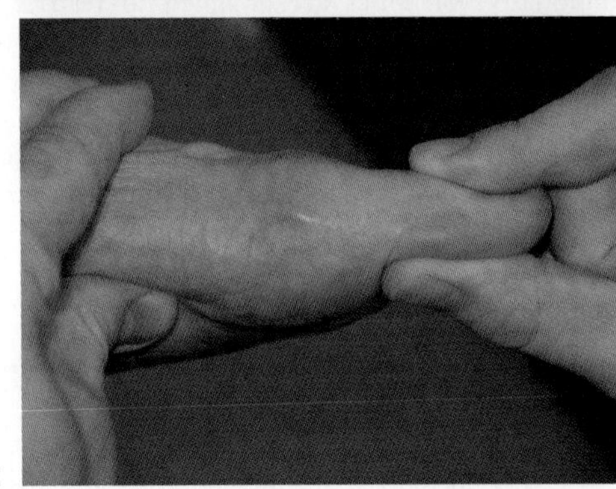

FIG 4 • Assessing first MTP joint motion in patient with hallux rigidus. **A.** Dorsiflexion produces symptomatic impingement. **B.** Often, plantarflexion is also painful, with traction of the dorsal soft tissue structures over the dorsal osteophyte. **C.** Neutral position demonstrating dorsal osteophyte.

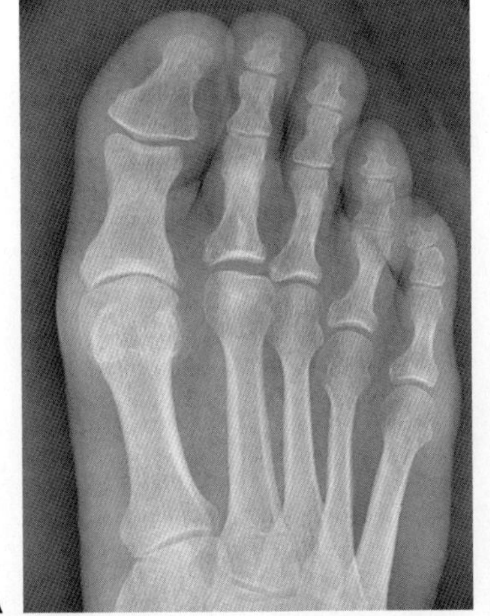

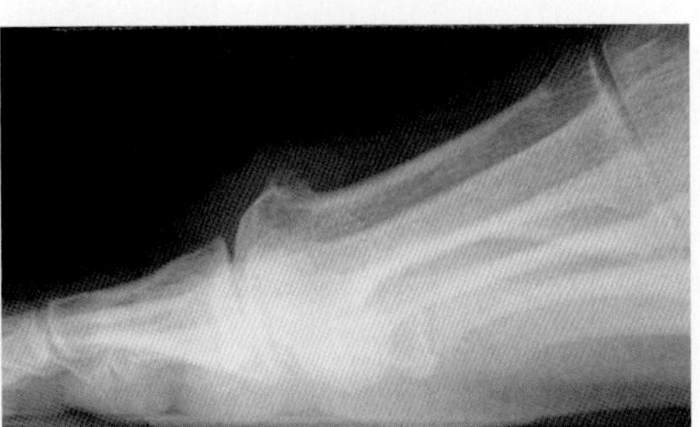

FIG 5 • Radiographs of patient with hallux rigidus. **A.** AP view demonstrating joint space narrowing. **B.** Lateral view with dorsal osteophyte on first metatarsal head.

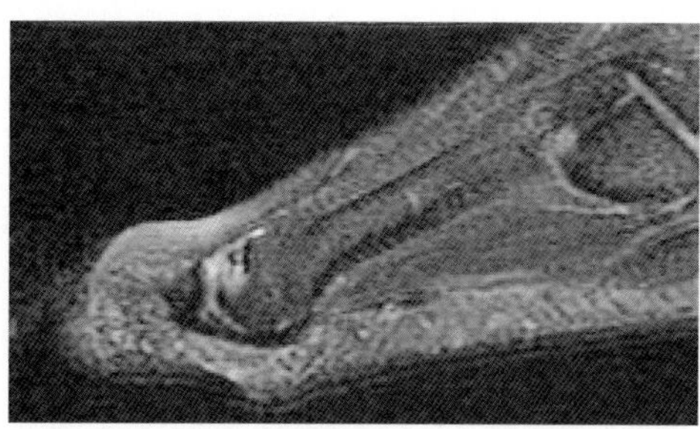

FIG 6 • MRI is not required in the evaluation of hallux rigidus but provides detail if the degree of degenerative change is mild and an osteochondral defect is suspected.

NONOPERATIVE MANAGEMENT

- Nonoperative treatment consists of the institution of NSAIDs, accommodative orthotics, and, rarely, physical therapy if gait abnormality is present.
- Accommodative orthotics are designed to restrict sagittal range of motion of the hallux and to redistribute weightbearing stresses across the first MTP joint with the use of a Morton's extension.
- If sesamoid inflammation is present, protective padding is added around the sesamoids and the orthotic is welled out under the sesamoids to provide stress relief.

SURGICAL MANAGEMENT

Preoperative Planning

- Preoperatively, patients are assessed for whether they are appropriate candidates for cheilectomy, or for fusion if there are symptoms of more global arthritis of the first MTP joint.
- Cheilectomy is performed for predominantly dorsal arthritic symptoms and for failure to respond to nonoperative means of treatment, as outlined in the previous section.

Positioning

- Preoperatively, patients receive a regional ankle block consisting of a 1:1 mixture of 0.5% bupivacaine and 1% lidocaine, without epinephrine.
- Intravenous antibiotics are administered in the holding area, 30 to 45 minutes before the procedure.
- The patient is placed supine on the operating room table, with the foot at the distal edge of the table to allow for easier fluoroscopic access.
- The foot, ankle, and lower leg are prepped and draped to the lower calf with the use of a leg holder.

Approach

- The first MTP joint is approached dorsally, starting distally from the midportion of the proximal phalanx, and extending proximally 3 cm proximal to the joint.

TECHNIQUES

INCISION AND EXPOSURE

- The incision is made medial to the extensor hallucis longus tendon, taking care to preserve the tendon within its sheath (**TECH FIG 1A**).
- Once the tendon is brought laterally and protected, the incision is carried down through the dorsal capsule and distally past the base of the proximal phalanx.
- Loose bodies and proliferative synovium are excised.
- The dorsal aspect of the collateral ligaments is reflected to allow for exposure of the medial and lateral aspects of the joint. Care must be taken to avoid inadvertently destabilizing the joint.
- Hohmann or Senn retractors are placed medially and laterally to protect the soft tissues. Particular attention is paid to protect the extensor hallucis longus tendon distally (**TECH FIG 1B,C**).
- The dorsal osteophyte from the base of the proximal phalanx is resected with a flexible chisel. The hallux is maximally dorsiflexed during this maneuver to protect the central and plantar cartilage of the first metatarsal head.
- The hallux is maximally plantarflexed to allow for examination of the cartilage of the metatarsal head.

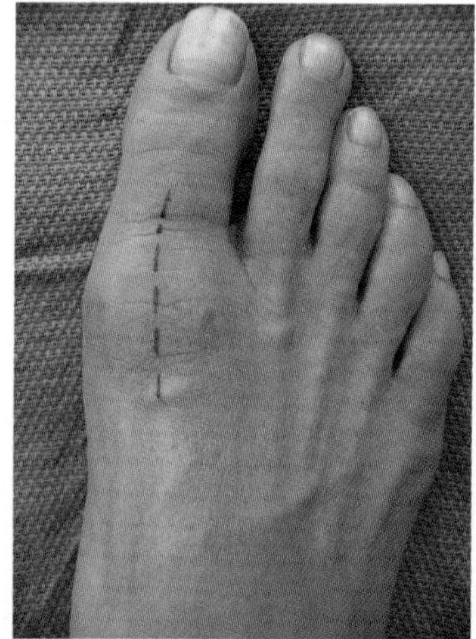

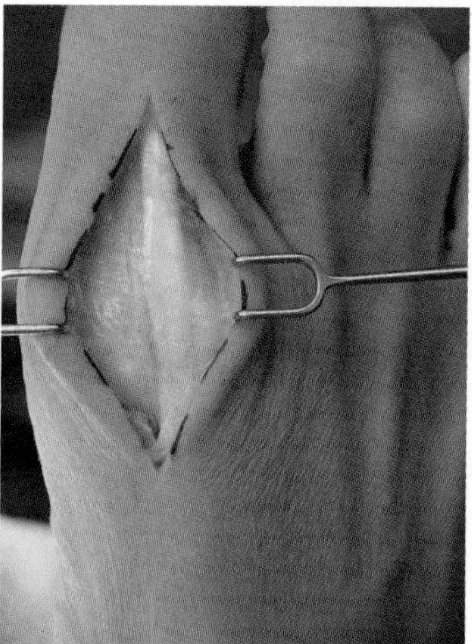

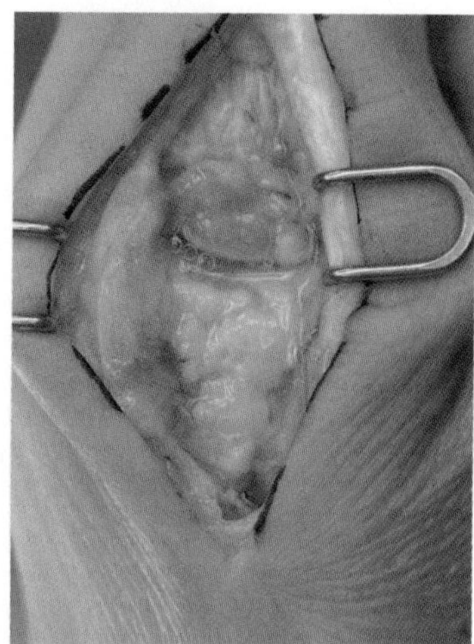

TECH FIG 1 • Approach. **A.** Dorsomedial incision. **B.** Identify and protect the dorsomedial sensory nerve to the hallux and the EHL tendon. **C.** Longitudinal capsulotomy after nerve and tendon are retracted.

RESECTION (TECH FIG 2A–I)

- The dorsal 25% to 30% of the metarsal head articular surface is resected with a flexible chisel, beginning distally and angled proximally to exit at the metaphyseal–diaphyseal junction of the metatarsal. The extent of articular surface resection frequently corresponds to the wear pattern of the cartilage. Avoid exiting too far proximal in the diaphyseal bone, which might weaken the metatarsal.
- Alternatively, a microsagittal saw can be used to resect bone from a proximal to distal direction, but care must be taken to avoid excessive articular cartilage resection. I prefer to start the cartilage resection from the metatarsal head distally.
- Medial and lateral osteophytes are resected, taking care to avoid destabliization of the collateral ligaments.

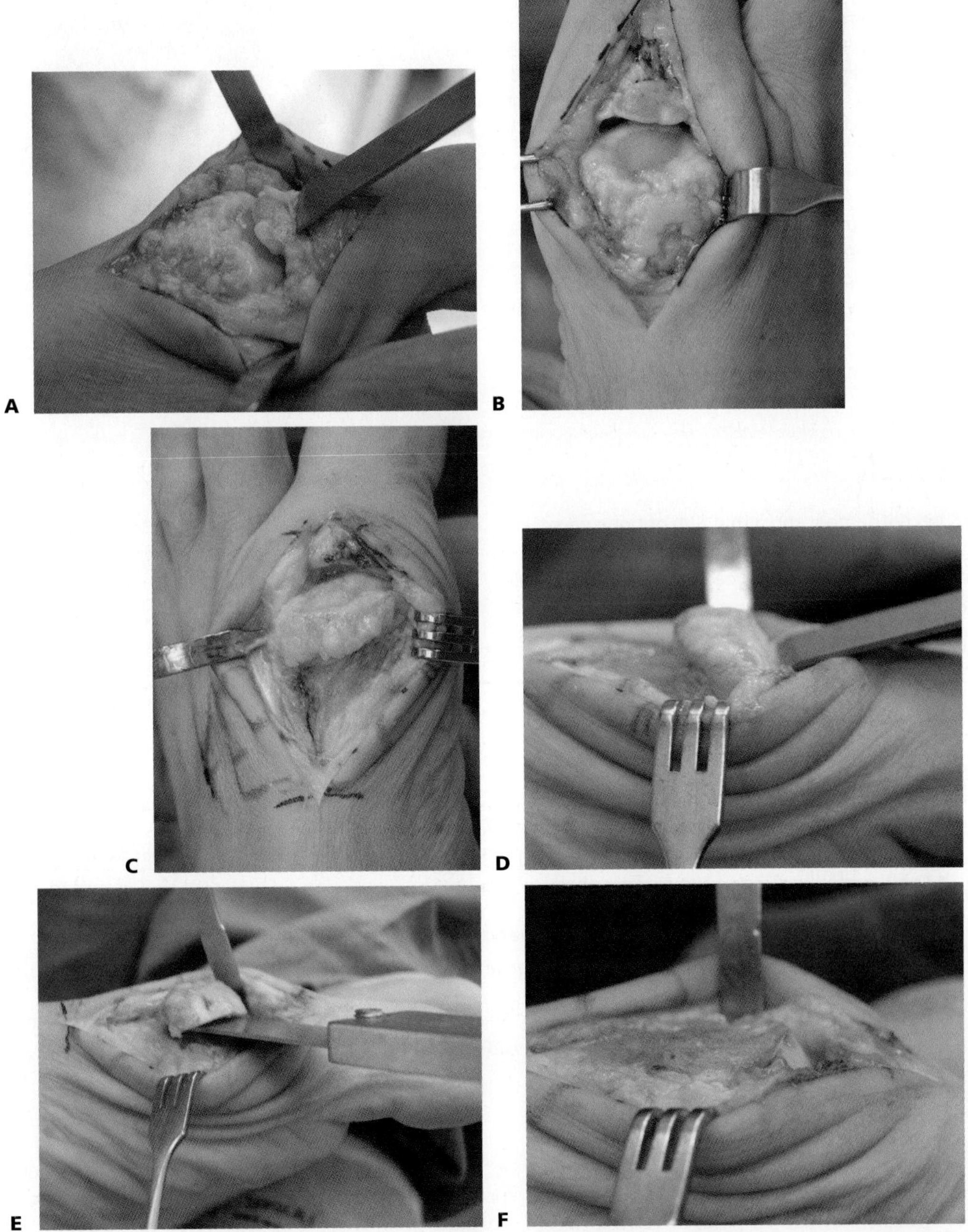

TECH FIG 2 • A–F. Resection. **A.** Removing dorsal osteophyte on proximal phalanx. **B.** Joint exposed, demonstrating typical degenerative wear pattern. Note medial and lateral osteophytes. **C.** Dorsal view of dorsal osteophyte. **D.** Sagittal view of large dorsal osteophyte and chisel positioned for resection. **E.** Chisel to resect osteophyte and dorsal ¼ to 1/3 of residual articular surface. **F.** After osteophyte resection. *(continued)*

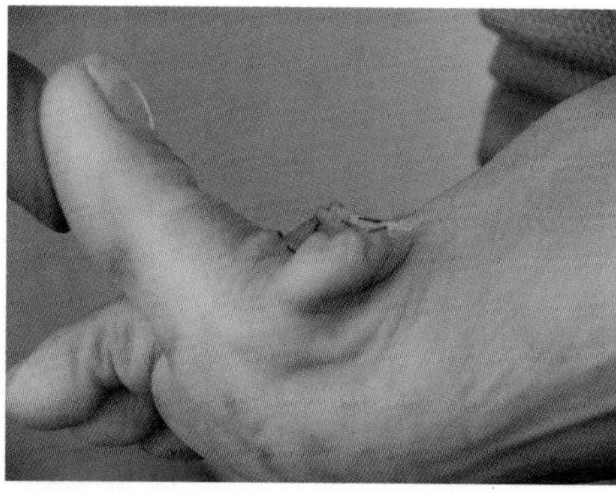

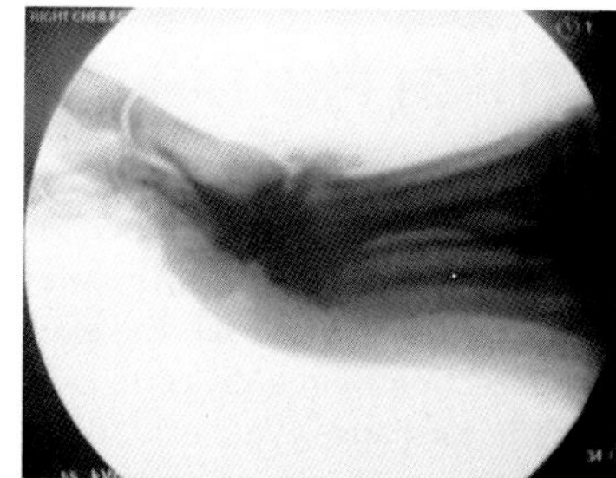

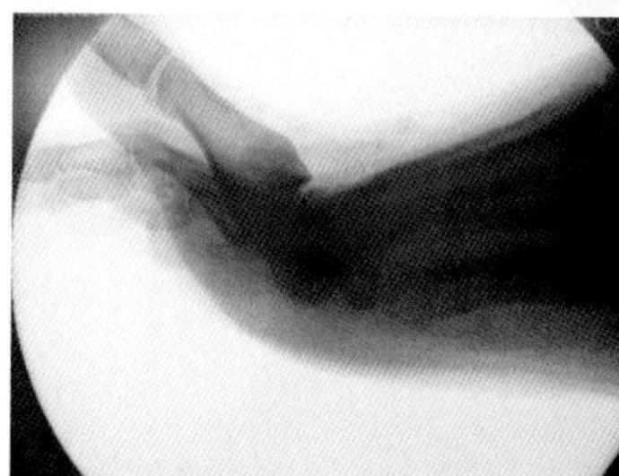

TECH FIG 2 • *(continued)* **G–I.** Checking first MTP joint range-of-motion after resection. **G.** Passive dorsiflexion of the toe relative to the metatarsal shaft axis should approach 90 degrees. **H.** Fluoroscopy prior to osteophyte resection. **I.** Fluoroscopy after osteophyte resection.

- The hallux is maximally dorsiflexed and inspected for any residual impingement. If necessary, additional bone is resected and motion re-evaluated.
- Fluoroscopy can be used to verify adequacy of bone resection, in both the AP and sagittal planes.
- If discrete osteochondral defect is noted, the base of the defect is drilled in multiple directions with a 0.045-inch Kirschner wire to facilitate bleeding into the defect and formation of fibrocartilage.

COMPLETION

- The wound is irrigated, and a thin film of bone wax is applied to the cancellous bone of the dorsal metatarsal.
- Closure of the capsule is performed with a 2-0 absorbable suture. If necessary, the extensor mechanism is centralized to prevent valgus drift of the hallux postoperatively.
- Subcutaneous closure is performed with either 2-0 or 3-0 absorbable suture, and the skin is closed with simple 4-0 nylon suture. A sterile compressive dressing is applied.

PEARLS AND PITFALLS

Indications	▪ Verify that the patient is experiencing symptoms of mechanical dorsal impingement. ▪ Global arthitis with a positive grind test and pain at rest is a contraindication for cheilectomy.
Approach	▪ Avoid destabilization of the extensor hallucis longus. Medial and lateral exposure should preserve the collateral ligaments. ▪ Avoid injury to the dorsomedial cutaneous branch of the superficial peroneal nerve.
Bone resection	▪ To protect the articular surface of the metatarsal, maximally dorsiflex the hallux while performing resection of the dorsal base of the proximal phalanx. ▪ Twenty-five to 30% of the articular surface of the metatarsal head needs to be resected to avoid residual impingement. Inadequate bone resection is responsible for most failures.

POSTOPERATIVE CARE

- Patients are instructed to elevate the operative leg for the first 10 days, with heel weight bearing in a postoperative shoe (**FIG 7A,B**).
- At 10 days, sutures are removed and Steri-Strips applied. Postoperative radiographs are obtained at this visit.
- At this point, weight bearing as tolerated is permitted in a postoperative shoe. The patient weans to a sneaker or comfortable shoe over the successive 10 to 14 days.
- Physical therapy is also instituted at 10 days, concentrating on re-establishing range of motion, diminishing edema, and performing scar massage.

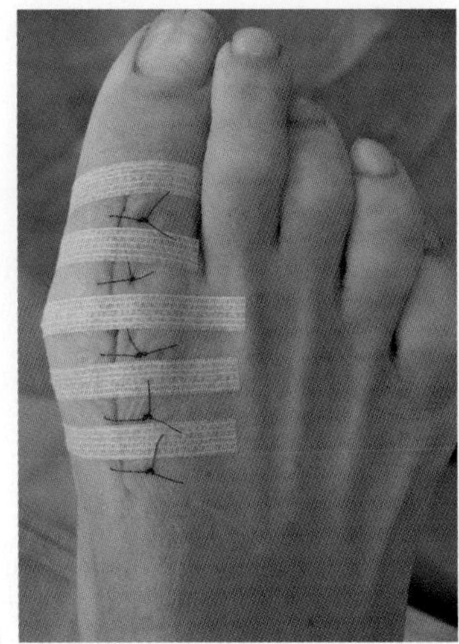
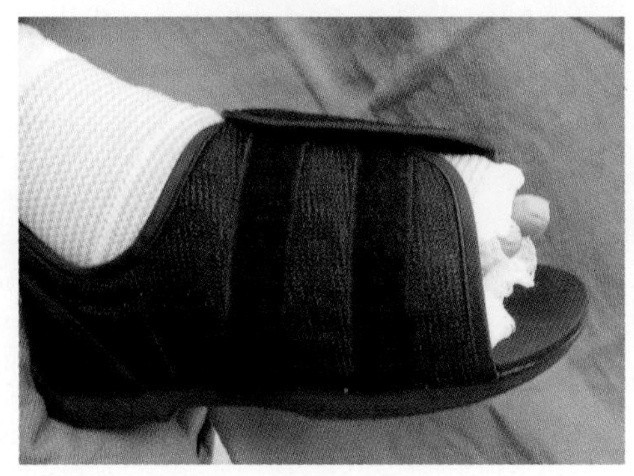

FIG 7 • Postoperative management. **A.** Closure. **B.** Immediate weight-bearing in a post-surgical shoe.

- Physical activity such as biking, swimming, and elliptical trainer and stairmaster usage is instituted shortly thereafter. Running activities are typically withheld until approximately 3 months after surgery.
- The use of an accommodative orthotic with a Morton's extension is occasionally prescribed for a period of time if patients complain of discomfort after activities, or continued weight bearing on the lateral aspect of the foot is necessary.

OUTCOMES

- Good to excellent outcomes after cheilectomy range from 72% to 92%.
- Better results are noted with grades I and II.
- Poorer outcomes are reported if there is over 50% loss of articular cartilage at time of surgery.
- No correlation is noted between postoperative radiographic deterioration of joint space and clinical outcome.
- Results do not tend to diminish with time.
- Less than 8% of patients subsequently require fusion.

COMPLICATIONS

- Inadequate bone resection
- Destabilization of the collateral ligaments
- Dorsomedial cutaneous nerve damage
- Progression of arthritis

REFERENCES

1. Coughlin MJ, Shurnas PS. Hallux rigidus: demographics, etiology, and radiographic assessment; Foot Ankle Int 2003;24:731–743.
2. Coughlin MJ, Shurnas PS. Hallux rigidus: grading and long-term results of operative treatment. J Bone Joint Surg Am 2003;85A: 2072–2088.
3. Feltham GT, Hanks SE, Marcus RE. Age-based outcomes of cheilectomy for the treatment of hallux rigidus. Foot Ankle Int 2001; 22:192–197.
4. Hattrup SJ, Johnson KA. Subjective results of hallux rigidus following treatment with cheilectomy. Clin Orthop Rel Res 1998;226: 182–191.
5. Mann RA, Clanton TO. Hallux rigidus: treatment by cheilectomy; J Bone Joint Surg Am 1988;70A:400–406.
6. Mulier T, Steenwerckx A, Thienpont E, et al. Results after cheilectomy in athletes with hallux rigidus. Foot Ankle Int 1999;20:232–237.

Chapter 19

Dorsal Cheilectomy, Extensive Plantar Release, and Microfracture Technique

Hajo Thermann and Christoph Becher

DEFINITION

- Hallux rigidus, osteoarthrosis of the first metatarsophalangeal joint (MTP), was first described by Cotterill[8] and Davies-Colley[12] in 1887.
- Pain and restriction in range of motion (ROM) in the first MTP joint are the major characteristics of hallux rigidus.[41]
- After hallux valgus, hallux rigidus is the second most common deformity of the first MTP joint. The big toe is the location in the foot with the highest incidence of osteoarthrosis; estimates suggest that nearly 10% of the adult population is affected by hallux rigidus.[18,19]
- The incidence of hallux rigidus is higher in women than in men.[5,6]

ANATOMY

- The first MTP joint is a stable joint formed by the rounded head of the first metatarsal bone fitting into the concave proximal facet of the proximal phalanx.
- The joint is enhanced by the plantar and collateral ligaments. The deep transverse metatarsal ligament is connected to the second ray.
- The sesamoid bones are embedded in the flexor hallucis brevis tendon. They are accommodated at the underside of the first metatarsal in two longitudinally oriented grooves. In a normal relationship, the sesamoids glide distally and proximally within the grooves by a combination of active and passive forces.
- The extensor hallucis longus tendon covers the dorsal side of the first MTP joint and inserts into the base of the distal phalanx.
- The dorsomedial cutaneous nerve is in danger when using a dorsomedial approach to the joint. It is the most medial branch of the superficial peroneal nerve. An anatomic study has shown that the minimum distance from the medial edge of the extensor hallucis longus tendon is 6 mm.[36]

PATHOGENESIS

- The mechanism responsible for developing hallux rigidus remains unclear.
- In theory, damage to the cartilage surface of the first MTP joint, ie, osteochondral fractures or chondral defects, may lead gradually to posttraumatic arthrosis.
- Alternatively, repetitive microtrauma to the first MTP joint, with eccentric overload and stresses that exceed physiologic stresses, may result in hallux rigidus, as seen in football players and ballet dancers.
- The contact distribution shifts dorsally with increasing degrees of extension.[1] This is consistent with the observation that chondral erosions often initially affect the dorsal aspect of the articular surface of the first metatarsal.
- Various factors, in isolation or in combination, have been suggested as contributing to the development of first MTP joint arthrosis: (1) hyperextension injury (ie, turf toe injury) to the hallux; (2) metatarsus primus elevatus; (3) osteochondral lesions; (4) a long first metatarsal; or even (5) wearing inappropriate shoes.[6,23,27,29,32,40,41]
- In 2003, Coughlin et al[9] evaluated 114 patients treated operatively for hallux rigidus over a 19-year period in a single surgeon's practice for demographics, etiology, and radiographic findings associated with hallux rigidus.
  - The disease was not associated with metatarsus primus elevatus, first ray hypermobility, increased first metatarsal length, Achilles or gastrocnemius tendon tightness, abnormal foot posture, symptomatic hallux valgus, adolescent onset, footwear, or occupation.
  - Hallux rigidus was associated with hallux valgus interphalangeus, female gender, and a positive family history in bilateral cases.
  - In most cases the problem was bilateral, except when trauma was involved—if trauma had occurred, then the problem was unilateral.
  - Metatarsus adductus was more common in patients with hallux rigidus than in the general population, but no significant correlation was found.
  - A flat or chevron-shaped MTP joint was more common in patients with hallux rigidus.

NATURAL HISTORY

- The natural history of hallux rigidus is similar to that of degenerative arthritis in any joint. Once the process has started, the articular cartilage is more susceptible to injury resulting from shear and compressive forces. The subchondral bone shares these stresses, which subsequently lead to increased subchondral bone density and formation of periarticular osteophytes. The osteophytes limit first MTP joint motion and further compromise the normal mechanics of this joint. This effect can accelerate the degenerative process.
- The natural history is, at the endpoint, stiffness and constant pain. The length of time that elapses from initial symptoms to constant pain varies widely. The standard time frame over which daily or recreational sports activities become painful is about 5 to 10 years, whereas athletes (eg, tennis and basketball players) who experience constant and repetitive impacts develop constant symptoms in a shorter period of time. In most patients, stiffness is not an issue.
- Outcomes in 22 patients with hallux rigidus representing 24 feet treated nonoperatively at an average follow-up of 14.4 years showed that the pain remained about the same in 22 feet, improved with time in 1 foot, and became worse in 1 foot. There was measurable loss of cartilage space

radiographically over time in 16 of 24 feet, and in 8 of the 16 feet, the loss of cartilage space was dramatic.[16]

PATIENT HISTORY AND PHYSICAL FINDINGS

- Hallux rigidus is associated with a positive family history of great toe problems in almost two thirds of patients.[9]
- The standard history is a trauma at the MTP joint several years earlier, but more often we find active persons—mostly former athletes—who are performing high-impact sports such as tennis, golf, or basketball. Starting with "feeling the joint" after exercising, it becomes a progressively limiting factor that prevents them from performing their sport at their normal level.
- The true etiology of hallux rigidus is often not known.
- In the early stages, the patient complains of pain only on dorsiflexion of the great toe; the ROM is unaffected or only moderately restricted. In the mid-stage of hallux rigidus, the patient complains of motion-dependent pain. Dorsiflexion of the great toe is restricted. Osteophytes may occur dorsal to the first metatarsal head and may be palpable, the plantar structures become tight, plantarflexion becomes painful at the sesamoid–metatarsal joint (mostly medial), and the ROM also is restricted. A dynamic stress test in dorsiflexion (ie, pressure with the thumb on the medial or lateral sesamoid) can distinguish between sesamoid–MT head pain and MTP pain. Unfortunately, this test is not clear in the presence of ongoing stiffness and arthritic changes of the MTP joint. The late stages present with reduced to complete inhibited dorsiflexion and plantarflexion of the toe, with palpable osteophytes dorsal (medial and lateral) to the metatarsal head and especially around the entire phalangeal base.
- The most striking physical manifestation of hallux rigidus noticed by patients is the bony prominence at the dorsum of the metatarsal head, which is disturbing and painful, especially in firm leather shoes.
- Methods for examining the first MTP joint are as follows:
  - ROM, dorsiflexion, and plantarflexion are checked. In the early stages, restriction of dorsiflexion ("dorsal impingement") is found. In later stages, restriction of plantarflexion and pain at the midrange of the motion arc (indicative of global first MTP joint degenerative joint disease) also are found.
  - Palpation of the first MTP joint. In later stages, palpable and painful osteophytes are present as a symptom of ongoing osteoarthritis.
  - Inspection for clinical changes in form or color of the first MTP joint

IMAGING AND OTHER DIAGNOSTIC STUDIES

- Standard weight-bearing AP (**FIGS 1** and **2**) and lateral radiographs of the foot as well as weight-bearing radiographs of the metatarsals and, in cases of sesamoid pathologies, a sesamoid special radiograph, should be performed.
- Coughlin and Shurnas[10] proposed a classification system based on the radiographic system of Hattrup and Johnson[20] that is representative of the natural history. It includes ROM, as well as radiographic and examination findings, as follows:
  - Grade 0: Dorsiflexion (DF) of 40 to 60 degrees (ie, 20% loss of normal motion), normal radiographic results, and no pain

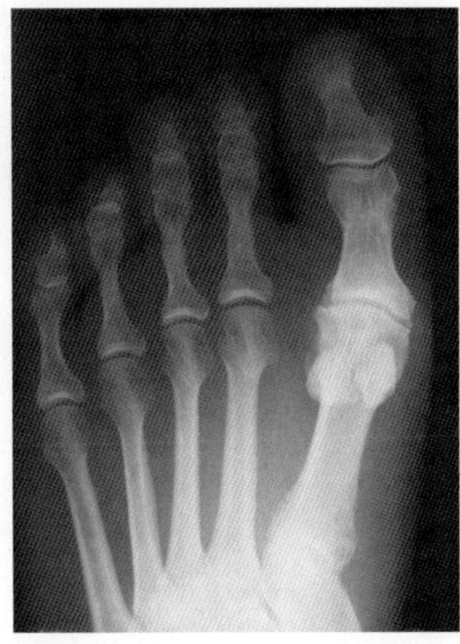

FIG 1 • Hallux rigidus grade 2 on AP weight-bearing radiograph.

  - Grade 1: DF of 30 to 40 degrees, dorsal osteophytes, and minimal to no other joint changes
  - Grade 2: DF of 10 to 30 degrees, mild flattening of the MTP joint, mild to moderate joint narrowing or sclerosis, and dorsal, lateral, or medial osteophytes
  - Grade 3: DF of less than 10 degrees, often less than 10 degrees plantarflexion, severe radiographic changes with hypertrophied cysts or erosions or with irregular sesamoids, constant moderate to severe pain, and pain at the extremes of the ROM
  - Grade 4: stiff joint, radiographs showing loose bodies or osteochondritis dissecans, and pain throughout the entire ROM
- Indications for MRI in MTP–sesamoid pathology include:
  - Severe pain in the MTP complex unrelated to radiographic results
  - Absence of visible joint space narrowing on radiography
  - Suspected osteochondral lesion in the MT head on radiography
  - Suspected sesamoid arthritis or necrosis on radiography
- The MRI examination should include sagittal, axial, and coronal views with T1-weighted (TR 35 ms, TE 16 ms) and

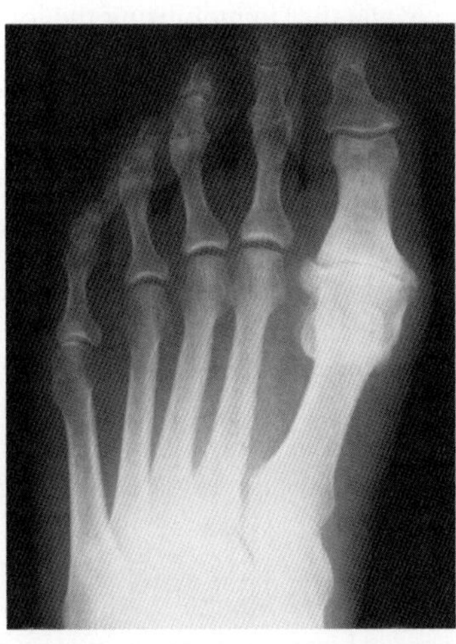

FIG 2 • Hallux rigidus grade 3 on AP weight-bearing radiograph.

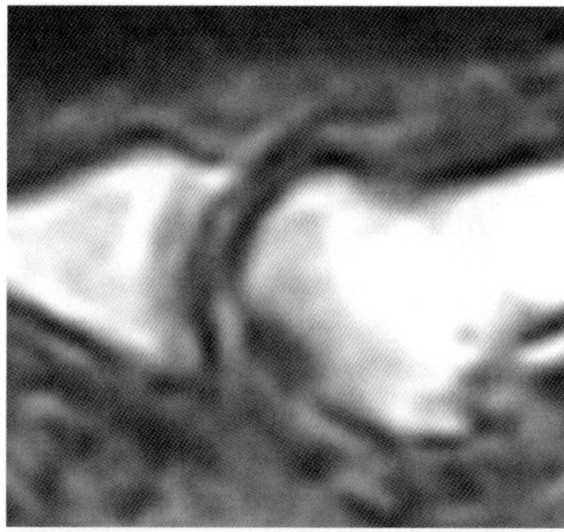

FIG 3 • MRI scan showing an osteochondral lesion of the metatarsal head.

high-resolution gradient echo (TR 1060 ms, TE 16 ms) images (**FIG 3**).

DIFFERENTIAL DIAGNOSIS

- Gout
- Rheumatoid arthritis
- Psoriatic arthritis
- Reiter's syndrome
- Infectious arthritis
- Sesamoid osteonecrosis

NONOPERATIVE MANAGEMENT

- The primary nonoperative treatments of hallux rigidus are anti-inflammatory therapy and pain relief by orthotic devices.
  - Anti-inflammatory drugs (eg, diclofenac) may be used systemically and locally.
  - Injections in the joint should be restricted to single cases. A single shot of corticosteroids may lead to pain relief.
  - Cooling devices also inhibit the inflammation process.
  - Orthotic devices such as stiff inserts for shoes or rocker bottom soles take pressure from the MTP joint by facilitating the scrolling process. To further alleviate pressure on the joint, a shoe with a roomy toe box should be worn, and high heels should be avoided.
  - Physical therapy helps keep the joint mobile.
- The question is whether immobilizing the joint by orthotics or stiff insoles in early arthritis is a reasonable approach, because doing so results in the functional breakdown of the MTP joint. In our practice, we prefer to keep the joint mobile by physical therapy and manual therapy and by having the patient perform exercises for dorsiflexion and plantarflexion daily (eg, aqua jogging on tiptoes).
- We have found that chondroitin and glucosamine sulfate, slow-acting drugs for the treatment of osteoarthritis,[21,34] have comparable success in improving the pain and symptoms of osteoarthritis.
- Additional nonsteroidal anti-inflammatory drugs and icing can be applied to support progress at the beginning of the physical therapy program.

SURGICAL MANAGEMENT

- The goal of surgical treatment is to achieve a pain-free joint.
- Several surgical approaches have been proposed in the literature, including resection arthroplasty,[7,22,23,30] interpositional arthroplasty,[2,19,24] MTP replacement (implant arthroplasty),[11,39] arthrodesis,[18,28,32] and cheilectomy.[13,18,20,25,27]
- After its first description by DuVries[13] in 1959, cheilectomy emerged as the most popular choice for surgical intervention. Indications for performing a cheilectomy are controversial.[10,14] Some authors recommend cheilectomy as a treatment for lower grades only,[17,18,20,31] whereas others have reported successful results even for higher grades of the disease.[14,15,27]
  - Cheilectomy resects the dorsal obstacle, but does not address the plantar pathology, which includes tremendous shortening of the plantar capsular, as well as the short flexors and plantar osteophytes of the phalangeal base.
  - Cheilectomy alone without plantar release, in our opinion, cannot be successful.
- A remaining cartilage lesion also may be responsible for persistent symptoms. This observation led to our idea of stimulating fibrocartilage regeneration by microfracturing the subchondral bone with a specially designed awl to open the zone of vascularization.
- Steadman[37] has developed a microfracture technique for the knee that creates fibrocartilage in chondral lesions.
  - It has been shown to be effective in comparison to untreated lesions in experimental studies in horses[16] and in clinical studies of the knee[33,37,38] and talus.[4]
- Coughlin and Shurnas type 2 and 3 lesions are indications for the microfracture technique.
  - In type 3 lesions, the patient must be informed that the surgery has only limited success.
- A contraindication for cheilectomy with microfracture is the stiff joint of types 3 and 4 osteoarthritis. In this case, in patients with a low activity level who want good range of motion, a resurfacing-type prosthesis (not a "head resection" type) is a good alternative and is being used with increasing frequency (**FIG 4**).
- Patients with isolated, painful osteochondral lesions without degenerative joint disease may be considered in rare cases for microfracture alone (for a small, contained lesion) or for an osteochondral transplantation from the plantar medial talus (**FIGS 5 AND 6**).

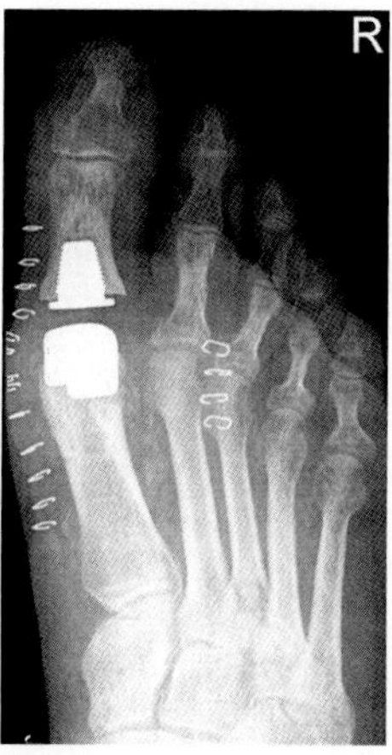

FIG 4 • Postoperative radiograph of first MTP joint prosthesis.

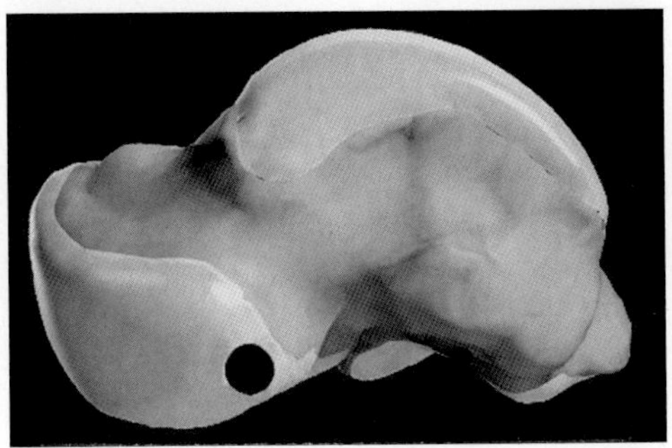

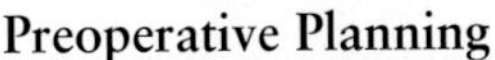

FIG 5 • Osteocondral autograft transplantation from the plantar medial talus.

Preoperative Planning

- Standard weight-bearing AP and lateral radiographs as well as, in some cases, MRI evaluation should be performed for grading the patient according to the Coughlin and Shurnas classification, and the cartilage damage should be assessed.
- The clinical examination should include measurement of active and passive ROM and determination of power in extension and plantarflexion, along with a dynamic stress test for evaluation of sesamoid pathology.

Positioning

- The patient is placed supine on the operating table.
- General or local anesthesia may be used, according to the setup and the surgeon's preference.
- A pneumatic tourniquet or Esmarch bandage should be used.

Approach

- A 4- to 5-cm incision is made anteromedially (**FIG 7**), being careful to protect the dorsal nerve above the first metatarsal head.

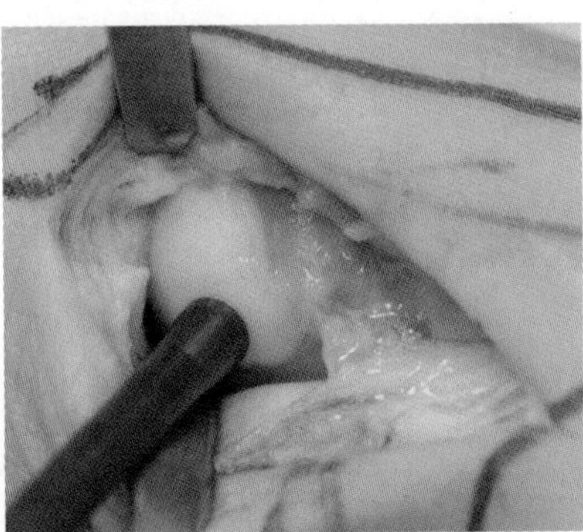

FIG 6 • Osteochondral autograft transplantation from the plantar medial talus.

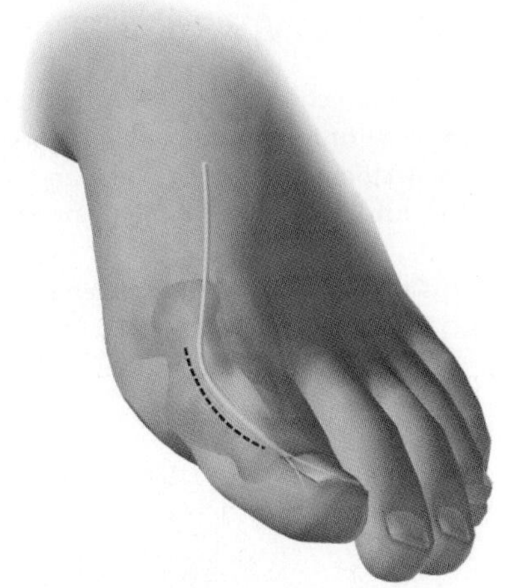

FIG 7 • Anteromedial approach.

- The fatty tissue and the subcutaneous tissue are dissected, and the joint capsule is prepared.
- The extensor hallucis longus tendon is retracted and the joint exposed (**FIG 8**).
- The joint is then inspected by flexing the great toe in the plantar direction.

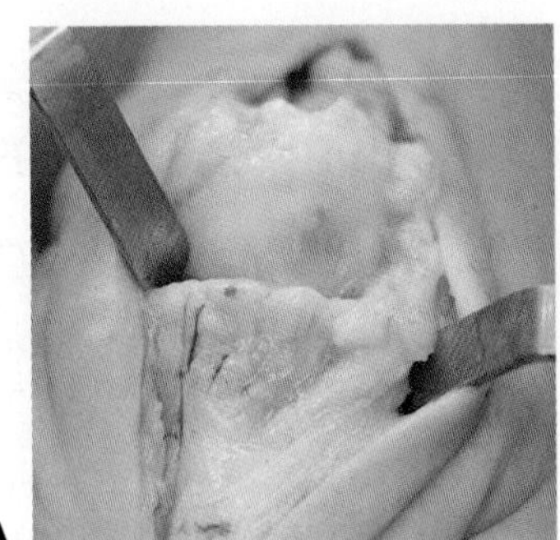

A

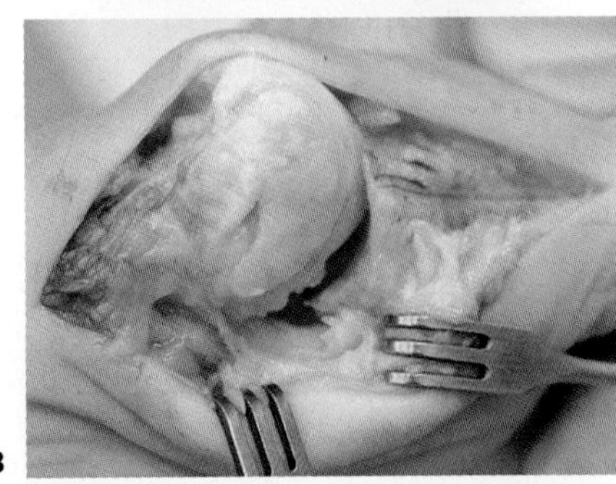

B

FIG 8 • Joint exposure from the lateral side showing the restriction in plantarflexion.

CHEILECTOMY

- After inspection of the joint, the dorsal osteophytes on the base of the proximal phalanx are removed.
- Cheilectomy is performed with an oscillating saw.
- The cut is performed in line with the dorsal metatarsal shaft.
  - The resection must not exceed about 15% to 20% of the metatarsal head (**TECH FIG 1**), because this leads to a jerking motion of the toe.
- Osteophytes remaining on the medial and lateral facet of the joint are removed with a sharp rongeur, plantarflexing the proximal phalanx (**TECH FIG 2**).
  - The rims are smoothed with a rasp.

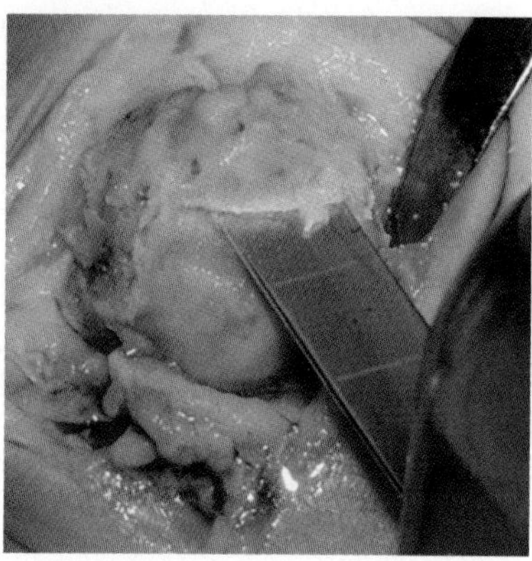

TECH FIG 1 • Cheilectomy

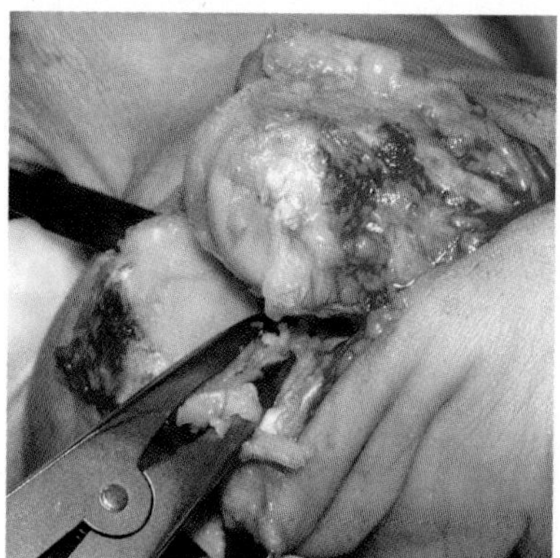

TECH FIG 2 • Resection of remaining osteophytes.

EXTENSIVE PLANTAR RELEASE

- Release of the plantar structures is very important for improving the ROM.
  - Because of the inhibition of dorsiflexion in the first MTP joint, contracture of the plantar structures (joint capsule, short toe flexors) has taken place.
- The joint capsule and the short flexors with the sesamoid bones are released subperiosteally using a McGlamry elevator (**TECH FIGS 3 AND 4**).
- The phalangeal attachment of the plantar capsule and the insertion of the short flexor muscles are released (**TECH FIG 5**).
  - This maneuver must be performed cautiously so as not to detach the tendons from their insertion.
- The joint is inspected again for plantar osteophytes of the phalangeal base and unstable cartilage parts, which will be resected.
  - Further resection to the metatarsal head must be avoided to prevent joint instability.
  - The rims are smoothed again with a rasp.
  - Osteophytes at the proximal sesamoid site must be resected, because this also is a source for plantar pain and restricted dorsiflexion. (**TECH FIG 6**)

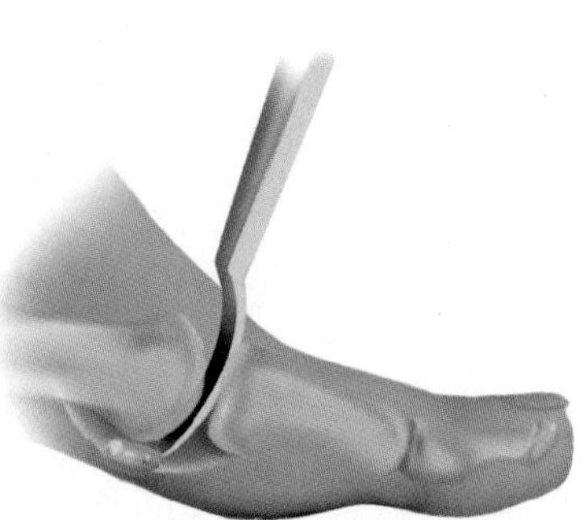

TECH FIG 3 • Plantar release using a McGlamry elevator.

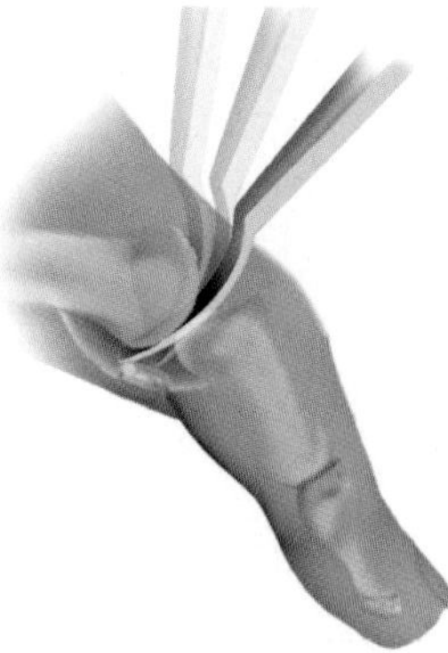

TECH FIG 4 • Plantar release using a McGlamry elevator.

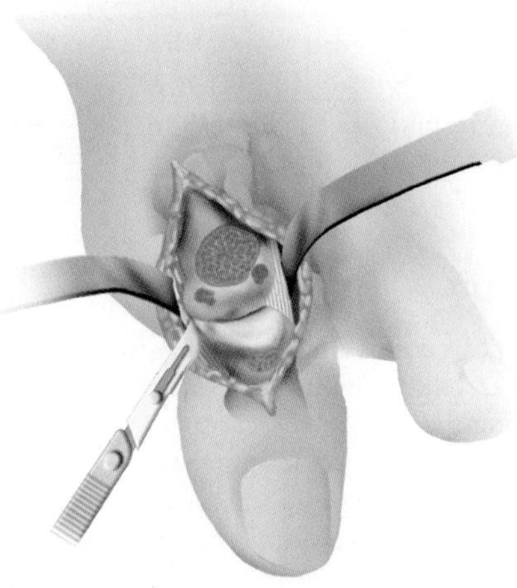

TECH FIG 5 • Release of the distal capsule and short flexors using a scalpel.

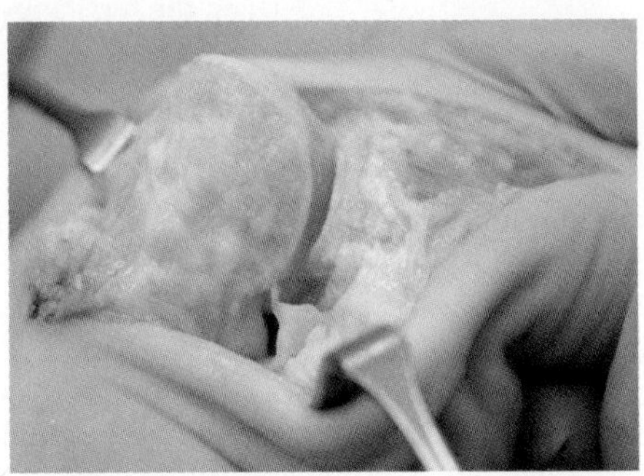

TECH FIG 6 • Plantarflexion after plantar release and resection of osteophytes.

MICROFRACTURE

- The remaining cartilage lesions at the first MTP joint or the proximal phalanx must be débrided of all remaining unstable cartilage and fibrous tissue.
  - The calcified cartilage layer must be completely removed.
- Using an awl, the microfractures are placed approximately 1 to 2 mm apart and about 2 to 4 mm deep (TECH FIG 7).

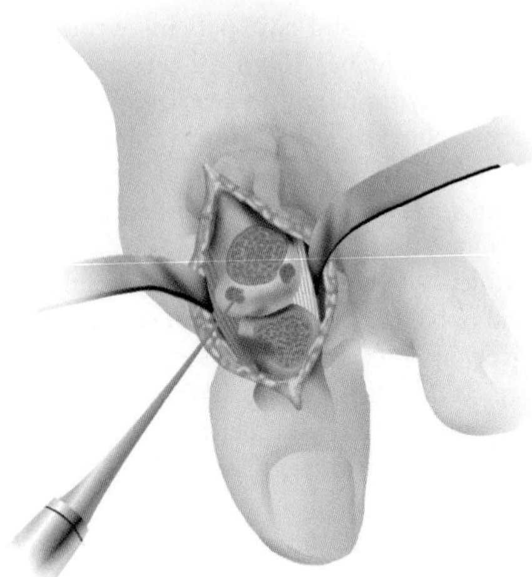

TECH FIG 7 • Microfracturing of the metatarsal head.

WOUND CLOSURE

- The joint capsule is closed with interrupted absorbable sutures, and a 0.8-mm drain is placed between the capsule and the continuous subcutaneous suture.
- The skin is sutured intracutaneously.
- Infiltration of the skin with bupivacaine and morphine decreases pain and need for pain killers after surgery.
- A small splint, which fixes the joint in dorsiflexion, is important to stretch the released shortened plantar structures (TECH FIG 8).

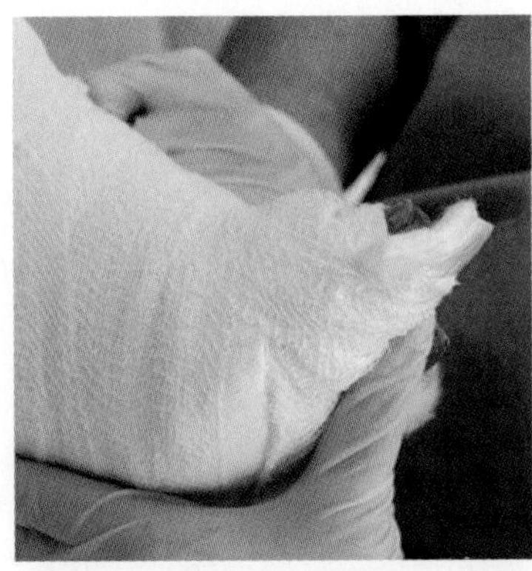

TECH FIG 8 • Splint in 40 degrees dorsiflexion.

PEARLS AND PITFALLS

Resection of the metatarsal head	■ Do not exceed 20% of the metatarsal head circumference. ■ Too much resection may lead to instability of the joint.
Plantar release of flexor tendons	■ Rough detachment of the short flexors may result in weak plantarflexion. ■ Using the McGlamry raspatory, a distinct sound must be heard and felt.

POSTOPERATIVE CARE

- After surgery a gauze-and-tape compression dressing is applied to the wound, and the hallux is fixed in 30 to 40 degrees dorsiflexion with a plantar cast for 2 days to support plantar release and to improve immediate ROM after surgery.
- A second-generation cephalosporin is prescribed for 5 days. Dexamethasone is given for 4 days, according to this schedule: day 1, 4 mg; day 2, 8 mg; day 3, 4 mg; and day 4, 2 mg.
  - This regimen provides protection from infection, and the dexamethasone provides significant reduction of pain and swelling, which helps to restore range of motion.
  - It also prevents excessive scar formation, which may result in recurrent loss of motion.
- The first dressing change, with removal of the drain, occurs on the second postoperative day.
- In our practice, from the second day, patients wear a postsurgical shoe with full weight bearing for 2 weeks to reduce loading and its accompanying pain and swelling. This allows the patient to become pain-free more quickly and makes it possible to regain dorsiflexion earlier (**FIG 9**).
  - The shoe permits good mobility and excellent conditions for decreased swelling and improved wound healing.
- "Aggressive" treatment of pain and swelling is crucial for the success of the surgical procedure, because regaining and stabilizing the intraoperatively attained ROM is the postsurgical goal.
- Passive and active ROM exercises are started from the second day if wound conditions and pain permit.
  - After removal of skin sutures, aggressive stretching is necessary to maintain ROM.
  - At this point, the patient should walk without the postsurgical shoe, focusing on a normal gait.
  - The rehabilitation program also includes isometric and proprioceptive training.
- Cooling, nonsteroidal anti-inflammatory drugs and physical therapy with joint distraction support the daily self-guided dorsiflexion exercises.
- At 3 to 4 months, the maximum ROM usually has been achieved. The patient must be aware that there is only a limited time frame for achieving good motion.

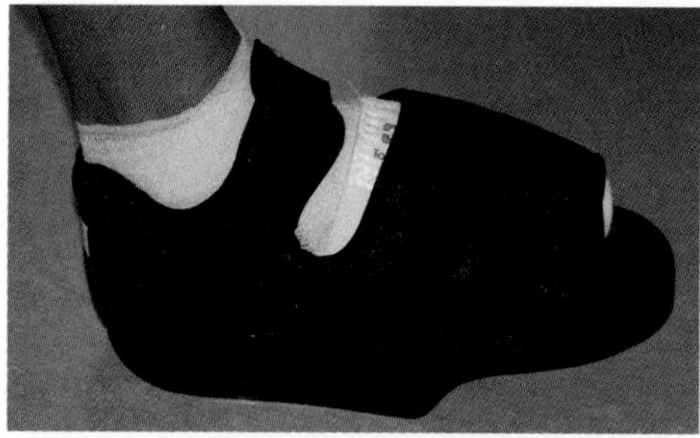

FIG 9 • This shoe reduces load to the forefoot.

OUTCOMES

- In a prospective study, 36 patients (26 women and 10 men) with 37 cases of hallux rigidus were operated by the senior author (HT) using the described technique.
  - Patients were examined and interviewed preoperatively as well as 1 year (mean 12m; 28 cases) and 2 years (mean 23m; 22 cases) postoperatively and rated using the American Orthopaedic Foot and Ankle Society (AOFAS) Hallux Metatarsophalangeal-Interphalangeal Score[31] and by a visual analog scale (VAS, not scaled 10 cm, where 0 is very poor and 10 is excellent).
  - The average age of the 36 patients at the time of surgery was 50 years (range 31 to 64 years).
  - Preoperative radiographs following Hattrup and Johnson's classification revealed 25 cases of grade 2 and 12 of grade 3. No patient was classified as grade 1.
  - Two patients, both grade 3, refused the follow-up examination.
- According to the AOFAS score, the results revealed a significant improvement: from 43 points preoperatively to an average of 78 points (range 35–100 points) after both 1 and 2 years postoperatively.
  - The average outcome on the VAS after 2 years was 7.1 for pain (preoperatively: 2.2; after 1 year: 7.0); 7.1 for function (preoperatively: 2.8; after 1 year: 6.7); and 7.4 for satisfaction (preoperatively: 1.1; after 1 year: 6.6).
  - Clinical examination showed an average improvement in ROM of 22 degrees.[3]
  - Patients classified as grade 3 were found to have significantly poorer results on average than grade 2.
  - Retrospectively, several of our patients would have been classified as grade 4 and, we now believe, should not have been considered for cheilectomy. We believe grade 3 is an indication if microfracturing and plantar release are added for treatment and the joint was not stiff before surgery.

COMPLICATIONS

- In patients with coexisting hallux valgus deformity, correction of the axis with a soft tissue release is essential for a successful result. However, the obligatory immobilization of the osteotomy reduces the options for postoperative management, and results sometimes are less successful in regaining ROM.
- If too much metatarsal head is resected with the cheilectomy, first MTP joint instability may ensue.
- Rough detachment of the short flexors may result in weak plantarflexion.

REFERENCES

1. Ahn TK, Kitaoka HB, Luo ZP, et al. Kinematics and contact characteristics of the first metatarsophalangeal joint. Foot Ankle Int 1997;18:170–174.
2. Barca F. Tendon arthroplasty of the first metatarsophalangeal joint in hallux rigidus: Preliminary communication. Foot Ankle Int 1997;18: 222–228.

3. Becher C, Kilger R, Thermann H. Results of cheilectomy and additional microfracture technique for the treatment of hallux rigidus. Foot Ankle Surg 2005;3:155–160.
4. Becher C, Thermann H. Results of microfracture in the treatment of articular cartilage defects of the talus. Foot Ankle Int 2005;26: 583–589.
5. Bingold AC, Collins DH. Hallux rigidus. J Bone Joint Surg Br 1950;32B:214–222.
6. Bonney G, Macnab I. Hallux valgus and hallux rigidus; a critical survey of operative results. J Bone Joint Surg Br 1952;34B:366–385.
7. Brandes M. Zur operativen Therapie des Hallux valgus. Zbl Chir 1929;56:2434–2440.
8. Cotterill JM. Condition of stiff great toe in adolescents. Edinburgh Med J 1887;33:459–462.
9. Coughlin MJ, Shurnas PS. Hallux rigidus: Demographics, etiology, and radiographic assessment. Foot Ankle Int 2003;24:731–743.
10. Coughlin MJ, Shurnas PS. Hallux rigidus. Grading and long-term results of operative treatment. J Bone Joint Surg Am 2003;85A: 2072–2088.
11. Cracchiolo A III, Swanson A, Swanson GD. The arthritic great toe metatarsophalangeal joint: A review of flexible silicone implant arthroplasty from two medical centers. Clin Orthop Relat Res 1981;157:64–69.
12. Davies-Colley N. Contraction of the metatarsophalangeal joint of the great toe. Br Med J 1887;1:728.
13. DuVries HL. Surgery of the Foot. St. Louis: Mosby, 1959.
14. Easley ME, Davis WH, Anderson RB. Intermediate to long-term follow-up of medial-approach dorsal cheilectomy for hallux rigidus. Foot Ankle Int 1999;20:147–152.
15. Feltham GT, Hanks SE, Marcus RE. Age-based outcomes of cheilectomy for the treatment of hallux rigidus. Foot Ankle Int 2001; 22:192–197.
16. Frisbie DD, Trotter GW, Powers BE, et al. Arthroscopic subchondral bone plate microfracture technique augments healing of large chondral defects in the radial carpal bone and medial femoral condyle of horses. Vet Surg 1999;28:242–255.
17. Geldwert JJ, Rock GD, McGrath MP, et al. Cheilectomy: still a useful technique for grade I and grade II hallux limitus/rigidus. J Foot Surg 1992;31:154–159.
18. Gould N. Hallux rigidus: Cheilotomy or implant? Foot Ankle 1981;1:315–320.
19. Hamilton WG, O'Malley MJ, Thompson FM, et al. Capsular interposition arthroplasty for severe hallux rigidus. Foot Ankle Int 1997; 18:68–70.
20. Hattrup SJ, Johnson KA. Subjective results of hallux rigidus following treatment with cheilectomy. Clin Orthop Relat Res 1988;226: 182–191.
21. Hua J, Sakamoto K, Kikukawa T, et al. Evaluation of the suppressive actions of glucosamine on the interleukin-1beta-mediated activation of synoviocytes. Inflamm Res 2007;56:432–438.
22. Keller WL. Surgical treatment of bunions and hallux valgus. New York Med J 1904;80:741.
23. Kessel L, Bonney G. Hallux rigidus in the adolescent. J Bone Joint Surg Br 1958;40B:669–673.
24. Lau JT, Daniels TR. Outcomes following cheilectomy and interpositional arthroplasty in hallux rigidus. Foot Ankle Int 2001;22: 462–470.
25. Mann RA, Clanton TO. Hallux rigidus: Treatment by cheilectomy. J Bone Joint Surg Am 1988;70A:400–406.
26. Mann RA, Coughlin MJ, eds. Surgery of the Foot and Ankle. St. Louis: Mosby, 1993.
27. Mann RA, Coughlin MJ, DuVries HL. Hallux rigidus: A review of the literature and a method of treatment. Clin Orthop Relat Res 1979;142:57–63.
28. McKeever DC. Arthrodesis of the first metartarsophalangeal joint for hallux valgus, hallux rigidus, and metatarsus primus varus. J Bone Joint Surg Br 1952;34B:129–134.
29. Meyer JO, Nishon LR, Weiss L, et al. Metatarsus primus elevatus and the etiology of hallux rigidus. J Foot Surg 1987;26:237–241.
30. Moberg E. A simple operation for hallux rigidus. Clin Orthop Relat Res 1979;142:55–56.
31. Mulier T, Steenwerckx A, Thienpont E, et al. Results after cheilectomy in athletes with hallux rigidus. Foot Ankle Int 1999;20: 232–237.
32. Ogilvie-Harris DJ, Carr MM, Fleming PJ. The foot in ballet dancers: the importance of second toe length. Foot Ankle Int 1995;16: 144–147.
33. Pässler HH. Die Technik der Mikrofrakturierung für die Behandlung von Knorpelschäden. Zentralbl Chir 2000;125:500–504.
34. Reginster JY, Deroisy R, Rovati LC, et al. Long-term effects of glucosamine sulphate on osteoarthritis progression: a randomised, placebo-controlled clinical trial. Lancet 2001;357:251–256.
35. Smith RW, Katchis SD, Ayson LC. Outcomes in hallux rigidus patients treated nonoperatively: a long-term follow-up study. Foot Ankle Int 2000;21:906–913.
36. Solan MC, Lemon M, Bendall SP. The surgical anatomy of the dorsomedial cutaneous nerve of the hallux. J Bone Joint Surg Br 2001;83B:250–252.
37. Steadman JR. Microfracture technique for full-thickness chondral defects: Technique and clinical results. Operative Techniques in Orthopaedics 1997;7:300–304.
38. Steadman JR, Briggs KK, Rodrigo JJ, et al. Outcomes of microfracture for traumatic chondral defects of the knee: Average 11-year follow-up. Arthroscopy 2003;19:477–484.
39. Swanson AB. Implant arthroplasty for the great toe. Clin Orthop Relat Res 1972;85:75–81.
40. Vilaseca RR, Ribes ER. The growth of the first metatarsal bone. Foot Ankle 1980;1:117–122.
41. Wülker N. Hallux rigidus. Orthopäde 1997;26:731–740.

Chapter **20**

Capsular Interpositional Arthroplasty

Andrew J. Elliott, Martin J. O'Malley, Timothy Charlton, and William G. Hamilton

DEFINITION

- Hallux rigidus refers to degenerative arthritis of the first metatarsophalangeal (MTP) joint that is characterized by pain, decreased range of motion (ROM), and proliferative osteophyte formation.

ANATOMY

- The first MTP joint is composed of the dorsal joint capsule, the medial and lateral collateral ligaments, the plantar plate–sesamoid–flexor hallucis brevis (FHB) tendon complex, the first metatarsal head, and the proximal articulating end of the proximal phalanx.
- Pathology is limited primarily to the first MTP joint, with prominent dorsal osteophyte on the metatarsal head.

PATHOGENESIS

- The origin of progressive first MTP joint cartilage degeneration is uncertain. Most attribute hallux rigidus to biomechanical disturbance or local pathology that leads to repetitive stress on articular cartilage and subsequent deterioration of the cartilage surface.
- Trauma
- Inflammatory arthridities (eg, rheumatoid arthritis, gout)
- Primary osteoarthritis
- Associated factors such as long first metatarsal, flat metatarsal head, metatarsus primus elevatus, pronated feet, or hallux valgus interphalangeus are often found in patients with arthritis of the first MTP joint.
- Long first metatarsal may be correlated with development of hallux rigidus.

NATURAL HISTORY

- Initially pain is localized to the dorsal aspect of the great toe MTP joint. Loss of motion is minimal but can be seen with activities that require maximum dorsiflexion. Over time, generally several years, the degree of involvement and loss of motion increase. Eventually, in the end stage of the process, the first MTP joint will lose nearly all motion. A varus or valgus deformity is usually not associated with this process.
- Pain may or may not progress as osteophytes form to stabilize the joint.
- Progression of osteophytes and joint space narrowing on radiographs may or may not correlate with symptoms.

PATIENT HISTORY AND PHYSICAL FINDINGS

- Typical history is swelling around the first MTP joint. Patients will complain frequently of a progressive increase in the size of the MTP joint and attribute this to a bunion type deformity.
- Occasionally, avoidance gait can result and cause an increased weight-bearing load on the lateral aspect of the foot.
- Initially, a tender dorsal osteophyte will be noted with MTP joint flexion retrograde elevation and uncovering of the dorsal portion of the articulation. Pain may be associated with local dorsal cutaneous nerve irritation caused by the osteophyte.
- Limited dorsiflexion with abutment of articular surfaces of the phalanx onto the metatarsal head can be seen. Periarticular osteophytes can be noted, particularly laterally.
- Compensatory hyperextension of the hallucal interphalangeal joint can be seen with longstanding disease.
- Axial compression of the MTP joint with pain can often differentiate the level of involvement of the degenerative process.
- Pain is felt with dorsiflexion activities (wearing high-heeled shoes, running, yoga).
- Progressive proliferation of osteophytes about the joint occurs and pain is felt with small–toe box shoes.
- Decreased dorsiflexion and plantarflexion motion of the joint is seen and pain is elicited with attempting these motions.
- Physical examination includes the following:
  - Visualize the dorsal osteophyte to check for swelling.
  - For lesser toe evaluation, examine for hammer toe formation or evidence of a more systemic process: Presence of multiple hammer toe formation with hallux rigidus suggests rheumatoid arthritis.
  - Evaluate ROM for dorsal based blocking of dorsiflexion.
  - Check axial compression by stabilizing the first metatarsal while compressing the proximal phalanx against the metatarsal head. Increasing levels of pain are associated with more complete joint involvement.
  - Tomassen's sign: With the ankle held in neutral, dorsiflexion of the MTP joint is measured. A positive result is suggestive of a stenosing flexor hallucis longus (FHL) tenosynovitis and not a static dorsal osteophyte.
  - Pain at the mid range of the motion arc implies a global first MTP joint arthritis that may not be amenable to dorsal cheilectomy alone but instead is better treated with interpositional arthroplasty or arthrodesis.

IMAGING AND OTHER DIAGNOSTIC STUDIES

- Standard weight-bearing anteroposterior (AP), oblique, and lateral radiographs of the foot
  - Grade 1: small lateral spurs with joint space preservation
  - Grade 2: metatarsal and phalangeal osteophytes with dorsal joint space narrowing and subchondral sclerosis
  - Grade 3: marked osteophyte formation with loss of joint space and subchondral cyst formation (**FIG 1**).
- Laboratory studies if serologic etiology suspected

DIFFERENTIAL DIAGNOSIS

- Trauma
- Primary osteoarthritis
- Degenerative arthritis

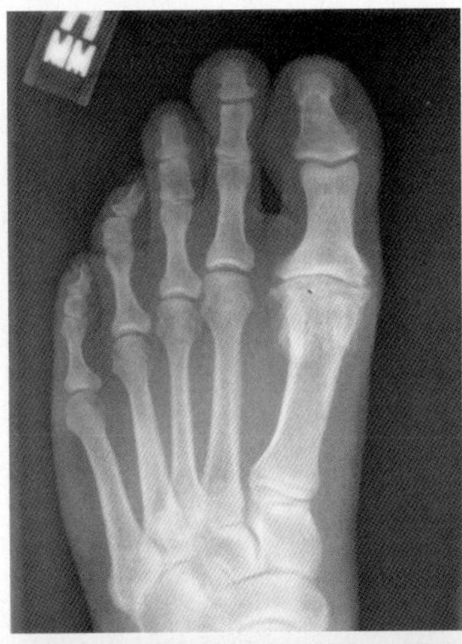

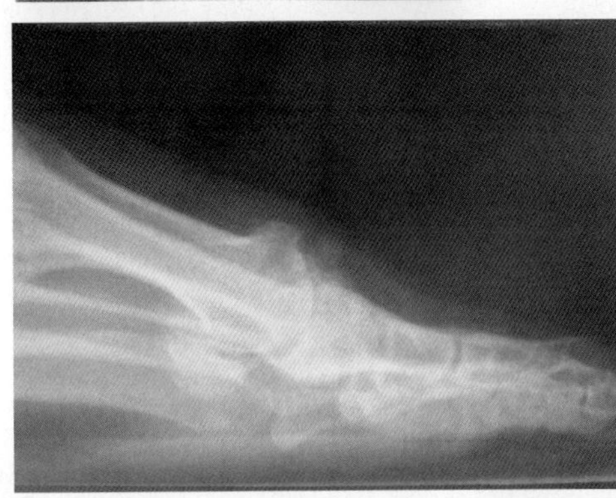

FIG 1 • **A.** AP view of a foot with hallux rigidus with a relatively longer second metatarsal and the suggestion of second metatarsal overload with flattening of the metatarsal head. **B.** Lateral view of the foot demonstrating dorsal osteophytes and joint space narrowing.

- Rheumatoid arthritis
- Seronegative arthropathy
- Gout
- Stenosing FHL tendon[9]

NONOPERATIVE MANAGEMENT

- Low-heeled shoes
- Steel shanks
- Stiff Morton's extension orthoses
- Nonsteroidal anti-inflammatory drugs
- Cortisone injection
- Rocker-sole shoe or over-the-counter rocker shoe

SURGICAL MANAGEMENT

- Grade I: cheilectomy to address mild osteophyte formation, joint space intact, minimal dorsal spur formation
- Grade II: cheilectomy with Moberg dorsal phalangeal osteotomy to address moderate osteophyte formation, joint space narrowing, subchondral sclerosis, bony proliferation on metatarsal head and phalanx on radiograph or significant intraoperative joint involvement
- Grade III: interposition arthroplasty or fusion to address marked osteophyte formation, loss of visible joint space, extensive bony proliferation[2,3]

Preoperative Planning

- Standing AP and lateral foot radiographs to anticipate level of intervention
- Consider consent for cheilectomy, Moberg dorsal osteotomy, and interposition arthroplasty. While arthrodesis could be considered as well, the goal of interpositional arthroplasty is to preserve motion in end-stage first MTP joint arthritis.
- Patients who do well with interpositional arthroplasty typically are moderately but not extremely active athletes who wish for retention of dorsiflexion of the toe for activities of daily living such as sports or use of certain shoe wear.
- Relative contraindications to interpositional arthroplasty include cases in which first MTP joint arthrodesis may be favored:
  - Long second metatarsal (potential risk for development of transfer metatarsalgia) (see **FIG 1A**)
  - Hallux valgus
  - Sesamoid arthritis
  - First tarsometatarsal instability: inflammatory arthridities
  - High-demand patients (athletes, dancers) present a challenge as we believe that they should be discouraged from this procedure yet are also not ideal candidates for first MTP joint arthrodesis.[6]
- Poor vascular status, neuropathy, and infection are absolute contraindications to this procedure.

Positioning

- The patient is placed supine with a bump under the contralateral lumbar region if needed to evert the foot for better exposure.
- The foot is placed at the bottom corner of the bed.
- A bolster is placed under the greater trochanter of the ipsilateral hip to avoid external rotation of the operated extremity.
- A mini C-arm is placed on the ipsilateral side of the bed, about 6 feet past the corner of the operating room table and at a 45-degree angle. In our experience, this positioning affords the best access to the foot and simplifies intraoperative imaging. Blankets or sheets are used to elevate the operated extremity to facilitate lateral fluoroscopic imaging unobstructed by the contralateral lower extremity.

Approach

- Two approaches are commonly used, dorsal and medial.
- The dorsal approach allows for easier access to the lateral osteophyte. This approach makes suturing the interposition tissue to plantar surface of the joint difficult, however.
- In contrast, the medial incision allows for easier access to the plantar surface and is the approach used by the senior author (W.G.H.). The capsule is carefully protected, with particular attention given to protecting the plantar nerve (Joplin's nerve) as well as the dorsal cutaneous branch.
- Protect the extensor hallucis longus (EHL) tendon and the dorsal and plantar digital nerves. Identify the extensor hallucis brevis (EHB) and the joint capsule.
- Ankle block anesthesia is used, plus an Esmarch ankle tourniquet with three wraps approximating 300 mg Hg, incorporating a full roll of Webril wrapped around the ankle to protect the skin overlying the Achilles tendon.

EXPOSURE AND CAPSULOTOMY

- A longitudinal midaxial medial approach to the first MTP joint is performed (**TECH FIG 1A**).
- The dorsomedial sensory cutaneous nerve to the hallux is identified and protected throughout the procedure.
- A thin layer of adventitial tissue may be mobilized to later be closed over the interpositional arthroplasty to further support the toe.
- The EHL tendon is identified (**TECH FIG 1B**), and the interval between the EHL and the underlying EHB is developed (**TECH FIG 1C**).
- The EHL and FHL tendons are identified and must remain protected throughout the procedure, not only from being transected but from being tethered by suture.
- A longitudinal medial capsulotomy is performed to expose the arthritic joint.
- The capsule is reflected from the proximal phalanx (**TECH FIG 1D,E**).
- We often use a towel clamp to carefully mobilize the base of the proximal phalanx (**TECH FIG 3F,G**).

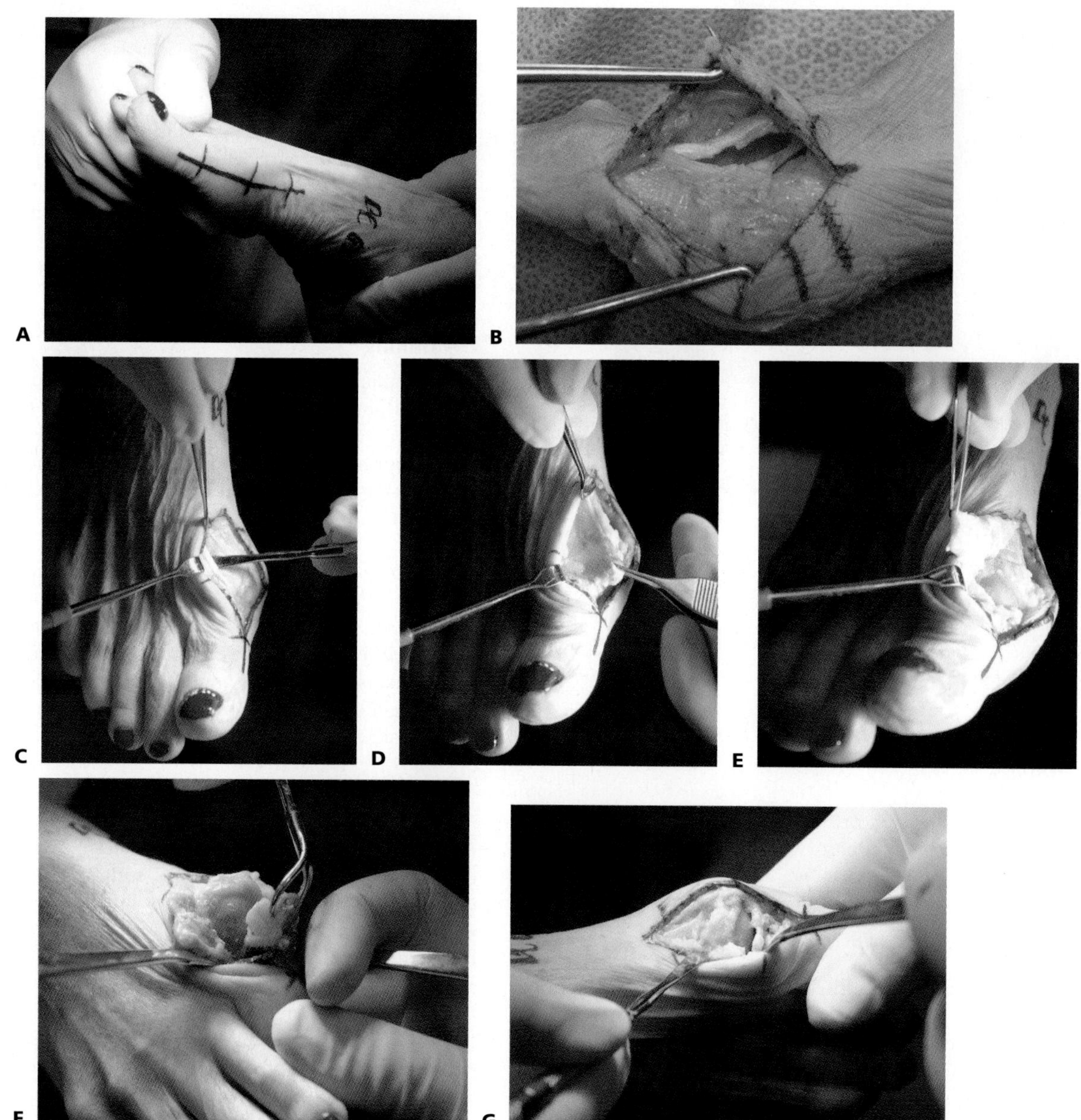

TECH FIG 1 • **A**. Midaxial incision centered over the medial first MTP joint. **B.** Cadaveric specimen demonstrating medial approach with the adventitial tissue over the medial joint capsule exposed and the EHL tendon and dorsomedial sensory cutaneous nerve identified. **C.** First MTP joint capsule being defined while elevating the EHL tendon. **D,E**. Dorsal capsule being reflected off the proximal phalanx. **F,G**. Use of a towel clip to mobilize the proximal phalanx.

CHEILOTOMY AND PHALANGEAL OSTEOTOMY

- Inspect joint and if over 50% of joint cartilage remains, consider proceeding with cheilectomy with or without dorsal (Moberg) closing wedge osteotomy of the phalanx.[2,3]
- If less than 50% of joint cartilage remains, perform cheilectomy of the dorsal third of the metatarsal head.
- Subperiosteally release the dorsal capsule, the EHB tendon insertion, and the plantar plate–FHB from the proximal phalanx base (TECH FIG 2A).
- Resect 25% (roughly 8 mm) of the proximal phalanx with a sagittal saw, protecting the EHL and FHL (TECH FIG 2B,C).
- We recommend that no more than this is resected from the proximal phalanx to avoid potential postoperative instability of the residual first MTP joint (TECH FIG 2D,E).

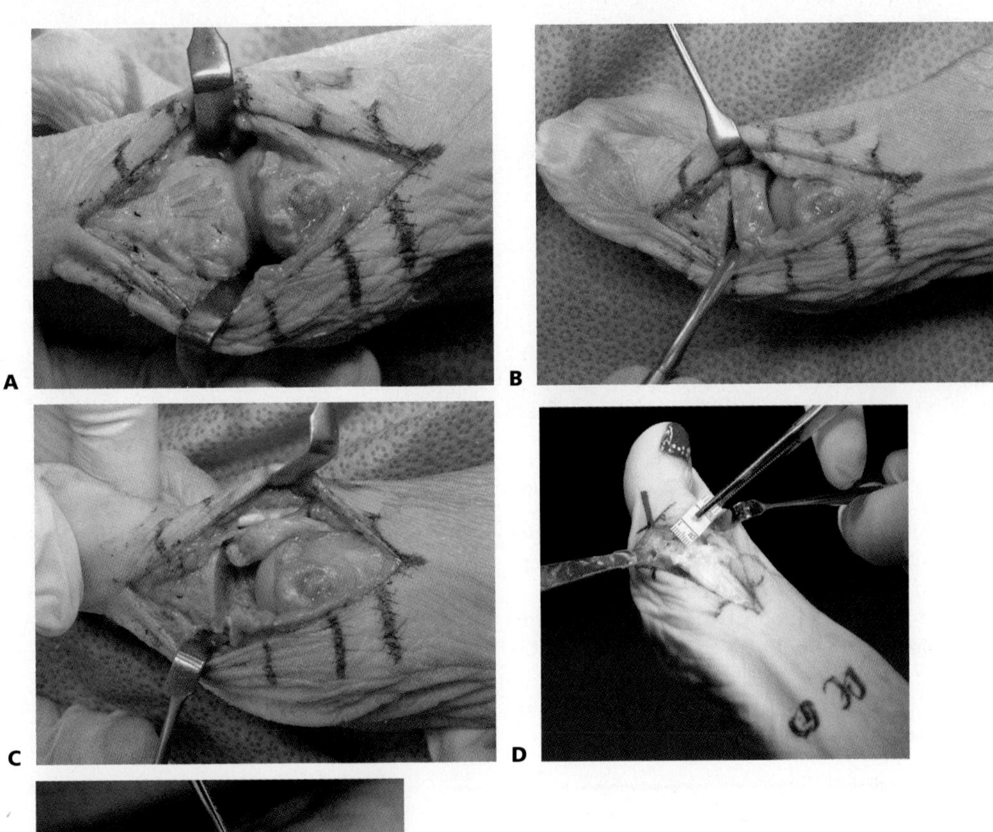

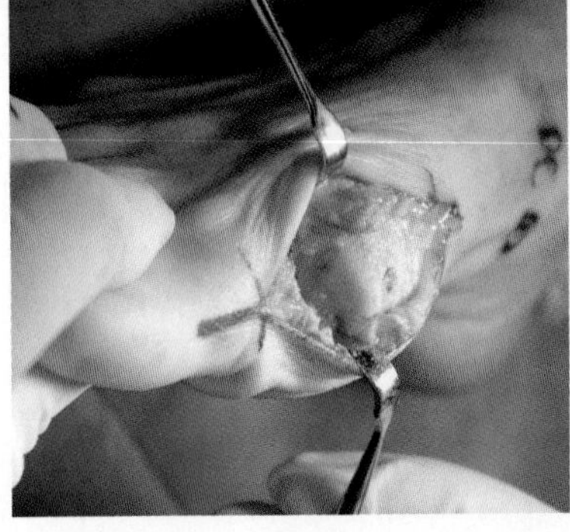

TECH FIG 2 • **A**. Cadaveric specimen with exposed first MTP joint. **B,C**. Cadaveric specimen demonstrating 25% resection of proximal phalanx base. Excessive resection of the proximal phalanx base must be avoided to maintain joint stability. **D**. Measuring planned resection from base of proximal phalanx. **E**. Gap created after dorsal cheilectomy and proximal phalanx resection.

INTERPOSITION ARTHROPLASTY

- Transect EHB tendon approximately 3 cm proximal to the joint. This prevents the capsular tissue from being retracted during gait. Moreover, the EHB tendon may then be used to augment the soft tissue interposition. Mobilize the EHB into the joint space (TECH FIG 3A,B).
- Suture capsular tissue to stumps of the FHB tendon with 0-0 nonabsorbable suture.
- The dorsal capsule is mobilized into the joint and approximated with the FHB tendon in a balanced fashion.
- Should the capsule not mobilize adequately, the dorsal cheilectomy may need to be increased.
- Protect the FHL tendon and the plantar nerves during suturing.

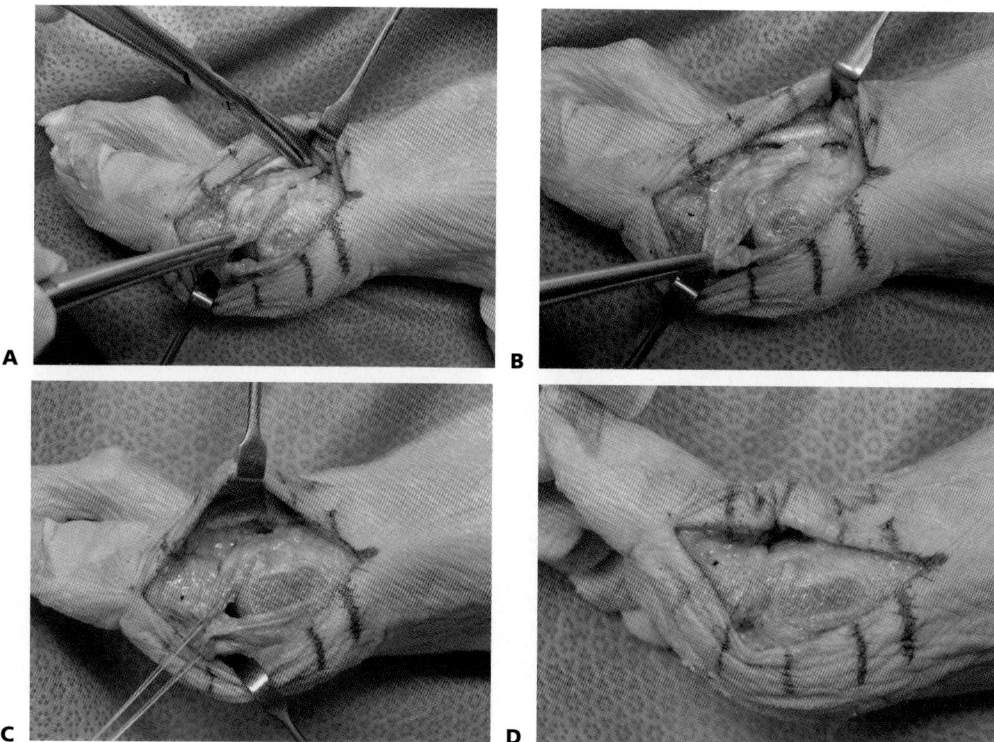

TECH FIG 3 • Cadaveric specimen. **A.** Dorsal capsule with EHB. **B.** EHB transected and tendon–capsule complex mobilized into joint. **C.** Capsule sutured to plantar plate. **D.** Toe taken through ROM.

- Typically, there remains a thin layer of adventitial tissue that is superficial to the capsule that can be carefully approximated to further support the toe.
- Evaluate balance and motion of the toe. Dorsiflexion should be uninhibited throughout the motion arc (TECH FIG 3C,D).
- Although originally described, we rarely use a K-wire to support the reconstruction.
- In our experience, the EHL tendon needs to be lengthened in less than 5% of these surgeries, or almost never. However, when necessary, we prefer to perform the lengthening through a horizontal Z pattern.
- The capsule is cut proximally such that it can be rotated down over the top of the metatarsal head. The capsule is mobilized and secured with 2-0 nonabsorbable suture. Repair is done via 2-0 or 3-0 Vicryl.

PEARLS AND PITFALLS

Insufficient capsular tissue	▪ Allograft (gracilis or hamstring) or autograft (plantaris[1] or hamstring) may be used for insufficient capsule. These can be placed into a cavity prepared by use of MTP joint fusion reamers[4] or a burr[1] instead of proximal phalanx resection.
Push-off weakness	▪ Perform oblique osteotomy of the proximal phalanx to decompress the MTP joint but leave the FHB–sesamoid complex attachment intact.[11]
"Floppy" toe	▪ Take care not to resect too much proximal phalanx. ▪ Place a K-wire at resection site, confirm with fluoroscopy, and cut along the wire.
Toe sits in dorsiflexion	▪ Lengthen the EHL if the toe sits in an extended position after reconstruction. ▪ Consider pinning with 0.062-inch K-wire for 3 weeks.
Anatomic considerations	▪ Avoid tethering the FHL tendon with the permanent sutures. ▪ Avoid injury to the plantar or dorsal medial digital nerves.
Relative lengths of the first and second metatarsals	▪ A long second metatarsal may be subject to transfer metatarsalgia with a capsular interpositional arthroplasty. We view a long second metatarsal as a relative contraindication to first MTP joint interpositional arthroplasty. Consider second metatarsal shortening osteotomy for patients with long second metatarsal to prevent transfer metatarsalgia.
Achieving optimal soft tissue balancing of the first MTP joint	▪ Balance the capsule when attaching it to the plantar plate. Then balance the toe relative to the first metatarsal by reapproximating the residual adventitial tissue. Although originally described, pinning should not be necessary.
Suture placement	▪ Use of a Hintermann retractor or lamina spreader with a K-wire hole attachment allows for excellent distraction of the joint to facilitate suture placement.

POSTOPERATIVE CARE

- Weight bearing as tolerated in postoperative shoe for 4 to 6 weeks. Begin gentle passive ROM at home.
- Sutures are removed at 10 to 14 days.
- If a pin is used temporarily, it is removed at 3 to 4 weeks.
- Patients should be made aware before surgery that they will have a "floppy" toe for several months until the the joint tissues and tendons stabilize with time.

OUTCOMES

- Between 73% and 94% of patients report good to excellent results.[1,4,6–8,10,11]
- In our experience, transfer metatarsalgia develops to some degree in 30% of patients.[6] These patients can be successfully managed with orthoses, lesser metatarsal shortening osteotomy, or lesser metatarsal plantar condylectomy.

COMPLICATIONS

- Transfer metatarsalgia, particularly with a long second metatarsal
- Resecting too little bone, leading to impingement and pain
- Cock-up deformity
- Hallux valgus or varus
- Floppy toe or stiffness
- Weakness of push-off with the first toe
- Injury to the dorsal and plantar digital nerves
- Tethering of the FHL tendon by the capsular sutures
- Floating great toe (rare and observed when EHL contracture is present and EHL is not lengthened)

REFERENCES

1. Barca F. Tendon arthroplasty of the first metatarsophalangeal joint in hallux rigidus: preliminary communication. Foot Ankle Int 1997;18: 222–228.
2. Coughlin MJ, Shurnas PS. Hallux rigidus: demographics, etiology, and radiographic assessment. Foot Ankle Int 2003;24:731–743.
3. Coughlin MJ, Shurnas PS. Hallux rigidus: grading and long-term results of operative treatment. J Bone Joint Surg Am 2003;85A: 2072–2088.
4. Coughlin MJ, Shurnas PJ. Soft-tissue arthroplasty for hallux rigidus. Foot Ankle Int 2003;24:661–672.
5. Hahn MP, Gerhardt N, Thordarson DB. Medial capsular interpositional arthroplasty for severe hallux rigidus. Foot Ankle Int 2009;30: 494–499.
6. Hamilton WG, Hubbard CE. Hallux rigidus: excisional arthroplasty. Foot Ankle Clin 2000;5:663–671.
7. Hamilton WG, O'Malley MJ, Thompson FM, Kovatis PE. Capsular interposition arthroplasty for severe hallux rigidus. Foot Ankle Int 1997;18:68–70.
8. Kennedy JG, Chow FY, Dines J, et al. Outcomes after interposition arthroplasty for treatment of hallux rigidus. Clin Orthop Rel Res 2006;445:210–215.
9. Kirane YM, Michelson JD, Sharkey NA. Contribution of the flexor hallucis longus to loading of the first metatarsal and first metatarsophalangeal joint. Foot Ankle Int 2008;29:367–377.
10. Lau JTC, Daniels TR. Outcomes following cheilectomy and interpositional arthroplasty in hallux rigidus. Foot Ankle Int 2001;22: 462–470.
11. Mroczek KJ, Miller SD. The modified oblique Keller procedure: a technique for dorsal approach interposition arthroplasty sparing the flexor tendons. Foot Ankle Int 2003;24:521–522.

Chapter 21 Arthrosurface HemiCAP Resurfacing

Thomas P. San Giovanni

DEFINITION

- Hallux rigidus is an arthritic condition of the first metatarsophalangeal (MTP) joint. It is the most common form of arthritis affecting the foot.
- An estimated 2% to 10% of the general population displays varying grades of hallux rigidus.[1,7,9]

ANATOMY

- Hallux rigidus involves the first MTP joint, which comprises the articulation between the first metatarsal head, the proximal phalangeal base, and the sesamoid complex.
- Although the proximal phalanx is often involved, the predominant disease involves the dorsal aspect of the metatarsal head with articular cartilage loss and dorsal osteophyte formation (**FIG 1**).

PATHOGENESIS

- The cause of hallux rigidus is controversial and is likely multifactorial.
- Predisposing or associated factors cited in the literature include flat, square-shaped metatarsal head morphology; metatarsus adductus; hallux valgus interphalangeus; positive family history with bilateral condition; and trauma.[1,9]
- Isolated or repetitive injury may cause damage to the dorsal aspect of the joint, which leads to altered mechanics (compressive and shear forces increased dorsally). Progressive deterioration of the articular surface, osteophyte formation, and joint contracture ensue.

NATURAL HISTORY

- In its early stages, articular cartilage loss is present along the dorsal aspect of the first metatarsal head. As the condition progresses, articular cartilage loss extends to the central aspects of the metatarsal head and lastly the plantar aspect (**FIG 2**).
- Although less involved, the proximal phalanx will exhibit varying degrees of articular cartilage loss and dorsal osteophyte formation.
- The natural history of hallux rigidus is one of gradual, progressive worsening.[9]

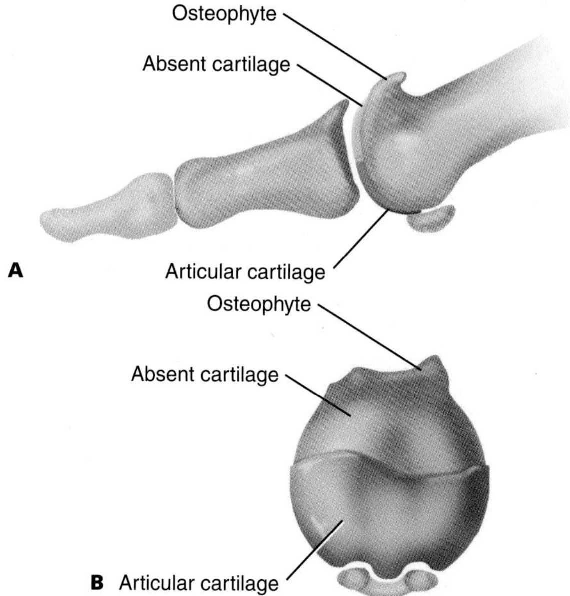

FIG 1 • **A.** Lateral diagram depicting articular cartilage loss and osteophyte along the dorsal aspect of the first metatarsophalangeal joint. **B.** Frontal view showing dorsal articular cartilage loss extending into the central aspect.

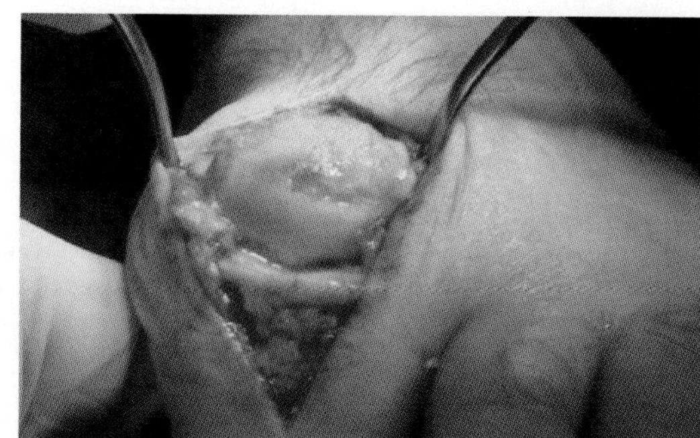

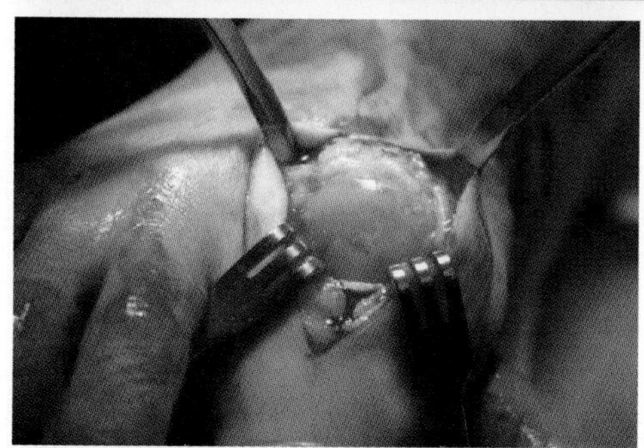

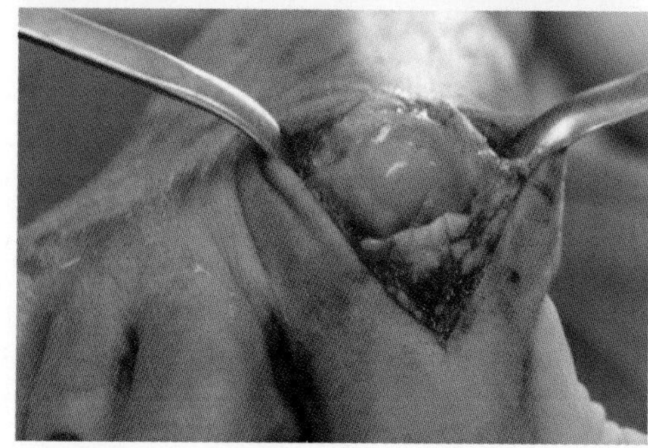

FIG 2 • Varying degrees of articular cartilage loss of the first metatarsal head in hallux rigidus. Radiographic findings often underestimate the extent of disease seen intraoperatively.

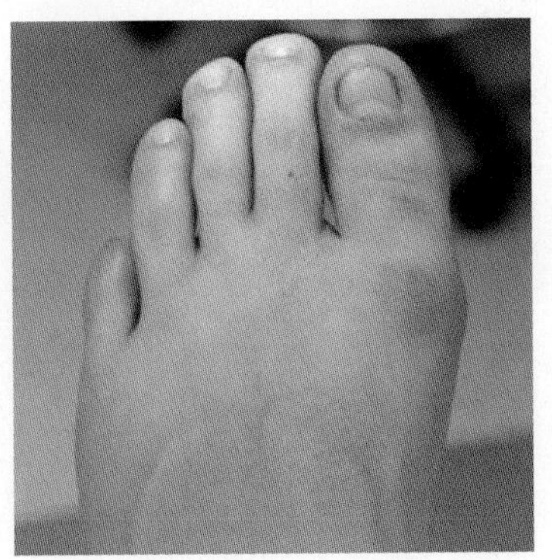
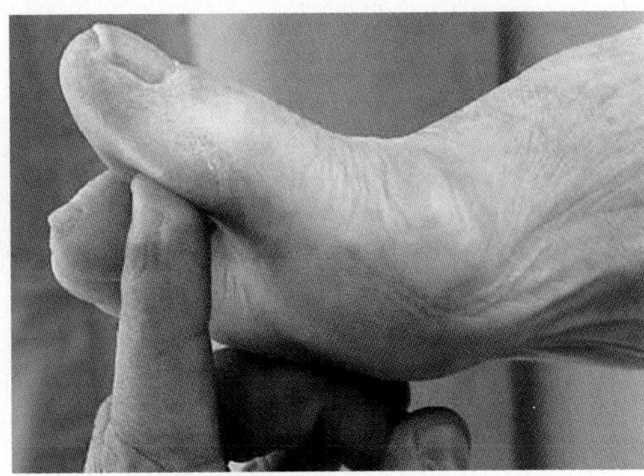

FIG 3 • A. Dorsal view of foot in hallux rigidus. Shoe wear may cause irritation over the dorsal bony prominence. B. Limited dorsiflexion is noted on the clinical examination.

PATIENT HISTORY AND PHYSICAL FINDINGS

- Patients present with complaints of dull, aching, and at times sharp pain along the dorsal aspect of the joint associated with weight-bearing activities.
- Complaints of stiffness and development of a painful dorsal bony prominence are characteristic of the condition.
- The physical examination reveals tenderness overlying the first MT head with a notable dorsal bony prominence, along with limited range of motion of the first MTP joint, particularly dorsiflexion (**FIG 3**).
- The examiner should assess for pain on midmotion, crepitus, positive first MTP grind test, and plantar tenderness overlying the sesamoids, which represents more extensive disease.

IMAGING AND OTHER DIAGNOSTIC STUDIES

- Weight-bearing AP, lateral, and oblique views are obtained. The examiner should assess for joint space narrowing, presence of dorsal osteophytes, and joint congruity.
- In a radiographic grading system often used in the literature, grades 1, 2, and 3 signify the percentage of joint space narrowing, the presence or absence of subchondral sclerosis or subchondral cyst, and the degree of osteophyte formation (Table 1, **FIG 4**).[4]
- CT and MRI advanced imaging studies are generally not obtained. Evaluation with MRI may occasionally be indicated if the radiographs appear normal but suspicion remains for a central osteochondral defect of the metatarsal head. CT scan is occasionally obtained to assess or confirm the presence of severe metatarsosesamoid involvement, signifying advanced disease.

DIFFERENTIAL DIAGNOSIS

- Gout
- Other systemic arthritides (rheumatoid arthritis, psoriatic arthritis, seronegative arthropathy)
- Posttraumatic arthritis
- Arthritis associated with severe hallux valgus or sequelae status post hallux valgus surgery
- Central osteochondral defect, first metatarsal head
- Avascular necrosis of the metatarsal head
- Sesamoiditis or sesamoid-related pathology
- Septic arthritis
- Soft tissue or bone neoplasm

NONOPERATIVE MANAGEMENT

- Nonoperative management of hallux rigidus includes shoe wear modifications, use of anti-inflammatories, orthotics with a Morton extension or carbon fiber plate orthotic, and rarely intra-articular cortisone injections.

SURGICAL MANAGEMENT

- When nonoperative management fails to provide adequate symptom relief, the patient and surgeon are faced with choosing from an array of surgical procedures.

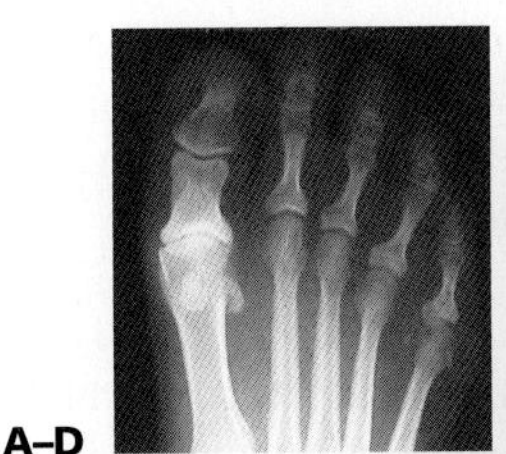
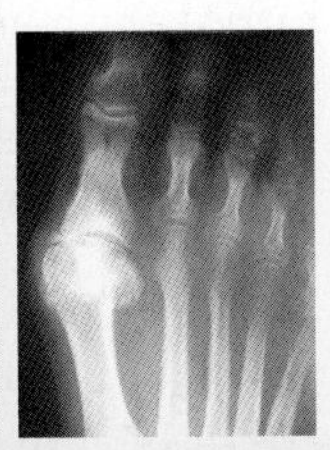
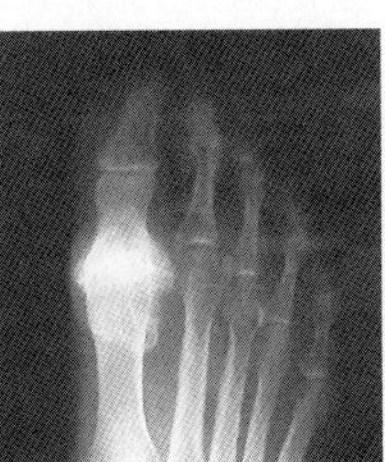
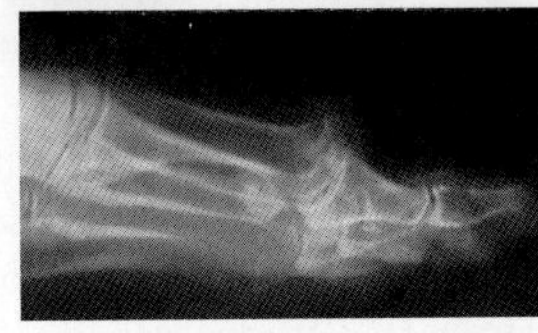

FIG 4 • A. Grade 1 hallux rigidus. B. Grade 2 hallux rigidus. C. Grade 3 hallux rigidus. D. Lateral view of hallux rigidus.

Table 1 Radiographic Grading System for Hallux Rigidus

Grade	Dorsal osteophyte	Joint space	Subchondral bone
1	Mild to moderate	Space preserved	Normal appearance
2	Moderate	<50% narrowing	Subchondral sclerosis
3	Marked	>50% narrowing	Subchondral sclerosis with or without bone cyst formation

Hattrup SJ, Johnson KA. Subjective results of hallux rigidus following treatment with cheilectomy. Clin Orthop Relat Res 1988;226:182–191.

- The most common performed procedure for hallux rigidus is a cheilectomy.
- Simple cheilectomy has been proven successful for early stages of hallux rigidus,[1,2,4,9] although cheilectomy outcomes are less promising with advanced disease, particularly grade 3.[1,7,8] As articular cartilage loss extends to the central and plantar aspects of the joint, the joint deterioration progresses beyond that which a cheilectomy would be expected to adequately treat.
- Alternative or adjunctive procedures to cheilectomy include:
  - Moberg dorsal closing wedge phalange osteotomy[10,14,15]
  - Various first metatarsal decompression osteotomies[14]
  - Soft tissue interpositional arthroplasties and modified oblique Keller resection[3,7]
  - Proximal phalangeal base hemiarthroplasty[11,16]
  - Metatarsal head resurfacing hemiarthroplasty[5,12,13]
  - Total great toe arthroplasty[6]
  - First MTP arthrodesis[1,9,11]
- Historically, a first MTP arthrodesis has proven to be the most reliable procedure for providing pain relief in advanced stages (grade 3).[1,11] However, many patients find the thought of complete motion loss in exchange for pain relief unacceptable and prefer not to undergo a fusion procedure for this reason alone.
- Alternative surgical solutions that maintain some degree of motion and provide pain relief have been sought in an effort to address this patient subset with advanced disease who refuse to undergo fusion. This has led to the development of various arthroplasty techniques, including soft tissue interposition or implant arthroplasty.
- One such implant is the Arthrosurface HemiCAP with the technique described below.

Preoperative Planning

- History and physical examination are performed with particular attention to the location of pain, mid-range motion pain, or significant symptomatic sesamoid involvement.
- Range of motion and active and passive dorsiflexion and plantarflexion are recorded preoperatively.
- Routine weight-bearing radiographs are assessed for the presence of dorsal osteophytes, the degree of joint space narrowing, joint alignment and congruency, metatarsal length, and sesamoid pathology.
- Careful preoperative discussion regarding the patient's goals and expectations are paramount in determining whether individual goals will be met by the procedure. A discussion of the risks and alternative procedures, in particular discussion regarding arthrodesis, is important.

Positioning

- The patient is positioned supine with a bump under the ipsilateral hip to rotate the foot to neutral.
- A tourniquet is applied; however, we prefer not to use a tourniquet during the case if possible. Excellent hemostasis is achieved on the approach and leads to a drier wound on closure. We believe that postoperative swelling from hemarthrosis or hematoma formation contributes to the early motion loss seen during the early postoperative period.

Approach

- A dorsal longitudinal incision is made centered over the first MTP joint.

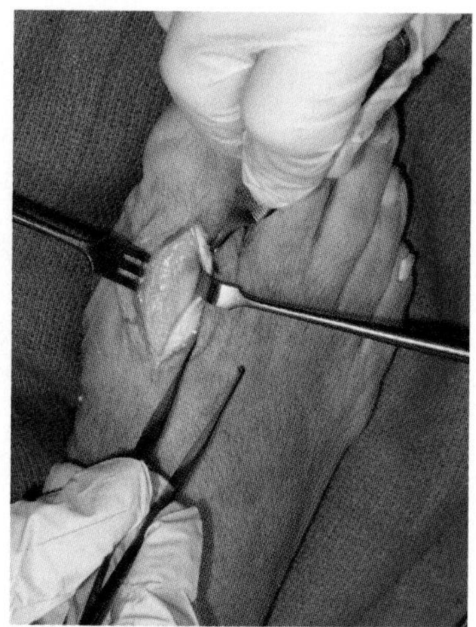

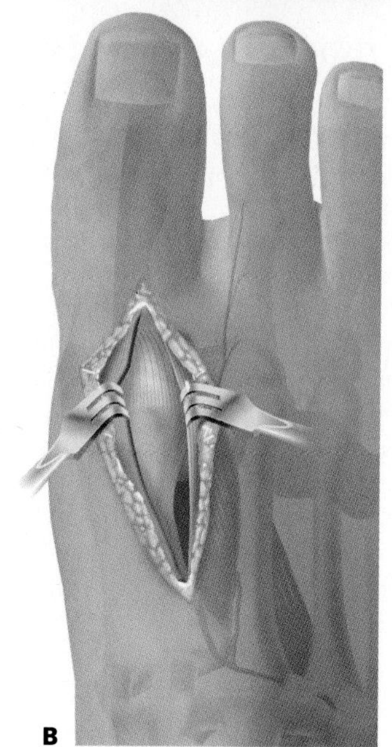

FIG 5 • Dorsal longitudinal incision. The capsulotomy is done medial to the extensor hallucis longus tendon and the tendon is retracted laterally.

- The extensor hallucis longus tendon is identified and retracted laterally (**FIG 5**).
- Sharp dissection is carried down just medial to the extensor hallucis longus tendon and a dorsal longitudinal capsulotomy is performed with soft tissue dissection performed subperiosteally along the medial and lateral aspects of the first metatarsal head.
- If a large proximal phalangeal base dorsal osteophyte is encountered upon approach, the phalangeal osteophyte is excised at this time. The metatarsal head osteophyte may be left until the implant is placed for excision at the end of the procedure.
- Plantarflexion of the hallux exposes the metatarsal head, and extensive articular cartilage loss is assessed.
- To release the plantar capsular joint contracture, a curved (McGlamry or similar) elevator can be passed between the sesamoids and plantar metatarsal head as long as this can be performed carefully without causing iatrogenic injury.

GUIDE PIN PLACEMENT FOR HEMICAP

- Obtain complete visualization of the metatarsal head with hallux plantarflexion.
- Place the centering spherical guide for the 15-mm HemiCAP on the metatarsal head with the feet of the guide in a superior–inferior position. A 15-mm guide is used typically; only on rare occasions is a 12-mm guide used as an alternative with an anatomically small head.
- The perimeter of the guide should not violate the metatarsal–sesamoid complex, and its inferior border is generally seated just above the crista. Avoid malplacement of the guide pin by plantarflexing the guide as necessary to adjust for normal inclination of the metatarsal shaft.
- Place the centering guide pin on the metatarsal head in line with the long axis of the metatarsal shaft and verify its position on AP and lateral fluoroscopic views. Adjust the guide pin as necessary to obtain correct placement (TECH FIG 1A–C). Pay particular attention to the guide pin lateral view, for there is a tendency to underestimate the degree of inclination of the metatarsal shaft; parallel to the long axis of the shaft is the desired position. Adjust the pin before proceeding.
- Use a cannulated drill over the guide pin and drill to depth so that the proximal shoulder of the drill bit is flush with the articular surface (TECH FIG 1D–G).

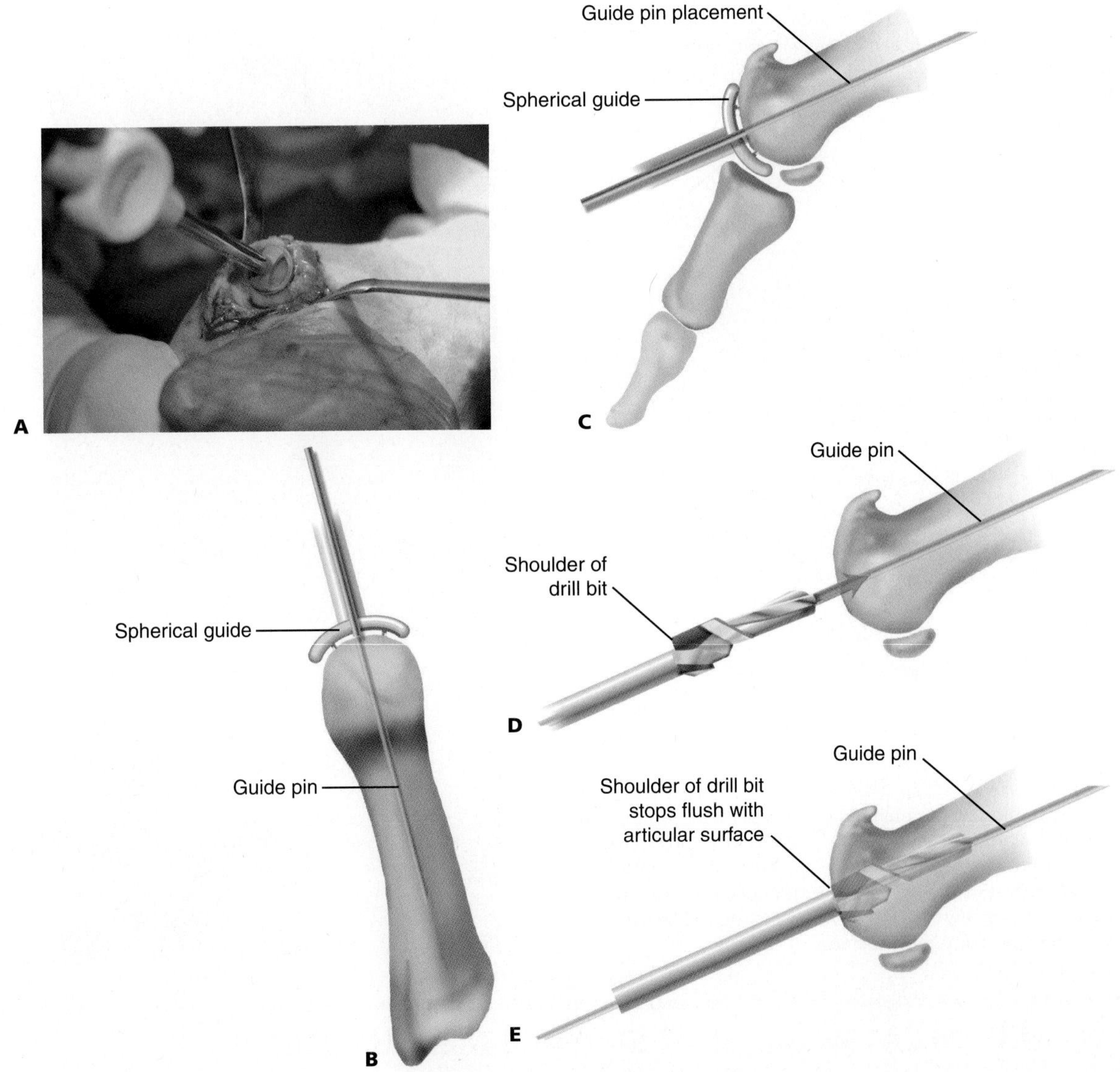

TECH FIG 1 • Guide pin placement. **A.** Intraoperative picture of spherical guide placement just above the crista of the first metatarsal. **B.** AP view of pin placed in line with the long axis of the first metatarsophalangeal shaft. **C.** Lateral image of pin placed parallel to the long axis of the metatarsophalangeal shaft. The surgeon can drop his or her hand as necessary to match the inclination of metatarsal and midline within the shaft. **D.** A cannulated drill is used over the guide pin. **E.** The proximal end of the drill bit should stop flush with the remaining articular surface. *(continued)*

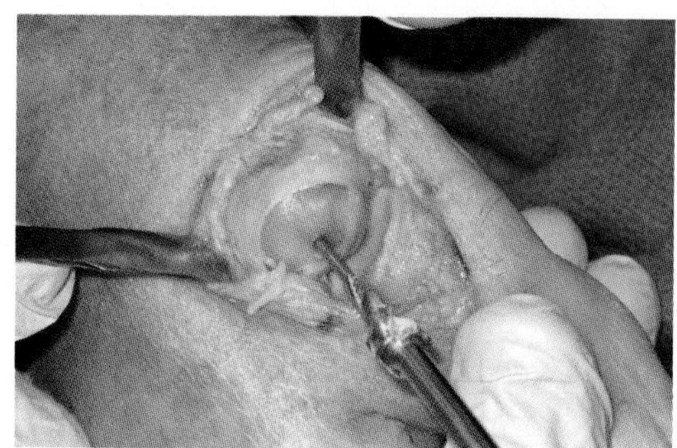

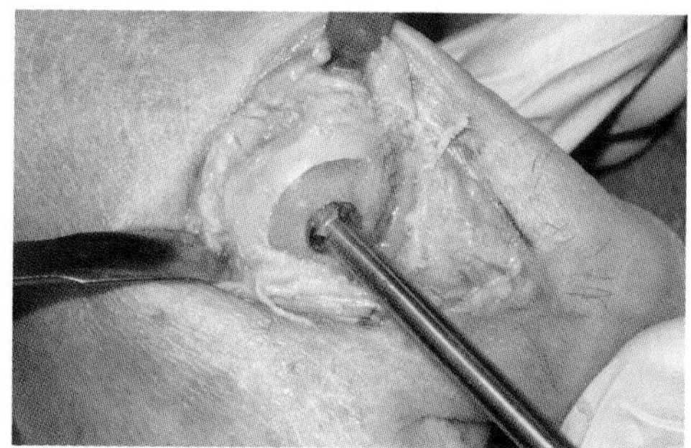

TECH FIG 1 • *(continued)* **F.** Intraoperative view of cannulated drill. **G.** Intraoperative view of drill's proximal end stopping flush with remaining joint line surface.

DRILL HOLE AND PLACEMENT OF TAPER POST SCREW

- Tap the drill hole to the etched line.
- Place the tapered screw of the HemiCAP implant, gaining purchase within the distal metatarsal bone. Bring the line indicator on the screwdriver just flush with the depth of the remaining articular surface level (**TECH FIG 2**).

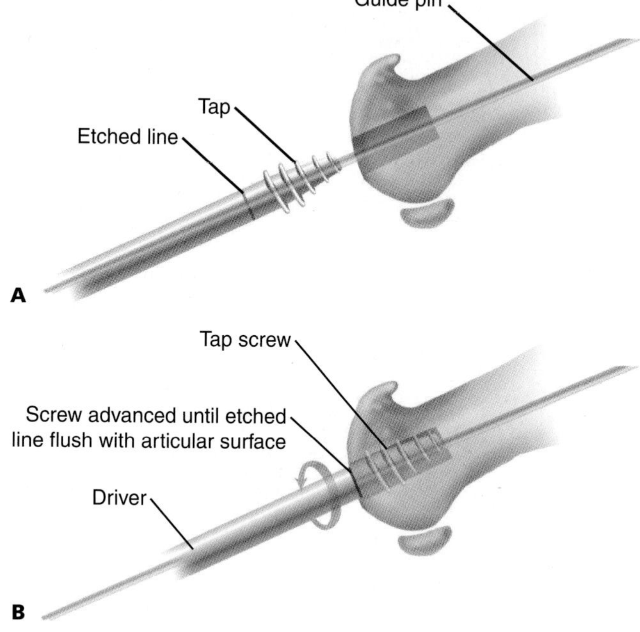

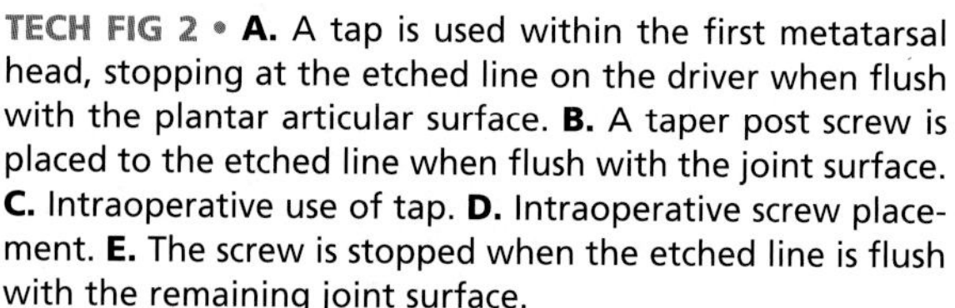

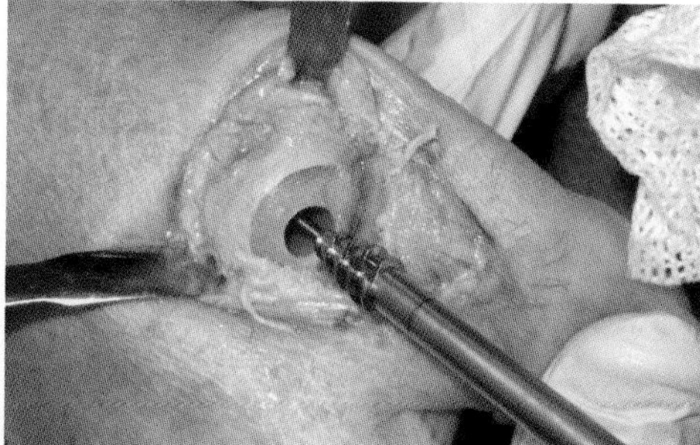

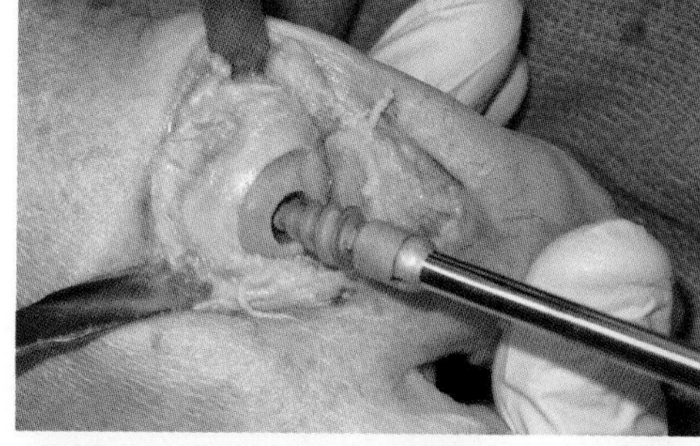

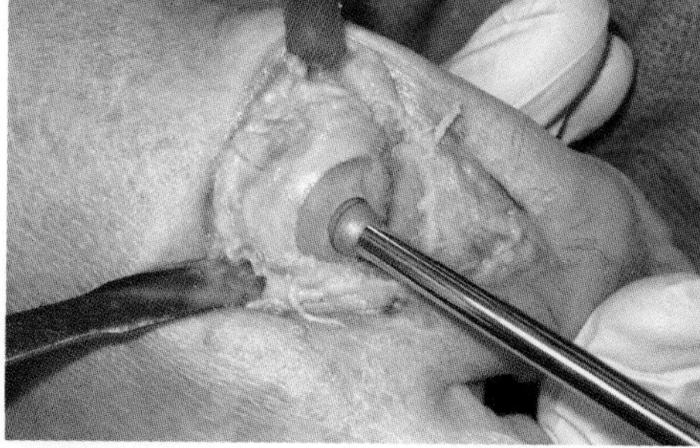

TECH FIG 2 • **A.** A tap is used within the first metatarsal head, stopping at the etched line on the driver when flush with the plantar articular surface. **B.** A taper post screw is placed to the etched line when flush with the joint surface. **C.** Intraoperative use of tap. **D.** Intraoperative screw placement. **E.** The screw is stopped when the etched line is flush with the remaining joint surface.

DEPTH AND METATARSAL HEAD SURFACE MEASUREMENTS

- Remove the guide pin and place the trial button cap to confirm the correct depth of the screw. Place the peak height of the trial cap flush or slightly countersunk to the level of the existing articular cartilage surface. The depth can be adjusted simply by either advancing or backing out the screw, with each quarter-turn accounting for 1 mm.
- Place the centering shaft pin through the cannulated portion of the screw to act as a centering point for measuring the radii of curvature of the metatarsal head at

four index points. This measures the geometric shape of the metatarsal head, assessing superior, inferior, medial, and lateral dimensions.

- Slide the contact probe device through the centering pin; this measures the distance at these four points pivoting at 90-degree intervals (TECH FIG 3). Record the numbers and choose the closest match to the provided implant size. Note: Choose the largest number measured in the superior and inferior and medial and lateral directions.
- Remove the centering shaft pin and place a standard guide pin back within the cannulated portion of the screw.

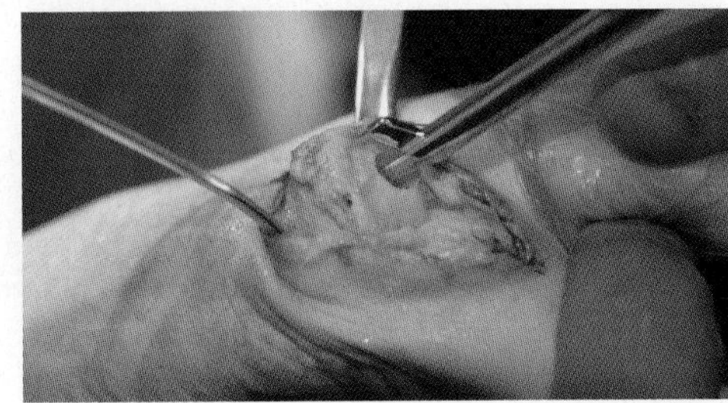

TECH FIG 3 • The guide pin is replaced with a wider centering shaft pin. A contact probe is then used to measure the dimensions of the metatarsal head so the proper implant size can be chosen.

SURFACE PREPARATION OF METATARSAL HEAD

- A circular surface reamer is then used (TECH FIG 4). The proper size is the largest size measured in either the superior–inferior or mediolateral directions. For example, if superior–inferior measures 3.0 mm and mediolateral 2.0 mm, then use a 3.0-mm circular reamer. Note: It is important to start the reamer before contacting the bone to avoid the remote chance of uncontrolled metatarsal bone blowout if poor bone quality is noted. The depth of the reamer is controlled, for it will stop on its own when contacting the screw.

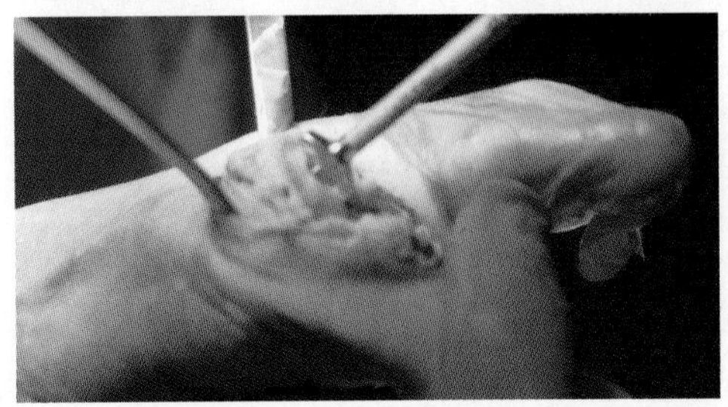

A

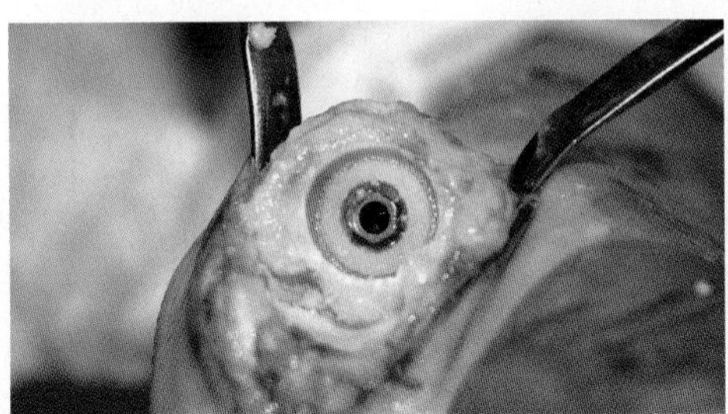

B

TECH FIG 4 • **A.** A circular reamer is used over the guide pin. There is a built-in stop when it reaches the edge of the screw. **B.** View after reaming for bone preparation for the HemiCAP. The screw is seen within the metatarsal head, for which the cap will mate with the Morse taper interlock.

PLACEMENT OF FORMAL CAP COMPONENT

- Confirm the trial size component so that it is congruent with the edge of the surrounding articular cartilage or slightly recessed.
- Place the formal HemiCAP component to resurface the arthritic metatarsal head by tamping the cap into position as it forms a Morse taper interlock with the neck of the seated screw (TECH FIG 5).

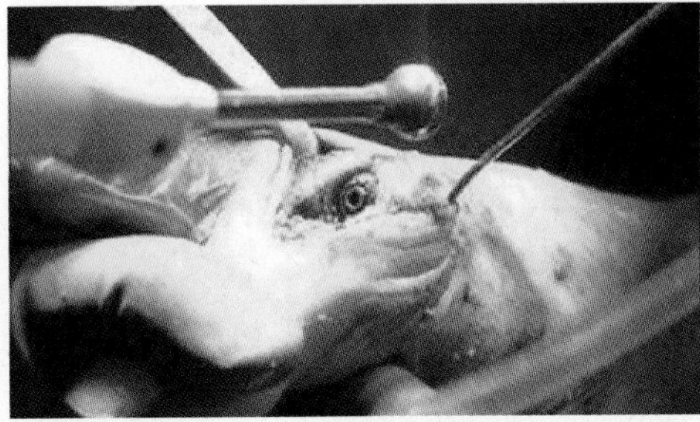

A

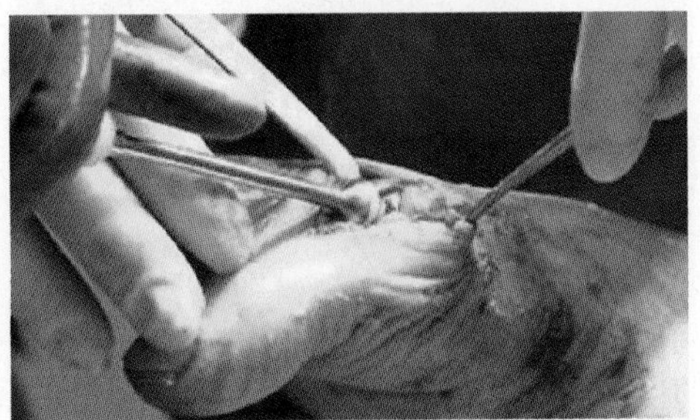

B

TECH FIG 5 • **A.** The HemiCAP implant is placed in the suction delivery device. **B.** Formal HemiCAP implant is tamped into place, forming a Morse taper interlock with the previously seated screw.

BONE EXCISION AND MOTION ASSESSMENT

- Remove dorsal osteophytes at this time with a microsagittal saw blade, osteotome, or rongeur. Any prominent bone along the dorsal, dorsomedial, and dorsolateral aspects is removed in an effort to eliminate any source of bony impingement as the hallux is brought into dorsiflexion (**TECH FIG 6**).
- Assess dorsiflexion of the hallux with passive motion. If motion still appears restricted, where the hallux cannot be dorsiflexed to 70 degrees relative to long axis of the first metatarsal, then consider performing an additional soft tissue or bony procedure.
- Consider a soft tissue procedure with release of plantar joint contracture (**TECH FIG 7**). This must be performed carefully so as not to cause any iatrogenic injury to the flexor hallucis brevis tendon or sesamoids. This may be performed with a Freer or McGlamry elevator or a small Beaver blade along the plantar capsule to elevate a few millimeters off the proximal phalangeal base or the plantar aspect of the first metatarsal.
- After soft tissue release, perform a slow, gentle dorsiflexion stretch of the hallux in a controlled manner in an effort to stretch the joint contracture.
- If after the soft tissue procedure more dorsiflexion is required, perform a simple Moberg closing wedge osteotomy of the proximal phalanx to improve dorsiflexion. Fixation of the Moberg phalangeal osteotomy may be achieved per the surgeon's preference. An Akin or biplanar (Mo-Akin) osteotomy may be performed in certain cases to address any concomitant mild hallux valgus (**TECH FIG 8**). Note: Avoid the Moberg procedure if there is no preoperative passive plantarflexion beyond neutral.
- Obtain final AP and lateral fluoroscopic images to confirm alignment of the HemiCAP device (**TECH FIG 9**).

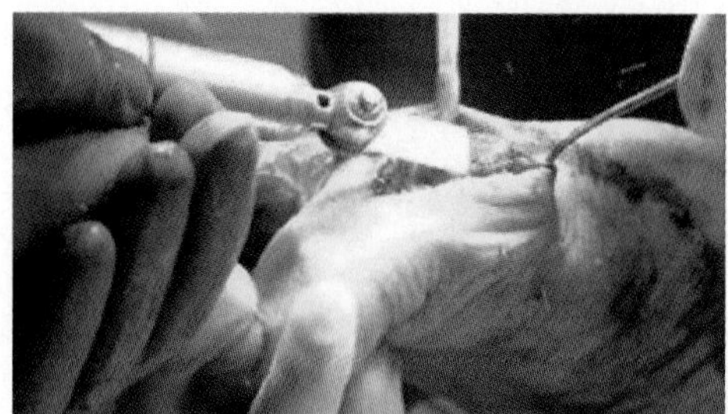
A

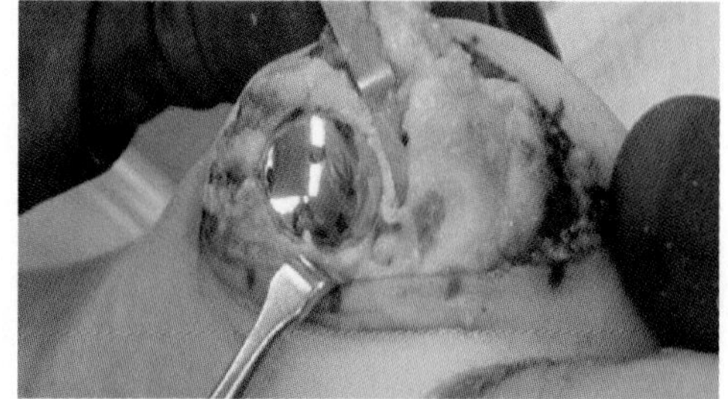
B

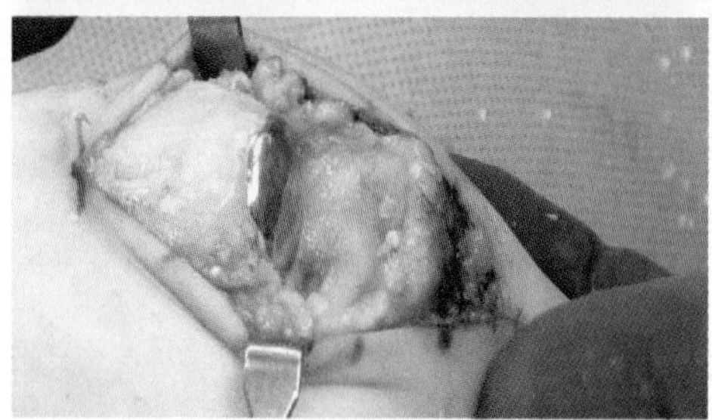
C

TECH FIG 6 • **A.** Excess bone along the dorsal, medial, and lateral aspects is removed with a microsagittal saw, osteotome, or rongeur, leaving an area of perimeter of bone to enclose the implant. **B, C.** Before and after decompression of surrounding bone around the HemiCAP.

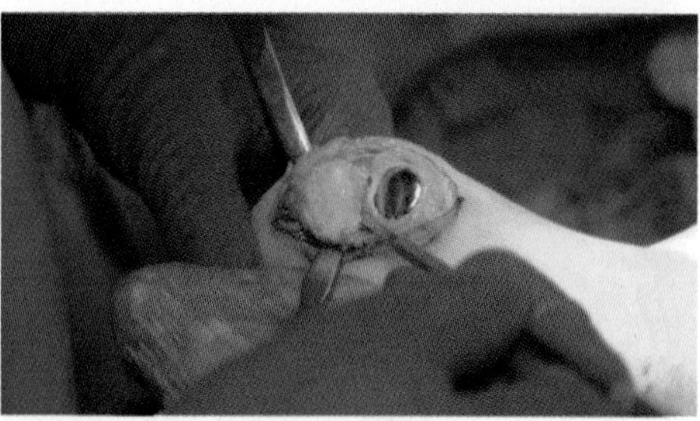

TECH FIG 7 • Plantar soft tissue release is performed along with subchondral drilling of the dorsal area of proximal phalanx articular cartilage loss.

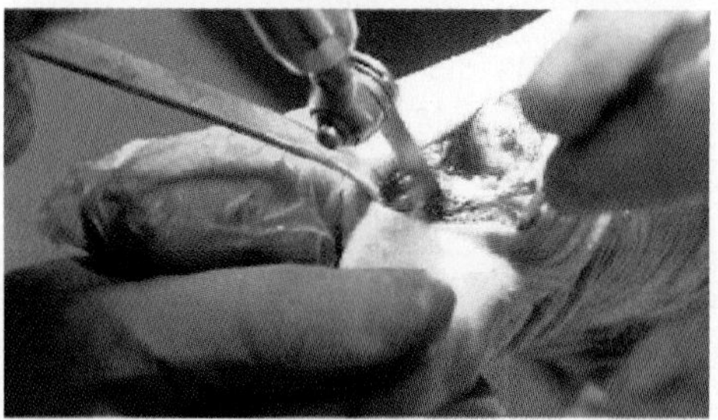
A

TECH FIG 8 • **A.** Moberg osteotomy is added by performing a dorsal closing wedge osteotomy of the proximal phalanx in certain cases for additional dorsiflexion. *(continued)*

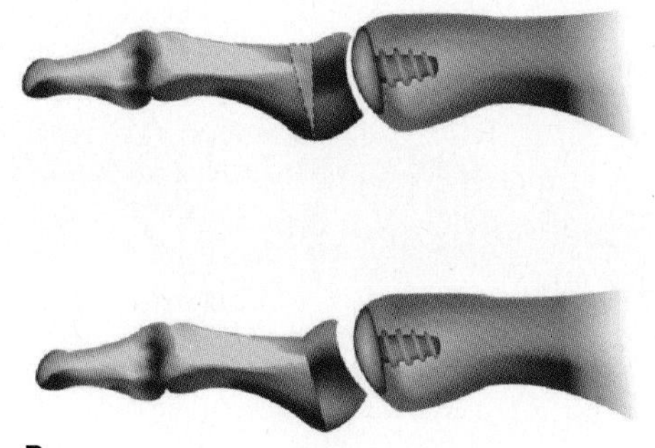

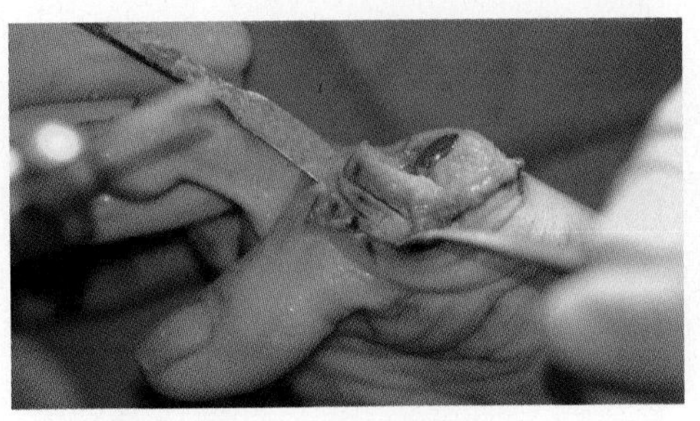

TECH FIG 8 • *(continued)* **B.** HemiCAP with Moberg osteotomy. **C.** Akin osteotomy or biplanar Mo-Akin osteotomy may be added at times to address concomitant mild hallux valgus.

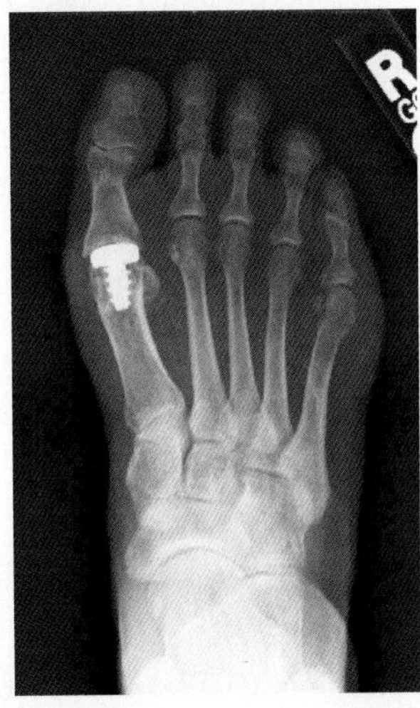

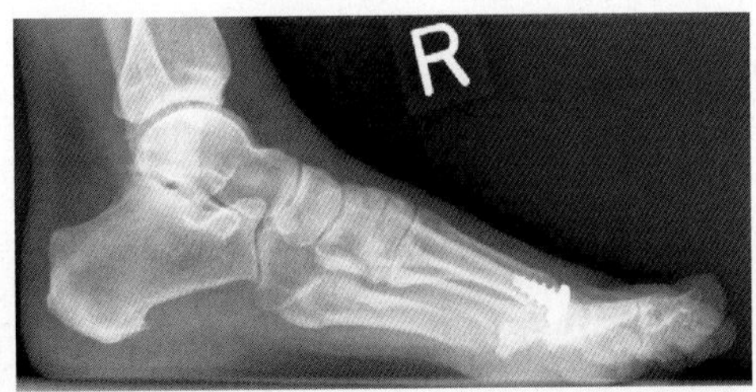

TECH FIG 9 • AP and lateral radiographs after HemiCAP resurfacing.

PEARLS AND PITFALLS

Indications	■ Evaluate for advanced arthritis of the metatarsal–sesamoid articulation. Failure to recognize this may lead to a poor result with persistent plantar joint pain. This patient would be a better candidate for arthrodesis. ■ Carefully review the patient's expectations preoperatively. If the patient cannot accept the possibility of reduced yet residual pain, he or she may be a better candidate for arthrodesis.
Guide pin placement	■ Avoid malposition of the implant by verifying that the guide pin placement is in line and parallel to the first metatarsal shaft axis on AP and lateral fluoroscopic views before drilling and placing the taper post screw. A common tendency is to underestimate the metatarsal inclination on the lateral view.
Intraoperative motion	■ Soft tissue contracture: Release a plantar joint contracture with a curve elevator between the sesamoid and metatarsal region. Avoid iatrogenic injury to the sesamoid articular surface. Consider subperiosteal release along plantar base of proximal phalanx with beaver blade and/or small elevator. ■ Peri-implant bone excision: After placement of the HemiCAP, carefully excise all surrounding bone around the dorsal, medial, and lateral aspects of the implant for thorough bony decompression in an effort to lessen the chances of residual bony impingement against the proximal phalanx. Leave a small rim of bone along the implant perimeter for cap stability. ■ Consider decompression of extremely tight joints with a concave conical reamer from an arthrodesis set (**FIG 6**). At the very start of the procedure, slightly decompress the joint by removing 2 to 3 mm of the metatarsal head (using either an 18- or 20-mm reamer). This tends to create joint space and a spherical head morphology. Some degree of joint decompression is beneficial. Avoid an overly aggressive decompression, which may create too much shortening, leading to altered sesamoid mechanics or lateral transfer metatarsalgia. ■ Consider adding a Moberg phalangeal osteotomy if additional dorsiflexion is desired (if unable to obtain at least 70 degrees intraoperatively after placement of the implant and soft tissue releases or decompression). Avoid the Moberg procedure if the patient preoperatively had no passive plantarflexion beyond neutral.

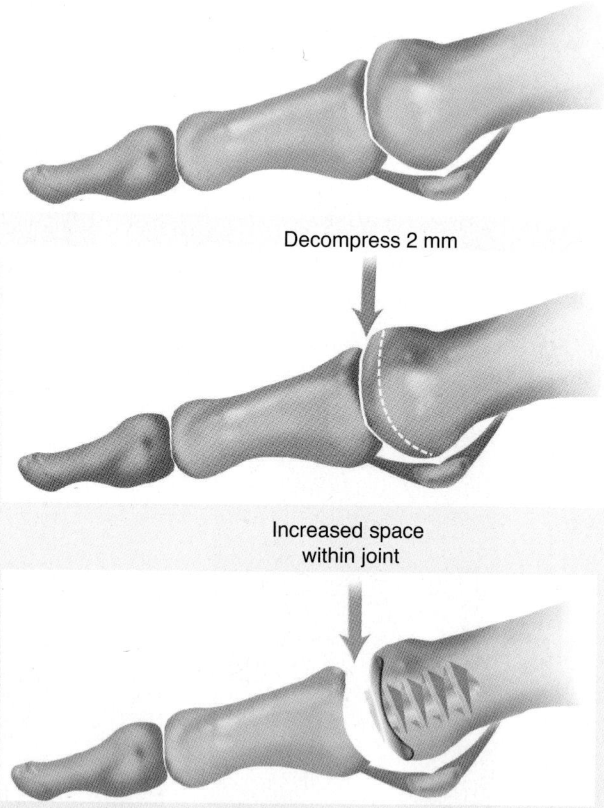

FIG 6 • **A.** Use of a conical reamer at the start of the case for a severely tight joint. Only 2 to 3 mm is decompressed in an effort to add space without adversely affecting the sesamoid mechanism. **B.** After decompression. **C.** Decompression with HemiCAP.

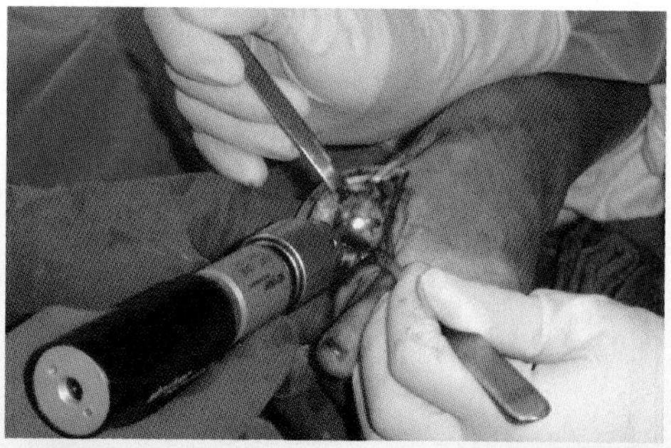

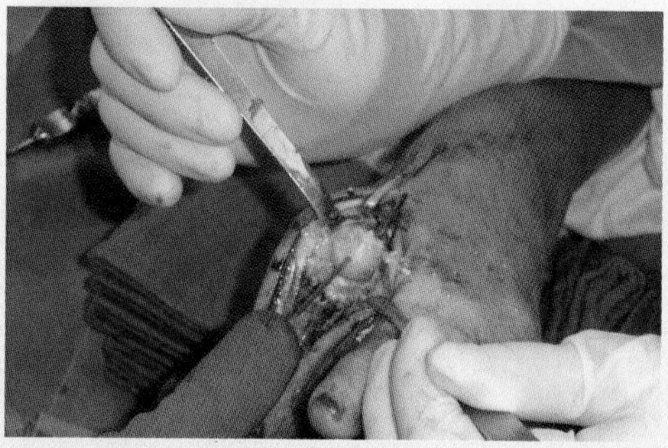

Postoperative swelling and hemarthrosis	■ No tourniquet: Postoperative swelling and hemarthrosis tend to restrict early joint motion. Performing the case without a tourniquet forces the surgeon to obtain excellent hemostasis upon the approach and leads to a drier wound on closure. Less postoperative swelling may reduce the degree of motion lost commonly seen postoperatively by allowing for improved early range of motion. ■ Consider using platelet-rich plasma for improved hemostasis of the wound with reduced postoperative swelling.
Postoperative motion	■ Early range-of-motion exercises are initiated within days. ■ Exchange the initial postoperative dressing for a light waterproof Op-Site dressing within 2 to 3 days postoperatively. Apply it along the dorsal incision site only so as not to hinder early motion due to a bulky restrictive dressing.

POSTOPERATIVE CARE

- A compressive dressing is placed intraoperatively.
- The dressing is changed at 2 to 3 days postoperatively for a light dressing along the dorsal incision only with a waterproof Op-Site (**FIG 7**). This allows for less restriction due to the bandage and encourages early range of motion.
- Early range-of-motion exercises are emphasized in an effort to preserve the motion gained intraoperatively. Some degree of motion loss is anticipated postoperatively from its intraoperative measurements, although every effort is made to minimize this amount.
- We have found the first 2 to 3 weeks to be a critical period for maintaining motion. Swelling, hematoma, or hemarthrosis that occurs within the joint postoperatively contributes to the loss of motion seen after surgery. Recent attempts to minimize this with strict hemostasis and an early motion protocol are encouraged. Patients are instructed to begin toe motion

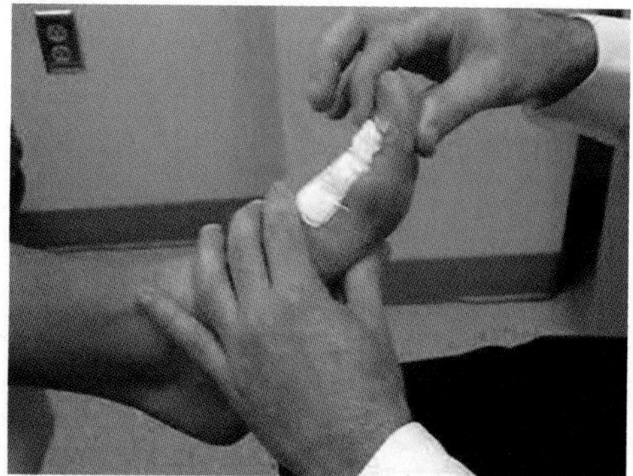

FIG 7 • The initial dressing is changed to a light dorsal postoperative dressing so as not to restrict early motion. A waterproof sealed Op-Site is used.

exercises early at home several times per day, in addition to formal physical therapy. The only restriction is that no passive plantarflexion be performed beyond neutral for the first 4 weeks if a Moberg proximal phalangeal osteotomy was performed. Physical therapy and rehabilitation continue until the patient reaches a normal gait pattern and range of motion is maximized.

- Patients are allowed to bear weight immediately on the heel of a rigid postoperative shoe or sandal. Between 3 and 4 weeks, the patient is transitioned to a running or jogging type of sneaker with a solid supportive sole.
- Radiographs are obtained at 1 week, 6 weeks, and 12 weeks postoperatively. Subsequent radiographs are obtained at 6 months, 1 year, and 2 years postoperatively.
- The patient should avoid placing high-impact stress on the joint, such as running, jogging, or sports involving pivoting and cutting, for at least the first 3 to 4 months postoperatively.

OUTCOMES

- A study by Hasselman and Shields[5] reported on 25 of their first 30 patients. At 20 months follow-up the patients showed a postoperative motion increase of 42 degrees (from 23 degrees preoperatively to 65 degrees postoperatively). Significant improvement in visual analog, AOFAS, and SF-36 scores were noted. All patients in this series claimed to be very satisfied with their results. Of note, an unspecified number of patients in this HemiCAP series underwent concomitant interpositional soft tissue grafting of the phalangeal side.
- The results of our follow-up study[13] on 36 patients at an average of 45 months were less favorable than those of the previously cited study, although fair satisfaction rates were achieved in this patient population that had refused to consider fusion. Good to excellent results were noted in 76% of patients, 12% fair, and 12% poor. We found a modest increase in dorsiflexion motion averaging 26 degrees (from 20 degrees preoperatively to 46 degrees postoperatively), along with improvement in visual analog scores from an average before surgery of 6.3 to an average of 2.2 after surgery. Although complete pain relief was not noted in most patients, the reduction of pain in the majority of the patients led to an overall satisfaction rate of 80% for the procedure at a follow-up of nearly 4 years. Intermediate-term radiographic evaluation of the HemiCAP prosthesis in 56 patients demonstrated no significant evidence of loosening; it appeared to show superior radiographic results compared to those of other metallic implants using a stemmed design.[13]
- Occasional evidence of regrowth of bony osteophytes along the dorsal perimeter of the implant was noted, whereas several patients displayed some degree of progressive chondral surface loss on the apposing proximal phalangeal base. These two issues may be factors associated with significant persistent pain and less-than-satisfactory results.
- When pain relief is the foremost goal of the patient, first MTP joint arthrodesis is the most predictable procedure for complete pain relief in advanced stages of hallux rigidus.
- When pain relief and preservation of some degree of joint motion are the desired goals, metatarsal head HemiCAP resurfacing can provide a reduction in pain and satisfactory outcome when patients understand the modest expectations—namely that complete pain relief may not be achieved with this procedure, rather a reduction in pain and maintenance of motion.

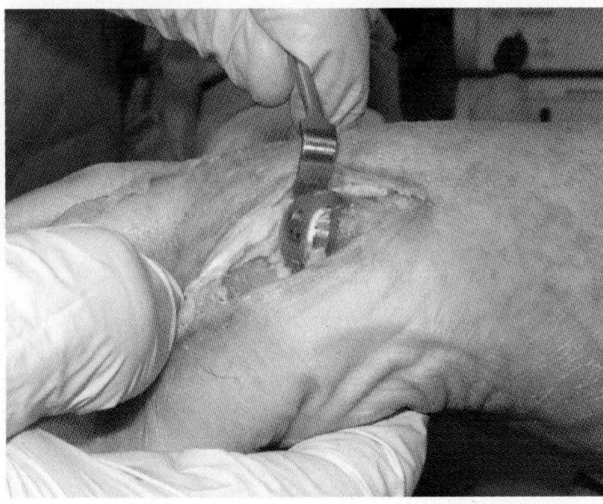

FIG 8 • Second-generation HemiCAP design with dorsal flange.

- It is critical to clearly explain this to the patient preoperatively so that the proper procedure can be chosen. As with all arthroplasty procedures (whether soft tissue interposition or implant), if the patient is unwilling to accept less-than-complete pain relief as a risk, then continued nonoperative treatment should be considered until a more predictable option becomes available or the patient accepts a fusion.
- Unlike other metallic prosthetic implants or Silastic implants, the HemiCAP did not display evidence of loosening. Rather, the mode of failure in cases in which patients were not satisfied proved to be secondary to persistence of pain or lack of adequate pain relief. Reformation of dorsal osteophytes and crepitus of the joint around the prosthetic implant or progressive chondral wear of the apposing phalangeal base may account for the residual pain seen in some patients.
- Given the lack of loosening seen in this implant, future design changes addressing dorsal periprosthetic bone formation and progressive arthritic changes of the proximal phalanx may provide a more predictable procedure with higher satisfaction rates. Design changes have been made for a second-generation HemiCAP with a dorsal flange and a more gradual dorsal curvature to the implant (**FIG 8**). These design modifications have been made in an effort to avoid recurrent periprosthetic dorsal osteophytes and improve the passive dorsiflexion gliding mechanism of the proximal phalanx on the metatarsal head during gait.
- The lack of radiographic loosening is encouraging with this design, and it may serve as a model for future development. Design improvements are under way to address specific issues in an effort to improve the predictability of pain relief and satisfaction rates.

COMPLICATIONS

- Joint stiffness
- Periprosthetic dorsal osteophyte formation
- Progressive arthritic changes, proximal phalangeal base
- Sesamoiditis
- Hallux valgus deformity

- Lateral transfer metatarsalgia
- Deep infection
- Metallosis

REFERENCES

1. Coughlin MJ, Shurnas PJ. Hallux rigidus: grading and long-term results of operative treatment. J Bone Joint Surg Am 2003;85A: 2072–2088.
2. Easley ME, Davis WH, Anderson RB. Intermediate to long-term follow-up of medial-approach dorsal cheilectomy for hallux rigidus. Foot Ankle Int 1999;20:147–152.
3. Hamilton WG, O'Malley MJ, Thompson FM, et al. Capsular interpositional arthroplasty for severe hallux rigidus. Foot Ankle Int 1997;18:68–71.
4. Hattrup SJ, Johnson KA. Subjective results of hallux rigidus following treatment with cheilectomy. Clin Orthop Relat Res 1988;226: 182–191.
5. Hasselman C, Shields N. Resurfacing of the first metatarsal head in the treatment of the hallux rigidus. Tech Foot Ankle Surg 2008;7: 31–40.
6. Konkel KF, Menger AG, Retzlaff SA. Mid-term results of Futura Hemi-great toe implants. Foot Ankle Int 2008;29:831–837.
7. Lau JTC, Daniels TR. Outcomes following cheilectomy and interpositional arthroplasty and hallux rigidus. Foot Ankle Int 2001;22: 462–470.
8. Mann RA, Clanton TO. Hallux rigidus: treatment by cheilectomy. J Bone Joint Surg Am 1988;70A:400–406.
9. Mann RA, Coughlin MJ, DuVries HL. Hallux rigidus: a review of literature and a method of treatment. Clin Orthop Relat Res 1979; 142:57–63.
10. Moberg E. A simple operation for hallux rigidus. Clin Orthop Relat Res 1979;142:55–56.
11. Raikin SM, Ahmad J, Pour AE, et al. Comparison of arthrodesis and metallic hemiarthroplasty of the hallux metatarsophalangeal joint. J Bone Joint Surg Am 2007;89A:1979–1985.
12. San Giovanni TP, Botto-Van Bemden A. First metatarsal head resurfacing: a new technique for surgical management of advanced hallux rigidus. Presented at American Academy of Orthopedic Surgery Annual Meeting, 2006.
13. San Giovanni TP, Marx R, Botto-Van Bemden A, et al. Presented at American Orthopedic Foot and Ankle Society Specialty Day at American Academy of Orthopedic Surgeons Annual Meeting, May 2010, New Orleans, Louisiana.
14. Seibert NR, Kadakia AR. Surgical management of hallux rigidus: cheilectomy and osteotomy phalanx and metatarsal. Foot Ankle Clin 2009;14:9–22.
15. Thomas PJ, Smith RW. Proximal phalanx osteotomy for surgical treatment of hallux rigidus. Foot Ankle Int 1999;20:3–12.
16. Townley CA, Taranow WS. A metallic hemiarthroplasty resurfacing prosthesis for the hallux metatarsophalangeal joint. Foot Ankle Int 1994;15:575–580.

Chapter 22

First Metatarsophalangeal Joint Hemiarthroplasty

Michael S. Aronow

DEFINITION

- Hallux rigidus is arthritis of the first metatarsophalangeal (MTP) joint.
- The amount of arthritis can range from focal areas of cartilage injury or osteophyte formation without joint space narrowing to ankylosis with complete loss of the joint space. In one classification system proposed by Hattrup and Johnson, grade I is osteophyte formation without joint space narrowing, grade II is narrowing of the joint space, and grade III is loss of visible joint space.

ANATOMY

- The joint consists of the articulation of the first metatarsal head with the hallux proximal phalanx and the medial and lateral sesamoids (**FIG 1**).
- The flexor hallucis brevis contains the two sesamoids within its medial and lateral heads and inserts on the plantar base of the hallux proximal phalanx.
- The flexor hallucis longus runs between the medial and lateral sesamoids and inserts on the plantar base of the hallux distal phalanx.
- The extensor hallucis longus and the more lateral extensor hallucis brevis insert into the extensor mechanism of the great toe.
- The abductor hallucis and adductor hallucis insert on the medial and lateral sesamoids respectively, along with the plantar base of the hallux proximal phalanx.

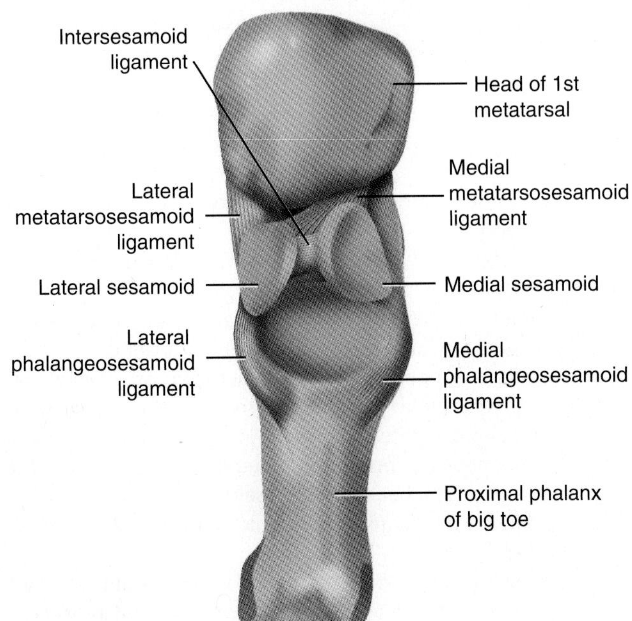

FIG 1 • Anatomy of the first metatarsophalangeal joint.

PATHOGENESIS

- Hallux rigidus may be secondary to primary osteoarthritis, systemic inflammatory arthritis, or less commonly septic arthritis.
- It may also be posttraumatic in nature, developing after a previous intra-articular fracture or significant turf toe injury to the ligamentous structures of the first MTP joint.
- Biomechanical factors such as a long, hypermobile, or dorsally elevated first metatarsal may lead to dorsal impingement of the proximal phalangeal base on the first metatarsal head with first MTP dorsiflexion.

NATURAL HISTORY

- The extent of arthritis often progresses with time, leading to increased osteophyte formation and joint space narrowing. This may occur with or without joint-sparing surgical intervention.

PATIENT HISTORY AND PHYSICAL FINDINGS

- Patients often complain of pain and stiffness in their first MTP joint. Symptoms may be exacerbated by shoes with a restrictive toe box and by walking barefoot or in shoes with a flexible forefoot.
- On examination there may be a prominent first metatarsal head, a swollen first MTP joint, and tender osteophytes of the metatarsal head and phalangeal base. First MTP joint motion may be limited and painful. Dorsiflexion range of motion should also be assessed with the patient bearing weight or with dorsal translation applied to the first metatarsal head to simulate weight bearing to assess for "functional hallux rigidus." In mild to moderate hallux rigidus (Hattrup and Johnson grade I and II), pain is principally with maximum joint dorsiflexion or plantarflexion secondary to dorsal osteophytes causing bone impingement or soft tissue tenting, respectively. With severe arthritis (Hattrup and Johnson grade III), there is usually pain throughout the entire arc of motion and a positive "grind test," in which mid-range of motion with axial compression applied to the first MTP joint is painful.

IMAGING AND OTHER DIAGNOSTIC STUDIES

- AP, lateral, oblique, and sesamoid views of the foot should be obtained to assess the extent of arthritis in the first MTP and in the adjacent first tarsometatarsal and hallux interphalangeal joints. An assessment is also made for any concurrent hallux valgus or hallux varus deformity, osteopenia, avascular necrosis, or occult sesamoid fracture.
- If needed, MRI and CT scan can provide more detailed information on the above, particularly sesamoid pathology, which is important as this procedure leaves the metatarsosesamoid joint intact.

DIFFERENTIAL DIAGNOSIS

- Osteochondral lesion
- Avascular necrosis
- Occult fracture

NONOPERATIVE MANAGEMENT

- Conservative treatment should always be offered before performing first MTP joint arthroplasty.
- The principal goal is to limit painful motion of the first MTP joint and pressure on prominent osteophytes. An accommodative shoe with a soft upper and a rigid forefoot rocker may be worn. A rigid turf-toe plate may be placed under a removable soft insole or an orthotic with a Morton's extension may be worn. Doughnut pads may be placed over tender osteophytes.
- Medications such as nonsteroidal anti-inflammatories, glucosamine and chondroitin sulfate, and acetaminophen may be taken.
- Corticosteroid and possibly hyaluronic acid injections may be performed.

SURGICAL MANAGEMENT

- There are many surgical options for hallux rigidus, including cheilectomy, metatarsal osteotomy, proximal phalangeal osteotomy, distraction arthroplasty, tissue interposition arthroplasty, implant arthroplasty, and arthrodesis.
- Of the many implants available, our preference is a cobalt chrome proximal phalangeal hemiarthroplasty made by BioPro (**FIG 2**). The material does not break down with associated extensive bone destruction like the silicone total and hemi implants, there are good long-term results published in the literature, and the amount of bone removed is small, making salvage of a failed prosthesis less challenging.
- Our potential indications for performing a first MTP hemiarthroplasty are symptomatic grade II arthritis with loss of greater than 50% of the metatarsal head articular cartilage and grade III arthritis without severe involvement of the articulation between the metatarsal head and the sesamoids.

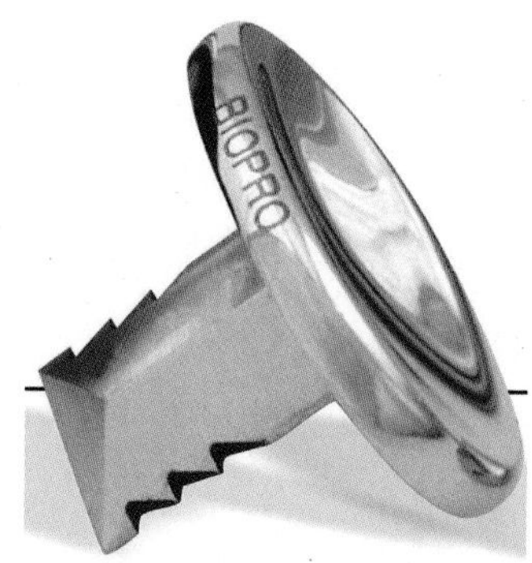

FIG 2 • BioPro first metatarsophalangeal hemiarthroplasty implant.

Preoperative Planning

- History, physical examination, and radiographs are reviewed to confirm the appropriate indications for the procedure and determine if there are any concurrent deformities or biomechanical abnormalities that also need to be addressed.
- The patient needs to be told that based on the intraoperative findings a decision may be made that hemiarthroplasty is not the best option and that a simple cheilectomy, arthrodesis, or tissue interposition arthroplasty may be preferable.
- The equipment to perform the hemiarthroplasty and the above alternatives should be readily available in the operating room.

Positioning

- The patient is placed in the supine position with a leg or thigh tourniquet.

Approach

- A dorsomedial approach is preferable, although a medial longitudinal approach can also be used in the presence of a previous incision there.

TECHNIQUES

FIRST MTP JOINT HEMIARTHROPLASTY USING THE BIOPRO PROSTHESIS

- Perioperative antibiotics and a regional anesthetic block are given.
- Make a longitudinal dorsomedial incision over the first MTP joint.
- Protecting the dorsomedial sensory nerve, expose the extensor digitorum longus tendon and dorsomedial joint capsule.
- Leaving a sufficient cuff of capsular tissue for subsequent repair, make a longitudinal capsulotomy medial to the extensor digitorum longus tendon.
- Using subperiosteal dissection and preserving the collateral ligaments, expose the dorsal aspect of the proximal phalanx and the dorsal, medial, and, if prominent, lateral aspect of the metatarsal head (**TECH FIG 1**).
  - Release any adhesions between the sesamoids and the metatarsal head.
- Inspect the joint to determine the extent of articular cartilage damage.
  - If there is severe ankylosis and arthritis of the metatarsosesamoid joints, then a first MTP joint arthrodesis or tissue interposition arthroplasty is probably a better option.
  - If the cartilage of the proximal phalanx and the plantar half of the metatarsal head is in good condition, then a cheilectomy with or without a metatarsal or phalangeal osteotomy is usually sufficient.
- Using a rongeur or sagittal saw, remove osteophytes from the metatarsal head, proximal phalangeal base, and also circumferentially about the sesamoids.
  - Remove a prominent medial eminence of the metatarsal head if it is present.
- Make an adequate dorsal cheilectomy of the metatarsal head.
  - With dorsal stress applied to the metatarsal head, there should be at least 70 degrees and preferably 90 degrees of first MTP dorsiflexion relative to the axis of the first metatarsal shaft.
  - Make an initial cut parallel to the dorsal cortex of the first metatarsal head. However, after the trial and final prostheses have been inserted, range of motion

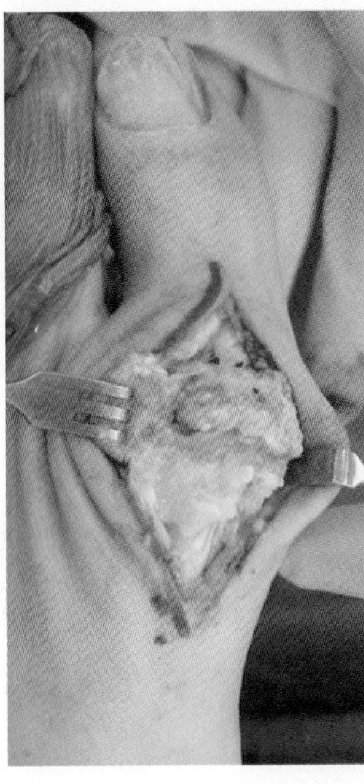

TECH FIG 1 • Exposure of dorsal osteophytes after capsular incision.

is reassessed and usually additional dorsal bone resection (up to 25% to 40% of the normal metatarsal head) is required. My experience with this procedure and with isolated cheilectomy is that there is a higher rate of recurrent symptoms if less than 30% of the dorsal metatarsal head is removed.

- Débride loose chondral flaps and drill or microfracture areas of visible subchondral bone on the remaining metatarsal head to promote fibrocartilage ingrowth.
- Remove the base of the proximal phalanx using a sagittal saw, with the cut perpendicular to the axis of the proximal phalanx.
  - Take care to avoid injuring the flexor hallucis brevis insertion, which may occur with resection of too much bone (>6 mm or 20% of the total proximal phalangeal length) or overpenetration of the saw blade.
- The implant sizer is the same thickness as the prosthesis (2 mm) and can be used to guide the amount of bone resection.
  - If only 2 mm of bone is removed, then the joint is usually too tight and postoperative motion is restricted.
  - Usually 3 to 4 mm of bone resection is required for adequate motion; this can be assessed by the amount of "shuck" with the trial implant inserted.
  - Ideally, the space between the trial or final implant and the metatarsal head should distract at least 3 mm with applied force.
  - Visualization of the plantar aspect of the joint may be easier after this cut has been made.
- Available BioPro implant diameters are 17 mm (small), 20 mm (medium), 21.5 mm (medium/large), and 23 mm (large); these implants are either porous coated and nonporous coated.
  - With the toe plantarflexed 90 degrees to improve exposure, use the sizer guide to determine the largest size implant that does not extend beyond the margins of the proximal phalangeal cut.
  - With respect to orientation, the prosthesis is slightly wider in the mediolateral dimension than the dorsal–plantar dimension.
  - There is a hole in the center of the sizer that is drilled to accommodate the stem of the trial prosthesis.
- Insert the trial stem and evaluate the extent of phalangeal base coverage and joint range of motion and stability. If as noted above there is insufficient joint distraction or dorsiflexion, more bone can be removed from the phalangeal base or dorsal metatarsal head, respectively.
- Once you are satisfied with the implant size and bone cuts, center the chisel with its longer end in the mediolateral dimension on the trial hole and use it to create a channel for the stem of the final prosthesis.
- Impact the prosthesis into position.
  - It should be flush with the phalangeal base and should not extend beyond its margins (TECH FIG 2).
  - Joint motion should be smooth with dorsiflexion and there should be at least 3 mm of "shuck," as noted above.
- Use AP and lateral fluoroscopy or plain radiographs to confirm acceptable prosthesis position (TECH FIG 3).
  - If the patient is not allergic, place bone wax on the cut dorsal surface of the metatarsal head and irrigate the joint.
- Close the joint capsule with absorbable suture.
  - If a large dorsal and medial eminence has been resected, then sometimes the capsule needs to be imbricated or partially removed. However, take care not to make the closure too tight, which may restrict postoperative motion.
  - Close the subcutaneous tissue and skin in layers and apply a sterile compressive dressing.

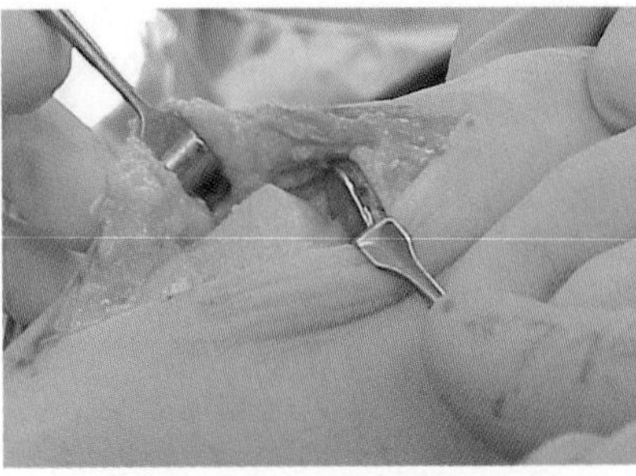

TECH FIG 2 • Cheilectomy has been performed and implant inserted.

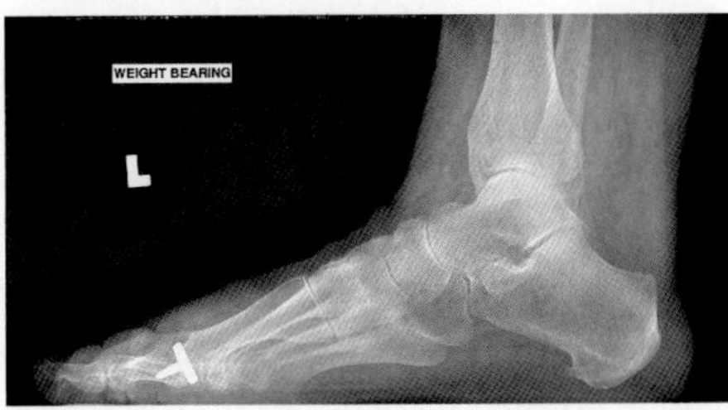

TECH FIG 3 • Postoperative lateral radiograph showing component in place.

PEARLS AND PITFALLS

- Failure to recognize and address concurrent deformity or potential causative biomechanical abnormalities may lead to progressive arthritis of the remaining metatarsal head and sesamoids, component loosening, and postoperative pain and stiffness.
- An adequate cheilectomy must be performed, particularly if there is residual elevation of the metatarsal head or hypermobility of the first tarsometatarsal joint. If not, there is more likely to be recurrent dorsal osteophyte formation and decreased postoperative range of motion.
- Sufficient bone must be removed from the proximal phalangeal base to decompress the joint without damaging the flexor hallucis brevis insertion.
- The stem of the prosthesis needs to press-fit tightly and be centered within the proximal phalangeal canal. An attempt to remove more dorsal than plantar phalangeal bone to "increase relative toe dorsiflexion" or protect the flexor hallucis brevis insertion risks having the tip of the stem abut or penetrate the plantar cortex and may lead to poorer results.

POSTOPERATIVE CARE

- Postoperatively, the patient may be weight bearing as tolerated in an orthopaedic or regular shoe.
- Aggressive early first MTP joint range-of-motion and strengthening exercises should be initiated within the first few days after surgery.
- Sutures are removed at 10 to 15 days postoperatively.

OUTCOMES

- The developer of the prosthesis reported his results for 279 procedures with follow-up of 8 months to 33 years as 93.1% excellent, 2.2% good, and 4.7% unsatisfactory results.[7]
  - Twelve of the 13 unsatisfactory results underwent revision, including prosthesis removal.
  - A subsequent update on 468 procedures with follow-up of 2 months to 38 years noted no additional revisions and one case of radiographic loosening.[2]
- In another study, seven patients (nine feet) underwent a BioPro resurfactin endoprosthesis and at 1-year follow-up noted an average increase on a modified American Orthopaedic Foot and Ankle Society Hallux Metatarsophalangeal-Interphalangeal 100-point scale from 51.1 to 77.8, an average increase in first MTP joint dorsiflexion range of motion from 11.9 to 17.9 degrees, and no change in first MTP join plantarflexion range of motion.[5]
- In a different study, 23 patients completed 1-year follow-up after BioPro hemiarthroplasty with an average ACFAS score increase from 41.2 to 80, average first MTP joint dorsiflexion increase from 12.6 to 50 degrees, and an average first MTP joint plantarflexion increase from 8 to 17.5 degrees.[3]
- Another study evaluated 32 procedures in 28 patients with an average follow-up of 33 months.[6]
  - Foot Function Index Pain, Disability, and Activity Scores improved; 82% of patients were completely satisfied and 11% were satisfied with reservations.
  - There were three cases of radiographic loosening or subsidence.
- In a retrospective comparison study, 21 BioPro hemiarthroplasties and 27 first MTP arthrodeses were evaluated at mean final follow-up of 79.4 and 30 months, respectively. Five (24%) of the hemiarthroplasties failed; one of them was revised, and four were converted to an arthrodesis. Eight of the feet in which the hemiprosthesis had survived had evidence of plantar cutout of the prosthetic stem on the final follow-up radiographs. The satisfaction ratings in the hemiarthroplasty group were good or excellent for 12 feet, fair for 2, and poor or failure for 7, with a mean pain score of 2.4 out of 10.[4]
- In the 16 procedures in 15 patients that we performed (average follow-up of 49 months), there was a 92% satisfaction rate and an 83% incidence of no or mild, occasional pain for index procedures and a 50% satisfaction rate and 25% incidence of no or mild, occasional pain for patients having had a previous failed first MTP joint cheilectomy or tissue interposition arthroplasty.[1]
  - There were three revision procedures—one implant removal for postoperative infection and two revision cheilectomies for recurrent osteophytes, possibly secondary to inadequate initial cheilectomy.

COMPLICATIONS

- Infection
- Nerve injury
- Component loosening
- Recurrent pain and loss of motion

REFERENCES

1. Aronow MS, Leger R, Sullivan RJ. The results of first MTP joint hemiarthroplasty in grade 3 hallux rigidus. Presented at the American Orthopaedic Foot and Ankle Society 22nd Annual Summer Meeting, La Jolla, CA, July 15, 2006.
2. Goez JC, Townley CO, Taranow WS. An update on the metallic hemiarthroplasty resurfacing prosthesis for the hallux. Presented at the 56th Annual Meeting and Scientific Seminar of the American College of Foot and Ankle Surgeons, Orlando, FL, February 1998.
3. Kissel CG, Husain ZS, Wooley PH, et al. A prospective investigation of the BioPro hemi-arthroplasty for the first metatarsophalangeal joint. J Foot Ankle Surg 2008;47(6):505–509.
4. Raikin SM, Ahmad J, Pour AE, et al. Comparison of arthrodesis and metallic hemiarthroplasty of the hallux metatarsophalangeal joint. J Bone Joint Surg Am 2007;89(9):1979–1985.
5. Roukis TS, Townley CO. BIOPRO resurfacing endoprosthesis versus periarticular osteotomy for hallux rigidus: short-term follow-up and analysis. J Foot Ankle Surg 2003;42(6):350–358.
6. Taranow WS, Moutsatson MJ, Cooper JM. Contemporary approaches to stage II and III hallux rigidus; the role of metallic hemiarthroplasty of the proximal phalanx. Foot Ankle Clin North Am 2005;10:713–728.
7. Townley CO, Taranow WS. A metallic hemiarthroplasty resurfacing prosthesis for the hallux metatarsophalangeal joint. Foot Ankle Int 1994;15:575–580.

Chapter 23

First Metatarsophalangeal Joint Arthrodesis: Perspective 1

Michael M. Stephens and Ronan McKeown

DEFINITION

- Arthrosis of the first metatarsophalangeal (MTP) joint is commonly seen in osteoarthritis (hallux rigidus), rheumatoid disease, and gout.
- The indication for surgical treatment of the first MTP joint is pain where conservative treatment has failed.
- Arthrodesis of the first MTP joint is the surgical treatment of choice in rheumatoid disease and is indicated in hallux rigidus when the disease is advanced.
- Many techniques in preparation of the joint exist to provide good cancellous apposition:
  - Flat cuts: these make accurate positioning of the toe difficult
  - Cone or peg socket: this leads to excessive shortening
  - Ball and socket: this results in minimal shortening and has the additional benefit of ease of adjustment in positioning the toe
- Various methods of fixation have been described. The most biomechanically advantageous method of fixation has been shown to be a dorsal plate and compression screw.[2,3]

ANATOMY

- The first MTP joint is a ball-and-socket joint.
- The normal hallux valgus angle is less than 15 degrees.
- The metatarsal inclination angle relative to weight bearing is usually 25 to 30 degrees but varies with foot type (greater for cavus, less for planus) (**FIG 1**).
- The final position of the arthrodesed first MTP joint must allow for heel rise during the late stance phase of gait.
- The position can be checked by applying a flat surface to the sole of the foot. The tip of the toe should clear the surface with the interphalangeal joint in full extension and should touch the surface with the interphalangeal joint in 45 to 60 degrees of flexion.

PATHOGENESIS

- Primary osteoarthritis (hallux rigidus) and the inflammatory arthritides (rheumatoid, gout, psoriatic arthritis) account for the majority of causative factors.

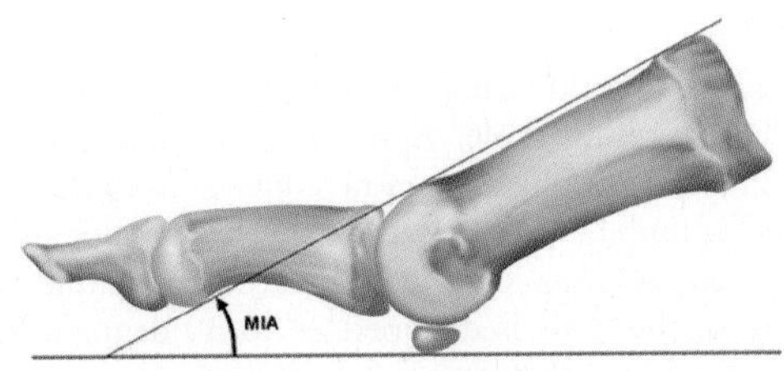

FIG 1 • Metatarsal inclination angle.

- Secondary osteoarthritis arises from mechanical abnormalities (hallux valgus and varus) and trauma resulting in joint incongruity and excessive cartilage wear.

NATURAL HISTORY

- The natural history of first MTP joint arthrosis is related to its cause.
- Hallux rigidus is a progressive disease process and the joint will deteriorate with time, but the patient's symptoms may not show the same deterioration.
- Progression of arthrosis secondary to the inflammatory arthritides will be related to the activity of the disease.

PATIENT HISTORY AND PHYSICAL FINDINGS

- In true hallux rigidus, patients experience an insidious onset of pain, swelling, and stiffness in the first MTP joint that is aggravated by activity (eg, walking, running).
- Lateral forefoot pain due to overload may develop as the foot supinates to avoid dorsiflexion of the first ray just before and immediately after heel rise.
- A comprehensive physical examination is required to enable diagnosis and selection of correct surgical procedure.
- The physician should palpate the MTP joint for tenderness; dorsal or dorsolateral osteophytes (cheilus) may be palpable and tender.
- The physician should examine the range of motion of the MTP and interphalangeal joints. Restriction in dorsiflexion but full plantarflexion may indicate that dorsiflexion osteotomy of proximal phalanx may improve the dorsiflexion arc.
- The grind test is not normally painful unless an osteochondral defect is present or degeneration is advanced. If painful, then arthrodesis is indicated.
- The physician should observe the patient's walking gait. Avoidance of weight bearing on the hallux implies pain. Callus may be present under the lesser metatarsals.
- The physician should palpate for posterior tibial and dorsalis pedis pulses. Peripheral vascular disease is a contraindication to surgery. If suspected, vascular assessment and treatment is required first.
- The physician should palpate and move the tarsometatarsal joint. Arthrosis of the tarsometatarsal joint is a relative contraindication to arthrodesis of the first MTP joint. The examiner should also palpate and move the interphalangeal joint. Arthrosis of the interphalangeal joint is a contraindication to arthrodesis of the first MTP joint.

Table 1 Grading of Hallux Rigidus

Grade	Dorsiflexion	Radiologic Findings	Clinical Findings	Treatment
0	> 40 degrees, minimal loss compared to normal side	Normal	No pain; stiffness with decreased range of movement only	Conservative
1a	30 to 40 degrees, < 50% loss compared to normal side but 40 degrees or more painless plantarflexion	Dorsal osteophyte, minimal joint space narrowing	Painful, limited dorsiflexion but large painless and normally unused plantarflexion arc	Moberg osteotomy and cheilectomy
1b	As above but minimal plantarflexion arc	As above	Occasional dorsal or dorsolateral pain; pain at extreme dorsiflexion (impingement) or plantarflexion (capsular tightening)	Cheilectomy
2a	10 to 30 degrees, < 75% loss compared to normal side	Dorsal, lateral, and medial osteophytes; only the dorsal 25% joint space is narrowed on the lateral radiograph.	Moderate dorsal or dorsolateral pain, just before maximum dorsiflexion or plantarflexion	Cheilectomy
2b	As above	As above	Dorsal or dorsolateral pain throughout arc of motion (positive grind test)	Arthrodesis
3	<10 degrees, >75% compared to normal side	Cyst formation; on the lateral radiograph, >25% joint space is narrowed; sesamoid involvement	Stiffness and constant pain; extreme pain at end of plantarflexion and dorsiflexion but not at midrange	Arthrodesis
4	As grade 3	As grade 3	As grade 3 plus pain in mid range of motion	Arthrodesis

This grading system is an adaptation by the authors (Stephens and McKeown) from Coughlin and Shurnas.[1]

IMAGING AND OTHER DIAGNOSTIC STUDIES

- Weight-bearing anteroposterior and lateral radiographs should be obtained before surgery.
  - The severity of the arthrosis can be assessed and any coexisting forefoot pathology identified and addressed at the time of surgery.
  - The hallux valgus angle and the metatarsal inclination angle should be measured accurately.
  - The lateral radiograph shows the cheilus and any narrowing of the joint space (either dorsally or throughout).
- Hallux rigidus can be graded using the clinical and radiologic information obtained.
- We have created a seven-point clinicoradiologic grading system (adapted from Coughlin and Shurnas[1]) that correlates the severity of the disease (symptoms, clinical examination, and radiologic findings) with the appropriate surgical procedure (Table 1).

NONOPERATIVE MANAGEMENT

- Nonoperative management encompasses activity modification, weight loss, analgesic and anti-inflammatory medication (oral and intra-articular), physiotherapy (tendo Achilles and hamstring stretching), and shoe modification.
- Shoe modification can involve a carbon fiber extended insole with cutouts for the lesser toes, metal stiffeners in the last, and a forefoot rocker sole.

SURGICAL MANAGEMENT

- Arthrodesis of the first MTP joint does not restore normal anatomy or gait pattern. The patient should be counseled as to the surgical goals and optimal outcome in order to have realistic expectations of the surgery.
- Absolute contraindications to first MTP joint fusion include active infection, peripheral vascular disease, and arthrosis of the interphalangeal joint.
- Relative contraindications to first MTP joint fusion include degeneration of the first tarsometatarsal joint and peripheral neuropathy.

Preoperative Planning

- Initial assessment should include examination of circulation, sensation, the first tarsometatarsal joint, the interphalangeal joint, and any previous surgical incisions about the foot.
- It may be necessary to consult with the patient's rheumatologist to reduce or stop immunosuppressant drugs before surgery.
- Preoperative weight-bearing AP and lateral radiographs should be obtained.

Positioning

- We prefer to position the patient supine with the heels at the end of the operating table. A thigh tourniquet is inflated to 350 mm Hg after prophylactic intravenous antibiotics have been given and the limb has been exsanguinated. The foot and leg are then prepared and draped above the knee in a routine manner.
- The end of the table is dropped 20 to 30 degrees. The surgeon sits at the end of the table.

Approach

- A dorsal approach is recommended regardless of previous scars. Care should be taken to avoid the dorsal cutaneous nerve and extensor hallucis longus. The former is retracted medially and the latter laterally, so they are protected.

ARTHRODESIS OF THE FIRST METATARSOPHALANGEAL JOINT USING A DORSAL TITANIUM CONTOURED PLATE (HALLU-S PLATE)

Exposure

- Make a dorsal slightly curved incision just medial to the extensor hallucis longus tendon and lateral to the dorsal cutaneous nerve, extending from the middle of the shaft of the first metatarsal to the interphalangeal joint.
- Retract the extensor hallucis longus tendon laterally.
- Make a capsulotomy in the same plane and expose the joint.
- Perform a synovectomy.
- Release the medial and lateral soft tissues to allow maximum plantarflexion of the proximal phalanx, exposing both articular surfaces.

Joint Preparation

- Excise any large medial eminence or osteophyte with an oscillating saw.
- Excise osteophytes on the proximal phalanx to find the true center and size of the articular surface.
- Size the articular surface of the proximal phalanx to determine the correct convex reamer required.
- Insert a 1.6-mm Kirschner wire through the center of the articular surface of the proximal phalanx and pass it in line with its long axis. In osteoporotic bone the wire should cross the interphalangeal joint into the distal phalanx to prevent toggling of the wire, leading to eccentric reaming.
- Guide the sized convex reamer over the Kirschner wire and ream the surface sparingly to expose subchondral cancellous bone (TECH FIG 1).
- Remove the Kirschner wire. Remove any fine collar of cartilage remaining around the wire entry hole. Insert the wire into the center of the articular surface of the first metatarsal and advance it along its long axis. If the bone is osteoporotic then the wire should cross the tarsometatarsal joint.
- Use the matched-sized concave reamer in a similar fashion to expose the subchondral cancellous bone of the metatarsal head (TECH FIG 2). Remove the wire and retain all fragments of bone in the reamer.

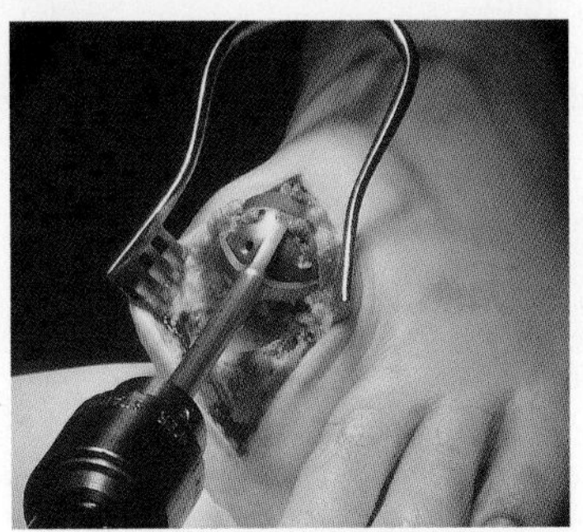

TECH FIG 2 • Reaming the articular surface of the metatarsal head.

Positioning

- Approximate the position of the hallux in relation to the first metatarsal and fix the position temporarily with an obliquely directed Kirschner wire. The ideal position is 20 to 25 degrees of dorsiflexion of the proximal phalanx in relation to the first metatarsal axis. The valgus angle should be 10 to 15 degrees. However, a gap of 3 to 5 mm must be left between the hallux and the second toe. The rotation of the hallux should be neutral so that the arc of rotation of the interphalangeal joint is at 90 degrees to the weight-bearing surface.
- Confirm the correct position of the hallux by placing a flat surface against the sole of the foot and bringing the ankle to 90 degrees. In this position, with the interphalangeal joint in full extension, the tip of the hallux lies about 1 cm from the flat surface. When the interphalangeal joint is flexed to 45 to 60 degrees, its tip comes in contact with the plantar surface. This enables the foot to rock at the MTP joint on heel rise (TECH FIG 3).

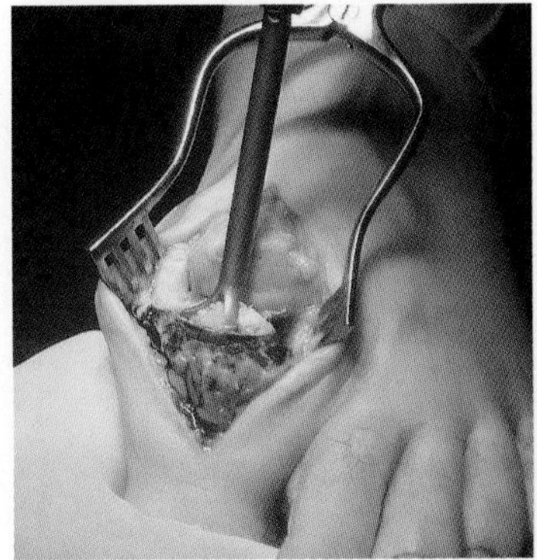

TECH FIG 1 • Reaming the articular surface of the proximal phalanx.

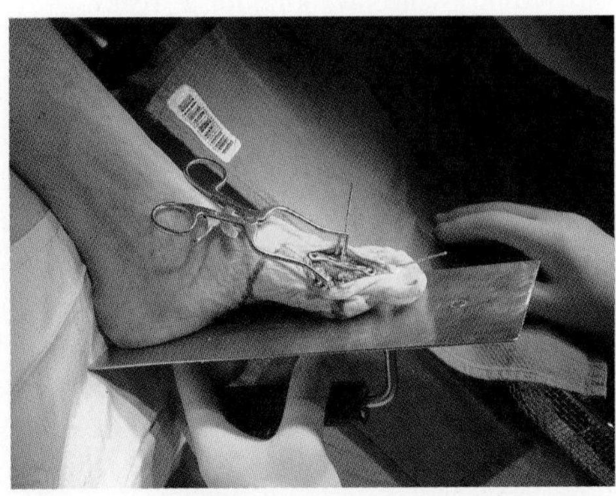

TECH FIG 3 • Foot plate to check arthrodesis position.

Fixation

- Insert an oblique 2.7-mm compression screw of appropriate length from distal medial to proximal lateral across the MTP joint.
- Size and secure the plate on the dorsal aspect of the joint with a Kirschner wire and fix it with six 2.7-mm self-tapping screws (**TECH FIGS 4 AND 5**). The plate is available in three side-specific (left and right) sizes (small for a small hallux, medium for a larger hallux, large for revision arthrodesis).
- Close the wound in layers over a drain.
- Apply a compression dressing.

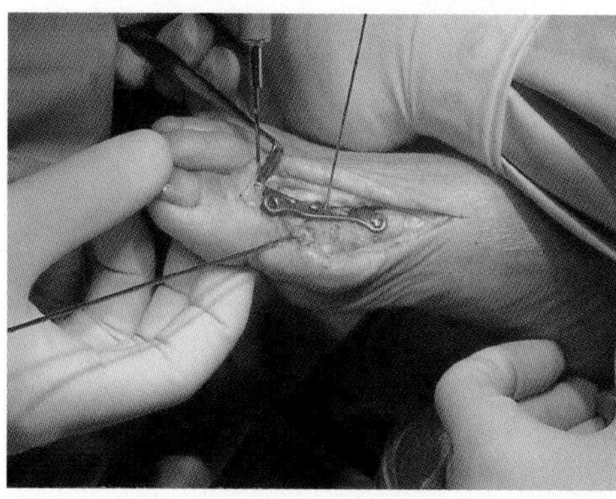

TECH FIG 4 • Plate secured with temporary Kirschner wire.

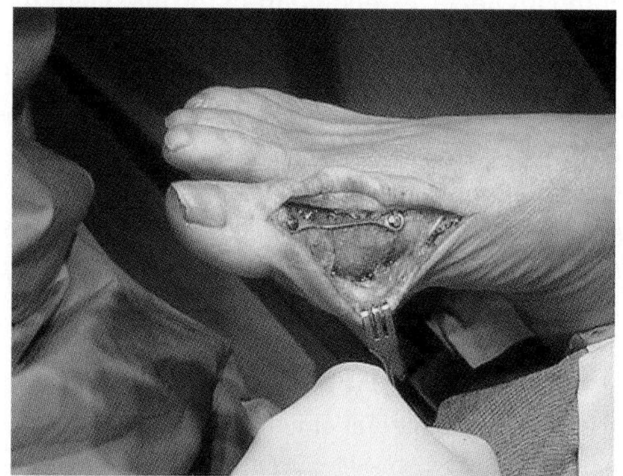

TECH FIG 5 • Screw fixation of plate.

PEARLS AND PITFALLS

Clinical examination	■ Coexisting arthritis of the tarsometatarsal and interphalangeal joints should be excluded. ■ Plantarflexion of the first MTP joint is functionless in bipedal gait. When painless, a Moberg osteotomy is helpful in patients with a good plantarflexion arc, especially in athletes.
Most problems arise from the final arthrodesis position.	
Too dorsiflexed	■ A painful corn develops on the dorsum of the interphalangeal joint.
Too plantarflexed	■ Callosities may form under the condyles of the proximal phalanx. With time, a hyperextension deformity can arise in the interphalangeal joint (recurvatum).
Too varus	■ Not a major concern but can cause problems with footwear
Too valgus	■ This can be a major problem and cause great irritation of the second toe due to impingement and the inability to cleanse the web space.

POSTOPERATIVE CARE

- If this technique is performed as an isolated procedure we do not use a cast but a compressive dressing and a postoperative stiff-soled shoe to allow early mobilization.
- Patients are kept non–weight-bearing for 2 weeks and then encouraged to bear weight by heel walking for 2 weeks.
- Four weeks after surgery a radiograph is taken (**FIG 2**). If there is evidence of consolidation, forefoot weight bearing is commenced in the postoperative shoe. Progression to full forefoot loading, assisted by crutches, follows over the next 4 weeks.
- Radiographs taken 8 weeks after surgery usually confirm consolidation. At this stage flat shoes with cushioned, shock-absorbing soles are worn.

OUTCOMES

- Union rates for arthrodesis are quoted in the literature ranging from 80% upward. Using this technique, we have achieved 100% union. The average time for union to be visible radiologically is 6 weeks. All patients experienced significant increases in their outcome scores.[3]

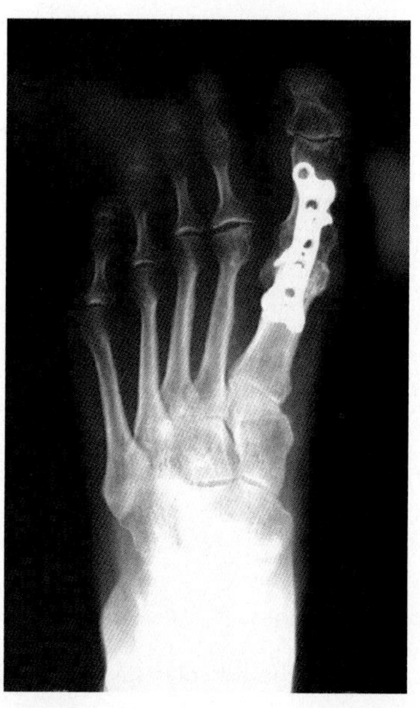

FIG 2 • Radiograph taken 4 weeks after surgery.

COMPLICATIONS

- Potential complications of first MTP joint arthrodesis include malunion, infection, delayed union, interphalangeal joint stiffness, extensor hallucis longus tenodesis (secondary to scarring), dorsal cutaneous nerve damage, and hardware problems.
- The incision described in this technique minimizes the risk to the extensor hallucis longus and dorsal cutaneous nerve while facilitating maximal plantarflexion to allow reaming.
- The ball-and-socket bone-end preparation minimizes shortening and provides a large congruent cancellous area of contact, enabling easy positioning of the hallux and reducing consolidation time. Temporary Kirschner wire fixation facilitates correct alignment.
- Use of the compression screw and dorsal plate ensures maximum stability.
- The low-profile precontoured titanium plate has inbuilt dorsiflexion and hallux valgus angles and is contoured to the specific shapes of the proximal phalanx and the first metatarsal. It acts as a neutralization plate and facilitates correct positioning. The differing screw axes increase pullout strength.
- These mechanical factors significantly reduce the risk of delayed union and nonunion.

REFERENCES

1. Coughlin M, Shurnas P. Hallux rigidus: grading and long-term results of operative treatment. J Bone Joint Surg Am 2003;85A:2072–2088.
2. Politi J, Hayes J, Njus G, et al. First metatarsal-phalangeal joint arthrodesis; a biomechanical assessment of stability. Foot Ankle Int 2003;24:332–337.
3. Stephens MM, Flavin R. Arthrodesis of the first metatarsophalangeal joint using a dorsal titanium contoured plate. Foot Ankle Int 2004;25:783–787.

Chapter 24 First Metatarsophalangeal Joint Arthrodesis: Perspective 2

Bertil W. Smith and Michael J. Coughlin

DEFINITION

- The term *hallux rigidus* refers to a painful condition of the first metatarsophalangeal (MTP) joint of the great toe that is characterized by restricted motion (mainly dorsiflexion) and periarticular bone formation.
- The basic pathologic entity is that of degenerative arthritis.
- Initially, hallux rigidus is characterized by pain, swelling, and MTP joint synovitis.
- As the degenerative process proceeds, proliferation of bony osteophytes on the dorsal and dorsolateral aspect of the first metatarsal head develop.
- With advanced disease, near-complete bony ankylosis may occur.

ANATOMY

- The round, cartilage-covered first metatarsal head articulates with the somewhat smaller, concave base of the proximal phalanx.
- Articulating on the plantar surface of the metatarsal head are the two sesamoids, which are contained in the tendon of the flexor hallucis brevis.
- Distally, the two sesamoids are attached by the plantar plate to the base of the proximal phalanx.
- The sesamoids are connected by the intersesamoidal ligament and protect, on their plantar surface, the tendon of the flexor hallucis longus within its tendon sheath.
- Dorsally, the extensor hallucis longus is anchored medially and laterally by the dorsal capsule and MTP joint hood ligaments.
- The tendons of the abductor and adductor hallucis pass medially and laterally, but much closer to the plantar surface of the MTP joint (**FIG 1** and **2**).

PATHOGENESIS

- The cause of hallux rigidus has not been determined, but joint trauma often is cited as a predisposing factor.
  - This may occur as a single episode, such as an intra-articular fracture, as a crush injury, or with repetitive microtrauma.
  - In a patient who sustains an acute injury to the MTP joint, forced hyperextension or plantarflexion may lead to an acute chondral or osteochondral injury.
- The only documented factors associated with the cause of hallux rigidus are a flat or chevron-shaped metatarsal articular surface, bilaterality in those with a positive family history, and female gender.
- Metatarsus primus elevatus typically is a secondary phenomenon related to the severity of the disease and restricted MTP joint motion, and is not a primary cause of hallux rigidus (**FIG 3**).

NATURAL HISTORY

- A patient with hallux rigidus typically complains of stiffness with ambulation and pain localized to the dorsal aspect of the first MTP joint that is aggravated by walking, especially during toe-off.
- Patients tend to ambulate with an inverted foot posture to prevent stress on the first MTP joint.
- With time and further osteophyte formation, increased bulk around the MTP joint periphery can lead to substantial discomfort with constricting footwear.
- More than 80% of patients, if followed long enough, will develop bilateral symptoms.
- Ninety-five percent of patients with bilateral symptoms have a positive family history.

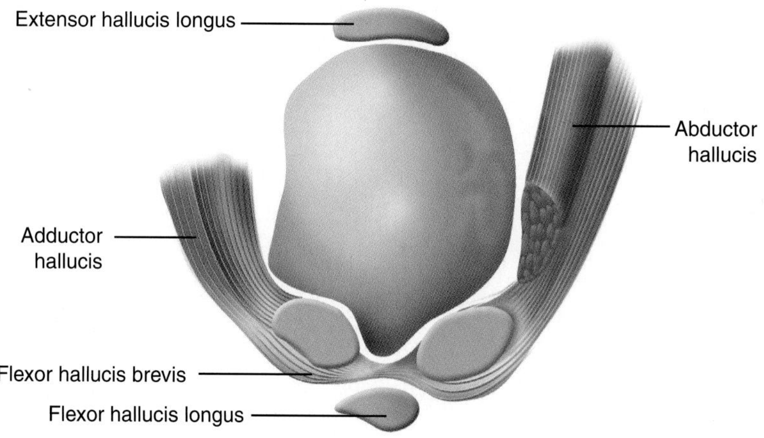

FIG 1 • Axial drawing of the first metatarsophalangeal (MTP) joint.

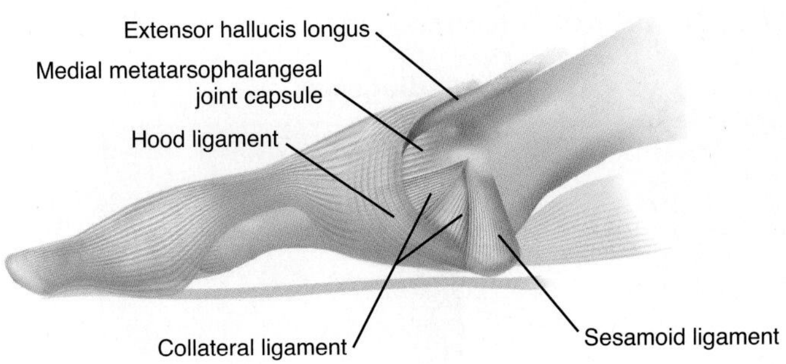

FIG 2 • Lateral drawing of the first MTP joint.

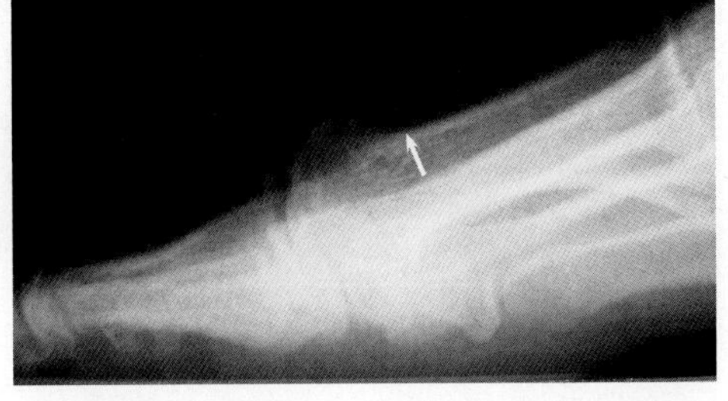

FIG 3 • Lateral radiograph of a patient with hallux rigidus and notable metatarsus primus elevatus (MPE). The arrow shows the elevation of the first metatarsal relative to the second.

PATIENT HISTORY AND PHYSICAL FINDINGS

- A complete examination to evaluate for associated forefoot pathology should include the following.

Interdigital Neuroma

- The interdigital spaces should be palpated for any tenderness.
- A Mulder's test should also be performed.
- The second and third interspaces are the most common locations for an interdigital neuroma.

Hammer Toe or Mallet Toe

- The patient should be examined while standing to evaluate for the presence of a hammer or mallet toe deformity.

Crossover Toe

- Inspection may reveal either medial or lateral deviation of the lesser toes. The MTP joints of the lesser toes should be palpated for plantar tenderness as well as thickening of the joint capsule. A drawer test of the lesser MTP joints also should be performed. Crossover toes usually affect the second and third digits.

Gastrocnemius Contracture

- A Silfverskiöld test should be performed to assess for a gastrocnemius contracture. This is rarely of clinical significance in patients with hallux rigidus.

IMAGING AND OTHER DIAGNOSTIC STUDIES

- Weight-bearing radiographs (AP, lateral, and seamoid views) are obtained to evaluate the first MTP joint.
- The Coughlin/Shurnas classification of hallux rigidus (Table 1) is used to grade the severity of joint arthrosis.
- The AP radiograph often demonstrates nonuniform joint space narrowing with widening and flattening of the first metatarsal head.
- An oblique radiograph may demonstrate a well-preserved joint space, which is obscured on the AP radiograph by overlying osteophytes.

Table 1 Coughlin/Shurnas Classification of Hallux Rigidus

Grade	Characteristics	Radiograph
0	Loss of 10%–20% dorsiflexion compared to the normal side. Normal or minimal radiographic findings.	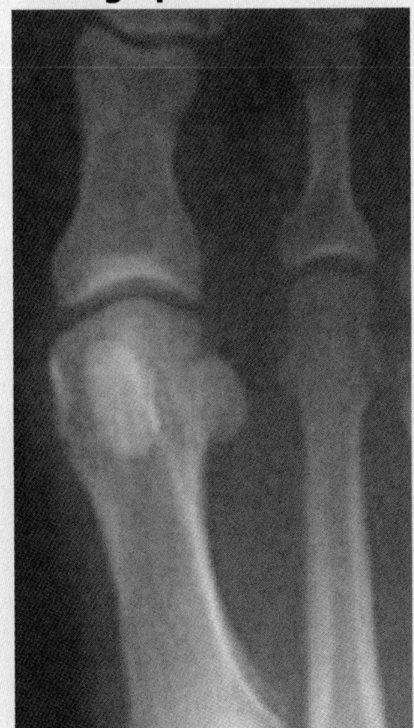

(continued)

Table 1 Coughlin/Shurnas Classification of Hallux Rigidus *(continued)*

Grade	Characteristics	Radiograph
1	Loss of 20%–50% dorsiflexion. Dorsal spur present with minimal joint space narrowing.	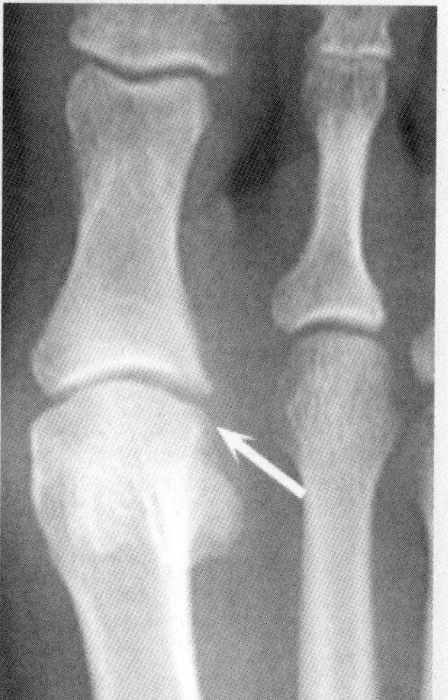 Arrow points to early osteophyte formation
2	Loss of 50%–75% dorsiflexion. Dorsal and lateral osteophytes present with less than 25% loss of joint space.	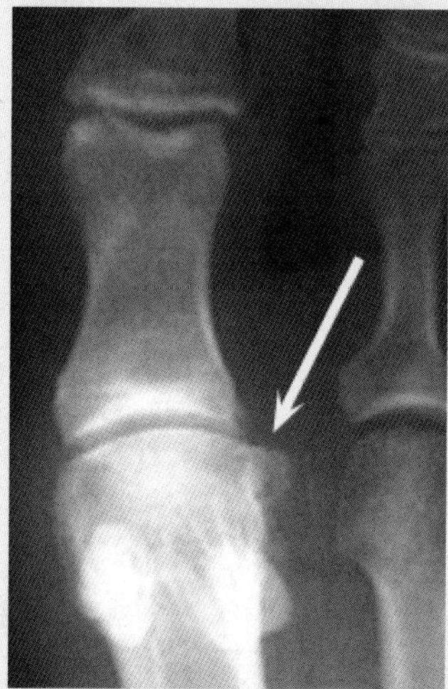 Arrow indicates dorsolateral osteophyte
3	Loss of 75%–100% dorsiflexion. Large dorsal and lateral osteophytes with substantial joint space narrowing.	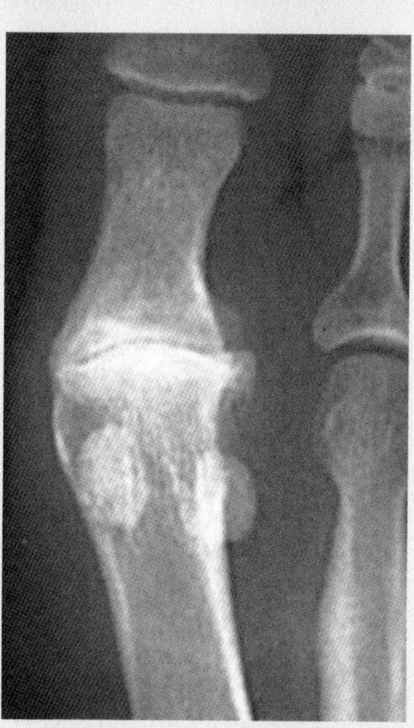

Table 1 Coughlin/Shurnas Classification of Hallux Rigidus *(continued)*

Grade	Characteristics	Radiograph
4	As in grade 3, but with advanced degenerative joint disease	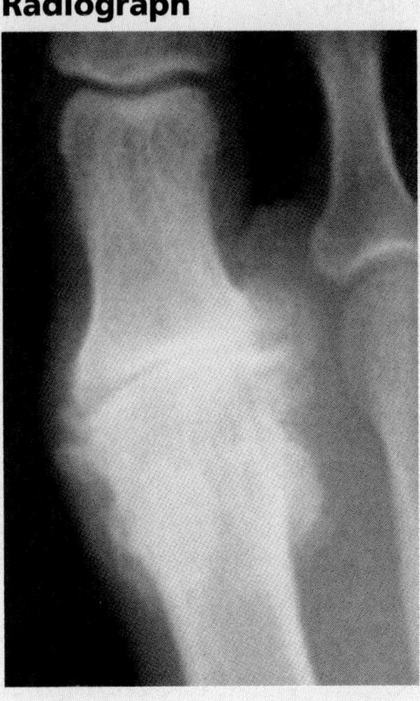

- On the lateral radiograph, with more severe disease, the dorsal metatarsal osteophyte resembles "dripping candle wax" as it courses proximally along the first metatarsal (**FIG 4**).
- The lateral radiograph also may be used to evaluate for the presence of an elevated first metatarsal in relation to the lesser metatarsals. Up to 5 mm of elevation is considered normal (see Fig 3).
- Dorsal proximal phalangeal osteophytes and loose bodies also may be seen.
- Subchondral cysts and sclerosis in the first metatarsal head, widening of the base of the proximal phalanx, and hypertrophy of the sesamoids are characteristic findings in more advanced stages of hallux rigidus.
- Rarely, an MRI scan may be necessary to identify an occult chondral or osteochondral injury in a younger patient with a history of an acute injury.

DIFFERENTIAL DIAGNOSIS

- MTP joint synovitis
- Osteochondral injury or loose body
- Gouty arthropathy
- Hallux rigidus
- Rheumatoid arthritis
- Turf toe or capsular ligamentous injury

NONOPERATIVE MANAGEMENT

- Conservative management of symptomatic hallux rigidus depends on a patient's symptoms and the magnitude of the articular degenerative process (see Table 1).
- NSAIDs and a graphite insole or Morton's extension to reduce MTP motion are the mainstays of conservative treatment (**FIG 5**).
- Several commercially prefabricated orthoses provide rigidity to the forepart of the shoe and can be moved from shoe to shoe.
- The addition of an extended steel or fiberglass shank placed between the inner and outer sole may be effective in reducing MTP joint motion as well.
- Custom-made orthoses may be fabricated to reduce midfoot pronation, which also may help to reduce symptoms.
- Unfortunately, orthoses also diminish available room in the toe box of the shoe, which may, in turn, increase pressure on the dorsal exostosis.
- Occasionally, judicious use of an intra-articular corticosteroid injection may provide temporary relief of pain.

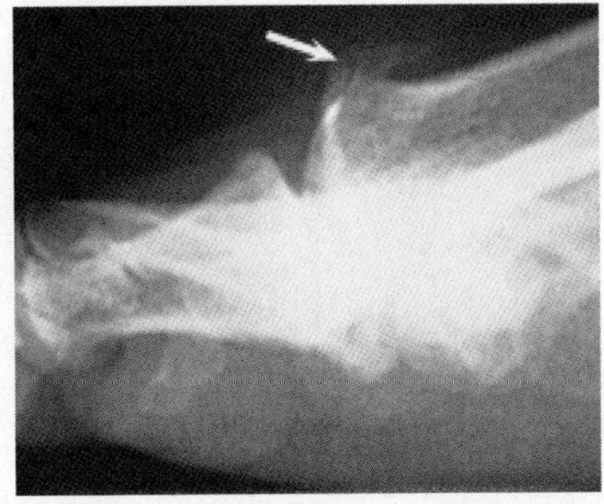

FIG 4 • Lateral radiograph of a patient with hallux rigidus. The arrow points to a large dorsal metatarsal osteophyte.

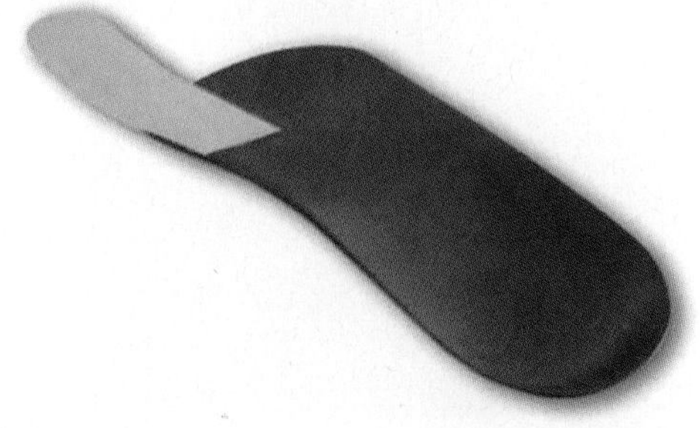

FIG 5 • Morton's extension used to restrict first MTP joint motion.

Table 2 Indications and Contraindications for Surgery

Indications	Contraindications
Grade 4 hallux rigidus	Active infection
Grade 3 hallux rigidus with less than 50% metatarsal articular cartilage remaining at the time of surgery	Significant interphalangeal (IP) joint degenerative arthritis
Deformity associated with severe hallux valgus, recurrent hallux valgus, traumatic arthritis, and rheumatoid arthritis	Grade 1, 2, and 3 hallux rigidus (with > 50% metatarsal articular cartilage remaining at the time of surgery) in younger athletic patients, in which case a cheilectomy is preferable[8,12,13]
Neuromuscular disorder with instability	Severe osteoporosis, which can make it difficult to stabilize a fusion site with routine methods of internal fixation
Failed implant surgery of the first MTP joint	

Repeated injections, however, may accelerate the degenerative process and are discouraged.

- Synovitis and limited MTP joint motion without radiographic changes should be evaluated by ruling out an inflammatory or erosive joint process with the following laboratory tests: serum CBC, ESR, CRP, ANA, RF, HLA-B27, and uric acid tests.

SURGICAL MANAGEMENT

- Indications and contraindications for surgery are presented in Table 2.

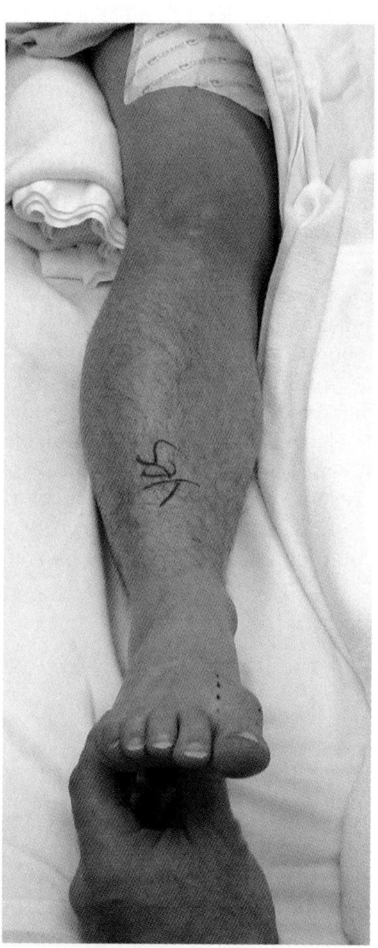

FIG 6 • Patient is positioned supine with a bump under the ipsilateral hip allowing the foot to rest in a neutral position.

Preoperative Planning

- All imaging studies must be carefully evalutated.
- An arthrodesis provides stability to the first MTP joint, maintains length of the first ray, relieves pain, achieves permanent correction of any deformity of the hallux, and allows the use of ordinary shoes.
- For grade 4 hallux rigidus, salvage procedures in addition to MTP joint arthrodesis include excisional arthroplasty,[6,13] soft tissue interpositional arthroplasty,[7,13] and prosthetic replacement.[13]
- The Keller procedure may be considered in more sedentary patients or the household ambulator with a grade 3 or 4 hallux rigidus. However, Coughlin and Mann[6] reported significant postoperative metatarsalgia after excisional arthroplasty.

Positioning

- The patient is placed supine on the operating table with a bump beneath the ipsilateral buttock to align the foot in a neutral position (**FIG 6**).
- A popliteal, sciatic, or ankle block is used for anesthesia.
- An Esmarch bandage is used to exsanguinate the foot and ankle. It is applied as an ankle tourniquet and wrapped just above the malleoli with a thin layer of padding beneath the bandage (**FIG 7**).

Approach

- Numerous surgical techniques have been proposed describing various approaches, techniques of joint preparation, and methods of internal fixation to improve both the alignment and the success rate of arthrodesis.

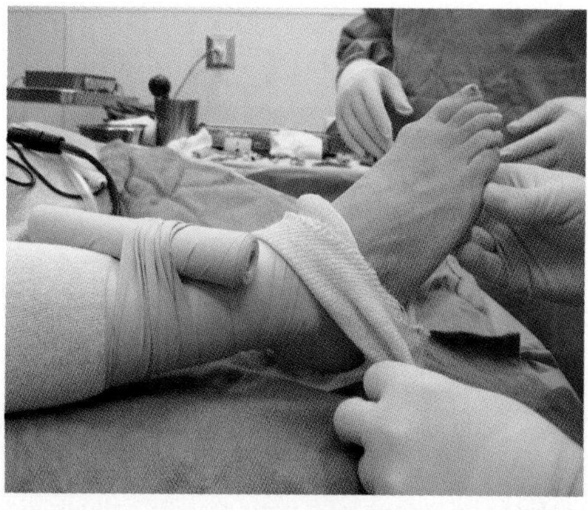

FIG 7 • An Esmarch bandage is used as a tourniquet.

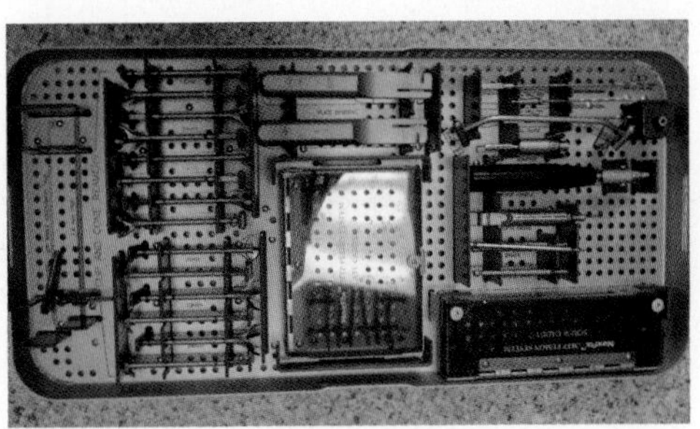

FIG 8 • The first MTP joint arthrodesis set.

- While the use of flat surfaces for MTP joint arthrodesis has been popular because of the simplicity of creating horizontal osteotomies of the proximal phalanx and metatarsal articular surfaces, this technique requires utter precision to obtain the desired alignment.
- The joint is prepared with a power reaming system coupled with internal fixation with a dorsal plate, providing a strong construct that actually "brings the bones to the plate," usually ensuring correct alignment (**FIG 8**).
- The convex male reamer excavates the proximal phalanx to a concave congrous surface, while the concave female portion of the reamer shapes the metatarsal surface to a matching uniform, curved hemisphere (**FIG 9**).
- The cup-shaped surfaces tend to resect less bone, reducing shortening of the first ray.

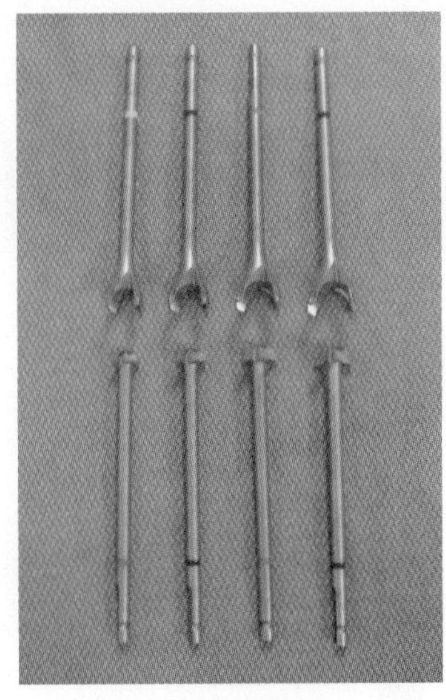

FIG 9 • Four sizes of matched metatarsal and phalangeal reamers.

- The curved nature of the cup-shaped surfaces allows preparation without predetermination of the dorsiflexion or plantarflexion, rotation, and varus and valgus alignment.
- After the joint preparation is completed, the surgeon can then select the appopriate alignment for the MTP joint arthrodesis.

JOINT EXPOSURE

TECHNIQUES

- A dorsal longitudinal incision is centered directly over the MTP joint in an interval between the medial and lateral common digital nerves.
- The incision is extended from a point just proximal to the interphangeal joint of the hallux to a point 3 to 4 cm proximal to the MTP joint.
- The dissection is deepened along the medial aspect of the extensor hallucis longus tendon through the extensor hood and the joint capsule (TECH FIG 1A).
- A thorough synovectomy is performed, and the MTP joint is inspected to locate osteophytes or loose bodies and to assess the extent of the articular cartilage damage (TECH FIG 1B).

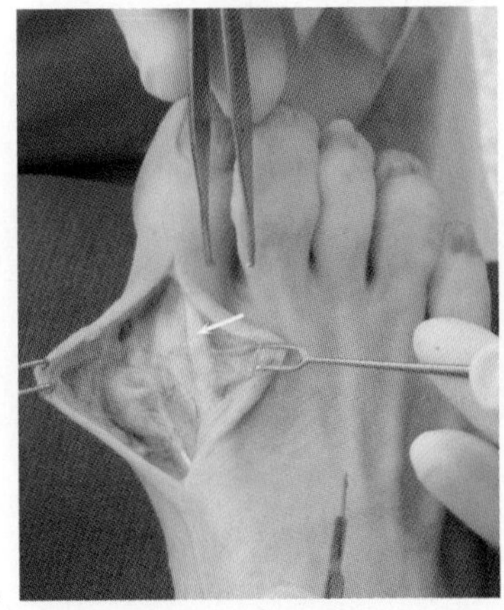

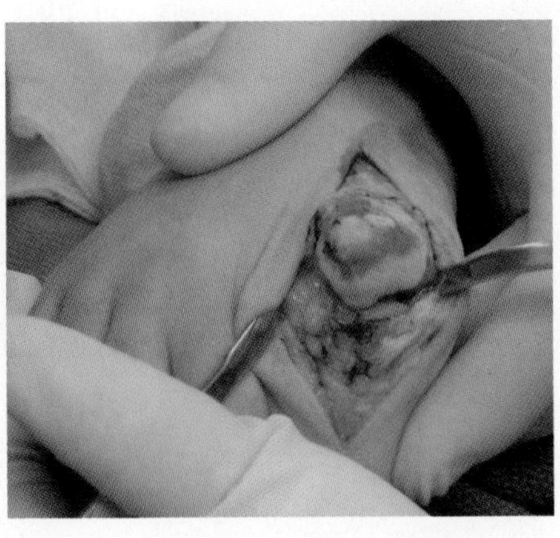

TECH FIG 1 • **A.** Dissection is carried out medial to the extensor hallucis longus (EHL) tendon (*arrow*). **B.** The EHL tendon has been retracted medially and a capsulotomy performed.

JOINT RESECTION AND DECOMPRESSION

- A thin section of the articular surfaces of the distal first metatarsal and proximal phalanx is removed using a sagittal saw (TECH FIG 2A,B).
- If further shortening of the first ray is desired, more bone may be resected from the metatarsal head.
- By decompressing the MTP joint, increased exposure is achieved for the MTP joint surface preparation.
- A sagittal saw is also used to resect the medial eminence if the fusion is performed for a hallux valgus deformity (TECH FIG 2C).

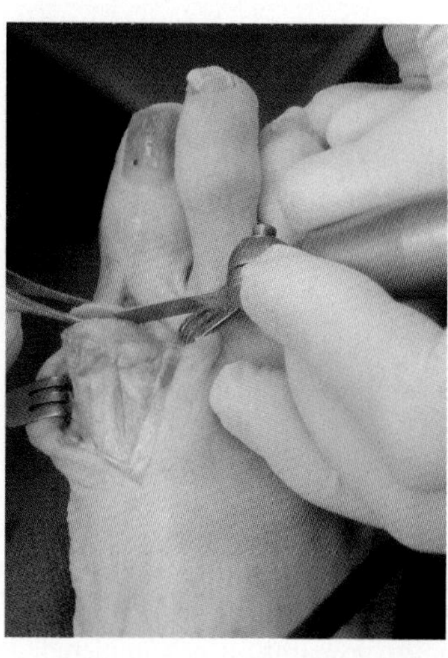

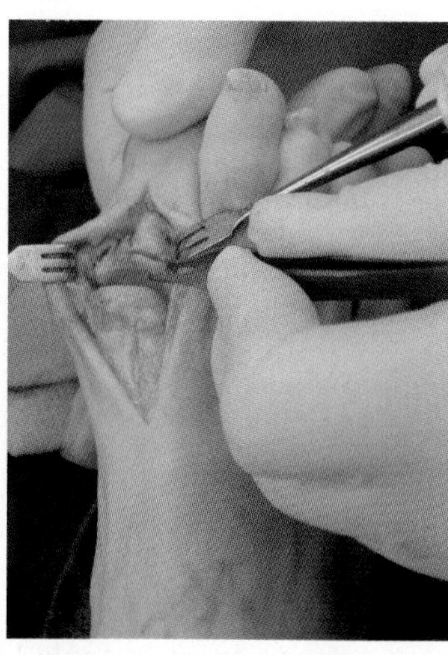

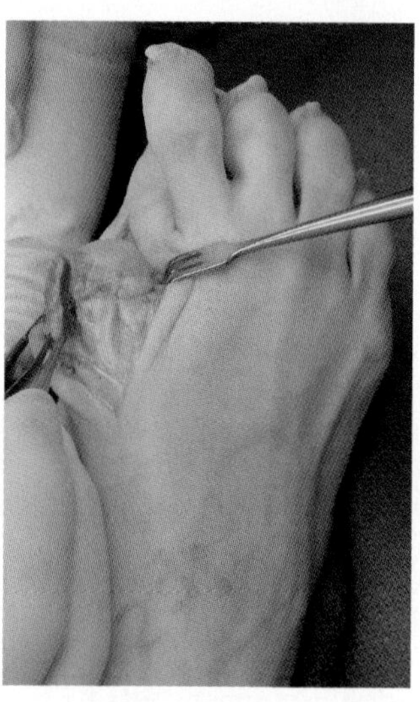

TECH FIG 2 • **A.** A wafer of the distal first metatarsal is removed. **B.** A thin section of the base of the proximal phalanx is resected. **C.** The medial eminence is resected in a patient with a hallux valgus deformity.

METATARSAL HEAD PREPARATION

- A 0.062-Kirschner wire (K-wire) is driven in a proximal direction at the center of the metatarsal head (TECH FIG 3A).
- The appropriate size of the reamer is chosen by comparing the diaphyseal width of the metatarsal to the inner size of the metatarsal reamer.
- The power reamer engages the K-wire and is then driven in a proximal direction, shaving the metatarsal subchondral surface and metaphysis to a cup-shaped convex surface (TECH FIG 3B).
- Any debris or excess bone along the periphery is removed with a rongeur.
- The K-wire is then removed and used to perforate the prepared metatarsal head in multiple places to increase the surface area for arthrodesis (TECH FIG 3C).

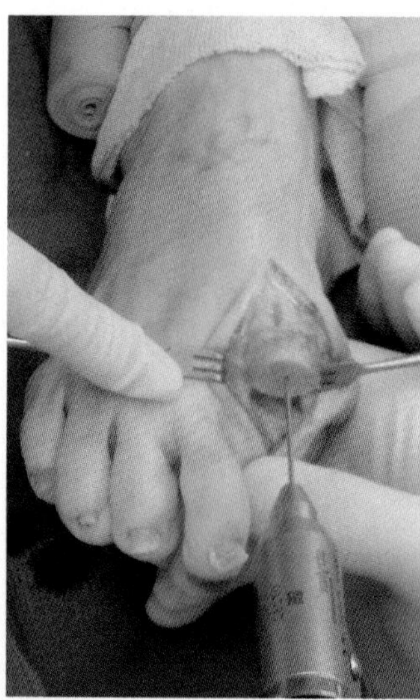

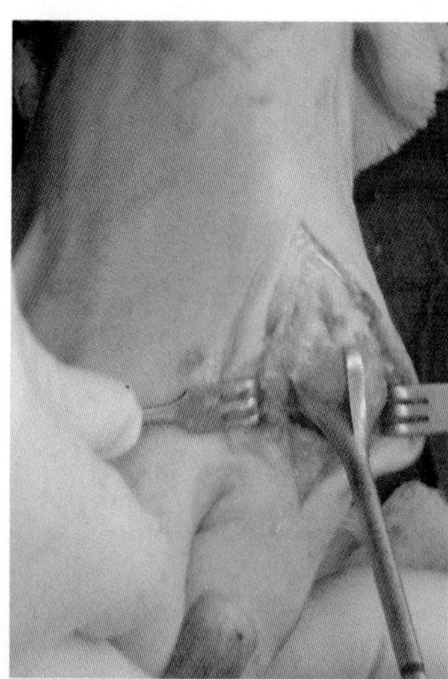

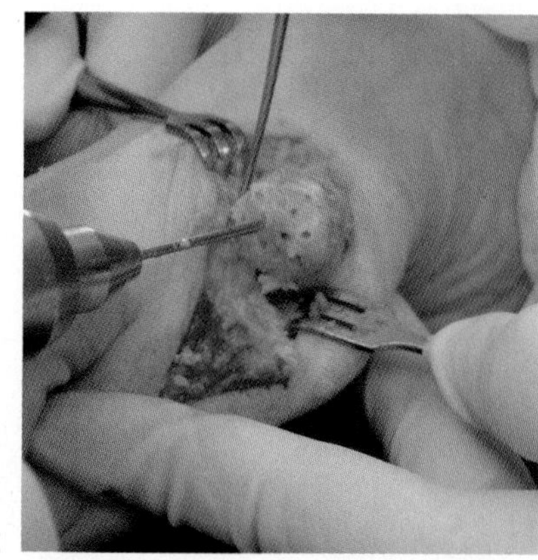

TECH FIG 3 • **A.** A K-wire is placed in the center of the metatarsal head. **B.** Power reamers prepare the metatarsal joint surface. **C.** Multiple perforations in the prepared metatarsal head.

PROXIMAL PHALANGEAL PREPARATION

- A 0.062-inch K-wire is centered on the base of the proximal phalanx and driven distally (TECH FIG 4A).
- The smallest of the convex cannulated phalangeal reamers is then chosen to prepare the phalangeal surface.
- Each successively larger reamer is used to enlarge the phalangeal surface until it matches the size of the prepared metatarsal surface (TECH FIG 4B).
- The K-wire is then removed and used to perforate the prepared phalangeal surface in multiple places to increase the surface area for arthrodesis (TECH FIG 4C).
- Cancellous bone shavings are collected throughout the joint preparation process and saved in a small cup to form a slurry for use as an autograft as the surfaces are coapted.

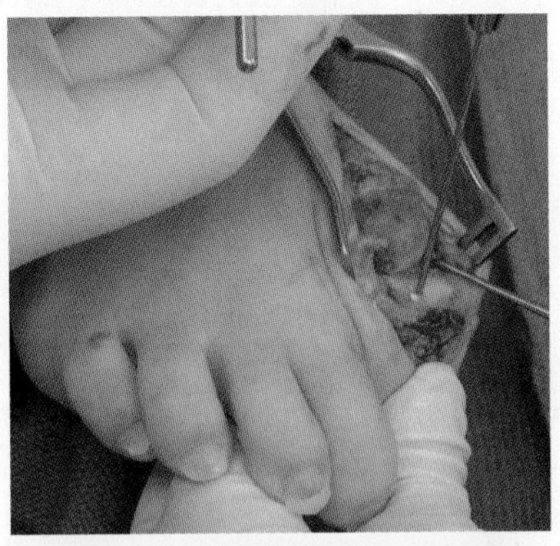

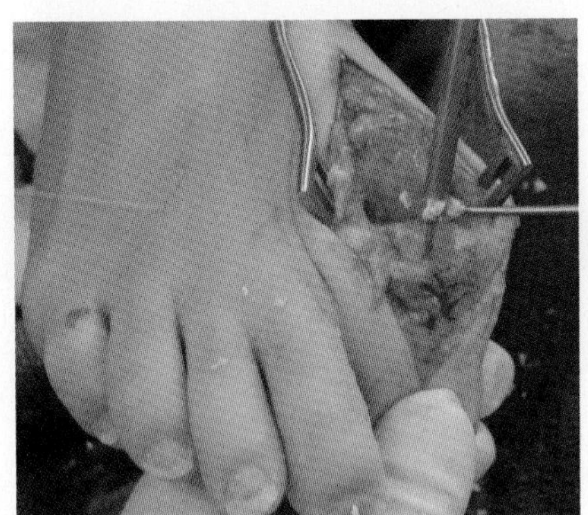

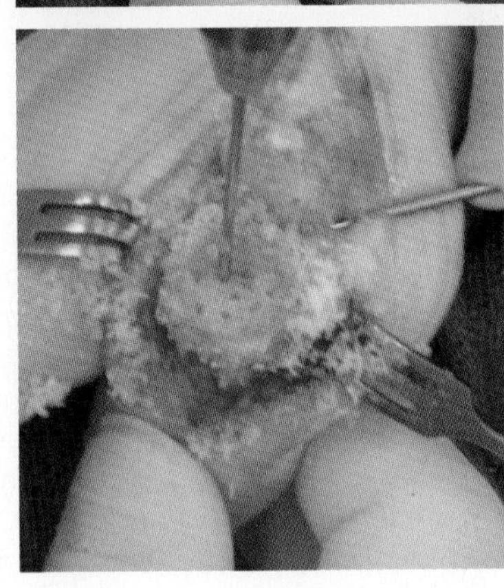

TECH FIG 4 • **A.** A K-wire is placed in the center of the base of the proximal phalanx. **B.** Power reamers prepare the proximal phalangeal joint surface. **C.** Multiple perforations in the prepared base of the proximal phalanx.

JOINT ALIGNMENT

- The bone slurry saved from the reamings is placed between the joint surfaces (TECH FIG 5).
- The congruous cancellous joint surfaces are coapted in the desired amount of varus and valgus, dorsiflexion and plantarflexion, and rotation.
- The desired position is 20 to 25 degrees of dorsiflexion, 10 to 15 degrees of valgus, and neutral rotation. For women who prefer high-heeled shoes, increased dorsiflexion at the fusion site may be desirable.
- All angular measurements relate to the axis of the first metatarsal shaft.
- An advantage of using the cup-shaped surface preparation technique is that any dimension may be adjusted without disturbing the other alignment variables.

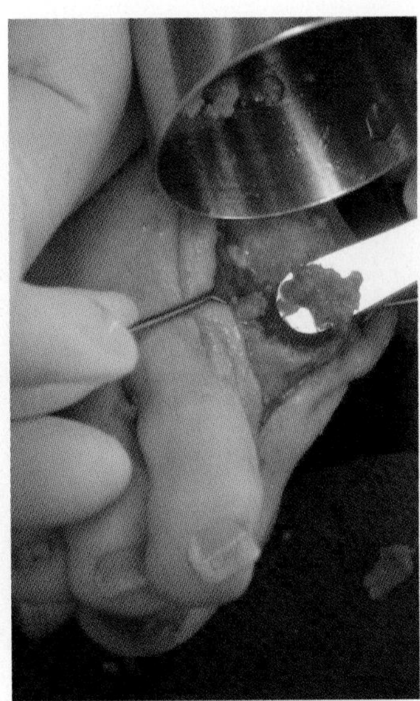

TECH FIG 5 • Cancellous autograft bone reamings are placed between the prepared joint surfaces before fixation.

INTERNAL FIXATION

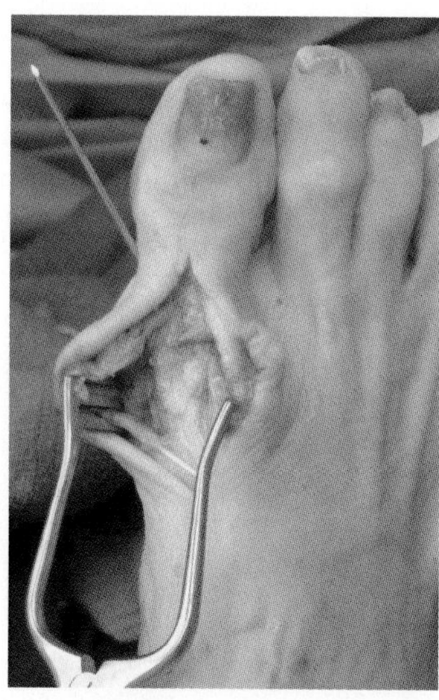

TECH FIG 6 • Temporary fixation with a 0.062-inch K-wire.

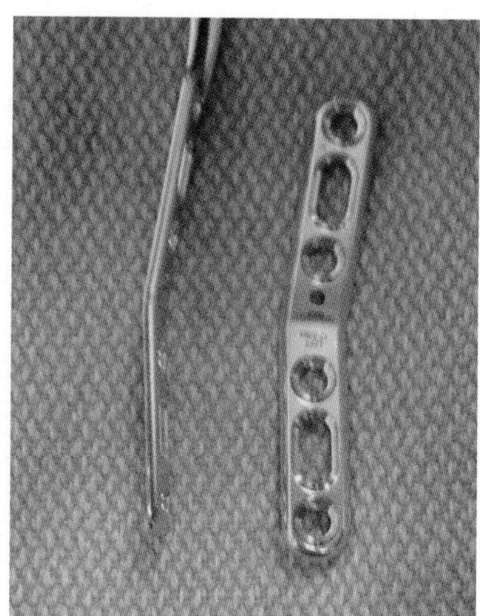

TECH FIG 7 • Precontoured primary arthrodesis plates.

- After obtaining proper alignment, the arthrodesis site is temporarily stabilized with one or two crossed 0.062-inch K-wires (TECH FIG 6).
- A rongeur is used to smooth the dorsal aspect of the first metatarsal and proximal phalanx to allow the plate to sit flush against the bone.
- The primary arthrodesis plate comes pre-bent to the desired dorsiflexion and valgus angles and is placed over the dorsal aspect of the prepared metatarsal and proximal phalanx (TECH FIG 7).
- If more or less dorsiflexion is desired, the plate may be bent further to the desired dorsiflexion.
- If more or less valgus is desired, the plate may be offset slightly to accommodate MTP joint angulation.
- Bicortical self-tapping screws are used first to fix the plate to the metatarsal. Locking screws may be used in the presence of osteopenic bone.
- The plate is then affixed to the proximal phalanx, with the first screw placed in compression.
- The K-wire is then removed, and a cross-compression screw is placed to augment the fixation construct (TECH FIG 8A).
- The general philosophy is that in most cases, the plate can be trusted for appropriate alignment of the arthrodesis.
- Using the flat surface of an instrument cover is helpful to ensure the hallux is in appropriate and acceptable dorsiflexion alignment.
- The capsule and skin are then closed in a routine manner (TECH FIG 8B).

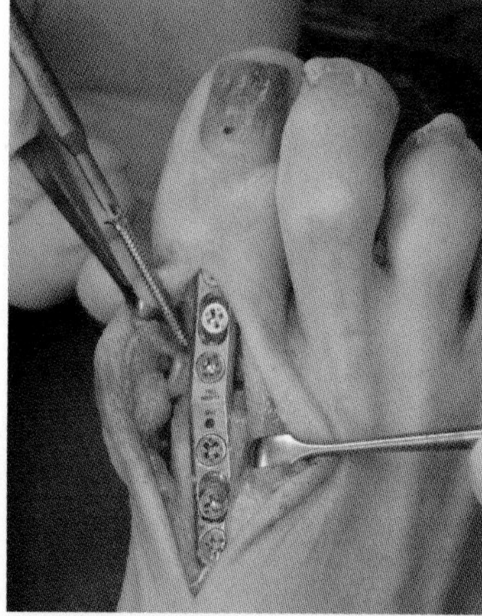

A

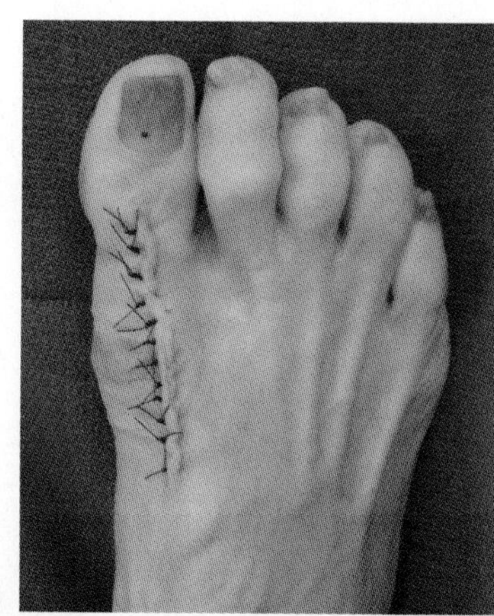

B

TECH FIG 8 • **A.** Dorsal plate in place. The compression screw will augment the fixation construct. **B.** Final wound closure with interrupted mattress sutures.

PEARLS AND PITFALLS

Joint preparation	■ Results vary depending on the selected method of joint preparation. ■ An enlarged surface area is created by using the cup-shaped reamers. ■ Coupled with this, multiple perforations of the prepared surfaces and the use of a bony slurry aid in increasing the rate of successful joint fusion.
Alignment	■ If the MTP joint is fixed in a straight position (minimal valgus or slight varus), the medial border of the hallux may impact the toe box of the shoe. ■ Dorsiflexion of less than 10 degrees may cause a complaint of pressure at the tip of the toe. ■ Malrotation in either pronation or supination is poorly tolerated (**FIG 10**). ■ The use of precontoured plates helps to minimize this type of complication.
Internal fixation	■ A variety of methods can be used to stabilize the arthrodesis, including K-wires, single or cross screws, staples, wire sutures, and plates. ■ We have demonstrated a high rate of successful fusion with dorsal plates and a cross-compression screw.
Radiographic parameters	■ Although preoperative radiographs may demonstrate an abnormally widened 1–2 intermetatarsal angle, a first metatarsal osteotomy is rarely if ever indicated in combination with a first MTP joint arthrodesis. ■ Typically, following decompression and arthrodesis of the first MTP joint, the 1–2 intermetatarsal angle will reduce substantially.

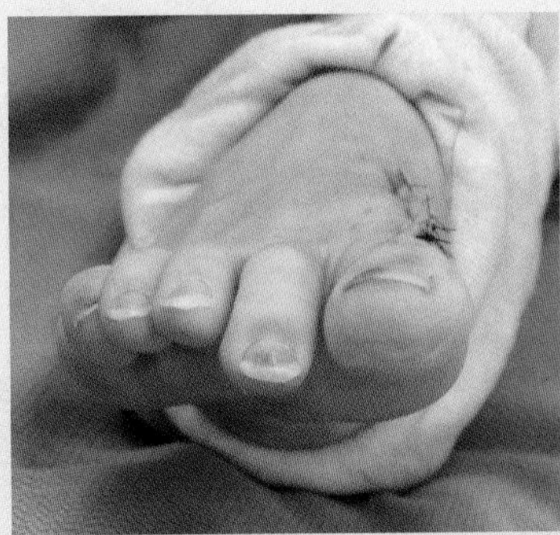

FIG 10 • Neutral rotation of the final arthrodesis. Note that the toenail is parallel to the plantar surface of the foot.

POSTOPERATIVE CARE

- The foot is wrapped in a gauze-and-tape compression dressing following the surgery, and the dressing is changed weekly.
- The patient is allowed to ambulate in a wooden-soled postoperative shoe or short walking boot.
- Weight initially is borne on the heel and lateral aspect of the foot.
- If the patient is considered unreliable, a below-knee cast is applied.
- Dressings or casts are discontinued at 12 weeks after surgery with radiographic evidence of a successful MTP joint arthrodesis (**FIG 11**).

OUTCOMES

- In seven published series on the use of conical joint preparation and dorsal plate fixation for MTP joint arthrodesis, we have achieved a 95% fusion rate (268/281 first MTP joint arthrodeses).[2,3,4,5,8,10,11]
- The preoperative diagnoses of this multiseries cohort included patients with hallux rigidus (28%); hallux valgus, as a primary, recurrent, or postoperative complication (41%); and rheumatoid arthritis (31%).
- Of the 13 nonunions in this multiseries analysis, only five were symptomatic.
- While the concept of cup-shaped preparation of joint surfaces has changed little over the last two decades except for refinement of power reamer design,[1,2,4,9,10,13] the techniques and design of the dorsal plate fixation have changed dramatically.
- Our initial use of a stainless steel mini-fragment plate witnessed a 34% hardware removal rate (12/35) after fusion, and occasional hardware failure.[2]

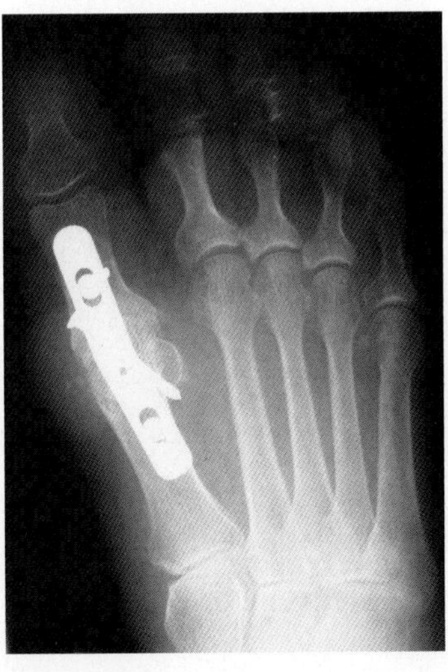

FIG 11 • AP radiograph of a healed first MTP joint fusion.

- More recently, the use of a precontoured low-profile titanium plate has demonstrated a significant reduction in the incidence of hardware removal, to 4% (2/53 cases).[10]
- Subjective good and excellent results were noted in 92% of cases (260/281 feet).
- Overall, 48 patients were noted to have slight progression of interphalangeal joint arthritis, but only six were symptomatic.

COMPLICATIONS

- Nonunion
- Malunion
- Hardware failure
- Interphalageal joint arthritis

REFERENCES

1. Coughlin MJ. Arthrodesis of the first metatarsophalangeal joint. Orthopaedic Review 1990;19:177–186.
2. Coughlin MJ. Arthrodesis of the first metatarsophalangeal joint with mini-fragment plate fixation. Orthopaedics 1990;13:1037–1048.
3. Coughlin MJ. Rheumatoid forefoot reconstruction. A long-term follow-up study. J Bone Joint Surg Am 2000;82A:322–341.
4. Coughlin MJ, Abdo RV. Arthrodesis of the first metatarsophalangeal joint with Vitallium plate fixation. Foot Ankle 1994;15:18–28.
5. Coughlin M, Grebing B, Jones C. Arthrodesis of the metatarsophalangeal joint for idiopathic hallux valgus: intermediate results. Foot Ankle Int 2005;26:783–792.
6. Coughlin MJ, Mann RA. Arthrodesis of the first metatarsophalangeal joint as salvage for the failed Keller procedure. J Bone Joint Surg Am 1987;69A:68–75.
7. Coughlin MJ, Shurnas P. Soft-tissue arthroplasty for hallux rigidus. Foot Ankle Int 2003;24:661–672.
8. Coughlin M, Shurnas P. Hallux rigidus. Grading and long-term results of operative treatment. J Bone Joint Surg Am 2003;85A:2072–2088.
9. Coughlin M, Shurnas P. Hallux rigidus. Surgical techniques (cheilectomy and arthrodesis). J Bone Joint Surg Am 2004;86A (Suppl 2): 119–130.
10. Goucher N, Coughlin M. Hallux metatarsophalangeal joint arthrodesis using dome-shaped reamers and dorsal plate fixation: a prospective study. Foot Ankle Int 2006;27:869–876.
11. Grimes JS, Coughlin M. First metatarsophalangeal joint arthrodesis as a treatment for failed hallux valgus surgery. Foot Ankle Int 2006;27:887–893.
12. Mann RA, Coughlin MJ, DuVries H. Hallux rigidus: A review of the literature and a method of treatment. Clin Orthop Relat Res 1979;142:57–64.
13. Shurnas P, Coughlin M. Arthritic conditions of the foot. In: Coughlin M, Mann R, Saltzman C, eds. Surgery of the Foot and Ankle, ed 8. Philadelphia: Elsevier, 2007:805–922.

Chapter 25 First Metatarsophalangeal Joint Arthrodesis: Perspective 3

John T. Campbell and Kevin L. Kirk

DEFINITION

- Disorders of the first ray are a common cause of foot and ankle problems. Arthrodesis of the hallux metatarsophalangeal (MTP) joint is a utilitarian technique in contemporary foot and ankle surgery.
- Arthrodesis can effectively address a variety of conditions affecting the hallux, including deformity, inflammatory and degenerative arthritides, spasticity and neuromuscular disorders, and salvage of failed surgeries.
- The most important aspect of this procedure is optimal positioning of the toe during first MTP joint arthrodesis.

ANATOMY

- The bony anatomy of the first MTP joint includes the rounded first metatarsal head, which articulates with the concave, elliptically shaped base of the proximal phalanx.
- Two longitudinal grooves separated by the crista, a central prominence, are located on the plantar surface of the metatarsal head. The two sesamoid bones contained in the medial and lateral tendon slips of the flexor hallucis brevis articulate with their corresponding longitudinal grooves on the inferior surface of the first metatarsal head. The flexor hallucis longus tendon runs between the two sesamoids, bypassing the MTP joint to insert distally onto the distal phalangeal base.
- The extensor hallucis brevis tendon inserts into the dorsal MTP capsule and the extensor hallucis longus runs distally to insert onto the distal phalanx.
- The strong, fan-shaped collateral ligaments of the MTP joint originate medially and laterally from the metatarsal head and run distally and plantarward to the base of the proximal phalanx. The metatarsosesamoid ligaments fan out in a plantar direction to the margin of the sesamoid and the plantar pad.
- Distally, the two sesamoids are attached by the fibrous plantar plate to the base of the proximal phalanx, stabilizing the joint plantarly (**FIG 1**).

PATHOGENESIS

- Common forms of degenerative arthritis that affect the hallux MTP joint include hallux rigidus and posttraumatic arthritis. Hallux rigidus may be the result of isolated trauma, with forced hyperextension and resultant chondral injury, or the result of repetitive microtrauma of the articular cartilage. Pathologic alteration in the kinematics of the first MTP joint also may lead to degenerative changes.
- Chondral erosion or loss is seen dorsally on the metatarsal head and phalangeal base.
- Inflammatory arthropathies can affect the hallux MTP joint, necessitating fusion. Common causes include rheumatoid

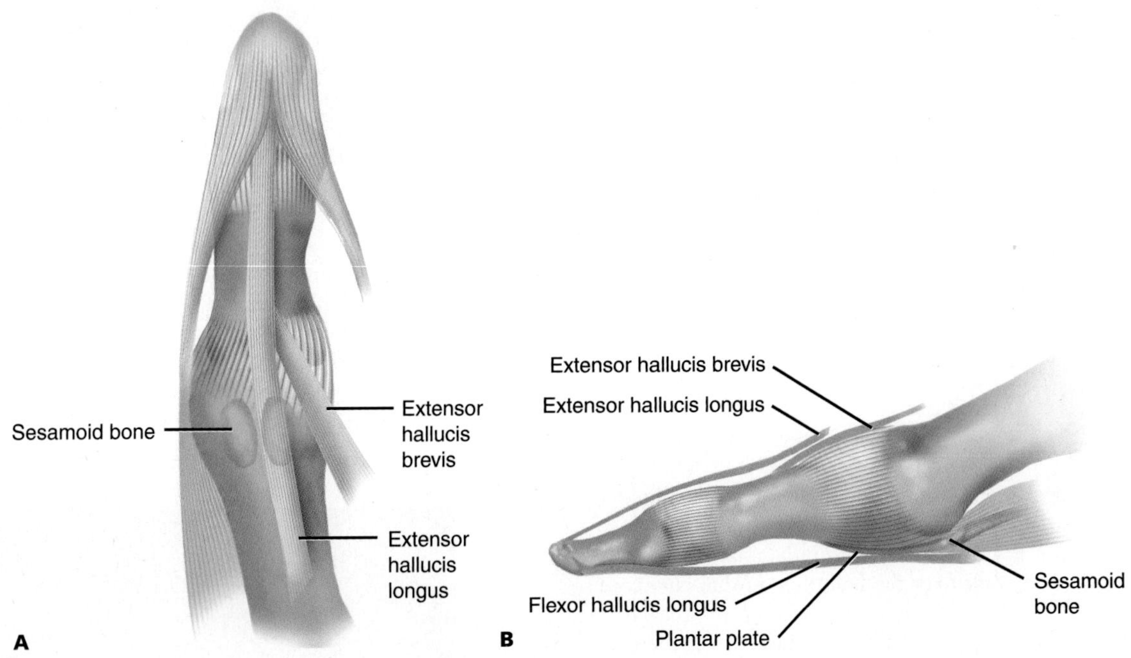

FIG 1 • **A.** Anterior and **(B)** lateral views of the first metatarsophalangeal joint.

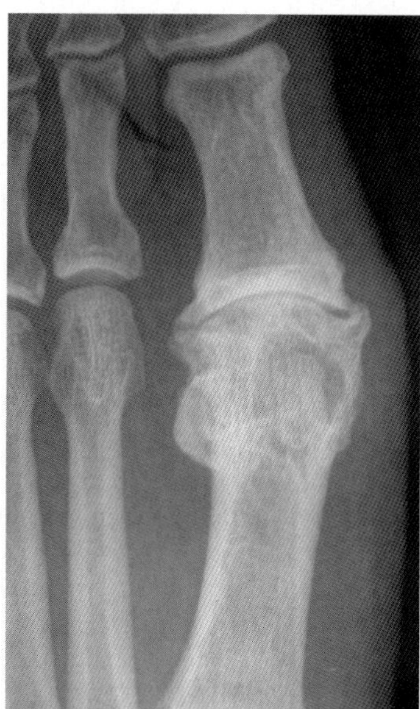

FIG 2 • AP weight-bearing radiograph of the first metatarsophalangeal joint. Note the joint narrowing, extensive osteophytes, and the medial subchondral cyst.

arthritis, gouty arthropathy, lupus, and seronegative spondyloarthropathies. Repetitive episodes of synovitis lead to chondral loss and joint narrowing.

- Progressive hallux valgus or hallux varus with severe deformity, spasticity (secondary to neurologic conditions), soft tissue contracture, or arthritis, or that occurring in elderly patients, also may benefit from MTP arthrodesis.

NATURAL HISTORY

- Hallux rigidus and degenerative arthritis present with progressive pain, stiffness, and osteophyte formation of the MTP joint.
- Initial symptoms of inflammatory arthritides include pain and swelling from MTP synovitis; progressive disease is marked by worsening stiffness, pain, and deformity.
- Hallux valgus or hallux varus deformities typically are flexible in the early stage, but over time these deformities tend to become progressively more rigid secondary to joint contracture.
- All of these conditions can produce pain, difficulty with ambulation, and transfer metatarsalgia to the lesser toes.

PATIENT HISTORY AND PHYSICAL FINDINGS

- Patient history
  - Pain and mechanical symptoms on ambulation in hallux rigidus and degenerative arthritis
  - Pain at rest or in the morning with inflammatory arthritis
  - Pain with shoe wear over the hallux or medial eminence (bunion)
  - Some patients complain of the prominence over the first MTP joint.
- Physical findings
  - Careful interview of the patient to identify contributing medical conditions, shoe wear history, previous treatment methods, and previous surgical procedures
  - Standing examination of the foot to assess for malalignment of the toe, including varus, valgus, or claw deformity
  - Gait examination to identify dynamic deformity of the foot, including forefoot supination or generalized pes planovalgus
  - Visible shortening of the hallux, failure of the toe to engage the ground, and lesser toe metatarsalgia or keratosis (callus) indicate mechanical unloading of the first ray.
  - Examination of the seated patient allows observation for callus, skin irritation, or presence of dorsal or medial bunion.
  - Palpation elicits tenderness about the joint. Hallux rigidus typically is tender dorsally, whereas the pain with hallux valgus is located medially over the bunion. Generalized degenerative or inflammatory arthritides exhibit diffuse tenderness about the MTP joint, and axial grinding of the phalanx against the metatarsal elicits pain.
  - Manipulation of the joint is performed to assess stability of the collateral ligaments and the relative flexibility or rigidity of varus or valgus toe deformity.
  - Range-of-motion examination often shows limited passive MTP dorsiflexion, with normal or reduced plantarflexion.
  - Skin irritation may be present over the dorsal exostosis or medial bunion.
  - Tingling, hypesthesias, or a positive Tinel (percussion) sign over the dorsal hallucal nerve may indicate nerve compression from synovitis or dorsal osteophytes.

IMAGING AND OTHER DIAGNOSTIC STUDIES

- Standing AP, lateral, and oblique radiographs are the standard views for evaluation. Additional views, such as an oblique or sesamoid view, sometimes are indicated.
  - The weight-bearing AP view is obtained to determine the overall alignment of the MTP joint. It also can be assessed for the extent of arthritic involvement, including joint narrowing, flattening of the metatarsal head, and the presence of subchondral sclerosis, erosions or cystic changes within the metatarsal head, osteopenia, or bone loss (**FIG 2**). This view can also facilitate evaluation of shortening of the first ray relative to the lesser metatarsals. The oblique view also can illuminate these findings.
  - The lateral weight-bearing view can show dorsal metatarsal or phalangeal osteophytes and can be used to evaluate the degree of joint narrowing (particularly plantarly) and the presence of an elevated first metatarsal (**FIG 3**). However, the plantar two thirds of the joint can be obscured by overlapping shadows of the lesser metatarsals.
  - An axial sesamoid view can be an adjunctive radiograph for evaluating the metatarsal–sesamoidal articulation for

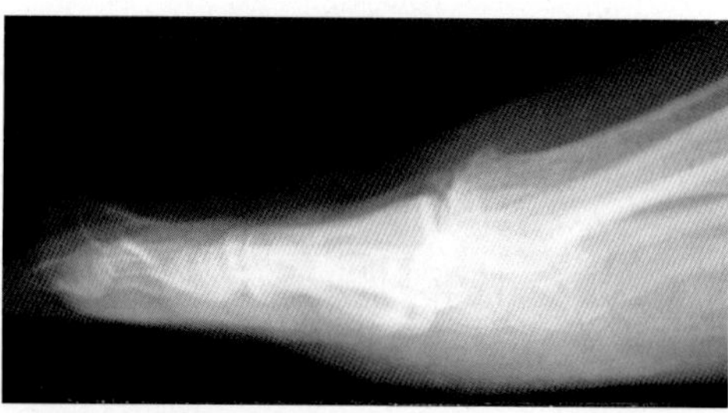

FIG 3 • Lateral weight-bearing view of the first metatarsophalangeal joint. A large dorsal osteophyte and plantar joint space narrowing are noted.

narrowing or cystic changes, although involvement of the metatarsosesamoid joint occurs infrequently, except with severe arthrosis.

- Additional imaging studies, such as CT or MRI, rarely are necessary. However, such scans may be useful for defining the degree of cyst involvement or avascular necrosis of the metatarsal head, which indicates the need for intraoperative bone grafting.

DIFFERENTIAL DIAGNOSIS

- Arthrodesis is appropriate for surgical correction of the following conditions:
  - Osteoarthritis or posttraumatic arthritis
  - Hallux rigidus
  - Severe hallux valgus, particularly in elderly patients
  - Hallux varus caused by inflammatory disorders, iatrogenic deformity after previous surgery, or idiopathic involvement
  - Inflammatory arthropathies, including rheumatoid arthritis, lupus, gout, and seronegative spondyloarthropathies
  - Soft tissue contracture, as in scleroderma
  - Deformity secondary to neurologic conditions or spasticity, such as that occurring in patients with diabetes or those who have experienced a stroke

NONOPERATIVE MANAGEMENT

- Nonoperative measures to be attempted before MTP arthrodesis include:
  - Nonsteroidal anti-inflammatory drugs to decrease joint pain and inflammation
  - Judicious use of corticosteroid injections into the hallux MTP joint to relieve synovitis, although repeated injections are not advised
  - The use of silicone gel, cotton wool, or felt pads to relieve pressure from calluses or impingement against the shoe or adjacent toe
  - Strapping or taping of the hallux may be useful for flexible deformities.
  - Comfortable shoe wear with low heels and wide toe box; extra-depth shoes may allow use of an orthotic device. Shoe modifications, such as a stiff sole or metatarsal bar, may unload the forefoot during push-off.
  - A full-length orthotic insole with a carbon fiber or stainless steel extension may limit the motion of a painful MTP joint in hallux rigidus.
  - Custom accommodative orthotic insole with a build-up under the hallux may improve weight bearing of a shortened or dorsiflexed first ray to diminish transfer metatarsalgia.

SURGICAL MANAGEMENT

- In situ hallux MTP arthrodesis is a utilitarian technique with a wide range of indications.[1–8,13,15–19,22]
- Absolute contraindications include active infection of the MTP joint, severe peripheral vascular disease, and poor soft tissue envelope secondary to systemic disease or scar tissue. In such patients, a joint-sparing procedure would be more appropriate.
- A relative contraindication to MTP arthrodesis is symptomatic interphalangeal joint arthritis; however, concurrent arthrodesis of both joints has been described.[20]

Preoperative Planning

- Radiographs are assessed for extensive bony lysis, erosions, or cysts that may require bone grafting.
- Severe bone loss, shortening, or failed implant arthroplasty may require distraction MTP arthrodesis with bulk bone graft, discussed elsewhere.
- Standard arthrodesis can be performed under general, spinal, or regional anesthesia, such as a popliteal or ankle block.
  - We prefer to administer an ankle block in conjunction with sedation, using a 1:1 mixture of 2% lidocaine and 0.5% ropivacaine, via a 26-gauge needle.

Positioning

- The patient is positioned supine with a roll under the ipsilateral hip.
- The procedure can be performed without a tourniquet or with a pneumatic calf or thigh tourniquet. Alternatively, an Esmarch tourniquet can be applied at the supramalleolar ankle over cotton padding, which is our preferred technique.

Approach

- Our preferred approach is a dorsal incision centered over the MTP joint.
- An alternate approach is the medial midline incision, based on the surgeon's preference or whether a previous surgical scar exists.

TECHNIQUES

IN SITU ARTHRODESIS OF THE HALLUX MTP JOINT WITH CROSSED-SCREW FIXATION

Incision and Exposure

- Make a dorsal incision over the MTP joint just medial to the extensor hallucis longus tendon.[1,4–8,10,17,18]
- Carry the dissection down to the joint capsule, avoiding the dorsomedial cutaneous nerve, a terminal branch of the superficial peroneal nerve.[3]
- Retract the extensor hallucis longus tendon laterally and perform an arthrotomy directly over the MTP joint.
- Perform subperiosteal dissection to raise medial and lateral flaps off the metatarsal head and base of the proximal phalanx, exposing the joint (**TECH FIG 1**).[3,5–7,16–18]
- Release the collateral ligaments and the plantar portion of the joint by releasing the plantar plate with a Freer elevator.
- Remove large osteophytes and loose ossicles with a rongeur.
- Resect the medial eminence from a dorsal approach with a microsagittal saw or chisel.[4,7,17,18]

Joint Preparation

- Prepare the joint surfaces for arthrodesis with a power burr or specialized reamers.

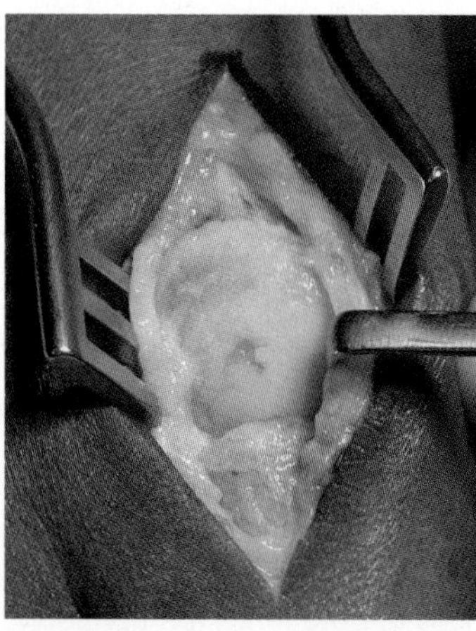

TECH FIG 1 • Exposure of metatarsal head through dorsal approach. The extensor hallucis longus tendon is retracted laterally with the exposed metatarsal head, showing a large dorsal osteophyte and loss of articular cartilage.

- Biomechanically, spherical surfaces provide for improved stability compared with flat cuts.[9] Hemispherical surfaces also provide more freedom for positioning the arthrodesis compared with flat saw cuts.
- Using a power burr, prepare the joint surfaces in a ball-and-cup fashion by removing the chondral surfaces.
- Shape the subchondral surface hemispherically, with the metatarsal head convex and the phalangeal base concave (TECH FIG 2).[22]
- Carefully avoid excessive bony resection, particularly in osteopenic or rheumatoid patients, to prevent additional shortening of the toe.

- An alternative method of joint preparation is to use specialized reamers that produce similar hemispheric surfaces (TECH FIG 3).
  - Using concentric reamers, plantarflex the proximal phalanx and insert a Kirschner wire axially in the center of the metatarsal head.
  - Use a cannulated, concave-shaped reamer to prepare the metatarsal head.
  - Remove the wire and then insert it in the proximal phalanx, and use a cannulated convex reamer.[1,3–6]
- A final method of joint preparation is with flat cuts using a saw blade.

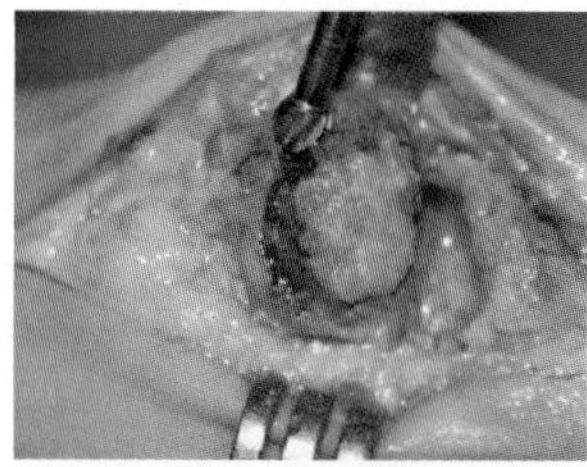

TECH FIG 2 • Joint preparation with power burr. The metatarsal head is shaped hemispherically in a convex manner to fuse with the concave base of the proximal phalanx.

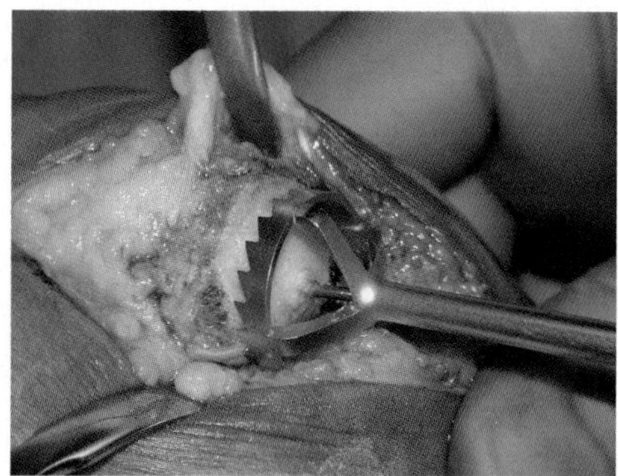

TECH FIG 3 • Alternative technique for joint preparation with specialized reamers. The Kirschner wire is placed in the center of the head to ensure concentric joint preparation.

  - Resect the ends of the metatarsal head and base of the phalanx, incorporating the chondral surfaces, with the cuts angled appropriately to produce the proper angles for subsequent positioning.[3–5,7]
- Create multiple drill holes in the metatarsal head and phalangeal base with a Kirschner wire or small drill bit to augment bleeding and bony ingrowth.

Arthrodesis Positioning and Fixation

- After preparing the joint surfaces, position the arthrodesis in 10 to 15 degrees of valgus, 15 degrees of dorsiflexion relative to the sole of the foot, and neutral pronation–supination.
- Because it can be difficult to determine the plane of the sole with the patient on the table, a more predictable method of positioning the toe is to determine dorsiflexion relative to the first metatarsal axis. In most cases, the appropriate angle is about 25 to 30 degrees of dorsiflexion.[1,3,6,7,11,12,14,16–19]
- The hallux is held provisionally with Kirschner wires or partially threaded guidewires from a cannulated screw set.
  - Confirm the positioning radiographically with a minifluoroscopy unit and clinically with use of a flat surface to simulate weight bearing (the cover of the screw set tray works nicely).
  - The hallux should be slightly off the surface with the heel on the cover (TECH FIG 4).
  - Placing a screwdriver handle under the heel simulates a shoe with a small heel; in this case, the pulp

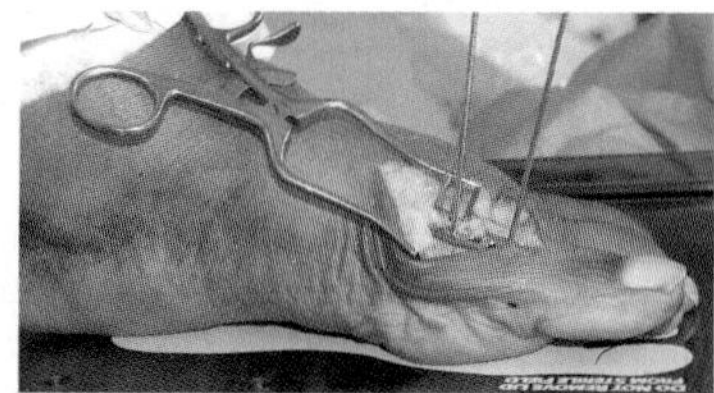

TECH FIG 4 • Positioning of the first metatarsophalangeal joint. A flat surface is used to position the toe properly. Note the positioning of the toe to allow for adequate clearance during gait.

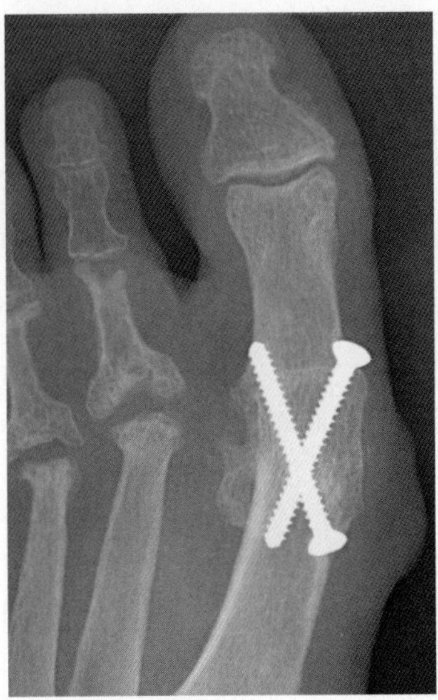

TECH FIG 5 • Postoperative radiograph shows the crossed-screw technique.

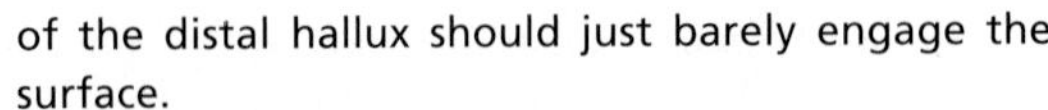

of the distal hallux should just barely engage the surface.

- Cannulated or solid screws can be used per the surgeon's preference. We use 4.0-mm cannulated screws in most patients; however, in some situations, such as for very large individuals, 4.5-mm screws can be used. Solid 3.5-mm cortical screws are an alternative (**TECH FIG 5**).
- Insert one guidewire from the medial aspect of the phalangeal base just distal to the metaphyseal flare and advance it across the arthrodesis site through the dorsolateral cortex of the metatarsal neck.
- Place the second wire from the medial aspect of the metatarsal neck, just proximal to the flare of the medial eminence; advance this wire distally and slightly plantarly across the arthrodesis site to engage the plantar–lateral cortex of the phalanx.
- Check wire position and length with fluoroscopy.
- Measure the wires percutaneously with the cannulated depth gauge and overdrill them with the cannulated drill bit. Then, countersink the cortex carefully to prevent subsequent cracking with screw placement.[3]

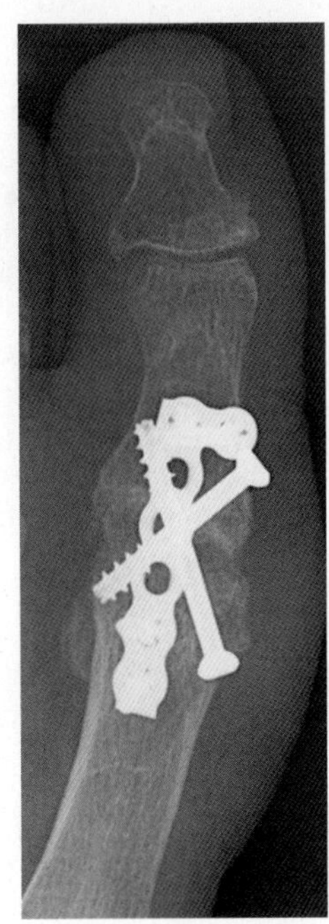

TECH FIG 6 • Alternative technique of fixation secondary to poor bone quality. Dorsal plating is used to augment the fixation.

- Place the partially threaded cannulated screws over the guidewires while compressing the hallux manually.
  - Alternatively, insert solid lag screws under fluoroscopic guidance.
- In the event of suboptimal fixation or in patients with osteopenic bone (eg, secondary to rheumatoid arthritis or chronic oral corticosteroid usage), a dorsal plate can be used for augmented fixation.
  - This plate can be a precontoured, commercially available hallux MTP fusion plate or a standard minifragment plate that is cut and contoured to fit, and then affixed to the dorsal surface of the metatarsal and phalanx with small-diameter screws (eg, 2.7 mm) (**TECH FIG 6**).
- Close the incision in layers with absorbable suture for the arthrotomy and subcutaneous layers and nonabsorbable monofilament for the skin.

ALTERNATIVE TECHNIQUE

- A medial incision over the hallux MTP joint can be used in the presence of a previous surgical scar or at the surgeon's preference.
- Carry out dissection at the level of the joint capsule, taking care to avoid the dorsomedial branch of the superficial peroneal nerve with elevation of the flap.
- Perform a midline arthrotomy to expose the metatarsal head and base of the proximal phalanx.[21]
- Prepare the joint surfaces with a saw blade.[21]
- To allow for correct positioning, make the cut on the metatarsal head perpendicular to the sole of the foot, and avoid resecting excessive bone when making the cut on the proximal phalanx. Then, position the hallux, with attention to all three planes as described above.
- Perform fixation with the crossed-lag-screw technique as described above, with supplemental dorsal plate fixation as needed.

PEARLS AND PITFALLS

Arthrodesis preparation	▪ To prevent shortening, avoid excessive bone resection.
Hallux positioning	▪ Intraoperatively, the position of the hallux is assessed fluoroscopically and clinically with a flat surface to simulate weight bearing. Proper positioning includes valgus of 10 to 15 degrees, dorsiflexion of 25 to 30 degrees relative to the metatarsal shaft (or 15 degrees relative to the sole of the foot), and neutral rotation. Clinically, the hallux should not impinge on the second toe and the nail plate should be aligned with the same plane as the lesser toes.
Guide pin breakage	▪ Maintain correct positioning of the hallux during insertion of the guide pin. Avoid bending and shearing of the wire during cannulated drilling.
Fixation problems	▪ When arthrodesis is performed on osteopenic bone, requiring additional fixation with a dorsal plate,[5] additional Kirschner wires or threaded pins[1,3] may be necessary to supplement standard crossed screws. Before the patient leaves the operating room, intraoperative fluoroscopy must be used in a biplanar fashion to identify fixation problems.

POSTOPERATIVE CARE

- In patients with an isolated arthrodesis that has good bone quality and solid fixation, weight bearing as tolerated on the heel and lateral border of the foot is allowed in a postoperative hard-soled shoe or fracture boot, restricting weight bearing on the forefoot.
- If there are concerns about bone quality, suboptimal fixation, or potential noncompliance by the patient, strict non–weight-bearing in a below-the-knee cast is maintained for 6 to 8 weeks.
- After 6 to 8 weeks, partial weight bearing is advanced, based on evidence of clinical and radiographic healing.
- Full weight bearing usually is achieved by 10 to 12 weeks, at which time the patient transitions from the postoperative shoe or boot into sneakers or comfortable, low-heeled walking shoes.
- At 14 to 16 weeks, with additional reduction in swelling, most patients can transition into unrestricted shoe wear; however, some individuals have permanent difficulty wearing fashion shoes or high heels.
- Prolonged walking and athletic activities usually resumes at 4 to 5 months.
- Custom-made orthotics with a build-up under the hallux to improve weight bearing of the first ray may dissipate forefoot stresses.

OUTCOMES

- The clinical results after hallux MTP arthrodesis usually are excellent, with high rates of bony union, patient satisfaction, and pain relief.
  - Union rates for in situ arthrodesis range from 77% to 100%.[4–8,11,13,16–18]
  - Patient satisfaction rates also are high, regardless of the indications.[5–8,10,11,13,16–18]
- MTP arthrodesis causes a rigid lever arm, resulting in an earlier toe-off in the gait cycle and decreasing the stress on the lesser metatarsals.[6,8,14,16–18] This stiffness may result in increased stress across the hallux interphalangeal joint.[14]
- After arthrodesis, the first ray shows improved weight-bearing capacity, with the foot compensating for the relative stiffness during stance phase.[10]

COMPLICATIONS

- Nonunion rates range from 5% to 10%.[5,10,13,17,18] Nonunion may not be symptomatic and may not require revision surgery.[13]
- Malunion after MTP arthrodesis can result in mild malalignment that is tolerated, but more severe malposition may be symptomatic.
  - Excessive dorsiflexion leads to unloading of the hallux and lesser toe transfer metatarsalgia.[1]
  - Positioning the hallux in relative plantarflexion may lead to interphalangeal joint irritation, callus formation, and later interphalangeal arthritis.[1,22]
  - Valgus positioning can lead to painful impingement on the second toe,[11] whereas varus positioning causes impingement of the hallux against the toe box of the shoe.
- Subsequent arthritis of the interphalangeal joint may occur in one third of cases.
  - Arthritis in the interphalangeal joint is more common than that of the first tarsometatarsal or other midfoot joints.
  - However, symptoms may be mild despite radiographic involvement and may take 10 years to develop.[11,16]
  - Severe symptoms may require secondary interphalangeal arthrodesis, which leads to extreme stiffness of the hallux.
- Iatrogenic nerve injuries of the dorsomedial cutaneous nerve are more common than injuries to the plantar nerves.
  - These may result in neuroma formation, mild numbness, or persistent dysethesias that compromise an otherwise successful arthrodesis.
  - Prevention by proper incision placement and meticulous surgical dissection remains the best strategy.

REFERENCES

1. Alexander IJ. Arthrodesis of the metatarsophalangeal and interphalangeal joints of the hallux. In Myerson M, ed. Current Therapy in Foot and Ankle Surgery. St. Louis: Mosby-Year Book, 1993:81–90.
2. Castro MD, Klaue K. Technique tip: revisiting an alternative method of fixation for first MTP joint arthrodesis. Foot Ankle Int 2001;22: 687–688.
3. Conti SF, Dhawan S. Arthrodesis of the first metatarsophalangeal and interphalangeal joints of the foot. Foot Ankle Clin 1996;1:33–53.
4. Coughlin MJ. Arthrodesis of the first metatarsophalangeal joint. Orthop Rev 1990;19:177–186.
5. Coughlin MJ. Arthrodesis of the first metatarsophalangeal joint with mini-fragment plate fixation. Orthopedics 1990;13:1037–1044.
6. Coughlin MJ. Rheumatoid forefoot reconstruction: a long-term follow-up study. J Bone Joint Surg Am 2000;82:322–341.
7. Coughlin MJ, Abdo RV. Arthrodesis of the first metatarsophalangeal joint with Vitallium plate fixation. Foot Ankle Int 1994;15: 18–28.
8. Coughlin MJ, Mann RA. Arthrodesis of the first metatarsophalangeal joint as salvage for the failed Keller procedure. J Bone Joint Surg Am 1987;69:68–75.

9. Curtis MJ, Myerson M, Jinnah RH, et al. Arthrodesis of the first metatarsophalangeal joint: a biomechanical study of internal fixation techniques. Foot Ankle 1993;14:395–399.
10. DeFrino PF, Brodsky JW, Pollo FE, et al. First metatarsophalangeal arthrodesis: a clinical, pedobarographic and gait analysis study. Foot Ankle Int 2002;23:496–502.
11. Fitzgerald JAW. A review of long-term results of arthrodesis of the first metatarso-phalangeal joint. J Bone Joint Surg Br 1969;51:488–493.
12. Harper MC. Positioning of the hallux for first metatarsophalangeal joint arthrodesis. Foot Ankle Int 1997;18:827.
13. Kitaoka HB, Patzer GL. Arthrodesis versus resection arthroplasty for failed hallux valgus operations. Clin Orthop Relat Res 1998;347: 208–214.
14. Mann RA. Surgical implications of biomechanics of the foot and ankle. Clin Orthop Relat Res 1980;146:111–118.
15. Mann RA, Katcherian DA. Relationship of metatarsophalangeal joint fusion on the intermetatarsal angle. Foot Ankle 1989;10:8–11.
16. Mann RA, Oates JC. Arthrodesis of the first metatarsophalangeal joint. Foot Ankle 1980;1:159–166.
17. Mann RA, Schakel ME II. Surgical correction of rheumatoid forefoot deformities. Foot Ankle Int 1995;16:1–6.
18. Mann RA, Thompson FM. Arthrodesis of the first metatarsophalangeal joint for hallux valgus in rheumatoid arthritis. J Bone Joint Surg Am 1984;66:687–692.
19. McKeever DC. Arthrodesis of the first metatarsophalangeal joint for hallux valgus, hallux rigidus, and metatarsus primus varus. J Bone Joint Surg Am 1952;34:129–134.
20. Mizel MS, Alvarez RG, Fink BR, et al. Ipsilateral arthrodesis of the metatarsophalangeal and interphalangeal joints of the hallux. Foot Ankle Int 2006;27:804–807.
21. Rydholm A, Rooser B. Surgical margins for soft-tissue sarcoma. J Bone Joint Surg Am 1987;69:1074–1078.
22. Trnka HJ. Arthrodesis procedures for salvage of the hallux metatarsophalangeal joint. Foot Ankle Clin 2000;5:673–686.

Chapter 26 Revision First Metatarsophalangeal Joint Arthrodesis

Michael M. Stephens and Ronan McKeown

DEFINITION

- Revision first metatarsophalangeal joint (MTPJ) arthrodesis is performed for pain or deformity following failed hallux valgus surgery, excisional arthroplasty, of prosthetic arthroplasty, and for nonunion or malunion following primary first MTPJ arthrodesis, when a trial of conservative treatment has been unsuccessful.
- As is the case for a primary arthrodesis, many techniques for preparation of the joint exist, all designed to provide good cancellous apposition. If possible, in revision surgery, it is better not to shorten and reduce the remaining bone stock.
  - Ball-and-socket preparation with reamers should be considered for failed hallux valgus surgery and nonunion of the first MTPJ as a way to achieve cancellous congruency with a large contact surface area. However this may not be possible: e.g., in the case of malunions, flat cuts should be performed.
  - In cases of failed Silastic (Dow Corning, Midland, MI) arthroplasty, the defect should be curettaged until normal bone is reached. This creates a defect that will require a ball-shaped interposition cancellous graft.
  - After a previous excisional arthroplasty with a large resection of the proximal phalanx, a tricortical interposition graft can be used to try to regain length.
- Many techniques exist for achieving fixation of the MTPJ. The use of a low-profile precontoured titanium plate and, when possible, a compression screw achieves a very stable construct, without the need to traverse the interphalangeal (IP) joint with threaded pins,[1–3] which can produce postoperative stiffness in that joint. Such a plate must have the facility to give strong stable fixation to the remaining short proximal phalanx and allow fixation of an interposition graft.

ANATOMY

- In revision surgery, normal anatomy may be severely disrupted. The first metatarsal length may be lost, the metatarsal head may be avascular, and the proximal phalanx may be short or have poor bone stock.
- The aim in revision arthrodesis is to create a painless and solid medial column, of a length that is appropriate to the foot, that provides a stable medial arch and a plantigrade foot that prevents load transfer to the lesser rays.
- Complex foot deformities may have additional problems with the alignment of the lesser toes. These should be corrected first, before the final hallux valgus arthrodesis angle is set.
- As in primary arthrodesis, the final position of the arthrodesed first MTPJ must allow for heel rise during the late stance phase of gait. Therefore, the tip of the toe should be clear of the weight-bearing surface with the IP joint in full extension. The tip of the hallux also should be able to touch the ground in midstance, simulated at surgery with the ankle at 90 degrees and a flat surface applied to the sole of the foot. In this position, the tip of the toe should be able to touch the flat surface with the IP joint in 45 to 60 degrees of flexion. In addition, a gap of 3 to 5 mm should be left between the first and second toes.

PATHOGENESIS

- Failed hallux valgus surgery may result in recurrent deformity, avascular necrosis of the metatarsal head, or pain and stiffness secondary to accelerated degeneration of the first MTPJ.
- Failed resection arthroplasty may result in recurrent valgus deformity, a cock-up deformity, or a flail toe[4] (**FIGS 1 AND 2**).
- Failed Silastic arthroplasty may result in an aggressive foreign body reaction with bone loss on one or both sides of the joint, depending on whether a single- or double-stemmed implant was used.
- Failed primary arthrodesis can lead to a painful deformity and hardware impingement. A fusion that is too straight leads to a painful callus under the condyles of the proximal phalanx; one that is too dorsiflexed leads to a painful callus on the dorsum of the IP joint.

PATIENT HISTORY AND PHYSICAL FINDINGS

- A thorough physical examination of the foot and ankle is necessary before a first MTPJ revision arthrodesis is begun.
- Any history of cigarette smoking should be documented and the patient cautioned about nonunion.
- Peripheral circulation and sensation must be tested.
- The age and site of previous scars should be noted so the safest approach may be planned.
- The IP joint, MTP joint, and first tarsometatarsal (TMT) joint should be examined as for primary arthrodesis.

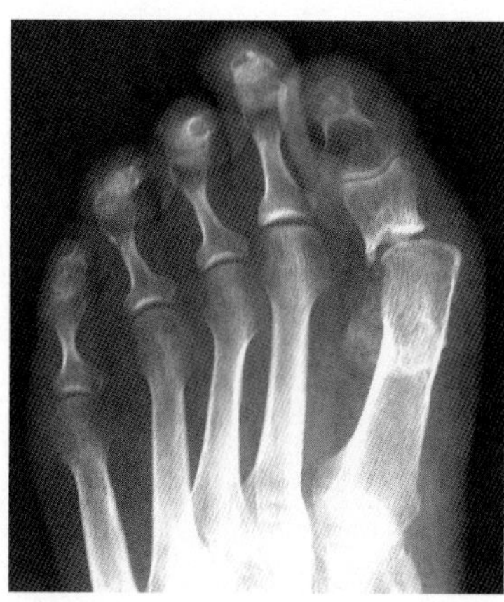

FIG 1 • A failed Keller's resection arthroplasty.

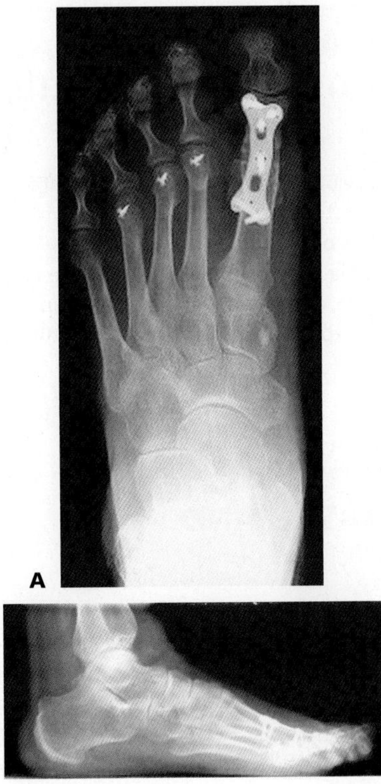

FIG 2 • **A.** AP radiograph following revision arthrodesis with tricortical iliac crest graft for failed excision arthroplasty. **B.** Lateral radiograph following revision arthrodesis with tricortical iliac.

IMAGING AND OTHER DIAGNOSTIC STUDIES

- If infection is suspected, it should be ruled out before surgery. A differential white cell count, C-reactive protein level, and erythrocyte sedimentation rate should be obtained. An isotope bone scan may be helpful, but it can be hot for nonunion or infection.
- Weight-bearing anteroposterior (AP) and lateral radiographs should be obtained for preoperative planning. Particular attention should be paid to the extent of bone loss from the proximal phalanx and metatarsal head, where an oblique radiograph may give more information. The severity of any deformity should be noted and any coexisting forefoot pathology identified and addressed at the time of surgery.
- If avascular necrosis is suspected, an MRI may be useful as long as the patient has no metallic implants.

NONOPERATIVE MANAGEMENT

- Nonoperative management encompasses activity modification, weight reduction, analgesic and anti-inflammatory medication (oral and intra-articular), physical therapy (e.g., tendo Achilles and hamstring stretching), functional foot orthoses, and customized shoes.
- Functional foot orthoses may include a stiffened insole with a Morton's extension to limit dorsiflexion of the hallux, a medial arch support, and a metatarsal dome.
- Customized shoes may include an extra-deep toe box, bunion pockets, or a stiffened sole with a metatarsal rocker.

SURGICAL MANAGEMENT

- Revision arthrodesis of the first MTPJ does not restore normal anatomy or gait pattern. The risks of nonunion, infection, neuroma formation, and vascular complications are greater than for primary arthrodesis. Time to union increases in proportion to the size of interposition graft required (i.e., a larger graft takes longer to become incorporated). The patient should be counseled toward realistic outcomes.
- Absolute contraindications to revision first MTPJ fusion include active infection and peripheral vascular disease.
- Relative contraindications to first MTPJ fusion include degeneration of the first TMT and IP joints or peripheral neuropathy.

Preoperative Planning

- Following a thorough examination to assess circulation, sensation, the first TMTJ, the IP joint, the lesser toes, and the skin (for previous surgical incisions or callus under the metatarsal heads), weight-bearing AP and lateral radiographs of the forefoot should be obtained.
- The extent of bone loss should be noted and the patient prepared and draped for harvesting iliac crest bone graft. We prefer to use the ipsilateral crest to limit postoperative disability to one side only.
- Any lesser toe deformity should be addressed before performing the arthrodesis so that the hallux may be set at the correct valgus angle to the neighboring toes and painful transfer lesions alleviated. The lesser toes may be clawed or hammered with subluxation or dislocation of the MTPJs. Provision should be made to perform proximal interphalangeal joint arthrodesis, MPTJ capsulotomy, extensor digitorum longus lengthening, plantar condylectomy, or Weil's osteotomies, as required. A Weil's osteotomy of the second metatarsal head should never be performed in isolation: an osteotomy of the third metatarsal head must accompany it to prevent transfer metatarsalgia to the third metatarsal head.
- A rheumatology consultation or preoperative anesthetic assessment should be done if necessary.

Positioning

- We prefer to position the patient supine with the heels at the end of the operating table. If bone graft is required, a sandbag is placed under the ipsilateral buttock.
- Prophylactic intravenous antibiotics are administered at induction of anesthesia. A thigh tourniquet is put in place after the limb has been exsanguinated. The iliac crest and leg are then prepared and draped in a routine manner.
- The end of the table is dropped 20 to 30 degrees, and the surgeon sits at the end of the table.

Approach

- A dorsal approach incorporating previous dorsal scars is recommended. The tissues should be handled carefully. Self-retaining retractors should be positioned under low tension for short periods of time only, particularly if the hallux is then held in forced plantarflexion. Excessive retraction with bone levers must be avoided.
- Because previous surgery may have caused intense scarring of the tissues, when possible, full-thickness flaps are raised off the metatarsus and proximal phalanx. Care should be taken to protect the dorsal cutaneous nerve and extensor hallucis longus and the terminal branch of the deep peroneal nerve in the first web space.

REVISION ARTHRODESIS OF THE FIRST METATARSOPHALANGEAL JOINT USING A DORSAL TITANIUM CONTOURED PLATE (HALLU-S PLATE; NEWDEAL, SAINT PRIEST, FRANCE)

- Ideally, a dorsal, slightly curved incision is made just medial to the extensor hallucis longus tendon and lateral to the dorsal cutaneous nerve, extending from the middle of the shaft of the first metatarsal to the interphalangeal joint.
- The extensor hallucis longus tendon is retracted laterally.
- A capsulotomy is made in the same plane, and the joint exposed.
- Any previous metalwork or implants are removed.
- A synovectomy is performed, along with excision of any avascular bone.
- The medial and lateral soft tissues are released to allow maximum plantarflexion of the proximal phalanx so as to fully expose both surfaces to be arthrodesed.

PREPARATION OF THE DISTAL FIRST METATARSAL AND PROXIMAL PHALANX

- Preparation of the surfaces and graft techniques vary according to the nature of revision.
  - Revision of nonunion of a primary arthrodesis, failed hallux valgus surgery, or failed excision arthroplasty (where there has been minimal resection of the proximal phalanx)
  - In these cases, where bone graft is not required, the arthrodesis site can be prepared with ball-and-socket reamers in a fashion similar to that for a primary arthrodesis. Osteophytes are excised, and the proximal phalanx is sized to determine the correct convex reamer. The proximal phalanx is reamed over a 1.6-mm guidewire. A size-matched concave reamer is used to prepare the metatarsal head in a similar manner (TECH FIG 1).
- Revision of malunion of primary arthrodesis
  - These cases are revised because the hallux is either too dorsiflexed or too plantarflexed. A simple closing wedge with flat cuts can be performed with the apex at the original arthrodesis site (TECH FIG 2).

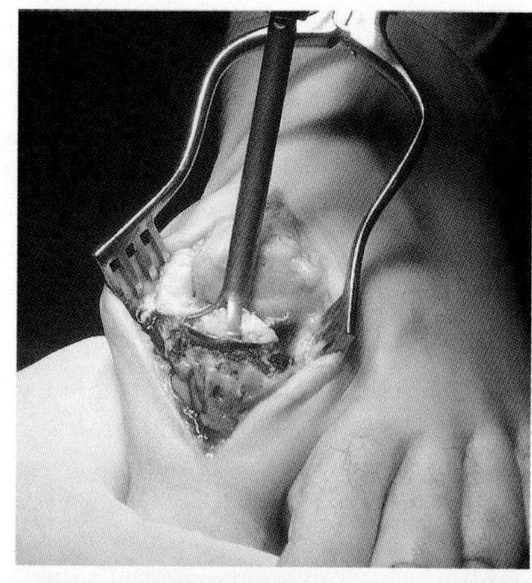

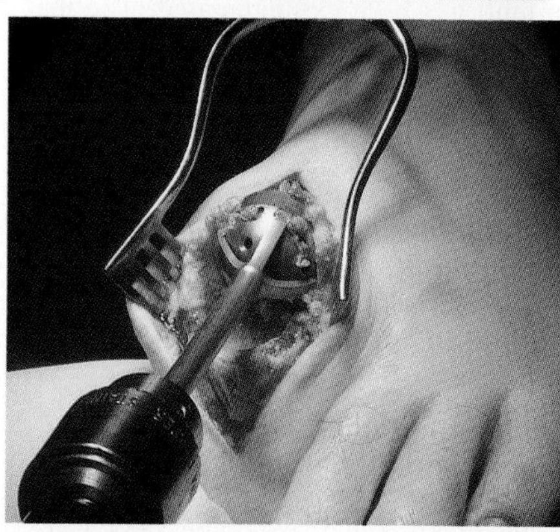

TECH FIG 1 • **A.** Reaming the articular surface of the proximal phalanx. **B.** Reaming the articular surface of the metatarsal head.

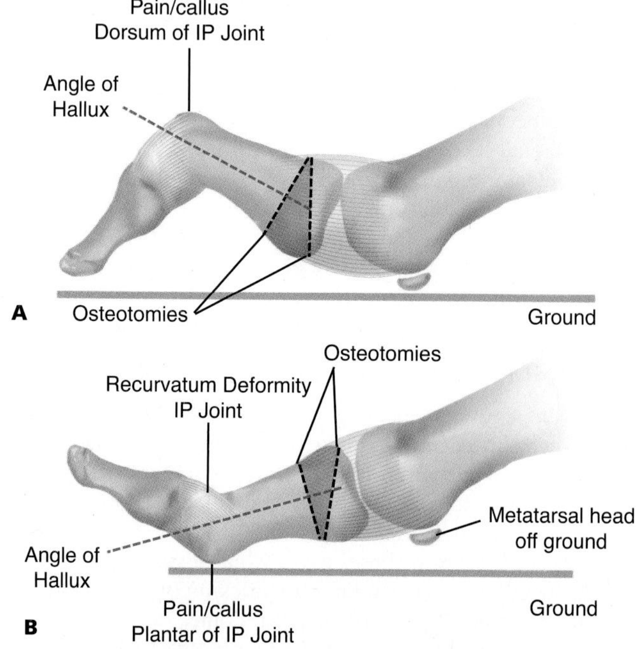

TECH FIG 2 • Revision of malunion.

COMPLEX REVISION CASES

- When the residual deficit in bone stock is such that the first ray is short and defunctioned, then either a tricortical iliac crest bone graft or a ball-shaped cancellous graft is required.
- The aim is to arthrodese the hallux in the best functional position. This position is determined as follows.
  - The geometry of the hallux is assessed by placing a flat surface against the sole of the foot and bringing the ankle to 90 degrees.
  - In this position, with the IP joint in full extension, the tip of the hallux should lie about 1 cm from the flat surface.
  - When the IP joint is flexed to 45 to 60 degrees, its tip comes in contact with the plantar surface. There should be a gap of 3 to 5 mm between the hallux and the second toe.
  - The rotation of the hallux should be neutral so that the arc of rotation of the IP joint is at 90 degrees to the weight-bearing surface.
- Revision for failed excision arthroplasty
  - Bone from the distal first metatarsal is resected back to vascular cancellous bone with an oscillating saw. A flat surface is placed on the sole of the foot. The osteotomy is performed in the coronal plane and in the sagittal plane, at 90 degrees to the flat surface.
  - Bone from the proximal phalanx is resected back to vascular cancellous bone with an oscillating saw, perpendicular to its long axis (TECH FIG 3).
  - The hallux is held in an estimated best position. The gap between the flat surfaces of the proximal phalanx and metatarsal head is measured. An appropriately sized tricortical iliac crest bone graft is harvested from the ipsilateral crest in a standard fashion.
- Revision for avascular necrosis following hallux valgus surgery
  - The distal first metatarsal and distal phalanx are prepared as previously described.
  - A retrograde 1.6-mm K-wire is passed through the proximal phalanx and retrieved distally. The hallux is held in the estimated correct position and the K-wire driven into the remaining metatarsal shaft.
  - A trough is cut out of the dorsum of each bone using the underlying K-wire as an alignment guide. The dimensions of the trough are measured, and the K-wire is then removed.

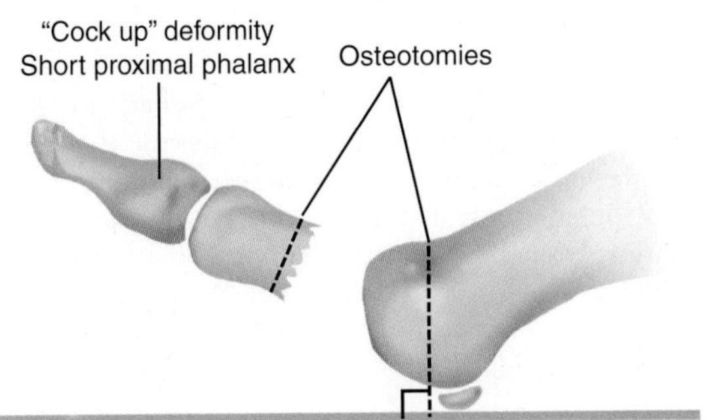

TECH FIG 3 • Revision of failed excision arthroplasty.

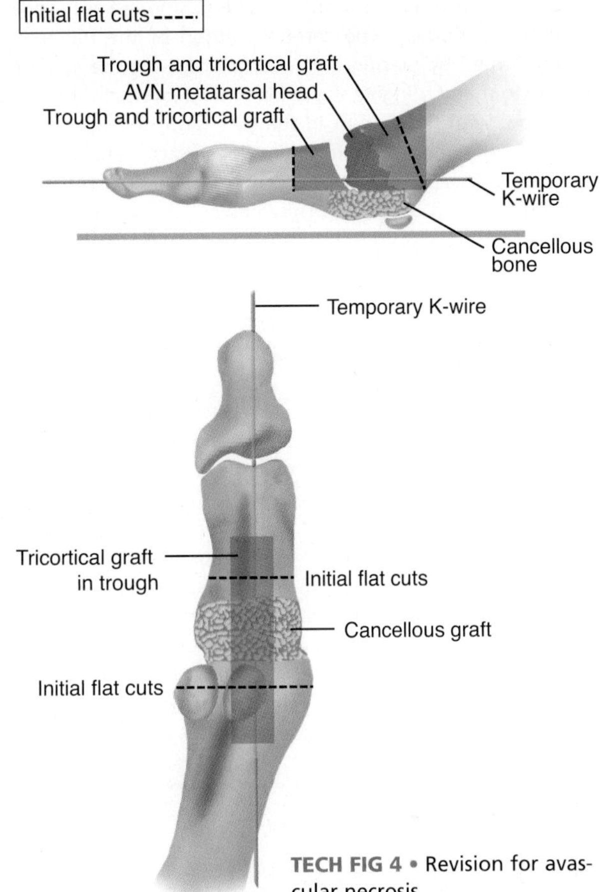

TECH FIG 4 • Revision for avascular necrosis.

  - An appropriately sized tricortical graft is harvested and inserted into the trough in each bone. The remaining defect is packed with cancellous graft (TECH FIG 4).
- Revision of failed prosthetic arthroplasty
  - Following curettage to normal bone, a considerable champagne-glass defect usually is present in each bone.
  - The defects are impaction grafted to create concave surfaces.
  - The hallux is again held in an estimated best position. A ball-shaped cancellous graft of sufficient size to fill the defect is prepared (TECH FIG 5).

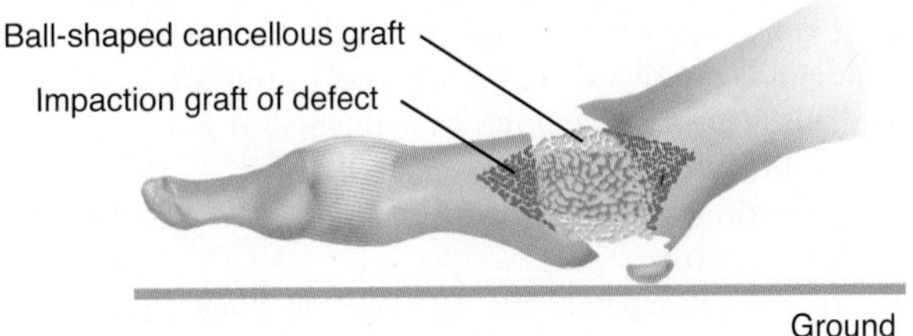

TECH FIG 5 • Revision for silicone foreign body reaction.

TECHNIQUES

POSITIONING OF THE HALLUX

- In simple revision cases, the hallux is positioned as for primary arthrodesis. The correct position of the hallux is confirmed by placing a flat surface against the sole of the foot and bringing the ankle to 90 degrees. In this position, with the IP joint in full extension, the tip of the hallux lies about 1 cm from the flat surface. When the IP joint is flexed to 45 to 60 degrees, its tip comes in contact with the plantar surface. This enables the foot to rock at the MTPJ on heel rise.
- If a graft is used, it is positioned in the arthrodesis site and the alignment of the hallux is reassessed using a flat surface against the sole of the foot, as described earlier. The interposition graft is trimmed as required to achieve the correct position of the hallux and the whole construct held with temporary K-wires.

FIXATION OF THE ARTHRODESIS

- When bone graft is not required, an oblique 2.7-mm compression screw of appropriate length is inserted from distal medial to proximal lateral across the MTPJ before a dorsal titanium precontoured low profile plate is secured.
- When an interposition graft is used, it may be necessary to reposition the temporary K-wire fixation to allow positioning of a trial plate. The plate is available in three side-specific sizes (small, medium, and large). In revision arthrodesis the large size usually is required for men, medium for women, and small if no interposition graft is used.
- The dorsum of the MTP joint may require feathering down with the oscillating saw to enable a flush fit, or the plate may need slight adjustment. If the hallux length has not been fully restored, then the plate needs to be straightened.
- The plate is now secured on the dorsal aspect of the joint with a K-wire and fixed with six to seven 2.7-mm–diameter self-tapping screws. The interposition graft is secured to the plate with one screw (see Fig 2).
- If the bone quality is poor and screw purchase is insufficient, 3-mm–diameter rescue screws can be used.
- The wound is closed in layers over a drain.
- A compression dressing is applied.

PEARLS AND PITFALLS

Silicone synovitis	▪ The centers of the defects are packed with loose cancellous graft to create a shallow, saucer-like deficiency. The iliac crest graft should then be shaped to form a ball.
Failed Keller-Brandes procedure	▪ Tricortical graft is required.
Avascular necrosis	▪ A trough is created and tricortical inlay graft is used.

POSTOPERATIVE CARE

- We prefer to use a compressive dressing and a postoperative stiff-soled shoe to allow early mobilization with careful heel weight bearing only.
- Early stretching of the tendo Achilles and range-of-motion exercises of the IP joint are encouraged.
- In revision cases, patients are kept non–weight-bearing for 4 weeks and then encouraged to bear weight by heel-walking for 4 weeks. Radiographs at this stage may show consolidation if bone graft has not been used.
- At 8 weeks post surgery, a radiograph is obtained. If there is evidence of consolidation, forefoot weight bearing is commenced in the postoperative shoe. Progression to full forefoot loading, assisted by crutches, follows over the next 4 weeks.
- Radiographs are taken 12 weeks post surgery. If these confirm consolidation, flat shoes with cushioned or shock-absorbing soles are worn.
- The time to union depends on the size of bone graft. Forefoot loading should commence only when there is some evidence of consolidation. Patients should be informed that the entire process can take up to 6 months, particularly if there has been a large defect filled with graft or there has been avascular necrosis.

OUTCOMES

- Time to union varies according to the patient's underlying medical condition and smoking habits, and in direct relationship to the size of graft used.
- The precontoured low-profile titanium plate used was originally designed to obtain the maximum possible purchase in a shortened proximal phalanx, following a Keller's procedure. In both the metatarsal and phalangeal ends, the three screws are on three different axes, to maximize pull-out strength. Additional holes are available to purchase the central graft. This fixation strength cannot be equalled with a single-axis dorsal plate.

COMPLICATIONS

- Infection
- IP joint stiffness

- Delayed union or nonunion
- Extensor hallucis longus tenodesis
- Dorsomedial sensory cutaneous nerve injury

REFERENCES

1. Mann RA, Thompson FM. Arthrodesis of the first metatarsophalangeal joint for hallux valgus in rheumatoid arthritis. J Bone Joint Surg Am 1984;66A:687–692.
2. Flavin R, Stephens MM. Arthrodesis of the 1st metatarsal phalangeal joint using a dorsal titanium contoured plate. Foot Ankle Int 2004; 25:783–787.
3. Stephens MM, ed. An Atlas of Foot and Ankle Surgery, ed 2. London: Martin Dunitz, 2001.
4. Machacek F, Easley M, Gruber F, et al. Salvage of the failed Keller resection arthroplasty. J Bone Joint Surg Am 2004;86A:1131–1138.

Chapter 27

Bone-Block Distraction of the First Metatarsophalangeal Joint

Hans-Joerg Trnka and Stefan G. Hofstaetter

DEFINITION

- First metatarsophalangeal arthrodesis is a reasonable alternative to a joint-sparing procedure in salvage of various great toe deformities.
- These deformities comprise failed hallux valgus procedures, avascular necrosis of the metatarsal head, failed first metatarsophalangeal (MTP) joint arthroplasty, prior infection, rheumatoid arthritis, posttraumatic conditions, hallux rigidus, severe hallux valgus deformities, and neuromuscular disorders.
- With minimal to moderate bone loss, we perform hallux MTP joint arthrodesis in situ, accepting slight shortening of the hallux. In our opinion, the slight shortening creates minimal cosmetic concerns and affords satisfactory functional improvement in a majority of cases.
- With marked shortening of the hallux and associated lesser metatarsalgia, an in-situ hallux MTP joint arthrodesis may fail to restore satisfactory function.
- We favor interposition structural bone graft to restore first ray length, which, in turn, should improve the weight bearing of the first metatarsal and hallux while alleviating lesser metatarsalgia.
- Sources for structural interposition bone block arthrodesis include (a) structural allograft (usually contoured from a donor femoral head or iliac crest) or (b) structural autograft (typically obtained from the patient's iliac crest). In our hands, ipsilateral anterior iliac crest harvesting is ideal for foot and ankle surgery because this site is readily accessible in the patient positioned supine on the operating table.
- Several configurations have been described for contouring the interpositional graft. We prefer the ball-and-socket technique, which affords three advantages over flat cuts or a conical preparation: (a) minimal resection of residual host bone, (b) optimal surface area at both ends of the graft for healing, and (c) relative ease of positioning the toe after preparing the arthrodesis without forfeiting contact area for fusion.

PATHOGENESIS

- In our referral practice, we most commonly use the ball-and-socket interpositional bone block distraction technique for severe bone loss after:
- Keller-Brandes procedure (**FIG 1A**), resection of the base of the proximal phalanx (this generally creates bone loss isolated to the hallux and not globally in the first ray)
- Mayo procedure (**FIG 1B**), resection of the first metatarsal head (creates a more global bone loss in the first ray)
- The Keller-Brandes and Mayo procedures have for the most part been abandoned because of their detrimental effects on forefoot function and the introduction of modern procedures that preserve anatomy.
- Avascular necrosis of the first metatarsal head (**FIG 1C**), a relatively rare complication of a distal chevron osteotomy
- Bone destruction after first MTP joint arthroplasty, particularly silicone implants (**FIG 1D**)

NATURAL HISTORY

- The natural history after failure of the aforementioned procedures is one of functional imbalance of the forefoot. The first ray fails to provide physiologic support, creating an overload phenomenon, or transfer metatarsalgia, to the lesser metatarsal heads. While the lesser metatarsals may be shortened to compensate for the loss of first ray length, this is often undesirable because there is no pathology at the lesser toes.

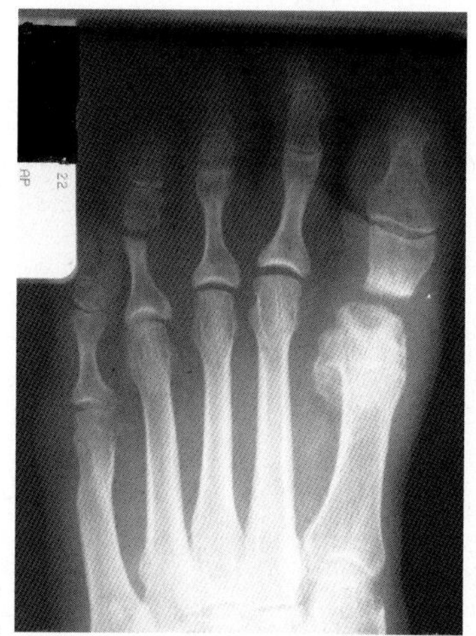

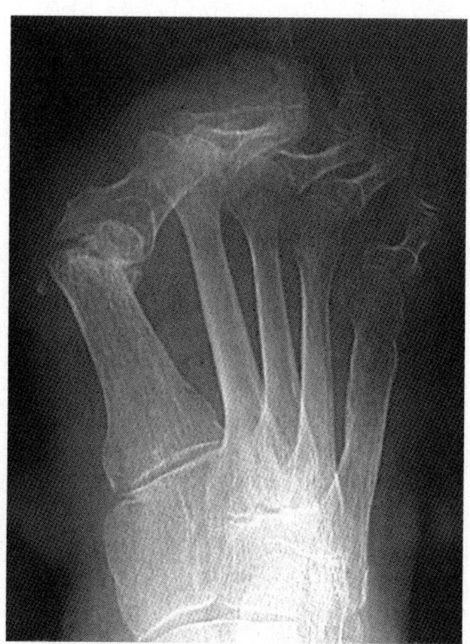

FIG 1 • **A.** Bone loss after Keller-Brandes procedure. **B.** Bone loss after Mayo resectional arthroplasty. *(continued)*

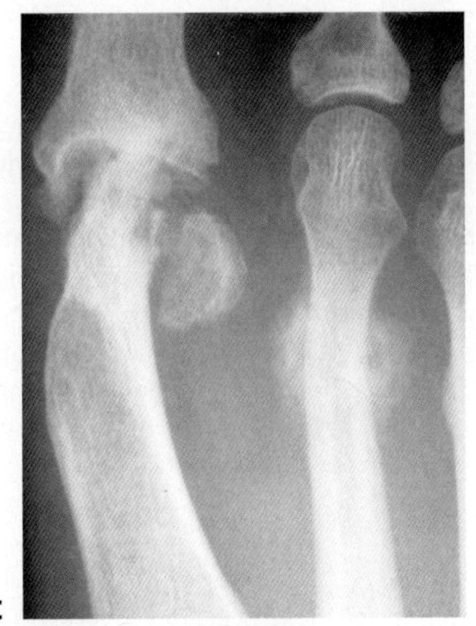
C

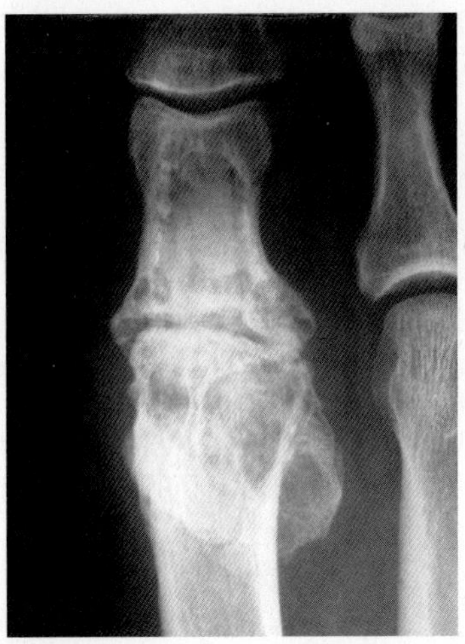
D

FIG 1 • *(continued)* **C.** Bone loss after avascular necrosis following a chevron osteotomy. **D.** Bone loss after failed silicon implant.

PATIENT HISTORY AND PHYSICAL FINDINGS

- The patient typically complains of pain and deformity in the hallux MTP joint and pressure and pain under the lateral forefoot.
- Typical physical examination findings include:
  - Short hallux or first ray (bone loss at the hallux only is typical with bone loss on the phalangeal or metatarsal head side; more global first ray bone loss occurs after the Mayo procedure, avascular necrosis of the metatarsal head, or a failed great toe implant)
  - Cock-up deformity of the hallux
  - Residual hallux valgus deformity and occasional hallux varus deformity
  - Pain and crepitance with range of motion of hallux
  - Pain and tenderness (and occasionally plantar callus formation) under the lesser metatarsal heads
- The potential iliac crest harvest site should also be inspected for unanticipated soft tissue concerns or to confirm that no prior graft harvest has been performed.

IMAGING AND OTHER DIAGNOSTIC STUDIES

- Weight-bearing foot radiographs, including AP, lateral, and oblique views
- With avascular necrosis of the first metatarsal head, an MRI of the forefoot may prove useful in estimating the extent of necrotic bone and predicting the size of the interpositional graft.

NONOPERATIVE MANAGEMENT

- In our experience, nonoperative treatment of the painful, shortened, and cocked-up hallux is generally unsuccessful. The shoe's toe box may be enlarged and an accommodative orthotic to post under the hallux may be considered, but this is generally of limited value.
- Metatarsal support, however, may relieve the symptoms related to transverse metatarsalgia by unloading the lesser metatarsal heads. If metatarsal pads are effective, then a custom orthotic with metatarsal support may prove beneficial as well.

SURGICAL MANAGEMENT

Preoperative Planning

- The decision to perform a structural femoral head or iliac crest allograft or an anterior iliac crest autograft must be made preoperatively. However, we recommend having the flexibility to use either method, with the patient's consent, if one graft proves ineffective based on intraoperative assessment. The patient should be aware of the risks of iliac crest graft harvest and the use of allograft bone.
- Myerson et al[5] in 2005 investigated the use of structural allografts in foot and ankle surgery and discussed the risks of using a structural allograft. One concern with the use of structural allograft is the possible transmission of disease and malignancy, but with the use of processed allografts the risk is practically zero. The risk of iliac crest bone harvest is donor-site morbidity, which includes local hematoma, local infection, and in rare cases local nerve irritation.
- We routinely draw a preoperative plan for the structural graft, determining the approximate amount of bone resection required and the length of graft that needs to be acquired.

Positioning

- The patient is positioned supine on the operating table, with a bump placed beneath the hip ipsilateral to the foot that will be operated on. This not only positions the foot in an ideal position (to allow improved assessment of proper hallux alignment) but also facilitates harvest of the iliac crest graft by making the anterior crest more accessible.

Approach

- First MTP joint: A standard dorsal approach is recommended, starting about 4 cm proximal to the MTP joint and extending to the interphalangeal joint. When possible, previous incisions should be incorporated into the approach, to avoid a skin bridge that may be at risk, particularly when the toe will be distracted with the interpositional graft.
- Iliac crest: An incision is made parallel and inferior to the anterior iliac crest, about 3 cm posterior to the anterior-superior iliac spine, to avoid injuring the lateral femoral cutaneous nerve.

PREPARATION OF THE MTP JOINT

- Start the dorsal skin incision about 4 cm proximal to the first MTP joint and extend it to the interphalangeal joint (TECH FIG 1).
- The extensor hallucis longus (EHL) tendon can be simply retracted if the first ray has minimal shortening. With moderate to severe shortening, particularly with associated cock-up toe deformity, the EHL tendon may need to be Z-lengthened to allow restoration of toe length and to avoid hyperextension at the hallux interphalangeal joint.
- Divide the first MTP joint capsule, scar tissue from prior surgery, and periosteum of the proximal phalanx and distal first metatarsal longitudinally and reflect them. While we subscribe to the principle of minimal soft tissue stripping, we believe that subperiosteal preparation is mandatory to afford sufficient mobilization of the hallux. However, we leave the plantar soft tissues to maintain the blood vessels supplying the residual metatarsal head and proximal phalanx (TECH FIG 2).
- We routinely remove any osteophytes and additional soft tissue adhesions.

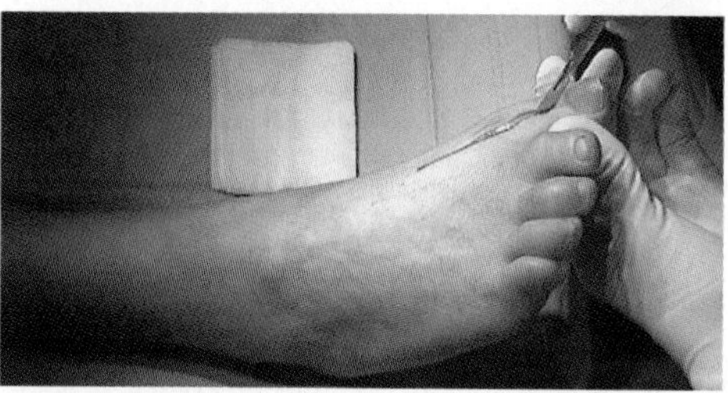

TECH FIG 1 • The joint capsule and the soft tissue coverage of the metatarsal and the phalanx are incised longitudinally straight down to the bone and then opened as an envelope. Subperiosteal preparation is mandatory to ensure sufficient release from the lateral soft tissue and scar adhesions.

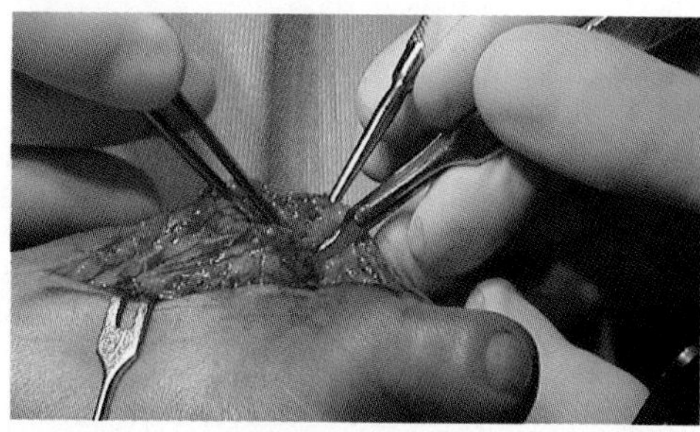

TECH FIG 2 • After the articular surfaces of the first metatarsophalangeal joint have been adequately freed, the big toe is brought into maximal plantarflexion.

REAMING OF THE METATARSAL HEAD AND BASE OF THE PROXIMAL PHALANX

- After mobilizing the articular surfaces of the first MTP joint, maximally plantarflex the hallux (TECH FIG 3).
- Insert a guidewire for the reamer set into the center of the metatarsal head. Place the appropriately sized "female" reamer over the guidewire (TECH FIG 4). Remove the sclerotic bone surface with the reamer down to cancellous bleeding bone.
- Expose the base of the proximal phalanx (TECH FIG 5) and place a guidewire for the reamer set (TECH FIG 6).
- In a similar manner, prepare the proximal phalanx with the "male" reamer counterpart (TECH FIG 7). Distract the toe to the desired length and measure the gap (TECH FIG 8).

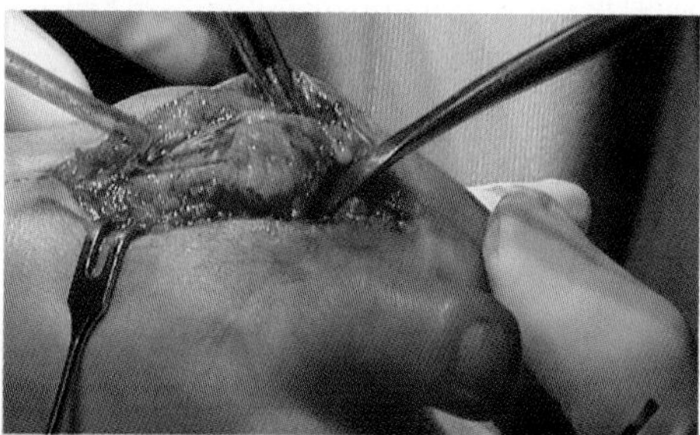

TECH FIG 3 • After the articular surfaces of the first metatarsophalangeal joint have been mobilized, the hallux is maximally plantarflexed.

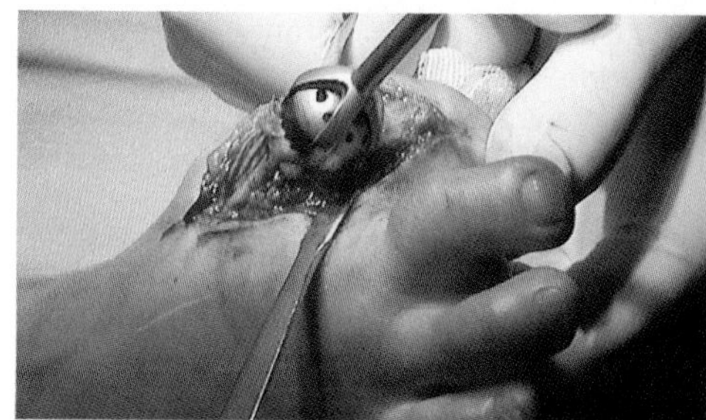

A

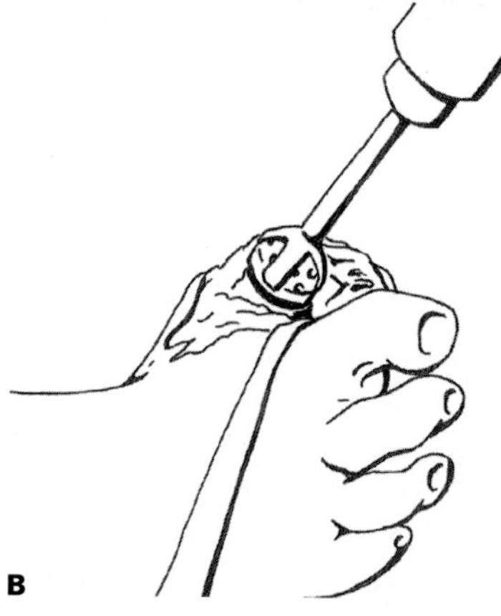

B

TECH FIG 4 • The adequately sized female reamer is then used to remove the sclerotic bone surface of the metatarsal head down to the cancellous bleeding bone.

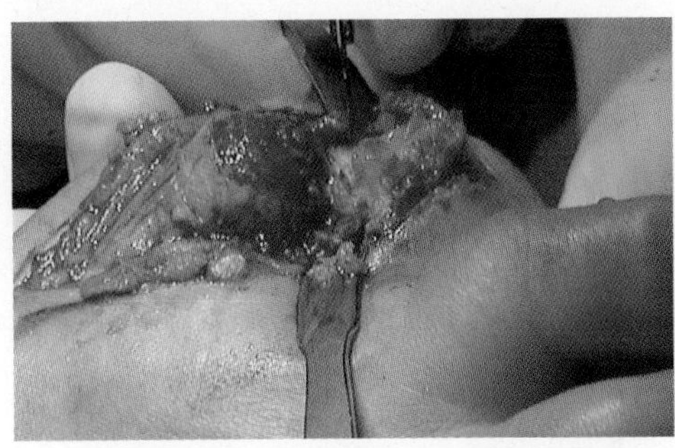

TECH FIG 5 • Exposure of the base of the proximal phalanx.

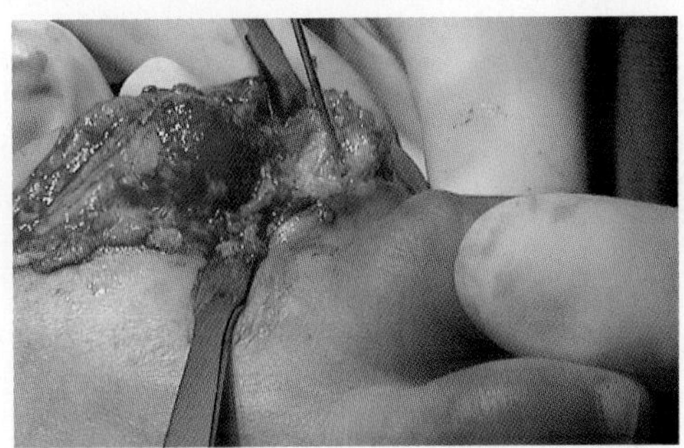

TECH FIG 6 • Placement of the guidewire of the reamer set.

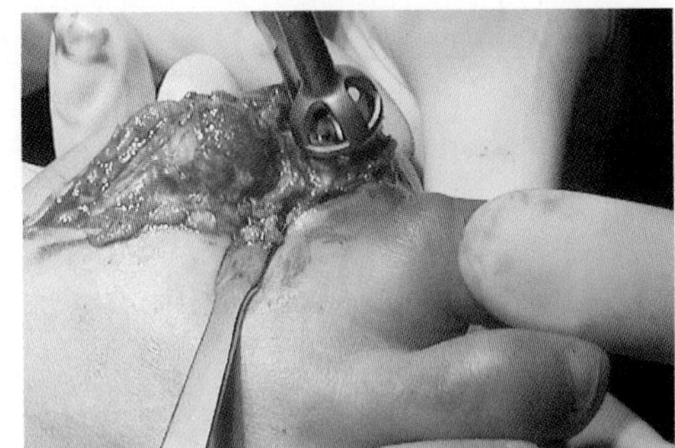

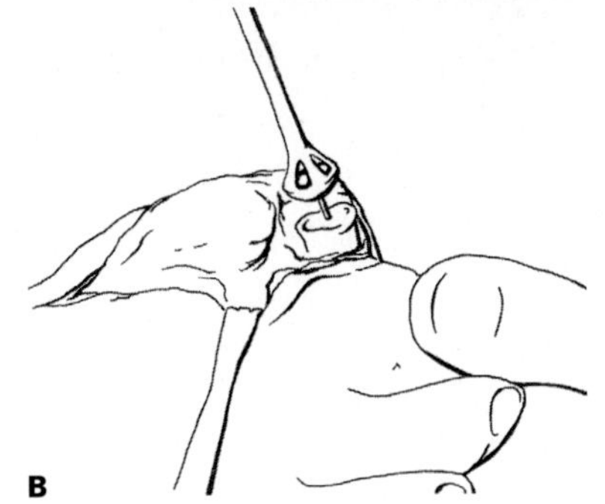

TECH FIG 7 • The male reamer is now used to remove the sclerotic bone surface of the metatarsal head down to the cancellous bleeding bone.

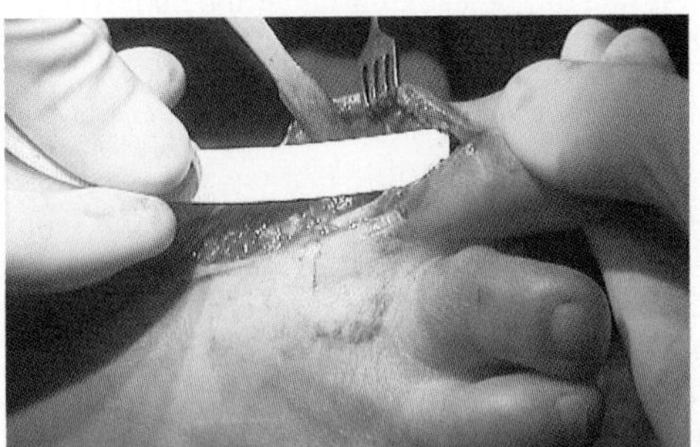

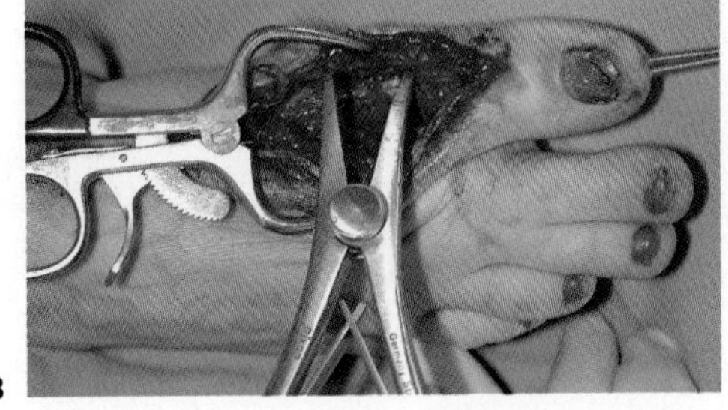

TECH FIG 8 • The toe can then be pulled into position of the desired length, and the exact extent of the gap in the joint is measured.

HARVEST OF THE ILIAC CREST BONE BLOCK

- Make the incision for the tricortical iliac crest block 3 cm posterior to the anterior-superior iliac spine (TECH FIG 9). Carry dissection down to the intermuscular plane using electrocautery for hemostasis. Reflect the periosteum from the superior crest. Insert a Hohmann retractor on the inner and outer aspects of the iliac crest, deep to the periosteum (TECH FIG 10). Based on

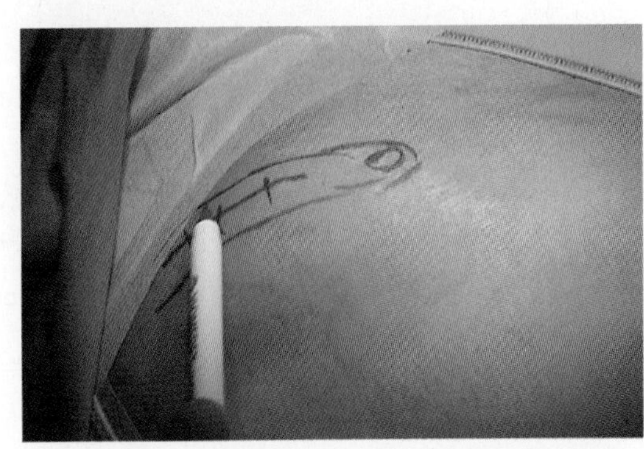

TECH FIG 9 • The incision for the tricortical iliac crest block is made 2 to 3 cm posterior to the anterior-superior iliac spine.

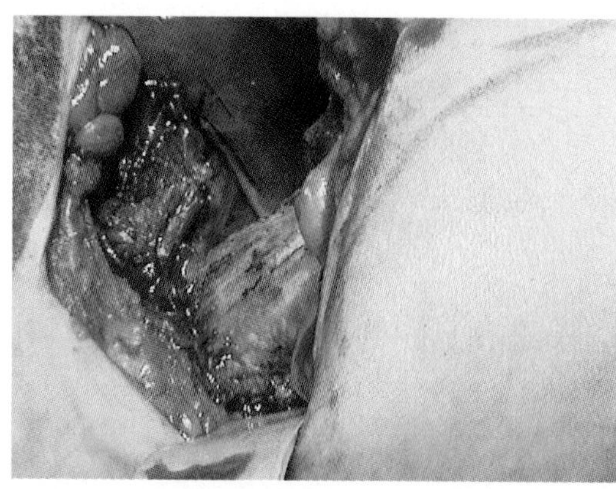

TECH FIG 10 • A Hohmann retractor is inserted on the inner and outer side of the iliac crest under the periosteum.

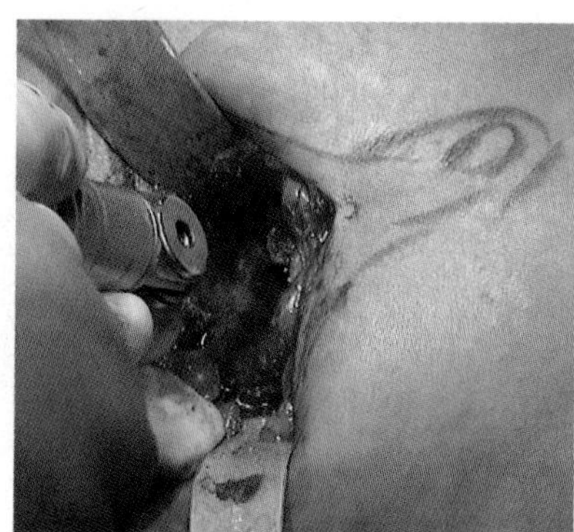

TECH FIG 11 • A saw is used to osteotomize the ends of the tricortical bone block.

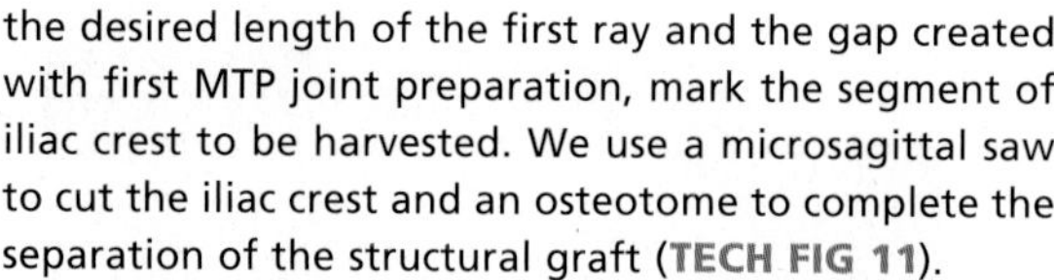

the desired length of the first ray and the gap created with first MTP joint preparation, mark the segment of iliac crest to be harvested. We use a microsagittal saw to cut the iliac crest and an osteotome to complete the separation of the structural graft (**TECH FIG 11**).

- Harvest the iliac crest structural graft (**TECH FIG 12**).
- The defect in the iliac crest may be backfilled with allograft bone chips. Close the periosteum after placing a drain. Reapproximate the subcutaneous tissues and close the skin.

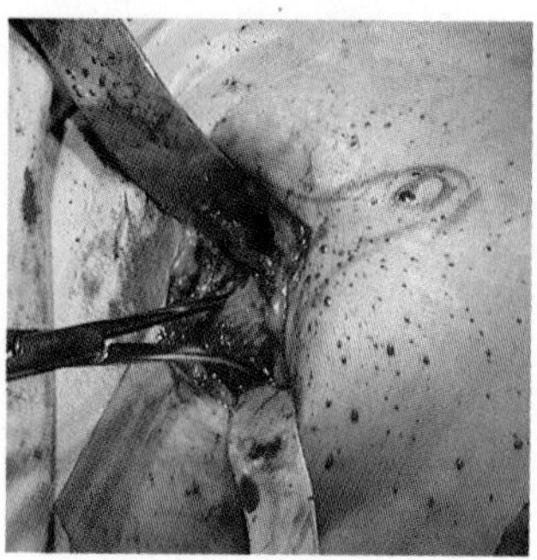

TECH FIG 12 • The iliac crest bone block is retrieved.

CONTOURING OF THE GRAFT

- Secure the graft (either the harvested iliac crest graft or a femoral head graft) on the back table using a forceps, to be shaped into the desired length (**TECH FIG 13**).
- Place a guidewire for the reamer set in the center of the graft's long axis. Use the same reamers that were used to prepare the first MTP joint to contour the ends of the graft. One end is prepared with the "female" reamer and the other using the "male" reamer to create optimal contact to the host bone (**TECH FIG 14**).

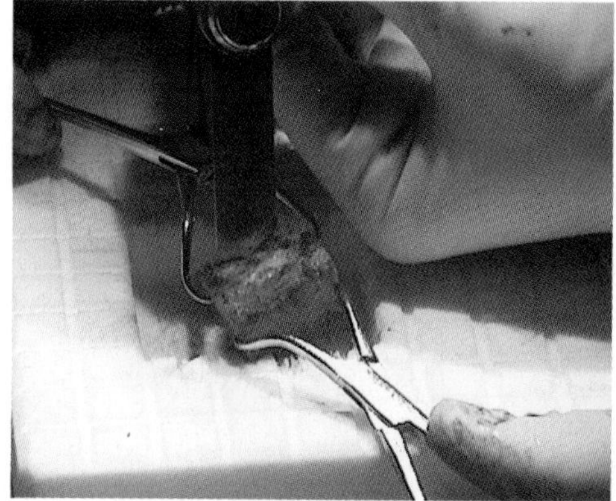

A

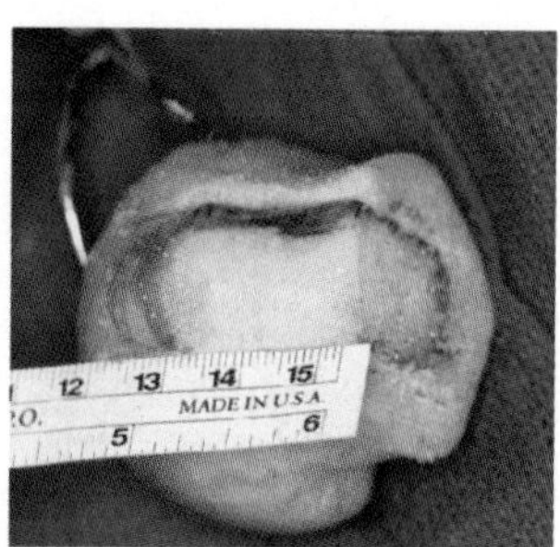

B

TECH FIG 13 • **A.** The graft is held on the table with a forceps and shaped into the desired length. **B.** The graft margins are marked on an allograft femoral head.

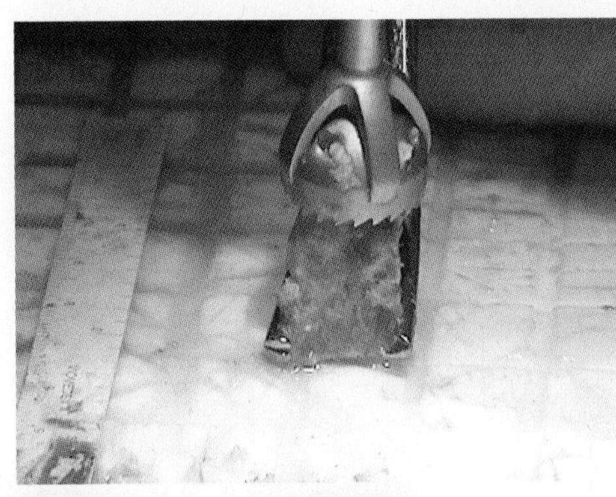

A

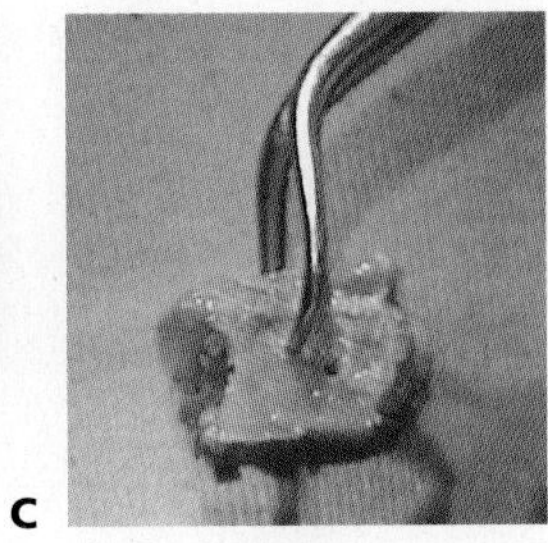

C

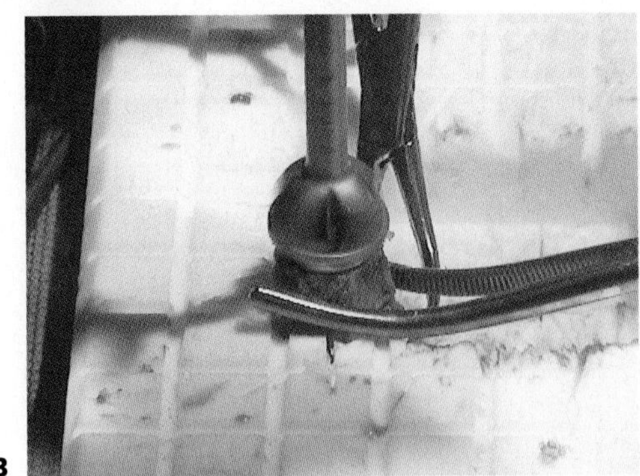

B

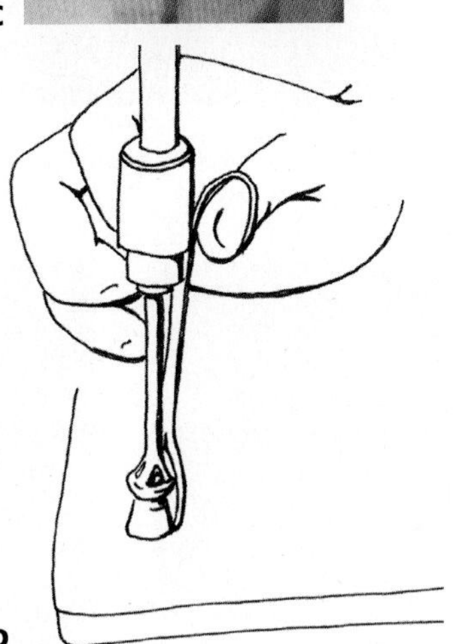

D

TECH FIG 14 • The same-sized female and male reamers are used to mold the two surfaces on the sides of the block, one as a ball and the other as a socket to fit to the ends of the proximal phalanx and the metatarsal head respectively.

INSERTION OF THE GRAFT AND FIXATION

- Insert the contoured graft (TECH FIG 15) into the prepared gap between metatarsal and phalanx. With a ball-and-socket shape on either end of the prepared gap, the alignment of the lengthened hallux may be seamlessly adjusted in any direction. Place either a standard plate or a special revision plate dorsally (TECH FIG 16). Place temporary pins to maintain the reduction, and confirm proper arthrodesis and plate positions fluoroscopically.
- In our experience, optimal hallux position for arthrodesis is (a) neutral rotation (no pronation or supination), (b) about 15 degrees of dorsiflexion (relative to the plantar surface of the foot), and (c) 5 degrees of valgus with respect to the first metatarsal (TECH FIG 17).
- To determine optimal sagittal plane position, a lid from an instrument tray may be used to simulate weight bearing. Ideally, the distal hallux tuft is 1 to 2 mm elevated from the plate when the ball of the foot and heel are contacting the instrument tray lid (TECH FIG 18).
- Place a 3.0-mm or 3.5-mm screw from the medial aspect of the residual proximal phalanx across the graft to the lateral aspect of the residual metatarsal (TECH FIG 19).
- Secure the plate to the construct, with screws in the proximal phalanx, graft, and metatarsal, while avoiding the initial screw (TECH FIG 20). Three or four absorbable deep sutures are generally adequate to cover the plate. We advocate the use of a small-diameter drain for 2 days postoperatively to reduce the risk of hematoma formation.
- Reapproximate the subcutaneous layer and skin in a tension-free manner; perform the closure carefully since the soft tissues are already under some tension due to lengthening of the first ray.
- After sterile dressings are placed on the wound, we routinely apply a well-padded short-leg cast that extends beyond the toes. We recommend univalving the cast.

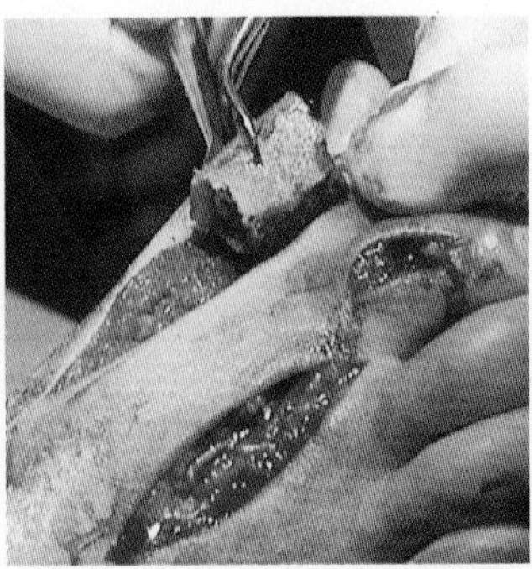

TECH FIG 15 • The molded graft is inserted into the gap between metatarsal and phalanx.

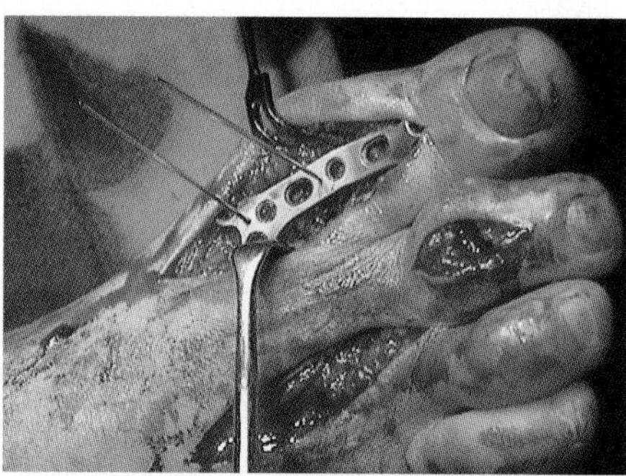

TECH FIG 16 • The special revision plate is placed dorsally.

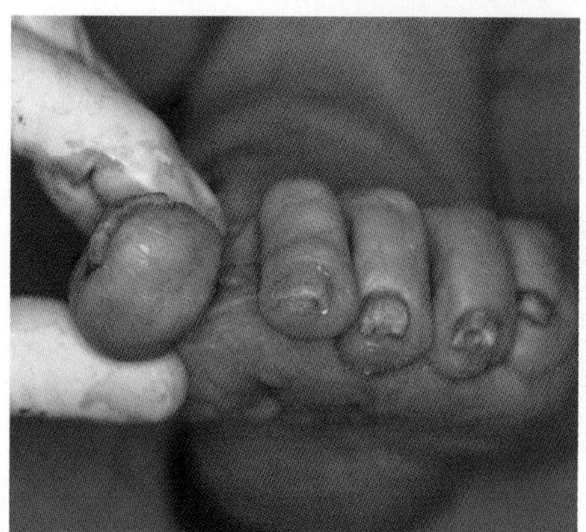

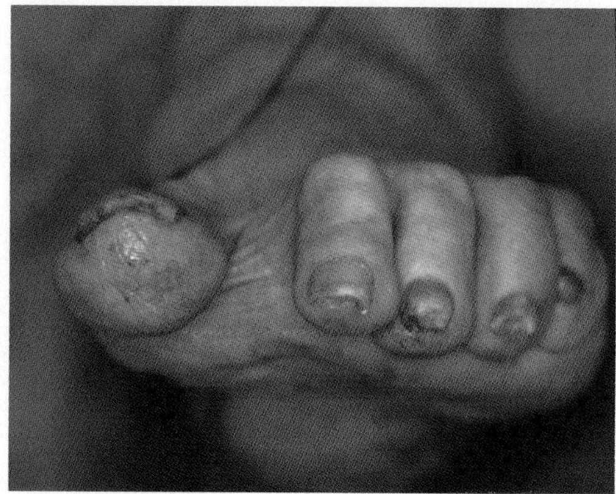

TECH FIG 17 • The hallux is positioned in neutral rotation, with special attention paid to the position of the toenail.

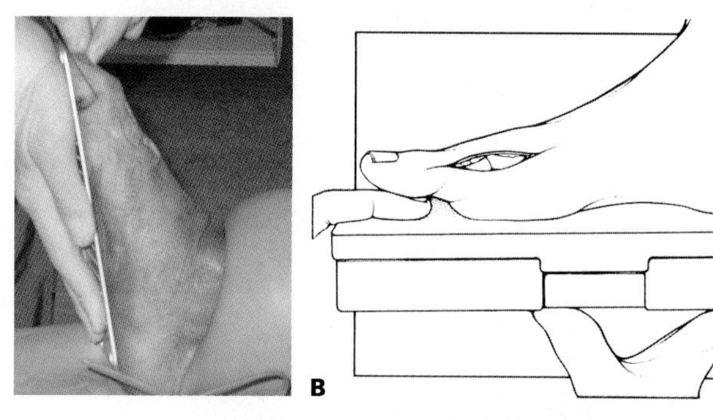

TECH FIG 18 • For the optimal extension, a lid of the instrument tray may be used to simulate floor contact.

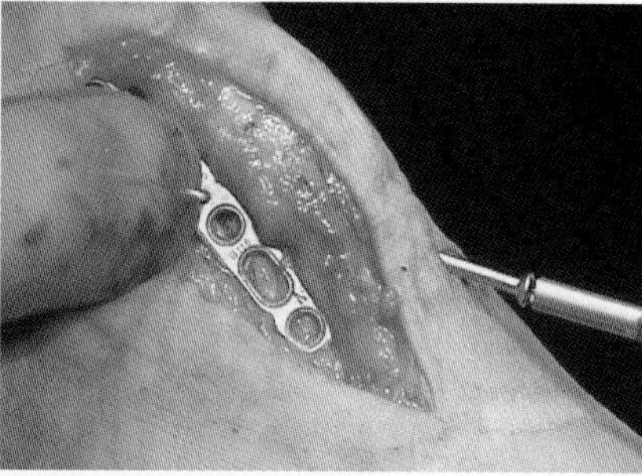

TECH FIG 19 • To add additional stability, a 3.0 AO screw is inserted from the medial aspect of the proximal phalanx of the great toe across the graft to the lateral side of the metatarsal.

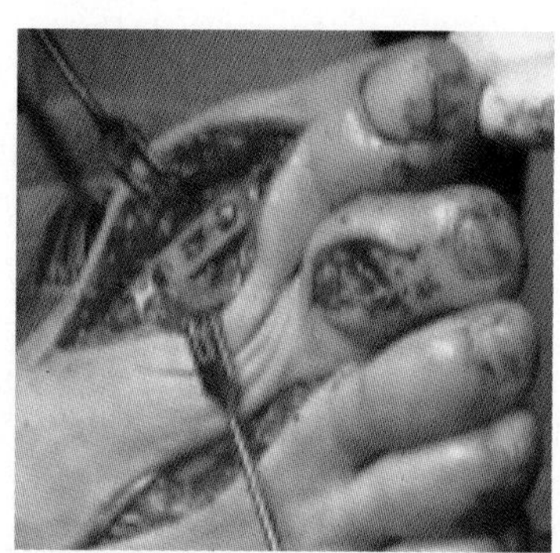

TECH FIG 20 • The plate is fixed with adequate screws.

PEARLS AND PITFALLS

- Avoid excessive dorsiflexion of the arthrodesis. Use the lid of an instrument tray to simulate the floor with weight bearing. Excessive elevation may lead to sesamoid overload, symptomatic irritation of the hallux in the shoe, and a poor cosmetic appearance.
- Avoid excessive plantarflexion of the arthrodesis. Use the lid of an instrument tray to simulate the floor with weight bearing. A plantarflexed toe position will result in symptoms during push-off in the gait cycle and eventual interphalangeal arthrosis from excessive stress of the hallux interphalangeal joint.
- Avoid being overzealous in lengthening; the soft tissues may be put on excessive tension, resulting in vascular compromise. One trick is to distract the hallux with a laminar spreader and deflate the tourniquet while harvesting or preparing the graft. If after 5 to 10 minutes the toe is still not well perfused, then the distraction may be too great and a shorter graft should be used.
- While varus position makes shoe wear difficult, excessive valgus is also poorly tolerated since the hallux impinges on the second toe. Slight valgus relative to the metatarsal is acceptable, but a neutral position, in our hands, is usually ideal.
- Residual pronation is poorly tolerated after first metatarsal arthrodesis and leads to a symptomatic medial toe callus. Be sure to align the hallux nail with the same orientation as the second and third toenails.

POSTOPERATIVE CARE

- We recommend placing the patient in a short-leg cast that extends beyond the toes for a full 6 to 8 weeks. The patient should be touch-down weight bearing until suture removal and then weight bearing on the heel until 6 to 8 weeks.

OUTCOMES

- Myerson et al[4,5] treated 24 patients with hallux MTP joint arthrodesis using bone graft to restore first ray length (**FIG 2**).
- This procedure was performed after bone loss subsequent to previous surgeries for the correction of hallux valgus and hallux rigidus with Silastic arthroplasty (n = 11), bunionectomy and distal metatarsal osteotomy (n = 6), Keller resection arthroplasty (n = 5), and total joint replacement (n = 2).
- All patients were examined clinically and radiographically at a mean interval of 62.7 months after surgery (range 26 to 108 months).
- Successful fusion was observed in 19 of the 24 patients (79.1%) at a mean of 13.3 weeks (range 11 to 16 weeks),

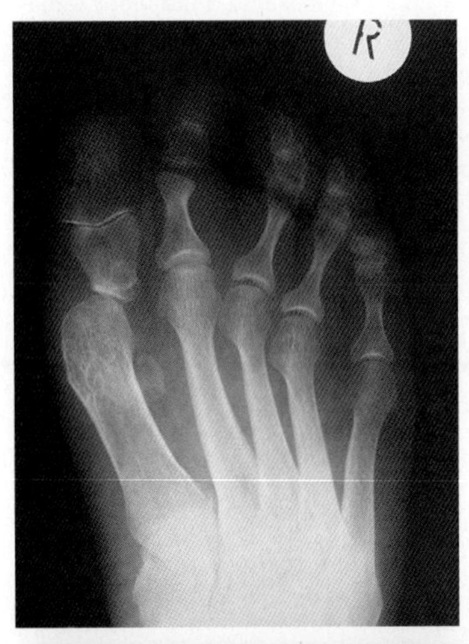

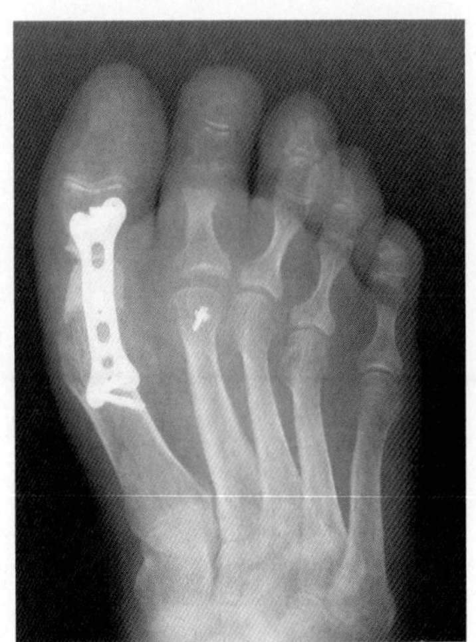

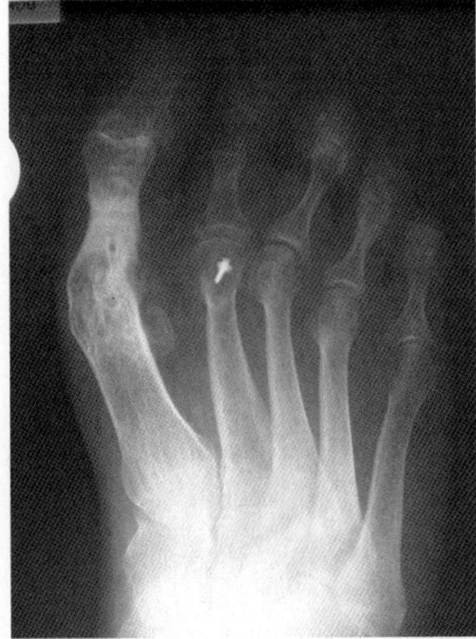

FIG 2 • **A.** A 45-year-old woman after Keller-Brandes arthroplasty. **B.** Postoperative photograph of a first metatarsophalangeal bone block fusion. **C.** 2-year follow-up after hardware removal.

and the first ray was lengthened by a mean of 13 mm (range 0 to 29 mm).

- Of the five nonunions noted radiographically, two were asymptomatic and three were managed successfully with further surgery.
- Complications included one deep infection requiring intravenous antibiotics and irrigation and débridement of the graft repeat surgery for treatment of osteomyelitis and two minor superficial wound infections managed effectively with oral antibiotics and local wound care.
- The mean AOFAS score improved from 39 points (range 22 to 60 points) to 79 points (range 64 to 90 points).

- Brodsky et al[1] reviewed 12 patients (12 feet) who underwent salvage first MTP arthrodesis with structural interposition autologous iliac crest bone graft.
  - Eight patients had a bony defect secondary to failed first MTP joint implant arthroplasties, two had avascular necrosis after failed bunion surgery, one had a nonunion of an attempted arthrodesis for failed bunion surgery, and one had been treated for osteomyelitis after cheilectomy.
  - Eleven cases had a single dorsal plate secured by screws and one case had two plates, one dorsal and one medial.
  - A plate, crossed screw(s), or Kirschner wire combinations were used in four cases.
  - Clinical arthrodesis was achieved after an average of 12 weeks (range 4 to 20).
    - Radiographic arthrodesis was achieved in 11 of 12 feet at an average of 15 weeks (range 8 to 28), with one pseudarthrosis.
  - The AOFAS forefoot clinical rating score averaged 70 points (maximum 90 after first MTP arthrodesis) at an average follow-up of 22 months (range 5 to 70).
  - Sesamoiditis, prominent hardware, and scar sensitivity were complaints in four patients postoperatively. Two cases required flap coverage for skin necrosis. There was no symptomatic progression of interphalangeal degenerative change postoperatively.

COMPLICATIONS

- Pseudarthrosis
- Wound dehiscence or infection
- Nerve irritation
- Poor alignment

REFERENCES

1. Brodsky JW, Ptaszek AJ, Morris SG. Salvage first MTP arthrodesis utilizing ICBG: clinical evaluation and outcome. Foot Ankle Int 2000;21:290–296.
2. Machacek F Jr., Easley ME, Gruber F, et al. Salvage of a failed Keller resection arthroplasty. J Bone Joint Surg Am 2004;86A:1131–1138.
3. Machacek F Jr., Easley ME, Gruber F, et al. Salvage of the failed Keller resection arthroplasty: surgical technique. J Bone Joint Surg Am 2005;87A(Suppl 1):86–94.
4. Myerson MS, Schon LC, McGuigan FX, et al. Result of arthrodesis of the hallux metatarsophalangeal joint using bone graft for restoration of length. Foot Ankle Int 2000;21:297–306.
5. Myerson MS, Neufeld SK, Uribe J. Fresh frozen structural allografts in the foot and ankle. J Bone Joint Surg Am 2005;87A:113–120.
6. Trnka HJ. Arthrodesis procedures for salvage of the hallux metatarsophalangeal joint. Foot Ankle Clin 2000;5:673–686.

Chapter 28 Surgical Management of Turf Toe Injuries

Christopher W. Nicholson and Robert B. Anderson

DEFINITION

- Turf toe injuries involve the capsular–ligamentous–sesamoid complex of the hallux metatarsophalangeal (MP) joint.[1,2] They fall within a spectrum ranging from stable capsular sprains to unstable disruptions of the complex.
- Turf toe injuries have become more prevalent with more rigid playing surfaces (ie, artificial turf) and less rigid shoe wear[7,10] and may be considered more disabling than ankle sprains.[5,9]
- Turf toe can result in significant disability and loss of playing time in athletes, so it must be diagnosed early and evaluated properly to restore function.

ANATOMY

- The hallux MP joint is stabilized by adjacent capsular, ligamentous, tendinous, and osseous structures (**FIG 1**). Disruption of a part of this complex results in a turf toe injury.
- The plantar plate is composed of the joint capsule, with attachments to the transverse head of the abductor hallucis, to the flexor tendon sheaths, and to the deep transverse intermetatarsal ligament.
- The tibial and fibular sesamoids articulate with the metatarsal head. They are contained within the medial and lateral portions of the flexor hallucis brevis (FHB) tendons, respectively. Their relationship to one another is maintained by the intersesamoid ligament. Ligamentous attachments also run between the sesamoids and the metatarsal head and proximal phalanx. The sesamoids may be bipartite.
- The FHB is located within the third plantar layer of the foot. It originates from the lateral cuneiform and the cuboid. It inserts into the proximal phalanx of the hallux and is innervated by the medial plantar nerve.
- Medially, in the first plantar layer of the foot, the abductor hallucis muscle originates from the medial process of the os calcis tuberosity. It inserts with the medial tendon of the FHB into the medial aspect of the base of the hallux proximal phalanx. It also is innervated by the medial plantar nerve.
- Laterally, also in the third plantar layer of the foot, the adductor hallucis has two heads. The oblique head originates from the base of metatarsals two through four, while the transverse head takes origin from the lateral fourth MP joint. The two heads unite and insert through the fibular sesamoid into the lateral aspect of the base of the hallux proximal phalanx. Both heads are innervated by the lateral plantar nerve.

PATHOGENESIS

- The primary mechanism of injury involves a hyperextension force to the hallux MP joint. Most commonly, an axial load is applied to the heel of a foot fixed in equinus (**FIG 2**).
- The most common variation is that created by a valgus-directed force, resulting in an injury to the plantar medial complex or tibial sesamoid that, if left untreated, may lead to a traumatic bunion and hallux valgus. A varus-directed force is less common but can lead to a traumatic varus deformity.
- In our experience, limited ankle dorsiflexion places the hallux MP joint at greater risk for injury, although the literature is controversial on this mode of pathogenesis.

NATURAL HISTORY

- The natural history of turf toe depends on the degree of injury to the capsular–ligamentous–sesamoid complex. Simple, stable sprains usually heal uneventfully. Missed or untreated unstable injuries may lead to hallux limitus or rigidus and chronic pain and push-off weakness.

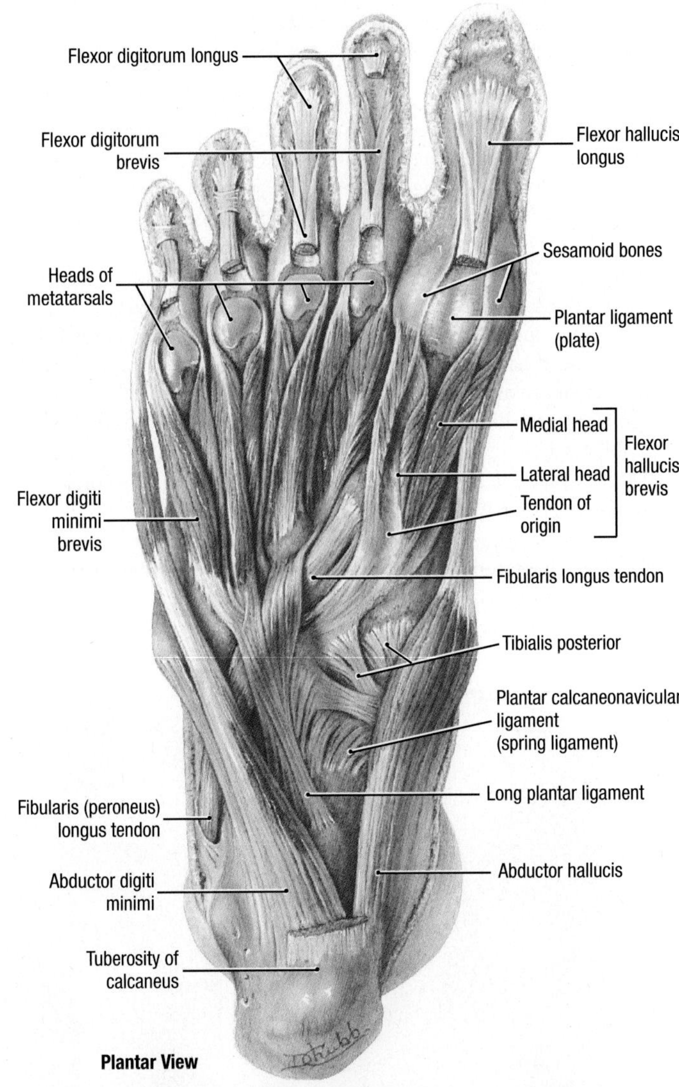

FIG 1 • Normal plantar anatomy of the hallux metatarsophalangeal joint. (From Agur AMR, Dalley AF. Grant's Atlas of Anatomy, 11th ed. Baltimore: Lippincott Williams & Wilkins, 2005.)

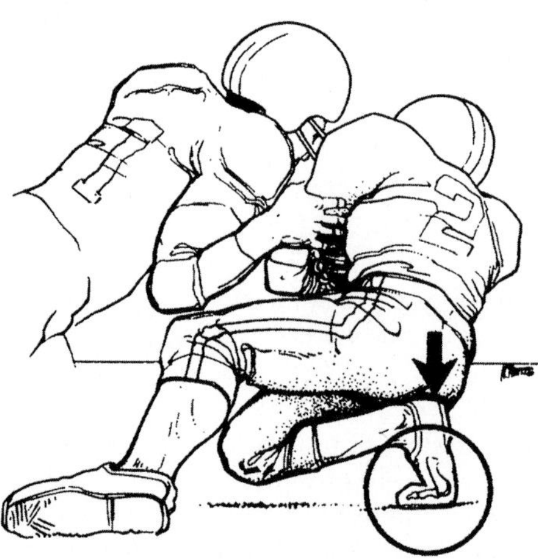

FIG 2 • Typical mechanism of turf toe injury: a foot fixed to the ground is subjected to an axial load and creates a hyperextension force at the hallux metatarsophalangeal joint.

PATIENT HISTORY AND PHYSICAL FINDINGS

- The history of this injury is particularly important. Useful information includes the type of shoe the patient was wearing, the circumstances of the injury (ie, the position of the foot at the time of injury, the direction of applied force, the type of athletic surface and shoe, any perceived "pop," and any initial obvious deformity, such as a dislocation that may have reduced spontaneously or required manual manipulation).
- In our experience, a regional anesthetic, such as a digital anesthetic block of the hallux, may be required to perform a satisfactory examination of the acute turf toe injury. However, significant swelling, as seen in the acute setting, will make this problematic.
- Relevant clinical findings include plantar swelling and ecchymosis about the hallux MP joint. Alignment of the hallux MP joint is noted and compared to the contralateral side. Asymmetric hallux valgus suggests a traumatic bunion, and asymmetric hallux varus implies traumatic injury to the lateral sesamoid complex. Dorsal dislocation of the first MP joint is an obvious finding and may involve severe injury to the sesamoid complex.
- The examination can include the following:
  - Active and passive hallux MP range of motion. Hallux MP motion varies widely among individuals, with reported plantarflexion from 3 to 40 degrees and dorsiflexion from 40 to 100 degrees. The best method is to compare to the noninjured contralateral side.
  - The examiner should observe the patient's gait (specifically, the time between heel rise and toe-off). The patient will shorten time spent after heel rise since this concentrates pressure onto the injured hallux MP joint.
  - Vertical Lachman test. A positive test is any laxity greater than the contralateral side.
- Turf toe classification
- A. Hyperextension (turf toe)
- Grade 1: Stretching of the plantar complex; localized tenderness, minimal swelling, no ecchymosis
- Grade 2: Partial tear; diffuse tenderness, moderate swelling, ecchymosis, restricted movement with pain
- Grade 3: Complete tear; severe tenderness to palpation, marked swelling and ecchymosis, limited movement with pain, positive vertical Lachman test; associated injuries possible (medial–lateral injury; sesamoid fracture/bipartite diastasis; articular cartilage–subchondral bone bruise)
- B. Hyperflexion (sand toe)
- C. Dislocation
- Type I: Dislocation of the hallux with the sesamoids; no disruption of the intersesamoid ligament; usually irreducible
- Type II: IIA (associated disruption of intersesamoid ligament; usually reducible); IIB (associated transverse fracture of one of the sesamoids; usually reducible); IIC (complete disruption of intersesamoid ligament with fracture of one of the sesamoids; usually reducible)

IMAGING AND OTHER DIAGNOSTIC STUDIES

- A thorough radiographic evaluation is mandatory (including weight-bearing views of the foot in the AP, lateral, and oblique planes) (**FIG 3**).

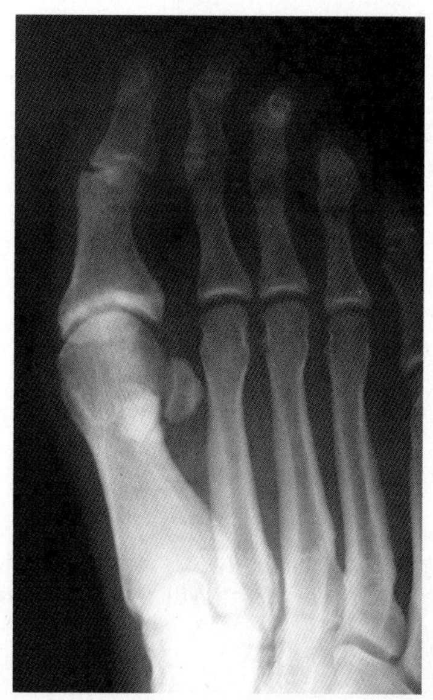

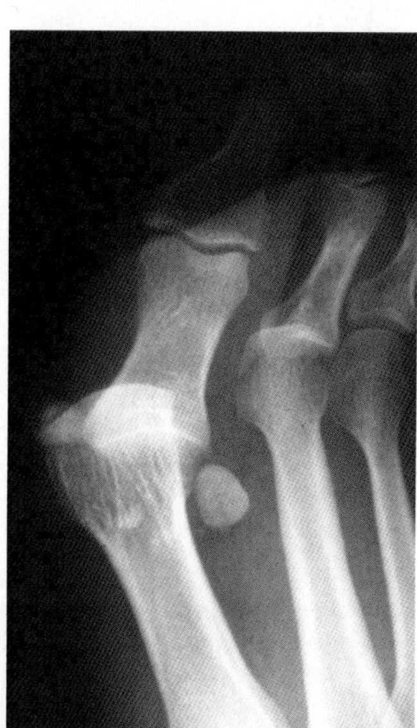

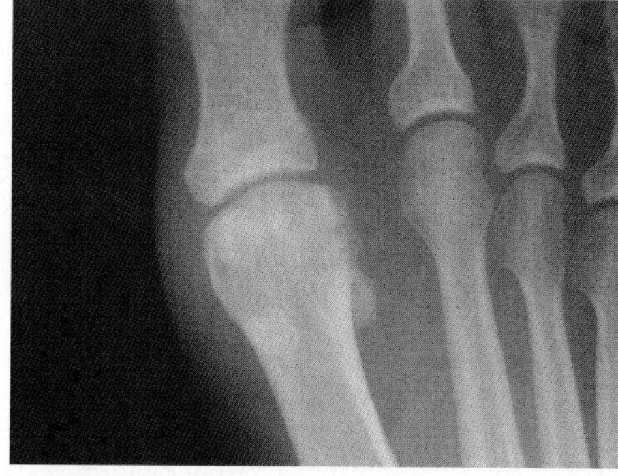

FIG 3 • **A.** AP foot radiograph showing proximal migration of the tibial sesamoid suggestive of an unstable turf toe injury. **B.** AP foot radiograph showing a hallux metatarsophalangeal dislocation with an associated sesamoid fracture.

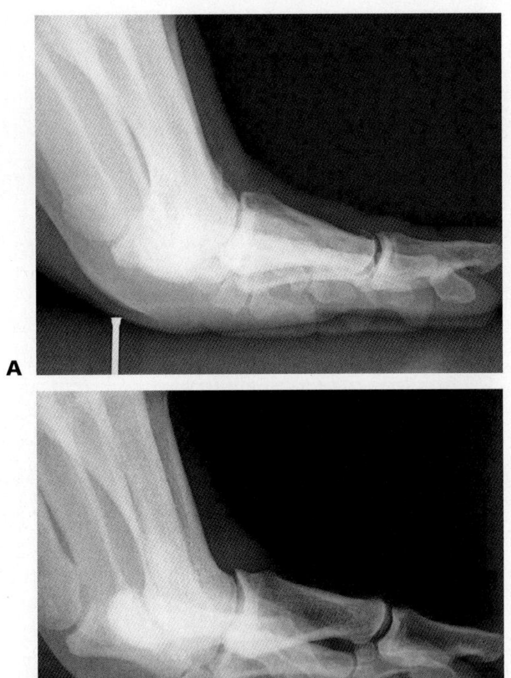

FIG 4 • Dorsiflexion stress lateral radiographs. **A.** Normal. Note the position of the sesamoids. **B.** Abnormal. Note the proximal migration of the sesamoid complex.

- Bilateral standing AP views are recommended for comparison.
- Forced (stress) dorsiflexion lateral views are helpful to diagnose diastasis of a bipartite sesamoid or a sesamoid fracture (**FIG 4**). It will also suggest distal disruption of the FHB if the sesamoid complex migrates proximally. Studies suggest that more than 10.4 mm from the tip of the tibial sesamoid to the phalanx or more than 13.3 mm from the fibular sesamoid equates to a 99.7% chance for plantar complex rupture.[11]
- Fluoroscopic evaluation has proven invaluable and is highly recommended when available. The hallux is dorsiflexed and if the sesamoids do not migrate distally, a plantar plate disruption can be inferred.
- MRI is recommended for any patient with radiographic abnormalities and for those with significant swelling, any ecchymosis or limitation of motion, or a positive vertical Lachman test (**FIG 5**). Osteochondral lesions and edema in the metatarsal head are often present and may be prognostic.

DIFFERENTIAL DIAGNOSIS

- Chondral or osteochondral lesion of the hallux metatarsal head
- Hyperflexion injury (sand toe)[6]
- Fracture of the proximal or distal phalanx of the hallux

NONOPERATIVE MANAGEMENT

- Rest, ice, elevation, and nonsteroidal anti-inflammatories[4]
- Immobilization with a boot or cast. A toe spica cast with the hallux in plantarflexion relieves tension on the injured plantar complex (**FIG 6**).

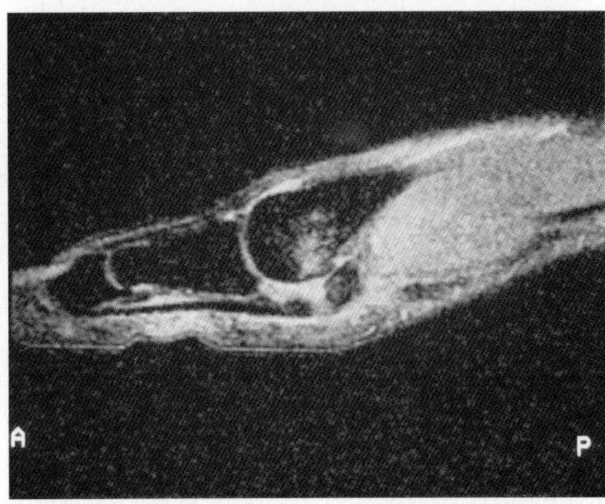

FIG 5 • Sagittal T2-weighted MR image showing distal soft tissue defect and proximal position of the sesamoid.

- Corticosteroid injections are avoided, especially in the athlete, to avoid rupture or further weakening of the capsular–ligamentous complex. Corticosteroids can mask unstable injuries that, if not addressed, can lead to hallux deformity and permanent loss of push-off strength.
- Taping of the hallux with a dorsal band to prevent excessive dorsiflexion
- Inserts, including off-the-shelf orthotics and custom devices that include the Morton extension to stiffen the first ray

SURGICAL MANAGEMENT

- Operative treatment should be considered for large capsular avulsions with an unstable joint; diastasis of a bipartite sesamoid or a sesamoid fracture; retraction of the sesamoids (single or both), traumatic bunion, or progressive hallux valgus; a positive vertical Lachman test; and the presence of a loose body or chondral injury.
- Serial examinations may be needed to document progressive varus–valgus or cock-up deformities, but ideally early diagno-

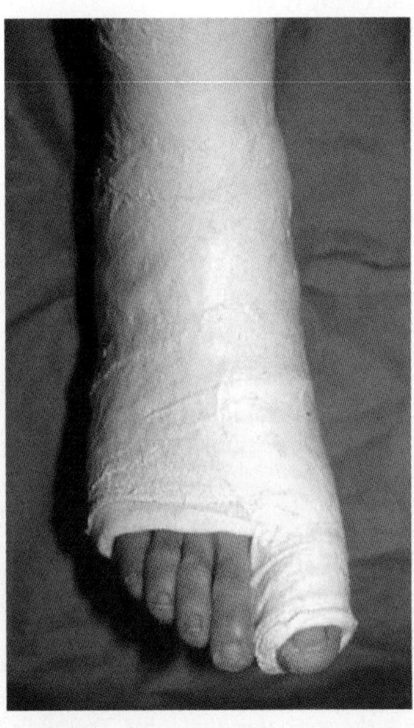

FIG 6 • Plaster toe spica cast for conservative or postoperative care of a turf toe injury.

sis and appropriate surgical repair of the injury are performed before these late sequelae develop.

Preoperative Planning

- The degree and exact location of the injury are determined before surgery. MRI is a useful preoperative tool to ascertain the area of involvement but may exaggerate the true extent of the injury by revealing adjacent edema.

Positioning

- While the patient may be placed prone for direct access to the sesamoid complex, we routinely perform surgical repair of turf toe injuries with the patient in the supine position. It is ideal to have the operative extremity in slight external rotation since the approach is largely medial. If the patient's natural tendency is not external rotation, then a bump can be placed under the contralateral hip or the table can be tilted toward the operative side.

Approach

- Described approaches include a plantar-medial, medial and plantar-lateral, and the J configuration. Over the past 3 years, we have employed the combined medial and plantar-lateral approach in patients suspected of having a complete plantar plate disruption. This approach allows for a more direct repair of the lateral structures without extensive skin and neurovascular dissection and retraction. Improved wound healing has been noted anecdotally (**FIG 7**).

A

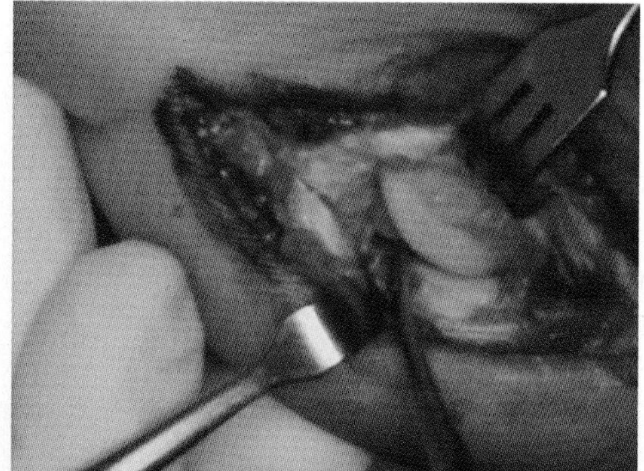

B

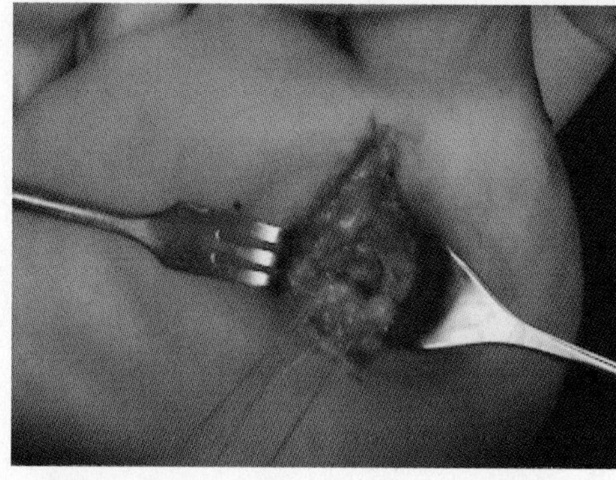

FIG 7 • Intraoperative photograph of the medial (**A**) and plantar-lateral (**B**) incisions about the hallux metatarsophalangeal joint used for exposure and repair of the plantar plate rupture.

TECHNIQUES

INCISION

- In this example, the surgeon has elected to use the J incision, which extends plantar-medial and then crosses plantarly along the flexor crease at the base of the phalanx (TECH FIG 1).
- Take extreme care to identify and protect the plantar-medial digital nerve (TECH FIG 2).
- Make a longitudinal incision at the level of the abductor hallucis tendon (TECH FIG 3). This allows both intra- and extra-articular examination of the plantar complex.
- Fully define the extent of the injury (TECH FIG 4).
- Once the defect has been fully defined, distally mobilize the plantar plate and sesamoid complex.

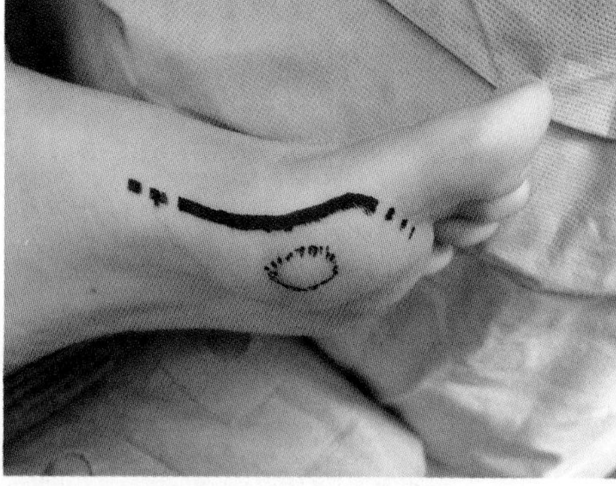

TECH FIG 1 • Planned hallux incision. This hockey-stick or J incision allows full exposure of the medial and plantar aspect of the metatarsophalangeal joint. The tibial sesamoid is outlined.

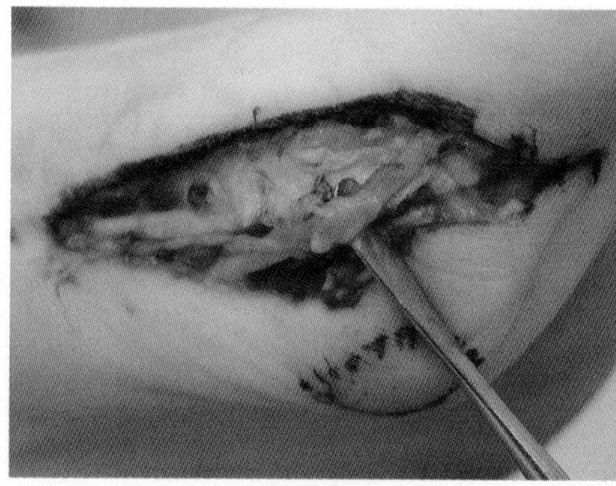

TECH FIG 2 • Intraoperative photograph showing identification and mobilization of the plantar-medial digital nerve.

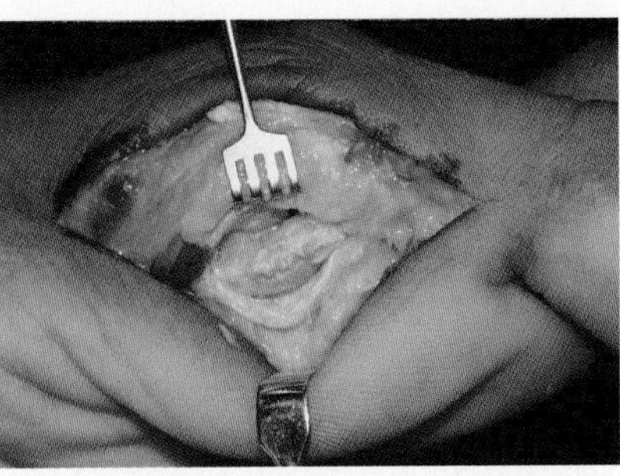

TECH FIG 3 • Longitudinal incision at the abductor hallucis and capsule allows visualization of the joint.

- In complete plantar ruptures, both sesamoids will be proximally retracted but will slide distally around the flexor hallucis longus (FHL) tendon.
- In chronic cases, this requires removal of fibrous scar tissue. Protect the FHL tendon while débriding scar tissue.
- Thoroughly examine the FHL tendon for longitudinal tears (TECH FIG 5). In our experience, longitudinal tears of the FHL tendon are most commonly associated with a late presentation of turf toe injury in which the FHL is subjected to frequent greater-than-physiologic stretching as a result of the lack of plantar restraint of the MP joint.

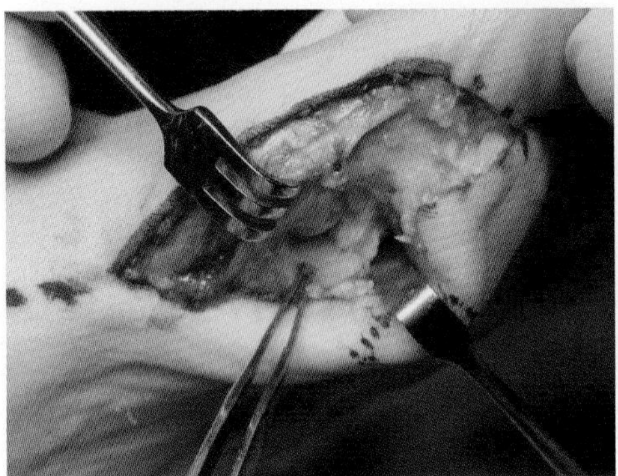

TECH FIG 4 • After exposure, the extent of the injury must be defined. This involves identifying each element of the plantar complex to determine its integrity.

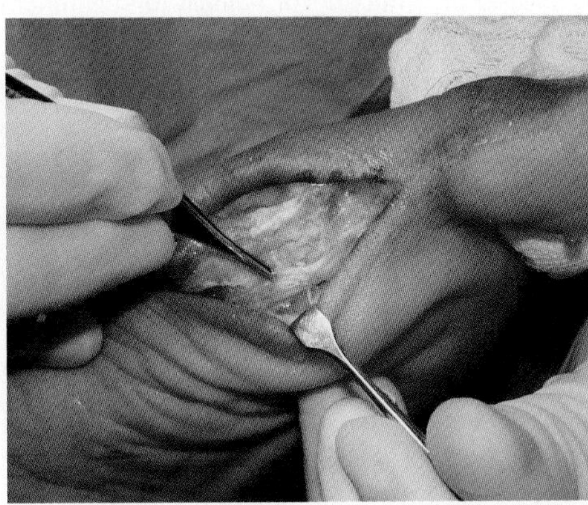

TECH FIG 5 • The flexor hallucis longus tendon is inspected for longitudinal tears and repaired primarily if necessary.

REPAIR OF DISTAL RUPTURES

- Make the J incision and identify the plantar-medial digital nerve where it crosses obliquely immediately deep to the planned incision. Once the nerve is identified, carefully retract it throughout the surgery, but with intermittent relaxation to limit the risk of a traction neuralgia.
- Make an incision at the level of the abductor hallucis tendon to allow examination of the MP joint.
- Identify the components of the plantar complex, including FHB, FHL, sesamoids, intersesamoid ligament, transverse and oblique heads of adductor hallucis, and plantar capsule. This step may take some time, depending on the degree of disruption and the time from injury.
- In acute cases, a rim of stout capsule typically remains on the base of the proximal phalanx. In the chronic situation, the sesamoid complex may appear redundant, often due to intervening scar tissue or elongated, weakened soft tissues at the site of injury (TECH FIG 6). We recommend excising the redundant scar tissue sharply and advancing the proximal intact and healthy portion of the complex (TECH FIG 7).

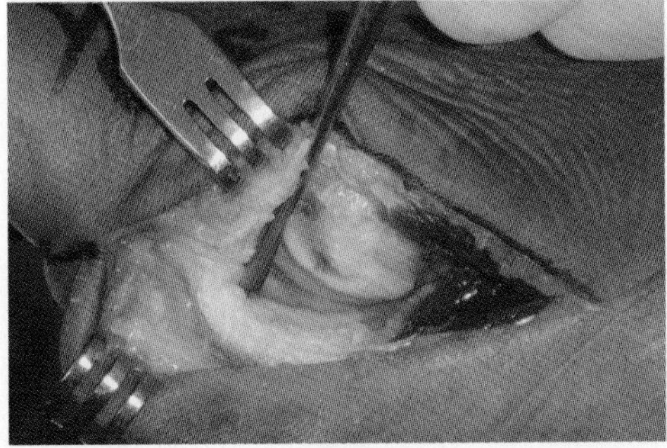

TECH FIG 6 • Turf toe variant with intact but redundant plantar complex.

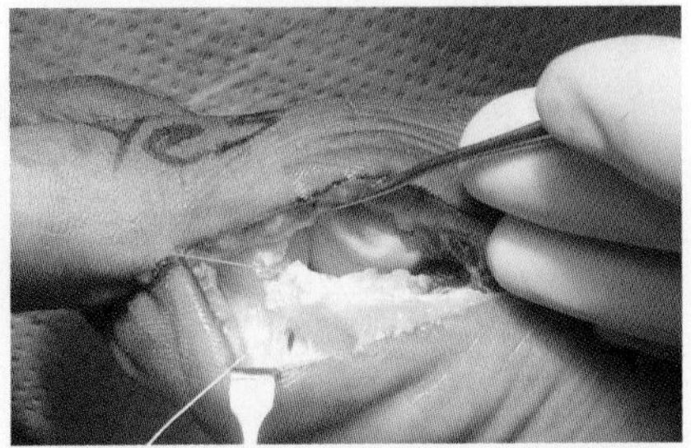

TECH FIG 7 • Redundant tissue is transversely excised and the remaining defect is repaired primarily.

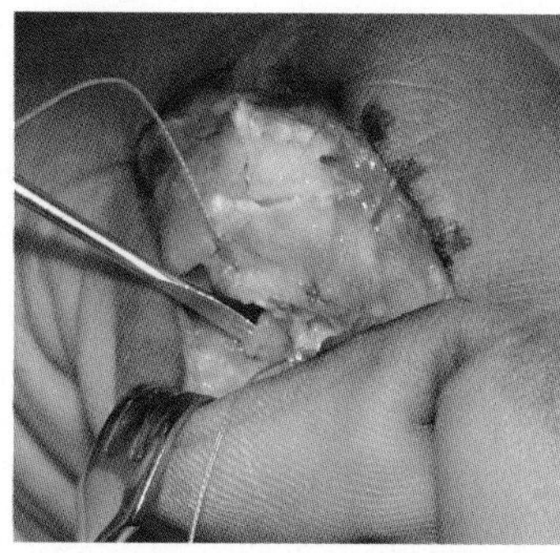

TECH FIG 8 • Repair proceeding from lateral to medial and working around the intact flexor hallucis longus tendon.

- Distal ruptures require primary repair of remnants from lateral to medial, working around the FHL tendon (TECH FIG 8).
- If the soft tissue is contracted and cannot be advanced to allow a primary repair, the FHB and abductor hallucis may be fractionally lengthened.
- If soft tissues are inadequate, suture anchors or drill holes to the plantar aspect of the base of the proximal phalanx may be used (TECH FIG 9). A drill hole can also be created in the distal pole of the tibial sesamoid if there is an absence of soft tissue for repair on the proximal aspect.
- Close the wound using standard techniques.

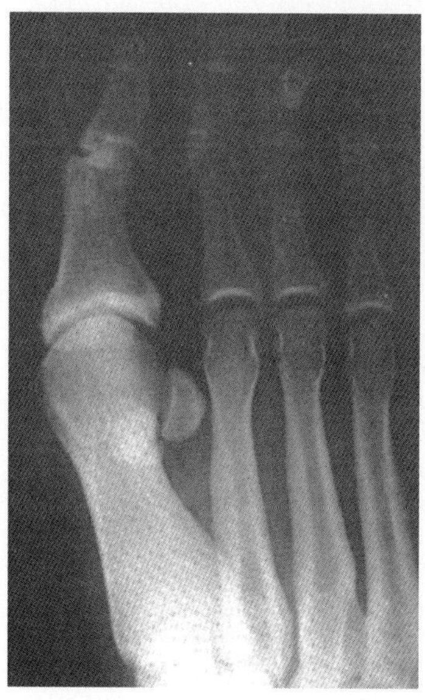

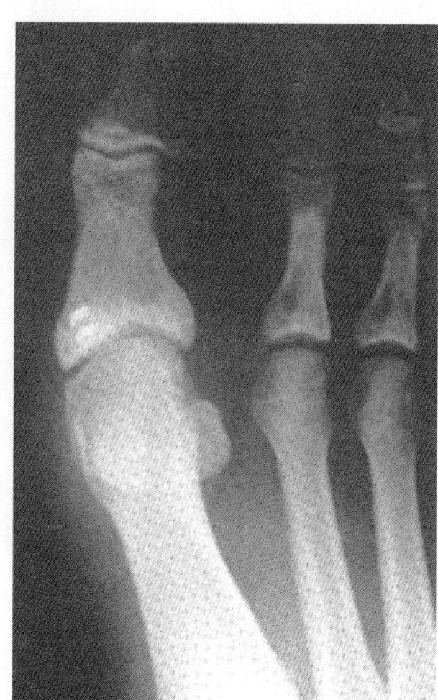

TECH FIG 9 • **A.** In the absence of healthy tissue at the base of the proximal phalanx, suture anchors can be used to advance the plantar complex. **B.** Radiograph showing anchors in the proximal phalanx.

REPAIR OF DIASTASIS OR FRACTURE OF THE TIBIAL SESAMOID

- Make a J incision, and protect the plantar-medial digital nerve. Retract the abductor superiorly.
- Identify the FHB with the associated tibial sesamoid.
- Diastasis or fracture of the tibial sesamoid may occasionally be repaired with a small-diameter cannulated screw. However, often comminuted fractures, particularly those in chronic injuries, are, in our opinion, better treated with excision of both poles of the fractured sesamoid. Sharply excise each osseous fragment from the FHB tendon. Repair the resulting soft tissue defect primarily (TECH FIG 10). A grasping tendinous stitch or simply a figure 8 stitch will usually suffice. Take care to avoid incorporating the FHL tendon in the repair.

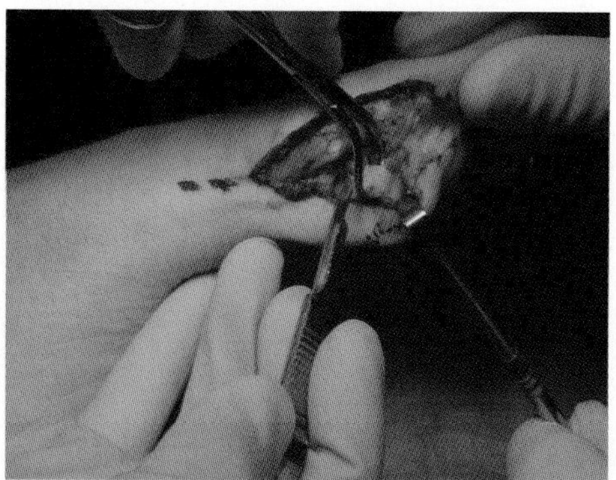

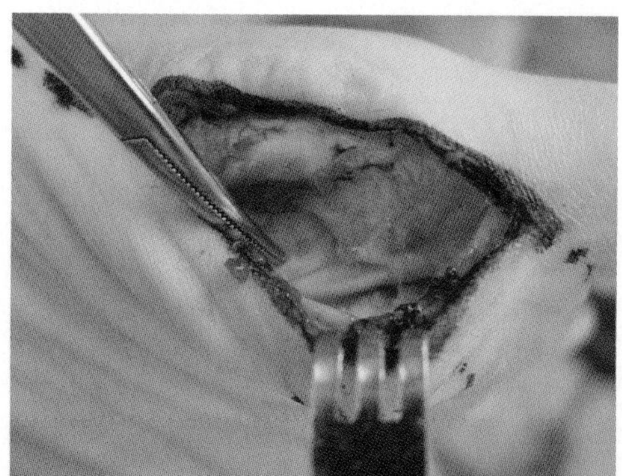

TECH FIG 10 • Repair of injury involving a tibial sesamoid fracture. **A.** The fragments are excised. **B.** The remaining void is often significant. *(continued)*

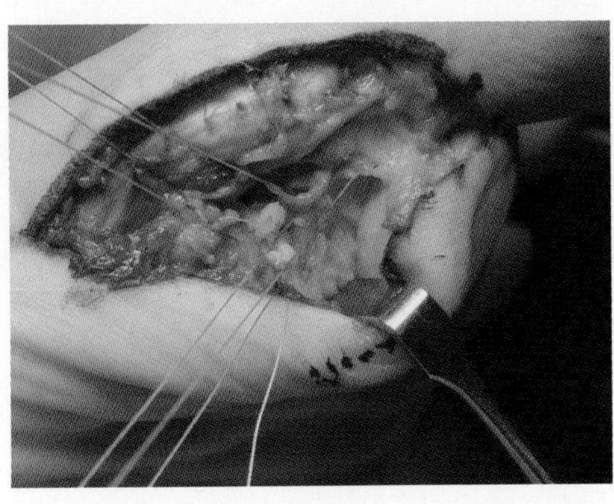

TECH FIG 10 • *(continued)* **C.** An attempt is made to close the void primarily with approximation of adjacent tissue.

- We maintain a low threshold to transfer the abductor hallucis tendon to the resulting plantar defect (**TECH FIG 11**). The distal aspect of the abductor hallucis tendon is easily elevated from its attachment on the proximal phalanx and rotated plantarly into the defect created by tibial sesamoid excision, where it is secured to the FHB tendon. This transfer affords not only an improved soft tissue closure of the defect but also, we believe, a dynamic component to strengthen the repair.
- Perform routine closure.

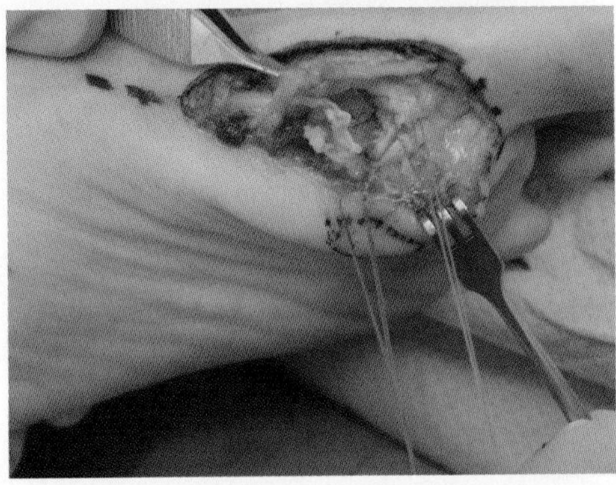

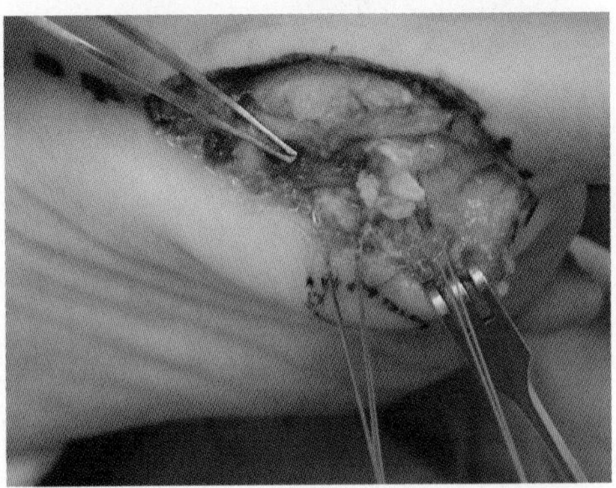

TECH FIG 11 • **A.** Advancement of the abductor hallucis tendon into the defect after sesamoid excision. The rerouted abductor tendon now serves as a flexor tendon. **B.** The abductor tendon has been advanced and secured.

REPAIR OF BOTH FIBULAR AND TIBIAL SESAMOIDS

- Use the standard J incision and the aforementioned approach.
- Isolate each fragment of both the tibial and fibular sesamoids. Reduce the corresponding fragments with a pointed reduction forceps.
- Due to the small size of the sesamoids and because comminution is often present, internal fixation can be difficult, with resultant further fragmentation of the sesamoids.
- Therefore, Cerclage the proximal and distal poles of the sesamoids using nonabsorbable suture (**TECH FIG 12**). Then repair the adjacent soft tissue.
- If the articular surface of the sesamoid is damaged or demonstrates significant cystic change or fragmentation within the sesamoid body, excise it. The defect is managed with an abductor tendon transfer as described above.
- If at all possible, avoid excising both sesamoids, as it may lead to a cock-up hallux toe deformity. If both sesamoids are painful and pathologic, it is best to stage the sesamoidectomies to lessen the risk for this complication.

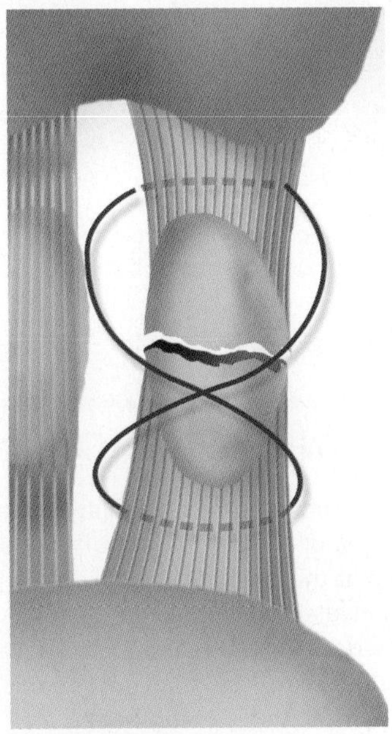

TECH FIG 12 • Standard cerclage technique used to repair a fractured or diastased sesamoid.

REPAIR OF TRAUMATIC BUNION

- In essence, this repair is a modified McBride bunionectomy or distal soft tissue procedure. Release the adductor hallucis tendon via a longitudinal incision in the dorsum of the first web space (**TECH FIG 13**). Transect it and elevate it off the lateral sesamoid.
- Make a medial incision and perform a longitudinal capsulotomy (**TECH FIG 14**).
- Perform a conservative excision of the bunion exostosis (**TECH FIG 15**). This assists with scarring of the medial structures.
- Identify the medial defects and repair them primarily as described above, followed by routine closure (**TECH FIG 16**).

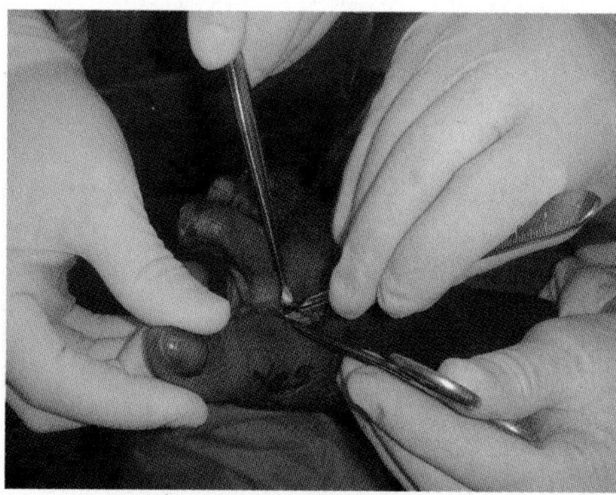

TECH FIG 13 • Incision and release of adductor hallucis in a traumatic bunion.

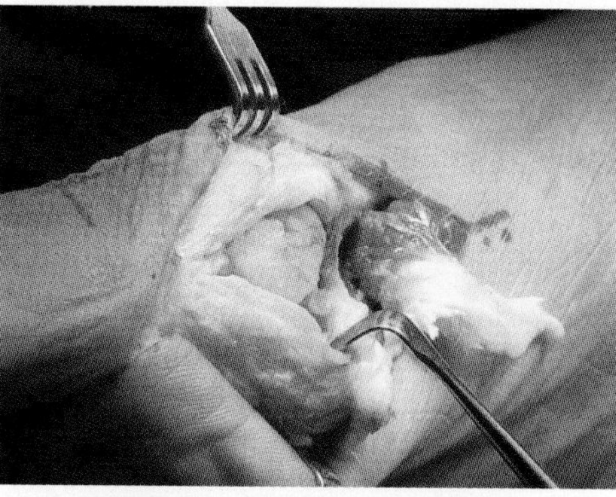

TECH FIG 14 • Standard J incision is performed followed by capsulotomy to expose the medial eminence.

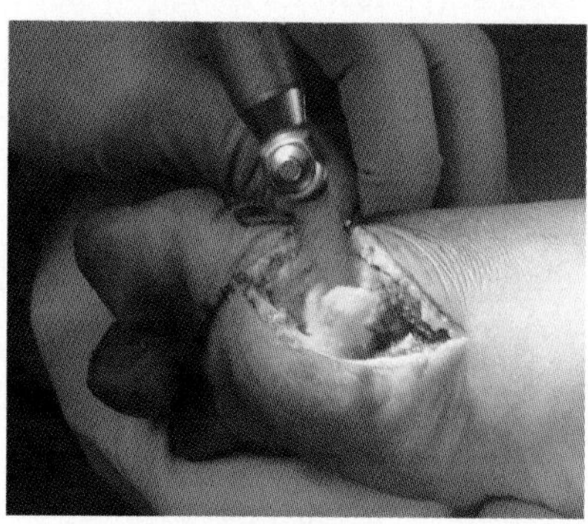

TECH FIG 15 • Intraoperative picture of a conservative medial eminence resection for a traumatic bunion.

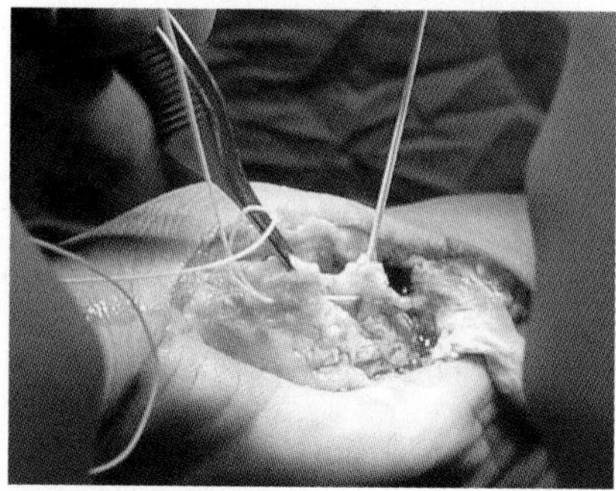

TECH FIG 16 • Primary capsular repair and advancement after medial eminence resection for a traumatic bunion.

CORRECTION OF LATE COCK-UP HALLUX DEFORMITY

- A sequela of untreated turf toe injury is the cock-up hallux deformity, or hyperextension of the hallux MP joint and flexion at the hallux IP joint.
- Perform a medial incision.
- Often, the dorsal capsule and extensor hallucis longus and brevis are contracted and must be released. The extensors may need to be Z-lengthened.
- Release the FHL as far distal as possible at its insertion into the distal phalanx. Make a dorsal-to-plantar drill hole in the proximal phalanx toward its base. Route the FHL tendon from plantar to dorsal through the osseous tunnel and secure it dorsally. A small interference screw may be used, or the tendon can simply be secured with a nonabsorbable suture.

PEARLS AND PITFALLS

Proper diagnosis	■ Attention to history and physical examination is paramount. An MRI is ordered if any concern for an unstable situation exists.
Progressive deformity	■ With injuries managed nonsurgically, serial examinations allow the physician to appreciate a tendency for progressive deformity. Surgical repair is recommended before the deformity leads to late sequelae such as traumatic bunion or cock-up deformity.
Plantar-medial soft tissue defects	■ These defects, typically noted after medial sesamoid excision, may be augmented with transfer of the abductor hallucis tendon into the defect.

POSTOPERATIVE CARE

- Postoperative care is a delicate balance between soft tissue protection and early hallux MP range of motion, avoiding arthrofibrosis of the sesamoid–metatarsal articulation.
- Gentle passive range of motion (plantarflexion) is initiated under supervision at 7 to 10 days after surgery.
- The patient remains non–weight-bearing in a removable splint or boot with the hallux protected for 4 weeks.
- At 4 weeks the patient is allowed to initiate active motion of the joint and ambulate in a boot.
- Modified shoe wear consisting of a turf toe plate (aluminum, steel, or carbon fiber) is instituted at 2 months.
- Return to contact activity occurs at 3 to 4 months, with protection from excessive dorsiflexion. Return to play depends on the player's position, level of discomfort, and healing potential.
- Full recovery is expected to take 6 to 12 months. Shoe modifications are generally needed for at least 6 months after return to play. In general, this correlates to the presence of 50 to 60 degrees of painless passive range of motion of the hallux MP joint.

OUTCOMES

- Clanton et al[3] found that half of 20 athletes had persistent symptoms, including stiffness and pain, at 5-year follow-up.
- Anderson et al[11] report that 17 of 19 college and professional athletes returned to full athletic activity with minimal residual discomfort after surgical repair of a turf toe injury.

COMPLICATIONS

- As with any surgery, infection and wound problems are potential complications. Athletes may be at increased risk if they attempt to initiate rehabilitation too early.
- Transient neuritis of the plantar-medial digital nerve at the level of the hallux MP joint is common due to retraction of the nerve during surgery. However, a transection and secondary neuroma may result in significant discomfort and difficulty with shoe wear and push-off.
- Disruption of the repair may result with excessive dorsiflexion during the early rehabilitation process.
- Inadequate rehabilitation or prolonged immobilization can cause significant hallux MP stiffness.

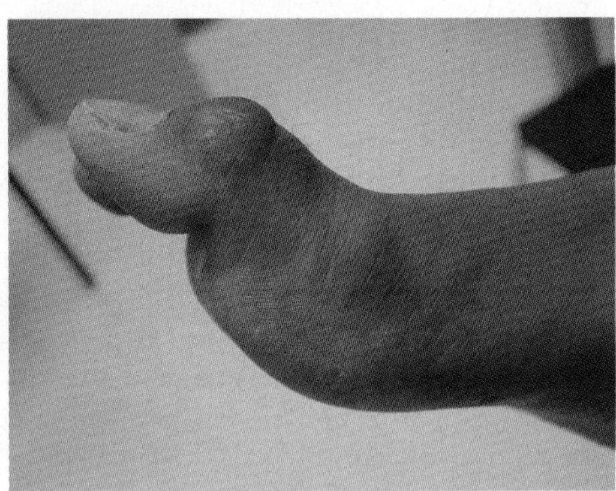

FIG 8 • Hallux claw toe after a missed turf toe injury.

- A missed or delayed diagnosis can lead to progressive hallux varus or valgus or cock-up deformity (**FIG 8**).

REFERENCES

1. Anderson RB. Turf toe injuries of the hallux metatarsophalangeal joint. Tech Foot Ankle Surg 2002;1:102–111.
2. Bowers KD Jr, Martin RB. Turf-toe: a shoe-surface related football injury. Med Sci Sports Exerc 1976;8:81–83.
3. Clanton TO, Butler JE, Eggert A. Injuries to the metatarsophalangeal joints in athletes. Foot Ankle 1986;7:162–176.
4. Clanton TO, Ford JJ. Turf toe injury. Clin Sports Med 1994;13: 731–741.
5. Coker TP, Arnold JA, Weber DL. Traumatic lesions of the metatarsophalangeal joint of the great toe in athletes. Am J Sports Med 1978;6:326–334.
6. Frey C, Andersen GD, Feder KS. Plantarflexion injury to the metatarsophalangeal joint ("sand toe"). Foot Ankle 1996;17:576–581.
7. Jones DC, Reiner MR. Turf toe. Foot Ankle Clin 1999;4:911–917.
8. McCormick JJ, Anderson RB. The great toe: failed turf toe, chronic turf toe, and complicated sesamoid injuries. Foot Ankle Clin 2009; 14:135–150.
9. Rodeo SA, O'Brien S, Warren RF, et al. Turf-toe: an analysis of metatarsophalangeal joint sprains in professional football players. Am J Sports Med 1990;18:280–285.
10. Rodeo SA, Warren RF, O'Brien SJ, et al. Diastasis of bipartite sesamoids of the first metatarsophalangeal joint. Foot Ankle 1993; 14:425–434.
11. Watson T, Anderson R, Davis W. Periarticular injuries to the hallux metatarsophalangeal joint in athletes. Foot Ankle Clin 2000;5: 687–713.

Chapter 29

Internal Fixation of Sesamoid Fractures

Geert I. Pagenstert, Victor Valderrabano, and Beat Hintermann

DEFINITION

- *Hallux sesamoid bone fracture* is a break through the sesamoid bone or cartilage. Medial sesamoid bone fractures are more common than lateral sesamoid bone fractures.[1,15]
- Fractures usually occur about perpendicular to the long axis of the elliptically shaped bone. Longitudinal and comminuted fractures are less common.[5,17]
- In partite or bipartite sesamoid bones, the fracture always occurs in the fibrocartilaginous junctional zone (most often perpendicular to the long axis), which can disguise the fracture.[15]

ANATOMY

- The hallux sesamoid bones usually are 13.5 ± 3 mm long. The sesamoid bones are larger in men than in women, and the medial sesamoid is more elliptically shaped and larger compared to the more circularly shaped lateral sesamoid.[14]
- The hallux sesamoid bones are invested in the tendon sheath of the flexor hallucis brevis. They connect with the intersesamoid ligament to form a solid pedestal to elevate the first ray and absorb stress during gait[2,3,14] (**FIG 1A**).
- The sesamoid complex acts as a fulcrum to the flexor hallucis brevis and longus tendons, increasing their lever arms and big toe push-off power, e.g., the patella to the quadriceps tendon[2,3] (**FIG 1B**).
- Failure of the bone to ossify completely during childhood results in a multi-part sesamoid bone. Bipartite sesamoids are much more common than those with three or more parts. Despite incomplete ossification, the sesamoid parts are firmly connected with fibrocartilaginous tissue to act as one bone. Spontaneous fusion can occur later in life.[10]
- Partite sesamoid bones are bilateral in only about 25% of cases; therefore, unilaterality cannot be relied upon as a criterion of fracture.[10]
- The main blood supply is provided over the posterior tibial to the medial plantar artery to the sesamoids. Considerable variation exists, however, such as the main blood supply from the lateral plantar artery or even the dorsal arterial arch.[7,14]
- In general, only one major artery pierces the cortex of the sesamoid bone at the plantar aspect of the proximal pole. Small vessels also enter from the plantar nonarticular side and over the capsular attachments as a second source of vascularity.[7,14]

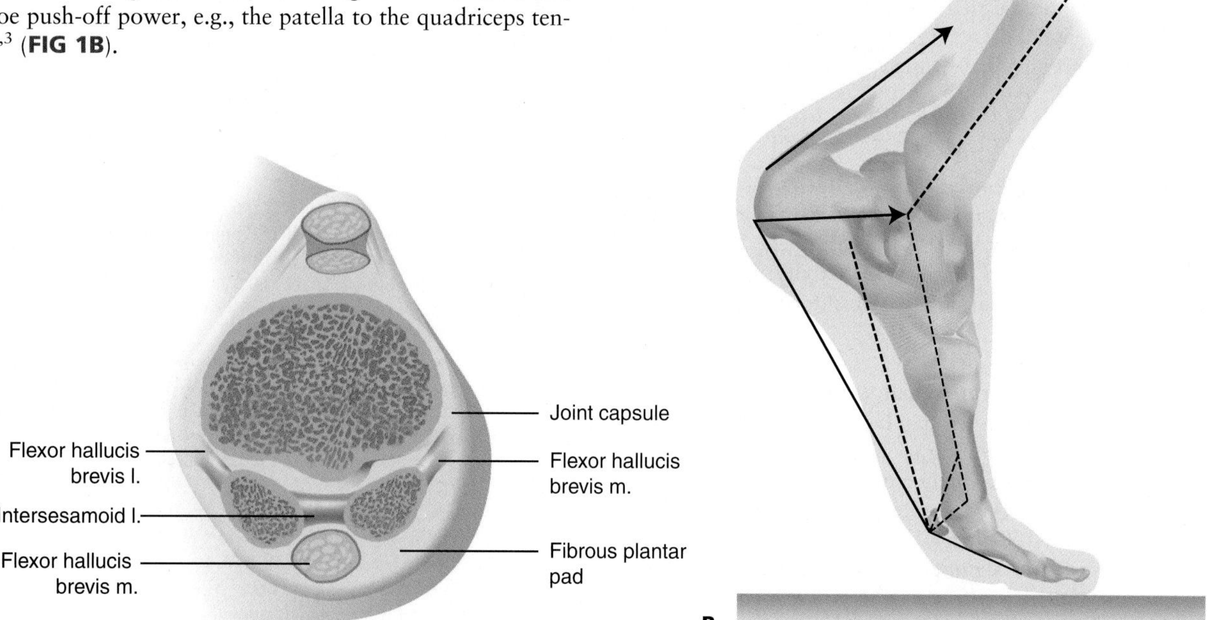

FIG 1 • Anatomy and biomechanics of the hallux sesamoid complex. **A.** The sesamoids elevate the first metatarsal bone. Fifty percent or more of body weight is transferred over the first ray. With sesamoid excision, preloading of the metatarsal bone is decreased, transferring the load to the lesser toes. **B.** Sesamoid bones increase the lever arm of the hallucis brevis and hallucis longus flexor tendons. Sesamoid excision reduces this lever and subsequently reduces push-off power of the big toe. (**A:** From Aper RL, Saltzman CL, Brown TD. The effect of hallux sesamoid resection on the effective moment of the flexor hallucis brevis. Foot Ankle Int 1994;15:462–470; **B:** From Aper RL, Saltzman CL, Brown TD. The effect of hallux sesamoid excision on the flexor hallucis longus moment arm. Clin Orthop Relat Res 1996;325:209–217.)

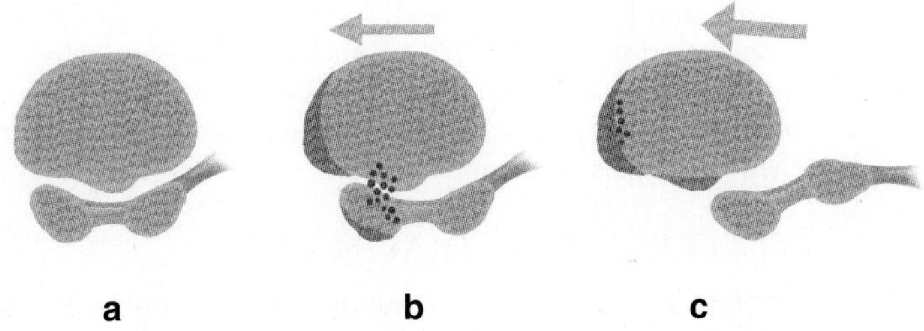

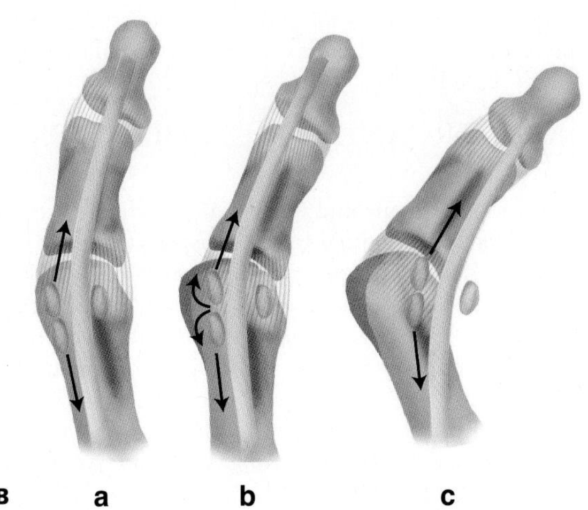

FIG 2 • Biomechanics of the sesamoid complex in hallux valgus deformity. **A.** Varus subluxation of the first metatarsal bone causes pressure concentration to the medial sesamoid bone. The intersesamoid crista enhances friction to the sesamoid joint surface. **B.** After stress fracture occurs, hallux deviation will cause constant fragment displacement. Therefore, immobilization may not suffice. Sesamoid excision will enhance hallux deviation if the deformity is not addressed. (**A,B:** From Pagenstert GI, Valderrabano V, Hintermann B. Medial sesamoid nonunion combined with hallux valgus in athletes. Foot Ankle Int 2006;27:135–140.)

PATHOGENESIS

- Acute trauma or chronic overuse leads to acute or stress fractures, respectively, of the sesamoid bones.[1,15]
- In the acute setting, the typical mechanism is excessive hyperextension of the big toe, also referred to as the "turf toe" injury seen in American football players. Disruption of the plantar joint capsule occurs as a trans-sesamoidal fracture–dislocation of the first metatarsophalangeal (MTP) joint.[15]
- Typically, in the chronic setting, no trauma is remembered. Pain and swelling increase insidiously over weeks, months, or years. Diagnosis is significantly delayed. Endurance sports such as running and dancing have shown to be associated with chronic stress fractures of the hallux sesamoid bones.[5,12]
- Foot deformities that concentrate pressure to the sesamoids increase the chance of suffering sesamoid stress fractures in both athletic and nonathletic persons. Cavus foot deformities with a steep plantar flexed first ray stress both sesamoid bones. Hallux valgus deformity with varus dislocation of the metatarsal head leads to pressure concentration at the medial sesamoid bone only[12,13] (**FIG 2**).

NATURAL HISTORY

- Acute fractures without mild dislocation heal normally with little or even no treatment.[15]
- Chronic stress fractures usually do not heal without surgery, which is explained by the typical pathogenesis described earlier. During the prolonged time to diagnosis and the constant friction of fracture fragments, necrotic tissue accumulates at the fracture site and prevents healing. Brodsky et al,[6] Van Hal et al,[17] and Saxena and Krisdakumtorn[16] independently reported on consecutive series of athletes with chronic sesamoid fractures. None of the sesamoid fractures in their series healed, even with prolonged nonsurgical regimens. Histologic examination after sesamoid excision revealed accumulation of necrotic tissue at the fracture site.[6]
- Foot deformities can cause fragment separation and may prevent healing with immobilization.[12]

PATIENT HISTORY AND PHYSICAL FINDINGS

- The patient history and physical examination must rule out the differential diagnoses.
  - The typical patient history is discussed in the section Pathogenesis.
- The physical examination includes examination of areas of localized pain and swelling, and hyperextension testing of the big toe.
- Patients have localized pain and swelling around the first MTP joint (**FIG 3**).

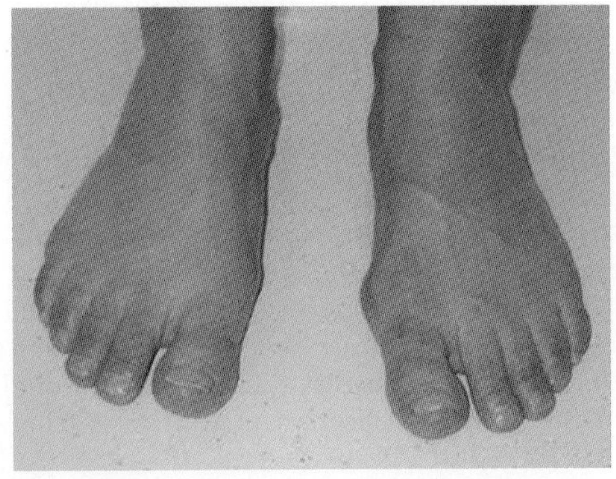

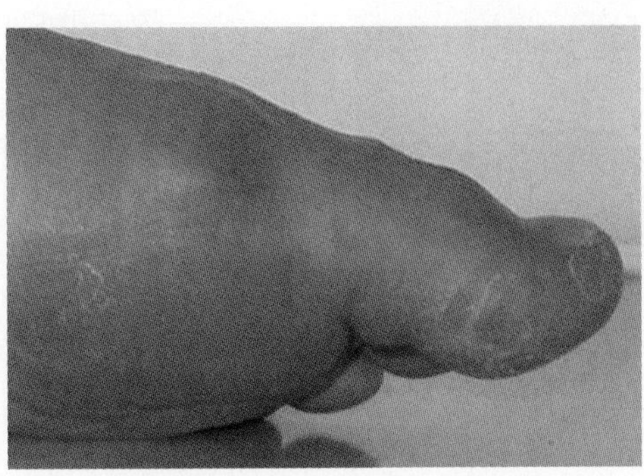

FIG 3 • Clinical appearance of sesamoid stress fracture. **A.** Swelling of the MTP joint with localized tenderness at the medial sesamoid bone. **B.** Evaluate the hallux valgus deformity on the left. Progression of the deformity was noted by the patient within the preceding 3 months.

- A complete examination of sesamoid status includes examination of the whole foot and ankle, with special attention to cavus deformity with a flexed first ray or hallux valgus deformity [12] (see Fig 2B).

IMAGING AND OTHER DIAGNOSTIC STUDIES

- Sesamoid oblique and tangential ("skyline") views are useful to evaluate sesamoid fracture displacement (**FIG 4A**).
- Partite sesamoid bones are bilateral in only about 25% of cases.[10] Therefore, radiographs of the contralateral foot do not rule out fracture. In addition, fractures of bipartite sesamoid bones occur at the fibrocartilaginous junctional zone.[15]
- A longitudinal CT scan of the foot has been shown to be very effective in demonstrating sesamoid stress fracture in difficult settings[4] (**FIG 4B**).
- MRI[11] and bone scans[8] are nonspecific for diagnosing stress fracture or distinguishing between a traumatized bipartite sesamoid and a stress fracture. Bone edema is seen on MRI in bone contusion, inflammatory disease, avascular necrosis, and infection.[11] Localized sesamoid scintigraphic activity has been demonstrated in about 26% to 29% of cases in asymptomatic active and sedentary populations.[8]
- On full weight-bearing radiographs of the lateral whole foot, the angle between the talus and the first metatarsal is evaluated. In a normal foot, it is straight or in up to 10 degrees of flexion. A greater amount of flexion demonstrates a flexed first ray, whereas flexion of less than 0 degrees demonstrates medial arch insufficiency, which is connected with hallux valgus formation.
- On full weight-bearing dorsoplantar radiographs of the foot, the hallux valgus, sesamoid position, metatarsus primus varus, and talo–first metatarsal angle are evaluated for stress concentration to the medial sesamoid bone. The talonavicular joint congruence is examined to identify excessive forefoot abduction with pes plano valgus or excessive adduction with neurogenic pes cavo varus.

A
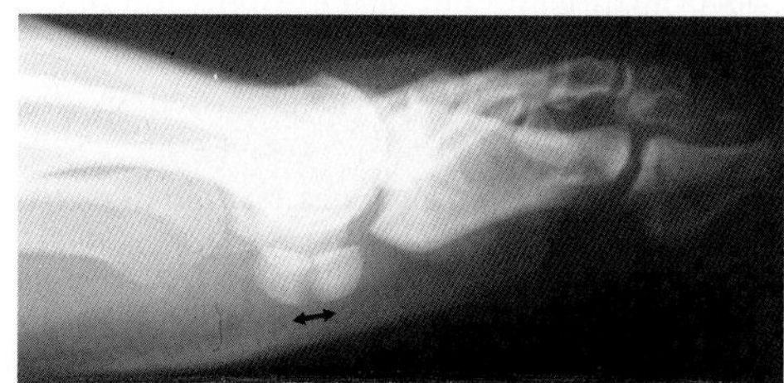
B
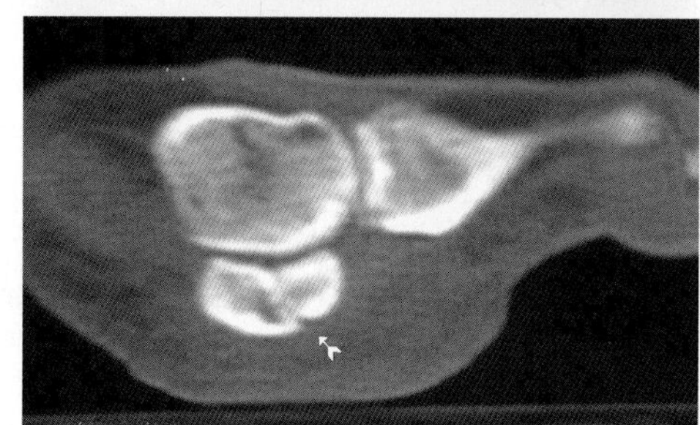

FIG 4 • Radiologic examination of sesamoid fractures. **A.** Conventional radiographs demonstrating horizontal sesamoid fracture dislocation. **B.** CT scan shows fracture line of chronic painful sesamoid, which was not visible on conventional radiographs.

DIFFERENTIAL DIAGNOSIS

- Hallux rigidus or sesamoid–first metatarsal bone osteoarthritis
- Hallux valgus
- First MTP joint capsuloligamentous disruptions (turf toe)
- Osteomyelitis and septic arthritis
- Podagra of gout and pseudogout
- Inflammatory arthritis
- Avascular necrosis of sesamoid or metatarsal head

NONOPERATIVE MANAGEMENT

- Acute fractures with up to 5 mm dislocation are treated with a forefoot immobilization shoe (stiff and convex sole) for 6 to 8 weeks.[15]
- Treatment of chronic fractures is controversial. Despite frequent failure after nonsurgical treatment attempts[5,6,12,13,16,17] and the already long time it takes to establish diagnosis, many physicians try immobilization with a shoe or cast, sometimes with the patient non–weight-bearing on crutches. Recommendations for the duration of this approach before surgery is advocated range from 6 to 12 weeks.[16,17]
- If the diagnosis of stress fracture was established soon after the symptoms began, activity modification and use of a stiff-soled shoe for 6 weeks may be successful. Modification in athletic training and eating habits, with running on soft ground only, a change of sole stiffness in the athletic shoe, and increased intake of calcium and vitamin D_3 may be reasonable adjuncts in the future.

SURGICAL MANAGEMENT

- Severe (>5 mm) acute trans-sesamoidal fracture dislocations of the first MTP joint require open repair of the capsule and flexor muscles.[15] The sesamoid bone fixation can be done with a compression screw or heavy no. 1 suture.
- Indications for percutaneous compression screw fixation include a transverse sesamoid stress fracture, transverse nonunion, or transverse symptomatic bipartite sesamoid. Fragments must be at least 3 mm to allow screw fixation.[13]
- Contraindications include infection, longitudinal sesamoid fractures, and comminuted fractures with multiple fragments that are too small for screw fixation. In these cases, partial or total sesamoid resection is indicated.
- Combined medial sesamoid fracture and hallux valgus deformity are best treated with conventional open correction of the hallux and open reduction and fixation of the sesamoid fracture by heavy no. 1 suture or compression screw.[12] Débridement of the necrotic fracture zone and grafting can be done to enhance healing.[1] In cases with less than 2 mm dislocation, the fracture zone can be stabilized by grafting only. The flexor brevis tendon sheath acts as tension band fixation.[1]

- In patients who are likely to be noncompliant, a temporary 2.5-mm K-wire can be placed through the first MTP joint to prevent hallux dorsiflexion and stress to the fragments.
- Combined hindfoot and first ray deformities with chronic sesamoid fractures must be addressed in the same surgery.[12]

Preoperative Planning

- Acute transsesamoidal fracture dislocations of the first MTP joint require open stabilization sometimes with an extended medioplantar L-shaped incision to reach the lateral aspect of the joint. Sesamoid fracture fixation is part of the plantar capsule or plate repair.[15]
- In chronic sesamoid fracture, preoperative planning should incorporate treatment of any underlying foot deformities.
  - A metatarsus primus flexus is treated with a dorsal extension osteotomy or arthrodesis.
  - A metatarsus primus varus and hallux valgus are addressed with appropriate osseous or soft tissue procedures.
  - Reduction of mechanical stress to the sesamoid bones is thought to be the main factor contributing to fracture healing. Surgical stress reduction alone may result in fracture healing even without sesamoid osteosynthesis in marked foot deformities.
- In the combined setting, medial sesamoid stress fractures are treated open because deformity correction is done at the same time as arthrotomy of the first MTP joint. Lateral sesamoid stress fractures are treated percutaneously, because deformity correction does not include arthrotomy of the first MTP joint.
- The least invasive approach can be used in the absence of foot deformities.
  - Chronic sesamoid fractures can be addressed by percutaneous compression screw fixation alone.
  - Surgery can be performed under local anesthesia, and the stab incision of the skin can be closed with Steri-Strips.
  - Healing is thought to occur because of reaming (vitalizing) of the fracture zone and fracture stabilization. Ossification of the bipartite sesamoids occurs.[13]
- Grafting of sesamoid nonunions (bipartite sesamoids) is inherently stabilized by the flexor brevis tendon sheath.[1] In cases of persistent instability after grafting, additional suture or screw fixation is advisable.

Positioning

- The patient is placed in the supine position for isolated sesamoid bone fixation or combined deformity corrections. A tourniquet is needed, except in percutaneous fixation.

Approach

- A medial internervous or medioplantar L-shaped approach to the lateral aspect of the first MTP joint is used for acute turf toe repair, including sesamoid fracture fixation or partial removal.[15]
- A standard medial internervous approach is used for grafting of medial sesamoid nonunions and combined hallux correction.[12]
- In the case of percutaneous fixation, a stab incision is made distal to the pole of the fractured sesamoid bone and distal to the weight-bearing area of the first MTP joint. Lateral sesamoid fractures usually are treated with percutaneous screw fixation.[13]

ANDERSON-MCBRYDE TECHNIQUE OF GRAFTING SESAMOID NONUNIONS[1]

- A medial internervous skin incision is made over the first MTP joint (TECH FIG 1A).
- Longitudinal capsulotomy and subperiosteal limited exposure of the medial sesamoid wall are done.
- Débridement of the necrotic tissue at the fracture site is performed with a small curette from an extra-articular medial approach (TECH FIG 1B).
- Fenestration of the MT head is performed to enable autologous bone harvesting (TECH FIG 1C).
- The sesamoid fracture zone is grafted and stuffed, with care not to disrupt the fracture line in the joint surface.
- If stability is in doubt, fixation with no. 1 resorbable suture is performed to leave the least amount of foreign material in situ. Cannulated compression screws are used as well and may provide higher compression. (Screw placement is described in the next section.)
- The suture needle is introduced from the proximal lateral pole along the internal lateral cortex to the distal lateral pole. Backstitching is done outside the bone under the medial sesamoid suspensory (capsule) ligament, back to the proximal medial pole, and knotted tight to stabilize the sesamoid joint line (TECH FIG 1D).
- The capsule and skin are closed as usual.
- A compressive dressing is applied with the foot in the neutral hallux position.

A

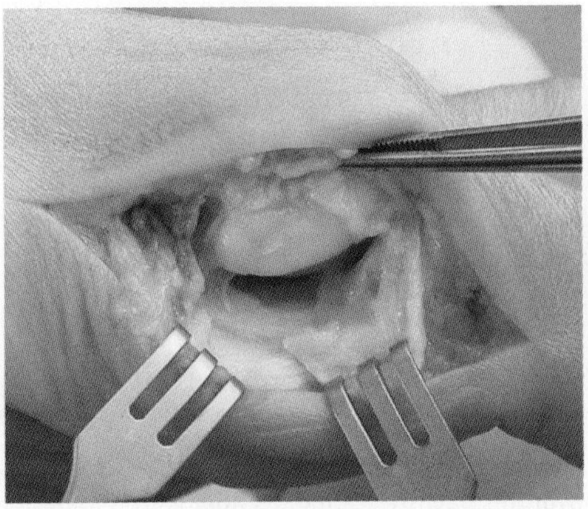

TECH FIG 1 • Anderson-McBryde technique. **A.** Medial internervous approach. *(continued)*

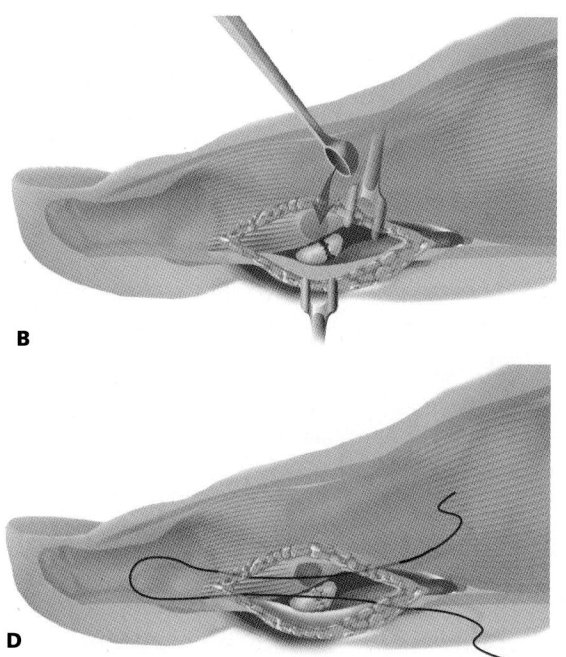

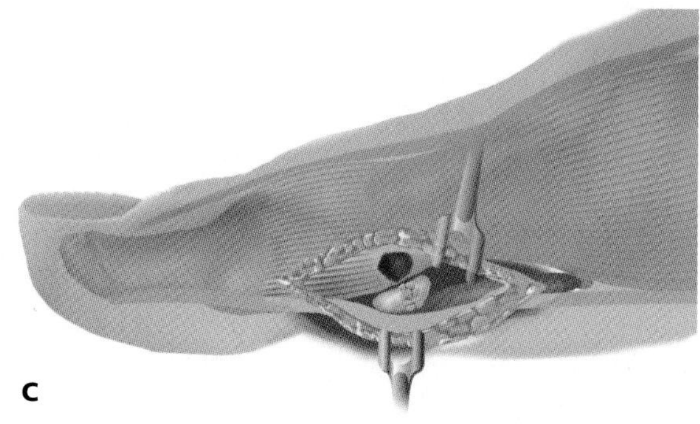

TECH FIG 1 • *(continued)* **B.** Débridement of the fracture with a small curette using an extra-articular approach to the necrotic tissue. **C.** Harvesting of autologous bone from the first metatarsal head. **D.** Suture cerclage of the fractured sesamoid.

PREFERRED TECHNIQUE OF PERCUTANEOUS SESAMOID SCREW FIXATION[13]

- The hallux is held in dorsiflexion, and the sesamoid bone is pressed against the MT head to level the fracture fragments against the joint line of the MT head (TECH FIG 2A).
- One 3-mm stab incision is done distal to the fractured sesamoid bone and distal to the weight-bearing area of the first MTP joint (TECH FIG 2B).
- The guidewire (1.5-mm wire for 2.4-mm self-tapping Bold screws [Newdeal, Lyon, France]) is introduced under fluoroscopic control from the distal pole, perpendicular to the fracture line and subchondral to the sesamoid joint line (TECH FIG 2C).

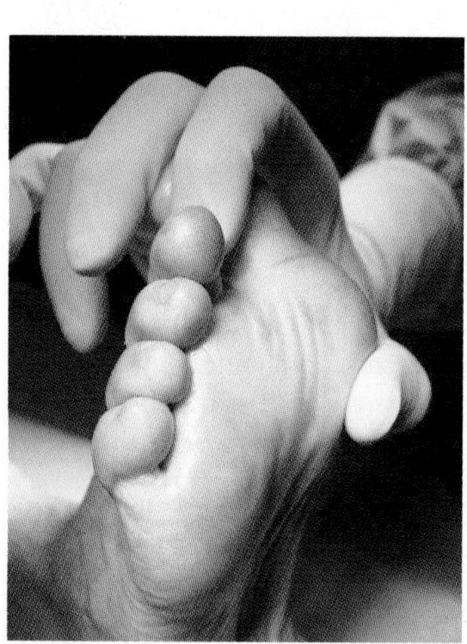

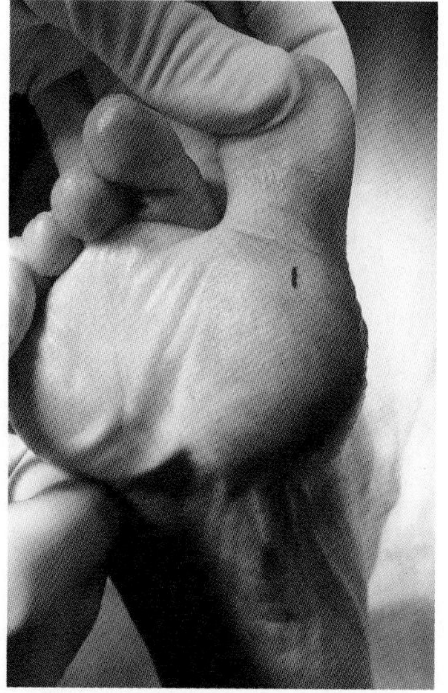

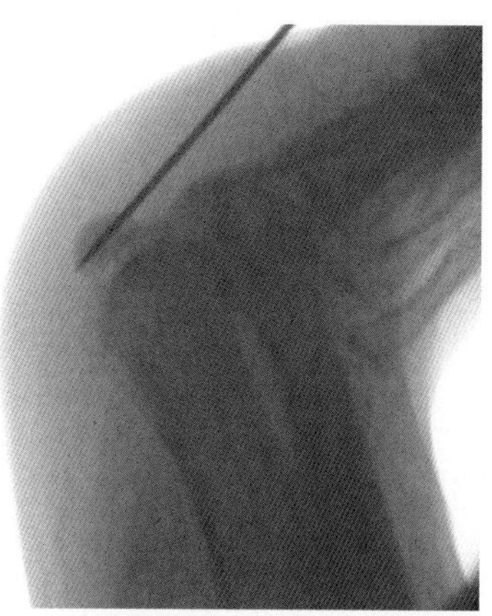

TECH FIG 2 • Preferred technique for percutaneous sesamoid screw fixation. **A.** Fixation of the hallux in hyperextension. Compress the sesamoid against the metatarsal head to level the fracture fragments against the joint line. **B.** Place the stab incision distal to the sesamoid outside the weight-bearing area of the MTP joint. **C.** Place the guidewire perpendicular to the fracture line, subchondral from proximal to distal. *(continued)*

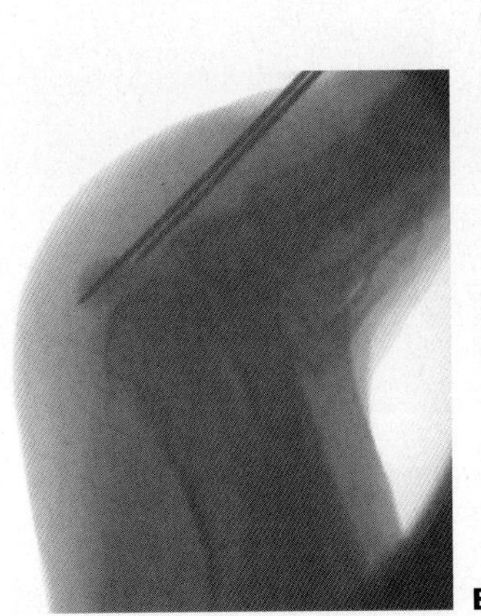

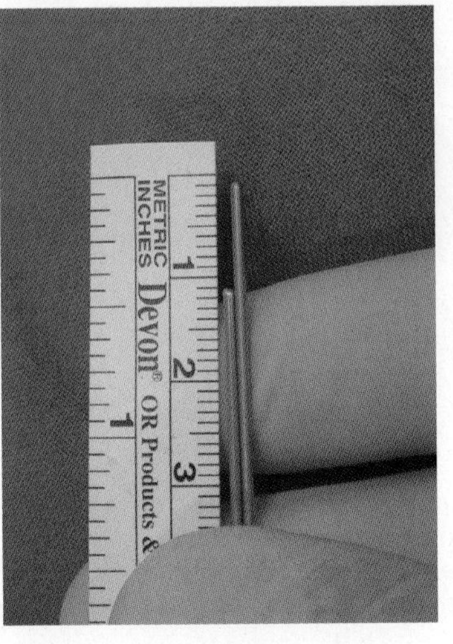

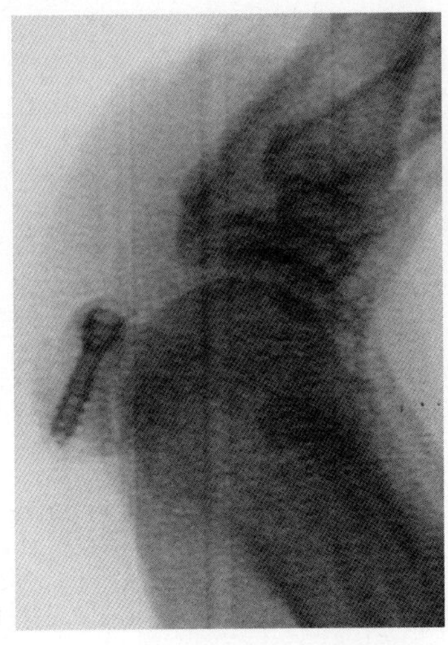

D E F

TECH FIG 2 • *(continued)* **D.** The guidewire should just pierce the proximal cortex. The second guidewire is advanced to the distal cortex for exact measurement. **E.** Measurement using two K-wires. **F.** The definitive screw should incorporate both cortices for optimal compression. The usual length of the screw ranges between 12 and 16 mm.

- The length of the headless cannulated compression screw is measured as the difference to a second guidewire that is held next to the first and is advanced to the sesamoid cortex. The usual range is between 12 and 16 mm. The shortest screw available is 10 mm (Bold screws; TECH FIG 2D and E).
- The screw should pierce the proximal cortex to enhance stability (TECH FIG 2F).
- The stab incision is closed with sterile strips.
- Apply compression dressing in neutral hallux position.

PEARLS AND PITFALLS

Indications	▪ Look for foot deformities causing excessive stress to the sesamoid bones. Correction will promote sesamoid healing and prevent treatment failure.[12] ▪ With late diagnosis of sesamoid stress fracture, early surgery will save time for the athlete.[12]
Postoperative management	▪ In cases of uncertain patient compliance, temporary K-wire fixation of the first MTP joint will protect against early excessive MTP joint dorsiflexion.

POSTOPERATIVE CARE

- Full weight bearing over the heel is allowed immediately after surgery.
  - A shoe with a stiff and convex sole is used to prevent dorsiflexion of the first MTP joint for 6 weeks after surgery, after which time conventional shoes are allowed.
  - Return to full athletic activity is not recommended before 12 weeks after surgery.
- Anderson and McBryde[1] treated their patients with 4 weeks non–weight-bearing and another 4 weeks with a weight-bearing cast. In our experience with the Anderson-McBryde procedure, hallux correction or turf toe repair requires no adaptations to the postoperative program outlined earlier.
- No suture removal or wound care is needed with percutaneous sesamoid fixation, because the stab incision has been closed by a sterile strip.
- With combined deformity correction, the type of correction performed dictates postoperative management.

OUTCOMES

- Blundell and colleagues[5] repaired nine sesamoid fractures in athletes with percutaneous cannulated screws and achieved excellent results. All of the athletes returned to their previous level of activity, with no complications reported. Blundell et al concluded that percutaneous screw fixation is a safe and fast procedure. They also questioned the importance of diagnosing the etiology of painful sesamoid fragments, because treatment is the same regardless of the cause.
- Anderson and McBryde[1] performed autogenous bone grafting of medial sesamoid nonunions in 21 athletic and nonathletic patients. Of these, 19 grafts healed, whereas 2 grafts failed because the initial fracture dislocation was greater than 2 mm. These two sesamoids were excised. All patients returned to their preinjury activity levels. No hallux deviations have been reported.
- At our institution, we performed screw fixation in eight athletes and suture fixation with grafting in two nonathletic women and had excellent results with full recovery.

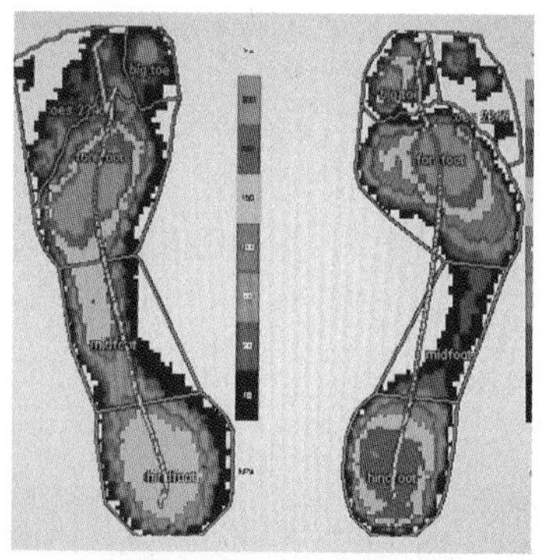
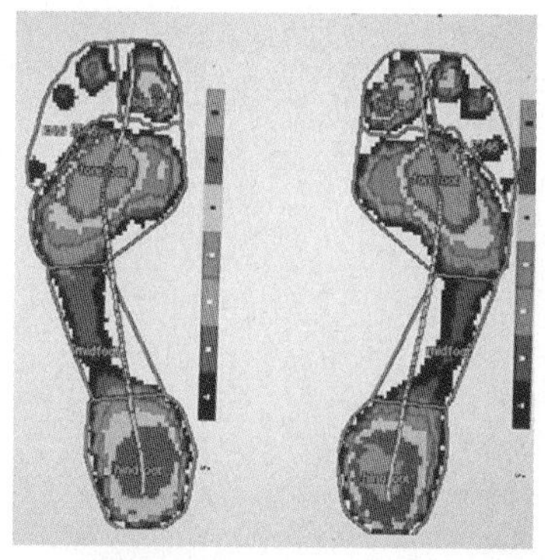
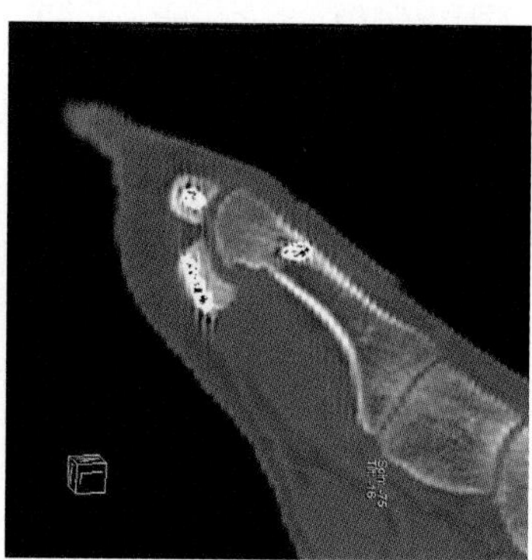

FIG 5 • Postoperative clinical and radiographic results. **A.** Preoperative pedobarogram shows functional amputation of the first MTP joint as a result of painful sesamoid nonunion in the left foot. **B.** Pedobarogram 8 weeks postoperatively shows normalization of pressure distribution of the left foot after sesamoid screw fixation. **C.** CT scan 8 weeks postoperatively shows the healed sesamoid fracture with a screw in place.

- The "athletic group" included six women and two men, all of whom were endurance athletes (eg, running, dancing).
- We treated two lateral and eight medial sesamoid bone nonunions.
  - In one patient, an accompanying forefoot-driven pes cavovarus was corrected with extension osteotomy of the first metatarsus.
  - In four patients, concomitant hallux valgus deformity was corrected in combined open surgery. In two of these patients, screws were used, and in two other patients sutures were used to stabilize the sesamoid bone during the open approach.
  - The rest of the patients were treated percutaneously. Local anesthesia was sufficient in one of these cases.
- All of the patients returned to their preinjury athletic or occupational activity level within 12 weeks after surgery.
- Clinical healing was documented with pedobarography (**FIG 5A,B**), and osseous healing of the fractures was proved by CT scan in three cases (**FIG 5C**). One screw had to be removed because of intermittent pain with exercise 1 year after surgery.
- Since then, we have used suture cerclage in open approaches, but we also continue to use percutaneous screw fixation.
  - No sesamoid has had to be excised, and no hallux deformity has occurred.

COMPLICATIONS

- Persistent sesamoid pain may be caused by:
  - Unrecognized foot deformity and continuous stress to the hallux sesamoids
  - Development of arthritis or avascular necrosis
  - Screw irritation
  - Focused therapy (eg, deformity correction, screw removal) may prevent total excision as a definitive treatment of persistent sesamoid pain.
- Hallux varus after lateral sesamoid excision, hallux valgus after medial sesamoid excision, and cock-up deformity after both sesamoids were excised have been consistently described in 10% to 20% of cases in the current literature.[6,16,17] No hallux deviation has been described after fixation of sesamoid bone fractures.[1,5,12,13]
- A lever arm for flexor tendons and consecutive hallux push-off can be reconstructed with sesamoid fixation and may be important for the running athlete.[2,3]
- This biomechanical advantage has been proven in vitro[2,3] but has an uncertain use in praxis, given the excellent functional results if only one sesamoid bone is excised.[6,15,16,17]

REFERENCES

1. Anderson RB, McBryde AM. Autogenous bone grafting of hallux sesamoid nonunions. Foot Ankle Int 1997;18:293–296.
2. Aper RL, Saltzman CL, Brown TD. The effect of hallux sesamoid resection on the effective moment of the flexor hallucis brevis. Foot Ankle Int 1994;15:462–470.
3. Aper RL, Saltzman CL, Brown TD. The effect of hallux sesamoid excision on the flexor hallucis longus moment arm. Clin Orthop Relat Res 1996;325:209–217.
4. Biedert R. Which investigations are required in stress fracture of the great toe sesamoids? Arch Orthop Trauma Surg 1993;112: 94–95.
5. Blundell CM, Nicholson P, Blackney MW. Percutaneous screw fixation for fractures of the sesamoid bones of the hallux. J Bone Joint Surg Br 2002;84B:1138–1141.
6. Brodsky JW, Robinson AHN, Krause JO, et al. Excision and flexor hallucis brevis reconstruction for the painful sesamoid fractures and non-unions: Surgical technique, clinical results and histo-pathological findings. J Bone Joint Surg Br 2000;82B:217.
7. Chamberland PDC, Smith JW, Fleming LL. The blood supply to the great toe sesamoids. Foot Ankle Int 1993;14:435–442.
8. Chisin R, Peyser A, Milgrom C. Bone scintigraphy in the assessment of the hallucal sesamoids. Foot Ankle Int 1995;16:291–294.
9. Coleman SS, Chestnut WJ. A simple test for hindfoot flexibility in cavovarus foot. Clin Orthop Relat Res 1977;123:60–62.
10. Inge GAL, Ferguson AB. Surgery of sesamoid bones of the great toe. Arch Surg 1933;27:466–489.
11. Karasick D, Schweitzer ME. Disorders of the hallux sesamoid complex: MR features. Skeletal Radiol 1998;27:411–418.
12. Pagenstert GI, Valderrabano V, Hintermann B. Medial sesamoid nonunion combined with hallux valgus in athletes. Foot Ankle Int 2006;27:135–140.
13. Pagenstert GI, Valderrabano V, Hintermann B. Percutaneous screw fixation of hallux sesamoid fractures. In: Scuderi GR, Tria AJ, eds. Minimally Invasive Orthopaedic Surgery. In press.
14. Prettenklieber ML. Dimensions and arterial vascular supply of the sesamoid bones of the human hallux. Acta Anat 1990;139:86–90.
15. Rodeo SA, Warren RF, O'Brien SJ, et al. Diastasis of bipartite sesamoids of the first metatarsophalangeal joint. Foot Ankle Int 1993;14:425–434.
16. Saxena A, Krisdakumtorn T. Return to activity after sesamoidectomy in athletically active individuals. Foot Ankle Int 2003;24: 415–419.
17. Van Hal ME, Keene JS, Lange TA, et al. Stress fractures of the great toe sesamoids. Am J Sports Med 1982;10:122–128.

Chapter **30** Tibial Sesamoidectomy

Simon Lee, Johnny Lin, and George B. Holmes, Jr.

DEFINITION

- Sesamoiditis is a general term that indicates an injury to the sesamoid bone. There are multiple possible causes, such as trauma (fracture, contusion, repetitive stress), infection, arthrosis, osteonecrosis, and osteochondritis dissecans.[3,5,13–15]
- There are two sesamoid bones located plantar to the metatarsal head of the hallux: the lateral or fibular and the medial or tibial sesamoid. The tibial sesamoid typically bears more stress than the fibular sesamoid and is more likely to be injured.[4]

ANATOMY

- The two sesamoid bones are located plantar to the metatarsal head within the tendon of the flexor hallucis brevis (FHB). They are held together by the intersesamoid ligament and plantar plate. The two sesamoids' dorsal surface articulates with the head of the first metatarsal facets, and they are separated by a crista. The sesamoids function to absorb the weight-bearing stress across the medial ray as well as protecting the flexor hallucis longus (FHL) tendon that passes between them. The tibial sesamoid is typically larger and located slightly more distal than the fibular sesamoid (**FIG 1**).
- During the stance phase of gait the sesamoids are slightly proximal to the metatarsal head, but with dorsiflexion of the hallux the sesamoids are pulled distally, protecting the exposed surface of the metatarsal head (**FIG 2**). During the act of toe raising, the sesamoids bear a significant amount of stress. This stress is typically concentrated more medially over the tibial sesamoid, thus accounting for the increased incidence of tibial sesamoid injuries.
- Biomechanically the sesamoids function as a fulcrum to provide a mechanical advantage to the FHB tendon during metatarsal phalangeal joint plantarflexion.[7]
- Ossification of the sesamoids typically occurs from multiple centers and occurs during the seventh to tenth years of life. The multiple ossification centers may account for the incidence of bipartite and tripartite sesamoids.[5]
- The tibial sesamoid is bipartite in about 19% of the population and bilateral in 25% of patients (**FIG 3**).[6]

PATHOGENESIS

- Symptoms can arise from a single acute traumatic event, or more commonly there is a history of minor or repetitive trauma as the cause of sesamoid pain.
- Acute injuries typically occur with a similar mechanism to a turf toe injury, acute hyperextension to the hallux metatarsophalangeal (MTP) joint, or a direct contusion to the sesamoid region of the forefoot. This can also result in a fracture or an injury to a bipartite sesamoid.
- In nonacute injuries the patient often cannot remember a specific incident or injury and can only initially recall activity-related discomfort to the forefoot. This history is typically noted in cases of repetitive stress, osteochondritis dissecans, and arthrosis. A bipartite sesamoid can similarly be injured in this case.
- Neuritic pain has also been described with compression to the plantar medial cutaneous nerve underlying the tibial sesamoid.

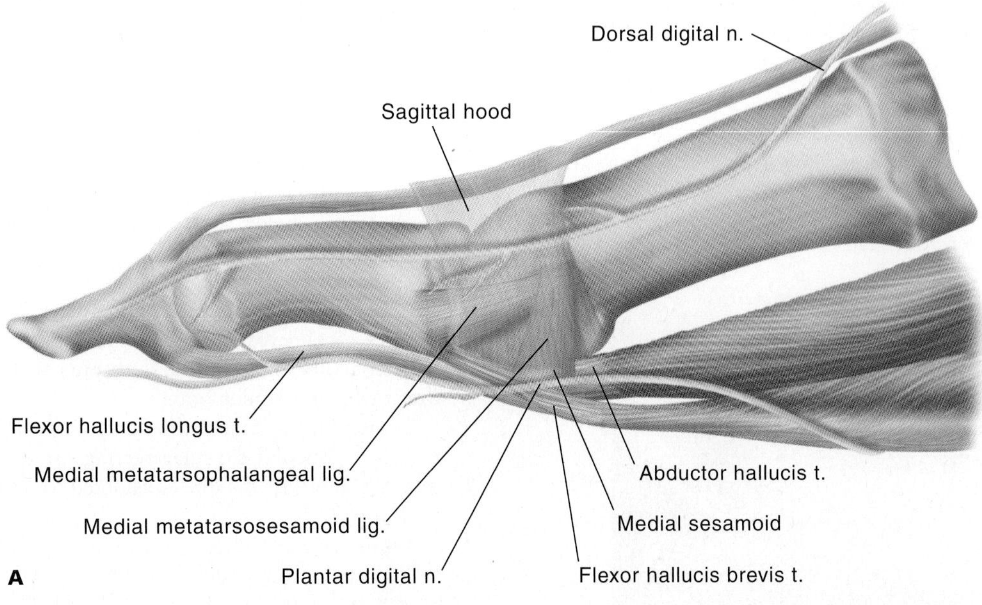

FIG 1 • **A.** Medial view of relevant anatomy with special note of the adductor hallucis brevis and the relationship to the plantar cutaneous nerve. *(continued)*

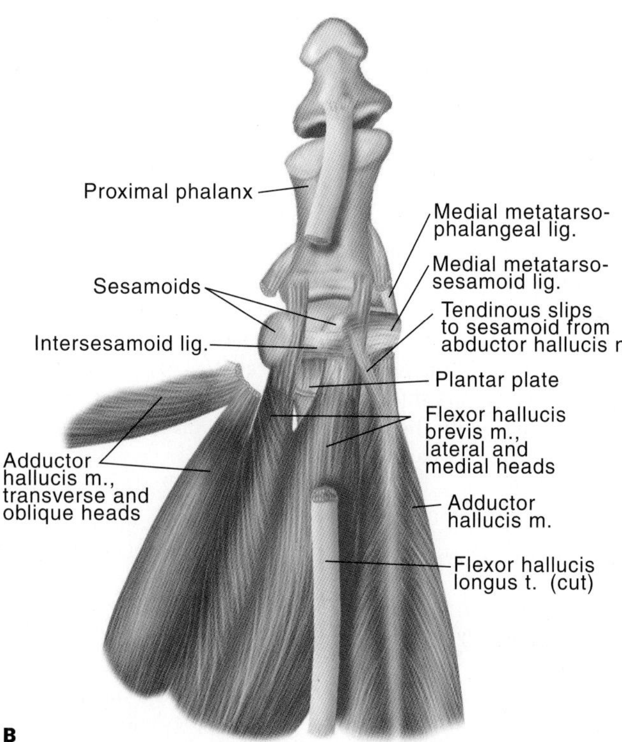

FIG 1 • *(continued)* **B.** Plantar view of the sesamoid complex and the investing structures.

NATURAL HISTORY

- Most sesamoid injuries resolve with appropriate nonoperative treatment.
- Sesamoiditis that does not resolve with conservative treatment is unlikely to improve significantly after 3 to 12 months.
  - As a result, patients often have pain that prevents them from participating in athletic activities.
  - Performing everyday activities that involve a dorsiflexed MTP joint such as stair climbing, toe raising, and in women wearing heels also can become bothersome.

PATIENT HISTORY AND PHYSICAL FINDINGS

- Most patients cannot remember a specific incident or injury, unless it was acute, and can only recall a gradual onset of discomfort to their forefoot. This pain is often generalized and localized to the great toe region. It is localized more plantarward and is worse with weight-bearing activity. Patients will often prefer cushioned shoe wear versus barefooted activity.

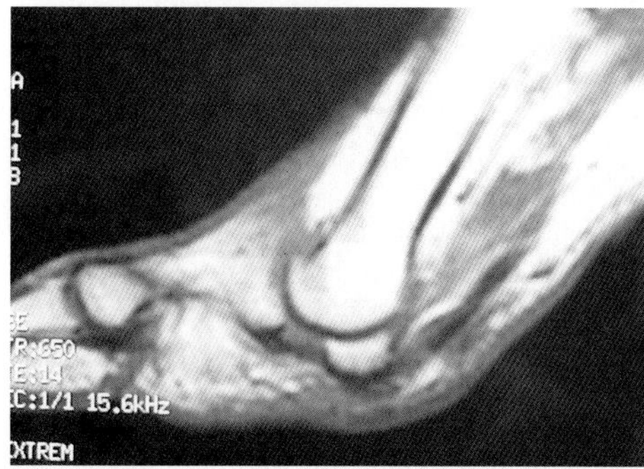

FIG 2 • A sagittal MRI view of the sesamoid–metatarsophalangeal complex showing the increased stress across the tibial sesamoid in metatarsophalangeal dorsiflexion.

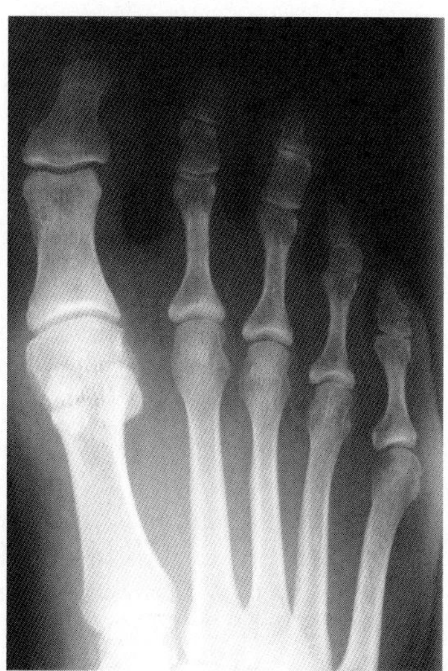

FIG 3 • AP view of the foot showing a bipartite sesamoid. (From Lee S. Technique of isolated tibial sesamoidectomy. Techn Foot Ankle Surg 2004;3:85–90, with permission.)

- Performing activities that require a dorsiflexed MTP joint such as running, jumping, toe raising, or stair climbing can become very irritating to this region.
- Gait can be antalgic, specifically in the toe-off phase, and can also reveal evidence of medial off-loading and lateral foot overload as the patient walks with the foot externally rotated.
- Clinical inspection will reveal swelling over the plantar aspect of the hallux MTP joint as well as tenderness to palpation under the tibial sesamoid. This pain can be exacerbated with forced dorsiflexion of the hallux MTP joint. There may be evidence of loss of dorsiflexion and less commonly plantarflexion of the MTP joint. Plantarflexion strength against resistance or with a single-limb toe raise may also be affected due to pain.
- In acute injuries or in patients with a bipartite sesamoid a drawer test of the hallux MTP joint may also reveal laxity, indicating a fracture of the sesamoid or disruption of the synchondrosis of a bipartite sesamoid.
- Direct palpation over the tibial sesamoid may also reveal a positive Tinel sign or paresthesia distally, indicating a compression over the plantar medial cutaneous nerve.
- Assessment of hallux alignment is critical.
  - Evidence of pre-existing hallux valgus or a cavus foot requires careful planning to identify patients who may require concomitant procedures to prevent further migration after tibial sesamoidectomy.
  - Augmenting a tibial sesamoidectomy with a lateral capsular release, medial capsular reefing, or metatarsal or phalangeal osteotomy may be considered to prevent progressive deformity.[5]
- Methods for examining the tibial sesamoid include:
  - Direct palpation under the tibial sesamoid with the foot in neutral and with dorsiflexion of the MTP joint
  - Range of motion (ROM): One hand should be placed on the proximal phalanx with the other stabilizing the metatarsal. Dorsiflexion and plantarflexion ROM should be assessed. Symmetry between the right and left side should be noted.

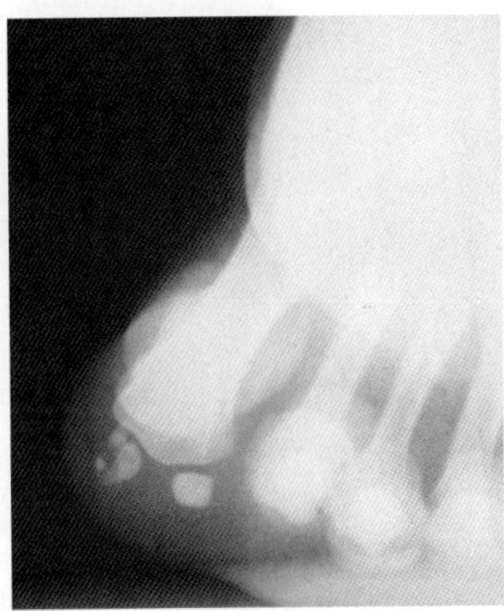

FIG 4 • A sesamoid view of the foot. Note the significant fragmentation of the tibial sesamoid. (From Lee S. Technique of isolated tibial sesamoidectomy. Techn Foot Ankle Surg 2004;3: 85–90, with permission.)

- Drawer test: The examiner grasps the proximal phalanx in one hand and the metatarsal head in the other and performs a dorsal to plantar stress of the MTP joint.
- Toe raise: The patient is asked to do double-limb and single-limb toe raises.

IMAGING AND OTHER DIAGNOSTIC STUDIES

- Routine radiographs should consist of standing anteroposterior (AP), lateral, oblique, and axial sesamoid views.
  - Plain radiographs will often be diagnostic in cases of arthrosis and osteochondritis dissecans if fragmentation is present (**FIG 4**).
  - A bipartite tibial sesamoid (Fig 3) occurs in up to 19% of the population, and differentiating it from a fracture or injury to the bipartite sesamoid can be difficult.[6]
    - A fractured sesamoid may have a sharp radiolucent line that may assist in differentiation.
    - AP radiographs in neutral and dorsiflexion may assist in evaluating separation of the sesamoid segments.
- A triple-phase bone scan or MRI is often required to confirm the diagnosis.
  - A triple-phase bone scan, with collimated views of the MTP joint, is very sensitive and may demonstrate increased uptake before radiographic changes become present (**FIG 5**).

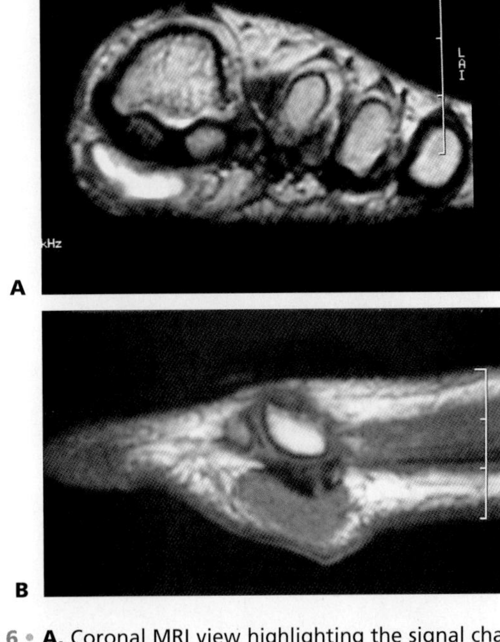

FIG 6 • **A.** Coronal MRI view highlighting the signal change of the tibial sesamoid, and reactive plantar bursitis, compared to the fibular sesamoid, indicating tibial sesamoid avascular necrosis. **B.** Sagittal MRI view of a tibial sesamoid fracture and subsequent reactive plantar bursitis. (From Lee S. Technique of isolated tibial sesamoidectomy. Techn Foot Ankle Surg 2004;3: 85–90, with permission.)

- MRI is more expensive but allows the examiner to identify most causes of hallux MTP pathology in addition to sesamoiditis (**FIG 6**).

DIFFERENTIAL DIAGNOSIS

- Infection, sesamoid–metatarsal or MTP arthrosis or chondromalacia, bursitis, flexor tendinosis, fracture, osteochondritis dissecans, intractable plantar keratosis, nerve compression, bi- or tripartite sesamoid, turf toe injury

NONOPERATIVE MANAGEMENT

- Most patients will respond to conservative therapy. This consists of rest or immobilization for 2 to 4 weeks, followed by protected weight bearing with an orthotic, walker boot, or cast for an additional 4 to 6 weeks.

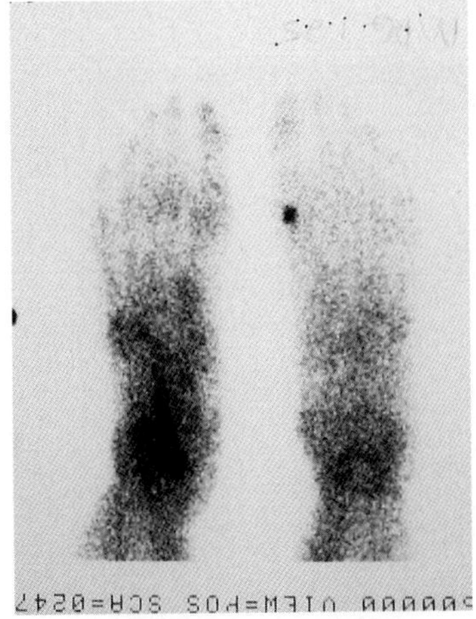

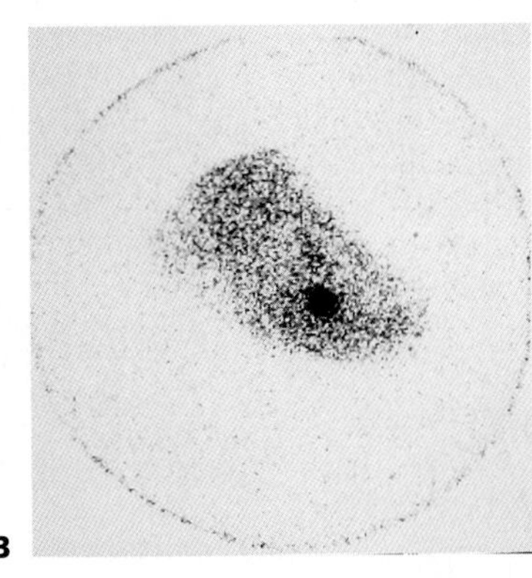

FIG 5 • **A.** Triple-phase bone scan showing increased uptake of the tibial sesamoid region in an AP view of bilateral feet. **B.** Collimated view showing the increased uptake of the tibial sesamoid. (From Lee S. Technique of isolated tibial sesamoidectomy. Techn Foot Ankle Surg 2004;3:85–90, with permission.)

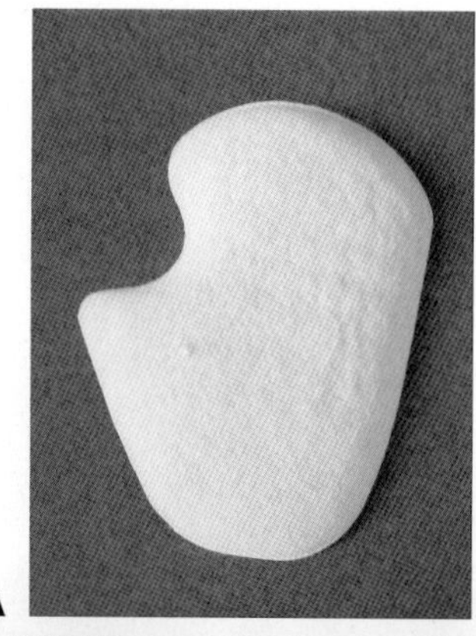

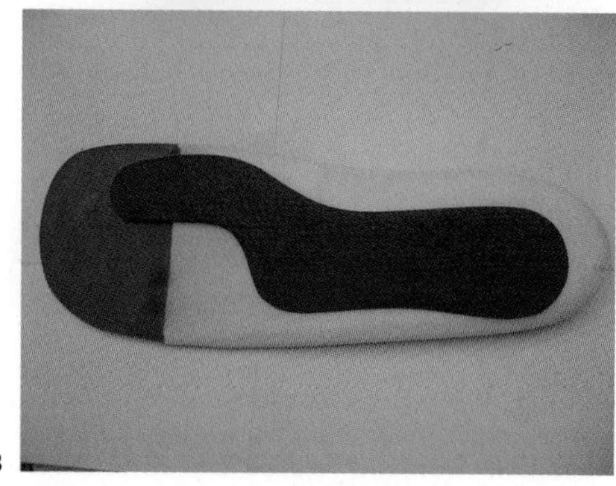

FIG 7 • **A.** Dancer's pad with sesamoid cut-out. **B.** Example of a Morton extension in an orthotic.

- Typically a hard-soled shoe will decrease the dorsiflexion stresses across the MTP joint, and a negative-heel shoe will decrease forefoot loading.
- An orthosis such as a turf-toe plate or dancer's pad with a medial longitudinal arch support will decrease the stresses across the sesamoids (**FIG 7**).
- In athletes, taping the MTP joint to prevent dorsiflexion may allow continued participation.
- The use of nonsteroidal anti-inflammatory medication may augment treatment.
- The judicious use of steroid injections for chronic sesamoiditis is also indicated.

SURGICAL MANAGEMENT

- Pain under the tibial sesamoid that is not responsive to conservative treatment is the main indication for operative intervention. The presence of hallux MTP malalignment, a cavus foot, or stiffness requires careful evaluation and may require additional surgical procedures to improve clinical results.
- Previous excision of the fibular sesamoid or absence of the fibular sesamoid is the main contraindication to a tibial sesamoidectomy.[1,2] A history of peripheral vascular disease, soft tissue or wound healing problems, diabetes mellitus, and smoking are also relative contraindications that require proper evaluation and discussion with the patient before operative intervention.

Preoperative Planning

- The initial evaluation of hallux alignment is of utmost importance.
- Although there is little literature in regard to the appropriate criteria for the addition of a hallux realignment procedure in an isolated tibial sesamoidectomy, the surgeon needs to keep in mind that any failure of reconstruction of the tibial FHB complex or failure to address pre-existing hallux malalignment will compromise patient outcome.
- In general, any patient whose hallux alignment would be considered for surgical realignment without tibial sesamoiditis should have the malalignment corrected during the tibial sesamoidectomy.

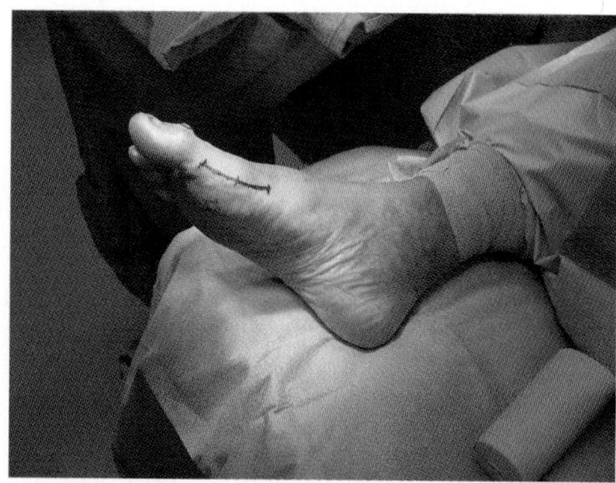

FIG 8 • Intraoperative picture showing the planned incision and the natural externally rotated view of the foot.

Positioning

- Anesthesia should be similar to a bunion procedure.
- An ankle block with some mild sedation is typically well tolerated.
- A well-padded supramalleolar Esmarch tourniquet is also used and is well tolerated.
- The patient should be placed on the operating table in a supine position.
- The natural external rotation of the lower extremity allows excellent exposure to the medial aspect of the forefoot (**FIG 8**).

Approach

- Dorsomedial, straight medial, and plantar medial incisions to approach the tibial sesamoid have all been described. The most commonly used incision is a longitudinal medial skin incision that is slightly plantar to the standard incision for a bunion excision (**FIG 9**). With the dorsomedial incision, it is very difficult to obtain adequate exposure of the plantar aspect of the foot, while the plantar medial incision is typically directly over the plantar cutaneous nerve and near the weight-bearing surface of the foot, increasing wound complications.

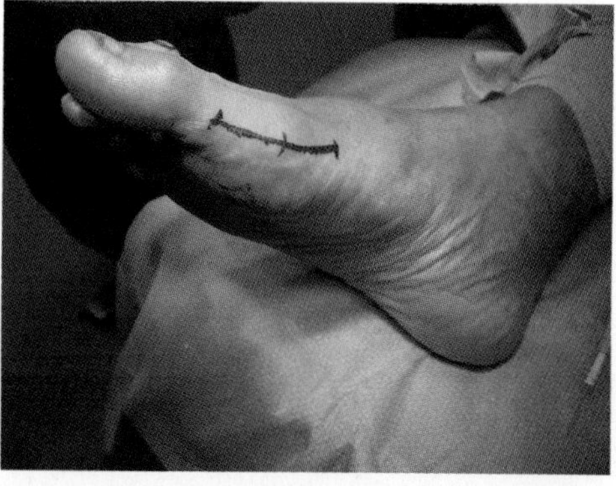

FIG 9 • Note the slightly plantar incision line.

TIBIAL SESAMOIDECTOMY

- The most commonly used incision is a longitudinal medial skin incision that is slightly plantar to the standard incision for a bunion excision.
- The plantar cutaneous nerve must be identified and mobilized for protection during the procedure (**TECH FIG 1**).
  - The nerve can usually be found along the inferior border of the abductor hallucis brevis tendon alongside the MTP joint.
  - Typically the nerve is mobilized inferior to the surgical dissection, although dorsal retraction has been described as well.
  - A vessel loop can also be placed around the nerve to protect it.
- Perform initial evaluation of the tibial sesamoid and metatarsal head articulation through an intra-articular exposure.
- Make a longitudinal incision in the capsule in line with the skin incision.
  - This incision is usually dorsal to the fibers of the insertion of the abductor hallucis tendon.
- Assess the sesamoid articular surface for significant displacement or step-off in acute fractures or bipartite sesamoids. In chronic cases, assess the resultant articular cartilage injury to the sesamoid or metatarsal head articulation of the hallux from osteonecrosis, osteochondritis dissecans, or arthrosis (**TECH FIG 2**).
- At this stage, when the decision is made to remove the sesamoid, the use of a Beaver mini-blade to outline the tibial sesamoid from the intra-articular approach will assist in its later removal.
- In an acute fracture or a bipartite sesamoid without articular damage, consider using bone grafting of the defect as opposed to performing a sesamoidectomy.
- Repair the capsulotomy with a 2-0 nonabsorbable suture before proceeding with the sesamoidectomy exposure (**TECH FIG 3**).
- Expose the sesamoid through an extra-articular plantar medial incision in line with the FHB fibers.
  - The sesamoid is embedded within a dense fibrous sheath, and careful dissection out of the FHB and its soft tissue attachments is required (**TECH FIG 4**).
  - This can be facilitated by the use of a Beaver mini-blade, using a pushing technique rather than a cutting motion, as well as grasping the sesamoid with a small towel clamp or Köcher clamp for stability.
  - Take utmost care to protect the nerve medially as well as the FHL laterally to prevent injury.
- Once the sesamoid is removed, carefully assess the continuity of the FHB complex. Typically there are some remaining fibers of the FHB complex.

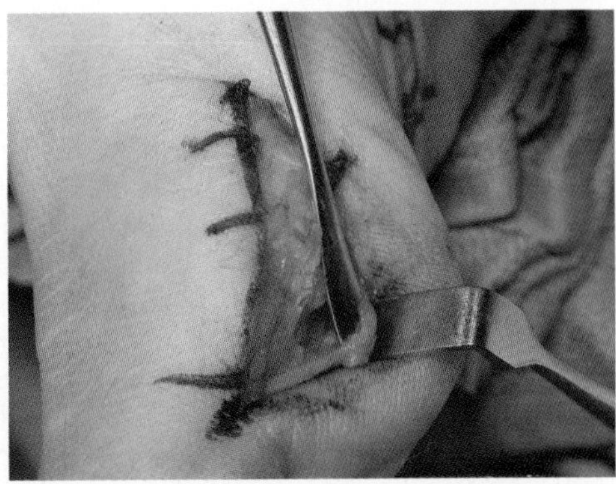

TECH FIG 1 • Intraoperative picture; the Freer elevator is underneath the plantar cutaneous nerve.

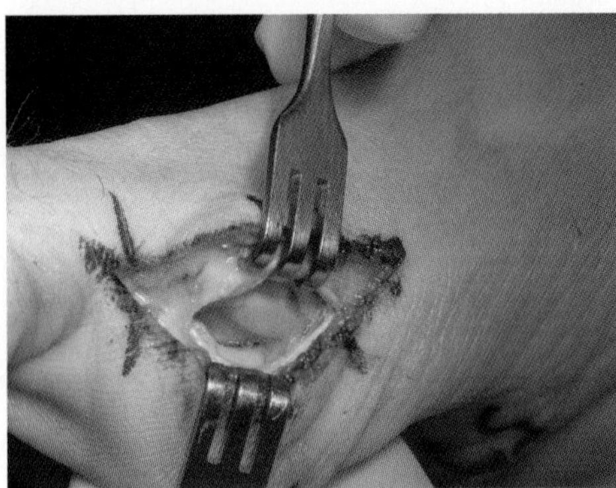

TECH FIG 2 • Intracapsular view showing the articulation of the tibial sesamoid and the metatarsal head. (From Lee S. Technique of isolated tibial sesamoidectomy. Techn Foot Ankle Surg 2004;3:85–90, with permission.)

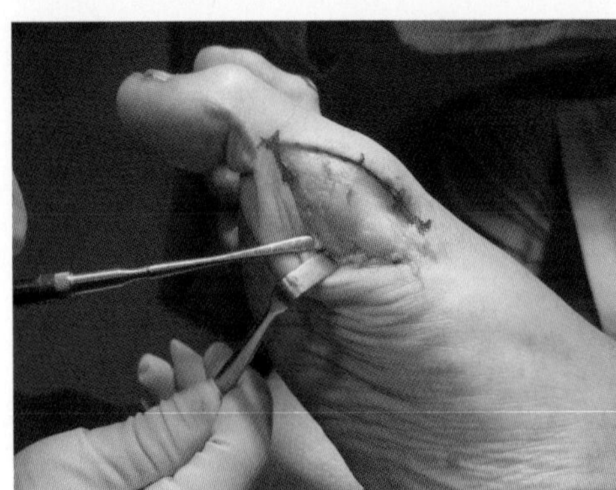

TECH FIG 3 • The tip of the Freer elevator is underneath the tibial sesamoid before dissection of the flexor hallucis brevis complex. Also note the longitudinal capsulotomy and repair.

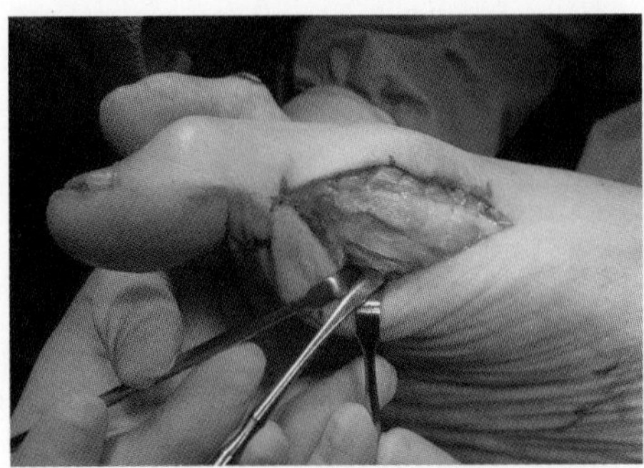

TECH FIG 4 • After the initial incision to separate the flexor hallucis brevis in line with its fibers.

TECHNIQUES

- In all patients, repair the defect with a 2-0 nonabsorbable suture in a triangular, figure 8 or pursestring fashion, with careful reapproximation of the FHB complex (**TECH FIG 5**). The use of a UCL taper needle is recommended due to its non-cutting aspect as well as a needle with a smaller radius of curvature, allowing easier manipulation.
- The FHL tendon can often be seen during this stage. Also assess the tendon at this time.
- Once the FHB complex is reapproximated, take the hallux through ROM to confirm that the FHB is intact and that the FHL tendon has not been inadvertently sutured.
- Complete the closure in standard fashion for a bunion procedure.
- Reapproximate the skin edges with a 3-0 nylon suture and dress the wound with a bunion dressing, with the hallux protected in plantarflexion and in mild varus.
- The patient is provided with a firm-soled postoperative shoe and allowed immediate heel weight bearing.

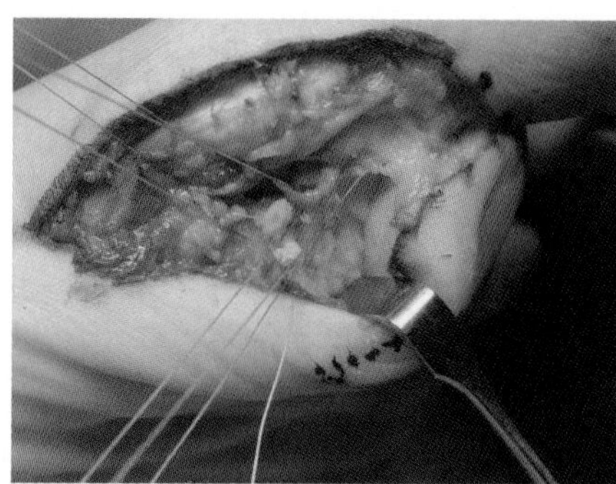

TECH FIG 5 • Note the flexor hallucis longus tendon deep to the operative incision as well as the subsequent pursestring repair of the flexor hallucis brevis complex.

PEARLS AND PITFALLS

Hallux malalignment	▪ The presence of a cavus foot, hallux valgus, claw toe, cock-up deformity, or stiffness requires careful evaluation and may require additional surgical procedures to improve clinical results.
Plantar cutaneous nerve	▪ The nerve is most commonly located plantar to the inferior border of the abductor hallucis brevis tendon. This nerve should be visualized and protected throughout the case.
Flexor hallucis brevis repair	▪ A UCL taper needle, with its smaller radius of curvature, is easier to use in the limited surgical field. Careful and meticulous repair of the FHB complex is required to prevent the development of malalignment.

POSTOPERATIVE CARE

- Patients are limited to heel weight bearing for 2 weeks.
- At the 2-week follow-up visit stitches are removed, a toe spacer is placed, and patients are allowed to bear weight as tolerated in a postoperative shoe or a short walker boot.
- Standing radiographs should be performed to confirm maintenance of hallux alignment (**FIG 10**).
- The toe spacer should remain in place for 6 to 8 weeks postoperatively to prevent hallux valgus deformity.
- If a hallux realignment procedure was also performed, we use a taping technique for 4 to 6 weeks similar to a bunion procedure.
- Patients are encouraged to begin active and passive ROM exercises for the hallux MTP joint after stitches are removed.
- In active patients, formal physical therapy is warranted to monitor patient progress and to assist in ROM and soft tissue modalities.
- Patients return at 6 weeks postoperatively and are then allowed to progress to accommodative shoe wear and activity as tolerated.
- Patients may occasionally require continued short-term use of a sesamoid relief orthotic while returning to activity.

OUTCOMES

- Hallux malalignment with resultant claw toe and cock-up and hallux valgus deformity after tibial sesamoid excision have been described.[8,9,11,12]
  - Historical studies have found a 10% to 42% incidence of hallux valgus and a 33% to 60% incidence of loss of motion on follow-up.[8,11,12]
  - Kaiman and Piccora[9] also reviewed tibial sesamoidectomies and concluded that assessment of the osseous relationship was crucial to prevent hallux valgus deformity. Their average follow-up was only 13.2 months and they found no evidence of valgus drift, but they recommended tendon balancing or capsulorrhaphy in conjunction with the tibial sesamoidectomy.
  - Van Hal et al[15] found no evidence of deformity or diminished range of motion.
  - Lee et al[10] reported on 20 patients without preoperative malalignment and noted no significant difference in postoperative ROM or the development of subsequent hallux malalignment.
- Saxena and Krisdakumtorn[14] reported on active individuals who had isolated tibial sesamoidectomies.
  - One patient developed loss of hallux flexion after surgery.
  - Two patients with hallux valgus deformity were identified before surgery. One patient had a concomitant distal metatarsal osteotomy with no further drift, while the other patient did not have a concomitant procedure at the same time and went on to a bunion correction at a later date.
- Inge and Ferguson[8] and Mann et al[11] found that 41% to 50% of their patients continued to have mild to severe pain after a tibial sesamoidectomy. More recently, however, Van Hal et al,[15] Saxena and Krisdakumtorn,[14] and Lee et al[10] have reported excellent pain relief in the majority of their patients with tibial sesamoidectomies in their athletic population.
- Aper et al[1] showed in two cadaveric studies that the FHB effective tendon moment arms are significantly decreased with

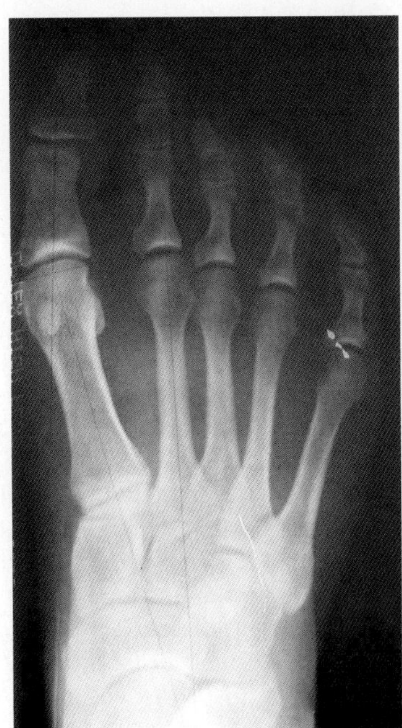

A

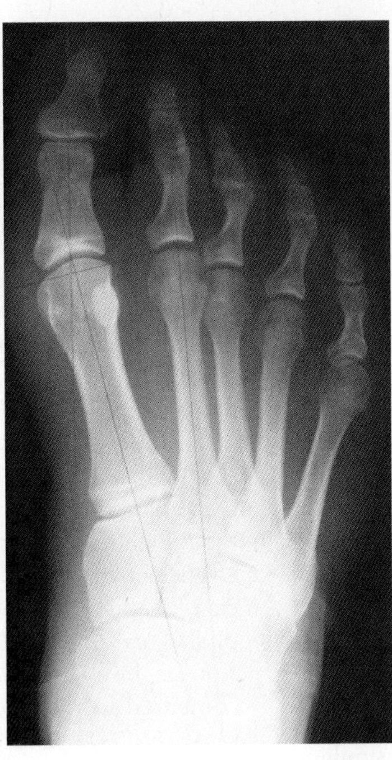

B

FIG 10 • Preoperative (A) and postoperative (B) standing radiographs of the foot showing no change in the clinical alignment of the metatarsophalangeal joint after tibial sesamoidectomy. (From Lee S. Technique of isolated tibial sesamoidectomy. Techn Foot Ankle Surg 2004;3:85–90, with permission.)

the excision of both hallux sesamoids. However, FHL effective tendon moment arms are noted to be diminished with isolated sesamoid excisions as well.[2] These studies may help to explain the functional weakness reported by Mann et al.[11] However, Van Hal et al[15] and Saxena and Krisdakumtorn[14] have not found any functional weakness of plantarflexion in any of their patients. Their patients were also able to return to their previous level of athletic participation with no functional deficit. Lee et al[10] also reported that 30% of their patients could not do a single-limb toe raise, indicating some plantarflexion weakness, but this did not affect any subsequent athletic activity.

COMPLICATIONS

- Complications related to tibial sesamoid excisions can be separated into intraoperative complications, insufficient pain relief, functional weakness, and hallux malalignment.
- The most common intraoperative complication reported is injury to the plantar digital nerve.
  - Patients typically complain of nerve irritation postoperatively. This generally responds well to observation or localized steroid injections. It occurs more commonly with fibular sesamoid excisions.
  - Complete laceration of the nerve has never been reported, and this nerve irritation appears to be the result of aggressive retraction during surgery. This can be avoided by using meticulous technique with identification and protection of the plantar digital nerve during surgery.
- Isolated complete sesamoidectomies are thought to alter the mechanical balance of the hallux MTP joint. Clinical studies have described stiffness, functional loss, cock-up deformity, claw toe deformity, and the development of a hallux valgus deformity after isolated tibial sesamoidectomies.[8,9,11,12]
  - As noted earlier, identifying and addressing any significant malalignment of the hallux MTP can decrease the rate of future deformities.
- The loss of single-limb toe raise has also been reported and may be related to the decreased moment arm and inadequate repair of the FHB complex.[10]

REFERENCES

1. Aper RL, Saltzman CL, Brown TD. The effect of hallux sesamoid resection on the effective moment of the flexor hallucis brevis. Foot Ankle Int 1994;15:462–470.
2. Aper RL, Saltzman CL, Brown TD. The effect of hallux sesamoid excision on the flexor hallucis longus moment arm. Clin Orthop Relat Res 1996;325:209–217.
3. Beaman DN, Nigo LJ. Hallucal sesamoid injury. Oper Tech Sports Med 1999;7:7–13.
4. Bizzaro AH. On the traumatology of the sesamoid structures. Ann Surg 1921;74:783.
5. Coughlin MJ. Sesamoid pain: causes and surgical treatment. AAOS Instructional Course Lectures 1990;39:23–35.
6. Dobas DC, Silvers MD. The frequency of partite sesamoids of the first metatarsal phalangeal joint. J Am Podiatry Assoc 1977;67:880–882.
7. Helal B. The great toe sesamoid bones: the lus or lost souls of the Ushaia. Clin Orthop Relat Res 1981;157:82–87.
8. Inge GAL, Ferguson AB. Surgery of the sesamoid bones of the great toe: an anatomic and clinical study, with a report of forty-one cases. Arch Surg 1933;27:466–489.
9. Kaiman ME, Piccora R. Tibial sesamoidectomy: a review of the literature and retrospective study. J Foot Surg 1983;22:286–289.
10. Lee S, William JC, Cohen BE, et al. Evaluation of hallux alignment and functional outcome after isolated tibial sesamoidectomy. Foot Ankle Int 2005;26:803–809.
11. Mann RA, Coughlin MJ, Baxter D, et al. Sesamoidectomy of the great toe. Presented at the 15th Annual Meeting of the American Orthopaedic Foot and Ankle Society, Las Vegas, Jan. 24, 1985.
12. Nayfa TM, Sorto LA. The incidence of hallux abductus following tibial sesamoidectomy. J Am Podiatr Assoc 1982;72:617–620.
13. Richardson EG. Hallucal sesamoid pain: causes and surgical treatment. J Am Assoc Orthop Surg 1999;7:270–278.
14. Saxena A, Krisdakumtorn T. Return to activity after sesamoidectomy in athletically active individuals. Foot Ankle Int 2003;24:415–419.
15. Van Hal ME, Keene JS, Lange TA, et al. Stress fractures of the great toe sesamoid. Am J Sports Med 1982;10:122–128.

Chapter 31

Flexor-to-Extensor Tendon Transfer for Flexible Hammer Toe Deformity

Emilio Wagner

DEFINITION

- A hammer toe deformity is defined by a flexion deformity of the proximal interphalangeal (PIP) joint, typically with associated metatarsophalangeal (MTP) joint hyperextension. The distal interphalangeal joint (DIP) may be flexed, extended, or in a neutral position.[3]

ANATOMY

- The plantar plates of the MTP and PIP joints of the toes provide insertion points for ligaments, tendons, and soft tissue septa.
  - At the MTP joint the plantar plate originates from the periosteum of the shaft of the metatarsal and it inserts onto the base of the proximal phalanx. Plantar plate dysfunction has been associated with hammer toes and claw toes.[7]
  - At the PIP joint the plantar plate also attaches in a similar way as in the MTP joint, lying immediately plantar to the joint.
  - The collateral ligaments insert to the plantar plate at both the PIP and MTP joints.
  - The final position of the toe depends on the delicate balance between the static stabilizers of the MTP and PIP joints (plantar plate, collateral ligaments) and the dynamic stabilizers (extrinsic and intrinsic tendons).
- The extensor digitorum longus (EDL) tendon is the primary extensor of the MTP joint; it attaches to the lateral four toes. The extensor digitorum brevis (EDB) tendon is the only dorsal intrinsic muscle of the foot, and it attaches to the medial four toes.
  - These two tendons maintain their orientation in part due to the fibroaponeurotic extensor hood.
    - Its proximal segment, called the extensor sling, attaches to the plantar base of the proximal phalanx. It receives contributions from the interossei muscles. Its distal segment or extensor wing receives the insertion of the lumbrical muscles.
  - Extension of the PIP and DIP joints is achieved by the coordinated action of the extrinsic extensor tendons and the intrinsic flexor muscles; with paralysis of the intrinsic muscles, the extensor muscles would extend only the MTP joints.
- The extrinsic flexors are the flexor digitorum brevis (FDB) and longus (FDL) muscles. The FDB and FDL tendons unite to the base of the middle and distal phalanx, respectively. They flex the PIP and DIP joints and are weak flexors of the MTP joint.
- The intrinsic flexors are the interossei and lumbrical muscles. The lumbricals flex the MTP joints and extend the interphalangeal joints; they have a stronger effect over the extension of the PIP and DIP joints due to their distal attachment compared to the interossei, which are weak extensors of the toes[7] (**FIG 1**).

PATHOGENESIS

- Any disruption of the foot's complex and delicate balance between the static stabilizers (ligaments, plantar plate) and dynamic stabilizers (intrinsic and extrinsic tendons) creates a lesser toe deformity.
  - With diminished intrinsic muscle flexion power, the extrinsic extensor tendons will extend the MTP joints. With MTP joint extension, the long flexor tendons flex the PIP and DIP joints, resulting in the intrinsic tendons being insufficient in flexing the MTP joint or extending the PIP or DIP joints. This imbalance creates deformity.
  - Plantar plate disruption may also compromise the balance of the toes and promote MTP joint hyperextension, thus leading to a similar chain of events to that described above (**FIG 2**).
- The pathologic anatomy of claw toes and hammer toes has been investigated in cadaveric dissections.

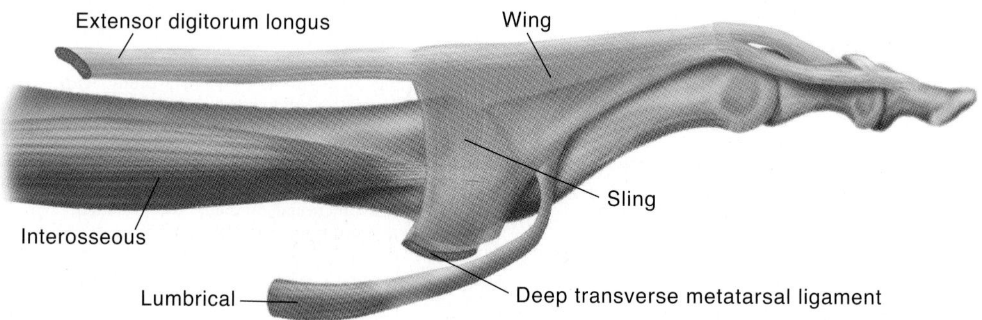

FIG 1 • Lateral view of the normal anatomy of the metatarsophalangeal and proximal interphalangeal joints of the lesser toes.

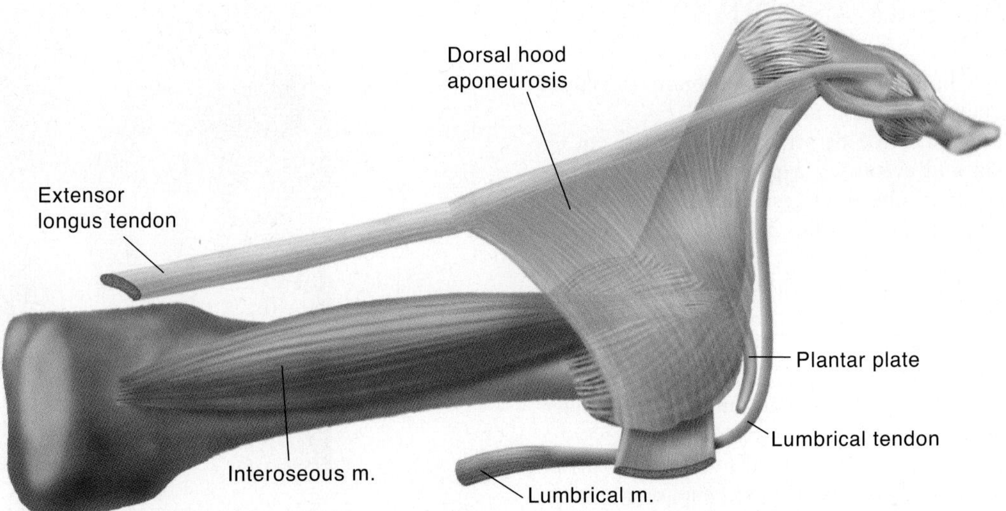

FIG 2 • Lateral view of the pathologic anatomy of a hammer toe. Notice how the metatarsophalangeal extension renders insufficient the lumbricals and dorsally subluxates the interosseous tendon. The proximal interphalangeal flexion subluxates the extensor tendon, and continued pull of the extensor digitorum will increase the proximal interphalangeal flexion.

- In one of these studies,[8] contributions of various anatomic structures to the deformity were determined:
  - For MTP joint hyperextension deformity, the skin provided about 9% of total deformity, the extensor tendons (EDL+EDB) 25%, the dorsal capsule 19%, and the collateral ligaments 47%.
  - For PIP joint flexion deformity, the skin accounted for about 20% of deformity, the FDB tendon 40%, and the plantar capsule 40%; the FDL tendon had no contribution.
  - These numbers show the relative importance of the different anatomic structures in the deformity and suggest which structures to release in surgery.
- With clawing (hyperextension of the MTP joint) the interossei become subluxated in relation to the MTP joint and their line of pull becomes dorsally situated in relation to the joint axis and center of MTP joint rotation.
  - This results in an increased deformity with interossei activity: instead of plantarflexion, they provide dorsiflexion at the MTP joint.
  - The lumbricals normally have an angle of 35 degrees with respect to the metatarsal axis. With clawing, they can subtend an angle of 90 degrees with the metatarsal axis, rendering them insufficient to flex the MTP joint.[8]
- Causes for lesser toe deformity are posttraumatic, inflammatory, neurologic, congenital, postsurgical, and nonspecific in nature.
  - Posttraumatic deformities include sequelae of leg injuries, fractures, soft tissue injuries, and compartment syndromes.
    - In these cases a scarring or contracture of the deep compartment of the leg can lead to flexion deformities of the toes.
    - A compartment syndrome after a calcaneal fracture, affecting the calcaneal compartment, will compromise the quadratus plantae muscle, thereby shortening the intrinsic musculature.
    - Damage to the tibial nerve due to these same reasons may also be responsible for loss of intrinsic flexor action, resulting in an MTP joint extension deformity.
  - Inflammatory: in rheumatoid arthritis due to capsular inflammation and disruption
    - Plantar plate attenuation may lead to MTP joint hyperextension and nonphysiologic PIP joint flexion.
  - Neuromuscular and congenital causes may alter the foot's intrinsic and extrinsic muscle balance.
    - Neuromuscular causes of lesser toe deformities include cerebral palsy, Charcot-Marie-Tooth disease, Friedreich ataxia, spinal dysraphism, and polio, among others.
    - Congenital causes include idiopathic cavovarus foot, clubfoot sequelae, and arthrogryposis.[7]
- Postsurgical causes
  - Dorsiflexion of the metatarsal head after distal metatarsal osteotomies (to relieve metatarsalgia, or synovitis)
  - Proximal metatarsal osteotomies with elevation of the distal fragment and secondary overpull of the flexor tendons[5]
  - Secondary to metatarsal lengthening due to undesired lengthening of the flexor and extensor tendons
- Nonspecific causes
  - Muscular imbalance, ineffectiveness of the intrinsic flexors, and age-related deficiencies of plantar structures[7]
  - Shoe wear has been implicated because of the buckling effect of the toes inside a short toe box, with resulting flexion of the PIP joint.

NATURAL HISTORY

- The natural history of this deformity is a slow progression to a claw toe, where extension of the MTP joint increases with an increase in PIP flexion.
- If the deformity is flexible, the prognosis is good, as a conservative option may be successful, or if surgery is deemed necessary, simple techniques typically meet with satisfactory outcomes.
- As the lesser toe deformity becomes fixed, the chance of a successful nonsurgical treatment decreases, and surgical treatment generally involves more complex reconstructive procedures with an increased risk for postoperative stiffness.

PATIENT HISTORY AND PHYSICAL FINDINGS

- The chief complaint is pain and tenderness on the dorsal PIP joint, typically due to pressure from the shoe.
- A progressive hammer toe deformity may lead to an extended MTP joint and eventually a plantar callus under the corresponding metatarsal head. Occasionally, with associated PIP and DIP flexion, a plantar callus at the tip of the toe will develop.
- Toe position must be evaluated with weight bearing to appreciate the full extent of the deformity. With the patient seated, the range of motion of the ankle and subtalar, transverse tarsal, and metatarsophalangeal joints is inspected.
- Flexibility of the MTP, PIP, and DIP joints must be determined as it influences surgical decision making.
- Inspection and palpation of the plantar foot may reveal calluses under the metatarsal heads and tips of the toes.
- A comprehensive neurovascular examination is performed. Correction of lesser toe deformities will place digital vessels and nerves on stretch; preoperative neurovascular compromise to the toes must be identified, particularly if surgical correction is considered.
- Examinations of the lesser toes' MTP and IP joints may include:
  - Push-up test (MTP): If the deformity is flexible, with the push-up test the MTP joint will flex to its normal position. If not, it will remain extended, defining a fixed deformity. Semiflexible deformities are those that correct partially with the push-up test.
  - Evaluation of PIP joint stiffness: Fixed deformities are present if it is not possible to obtain full extension of the PIP joint. Flexible deformities allow the PIP joint to extend fully.
  - Evaluation of MTP joint stability: Stage 0, no laxity to dorsal translation; stage 1, the base of the proximal phalanx can be subluxated with the dorsal stress; stage 2, the proximal phalangeal base can be dislocated and relocated; stage 3, the base of the proximal phalanx is fixed in a dislocated position.[10]

IMAGING AND OTHER DIAGNOSTIC STUDIES

- Plain radiographs
  - Inflammatory arthritis may be associated with periarticular erosions, and this may influence surgical management.
  - The extent of the deformity is characterized on plain radiographs: subluxation, dislocation, or medial or lateral deviation. Dislocation of the MTP joint is characterized by an overlap of the base of the proximal phalanx on the head of the metatarsal on the AP view and complete dorsal displacement of the proximal phalanx relative to the metatarsal head on the lateral view (**FIG 3**).

DIFFERENTIAL DIAGNOSIS

- Fixed hammer toe or claw toe deformities (not amenable to treatment with tendon transfer alone)
- Metatarsophalangeal synovitis (absence of deformity warranting tendon transfer)
- Posttraumatic toe deformities
- Soft tissue tumors of the toes

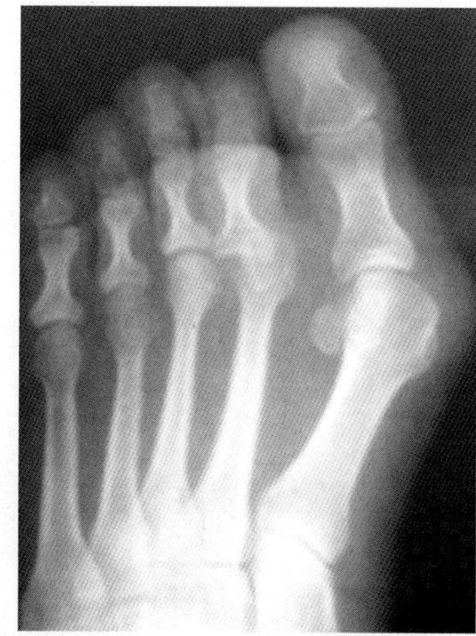

FIG 3 • AP view of a foot with hammer toe deformity with metatarsophalangeal joint subluxation. Notice the overlap between the base of the proximal phalanx and the metatarsal head.

NONOPERATIVE MANAGEMENT

- For flexible deformities, an initial conservative approach is recommended.
- Stretching exercises may help but have little proven benefit as they do not alter the imbalance of extrinsic and intrinsic tendons.
- Shoe wear modifications: wider, deeper toebox to give more room to the toes
- Metatarsal pads to relieve metatarsal head pressure and toe sleeves to cushion pressure on the dorsum of the PIP joints. Orthotics with metatarsal padding must be used judiciously since they elevate the toes and may lead to greater dorsal PIP joint pressure.
- Hammer toe sling orthoses (or taping) are available that hold the proximal phalanx in a more physiologic position (**FIG 4**).
- The value of these measures depends to some degree on the degree of flexibility remaining in the deformity.

SURGICAL MANAGEMENT

- A toe flexor-to-extensor tendon transfer is rarely performed in isolation; typically, it is an adjunct to a more comprehensive correction of hammer toe and claw toe deformities.
- The goal of a flexor-to-extensor tendon transfer is to reposition the proximal phalanx into a more physiologic alignment, with realignment of the MTP and PIP joints. It is essentially

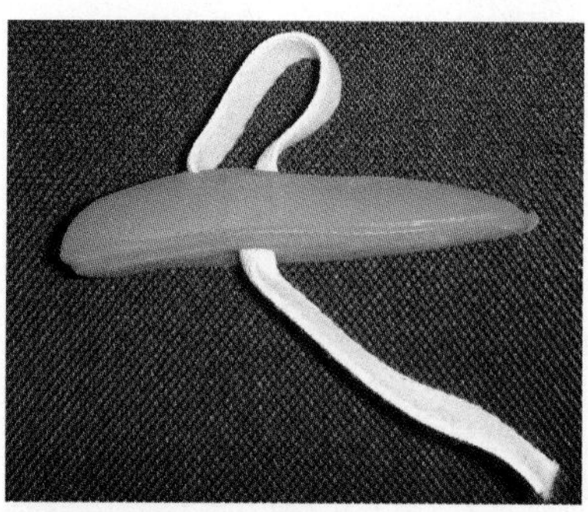

FIG 4 • Hammer toe orthosis designed to hold the proximal phalanx in a plantarflexed position.

"taping of the toe under the skin." Despite flexible deformity, tendon transfer may need to be performed with dorsal capsulotomy and collateral ligament release of the MTP joint. As the deformity becomes more fixed, a PIP arthroplasty–arthrodesis with or without metatarsal shortening osteotomy would typically be warranted, but a flexor-to-extensor tendon transfer may need to be added to avoid residual elevation of the toe ("floating toe"), one that does not touch the floor with weight bearing.

Preoperative Planning

- For MTP joint hyperextension deformity, a bone-shortening procedure can be performed; We are currently evaluating this procedure.
  - Generally a soft tissue procedure is chosen; the choice will vary depending on the amount of release needed.
  - Progressive releases have to be made, starting with the dorsal skin, followed by extensor tendons (tenotomy or lengthening), the dorsal capsule, and collateral ligaments, until an aligned MTP joint is obtained.
  - For further correction and stabilization, a flexor-to-extensor transfer should be added. In this case, the transfer should be done suturing the FDL to the EDL proximal to the middle of the proximal phalanx, to obtain more flexion power over the MTP joint.
- For PIP joint flexion deformities, FDB releases are considered if the flexion contracture is not solved percutaneously.
  - If FDB tenotomy is not enough to treat the PIP deformity, a PIP joint arthroplasty or arthrodesis should be added.
  - A bone-shortening procedure can be also considered, typically a metatarsal-shortening osteotomy. In our opinion, a resection of the proximal aspect of the proximal phalanx should be avoided due to a high prevalence of postoperative MTP joint instability.
  - The flexor-to-extensor transfer will correct the PIP joint flexion if flexible and will also stabilize the deformity if a FDB tenotomy or a PIP joint arthroplasty was performed. In this case, the transfer should be done suturing the FDL to the EDL distal to the middle of the proximal phalanx to obtain more extension power over the PIP joint.

Positioning

- A supine position is preferred, with the involved foot on the same side as the surgeon.
- When performing the flexor-to-extensor transfer, as a plantar approach is needed, enough distance between the foot and the distal end of the table has to be available so that the surgeon can work comfortably (**FIG 5**).

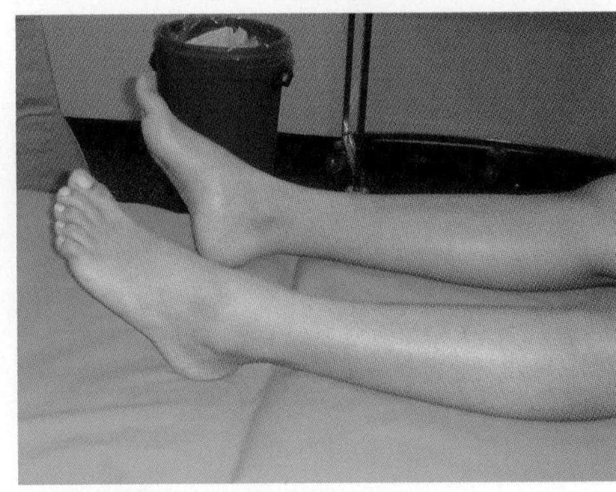

FIG 5 • Positioning of the patient with adequate room for the surgeon to comfortably approach the toe distally.

Approach

- For the MTP approach, a longitudinal dorsal incision over the involved MTP joint is performed.
  - The incision can be performed in a curvilinear fashion to avoid skin contractures (in our experience a rare complication).
- For the PIP joint approach, a dorsal transverse approach over the PIP joint is performed, removing the hyperkeratotic skin with the incision.
  - It is also possible to perform a longitudinal incision after the tendon transfer incision, which may include the MTP incision when an additional procedure has been performed over the MTP joint.
- For the flexor-to-extensor transfer, a dorsal approach over the proximal phalanx must be made.
  - In our experience, an extension deformity at the MTP joint is virtually always present, and therefore a procedure over the MTP joint is commonly performed. This MTP approach can be used, extending it distally.
  - To gain access to the flexor tendons, two plantar incisions have to be made, one transverse along the proximal skin crease of the toe and the second oblique over the DIP joint.
  - This last incision can be made transverse and a percutaneous FDL tenotomy can be performed.
  - There is a risk of damaging the plantar plate of the DIP joint and hyperextension of the joint can be observed.

FLEXOR-TO-EXTENSOR TENDON TRANSFER

TECHNIQUES

- Make a plantar incision in a short transverse fashion along the proximal skin crease of the involved toe.
  - Carry the dissection through the subcutaneous layer. Identify the flexor tendon sheath and open it longitudinally with a blade (**TECH FIG 1**).
  - This incision can also be made longitudinally, as shown by Boyer and DeOrio,[2] which helps to avoid damage to the neurovascular structures.

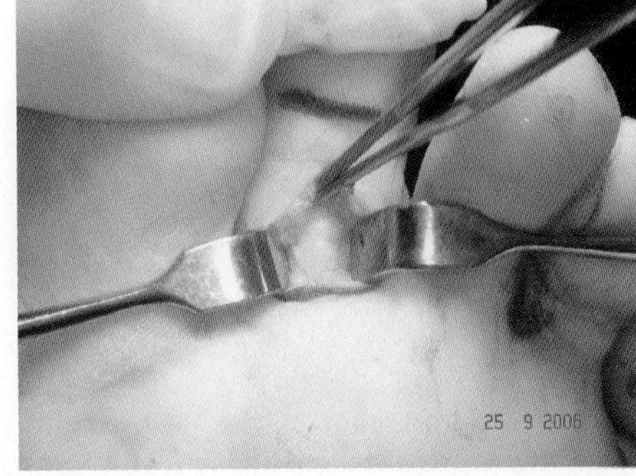

TECH FIG 1 • Plantar view of the proximal plantar incision: flexor tendon sheath identification.

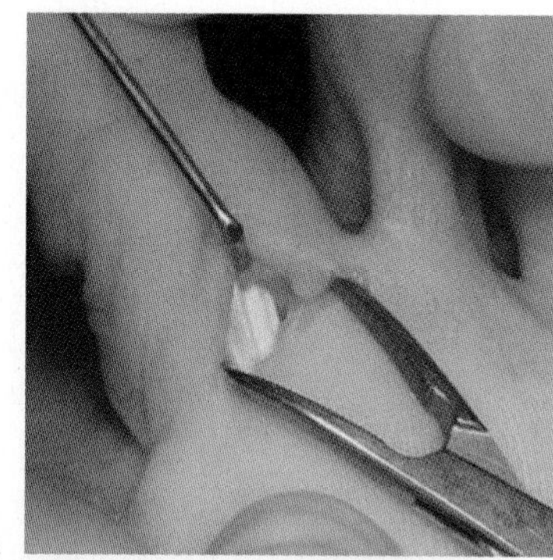

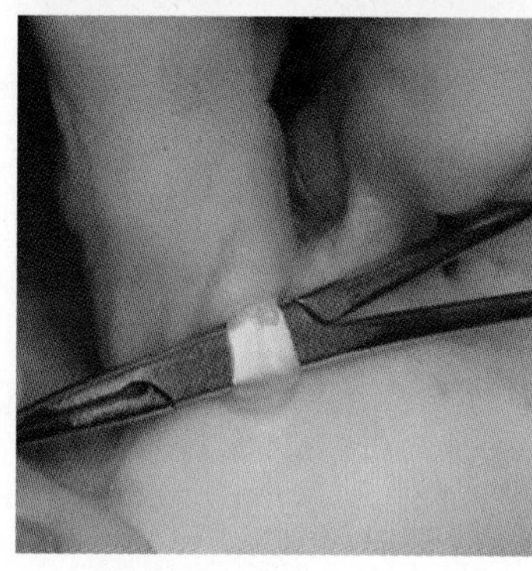

TECH FIG 2 • **A.** The flexor digitorum brevis appears dividing itself in two slips, and the flexor digitorum longus (FDL) rests in between. The FDL possesses a midline raphe, which helps to identify it. **B.** The FDL is identified with a small hemostat, and traction is being placed on it.

- Identify the FDL tendon between the slips of the FDB (**TECH FIG 2A**) and retract it with a hemostat to the surface of the wound, placing it into traction (**TECH FIG 2B**). Keep the dissection central to avoid excursion to the adjacent medial and lateral digital neurovascular bundles.
- Place a second plantar incision oblique in orientation over the DIP, just proximal to the fat pad, and identify the plantar capsule of the joint to protect it. Detach the FDL from its insertion to the distal phalanx. As noted before, this incision can be made transversely and the FDL can be detached percutaneously (**TECH FIG 3**). Keep the stab incision central to avoid damage to the digital neurovascular bundles. Although the incision is at the distal crease, direct the scalpel proximally at a 45-degree angle

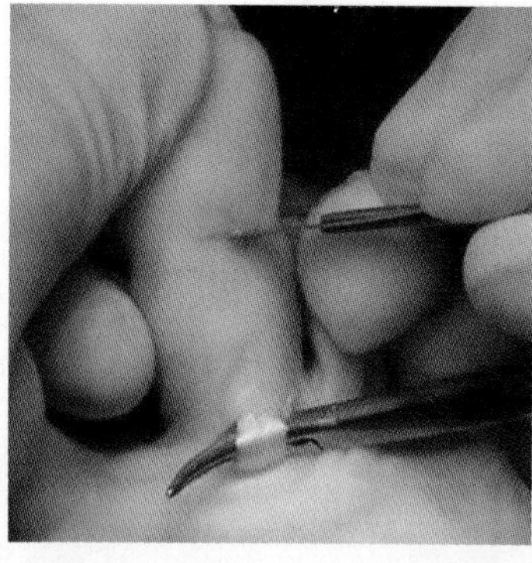

TECH FIG 3 • Detachment of the flexor digitorum longus through a transverse distal incision in a percutaneous way.

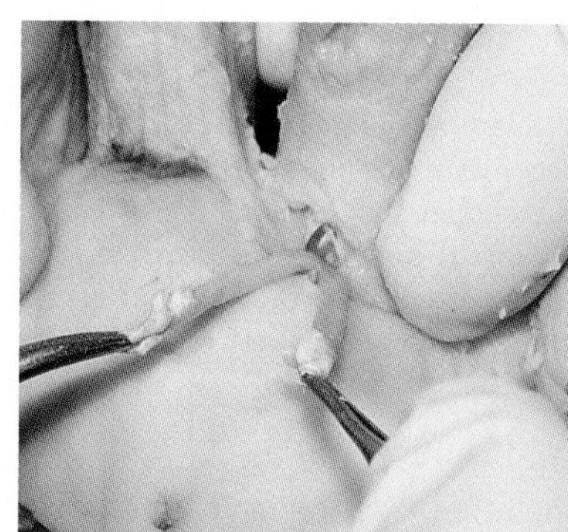

TECH FIG 4 • Splitting of the flexor digitorum longus in two following the midline raphe.

to ensure that the FDL tendon is transected and the DIP plantar plate is avoided.
- Pull the FDL tendon from the proximal incision and separate it into two slips along its midline raphe. Hold each half with a hemostat (**TECH FIG 4**).
- Place a dorsal longitudinal incision over the dorsum of the proximal phalanx just distal to its midpoint to the proximal metaphyseal flare.
  - Perform superficial dissection, and identify the extensor tendon and split it in line with the long axis of the phalanx (**TECH FIG 5**). Carry the dissection in a subperiosteal manner deep to the neurovascular bundle.
  - Identify the tip of the hemostat in the plantar incision. Take care to avoid pinching the bundle. The tip

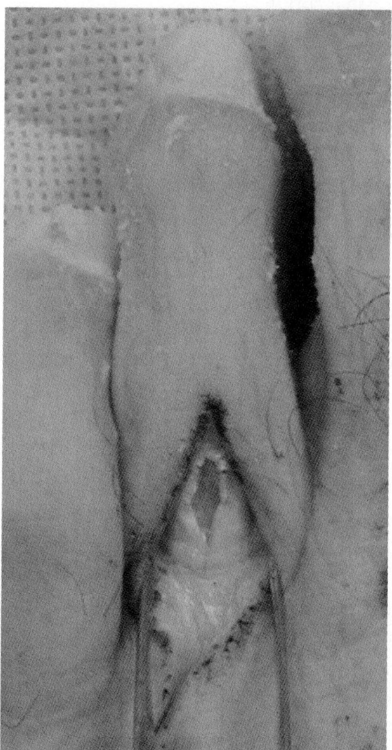

TECH FIG 5 • Dorsal incision over the proximal phalanx, identifying the extensor tendon and splitting it following the longitudinal axis.

of the hemostat must be passed through the slips of the FDB tendon (TECH FIG 6).

- First, pull half of the FDL tendon from the plantar aspect of the toe to the dorsal aspect, keeping their relative position—in other words, the lateral one is pulled to the lateral dorsal aspect of the phalanx and vice versa.
  - With the ankle held in a neutral position, the MTP joint in 20 degrees of plantarflexion, and the PIP joint in neutral, secure both slips of the FDL over the extensor tendon with two or three separate stitches of 4-0 absorbable suture.
- Evaluate the MTP joint at this time to observe for continued extension at that joint. If any is present, alternative procedures will need to be performed.
- Close the wound with absorbable stitches on the plantar incisions and nylon dorsally.
- Before breaking sterility, deflate the tourniquet to ensure revascularization of the toe.

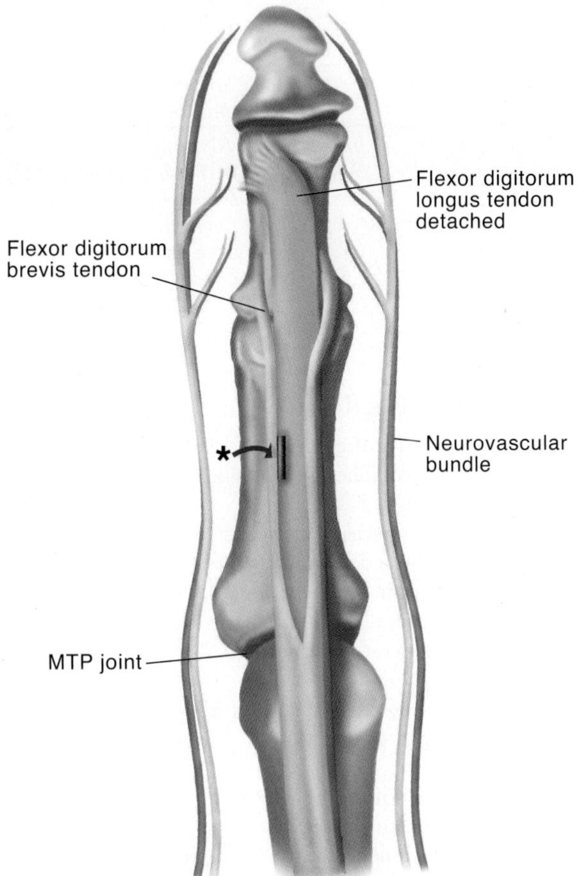

TECH FIG 6 • Plantar view of the toe showing a small hemostat passing through the dorsal incision, deep to the neurovascular bundle and through the slips of the flexor digitorum brevis tendon to hold one of the slips of the flexor digitorum longus tendon.

FLEXOR-TO-EXTENSOR TENDON TRANSFER THROUGH A DRILL HOLE

- The technique is as above up to the step where the FDL is brought through the plantar aspect of the toe.
- Make a dorsal longitudinal incision over the proximal phalanx from just proximal to its midpoint to the distal metaphyseal flare.
  - Take the dissection down to the extensor sheath and split the sheath and periosteum in line with the incision, exposing the dorsum of the phalanx.
- Place a drill hole dorsal to plantar large enough to allow passage of the tendon, in the junction of the middle and distal third of the proximal phalanx.
  - Generally we use a 2.0-mm drill and take care to avoid making a hole larger than one third of the diameter of the bone.
- Pass the tendon between the short flexors and through the hole. Position the foot as above and suture the tendon with 4-0 absorbable sutures to the extensor sheath.
- The rest of the procedure remains the same as described above.

PEARLS AND PITFALLS

Indications	■ Evaluate the stiffness of the deformity preoperatively. It is important to inform the patient about the possible additional procedures needed and the corresponding outcome. The surgery for hammer toes is a step-by-step procedure: additional surgery is commonly needed as the alignment is being corrected. Soft tissue procedures will be followed if needed by bone-shortening procedures and tendon transfers, depending on the alignment we obtain.
Preoperative planning	■ Always correct the deformity going proximal to distal. Deciding to add a bone procedure is not always easy; it depends on how stiff the deformity is. A Weil osteotomy will most probably correct the extension component of the MTP joint and some of the flexion component at the PIP joint. The problem is the resulting soft tissue balance, where an MTP joint that is too unstable may lead to a floating toe. Therefore, if there is not metatarsalgia, we prefer to do soft tissue procedures before adding a bone shortening.

PIP resection arthroplasty or arthrodesis	▪ This is a common adjunct in hammer toe surgery. Failure to resect enough of the head of the proximal phalanx can lead to postoperative pain or recurrence of the deformity. Failure to perform the tenodesis and dermodesis adequately to stabilize the joint may also result in a recurrence.
Flexor-to-extensor transfer	▪ When performing the transfer, hold down the toe to 20 degrees of plantarflexion at the MTP joint and the ankle at 90 degrees. Adequate traction on the tips of the tendon will suffice to hold down the toe. Sometimes half of the tendon can be stripped off before performing the transfer. In this case it is possible to perform the transfer through a drill hole to achieve an adequate balance with just one slip of the tendon. If the tissues are of bad quality, then a Kirschner wire may be used to fix the joint and protect the repair.

POSTOPERATIVE CARE

- Individual soft compressive dressings are placed over each operated toe; sterile strips of adhesive bandage are commonly used to keep each toe aligned.
- Small "tie-down" straps are used to hold each toe in plantarflexion (the straps are placed around the proximal phalanx of each toe). These are kept in place for 6 weeks.
- A soft compressive dressing is placed over the foot, and the foot is placed in a postoperative shoe with a rigid rocker-bottom sole.
- Immediate weight bearing as tolerated is allowed, with a plantigrade foot, keeping the MTP joints neutral inside the postoperative shoe.
- From week 2 to 4, once soft tissues allow mobilization and the stitches are removed, passive plantar flexion exercises at the level of the MTP joint are done to stretch the dorsal structures.
- From the sixth week on, depending on comfort and edema, a return to normal shoes is permitted.

OUTCOMES

- The first reports of this technique used both the FDL and FDB tendons in the transfer.
  - Parrish[9] in 1973 described the technique shown in this chapter, using only the FDL and splitting the tendon longitudinally and suturing each half to each other under the extensor tendon. Fifteen of 18 patients had good to excellent results (83%).
  - Barbari and Brevig[1] reported 89% patient satisfaction in 39 cases.
  - Cyphers and Feiwell[4] reported 95% good to excellent results in 20 patients with residual paralysis from myelomeningocele.
  - Boyer and DeOrio[2] recently reported an 89% satisfaction rate, using the technique in fixed and flexible hammer toes. They reported better results for fixed deformities where a concomitant resection of the head of the proximal phalanx was performed.
- Our experience with this technique over the past 6 years has yielded a good to excellent result in 83% of the 40 cases (unpublished data).
  - Most postoperative complaints are due to stiffness of the PIP joint, and in relation to the MTP joint when a procedure was added at this level (osteotomy, tenotomy, or capsulotomy).
  - Recurrence of deformity has been noted in 9% of the cases.
  - Retrospective evaluation of our results has shown that incomplete evaluation of the preoperative stiffness at the MTP joint may explain most of the recurrences.

COMPLICATIONS

- Swelling and numbness
  - These complications usually subside with time.[3]
  - Loss of vascularity can occur due to traction on the neurovascular bundle or compression due to the transfer.
    - Waiting, using a warm gauze, modifying or removing the Kirschner wire if used, and redissecting to ensure that the neurovascular bundle is not compressed are useful measures to solve this problem.
    - A small amount of lidocaine around the bundle can assist in smooth muscle relaxation. Nitro paste can be applied to the toe too.
- PIP stiffness
  - This has been reported in up to 60% of cases[6] (excluding joint arthrodesis or arthroplasties).
  - It is one of the main reasons for dissatisfaction, specifically in flexible hammer toe deformity correction.[4]
  - In earlier studies, no mention was made of preoperative stiffness, so it is difficult to quantify the relative contribution of previous stiffness (in fixed hammer toes) versus stiffness due to the transfer itself.
- Hyperextension deformities
  - Hyperextension deformities at the DIP joint are the infrequent result of excessive dissection in the volar aspect of the DIP joint when harvesting the FDL tendon.
    - They can be avoided with careful dissection.
  - These deformities at the MTP joint are due to inadequate positioning of the transfer (too distal over the proximal phalanx) or preoperative stiffness not adequately evaluated, which may need, besides additional MTP joint releases, bone-shortening procedures.
- Recurrence of the deformity
  - This has been reported in up to 20% of cases.
  - Recurrence is due to inadequate tension of the transfer, preoperative stiffness not adequately evaluated requiring additional soft tissue releases or bone-shortening procedures, underlying neurologic causes, excessive dorsal soft tissue scarring, or failure of the transfer.

REFERENCES

1. Barbari SG, Brevig K. Correction of clawtoes by the Girdlestone-Taylor flexor-extensor transfer procedure. Foot Ankle 1984;5:67–73.
2. Boyer ML, DeOrio JK. Transfer of the flexor digitorum longus for the correction of lesser-toes deformities. Foot Ankle 2007;28:422–430.
3. Coughlin M. Lesser toes abnormalities. J Bone Joint Surg Am 2002;84A:1446–1469.
4. Cyphers SM, Feiwell E. Review of the Girdlestone-Taylor procedure for clawtoes in myelodysplasia. Foot Ankle 1988;8:229–233.

5. Hurwitz S. Hammertoe deformity following forefoot surgery. Foot Ankle Clin 1998;3:269–277.
6. Kirchner J, Wagner E. Girdlestone-Taylor flexor-extensor tendon transfer. Tech Foot Ankle Surg 2004;3:91–99.
7. Marks R. Anatomy and pathophysiology of lesser toes deformities. Foot Ankle Clin 1998;3:199–213.
8. Myerson M, Shereff M. The pathological anatomy of claw and hammer toes. J Bone Joint Surg Am 1989;71A:45–49.
9. Parrish TF. Dynamic correction of clawtoes. Orthop Clin North Am 1973;4:97–102.
10. Thompson F, Hamilton W. Problem of the second metatarsophalangeal joint. Orthopedics 1987;10:83–89.

Chapter 32 Hammer Toe Correction

Lloyd C. Briggs, Jr.

DEFINITION

- Hammer toe deformity is one of the most common lesser toe disorders. Its severity can range the gamut from asymptomatic to disabling.
- Appropriate treatment of lesser toe disorders begins with determination of the exact joints involved and the plane of the primary and secondary deformities.
- Sagittal plane deformities of the lesser toes are generally classified as hammer toes (**FIG 1**), claw toes (**FIG 2**), and mallet toes (**FIG 3**).
- Specifically, a hammer toe is a lesser toe deformity in which a sagittal plane, flexion contracture of the proximal interphalangeal (PIP) joint is the primary deformity.
- A secondary, slight extension deformity of the metatarsophalangeal (MTP) joint may be present with a hammer toe, but this deformity is secondary and does not represent the primary deformity.
- The primary deformity being at the level of the PIP joint differentiates a hammer toe from a mallet toe or claw toe, in which case the primary deformity is located at the distal interphalangeal joint or the MTP joint, respectively.
- Hammer toe deformities are further classified as flexible or fixed depending on whether they completely correct with gentle, passive manipulation.

ANATOMY

- The lesser toes comprise three articulating phalanges (distal, middle, and proximal) that, at the proximal phalanx, articulate with the metatarsal head. The only exception to this pattern is the fifth toe, which in about 15% of individuals comprises just two phalanges (distal and proximal).
- The interphalangeal joints and their corresponding ligaments normally allow flexion but not extension past neutral, while the MTP joint complex allows both flexion and extension.
- Active motion of the toe and dynamic stability of the toe are achieved by both extrinsic muscles (originating in the leg) and intrinsic muscles (originating in the foot) (**FIG 4**).

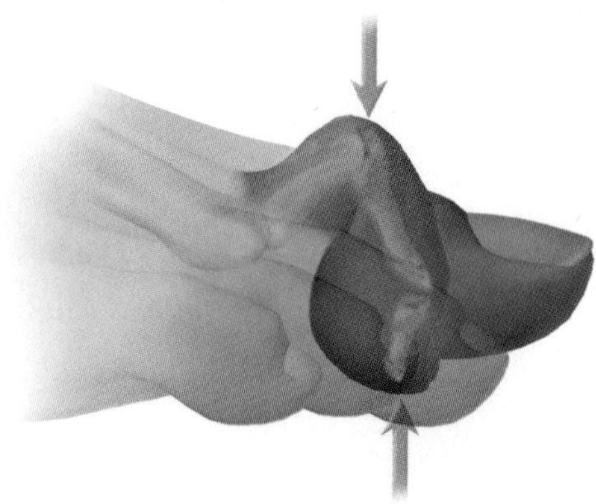

FIG 2 • Claw toe. The primary deformity is at the metatarsophalangeal joint.

- The extensor digitorum longus and flexor digitorum longus are the extrinsic muscles.
- The extensor digitorum longus invests the extensor hood over the proximal phalanx as well as inserting on the dorsal aspect of both the middle and distal phalanx (**FIG 5**), while the flexor digitorum longus inserts only on the distal phalanx.
- The intrinsic muscles of the toes include seven interosseous muscles, four lumbricals, the abductor digiti minimi, the flexor digitorum brevis, and the extensor digitorum brevis.

PATHOGENESIS

- Although the etiology of lesser toe deformities is multifactorial and includes neurologic, congenital, traumatic, and arthritic causes, the usual culprit for hammer toe deformity is restrictive shoe wear that does not provide sufficient room for the toes.
- Crowding of the toes in a shoe's toe box can be the result of poor shoe design, poor shoe fit, or a foot condition such as a hallux valgus deformity (and to a lesser degree bunionette deformity) that crowds the toe box so that pressure is applied

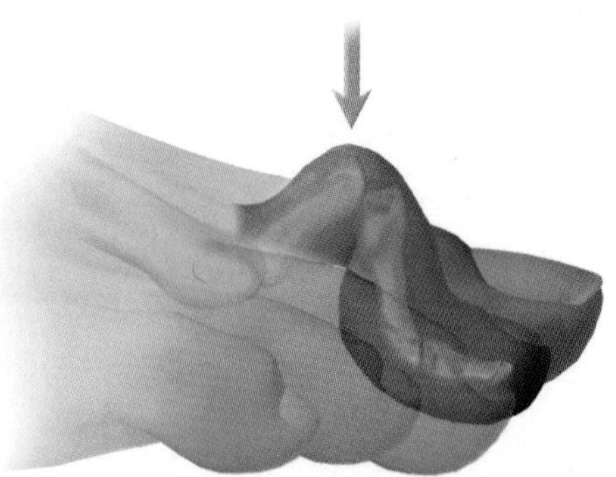

FIG 1 • Hammer toe. The primary deformity is at the proximal interphalangeal joint.

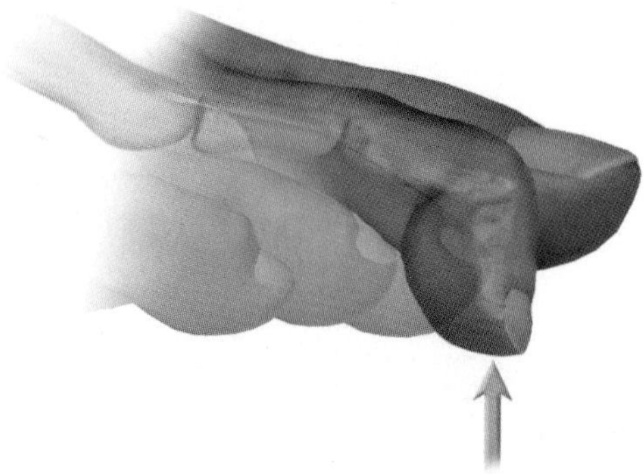

FIG 3 • Mallet toe. The primary deformity is at the distal interphalangeal joint.

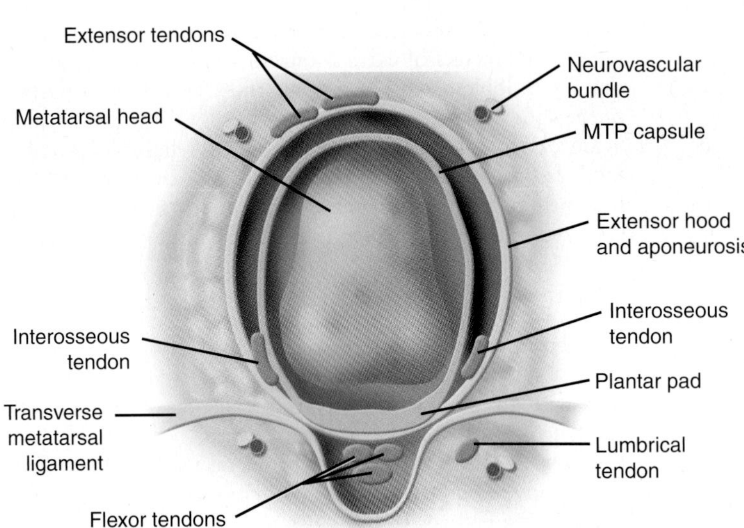

FIG 4 • Cross-sectional anatomy of the lesser toe at the level of the metatarsal head.

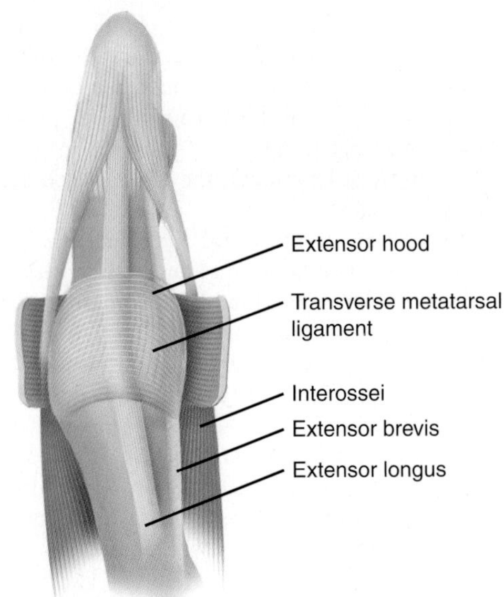

FIG 5 • Dorsal view of a right lesser toe.

to the tips of the lesser toes and causes them to be passively flexed within the shoe for prolonged periods.

- As the extensor digitorum longus, the primary extensor of the PIP joint, simultaneously inserts on the middle and distal phalanx, the flexion of the PIP joint by the pressure of the toe box is reinforced by the inability of the extensor digitorum longus tendon to extend the PIP joint when the proximal phalanx is not neutrally aligned (ie, the MTP joint is dorsiflexed).
- This passive dorsiflexion at the MTP joint can occur from the pressure of the toe box on the toe as well as from elevation of the heel (eg, high-heeled shoe wear).
- As flexible hammer toe deformity is generally well tolerated, the patient does not usually seek treatment during the initial development of a hammer toe.
- With time, unless the factors that are stressing the toe are eliminated, the hammer toe will progress to a symptomatic fixed deformity.

NATURAL HISTORY

- Hammer toe deformity generally worsens with time if the causative factors are not mitigated. Over time, the PIP joint flexion deformity will tend to increase and the toe will eventually progress from a flexible to a fixed deformity.

PATIENT HISTORY AND PHYSICAL FINDINGS

- The most important information to elicit from the patient's history is whether the patient's complaints are solely resulting from the hammer toe deformity or whether other sources of pain are present.
- Occasionally, patients will present requesting surgery, having already made the diagnosis on their own. They experience pain in the foot and because the hammer toe deformity is the only abnormality they can see, they may conclude, sometimes mistakenly, that the hammer toe is the source of their pain.
- A good patient history includes the conservative treatment measures that have been tried, the types of shoes the patient wants to wear, the sorts of shoes the patient needs to wear for his or her occupation (ie, steel-toed shoes), and other patient factors that might be relative contraindications for surgery (eg, peripheral vascular disease) or would encourage you to pursue operative intervention (eg, history of ulceration).
- Typically, patients with a hammer toe deformity present with a complaint of pain centered over the PIP joint that is relieved with removal of their shoes.
- The degree of deformity generally corresponds to the degree of symptoms.
- Symptoms of numbness and tingling in the foot, diffuse pain, pain that occurs at night, or pain that does not improve with removal of shoes or shoe modifications raises concerns that the pain may be nonmechanical or emanating from a source other than the hammer toe.
- Attempts by the patient to try different toe pads or different shoes should be noted in the history, as improvements in the patient's pain with more reasonable shoe wear helps to clarify the diagnosis as well as direct efforts for nonoperative care.
- A history of neuropathy, peripheral vascular disease, systemic arthritides, and diabetes is important to elicit to assess for operative risk as well as to screen for other confounding sources of foot and toe pain.
- Finally, a history of ulceration or infection needs to be elicited, as this may indicate a need for more urgent operative correction of the deformity to prevent recurrence.
- The physical examination for hammer toe deformity, as with all foot and ankle examinations, begins with inspection of foot posture. Calluses, scars, and previous surgical incisions should be noted, as should the degree of the toe deformity.
- Hallux valgus deformity and bunionette deformity need to be assessed as to their contribution to the crowding of the toe box.
- With the patient standing, there must be enough room for the hammer toe to lie in the corrected position if surgically corrected. If a coexistent hallux valgus deformity prevents the hammer toe from being fully corrected, then the bunion must be surgically addressed at the same time as the hammer toe to avoid recurrence of the lesser toe deformity.

- Palpation of the foot and toes should reveal a point of maximal tenderness over the PIP joint, and the ability or inability to passively correct the hammer toe to neutral should be recorded.
- Finally, as with all foot examinations, pulses and foot sensation area are assessed.
- Methods for examining the hammer toe deformity include the following:
  - Palpation of the distal interphalangeal, PIP, and MTP joints for points of maximal tenderness. The PIP joint should be the area of maximal tenderness, but the tip of the toe may be painful as well.
  - Gentle manual straightening of the toe to assess the ability of the toe to correct to neutral. If the toe completely corrects to neutral it is considered a flexible deformity. If the toe does not completely correct, it is considered a fixed deformity. A flexible deformity can be addressed with a soft tissue procedure such as a flexor-to-extensor tendon transfer, but a fixed deformity will require bone resection for surgical correction.
  - Push-up test: With the patient seated and knee flexed, the examiner dorsiflexes the ankle to neutral by applying pressure under the metatarsal heads. The correction of the toe deformity with this maneuver is noted. This will determine whether the deformity is fixed versus flexible and is also useful in the operating room to assess residual MTP joint contracture after the hammer toe has been corrected at the PIP joint. Residual MTP joint contracture necessitates additional surgical correction at the MTP joint such as extensor tendon lengthening, capsular release, or collateral ligament release.

IMAGING AND OTHER DIAGNOSTIC STUDIES

- Standing radiographs of the foot (AP standing, lateral standing, and an oblique view) are helpful to assess alignment of the toes as well as to rule out arthritis of the various toe joints.
- Vascular studies of the lower extremity (transcutaneous PO_2 readings and arterial Doppler studies with waveforms and toe pressures) are essential if surgical intervention is contemplated and there is any question of vascular compromise.

DIFFERENTIAL DIAGNOSIS

- Claw toe
- Mallet toe
- Crossover toe deformity
- Degenerative joint disease
- Morton neuroma
- Neuropathy
- Radiculopathy
- Vascular insufficiency
- Metatarsal stress fracture
- MTP joint instability or synovitis

NONOPERATIVE MANAGEMENT

- Ultimately, the treatment of a hammer toe deformity involves "making the shoe fit the foot, or the foot fit the shoe."
- Conservative treatment for a symptomatic hammer toe involves accommodating the deformity with a shoe the patient finds acceptable. Generally, an athletic-type shoe with a soft toe box will accommodate many mild deformities, whereas a prescription extra-depth shoe with an extra-wide toe box will be needed to accommodate others.
- Occasionally, softening of the leather upper of a shoe and stretching of the shoe over the area of the deformity will allow several millimeters of extra room for the toe, and in extreme cases a "bubble patch" or cut-out and elevation of a portion of the shoe toe box can give relief.
- Silicone toe sleeves or toe pads can help relieve symptoms in mild deformities, but they are not usually successful for the treatment of fixed deformities as they tend to "stuff" the already crowded toe box and make the deformity more symptomatic.

SURGICAL MANAGEMENT

- The primary indication for surgical correction of a hammer toe is a symptomatic (painful or preulcerative lesion) in a patient with adequate vascularity and realistic expectations who has failed to respond to conservative care.
- Generally, patients with these problems tend to present having already attempted some type of conservative treatment or change in shoe wear. If they have not, it is worthwhile to educate the patient concerning the nature of the problem and conservative treatment options.
- Generally, the most important determinant of postoperative patient satisfaction is a realistic preoperative expectation. When considering surgery, the patient should be told that by choosing surgery he or she is electing to trade a painful, thin, deformed toe with some voluntary motion for a less painful (ideally pain-free), short, scarred, possibly numb, swollen toe with little volitional control. The patient should not make the decision for surgery based on whether he or she wants a "normal" toe.
- If the patient's preoperative expectations are too high, he or she should be advised to maximize conservative care and avoid surgery, as most likely he or she would be disappointed with the surgical outcome.
- Preoperatively, the patient's shoe wear goals should be discussed, stressing that the goal of the operation is to allow the patient to wear "reasonable" shoes.
- A patient with a coexistent hallux valgus deformity that does not allow adequate space for the lesser toe to move down onto the floor with surgical correction will have to have the hallux valgus deformity corrected at the time of the lesser toe surgery to avoid recurrence of the hammer toe.
- In this situation the hallux valgus deformity will have to be corrected even if it is asymptomatic. The patient needs to be counseled that correction of an asymptomatic hallux valgus deformity, to provide space for the hammer toe, may lead to a painful or numb great toe ("It is difficult to make something that doesn't hurt better"). Patients need to be aware of this possibility before electing surgery and consider it in their decision to have surgery.
- With the decision made to proceed with fixed hammer toe deformity correction, there are primarily two surgical options: PIP joint resection arthroplasty and PIP joint arthrodesis.
- With either option, the fixed nature of the hammer toe deformity requires resection of bone to shorten the toe so that, as it is straightened, the contracted, plantar neurovascular structures are not injured, which would occur with simply forcibly straightening the toe and pinning it without bone resection.
- PIP joint resection arthroplasty involves resecting the distal condyles of the proximal phalanx, which relieves the deformity and often retains a small amount of motion at the PIP joint.

This procedure has almost universally good results and is generally regarded as the gold standard for the correction of the majority of hammer toe deformities.

- When it is desirable to have permanent, multiplanar stability at the PIP joint or to perform the procedure without the use of a postoperative stabilizing Kirschner wire, arthrodesis at the PIP joint may be a better option.
- PIP joint arthrodesis involves preparation of the adjacent middle and proximal phalanx articular surfaces and some type of fixation to create stability at the fusion site. Several methods of fixation have been advocated, including Kirschner wire fixation and preparing the bone so that it interdigitates, such as in a peg and dowel fusion,[1] intramedullary screw fixation,[4] or an interphalangeal implant such as the StayFuse™ implant (Nexa Orthopedics)[2] (**FIG 6**).
- The StayFuse implant is designed for PIP joint arthrodesis. It is composed of two matching titanium components that are individually inserted into the prepared middle and proximal phalanxes and then interlocked, creating stable PIP joint fixation.
- Arthrodesis is beneficial for patients for whom recurrence of deformity is likely, such as in severe deformity or revision hammer toe surgery. Situations in which a pin extending from the toe may pose an unacceptable infection risk, such as in a patient with diabetes mellitus, rheumatoid arthritis, or compliance issues, may benefit from arthrodesis with an implant spanning the PIP joint.
- Fusion is also useful for crossover toe deformity correction, when destabilizing the PIP joint with a resection arthroplasty may result in a symptomatic angular deformity at the PIP joint, as crossover toe deformity invariably recurs with time.
- Table 1 compares PIP joint resection arthroplasty versus arthrodesis.

A

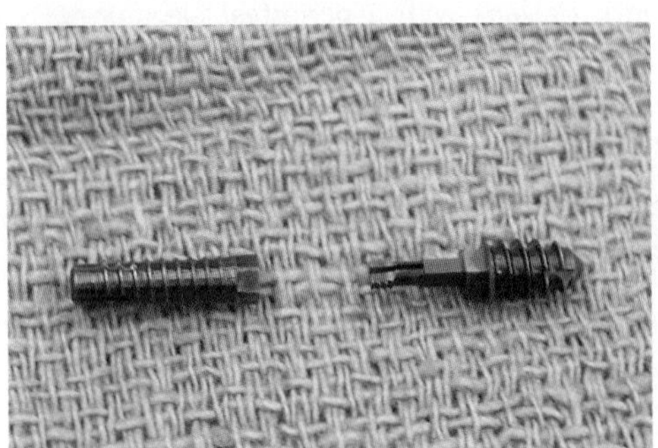

B

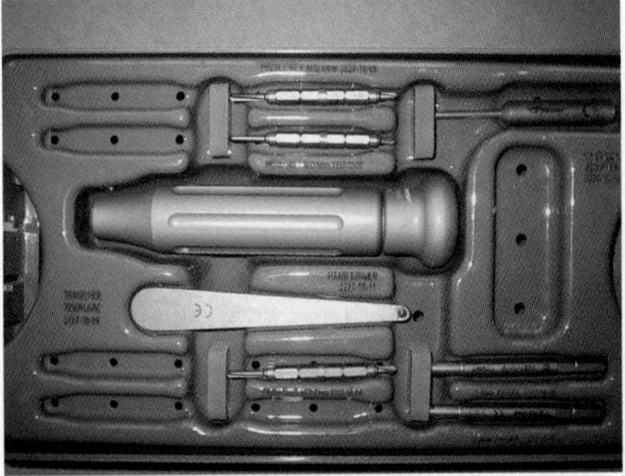

FIG 6 • **A.** StayFuse implant. **B.** StayFuse Inter-digital Fusion System: autoclavable case with (from top to bottom), 6-mm double-ended gray piloting bit, 1/8-inch chuck adapter, 5-mm double-ended gray piloting bit, universal driver handle, transfer template, double-ended blue piloting bit, large driver bit, and small driver bit. (From Briggs LC. Proximal interphalangeal joint arthrodesis using the StayFuse implant. Tech Foot Ankle Surg 2004;3:77–84.)

Table 1 PIPJ Resection Arthroplasty vs. Arthrodesis

Arthroplasty Indications

The gold standard. The procedure of choice unless there is a special circumstance.

Arthrodesis Indications

Situations with expected high recurrence rates (severe deformities and revision hammer toe surgery)

Unacceptable elevated infection risk with external pin (diabetes, rheumatoid arthritis, or anticipated noncompliance)

Need for multiplanar stability (crossover toe deformity)

Preoperative Planning

- With any toe surgery, adequate vascularity must be ensured before proceeding with surgery.
- With lesser toe surgery, especially in the revision situation or if the patient has systemic conditions that might impair toe circulation, vascular injury to the toe and loss of the toe are possibilities and need to be discussed with the patient before the surgery.
- For PIP joint arthrodesis with use of the StayFuse implant, a preoperative AP radiograph of the foot is useful to template the size of the implant. The proximal phalanx is templated first, keeping in mind that the bone will be a millimeter or two shorter after the bone resection and that the ideal implant fit would be to just engage the cortex of the phalanx.
- The proximal phalanx and middle phalanx are each individually templated to assess the size of the canal and the appropriate implant width and length (Table 2). This, in turn, determines the size of the hand drill bit, which is color-coded gray or blue.
- The goal is to find an implant that will fill the canal, but it is generally better to err on the side of a smaller and shorter implant to avoid breaking the phalanx cortex and decreasing fusion site stability.

Positioning

- Positioning of the patient is supine, with the patient's heel resting at the end of the operating table. A small padded bump may be placed under the ipsilateral greater trochanter of the hip to internally rotate the foot to give better access to the dorsum of the foot.

Table 2 StayFuse Implant Sizes

Proximal Phalanx Size	Middle Phalanx Size
2.8 mm × 11 mm (blue)	3.8 mm × 6 mm or 4.3 mm × 6 mm (blue)
3.3 mm × 14 mm or 3.8 mm× 14 mm (gray)	3.8 mm × 6 mm (gray) 4.3 mm × 6 mm (gray) 5.0 mm × 5 mm (gray) 5.0 mm × 6 mm (gray)

- The procedure can be easily performed with an ankle block or forefoot block with or without a tourniquet.
- We generally prefer an ankle block and use an ankle Esmarch tourniquet if there are no vascular issues with regard to the toes; otherwise we perform the procedure without a tourniquet.

Approach

- PIP joint resection arthroplasty and PIP joint arthrodesis are both performed through a dorsal approach to the PIP joint. We usually mark out a curvilinear incision over the MTP joint as well in case the extensor tendon or MTP joint capsule needs to be approached after the hammer toe correction to address any residual extension deformity at the MTP joint (**FIG 7**).

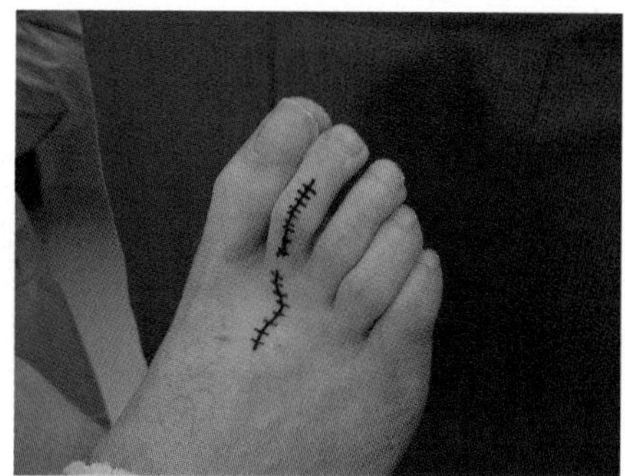

FIG 7 • Skin markings for hammer toe surgery.

TECHNIQUES

PROXIMAL INTERPHALANGEAL JOINT ARTHROPLASTY

- Make a straight longitudinal dorsal approach through the skin overlying the PIP joint, exposing the extensor tendon overlying the joint. The incision is about 1.5 cm long.
- Generally, for hammer toe surgery, I use a longitudinal incision, but a transverse incision can be used (**TECH FIG 1A**). With the toe flexed, remove a transverse-oriented ellipse of skin over the dorsum of the PIP joint. The size of the ellipse depends on the amount of redundant skin but is generally about 3 mm wide. This incision has the benefit of removing some of the redundant tissue overlying the PIP joint and may be more cosmetic, but it can make the hammer toe correction more difficult if the incision is not placed directly over the proximal phalanx condyles.
- With either initial incision, the remainder of the procedure for PIP joint arthroplasty is the same.
- Retract the skin, and expose the extensor tendon and cut it transversely over the joint as the toe is slightly flexed.
- Introduce a no. 15 blade into the joint between the collateral ligament and the underlying condyle of the proximal phalanx, releasing one side and then the other (**TECH FIG 1B**).
- Direct the knife blade proximally, staying along the bone and not penetrating below the level of the plantar plate. Progressively flexing the toe to keep the collateral ligaments under tension helps make them easier to cut.
- With the collateral ligaments released and the toe flexed, bluntly dissect the plantar plate off the neck of the proximal phalanx with a periosteal elevator to completely expose the proximal phalanx condyles (**TECH FIG 1C**).

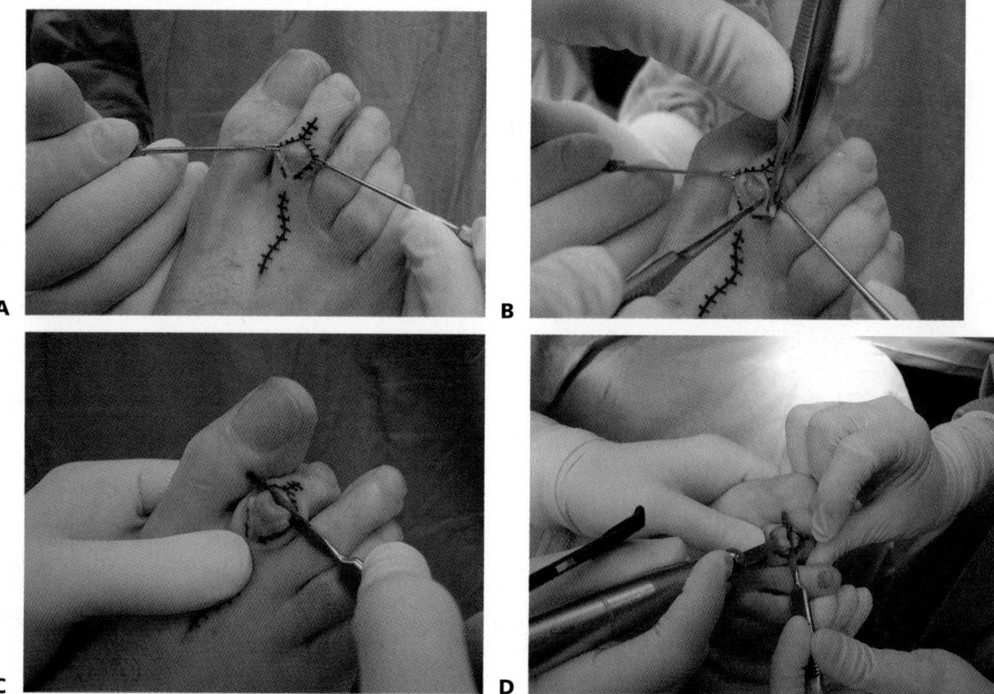

TECH FIG 1 • **A.** Dorsal approach for proximal interphalangeal joint arthroplasty exposing the extensor digitorum longus tendon. **B.** Releasing the collateral ligaments from the proximal phalanx with retraction of the extensor digitorum longus tendon. **C.** Releasing the plantar plate and exposing the proximal condyles. **D.** The proximal phalanx is cut at right angles while protecting the plantar soft tissues.

- Resect the condyles using a sagittal saw oriented at a 90-degree angle to the axis of the proximal phalanx in both the coronal and sagittal planes at the metaphyseal–epiphyseal junction. A Freer elevator is placed under the proximal phalanx condyles to aid exposure and protect the underlying soft tissues while the bone is being cut (**TECH FIG 1D**).
- Extend the toe to see if adequate bone has been resected. Ideally, gentle extension of the toe should bring the toe to neutral but not hyperextension. If the toe does not extend completely, if more than gentle extension is needed to do so, or if the toe seems to want to "spring back" to a more flexed position, additional bone can be resected, preferably a millimeter or two at a time until the toe is properly tensioned.
- The goal is to remove enough bone so that the toe straightens completely without residual tension on the plantar soft tissues so that the deformity is corrected and the soft tissues are balanced.
- Excessive resection of the bone can lead to postcorrection hyperextension at the PIP joint, which can make the patient symptomatic at the poorly padded plantar aspect of the PIP joint.
- In addition, excessive shortening of the bone will result in varus–valgus instability of the toe, especially as the proximal phalanx resection moves from the metaphysis into the shaft of the proximal phalanx.
- With adequate bone removed from the proximal phalanx, palpate the dorsal aspect of both the middle and proximal phalanges and smooth any bony prominences with a rongeur if necessary.
- Place a 0.045 Kirschner wire (a 0.062 Kirschner wire is used if the MTP joint is to be pinned) in the center of the articular surface of the middle phalanx and pass it across the middle phalanx through the distal phalanx and out the tip of the toe.
- Insert the Kirschner wire into the toe until it extends only a millimeter or two from the middle phalanx. Then reduce the PIP joint in its neutral position and drive the Kirschner wire into the proximal phalanx shy of the MTP joint.
- The pin position can be assessed with an AP fluoroscopic view (**TECH FIG 2**).
- Perform a push-up test and assess the corrected position of the toe at the MTP joint. If the MTP joint corrects to neutral, proceed to closure, but if there appears to be extension at the MTP joint, that is addressed with a MTP joint soft tissue release.
- Make a curvilinear incision over the MTP joint about 2.5 cm long. Identify and lengthen the extensor hallucis longus tendon in a Z-fashion (**TECH FIG 3**).
- I lengthen the extensor hallucis longus tendon by dissecting out the tendon and placing a sterile tongue depressor under the tendon to both protect the underlying soft tissues and assure myself that an adequate length of tendon has been exposed (about 2 cm).
- First divide the tendon longitudinally in halves and then cut it proximally and distally to create a Z-pattern cut.
- Isolate the extensor digitorum brevis tendon, which travels laterally to the extensor digitorum longus tendon, and tenotomize it to further relieve any dorsiflexion contracture.
- Perform the push-up test again, and if additional extension of the proximal phalanx at the MTP joint remains, cut the capsule of the MTP joint transversely and release the dorsal third of the collateral ligaments on both sides of the metatarsal head in a similar fashion to how the PIP joint collateral ligaments were released in the initial part of the procedure (**TECH FIG 4**).

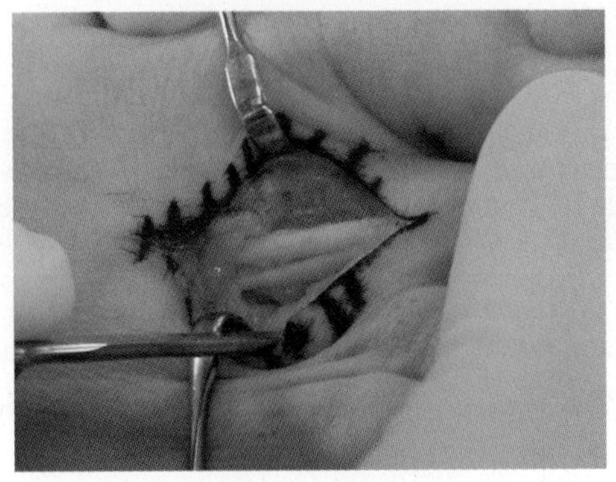

TECH FIG 3 • Exposure of the extensor digitorum longus and brevis over the metatarsophalangeal joint.

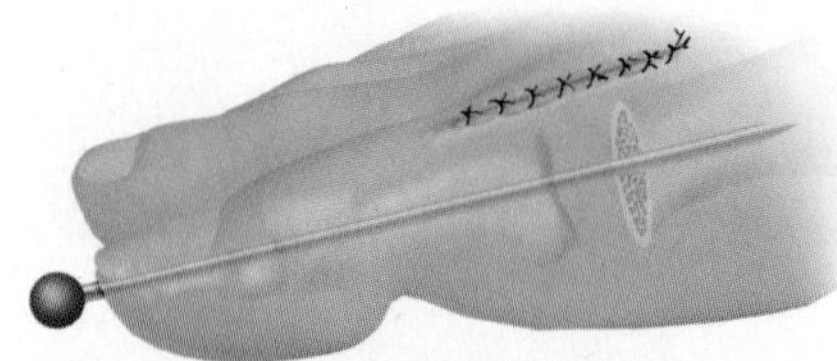

TECH FIG 2 • Completed proximal interphalangeal joint resection arthroplasty hammer toe deformity correction. (After Briggs LC. Proximal interphalangeal joint arthrodesis using the StayFuse implant. Tech Foot Ankle Surg 2004;3:77–84.)

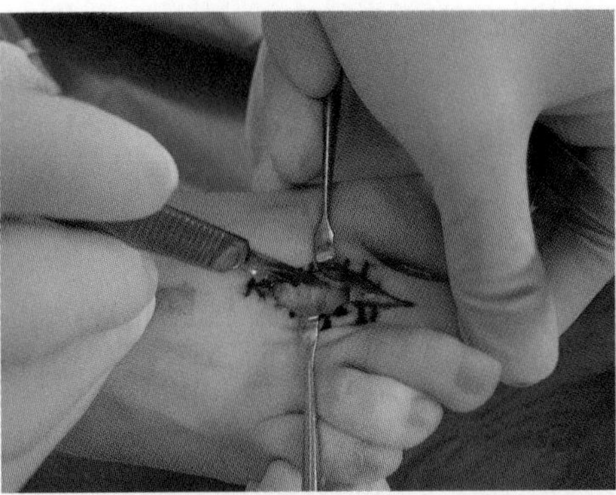

TECH FIG 4 • Release of the dorsal portion of the collateral ligaments of the metatarsophalangeal joint after the extensor digitorum brevis has been tenotomized, the extensor digitorum longus Z-lengthened, and the metatarsophalangeal joint capsule released.

- If the MTP joint has to be addressed, use a 0.062 Kirschner wire, instead of the 0.045 Kirschner wire, to pin the PIP joint and the MTP joint. The wire is usually placed 2 cm or more into the metatarsal, across the MTP joint to stabilize the joint. Pin the MTP joint while the ankle is held in neutral flexion and the toe is held in 5 degrees of flexion at the MTP joint.
- Close the PIP joint using a 4-0 plain suture to close the extensor tendon in one layer; then close the skin with simple 4-0 plain suture.
- Close the extensor tendon at the MTP joint with a 2-0 nonabsorbable suture, followed by a 4-0 subcuticular closure and 4-0 nylon skin closure.

PROXIMAL INTERPHALANGEAL JOINT ARTHRODESIS

- The surgical technique for the arthrodesis is identical to that for the arthroplasty with regard to joint exposure.
- After exposing the proximal phalanx condyles, use a sagittal saw to resect the proximal phalanx at the junction of the metaphyseal–epiphyseal junction as described previously.
- In addition to exposing the proximal phalanx, arthrodesis requires exposure of the middle phalanx. This is exposed using sharp dissection to remove the soft tissue for a millimeter or two along the dorsal, medial, and lateral aspects of the middle phalanx (**TECH FIG 5**).
- With the middle phalanx exposed, use a narrow sagittal saw blade to resect the articular cartilage and a millimeter or so of the subchondral bone. Be careful not to leave bony fragments or ledges in the depths of the wound, as these may later be prominent when the toe is fused.
- With both the proximal phalanx and the middle phalanx exposed, bring the toe into extension to see if the bony surfaces adequately align and if overall toe alignment is acceptable. Additional bony resection can be performed at this time. Make sure enough bone has been removed to avoid excessive tension on the contracted plantar neurovascular bundles once the toe is realigned. Once the implant is engaged, it is difficult to remove it should the toe not "pink up" after the removal of the tourniquet. However, although adequate bony resection is necessary, excessive bony resection should be avoided as it will lead to a cosmetically displeasing short toe.
- After the bone resection, place a 0.062 Kirschner wire down the center of the proximal phalanx to find the central axis of the bone. Use an AP fluoroscopic picture to confirm that the Kirschner wire is centrally placed and perpendicular to the cut surface.
- Remove the Kirschner wire and use the hand drill to create a channel for the implant in the proximal phalanx (**TECH FIG 6**). Preoperatively, using the radiographic template, determine the appropriate size implant for both the proximal and middle phalanges. Generally, if there is a question about whether a larger or smaller implant best fits the canal of the phalanx, it is best to err on the side of the smaller implant to avoid breaking the cortex and making the implant less stable.
- After making the channel in the proximal phalanx, place a double-sided punch (transfer template) in the channel. Reduce the cut surface of the middle phalanx and press it onto the exposed side of the double-sided punch (**TECH FIG 7A**). This scores the middle phalanx and indicates the proper insertion point for the middle phalanx implant.
- Pay special attention to assessing the mediolateral translation of the middle phalanx on the proximal phalanx when scoring the middle phalanx. Ideally, the medial and lateral cortices of the adjacent phalanges should align to avoid symptomatic bony prominences once the joint is fused.

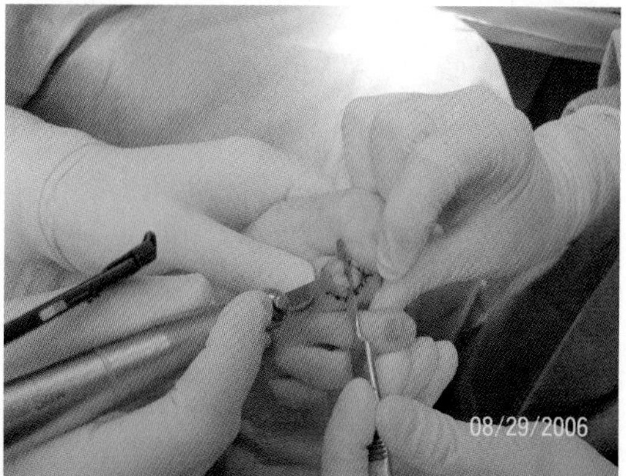

TECH FIG 5 • Preparation of the middle phalanx with sagittal saw.

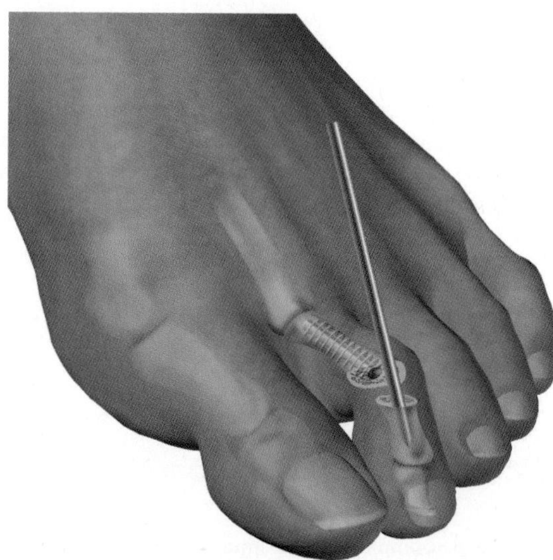

TECH FIG 6 • Middle phalanx is prepared with the hand drill. (After Briggs LC. Proximal interphalangeal joint arthrodesis using the StayFuse implant. Tech Foot Ankle Surg 2004;3:77–84.)

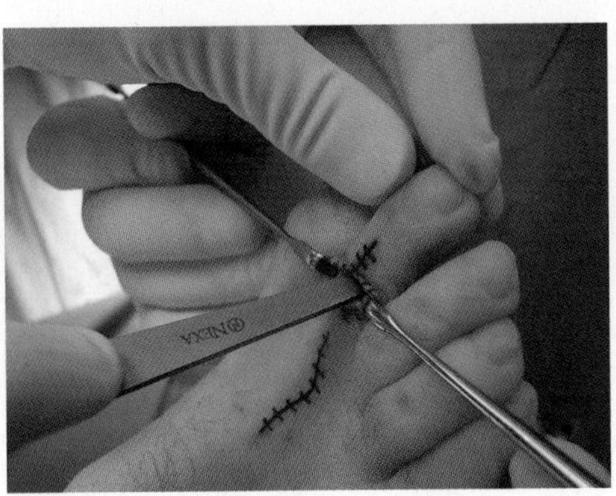

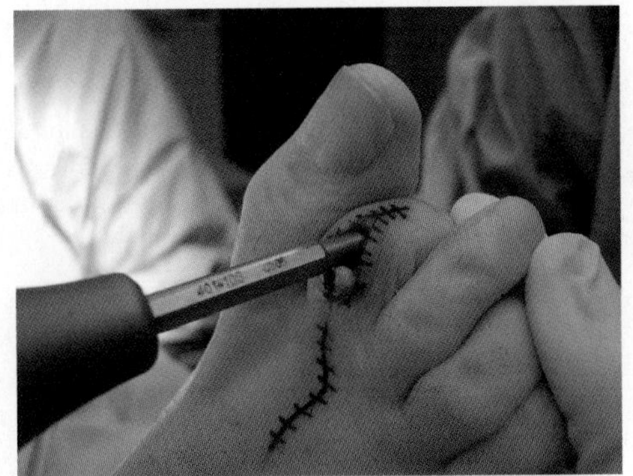

TECH FIG 7 • **A.** Transfer template is used to line up middle and proximal phalanx drill starting points. **B.** Channel made in the middle phalanx.

- After the middle phalanx has been scored, use the hand drill to prepare the implant channel for the middle phalanx (TECH FIG 7B).
- With both sides prepared, insert the proximal phalanx implant first to avoid interference with its placement by the protruding flutes of the middle phalanx implant once it is inserted (TECH FIG 8A). Insert the proximal phalanx implant flush with the cut surface. The driver bit, which is used to insert the implant, is designed to disengage once the implant is flush with the level of the bone cut (TECH FIG 8B,C).
- Place the middle phalanx implant with the body of the implant flush with the cut surface of the bone and the flutes of the implant exposed. The slot between the tines should be oriented in the sagittal plane as opposed to the horizontal plane to reduce the chance of the flutes bending as the implants are engaged (TECH FIG 9A).
- The implants are then ready to be engaged. They are distracted and brought together, engaging the two components as horizontally as possible to avoid bending the flutes of the middle phalanx implant (TECH FIG 9B). It is very important not to lever the two components together, as this can lead to bending the implants, which can make it impossible to engage the two components. It is recommended to grasp the toe with a 4×4 dressing sponge to give better hold of the toe as you manipulate it.[6]
- As the flutes of the one implant engage the other, a ratcheting sound will be audible. Once the middle phalanx is sufficiently engaged in the proximal phalanx, the hexagonal base of the fluted component will attempt to engage the proximal phalanx component. Slight gentle rotation of the tip of the toe may be necessary to subtly rotate the middle phalanx implant and allow the hexagonal portions of the implants to engage (TECH FIG 10A).

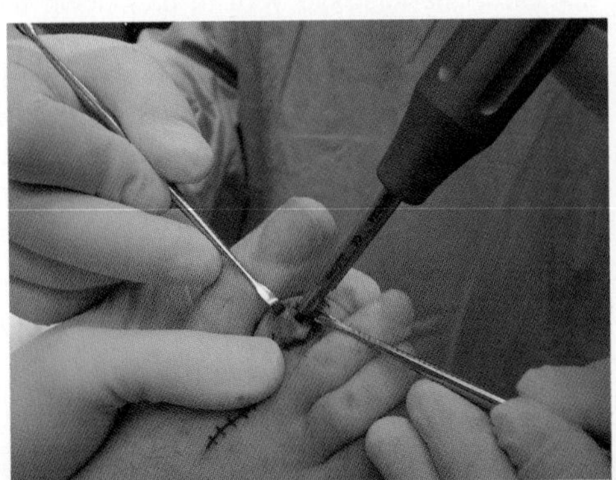

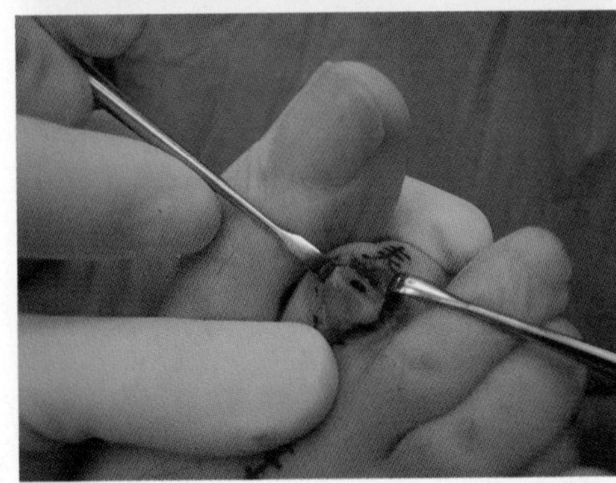

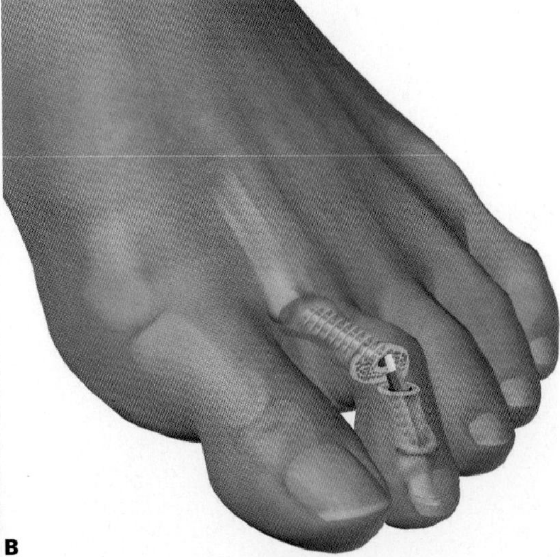

TECH FIG 8 • **A.** Insertion of the proximal phalanx implant. **B.** Fully inserted implant **C.** Seating of the implant flush with the cut bony surface. (After Briggs LC. Proximal interphalangeal joint arthrodesis using the StayFuse implant. Tech Foot Ankle Surg 2004;3:77–84.).

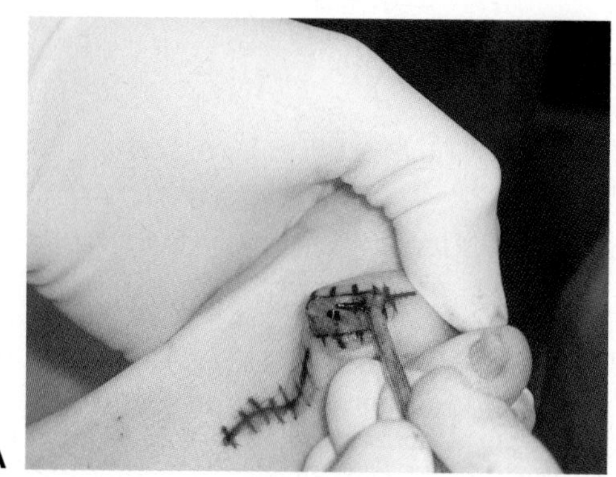

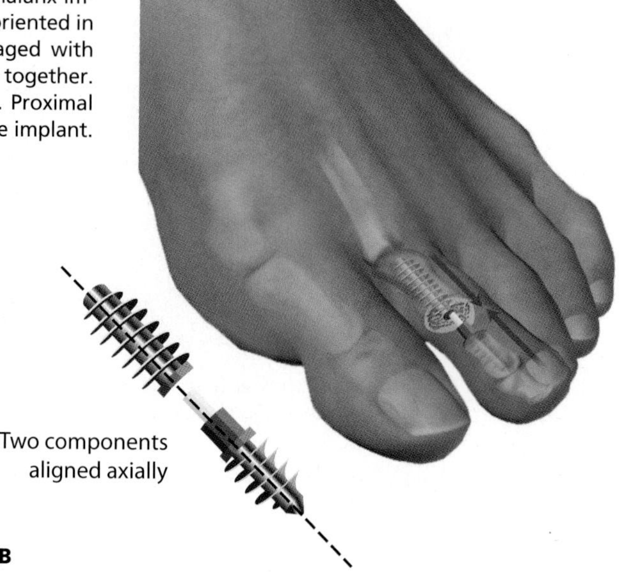

TECH FIG 9 • A. Both the proximal and middle phalanx implants are seated. The space between the flutes is oriented in the sagittal plane. **B.** The two implants are engaged with axial compression rather than levering the implants together. This avoids bending the implant. (After Briggs LC. Proximal interphalangeal joint arthrodesis using the StayFuse implant. Tech Foot Ankle Surg 2004;3:77–84.)

- If some twisting of the toe is necessary, after the hexagonal portions of the implants first engage, "derotate" the toe before the final compression is achieved so that the final compression of the toe is in the properly aligned position.
- As the implant is fully interdigitated, the ends of the bones should visually come to rest together and the implant should fully engage, as evident on an AP fluoroscopic view (TECH FIG 10B).
- A C-arm is usually used to confirm that the component is properly engaged and the toe is well aligned.
- If the implants engage, but not fully, as long as a portion of the hexagonal section of the implant is engaged, this is acceptable. If there is only a slight gap at the bone fusion site, this is acceptable as well, but I usually place some bone graft from the resected condyles to fill the gap.
- With the toe implant inserted, palpate the bony dorsal surface of the toe to make sure that there are no protrusions; remove any with a rongeur to create a smooth surface.
- The remainder of the arthrodesis procedure is identical to the PIP joint arthroplasty, with the exception being that if the MTP joint must be addressed, it is done so without fixing it with a Kirschner wire, as the StayFuse implant will not allow the Kirschner wire to pass down the toe. In these cases, I extend the dressing sponges or ABD pads out over the toe with the dressing to provide a block to dorsiflexion of the toe. In the immediate postoperative period, I initiate taping of the toe in neutral position at the first postoperative visit and continue it for up to 3 months.

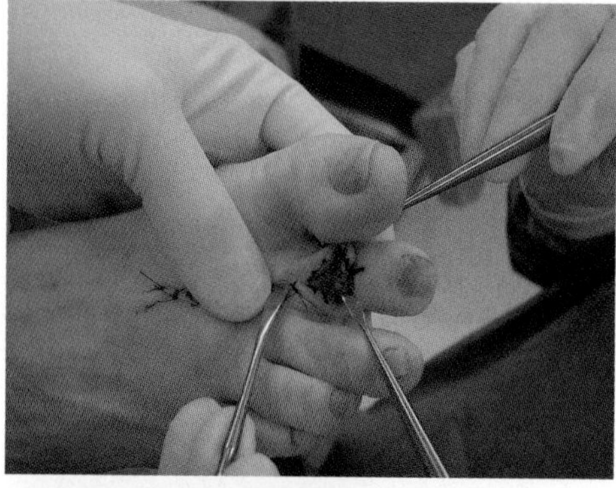

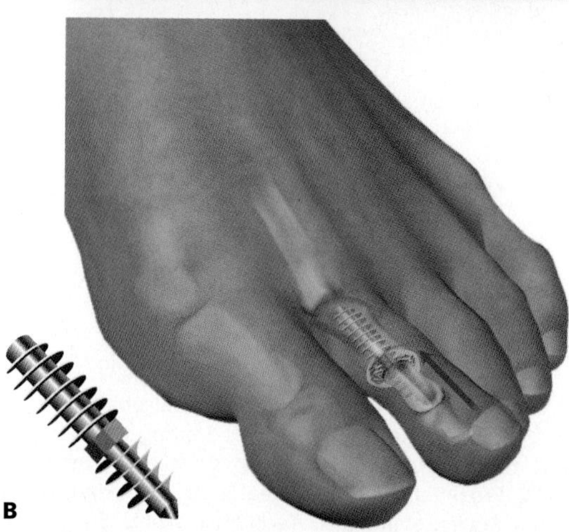

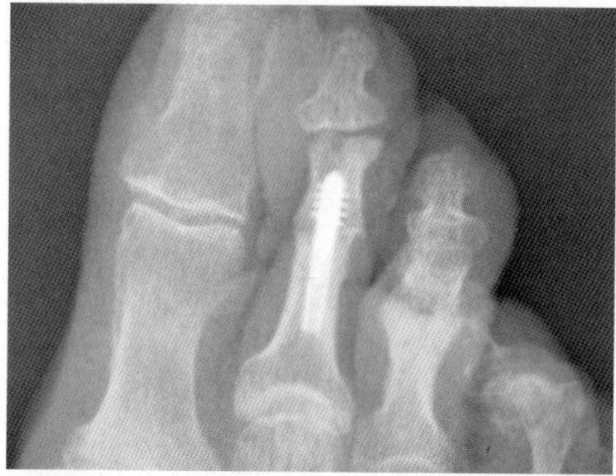

TECH FIG 10 • A. Toe with implant properly seated. **B.** Implant securely engaged. (After Briggs LC. Proximal interphalangeal joint arthrodesis using the StayFuse implant. Tech Foot Ankle Surg 2004;3:77–84.)

PEARLS AND PITFALLS

Avoid vascular compromise	▪ Assess the circulation preoperatively. ▪ Keep all dissection around the phalanxes subperiosteal. ▪ Make sure there is adequate resection of bone at the PIP joint. The implant or Kirschner wire should only hold the correction that was obtained with the bone resection. ▪ If the toe does not "pink up" at the end of the case after the tourniquet is let down, wait 10 minutes for reperfusion. If this does not resolve the problem, check to see if all constrictive dressings have been removed. ▪ Next, apply warm saline-soaked sponges to the toe. ▪ If this does not allow the toe to pink up, 1% lidocaine without epinephrine can be lavaged over the neurovascular structures. ▪ Nitropaste applied to the toe has also been advocated in this situation. ▪ Finally, in the case of PIP joint arthroplasty, removal of the Kirschner wire may be necessary. Slight bending (5 to 10 degrees) of the Kirschner wire to flex the PIP joint more or dorsiflex the MTP joint slightly is acceptable, although it makes taking the Kirschner wire out more difficult postoperatively. In the case of PIP joint arthrodesis the implant might have to be removed, although we have not found this be necessary.
Avoid pinning the toe too straight (PIP joint arthroplasty)	▪ When pinning the toe, try to start more plantarly on the middle phalanx and then exit the tip of the toe. When the pin is then driven back in a retrograde fashion there is a slight flex at the PIP joint.
Removing the implant (PIP joint arthrodesis)	▪ If after insertion the implant has to be removed, the dorsal cortex of either middle or proximal phalanx must be partially removed. Whichever side of the implant is the narrower in relation to the canal diameter should be teased out by removing as little of the dorsal cortex as necessary. ▪ After one end of the implant is removed the implant can be grabbed and used to unscrew the implant from the opposite side. After this, one option is to insert another implant using one with a slightly larger diameter in the portion that has had the dorsal cortex partially removed. ▪ The larger diameter of the implant will allow the implant to have some purchase in this situation.
Avoid bending the implant (PIP joint arthrodesis)	▪ Do not lever the implant together, but distract, engage, and then bring the implant together with it axially aligned. It is critical to position the middle phalanx implant's flutes so that the space between them is oriented in the sagittal plane. This will help keep the implant from bending as it is initially engaged.
Selecting the proper-sized implant (PIP joint arthrodesis)	▪ When using the radiographic template, remember to take into account the bone resection. Preoperatively, make sure the implant will not be too large for the toes. While we have occasionally used the StayFuse implant for the fifth toe, most of the fifth-toe phalanxes are too small for an implant.
Avoid incomplete engagement of the StayFuse implant (PIP joint arthrodesis)	▪ Make sure the base of the middle phalanx implant and the proximal phalanx implant are flush with the bone cut. The insertion device is designed to disengage once the implant is at the proper depth, but occasionally it will bury the implant too deeply. ▪ If the implant only partially engages, but a portion of the hexagonal interface is engaged, this is acceptable if the bone has been brought into proper apposition.

POSTOPERATIVE CARE

- Immediately postoperatively, the patient is advised to heel weight bear in a postoperative shoe.
- For the first 2 days activity is limited as the patient is advised to spend the majority of time with the foot up and elevated above the heart.
- After this, activity and elevation should be guided by swelling.
- Sutures are removed at 2 to 3 weeks and any pins are removed at 3 weeks.
- At 3 weeks, the patient can attempt to get into a loose tennis shoe but should be encouraged to wear the postoperative shoe as needed for comfort.
- At 6 weeks the patient can resume vigorous activity as tolerated.
- In the case of an arthrodesis with an implant, radiographs are obtained at the first postoperative visit and at 6 weeks. If the patient is asymptomatic at that time and radiographs do not show signs of arthrodesis, further radiographs are probably unnecessary.
- If the MTP joint has been addressed, we will strap the toe in a neutral position with cloth tape or a Budin splint for up to 12 weeks. We start this after the pin has been removed at week 3 or at the first postoperative visit if a pin has not been used.

OUTCOMES

- Large long-term studies[3,5] on excisional arthroplasty and arthrodesis have shown high satisfaction rates, in the range of 80% to 90%. There are no published studies involving the use of the StayFuse implant, but with the rigid fixation that the implant provides one would expect similar if not better results than have been reported with other forms of PIP joint arthrodesis.

COMPLICATIONS

- Neurovascular compromise
- Prolonged
- Loss of volitional control
- Swelling
- Recurrence
- Toe "too straight"
- Infection
- Transfer lesion
- Nonunion

REFERENCES

1. Alvin F, Garvin K. Peg and dowel fusion of the proximal interphalangeal joint. Foot Ankle 1980;1:90–94.
2. Briggs LC. Proximal interphalangeal joint arthrodesis using the StayFuse implant. Tech Foot Ankle Surg 2004;3:77–84.
3. Coughlin MJ, Dorris J, Polk E. Operative repair of fixed hammer toe deformity. Foot Ankle Int 2000;21:94–104.
4. Jones S, Hussainy HA, Flowers MJ. Arthrodesis of the toe joints with intramedullary cannulated screw for correction of hammer toe deformity. Foot Ankle Int 2004;25:256–261.
5. O'Kane C, Kilmartin T. Review of proximal interphalangeal joint excisional arthroplasty for the correction of second toe hammer toe deformity in 100 cases. Foot Ankle Int 2005;26:320–325.
6. Surgical Technique StayFuse Implant. Nexa Orthopedics.

Chapter 33 Weil Lesser Metatarsal Shortening Osteotomy

Stefan G. Hofstaetter and Hans-Joerg Trnka

DEFINITION

- Subluxation or dislocation of the metatarsophalangeal (MTP) joints results in a disruption of the fibers of the plantar plate, which is the central structure of the MTP joint dislocation. The plate provides a cushion to the joint and weight-bearing forces.
- The key point in deciding how to treat this pathology is to determine whether the pathology leads to abnormal pressure distribution in the forefoot.

ANATOMY

- The proximal phalanx and the fibrocartilaginous plantar plate form an anatomic and functional unit at the MTP joint.
- The plate is the major factor of dorsoplantar stability.
- The plantar plate attaches to the proximal phalanx and the plantar fascia, but except for the two collateral ligaments, it is without substantial fibrous attachment to the metatarsal head.[14]
- The extensor digitorum longus tendon extends to the proximal phalanx and the proximal interphalangeal joint.
- Antagonists of the extensor mechanism are the flexor tendons and the plantar plate.
- The function of the interossei and lumbrical muscles is to hold the proximal phalanx in a neutral position.

PATHOGENESIS

- High functional stresses of weight bearing and repetitive hyperextension of the MTP joint can lead to attenuation or rupture of the plantar plate, followed by subluxation or dislocation of the toe.
- A hallux valgus deformity is often associated with a subluxated second MTP joint.[5,10]
- The hallux pushes the second toe lateral, which may lead to instability and maybe to subluxation.
- It may also result from an excessive length of the second or third metatarsal relative to the first metatarsal.
- The second MTP joint is then biomechanically more subject to the pressure of tight stockings or shoes.
- Once the plantar plate is elongated and ruptured, the dorsal capsule and the extensor tendon become contracted, leading to a chronically dislocated MTP joint.[14]

NATURAL HISTORY

- Weil presented in 1992 in Europe a joint-preserving, intra-articular shortening osteotomy, and Barouk first published it in 1996.[1]
- Researchers from Europe have shown in anatomic, clinical, and radiologic studies the advantages of the Weil osteotomy compared to alternative procedures.[9,14,15]
- A dorsal soft tissue release with pin fixation,[3] silicone implants,[4] metatarsal neck osteotomies without fixation (Helal osteotomy),[8,12] and MTP joint excisional arthroplasties[6] have been reported in the literature as surgical alternatives. However, a high rate of complications such as nonunions, malalignments, and transfer lesions are associated with these alternative surgical procedures.

PATIENT HISTORY AND PHYSICAL FINDINGS

- Physical examination methods include the following:
  - Determining circulatory status is necessary to assess not only the feasibility of an individual procedure but also whether multiple procedures can be performed, if necessary.
  - Clinical examination of cutaneous sensory response may indicate a systemic disease such as diabetes.
  - The drawer test is used to evaluate the stability of all the MTP joints and the reducibility of lesser toe deformities in plantarflexion. How stable overall is the first ray?
  - Passive range of motion: Normal range of motion is 60 to 80 degrees full extension to 40 degrees full flexion; loss of flexion may be a result of the contracted extensor tendons or because the proximal phalanx lies dorsal to the second metatarsal head.
- Each patient must be analyzed individually, with attention to a detailed history and a careful clinical examination. Ruling out differential diagnosis is mandatory.
- History of painful forefeet over a long period of months or years
- The pain usually occurs dorsally over the toe and on the plantar side of the metatarsal head.
- Plantar keratosis: This callus is a circumscribed keratotic area under the metatarsal head that usually corresponds with the patient's complaints (**FIG 1**).
- Hammer toe: A hammer toe deformity may lead to MTP joint subluxation, dislocation, or both. However, MTP joint subluxation and dislocation can also lead to a hammer toe deformity.

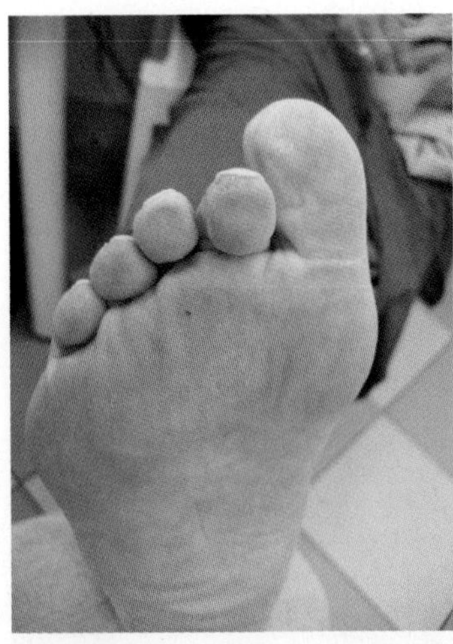

FIG 1 • Plantar aspect of the foot with a hyperkeratotic area under the second metatarsal head.

- A simultaneous hallux valgus deformity may lead to dorsiflexion forces in the second MTP joint. The great toe may cross under the second toe ("crossover toe deformity").
- A prominent dorsal base of the proximal phalanx is easily palpated.
- Tightness of extensor tendons: The toe cannot be plantarflexed due to pain and to shortening of the extensor muscle and interossei dorsalis muscle.
- Rarely a third or fourth toe is subluxated.

IMAGING AND OTHER DIAGNOSTIC STUDIES

- Dorsoplantar and lateral weight-bearing radiographs should be obtained to rule out fractures or associated injuries and degenerative arthritic changes.
- All radiographs are examined for the length of the second and third toe relative to the first and the alignment (Maestro line).
- Radiographs must be obtained for subluxation or dislocation to assess joint congruency of the lesser MTP joints (**FIG 2**).
- A "gun barrel" sign may be seen on the AP radiograph. The diaphysis of the proximal phalanx projects as a round hole in the area of the distal condyle of the proximal phalanx.
- The articular cartilage of the adjoining surfaces leaves a "clear space" of 2 to 3 mm. This clear space diminishes with progression of the hyperextension of the MTP joint.
- Avascular necrosis of a lesser metatarsal head with infraction (Freiberg infraction) may be seen.
- The hallux valgus angle and the intermetatarsal angle are measured.
- Pedobarography is highly sensitive to peak pressures in the foot. It allows static and dynamic qualitative measurement of pedal pressures and load distribution for specific areas of the foot. Load imbalance may also be detected, as well as insufficiency of the first ray.

DIFFERENTIAL DIAGNOSIS

- Morton neuroma
- Freiberg infraction (avascular necrosis of the metatarsal head)
- Rheumatoid arthritis
- Nonspecific synovitis
- Metatarsal head fracture

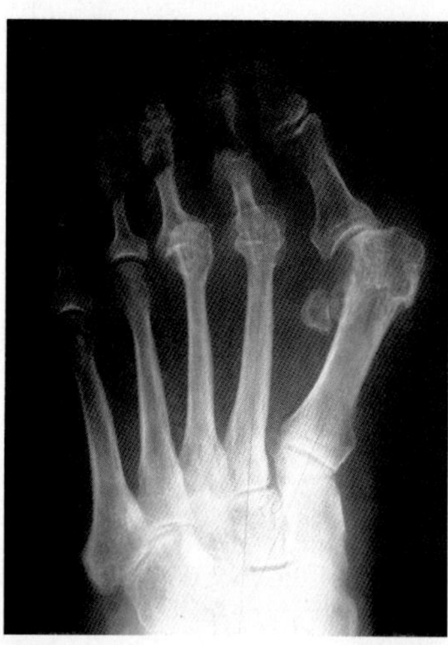

FIG 2 • Severe subluxated second and third metatarsophalangeal joint with an associated hallux valgus deformity.

NONOPERATIVE MANAGEMENT

- Initial treatment options for metatarsalgia include shoe wear modifications, metatarsal pads, and custom-made orthoses.
- Trimming of the callus mechanically
- Orthotics for the foot
  - Reduce forefoot pressure
  - Lower heel to reduce metatarsal head pressure (avoid high-heeled shoes)
  - Carefully placed metatarsal pad proximal to painful metatarsal head
- If metatarsalgia is due to a ruptured volar plate (such as in rheumatoid arthritis), often a stiff, full-length insole that limits MTP hyperextension of the foot is useful.
- However, conservative treatment in an already existing dislocation is of no benefit, and surgical intervention is indicated.[11]

SURGICAL MANAGEMENT

- The Weil osteotomy is a joint-preserving, intra-articular shortening osteotomy and has been recommended for the treatment of metatarsalgia resulting from a dislocated or subluxated MTP joint.
- The goal of the Weil osteotomy is first to alter load transmission through the forefoot by shifting the plantar fragment proximal to the area of the lesion, where thicker and more compliant soft tissue is still present, and second to resolve the hammer toe deformity or MTP subluxations that are increasing or resulting in metatarsalgia.

Preoperative Planning

- All radiographic images are reviewed for subluxation or dislocation, alignment of the metatarsal heads, hallux valgus deformity, degenerative changes of the joints, and claw toes.
- If there is a hallux valgus deformity or a hypermobile first tarsometatarsal joint, this pathology should be corrected to achieve a satisfying result.
- The length of shortening is measured on the plain radiographs. The second metatarsal should be even with or shorter than the first, and the third should be shorter than the second metatarsal.
- During the preoperative physical examination the surgeon must look for plantar keratotic disorders.
- The tightness of the extensor tendon is palpated.
- A drawer test of the dislocated MTP joint should be included in the examination under anesthesia (**FIG 3**).

Positioning

- The patient is positioned supine on the operating table.
- The surgery is performed either under general anesthesia or using a regional ankle block supplemented with intravenous or oral sedation.
- An Esmarch tourniquet may be used to obtain a bloodless field.

Approach

- A 3-cm longitudinal incision is made dorsal over the metatarsal for a single osteotomy, over the web space for a double osteotomy, and over two metatarsals for a triple osteotomy.
- A small amount of soft tissue dissection is done to identify the extensor tendons, which are lengthened in a Z fashion.
- A transverse or longitudinal capsulotomy of the MTP joint is used to identify the junction of the head and neck.

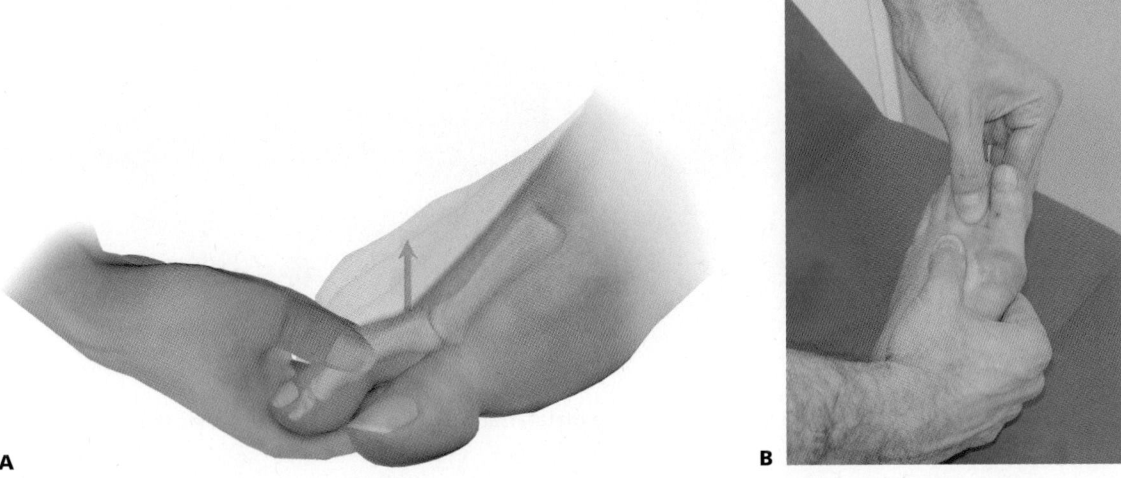

FIG 3 • **A, B.** The surgeon grasps the base of the proximal phalanx and attempts to sublux or dislocate the joint with a dorsally directed force.

EXPOSURE OF METATARSAL

- Make a 3-cm longitudinal incision dorsal over the metatarsal for a single osteotomy (TECH FIG 1A,B) or over the web space for a double osteotomy.
- Perform a small amount of soft tissue dissection to identify the extensor tendons, and lengthen them in a Z fashion (TECH FIG 1C–E).
- Incise the joint capsule in a transverse fashion and release the collateral ligaments if necessary.

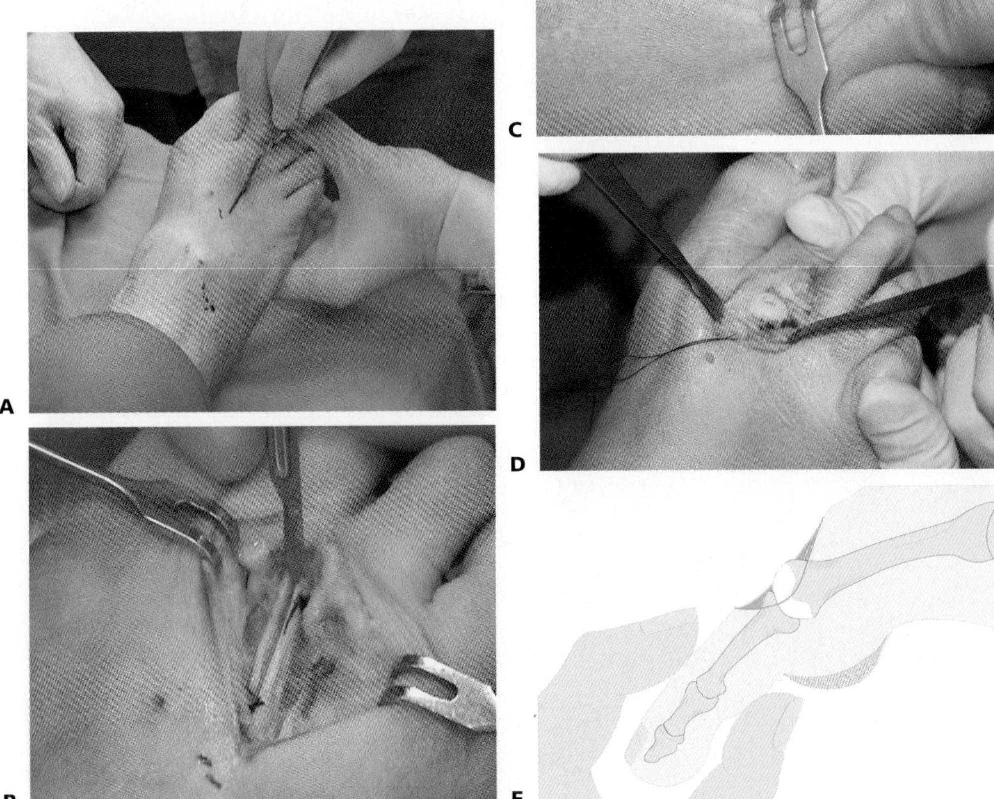

TECH FIG 1 • **A, B.** Dorsal skin incision. **C–E.** Z lengthening of the extensor digitorum longus tendon; the extensor digitorum brevis tendon is usually cut. *(continued)*

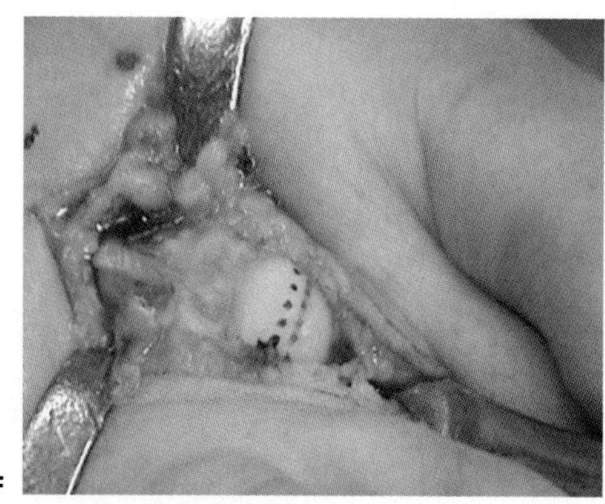

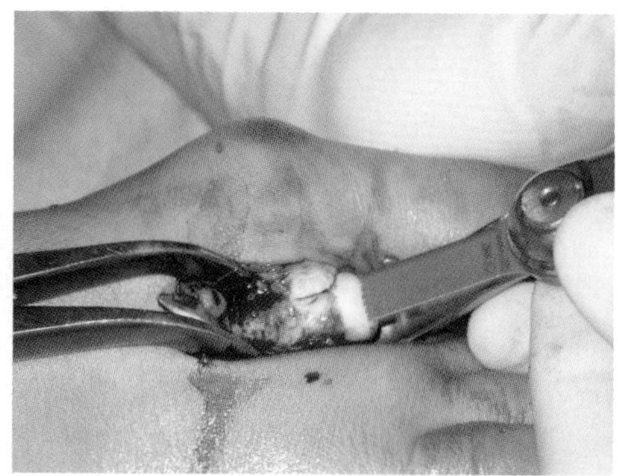

TECH FIG 1 • *(continued)* **F, G.** Exposure of the metatarsal with two Hohmann retractors; the head is exposed using an elevator.

- Expose the metatarsal head with two small Hohmann retractors. Maximally plantarflex the toe and expose the metatarsal head with the help of an elevator (**TECH FIG 1F,G**).
- Take care not to strip the plantar soft tissue attachments to aid in stabilizing the osteotomy and maintain vascularity to the head.

OSTEOTOMY AND BONY SLICE EXTRACTION

- Use a 2-mm bony slice extractor to lift the plantar fragment because the axis of motion of the MTP joint has changed with plantarflexion of the metatarsal head.
- Expose the metatarsal head and mark the osteotomies (**TECH FIG 2A**).
- Use an oscillating saw to perform the osteotomy at the dorsal portion of the metatarsal head without finishing the second cortex totally to avoid a free-gliding plantar fragment (**TECH FIG 2B**).
- The second osteotomy through both cortices is 2 mm under the dorsal cut (**TECH FIG 2C,D**).
- The bony slice can now be easily removed (**TECH FIG 2E,F**).

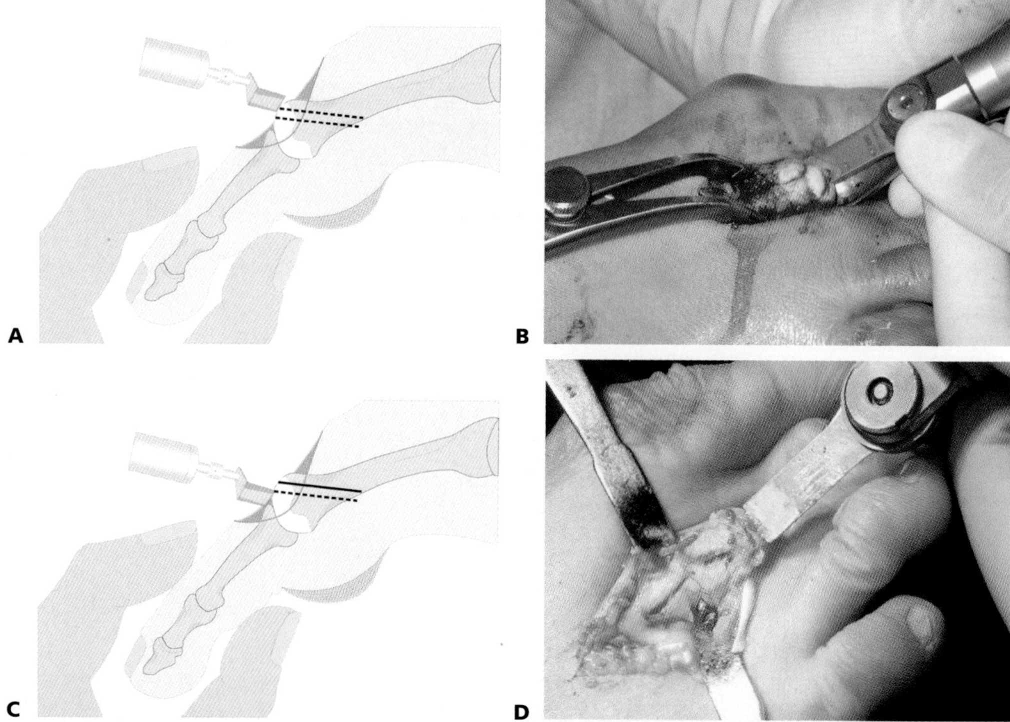

TECH FIG 2 • **A.** Exposure of the metatarsal head and marking of the two osteotomy levels. **B.** Osteotomy at the dorsal aspect of the metatarsal head. **C, D.** Plantar osteotomy of the metatarsal head. *(continued)*

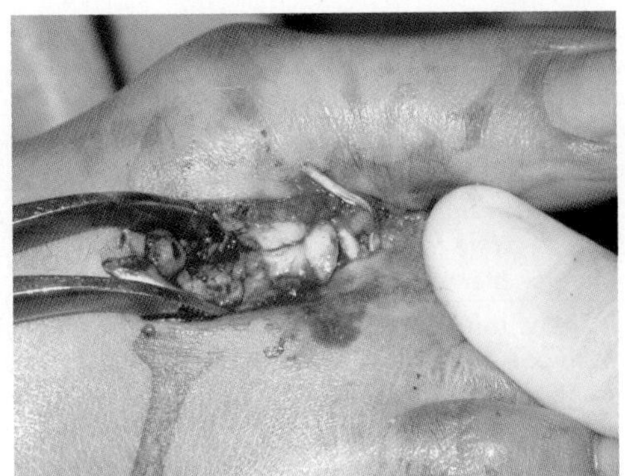

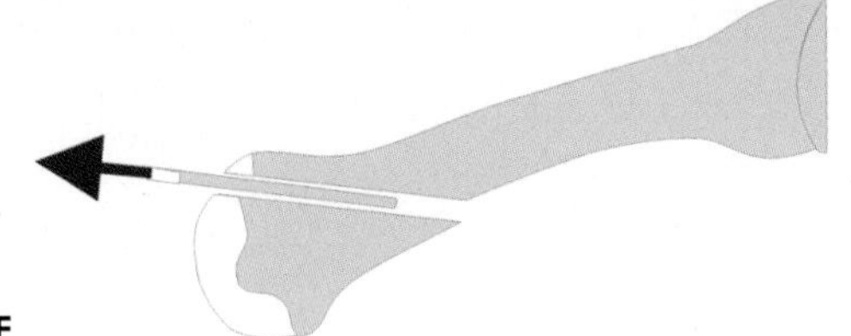

TECH FIG 2 • *(continued)* **E, F.** Removal of the bony slice after the osteotomies.

FIXATION OF THE MOBILE FRAGMENT

- Grasp the plantar mobile fragment with a pointed reduction clamp and shift it proximally to achieve the requisite amount of shortening that was measured preoperatively on the dorsoplantar radiographs (TECH FIG 3A).
- The second metatarsal should be even with or shorter than the first, and the third should be shorter than the second metatarsal.
- The plane of the osteotomy should be as parallel to the ground surface as possible. Secure the osteotomy with a special 2-mm titanium "snap off screw" (Wright Medical Technology) (TECH FIG 3B). Use a 12-mm length for the second metatarsal and 11 mm for the other metatarsals.
- Remove the resulting dorsal protuberance over the metatarsal head remnant with a rongeur or the edge of the saw blade (TECH FIG 3C,D).
- Repair the overlying Z-lengthened extensor tendon and suture the skin.

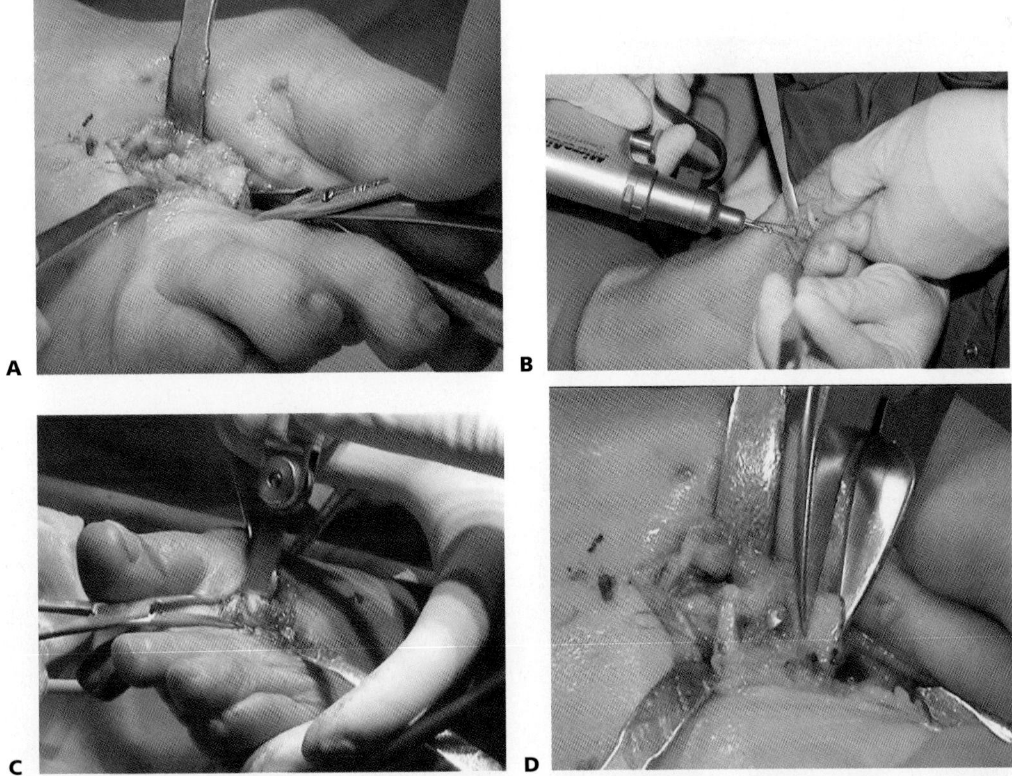

TECH FIG 3 • **A.** Positioning of the plantar fragment. **B.** Fixation of the Weil osteotomy with a snap off screw (Wright Medical Technology). **C, D.** Modeling of the dorsal protuberance with a rongeur or the edge of the saw blade.

PEARLS AND PITFALLS

Collateral ligaments	■ We do not routinely release the collateral ligaments when performing a Weil osteotomy. A substantial portion of the metatarsal head blood supply courses via delicate arteries in the collateral ligaments.
Orientation of the saw blade	■ We dorsiflex the ankle and use the plantar heel as a guide to orient the saw blade in the sagittal plane and look at the whole forefoot to get the orientation in the transverse plane.
Wedge resection	■ We excise a wedge within the osteotomy in lieu of creating a single cut. Elevation is not important regarding loading of the head, but elevating the head will maintain a favorable center of rotation for the head. In theory, this will keep the intrinsic flexor tendons plantar to the center of rotation, thereby reducing the risk for postoperative toe elevation ("floating toe").

POSTOPERATIVE CARE

- Dressings and a tight bandage are used to protect the suture and to prevent swelling.
- The patient's toes are taped in slight plantarflexion.
- Weight bearing with a postoperative shoe is allowed after the first postoperative day (**FIG 4A**).
- Patients should wear the postoperative shoe for 6 weeks.
- Postoperative imaging includes dorsoplantar and lateral radiographs (**FIG 4B–D**).
- Passive motion (starting on the 5th postoperative day) of the MTP joint is indicated and necessary to prevent postoperative extension contracture.
- If swelling occurs, foot elevation, cryotherapy, and elastic stockings may keep the swelling down.

OUTCOMES

- Clinical results of the Weil osteotomy have been promising. Outcomes include a significant reduction of pain, a significant reduction in plantar callus formation, a low dislocation rate, and increased ambulatory capacity.
- No malunion or pseudarthrosis was documented in the literature.
- Bony and soft tissue modifications such as lengthening of the extensor tendon, 2-mm bony slice extraction, and inser-

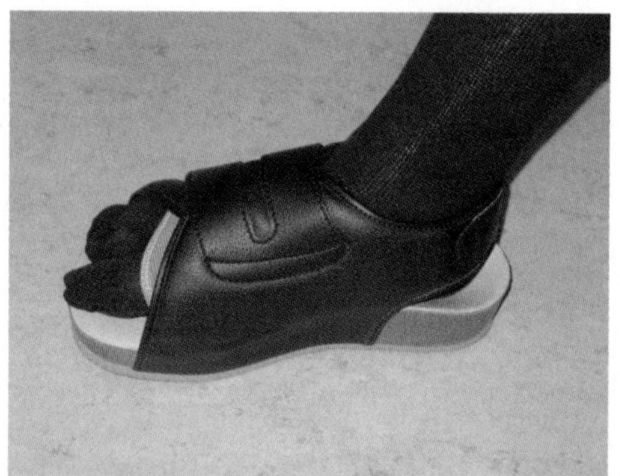

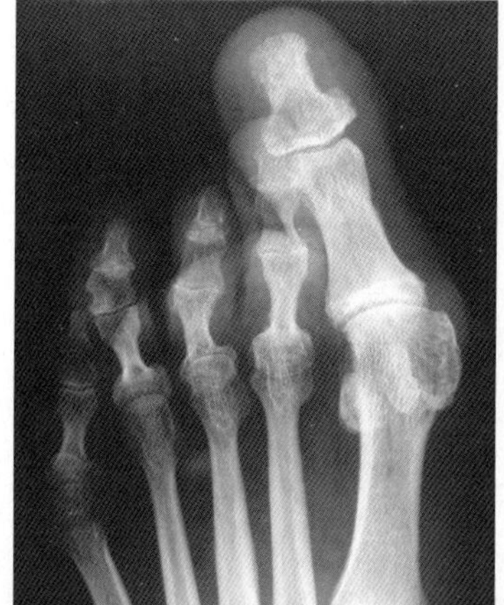

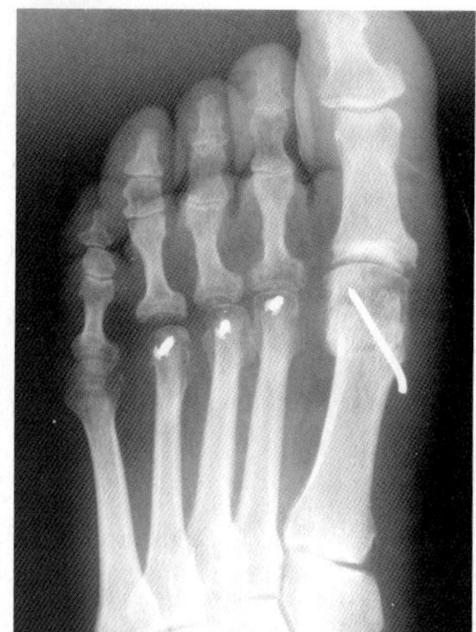

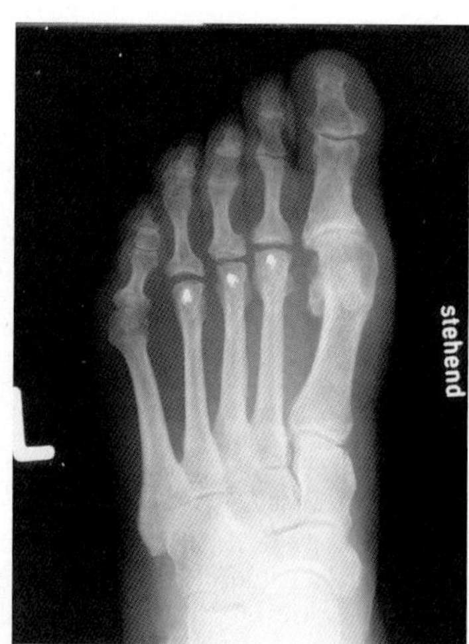

FIG 4 • **A.** Postoperative shoe. **B.** Preoperative radiographs with hallux valgus deformity and subluxation of second and third metatarsophalangeal joint. **C.** Chevron osteotomy with pin fixation along with a Weil osteotomy on the second, third, and fourth rays. **D.** Seven-year radiograph showing maintenance of corrected lesser metatarsophalangeal joints.

tion of a Kirschner wire from the tip of the toe across the MTP joint and the osteotomy into the metatarsal, in a position of 5 degrees plantarflexion (in severely subluxated contracted cases), may prevent postoperative dorsiflexion contracture.

▪ Boyer and DeOrio[2] described good results of a single-pin fixation for a combined metatarsal neck osteotomy with proximal interphalangeal joint resection arthroplasty and flexor digitorum longus transfer in severely dislocated MTP joints and severe hammer toe deformities.

COMPLICATIONS

▪ Reported complications in the literature are floating or stiff toes, a high rate of postoperative dorsiflexed contracture and transfer metatarsalgia in cases of excessive shortening with variable rates, and a limitation of the range of motion in the MTP joint.[7,9]

REFERENCES

1. Barouk LS. [Weil's metatarsal osteotomy in the treatment of metatarsalgia.] Orthopade 1996;25:338–344.
2. Boyer ML, DeOrio JK. Metatarsal neck osteotomy with proximal interphalangeal joint resection fixed with a single temporary pin. Foot Ankle Int 2004;25:144–148.
3. Coughlin MJ. Subluxation and dislocation of the second metatarsophalangeal joint. Orthop Clin North Am 1989;20:535–551.
4. Cracchiolo A III, Kitaoka HB, Leventen EO. Silicone implant arthroplasty for second metatarsophalangeal joint disorders with and without hallux valgus deformities. Foot Ankle 1988;9:10–18.
5. Davies MS, Saxby TS. Metatarsal neck osteotomy with rigid internal fixation for the treatment of lesser toe metatarsophalangeal joint pathology. Foot Ankle Int 1999;20:630–635.
6. DuVries HL. Dislocation of the toe. JAMA 1956;160:728.
7. Hart R, Janecek M, Bucek P. [The Weil osteotomy in metatarsalgia.] Z Orthop Ihre Grenzgeb 2003;141:590–594.
8. Helal B, Greiss M. Telescoping osteotomy for pressure metatarsalgia. J Bone Joint Surg Br 1984;66:213–217.
9. Hofstaetter SG, Hofstaetter JG, Gruber F, et al. The Weil osteotomy: a seven-year follow-up. J Bone Joint Surg Br 2005;87B:1507–1511.
10. Kitaoka HB, Patzer GL. Chevron osteotomy of lesser metatarsals for intractable plantar callosities. J Bone Joint Surg Br 1998;80:516–518.
11. Mann RA. Metatarsalgia: common causes and conservative treatment. Postgrad Med 1984;75:150–163.
12. Trnka HJ, Kabon B, Zettl R, et al. Helal metatarsal osteotomy for the treatment of metatarsalgia: a critical analysis of results. Orthopedics 1996;19:457–461.
13. Trnka HJ, Mühlbauer M, Zettl R, et al. Comparison of the results of the Weil and Helal osteotomies for the treatment of metatarsalgia secondary to dislocation of the lesser metatarsophalangeal joints. Foot Ankle Int 1999;20:72–79.
14. Trnka HJ, Nyska M, Parks BG, et al. Dorsiflexion contracture after the Weil osteotomy: results of cadaver study and three-dimensional analysis. Foot Ankle Int 2001;22:47–50.
15. Vandeputte G, Dereymaeker G, Steenwerckx A, et al. The Weil osteotomy of the lesser metatarsals: a clinical and pedobarographic follow-up study. Foot Ankle Int 2000;21:370–374.
16. Winson IG, Rawlinson J, Broughton NS. Treatment of metatarsalgia by sliding distal metatarsal osteotomy. Foot Ankle 1988;9:2–6.

Chapter 34 Angular Deformity of the Lesser Toes

Adolph S. Flemister, Jr., and Brian D. Giordano

BACKGROUND

- Varus or valgus angulation of the lesser toes can result in significant pain and disability and can be grouped broadly into the following subcategories:
  - Crossover or crossunder second toe
  - Congenital crossover fifth toe
  - Curly toe deformity
  - Isolated metatarsophalangeal (MTP) joint angular deformity
  - Clinodactyly
- Understanding the etiology behind each type of angular toe deformity is crucial for determining whether surgical or nonsurgical management is appropriate.
- Angular toe deformities can occur as the result of a variety of intrinsic or extrinsic factors, including inflammatory arthritis, trauma, congenital abnormalities, neuromuscular disorders, and poorly fitting shoe wear.
- Surgical management options are based on the severity of the deformity, degree of response to nonsurgical management, and underlying cause of the deformity. A variety of surgical procedures have been proposed to address angular deformity of the lesser toes:
  - Tenodesis
  - Tenotomy
  - Tendon transfer
  - Soft tissue release
  - Soft tissue lengthening
  - Proximal basilar osteotomy
  - Resection arthroplasty
  - Interphalangeal fusion
- Outcomes are predicated on the degree of return to full activity, pain relief, and recurrence of deformity.

DEFINITIONS

- *Crossover second toe deformity* (**FIG 1A**) is characterized by a second toe that lies dorsomedially relative to the hallux.
- *Congenital crossover fifth toe* (**FIG 1B**) represents a variable congenital anomaly involving the fifth MTP joint in which the small toe deviates medially and superiorly relative to the fourth toe. Patients typically complain of discomfort and irritation over the dorsum of the fifth toe, especially when wearing constrictive footwear.
- *Curly toe deformity* (**FIG 1C**) is a relatively common congenital anomaly, usually found in children, that may be related to intrinsic muscle paresis, although this relationship has not been clearly established. The deformity usually involves the fourth or fifth toe, or both, and is characterized by a flexible

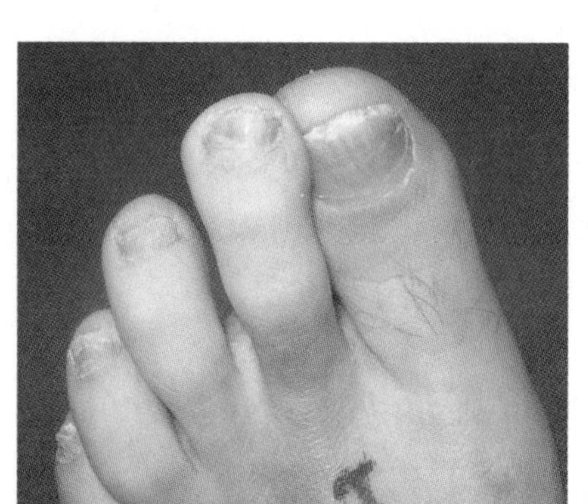
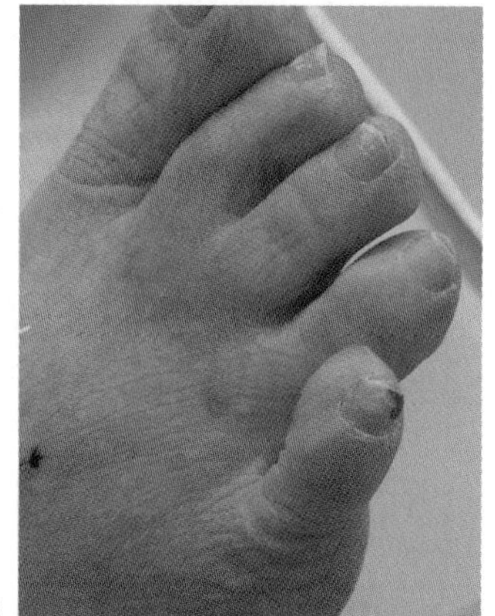
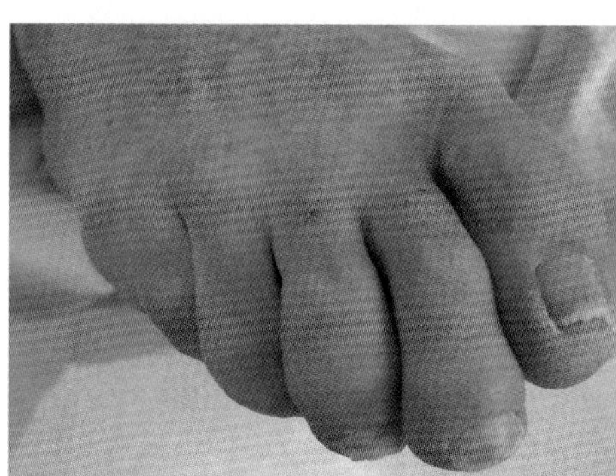
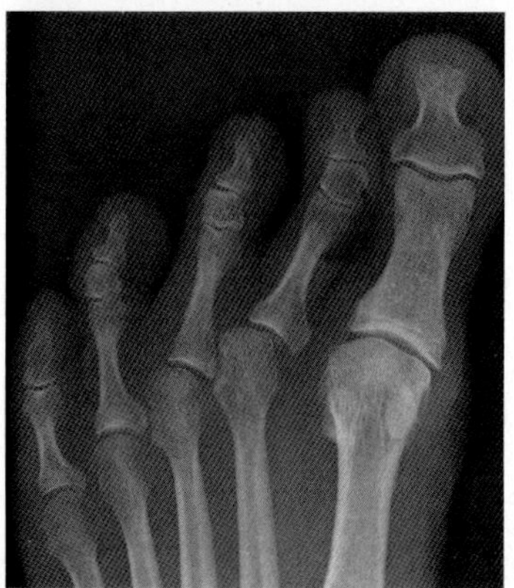
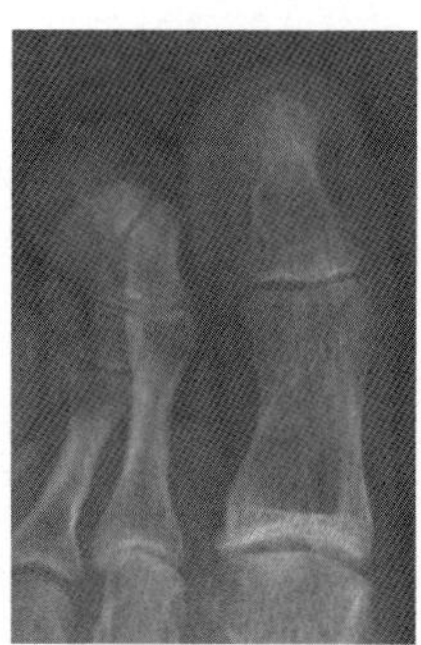

FIG 1 • **A.** Crossover second toe deformity. **B.** Congenital crossover of the fifth toe. **C.** Curly toe deformity. **D.** Isolated metatarsophalangeal angular deformity. **E.** Clinodactyly.

flexion deformity of the proximal interphalangeal (PIP) and distal interphalangeal (DIP) joints with underlapping of the fourth toe on the third and of the fifth toe on the fourth.

- *Isolated MTP angular deformity* (**FIG 1D**) is varus or valgus angulation of the lesser toes occurring solely through the MTP joint. This often occurs in conjunction with great toe varus or valgus deformity.
- *Clinodactyly* (**FIG 1E**) is varus or valgus deviation of a toe caused by angulation within the phalanx itself. This condition is more commonly seen in the fingers and is often associated with a syndrome (eg, symphalangism) or chromosomal disorder.

ANATOMY

- The extensor digitorum longus (EDL) forms three tendinous slips on the dorsum of each toe; the first inserts into the middle phalanx, and the remaining two merge and insert on the distal phalanx.
- In concert, the EDL and extensor digitorum brevis (EDB) extend the MTP, PIP, and DIP joints through their pull on the extensor hood.
- The flexor digitorum longus (FDL) courses deep to the flexor digitorum brevis (FDB) on the plantar surface of the toe and acts as a powerful flexor at the DIP joint.
- The PIP and MTP joints are flexed through the combined action of the FDL and FDB tendons as well as the lumbrical and interosseous muscles.
- The intrinsics first pass plantar to the axis of MTP joint rotation and then dorsal to the axis of motion of the PIP and DIP joints. This anatomic relationship allows the intrinsics to act as flexors at the MTP joint and extensors at the PIP and DIP joints.
  - Disruption of this delicate balance can lead to problematic disequilibrium between the intrinsics and extrinsics, which in turn can result in characteristic lesser toe deformities and associated pressure phenomena.
- The medial collateral ligament (MCL) and lateral collateral ligament (LCL) play a vital role in stabilizing the MTP joint by acting as static constraints to joint subluxation or dislocation. The collaterals originate from the dorsal aspect of the metatarsal head and insert distally both at the base of the proximal phalanx and at the plantar plate.
- In addition to providing stability in the transverse plane, the collaterals resist dorsal subluxation of the proximal phalanx on the metatarsal head. Laxity of the collaterals is commonly noted intraoperatively with angular lesser toe deformities and, in some cases, is thought to play an causative role in the development of these deformities.

CROSSOVER DEFORMITY OF THE SECOND TOE

PATHOGENESIS

- Crossover second toe deformity most commonly occurs as the result of attritional rupture of the LCL and lateral capsule of the second toe.
- Frequently, this specific type of lesser toe deformity occurs in association with longstanding hallux valgus.
- Association with a long second metatarsal and attenuation of the first dorsal interosseous tendon and plantar plate are also common.
- Destabilization of the second MTP joint can also occur as the result of trauma, synovitis related to underlying inflammatory arthritides such as rheumatoid arthritis, nonspecific or chronic synovitis, constriction from narrow-toebox shoes, or connective tissue diseases such as systemic lupus erythematosus.
- Neuromuscular disorders such as diabetic neuropathy, Charcot-Marie-Tooth disorder, poliomyelitis, or Friedreich's ataxia can also disrupt the dynamic stability of the foot and, subsequently, that of the lesser toes.
- Often, medial soft tissue such as the MCL, medial capsule, and interosseous and lumbrical tendons are contracted at the MP joint.

NATURAL HISTORY

- Early synovitis, then subluxation, and finally dorsomedial or inferomedial dislocation are the characteristic stages in the natural progression of this coronal plane deformity.

PATIENT HISTORY AND PHYSICAL FINDINGS

- Crossover second toe deformity presents either as a dorsomedially subluxated second toe that crosses up and over the hallux or as an inferomedially subluxated second toe that crosses under the great toe.
- There is often associated hyperextension or hyperflexion at the proximal phalanx at the MTP joint and adduction of the second ray from the midline.
- A painful intractable plantar keratotic lesion beneath the second metatarsal head or dorsal corn over any portion of the second phalanges (particularly over the PIP joint) may be due to impingement of the toebox of the shoe.
- Instability of the plantar plate can be evaluated by the drawer test applied in the sagittal plane.

IMAGING AND DIAGNOSTIC STUDIES

- All angular deformities involving the lesser toes can be appropriately studied by examining standard anteroposterior (AP), lateral, and oblique radiographs of the affected foot.

NONOPERATIVE MANAGEMENT

- In general, conservative measures are more effective for treatment of subluxation of the second MTP joint versus dislocation.
- Activity modification is usually necessary to resolve underlying second MTP synovitis.
- Some degree of relief is usually afforded by avoidance of shoes with a tight, narrow toebox and by modification of shoe wear to include a broad toebox with extra depth.
- Splinting or taping the second toe in plantarflexion may relieve symptoms but does not correct deformity.
- Placing a metatarsal pad in the shoe may help relieve pressure on the plantar plate.
- Wearing a shoe with a firm sole may prevent propagation of synovitis and further attenuation of the plantar plate.
- Metatarsal bars or a full-length rocker bottom sole with metal inlay may provide additional means of relieving pressure at the second MTP joint.

SURGICAL MANAGEMENT

Preoperative Planning

- All radiographs should be carefully examined to evaluate the degree of deformity of the hallux and surrounding lesser toes.
- Clinical examination should determine whether the deformities at the interphalangeal and MTP joints are flexible or rigid.

- Hallux valgus deformity, which does not allow for correction of the second toe, must be corrected.
- PIP deformity should be corrected with an interphalangeal joint fusion or arthroplasty.

Surgical Options and Indications

- Dorsal capsular release and repair of the lateral collateral ligament is a soft tissue realignment procedure that is indicated for mild crossover toe deformities.
- The Girdlestone-Taylor procedure, or transfer of the split FDL tendon to the dorsum of the proximal phalanx, is a well-established procedure.[3,13] All grades of second toe deformity may benefit from it.
  - Initially described for the correction of flexible lesser toe deformities in patients with underlying neuromuscular disorders, this procedure has undergone various modifications throughout the years.
  - A PIP resection can be performed simultaneously for correction of rigid deformity.
- The EDB tendon transfer was originally described by Haddad et al and is most appropriate in patients with mild to moderate deformity.[4] Benefits include better control of sagittal plane motion and less stiffness than is associated with an FDL transfer.
- A recent modification of the EDB transfer, as popularized by Lui and Chan, attempts to reduce the supination force of the transferred EDB, as well as to provide a more robust side-to-side suture repair.[8]
- Proximal phalanx basilar osteotomy is indicated for resistant angular deformities of the lesser toes and for failure to achieve multiplanar correction after complete soft tissue release at the MTP joint.
- The Weil osteotomy can be used to shorten the second metatarsal as well as to decrease the overall prominence of the second metatarsal head (**FIG 2**).
  - This procedure is used for persistent subluxation of the second MTP joint after adequate soft tissue procedures have been performed.
  - It may be used as an alternative to a flexor to extensor transfer.
  - A flexor to extensor transfer can be performed simultaneously for additional correction in refractory cases.

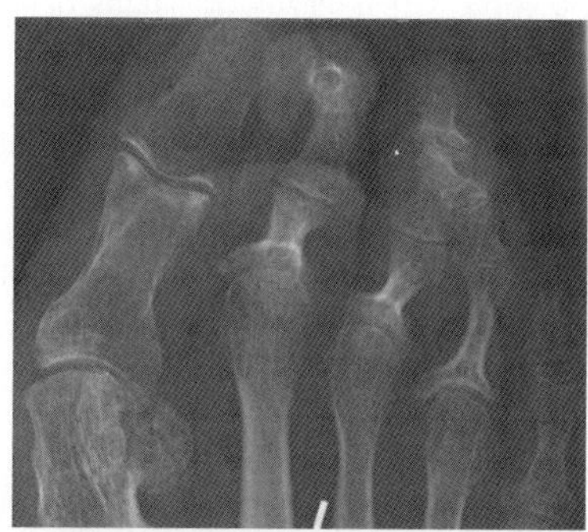
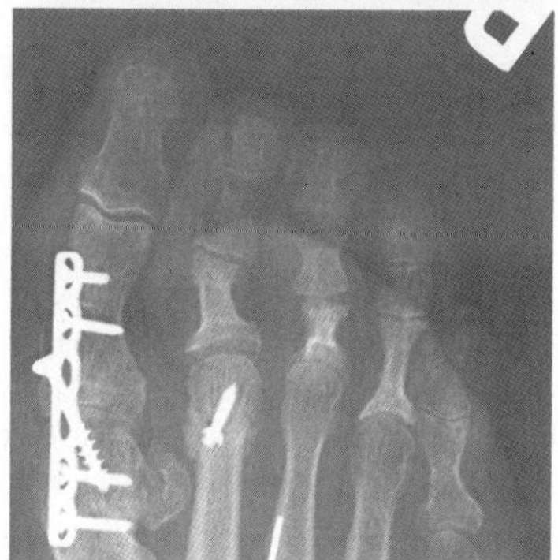

FIG 2 • The Weil osteotomy can be used to shorten the second metatarsal as well as to decrease the overall prominence of the second metatarsal head.

TECHNIQUES

DORSAL CAPSULAR RELEASE AND REPAIR OF THE LATERAL COLLATERAL LIGAMENT

- The second MTP joint is approached via a 3-cm longitudinal, curved, or Z-shaped incision.
- A dorsal incision in the adjacent web space is also appropriate.
- The EDL and EDB are sectioned and the dorsal capsule is opened (**TECH FIG 1A**).
- Release of the EDL, EDB, and dorsal capsule allows the sagittal plane deformity to be addressed (**TECH FIG 1B**).

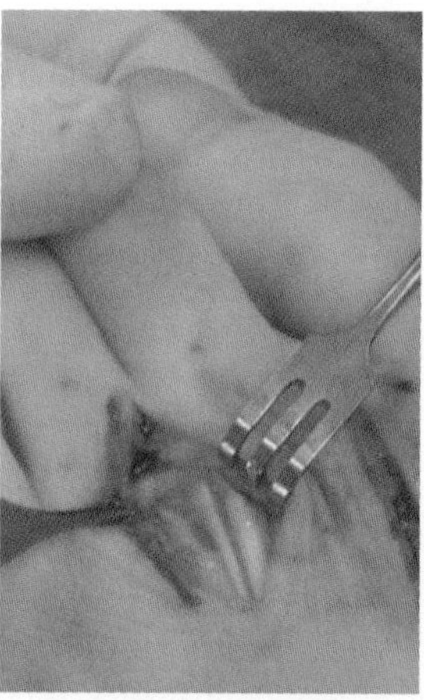
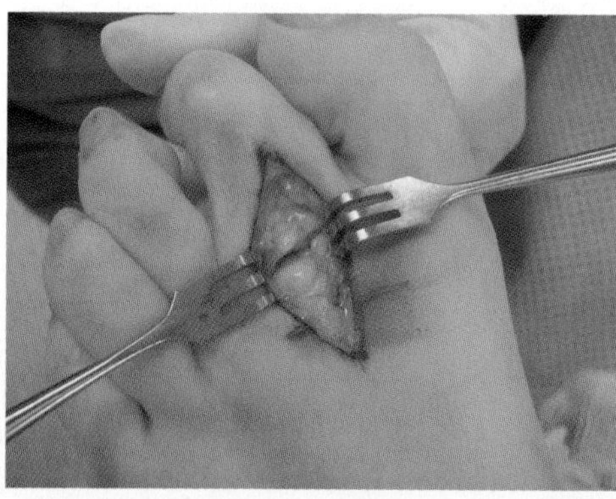

TECH FIG 1 • **A.** The extensor digitorum longus (*EDL*) and the extensor digitorum brevis (*EDB*) are sectioned and the dorsal capsule is opened. **B.** The EDL, EDB, and dorsal capsule are released. *(continued)*

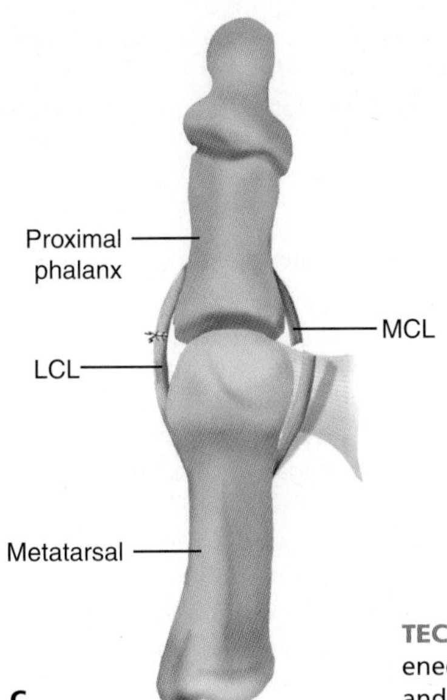

- Balancing the MCL and the LCL is required to address coronal plane deformity.
  - The contracted MCL is released off the metatarsal and the phalanx from dorsal to plantar.
  - The attenuated LCL is then repaired in a shortened fashion (**TECH FIG 1C**).
- For added stabilization, the MTP joint is pinned from distal to proximal using a 0.054- or 0.062-inch K-wire.

TECH FIG 1 • *(continued)* **C.** Repair of the lateral collateral ligament (*LCL*) in a shortened fashion and release of the medial collateral ligament (*MCL*) off the metatarsal and phalanx.

FLEXOR-TO-EXTENSOR TENDON TRANSFER (GIRDLESTONE-TAYLOR PROCEDURE)

- The second MTP joint is approached through a dorsal longitudinal incision extending from the MTP joint to the PIP joint.
- The extensor tendons are retracted laterally, and the MTP joint is entered through a dorsal capsulotomy.
- The MCL is then sectioned.
- In patients with more advanced deformity, further correction may be obtained with EDL lengthening and EDB tenotomy as well as a release of the interosseous and lumbrical tendons.
- A small transverse plantar incision is then made at the level of the proximal flexion crease, and the FDL tendon is identified using blunt dissection (**TECH FIG 2A**).
- The FDL tendon is released from its insertion onto the distal phalanx via a percutaneous tenotomy at the level of the DIP joint.
- The released FDL tendon is brought into the proximal wound and split centrally along the median raphe (**TECH FIG 2B**).
- Each limb is then passed from plantar to dorsal on either side of the proximal phalanx, avoiding injury to adjacent neurovascular structures.
- When a fixed contracture of the PIP is present, resection of the distal one fourth of the proximal phalanx can be performed after the extensor hood and collateral ligaments are incised.

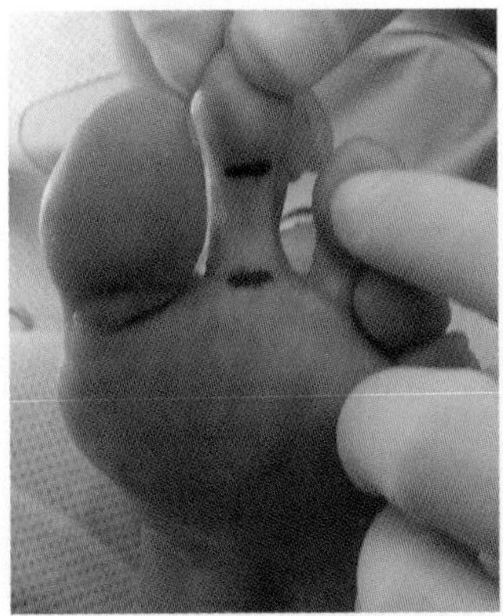
A

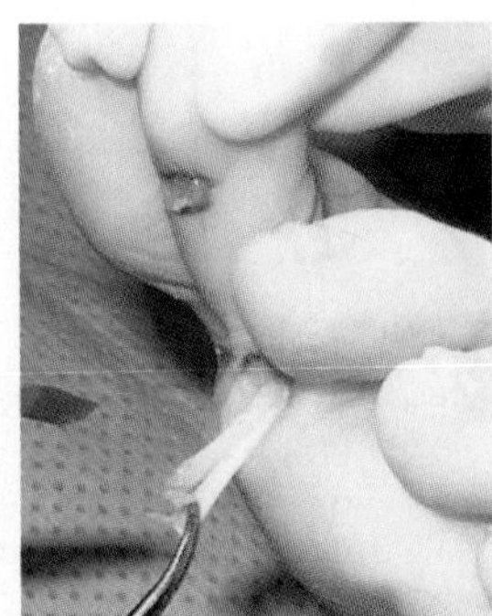
B

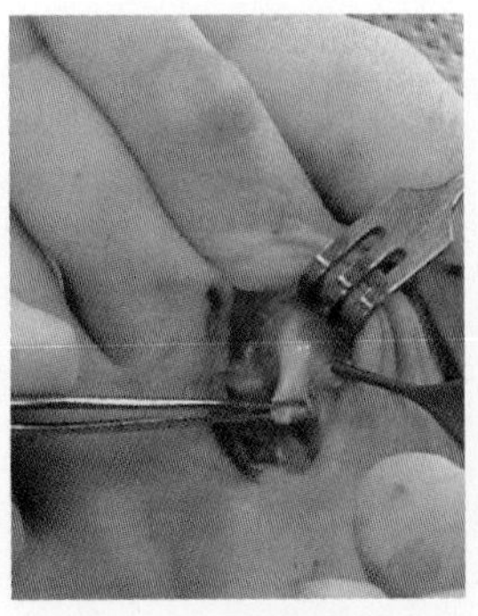
C

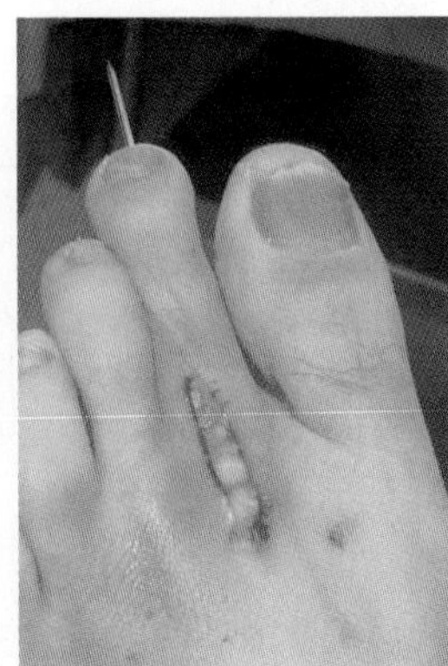
D

TECH FIG 2 • **A.** A small transverse plantar incision is then made at the level of the proximal flexion crease. **B.** The released flexor digitorum longus (FDL) tendon is brought into the proximal wound and split centrally along the median raphe. **C.** The limbs of the split FDL are passed over the extensor hood, tensioned, and sutured. **D.** The incisions are then closed in a layered fashion.

- The limbs of the split FDL are then passed over the extensor hood, tensioned (with the ankle held in a neutral or slightly dorsiflexed position), and sutured to each other with 4-0 nonabsorbable sutures (**TECH FIG 2C**).
- Manual manipulation of the proximal phalanx can be performed to assess the tensioning of the transferred tendons. The MTP joint should remain slightly mobile, not overly tight, when correct tensioning is achieved.
- A 0.062-inch K-wire is driven, in retrograde fashion, from the base of the proximal phalanx distally through the tip of the toe and then antegrade across the MTP joint with the toe held parallel to the floor or weight-bearing surface of the foot.
- The incisions are then closed in a layered fashion (**TECH FIG 2D**).

EXTENSOR DIGITORUM BREVIS TENDON TRANSFER

- A dorsal approach similar to that used for a flexor-to-extensor transfer is used to perform an EDB tendon transfer.
- The EDB tendon is identified and freed proximally after dissection and release of the MTP joint capsule and lengthening of the EDL tendon.
- After two 4-0 stay sutures have been placed longitudinally into the tendon 4 cm proximal to the MTP joint, the tendon is transected between these two sutures (**TECH FIG 3A**).
- Care is taken to maintain the integrity of the distal EDB tendon insertion, and the distal EDB tendon stump is then passed from distal to proximal underneath the transverse metatarsal ligament and lateral to the MTP joint (**TECH FIG 3B**).
- A 0.062-inch K-wire is placed across the MTP joint with the toe held in a corrected position.
- The passed distal limb of the EDB is then tensioned and secured by a direct end-to-end tendon repair to the proximal stump, with the joint held in congruity (**TECH FIG 3C**).

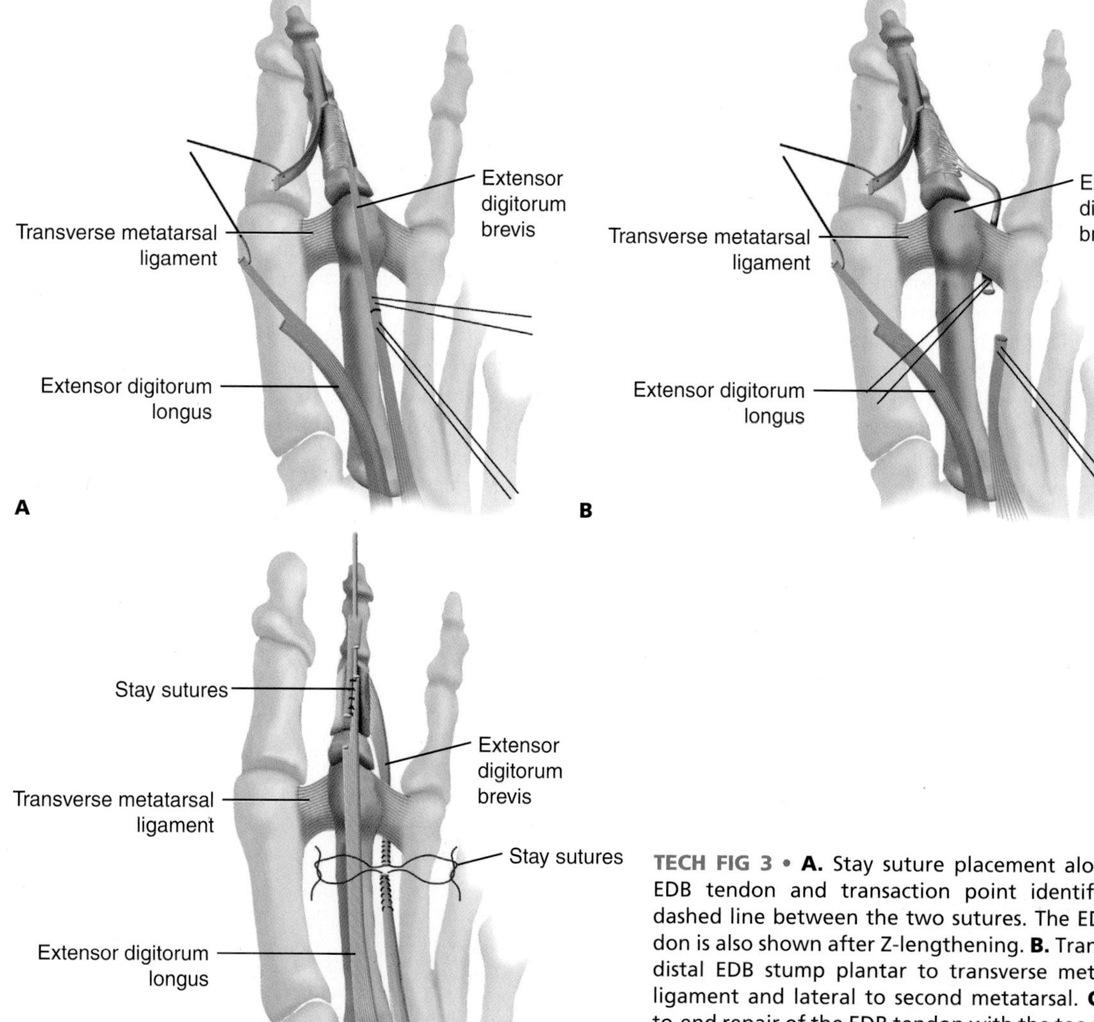

TECH FIG 3 • **A.** Stay suture placement along the EDB tendon and transaction point identified by dashed line between the two sutures. The EDL tendon is also shown after Z-lengthening. **B.** Transfer of distal EDB stump plantar to transverse metatarsal ligament and lateral to second metatarsal. **C.** End-to-end repair of the EDB tendon with the toe pinned in a corrected position. The Z-lengthened EDL tendon is also shown following repair.

MODIFIED EXTENSOR DIGITORUM TENDON TRANSFER

- Under tourniquet control, a lazy S incision is used to expose the EDL and EDB of the second toe.
- A long Z incision of the EDL is made, and the EDB is released at the distal metatarsal level (**TECH FIG 4A**).
- The MTP joint is entered transversely, and the MCL is sectioned.
- A transverse bone tunnel is placed through the proximal aspect of the proximal phalanx using a 2.5-mm drill.
- The distal stump of the EDL is passed through the bone tunnel from medial to lateral. The passed tendon is then shuttled from distal to proximal, plantar to the transverse metatarsal ligament between the second and third metatarsals.
- The transferred tendon is tensioned, and a 0.062-inch K-wire is inserted across the MTP joint to hold the toe in a corrected position (**TECH FIG 4B**).
- The distal stump of the EDL is then repaired side to side with the proximal stump of the EDB.
- The proximal stump of the EDL is then sutured to the distal stump of the EDB in side-to-side fashion.

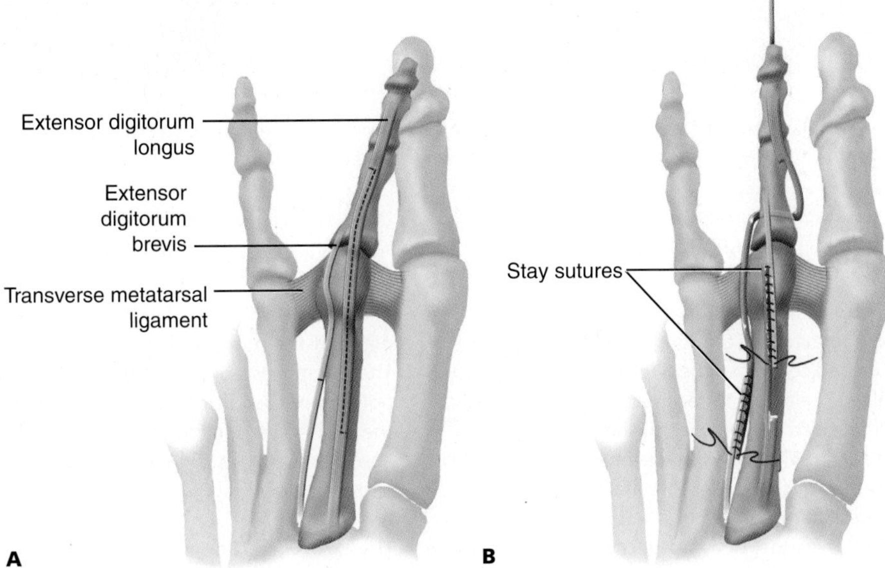

TECH FIG 4 • **A.** Long Z incision through the EDL tendon. EDB transected at the level of the distal metatarsal shaft. **B.** Correction of deformity and pinning. The distal EDL stump has been shuttled through the transverse drill tunnel and anastamosed to the proximal stump of the EDB tendon. The proximal stump of EDL has been repaired side to side with the distal stump of the EDB. (Adapted from Lui TH, Chan KB. Technique tip: modified extensor digitorum brevis tendon transfer for crossover second toe correction. Foot Ankle Int 2007; 28:521–523.)

PROXIMAL PHALANX BASILAR OSTEOTOMY

- An oblique incision is made over the MTP joint extending longitudinally onto the dorsum of the base of the proximal phalanx.
- Extensor tenotomy or lengthening and dorsal capsular incision with collateral release can all be added for further soft tissue correction.
- If complete correction is not attainable following these soft tissue releases, the approach can be extended to the base of the proximal phalanx, where a proximal phalanx basilar osteotomy can subsequently be performed.
- Davis et al described using a small awl to make multiple perforations at the base of the proximal phalanx opposite the direction of toe deviation[2] (**TECH FIG 5A**).
- After penetrating the appropriate cortex multiple times, taking care not to perforate the opposite cortex, finger pressure alone is used to complete the osteotomy and correct the underlying deformity (**TECH FIG 5B**).
- A 0.045-inch K-wire is placed percutaneously if added stability is needed.

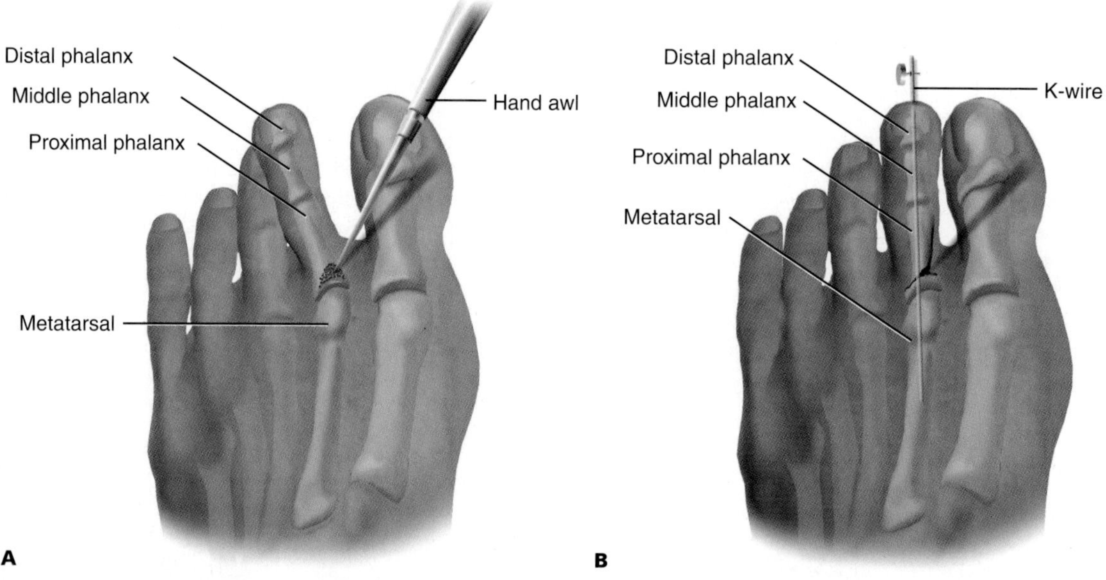

TECH FIG 5 • A. A hand awl is used to make multiple perforations in the medial cortex of the proximal phalanx. **B.** K-wire stabilization after osteotomy completion and positional correction.

DISTAL HORIZONTAL METATARSAL OSTEOTOMY (WEIL OSTEOTOMY)

- A dorsal 3-cm longitudinal incision is made over the second MTP joint, the extensor tendons are retracted, and the capsule is incised to expose the MTP joint.
- Collaterals are then released to facilitate delivery of the second metatarsal head dorsally out of the wound.
- Plantar flexion at the MTP allows for optimal exposure of the articular surface of the second metatarsal.
- With use of an oscillating saw, a cut is initiated at the articular surface of the most dorsal aspect of the second metatarsal head.
- The cut is carried proximally and parallel to the plantar plane of the foot (TECH FIG 6A).
- The plantar osteotomy fragment is then grasped with a pointed reduction clamp and slid proximally to achieve the desired amount of shortening (TECH FIG 6B).
- The osteotomy is finally secured with a compression screw placed in lag fashion from dorsal to plantar (TECH FIG 6C).
- The excess dorsal bony prominence is shaved to a smooth surface.

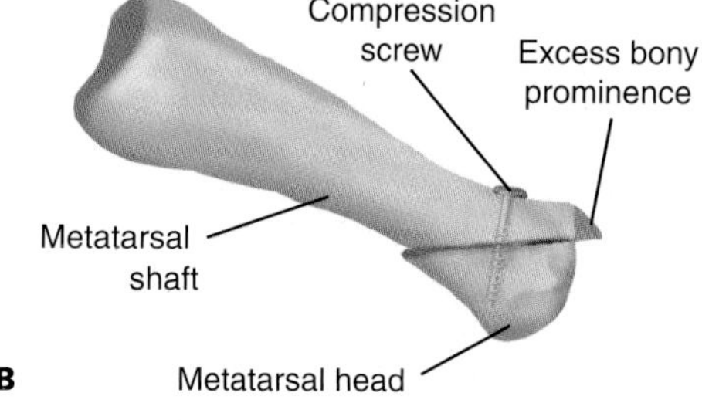

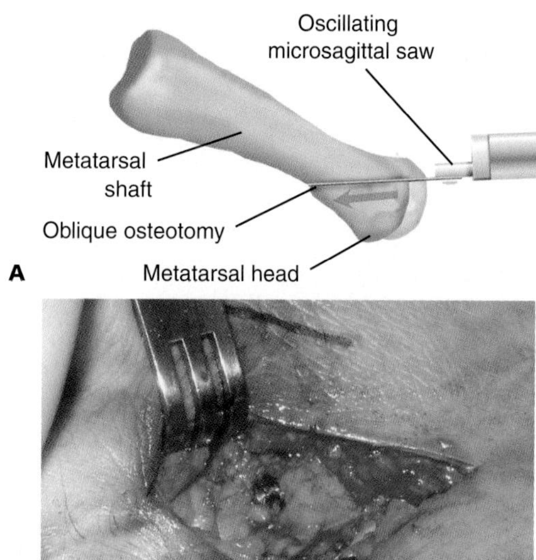

TECH FIG 6 • A. Diagram of osteotomy plane, made using an oscillating saw. Care must be taken to initiate the saw cut at the dorsalmost aspect of the second metatarsal head. **B.** The osteotomy is slid proximally and fixed with a compression screw from dorsal to plantar. **C.** The osteotomy is finally secured with a compression screw placed in lag fashion from dorsal to plantar.

PEARLS AND PITFALLS

Dorsal capsular release and repair of the lateral collateral ligament	▪ Procedure is best used to correct mild or early deformities. ▪ Before pinning the second toe, the surgeon should ensure that the toe is able to passively lie in a corrected position after adequate dorsal capsular release and LCL repair. There is a high probability that if the surgeon has to rely on pin fixation to maintain the second toe in a corrected position, this correction will be lost over time.
Flexor-to-extensor tendon transfer	▪ Procedure should be used for correction of moderate crossover toe deformity or for toes that display a tendency to resublux after initial correction. ▪ When passing the FDL through the proximal plantar incision, flexing the toe will further relax the flexor and facilitate delivery of the tendon to the proximal plantar incision. ▪ Overtensioning either limb of the FDL prior to repair can result in further malalignment of the toe and shift the toe into even greater varus or valgus deformity. ▪ Rapid postoperative mobilization and early K-wire removal (2 weeks postoperatively) are crucial to preventing uncomfortable postoperative stiffness.
EBD tendon transfer	▪ Rapid postoperative mobilization and K-wire removal (2 weeks postoperatively) are crucial to preventing uncomfortable postoperative stiffness. ▪ For advanced deformity (rigid stage 3 or 4), FDL transfer may be more appropriate. ▪ Anchoring the brevis tendon into a metatarsal head drill hole may lead to a higher recurrence rate than an end-to-end transfer. ▪ Supination of the second toe may result from overpull of the EDB.
Modified EBD tendon transfer	▪ The Z-lengthening of the EDL should be long enough to permit passage through the bone tunnel and eventual anastomosis of the transfer. ▪ The EDB is cut at the distal MT level to preserve adequate length to facilitate the transfer. ▪ Drill tunnel placement is critical. The tunnel should be placed close to the longitudinal axis of the proximal axis and not too dorsal or plantar. ▪ Correction of the hyperextension deformity relies mainly on adequate soft tissue release. Reflection of the plantar capsule and plate off the metatarsal head using an elevator may be necessary to accomplish adequate soft tissue release. ▪ Placing the drill tunnel too dorsal will lead to residual supination; locating it too plantar will lead to hyperextension of the MTP joint.
Proximal phalanx basilar osteotomy	▪ If complete correction of the crossover toe deformity is not attainable following initial soft tissue releases, the approach can be extended to the base of the proximal phalanx, where a proximal phalanx basilar osteotomy can be performed. ▪ Care should be taken to prevent perforation of the far cortex when performing the osteotomy, or instability and delayed bony union may result.
Weil osteotomy	▪ The distal fragment of the osteotomy can be preliminarily secured with a K-wire prior to completion of the dorsal-to-plantar compression screw fixation. ▪ Pinning across the MTP joint will decrease the risk of floating toe deformity. ▪ Avoid securing the distal osteotomy fragment in plantarflexion; if anything, err on the side of dorsiflexion if accepting mild angular deformity in the sagittal plane.

POSTOPERATIVE CARE

- Dorsal capsular release and repair of the lateral collateral ligament
  - The pin is left in for approximately 3 to 4 weeks.
  - Immediate ambulation is allowed in a stiff postoperative shoe.
  - Once the pin is removed, the toe is taped in plantarflexion for another 3 to 4 weeks.
  - The patient is progressed into normal shoe wear once the pin is removed.
- Girdlestone-Taylor procedure
  - Ambulation in a hard-soled shoe using only the heel is permitted immediately following surgery.
  - The K-wire is removed between 2 and 3 weeks postoperatively.
  - The patient is instructed to adhere to 6 additional weeks of taping the toe in slight plantarflexion and lateral deviation.
- EDB tendon transfer
  - Postoperative care is essentially identical to that used for a flexor-to-extensor transfer.
  - The percutaneously placed K-wire is maintained for 2 to 3 weeks, followed by an additional 6 weeks of taping the corrected toe to maintain alignment.
- Modified EDB tendon transfer: The pin is kept in place for 3 to 6 weeks followed by 6 additional weeks of toe taping.
- Proximal phalanx basilar osteotomy
  - After surgery, dressings are placed with the toe maintained in an overcorrected position.
  - The patient is placed in a hard-soled shoe, and dressing changes are performed weekly.
  - At 6 weeks postoperatively, the patient is advanced to a soft-soled shoe as tolerated.
  - K-wire is removed at 4 weeks postoperatively.
  - Postoperative radiographs are assessed at 4 to 6 weeks to evaluate for bony healing at the osteotomy site.
- Weil osteotomy
  - Sterile dressings are placed intraoperatively, and the toe is taped down in an overcorrected position.
  - Dressings are changed weekly until drainage ceases.
  - Weight bearing in a postoperative shoe is resumed immediately after surgery.

OUTCOMES

- Girdlestone-Taylor procedure
  - Thompson and Deland performed FDL flexor-to-extensor tendon transfers on 13 feet in 11 patients and reported that at an average follow up of 33.4 months all patients had substantial pain relief, with 8 of 13 becoming completely pain-free.[14]
  - They concluded that while flexor-to-extensor tendon transfer is successful in re-establishing MTP joint congruity and relieving pain due to instability, rapid postoperative mobilization and early K-wire removal (2 weeks postoperatively) are crucial to preventing uncomfortable postoperative stiffness.
- EDB tendon transfer
  - Haddad and colleagues performed either flexor-to-extensor or EDB tendon transfer on 38 patients (42 feet) with an average follow-up of 51.6 months.[4]
  - Of the 31 patients (35 feet) followed until their final examination, 24 were satisfied with their surgical correction, 6 were satisfied with reservations, and 1 was dissatisfied.
  - No statistical significance in clinical outcome was demonstrated between patients who underwent FDL tendon transfer and those who underwent EDB tendon transfer; but Haddad et al recommended the technique because they believed that it demonstrated better patient satisfaction and improved flexibility compared with the FDL transfer.
  - Other advantages favoring EDB transfer over FDL transfer that were cited were better postoperative range of motion (78 degrees for EDB versus 62 degrees for FDL) and hence better patient satisfaction, decrease in recurrence of deformity (14%), and better pain control (71% asymptomatic; 26% mild pain).
- Weil osteotomy
  - Hofstaetter and colleagues analyzed their results at 1 and 7 years in 25 feet using the Weil osteotomy for treatment of instability at the MTP joint.[6]
  - Good to excellent results were obtained in 21 feet (84%) after 1 year and in 22 (88%) after 7 years.
  - The authors demonstrated marked improvement in pain, diminished plantar callus formation, and an increase in walking capacity.
  - Adverse results included recurrent instability, floating toes, and restricted motion at the MTP joint, but these complications were often not clinically significant.

COMPLICATIONS

- Dorsal capsular release and repair of the lateral collateral ligament
  - Recurrence
  - MTP stiffness
  - Persistent swelling
  - Failure to achieve correction
- Girdlestone-Taylor procedure
  - Swelling
  - Recurrent deformity
  - Stiffness
  - Hyperextension
- EDB tendon transfer
  - Recurrent crossover toe deformity or failure to achieve complete correction of deformity
  - Infection
  - Symptomatic incisional scar formation
  - Stiffness of the MTP joint, especially with flexor-to-extensor tendon transfer
- Proximal phalanx basilar osteotomy
  - Infection
  - Loss of correction with persistent angular deformity
  - Failure of union at the osteotomy site
- Weil osteotomy
  - Persistent dorsiflexion at the MTP joint (floating toe deformity)
  - Claw toe
  - Nonunion or malunion at the osteotomy site
  - Stiffness at the MTP joint due to incorporation of articular surface into osteotomy cut
  - Overcorrection with excessive shortening of the second metatarsal
  - Hardware failure or prominence
  - Infection
  - Neurovascular insult

ISOLATED METATARSOPHALANGEAL ANGULAR DEFORMITY

PATHOGENESIS

- Isolated MTP angular deformity of the lesser toes is defined as varus or valgus deformity exclusively at the MTP joint relative to the normal anatomic axis of the toe.
- Toes 2, 3, 4, and 5 are usually involved.
- This type of deformity characteristically follows abnormal deviation of the hallux, which is frequently in a position of varus or valgus.

SURGICAL MANAGEMENT

- To achieve successful correction of the lesser toes, it is usually necessary to address any varus or valgus deformity of the hallux concomitantly.
- Procedures that are used to correct isolated MTP angular deformity are similar to those used for surgically treating mild or moderate crossover second toe deformities and are described earlier in this chapter.

PEARLS AND PITFALLS

- Deviations in the lesser toes tend to follow angular deformities of the hallux. To create lasting correction of the lesser toes, the surgeon must address deformity of the hallux concomitantly.
- Failure to address associated deformity of the hallux can result in early loss of successful lesser toe correction.

CLINODACTYLY

PATHOGENESIS

- Clinodactyly refers to the medial or lateral deviation of a toe caused by true angulation within a phalanx.
- This type of lesser toe deformity is thought to result from a failure of segmentation between the normally transverse epiphysis and metaphysis.
- Often bilateral and familial, clinodactyly most frequently involves the DIP joint of the fourth and fifth digits, although any digit may be involved.

- There is also a strong predilection for involvement of the fingers with this lesser toe deformity.
- A variety of syndromes and chromosomal disorders have been linked to clinodactyly of the lesser toes (symphalangism, brachydactyly, trisomy 21, Turner syndrome, Holt-Oram syndrome, Marfan syndrome).
- An associated "delta phalanx," or a triangular middle phalanx, is sometimes associated with clinodactyly.

NATURAL HISTORY

- Clinodactyly is usually nonprogressive and no more than a cosmetic concern, although overlapping or underlapping of adjacent toes may occur.
- If significant overlap or underlap is present, impingement on adjacent digits may cause the patient to be symptomatic.

PATIENT HISTORY AND PHYSICAL FINDINGS

- The affected toe is deviated medially or laterally relative to the normal longitudinal axis of the toe.
- The DIP of the involved toe is the most common site of angulation.
- A complete physical examination should be performed because of the prevalence of clinodactyly with associated syndromes and chromosomal disorders.
- Impingement on adjacent toes due to overlapping or underlapping may cause indentation on the toes, local irritation, corns, or callosities at variable locations from associated pressure phenomenon.

IMAGING AND DIAGNOSTIC STUDIES

- All angular deformities involving the lesser toes can be appropriately studied by examining standard AP, lateral, and oblique radiographs of the affected foot.

NONOPERATIVE MANAGEMENT

- For symptomatic toes, strategic padding, stretching, taping, and accommodative shoe wear may temporarily alleviate certain components of a patient's discomfort. These conservative approaches are often ineffective, however.

SURGICAL MANAGEMENT

- Surgical options include wedge osteotomies, arthrodesis, and soft tissue–lengthening procedures.[9]
- Both opening and closing wedge osteotomies can effectively address angulation at the affected joint.
- Closing wedge osteotomy or arthrodesis is indicated for the treatment of symptomatic clinodactyly of any severity grade.
- A closing wedge osteotomy can be performed at the middle or distal phalanx through a small transverse dorsal incision.
- Intercalary allograft can be used to perform an opening wedge osteotomy and thereby preserve much of the length of the digit, but Z-plasty of the skin must also be performed for added soft tissue correction.
- A closing wedge arthrodesis of the affected joint is an acceptable treatment method provided that excessive shortening of the digit is not present.
- Skin dermodesis may be added for further acceptability of correction.

TECHNIQUES

CLOSING WEDGE OSTEOTOMY OR ARTHRODESIS

- The skin over the affected middle or distal phalanx is incised through a dorsal incision. Redundant skin, equal to the planned osteotomy, is carefully removed (TECH FIG 7A).
- Subperiosteal exposure is obtained at the apex of the deformity (TECH FIG 7B).
- A microsagittal saw is used to create the desired cut at an appropriate angle to facilitate a satisfactory correction.
- Care should be taken to preserve a small bridge of bone at the far cortex.
- The osteotomy fragment is removed, and the wedge is closed with manual manipulation (TECH FIG 7C).
- If an arthrodesis is desired, the closing wedge may be removed through the interphalangeal joint.
- Dermodesis is then performed, incorporating skin into the closure.
- Alternatively, a K-wire can be placed percutaneously, in retrograde fashion, for added stability.
- Sterile dressings are placed, emphasizing overcorrection of the affected toe.

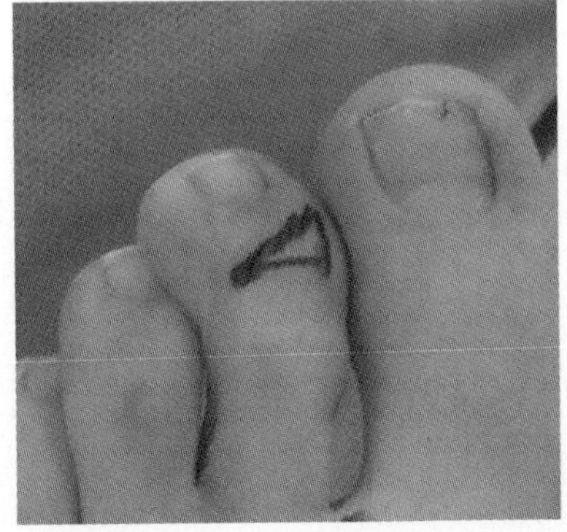
A

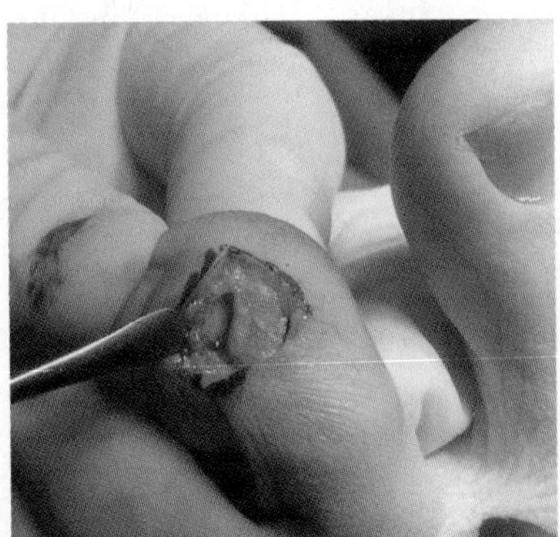
B

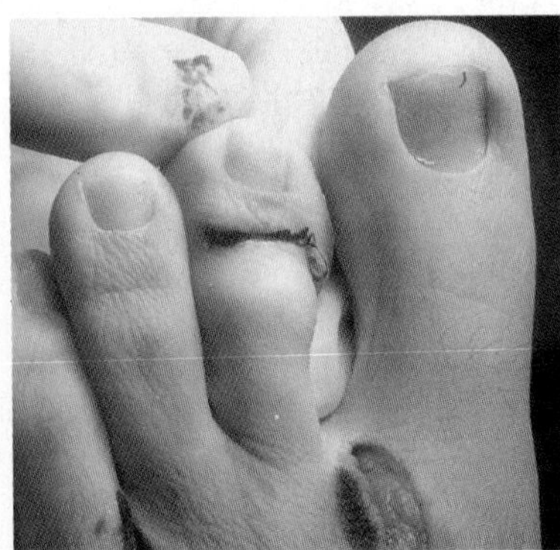
C

TECH FIG 7 • A. The affected middle or distal phalanx is approached through a dorsal incision. **B.** Subperiosteal exposure is obtained at the apex of the deformity. **C.** The osteotomy fragment is removed, and the wedge is closed with manual manipulation.

POSTOPERATIVE CARE

- If a K-wire is placed, it should be removed by 4 weeks postoperatively.
- Weight bearing in a postoperative shoe is permitted to tolerance immediately after surgery.
- Dressings should be changed until drainage subsides, with continued emphasis on maintaining an overcorrected position of the toe.

OUTCOMES

- Reports are largely anecdotal but overall have been favorable and support the continued use of the procedure.

COMPLICATIONS

- Neurovascular insult due to an overaggressive exposure
- Loss of reduction due to inadequate stabilization
- Wound healing problems
- Violation of the dorsal extensor structures
- Failure of bony healing at the osteotomy site

CONGENITAL CROSSOVER FIFTH TOE DEFORMITY

PATHOGENESIS

- Although the underlying cause is unknown, congenital crossover fifth toe is widely recognized as a familial problem with an equal gender predilection.
- Often bilateral (20% to 30% of cases), congenital crossover fifth toe (or congenital overriding fifth toe) deformity causes pain with restrictive shoe wear and other symptoms in about half of all patients.[9]
- Pathoanatomy includes dorsomedial subluxation and adduction at the fifth MTP joint, with external rotation of the toe.
- There is associated contracture of the fifth toe EDL tendon, skin of the dorsal fourth web space, MCL, and dorsomedial MTP joint capsule.
- Often, impingement lesions at the base of the adjacent fourth toe identify the compressive influence of the overriding fifth toe due to its subluxated position.
- Furthermore, dorsal subluxation of the fifth toe at the MTP joint causes excessive pressure on the metatarsal head. This abnormal pressure distribution can lead to painful plantar callosity under the metatarsal head.
- When the fifth toe crosses *under* the fourth toe, painful callosity may develop under any portion of the toe that comes in abnormal contact with the ground surface during weight bearing.

NATURAL HISTORY

- Crossover fifth toe deformity is almost always present from birth and therefore is usually nonprogressive with respect to its degree of deformity.
- As stated, a painful callosity of either the fourth or fifth toes may develop over time because of pressure phenomenon in cases of longstanding deformity.
- Also, abnormal pressure distribution due to subluxation at the fifth MTP joint can eventually lead to pain at the plantar surface of the fifth metatarsal head and metatarsalgia.
- Approximately half of all patients experience symptoms due to an overriding fifth toe.

PATIENT HISTORY AND PHYSICAL FINDINGS

- On examination, the fifth toe is noted to override the fourth toe to a variable degree.
- The interphalangeal joints are usually in normal full extension.
- There is often mild dorsiflexion at the MTP joint as well as malalignment and contracture of the skin at the fourth web space.
- In patients with longstanding deformity, the toe may assume a flattened, paddle-shaped appearance in the AP plane that is usually the result of years of compression by constrictive shoe wear.
- The toenail usually appears normal, and the toe is able to participate in active flexion and extension.
- A hard corn of the fifth toe or a soft corn between the fourth and fifth toes may also develop because of pressure phenomenon.

IMAGING AND DIAGNOSTIC STUDIES

- All angular deformities involving the lesser toes can be appropriately studied by examining standard AP, lateral, and oblique radiographs of the affected foot.
- Radiographs show dorsolateral subluxation at the MTP joint.

NONOPERATIVE MANAGEMENT

- Reliably ineffective, conservative treatment modalities include splinting, taping, accommodative shoe wear, and protective padding.

SURGICAL MANAGEMENT

- Many surgical approaches have been advocated for correction of crossover fifth toe deformity, and many modifications of these have been subsequently developed.
- The type of procedure selected is based on the severity of deformity encountered.
- Soft tissue procedures such as dorsal skin lengthening with Z-plasty of contracted skin, dermodesis of redundant skin, EDL tendon transfer, EDL lengthening or release, syndactylization of the fourth and fifth toes, and dorsal and medial capsular release have all been described and proved effective.[1,5,7–12,15,16]
- Bony resection, performed in isolation or in conjunction with any of the aforementioned soft tissue procedures, has also been successful in correcting crossover fifth toe deformity.
- Proposed salvage operations include the so-called Ruiz-Mora procedure (proximal phalangectomy via a plantar elliptical incision with soft tissue realignment and plantar dermodesis) with or without syndactylization of the fifth toe to the fourth, and even amputation.
- The DuVries technique can be used to correct mild to moderate deformities.
- The Lapidus procedure can be used to address moderate to severe deformities.
  - In this technique, the EDL is isolated and rerouted under the MTP joint and attached to the abductor digiti quinti muscle or lateral joint capsule.
  - Unlike other procedures, the Lapidus technique allows for rotational correction, expanding the indications for its use.

DUVRIES TECHNIQUE FOR CORRECTION OF CROSSOVER FIFTH TOE DEFORMITY

- A longitudinal incision is made over the fourth web space.
- An extensor tenotomy is performed, followed by dorsal capsulotomy and medial collateral ligament release (TECH FIG 8A).
- The toe is plantarflexed, bringing the skin along the lateral margin of the incision distally (TECH FIG 8B).
- Layered suture closure is performed with the toe held in an overcorrected position of plantarflexion and lateral deviation to maximize the degree of soft tissue correction afforded by this technique (TECH FIG 8C).
- Soft tissue release and skin advancement alone are usually sufficient to hold the toe in an adequately corrected position. Otherwise, a K-wire can be placed percutaneously for added stabilization and correction.

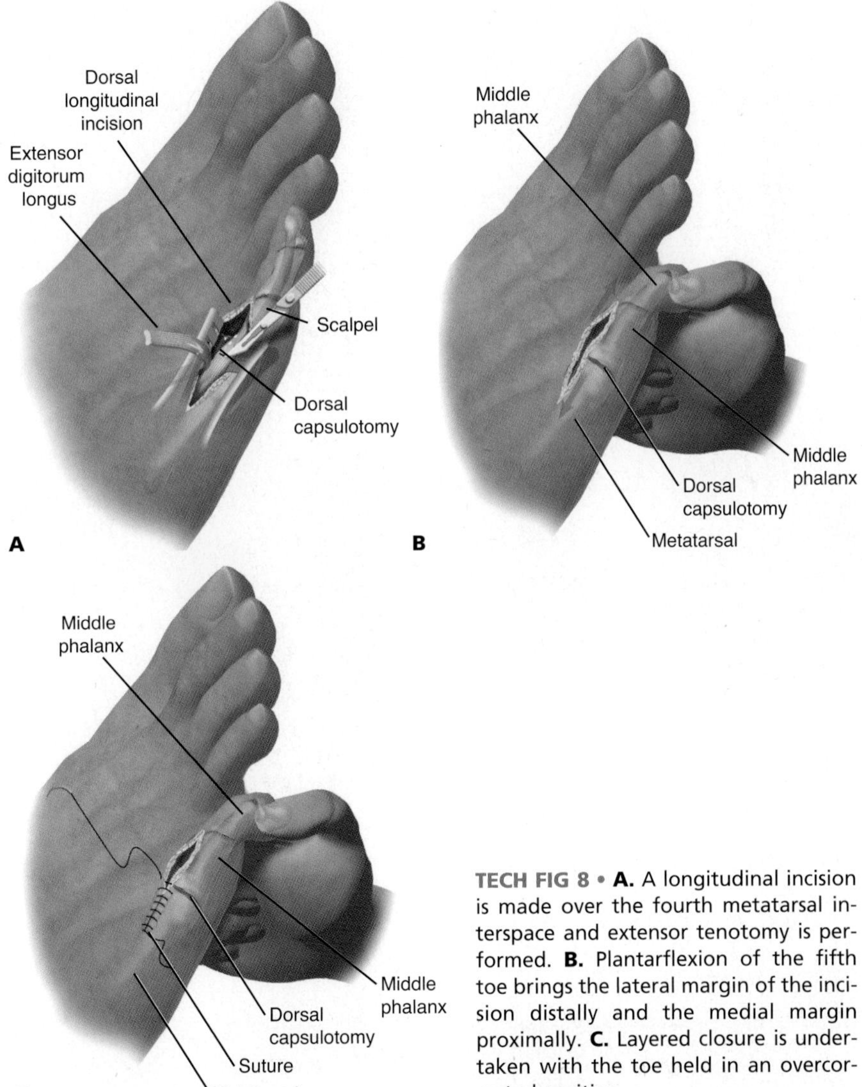

TECH FIG 8 • **A.** A longitudinal incision is made over the fourth metatarsal interspace and extensor tenotomy is performed. **B.** Plantarflexion of the fifth toe brings the lateral margin of the incision distally and the medial margin proximally. **C.** Layered closure is undertaken with the toe held in an overcorrected position.

LAPIDUS PROCEDURE

- A longitudinal hockey stick–shaped or curvilinear incision is carried along the dorsomedial border of the fifth toe, from the level of the medial DIP joint distally to the fourth web space proximally.
- Through this incision, a thorough dorsomedial capsulotomy of the fifth MTP joint is made.
- Any adhesions encountered between the plantar capsule and metatarsal head should be released with a curved elevator to prevent hyperextension deformity of the MTP joint after capsular release.
- The hook of the hockey stick incision is then created by extending the incision over the dorsum of the fifth MTP

joint laterally and proximally to the lateral aspect of the fifth MTP head.

- The extensor tendon is carefully exposed, maintaining the extensor hood expansion, and the fifth toe is forcibly plantarflexed, causing the extensor tendon to become taut.
- A second, 1-cm incision is made transversely over the taut EDL tendon at the mid-diaphyseal level of the fifth metatarsal (TECH FIG 9A).
- Using this incision, an EDL tenotomy is performed (TECH FIG 9B).
- The distal limb of the EDL tendon is retrieved and then passed beneath the plantar aspect of the fifth toe from the dorsomedial DIP joint to the lateral aspect of the fifth MTP joint.
- The passed extensor tendon is then sutured to the conjoined tendon of the abductor and short flexor of the fifth toe (TECH FIG 9C).
- The fifth toe is held in an overcorrected position, and the transplanted extensor tendon is placed under slight tension prior to suture fixation.
- Skin is closed with interrupted sutures or with advancement techniques if significant skin contractures are present.

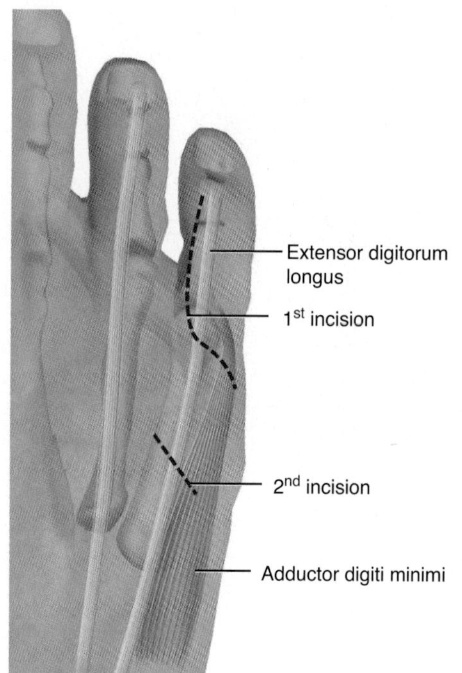

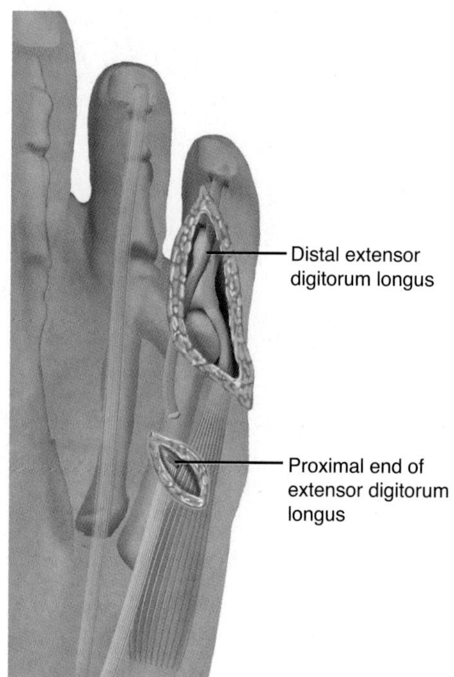

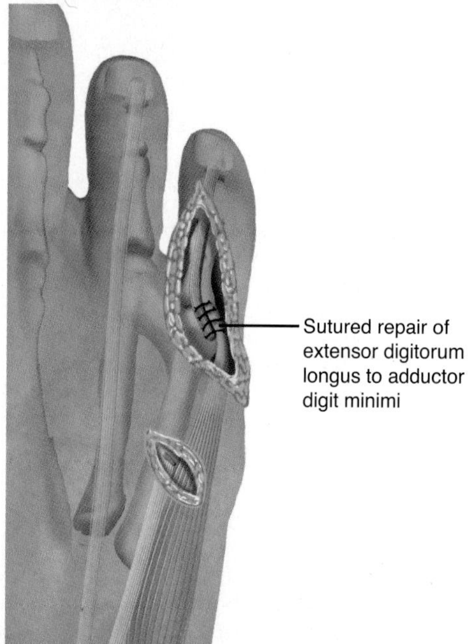

TECH FIG 9 • **A.** Incisions for the Lapidus technique. **B.** EDL tenotomy using the more proximal of the two incisions. **C.** Transfer of the distal EDL limb beneath the fifth toe and repair to the conjoined tendon.

PEARLS AND PITFALLS

DuVries technique	■ Procedure is best used for mild deformities without associated rotational deformity of the toe. If any substantial rotational deformity is present, the Lapidus procedure is a more appropriate surgical solution. ■ Failure to hold the toe in an overcorrected position while performing soft tissue advancement and layered closure will result in a higher recurrence rate.
Lapidus procedure	■ Following dorsomedial capsulotomy, any adhesions encountered between the plantar capsule and metatarsal head should be released with a curved elevator to prevent hyperextension deformity of the MTP joint after capsular release. ■ If the toe is not held in an overcorrected position during repair, or if transplanted extensor tendon is incorrectly tensioned, early recurrence is common.

POSTOPERATIVE CARE

- DuVries technique
  - The toe is taped in a slightly overcorrected (plantarflexed and lateral) position for 6 weeks in a hard-soled postoperative shoe, after which unrestricted weight bearing is permitted.
  - If a pin is placed, it should be removed at 4 weeks postoperatively and the toe taped for a total of 6 weeks.
- Lapidus procedure
  - Postoperatively, the toe is dressed in a corrected position and weight bearing in a postoperative shoe is allowed. Sutures are removed at 2 weeks, and the toe is then taped in a corrected position for another 4 to 6 weeks. Regular shoe wear is allowed at 4 to 6 weeks.
  - Alternatively, if there is concern about the strength of the repair, the operative foot is maintained in a splint for a total of 3 to 4 weeks, and progression to full weight bearing and activity in a wide toebox shoe is gradually allowed.

OUTCOMES

- In his original description, Lapidus notes that his experience with the procedure that bears his name resulted in satisfactory outcomes in all cases.[7]

COMPLICATIONS

- A 5% to 10% recurrence rate has been reported using the DuVries technique. Mild swelling and clinically insignificant postoperative edema have also been reported.
- Circulatory insult and wound healing problems are potential risks of the Lapidus procedure but were not reported by Lapidus in his original description. Recurrence of deformity has also been reported.

CROSSUNDER FIFTH TOE DEFORMITY (CONGENITAL CURLY TOE OR UNDERLAPPING FIFTH TOE)

PATHOGENESIS

- Although the cause of curly toe deformity is unknown, it is thought to be familial in nature, with a high instance of bilaterality.
- Frequently, this type of lesser toe deformity involves both fourth *and* fifth toes and is usually symmetric.
- Hypoplasia of the intrinsic musculature has been proposed as a causative influence on the development of curly toe deformity, but this notion has not been substantiated in the literature.
- The fifth toe is flexed, deviated plantarward in varus, and is laterally rotated at the DIP joint.
- The EDL and dorsal capsule are often attenuated, in contrast to overlapping fifth toe deformity.
- The plantar MTP joint capsule and FDL tendon are often contracted and shortened also.

NATURAL HISTORY

- As curly toe deformity is frequently congenital, progression is limited, and cosmesis is the major concern of parents and caretakers.
- The deformity is often asymptomatic in children and may improve without intervention.
- With initiation of weight bearing and different stages of shoe wear, chronic skin irritation can develop, the toenail may become short and flattened, and other pressure phenomena such as corns and callosities may develop.

PATIENT HISTORY AND PHYSICAL EXAMINATION

- As previously stated, the fifth toe is flexed, deviated plantarward in varus, and laterally rotated at the DIP joint.
- The distal phalanx or the distal and middle phalanges underride the more medial toe as a result of these anatomic abnormalities.
- The deformity is usually flexible in childhood but may become rigid as an adult.
- In contrast to crossover fifth toe deformity, the skin in the web spaces is normally aligned, but it can become hyperemic from chronic irritation.
- Patients usually present with varying degrees of symptoms caused by pressure on the weight-bearing surface of the curly toe.
- Callosities, corns, or nail deformities can all develop and cause discomfort with curly toe deformities.

IMAGING AND DIAGNOSTIC STUDIES

- All angular deformities involving the lesser toes can be appropriately studied by examining standard AP, lateral, and oblique radiographs of the affected foot.
- Imaging of the curly toe is usually unnecessary and does not contribute significantly to management strategies.

NONOPERATIVE MANAGEMENT

- Conservative treatment modalities, including splinting, taping, accommodative shoe wear, and protective padding, may relieve symptoms but are usually ineffective for correcting the deformity.

SURGICAL MANAGEMENT

- For flexible deformities, FDL and FDB tenotomy have been recommended in the pediatric population.
- Flexor-to-extensor transfer, syndactylization with or without partial proximal phalangectomy, middle phalangectomy, and derotational procedures have all been proposed as surgical options to address the underlying pathoanatomy.
- A simple flexor tenotomy can be used to correct mild underlapping fifth toe deformity.
- Originally described by Taylor and credited to Girdlestone in 1951, the flexor-to-extensor tendon transfer is based on the premise that curly toe deformity results from weakness of the intrinsic musculature.[13] This technique was described earlier in this chapter.
- The Thompson technique uses resection arthroplasty of the proximal phalanx in combination with Z-plasty of the skin to achieve derotation of the toe and correction of the deformity.[15] This technique is useful for addressing more rigid, severe crossunder fifth toe deformities.

TECHNIQUES

FLEXOR TENOTOMY

- Various surgical incisions have been successfully used to perform open flexor tenotomy, including a longitudinal incision proximal to the proximal flexor crease, a longitudinal incision distal to the proximal flexor crease, and a transverse incision 1 mm from the proximal flexor crease.
- It is important not to violate the proximal flexor crease with the incision, or scar formation may occur and recurrent deformity can develop.
- The flexor sheath is incised longitudinally, long and short flexor tendons are carefully exposed, and tendons are then transected at the same level (**TECH FIG 10**).
- Manual manipulation may be used to improve the adequacy of correction.
- The wound is closed with interrupted 3-0 absorbable sutures.

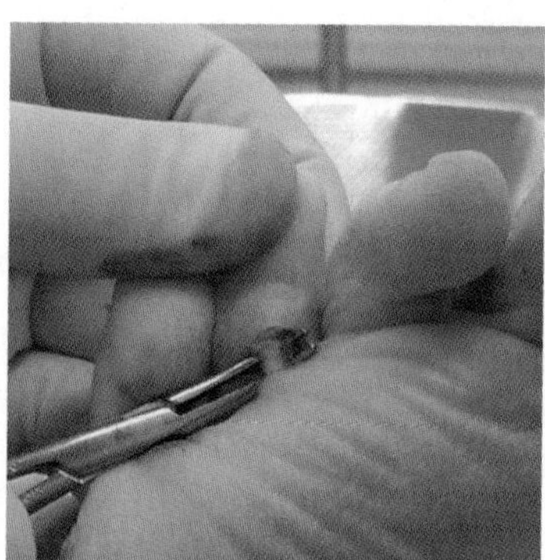

TECH FIG 10 • The flexor sheath is incised longitudinally, the long and short flexor tendons are carefully exposed, and the tendons are then transected at the same level.

THOMPSON PROCEDURE

- A laterally based Z-type or elliptical incision is made over the proximal phalanx.
- Subperiosteal dissection is used to expose the distal half of the proximal phalanx.
- Partial phalangectomy of the distal 25% to 50% of the proximal phalanx or complete phalangectomy is then performed using a microsagittal saw.
- If persistent flexion contracture exists at the level of the PIP, a flexor tenotomy can be added for further correction.
- The digit is manually derotated and a 0.045-inch K-wire is placed in a retrograde fashion across the PIP joint for stabilization.
- Additional soft tissue correction is obtained by using a reverse-Z closure with 4-0 nylon vertical mattress sutures.
- If an elliptical incision was used initially, full-thickness closure is performed with the toe derotated using a dermodesis.

PEARLS AND PITFALLS

Flexor tenotomy	▪ Failure to transect all three plantar tendons can lead to an incomplete correction of the deformity. ▪ It is important not to violate the proximal flexor crease with the incision, or scar formation may occur and recurrent deformity can develop.
Girdlestone-Taylor procedure	▪ Isolated flexor tenotomy and flexor-to-extensor transfer appear to be equally efficacious. However, it is thought that the long flexor tenotomy represents the essential portion of either procedure and that flexor-to-extensor transfer is unnecessary.
Thompson procedure	▪ If persistent flexion contracture exists at the level of the PIP, a flexor tenotomy can be added for further correction. ▪ Overresection of the proximal phalanx can lead to a "floppy," unstable toe as well as a transfer lesion beneath the fourth metatarsal.

POSTOPERATIVE CARE

- Flexor tenotomy: Sterile dressings and elastic straps are applied to maintain correction, and the wound is inspected 10 days postoperatively.
- Girdlestone-Taylor procedure: Sterile dressings are applied and full weight bearing is permitted in a short leg plaster splint with an extended toebox. Splinting is maintained for 4 to 6 weeks.
- Thompson procedure: The foot is placed in a hard-soled shoe postoperatively, and pins are removed at 4 weeks. Using taping techniques, the toe is maintained in a derotated position for 6 additional weeks.

OUTCOMES

- Flexor tenotomy
  - Ross and Menelaus reviewed their long-term outcome data on open flexor tenotomy performed in 62 children (188 toes) and found that at an average follow-up of 9.8 years, 95% of the toes examined had maintained satisfactory correction and no patients were aware of any loss of toe function.[11]
  - The fourth and fifth toes had significantly more fair and poor results, hypothesized to be due to greater rotational deformity of these toes, especially the fifth.
  - Overall, the authors concluded that open flexor tenotomy is a safe, reliable, and effective method for correcting curly toes in children and is preferable to flexor-to-extensor transfer.
- Girdlestone-Taylor procedure
  - In a double-blind, randomized, prospective trial, Hamer and colleagues studied long-term data from 46 toes (19 patients) randomly assigned to either flexor tenotomy or flexor-to-extensor tendon transfer for operative correction of curly toe deformity.[5]
    - In general, results were good, with all patients remaining symptom-free at final follow-up.
    - The authors concluded that neither procedure was clearly superior to the other, that long flexor tenotomy was the essential portion of either procedure, and that flexor-to-extensor transfer was unnecessary.
  - Biyani and colleagues reviewed 130 curly toes in 43 children that were treated with flexor-to-extensor tendon transfer over a period of 24 years.[1]
    - At an average follow-up of 8 years (range 1 to 25 years), good to excellent results were obtained in 95 toes (73%), fair results in 25 toes (19%), and poor results in 10 toes (8%).
- In general, results of the Thompson procedure have been acceptable.

COMPLICATIONS

- Flexor tenotomy
  - When performing longitudinal skin incision, care should be taken to avoid crossing the flexion creases because scar formation and skin contracture have been reported.
  - Ten of 188 patients in Ross and Menelaus' study were found to have tethering of the plantar skin as a result of violating some aspect of the flexor crease.[11]
  - Stiffness has also been reported as a complication of flexor tenotomy.
  - Neurovascular compromise has not been reported but, in theory, represents a significant potential complication with this procedure.
- Recurrent deformity, failure to achieve full correction, and infection are all potential complications of the Girdlestone-Taylor procedure.
- Thompson procedure
  - Digital edema from resection arthroplasty can result, as well as neurovascular insult to the digital bundle.
  - Recurrence in single or multiple planes can also result from attempts at derotation.
  - Overresection can lead to a "floppy," unstable toe as well as a transfer lesion beneath the fourth metatarsal.

REFERENCES

1. Biyani A, Jones DA, Murray JM. Flexor to extensor tendon transfer for curly toes: 43 children reviewed after 8 (1–25) years. Acta Orthop Scand 1992;63:451–454.
2. Davis WH, Anderson RB, Thompson FM, Hamilton WG. Technique tip: proximal phalanx basilar osteotomy for resistant angulation of the lesser toes. Foot Ankle Int 1997;18:103–104.
3. Girdlestone GR. Physiology for hand and foot. J Chart Soc Physiother 1947;32:167–169.
4. Haddad SL, Sabbagh RC, Resch S, et al. Results of flexor-to-extensor and extensor brevis tendon transfer for correction of the crossover second toe deformity. Foot Ankle Int 1999;20:781–788.
5. Hamer AJ, Stanley D, Smith D. Surgery for curly toe deformity: a double-blind, randomized, prospective trial. J Bone Joint Surg Br 1993;75B:662–663.
6. Hofstaetter SG, Hofstaetter JG, Petroutsas JA, et al. The Weil osteotomy: a seven-year follow-up. J Bone Joint Surg Br 2005;87B: 1507–1511.
7. Lapidus PW. Transplantation of the extensor tendon for correction of the overlapping fifth toe. J Bone Joint Surg Br 1942;24B:555–559.
8. Lui TH, Chan KB. Technique tip: modified extensor digitorum brevis tendon transfer for crossover second toe correction. Foot Ankle Int 2007;28:521–523.
9. Myerson MS. Foot and Ankle Disorders. Philadelphia: WB Saunders, 2000:322.
10. Paton RW. V-Y plasty for correction of varus fifth toe. J Pediatr Orthop 1990;10:248–249.
11. Ross ERS, Menelaus MB. Open flexor tenotomy for hammer toes and curly toes in childhood. J Bone Joint Surg Br 1984;66B:770–771.
12. Stamm TT. Minor surgery of the foot: elevated fifth toe. In: Carling ER, Ross JP, eds. British Surgical Practice, vol 4. London: Butterworth, 1948:161–162.
13. Taylor RG. The treatment of claw toes by multiple transfer of flexor into extensor tendons. J Bone Joint Surg Br 1951;33B:539–542.
14. Thompson FM, Deland JT. Flexor tendon transfer for metatarsophalangeal instability of the second toe. Foot Ankle 1993;14: 385–388.
15. Thompson TC. Surgical treatment of disorders of the fore part of the foot. J Bone Joint Surg Br 1964;46B:1117–1128.
16. Wilson JN. V-Y correction for varus deformity of the fifth toe. Br J Surg 1953;41:133–135.

Chapter 35 Surgical Correction of Bunionette Deformity

Johnny T.C. Lau, W. Bryce Henderson, and Gilbert Yee

DEFINITION

- A bunionette deformity is a painful prominence on the lateral aspect of the fifth metatarsal head. This is usually caused by a prominent lateral metatarsal condyle, bowing of the fifth metatarsal, or increased intermetatarsal angle.

ANATOMY

- The Coughlin classification[4] illustrates the pertinent anatomic differences between the different types of bunionette deformities:
  - In type 1, a prominent lateral condyle may be noticeable under the callus.
  - In type 2, a curvature in the metatarsal shaft may be evident.
  - In type 3, there is a wider-than-expected angle between the fourth and fifth metatarsal. All may be associated with an inflamed bursa or callus, depending on the chronicity of the problem.

PATHOGENESIS

- This was historically named a tailor's bunionette, because tailors spent long hours with crossed legs, causing pressure over the fifth metatarsal head and resulting in local pressure and formation of a callus and occasionally a painful bursa.
- Local pressure can also be increased by a larger-than-normal lateral metatarsal condyle, angulation in the shaft of the metatarsal, or a wide intermetatarsal space, resulting in local tissue inflammation, pain, and swelling.

NATURAL HISTORY

- It has a female-to-male ratio of between 1:1 and 10:1.[5]
- The natural history is increasing formation of painful callus and bursae over the area.
- It can result in ulceration if proper foot care is not instituted or if underlying neuropathy is present.
- It usually requires regular paring of callus, wide toe box shoe modifications, or surgical treatment.

PATIENT HISTORY AND PHYSICAL FINDINGS

- Patients complain of pain and tenderness over the lateral aspect of the foot over the fifth metatarsal head.
- Symptoms are usually worse with activity, especially any position causing increased pressure over the metatarsal head.
- Enclosed shoes will exacerbate symptoms when causing local pressure. Hence, it is often described as improved in the summer, with less restrictive footwear and perhaps reduced work hours.
- The examiner should view both feet simultaneously while standing.
- The examiner should look for a prominent lateral metatarsal condyle, an obvious curvature in the metatarsal shaft, or a wide intermetatarsal angle.
- The examiner should note any hard or soft callus over the lateral aspect of the metatarsal.
- The examiner should look for any ulceration over the callus or between the fourth and fifth toes.

IMAGING AND OTHER DIAGNOSTIC STUDIES

- Standing plain radiographs (AP, lateral, and oblique views) are necessary.
- For all views, the radiographs are evaluated for osteoarthritis, narrow joint space, subchondral sclerosis, osteophyte formation, enlarged metatarsal condyle, curvature of metatarsal shaft, or a wide intermetatarsal angle between the fourth and fifth metatarsal shafts.
- Oblique radiographs may give a better view of the metatarsal head.
- On the lateral radiograph, the surgeon should look for any flexion or extension of the interphalangeal joints suggestive of claw or hammer toes.

DIFFERENTIAL DIAGNOSIS

- Curly toe
- Claw toe
- Hammer toe
- Stress fracture of the fifth metatarsal
- Fifth metatarsal fracture with prominent fracture callus

NONOPERATIVE MANAGEMENT

- Nonoperative management focuses on decreasing pressure.
- It is very important for the patient to avoid sitting positions that place lateral-sided pressure on the fifth metatarsal.
- Placing lamb's wool or cotton between the fourth and fifth toes to reduce medial deviation of the fifth toe can reduce lateral-sided pressure.
- Proper-fitting wide toe box or orthopaedic shoes can alleviate pressure caused by footwear.

SURGICAL MANAGEMENT

Preoperative Planning

- The surgeon should take into consideration any previous scars, edema, or skin abnormalities that would affect incision placement.
- Plain weight-bearing films are reviewed to determine which type of bunionette is present. Soft tissue release or osteotomy is based on the type of deformity.
- Type 1 deformity is treated with excision of the lateral metatarsal condyle.
- Type 2 deformity is treated with a distal metatarsal osteotomy. We describe the chevron type of osteotomy to correct the lateral deviation in the distal metatarsal shaft. The lateral deviation angle measures the degree of lateral bowing and is measured off the medial aspect of the fifth metatarsal shaft

base to the center of the metatarsal head. The normal value is 2.6 degrees (range 0 to 7 degrees).[4]

- In type 3 deformity a wide intermetatarsal angle between the fourth and fifth metatarsal is noted, with the mean angle being 6.5 degrees (range 3 to 11 degrees).[7] This is best treated with a proximal Ludloff metatarsal osteotomy.

Positioning

- The patient s positioned supine on a radiolucent operating table. A small lift is placed under the buttock on the operative side. A tourniquet is placed on the upper thigh or a sterile Esmarch tourniquet is placed above the ankle.

Approach

- All skin incisions should be lateral, with caution to avoid any digital nerves on the lateral aspect of the fifth toe.
- This approach allows for bunionectomy and osteotomy of the shaft with screw, pin, or plate fixation, and the approach can be extended proximally or distally if needed.

LATERAL METATARSAL CONDYLECTOMY WITH CAPSULAR PLICATION

- Use a lateral approach, making an incision down to the capsule (TECH FIG 1).
- Free the soft tissue between the capsule and the overlying skin to expose the lateral aspect of the metatarsal head (TECH FIG 2A,B).

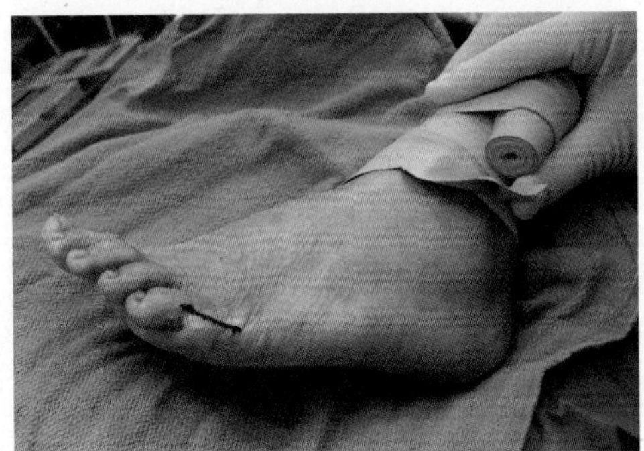

TECH FIG 1 • Lateral incision over bunionette.

- Make a V-shaped capsulotomy with the proximal apex to allow for plication on closure (TECH FIG 2C,D).
- Expose the enlarged lateral condyle of the fifth metatarsal. Place small Hohmann retractors below and above the metatarsal head to protect both flexor and extensor tendons (TECH FIG 3A).
- With a small saw, excise the prominent lateral condyle head parallel to the shaft of the metatarsal (TECH FIG 3B,C).
- Pull the distal part of the V capsulotomy proximally to the desired amount of tension and sew with a heavy nonabsorbable suture (TECH FIG 3D).
- Close the subcutaneous tissue with small absorbable suture and the skin with small nonabsorbable suture.
- Place a small amount of gauze between the fourth and fifth toes to keep the fifth toe from deviating medially while it heals.

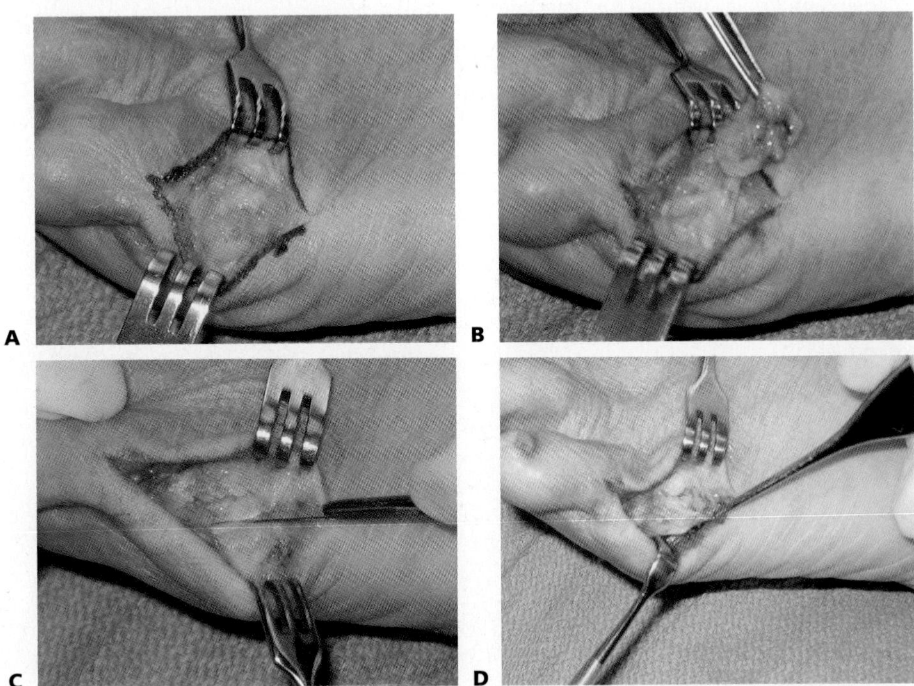

TECH FIG 2 • **A.** Dissection through subcutaneous tissue to bursa. **B.** Excision of bursa over bunionette. **C,D.** V-shaped capsulotomy performed to expose bunionette.

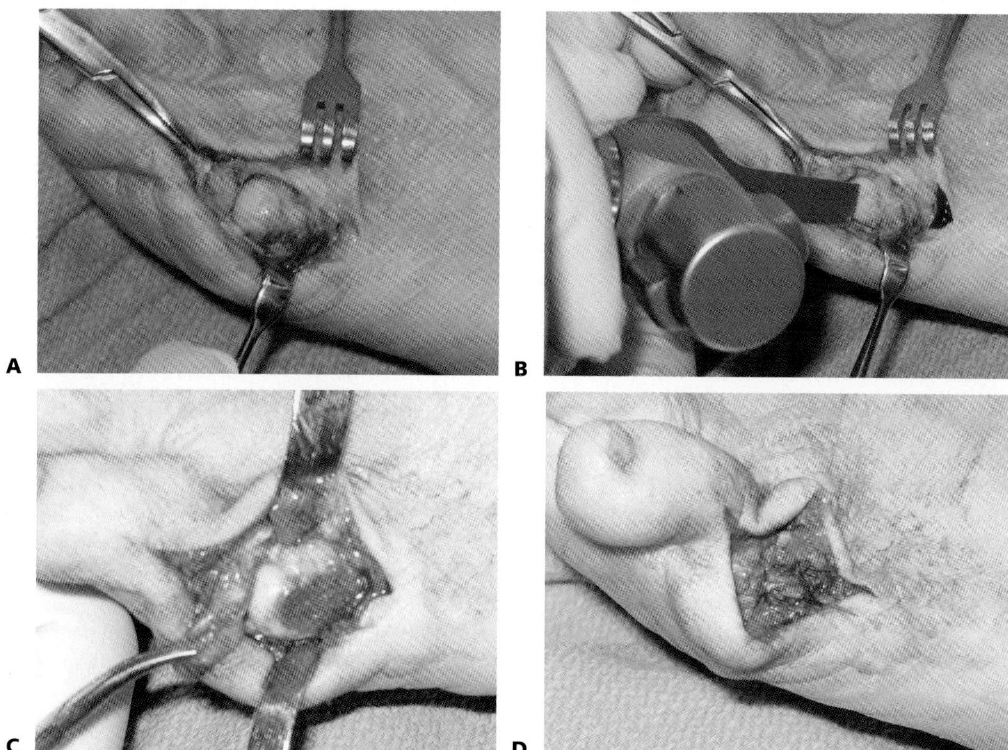

TECH FIG 3 • **A.** Bunionette exposed through capsulotomy. **B, C.** Bunionette excised with saw. **D.** V-shaped capsulotomy repaired with proximal advancement to correct deformity.

CHEVRON OSTEOTOMY OF THE FIFTH METATARSAL

- Make a lateral incision down to the capsule.
- Free the soft tissue between the capsule and the overlying skin to expose the lateral aspect of the metatarsal head.
- Make a V-shaped capsulotomy with the proximal apex to allow for plication on closure.
- Expose the enlarged lateral condyle of the fifth metatarsal and perform excision of the lateral metatarsal condyle as described previously (TECH FIG 4A–C).
- Mark the center of the freshly cut lateral aspect of the metatarsal head with a sterile marker (TECH FIG 4D).
- The limbs of the chevron osteotomy are 60 degrees.
- Use your free hand to palpate the plane of the metatarsal heads, and make the chevron osteotomy parallel to the plantar surface of the foot (TECH FIG 4E,F).

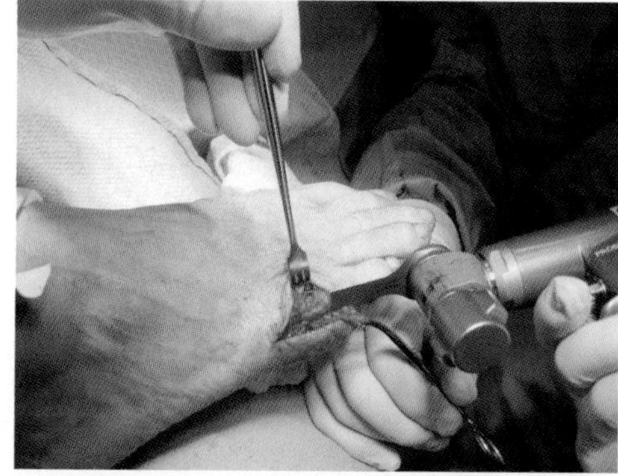

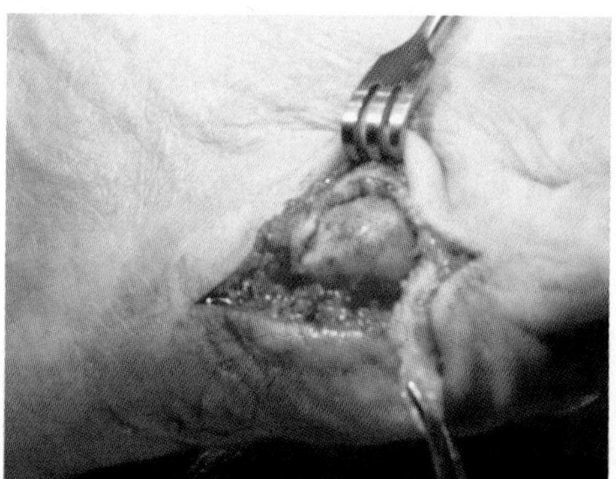

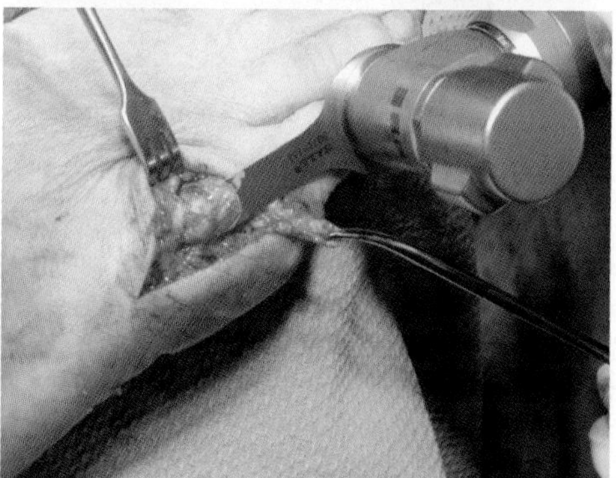

TECH FIG 4 • **A.** Bunionette exposed through lateral approach and V-shaped capsulotomy. **B, C.** Bunionette excision performed with saw. *(continued)*

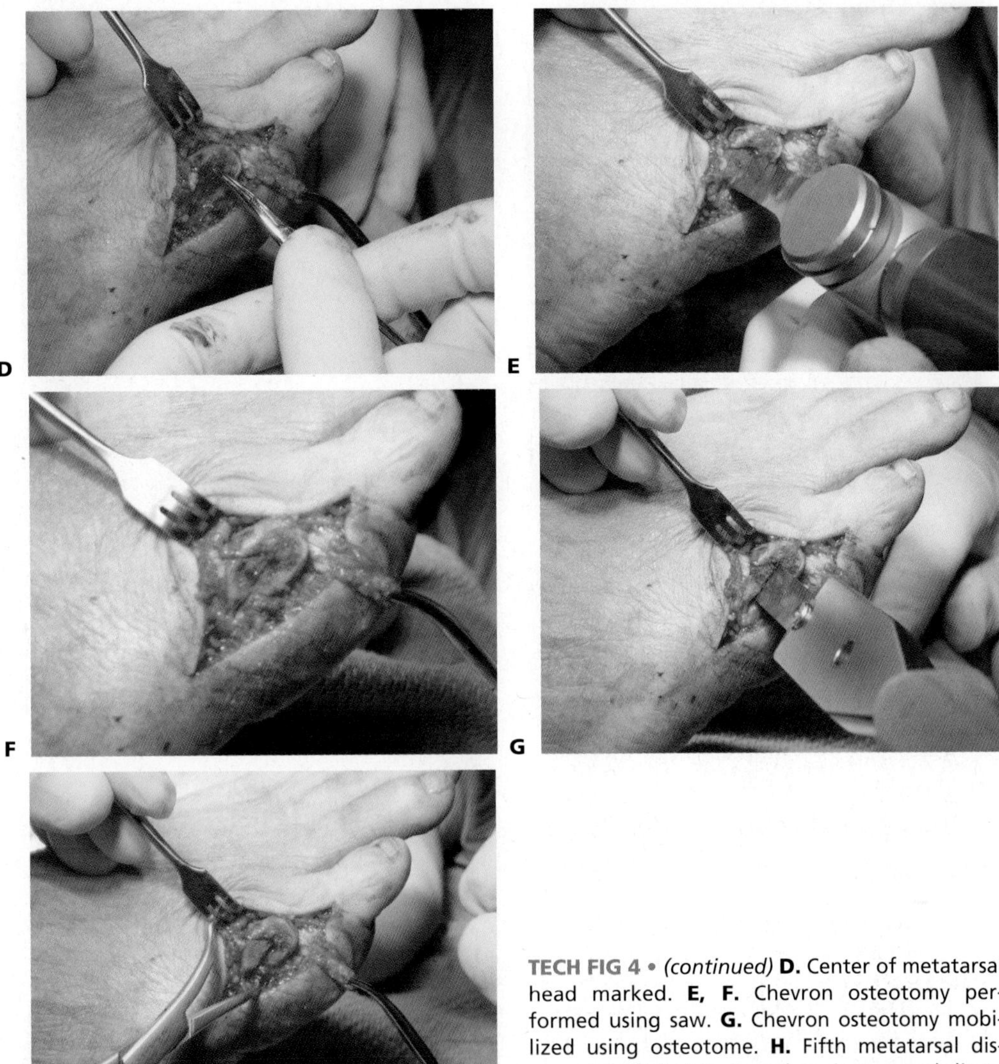

TECH FIG 4 • *(continued)* **D.** Center of metatarsal head marked. **E, F.** Chevron osteotomy performed using saw. **G.** Chevron osteotomy mobilized using osteotome. **H.** Fifth metatarsal displaced medially 3 to 4 mm by using a towel clip to pull the metatarsal shaft lateral and impacting the metatarsal head distally.

- Shift the metatarsal head medially, leaving 3 to 4 mm of exposed metatarsal shaft (TECH FIG 4G,H AND 5A,B).
- Cut the residual lateral bone with the saw again parallel to the metatarsal shaft.
- Secure the osteotomy with a mini-fragment screw inserted from proximal to distal fixing the osteotomy site. Alternatively, a Kirschner wire can be used to secure the osteotomy site (TECH FIG 5C,D).
- Close the capsule with a heavy nonabsorbable suture.
- Close the subcutaneous tissue with small absorbable suture and the skin with small nonabsorbable suture.

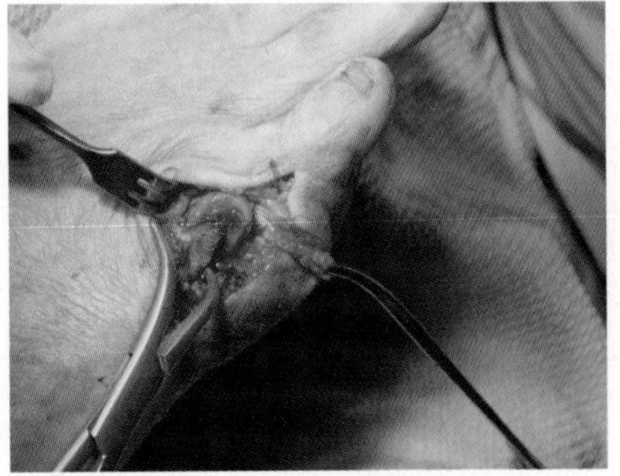

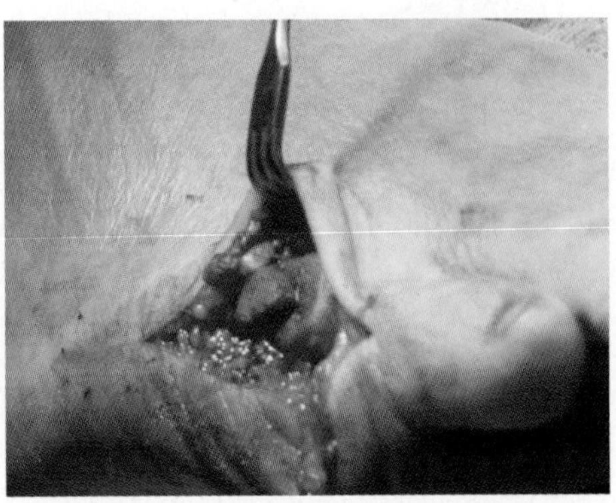

TECH FIG 5 • **A, B.** Amount of displacement of the chevron osteotomy. *(continued)*

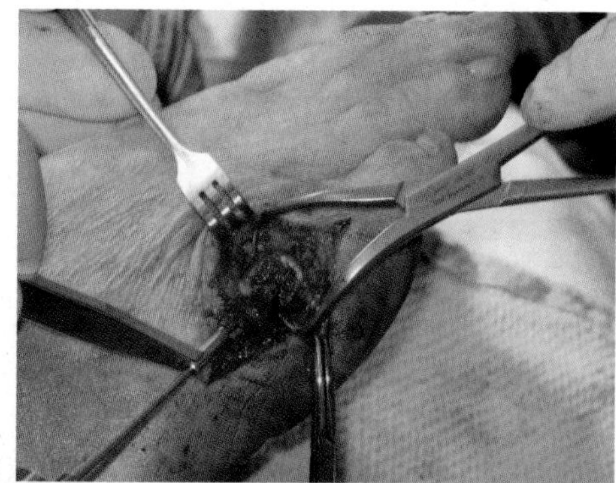
C

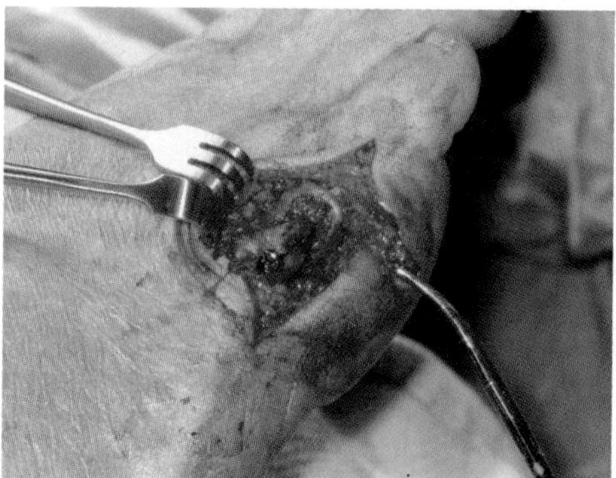
D

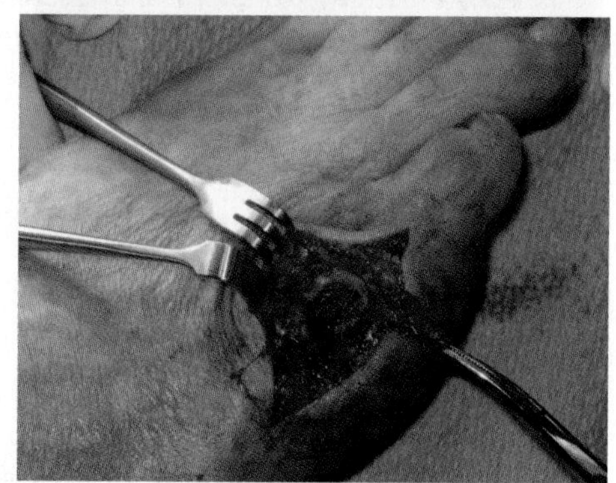
E

TECH FIG 5 • *(continued)* **C, D.** Metatarsal head is stabilized with a towel clip and fixed using a mini-fragment screw. **E.** Overhanging bone on the proximal and lateral aspect of the metatarsal shaft is excised.

OBLIQUE METATARSAL SHAFT OSTEOTOMY (COUGHLIN)

- Make a lateral skin incision and carry it down to the capsule.
- Free the soft tissue between the capsule and the overlying skin to expose the lateral aspect of the metatarsal head.
- With a sterile marker, mark the plantar aspect of the metatarsal where the capsule meets the metatarsal neck. Then mark the osteotomy on the dorsal proximal aspect.
- Place Hohmann retractors above and below to protect the extensor and flexor tendons.
- Cut the osteotomy two thirds of the way, leaving the plantar third intact.
- Insert a mini-fragment screw (2.0 or 2.7 mm) in the proximal portion of the osteotomy. Tighten the screw completely and then loosen it before completing the osteotomy.
- Complete the osteotomy.
- Swing the distal portion medially to the desired amount of correction and tighten the proximal screw. Insert another 2.0- or 2.7-mm screw more distally to supplement fixation.
- Cut the excess bone from the proximal osteotomy site with the saw.
- Close the subcutaneous tissue with small nonabsorbable suture and the skin with nonabsorbable suture.

PEARLS AND PITFALLS

Lateral metatarsal head excision	▪ Avoid excising too much metatarsal since it can result in joint instability. ▪ The osteotomy should be directed away from the metatarsal shaft to avoid splitting the metatarsal with the osteotomy.
Chevron osteotomy	▪ The apex of the osteotomy should be located in the center of the metatarsal head. If it is too distal, it can fracture the head. If it is too proximal, the location of the osteotomy is diaphyseal bone, which may take longer to heal. ▪ If the plane of the osteotomy is not parallel to the plantar aspect of the foot, it will prevent shifting of the metatarsal head.
Oblique osteotomy	▪ A long oblique osteotomy is needed to achieve better correction and more stable fixation. ▪ Screw placement for the osteotomy is important. If it is too close to the end of the osteotomy, it will fracture the osteotomy. If it is too distal to the end of the osteotomy, it limits the correction since the point of rotation is more distal than the apex of the osteotomy. ▪ Stable fixation is key to union and maintaining the correction.

POSTOPERATIVE CARE

- The wound is checked at 1 week postoperatively to examine for any evidence of infection.
- Sutures are removed at 2 weeks.
- If a pin was used, it is removed at 6 weeks.
- Heel walking only is permitted for 6 weeks.
- In the oblique metatarsal osteotomy a postoperative fiberglass splint is applied in the operating room and is changed to an air cast at 2 weeks. This is continued for 6 weeks.

OUTCOMES

- Although the bunionette deformity is common, it is rarely symptomatic enough to warrant surgical intervention. This is reflected by the small numbers found in case studies reported in the literature.
- Kitaoka and Holiday[5] reported results on 21 feet (16 patients) who underwent lateral condylar resection for bunionette. The overall results were considered good in 15 feet, fair in 3, and poor in 3. However, 23% of the patients had recurrent or persistent lateral forefoot pain. They attributed the failures to an inadequate amount of resection, MTP joint subluxation, and severe forefoot splaying. Limitations of the procedure included lack of deformity correction, a significant incidence of residual lateral forefoot pain, and difficulty treating bunionettes with intractable plantar keratosis.
- Several studies have reported good results in the surgical treatment of bunionette with chevron osteotomies.[2,6,7] Moran and Claridge[7] felt that stabilization of the osteotomy site with fixation was necessary to minimize the risk of displacement. One study reported that Kirschner wire fixation led to less dorsal displacement of the distal fragment.[8] In Kitaoka et al's[6] series of chevron osteotomies for bunionettes, they used Kirschner wire fixation in only 1 of 19 patients due to intraoperative instability at the osteotomy site; however, they did note postoperative displacement in another patient. No incidence of displacement was found in series that routinely used fixation.[2,7] Limited correction of the fourth–fifth intermetatarsal angle was seen, where 1 mm of translation results in a decrease of that angle of only 1 degree.[3,6] The fifth metatarsal head can be shifted only 33% to 40% of its width, generally in the range of 3 to 4 mm.[2,3,6,7] However, Kitaoka et al[6] noted that neither the preoperative nor the postoperative intermetatarsal fourth–fifth angle correlated with the postoperative foot score.
- Oblique metatarsal osteotomies have been shown to provide the biggest correction for a type II or III deformity with a high intermetatarsal angle.[4,9,12] Coughlin[4] found that the intermetatarsal angle decreased from an average of 16 degrees preoperatively to 0.5 degrees postoperatively. Results have shown a reliable improvement in postoperative subjective scores.[4,9,12] With the use of internal fixation, there was only one report of delayed union.[4,9,12] This is compared to other series reporting rates of delayed union of up to 11% without fixation.[11] However, prominent hardware can be an issue, and in one study 87% of patients required later removal.[4] Proximal osteotomies are not recommended due to the poor blood supply in the region and the higher risk of delayed or nonunion.[1,10]

COMPLICATIONS

- Infection
- Recurrent deformity
- Digital nerve injury
- Nonunion of the osteotomy
- Displacement of the osteotomy
- Avascular necrosis of the fifth metatarsal head
- Transfer metatarsalgia

REFERENCES

1. Baumhauer JF, DiGiovanni BF. Osteotomies of the fifth metatarsal. Foot Ankle Clin 2001;6:491–498.
2. Boyer ML, Deorio JK. Bunionette deformity correction with distal chevron osteotomy and single absorbable pin fixation. Foot Ankle Int 2003;24:845–857.
3. Cooper PS. Disorders and deformities of the lesser toes. In: Myerson MS, ed. Foot and Ankle Disorders. Philadelphia: WB Saunders, 2000:335–358.
4. Coughlin MJ. Treatment of bunionette deformity with longitudinal diaphyseal osteotomy with distal soft tissue repair. Foot Ankle 1991;11:195–203.
5. Kitaoka HB, Holiday AD. Lateral condylar resection for bunionette. Clin Orthop Relat Res 1992;278:183–192.
6. Kitaoka HB, Holiday AD, Campbell DC. Distal chevron metatarsal osteotomy for bunionette. Foot Ankle 1991;12:80–85.
7. Moran MM, Claridge RJ. Chevron osteotomy for bunionette. Foot Ankle Int 1994;15:684–688.
8. Pontious J, Brook JW, Hillstrom HJ. Tailor's bunion: is fixation necessary? J Am Podiatr Med Assoc 1996;86:63–73.
9. Radl R, Leithner A, Koehler W. The modified distal horizontal metatarsal osteotomy for correction of bunionette deformity. Foot Ankle Int 2005;26:454–457.
10. Shereff MJ, Yang QM, Krummer FJ. The vascular anatomy of the fifth metatarsal. Foot Ankle Int 1991;11:350–353.
11. Sponsel KH. Bunionette correction by metatarsal osteotomy. Orthop Clin North Am 1976;7:808–819.
12. Vienne P, Oesselmann M, Espinosa N. Modified Coughlin procedure for surgical treatment of symptomatic tailor's bunion: a prospective follow-up study of 33 consecutive operations. Foot Ankle Int 2006;27:573–580.

Chapter 36

Rheumatoid Forefoot Reconstruction

Thomas G. Padanilam

DEFINITION

- Rheumatoid arthritis is an inflammatory condition of synovial joints that usually presents as a symmetric polyarthropathy.
- Ninety percent of patients with chronic rheumatoid arthritis have involvement of the foot; the forefoot is the most commonly involved area of the foot.

ANATOMY

- The metatarsophalangeal (MTP) joint of the foot is stabilized by the plantar plate, the collateral ligaments, the capsule, and a dynamic balance between the intrinsic and extrinsic muscles of the foot.
- The intrinsic muscles are plantar to the MTP joint axis and help to plantarflex the joint.
- The proximal phalanx of the hallux has a valgus orientation of 0 to 15 degrees at the MTP joint.
- A plantar fat pad normally provides cushioning and protection for the metatarsal heads.

PATHOGENESIS

- Unrelenting synovitis leads to a painful and swollen joint. This causes a stretching of the ligamentous structures surrounding the MTP joint.
- Ligament stretching combined with forces of walking leads to soft tissue instability, articular cartilage destruction, and subchondral bone resorption.
- Residual laxity leads to subluxation and dislocation of the lesser MTP joints. This allows the metatarsal head to protrude through the plantar plate and capsule.
- The hallux most commonly develops a hallux valgus deformity, with an occasional hallux varus developing.
- MTP instability leads to intrinsic muscles becoming dorsal to the MTP axis, which leads to loss of active MTP flexion and interphalangeal extension. This leads to a claw-toe deformity.
- Dislocation of the metatarsal lesser MTP joints leads to a distal migration of the fat pad, which exposes the metatarsal heads, increasing pressure in this area.

NATURAL HISTORY

- Rheumatoid arthritis initially presents in the foot in about 17% of patients.
- It is a progressive disorder that may start as synovitis and progress to dislocations and degeneration of the joint.
- The longer active rheumatoid disease is present, the greater the likelihood the patient will develop deformities as a result of the associated synovitis.

PATIENT HISTORY AND PHYSICAL FINDINGS

- Initially, patients often complain of an insidious onset of poorly defined forefoot pain and difficulty with ambulation. As synovitis leads to deformity within the forefoot, the symptoms then become more localized.
- Patients will often have shoe wear-related irritation along the medial eminence of the hallux and along the dorsal aspects of the proximal interphalangeal joints of the lesser toes.
- With the development of the lesser-toe MTP dislocation, pain on the plantar aspect of the metatarsal heads is present.
- Hallux valgus: the examiner should look for the degrees of valgus orientation and its impingement on lesser toes. Patients often have pain along the medial eminence and from pressure on the toes (**FIG 1**).
- Lesser MTP dislocation and plantar callus: the examiner should inspect and palpate the dorsal and plantar aspects of the forefoot. MTP instability can vary from subluxation to dislocation. Increased pressure under the metatarsal heads is a common source of pain (**FIG 2**).
  - Examination should include range of motion for the ankle joint, subtalar joint, and MTP joints.
- The examiner should perform a complete vascular and neurologic examination of the foot.

IMAGING AND OTHER DIAGNOSTIC STUDIES

- Plain radiographs will often show periarticular osteopenia, symmetric joint space narrowing, marginal cortical erosions, and subchondral cysts (**FIG 3**).
- The severity of hallux valgus and the presence of MTP dislocation can be evaluated.

DIFFERENTIAL DIAGNOSIS

- Inflammatory arthritides such as psoriatic arthritis, Reiter syndrome (reactive arthritis), and ankylosing spondylitis
- Gout and pseudogout
- Connective tissue disorders (ie, lupus)

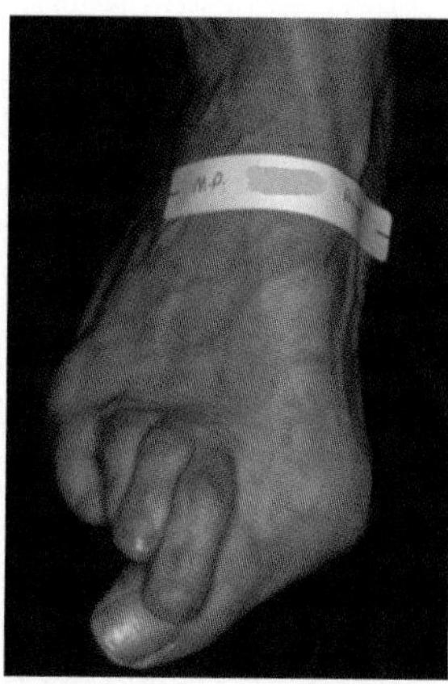

FIG 1 • Hallux valgus: the examiner should inspect the foot with the patient standing.

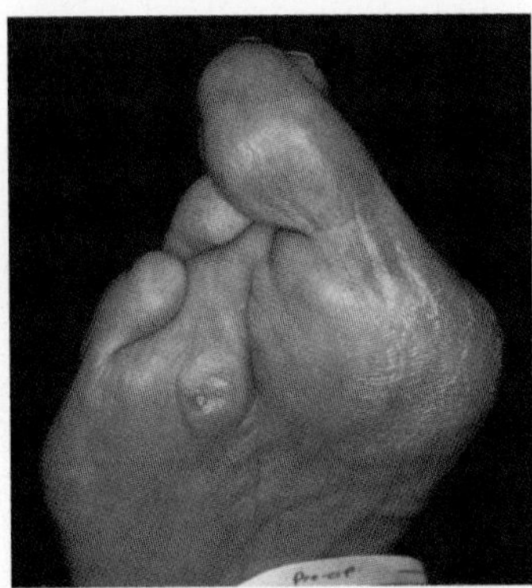

FIG 2 • Lesser metatarsophalangeal dislocation and plantar callus: the examiner should inspect and palpate the dorsal and plantar aspects of the forefoot.

- Inflammatory bowel disease (Crohn disease or ulcerative colitis)
- Neurologic disorders
- Osteoarthritis

NONOPERATIVE MANAGEMENT

- New pharmacologic agents that can control synovitis have the potential for minimizing the severity and frequency of deformities seen.
- Shoe wear modifications such as extra-depth shoes decrease shoe wear irritation.
- Custom inserts can help relieve pressure from painful areas.
- Plantar calluses may benefit from periodic shaving.

SURGICAL MANAGEMENT

- Surgical treatment is indicated for patients whose pain is unrelieved by nonoperative treatment or those with ulcerative lesions due to their deformity.
- The goals of surgical treatment include:
  - Restoration of the weight-bearing function of the first ray
  - Relocation of the plantar fat pad
  - Reduction of pressure under the lesser metatarsal heads
  - Correction of claw toe or hammer toe deformities
- A variety of methods have been described, but probably the most reliable method for accomplishing these goals is with fusion of the first MTP joint, resection of the lesser metatarsal heads, and either osteoclasis or open hammer toe repair.

Preoperative Planning

- These patients have a relatively poor soft tissue envelope, and this may compromise wound healing.
- There is no perioperative standard as to whether to continue the use of disease-modifying antirheumatic drugs.
- Consideration should be given regarding the need for cervical spine evaluation before general anesthesia.

Positioning

- The patient is placed supine on the operating table (**FIG 4**), with the foot positioned near the distal end of the table.

Approach

- The first MTP joint can be exposed through a dorsal or medial approach. Both provide adequate exposure, but the medial approach may provide a greater skin bridge between incisions. Incisions from previous procedures may dictate the approach used.
- Lesser metatarsal head resection can be performed through dorsal longitudinal incisions or a plantar incision. While the plantar approach may provide more direct access to the metatarsal head when the MTP joint has been dislocated for a while, there is more of a risk of problems with wound healing.

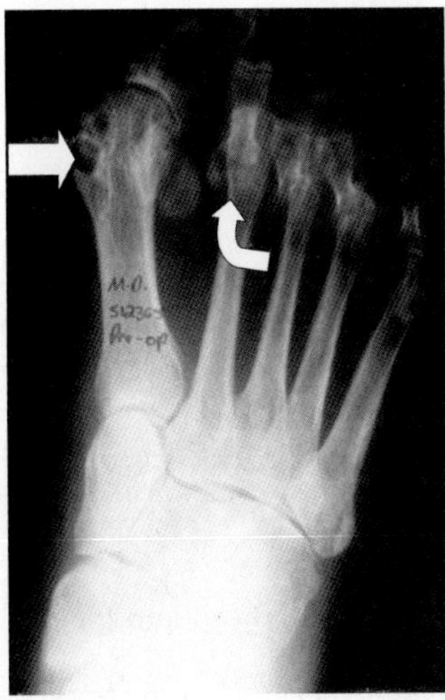

FIG 3 • Loss of joint space, severe hallux valgus, and associated osteopenia. The *straight arrow* shows marginal cortical erosion. The *curved arrow* shows the overlap between the proximal phalanx and the metatarsal head seen with dislocation of the joint.

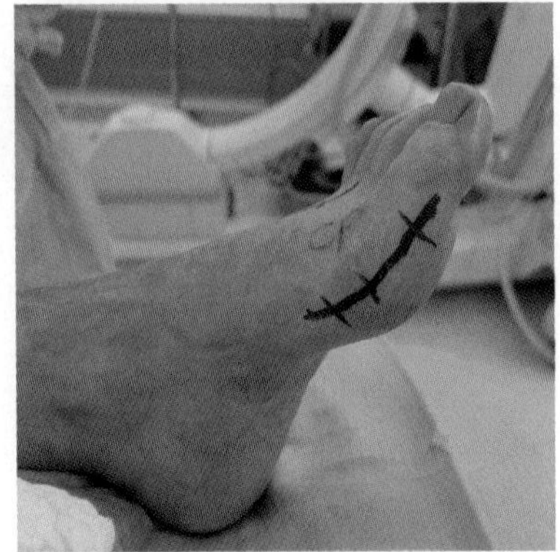

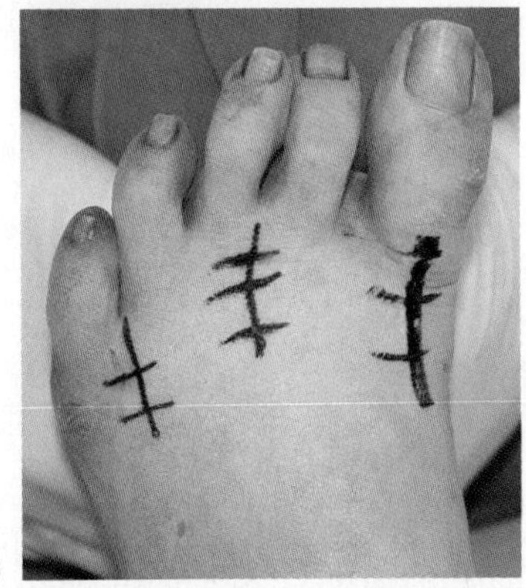

FIG 4 • **A.** The patient is placed supine with the foot near the distal end of the table. **B.** The foot is positioned so the dorsal aspect can be visualized. This may require the use of a blanket roll or sandbag under the ipsilateral hip.

TECHNIQUES

HAMMER TOE CORRECTION

- If the deformity at the proximal interphalangeal (PIP) joint of the lesser toes are not severe, then the contractures at the joint can be corrected by closed manipulation (TECH FIG 1).
  - Grasp the toe distal and proximal to the PIP joint and hyperextend it until the joint is resting in a neutral position.
- If the deformity is severe, an open hammer toe correction is performed (TECH FIG 2).
  - Make an elliptical incision along the PIP joint.
  - Remove an elliptical portion of skin over the PIP joint and open the capsule over the joint.
  - Release the collateral ligaments and expose the head of the proximal phalanx.
  - Resect the proximal phalanx at the metaphyseal–diaphyseal junction.
  - Stabilize the area with a Kirschner wire after performing metatarsal head resections.

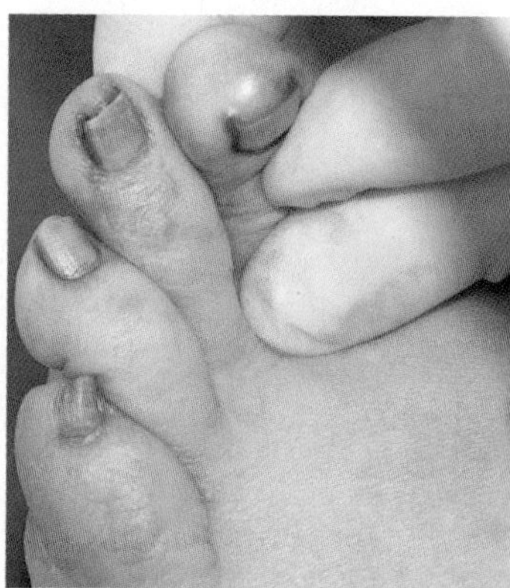

TECH FIG 1 • Performance of osteoclasis, in which the proximal interphalangeal joint is passively manipulated to break up contracture.

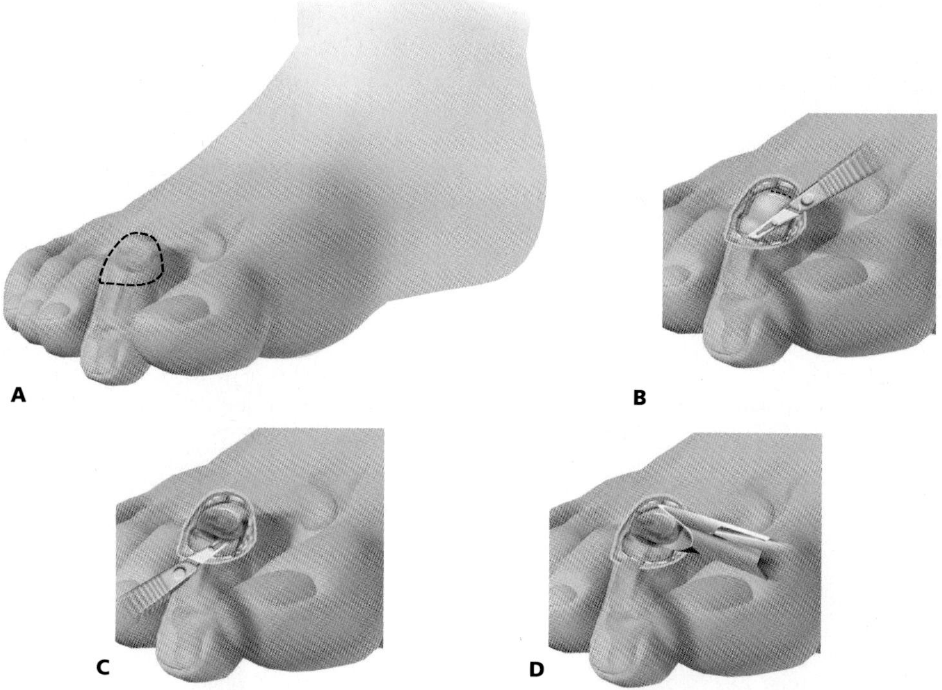

TECH FIG 2 • An open hammer toe repair is performed with an elliptical incision over the proximal interphalangeal joint (**A**), followed by capsular release (**B**), and exposure (**C**) and resection (**D**) of the head of the proximal phalanx. (Adapted from Coughlin M, Mann R, eds. Surgery of the Foot and Ankle, 7th ed. St. Louis: Mosby, 1999.)

LESSER METATARSAL HEAD RESECTION

- Make longitudinal incisions over the second and fourth intermetatarsal spaces (TECH FIG 3).
- Blunt dissection is recommended to minimize trauma.
- Identify the extensor digitorum longus and retract it to one side.
- Release the dorsal capsule and collateral ligaments off the metatarsal head.
- Bring the metatarsal head into the dorsal aspect of the incision.
- A curved retractor can be useful in obtaining exposure of the metatarsal head.
- Use a sagittal saw to resect the metatarsal head. The blade is oriented in an oblique fashion from dorsal–distal to plantar–proximal.

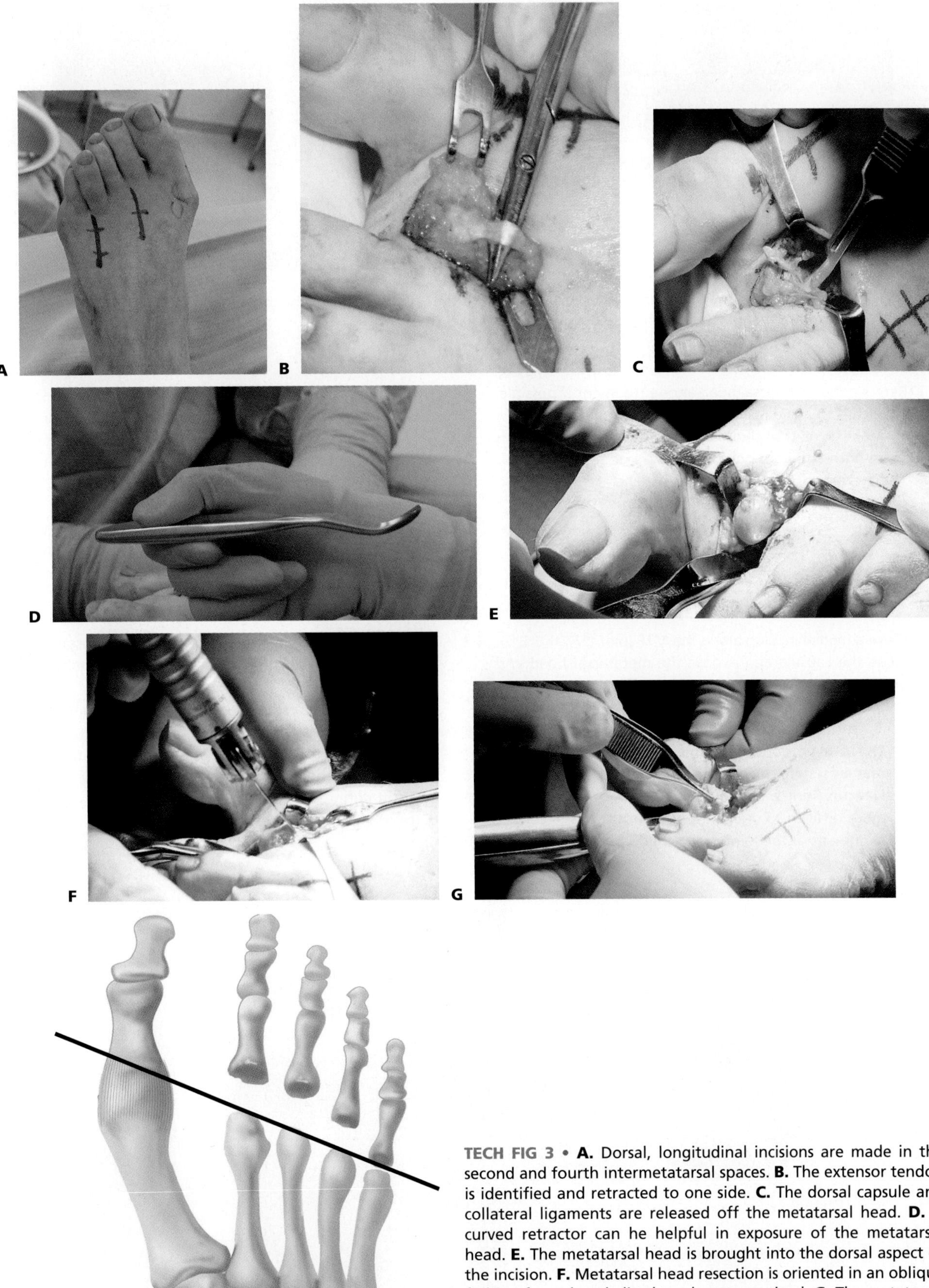

TECH FIG 3 • A. Dorsal, longitudinal incisions are made in the second and fourth intermetatarsal spaces. **B.** The extensor tendon is identified and retracted to one side. **C.** The dorsal capsule and collateral ligaments are released off the metatarsal head. **D.** A curved retractor can he helpful in exposure of the metatarsal head. **E.** The metatarsal head is brought into the dorsal aspect of the incision. **F.** Metatarsal head resection is oriented in an oblique fashion from dorsal–distal to plantar–proximal. **G.** The metatarsal head is removed as one fragment if possible. **H.** Progressive resection from the second to fifth metatarsal is performed, creating a smooth cascade. (Adapted from Coughlin M, Mann R, eds. Surgery of the Foot and Ankle, 7th ed. St. Louis: Mosby, 1999.) *(continued)*

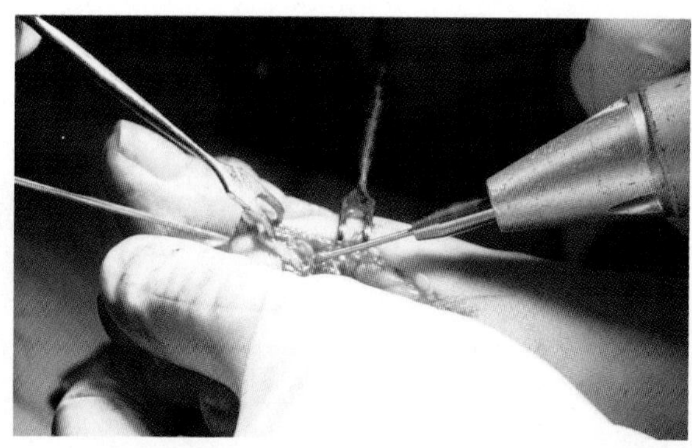

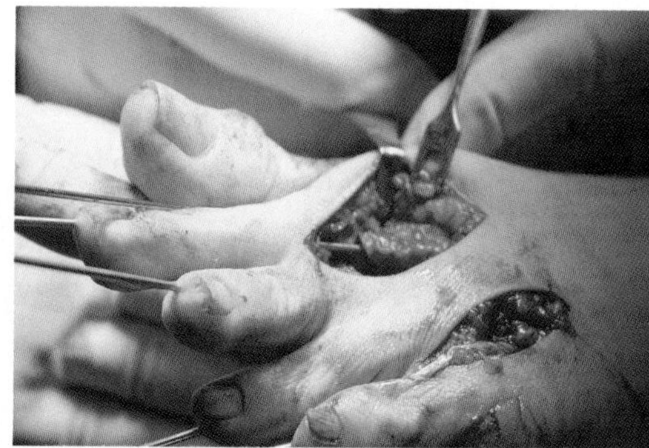

TECH FIG 3 • *(continued)* **I.** Kirschner wires are passed from the base of the proximal phalanx to the tip of the toes. **J.** The wires are then passed retrograde down the metatarsal shaft.

- Remove the metatarsal head as one fragment if possible. Take care to avoid leaving any bone fragments.
  - Make sure the plantar aspect of the metatarsal is smooth and does not have a sharp edge.
- The metatarsal head resection usually starts on the second metatarsal and moves laterally.
  - Leave the third metatarsal slightly shorter than the second and the fourth shorter than the third metatarsal. This creates a smooth cascade from medial to lateral.
- Pass 0.625-mm Kirschner wires from the base of the proximal phalanx to the tip of the toes.
- Pass the wires retrograde down the metatarsal shaft.

HALLUX MTP ARTHRODESIS

- Make a medial incision along the MTP joint (TECH FIG 4).
- Incise the capsule and expose the metatarsal head and proximal phalanx.
- Prepare the joint surfaces by removing the remaining articular cartilage and exposing the underlying bone.
  - This can be done with the use of a cup and cone reamer system or with rongeurs and curettes.
  - Flat cuts using a saw can also be used, but it is slightly more difficult to orient the cuts such that the correct alignment of the joint is obtained.
- Place the MTP joint in 10 to 15 degrees of valgus and 20 to 25 degrees of dorsiflexion relative to the metatarsal shaft.
  - The correct dorsiflexion can be approximated by using a flat tray as a guide and keeping the pulp of the hallux 5 to 10 mm off the surface of the tray.
- The position is held temporarily with a Kirschner wire.
- Perform definitive fixation with cross screws or a dorsal plate or, in salvage cases, threaded pins.
- Close the wounds and apply a forefoot dressing.

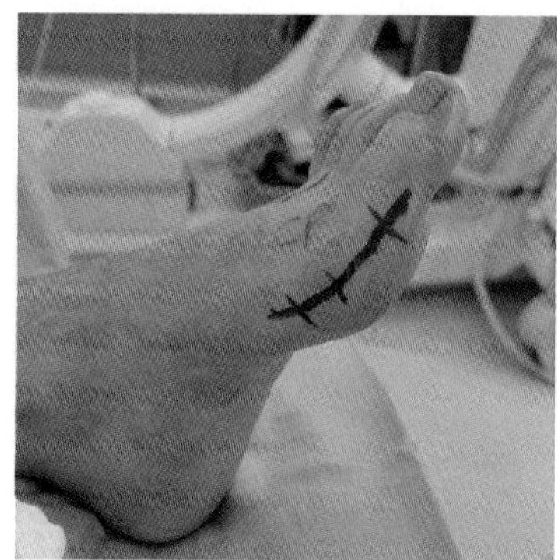

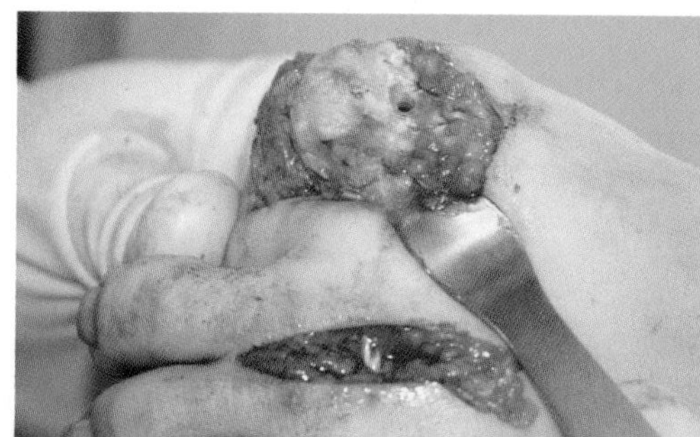

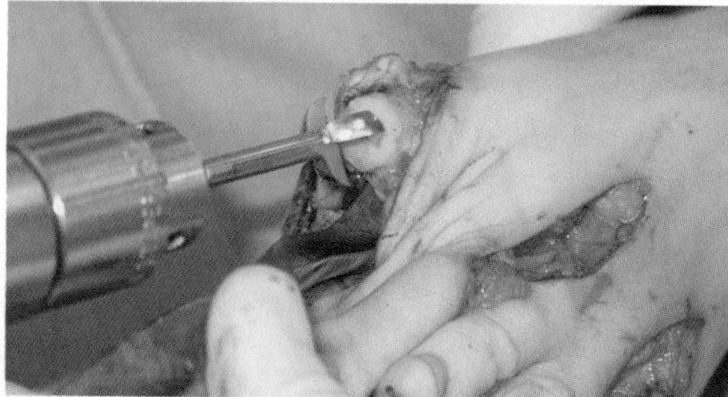

TECH FIG 4 • A. Medial incision for exposure of hallux metatarsophalangeal. **B.** The proximal phalanx and metatarsal head articular cartilage are exposed. **C.** Joint preparation using a cup and cone reamer. *(continued)*

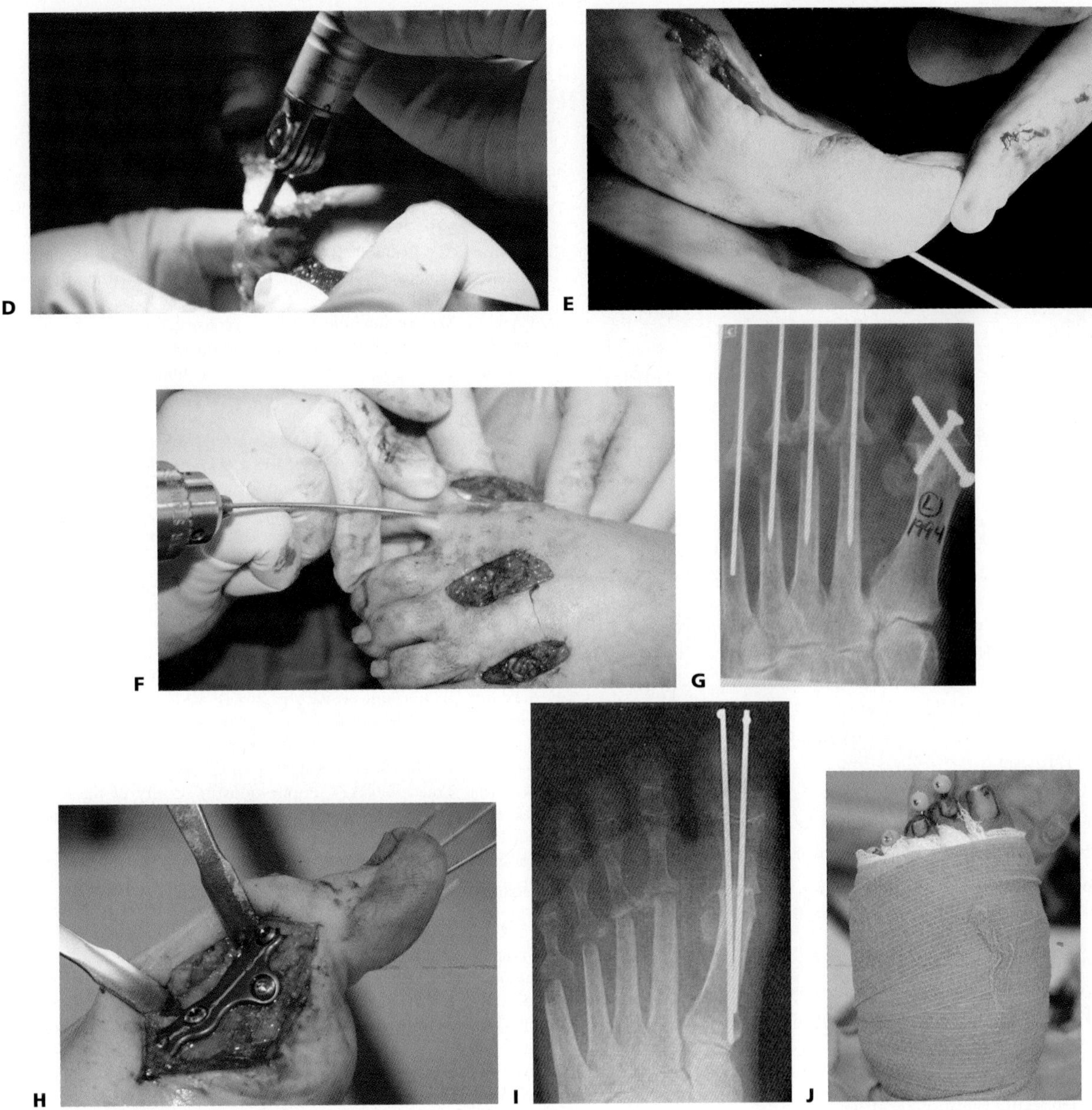

TECH FIG 4 • *(continued)* **D.** Joint preparation with flat cuts. **E.** A flat tray is used to guide dorsiflexion. The pulp of the hallux sits 5 to 10 mm off the tray. **F.** Temporary fixation with a Kirschner wire. **G.** Crossed-screw fixation of fusion. **H.** Dorsal plate fixation. **I.** Fixation with threaded pins. **J.** Postoperative forefoot dressing.

PEARLS AND PITFALLS

Hammer toe correction	■ Fixed deformities often require an open correction. ■ Failure to correct the deformity can lead to recurrent deformity.
Metatarsal head resection	■ Oblique orientation of the resection helps decrease plantar pressure and sharp plantar edges. ■ Loose fragments can lead to recurrent callus formation and should be avoided. ■ Adequate decompression of the lesser MTP joint is seen with about 1 cm of space between the base of the phalanx and remaining metatarsal. ■ Progressive shortening of the metatarsals from medial to lateral allows better stress transfer. ■ After pin fixation, check the vascularity of the toe, as compromise occasionally requires pin removal.
Hallux MTP fusion	■ This is performed after the lesser metatarsal head resection to prevent an excessively long first ray. ■ Excessive dorsiflexion can cause pain over the interphalangeal joint and under the metatarsal head. ■ Fusion in greater than 20 degrees of valgus can increase the incidence of interphalangeal joint arthritis. ■ Care must be taken to prevent excessive pronation or supination of the toe.

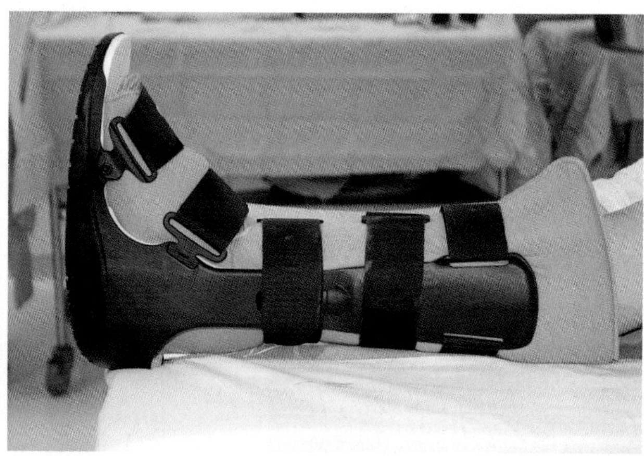

FIG 5 • Postoperative walking boot.

POSTOPERATIVE CARE

- After placement of the forefoot dressing, a walking boot is applied (**FIG 5**).
- Patients are instructed to bear weight on the heel of the foot.
- Sutures are removed 10 to 14 days after surgery.
- A forefoot dressing is used for the first 6 weeks.
- Kirschner wires are removed at 6 weeks.
- A walking boot is used for 8 to 10 weeks, based on healing of the first MTP fusion.

OUTCOMES

- Most studies have noted a significant improvement in ability to ambulate and in shoe wear options.
- Patient satisfaction rates are high and seem to hold up over time.
- Patients should be aware that the lesser toes are unlikely to touch the floor and can be floppy, there may be a change in shoe size, and toes may develop a rotational deformity.

COMPLICATIONS

- Recurrent intractable plantar keratosis
- Recurrent toe deformities
- Wound healing problems
- Nonunion of MTP fusion
- Infection

REFERENCES

1. Abdo RV, Iorio LJ. Rheumatoid arthritis of the foot and ankle. J Am Acad Orthop Surg 1994;2:326–332.
2. Beauchamp CG, Kirby T, Rudge SR. et al. Fusion of the first metatarsophalangeal joint in forefoot arthroplasty. Clin Orthop Relat Res 1984;190:249–253.
3. Clayton ML, Leidholt JD, Clark W. Arthroplasty of rheumatoid metatarsophalangeal joints: an outcome study. Clin Orthop Relat Res 1997;340:48–57.
4. Coughlin MJ. Rheumatoid forefoot reconstruction: a long-term follow-up study. J Bone Joint Surg Am 2000;82A:322–341.
5. Garner RW, Mowat AG, Hazleman BL. Wound healing after operations of patients with rheumatoid arthritis. J Bone Joint Surg Br 1973;55B:134–144.
6. Hamalainen M, Raunio P. Long-term followup of rheumatoid forefoot surgery. Clin Orthop Relat Res 1997;340:34–38.
7. Jaakkola JI, Mann RA. A review of rheumatoid arthritis affecting the foot and ankle. Foot Ankle Int 2004;25:866–874.
8. Lipscomb PR, Benson GM, Sones DA. Resection of proximal phalanges and metatarsal condyles for deformities of the forefoot due to rheumatoid arthritis. Clin Orthop Relat Res 1972;82:24.
9. Mann RA, Schakel ME II. Surgical correction of rheumatoid forefoot deformities. Foot Ankle Int 1995;16:1–6.
10. Mann RA, Thompson FM. Arthrodesis of the first metatarsophalangeal joint for hallux valgus in rheumatoid arthritis. J Bone Joint Surg Am 1984;66A:687–692.
11. McGarvey SR, Johnson KA. Keller arthroplasty in combination with resection arthroplasty of the lesser metatarsophalangeal joints in rheumatoid arthritis. Foot Ankle 1988;9:75–80.
12. Nassar J, Cracchiolo A. Complications in surgery of the foot and ankle in patients with rheumatoid arthritis. Clin Orthop Relat Res 2001;39:140–152.
13. Spiegel TM, Spiegel JS. Rheumatoid arthritis in the foot and ankle: diagnosis, pathology, and treatment: the relationship between foot and ankle deformity and disease duration in 50 patients. Foot Ankle 1982;2:318–324.
14. Thomas S, Kinninmonth AWG, Kumar S. Long-term results of the modified Hoffman procedure in the rheumatoid forefoot. J Bone Joint Surg Am 2005;87A:748–775.
15. Thordarson DB, Aval S, Krieger L. Failure of hallux MP preservation surgery for rheumatoid arthritis. Foot Ankle Int 2002;23:486–490.
16. Trieb K. Management of the foot in rheumatoid arthritis. J Bone Joint Surg Br 2005;87B:1171–1177.
17. Vandeputtee G, Steenwerckx A, Mulier T, et al. Forefoot reconstruction in rheumatoid patients: Keller-Lelievre-Hoffman versus arthrodesis MTP1-Hoffman. Foot Ankle Int 1999;20:438–443.

Chapter 37

Morton's Neuroma and Revision Morton's Neuroma Excision

David R. Richardson

DEFINITION

- A primary interdigital (Morton's) neuroma is in fact not a neuroma as it does not involve the haphazard proliferation of axons seen in a traumatic nerve injury.
  - Instead, this condition is best described as an interdigital perineural fibrosis.
- It was first described in 1845 by Lewis Durlacher, a chiropodist to the Queen of England.
- Recurrent neuromas are true histopathologic (haphazard proliferation of axons) amputation stump neuromas.
- Eighty-five to 90% of nontraumatic neuromas are found in the third web space. The rest are found in the second web space.

ANATOMY

- The medial plantar nerve supplies sensation to the first, second, and third digits and the medial aspect of the fourth digit. It emerges plantar and medial to the flexor digitorum brevis, coursing obliquely across the plantar surface of the muscle.
- The lateral plantar nerve supplies sensation to the lateral half of the fourth and the fifth digit.
- Both are branches of the tibial nerve and terminate with digital branches that course plantarly deep to the transverse metatarsal ligament (**FIG 1**).
- The lumbrical tendon appears lateral and superficial to the digital nerve as it attaches to the medial aspect of the extensor expansion of the digit and may be mistaken for nerve.
- In a cadaveric study, Levitsky et al[12] found that 27% of specimens had a communicating branch connecting the medial and lateral plantar nerves. They also noted that the second and third interspaces were significantly narrower than the first and fourth.
- Changes in the nerve itself involve perineural fibrosis, demyelinization and degeneration of nerve fibers, endoneural edema, and the absence of inflammatory changes.
- Plantar-directed nerve branches may tether the common digital nerve to the plantar skin.
- Theses nerve branches are present up to 4 cm proximal to the transverse metatarsal ligament.

PATHOGENESIS

- All histologic changes in a primary interdigital neuroma occur distal to the transverse metatarsal ligament, as shown in studies by Lassmann[11] and Graham et al.[7]
- The cause is unclear but is thought to evolve as an entrapment neuropathy.
- The second and third intermetatarsal spaces are narrower than the first and fourth.
- Mobility between the medial three rays and the lateral two rays may contribute to the high number of primary neuromas in the third interspace.
- In a limited number of patients (about 27%) the common digital nerve to the third interspace consists of branches from the medial and lateral plantar nerves, which perhaps increases the size of the nerve and predisposes it to entrapment (Fig 1).
- A "recurrent interdigital neuroma" may be due to several factors, including failure to make the correct diagnosis originally.
- Neurogenic pain may be due to causes other than perineural fibrosis, such as neuropathy and radiculopathy. Also, neuroma-like symptoms may be due to nerve irritation from local synovitis or bursitis.
- Beskin and Baxter[3] found that in patients with recurrent symptoms of interdigital neuroma, about two thirds presented within 12 months and one third had recurrence 1 to 4 years after primary surgery.
- Those with "recurrence" within the first 12 months probably represent patients who were originally misdiagnosed.

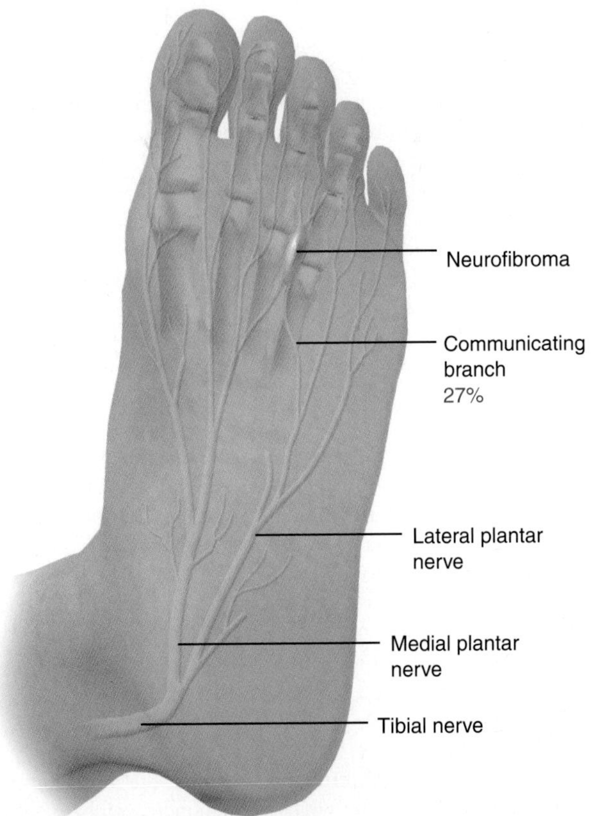

FIG 1 • Course of medial and lateral plantar nerve. A communicating branch of the lateral plantar nerve occurs in about 27% of patients.

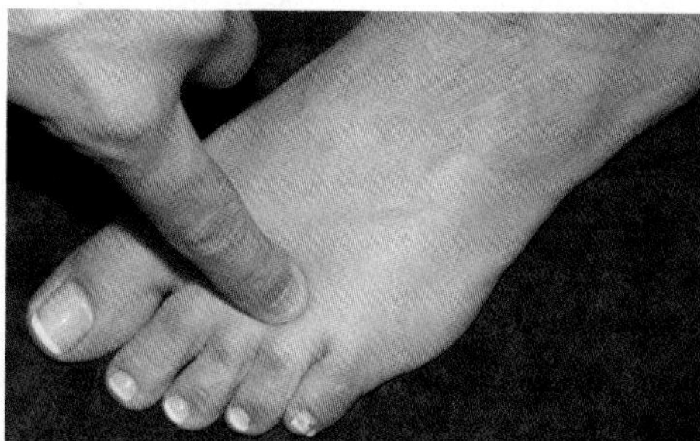

A

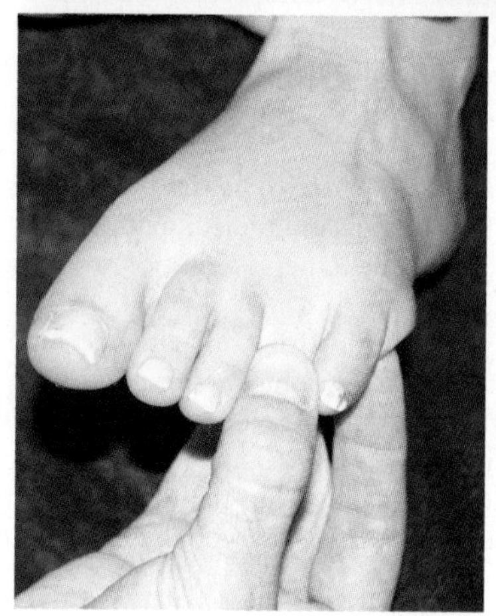

B

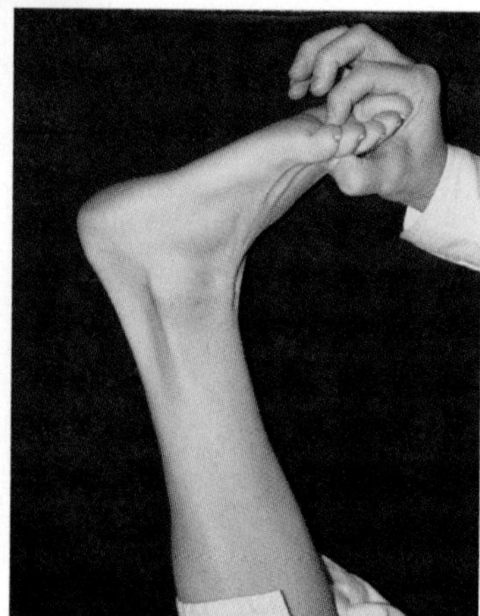

C

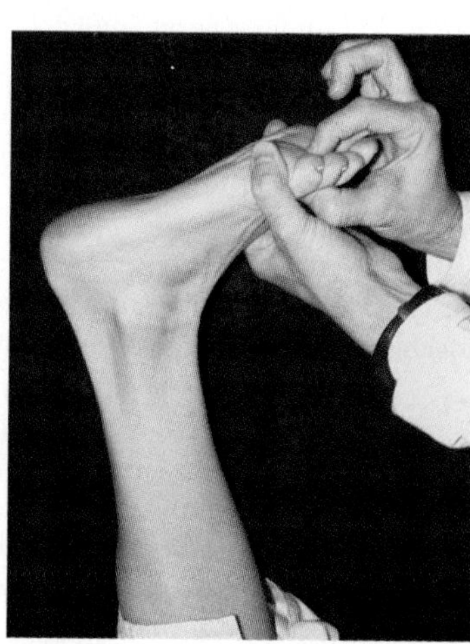

D

FIG 2 • **A.** Standing palpation of the web space. **B.** Metatarsophalangeal joint plantarflexion stress test. **C.** Mulder test: The examiner places the thumb on the dorsal surface and the index finger on the plantar surface in the affected web space and applies gentle pressure. **D.** With the opposite hand the examiner applies a gentle squeeze to the forefoot in a mediolateral direction. A clicking sensation that reproduces the patient's pain will often be appreciated.

- Those presenting after 12 months probably represent patients with a true bulb neuroma at the cut end of the common digital nerve. It probably requires at least this length of time for a neuroma to grow big enough to cause symptoms.
- Formation of a recurrent neuroma after primary surgery is usually due to inadequate resection.
- Plantar-directed nerve branches may tether the common digital nerve to the plantar skin and not allow for retraction of the nerve after it is cut. These nerve branches may occur up to 4 cm proximal to the transverse metatarsal ligament.

NATURAL HISTORY

- Interdigital neuromas occur more commonly in females.
- The primary symptom of an interdigital neuroma is pain, most often described as burning, aching, or cramping.
- The pain often radiates to the toes or proximally along the plantar aspect of the foot.
- Relief usually occurs with removing narrow toe-box shoes.
- Walking barefoot on soft surfaces often produces no symptoms.

PATIENT HISTORY AND PHYSICAL FINDINGS

- In patients with an interdigital neuroma, the most common complaint is plantar pain, which is often increased by walking.
- Pain is often relieved by resting and removing shoes.
- Often there are no symptoms with barefoot walking on a soft surface.
- About half of patients describe pain radiating to the toes.
- The duration of pain varies from a few weeks to many years.
- Plantar tenderness in the web space is the most common physical examination finding.
- The examiner should inspect for deviation or subluxation of the toes or fullness of the web space. This is best done with the patient standing (**FIG 2A**).
- Palpating the web space proximal to the metatarsal heads and proceeding distally will usually reproduce the patient's symptoms.
- It is often difficult to differentiate adjacent metatarsophalangeal (MTP) joint synovitis from a neuroma.
  - Plantarflexion of the corresponding MTP joint may help with the diagnosis (**FIG 2B**). This maneuver often causes little increased pain in those with an interdigital neuroma but is quite painful in those with MTP joint synovitis.
  - Difficulty in making a diagnosis may arise when primary synovitis causes secondary neuritic symptoms.
- The Mulder test is also useful.
  - Pain may be present on the asymptomatic contralateral side but is usually not as painful and the "click" not as striking.
  - This test is best performed with the patient lying prone and the knee flexed 90 degrees. The examiner places the thumb on the dorsal surface and the index finger on the plantar surface in the affected web space and applies gentle pressure (**FIG 2C**). With the opposite hand the examiner applies a gentle squeeze to the forefoot in a mediolateral direction (**FIG 2D**). A clicking sensation that reproduces the patient's pain will often be appreciated.

IMAGING AND OTHER DIAGNOSTIC STUDIES

- The diagnosis of an interdigital neuroma is most often made solely on the basis of the history and physical examination.

- Standing AP, lateral, and oblique radiographs are necessary to exclude osseous pathology and to assess the MTP joint.
- The use of nerve conduction testing has not been shown to be beneficial, as findings often are abnormal in patients without symptoms of an interdigital neuroma.
- Studies differ as to the benefit of ultrasonography or MRI. If necessary, ultrasonography appears to be more useful than MRI in cases with a questionable diagnosis.
- A diagnostic injection may be helpful, although other pathology in the area may improve with this local anesthetic.
  - 2 cc of lidocaine is placed in the symptomatic web space through a dorsal approach.
  - The needle must be plantar to the transverse metatarsal ligament.

DIFFERENTIAL DIAGNOSIS

- Adjacent web space neuroma
- MTP joint synovitis
- Freiberg osteochondrosis
- Stress fracture of the metatarsal neck
- Tarsal tunnel syndrome
- Peripheral neuropathy
- Lumbar radiculopathy
- Unrelated soft tissue tumor (eg, ganglion, synovial cyst, lipoma)

NONOPERATIVE MANAGEMENT

- Although reported results of conservative treatment vary, it is still worthwhile to try, as 30% to 40% of patients may avoid surgery.
- The patient should be fitted with a wide, soft, laced shoe with a low heel.
- A soft metatarsal support should be added just proximal to the metatarsal heads (**FIG 3A**).
- An injection of steroids with anesthetic may be both diagnostic and therapeutic. For there to be diagnostic value, however, the anesthetic must be directed to the common digital nerve in the affected web space and not into the MTP joint. A combination of 40 mg Depo-Medrol and 1 cc 0.25% Marcaine is used for the injection (**FIG 3B**). Thirty percent of patients may have relief for 2 years or longer. Steroids should be used with caution as fat pad atrophy, skin discoloration, or MTP joint capsule laxity may result and create a new problem for the patient.

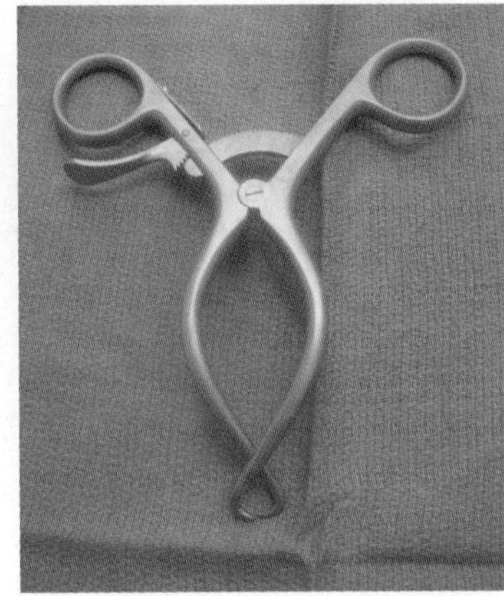

FIG 4 • A neuroma retractor may help with exposure during surgery.

SURGICAL MANAGEMENT

- The indication for surgery is failure of conservative treatment in a patient who is healthy enough to undergo forefoot surgery and who has appropriate vascular status.

Preoperative Planning

- A forefoot or ankle block may be used. Twenty to 30 cc of a 50% mixture of a short- and long-acting anesthetic (eg, lidocaine and Marcaine) without epinephrine is recommended.
- An examination under anesthesia allows for better appreciation of an interspace mass and often will produce a more striking Mulder click.
- Instruments needed include a Weitlaner or neuroma retractor (**FIG 4**), small tenotomy scissors, a Senn retractor, and a Freer elevator.
- An ankle tourniquet is used with cast padding and an Esmarch bandage.
- If a plantar approach is being used (recurrent neuroma), the surgeon should palpate and outline with a sterile marker the metatarsal heads corresponding to the web space being explored.

Positioning

- The patient is placed supine with a 3-inch bump under the distal leg just proximal to the heel. The heel should be floating just off the bed.

A

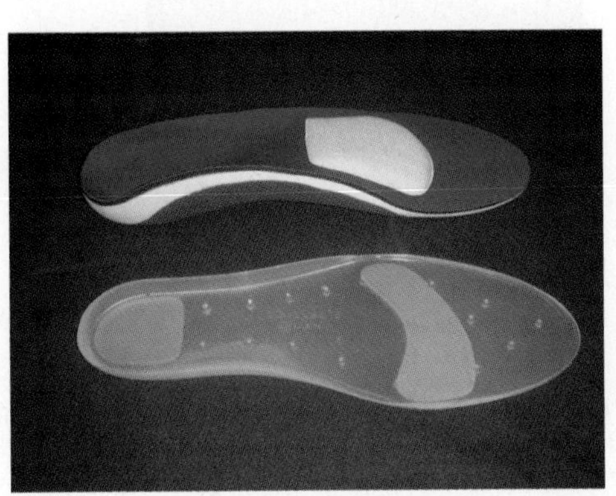

B

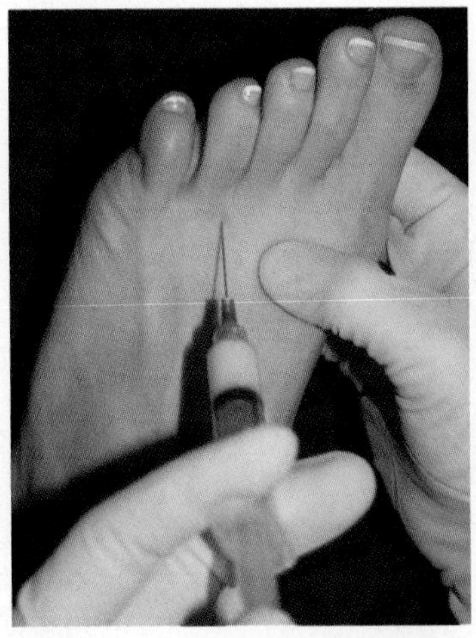

FIG 3 • **A.** Soft inserts and metatarsal support should be the first line of treatment. **B.** Steroid injection may improve symptoms and help with diagnosis.

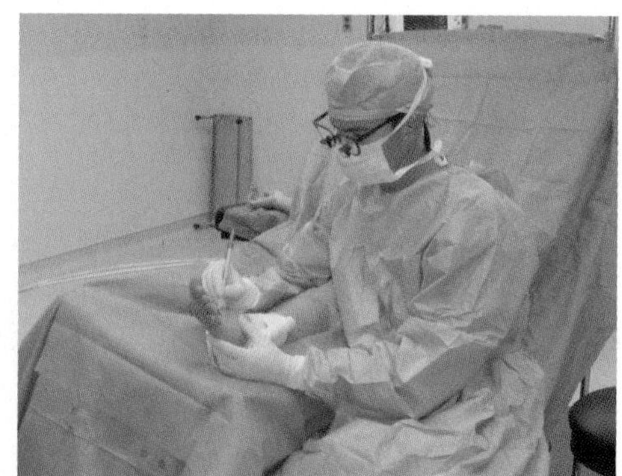

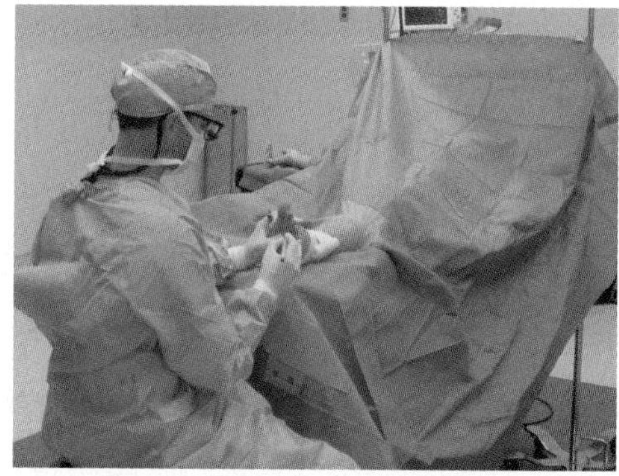

FIG 5 • **A.** Surgeon position for primary neuroma excision. Magnifying loupes are beneficial. **B.** Surgeon position for revision neuroma excision.

- For a primary interdigital neuroma the surgeon should sit proximal to the foot with the assistant positioned at the end of the table to assist with retraction (**FIG 5A**).
- A plantar approach is used for recurrent neuromas. The surgeon sits at the end of the table facing the plantar aspect of the foot (**FIG 5B**).

Approach

Primary Interdigital Neuroma

- A dorsal approach is used for primary neuromas.
- A dorsal incision is made 3 cm proximal to the web, extending distally to the edge of the web space (**FIG 6**).
- The incision is slightly oblique and medial to the extensor tendons. It is important not to follow the tendons themselves, as they will take a more lateral direction.
- The dissection is deepened and the dorsal sensory nerves are retracted to the side of least resistance.
- The lumbrical tendon is lateral to the dissection.
- The surgeon should proximally identify the dorsal interosseous fascia and muscle belly and follow it distally to the bursa overlying the transverse metatarsal ligament.
- The surgeon should place a Weitlaner or neuroma retractor between the metatarsals and spread them apart.
- The bursa is opened to identify the transverse metatarsal ligament.
- Web space fat is retracted using a Senn retractor and the distal aspect of the intermetatarsal ligament is identified.
- A Freer elevator is placed beneath the transverse metatarsal ligament from distal to proximal, protecting the underlying structures.
- The transverse metatarsal ligament is incised with a no. 15 blade knife, staying on top of the Freer elevator.
- The lumbrical tendon is in the lateral aspect of the dissection just plantar to the intermetatarsal ligament.
- The neurovascular bundle is identified medial and plantar to the lumbrical.

Recurrent Neuroma

Plantar Longitudinal Incision

- A longitudinal plantar incision is made 4 cm proximal to the web, extending distally to within 1 cm of the web space.
- The incision is made between the metatarsal heads (which have been identified and marked before making an incision) and proceeds just distal to this area (**FIG 7**).
- A small Weitlaner retractor is placed to retract the fat overlying the plantar aponeurosis.
- Using a no. 15 blade knife, the aponeurosis is incised in line with the skin incision.

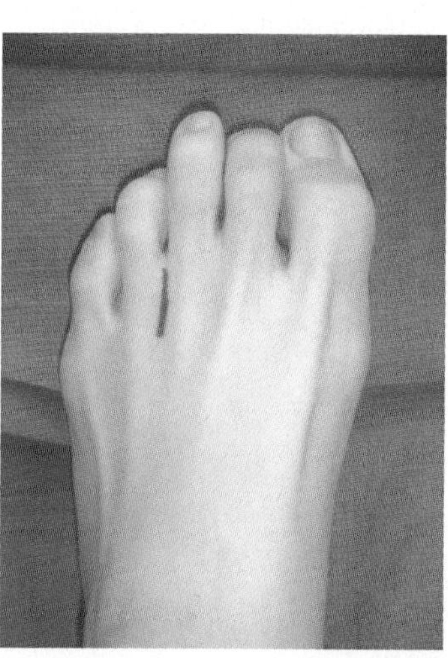

FIG 6 • For a primary interdigital neuroma, a 3-cm incision is made in the affected web space just medial to the extensor tendons.

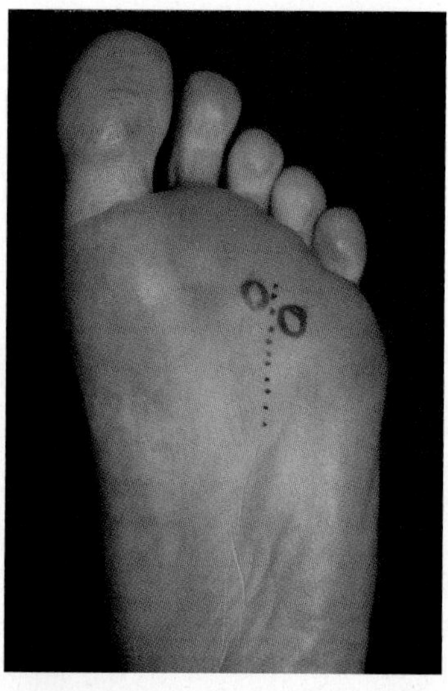

FIG 7 • For recurrent interdigital neuromas, a 4-cm longitudinal plantar incision is made proximal to the web extending distally to within 1 cm of the web space.

- A tenotomy scissors is used to bluntly spread until the common digital nerve is identified proximally.
- The surgeon dissects distally to identify the stump neuroma.

PLANTAR TRANSVERSE INCISION

- A 3- to 4-cm transverse plantar incision is made over the affected interspace just proximal to the weight-bearing pad and parallel to the natural crease (**FIG 8**).
- The metatarsal heads are continually palpated to provide a reference point to the appropriate interspace to be explored.
- The dissection is carefully deepened with scissors to expose the septa of the plantar fascia.
- The interval between the longitudinal limbs of the plantar fascia septa is opened with scissors.
- The bands of the plantar fascia are retracted medially and laterally with a Senn retractor and the interspace is carefully explored with blunt dissection to identify the common digital nerve and vessel.
- The nerve (neuroma) will lie superficial (plantar) to the flexor digitorum brevis muscle or tendon and immediately deep (dorsal) to the plantar fascia.
- The surgeon dissects distally to identify the stump neuroma.
- The neuroma is identified and dissected proximally 1 to 2 cm.

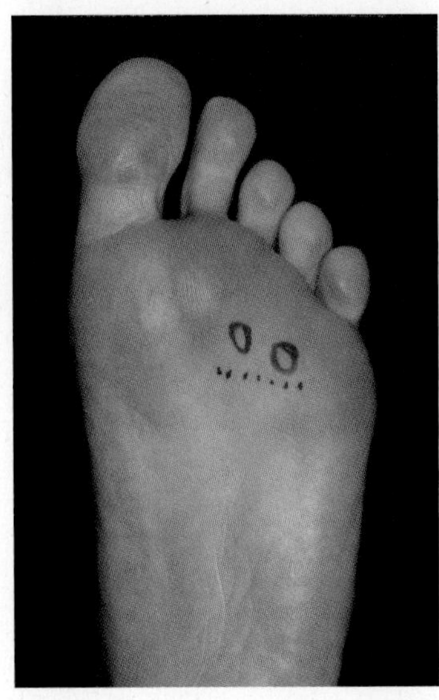

FIG 8 • Alternatively, one may use a 3- to 4-cm transverse plantar incision. The incision is placed over the affected interspace just proximal to the weight-bearing pad and parallel to the natural crease.

PRIMARY INTERDIGITAL NEUROMA EXCISION (DORSAL)

- Once the approach has been completed the nerve should be identified in the wound. It is usually easier to identify the nerve proximally and dissect distally (**TECH FIG 1A**).
- Manually palpate in the wound to be sure the transverse metatarsal ligament has been completely transected, as this is essential to a successful outcome.
- Despite the size of the nerve or the obvious presence of a neuroma, the nerve should be resected as planned.
- Structures that may be mistaken for the nerve include the lumbrical tendon, which passes to the medial portion of the adjacent proximal phalanx (extensor expansion) and therefore is lateral to the nerve. The common digital artery usually crosses proximal medial to distal lateral lying dorsally over the nerve. The artery often emerges from under the metatarsal neck and if identified needs to be dissected away from the nerve and preserved.
- Using gentle traction (**TECH FIG 1B**), transect the nerve about 4 cm proximal to the transverse metatarsal ligament.
- The transverse head of the adductor hallucis may need to be retracted dorsally to identify the plantar-directed

TECHNIQUES

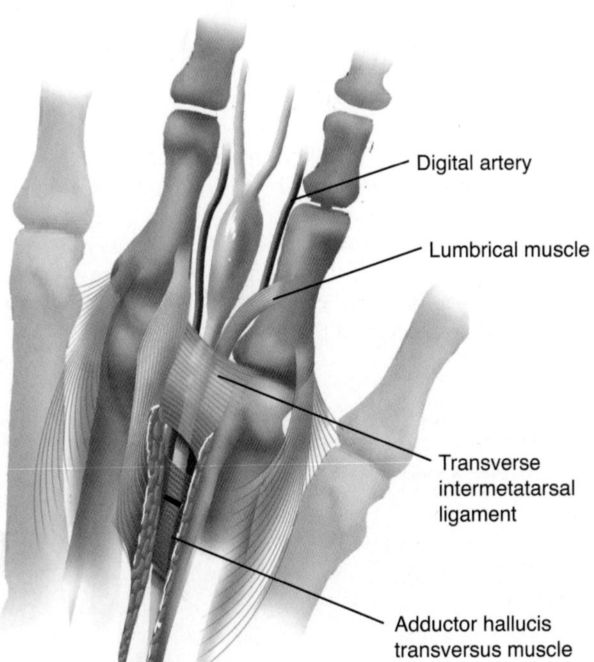

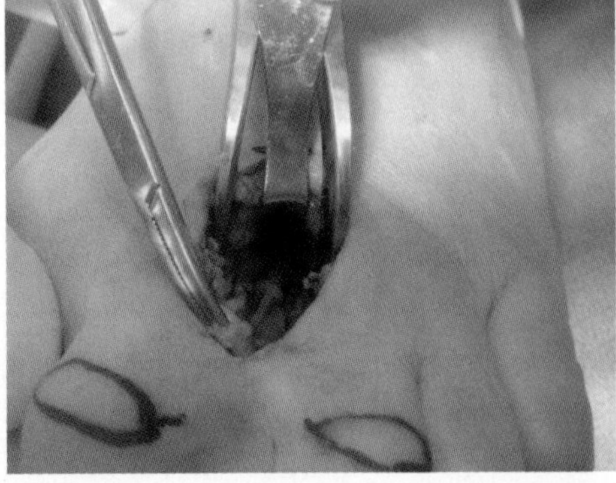

TECH FIG 1 • **A.** The transverse metatarsal ligament must be divided. **B.** The neuroma is visualized and the common digital nerve transected 4 cm proximal to the transverse metatarsal ligament and allowed to retract proximal to the weight-bearing pad of the forefoot. *(continued)*

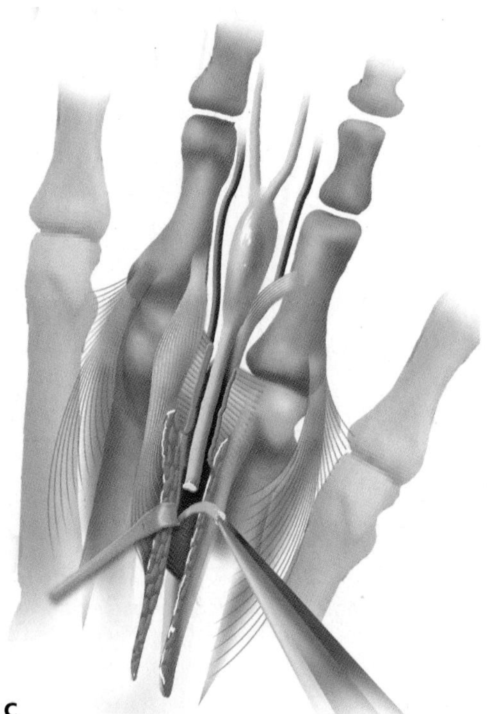

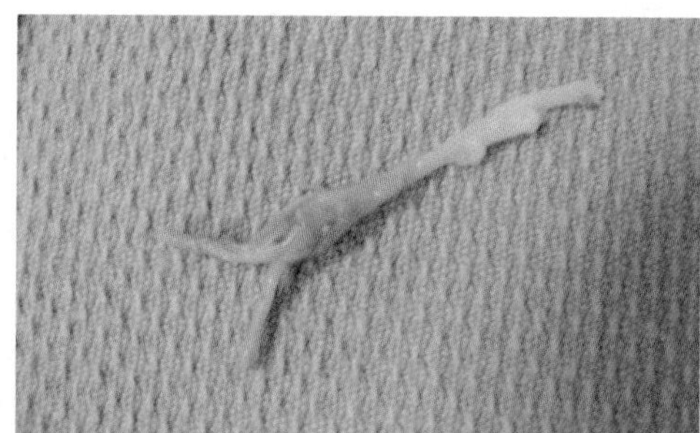

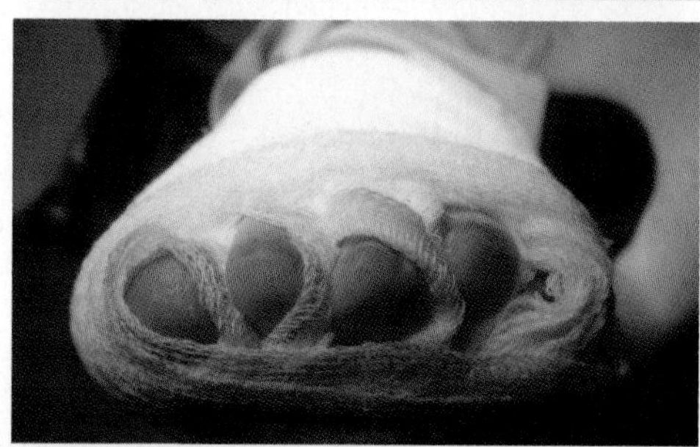

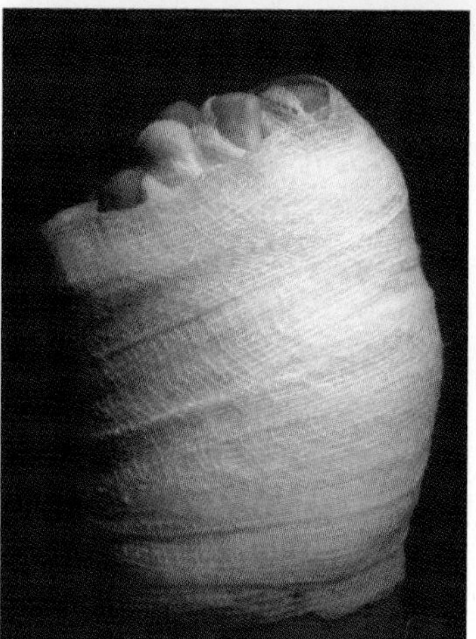

TECH FIG 1 • *(continued)* **C.** After transection of the intermetatarsal ligament, the nerve is transected proximally (the transverse head of the adductor hallucis muscle often must be retracted) and dissected distally past the bifurcation. **D.** The specimen is sent for pathologic examination. **E,F.** For a primary neuroma excision, a mildly compressive dressing is placed and the patient is allowed to bear weight as tolerated in a postoperative shoe.

branches of the common digital nerve. Divide these branches to allow the proximal aspect of the nerve to retract at least 1 to 2 cm proximal to the weight-bearing pad of the forefoot (TECH FIG 1C).

- Use a hemostat to place the remaining nerve stump well proximal and dorsal into the interosseous muscles.
- Circumferentially dissect the nerve distally to the bifurcation of the proper digital branches.
- Divide the proper digital nerve just distal to the bifurcation.
- Send the specimen (TECH FIG 1D) for pathologic examination.
- With the Weitlaner or neuroma retractor still in place, release the ankle tourniquet. Use cautery to obtain hemostasis.
- Irrigate the wound with sterile saline.
- Close the wound with 4-0 nylon suture in a running locking fashion.
- If subcutaneous suture is desired, use a 3-0 Monocryl, taking care not to include the dorsal sensory nerves.
- Place a mildly compressive dressing over a Xeroform gauze covering the wound (TECH FIG 1E,F).

REVISION INTERDIGITAL NEUROMA EXCISION (PLANTAR LONGITUDINAL INCISION)

- Once the approach has been completed, the neuroma is identified just deep to the distal extensions of the plantar fascia that fan out to attach to the plantar aspects of the MTP joints and just superficial (plantar) to the flexor digitorum brevis.
- The intermetatarsal ligament is often scarred in but does not need to be transected as it is distal and dorsal to the neuroma.
- Place gentle traction on the common digital nerve (TECH FIG 2A). Identify and excise the neuroma (TECH FIG 2B).

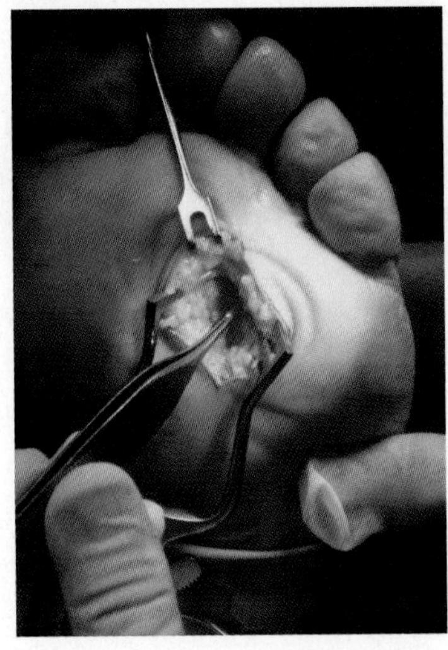

A

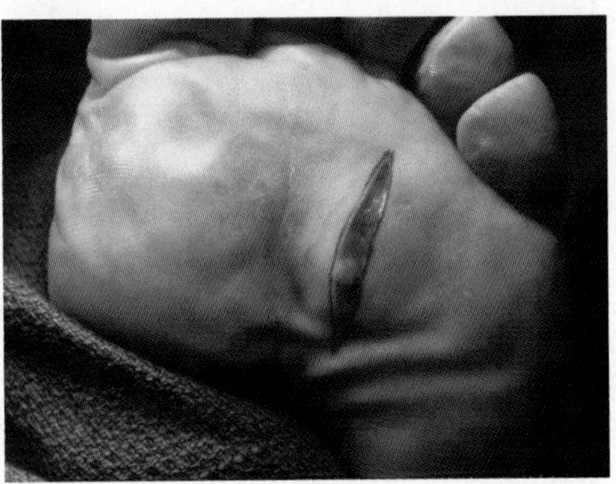

B

TECH FIG 2 • **A.** The plantar longitudinal incision is shown with gentle traction placed on the common digital nerve. **B.** Excision of the recurrent neuroma through a plantar longitudinal incision.

- Allow the common digital nerve to retract proximally as far as possible.
- Release the ankle tourniquet and obtain hemostasis.
- Irrigate the wound with sterile saline.
- Close the wound with interrupted 3-0 nylon suture in a vertical mattress fashion.
- Place a mildly compressive dressing over a Xeroform gauze on the wound.
- Place the patient in a short-leg posterior splint.

REVISION INTERDIGITAL NEUROMA EXCISION (PLANTAR TRANSVERSE INCISION)

- Once the plantar transverse approach is made, the technique is exactly the same as described above for the plantar longitudinal incision.

PEARLS AND PITFALLS

Always perform a thorough history and physical examination. This is the primary basis of diagnosis and treatment.	■ Perform standing, sitting, and prone examination of the foot and ankle.
Attempt conservative treatment before surgery.	
Discuss with the patient possible complications of surgery, especially incomplete relief and recurrence.	
Transect the common digital nerve at least 3 to 4 cm proximal to the transverse metatarsal ligament (Tech Fig 1C).	■ Grasp the nerve and with gentle traction pull it distally. Transect and allow the nerve to retract.
Release the tourniquet and obtain hemostasis before closure.	■ Hematoma formation increases the risk of slow wound healing and infection.

POSTOPERATIVE CARE

- For 24 hours the operative extremity is maximally elevated and the patient ambulates only for bathroom privileges.
- For a primary excision (dorsal approach), the patient is then allowed to ambulate with weight bearing as tolerated in a hard-soled postoperative shoe for 4 weeks.
- For a revision excision (plantar approach), the patient is kept non–weight-bearing on crutches for 2 weeks and then transitioned into a stiff-soled postoperative shoe for another 2 weeks with weight bearing as tolerated.
- Sutures are removed at 2 weeks and Steri-Strips are placed on the wound.
- At 4 weeks after surgery the patient is allowed into a wide toe-box, soft-vamp comfortable shoe and progressed as tolerated.

OUTCOMES

- Surgical excision of a primary neuroma has a reported success rate of 51% to 90%, although results tend to diminish with time. A recent study by Womack et al[22] suggests long-term pain relief is not as significant as once thought.

- These results seem to be similar for both second and third web space neuroma excisions.
- After re-exploration for a recurrent neuroma, less-than-complete satisfaction can be expected in 20% to 40% of individuals.

COMPLICATIONS

- Recurrence of symptoms: This may be due to incorrect diagnosis, incomplete resection, or true recurrence.
  - Recurrence of symptoms due to incorrect diagnosis and incomplete resection usually occurs within the first 12 months.
  - Recurrence after 1 year is more likely related to the formation of a stump neuroma.
- Significant wound complications are rare, but slow wound healing and superficial cellulitis are more common.
- Incisional tenderness after a plantar approach is less common than one may suppose but may occur if placed under a weight-bearing portion of the forefoot.

REFERENCES

1. Alexander IJ, Johnson KA, Parr JW. Morton's neuroma: a review of recent concepts. Orthopedics 1987;10:103.
2. Amis JA, Siverhus SW, Liwnicz BH. An anatomic basis for recurrence after Morton's neuroma excision. Foot Ankle 1992;13:153.
3. Beskin JL, Baxter DE. Recurrent pain following interdigital neurectomy—a plantar approach. Foot Ankle 1988;9:34.
4. Bradley N, Miller WA, Evans JP. Plantar neuroma: analysis of results following surgical excision in 145 patients. South Med J 1976;69:853.
5. Coughlin MJ, Pinsonneault T. Operative treatment of interdigital neuroma: a long-term follow-up study. J Bone Joint Surg Am 2001; 83A:1321.
6. Durlacher L. A Treatise on Corns, Bunions and Diseases of the Nails, and the General Management of the Feet. London: Simpkin, Marshall, 1845.
7. Graham CE, Johnson KA, Ilstrup DM. The intermetatarsal nerve: a microscopic evaluation. Foot Ankle 1981;2:150.
8. Guiloff RJ, Scadding JW, Klenerman L. Morton's metatarsalgia: clinical, electrophysiological, and histological observations. J Bone Joint Surg Br 1984;66B:586.
9. Johnson JE, Johnson KA, Unni KK. Persistent pain after excision of an interdigital neuroma. J Bone Joint Surg Am 1988;70A:651.
10. Kay D, Bennett GL. Morton's neuroma. Foot Ankle Clin 2003;8:49.
11. Lassmann G. Morton's toe: clinical, light and electron microscopic investigations in 133 cases. Clin Orthop Relat Res 1979; 142:73.
12. Levitsky KA, Alman BA, Jevsevar DS, et al. Digital nerves of the foot: anatomic variations and implications regarding the pathogenesis of interdigital neuroma. Foot Ankle 1993;4:208.
13. Mann RA. Interdigital neuroma. In Evarts MC, ed: Surgery of the Musculoskeletal System. New York: Churchill Livingstone, 1983.
14. Mann RA, Reynolds JC. Interdigital neuroma: a critical analysis. Foot Ankle 1983;3:238.
15. McElvenny RT. The etiology and surgical treatment of intractable pain about the fourth metatarsophalangeal joint (Morton's toe). J Bone Joint Surg 1943;25:675.
16. Morton TG. A peculiar and painful affection of the fourth metatarsophalangeal articulation. Am J Med Sci 1876;71:37.
17. Nissen KI. Plantar digital neuritis (Morton's metatarsalgia). J Bone Joint Surg Br 1948;30B:84.
18. Richardson EG, Brotzman SB, Graves SC. The plantar incision for procedures involving the forefoot: an evaluation of one hundred and fifty incisions in one hundred and fifteen patients. J Bone Joint Surg Am 1993;75A:726–731.
19. Sharp RJ, Wade CM, Hennessy MS, et al. The role of MRI and ultrasound imaging in Morton's neuroma and the effect of size of lesion on symptoms. J Bone Joint Surg Br 2003;85B:999.
20. Stamatis ED, Karabalis C. Interdigital neuromas: current state of the art—surgical. Foot Ankle Clin 2004;9:287.
21. Stamatis ED, Myerson MS. Treatment of recurrence of symptoms after excision of an interdigital neuroma: a retrospective review. J Bone Joint Surg Br 2004;86B:48.
22. Womack JW, Richardson DR, Murphy GA, et al. Long-term evaluation of interdigital neuroma treated by surgical excision. Foot Ankle 2008;29(6):574.

Chapter 38

Uniportal Endoscopic Decompression of the Interdigital Nerve for Morton's Neuroma

Steven L. Shapiro

DEFINITION

- Morton's neuroma is a nerve entrapment syndrome in which the intermetatarsal nerve in the second or third web space becomes compressed by the intermetatarsal ligament, enlarges, and undergoes perineural fibrosis.[2–4]

ANATOMY

- The most important soft tissue structure is the transverse intermetatarsal ligament (TIML), which is a continuation of the plantar plates. This structure becomes taut during the late midstance and push-off phases of gait.
- The TIML should be well visualized. It measures 10 to 15 mm long and 2 to 3 mm thick.[1]
- The lumbrical tendon is located on the plantar lateral aspect of the TIML. It is the most likely structure to be severed during endoscopic decompression of the intermetatarsal nerve, but with proper identification it can be spared. In my experience, inadvertent severing of the lumbrical tendon, however, has not resulted in any adverse sequelae.
- The plantar interossei muscles are superior to the TIML in the second, third, and fourth intermetatarsal spaces.
- The intermetatarsal nerve is plantar to the TIML and should not be visualized during endoscopic division of the TIML; the nerve, however, may be seen by rotating the cannula 180 degrees, to the 6 o'clock position. With the cannula in the proper position the nerve is protected.

PATHOGENESIS

- The clinical symptoms of this condition were first described by Durlacher in 1845 and later by Morton in 1876. It is Morton's name that has remained linked to this condition.
- The most recent literature attributes Morton's neuroma to nerve entrapment; this has been confirmed by electron microscopy.
- Perineural fibrosis has been identified at the level of nerve compression.

NATURAL HISTORY

- The symptoms of Morton's neuroma are dull, aching pain in the ball of the foot, often radiating into the second, third, or fourth toes.
  - This may be associated with tingling, burning, or numbness.
  - It may occur gradually over several months or progress more acutely.
- Overuse activities and compression by narrow-toed shoes and high heels have been implicated.
- 75% of patients are female.
- The average age of onset is 54.[5]
- Occasionally trauma can result in formation of an interdigital neuroma.
- Pain is sometimes relieved by removing the shoe.

PHYSICAL FINDINGS

- Classic findings include localized tenderness in the second or third web space. Subtle swelling may be present in the affected web spaces. The two adjacent toes may be slightly separated.
- Mulder's click (a palpable snap) may be elicited in the affected web space.
- The metatarsal compression test may be positive.
  - This is performed by grasping and squeezing the patient's forefoot. This maneuver is positive if it reproduces the patient's symptoms.

IMAGING AND DIAGNOSTIC STUDIES

- Plain films should routinely be performed to rule out other pathologies.
- If the diagnosis or correct web space is in doubt, sonographic imaging can be performed with a high degree of accuracy in experienced hands.
- MRI is not operator-dependent but yields a large percentage of false-negative and false-positive findings and is also much more costly than sonography.
- On ultrasound, a neuroma appears as a hypoechoic oval mass in the interspace at the level of the metatarsal heads. The size of the neuroma can be measured.[5]

DIFFERENTIAL DIAGNOSIS

- Metatarsal stress fracture
- Freiberg disease (avascular necrosis of the metatarsal head)
- Synovitis
- Intermetatarsal bursitis
- Metatarsophalangeal synovitis
- Peripheral neuropathy
- Lumbar radiculopathy
- Tarsal tunnel syndrome
- Vascular claudication
- Spinal stenosis

NONSURGICAL MANAGEMENT

- Conservative treatment may include metatarsal pads, orthotics, shoes with a wide toebox, steroid injections, and, more recently, alcohol injections.
- In our experience, conservative treatment has been successful in about 70% of patients.

SURGICAL MANAGEMENT

- Surgery is indicated when conservative treatment has failed to relieve pain after at least 6 months.
- The advantage of dividing the TIML without excising the interdigital neuroma is that there is no loss of sensation or possible formation of a stump neuroma, which may produce symptoms worse than those with which the patient originally presented. Barrett and Pignetti introduced endoscopic

decompression of the intermetatarsal nerve, a procedure that offers several advantages over an open procedure, including a smaller incision, faster postoperative recovery, and a reduced incidence of hematoma and infection.[1]

- Although these authors reported good and excellent results in 88% of patients, the original technique was difficult, with a steep learning curve.
- They have since modified their technique, changing from two portals to a single portal.

Preoperative Planning

- All patients should have plain films preoperatively to rule out other diagnoses, in particular stress fracture or Freiberg infraction.
- In our experience, preoperative ultrasound is valuable in confirming the diagnosis.
- Without ultrasound, simple palpation of the web space is typically accurate in determining which web space is most tender.
- Diagnostic lidocaine injection may also pinpoint the appropriate web space. However, if both the second and third web spaces are symptomatic, the surgeon should consider endoscopy on both spaces.

Positioning

- The patient should be positioned supine on the operating table.
- We use a bump under the ipsilateral buttock and thigh when the leg tends to externally rotate.
- The toes should extend just beyond the end of the table, with the heel firmly resting on the table.
- Anesthesia may be general or regional (popliteal or ankle block).
- Local anesthesia should be avoided, as it may distort the endoscopic anatomy.
- Prophylactic intravenous antibiotics are given when the patient comes to the operating room.
- We routinely use an ankle tourniquet inflated to 250 mm Hg. Equipment required includes the AM Surgical set and a 30-degree 4-mm scope. The AM Surgical system includes an elevator, slotted cannula and obturator, locking device, and disposable knife blade.

TECHNIQUES

SINGLE-PORTAL TECHNIQUE

- Presented here is a technique originally designed by Dr. Ather Mirza for endoscopic carpal tunnel release. I have adapted the instrumentation for uniportal endoscopic decompression of the intermetatarsal nerve (**TECH FIGS 1 AND 2**).[6]
- Make a 1-cm vertical incision in the appropriate web space and spread the subcutaneous tissue gently with blunt Stevens scissors.
- Use the AM Surgical elevator to palpate and separate the TIML from the surrounding soft tissues. Scrape the elevator both dorsal and plantar to the TIML.
- Place the slotted cannula and obturator through the same path, just plantar to and scraping against the TIML. The slot should face dorsally at the 12 o'clock position (**TECH FIG 3**).
- Remove the obturator from the cannula and remove any fat or fluid from the cannula with absorbent cotton-tipped applicators.
- Insert a short 4-mm 30-degree scope into the cannula.
- Visualize the entire TIML by advancing the scope. The ligament is dense and white. The lumbrical tendon can often be seen just lateral to the TIML.
- The intermetatarsal nerve can be visualized by rotating the cannula 180 degrees so that the slot is facing plantar at 6 o'clock. The nerve can often be seen unless obscured

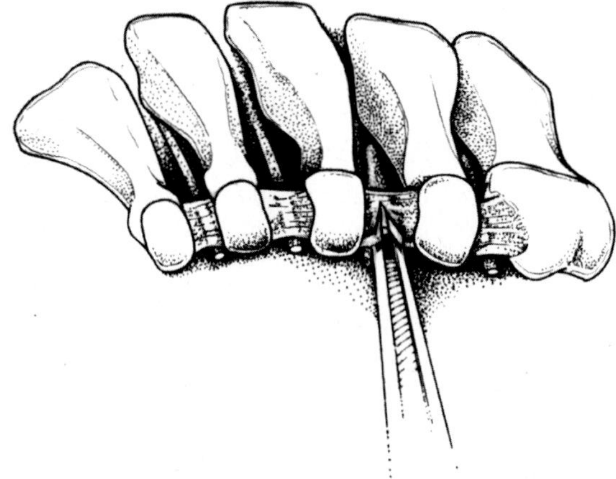

TECH FIG 1 • Surgical technique for uniportal endoscopic decompression of the intermetatarsal nerve. Cannula is in the interspace just plantar to the transverse intermetatarsal ligament and dorsal to the intermetatarsal (interdigital) nerve. The transverse intermetatarsal ligament is being transected from distal to proximal. (Courtesy of AM Surgical.)

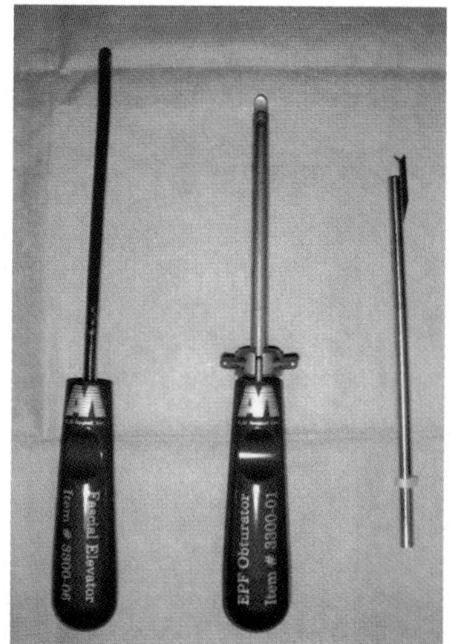

TECH FIG 2 • Instrumentation. From left to right: elevator, cannula and obturator, disposable knife.

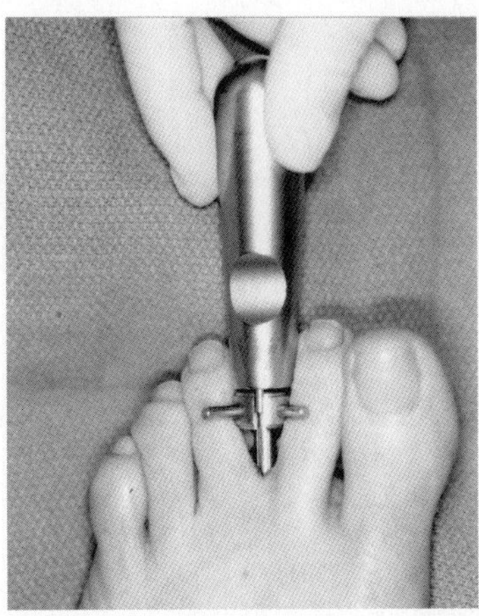

TECH FIG 3 • Intraoperative view of insertion of cannula and obturator into second web space, notch at 12 o'clock, positioned to view the transverse intermetatarsal ligament.

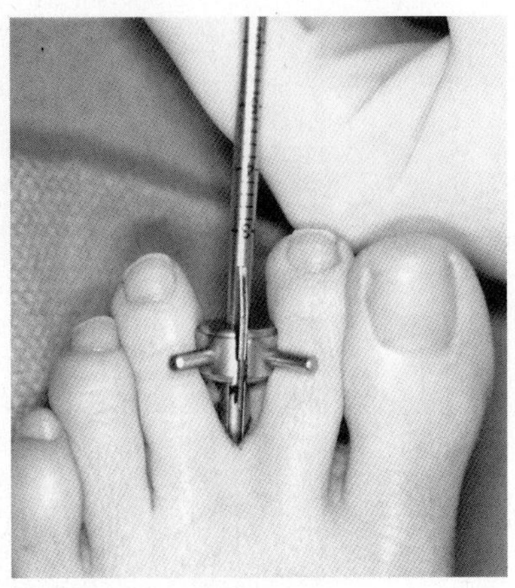

TECH FIG 5 • Intraoperative view of knife mounted to scope in position in cannula ready to enter second web space and transect the transverse intermetatarsal ligament.

by fat. It is often thickened distally, tapers, and becomes normal proximally (TECH FIG 4).

- Return the cannula to the 12 o'clock position and remove the scope from the cannula.
- Slide the disposable endoscopic knife onto the locking device with the lever in the open position.
- Insert the knife and locking device assembly into the scope and advance the knife blade until it nearly touches the lens. The blade should also be parallel to the lens. Push the lever of the locking device forward until finger tight (TECH FIG 5).
- Advance the scope and knife assembly through the cannula. Visualize the knife blade transecting the TIML from distal to proximal (TECH FIG 6). While cutting the TIML, maintain the cannula tight against the ligament. Place more tension on the TIML by placing a finger of the nondominant hand between the adjacent metatarsal necks.
- Withdraw the scope and knife assembly and remove the knife from the scope. Reinsert the scope to confirm complete transection of the TIML. The divided edge of the ligament can be observed to further separate by applying manual digital pressure between the adjacent metatarsal heads.
- Irrigate the wound through the cannula.
- Remove the cannula, insert the elevator into the wound, and palpate the interspace. The taut TIML should no longer be palpable.
- Deflate the tourniquet; irrigate and close the wound with one or two interrupted mattress sutures. Apply a soft compression dressing and postoperative shoe.
- If the surgeon chooses to perform a neurectomy in cases where the nerve is very large and bulbous, the incision can be extended proximally 1 to 2 cm and neurectomy can be performed in routine fashion.

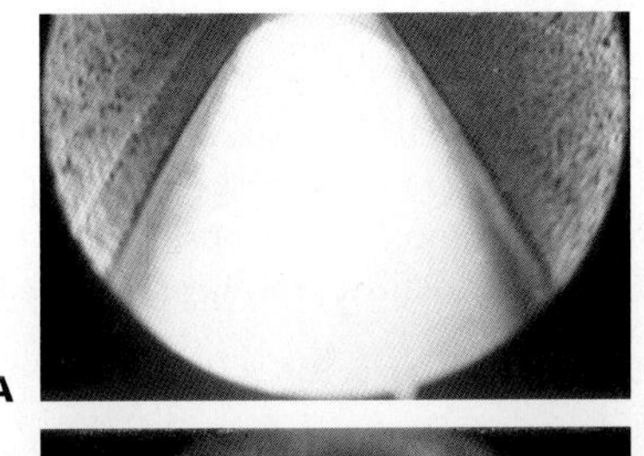

A

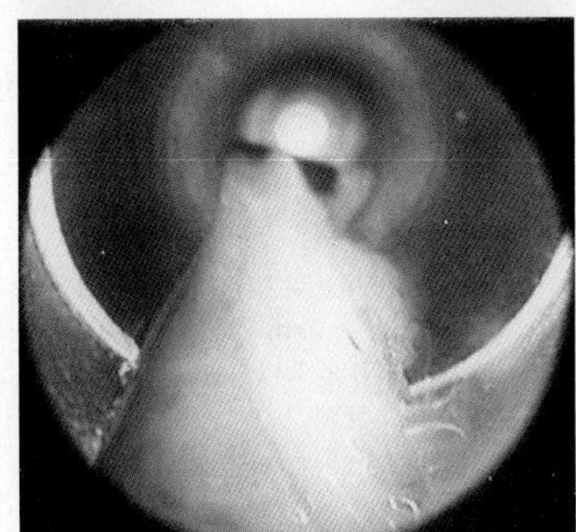

B

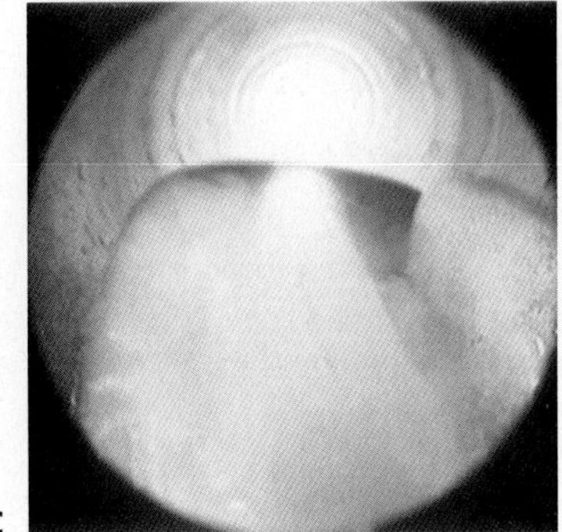

C

TECH FIG 4 • **A.** Endoscopic view of transverse intermetatarsal ligament. **B.** Normal interdigital nerve. **C.** Thickened interdigital nerve (neuroma).

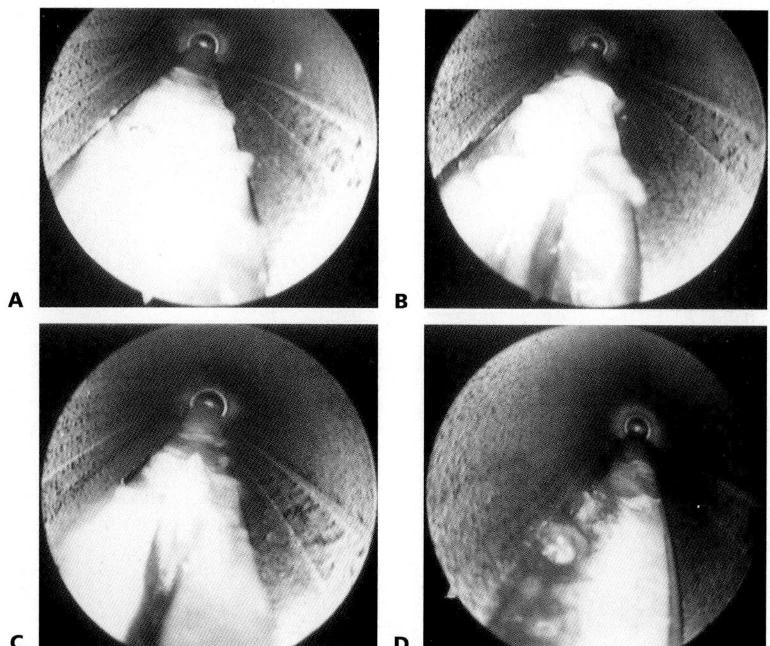

TECH FIG 6 • **A.** Endoscopic view of transverse intermetatarsal ligament. **B, C.** Endoscopic views of knife blade transecting the transverse intermetatarsal ligament. **D.** Endoscopic view after release of transverse intermetatarsal ligament.

PEARLS AND PITFALLS

- The key to the procedure is isolating and separating the TIML from the soft tissues. Developing these tissue planes with the elevator is the critical step; everything else follows.
- Hugging the TIML with the cannula while cutting is very important.
- If unable to visualize the TIML, abort the procedure and perform the procedure open.

POSTOPERATIVE CARE

- Ice and elevation are recommended for the first 48 to 72 hours.
- Weight bearing as tolerated is permitted in a surgical shoe. Crutches or a walker should be provided as needed.
- Sutures are removed in 12 to 14 days. A comfortable shoe or sandal may then be worn.
- Vigorous activities such as running or racquet sports should be avoided for 4 to 6 weeks.
- Patients should be advised that complete resolution of symptoms may take up to 4 months.

OUTCOMES

- Barrett and Pignetti reported 88% good and excellent results in over 40 patients.[1]
- In our first 24 patients, there were 82% good and excellent results at 6 months postoperatively.

COMPLICATIONS

- In the first 50 patients there have been no infections.
- Two wound dehiscences occurred that healed uneventfully.
- The postoperative protocol was then changed from suture removal at 10 to 14 days postoperatively.
- No further dehiscences have occurred.

REFERENCES

1. Barrett SL, Pignetti TT. Endoscopic decompression for routine neuroma: preliminary study with cadaveric specimen: early clinical results. J Foot Ankle Surg 1994;33:503–508.
2. Dellon AL. Treatment of Morton's neuroma as a nerve compression; the role for neurolysis. J Am Podiatr Med Assoc 1992;82:399–402.
3. Gauthier GT. Morton's disease: a nerve entrapment syndrome: a new surgical technique. Clin Orthop Relat Res 1979;142:90–92.
4. Graham CE, Graham DM. Morton's neuroma: a microscopic evaluation. Foot Ankle 1984;5:150–153.
5. Shapiro PS, Shapiro SL. Sonographic evaluation of interdigital neuroma. Foot Ankle 1995;16:604–606.
6. Shapiro SL. Endoscopic decompression of the intermetatarsal nerve for Morton's neuroma. Foot Ankle Clin North Am 2004;9:297–304.

Chapter 39 Plantarflexion Opening Wedge Medial Cuneiform Osteotomy

Jeffrey E. Johnson

DEFINITION

- Forefoot varus is a component of the multiplanar pes planovalgus deformity that occurs as a result of posterior tibial tendon insufficiency.
- In addition to being a component of adult acquired flatfoot deformity, forefoot varus is also present in some cases of congenital pes planus and posttraumatic deformities of the first tarsometatarsal joint.
- In 1936, F. J. Cotton described an adjunctive procedure for the operative treatment of flatfoot deformity using an opening wedge plantarflexion medial cuneiform osteotomy to restore what he termed the "triangle of support" of the static foot.[3]

ANATOMY

- Forefoot varus deformity may occur through a dorsiflexion angulation or rotation at the talonavicular, naviculocuneiform, or tarsometatarsal joints.
- These joints are supported by the spring ligament and the plantar intertarsal ligaments, including the long plantar ligament.
- In addition, the naviculocuneiform and tarsometatarsal joints are supported by their relatively constrained joint architecture, which in the normal state allows only a few degrees of motion in the sagittal plane.
- Medial displacement calcaneal osteotomy, lateral column lengthening, and subtalar fusion all provide correction of heel valgus; lateral column lengthening will correct forefoot abduction, but none of these procedures adequately addresses the fixed forefoot varus component of the pes planovalgus deformity.

PATHOGENESIS

- The pathogenesis of forefoot varus in association with an adult acquired flatfoot deformity secondary to posterior tibial tendon insufficiency is not well understood.
- Forefoot varus is presumed to develop when the posterior tibialis tendon can no longer provide dynamic support to the medial column of the midfoot. In the absence of the posterior tibialis tendon acting as a dynamic stabilizer, the static ligamentous stabilizers (spring ligament complex and the plantar supporting intertarsal ligaments) stretch out due to the repetitive dorsally directed weight-bearing forces on the medial column of the foot.
- Several patterns of medial column "sag" have been described, although the understanding of why some patients have dorsal instability at the first tarsometatarsal joint, the naviculocuneiform joint, or the talonavicular joint is not well understood. The differences in the magnitude and location of the dorsal "sag" may be related to bony anatomy, generalized ligamentous laxity, the presence or absence of gastroc–soleus contracture, and the existence of an underlying congenital pes planovalgus deformity.

NATURAL HISTORY

- The natural history of forefoot varus associated with an acquired adult flatfoot deformity has not been studied. It is presumed that the severity of the forefoot varus deformity progresses as the underlying pes planovalgus deformity progresses. Longstanding instability and subluxation at the first tarsometatarsal joint or naviculocuneiform joint may result in localized osteoarthritis of these joints.
- Some acquired adult flatfeet develop a fixed forefoot varus without osteoarthritis when the deformity has been longstanding and capsular stiffness holds the joint in the deformed position.

PATIENT HISTORY AND PHYSICAL FINDINGS

- Forefoot varus is one of the components of a pes planovalgus deformity that is determined primarily by radiographic and physical examination findings.
- In the patient history, there may be complaints of localized pain to the dorsal medial column of the midfoot, either the tarsometarsal joint or the naviculocuneiform joint.
- Patients may complain of pressure-related discomfort beneath the base of the first metatarsal or cuneiform due to excessive weight bearing at the apex of the plantar medial column sag.
- The presence and the magnitude of forefoot varus are determined on physical examination by placing the hindfoot into the "subtalar neutral" position with the patient seated (**FIG 1**). With the hindfoot held in neutral, with the talonavicular joint congruent, a dorsally directed force is applied to the fourth and fifth metatarsal heads until the ankle is dorsiflexed to the neutral position. If the first metatarsal head rests above the transverse plane of the fifth metatarsal, then forefoot varus is present. Forefoot varus is quantified clinically by the degree to which the first metatarsal rests above the transverse plane of the forefoot as a mild, moderate, or severe deformity.
- The deformity is also qualified by whether the forefoot varus deformity is passively correctable by manual pressure to bring the first ray back down to the level of the other metatarsals or whether it is fixed in this position.

IMAGING AND OTHER DIAGNOSTIC STUDIES

- Standing, AP, and lateral radiographs with a medial oblique view of the involved foot will determine the presence of subluxation or osteoarthritis at the first tarsometatarsal or naviculocuneiform joint.
- The lateral standing radiograph will quantify the amount of dorsiflexion based on the measurement of the lateral talo–first metatarsal angle.

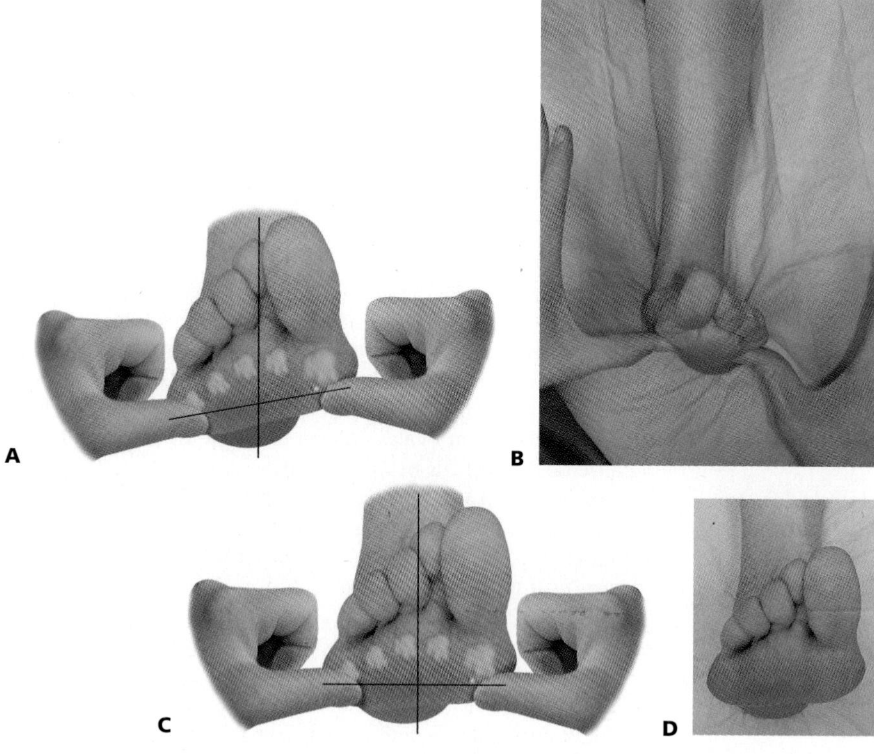

FIG 1 • Placing the hindfoot into the "subtalar neutral" position allows the examiner to determine the presence and the magnitude of a forefoot varus deformity that may accompany pes planovalgus. **A,B.** The forefoot is in varus alignment relative to the neutral heel as evidenced by the examiner visualizing and palpating the first metatarsal head dorsally translated relative to the fifth metatarsal head. **C,D.** The forefoot and hindfoot alignment are both in neutral with the first and fifth metatarsal heads in the same plane. This is the position desired after the appropriate-sized bone wedge has been placed into the first cuneiform osteotomy.

- The apex of the deformity may be at the talonavicular joint, the naviculocuneiform joint, or the first tarsometatarsal joint.
- In the case of an acquired flatfoot deformity superimposed on a congenital pes planovalgus deformity, comparison measurements of the opposite-foot standing radiograph may help determine what amount of deformity is a result of posterior tibial tendon insufficiency.
- A weight-bearing AP radiograph of the involved ankle will determine the presence of a valgus tilt of the talus within the ankle joint mortise secondary to deltoid insufficiency.
- Additional procedures to address medial ankle instability due to deltoid ligament insufficiency may be needed to fully correct the valgus hindfoot deformity.

DIFFERENTIAL DIAGNOSIS

- Forefoot varus secondary to instability or osteoarthritis at the first tarsometatarsal joint
- Global forefoot varus associated with supination of the first, second, and third metatarsals

NONOPERATIVE MANAGEMENT

- If the deformity is passively correctable, a custom-molded total contact foot orthosis is fabricated with posting under the medial aspect of the hindfoot and midfoot to correct heel valgus and additional posting placed under the lateral aspect of the forefoot to promote plantarflexion of the first ray with weight bearing.
- If the forefoot varus is fixed, an accommodative total contact foot orthosis would be fabricated with medial posting under the entire hindfoot and midfoot, or a medial wedge could be added to the sole of the shoe.
- If pain symptoms are not controlled with foot orthoses alone, a custom-made leather and polypropylene molded gauntlet-style brace or a polypropylene custom-molded short articulated ankle–foot orthosis would be indicated.[1,2]
- Since forefoot varus is only one component of a complex multiplanar pes planovalgus deformity, decision making about conservative versus operative treatment will most likely depend on the characteristics of the hindfoot valgus deformity rather than solely on the forefoot varus component alone.

SURGICAL MANAGEMENT

- The plantarflexion opening wedge medial cuneiform osteotomy for correction of fixed forefoot varus associated with a flatfoot deformity is rarely performed in isolation and typically is performed as a component of multiple procedures to correct a given flatfoot deformity.
- Typically, the surgeon begins with bony correction of the foot, followed by soft tissue reconstruction and tendon transfers.
- The reconstructive procedure begins in the proximal aspect of the foot and ankle and proceeds distally since each level of correction is determined by aligning it to the next-most-proximal segment. Therefore, the forefoot varus is often the last portion of the bony deformity to be corrected during the realignment portion of the procedure.
- Occasionally, once the hindfoot deformity correction has been performed, the apparent forefoot varus that was present preoperatively has been improved sufficiently that osteotomy of the first cuneiform is not required.

Preoperative Planning

- This opening wedge osteotomy requires interposition of some type of bone graft material. Therefore, the surgeon should be prepared to harvest a bone graft or have allograft or synthetic bone graft material available.

- We have used exclusively frozen tricortical iliac crest allograft bone for this interposition osteotomy without complication.

Positioning

- The patient is positioned supine with a small pad placed under the ipsilateral buttock to internally rotate the foot to the neutral position.

Approach

- The osteotomy opens dorsally; therefore, the approach is over the dorsal aspect of the first cuneiform.
- If procedures are performed on the medial side of the midfoot, the incisions should be kept at least 3 cm apart to minimize undermining.
- Performing this osteotomy through a medial approach would significantly increase the difficulty, would require significant additional soft tissue dissection, and would require retraction of the anterior tibialis tendon near its insertion.

PLANTARFLEXION OPENING WEDGE MEDIAL CUNEIFORM OSTEOTOMY FOR CORRECTION OF FIXED FOREFOOT VARUS (COTTON OSTEOTOMY)

- Under tourniquet control, make a dorsal longitudinal skin incision over the medial cuneiform and the base of the first metatarsal.
- Carry dissection through the skin and subcutaneous tissue to develop the interval between the extensor hallucis longus tendon (retracted medially) and the extensor hallucis brevis tendon (retracted laterally).
- Free up and retract any crossing cutaneous branches of the superficial peroneal nerve.
- Expose the dorsal portion of the medial cuneiform with identification of the first tarsometatarsal joint and the joint between the medial and middle cuneiform. It is not necessary to open the joint capsule of the first tarsometatarsal joint.
- With fluoroscopic guidance, identify the midportion of the cuneiform and draw a saw cut line on the bone. Usually this line is at or just proximal to the plane of the second tarsometatarsal joint (**TECH FIG 1**).
- With a small microsagittal saw, make a transverse osteotomy in the dorsal-to-plantar direction through the midportion of the medial cuneiform by cutting down to, but not through, the plantar cortex (**TECH FIG 2**).
- Use a thin osteotome to complete the osteotomy, leaving the plantar periosteum intact.
- Pull the osteotome distally to lever open the medial cuneiform osteotomy and plantarflex the first ray (**TECH FIG 3**).
- Using a ruler, measure the amount of opening of the cuneiform osteotomy needed to achieve the desired plantarflexion of the first ray.
- On average, a 4- to 6-mm wedge of bone graft is needed to plantar-displace the first metatarsal to the desired level of the other metatarsal heads (especially the fifth metatarsal) in order to restore Cotton's normal "tripod" configuration.
- A wedge of iliac crest bone graft is either harvested from the patient or obtained from the bone bank.
- Use a microsagittal saw to shape this bone into a wedge, with the dorsal cortex of the iliac crest wedge cut to the width of the dorsal opening gap that was measured

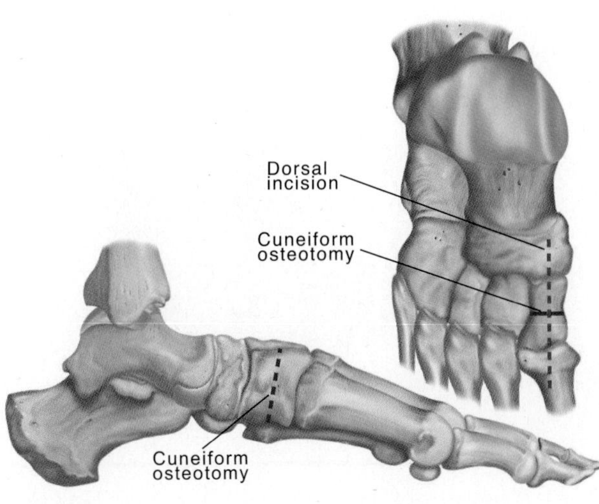

TECH FIG 1 • Location of first cuneiform osteotomy.

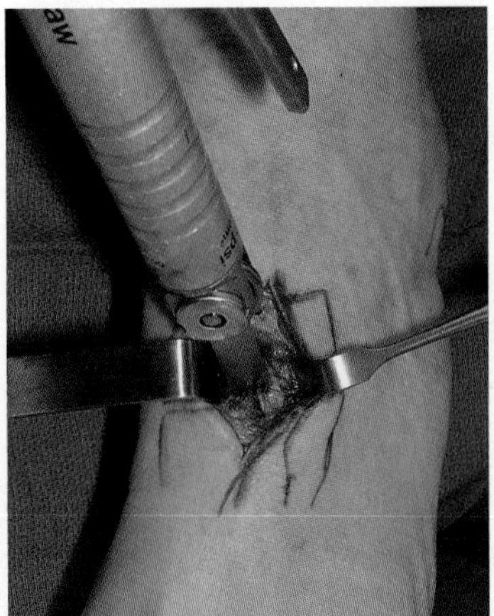

TECH FIG 2 • The osteotomy is made dorsal to plantar across the midportion of the first cuneiform. A narrow elevator or retractor is placed into the 1, 2 intercuneiform joint to prevent inadvertent osteotomy of the second cuneiform.

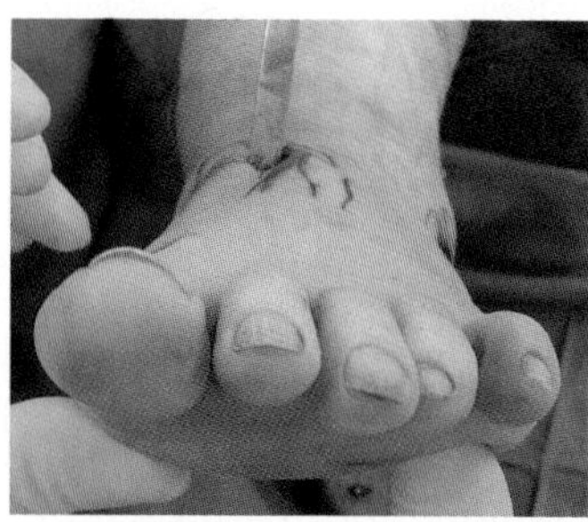

TECH FIG 3 • An assistant levers the osteotomy open to depress the first metatarsal head while the surgeon determines when the forefoot varus deformity has been adequately corrected.

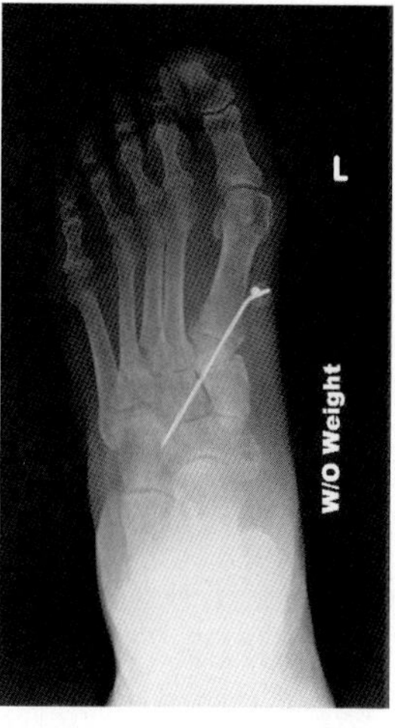

TECH FIG 5 • Fixation of the osteotomy with a 0.62-inch Kirschner wire placed from the distal portion of the first cuneiform obliquely into the second cuneiform.

previously and oriented so that the exposed cancellous bone surfaces of the iliac wedge will be adjacent to the exposed cancellous surfaces of the osteotomized cuneiform.

- Use a narrow osteotome to lever open the cuneiform osteotomy while an assistant places plantar-directed pressure on the first metatarsal to help open the osteotomy maximally while the bone graft wedge is impacted from dorsal to plantar into the medial cuneiform osteotomy using a bone tamp (**TECH FIG 4**).
- Place small amounts of morselized cancellous bone graft, either as autograft from adjacent osteotomies of the hindfoot or from the piece of allograft, medially and laterally around the bone wedge to fill whatever gap remains in the cuneiform.
- The osteotomy is stable due to the surrounding ligamentous support and the compression across the bone wedge created by tamping the bone wedge into the osteotomy. Use percutaneous fixation across the osteotomy to prevent dorsal displacement of the bone block until early healing has occurred (**TECH FIG 5**).
- Bend to 90 degrees the percutaneous pin protruding from the dorsal medial aspect of the first cuneiform and apply a pin cap.
- Irrigate the wound and close it in layers.

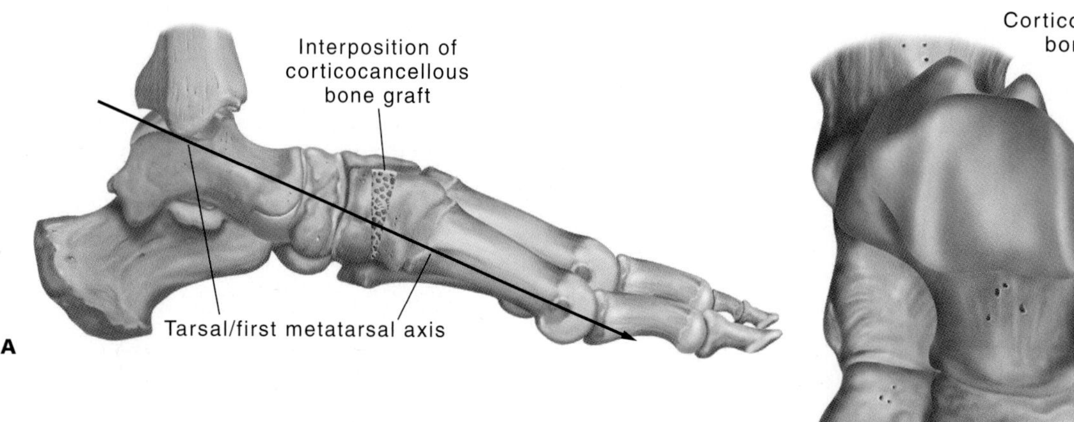

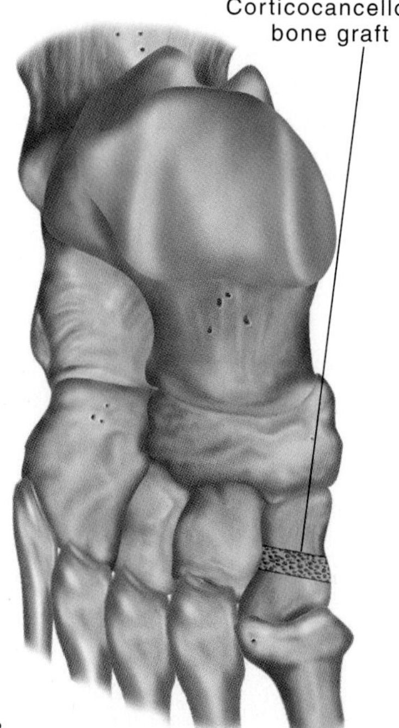

TECH FIG 4 • The interposition bone graft wedge is placed into the dorsal opening in the first cuneiform to depress the first metatarsal and correct the forefoot varus deformity.

PEARLS AND PITFALLS

Graft placement	■ Avoid placing the graft too far laterally, which would cause impingement of the graft against the second cuneiform.
Fixation problems	■ Dorsal screw fixation is not usually necessary, and the prominence of the dorsal screw head often requires hardware removal.
Contouring bone	■ After graft fixation, the microsagittal saw or a power rasp is used to smooth down any portions of the graft that extend beyond the surface of the cuneiform either medially or dorsally and to reduce any prominence of the cuneiform that may have been created by the distraction osteotomy.

POSTOPERATIVE CARE

- The pin site is dressed along with the other wounds and a compressive, bulky Robert Jones type of dressing is applied with medial lateral and posterior plaster slab splints covered with an elastic wrap.
- If a tendon transfer has been performed as part of the reconstructive procedure, the foot is positioned as needed for proper soft tissue healing.
- At 10 to 14 days after surgery, the splint, dressings, and sutures are removed.
- A dressing is placed around the pin site, which is then padded with a small felt doughnut, and a short-leg fiberglass cast is applied in neutral or whatever position is needed for proper soft tissue healing if a tendon transfer has been performed.
- The cast is removed at 6 weeks after surgery.
- Radiographs are obtained to ensure early incorporation of the graft without displacement.
- The percutaneous pin is removed and full weight bearing as tolerated is allowed in a removable walker boot (**FIG 2**). Joint and muscle rehabilitation, as indicated by the other operative procedures performed in addition to cuneiform osteotomy, is begun.

OUTCOMES

- Outcomes of this procedure have shown predictable healing. In review of 16 feet (15 patients) by Hirose and Johnson[4] there were no malunions or nonunions. All patients at follow-up described mild to no pain with ambulation.
- Average improvement in the first metatarsal–medial cuneiform angle as measured on the lateral radiograph was 9 degrees.[4]
- Because of the variety of hindfoot procedures performed in patients undergoing the cuneiform osteotomy, the degree of hindfoot correction contributed by the cuneiform osteotomy alone is difficult to determine.[4]
- This procedure combined with hindfoot reconstruction for flatfoot provides superior correction of the flatfoot deformity (as evidenced by the lateral talo–first metatarsal angle and the medial-cuneiform-to-floor distance) compared to flexor digitorum longus tendon transfer with subtalar joint arthrodesis or medial displacement calcaneal osteotomy.[4]

COMPLICATIONS

- No complications have been described in the few reports on this procedure except for the need for hardware removal due to a prominent screw head.
- Structures at risk during the exposure include the extensor hallucis longus or the extensor digitorum brevis tendon and the deep peroneal nerve.
- Although predictable healing has been noted, nonunion, overcorrection, and undercorrection could occur.
- When a dorsal screw is used for fixation, removal of the hardware is often required due to dorsal shoe pressure or irritation of the overlying nerve or tendon.

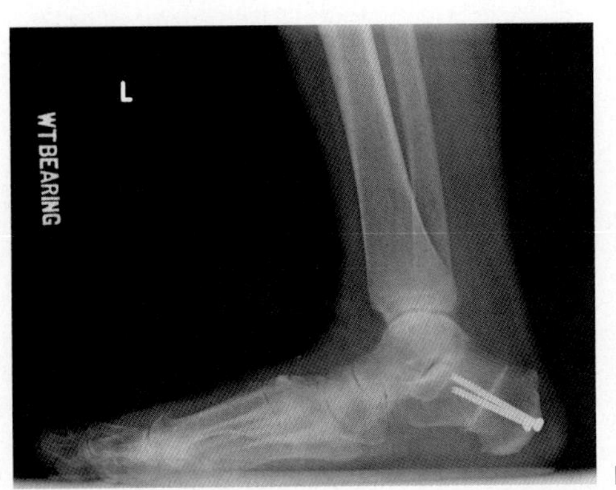

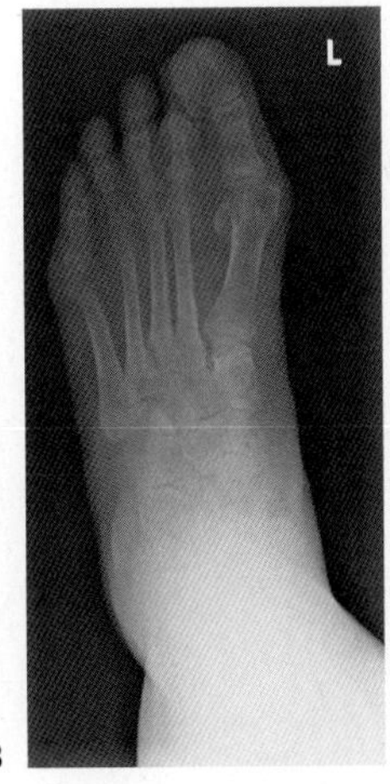

FIG 2 • Lateral (**A**) and AP (**B**) radiographs at 10 weeks after acquired flatfoot deformity correction with first cuneiform osteotomy. The allograft bone wedge has healed.

REFERENCES

1. Alvarez RG, Marini A, Schmitt C, et al. Stage 1 and II posterior tibial tendon dysfunction treated by a structured nonoperative management protocol: an orthosis and exercise program. Foot Ankle Int 2006:27:2–8.
2. Augustin JF, Sheldon SL, Berberian WS, et al. Nonoperative treatment of adult acquired flatfoot with the Arizona brace. Foot Ankle Clin North Am 2003;8:491–502.
3. Cotton FJ. Foot statics and surgery. N Engl J Med 1936;214:24–27.
4. Hirose CG, Johnson JE. Plantarflexion opening wedge medial cuneiform osteotomy for correction of fixed forefoot varus associated with flatfoot deformity. Foot Ankle Int 2004;25:568–574.
5. Johnson JE, Cohen BE, DiGiovanni BF, et al. Subtalar arthrodesis with flexor digitorum longus transfer and spring ligament repair for treatment of posterior tibial tendon insufficiency. Foot Ankle Int 2000;21:722–729.
6. Johnson JE. Plantarflexion opening wedge cuneiform osteotomy for correction of fixed forefoot varus. Tech Foot Ankle Surg 2004; 3:2–8.
7. Myerson MS, Corrigan J, Thompson FM, et al. Tendon transfer with calcaneal osteotomy for treatment of posterior tibial tendon insufficiency: a radiological investigation. Foot Ankle Int 1995; 16:712–718.

Chapter 40 Tarsometatarsal Arthrodesis

Ian L.D. Le and Mark E. Easley

DEFINITION

- Arthrodesis of the first, second, and third tarsometatarsal (TMT) joints is a relatively uncommon procedure used for the treatment of midfoot arthrosis.
- The majority of cases arise from either posttraumatic arthrosis or as part of a systemic inflammatory arthropathy.

ANATOMY

- The medial column of the foot is anatomically designed to be rigid and impart a strong lever arm for push-off, whereas the lateral column is mobile, allowing for forefoot accommodation to walking surfaces.
- Consequently, the first, second, and third TMT joints typically exhibit minimal axial or sagittal plane motion compared to the more mobile fourth and fifth TMT joints.
- Arthrosis of the first, second, and third TMT joints is best addressed surgically via arthrodesis; arthrosis of the fourth and fifth TMT joints is best addressed surgically with a motion-preserving operation including interposition or arthroplasty.
- The goal of foot surgery is to obtain a plantigrade position with normal underlying mechanical alignment to allow for weight bearing, shock absorption, accommodation, and power for efficient painless gait.
- The first TMT joint is typically 30 mm deep.
- The second TMT joint is recessed proximally in relation to the adjacent first and third TMT joints.

PATHOGENESIS

- Equinus is often an underlying pathologic feature.

NATURAL HISTORY

- There are no reported data regarding the natural history of TMT arthrosis, although it can be reasonably assumed that, with the exception of inflammatory arthropathy, most cases of midfoot arthrosis will progress at a variable rate over time, although symptoms may wax and wane.

PATIENT HISTORY AND PHYSICAL FINDINGS

- Pain is often well localized to the dorsum of the midfoot, although some patients may simply complain of a vague dorsal foot discomfort.
- Due to the lack of abundant subcutaneous tissue on the dorsum of the foot, inspection usually reveals localized swelling and osteophytic formation directly over the TMT joints.
- Palpation of the foot tenderness over the affected TMT joints that is exacerbated with motion is characteristic.
- Examination of the extensor tendons and subcutaneous tissue is done to rule out other pathology, including ganglions.
- Physical examination methods include the equinus or Silfverskiöld test. The examiner corrects the hindfoot to neutral subtalar position and checks dorsiflexion range of motion with the knee in straight extension and then flexed 30 degrees. An inability to obtain neutral dorsiflexion with the knee in straight extension that corrects with flexion is indicative of isolated gastrocnemius equinus.

IMAGING AND OTHER DIAGNOSTIC STUDIES

- Plain weight-bearing radiographs including AP, lateral, and oblique views of the foot should be obtained. Every effort should be made to obtain a true lateral radiograph with talar dome overlap.
- Seldom is a CT scan, MRI, or other imaging modality needed except to rule out a subtle Lisfranc injury.
- If there is question as to the cause of midfoot pain, a fluoroscopically guided injection of the suspected TMT joint can be both therapeutic and more importantly diagnostic.

DIFFERENTIAL DIAGNOSIS

- Lisfranc injury
- Metatarsal stress fracture
- Gout or other inflammatory arthropathy
- Ganglion
- Neuroma of the superficial or deep peroneal nerve

NONOPERATIVE MANAGEMENT

- Many patients with hallux valgus and hypermobility of the first TMT joint can be asymptomatic.
- However, once symptoms develop, progression is inevitable, in particular in patients with underlying equinus contractures.
- Initially management can be directed at resolving local symptoms, such as nonsteroidal anti-inflammatories, activity modification, rest, weight loss, shoe modifications, and orthotics.
- A stiff-soled rocker-bottom shoe or rigid orthotic minimizes motion across the midfoot, alleviating pain arising from the TMT arthrosis.
- In patients with equinus, a well-directed physiotherapy stretching protocol can be helpful.

SURGICAL MANAGEMENT

- Indication: persistent pain despite an adequate course of conservative management
- Contraindication: open physeal growth plates

Preoperative Planning

- AP foot plain radiographs are reviewed for the extent of involvement of midfoot joints and relative lengths of metatarsal heads.
- Lateral foot plain radiographs are reviewed for talar–first metatarsal angle and evidence of a cavus or planus foot.

- Based on the above, the surgeon templates an operative plan.
- The surgeon should intraoperatively assess for equinus and the need for percutaneous tendo Achilles lengthening or gastrocnemius slide.

Positioning

- Patients are placed supine on a radiolucent table with a padded wedge or bump under the ipsilateral hip to correct external rotation.
- The arm is placed across the chest and the ulnar nerve is padded.
- A tourniquet is applied either to the calf or the thigh. If proximal tibial bone graft is considered, the tourniquet should be applied on the thigh.
- The limb is exsanguinated with an elastic bandage and the tourniquet is inflated.

Approach

- Most commonly, two well-spaced longitudinal incisions are made to allow adequate exposure of the first, second, and third TMT joints.
- A 4-cm medial incision is centered over the lateral third of the first TMT joint. This allows exposure of the entire first TMT joint and the medial half of the second TMT joint.
- A 4-cm lateral incision is made over the third TMT joint. This allows exposure of the lateral half of the second TMT joint and the entire third TMT joint.
- Every effort is made to maximize the skin bridge between the two incisions to prevent wound necrosis or slough. Aggressive skin retraction must be minimized and done through deeper layers and not superficially.

TECHNIQUES

EXPOSURE OF THE FIRST AND SECOND TARSOMETATARSAL JOINTS

- Make the medial incision between the extensor hallucis longus and extensor hallucis brevis, roughly in line with the lateral third of the first TMT joint (**TECH FIG 1**).
- Carry dissection down with caution to avoid the dorsal cutaneous nerves.
- Identify the deep peroneal nerve with the accompanying dorsalis pedis artery just deep to the medial aspect of the extensor hallucis brevis tendon, coursing toward the first web space.
- Identify the first TMT joint by moving the first metatarsal, and cut the capsule transverse in line with the joint to minimize periosteal stripping.
- Carry the dissection up between the first and second metatarsal bases; the second TMT joint can be identified more proximally relative to the first TMT joint.
- Denude all joint surfaces of cartilage with a combination of an AO elevator, a quarter-inch osteotome, straight and curved curettes, and rongeur.
- Use a 2.0-mm drill bit to create a series of perforations in the arthrodesis surfaces to optimize surface area and blood flow. A lamina spreader can be helpful for distraction.
- In similar fashion, prepare the first TMT joint, the medial aspect of the second TMT joint, and the articulation between the first and second metatarsal bases.
- Avoid using an oscillating saw, as it can predispose to the risk of metatarsal shortening.
- It is imperative to remove cartilage all the way down to the plantar aspect of the first TMT joint to prevent excessive dorsiflexion. The first TMT joint is 28 to 30 mm deep.

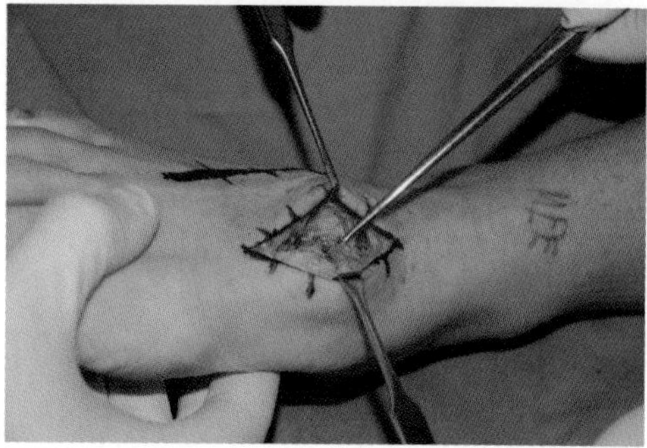

TECH FIG 1 • First and second tarsometatarsal joint exposure and preparation.

EXPOSURE OF THE SECOND AND THIRD TARSOMETATARSAL JOINTS

- Make the second longitudinal incision described above earlier over the third TMT joint.
- Carry dissection to the extensor digitorum brevis muscle belly, avoiding the dorsal cutaneous nerves (**TECH FIG 2**).
- Typically, the extensor digitorum brevis cannot be retracted plantar, so instead it is split in line with the incision to expose the underlying third TMT joint.
- Again, split the periosteum in line with the joint to avoid excessive periosteal stripping.
- Expose the lateral aspect of the second TMT joint and the space between the second and third metatarsal bases.
- Prepare these arthrodesis surfaces in a similar manner to that described earlier.

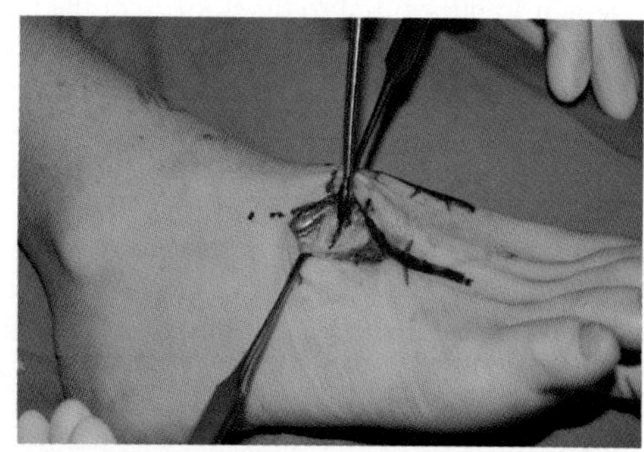

TECH FIG 2 • Third tarsometatarsal joint exposure and preparation.

TEMPORARY STABILIZATION

- Before stabilization, hold the foot in a reduced position and palpate the forefoot to ensure it is plantigrade.
- Two crossed 0.062 Kirschner wires are used to hold the first TMT joint in a reduced position. They should be placed where the final screws will ultimately be positioned (TECH FIG 3A).
- Place the first from the dorsal medial cuneiform to the plantar aspect of the first metatarsal base. Place the second from the dorsal first metatarsal shaft to the plantar aspect of the medial cuneiform.
- Reduce the second metatarsal to the middle cuneiform and the first metatarsal base. Again, palpate the forefoot to ensure the plantar metatarsal heads are level.
- Make a stab incision over the medial aspect of the medial cuneiform through the skin only. Dissect down to bone with retraction of the tibialis anterior.
- Hold the second metatarsal in place with a guide pin from the 3.0-mm cannulated screw set while protecting the tibialis anterior tendon (TECH FIG 3B).
- Aim the wire from the medial cuneiform to the base of the second metatarsal.
- Make a stab incision on the lateral forefoot to facilitate insertion of another guide pin from the 3.0-mm cannulated screw set to stabilize the third metatarsal to the cuneiforms in a reduced position (TECH FIG 3C).
- Examine the foot position to confirm plantigrade position before final stabilization.

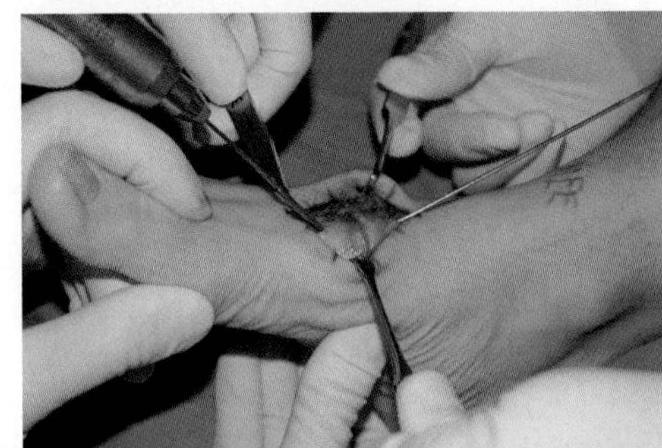
A

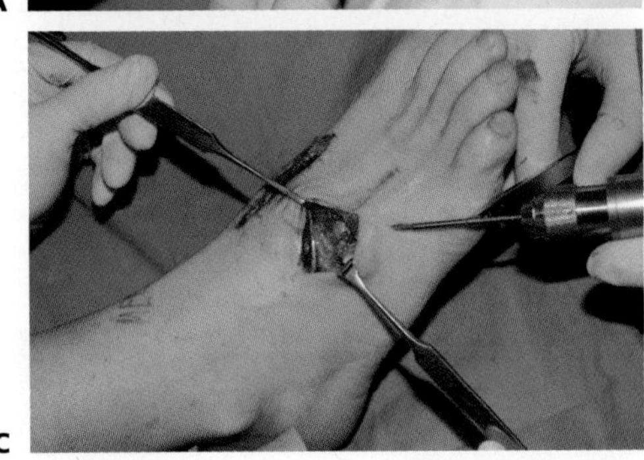
C

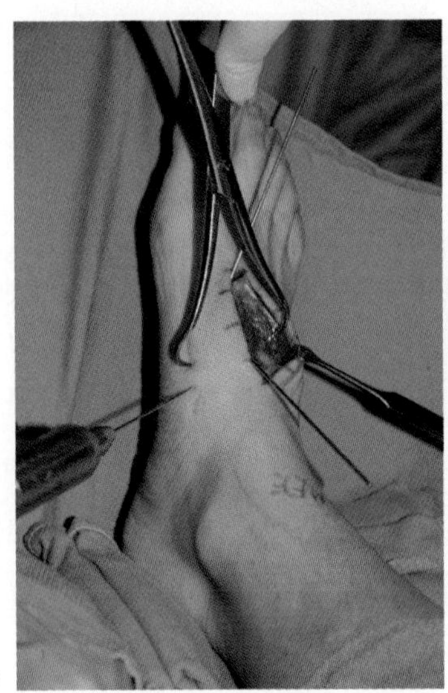
B

TECH FIG 3 • **A.** First tarsometatarsal joint temporary fixation. **B.** Second tarsometatarsal joint temporary fixation. **C.** Third tarsometatarsal joint fixation with screw.

FIRST TARSOMETATARSAL DEFINITIVE STABILIZATION

- The first TMT joint is stabilized first.
- Place a 3.5-mm drill sleeve over the 0.062 Kirschner wire from the medial cuneiform to the first metatarsal and use a cautery mark to mark the angulation of the wire.
- Back the 0.062 Kirschner wire out while maintaining the drill sleeve in a fixed position. Use a 3.5-mm drill followed by a 2.5-mm drill to allow insertion of a 3.5-mm cortical screw in a lag manner. Countersink the screw head before insertion.
- Use similar steps to place an additional lag screw from the first metatarsal to the cuneiform.

SECOND AND THIRD TARSOMETATARSAL DEFINITIVE STABILIZATION

- Drill the second metatarsal cannulated wire with a cannulated drill.
- Use a 3.5-mm drill followed by a 2.5-mm drill to allow insertion of a lag screw. A washer may be needed due to the softer cuneiform bone.
- Protect the tibialis anterior tendon during insertion of this screw.
- Use a similar technique to insert the screw from the third metatarsal to the middle cuneiform.
- Obtain further stabilization of the second and third TMT joints by placing compression staples (TECH FIG 4).

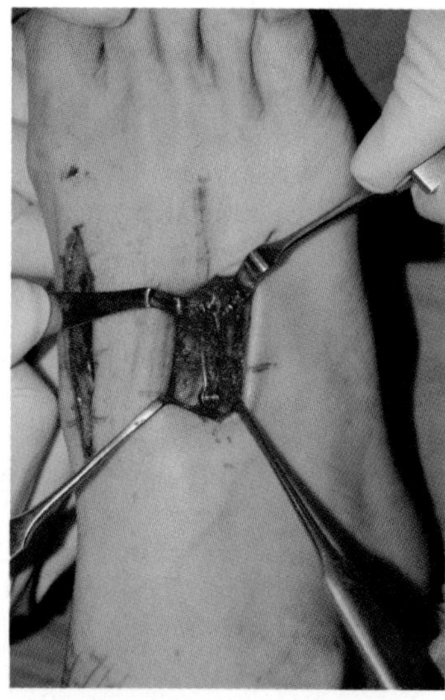

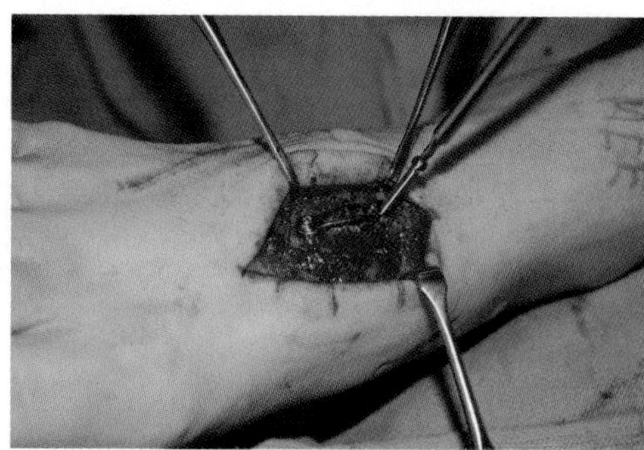

TECH FIG 4 • **A.** Third tarsometatarsal joint fixation with compression staple. **B.** Second tarsometatarsal fixation with additional compression staple.

BONE GRAFTING

- Bone graft is applied to the dorsal surfaces of all arthrodesis sites.
- Autograft or allograft may be used. We often use cancellous allograft mixed with a platelet-rich derivative to promote both osteoconduction and osteoinduction.
- Autograft may be harvested from the calcaneus, proximal or distal tibia, or iliac crest.

INTRAOPERATIVE FLUOROSCOPY

- Obtain AP, lateral, and oblique images to ensure adequate reduction and opposition of arthrodesis surfaces in addition to appropriate hardware positioning (TECH FIG 5).

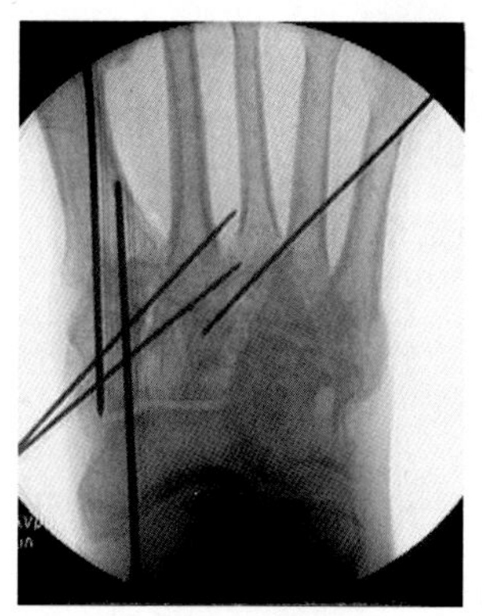

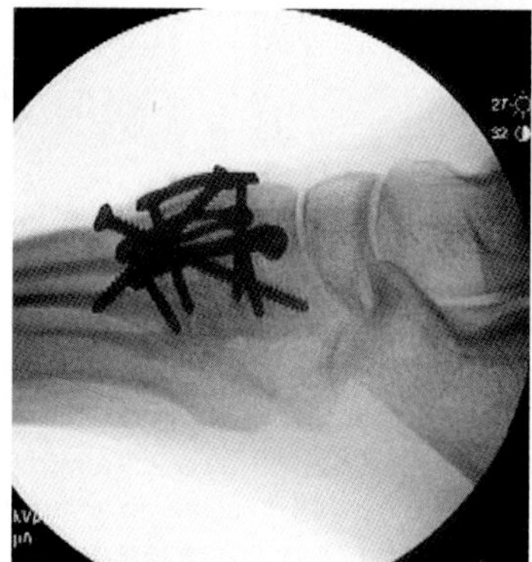

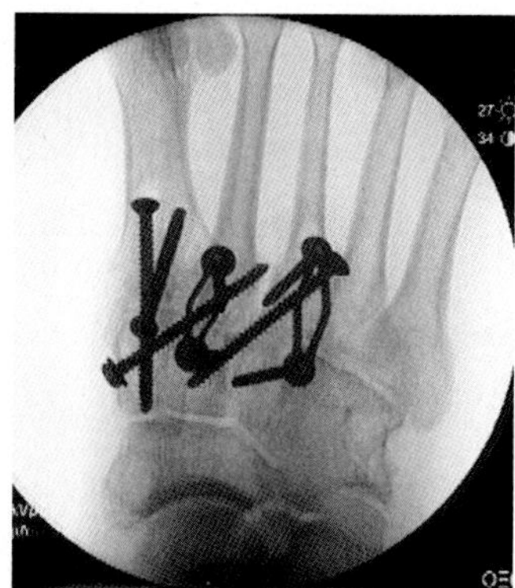

TECH FIG 5 • **A.** Intraoperative fluoroscopy of temporary stabilization. **B, C.** Final radiographic images.

WOUND CLOSURE

- Deflate the tourniquet as pressure is applied to the wound.
- Obtain hemostasis and insert a drain to prevent postoperative hematoma formation.
- Reapproximate the capsule over the TMT joints with an absorbable suture.
- Reapproximate subcutaneous tissue with interrupted buried absorbable sutures.
- Close the skin with horizontal or vertical mattress nylon sutures with minimal tension.

PEARLS AND PITFALLS

- Persistent dorsiflexed first metatarsal or lesser metatarsalgia
  - Failure to resect plantar aspect of the first TMT joint
- Prominent first, second, or third metatarsal heads
  - Failure to hold the metatarsals in a plantigrade position before definitive stabilization
- Nonunion
  - Inadequate joint preparation or inadequate fixation
  - Lack of bone graft
- Wound complication
  - Poor soft tissue handling
  - Excessive skin retraction
  - Poor incision placement

POSTOPERATIVE CARE

- A well-molded below-knee posterior splint is applied with toes exposed.
- Analgesic control is optimal with a local or regional anesthetic in addition to oral narcotics.
- The patient is mobilized on a knee scooter, non–weight-bearing.
- Progressive weight bearing is permitted between 6 and 12 weeks in a removable boot.
- The patient is weaned out of the removable boot into standard shoes at 12 weeks.

OUTCOMES

- Relatively little is published on outcomes of midfoot arthrodesis.
- With appropriate surgical indications, surgical technique, and patient compliance, patient satisfaction rates exceed 90%.

REFERENCES

1. Hansen ST. Functional Reconstruction of the Foot and Ankle. Philadelphia: Lippincott Williams & Wilkins, 2000:332–334.
2. Johnson JE, Johnson KA. Dowel arthrodesis for degenerative arthrodesis of the tarsometatarsal (Lisfranc) joints. Foot Ankle 1986;5:243–253.
3. Komenda GA, Myerson MS, Biddinger KR. Results of arthrodesis of the tarsometatarsal joints after traumatic injury. J Bone Joint Surg Am 1996;78A:1665–1676.
4. Mann RA, Prieskorn D, Sobel M. Mid-tarsal arthrodesis for primary degenerative osteoarthrosis or osteoarthrosis after trauma. J Bone Joint Surg Am 1996;78A:1376–1385.
5. Sangeorzan BJ, Veith R, Hansen ST. Fusion of Lisfranc's joint for salvage of tarsometatarsal injuries. Foot Ankle 1990;10: 193–200.
6. Vertullo CJ, Easley ME, Nunley JA. The transverse dorsal approach to the Lisfranc joint. Foot Ankle Int 2002;23:420–426.

Chapter 41 Midfoot Arthrodesis

Mark E. Easley

DEFINITION

- This is a procedure to definitively treat midfoot arthrosis with or without deformity.

ANATOMY

- Midfoot articulations include:
  - Tarsometatarsal joints
  - Naviculocuneiform joints
- In the coronal plane, the midfoot may be viewed as three columns:
  - Medial column (the first ray)
  - Middle column (the second and third rays)
  - Lateral column (the fourth and fifth rays)
- These articulations form an arch in both the longitudinal plane and the transverse plane.
- The second cuneiform is the keystone to the transverse arch.
- Anatomic alignment in the longitudinal plane is rather simple to assess on weight-bearing radiographs of the foot.
  - In both the AP and lateral planes, the talo–first metatarsal axis should be congruent.
- Physiologically, the medial and middle columns (first through third rays) have congruent joints and tight ligaments, leaving little motion.
  - This is important to ensure the midfoot serves as a rigid lever during the gait cycle's stance and push-off.
- In contrast, the lateral column (fourth and fifth rays) is relatively supple.
  - This is important to allow the foot to accommodate to various surfaces.
- Given that the midfoot's medial and middle columns are physiologically stiff, arthrodesis of these joints in physiologic alignment creates few functional deficits. However, arthrodesis of the lateral column is generally contraindicated, as the midfoot's ability to accommodate to various surfaces is forfeited.

PATHOGENESIS

- When the compact and stable midfoot anatomy is compromised, the talo–first metatarsal relationship is disrupted and the foot loses its mechanical advantage during the stance and push-off phases of gait.
- In the sagittal (lateral) plane this leads to loss of the longitudinal arch at the midfoot, with a midfoot sag.
  - In the extreme case the arch will reverse and become a "rocker-bottom deformity."
- In the coronal (AP) plane the forefoot drifts into abduction relative to the hindfoot.
- A plantigrade foot balances relatively evenly on the weight-bearing surfaces of the first and fifth metatarsals and the heel. When the midfoot collapses, this balance is disrupted and weight bearing eventually may be on the midfoot as well.
- With progressive midfoot deformity, the hindfoot may eventually lose its physiologic alignment, typically with greater-than-physiologic valgus.
  - This typically leads to shortening of the Achilles tendon and equinus contracture.
- In extreme cases, the ankle may become incongruent as well.
- Causes include:
  - Posttraumatic arthritis (chronic Lisfranc fracture-dislocation)
  - Primary arthritis
  - Inflammatory arthropathy (rheumatoid arthritis)
  - Charcot neuroarthropathy

NATURAL HISTORY

- An injury to the midfoot articulations or the ligaments, particularly the "Lisfranc ligament" between the base of the second metatarsal and the first cuneiform, leads to destabilization of the midfoot's architecture and a tendency toward gradual progressive arch collapse and forefoot abduction.

PATIENT HISTORY AND PHYSICAL FINDINGS

- History
  - Often (but not always) midfoot trauma is reported. Primary and inflammatory arthritis may be responsible without trauma. Also, a patient with neuropathy may develop midfoot destabilization but without recollection of trauma or with a history of what appeared to be only a minor trauma.
  - Patients experience pain with weight bearing, especially with push-off during the gait cycle.
  - They may also note a fallen arch and difficulty with shoe wear.
- Physical examination
  - The patient must be examined while weight bearing. Comparison to the uninvolved contralateral foot is sometimes useful as a baseline of the patient's physiologic alignment.
    - With advanced disease, loss of the longitudinal arch and forefoot abduction are present.
  - Midfoot tenderness and pain with stress
    - Tenderness is typically focused on the midfoot.
    - Stress of the midfoot produces midfoot pain.
    - The "piano key test" isolates the focus of the pathology to the specific tarsometatarsal joint.
- Neurologic examination
  - If there is a concern for neuropathy, the Semmes-Weinstein monofilaments should be used to determine protective sensation.
    - If the patient can sense the 5.07 monofilament, protective sensation is deemed intact.

IMAGING AND OTHER DIAGNOSTIC STUDIES

- Weight-bearing radiographs of the foot are obtained: AP, oblique, and lateral views.
- Rarely is CT required for assessment or preoperative planning.
- If there is a question of which midfoot articulations may be symptomatic, selective or diagnostic injections may be useful.

DIFFERENTIAL DIAGNOSIS

- See "Pathogenesis" on previous page.

NONOPERATIVE MANAGEMENT

- Activity modification
- Nonsteroidal anti-inflammatory agents (NSAIDs)
- Intra-articular corticosteroid injection
- Mechanical support
  - Longitudinal arch support
  - Stiffer-soled shoe with or without a slight or low-profile rocker-bottom modification
    - With limited deformity and midfoot arthritis, a rocker may be placed on a sensible regular shoe; it need not be a big cumbersome shoe.
    - However, with greater deformity, the shoe may need to be accommodative.
  - Bracing
    - Stiffer-soled shoe with rocker modification in combination with a double-upright brace or ankle–foot orthosis (AFO)
    - Diabetics with neuropathy or neuroarthropathy will require the above in combination with a total-contact insert.

SURGICAL MANAGEMENT

- Surgical management is warranted with failure of nonoperative measures.
- Procedures may include arthrodesis in situ or arthrodesis in combination with realignment midfoot osteotomy. Occasionally, adjunctive hindfoot procedures and Achilles tendon lengthening may be warranted.

Preoperative Planning

- Preoperative weight-bearing radiographs of the foot are essential to determine the preoperative plan.
  - The goal is to restore congruency in the AP and lateral talo–first metatarsal alignment.
  - The deformity must be studied to determine the optimal method for realignment.
  - The degree of destruction or distortion of the midfoot anatomy (particularly with erosive changes of an inflammatory arthropathy) is important and factors in how to best reconstruct the midfoot.
  - Associated hindfoot deformity may need to be addressed as well.
- Equinus contracture
  - The preoperative assessment should include the condition of the Achilles tendon.
  - Often Achilles lengthening, either with a triple cut or gastrocnemius-soleus recession, is necessary to realign the foot and may serve to unload stresses on the midfoot.
- Equipment
  - Various screw and plating systems, some even dedicated to the midfoot, are available.
  - Depending on the planned reconstruction, the following options exist:
    - Standard screws and plates
    - Locking midfoot plates
    - Intramedullary screws
    - Compression staples or compression plates

Positioning

- The patient is positioned supine on the operating table.
- I routinely use a tourniquet.

Approach

- Dual longitudinal approach over the midfoot
  - One dorsal and one medial
  - Most common
- Transverse approach
  - Has been used by many surgeons but is not universally accepted

SCREW AND COMPRESSION PLATE FIXATION

- This patient is a 38-year-old woman with post-traumatic arthritis after chronic Lisfranc fracture-dislocation. The patient also had a "nutcracker" injury to her cuboid with some lateral column degenerative change (**TECH FIG 1**).
- Approach
  - Dual dorsal longitudinal incisions with adequate skin bridge
  - Medial incision
    - Extensor hallucis brevis exposed (**TECH FIG 2A**)
    - Deep neurovascular bundle deep to extensor hallucis longus muscle–tendon (**TECH FIG 2B**)
  - First and second tarsometatarsal (TMT) joint preparation
    - Particularly deep joint (2.5 to 3.0 mm)
    - Essential to remove all plantar prominences and cartilage to avoid dorsiflexion malunion (**TECH FIG 2C**)
    - Important to remove scar tissue between base of second metatarsal and first cuneiform to allow reduction of second metatarsal base (**TECH FIG 2D**)
    - Penetrate the subchondral bone to promote fusion (**TECH FIG 2E**).
- Lateral incision (with adequate skin bridge) (**TECH FIG 2F**)
  - Protect the superficial peroneal nerve branch or branches (**TECH FIG 2G**).
  - Third TMT joint preparation: Remove residual cartilage and penetrate subchondral bone (**TECH FIG 2H,I**).
- Add bone graft as necessary.
- Reduce the deformity.
  - The "windlass" mechanism may be useful in reducing the TMT joints and particularly in avoiding dorsiflexion malunion. Moreover, it compresses the joints (**TECH FIG 3A**).

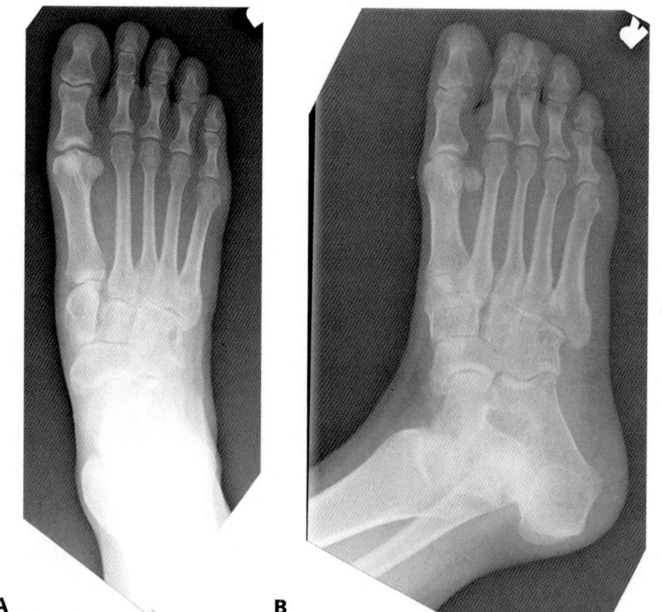

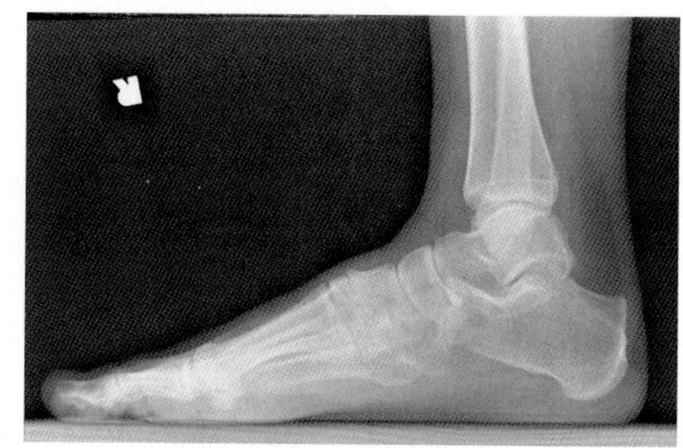

TECH FIG 1 • Preoperative radiographs of 38-year-old woman with postoperative midfoot arthritis secondary to chronic Lisfranc injury. **A.** AP view. **B.** Oblique view (note distortion to cuboid: chronic "nutcracker" injury). **C.** Lateral view.

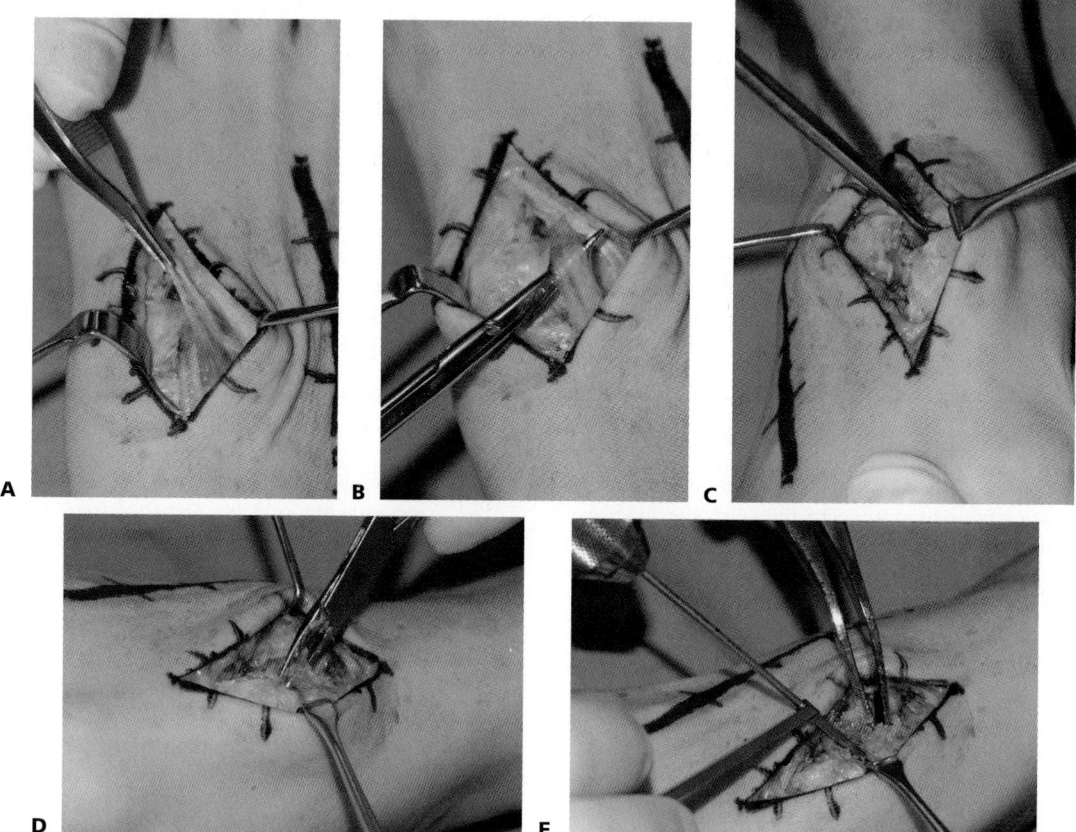

TECH FIG 2 • Dorsal medial approach. **A.** Extensor hallucis brevis (EHB) muscle elevated. **B.** Immediately deep to EHB is the deep neurovascular bundle. **C–E.** Preparing medial aspect of tarsometatarsal (TMT) joints. **C.** Sharp elevator for first TMT joint. (Note: toes at top of **A, B,** and **C.**) **D.** Rongeur in junction between base of second metatarsal and first cuneiform (it is important to be sure the second metatarsal fully reduces). **E.** Drill to penetrate subchondral bone. The second TMT joint is prepared in a similar manner. *(continued)*

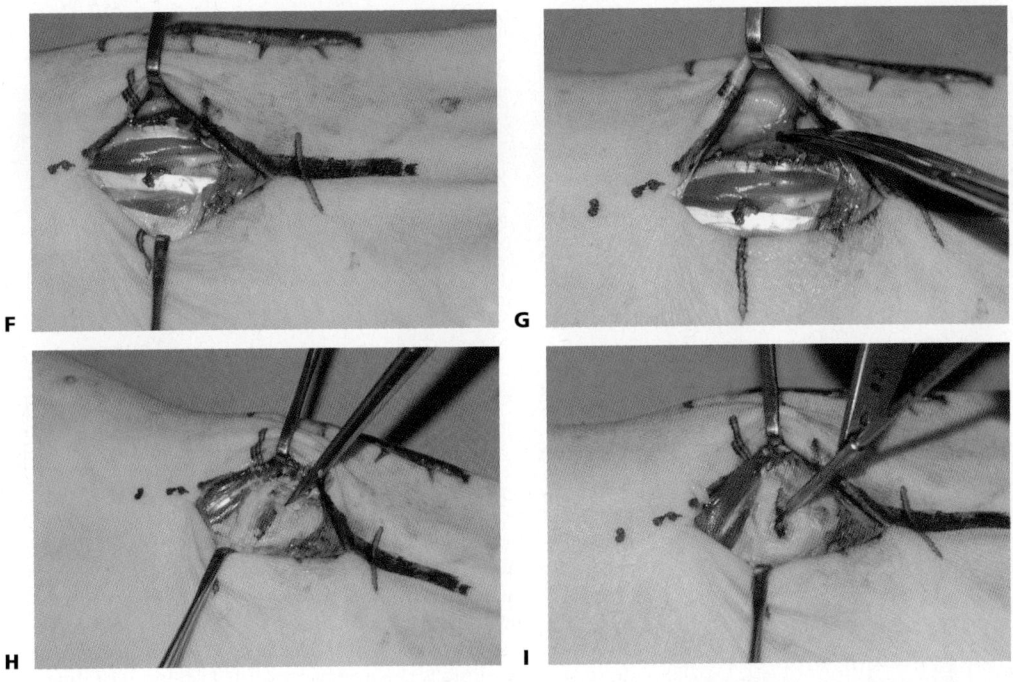

TECH FIG 2 • *(continued)* Dorsolateral approach. **F.** Interval identified. **G.** Superficial peroneal nerve branches are identified and protected. **H, I.** Preparation of third TMT joint. **H.** Sharp elevator to remove residual cartilage. **I.** Drilling subchondral bone. (Note: toes at right side of **F, G, H,** and **I.**)

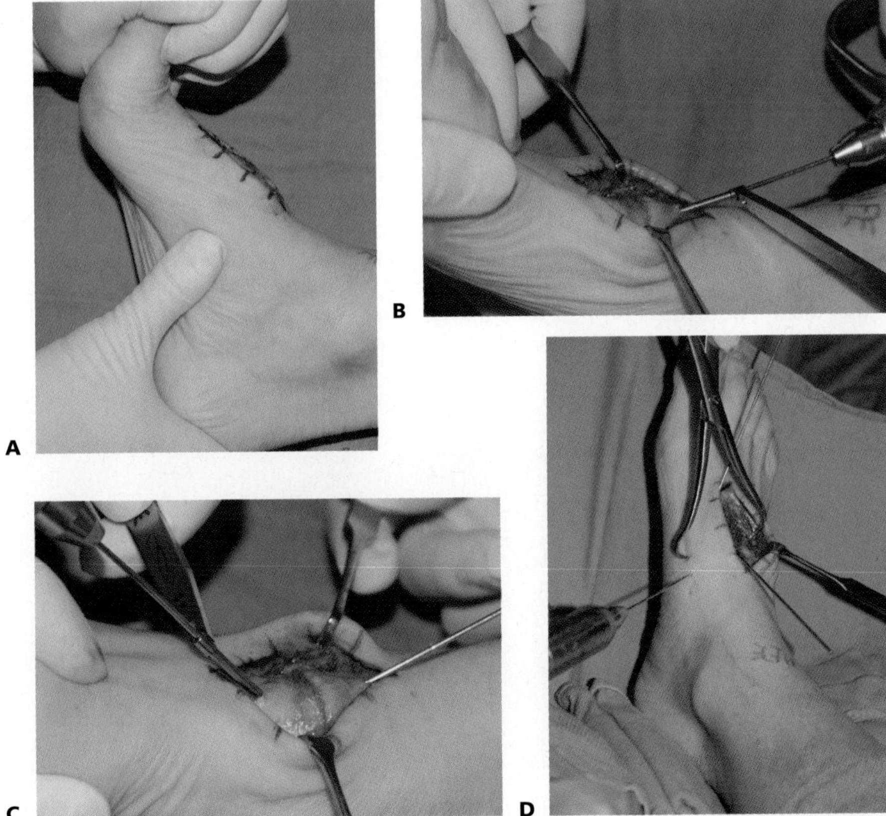

TECH FIG 3 • **A.** Using the windlass mechanism to assist in reduction and promote proper alignment of the tarsometatarsal (TMT) joints. Note dorsiflexion of the toes and ankle to tighten plantar soft tissues; this compresses the TMT joints and keeps them from dorsiflexing. **B, C.** Provisional fixation of first TMT joint. **B.** Proximal to distal pin. **C.** Distal to proximal pin. Note that the windlass mechanism is still being maintained with dorsiflexion of the toes. **D.** Large bone reduction clamp to ensure that the second metatarsal base is reduced, much like open reduction and internal fixation of an acute Lisfranc fracture-dislocation. Provisional pin to fix second metatarsal base.

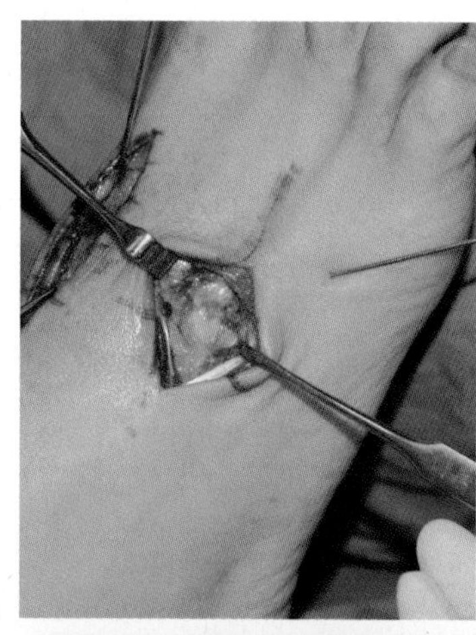

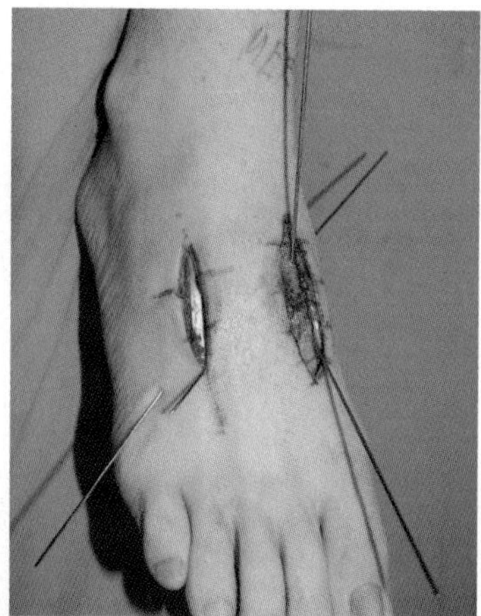

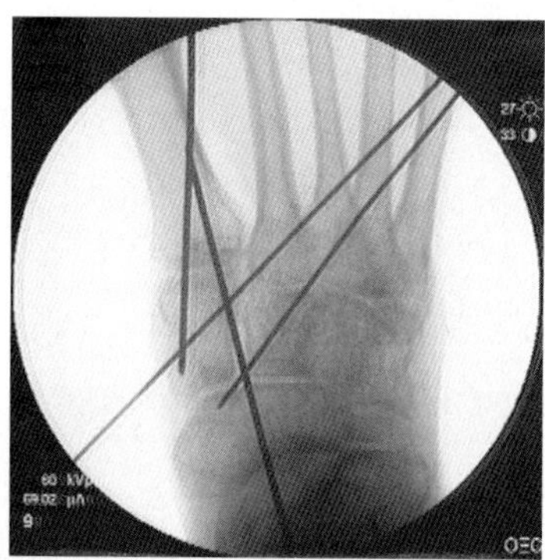

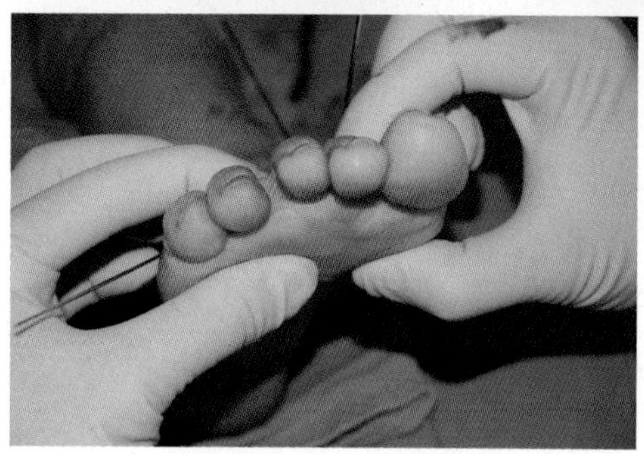

TECH FIG 4 • A. Provisional lateral fixation. **B,C.** Provisional fixation for second metatarsal is the guide pin for the drill for the screw to be placed from the first cuneiform to the second metatarsal base, a traditional "Lisfranc screw." **B.** Clinical view. **C.** Fluoroscopic view. Note that the guide pin position was checked on fluoroscopy and measured to determine optimal screw length, and then the guide pin was driven fully through the second metatarsal to exit the lateral wound. This way, when the guide pin is drilled and potentially sheared by the drill, both ends of the guide pin may still be retrieved. **D.** Before placing definitive fixation, the surgeon should check the balance of the forefoot (metatarsal heads). Metatarsal heads should be well balanced, with the sesamoids slightly more plantar than the second and third metatarsal heads.

  - I maintain dorsiflexion of the toes (activates windlass mechanism) while I place the provisional fixation (**TECH FIG 3B,C**).
  - Using a bone reduction clamp as for open reduction and internal fixation of an acute Lisfranc fracture-dislocation may be helpful. After the second metatarsal base is reduced, I place a guide pin to drill with a cannulated drill the path for a classic "Lisfranc screw" (**TECH FIG 3D**).
- Provisional fixation of middle column (**TECH FIG 4A**)
- Thin guide pins for cannulated drills are fragile. I measure the desired screw length and then pass the wires all the way through the foot. That way, if the guide pin should break, I can retrieve both ends and not leave a pin in the foot that may block my desired screws (**TECH FIG 4B,C**).
- Balance of the forefoot is essential. While performing provisional fixation, keep in mind that the metatarsal heads need to be balanced.
  - Typically, that means that the sesamoids are slightly more plantar than the second and third metatarsal heads (**TECH FIG 4D**).
- I routinely use solid screws but may initiate the drill hole with a cannulated system. For the placement of a solid "Lisfranc screw" from the first cuneiform to the base of the second metatarsal, I overdrill the guide pin, but only to the medial cortex of the second metatarsal base. Then I remove the guide pin and complete the drill hole through the second metatarsal base with a solid drill. I then overdrill the first cuneiform. Then I place the solid screw in lag fashion. I typically use a washer for this screw (**TECH FIG 5**).

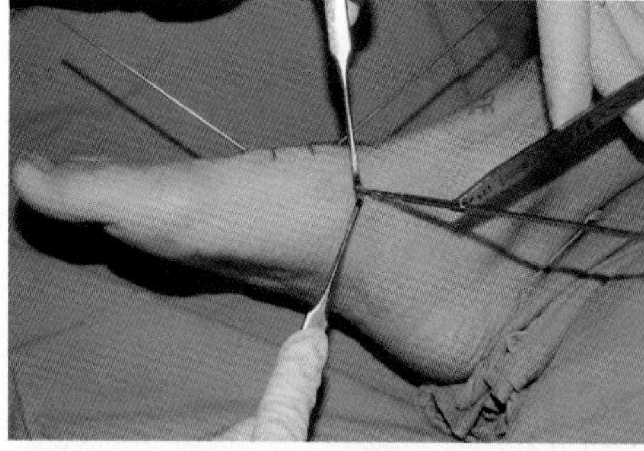

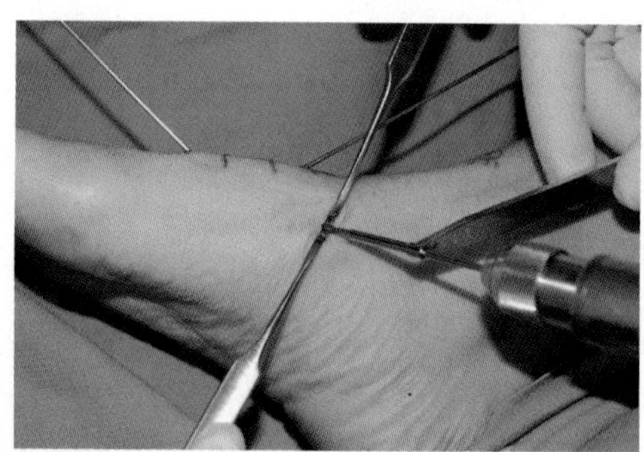

TECH FIG 5 • Placing the "Lisfranc screw." **A.** Initiating the drill hole with a cannulated drill over the guide pin. **B.** Guide pin is removed and drill hole completed with a solid drill. *(continued)*

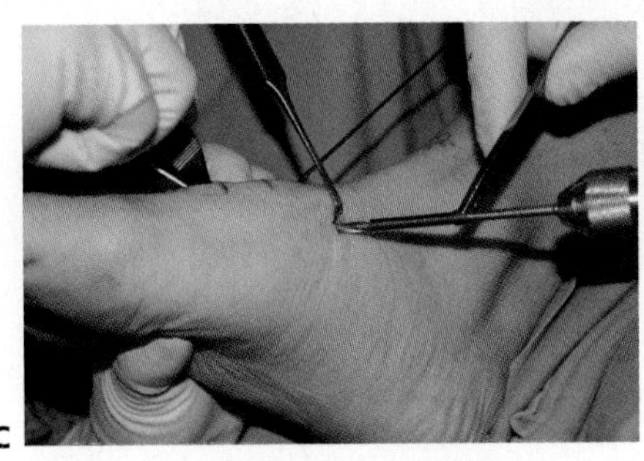

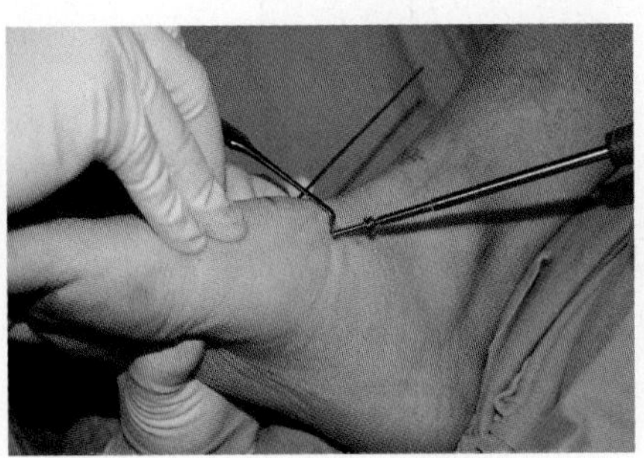

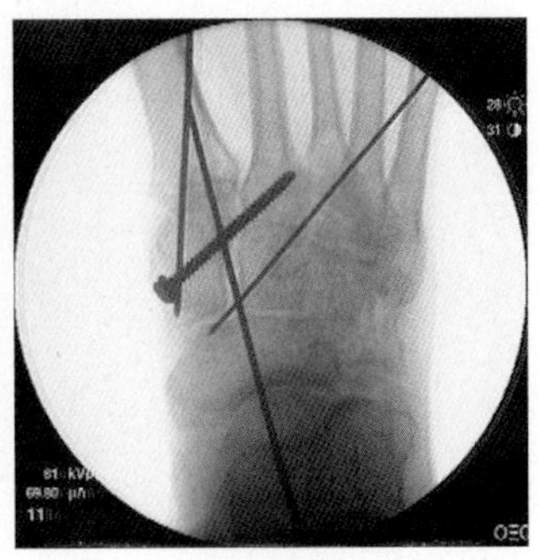

TECH FIG 5 • *(continued)* **C.** Proximal cortex (first cuneiform) is overdrilled to create lag effect. **D.** Solid screw is placed. **E.** Fluoroscopic view.

- The "Lisfranc screw" stabilizes the base of the second metatarsal and it will limit dorsiflexion of the second TMT joint if a compression plate is used dorsally.
- I routinely use two lag screws to stabilize the first TMT joint (**TECH FIG 6A–F**).
- It is important to use a countersink on the distal-to-proximal screws so that the dorsal cortex of the first metatarsal base does not fracture when the screw is fully seated (**TECH FIG 6E**).
- The middle column may be further stabilized with a lag screw (**TECH FIG 6G–J**).
- I secure the third TMT joint with a dorsal compression plate; with the lag screw already placed, excessive dorsiflexion of the third TMT joint is avoided (**TECH FIG 7A–F**).
- I also use a dorsal compression plate on the second TMT joint. Since the "Lisfranc screw" has already been placed, dorsiflexion can be avoided.

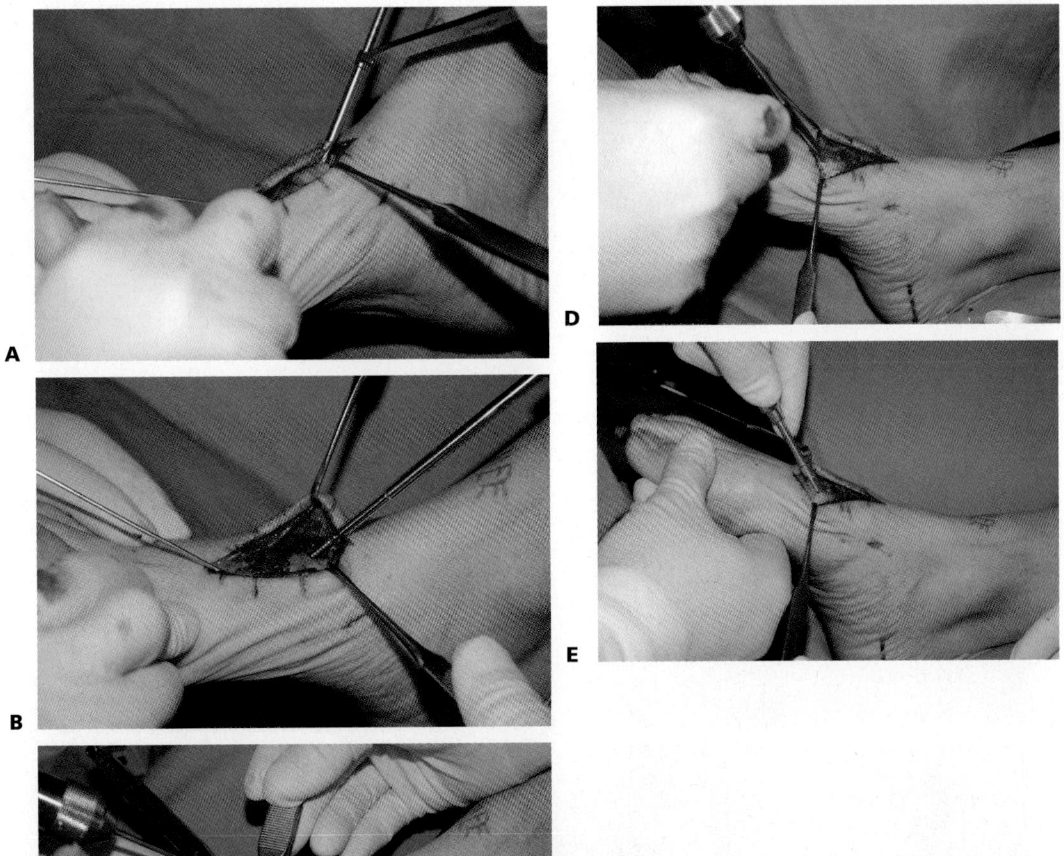

TECH FIG 6 • **A,B.** Proximal to distal lag screw across first tarsometatarsal (TMT) joint. **A.** After removal of provisional fixation, overdrilling proximal cortex. **B.** Solid screw placement. **C–F.** Distal to proximal screw across the first TMT joint. **C.** After removal of provisional fixation, solid drill. **D.** Overdrill near cortex (first metatarsal). **E.** Countersink (essential so that dorsal first metatarsal cortex does not fracture). *(continued)*

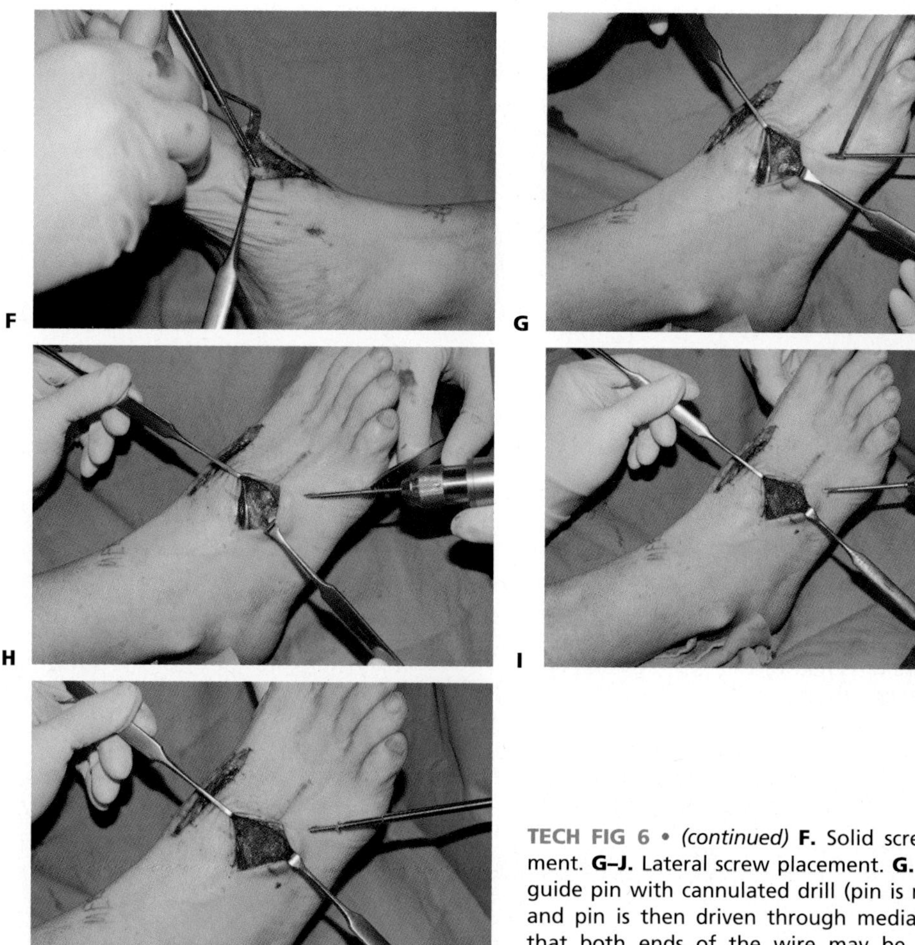

TECH FIG 6 • *(continued)* **F.** Solid screw placement. **G–J.** Lateral screw placement. **G.** Overdrill guide pin with cannulated drill (pin is measured and pin is then driven through medial foot so that both ends of the wire may be retrieved should the pin break). **H.** Drill with solid drill bit. **I.** Overdrill. **J.** Solid screw placed.

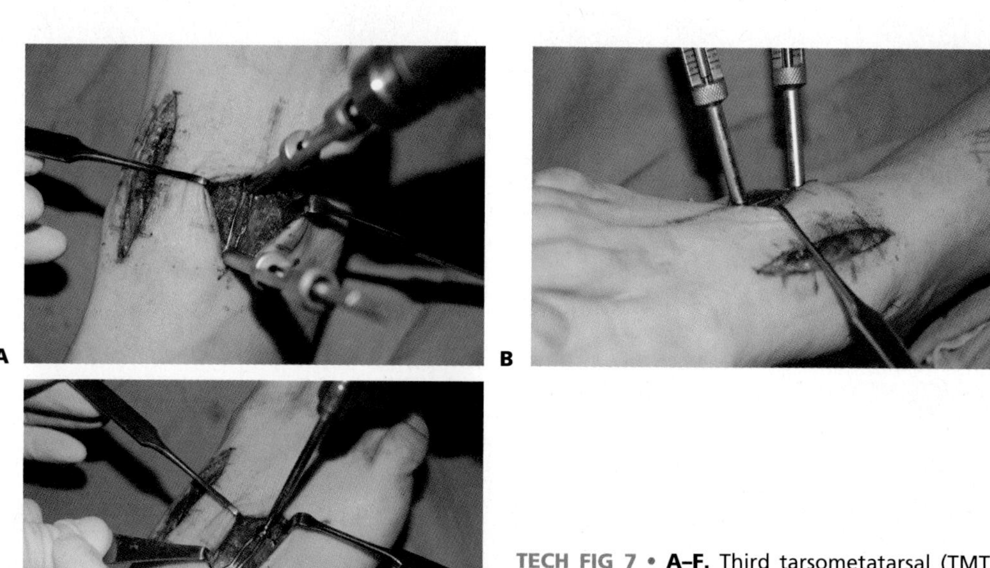

TECH FIG 7 • **A–F.** Third tarsometatarsal (TMT) joint compression plate. **A.** Plate positioned. **B.** Locking screws placed (surgeon must be sure plate is flush with the bone before locking the plate). **C.** View from medial side to show drill towers. *(continued)*

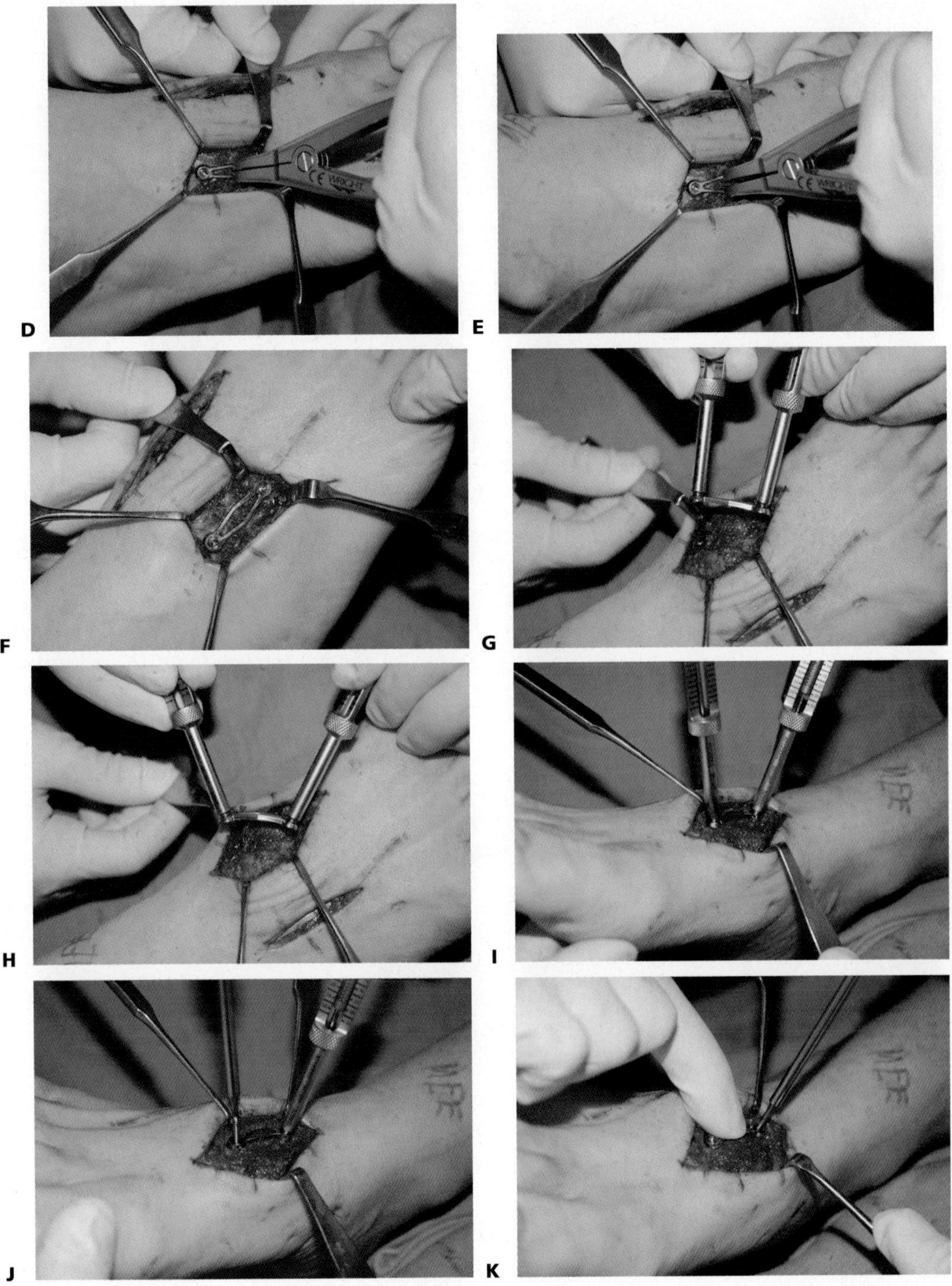

TECH FIG 7 • *(continued)* **D.** Compression device placed. **E.** Plate in position, now being compressed. **F.** Final plate position. **G–M.** Second TMT joint compression plate. **G.** Plate before contouring. **H.** Plate after contouring to match second TMT joint. **I.** Plate positioned, screw holes drilled. **J.** Locking screw being inserted. **K.** Surgeon must be sure that plate is flush with bone before fully seating the locking screws. *(continued)*

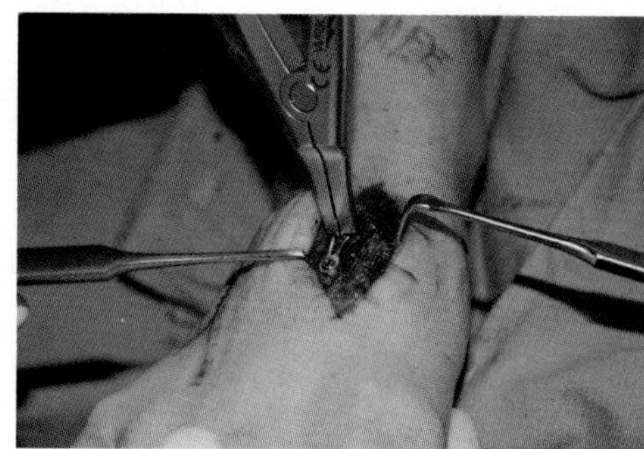

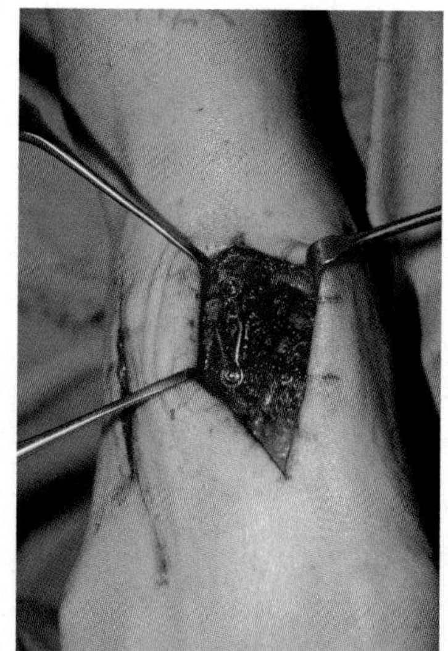

TECH FIG 7 • *(continued)* **L.** Compression device. **M.** Final plate position.

   - Precontouring the plate also prevents dorsiflexion (TECH FIG 7G–M).
- Intraoperative fluoroscopy of the construct confirms reduction and that dorsiflexion has been avoided (TECH FIG 8).
- The hardware is often close to the deep neurovascular bundle (TECH FIG 9A).
- I routinely use a drain for this procedure (TECH FIG 9B).
- Follow-up radiographs suggest satisfactory reduction. The patient had some residual lateral column symptoms, so I opted to add a subtalar arthroereisis implant to correct hindfoot alignment and perhaps unload some lateral column stress. Fortunately, that was a satisfactory solution in this case (TECH FIG 10).
   - The first through third TMT articulations have little physiologic motion, so arthrodesing them leaves little functional deficit.
   - To avoid loss of the midfoot's accommodative capacity, I rarely if ever fuse the lateral side.

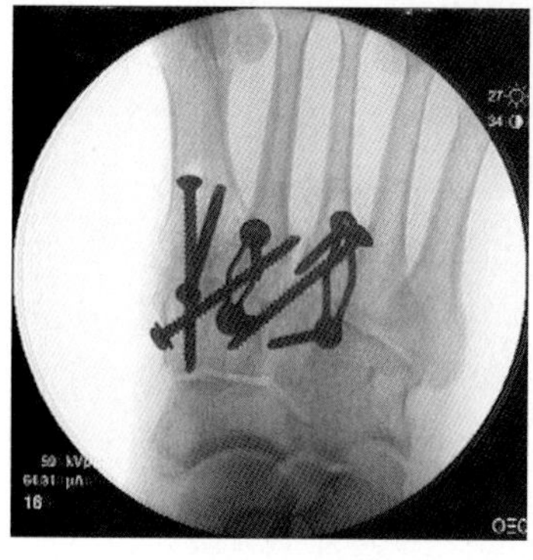

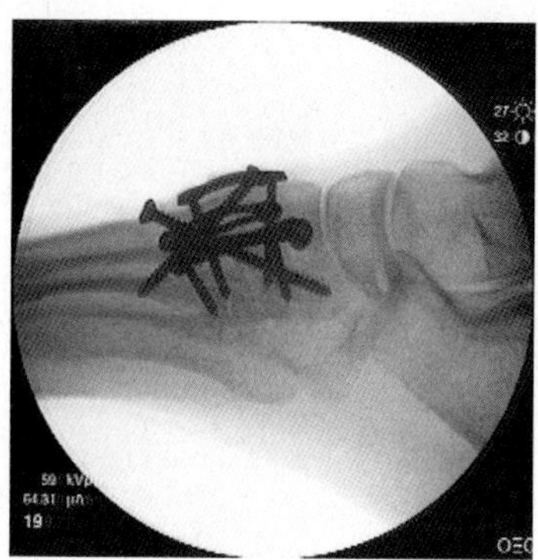

TECH FIG 8 • Fluoroscopic views of final construct. **A.** AP view. **B.** Lateral view. Note that first metatarsal is not elevated.

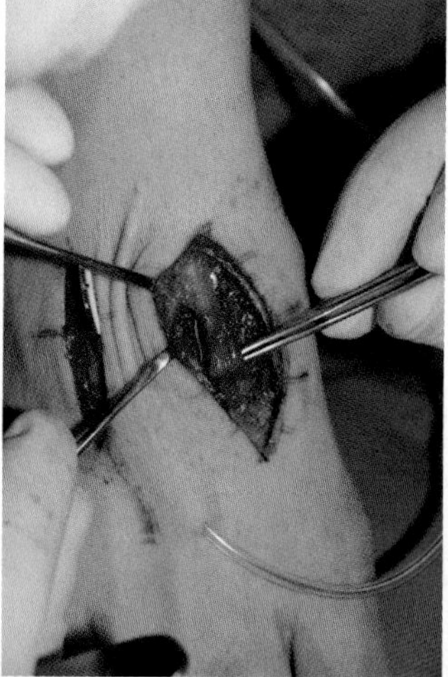

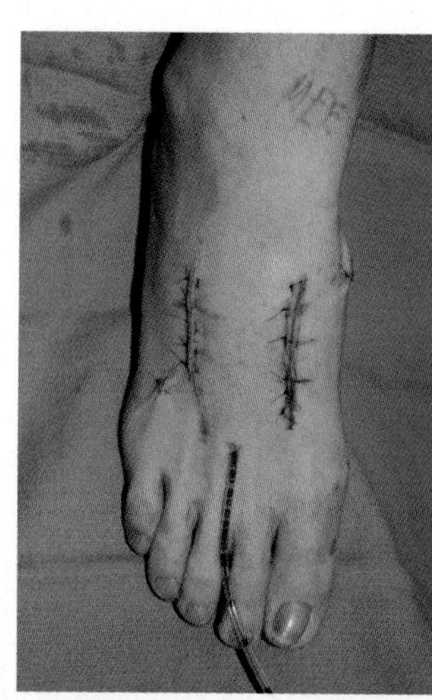

TECH FIG 9 • **A.** Deep neurovascular bundle intact but will lie directly on second tarsometatarsal (TMT) joint compression plate. Note use of a drain (my preference). **B.** Wounds closed without tension on skin bridge.

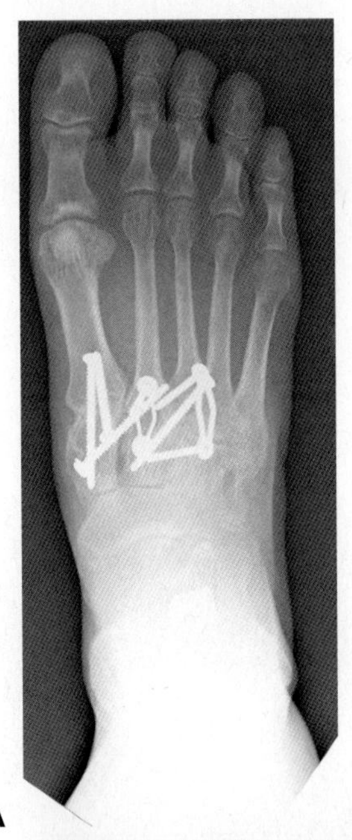

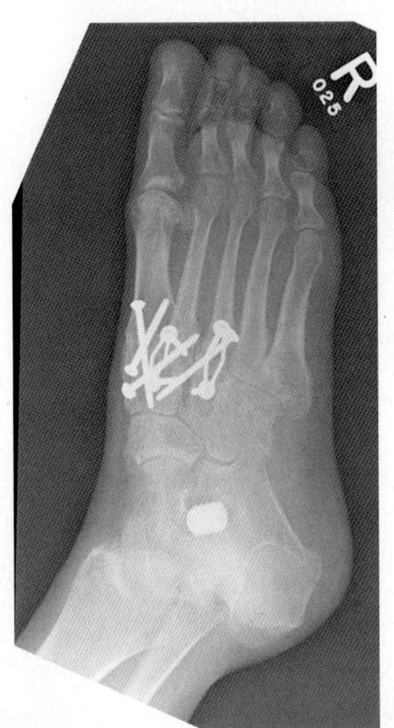

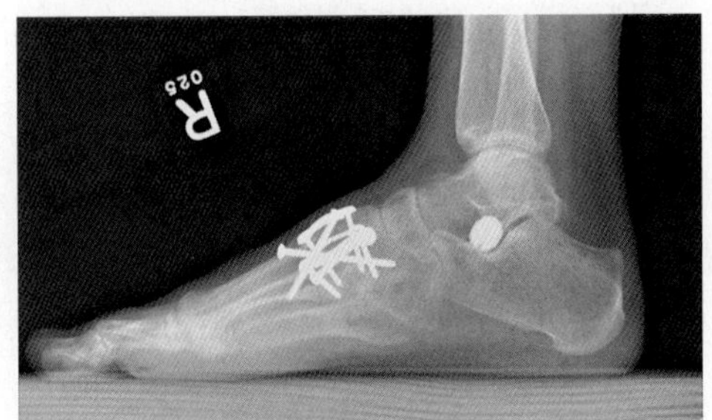

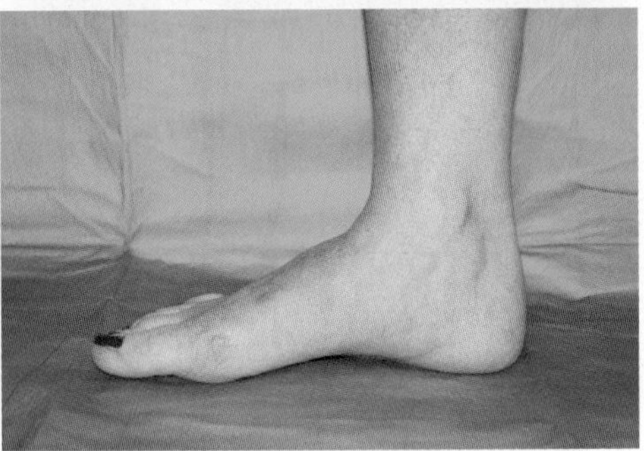

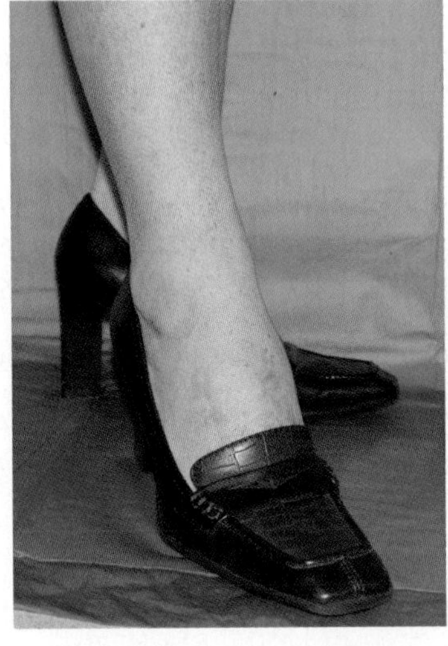

TECH FIG 10 • Final radiographs. **A.** AP view (note restoration of talo–first metatarsal axis). **B.** Oblique view. **C.** Lateral view (also with restoration of talar–first metatarsal axis). Note subtalar arthroereisis. This patient had some residual lateral foot pain and greater-than-physiologic hindfoot valgus, probably secondary to the injury to the cuboid. While subtalar arthroereisis does not address this directly, it reoriented the hindfoot adequately to relieve the lateral column stress. **D.** Clinical view of arch. **E.** The midfoot articulations normally have limited motion, so fusion of these joints does not restrict the foot substantially.

PLATE FIXATION WITH DEDICATED MIDFOOT PLATING SYSTEM

- More recently, midfoot-specific plating systems have been developed.
- This patient is a 48-year-old woman with midfoot Charcot neuroarthropathy failing bracing (TECH FIG 11). She had severe distortion of the midfoot anatomy and loss of the longitudinal arch.
- Approach
  - Medial midaxial approach to allow for medial plating (TECH FIG 12A–C)
    - Protect the tibialis anterior tendon.
    - However, should the tendon become detached, in my experience it can be sutured securely to the appropriate soft tissues during closure, and with prolonged immobilization to allow the midfoot to heal, the patient typically will retain full active dorsiflexion.
    - Joint preparation: Remove residual articular cartilage and penetrate the subchondral bone (TECH FIG 12D).
- Dorsal longitudinal approach
  - The deep neurovascular bundle is immediately deep to the extensor hallucis brevis tendon. The deep neurovascular bundle must be identified and protected throughout the procedure (TECH FIG 13).
  - Joint preparation: Often this is interesting, with the amount of distortion of the anatomy from the Charcot process.
  - Reduction: As for an acute Lisfranc fracture-dislocation, a bone reduction clamp from the first cuneiform to the base of the second or third metatarsal is helpful (TECH FIG 14). Once the reduction is confirmed fluoroscopically, provisional fixation can be placed.
- Medial plating (TECH FIG 15A-C)
  - Modern dedicated midfoot fusion plates have a contour that matches, for the most part, physiologic anatomy. If the plate fits well, then the reduction is typically acceptable.

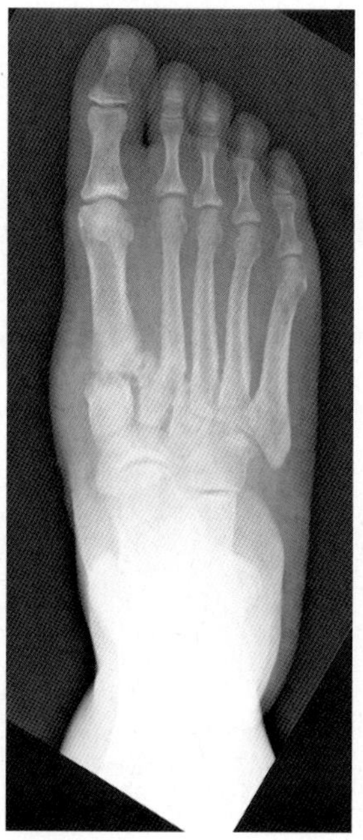

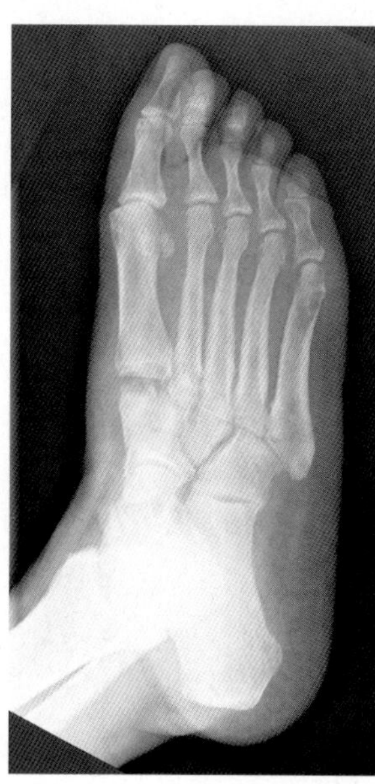

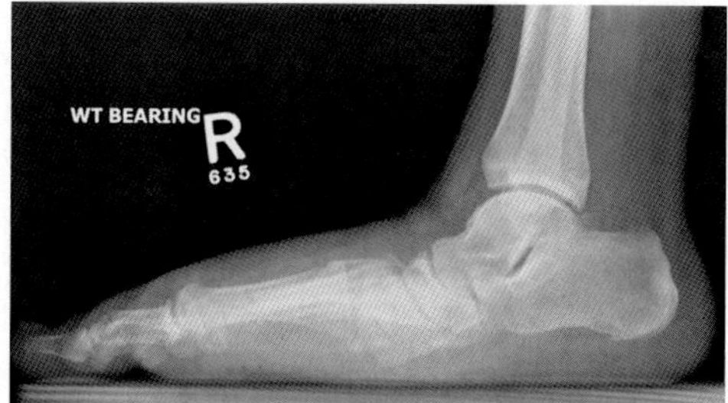

TECH FIG 11 • Preoperative weight-bearing radiographs of 48-year-old patient with midfoot Charcot neuroarthropathy. **A.** AP view. **B.** Oblique view. **C.** Lateral view.

- Also, if the plate is positioned properly on the first cuneiform, then the first metatarsal can be reduced to the plate and the reduction is typically satisfactory.
- A lag screw can be added to the medial column construct, but often there is little room for such a screw and the plate, unless a headless screw is placed deep to the plate.

- Dorsal plating (**TECH FIG 15D–G**)
  - Dedicated dorsal plating systems are now also available. These locking plates secure the first through third TMT joints.
  - Alternatively, individual plates may be used on each TMT joint; however, in my opinion, if a single plate can be used to stabilize all three TMT joints, the construct tends to be stronger.
  - With the distortion of anatomy from Charcot neuroarthropathy, these plates designed for physiologic anatomy sometimes are difficult to place perfectly on all three TMT joints.
  - Take care to protect the deep neurovascular bundle (in neuropathy, obviously the artery only matters) and the extensor tendons.
- Follow-up radiographs for the same patient (**TECH FIG 16**)

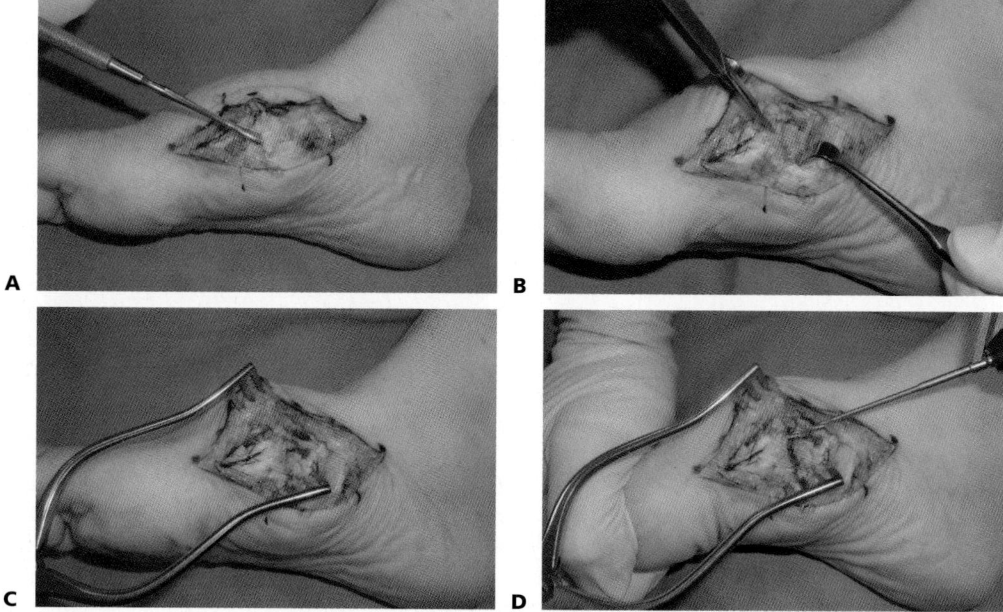

TECH FIG 12 • Direct medial midaxial approach. **A.** Exposure. **B.** Reflecting tibialis anterior tendon to expose first tarsometatarsal joint. **C.** Full exposure. **D.** After removing residual cartilage, subchondral bone is drilled to promote fusion.

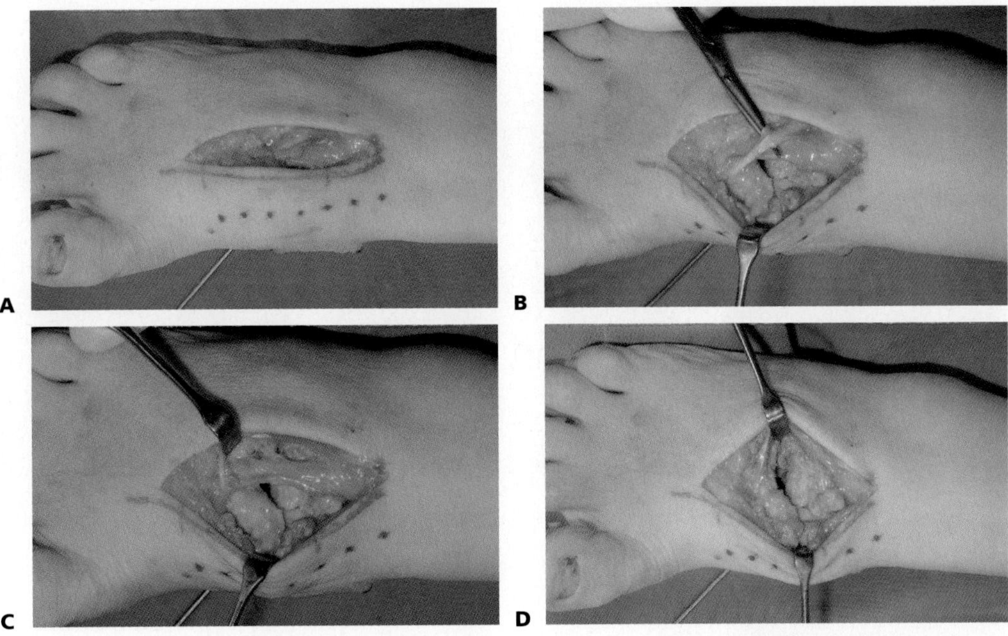

TECH FIG 13 • Dorsal approach. **A.** Approach. **B.** Extensor hallucis brevis (EHB) tendon directly over deep neurovascular bundle. **C.** EHB tendon retracted to expose deep neurovascular bundle. **D.** Neurovascular bundle protected and second and third TMT joints exposed to prepare for arthrodesis (note eccentric joint deformity secondary to Charcot neuroarthropathy).

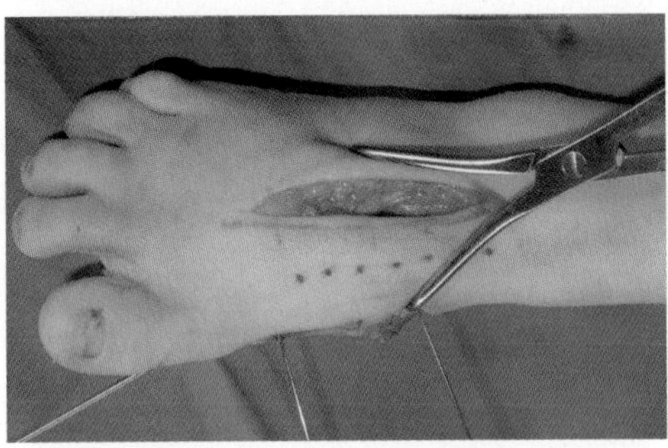

TECH FIG 14 • Bone reduction clamp used to reduce medial and middle columns of the foot after joint preparation (and bone grafting) performed.

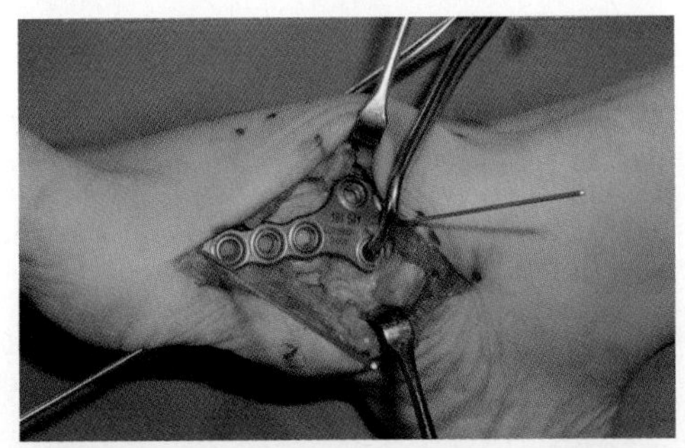

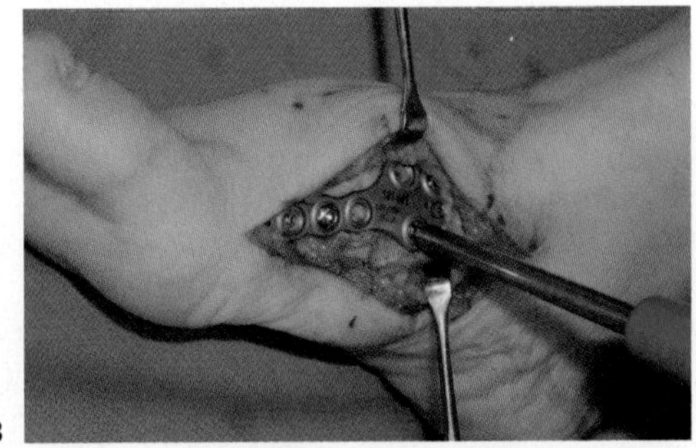

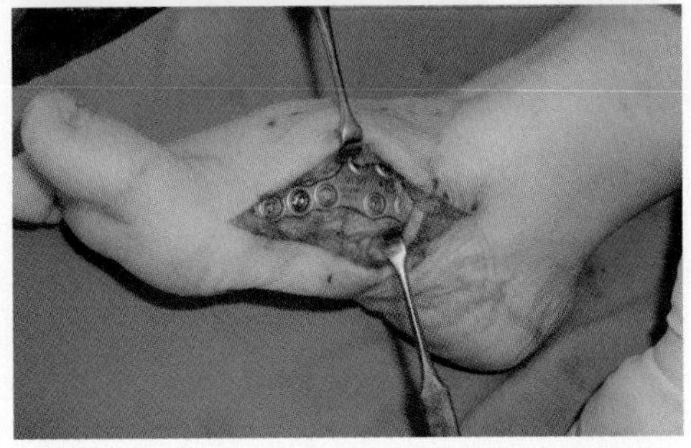

TECH FIG 15 • **A–C.** Medial plate. The plate is designed to restore physiologic alignment; therefore, it may be used as a reduction tool. Occasionally I fix the plate to the first cuneiform and then "bring" the first metatarsal to the plate. *(continued)*

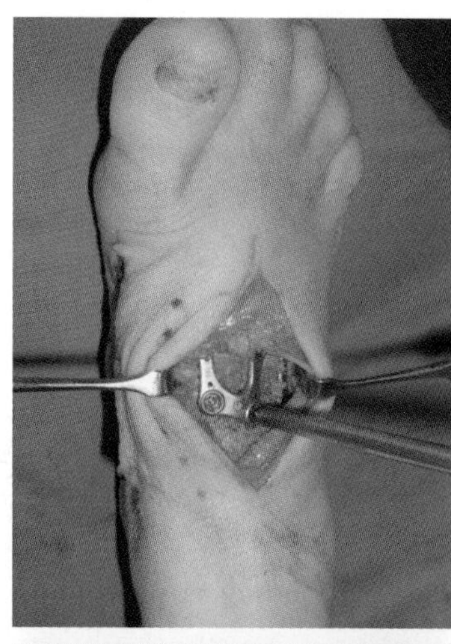
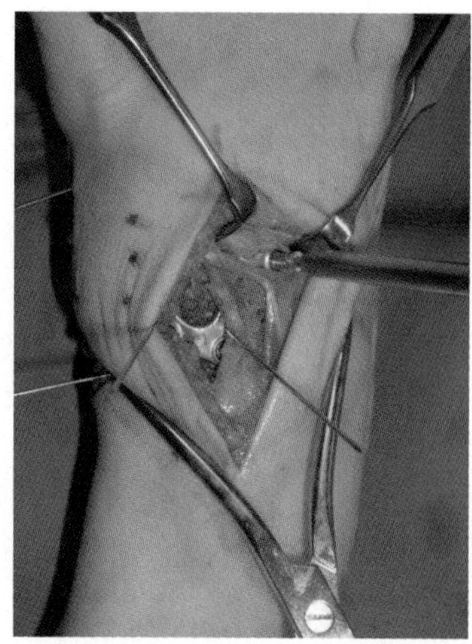
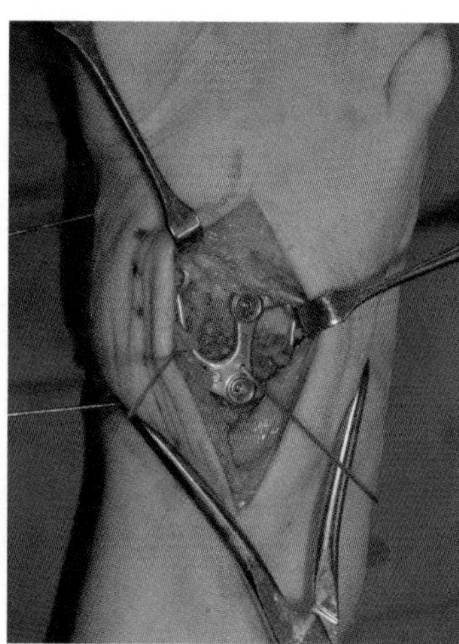
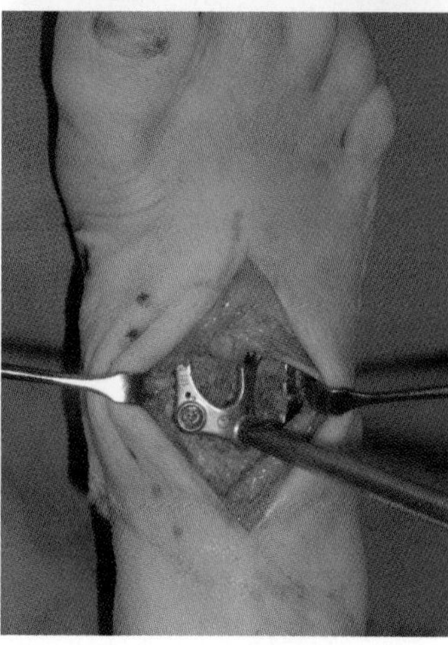

TECH FIG 15 • *(continued)* **D–G.** Dorsal plate. The plate extends from the first tarsometatarsal (TMT) joint to the third TMT joint, so it must be carefully positioned under the deep neurovascular bundle and the extensor tendons.

- In this case of Charcot neuroarthropathy and dislocation of the fourth and fifth TMT joints, I opted to also arthrodese the lateral column.
- Only in this situation of neuroarthropathy do I attempt to fuse the lateral column. Typically, I do not wish to sacrifice the midfoot's ability to accommodate.

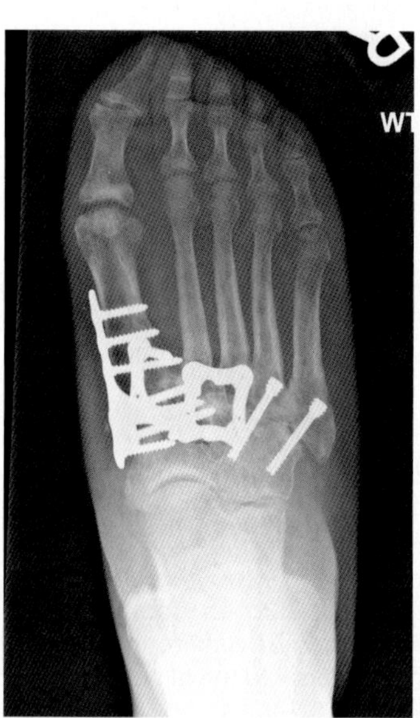
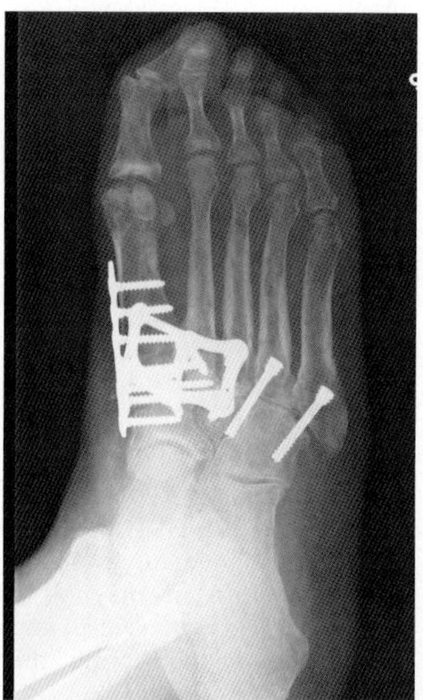
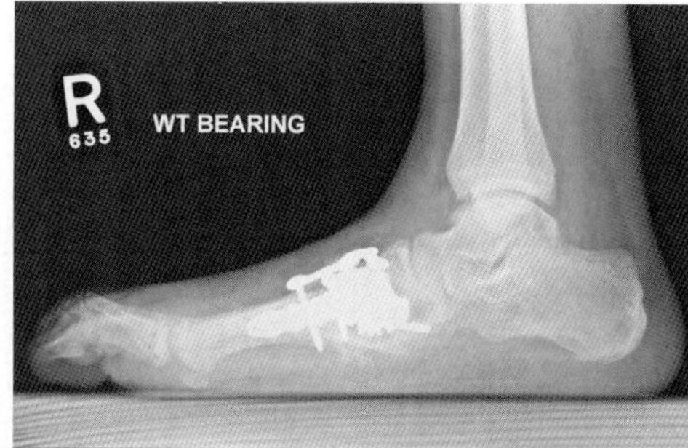

TECH FIG 16 • Follow-up radiographs. **A.** AP view. **B.** Oblique view. **C.** Lateral view. In this patient with Charcot neuroarthropathy, the lateral column of the foot was also arthrodesed. I do not routinely arthrodese the lateral column but make an exception in select cases of Charcot neuroarthropathy where added stability may be needed for preoperative 4-5 tarsometatarsal joint dislocation.

EXTERNAL FIXATION

- This patient is a 44-year-old woman with midfoot sag and forefoot abduction deformity failing nonoperative treatment (**TECH FIG 17**).
- Medial approach for midfoot biplanar osteotomy. Two reference pins serve to mark the desired osteotomy (confirmed fluoroscopically) (**TECH FIG 18**).
- Saw positioned for planned osteotomy; however, to maintain stability of the foot, I routinely apply the external fixator first and then complete the osteotomy (**TECH FIG 19A**).
- Application of the external fixator. In this case a "butt frame" construct is used.
- Hindfoot component
  - This portion of the frame stabilizes the hindfoot with two U-rings.
  - The frame is first secured with thin wires (**TECH FIG 19B,C**).
  - Next half-pins are added for further stability (**TECH FIG 19D**).
  - I usually tension the thin wires after the half-pins have been inserted. (**TECH FIG 19E,F**).
- Forefoot component
  - Add a partial ring to the forefoot and first stabilize it with three tensioned thin wires (**TECH FIG 19G**).
  - I typically add a half-pin to the forefoot–midfoot after I have performed the osteotomy and then know

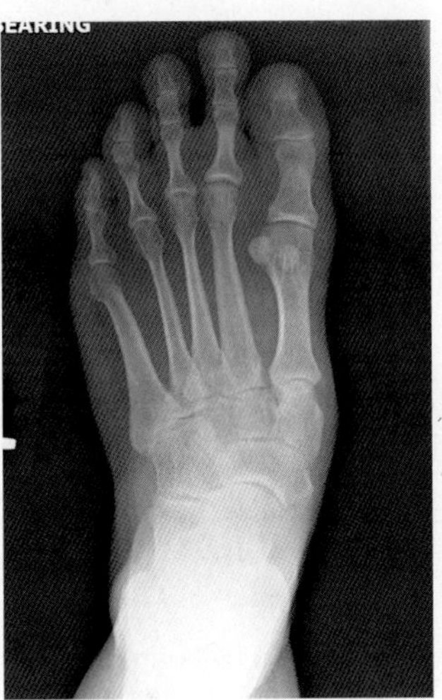

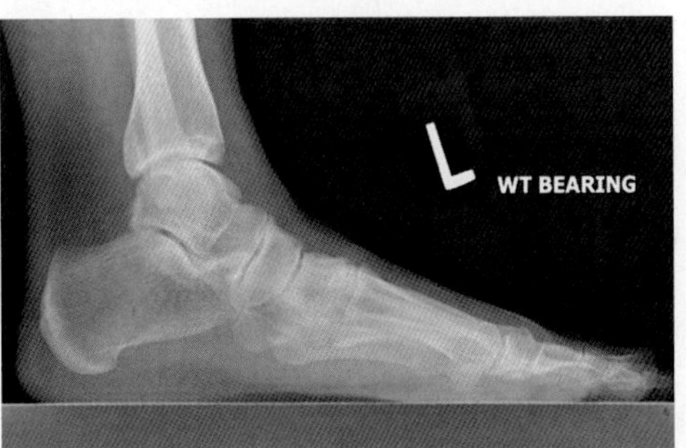

TECH FIG 17 • Preoperative weight-bearing radiographs of 44-year-old woman with midfoot deformity leading to forefoot abduction and midfoot sag, failing nonoperative measures. **A.** AP view. **B.** Lateral view.

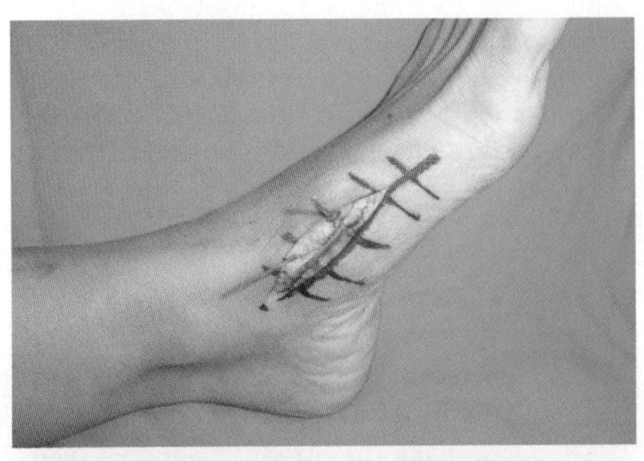

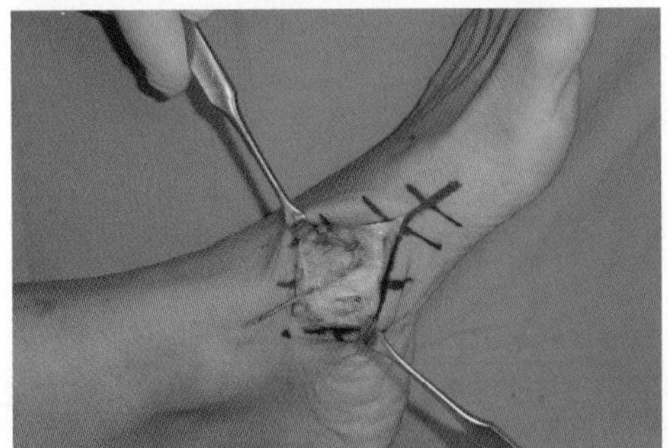

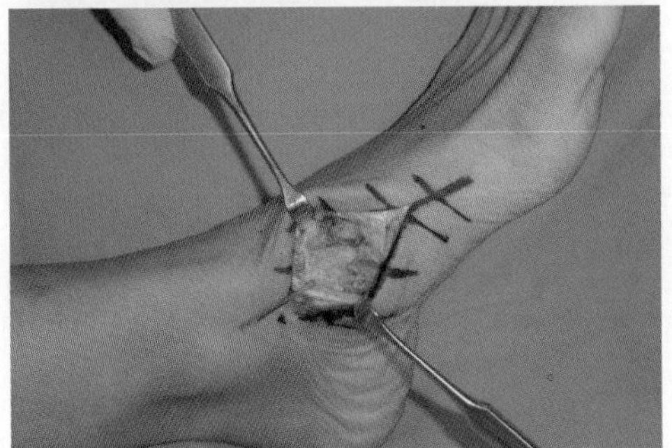

TECH FIG 18 • Medial midaxial approach. **A.** Exposure. **B.** Tibialis anterior tendon protected and guide pins in place to mark proposed midfoot biplanar osteotomy. **C.** Full exposure.

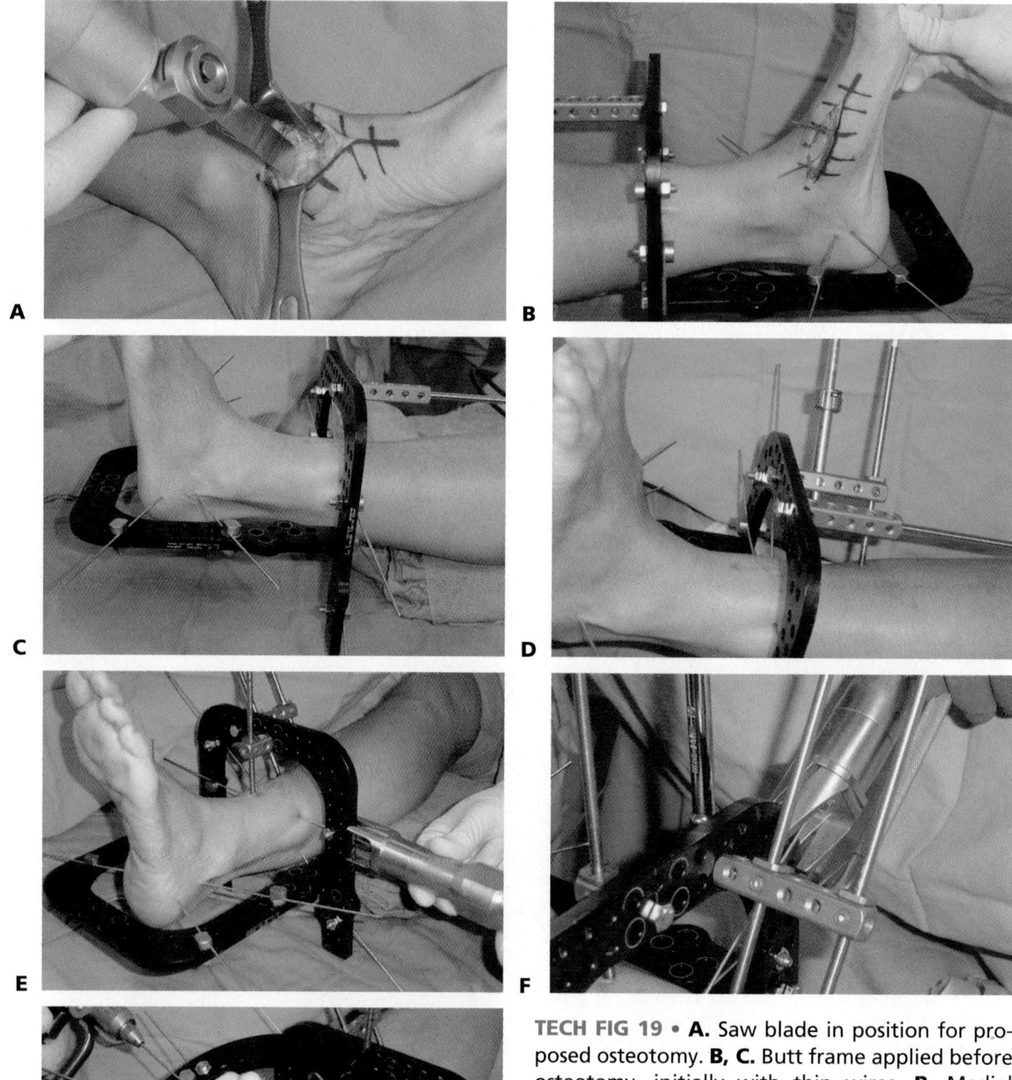

TECH FIG 19 • **A.** Saw blade in position for proposed osteotomy. **B, C.** Butt frame applied before osteotomy, initially with thin wires. **B.** Medial view. **C.** Lateral view. Note U-ring like a stirrup in coronal plane to stabilize hindfoot. Attached to this is second U-ring to provide further support in tibia. **D.** Frame stabilized further with half-pins from proximal U-ring into tibia. **E, F.** Tensioning thin wires. **G.** Applying the forefoot ring, primarily with tensioned thin wires, but I routinely add one small-diameter half-pin to augment the ring's stability.

exactly where the struts connecting the forefoot to the hindfoot rings will be positioned.

- Midfoot osteotomy
  - I use an oscillating saw, but a Gigli saw may be used as well (TECH FIG 20A).
  - I create a biplanar wedge with a medial and plantar base to correct abduction and promote plantarflexion in order to recreate the arch.
  - I complete the osteotomy with an osteotome (TECH FIG 20B).
  - Remove the wedge of bone (TECH FIG 20C).
  - The osteotomy can then be closed (TECH FIG 20D,E).
    - If it should not close congruently, protect the soft tissues, place the saw in the osteotomy, close the osteotomy as much as possible, and run the saw gently to remove any irregularities. This trick tends to make the osteotomy appose well.
  - Through this osteotomy, the forefoot may also be derotated.
    - I often "spin" the forefoot out of varus, a common forefoot deformity associated with a flatfoot.
- Place the struts to connect the hindfoot frame to the forefoot ring (TECH FIG 20F–I).
  - Add compression. With the system's computer program, further correction can be added now or even postoperatively.
  - I routinely reduce the deformity as much as possible intraoperatively, always ensuring appropriate bony

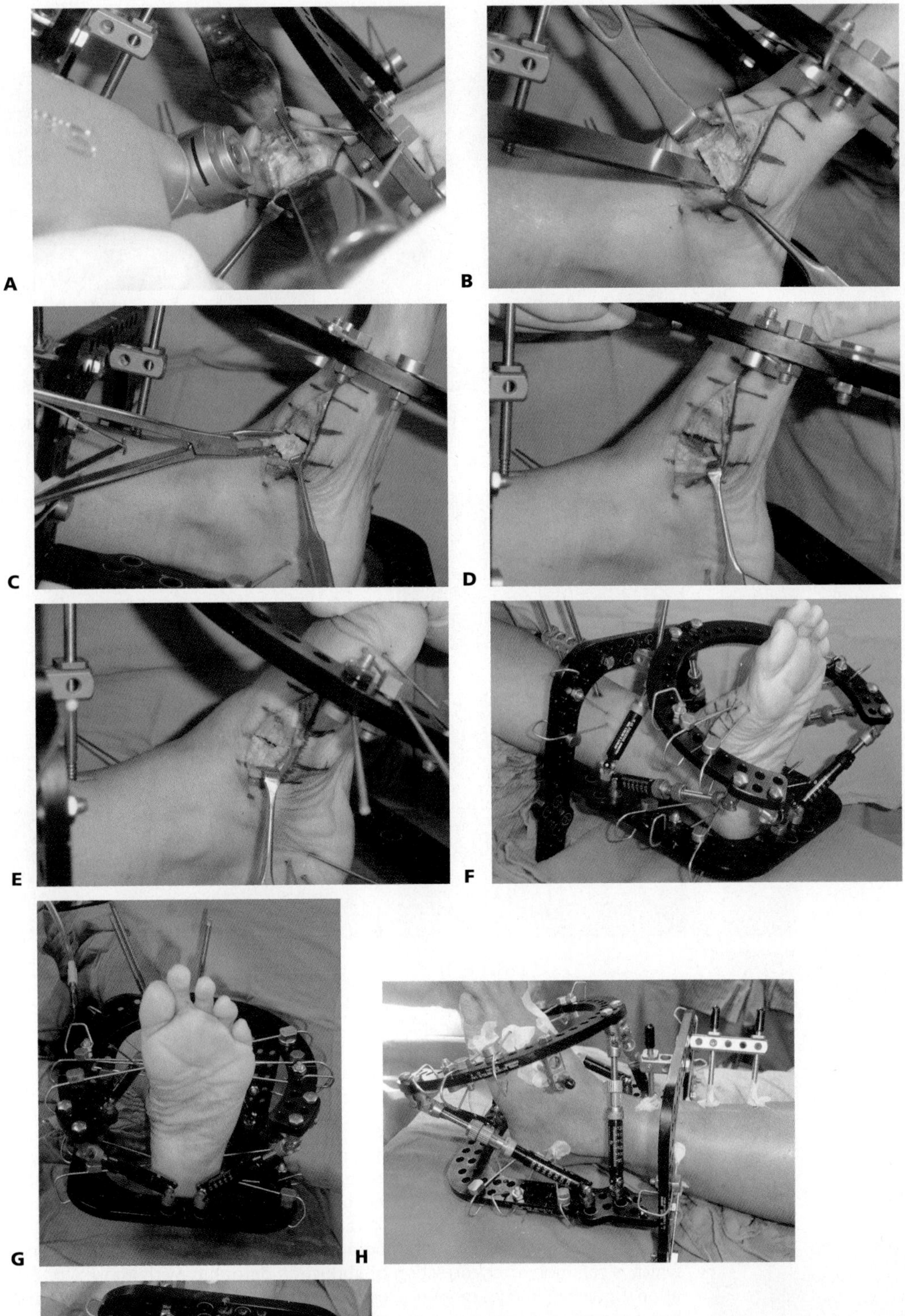

A B C D E F G H

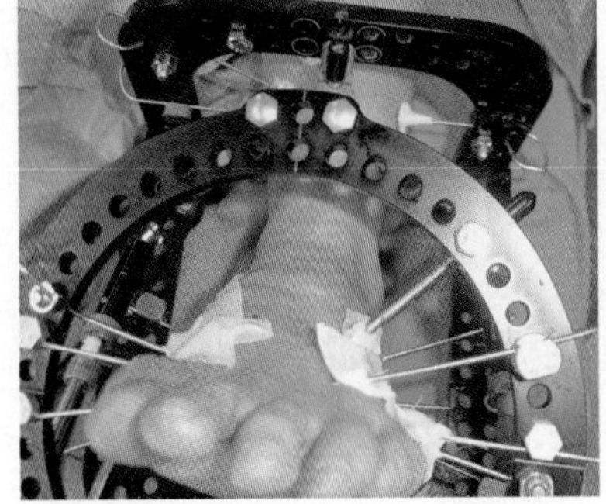

I

TECH FIG 20 • **A–C.** Midfoot biplanar osteotomy at planned osteotomy site after application of external fixator (butt frame). **A.** Saw cut. **B.** Completion of osteotomy with an osteotome. **C.** Removal of bone wedge with a rongeur. **D, E.** Reducing the deformity. **D.** Osteotomy open. **E.** Osteotomy closed medially and plantarly. **F, G.** Frame in place, with struts attached and osteotomy compressed. **F.** Medial view. **G.** Plantar foot view, demonstrating recreation of the arch and correction of abduction deformity. **H, I.** Dressings placed on wires and pins. Note the half-pin added to dorsolateral forefoot. **H.** Lateral view. **I.** AP view.

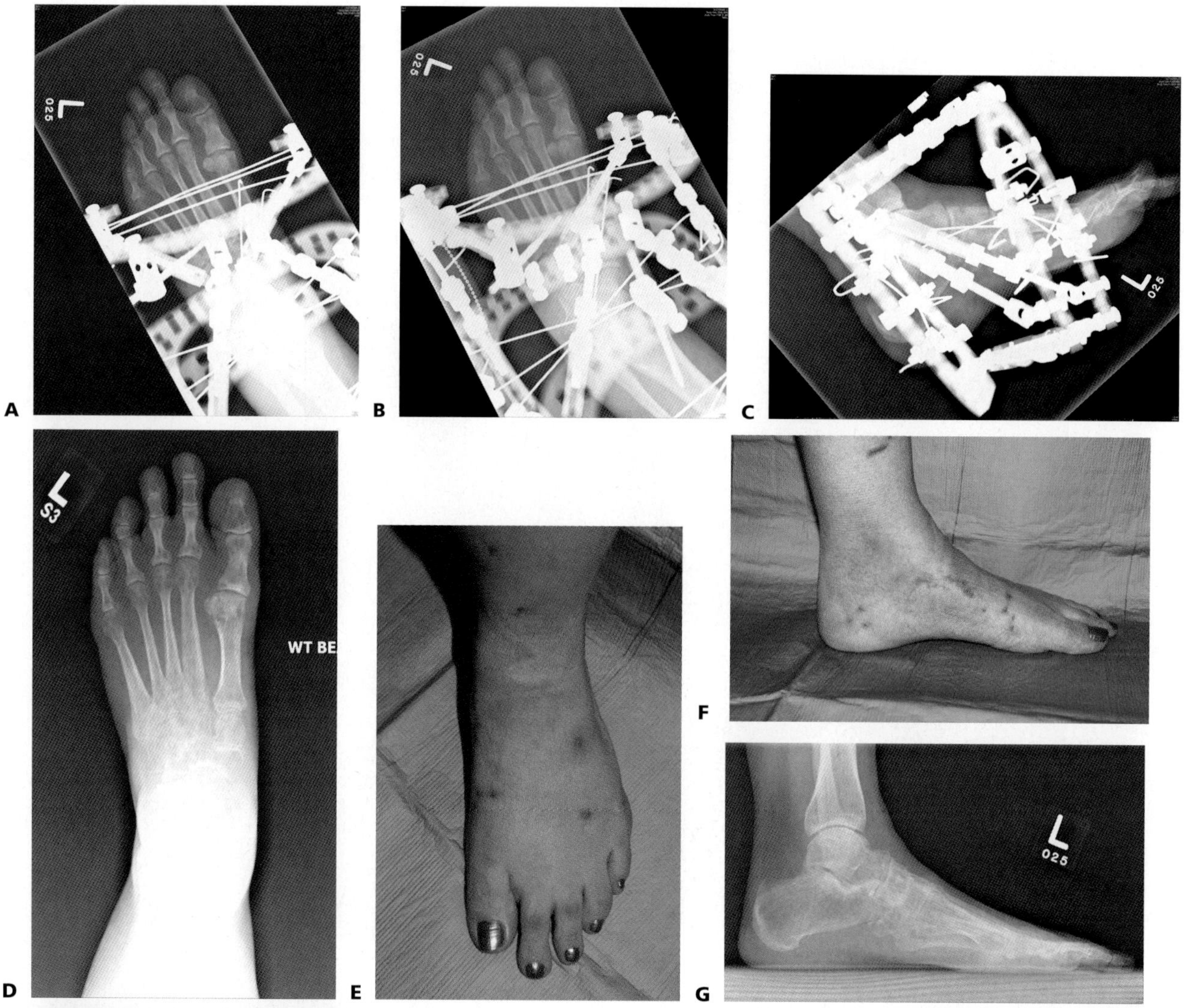

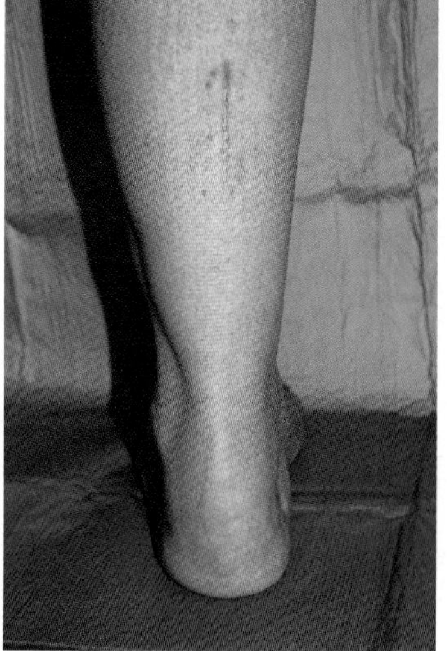

TECH FIG 21 • **A–C.** Postoperative radiographs. **A.** AP view. **B.** Oblique view. **C.** Lateral view. Note supplemental wires placed across osteotomy site for initial stabilization. With external fixation, further correction and compression may be performed after the index procedure. **D, E.** Clinical and radiographic follow-up after external fixator removal. **D.** Weight-bearing AP radiograph. **E.** Clinical view. The first ray appears short, which is common after correction of abduction deformity with internal or external fixation. However, in my experience, provided the first ray is adequately plantarflexed and bears weight, the foot functions well with little risk of transfer metatarsalgia despite a relatively long second metatarsal. **F–H.** Clinical and radiographic follow-up after external fixator removal. **F.** Lateral clinical view. **G.** Lateral weight-bearing radiograph (note restoration of arch). **H.** Hindfoot clinical view (note healed incision for gastrocnemius-soleus recession).

apposition at the arthrodesis site, and then compress further to promote stability and healing.

- Follow-up radiographs with frame in place are shown in **TECHNIQUE FIGURE 21A–C**.
- Final follow-up after frame removal is shown in **TECHNIQUE FIGURE 21D–H**.
- Often, after flatfoot correction for midfoot collapse, the first ray may appear short.
- In my experience, as long as I plantarflex the first ray adequately and avoid dorsiflexion of the medial column, transfer metatarsalgia is rarely a problem.

ADDITIONAL CASE

- This 32-year-old man had undergone open reduction and internal fixation of a Lisfranc fracture-dislocation and subsequent hardware removal at an outside institution (**TECH FIG 22**). He had failed further nonoperative measures.
- I performed a midfoot medial column plantar plating in combination with middle column dorsal plating after attempted deformity correction (**TECH FIG 23**).
- Follow-up radiographs (**TECH FIG 24**) show that while his longitudinal arch appears corrected, his forefoot still remains in abduction, and he remains symptomatic.
- Further nonoperative care failed.
- Re-revision surgery was performed.
  - Medial biplanar wedge osteotomy after hardware removal (**TECH FIG 25A–C**)

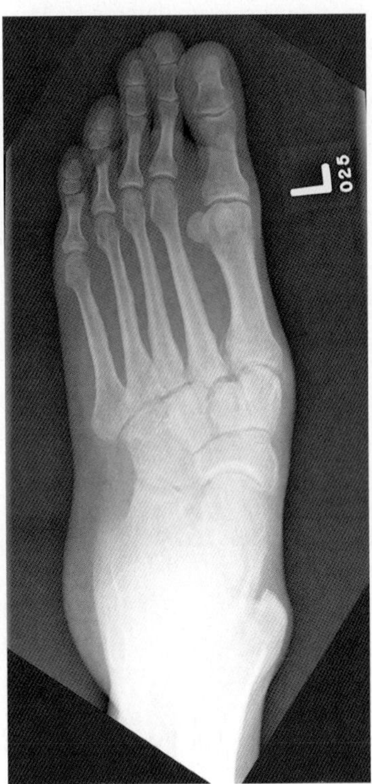

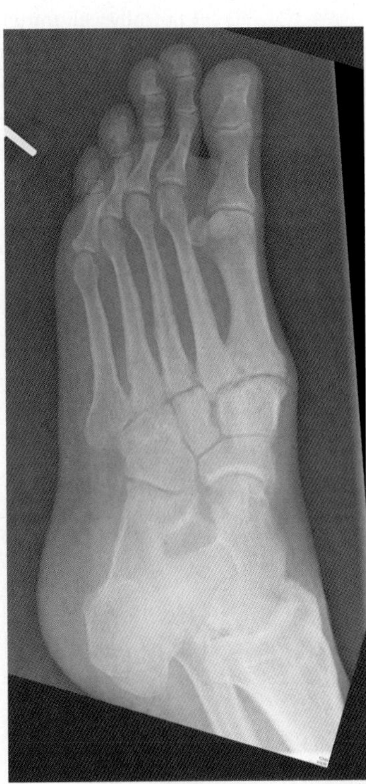

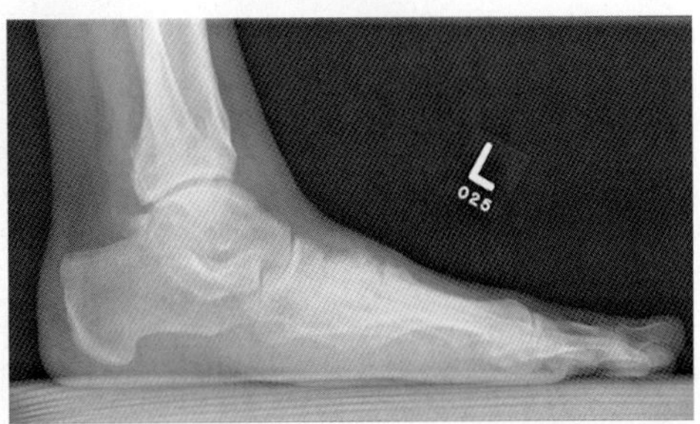

TECH FIG 22 • Preoperative weight-bearing radiographs of a 32-year-old man with chronic Lisfranc fracture-dislocation that had undergone prior open reduction and internal fixation of the injury and subsequent hardware removal. **A.** AP view. **B.** Oblique view. **C.** Lateral view.

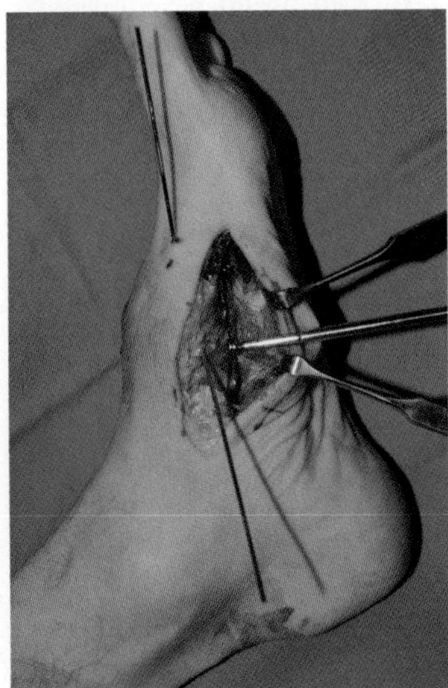

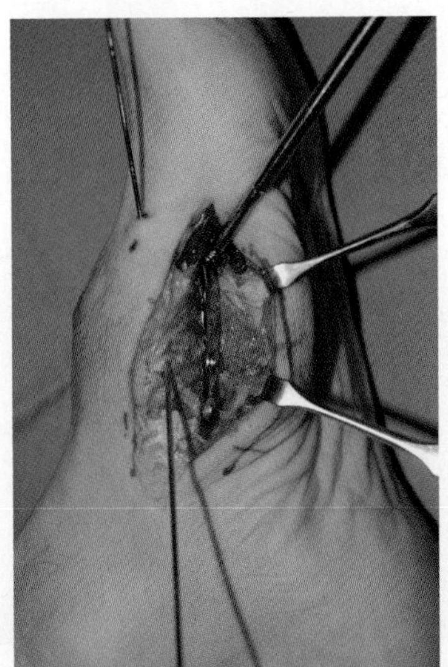

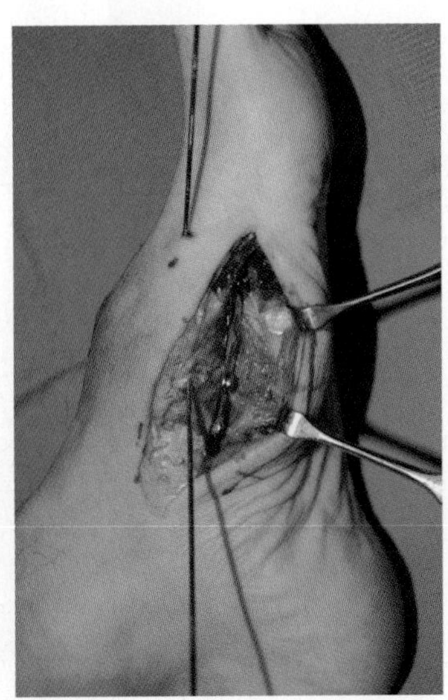

TECH FIG 23 • Revision surgery with medial plantar plating and middle column plating through dual longitudinal approaches after attempted reduction of severe abduction deformity and midfoot collapse. **A–C.** Screw fixation of medial column plantar plate. Note provisional wire fixation. *(continued)*

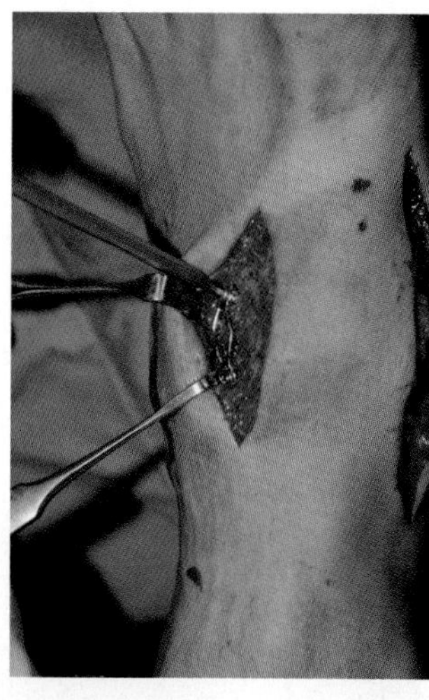

TECH FIG 23 • *(continued)* **D.** Dorsal approach to middle column for compression plating.

- Further correction of abduction deformity and more plantarflexion to the medial column
- I was able to reuse the plantar plate (**TECH FIG 25D,E**).
- I performed two adjunctive hindfoot procedures:
  - Medial displacement calcaneal osteotomy (**TECH FIG 25F**)
  - Subtalar arthroereisis (**TECH FIG 25G**)
- Follow-up weight-bearing radiographs suggest improved alignment, particularly with respect to the talo–first metatarsal axis in the AP plane (**TECH FIG 26A,B**).
- Clinically, alignment and function were improved. In fact, he has perhaps better alignment in his operated foot than his contralateral foot (remains to be seen if this is advantageous, but anecdotally appears to be the case) (**TECH FIG 26C–E**).

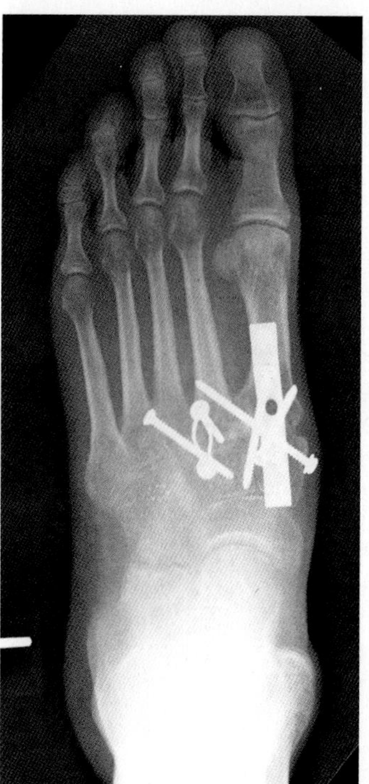

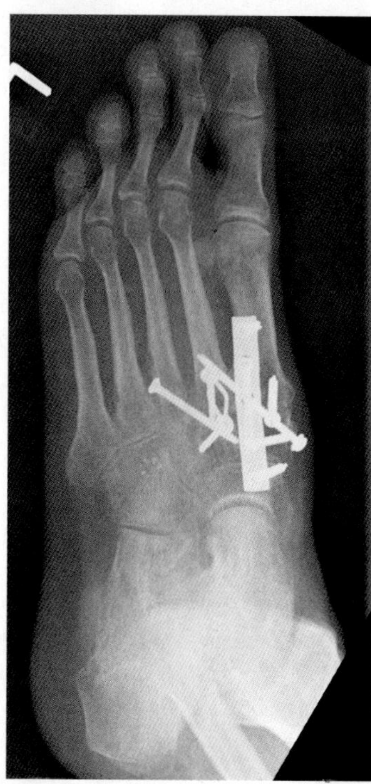

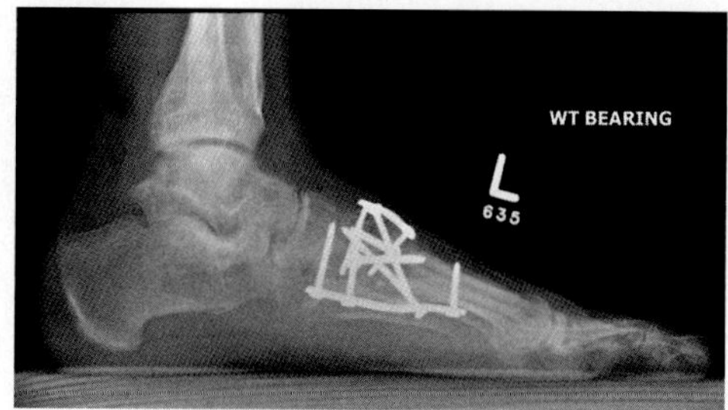

TECH FIG 24 • Follow-up weight-bearing radiographs. While arch is restored, forefoot abduction is incompletely corrected. **A.** AP view. **B.** Oblique view. **C.** Lateral view. Patient was improved but remained symptomatic and failed orthotic management.

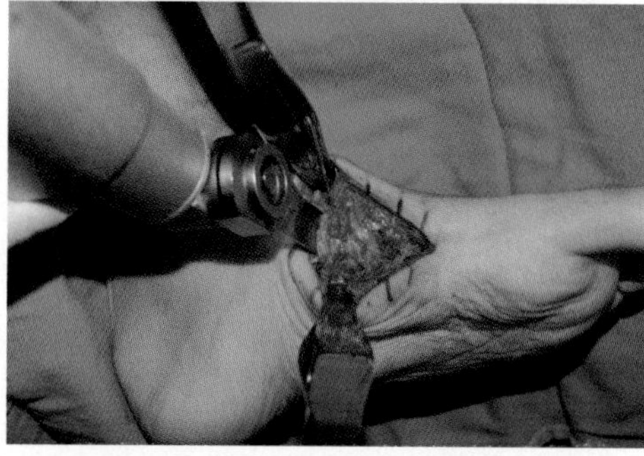

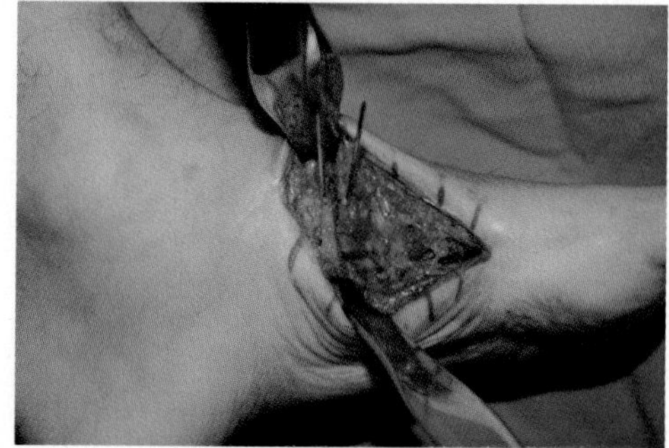

TECH FIG 25 • **A–C.** Re-revision surgery with removal of plantar plate and medial approach biplanar midfoot osteotomy to correct residual abduction deformity and promote even further plantarflexion of the medial column. **A.** Saw to create biplanar osteotomy along reference pins marking proposed osteotomy. **B.** Wedge resected. *(continued)*

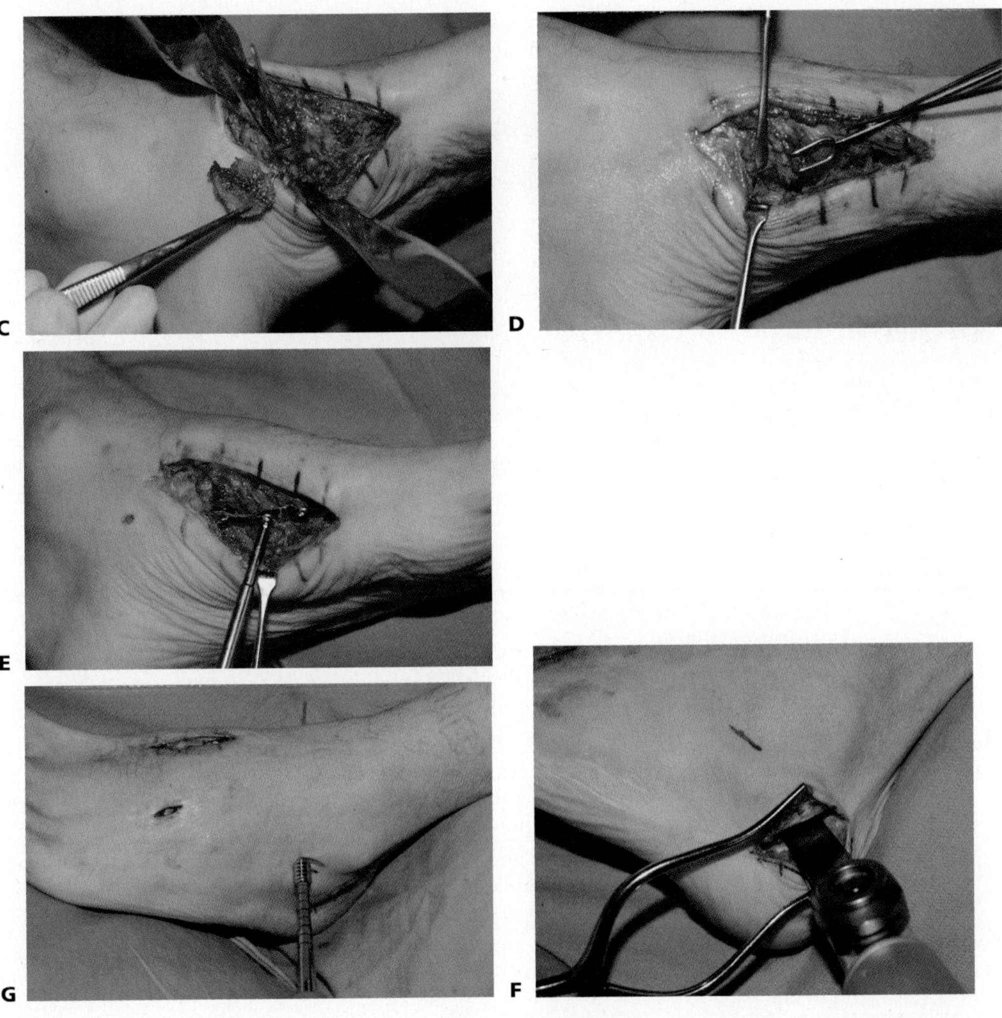

TECH FIG 25 • *(continued)* **C.** Wedge removed. **D.** Deformity reduced. **E.** Plantar plate reapplied. **F, G.** Supplemental hindfoot correction. **F.** Medial displacement calcaneal osteotomy. **G.** Subtalar arthroereisis.

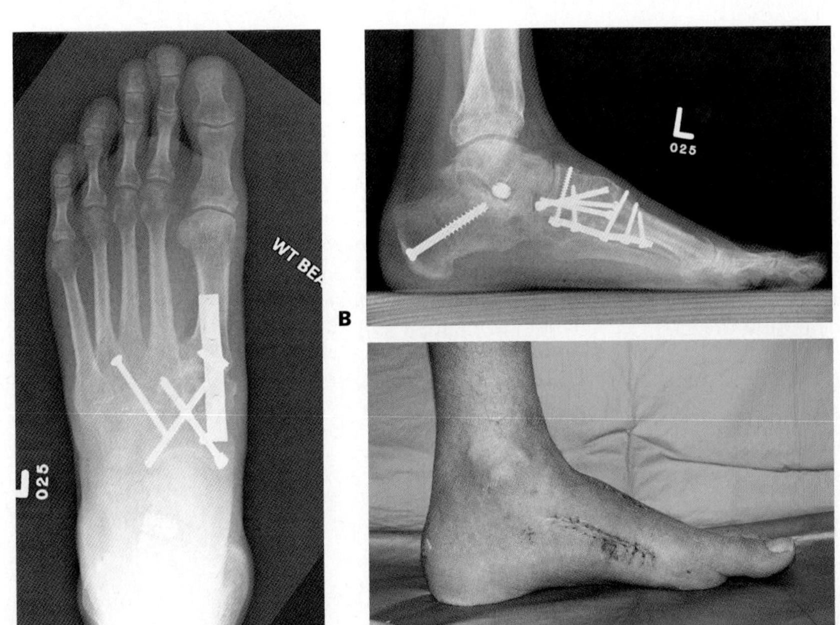

TECH FIG 26 • **A, B.** Follow-up weight-bearing radiographs. **A.** AP view (note correction of abduction) and near-anatomic restoration of congruent talo–first metatarsal axis. **B.** Lateral view, also with restoration of talo–first metatarsal axis. **C–E.** Clinical follow-up. **C.** Lateral view. *(continued)*

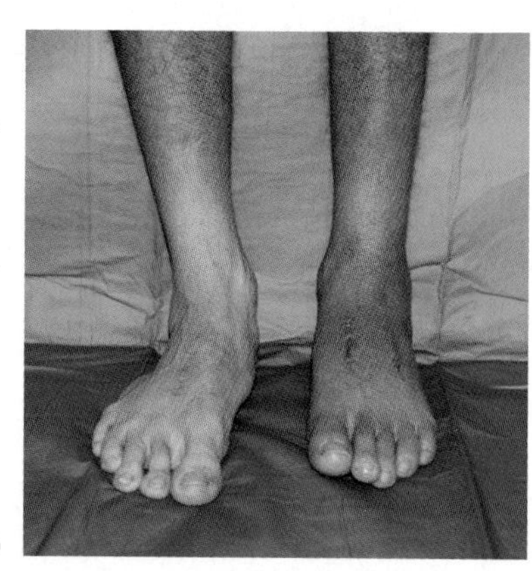

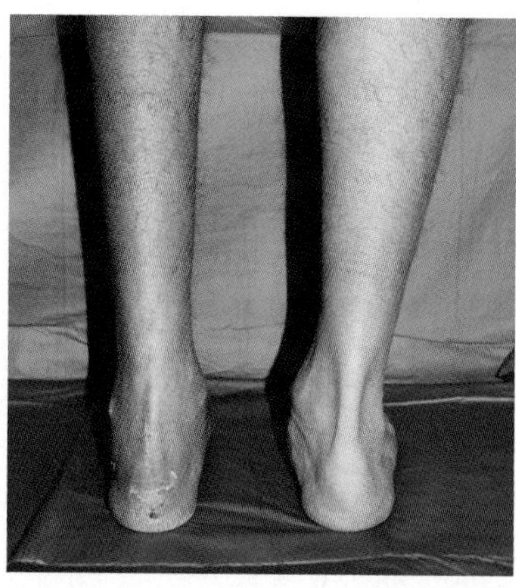

TECH FIG 26 • *(continued)* **D.** AP view. **E.** Hindfoot view. Operated foot is in a more physiologically normal position than contralateral foot.

PEARLS AND PITFALLS

Deformity correction	▪ Realign talo–first metatarsal axis in both the AP and lateral planes; undercorrection rarely leads to satisfactory outcome.
TMT joint anatomy	▪ The TMT joints are quite deep (2.5 to 3.0 cm).
Avoid dorsiflexion or elevated malpositioning	▪ Be sure to prepare the TMT joints to their bases; leaving plantar bone and cartilage will lead to a dorsiflexion malunion. Also, do not take any dorsal bone from the TMT joints.
Correct abduction	▪ The physiologically normal medial aspect of the medial column of the foot is relatively straight; with severe midfoot deformity the first metatarsal must really be swung around to align anatomically; then the lesser metatarsals should follow.
Forefoot balance	▪ When arthrodesing the TMT joints be sure to check the relative position of the metatarsal heads. The first metatarsal head and sesamoids should be slightly plantar to the lesser metatarsal heads. Palpate this balance as the midfoot is provisionally stabilized.
Tricks to correcting abduction	▪ (1) In severe deformity avoid first metatarsal elevation and attempt to reduce the abduction deformity. Fix the plate to the medial aspect of the first cuneiform, then reduce the first metatarsal to the plate. ▪ (2) As for a reduction of a Lisfranc fracture-dislocation, use a large bone reduction clamp to reduce the base of the second metatarsal by spanning the course of the first cuneiform–second metatarsal base.

POSTOPERATIVE CARE

- A splint is used that extends beyond the toes with the ankle in neutral position for 2 weeks.
- The patient returns to the clinic at 2 weeks for suture removal and application of a short-leg cast with the ankle in neutral position. Touch-down weight bearing only is permitted.
- The patient returns to the clinic at 6 weeks for radiographs out of plaster (three views of the foot). If progression toward healing is suggested by radiographs, the surgeon should consider placing the patient in a cam boot, but still only touch-down weight bearing is permitted.
- At 10 weeks, the patient returns for repeat radiographs (weight bearing, three views of the foot).
- If progression toward healing is suggested radiographically, weight bearing is gradually added over 3 weeks, in the cam boot. Then, the patient gradually transitions into regular shoes. I often recommend a longitudinal arch support and a relatively stiff sole.
- If no progression toward healing is seen, the patient is returned to the boot, with limited weight bearing, and the boot is used for 3 to 4 weeks.

OUTCOMES

- There are limited level IV studies for midfoot arthrodesis, but there are reasonable functional outcomes and improvement in pain scores for midfoot arthrodesis based on the weak literature.
- Results are generally better when restoration of physiologically normal alignment is achieved.
- There are virtually no reported outcomes for modern dedicated midfoot plating systems.
- More information and higher-level evidence are needed.

COMPLICATIONS

- Undercorrection
- Overcorrection
- Infection
- Wound dehiscence
- Nonunion
- Malunion
  - Greater-than-physiologic elevation of one or more metatarsals
  - Imbalance of the metatarsal heads

REFERENCES

1. Coetzee JC, Ly TV. Treatment of primarily ligamentous Lisfranc joint injuries: primary arthrodesis compared with open reduction and internal fixation—surgical technique. J Bone Joint Surg Am 2007;89A (Suppl 2 Pt 1):122–127.
2. Ferris LR, Vargo R, Alexander IJ. Late reconstruction of the midfoot and tarsometatarsal region after trauma. Orthop Clin North Am 1995;26:393–406.
3. Greisberg J, Assal M, Hansen ST Jr, et al. Isolated medial column stabilization improves alignment in adult-acquired flatfoot. Clin Orthop Relat Res 2005;435:197–202.
4. Horton GA, Olney BW. Deformity correction and arthrodesis of the midfoot with a medial plate. Foot Ankle 1993;14:493–499.
5. Jung HG, Myerson MS, Schon LC. Spectrum of operative treatments and clinical outcomes for atraumatic osteoarthritis of the tarsometatarsal joints. Foot Ankle Int 2007;28:482–489.
6. Komenda GA, Myerson MS, Biddinger KR. Results of arthrodesis of the tarsometatarsal joints after traumatic injury. J Bone Joint Surg Am 1996;78A:1665–1676.
7. Raikin SM, Schon LC. Arthrodesis of the fourth and fifth tarsometatarsal joints of the midfoot. Foot Ankle Int 2003;24: 584–590.
8. Rammelt S, Schneiders W, Schikore H, et al. Primary open reduction and fixation compared with delayed corrective arthrodesis in the treatment of tarsometatarsal (Lisfranc) fracture dislocation. J Bone Joint Surg Br 2008;90B:1499–1506.
9. Sammarco VJ, Sammarco GJ, Walker EW Jr, et al. Midtarsal arthrodesis in the treatment of Charcot midfoot arthropathy: surgical technique. J Bone Joint Surg Am 2010;92A(Suppl 1 Pt 1):1–19.
10. Sammarco VJ, Sammarco GJ, Walker EW Jr, et al. Midtarsal arthrodesis in the treatment of Charcot midfoot arthropathy. J Bone Joint Surg Am 2009;91A:80–91.
11. Suh JS, Amendola A, Lee KB, et al. Dorsal modified calcaneal plate for extensive midfoot arthrodesis. Foot Ankle Int 2005;26: 503–509.
12. Toolan BC. Midfoot arthrodesis: challenges and treatment alternatives. Foot Ankle Clin 2002;7:75–93.
13. Vertullo CJ, Easley ME, Nunley JA. The transverse dorsal approach to the Lisfranc joint. Foot Ankle Int 2002;23:420–426.

Chapter 42

Percutaneous Midfoot Osteotomy With External Fixation

Bradley M. Lamm, Ahmed Thabet, John E. Herzenberg, and Dror Paley

ANATOMY AND PATHOGENESIS

- The midfoot extends from the midtarsal joint to the Lisfranc joint and connects the hindfoot and forefoot.[2,3] Normal gait requires complex synergetic actions between the joints of the hindfoot and midfoot.[6]
- Midfoot deformities can be either stiff or flexible and can present as uniplanar or multiplanar deformities.
- Midfoot deformities have a severe impact on the pedal biomechanics by altering weight-bearing forces and pedal alignment.

PATIENT HISTORY AND PHYSICAL FINDINGS

- Preoperative clinical examination and radiographs(**FIG 1**) are used to determine the degree and location of deformity.
- Clinical examination is critical with midfoot deformities for assessment of the joint range of motion, flexibility, and the degree of rotation deformity (supination and pronation).

SURGICAL TREATMENT

- The goal of surgical intervention is to restore pedal alignment, to allow proper transfer of weight from hindfoot to forefoot during gait, to decrease pain, and to re-establish functional gait without affecting adjacent joint motion.[2]
- Conventional midfoot osteotomies are limited, as acute deformity correction can cause neurovascular compromise and requires extensive exposure, retained hardware can increase risk of infection, and wedge resection can sacrifice normal joints and alter anatomic realignment.[5]
- In the literature, many types of osteotomies have been described for correction of midfoot deformities, each one designed to correct a specific deformity or condition.[2,3,7,8]
  - Cavus: Cole, Japas, and Akron osteotomies
  - Relapsed clubfoot and metatarsus adductus: medial opening cuneiform wedge and lateral closing cuboid wedge osteotomies
- We present a percutaneous midfoot Gigli saw osteotomy technique for correction of uniplanar and multiplanar midfoot deformities.
  - This unique percutaneous saw technique was first described in 1894 by Italian obstetrician Leonard Gigli.
  - A Gigli saw is a twisted stainless steel cable that is a very effective cutting surface when used in a reciprocating fashion against bone.[1]
- Our technique has several major advantages:
  - It is minimally invasive, which decreases the risk of soft tissue injury and infection and improves osseous healing by preserving the periosteum and soft tissues. It minimizes the soft tissue insult, which is essential for the multiply operated foot.
  - It is not limited by the magnitude of the deformity, spares joints and growth plates, and allows for ease of uniplanar or multiplanar deformity correction.
  - Gradual external fixation produces regenerated bone, which is preferred to bone resection. The bone resection can increase foot stiffness.
  - Gradual external fixation also allows for accurate anatomic realignment of the foot, which re-establishes normal ligament and muscle function.[4,5]

Preoperative Planning

- Radiographic planning determines the center of rotation angulation (CORA) of the midfoot deformity.[4]
- The level of the CORA, together with clinical examination and radiographic assessment to determine the degree and location of deformity, determines the correct osteotomy level.

Positioning

- The patient is placed in a supine position on a radiolucent table.

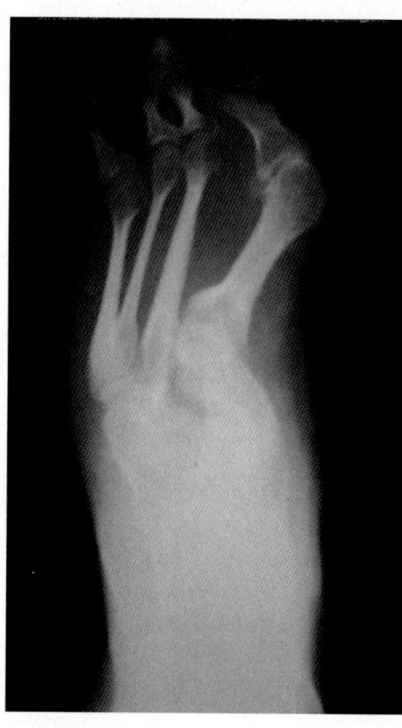

FIG 1 • Weight-bearing AP radiographic view shows a midfoot adduction deformity (35 degrees) in an adult patient with fibular hemimelia. In addition, she also has a hallux abductovalgus deformity. (Copyright 2008, Rubin Institute for Advanced Orthopedics, Sinai Hospital of Baltimore.)

- The leg is prepped just below a nonsterile thigh tourniquet, which allows for bending of the knee during surgery. The ability to flex the knee 90 degrees intraoperatively is advantageous in obtaining anteroposterior (AP) fluoroscopic imaging of the foot.
- A hemisacral bump is placed to obtain a foot-forward position.
- The patient is prepped and draped, and the tourniquet is elevated.

Approach

- Various levels of midfoot osteotomies can be performed (talocalcaneal neck or cuboid-navicular or cuboid-cuneiform bones) based on preoperative planning.
- The talocalcaneal neck osteotomy is used when the subtalar joint is stiff or fused.
- When the subtalar joint is a mobile, the level of the midfoot osteotomy is across the cuboid and navicular or cuboid and cuneiform.[4,5]

MIDFOOT OSTEOTOMY

- The midfoot osteotomy is performed before external fixation application or screw insertion.
- With the aid of fluoroscopy, the level of osteotomy is identified and marked (TECH FIG 1A).
- A 1.8-mm Ilizarov wire is placed on the foot under fluoroscopic guidance, and a marking pen is used to mark the exact level of the osteotomy on both the AP and lateral views.
- All midfoot osteotomies require four percutaneous transverse incisions.
- The first incision is made transversely at the plantar lateral border of the foot, and subperiosteal dissection with a periosteal elevator is performed across the plantar vault of the foot. This subperiosteal dissection creates a subperiosteal tunnel that protects the tendons and neurovascular bundle along the plantar aspect of the foot.
  - The periosteal elevator is then maneuvered in a rocking motion against the bone and across the entire plantar arch to the plantar medial foot (TECH FIG 1B).
- A second transverse incision is made where the skin is tented by the extension of the periosteal elevator, and the elevator is removed.
  - A no. 2 Ethibond suture is clasped with a curved tonsil hemostat and passed through the previously created subperiosteal tunnel from the lateral incision to the medial incision (TECH FIG 1C).
  - Once the suture is passed, the Gigli saw is tied to the suture and pulled from lateral to medial through in the same subperiosteal tunnel (TECH FIG 1D).
  - The position of the Gigli saw is checked by image intensifier to ensure that the level of osteotomy has been properly maintained.
  - Through the medial plantar incision, the periosteal elevator is passed across the dorsum of the foot subperiosteally below the tibialis anterior tendon so as to exit just lateral to this tendon.
- The third transverse incision is made lateral to the tibialis anterior tendon, where the elevator tents the dorsal skin.
  - The curved tonsil is then passed subperiosteally from the third incision to the second incision to clasp the Ethibond suture, which is pulled with the Gigli saw through the third incision (TECH FIG 1E).
  - Again the elevator is extended from the third incision across the dorsum of the foot laterally and subperiosteally below the extensor tendons to exit at the level just dorsal to the cuboid and the first incision.
- The fourth transverse incision is made where the elevator tents the lateral skin (TECH FIG 1F).
  - From the fourth to third incision, the curved tonsil grasps the suture attached to the Gigli saw and is pulled through the fourth incision.

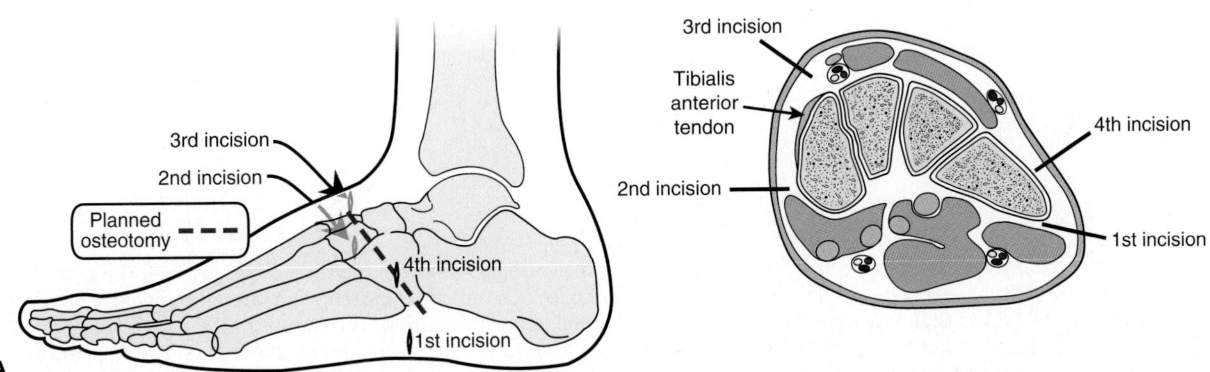

TECH FIG 1 • Percutaneous Gigli saw osteotomy of the midfoot. **A.** There are three levels in the midfoot at which a Gigli saw is passed percutaneously: the talocalcaneal neck, the cuboid-navicular bones, and the cuboid-cuneiform bones. The illustration shows a cuboid-cuneiform level osteotomy. Four small incisions are used to pass the saw: one medial plantar, one lateral plantar, and two dorsal incisions. *(continued)*

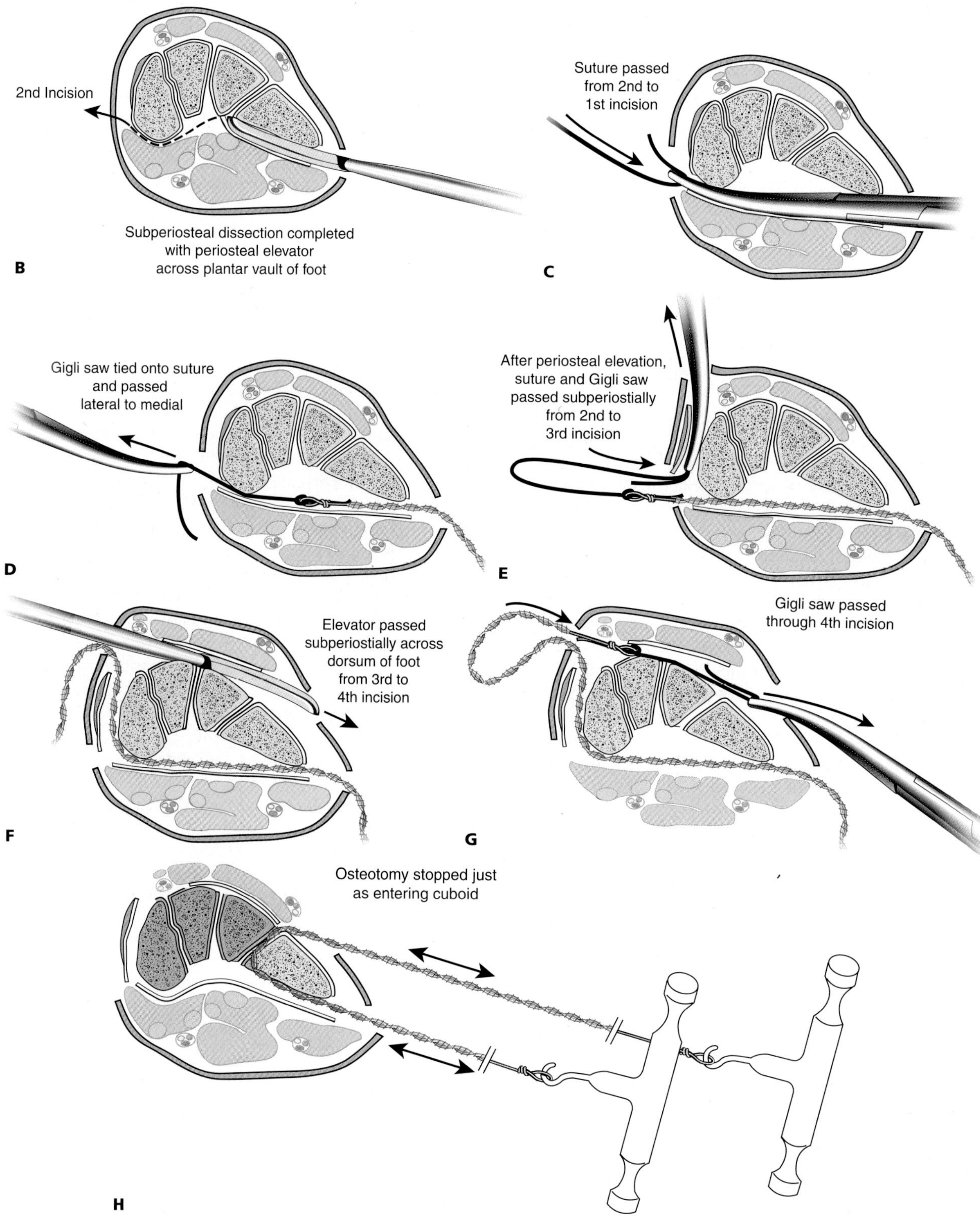

TECH FIG 1 • *(continued)* **B.** Because of the concavity of the transverse arch and the multiple bones present, the plantar periosteal elevation often weaves in and out of the subperiosteal space. **C.** A suture is passed from lateral to medial (the reverse can also be done). **D.** The Gigli saw is passed from lateral to medial under the foot. **E.** Through a third incision, which is made on the dorsomedial aspect of the foot, the suture and Gigli saw are passed to the dorsum of the foot. **F.** A fourth incision is made on the dorsolateral side, and the periosteum is elevated on the dorsum of the foot. **G.** The suture and Gigli saw are passed around the foot from plantar to dorsal, exiting on the dorsolateral side opposite the entrance site on the plantar lateral side. **H.** The bone is cut by the Gigli saw to the level of the cuboid. *(continued)*

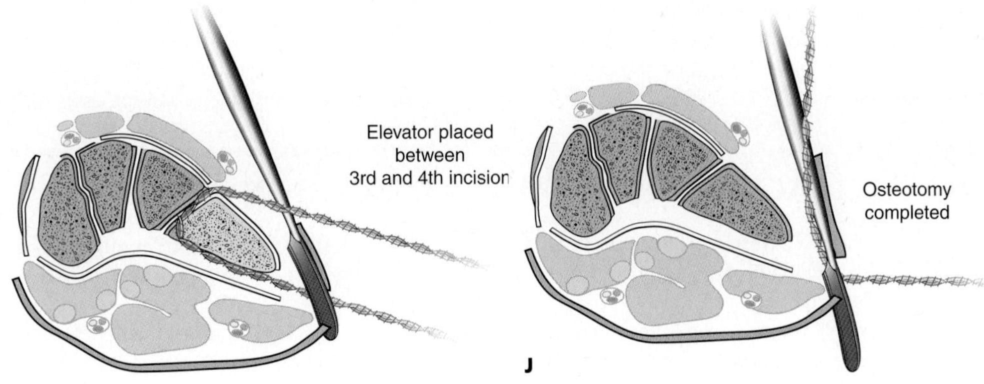

TECH FIG 1 • *(continued)* **I.** The lateral periosteal bridge is elevated and maintained to protect the skin crossing the Gigli saw. **J.** The cuboid bone is then cut, and the saw is cut and removed. (Copyright 2008, Rubin Institute for Advanced Orthopedics, Sinai Hospital of Baltimore.)

- The Gigli saw is now circumferentially around the bones of the midfoot (**TECH FIG 1G**). Care must be taken during the passage of the Gigli saw to maintain the correct level of the planned osteotomy.
- The two Gigli saw handles are now attached, and, using a reciprocating motion, the midfoot is cut from medial to lateral (**TECH FIG 1H**). The Gigli saw handles may need to be crossed while making the reciprocating cut to avoid lateral soft tissue injury.
- To avoid injury to the peroneal tendons and lateral skin, cutting is stopped just before the lateral bone is exited. A periosteal elevator is placed between the fourth and first incisions crossing the Gigli saw, and then the cut is continued (**TECH FIG 1I**).
  - When the cut is complete, the elevator will block further progression of the saw.
- After completion of the cut, the osteotomy is checked with the image intensifier.
- The Gigli saw is then cut and withdrawn from the foot (**TECH FIG 1J**).
- The tourniquet is deflated, and the incisions are closed.[4,5]

EXTERNAL FIXATION APPLICATION

- External fixation allows for gradual correction of deformity and lengthening, which can be accomplished by the Ilizarov external fixator or the Taylor spatial frame.
- Stirrup wires placed just proximal and distal to the midfoot osteotomy are used.
  - As a rule, forces tend to take the passage of least resistance, which in the foot are the joints and growth plates, so it is essential to add these two stirrup wires adjacent to each side of the osteotomy. Each wire is carefully inserted on either side of the osteotomy under fluoroscopic guidance (**TECH FIG 2**).
- Then proceed to build the frame according to the deformity, fixing the tibia, talus, calcaneus, and proximal midfoot with the proximal fixation block and the distal midfoot and forefoot with the distal fixation block.
- Finally, the stirrup wires are attached to the frame distally and proximally as appropriate.
- Stirrup wires do not need to be tensioned.
- Olive stirrup wires are used to limit osseous transverse plane deviation during gradual external fixation correction.

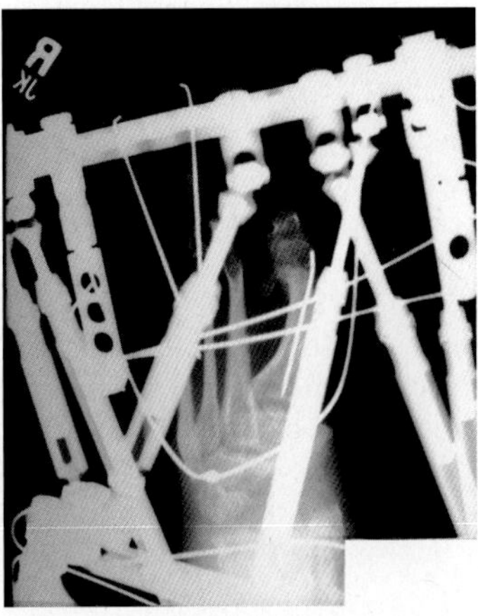

TECH FIG 2 • Opening medial wedge and normotrophic regenerate bone formation during distraction treatment of the patient in Figure 1 with the Taylor spatial frame. The stirrup wires are adjacent to the percutaneous midfoot Gigli saw osteotomy. A lateral olive wire is used to resist lateral forefoot translation during the distraction treatment. The hallux abductovalgus was acutely corrected. (Copyright 2008, Rubin Institute for Advanced Orthopedics, Sinai Hospital of Baltimore.)

ACUTE CORRECTION CONSIDERATIONS

- When performing a midfoot derotation (supination and pronation) correction, the medial muscle and fascia (abductor hallucis muscle) must be released from the osseous midfoot attachments.

- Wedge resection can be performed by using two separate Gigli saws passed simultaneously.
  - The distal cut is performed first, and the proximal cut is performed second.
  - Then the two medial percutaneous incisions are connected to remove the osseous wedge.
- Screw fixation, tension band wire, plates, staples, or static external fixation can also be used for fixation.

GRADUAL DISTRACTION THEN ACUTE CORRECTION

- When using the Ilivarov external fixator for small feet (pediatric patients), a valuable technique is gradual distraction then acute correction.
- Initial foot distraction for 2 or 3 weeks with external fixation is performed to disengage the bone segments and distract the soft tissue envelope.
- Then, under general anesthesia, the forefoot fixation is disconnected from the hindfoot frame and acute manipulation (derotation, angulation, or translation) of the forefoot is accomplished to achieve the correct position.
- The forefoot and hindfoot fixation is reattached in the corrected position and maintained until bone consolidation.
- This technique reduces the time the external fixator is needed.

PEARLS AND PITFALLS

Adjuvant procedures	▪ Adjuvant soft tissue procedures can be used with midfoot osteotomy to achieve full correction and address the associated deformities.
Flexion contracture	▪ Pinning of toes is done to avoid flexion contracture during distraction treatment. Digital pins should be attached to the foot frame, thereby increasing foot frame stability.
Tarsal tunnel decompression	▪ Tarsal tunnel decompression, either acute or gradual, should be considered for large deformity corrections. ▪ Acute corrections, patients with significant scarring, and posttraumatic foot injuries are all considerations for tarsal tunnel decompression. ▪ When the aforementioned situations are encountered, a prophylactic tarsal tunnel decompression is recommended.
Cavus deformity	▪ Plantar fascial release or partial or complete excision of the plantar fascia should be considered for cavus deformity correction.
Equinus contracture	▪ Gastrocnemius recession, gastrocnemius-soleus recession, or Achilles tendon lengthening should be performed for equinus contracture (either percutaneous or open) as deemed appropriate.
Proximal limb deformities	▪ Assess and correct if necessary.

OUTCOMES AND COMPLICATIONS

- We reviewed our series of midfoot deformities corrected with the percutaneous Gigli saw midfoot osteotomy and external fixation.
  - These patients achieved our goal of a plantigrade foot position with improvement in gait (**FIG 2**).
  - Minor complications included digital flexion contractures, which were treated by flexor tenotomy, and superficial pin tract infections, which were treated with oral antibiotics.
  - Major complications included premature consolidation, which required reosteotomy, and a tarsal tunnel syndrome, which developed during treatment and required surgical decompression.
- We also have performed a series of cadaveric midfoot Gigli saw osteotomies under fluoroscopy to determine the safety of this osteotomy.
- After completion of the osteotomy, the dissection revealed no neurovascular or tendon or muscle damage.

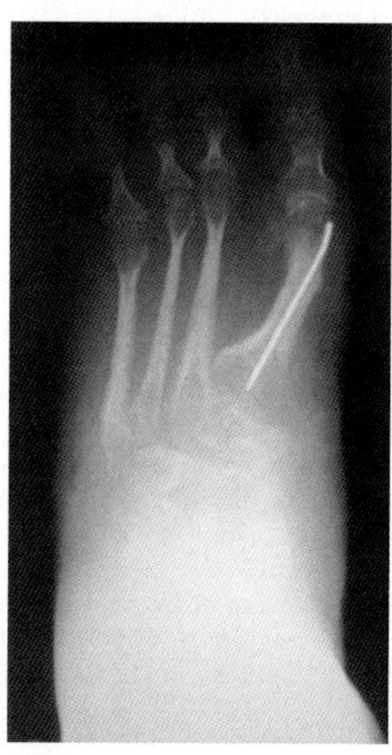

FIG 2 • Final weight-bearing AP radiographic view of the patient in Figure 1 and Techniques Figure 2 shows full correction of the adduction deformity (straight lateral border of the foot). (Copyright 2008, Rubin Institute of Advanced Orthopedics, Sinai Hospital of Baltimore.)

ACKNOWLEDGMENT

The authors thank Joy Marlowe, MA, for her excellent illustrative artwork and Alvien Lee for his photographic expertise.

REFERENCES

1. Brunori A, Bruni P, Greco R, et al. Celebrating the centennial (1894–1994): Leonard Gigli and his wire saw. J Neurosurg 1995;82: 1086–1090.
2. Conti SF, Kirchner JS, Van Sickle D. Midfoot osteotomies. Foot Ankle Clin 2001;6.
3. Dehne R. Osteotomy of the pediatric foot. Foot Ankle Clin 2001;6.
4. Paley D. Principles of Deformity Correction. New York: Springer, 2005.
5. Paley D. The correction of complex foot deformity using Ilizarov's distraction osteotomies. Clin Orthop Relat Res 1993;293:97–111.
6. Perry J. Gait analysis: Normal and Pathological Function. Thorofare, NJ: Slack, 1992.
7. Statler TK, Tullis BL. Pes cavus. J Am Podiatr Med Assoc 2005;95: 42–52.
8. Wilcox PG, Weiner DS. Akron mid tarsal dome osteotomy in the treatment of rigid pes cavus: a preliminary review. J Pediatr Orthop 1985;5: 333–338.

Chapter 43 Surgical Stabilization of Nonplantigrade Charcot Arthropathy of the Midfoot

Michael S. Pinzur

DEFINITION

- Charcot foot arthropathy is a destructive process that primarily affects the foot and ankle of patients with longstanding diabetes (10-plus years) and peripheral neuropathy (PN).[4,5,8]
- The resulting disabling deformity impairs walking, can be painful, and makes patients prone to develop overlying skin ulceration, leading to deep infection and eventual amputation. Outcome data derived from the AOFAS Diabetic Foot Questionnaire have revealed that Charcot foot arthropathy has a severe negative impact on health-related quality of life in affected individuals.[6]
- Historically, clinical management has been dictated by anecdotal observation, with little data that would stand up to current evidence-based medicine standards.
- Treatment has classically been passive and accommodative. Acute active-phase management has been accomplished with a non–weight-bearing total-contact cast until the active destructive phase has resolved. This has been followed by accommodative bracing with custom therapeutic shoes, accommodative foot orthoses, ankle–foot orthoses, and a special accommodative orthosis, the Charcot Restraint Orthotic Walker (CROW; **FIG 1**).
- Based on similar anecdotal observation and level IV scientific evidence, most recent publications in peer-reviewed literature recommend universal correction of deformity combined with arthrodesis.[7,14,22,23]
- This chapter will present an evidence-based algorithm for use in the management of Charcot foot arthropathy at the level of the midfoot.

ANATOMY

- The foot is a unique end organ adapted for weight bearing.
- The multiple linked small bones normally allow the uniquely durable soft tissue envelope of the plantar surface to be prepositioned to accept the load of weight bearing.
- The destructive process associated with Charcot foot arthropathy impairs the ability of this mechanism to orient the foot in an optimal position to take advantage of its durable soft tissue envelope.
- The ensuing deformity produces weight bearing through less durable tissues, leading to tissue failure, deep wound formation, destructive osteomyelitis, and systemic sepsis.

PATHOGENESIS

- The primary risk factor for the development of Charcot foot arthropathy is longstanding peripheral neuropathy as measured by insensitivity to 10 grams of applied pressure (**FIG 2**).
- While other causes of absence of protective sensation have been associated with the development of Charcot foot arthropathy, longstanding diabetes is present in well over 95% of affected individuals.
- The majority of diabetics who develop foot-associated morbidity are morbidly obese.[18] Glycemic management can be with insulin, oral medications, or diet. As with all of the morbidities associated with diabetes, the risk for foot-associated morbidity is decreased with tight glycemic management.
- Trauma appears to be an important inciting factor. The trauma can be significant, seemingly trivial, or due to repetitive mechanical stress.
- The neurotraumatic theory suggests that patients with longstanding PN and a loss of protective sensation develop a mechanical "stress" fracture. Due to the absence of protective sensation, they continue weight bearing, leading to a condition that mimics a hypertrophic nonunion.
- The neurovascular theory suggests that a vasomotor PN leads to high-flow arteriovenous shunting, causing bony depletion of calcium, leading to bone weakening and the well-known deformities.
- While the presence of sensory PN is well recognized, the accompanying motor and vasomotor neuropathies are often overlooked. The motor neuropathy affects the smaller nerves and muscles of the anterior leg (foot and ankle dorsiflexors) earlier in the disease process than the posterior leg compartments. This motor imbalance is currently appreciated as an

A

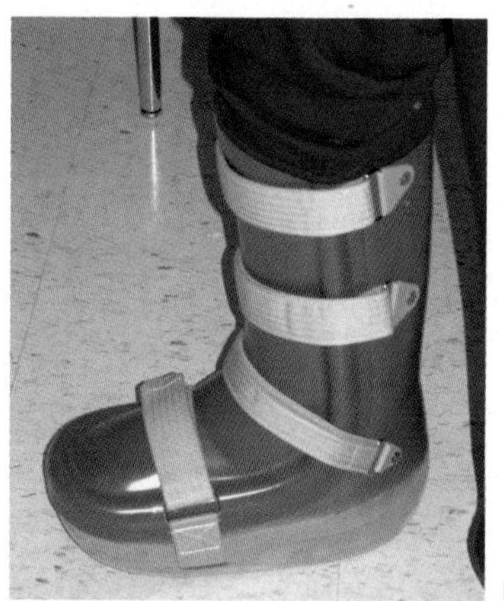

B

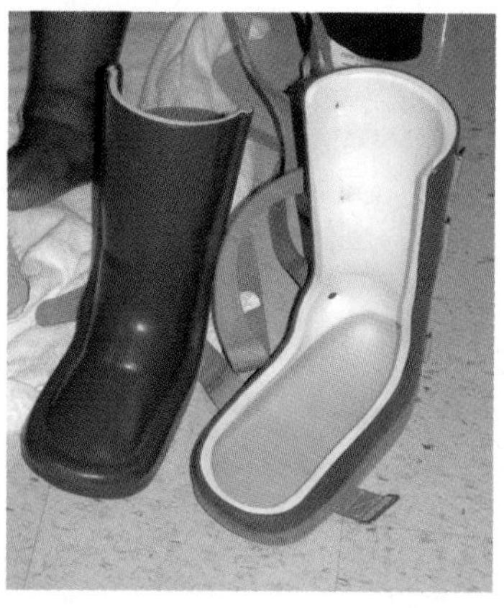

FIG 1 • Charcot Restraint Orthotic Walker (CROW). The custom-fabricated clamshell ankle–foot orthosis is lined with a pressure-dissipating material. It is designed to both optimize positioning of the deformed Charcot foot and dissipate local pressure to bony prominences over a wide surface area.

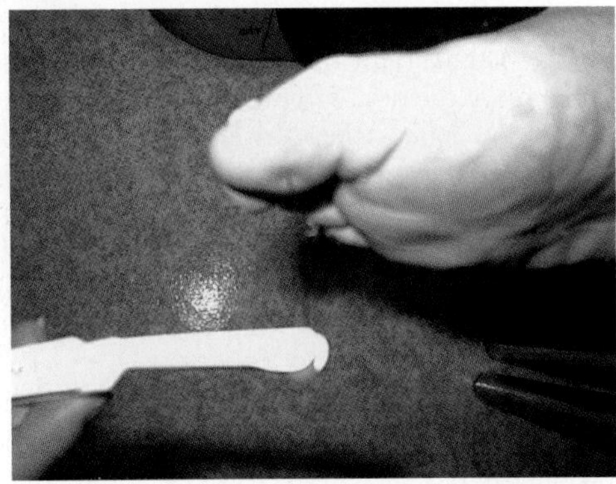

FIG 2 • The Semmes-Weinstein 5.07 monofilament applies 10 grams of pressure. The inability to "feel" this amount of pressure appears to be the threshold of peripheral neuropathy associated with the development of the two major foot morbidities associated with diabetes: diabetic foot ulcers and Charcot foot arthropathy.

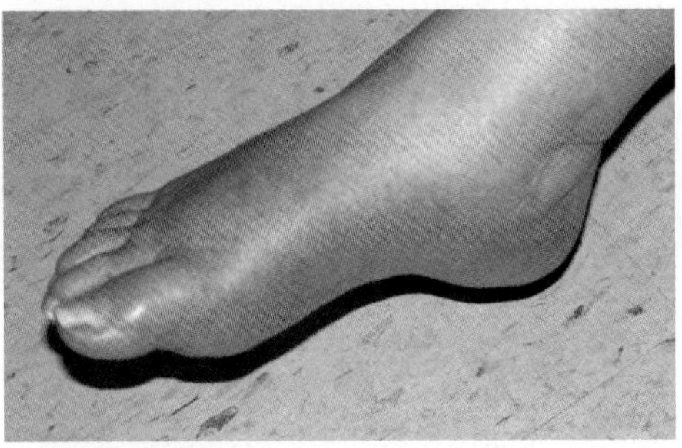

FIG 3 • Patients classically present with a grossly swollen, nonpainful foot without a history of trauma. In fact, most remember an episode of trauma, often trivial, and many are painful. Patients generally do not have a draining wound, supporting the presence of a diabetic foot abscess. The erythema is generally greatly lessened with elevation, which clinically differentiates it from infection.

important component leading to breakdown of the foot at the midfoot level during the terminal stance phase of gait. The autonomic neuropathy is likely involved as a component of the neurovascular theory.

- Baumhauer has demonstrated, via histochemical studies, the cytokines involved with the development of the destructive process, which resembles acute rheumatoid pannus.[2]
- The answer is likely a combination of both pathologic theories. Trauma, or some unknown inciting factor, initiates a process that releases specific cytokines. These cytokines lead to the development of destructive gray tissue that histologically resembles rheumatoid pannus.[2]

NATURAL HISTORY

- Most of the background observations in common orthopaedic textbooks are based on anecdotal observation, with little information that would comply with current evidence-based medicine standards.
- Eichenholtz[8] in 1966 published a detailed monograph based on his observations in 66 patients. This objective clinical, radiographic, and histologic information provides objective benchmark data. This monograph objectively describes the destructive disease process as well as the progression of deformity.
- The AOFAS Diabetic Foot Questionnaire provides objective data to support Eichenholtz's appreciation of the severe negative impact on health-related quality of life in affected individuals.[6]
- This very negative clinical observation has prompted many experienced clinical researchers to arbitrarily advise, without evidence-based medicine support, correction of deformity and arthrodesis at the onset of symptoms.[7,14,22,23]

PATIENT HISTORY AND PHYSICAL FINDINGS

- The classic presentation is a grossly swollen, painless foot, without a history of trauma, in a longstanding diabetic. In fact, better than half of patients will remember a specific traumatic event, although it might be trivial. Most patients are in their mid-50s to mid-60s, and most are obese (**FIG 3**).[15,17–20]
- Affected individuals generally have longstanding (10-plus years) diabetes with evidence of PN, as measured by insensitivity to the Semmes-Weinstein 5.07 (10-gram) monofilament (Fig 1).
- Patients often describe a feeling of "crunching" and instability at the involved site.
- On clinical examination, the foot is very swollen and warm. There is often gross nonpainful instability at the site of clinical involvement.

IMAGING AND OTHER DIAGNOSTIC STUDIES

- Treatment can generally be determined based on clinical examination and plain radiography.
- Weight-bearing biplanar radiographs of the foot and ankle are essential.
- Eichenholtz[8] arbitrarily categorized the timeline of the disease process into three stages.
  - Stage I is the early active stage of the disease process. Radiographs will be normal.
  - Stage II is entered when there is sufficient destruction of the ligamentous structures of the involved joints to allow joint dislocation or periarticular fracture. A healing response will often develop during this destructive phase of the disease process, prompting other authors to divide the disease process into more stages. This is when the radiographs take on the characteristic appearance of hypertrophic destruction with or without bony repair and the appearance of a hypertrophic nonunion.
  - Stage III is the consolidation of the destructive process, characterized by a "burning out" of the bony destruction. This is the stage when the foot assumes the characteristic deformities with hypertrophic reactive bone formation.
- Nuclear scanning is rarely helpful in distinguishing acute Charcot foot arthropathy from diabetic foot infection or abscess.
- MR imaging is occasionally beneficial when it demonstrates bony destruction contiguous to a wound.

DIFFERENTIAL DIAGNOSIS

- In the least destructive presentations of the disease process, patients are frequently misdiagnosed with a deep venous thrombosis, cellulitis, acute gout, or tenosynovitis.
  - Doppler ultrasound studies are normal, and patients do not respond to antibiotic therapy.

- The critical differential is foot abscess.
  - Patients with a diabetic foot abscess, or infective cellulitis, will feel ill.
  - The first sign of occult infection in the diabetic is increasing blood sugar or increasing insulin demand. White blood cell count may not increase, as these patients are often poor hosts and are not capable of mounting a normal immune response.
  - Patients with deep infection will generally have an entry portal for infection, which might be as simple as an infected ingrown toenail, or a crack or pinhole between the toes.
- Patients with acute Charcot foot arthropathy do not experience malaise, they have normal blood sugar levels (for the individual patient), and they do not have any purulent drainage. The erythema often disappears with elevation, in contrast to the patient with a diabetic foot infection.

NONOPERATIVE MANAGEMENT

- Classically, treatment has been accommodative with a non-weight-bearing total-contact cast during the acute phase.
- Long-term management has been accomplished with accommodative bracing.
- Surgery was only advised for bony infection or when orthotic management could not accommodate the acquired deformity.
- Based on clinical observations in patients who were not clinically plantigrade or would or could not use a CROW, we started to develop a clinical algorithm (**FIG 4**).
  - We defined a desired clinical outcome as remaining ulcer-free and maintaining walking independence with commercially available depth-inlay shoes and custom accommodative foot orthoses.
- It has been determined that patients who are clinically plantigrade at the time of presentation and have a colinear lateral talar–first metatarsal axis, as determined from weight-bearing dorsal–plantar radiographs, and have no bony prominences, can achieve the desired outcome without surgery.[3,15]
- Patients who meet the criteria for nonoperative treatment are initially treated with a weight-bearing total-contact cast.
  - The cast is changed every 14 days until the affected joint is clinically stable and the volume of the limb stabilizes.[19] The patient is then progressed to a commercially available pneumatic fracture boot.
  - When the foot volume reaches a plateau, the patient is evaluated for long-term management with commercially available depth-inlay shoes and custom accommodative foot orthoses (**FIG 5**).[1,21]
- The patient in **FIGURE 6** demonstrates the difficulties in long-term management of the nonplantigrade patient without correction of the deformity.
  - The acute destructive process can be managed with a total-contact cast.
  - This patient was very compliant, wearing the therapeutic footwear full time. She returned for routine visits to the physician and pedorthist.
  - Despite close monitoring, she developed an ulcer in the skin overlying the head of the talus. When multiple surgical attempts failed, a transtibial amputation was necessary because of infection.

SURGICAL MANAGEMENT

- There is disagreement whether the common midfoot location for the development of Charcot foot arthropathy is due to the mechanical forces produced by simple motor imbalance or to intrinsic contracture of the gastrocnemius–soleus muscle–tendon complex, which limits passive ankle dorsiflexion.[11,12]

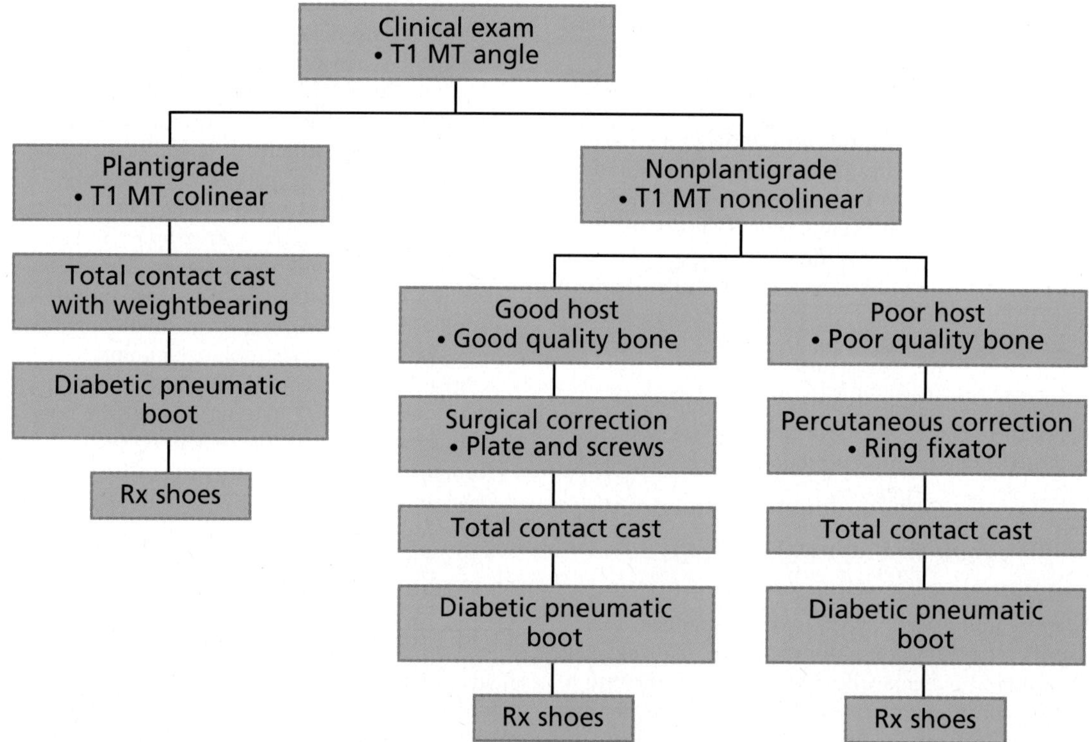

FIG 4 • Treatment algorithm for acute Charcot foot arthropathy.

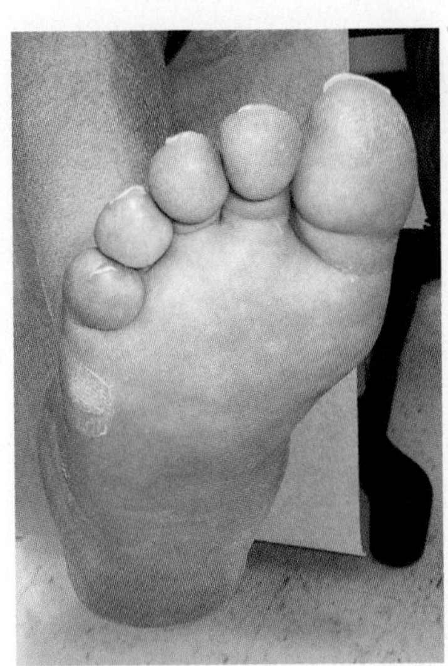
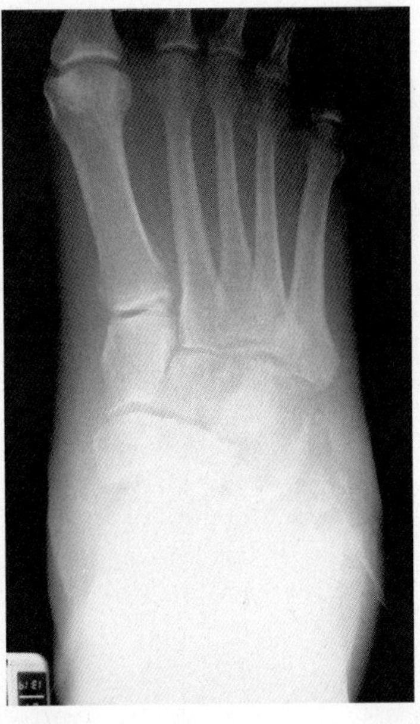
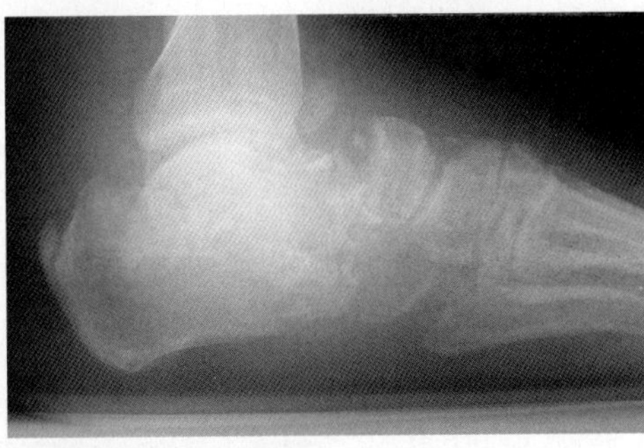

FIG 5 • **A.** This patient is clinically plantigrade with durable skin and connective tissue aligned for weight-bearing. **B,C.** Weight-bearing radiographs on presentation. Despite the deformity, treatment was accomplished with a weight-bearing total-contact cast until the acute destructive process subsided. Long-term management was accomplished with commercially available therapeutic footwear (depth-inlay shoes and custom accommodative foot orthoses).

- Most experts agree that the first step in surgical treatment is a lengthening of the gastrocnemius–soleus motor group to create balance between ankle flexors and extensors. Whichever theory one subscribes to, it has become apparent that lengthening of the gastrocnemius–Achilles tendon motor unit by gastrocnemius recession or percutaneous Achilles tendon lengthening is important.
- In most patients, the progressive deformity is biplanar. Correction of the bony deformity can generally be achieved by removing a sufficient wedge of bone at the apex of the deformity (ie, a partial tarsectomy) to create a plantigrade foot.
- In patients who are clinically good hosts, have no evidence of open wounds overlying bony deformity and no deep infection, and appear to have a reasonable quality of bone density, surgical stabilization can predictably be accomplished with internal fixation.[10]
- Crossed large fragment screws (cannulated or noncannulated), long posterior-to-anterior screws, and plate and screw constructs have been advocated for maintaining the surgical correction.
- Our preferred method of achieving surgical stabilization is with a tension-band 3.5-mm plate applied over the apex of the deformity. Due to the poor quality of local bone, 6.5-mm cortical bone screws are used to secure fixation (**FIG 7**).
- In patients who clinically appear to be poor surgical hosts or have wounds or skin ulceration overlying bony deformity, deep infection, or poor-quality osteopenic bone, surgical stabilization is accomplished with a three-level ring external fixator (**FIG 8**).[9,16]

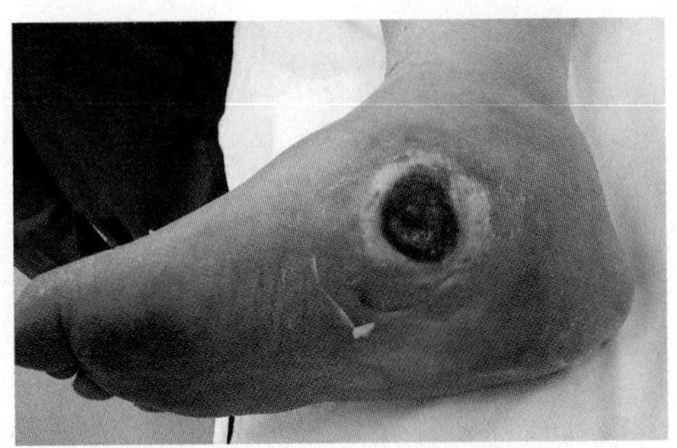
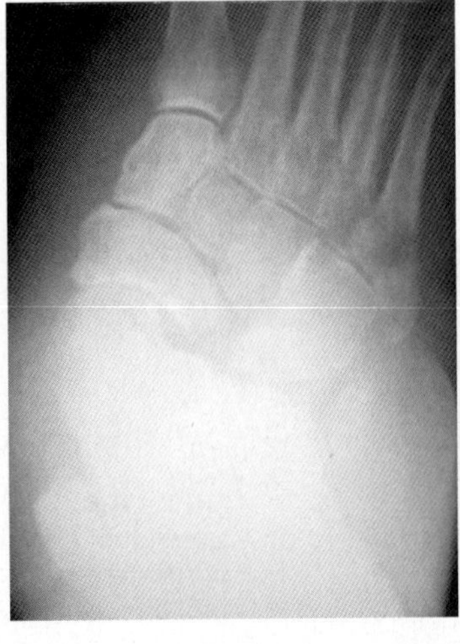

FIG 6 • This 55-year-old, extremely cooperative patient was successfully treated with a total-contact cast, progressing to therapeutic footwear. Despite very careful attention by the patient and close monitoring by her physicians, she developed this ulcer using therapeutic footwear 2.5 years after the development of a Charcot foot deformity.

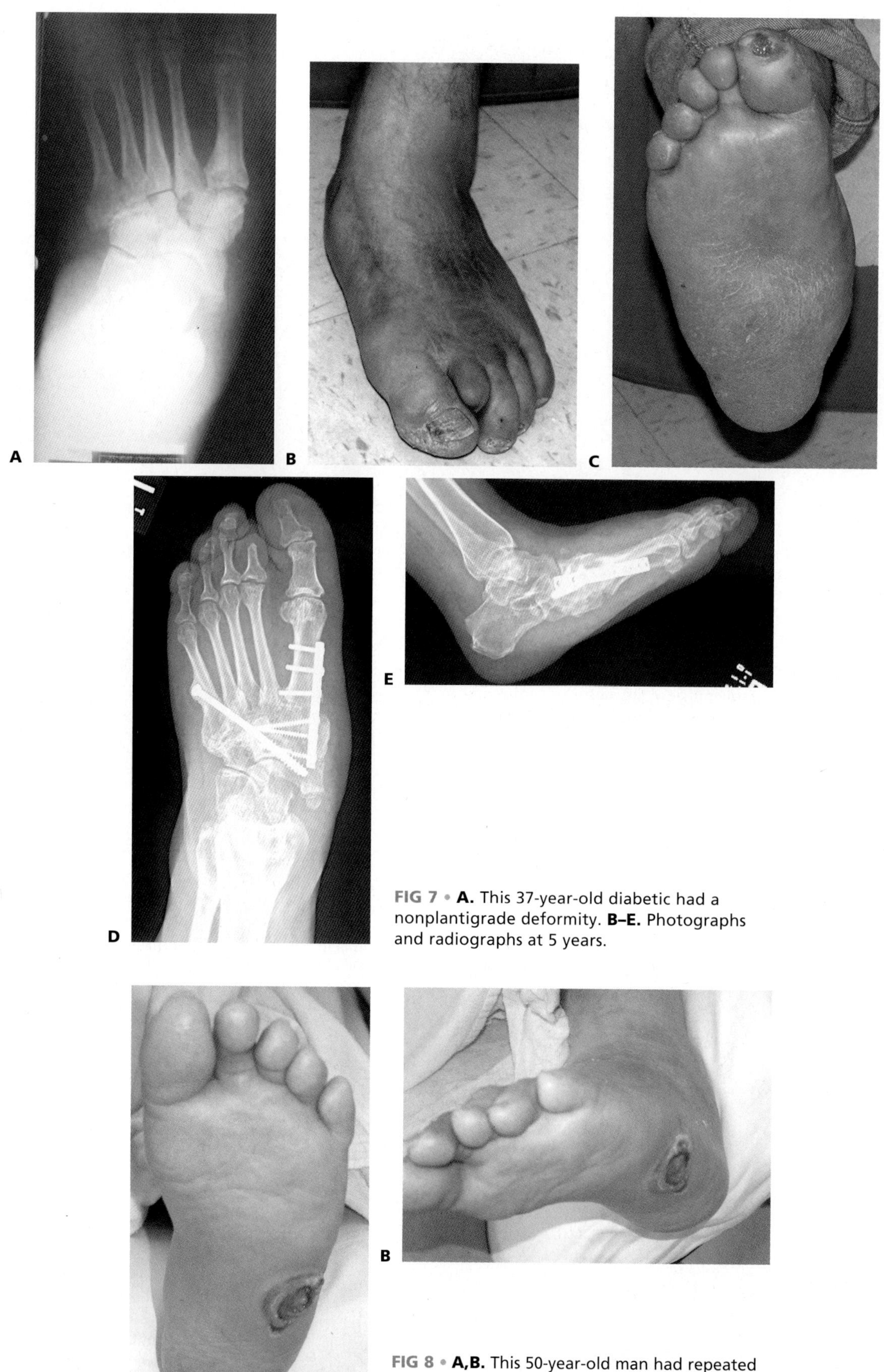

FIG 7 • **A.** This 37-year-old diabetic had a nonplantigrade deformity. **B–E.** Photographs and radiographs at 5 years.

FIG 8 • **A,B.** This 50-year-old man had repeated lateral foot infections despite resection of the fifth metatarsal. Note the rotational deformity of the forefoot relative to the hindfoot. *(continued)*

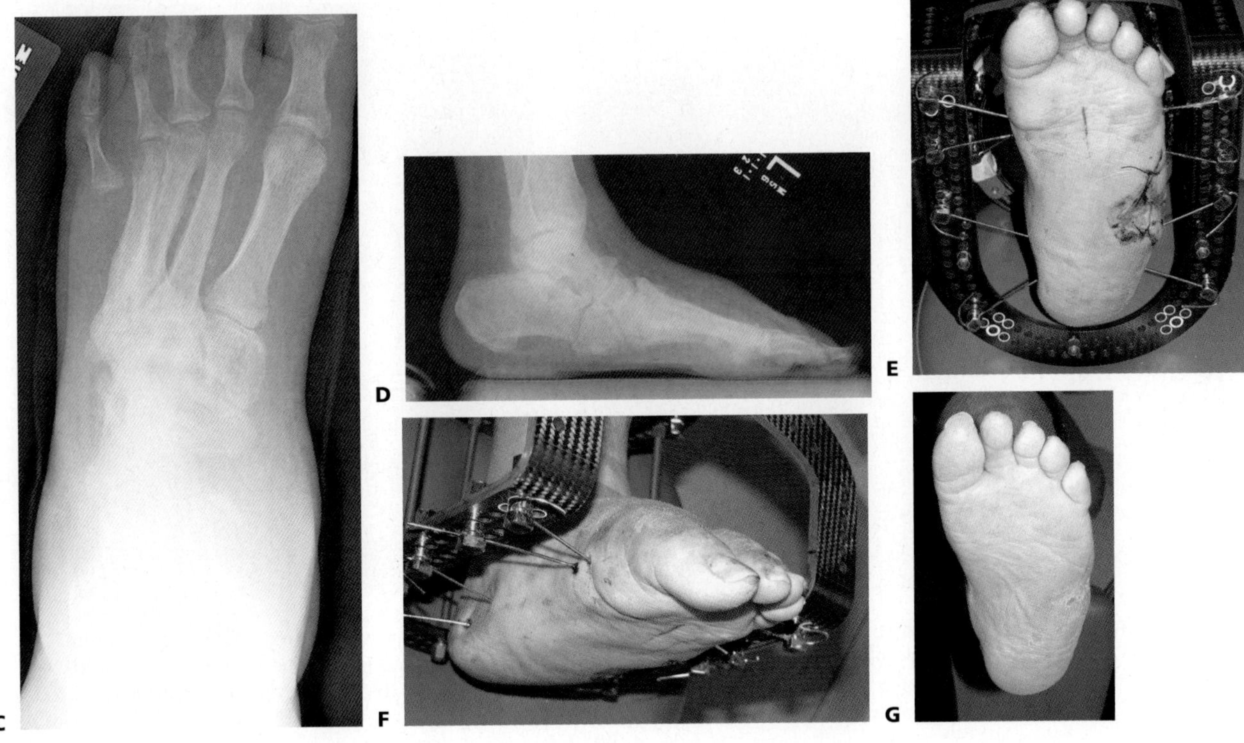

FIG 8 • *(continued)* **C,D.** Initial weight-bearing radiographs. **E,F.** Percutaneous tendon Achilles lengthening was followed by a wedge resection of sufficient bone, through the ulcer, to correct the deformity. **G.** Photograph at 1 year.

SURGICAL STEPS

- The first step is a lengthening of the gastrocnemius musculotendinous unit by either percutaneous triple hemisection of the Achilles tendon or fractional muscle lengthening of the gastrocnemius (Strayer procedure).
- Correction of the bony deformity is accomplished through an incision placed directly over or just inferior to the apex of the deformity. A biplanar wedge of bone is resected at the apex of the deformity, allowing correction of the deformity and creation of a plantigrade foot.

INTERNAL FIXATION

- When stabilization is accomplished with internal fixation, a tension-band 3.5-mm bone plate is used with large fragment screws to optimize screw fixation in osteopenic bone (Fig 7).

EXTERNAL FIXATION

- When surgical stabilization is accomplished with ring external fixation, a percutaneous smooth pin is sometimes valuable to establish temporary fixation while the ring external fixation frame is secured.
- A neutral ring external fixation frame is assembled before surgery. The frame has limited adjustability to increase frame stability and minimize the risk for bolt or screw loosening.
- The heel is safely positioned to avoid contact between the skin and the external fixator frame. Three oblique olive wire pins are initially applied through the calcaneus and then tensioned within the inferior ring. Three oblique olive wire pins are then placed through the metatarsal, with the forefoot aligned to the hindfoot in both plans, thus creating a plantigrade foot.
- The ring is then secured to the tibia, first through the proximal ring and then through the middle ring. The rings are safely positioned to maintain alignment of the foot to the leg and to avoid contact between the limb and the frame (**TECH FIG 1**).

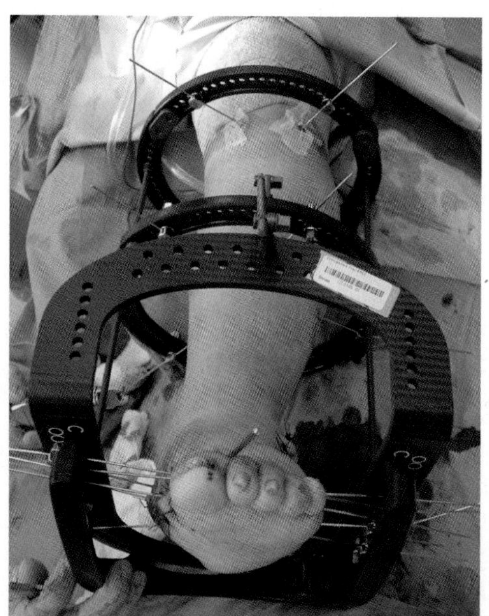

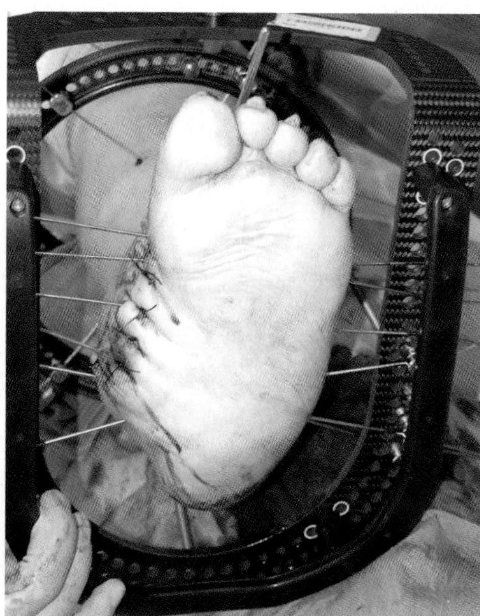

TECH FIG 1 • **A,B.** The hindfoot is initially secured to the frame with two or three 30-degree-oriented tensioned olive wires. Care is taken to avoid pressure between the skin and the frame. The forefoot is then secured in a similar fashion. Two upper levels are provided to dissipate the load. Patients are allowed to bear some weight for transfers.

PEARLS AND PITFALLS

- Many of these patients are obese and have poor balance due to their PN. It is virtually impossible for them to maintain a non–weight-bearing status. Every effort should be made to allow them to bear some weight in order to assist in transfers.
- Because of their diabetes, these individuals are poor surgical hosts. Large wounds with a great deal of soft tissue stripping should be avoided.

POSTOPERATIVE CARE

- Patients undergoing nonoperative treatment (ie, those who are clinically plantigrade and have a radiographic colinear lateral talar–first metatarsal axis) are initially treated with a weight-bearing total-contact cast.
  - The cast is changed every 2 weeks to ensure bony immobilization and to avoid pressure ulcerations from a poorly fitting cast.
    - The total-contact cast is maintained until the foot is clinically stable and the limb volume is reasonably stable. This usually can be accomplished in 6 to 8 weeks (three or four casts).
  - Patients are then transitioned to a commercially available pneumatic diabetic walking boot until limb volume is sufficiently stable to allow fitting with commercially available depth-inlay shoes and custom accommodative foot orthoses.
    - The shoe is generally modified with a cushioned heel and rocker sole.
    - In the occasional patient whose foot becomes nonplantigrade or who develops a noncolinear lateral talar–first metatarsal axis or a painful nonunion, surgical stabilization is advised.
- Patients undergoing surgical correction and maintenance with internal fixation are initially immobilized with a posterior plaster splint.
  - Weight bearing is initiated 7 to 10 days after surgery with a total-contact cast if the wound is secure.
  - The cast is maintained for 6 to 8 weeks, when patients are managed in a similar fashion to the nonoperative group.
- Patients treated with surgical correction and immobilization with a ring external fixator are allowed to bear about 30 pounds of weight during treatment.
  - The external fixator is removed at 8 to 12 weeks, at which point a weight-bearing total-contact cast is applied for 4 to 6 weeks.
  - Progression to therapeutic footwear is accomplished in a similar fashion to the other groups.

OUTCOMES

- During the past 10 years, only three patients treated nonsurgically developed a nonunion at the site of their Charcot arthropathy with sufficient pain to warrant surgical stabilization.[15]
- The initial complication rate in the surgical patients was high compared with current standards. Infection rates have been greatly reduced with the use of the ring external fixator in high-risk, poor-host patients with open wounds or deep bony infection.
- Mechanical failure and deep bony infection rates were high in the early experience with crossed-screw constructs, leading to a great deal of morbidity and three transtibial amputations.

- In patients with adequate bone quality, the screw-plate construct can achieve successful outcomes in more than 90% of patients.
- The absolute worst hosts undergo surgical correction through small incisions followed by immobilization with a ring external fixator. The complication rate in this group is surprisingly small.
- Surgical correction of the deformity is accomplished before application of the external fixator, so the frame need not be adjustable. This absence of multiple connections appears to be responsible for the limited frame-associated morbidity.

COMPLICATIONS

- Patients treated without surgery have had limited numbers of complications.
  - The rare cast-associated pressure ulcer generally resolves with local skin care and cast change. Changing the total-contact cast every 14 days appears to avoid cast-associated morbidity.
- Wound infection and mechanical failure were not uncommon during the early experience with internal fixation in this group. Wound infections are treated with surgical débridement, culture-specific parenteral antibiotics, and occasional management with a vacuum-assisted wound care system.
- Mechanical failure was also more common when internal fixation was accomplished with crossed large fragment screws. It has been uncommon when the tension-band plate–large fragment screw construct has been used to accomplish internal fixation.
- Stabilization of surgical correction with tensioned olive wires and ring external fixation has greatly decreased the incidence of wound infection and mechanical failure in the highest-risk group of patients.
- Two patients in the ring external fixation group developed stress fractures months after removal of the ring external fixators. One healed with simple cast immobilization. One progressed to a nonunion. Uneventful healing was accomplished after closed antegrade intramedullary nailing.

REFERENCES

1. American Diabetes Association. Clinical Practice Recommendations 2004. Diabetes Care 2004;27(Supplement 1).
2. Baumhauer JF, O'Keefe R, Schon L, et al. Free cytokine-induced osteoclastic bone resorption in Charcot arthropathy: an immunohistochemical study. Foot Ankle Int 2006;27:797–800.
3. Bevan WP, Tomlinson MP. Radiographic measure as a predictor of ulcer formation in midfoot Charcot. Paper presented at the Annual Meeting of the American Orthopaedic Foot and Ankle Society, Seattle, July 2004.
4. Charcot JM. Sur quelques arthropathies qui paraissant dependre d'une lesion du cerveau ou de la maelle epiniere. Arch Physiol Norm Path 1868;1:161–178.
5. Charcot JM. Lecons sur les maladies nerveux. New Sydenham Series, 4th Lesson, 1868.
6. Dwahan V, Spratt K, Pinzur MD, et al. The AOFAS Diabetic Foot Questionnaire: stability, internal consistency, and measurable difference. Foot Ankle Int 2005;26:717–731.
7. Early JS, Hansen ST. Surgical reconstruction of the diabetic foot. Foot Ankle Int 1996;17:325–330.
8. Eichenholtz SN. Charcot Joints. Springfield, IL: Charles C Thomas, 1966.
9. Farber DC, Juliano PJ, Cavanagh PR, et al. Single-stage correction with external fixation of the ulcerated foot in individuals with Charcot neuroarthropathy. Foot Ankle Int 2002;23:130–134.
10. Herbst SA, Jones KB, Saltzman CL. Pattern of diabetic neuropathic arthropathy associated with the peripheral bone mineral density. J Bone Joint Surg Br 2004;86B:378–383.
11. Ledoux WR, Shofer JB, Ahroni JH, et al. Biomechanical differences among pes cavus, neutrally aligned, and pes planus feet in subjects with diabetes. Foot Ankle Int 2003;24:845–850.
12. Mueller MJ, Sinacore DR, Hastings MK, et al. Effect of Achilles tendon lengthening on neuropathic plantar ulcers. J Bone Joint Surg Am 2003;85A:1436–1445.
13. Papa J, Myerson M, Eaton K, et al. The total contact cast for management of neuropathic plantar ulceration of the foot. J Bone Joint Surg Am 1992;74A:261–269.
14. Papa J, Myerson M, Girard P. Salvage, with arthrodesis, in intractable diabetic neuropathic arthropathy of the foot and ankle. J Bone Joint Surg Am 1993;75A:1056–1066.
15. Pinzur MS. Surgical vs. accommodative treatment for Charcot arthropathy of the midfoot. Foot Ankle Int 2004;25:545–549.
16. Pinzur MS. Ring fixation in Charcot foot and ankle arthropathy. Tech Foot Ankle Surg 2006;5:68–73.
17. Pinzur MS. Benchmark analysis of diabetic patients with neuropathic (Charcot) foot deformity. Foot Ankle Int 1999;20:564–567.
18. Pinzur MS, Freeland R, Juknelis D. The association between body mass index and diabetic foot disorders. Foot Ankle Int 2005;26: 375–377.
19. Pinzur MS, Lio T, Posner M. Treatment of Eichenholtz stage I Charcot foot arthropathy with a weight-bearing total-contact cast. Foot Ankle Int 2006;27:324–329.
20. Pinzur MS, Sage R, Stuck R, et al. A treatment algorithm for neuropathic (Charcot) midfoot deformity. Foot Ankle Int 1993;14: 189–197.
21. Pinzur MS, Slovenkai MP, Trepman E, et al. Guidelines for diabetic foot care: recommendations endorsed by the Diabetes Committee of the American Orthopaedic Foot and Ankle Society. Foot Ankle Int 2005;26:113–119.
22. Simon SR, Tejwani SG, Wilson DL, et al. Arthrodesis as an early alternative to nonoperative management of Charcot arthropathy of the diabetic foot. J Bone Joint Surg Am 2000;82A:939–950.
23. Weinfeld SB, Lew K. Surgical treatment of neuropathic hindfoot and ankle deformities. Paper presented at the Annual Meeting of the American Orthopaedic Foot and Ankle Society, Seattle, July 2004.

Chapter 44

Axial Screw Technique for Midfoot Arthrodesis in Charcot Foot Deformities

Vincent James Sammarco and G. James Sammarco

DEFINITION

- Fracture through the midfoot in the neuropathic patient may accompany minor or incidental trauma and if unchecked may lead to severe deformity or "rocker-bottom" foot deformity.
- This chapter will demonstrate a technique used for fusion of the unstable midfoot fracture dislocation.

ANATOMY

- Charcot fracture-dislocation of the midfoot may occur through the tarsometatarsal, intercuneiform, or transverse tarsal joints.
- Multiple patterns may exist and are often complicated by bony dissolution. Attempts to classify these dislocations have been described by Sammarco and Conti[11] and Schon et al[14] (**FIGS 1 AND 2**).

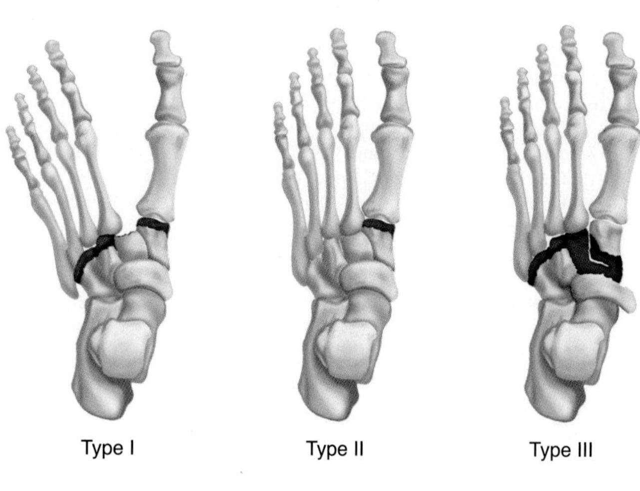

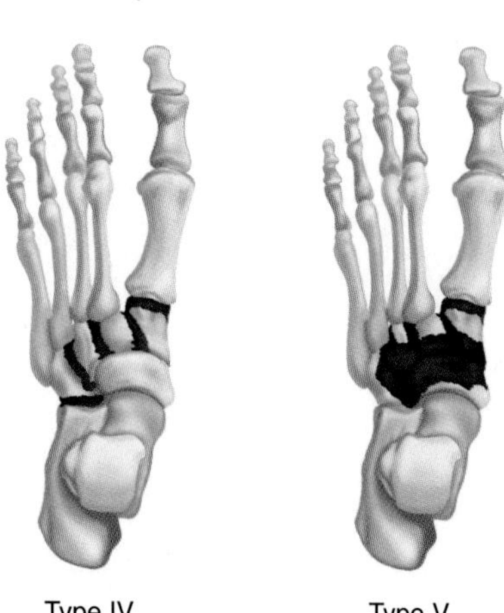

FIG 1 • Classification of Charcot midfoot fracture-dislocation as described by Sammarco and Conti.

PATHOGENESIS

- Peripheral neuropathy is most commonly related to diabetes but may occur with other neurologic disorders as well.
- Glycosylation and diminished blood supply to the peripheral nerves result in progressive loss of sensation, motor innervation, and autonomic function.
  - Longer nerves are more severely affected, resulting in the typical "stocking and glove" sensory deficit.
- Loss of protective sensation in the lower limb predisposes patients to ulceration and may make them oblivious to fractures or dislocations.
- Loss of motor function leads to intrinsic imbalance of muscles in the lower extremity and commonly leads to equinus contracture of the ankle and Achilles, which significantly increases the forces through the foot during gait.
  - Intrinsic imbalance in the foot musculature also results in clawing of the hallux and lesser digits.
- Autonomic sensory loss results in drying and cracking of the skin, which diminishes integumentary protection from pathogens.
  - Autonomic dysfunction also is responsible for loss of vasomotor control, which may lead to edema and stasis.

NATURAL HISTORY

- Midfoot fracture dislocation in the insensate patient may result acutely from direct trauma but more commonly is due to repetitive microtrauma in insensate joints. Once instability develops, bony deformity usually follows and worsens due to neurally stimulated vasomotor response, which increases blood flow to the area and leads to bony dissolution. Because the process is typically painless, the patient may be unaware or

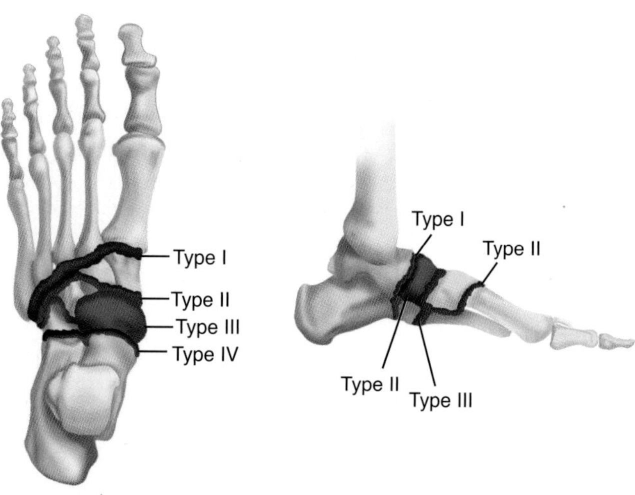

FIG 2 • Classification of Charcot midfoot fracture-dislocation by Schon and Weinfeld.

unconcerned that a problem is present until massive soft tissue swelling, gross deformity, ulceration, and infection are present.

- Fracture and dissociation through the midfoot may progress to a dorsal dislocation of the metatarsals. Once bony dissociation occurs, contracture of the soft tissue envelope makes reduction of the deformity difficult or impossible without surgical resection of bone at the fracture site.
- Charcot neuroarthropathy was staged by Eichenholz.[6]
  - Stage I is the inflammatory stage. The foot is hyperemic, swollen, and hot. Bony dissolution and fragmentation may be present on radiographs.
  - Stage II is the coalescence phase, where swelling and edema decrease, temperature decreases, and redness improves.
  - In Stage III, bony consolidation occurs, often with significant residual deformity.
- Deformity at the level of the midfoot is poorly tolerated and leads to a significant increase in localized plantar pressures at the apex of the deformity. Commonly these increased soft tissue pressures, combined with the previously mentioned loss of protective sensation and loss of normal integumentary function, may lead to ulceration and potentially deep infection. In diabetics, these problems are worsened by impaired circulation and immunologic function and can lead to amputation of the limb. If osteomyelitis develops, limb salvage may still be possible but the risk of amputation is greatly increased.
- This technique is one of a series of evolving techniques aimed at reconstructing these significant deformities.[1–5,8–13] Standard arthrodesis techniques often fail in these patients due to the poor bone quality and significant fragmentation that accompanies these cases.[15] The goals of this technique are to aid in reduction of deformity and to allow the fixation devices to bridge the area of dissolution at the apex of the deformity, achieving fixation in more normal bone proximally and distally.

PATIENT HISTORY AND PHYSICAL FINDINGS

- The patient with Charcot neuroarthropathy of the foot may present in any of the Eichenholz stages, but by far the most common presentation to the orthopaedist is the inflammatory stage, with presumed cellulitis and osteomyelitis.
- A history of trauma may or may not be present. Stage I and II patients will present with a swollen, red, and warm foot. Patients presenting to the orthopaedist in stage III will typically have a stable deformity that may or may not be amenable to bracing.
- Prognosis is significantly affected by four things for these patients: the presence of infection, the presence of adequate blood flow in the extremity to the level of the digits, the presence of chronic venous stasis with associated poor integument, and the ability for the patient to adequately control his or her medical comorbidities. Patients who are immunocompromised due to transplant or those receiving dialysis have a much worse prognosis than those with diabetes alone.
- The presence or absence of infection must be established at the onset of treatment. This may be difficult as many of the physical signs of stage I Charcot deformity are indistinguishable from an infection.
- Lack of constitutional symptoms does not preclude infection in diabetics, who may not be able to mount an adequate immune response, and patients are often started on antibiotics at presentation. At the time of consultation, the patient has often already been admitted to the hospital with the initiation of intravenous antibiotics, bed rest with elevation of the extremity, and a non–weight-bearing status, thus blurring the ability to distinguish whether the patient improved due to simple rest or medications.
- A history of fevers and chills, inability for diabetics to control their blood sugar levels, and a history of previous or current ulceration increase the likelihood of active infection at presentation.
- The physical examination should document the presence or absence of pulses.
- Neuropathy should be documented with a 5.07 Semmes-Weinstein monofilament, and the level of intact sensation should be noted in the patient's record.
- Protective sensation may be present even with Charcot neuroarthropathy. Any ulceration should be carefully documented, as well as its depth and Wagner grade.[16] The presence of fluctuance may be suspicious for abscess and crepitation of the skin may represent gas gangrene; both require prompt diagnosis and surgical treatment. It is important to evaluate the contralateral foot and ankle as well as the patient may have pathology that is unrecognized.
- Items in the history that suggest that surgical stabilization may be required include gross instability on physical examination, acute fracture-dislocation from trauma, and recurrent ulcerations despite appropriate nonoperative treatment (**FIG 3**).

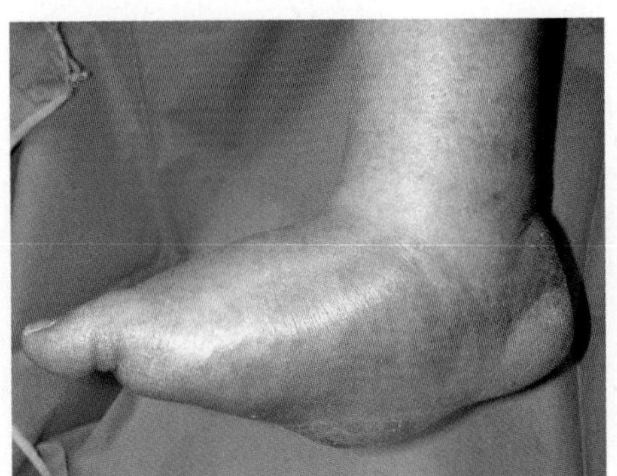
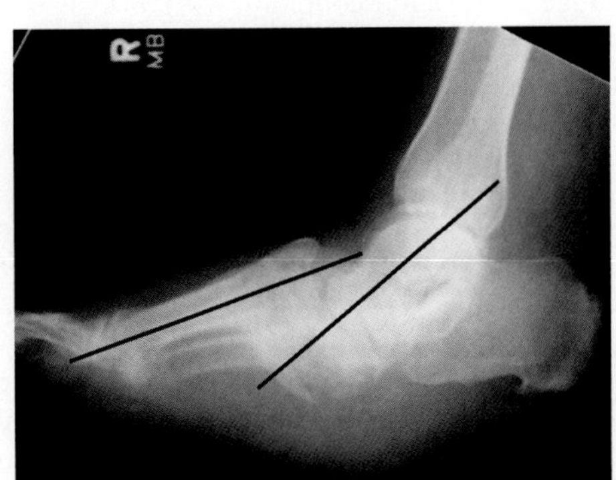

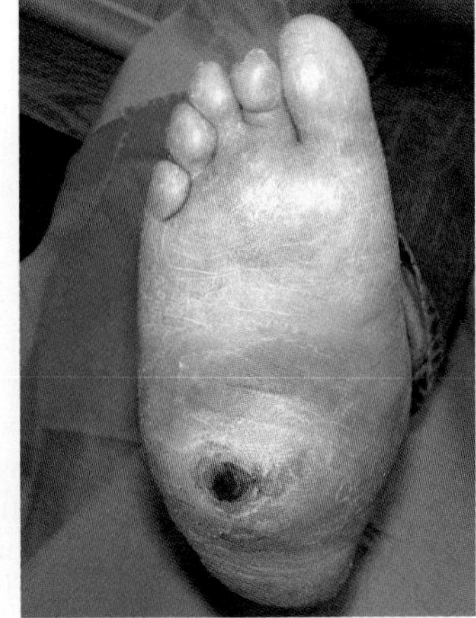

FIG 3 • A 54-year-old man with Charcot midfoot fracture-dislocation. **A.** Clinical deformity. **B.** Lateral radiograph showing midfoot fracture-dislocation. **C.** Plantar ulceration recalcitrant to extended contact casting. (Reprinted with permission. Copyright 2006 Cincinnati SportsMedicine Orthopaedic Center.)

IMAGING AND OTHER DIAGNOSTIC STUDIES

Radiographs

- Radiographs of the ankle and foot should be taken (weight bearing when possible) to help stage the deformity.
- Typical radiographic changes include fracture and dislocation, bony destruction, periosteal reaction, and malalignment.
- These findings are difficult to distinguish from acute or chronic osteomyelitis and alone are unreliable for determining the presence or absence of infection. Radiographs alone are sufficient for diagnosing the disease process, but other imaging studies are often necessary to determine the presence or absence of infection.

MRI

- MRI is frequently used to help determine the presence of osteomyelitis, but caution must be given to interpretation as the false-positive rate is very high. Bone destruction and bone and soft tissue edema may be present in Charcot neuroarthropathy without infection and alone should not be used to determine the presence of infection.
- Enhancement with intravenous gadolinium gives stronger support to the presence of infection.
- The presence of a fluid collection consistent with abscess formation or air associated with Charcot deformity and the above MRI findings should be considered diagnostic for deep infection.

CT

- CT scan may show extensive bony destruction, periosteal reaction, and malalignment.
- The use of CT is unnecessary for diagnosis, but it can be helpful in surgical planning.
- The presence of air on a CT scan is considered diagnostic for deep infection and may represent with gas gangrene, or more commonly communication with an ulcer.

Nuclear Imaging

- Nuclear imaging is particularly useful in helping differentiate an infected Charcot process from a noninfected process.
- A three-phase technetium bone scan alone will be of little value as increased uptake will usually be present in all three phases. However, when this study is immediately followed by a labeled white blood cell scan, the combined studies can be useful to decide whether the process is Charcot process alone, soft tissue infection, or osteomyelitis.
- Other isotopes may be useful in differentiating infection from a sterile Charcot process and include ^{99m}Tc sulfur colloid and combined bone and white cell "dual peak imaging." A detailed discussion of nuclear imaging is beyond the scope of this text and the reader is referred elsewhere for further study.[7]

Electrodiagnostic Testing

- This is usually unnecessary when peripheral neuropathy can be documented on physical examination.
- Electrodiagnostic testing can be useful in patients who have relatively normal sensory examination but whose radiographic and clinical findings are suggestive of neuropathic arthropathy. It is useful for documentation of deficits and also may be helpful in diagnosis of the underlying reason for neuropathy.

Vascular Testing

- We recommend rigorous workup of any suspected vascular insufficiency. This usually entails screening with noninvasive arterial examination in patients who do not have readily palpable pulses on physical examination.
- Arterial insufficiency is a relative contraindication to surgical reconstruction. Referral to a vascular surgeon should be considered for staged arterial reconstruction if significant insufficiency is present.

DIFFERENTIAL DIAGNOSIS

- Osteomyelitis, acute or chronic
- Abscess or gangrene
- Traumatic dislocation

NONOPERATIVE MANAGEMENT

- The majority of patients who develop noninfected Charcot arthropathy can be treated nonoperatively.
- Nonsurgical treatment typically entails a period of cast immobilization using a total-contact cast, and possibly a period of limited or non–weight-bearing.
- The goal of nonsurgical treatment with casting is to have the foot consolidate to a plantigrade structure without significant bony prominence.
- Once the foot has entered Eichenholz stage III, the patient is fitted for accommodative orthotics and shoe wear. Accommodative devices may be as simple as an off-the-shelf Plastazote orthotic if there is little residual deformity. More commonly, there is some deformity and the patient will require a custom-molded multidensity foam orthotic.
- A Charcot restraint orthotic walker (CROW) is necessary if there is severe deformity. Surgery is typically reserved for patients with acute fracture dislocations, those with progressive or unbraceable deformities, and those with recurrent ulceration despite multiple attempts at accommodative bracing.

SURGICAL MANAGEMENT

Preoperative Planning

- It is important to establish the absence of infection. Active infection or osteomyelitis is a contraindication for this technique as the hardware is typically permanent and difficult or impossible to remove without significant bony destruction. As noted previously, vascular workup is necessary before the procedure.
- The involvement of an astute internist is important in control of diabetes and medical comorbidities. The timing of surgery is important. Acute trauma without bony dissolution or significant swelling can be safely reduced and fused within a week or two of injury, providing the dislocation is recognized and the patient has not entered the inflammatory stage of the neuroarthropathy process.
- Once the patient enters the inflammatory phase, we prefer to cast the patient for 6 to 8 weeks to allow the edema to resolve and perform the reconstruction in a staged manner.

Indications

- This technique involves passing large-bore cannulated screws across the uninvolved metatarsal heads through the metatarsophalangeal (MTP) joints and is contraindicated in patients without significant sensory neuropathy.
- This technique is most useful for deformity at the tarsometatarsal level, and can be extended across the naviculocuneiform joints.

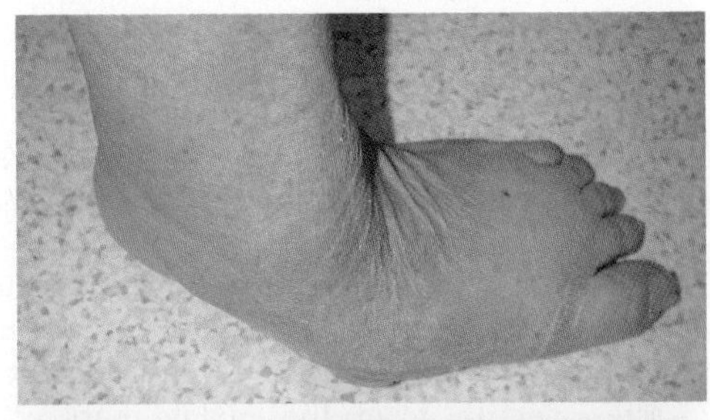
A

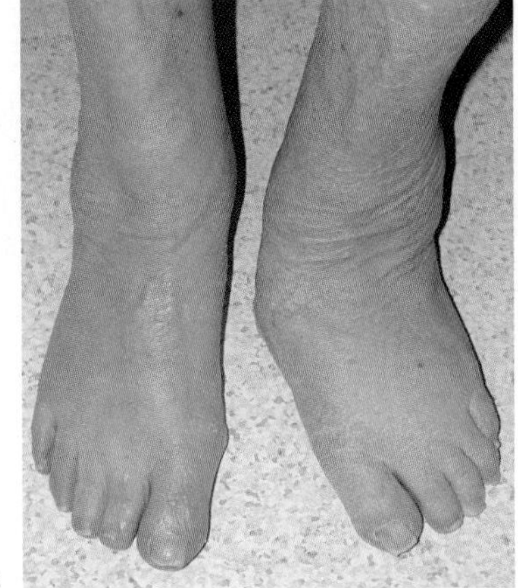
B

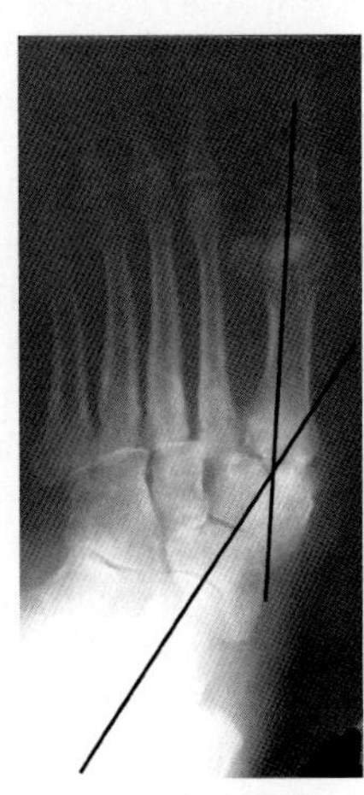
E

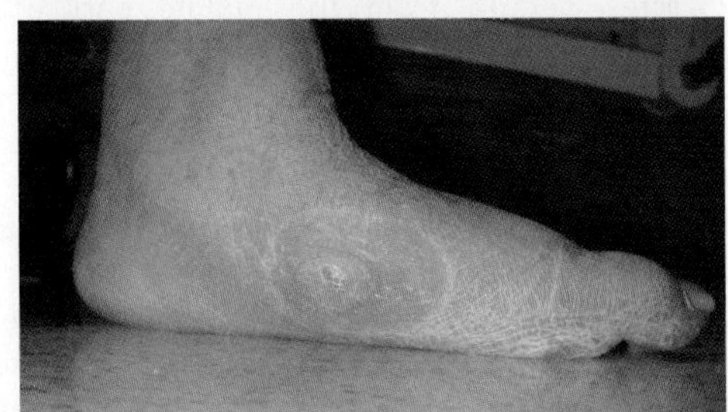
C

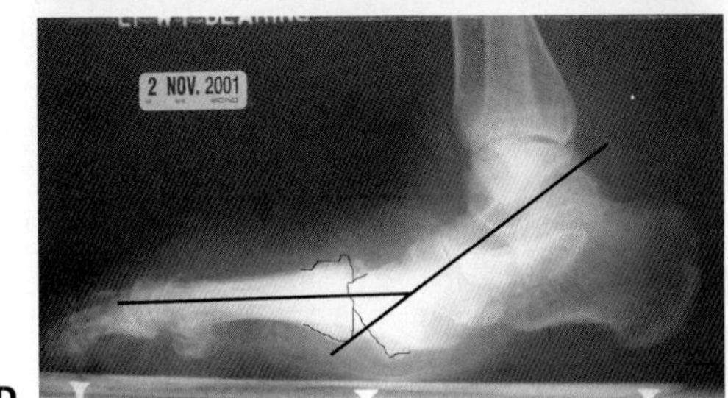

D

FIG 4 • Case example for technique demonstration: a 71-year-old woman with idiopathic neuropathy. **A, B, C.** Clinical photographs show midfoot deformity after spontaneous midfoot fracture-dislocation. Ulceration was present medially, which resolved after 6 weeks of contact casting. **D, E.** Preoperative clinical radiographs show dislocation at the tarsometatarsal joint. Gross instability was present on physical examination. (**A,** from Sammarco VJ, Sammarco GJ, Walker EW Jr, Guiao RP. Midtarsal arthrodesis in the treatment of Charcot midfoot arthropathy: surgical technique. J Bone Joint Surg Am 2010;92(Supplement 1 Part 1):1–19; printed with permission.)

- A higher rate of failure, screw breakage, and nonunion is associated with fusions that cross the transverse tarsal joint, and extended non–weight-bearing may be required to achieve fusion at this level (**FIG 4**).

Positioning

- The patient is positioned supine with a bump under the hip so that the toes face perpendicular to the operating table.
- A pneumatic tourniquet is used at the thigh.
- The patient is prepared and draped above the knee. A three-step tendo-Achilles lengthening, gastroc–soleus recession, or both is performed to achieve ankle dorsiflexion of 15 degrees before inflating the tourniquet.

Approach

- A two- or three-incision approach is used to reduce deformity and to prepare the arthrodesis bed. A medial approach is used to expose the medial column.
- The insertions of the tibialis anterior and posterior should be left undisturbed when possible, but they are often attached to fragmented or dislocated bone and should be secured with nonabsorbable suture placed in a locking fashion during the approach, for reattachment at closure.
- A subperiosteal dissection is carried out above and below the level of the deformity. The middle column of the foot is approached though a dorsal incision centered between the second and third metatarsal bases.
- Care should be taken to preserve the dorsalis pedis artery at this level. A third incision is usually necessary for exposure and reduction of the lateral column and is carried out dorsally at the level of the fourth and fifth tarsometatarsal joints.
- Care must be taken to provide an adequate skin bridge between the dorsal incisions or wound necrosis or dorsal slough may occur.

AXIAL SCREW TECHNIQUE FOR MIDFOOT ARTHRODESIS IN CHARCOT FOOT DEFORMITIES

Resection

- Perform bone resection with an oscillating saw at the level of deformity.
- Adequate bone resection is necessary to prevent excessive tension on the dorsal soft tissue envelope and vascular structures.
- Bone resection is at the level of the deformity and usually involves resection of some bone from the proximal and distal fragments. Carry out bone resection medially for the medial column, and dorsally for the middle and lateral columns.
- Remove bone from the dorsal incisions with a curved curette or pituitary rongeur. Adequate bone resection is indicated by the ability to manually reduce the deformity.
- Resect bone slowly so that a balanced reduction can be achieved between the metatarsal bases. It is possible to

resect so much bone that adequate bony apposition cannot be achieved for successful arthrodesis (TECH FIG 1A–C).

- Place guidewires in the metatarsal shafts without crossing the apex of the deformity. This can be done retrograde through the MTP joints under fluoroscopic control, although this can be quite time-consuming and technically demanding. To pass retrograde guidewires, hold the MTP joint in hyperdorsiflexion and pass the wire under fluoroscopic guidance across the joint and into the metatarsal head and into the shaft. Alternatively, pass the guidewires antegrade though the apex of the deformity. After bony resection, flex the foot through the middle and enter the metatarsal base with a curved curette, then a guidewire, which is passed into the metatarsal shaft. Then dorsiflex the MTP joint and drive the wire out through the plantar skin distally. The fifth metatarsal can usually not be fixed axially because the intramedullary canal typically aligns lateral to the cuboid (TECH FIG 1D–G).
- Ream the metatarsal shafts with cannulated drills. It is best to start with a small guidewire and a small cannulated drill and then change to a larger guidewire and larger cannulated drills. The medial column is usually drilled to 5.5 mm and a screw 6.5 mm or 8.0 mm in diameter is applied. The lesser metatarsals are usually drilled to 4.5 mm and a screw 4.5 mm or 5.0 mm is applied.
- Once the guidewires are in place in the reamed metatarsal shafts, hold the deformity reduced and advance the guidewires into the midfoot. Measure screw length from the middle part of the first metatarsal head in the medial column, and from the metaphyseal–diaphyseal junction of the lesser metatarsals. A counter-sink must be applied through the metatarsal head or it may fracture as the screw head is applied. Use screws with reduced-diameter heads (TECH FIG 1H,I).
- After applying the screws, sequentially tighten them to provide compression across the arthrodesis site.
- Perform a layered closure. Close the skin with 3-0 nylon suture applied with vertical mattress technique. A drain is usually not necessary.

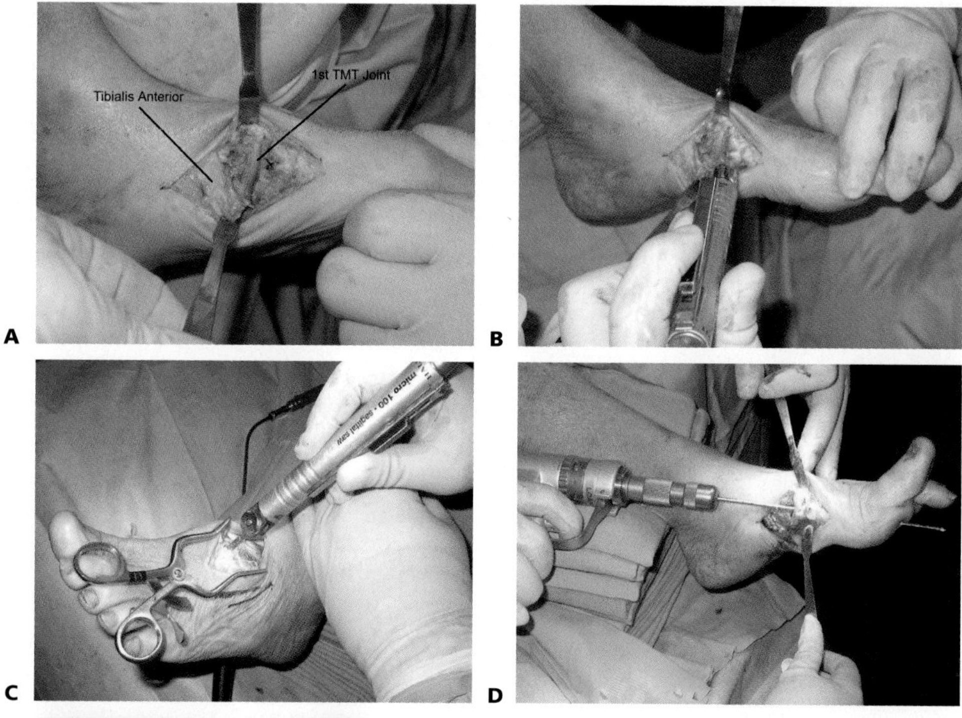

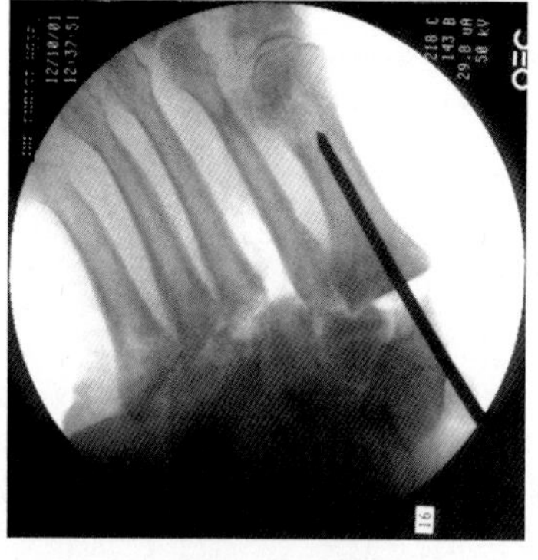

TECH FIG 1 • EUR Bone resection and exposure. **A–C.** Medial column is exposed: note the tibialis anterior tendon insertion, which must be reattached if it is released for reduction. The saw is used to resect bone plantarly and medially to restore axial alignment and to relieve soft tissue tension. **D–G.** Preparation of the intramedullary canals is done after the bone resection. Fluoroscopic control is used during wire placement and reaming. **D, E.** Medial column. (**D, E,** from Sammarco VJ, Sammarco GJ, Walker EW Jr, Guiao RP. Midtarsal arthrodesis in the treatment of Charcot midfoot arthropathy: surgical technique. J Bone Joint Surg Am 2010;92(Supplement 1 Part 1):1–19; reprinted with permission.) *(continued)*

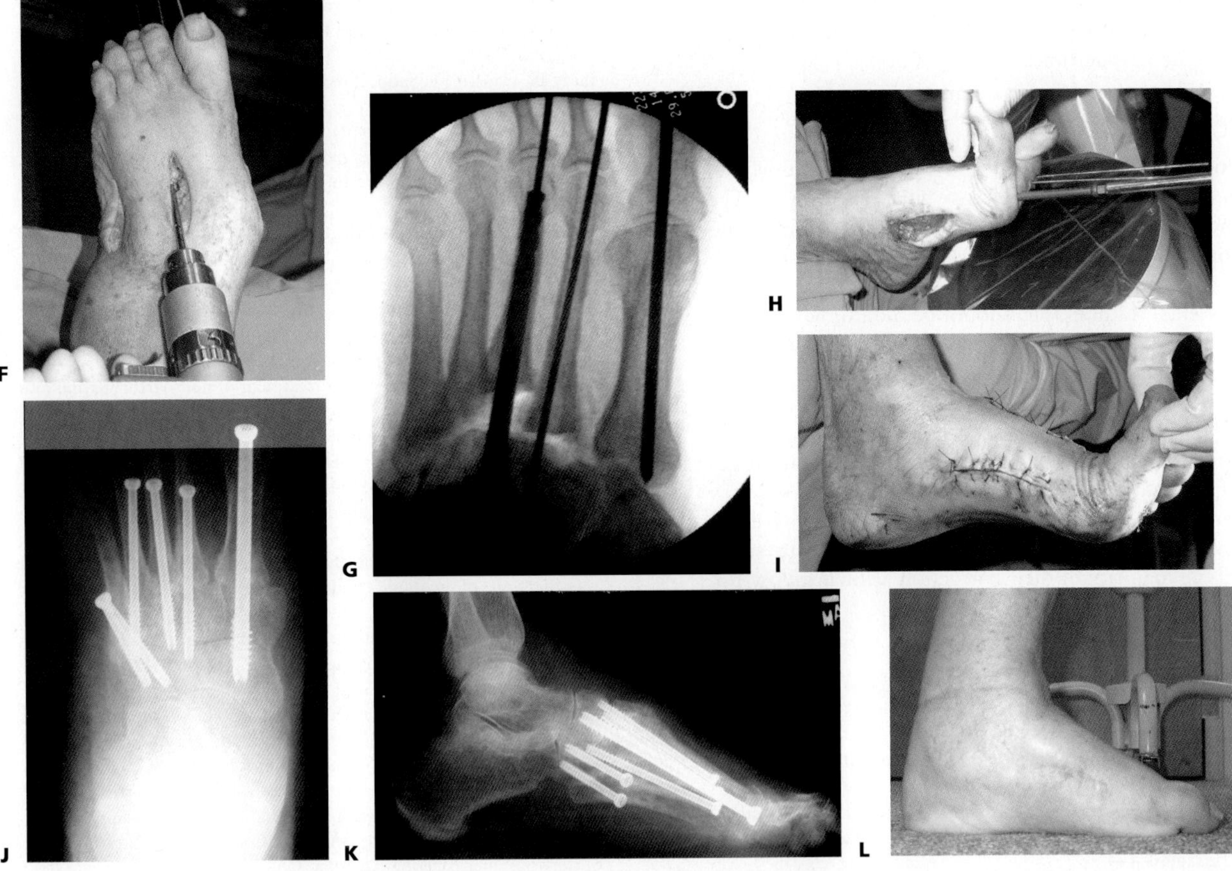

TECH FIG 1 • *(continued)* **F, G.** Middle and lateral columns. **H.** Application of the screws axially across the arthrodesis site after advancing the guidewires to the desired level. **I.** Intraoperative photograph of correction. **J, K.** Postoperative radiographs showing midfoot fusion without recurrence. **L.** Clinical photograph taken 1 year postoperatively. (**G, H, J–L,** from Sammarco VJ, Sammarco GJ, Walker EW Jr, Guiao RP. Midtarsal arthrodesis in the treatment of Charcot midfoot arthropathy: surgical technique. J Bone Joint Surg Am 2010;92(Supplement 1 Part 1):1–19; reprinted with permission.)

PEARLS AND PITFALLS

- Treatment of midfoot arthropathy is controversial and most cases can be managed nonoperatively by casting and bracing.
- Surgery is indicated for grossly instability, recurrent ulceration, a nonplantigrade foot and unbraceable deformity.
- When surgery is done: span the area of dissolution; adequate bone resection, use bigger, stronger implants; place implants where they offer mechanical advantage.
- Keys to success: do not operate on dysvascular limbs, eradicate infection/ulcer prior to applying internal fixation, aggressive surgical treatment of equinus, get a good correction.

POSTOPERATIVE CARE

- The patient is placed in a well-padded posterior splint postoperatively. This is typically changed within a few days of the surgery and switched to a cast.
- The patient is non–weight-bearing for 10 to 16 weeks, and may begin weight bearing in a pneumatic walking boot once bony consolidation is evident radiographically (average 12 weeks).
- Once edema and swelling are under control, the patient may be graduated to diabetic shoe wear with a custom multidensity foam orthotic.
- Techniques Figure 1J–L shows postoperative radiographs and a photograph.

OUTCOMES

- The authors reported on 20 patients followed for an average of 49 months (range 20 to 77 months).[17]
- Complete arthrodesis of all joints was noted in 75% of patients and partial fusion with stable correction was noted in all patients.
- There were five hardware failures and three patients required removal of screws that backed out partially.

- All patients returned to functional status with diabetic shoe wear and orthotics. None required above-ankle bracing.
- There were no amputations.

COMPLICATIONS

- Screw loosening, backing-out, and hardware failure may occur as fixation will sometimes cross uninvolved joints. The surgeon should avoid crossing the calcaneocuboid and talonavicular joints when possible. Crossing uninvolved joints is acceptable when necessary to achieve adequate fixation in neuropathic patients. Radiographs should be monitored carefully when weight bearing is initiated as screws will sometimes bend before failing and can be exchanged percutaneously. Screws that back out into the ankle or MTP joint should be removed or exchanged.
- Overcorrection can occur and may result in ulceration beneath the first metatarsal head.
- Partial nonunion may occur and does not need to be treated as long as the foot is plantigrade. All patients in our series maintained the majority of their correction at final follow-up.

REFERENCES

1. Alvarez RG, Barbour TM, Perkins TD. Tibiocalcaneal arthrodesis for nonbraceable neuropathic ankle deformity. Foot Ankle Int 1994;15:354–359.
2. Bono JV, Roger DJ, Jacobs RL. Surgical arthrodesis of the neuropathic foot: a salvage procedure. Clin Orthop Relat Res 1993;296:14–20.
3. Campbell JT. Intra-articular neuropathic fracture of the calcaneal body treated by open reduction and subtalar arthrodesis. Foot Ankle Int 2001;22:440–444.
4. Cooper PS. Application of external fixators for management of Charcot deformities of the foot and ankle. Foot Ankle Clin 2002;7:207–254.
5. Early JS, Hansen ST. Surgical reconstruction of the diabetic foot: a salvage approach for midfoot collapse. Foot Ankle Int 1996;17:325–330.
6. Eichneholz SN. Charcot Joints. Springfield, IL: Charles C Thomas; 1966.
7. Lewis P. Scintigraphy in the foot and ankle. Foot Ankle Clin 2000; 5:1–27.
8. Myerson MS, Henderson MR, Saxby T, et al. Management of midfoot diabetic neuroarthropathy. Foot Ankle Int 1994;15:233–241.
9. Papa J, Myerson M, Girard P. Salvage, with arthrodesis, in intractable diabetic neuropathic arthropathy of the foot and ankle. J Bone Joint Surg Am 1993;75A:1056–1066.
10. Pinzur MS. Charcot's foot. Foot Ankle Clin 2000;5:897–912.
11. Sammarco G, Conti SF. Surgical treatment of neuroarthropathic foot deformity. Foot Ankle Int 1998;19:102–109.
12. Schon LC, Easley ME, Weinfeld SB. Charcot neuroarthropathy of the foot and ankle. Clin Orthop Relat Res 1998;349:116–131.
13. Schon LC, Marks RM. The management of neuroarthropathic fracture-dislocations in the diabetic patient. Orthop Clin North Am 1995;26:375–392.
14. Schon LC, Weinfeld SB, Horton GA, et al. Radiographic and clinical classification of acquired midtarsus deformities. Foot Ankle Int 1998;19:394–404.
15. Simon SR, Tejwani SG, Wilson DL, et al. Arthrodesis as an early alternative to nonoperative management of Charcot arthropathy of the diabetic foot. J Bone Joint Surg Am 2000;82A:939–950.
16. Wagner FW. Transcutaneous Doppler ultrasound in the prediction of healing and the selection of surgical level for dysvascular lesions of the toes and forefoot. Clin Orthop Relat Res 1979;142:110–114.
17. Walker E, Sammarco VJ, Sammarco GJ. Surgical treatment of Charcot midfoot collapse with midtarsal arthrodesis using long intramedullary screw fixation. American Orthopaedic Foot and Ankle Society Summer Meeting, La Jolla, CA.

Chapter 45

Minimally Invasive Realignment Surgery of the Charcot Foot

Bradley M. Lamm and Dror Paley

BACKGROUND

- The aftereffects of Charcot joint disease include joint subluxation or dislocation, loss of bone quality, and osseous malalignment (**FIG 1**).
  - As a result of the deformed Charcot foot position, aberrant weight-bearing forces and altered muscle–tendon balance increase the risk for ulceration, infection, and amputation.
  - When treating the Charcot neuropathic foot, the best results are achieved when intervention is initiated as early as possible.
- In acute Charcot neuroarthropathy, the goal of treatment is to stabilize the foot. Total contact casting is the traditional treatment.
  - In this patient population, it is extremely difficult to maintain non–weight-bearing status for multiple reasons, including muscle atrophy, obesity, and diminished proprioception.
  - Non–weight-bearing immobilization for months produces osteopenia of the involved foot and increased weight-bearing forces on the contralateral limb.
  - The sequelae can make it difficult for subsequent surgery on the involved foot and can lead to ulceration and Charcot neuroarthropathy in the contralateral foot.
- In chronic Charcot neuroarthropathy, the goal of treatment is to realign the soft tissue and osseous structures. In general, surgeries are aimed at realignment, but in these extremely deformed feet, acute realignment is challenging.
  - Traditionally, acute realignment procedures such as Achilles tendon lengthening, ostectomy, débridement, osteotomy, arthrodesis, and open reduction with internal fixation (plantar plating) have been attempted.[4]
  - Acute correction via open reduction with application of static external fixation has also been reported.[2]
  - More recently, internal fixation methods have been augmented or replaced by external fixation as a means of static fixation of a Charcot reconstruction.[6]
- Here, we present a new two-stage minimally invasive gradual correction method with the use of external fixation for acute and chronic Charcot reconstruction, which was developed by the senior author (D.P.).[3]
- Gradual deformity correction with external fixation is preferred for large-deformity reductions of the dislocated Charcot joints of the foot. Correction with external fixation allows for gradual, accurate realignment of the dislocated or subluxated Charcot joints.

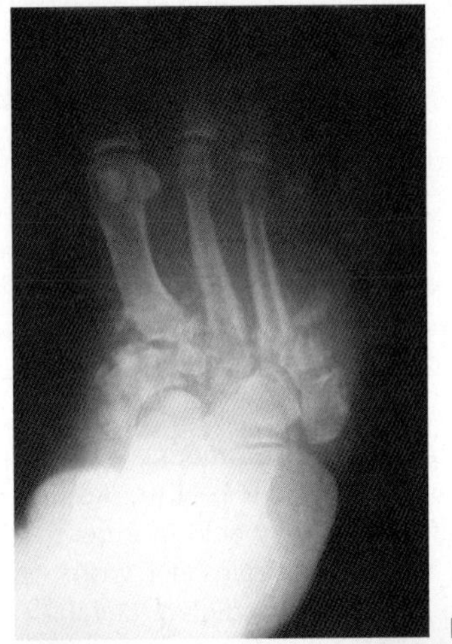
A

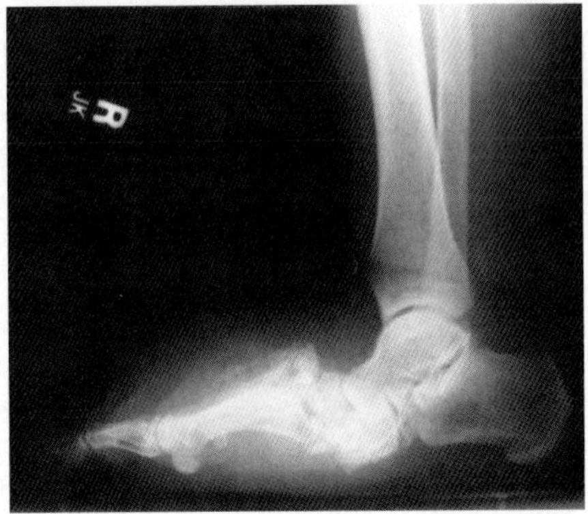

B

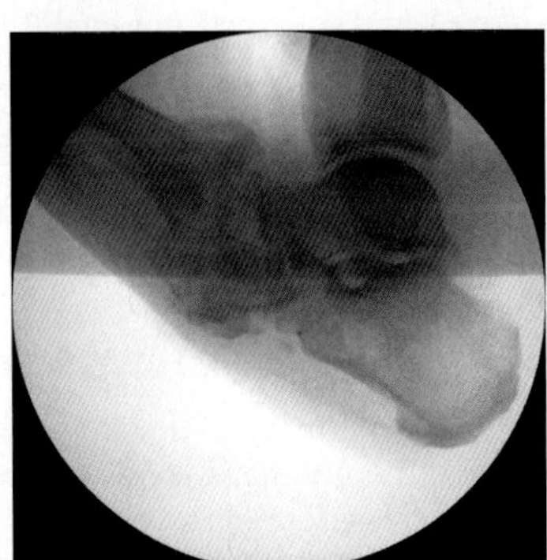
C

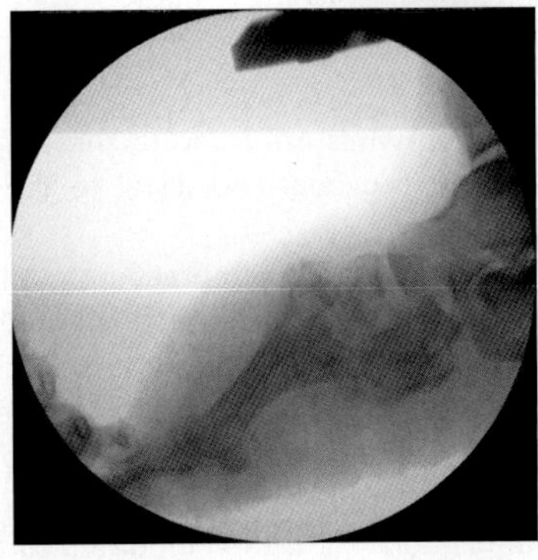
D

FIG 1 • Midfoot Charcot neuroarthropathy deformity (Eichenholtz stage II, unstable, with lateral ulceration and previous resection of the fourth and fifth metatarsals). **A.** AP radiograph shows midfoot adduction deformity. **B.** Lateral radiograph shows rocker-bottom and equinus deformities. Note the dorsal displacement of the forefoot and the break in Meary's angle. Lateral still images, obtained by using video fluoroscopy, confirm the instability of the midfoot Charcot deformity, demonstrating significant forefoot dorsiflexion (**C**) and plantarflexion (**D**). (Copyright 2008, Rubin Institute for Advanced Orthopedics, Sinai Hospital of Baltimore.)

SURGICAL TREATMENT

- The goals of surgical intervention for the Charcot foot are to restore anatomic alignment, impart stability, prevent amputation, prevent foot shortening, and allow the patient to be ambulatory.
- Historically, open reduction with internal fixation was the mainstay for treatment of Charcot foot deformities.
  - Large open incisions were made to remove the excess bone, reduce the dislocated bone, and stabilize with internal fixation (screw fixation or plantar plating).
  - These invasive surgical procedures typically resulted in shortening of the foot or incomplete deformity reduction and occasionally resulted in neurovascular compromise, incision healing problems, infection, and the use of non–weight-bearing casts and boots.
- In cases of tarsometatarsal Charcot deformity, open reduction is advantageous.
  - Typically, Charcot neuroarthropathy of the tarsometatarsal joints is associated with mild to moderate deformities because the tarsometatarsal joints are structurally interlocked.
  - Acute realignment is achieved by performing a wedge resection or open reduction with fusion and internal fixation to produce a stable foot.
- In acute Charcot neuroarthropathy, a static external fixation is placed to stabilize the Charcot process. The smooth wire fixation for the external fixation is applied so as to avoid the "hot," or Charcot, joint region of the foot.
  - The static fixator is applied strategically so gradual realignment can begin after the acute phase of Charcot has passed. Thus, the external fixator serves a dual purpose by stabilizing both the acute Charcot joint and the subsequent realignment of the dislocated osseous anatomy.
  - Once the bony anatomy is realigned, the external fixation is removed and a formal minimally invasive fusion of the Charcot joint is performed. Rigid intramedullary metatarsal screws are used to maintain the fusion.
- Chronic stable or coalesced Charcot foot deformities require an osteotomy for correction of the deformity. We prefer a percutaneous Gigli saw osteotomy technique.
  - Midfoot osteotomies can be performed across three levels (ie, talar neck and calcaneal neck, cubonavicular osseous level, and cuneocuboid osseous level).
  - Performing Gigli saw osteotomy across multiple metatarsals should be avoided because of the neurovascular injury.[3]
- For an unstable or an incompletely coalesced Charcot foot, correction can be obtained through gradual distraction.
  - Despite the radiographic appearance of coalescence (superimposition of the dislocated or fragmented pedal bone due to the Charcot process), most Charcot deformities can undergo distraction without osteotomy to realign the pedal anatomy.
  - An Achilles tendon lengthening is performed and held in a neutral position with the external fixation. This restores the normal calcaneal pitch and hindfoot position.
  - Then, under fluoroscopy, acute forefoot reduction is attempted and, if possible, fixation with intermedullary metatarsal screws is carried out.
  - Acute reduction of the forefoot is rarely successful, however. If the forefoot cannot be acutely reduced, an external fixator is used to hold the hindfoot position while the forefoot is lengthened and realigned.

Approach

- This first stage of the procedure consists of osseous realignment of the forefoot on a fixed hindfoot, which is achieved with an external fixator using distraction.
- After realignment, the correction is maintained by minimally invasive arthrodesis of the Charcot joint and is fixed with percutaneous intramedullary metatarsal screws.

TECHNIQUES

STAGE 1

Plate Fixation and Achilles Tendon Lengthening

- The first stage consists of osseous realignment achieved by performing an acute Achilles tendon lengthening and gradual soft tissue distraction with the Taylor spatial frame (TSF). Patient adjustments of the TSF (forefoot 6 × 6 butt frame) provide gradual relocation of the forefoot on the fixed hindfoot.
- The distal tibia, talus, and calcaneus are fixed with two U-plates joined and mounted orthogonal to the tibia in both the anteroposterior (AP) and lateral planes.
  - The U-plate is affixed to the tibia with one lateromedial 1.8-mm wire and two or three additional points of fixation (combination of smooth wires or half-pins).
  - For additional stability, a second distal tibial ring can be added, creating a distal tibial fixation block.
- It is essential to fix the hindfoot in a neutral position; an Achilles tendon lengthening typically is required to achieve a neutral hindfoot position. We prefer performing percutaneous Z-lengthening of the Achilles tendon.
- With the hindfoot manually held in a neutral position, the U-plate is fixed to the calcaneus with two crossing 1.8-mm wires. A 1.8-mm mediolateral talar neck wire also is inserted and fixed to the U-plate.

External Fixation Setup

- Two 1.8-mm stirrup wires are inserted through the osseous segment just proximal and distal to the Charcot joints.
- The stirrup wires are bent 90 degrees just outside the skin to extend and attach but are not tensioned to their respective external fixation rings distant from the point of fixation. Stirrup wires capture osseous segments that are far from an external fixation ring, thereby providing accurate and precise Charcot joint distraction.
- A full external fixation ring is then mounted to the forefoot by two 1.8-mm crossing metatarsal wires and the aforementioned distal stirrup wire.

- Digital pinning often is required whereby the digital wires (1.5 or 1.8 mm) are attached to the forefoot ring.
- Finally, the six TSF struts are placed and final radiographs obtained (AP and lateral views of the foot to include the tibia; **TECH FIG 1**).
- Orthogonal AP and lateral view fluoroscopic images are obtained of the reference ring; these images provide the mounting parameters that are needed for the computer planning.
- The choice of which ring (distal or proximal) to use as the reference ring is based on the surgeon's preference; typically, a distal reference is chosen for foot deformity correction.
  - Superimposition of the reference ring on the final films is critical for accurate postoperative computer deformity planning.
- Computer planning of the TSF is a critical part of this procedure. The surgeon enters the deformity and mounting parameters into an Internet-based software (www.spatialframe.com) that produces a daily schedule for the patient to perform adjustments on each of the six struts. The rate and duration of the patient's schedule is controlled by the surgeon's data entry.
- The patient returns for clinical and radiographic follow-up in the office weekly or biweekly.

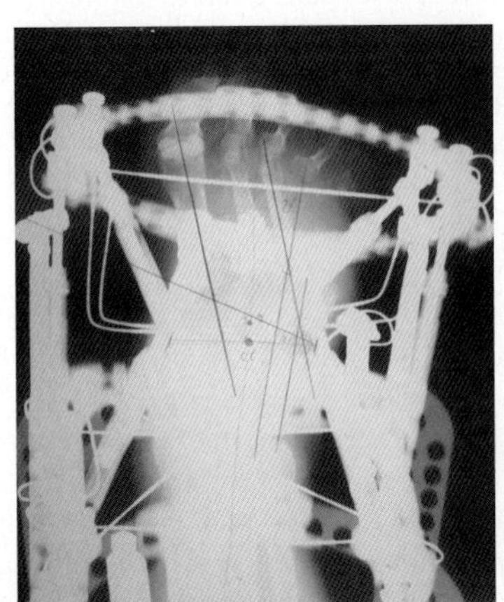
A

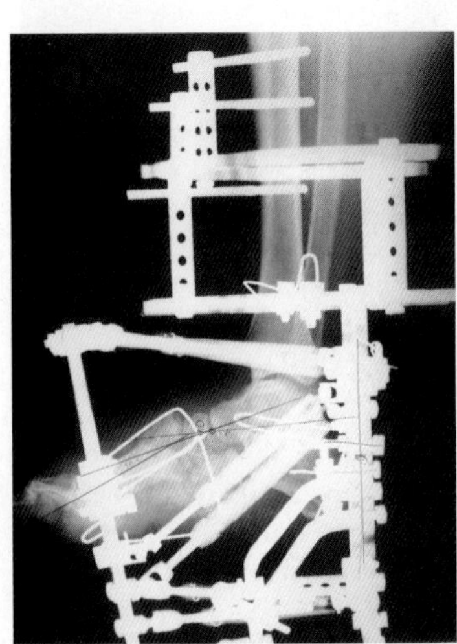
B

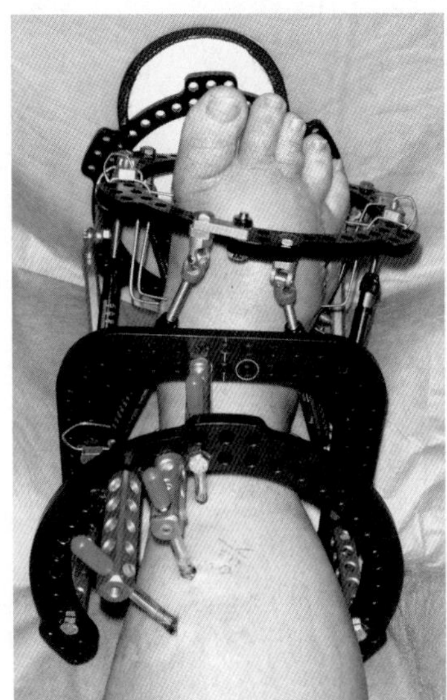
C

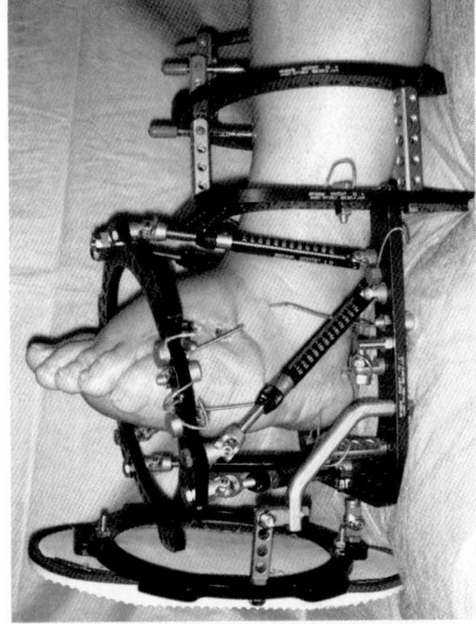
D

TECH FIG 1 • **A.** Immediate postoperative AP radiograph shows midfoot adduction (20 degrees) in the patient shown in Figure 1. **B.** Immediate postoperative lateral radiograph shows plantarflexion of the forefoot (10 degrees). The change in forefoot position as compared with the preoperative radiographs is due to the acute manipulation intraoperatively. The stirrup wires (90-degree bent wires that are not tensioned) are placed adjacent to the region of distraction and realignment (midfoot). These stirrup wires ensure focused distraction. Note the TSF planning lines and reference points. **C,D.** Clinical photographs show the TSF (forefoot 6 × 6 butt) applied. In **C**, note the delta configuration of the tibial half-pins and the build-out (two-hole plate) off the distal foot ring to allow for soft tissue clearance. In **D**, note the stirrup wires adjacent to the distraction region. (Copyright 2008, Rubin Institute for Advanced Orthopedics, Sinai Hospital for Baltimore.)

STAGE 2

Frame Removal and Arthrodesis

- Gradual distraction for realignment of the dislocated Charcot joints is obtained in approximately 1 to 2 months. After gradual distraction with the TSF has realigned the anatomy of the foot (**TECH FIG 2A**), the second stage of the correction is performed.
- The external fixator is removed simultaneously with performance of minimally invasive arthrodesis of the affected joints using percutaneous insertion of internal fixation (**TECH FIG 2B**).
- Before frame removal, small transverse incisions (2 to 3 cm in length) are made overlying the appropriate joints to perform cartilage removal and joint preparation for arthrodesis.

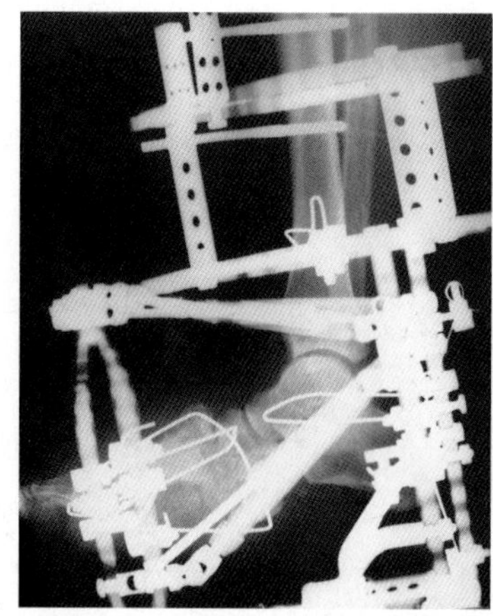

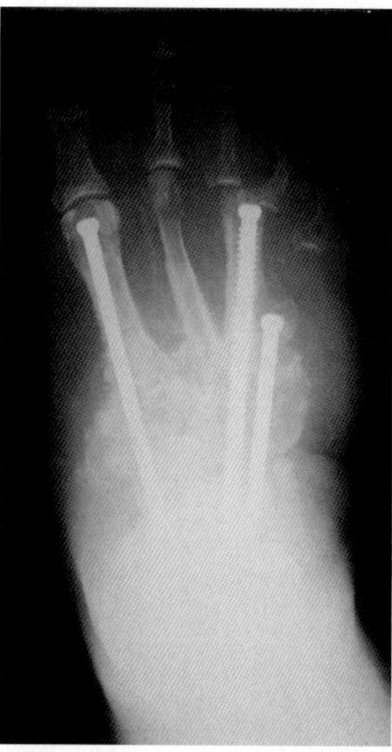

TECH FIG 2 • A. Lateral view radiograph after 1 month of gradual TSF correction shows a normal (or zero) Meary's angle and distraction of the midfoot in the same patient. The dorsal foot ulcer has healed and the foot is correctly positioned. **B.** Immediately after removal of the external fixator, a minimally invasive fusion of the midtarsal joint was performed to prevent future Charcot foot collapse. A weight-bearing AP radiograph shows two percutaneous intramedullary metatarsal screws and a lateral column screw that were inserted for stabilization of the fusion of the midtarsal joint. Note the accurate anatomic reduction. (Copyright 2008, Rubin Institute for Advanced Orthopedics, Sinai Hospital for Baltimore.)

- Minimally invasive arthrodesis is easily performed because the Charcot joints are already distracted.
- Under fluoroscopic guidance, the guidewires for the large-diameter cannulated screws are inserted percutaneously through the plantar skin incision into the metatarsal head by dorsiflexing the metatarsophalangeal joint.
- After the lateral and medial column guidewires (fourth, first, and second metatarsals) are inserted to maintain the corrected foot position, the frame is removed and the foot is reprepped.

Intramedullary Screw Fixation and Closure

- Typically, three large-diameter cannulated intramedullary metatarsal screws are inserted: medial and lateral column partially threaded screws for compression of the arthrodesis site and one central (second metatarsal) fully threaded screw for additional stabilization.
- These screws span the entire length of the metatarsals to the calcaneus and talus, provide compression across the minimally invasive arthrodesis site, and stabilize adjacent joints. The intramedullary metatarsal screws cross an unaffected joint, the Lisfranc joint, thereby protecting the Lisfranc joint from experiencing a future Charcot event.
- The minimally invasive incisions are then closed, and a well-padded L and U splint is applied.
- At the time of hospital discharge, the patient is placed in a non–weight-bearing short leg cast for 2 to 3 months, and then gradual progression to weight bearing is achieved. Thus, the entire treatment is completed in 4 to 5 months (**TECH FIG 3**).

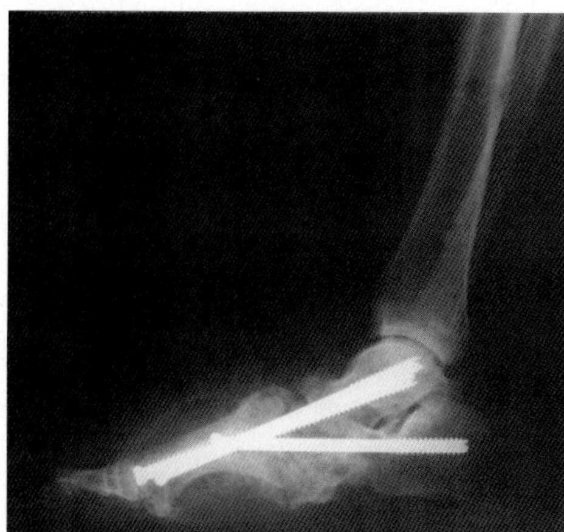

TECH FIG 3 • A postoperative lateral view radiograph from the same patient shows a healed plantigrade foot with intact intramedullary metatarsal screws. Note the accurate anatomic reduction, fusion of the involved Charcot joint (midtarsal joint), protection of the adjacent Lisfranc joints (stability via screw fixation), ridged internal stability, restoration of foot length, healed ulceration, and preservation of the subtalar and ankle joints. (Copyright 2008, Rubin Institute for Advanced Orthopedics, Sinai Hospital for Baltimore.)

PEARLS AND PITFALLS

- External fixation construction is challenging because of the small size of the foot. When applying the forefoot 6 × 6 butt frame, it is important to mount the U-plate on the hindfoot as posterior as possible and the forefoot ring as anterior as possible. The greater the distance between the forefoot and hindfoot ring, the more space for the TSF struts.
- Bone segment fixation is important; otherwise, failure of osteotomy separation or incomplete anatomic reduction occurs. Small wire fixation is preferred in the foot because of the size and consistency of the bones.
- When treating a patient with neuropathy, construction of extremely stable constructs is of great importance. External fixation for Charcot deformity correction should include a full distal tibial ring with a closed foot ring.

OUTCOMES

- We have performed this gradual distraction technique for the past 5 years and have achieved good to excellent success in more than a dozen feet.
- Feet were operated on at various stages of Charcot deformity (Eichenholtz stages I, II, and III).
- When comparing the average change in preoperative and postoperative radiographic angles, the transverse plane talar–first metatarsal angle, sagittal plane talar–first metatarsal angle, and calcaneal pitch angle were all found to be significantly altered.
- Most notably, no deep infection, no screw failure, and no recurrent ulcerations occurred and no amputations were necessary during the past 5 years.
- Gradual Charcot foot correction with the TSF plus minimally invasive arthrodesis has constituted a safe and effective treatment.
- Our results are promising. The advantages of our method when compared with the resection and plating method reported by Schon[4] or the resection and external fixation method reported by Cooper[1] are preservation of foot length (no bone resection), accurate anatomic realignment of soft tissues and bone, and a stable foot. Furthermore, our method is much less invasive and allows for partial weight bearing.

ACKNOWLEDGMENT

We thank Amanda Chase, MA, for her editing assistance, and Alvien Lee for his photographic expertise.

REFERENCES

1. Cooper PS. Application of external fixators for management of Charcot deformities of the foot and ankle. Foot Ankle Clin 2002;7:207–254.
2. Jolly GP, Zgonis T, Polyzois V. External fixation in the management of Charcot neuroarthropathy. Clin Podiatr Med Surg 2003; 20:741–756.
3. Paley D. Principles of Deformity Correction. Rev ed. Berlin: Springer-Verlag, 2005.
4. Schon LC, Easley ME, Weinfeld SB. Charcot neuroarthropathy of the foot and ankle. Clin Orthop Relat Res 1998;349:116–131.
5. Trepman E, Nihal A, Pinzur MS:.Current topics review: Charcot neuroarthropathy of the foot and ankle. Foot Ankle Int 2003;6:46–63.
6. Wang JC, Le AW, Tsukuda RK. A new technique for Charcot's foot reconstruction. J Am Podiatr Med Assoc 2002;92:429–436.

Chapter 46

Flexor Digitorum Longus Transfer and Medial Displacement Calcaneal Osteotomy

Gregory P. Guyton

DEFINITION

- The posterior tibial tendon undergoes tearing and degeneration, and as it fails the foot falls into a planovalgus configuration. Posterior tibial tendon dysfunction (PTTD) is the most common cause of an adult acquired flatfoot deformity.
- Most cases occur spontaneously without known antecedent trauma. Women are much more commonly affected than men, with a typical age range older than 50 years.
- With time, a rigid deformity develops. The degree and flexibility of the deformity play a key role in determining treatment.

ANATOMY

- The posterior tibialis typically degenerates in an area underneath the medial malleolus and distally to its insertion. The process is not inflammatory but is rather characterized by replacement of the normal collagen fibers with amorphous scar and mucinous degeneration.[6]
- As the arch falls, the hindfoot will fall into valgus relative to the leg, while the forefoot will abduct through the talonavicular joint. Uncovering of the talar head results as the forefoot pivots laterally.
- The sag of the arch and the abduction of the forefoot can be described in terms of the loss of alignment of the first metatarsal and the talus. The long axes of these bones should normally be colinear. A sag of the arch is seen by an angulation in this line on the standing lateral radiograph, while abduction of the forefoot is seen by lateral angulation of this line on the AP view.

PATHOGENESIS

- In most cases the cause of PTTD is unknown and is not associated with a clear antecedent trauma.
- The collapse of the arch is the result of a tendon imbalance. The antagonists to the posterior tibialis are the peroneals, and they must be functional for the deformity to develop.
- A single study has suggested a correlation of PTTD with the HLA B-27 genotype typically associated with seronegative arthropathies.[9]
- Cumulative mechanical factors likely play a role in the development of the disorder; a pre-existing planovalgus deformity presumably places extra stress on the tendon and is thought to be a risk factor for degeneration.
- The presence of an accessory navicular ossicle within the tendon substance at its insertion into the medial pole of the navicular is also a risk factor for tendon degeneration, likely from local mechanical stress (**FIG 1**).

NATURAL HISTORY

- Dysfunction of the posterior tibialis is thought to be the initiating event in the collapse of the arch.[2]
- Early in the course of the disease, pain along the course of the posterior tibialis or weakness of its function will be present without any arch collapse. This is called stage I disease.
- With time, a planovalgus foot deformity develops. Initially this deformity is flexible and is called stage II disease.
- A fixed deformity eventually results; this is called stage III disease. The first component of the deformity to become fixed is usually an elevation of the first ray relative to the fifth ray. This is the result of a compensation of the forefoot for the hindfoot valgus and is called a fixed forefoot varus. Later, the valgus alignment of the calcaneus through the subtalar joint becomes contracted and irreducible.
- Rarely, a secondary failure of the deltoid ligament along the medial aspect of the hindfoot develops as the mechanical stresses placed upon it by the flattened arch increase. This is called a stage IV deformity.
- Achilles tendon contracture is commonly seen in association with PTTD. As the planovalgus deformity develops, the foot collapses through the arch and the Achilles is no longer stretched to its normal length in a standing or walking posture.
- Table 1 details the PTTD stages.

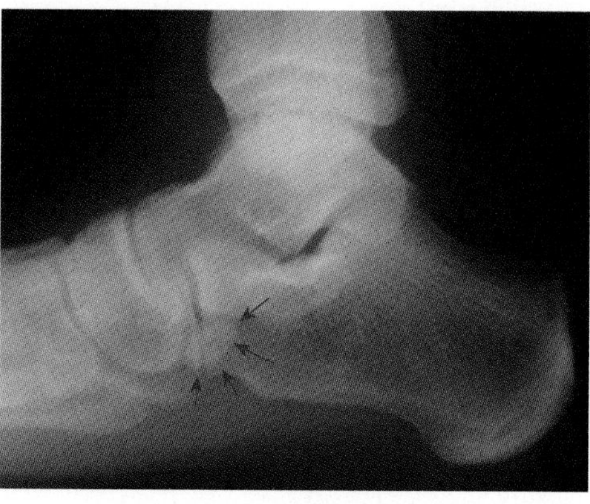

FIG 1 • The accessory navicular may be subtle and can usually be seen on the lateral or AP radiographs.

Table 1 Stages of Posterior Tibial Tendon Dysfunction

Stage I: Tenosynovitis and tear without arch collapse
Stage II: Tenosynovitis and tear with flexible deformity
Stage III: Fixed deformity present
Stage IV: Additional deltoid ligament insufficiency with tibiotalar tilt

PATIENT HISTORY AND PHYSICAL FINDINGS

- Most, but not all, patients present with pain along the medial arch.
- In some cases, lateral impingement develops as the valgus posture of the hindfoot becomes extreme. The calcaneus impinges against the inferior border of the fibula. This is usually a late finding and is often intractable to conservative management.
- The most painful phase of PTTD is usually as the tendon is actively degenerating. Some patients will note a history of intense pain that diminishes once the tendon finally ruptures completely. They may present with deformity or lateral pain as their primary complaint.
- Other deformities may coexist, most significantly hallux valgus or midfoot arthritis.
- Methods for examining the foot for PTTD include:
  - The single-leg toe rise. The examiner should note the ability to perform the maneuver, the presence of inversion, and the presence or absence of pain. This is a critical and sensitive screening test. Action of the posterior tibialis is required to invert and lock the hindfoot, allowing the foot to act as a rigid lever through which the Achilles powers the ankle into plantarflexion.
  - The "too many toes" sign. The examiner observes the standing patient from behind. The more abducted forefoot will show more toes visible on the lateral side of the leg. The examiner also notes the presence of forefoot abduction. Abduction of the forefoot occurs as the posterior tibialis fails and must be corrected in treatment.
  - Power of the posterior tibialis. The examiner isolates the tendon by resisted inversion past the midline with the foot held in plantarflexion. Typical muscle strength grading is used. The result can be normal early in the disease. The patient may attempt to substitute the anterior tibialis; it is also an invertor but will dorsiflex the ankle as well.
  - Fixed forefoot varus. The examiner holds the calcaneus in a neutral position (out of valgus) and notes any fixed elevation of the first ray relative to the fifth. The severity of deformity is noted in degrees. Fixed forefoot varus must be accounted for in any treatment algorithm and is usually the first component of the deformity to become rigid.
  - Achilles contracture. The examiner holds the calcaneus in a neutral position and notes dorsiflexion of the ankle with the knee both flexed and extended (the Silfverskiöld test). The result is measured in degrees of ankle dorsiflexion. A significant Achilles contracture limits the degree of correction possible with bracing and may require surgical correction.

IMAGING AND OTHER DIAGNOSTIC STUDIES

- Plain radiographs should be obtained with weight bearing to adequately describe the alignment of the foot. The talo–first metatarsal angle describes the sag of the arch when drawn on the lateral view and the abduction of the forefoot when drawn on the AP view.
- Plain foot radiographs should also be examined for the presence of hindfoot arthritis, midfoot arthritis or instability, and an accessory navicular.
- A standing ankle mortise view should be obtained to rule out deltoid laxity (stage IV disease).
- MRI is not routinely necessary and may underestimate the severity of disease, but it may be useful in ruling out other pathologies. Findings of PTTD typically include fluid in the sheath, dramatic thickening of the tendon, and a heterogeneous signal within the tendon substance indicating the presence of interstitial tears (**FIG 2**).

DIFFERENTIAL DIAGNOSIS

- Midfoot arthritis resulting in pes planus through tarsometatarsal joint collapse
- Medial ankle arthritis
- Medial osteochondral lesion of the talus
- Neurogenic failure of the posterior tibialis through spinal or central pathology

NONOPERATIVE MANAGEMENT

- The flatfoot that results from posterior tibial tendon failure is irreversible, but symptoms may be controllable in many patients by nonoperative means.
- A simple in-shoe semirigid or rigid foot orthotic may provide sufficient arch support to reduce symptoms in some patients.
- The gold standard for nonoperative management is the use of a cross-ankle brace. This allows direct control of the tendency of the calcaneus to fall into valgus. The most commonly used and best tolerated is a leather ankle lacer with an incorporated custom-molded plastic stirrup, often referred to as an Arizona brace after a common brand name.[1] Other options that may be suitable for higher-demand situations or patients with edema control problems include a hinged molded ankle–foot orthosis or a conventional double-metal upright ankle–foot orthosis with a leg strap.
- Steroid injections into the posterior tibial tendon sheath are contraindicated as they may directly or indirectly precipitate frank rupture and further collapse.
- No brace, physical therapy regimen, or medication has been shown to modify the course of the disease or the ultimate outcome for the tendon. These are all best thought of as modalities to control the symptoms.

SURGICAL MANAGEMENT

- Surgery is indicated when the symptoms cannot be controlled by a nonoperative means acceptable to the patient. An active patient in his or her 50s, for instance, may find the use of an Arizona brace for the remainder of his or her life to be intolerable and may choose to pursue a surgical remedy.

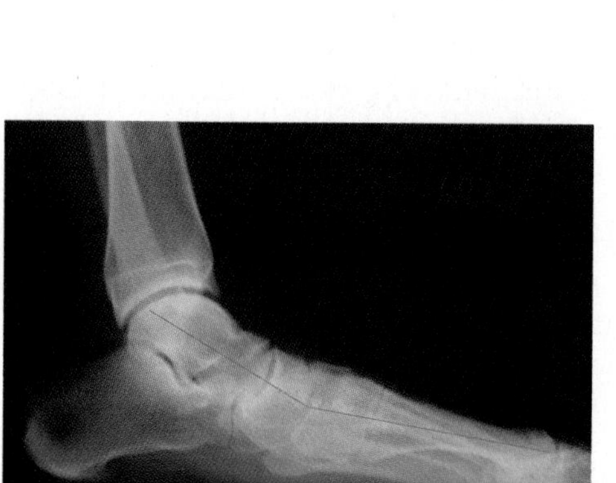

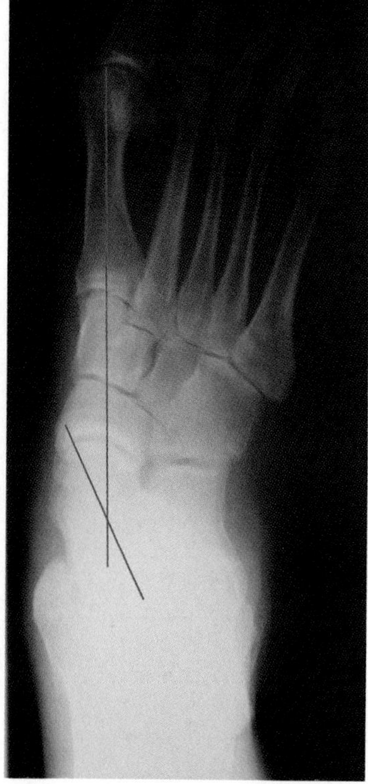

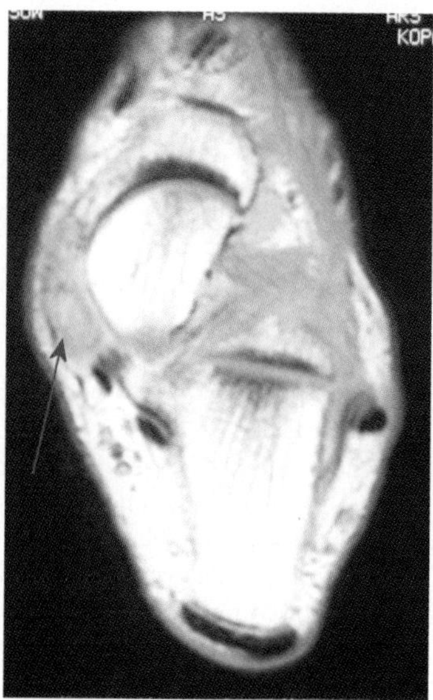

FIG 2 • The talo–first metatarsal angle is drawn down the long axis of the talus and the first metatarsal on both lateral (**A**) and AP (**B**) radiographs. Any break from a straight line demonstrates both sag and abduction of the arch. MRI findings (**C**) include the presence of edema within the tendon substance and enlargement. Normal absence of signal within the adjacent flexor digitorum longus and flexor hallucis longus tendons is visible on the image.

Preoperative Planning

- The patient's size must be considered before any motion-sparing tendon reconstruction in the hindfoot is considered. Although not rigorously proven in the literature, the morbidly obese patient with an acquired pes planus deformity is at greater risk to break down the repair and may be better served by a triple arthrodesis.
- The presence of hindfoot arthritis similarly requires a fusion rather than an osteotomy and tendon reconstruction.
- A fixed forefoot varus should be addressed, either as part of the procedure through a medial column osteotomy or by a triple arthrodesis if severe.
- Tightness of the gastrocnemius should also be assessed to determine if a fractional lengthening of the gastrocnemius (Strayer procedure) will be required.

Positioning

- The patient is positioned supine with a bolster under the ipsilateral hip. This internally rotates the leg to allow access to the lateral aspect of the calcaneus, which is addressed first. The bolster may then be removed to allow the leg to externally rotate and allow access to the medial aspect of the foot.
- A tourniquet is applied to the thigh.

Approach

- The posterior tibial tendon is débrided directly and augmented or replaced by transferring the flexor digitorum longus (FDL) to the navicular. This procedure alone was first described in the 1980s and proved quite effective at pain control in most cases, although static correction of the arch was minimal.[2,5]
- A medial displacement calcaneal osteotomy is then used to provide a measure of arch correction, directly addressing the hindfoot valgus. Indirectly, this raises the sag along the medial column of the foot as well and helps correct the talo–first metatarsal angle. Correcting the mechanics of the arch is thought to confer an element of protection to the FDL transfer.[3,7,8,11]
- If necessary, up to about 20 degrees of forefoot varus may be corrected by a plantarflexion osteotomy of the medial column through the medial cuneiform (the Cotton procedure). This allows the indications for a motion-sparing procedure to be expanded to a wider patient population, and the need for this step is assessed after the other components of the correction are complete.[4]
- Once the arch is corrected, a final check of the tightness of the gastrocsoleus complex is made to ensure that a lengthening is not required.

MEDIAL DISPLACEMENT CALCANEAL OSTEOTOMY

- Make a 4-cm oblique incision over the lateral aspect of the calcaneal tuberosity behind the peroneal sheath (**TECH FIG 1A**).
- Carefully avoid the sural nerve during dissection down to the periosteum (**TECH FIG 1B**).
- Pass a small elevator above and below the calcaneal tuberosity. Ensure that inferiorly the cut will be anterior to the origin of the plantar fascia.
- Place small retractors superiorly and inferiorly, and place a low-profile self-retainer in the center of the wound.
- Use a narrow microsagittal saw to cut the tuberosity from lateral to medial. Using a narrow handheld blade provides greater tactile feedback to avoid overpenetration on the medial side (**TECH FIG 1C**).
- Lever the osteotomy free with a large osteotome or elevator.
- Place a lamina spreader in the osteotomy and leave it for about 1 minute to allow for stress relaxation of the tissues on the medial side. If necessary, a Cobb elevator can be used to gently strip the area (**TECH FIG 1D,E**).
- Displace the tuberosity fragment medially, usually by about 1 cm. Fix it with one or two 5.0- to 6.5-mm screws placed percutaneously from the posterior tuberosity (**TECH FIG 1F**).
- Obtain lateral and axial calcaneal fluoroscopy shots to confirm displacement of the tuberosity and confinement of the screws within bone.
- With a rongeur, smooth any sharp step-off on the lateral side of the osteotomy (**TECH FIG 1G,H**).

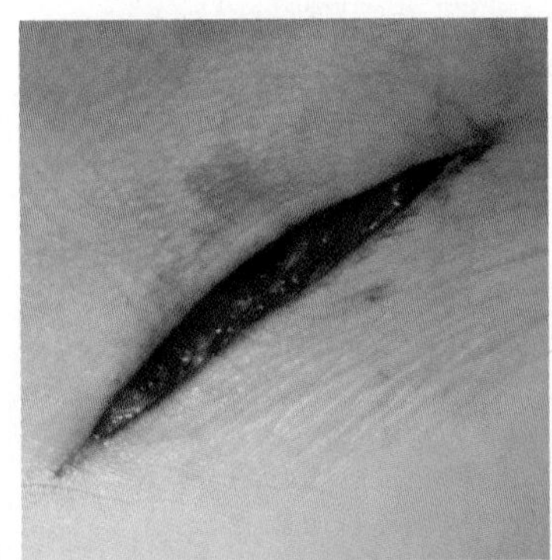
A

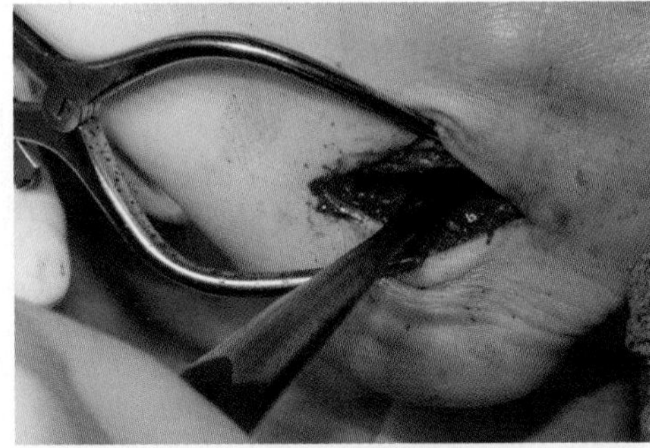
D

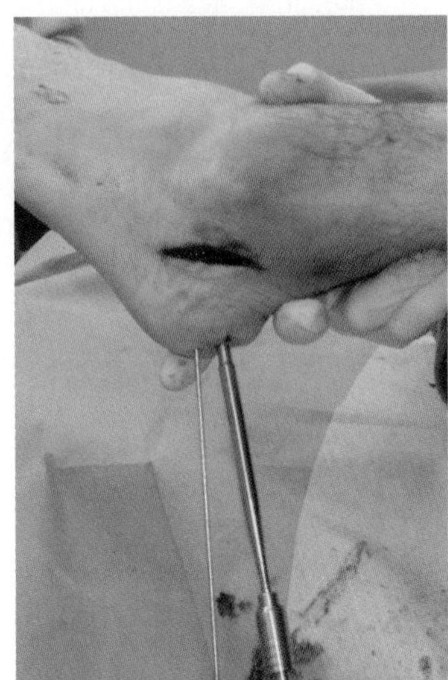
F

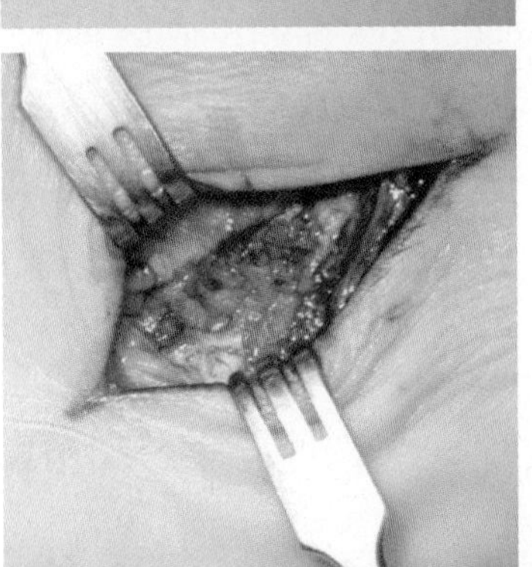
B

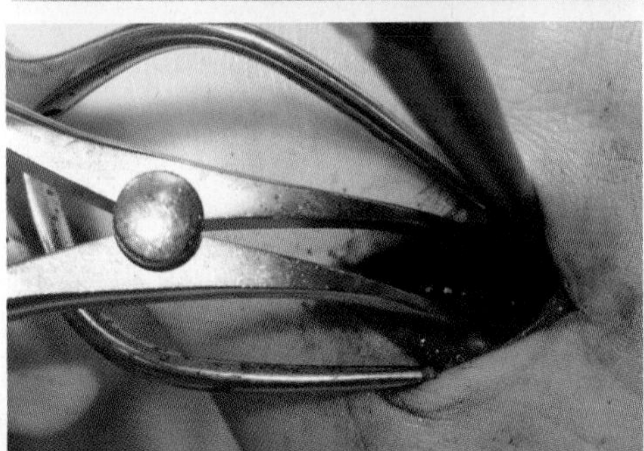
E

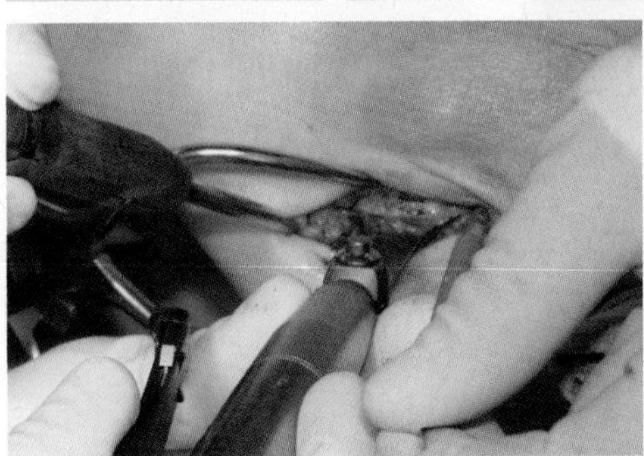
C

TECH FIG 1 • **A.** Oblique incision for the calcaneal osteotomy. **B.** Careful dissection to the periosteum is made, avoiding the sural nerve. **C.** Dorsal and plantar retractors are placed and a microsagittal saw is used to make the cut. **D.** A Cobb elevator is used to free up the osteotomy. **E.** A lamina spreader is placed to provide further stress relaxation of the tissues. **F.** After displacement, retrograde screws are used to provide fixation. *(continued)*

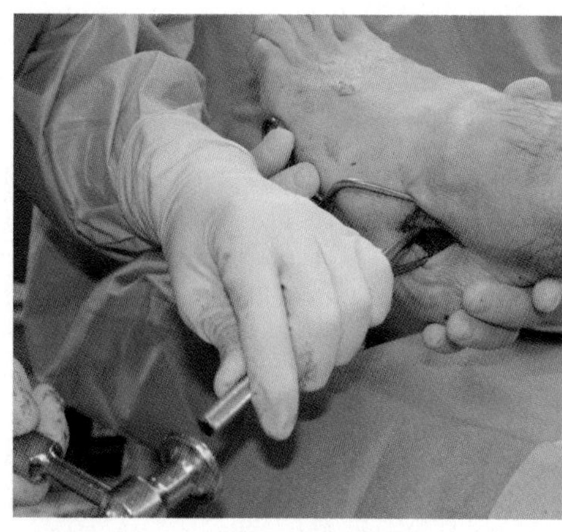

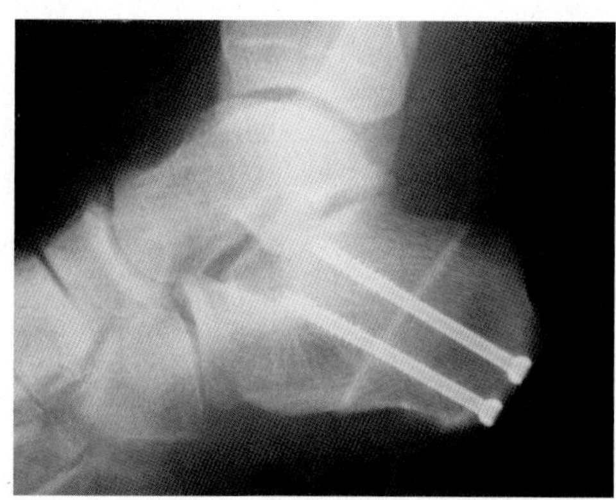

TECH FIG 1 • *(continued)* **G.** The sharp margin of the osteotomy is impacted to form a smooth contour. **H.** Radiographic appearance after fixation with two 5.0 screws.

POSTERIOR TIBIAL TENDON DÉBRIDEMENT AND FLEXOR DIGITORUM LONGUS TRANSFER

- Make a longitudinal incision down the medial column of the foot, beginning behind the medial malleolus, passing over the navicular tuberosity, and following the inferior border of the first metatarsal (**TECH FIG 2A**).
- Open the posterior tibialis sheath and débride the tendon. Complete tendon resection is appropriate in the vast majority of cases, as any remaining diseased tendon is a potential source of pain. Leave roughly a 1-cm stump of tendon attached to the navicular tuberosity to facilitate reconstruction (**TECH FIG 2B**).
- Identify the FDL sheath and open it just below the medial malleolus. It is located inferior to the posterior tibialis sheath and lies superficial to the sustentaculum tali (**TECH FIG 2C**).
- Trace the FDL sheath distally to about 2 to 3 cm distal to the navicular tuberosity. To achieve this, develop the plane between the abductor hallucis and the first metatarsal periosteum and take down a portion of the tendinous origin of the flexor hallucis brevis. This reveals the decussation of the flexor hallucis longus

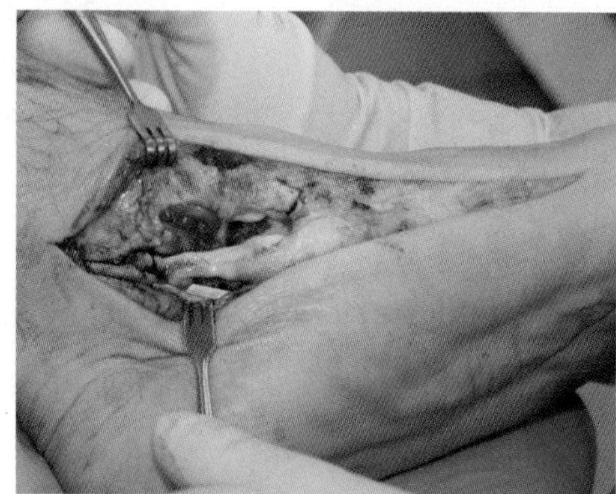

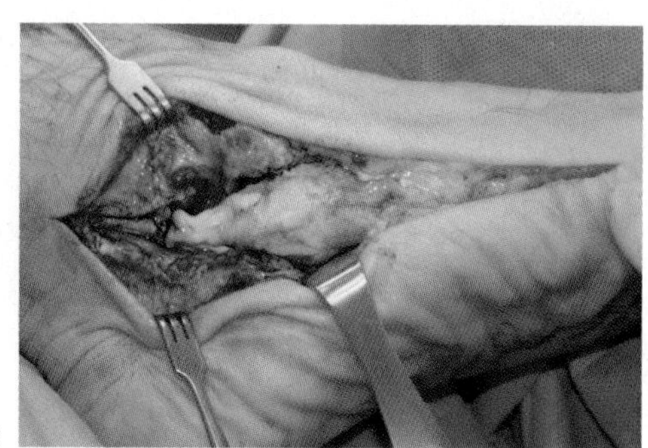

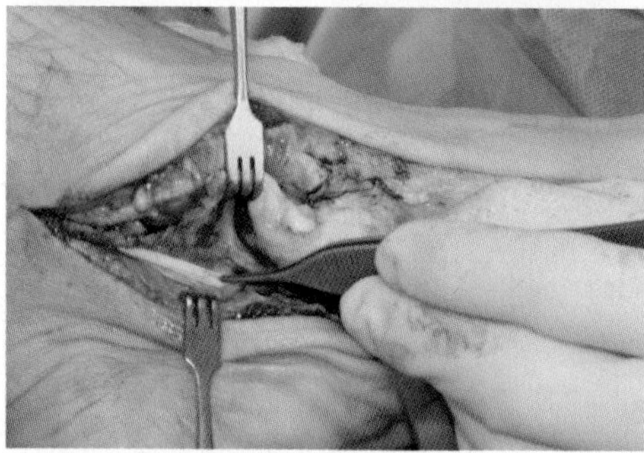

TECH FIG 2 • **A.** A longitudinal incision is made along the posterior tibialis sheath and medial midfoot. **B.** The posterior tibialis is found to be completely deficient and is débrided. **C.** The flexor digitorum longus (FDL) sheath is opened proximally behind the posterior tibialis sheath. *(continued)*

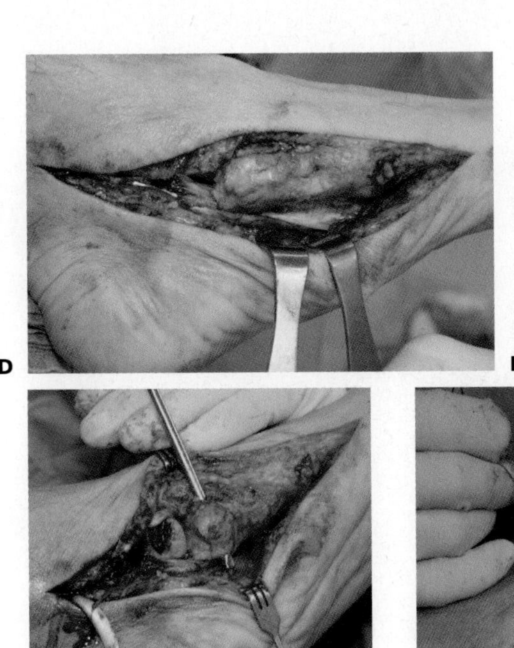
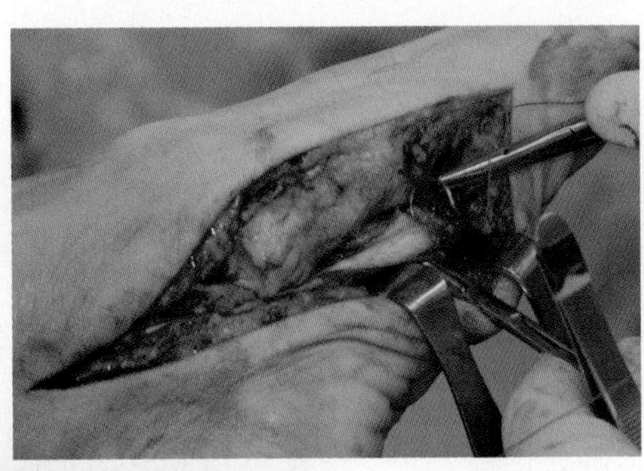
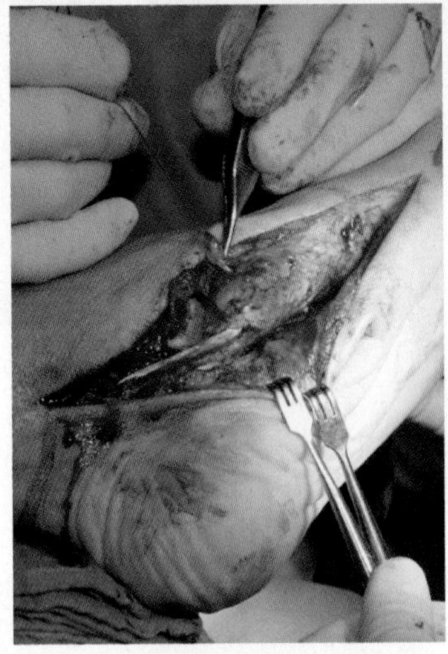
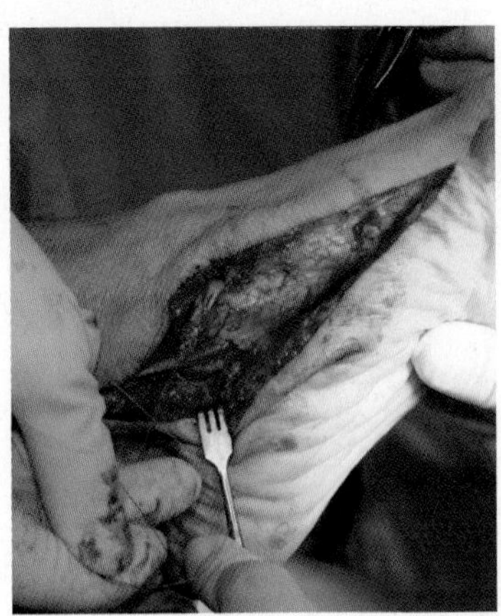
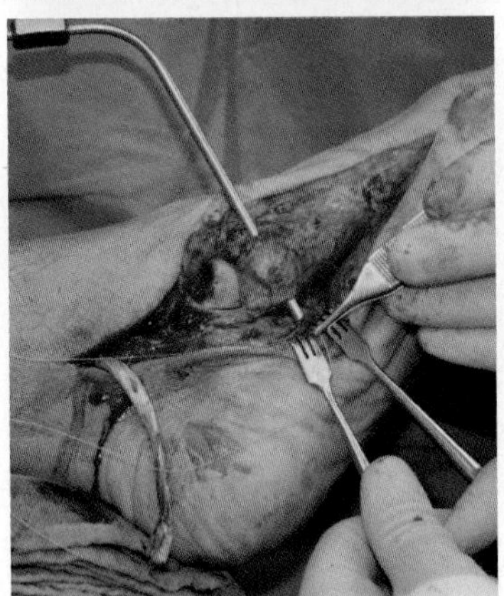

TECH FIG 2 • *(continued)* **D.** The FDL is followed and exposed to the knot of Henry. **E.** A distal tenodesis of the FDL and flexor hallucis longus is made; the FDL is then cut. **F.** A dorsal-to-plantar drill hole is made in the navicular tuberosity. **G.** Placing a sucker tip to suck the sutures through the drill hole allows for easy passage. **H.** The FDL is passed through the navicular from plantar to dorsal. **I.** The FDL is turned back upon itself and sutured in place, and the spring ligament is repaired.

(FHL) and FDL, also called the knot of Henry (TECH FIG 2D).

- The FDL is optionally tenodesed to the FHL at the distal aspect of the incision, and any evident juncturae between the two tendons are resected. While small toe function is theoretically aided by this tenodesis, there appears to be little clinically recognizable effect from its omission (TECH FIG 2E).
- Drill a 4- to 5-mm hole through the navicular tuberosity and apply a lead stitch to the FDL tendon. Pass it through the hole from plantar to dorsal and suture it into the deep periosteum at both entrance and exit. If possible, pass it back upon itself. Hold the foot in about 20 degrees of equinus and 20 degrees of inversion during this maneuver (TECH FIG 2F–I).
- Any evident defects or redundancy in the plantar talonavicular ligament (spring ligament) can be imbricated at this time.

PLANTARFLEXION OSTEOTOMY OF THE MEDIAL CUNEIFORM (COTTON PROCEDURE)

- Make a 4-cm incision centered over the medial cuneiform. This should be a separate incision from that used for the posterior tibialis reconstruction, and usually a 3- to 4-cm skin bridge can be achieved (TECH FIG 3A).
- Identify the central portion of the medial cuneiform, essentially even with the base of the second metatarsal. Drive a Kirschner wire in to template the desired location of the osteotomy (TECH FIG 3B,C).

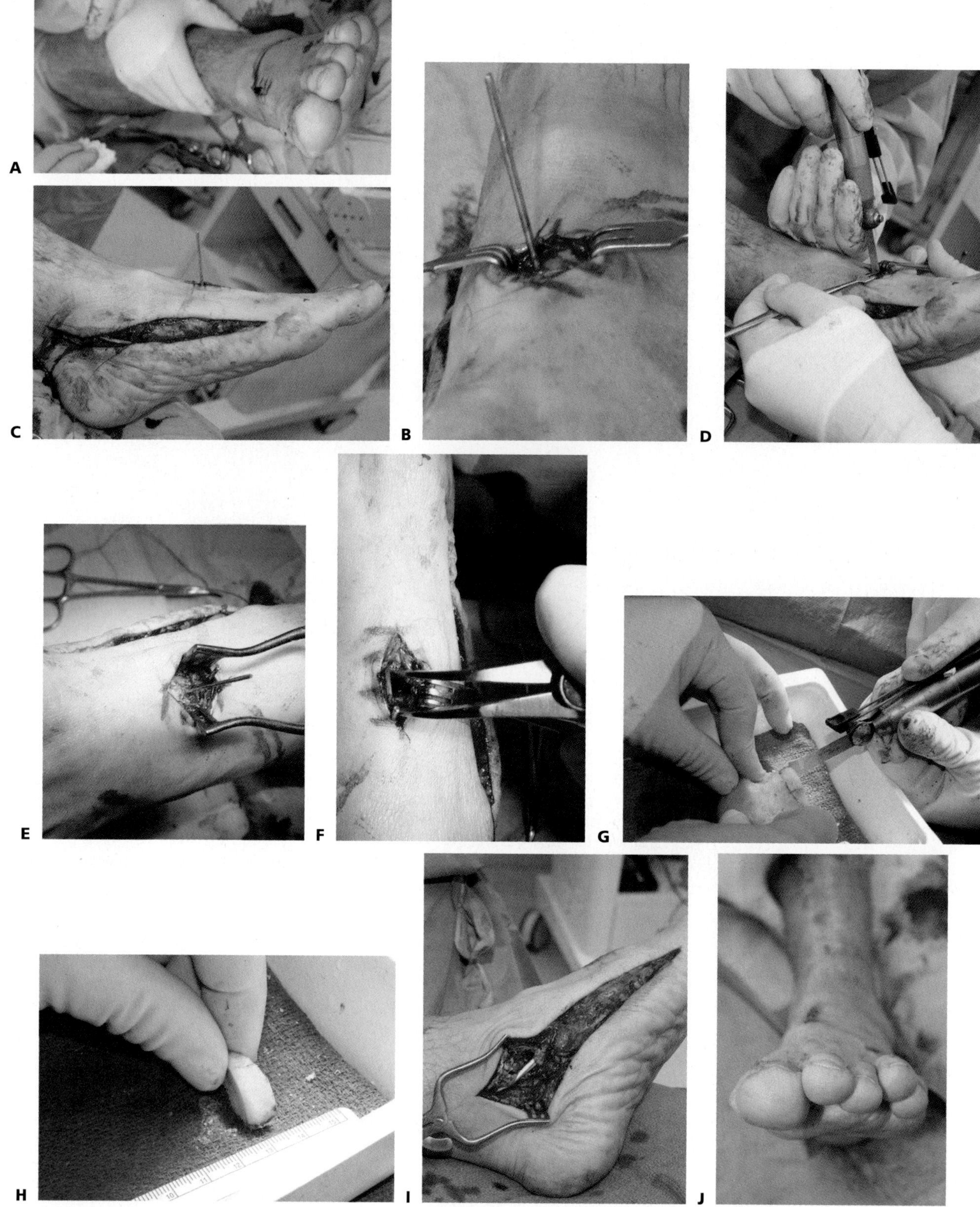

TECH FIG 3 • A. Residual forefoot varus is noted after the other components of the reconstruction are done. **B, C.** A longitudinal incision is made over the medial cuneiform and a Kirschner wire is placed to mark the center of the bone. The position is then checked fluoroscopically. **D.** A microsagittal saw is used to create the osteotomy, leaving the plantar cortex intact as a hinge. **E.** Temporary Kirschner wires are placed on either side of the osteotomy. **F.** A lamina spreader is used against them to lever the osteotomy open, dropping the medial column. **G.** A femoral head allograft is used to provide a wedge of bone, which (**H**) typically measures 5 to 7 mm at its base. **I, J.** After impaction of the allograft, the medial column has been plantarflexed and the forefoot varus has been corrected.

- Use a microsagittal saw to create a transverse osteotomy through the medial cuneiform only, taking care to avoid penetrating the plantar cortex (**TECH FIG 3D**).
- Hinge open the osteotomy with a small osteotome. Kirschner wires drilled on either side of the osteotomy spread with a lamina spreader can facilitate access (**TECH FIG 3E,F**).
- Insert a tapered piece of graft into the osteotomy to complete the correction. A piece from the calcar of a femoral head allograft or iliac crest allograft may be used. Proximal tibial autograft is also suitable. The piece is sized depending on the degree of correction required; typically a wedge measuring 5 to 7 mm at its base is used (**TECH FIG 3G,H**).
- Fixation is not usually necessary. If the graft is not felt to be stable, a dorsal three-hole 2.0-mm or 2.4-mm plate can be contoured to fit (**TECH FIG 3I,J**).

PEARLS AND PITFALLS

Indications	■ Excessive forefoot varus (over 30 degrees) cannot be accommodated. ■ Hindfoot arthritis must be carefully ruled out using weight-bearing films.
Medial displacement calcaneal osteotomy	■ The sural nerve must be carefully protected; sural neuritis is a common issue postoperatively. ■ Avoid placing the osteotomy cut too far posteriorly into the origin of the plantar fascia. ■ Adequate displacement is achievable only if the tuberosity can be adequately distracted before attempting the medial shift. ■ Confirm screw placement with an axial fluoroscopic image.
Posterior tibial tendon reconstruction	■ Have a low threshold for complete resection of the posterior tibial tendon. ■ Be prepared for vascular perforators overlying the approach to the knot of Henry. ■ Suture anchors may provide a salvage if the FDL is harvested too short or if tunnel problems occur.
Cotton osteotomy	■ Be sure the osteotomy will be parallel to the first tarsometatarsal joint by checking the templating Kirschner wire position on the lateral fluoroscopic image. ■ Slight overcorrection is usually well tolerated.

POSTOPERATIVE CARE

- A bulky postoperative splint is initially applied.
- The patient is transferred to a removable boot at 10 to 14 days and allowed gentle active foot motion only.
- Weight bearing may commence at 1 month for the calcaneal osteotomy alone, 6 weeks if a cuneiform osteotomy has been performed.
- Physical therapy for hindfoot motion and posterior tibialis strengthening commences with weight bearing and is continued for at least 6 weeks. Thera-Band exercises are particularly useful.
- Regular shoe wear is initiated at 2.5 to 3 months depending upon swelling. Postoperative compression stockings may be useful in some patients.
- Patients should be warned that the full effect of surgery may take up to 1 year to occur. This time is required for the small cross-sectional area of the transferred FDL tendon to hypertrophy into its new expanded role.

OUTCOMES

- Initial reports of FDL transfer with posterior tibialis débridement alone demonstrated excellent pain relief but little lasting correction of the arch.[2,5]
- The FDL transfer in combination with a calcaneal osteotomy has demonstrated lasting radiographic arch correction and the functional ability to perform a single-leg toe rise. Three-year to 5-year follow-up studies have shown success rates of 90% or greater.[3,7,8,11]
- Long-term follow-up of the medial cuneiform osteotomy in this setting is not yet available. One short-term study detailing its use in a variety of foot deformity corrections in adults demonstrated no nonunions in 16 feet.[4]
- Dramatic hypertrophy of the FDL muscle occurs over the first year after transfer.[10] No clinical difference in ultimate strength has been noted between patients in whom the diseased posterior tibialis was excised versus débrided and retained.

COMPLICATIONS

- Sural nerve injury
- Navicular tunnel failure or early FDL pullout
- Hardware tenderness from the posterior calcaneal screws
- Nonunion
- Deep venous thrombosis

REFERENCES

1. Augustin JF, Lin SS, Berbarian WS, et al. Nonoperative treatment of adult acquired flat foot with the Arizona brace. Foot Ankle Clin 2003;8:491–523.
2. Funk DA, Cass JR, Johnson KA. Acquired adult flat foot secondary to posterior tibial tendon pathology. J Bone Joint Surg Am 1986;68A:95–102.
3. Guyton GP, Jeng C, Krieger LE, et al. Flexor digitorum longus transfer and medial displacement calcaneal osteotomy for posterior tibial tendon dysfunction: a middle-term clinical follow-up. Foot Ankle Int 2001;22:627–632.

4. Hirose CE, Johnson JE. Plantarflexion opening wedge medial cuneiform osteotomy for correction of fixed forefoot varus associated with flatfoot deformity. Foot Ankle Int 2004;25:568–574.
5. Mann RA, Thompson FM. Rupture of the posterior tibial tendon causing flatfoot: surgical treatment. J Bone Joint Surg Am 1985;67A:556–561.
6. Mosier SM, Pomeroy G, Manoli A II. Pathoanatomy and etiology of posterior tibial tendon dysfunction. Clin Orthop Relat Res 1999;365:12–22.
7. Myerson MS, Badekas A, Schon LC. Treatment of stage II posterior tibial tendon deficiency with flexor digitorum longus tendon transfer and calcaneal osteotomy. Foot Ankle Int 2004;25: 445–450.
8. Myerson MS, Corrigan J. Treatment of posterior tibial tendon dysfunction with flexor digitorum longus tendon transfer and calcaneal osteotomy. Orthopedics 1996;19:383–388.
9. Myerson M, Solomon G, Shereff M. Posterior tibial tendon dysfunction: its association with seronegative inflammatory disease. Foot Ankle 1989;9:219–225.
10. Rosenfeld PF, Dick J, Saxby TS. The response of the flexor digitorum longus and posterior tibial muscles to tendon transfer and calcaneal osteotomy for stage II posterior tibial tendon dysfunction. Foot Ankle Int 2005;26:671–674.
11. Wacker JT, Hennessy MS, Saxby TS. Calcaneal osteotomy and transfer of the tendon of flexor digitorum longus for stage-II dysfunction of tibialis posterior: Three- to five-year results. J Bone Joint Surg Br 2002;84B:54–58.

Chapter **47** Lateral Column Lengthening

Donald R. Bohay and John G. Anderson

DEFINITION

- Posterior tibial tendon insufficiency is a common diagnosis in the foot and ankle surgeon's practice, and the most common cause of unilateral acquired flatfoot deformity.
- The constellation of presenting findings typically include painful flatfoot deformity, dorsolateral peritalar subluxation, and hindfoot valgus.
- The degree of hindfoot deformity and stiffness is variable and may be classified along the continuum described by Johnson and Strom (and Myerson) from stage I (mild posterior tibial tendinopathy without hindfoot deformity) to stage IV (severe posterior tibial tendon insufficiency, severe hindfoot deformity, and valgus talar tilt).
- Optimal treatment continues to be debated.
- Lateral column lengthening, either used in isolation or in combination with other procedures, is our preferred technique for the treatment of the posterior tibial tendon insufficient foot with supple deformity.[5]

ANATOMY

- The lateral column can be defined as the sum of the fourth and fifth tarsometatarsal joints, cuboid, calcaneocuboid joint, and calcaneus.
- The peroneus brevis inserts on the base of the fifth metatarsal and is the natural antagonist to the posterior tibial tendon.
- The calcaneocuboid joint is the primary motion segment of the lateral column.
- Fusion of the calcaneocuboid joint has no impact on subtalar joint motion and decreases talonavicular joint motion by one third.[1]

PATHOGENESIS

- As the posterior tibial tendon and secondary support structures (plantar medial ligaments, including the spring ligament) fail, the midfoot displaces laterally on the hindfoot.
- The contracted Achilles tendon and gastrocnemius muscles plantarflex the calcaneus.
- The navicular and medial cuneiform are displaced dorsal to the talus.
- The forefoot loses its ability to supinate.
- With this progressive deformity, the posterior heel shifts lateral to the axis of rotation through the talus, causing the contracted Achilles tendon or gastrocnemius muscles to function as strong hindfoot evertors, thereby worsening the alignment.
- The deformity increases as the lateral column is functionally shortened and the lateral talus creates impingement in the sinus tarsi,[3] and eventually on the anterior process of the calcaneus.
- We characterize this progressive deformity as dorsolateral peritalar subluxation.

NATURAL HISTORY

- A functionally shortened lateral column occurs in the patient with the supple deformity described in stage II of Johnson and Strom's classification system.
- As the deformity approaches its maximum, the static restraints of the medial column fail and it is effectively lengthened through collapse of the naviculocuneiform or first metatarsal–cuneiform joint.
- The sinus tarsi will close and lateral impingement will become a significant clinical finding.
- The peroneus brevis may become contracted and the Achilles and gastrocnemius contracture worsens.
- Over time a supple or flexible deformity may become rigid and irreducible.
- Generally, no radiographic evidence of calcaneocuboid joint arthritis is noted.
- A structurally shortened lateral column occurs as noted by virtue of calcaneocuboid joint arthritis.
- As the transition from stage II to stage III occurs, the deformity becomes rigid and the ability of the surgeon to correct the deformity with joint-sparing procedures and without arthrodesis of essential joints becomes limited and eventually impossible.

PATIENT HISTORY AND PHYSICAL FINDINGS

- As the patient moves through the clinical stages of posterior tibial tendon insufficiency, the complaints will vary from vague discomfort behind the medial malleolus and swelling to increasing deformity, lack of propulsion power, inability to single toe raise, and finally lateral-sided "ankle" pain.
- This lateral-sided "ankle" pain usually represents sinus tarsi impingement as the lateral shoulder of the talus impinges on the sinus tarsi.
- The deformity will continue to be supple in the early stages.
- Eventually the deformity will increase and become rigid, with the complaints ranging from a tired, weak foot with medial arch pain and lateral-sided "ankle" pain to increasing ankle deformity and joint pain and potentially ipsilateral knee and hip pain.

IMAGING AND OTHER DIAGNOSTIC STUDIES

- Plain radiographs should be obtained with weight bearing to adequately describe the alignment of the foot. The talo–first metatarsal angle describes the sag of the arch when drawn on the lateral view and the abduction of the forefoot when drawn on the AP view.
- Plain foot radiographs should also be examined for the presence of hindfoot arthritis, midfoot arthritis or instability, and the presence of an accessory navicular.

- A standing ankle mortise view should be obtained to rule out the possibility of deltoid laxity (stage IV disease).
- MRI is not routinely necessary and may underestimate the severity of disease, but it may be useful in ruling out other pathologies. Findings of posterior tibial tendon deformity typically include fluid in the sheath, dramatic thickening of the tendon, and a heterogeneous signal within the tendon substance, indicating the presence of interstitial tears.

DIFFERENTIAL DIAGNOSIS

- Midfoot arthritis resulting in pes planus through tarsometatarsal joint collapse
- Medial ankle arthritis
- Medial osteochondral lesion of the talus
- Neurogenic failure of the posterior tibialis through spinal or central pathology

NONOPERATIVE MANAGEMENT

- The resultant flatfoot after posterior tibial tendon failure is irreversible, but symptoms may be controllable in many patients by nonoperative means.
- A simple in-shoe semirigid or rigid foot orthotic may provide sufficient arch support to reduce symptoms in some patients.
- The gold standard for nonoperative management is the use of a cross-ankle brace. This allows direct control of the tendency of the calcaneus to fall into valgus. The most commonly used and best tolerated is a leather ankle lacer with an incorporated custom-molded plastic stirrup, often referred to as an Arizona brace after a common brand name.[2] Other options that may be suitable for higher-demand situations or patients with edema control problems include a hinged molded ankle–foot orthosis (MAFO) or a conventional double-metal upright AFO with a leg strap.
- Steroid injections into the posterior tibial tendon sheath are contraindicated as they may directly or indirectly precipitate frank rupture and further collapse.
- No brace, physical therapy regimen, or medication has been shown to modify the course of the disease or the ultimate outcome for the tendon. These are all best thought of as modalities to control the symptoms.

SURGICAL MANAGEMENT

Preoperative Planning

- The surgeon should obtain and review appropriate bilateral weight-bearing foot and ankle radiographs (**FIG 1**), assess comorbidities, and consider whether adjunctive procedures are needed.
- The surgeon should decide whether to use allograft or autograft.[2]
- The surgeon should note the presence or absence of calcaneocuboid joint arthritis. In our hands, symptomatic calcaneocuboid joint arthritis is an indication to perform the lateral column lengthening through the calcaneocuboid joint and not through the anterior process of the calcaneus.

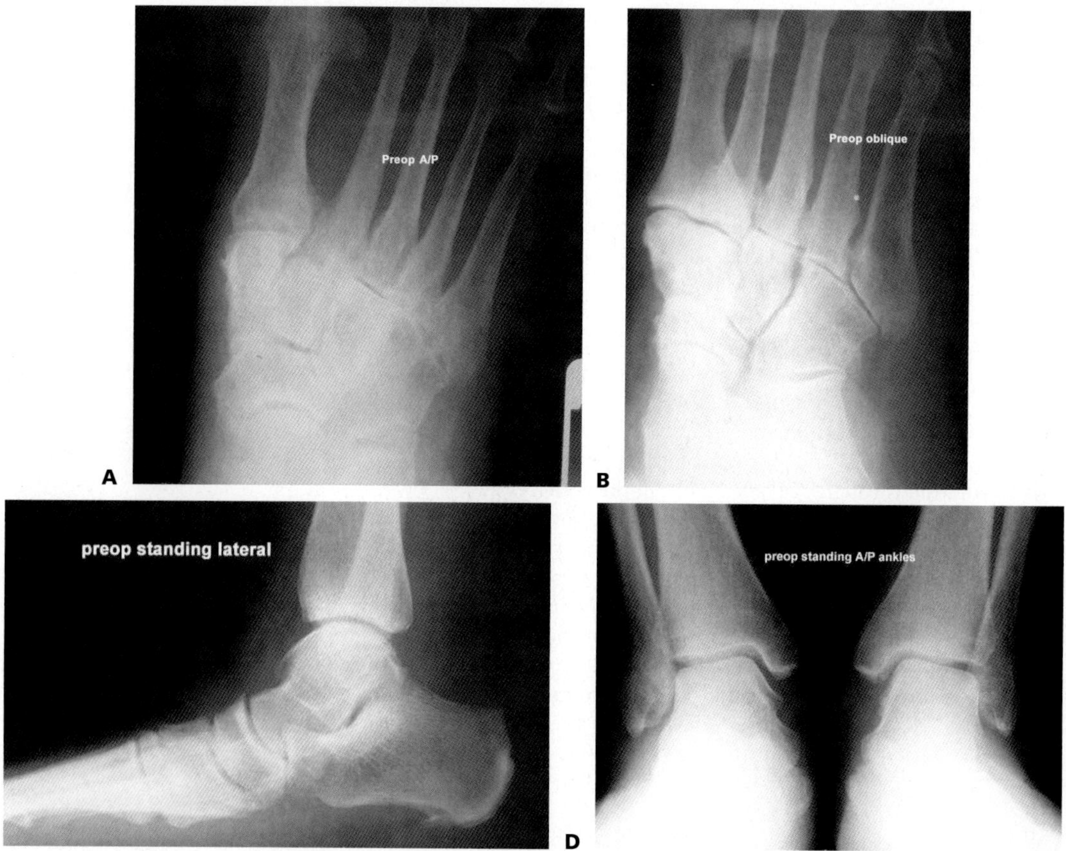

FIG 1 • Preoperative views of the foot: AP (**A**), oblique (**B**), lateral (**C**). **D.** Preoperative AP view of the ankle.

Positioning

- We position the patient supine with a sandbag bump under the ipsilateral hip (**FIGS 2 AND 3**).
- We routinely use a thigh tourniquet.
- We judiciously use fluoroscopy.

Approach

- While an Ollier incision may be used, we typically access the lateral column through a longitudinal lateral approach (**FIG 4**) or occasionally an extensile lateral approach.

A

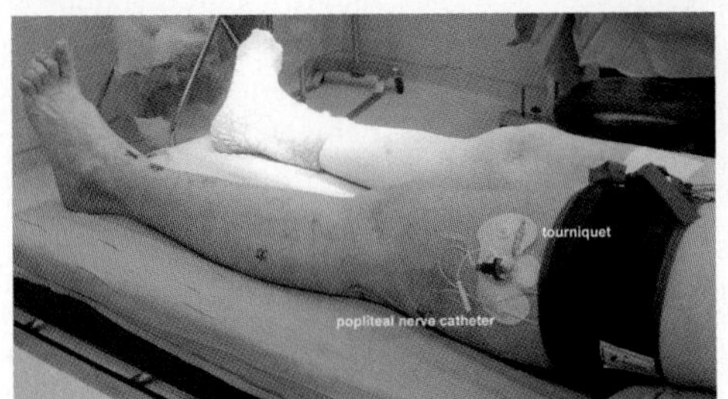

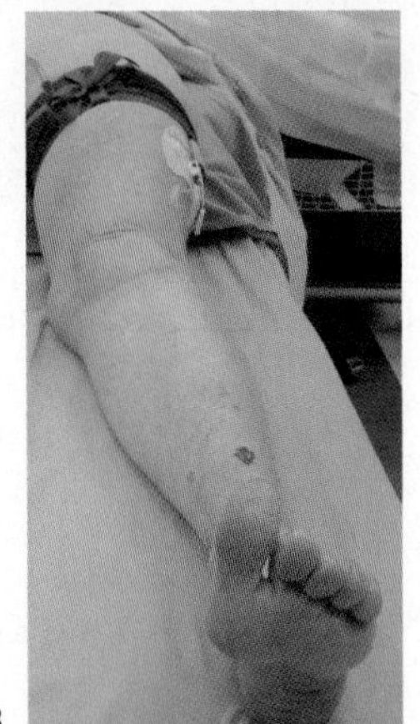

B

FIG 2 • Supine position with popliteal nerve catheter and thigh tourniquet.

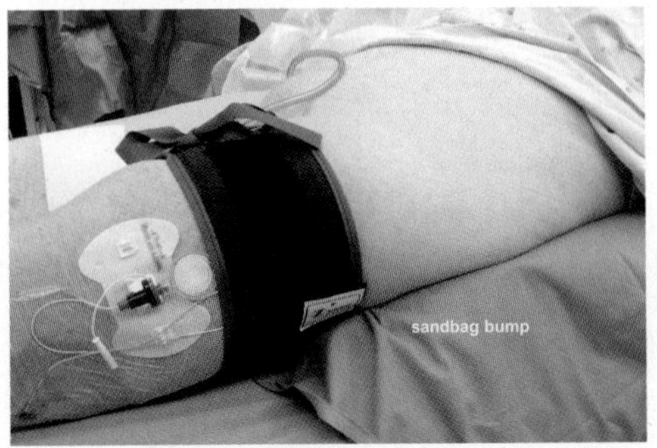

FIG 3 • Sandbag under ipsilateral hip.

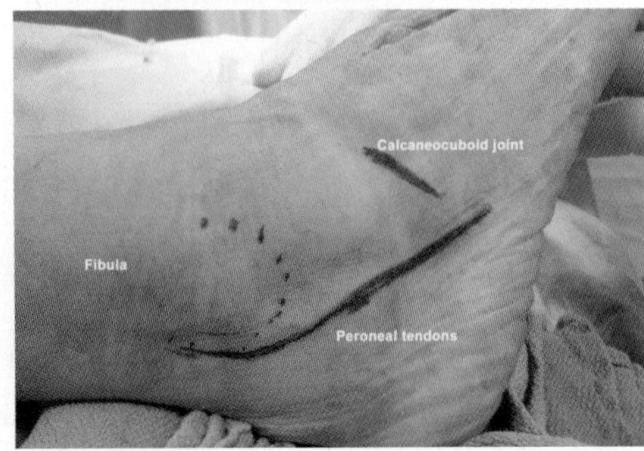

FIG 4 • Landmarks for lateral approach to the lateral column.

LATERAL COLUMN LENGTHENING VIA ANTERIOR CALCANEUS (EVANS)

Approach

- Our standard lateral incision is centered over the calcaneocuboid joint and extended proximally to the sinus tarsi (**TECH FIG 1A**).
- Make the incision about 6 to 8 cm long, parallel to the plantar foot, and perpendicular to the calcaneocuboid joint.
- Identify the sural nerve and peroneal tendons and carefully retract them plantarward (**TECH FIG 1B**).
- Elevate the extensor digitorum brevis muscle from the anterior process of the calcaneus to expose the superior corner of the calcaneocuboid joint and the sinus tarsi at the angle of Gissane (**TECH FIG 1C**).
- Place small Hohmann retractors, one in the sinus tarsi and the other plantar to the anterior calcaneus, after subperiosteal dissection enhances the exposure to the lateral column.

A

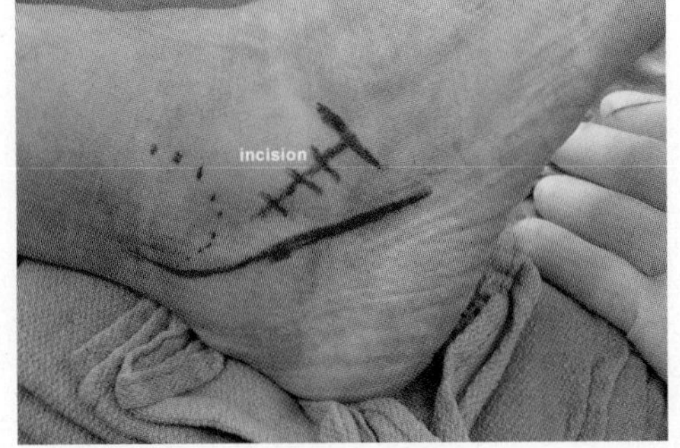

B

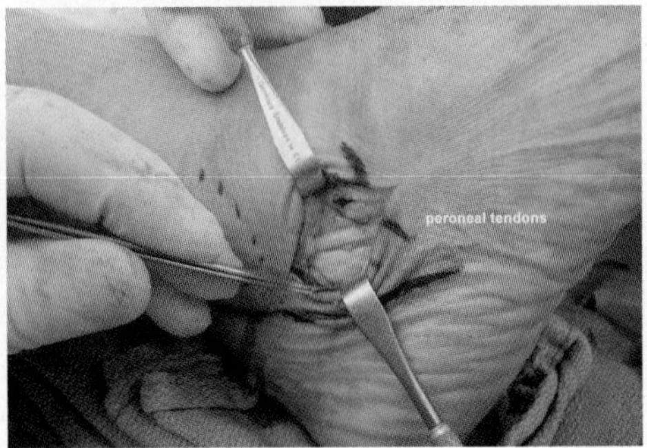

TECH FIG 1 • **A.** Incision site for the lateral approach. **B.** Lateral incision showing exposure of the peroneal tendons. *(continued)*

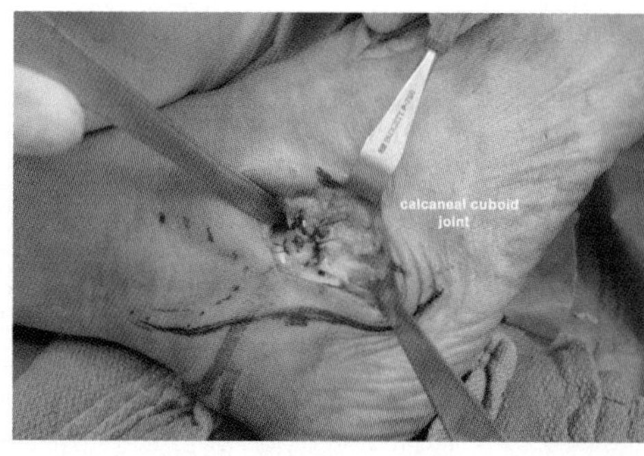

TECH FIG 1 • *(continued)* **C.** Elevation of the extensor digitorum brevis and retraction of the peroneal tendons with small Hohmann retractors.

Osteotomy

- With a Bovie electrocautery or a marking pen, mark a point on the lateral calcaneus 1.5 to 2.0 cm proximal to the superior corner of the calcaneocuboid joint (**TECH FIG 2A**).
- We perform the anterior calcaneal osteotomy with a small oscillating saw and routinely use irrigation to avoid thermal damage to the bone.
- Be sure to keep the saw blade perpendicular to the plantar foot.
- Take care to avoid injury to the peroneal tendons with the saw (**TECH FIG 2B**).
- Finish the osteotomy with an osteotome, leaving the medial hinge intact (**TECH FIG 2C**). You may need to obtain an intraoperative fluoroscopy image to confirm that the osteotome is approaching (but not violating) the medial bony hinge; AP and oblique fluoroscopy images typically demonstrate this best.
- Place a small lamina spreader in the osteotomy (**TECH FIG 2D**) and gently spread until the desired correction is achieved.
- An intraoperative AP fluoroscopy image of the foot with the lamina spreader in place is useful in determining the amount of correction by appreciating the restoration of talar head coverage by the navicular. The lateral radiograph confirms the lengthening of the lateral column.
- By removing the lamina spreader without changing the amount of "spread" on the lamina, the lamina spreader can be used as a caliper to measure the size of the graft (**TECH FIG 2E**).
- The distance between the teeth of the lamina determines the graft size (**TECH FIG 2F**).

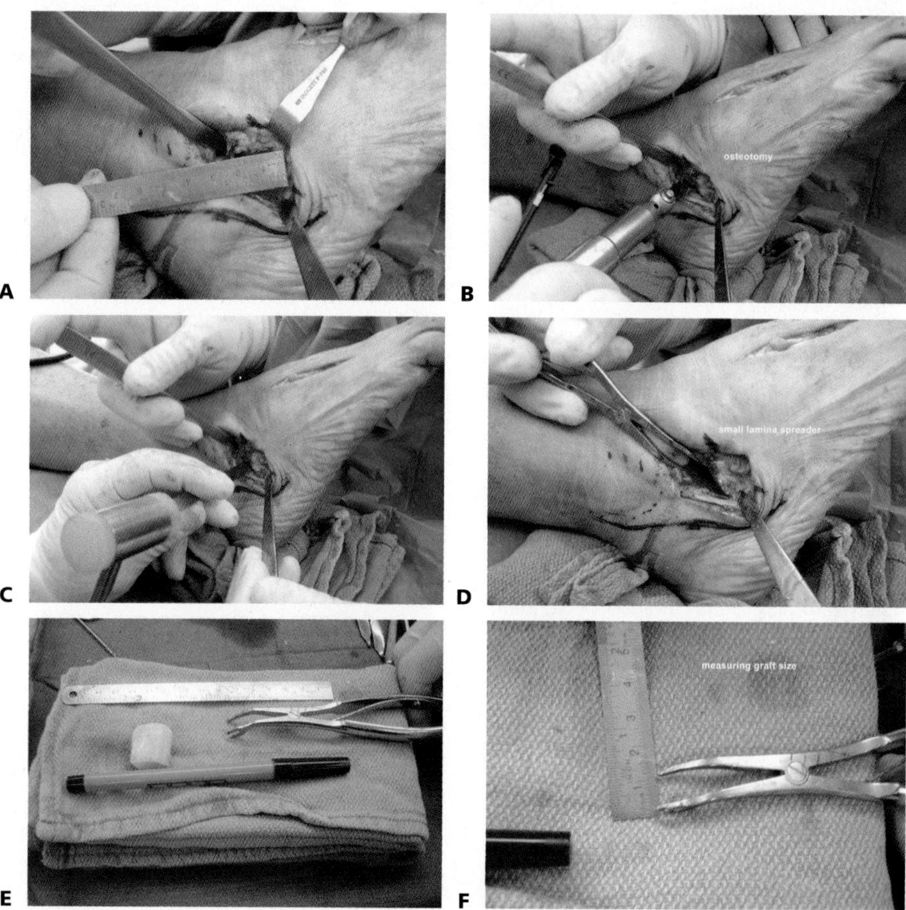

TECH FIG 2 • **A.** Measuring 1.5 to 2.0 cm proximal from the calcaneocuboid joint. **B.** Osteotomy of the anterior os calcis using a small oscillating saw. **C.** Completion of the osteotomy using an osteotome. **D.** Small lamina spreader is used to distract the osteotomy appropriately. **E.** Note the open lamina spreader on the back table, to be used as a caliper to measure the bone graft size. **F.** Measuring the distance between the teeth of the lamina spreader for bone graft size.

- When using allograft, use at least a 15-mm-wide iliac crest wedge or patellar wedge. Mark the wedge size from the measurement obtained above and then carefully cut the block in a "pie" or wedge shape, with the cortical side widest (**TECH FIG 3A,B**).
- When using autograft, use a standard approach to the iliac crest, avoiding the superficial branch of the femoral nerve, and make an incision about 6 cm long. Expose the anterior iliac crest using subperiosteal dissection and Taylor retractors. Mark the size of the graft from the measurement previously obtained and score the margins with a curved osteotome. Cut the block as a "pie" or wedge in situ, or remove a standard block and trim it to a "pie" or wedge on the back table.
- Place the block into the lateral column osteotomy and tamp it in securely with a bone tamp and mallet. The graft should be flush with the margins of the osteotomy (**TECH FIG 3C–E**).
- Use caution to avoid fracturing the graft. We use a small lamina spreader without teeth and place it in the far dorsal lip of the osteotomy and distract. The allograft comes in just plantar to that and usually can be tamped in with a few taps of the mallet. Avoid striking the allograft central but, rather, on the hard cortical edges.
- Avoid subluxation of the calcaneocuboid joint. Occasionally, we temporarily fix the calcaneocuboid joint in its anatomic position with a 0.062 Kirschner wire before implanting the graft.

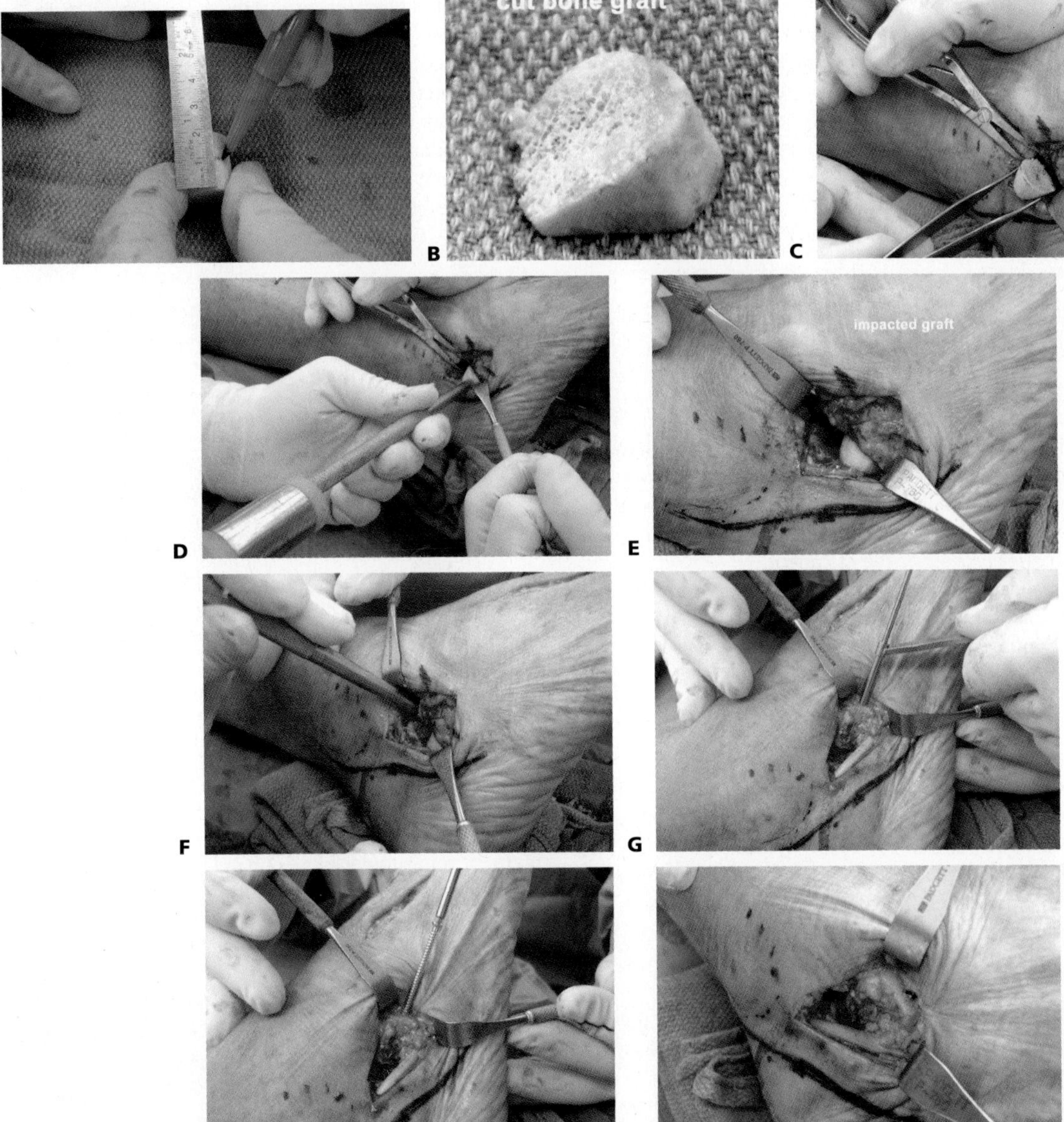

TECH FIG 3 • **A.** Marking the bone graft to the appropriate size. **B.** Bone graft wedge ready for implantation. **C.** Placing the bone graft into the osteotomy site. **D.** Tamping the bone graft into place. **E.** Impacted iliac crest wedge. **F–I.** Securing the graft with a single 3.5-mm screw from the anterosuperior corner of the calcaneocuboid joint through the graft and into the os calcis. *(continued)*

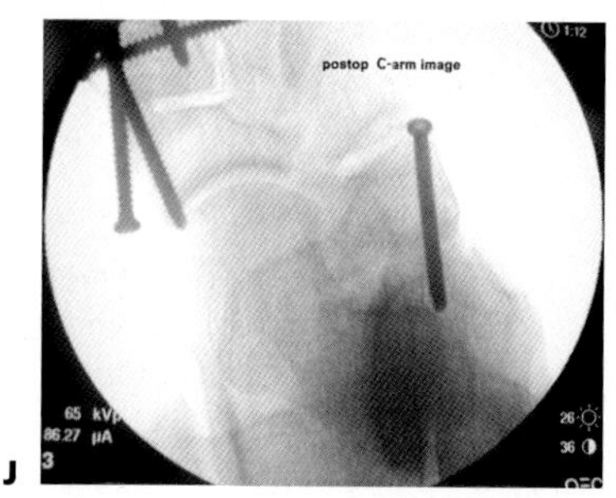

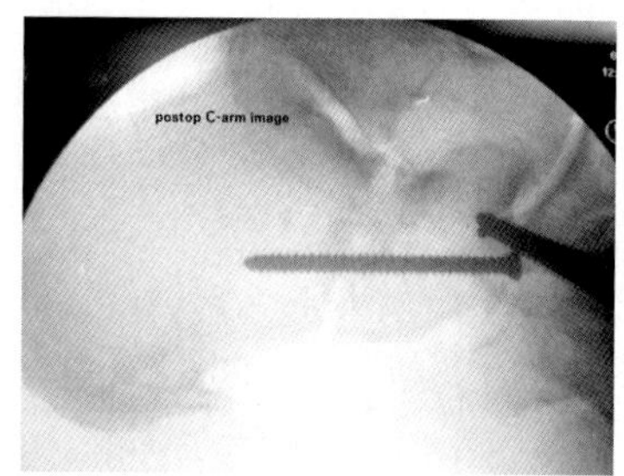

TECH FIG 3 • *(continued)* **J.** AP C-arm image after procedure to confirm graft and screw position. **K.** Lateral C-arm image.

- We secure the graft with a single 3.5-mm screw from the anterosuperior corner of the calcaneocuboid joint across the graft into the proximal calcaneus (**TECH FIG 3F–I**).
- In our opinion, a fully threaded positional screw is ideal and there is no need to apply compression since the graft is already under compression in the distracted osteotomy. In fact, lag technique may lead to crushing the graft.
- Supplement the lateral column osteotomy with remaining cancellous bone.
- Check clinical alignment.
- Use AP and lateral fluoroscopy images to confirm position and restoration of lateral column height, the talo–first metatarsal angle, and correction of dorsolateral peritalar subluxation (**TECH FIG 3J,K**).
- Undercorrection to residual deformity or overcorrection to an adductus deformity can be avoided by checking for desired alignment with the lamina spreader in place, before sizing and inserting the graft.
- We routinely close the deeper layers with 3-0 Maxon and the skin using 3-0 nylon.

LATERAL COLUMN LENGTHENING VIA CALCANEOCUBOID JOINT DISTRACTION ARTHRODESIS

Approach

- Approach the calcaneocuboid joint through a standard lateral approach centered over the calcaneocuboid joint and extending a total length of 6 to 8 cm, slightly more distal than the approach for lateral column lengthening via the anterior process of the calcaneus.
- Identify the peroneal tendons and sural nerve and retract them plantarward, and elevate the extensor digitorum brevis muscle dorsally.
- Distract the calcaneocuboid joint with a small lamina spreader and remove the articular cartilage from both sides of the joint.
- Drill the subchondral bone with a 2.0-mm drill or a 0.062 Kirschner wire to provide vascular channels.
- Distract the calcaneocuboid joint using the small lamina spreader until the desired correction is obtained.
- Check AP and lateral fluoroscopy images with the lamina spreader in place. The AP image confirms that the navicular is reduced on the talar head and the lateral view confirms that subluxation of the calcaneocuboid joint is avoided.
- Remove the lamina spreader without changing the amount of "spread" on the lamina so it can be used as a caliper to measure the size of the graft.
- The distance between the teeth of the lamina determines the graft size.
- When using allograft, use at least a 15-mm-wide iliac crest wedge or patellar wedge. Mark the wedge size from the measurement obtained above and then carefully cut the block in a "pie" or wedge shape, with the cortical side widest.
- When using autograft, use a standard approach to the iliac crest, avoiding the superficial branch of the femoral nerve, and make an incision about 6 cm long. Expose the anterior iliac crest using subperiosteal dissection and Taylor retractors. Mark the size of the graft from the measurement previously obtained and score the margins with a curved osteotome. Cut the block as a "pie" or wedge in situ, or remove a standard block and trim it to a "pie" or wedge on the back table.
- Insert the graft in the calcaneocuboid joint, as flush as possible with the lateral column of the foot, and confirm correction clinically and fluoroscopically.
- Maintain congruent alignment of the cuboid and calcaneus during graft insertion.
- Secure the arthrodesis with a small H-plate, cervical plate, or semitubular plate (**TECH FIG 4**).
- Avoid overcompression and shortening of the lateral column.
- Augment the fusion with further bone graft.
- Check overall clinical correction.
- AP and lateral fluoroscopy images serve to confirm restoration of lateral column height, talo–first metatarsal angle, and dorsolateral peritalar subluxation.
- By checking realignment with the lamina spreader before contouring or inserting the graft, overcorrection to adductus deformity and undercorrection with residual abduction is avoided.
- We routinely close the wound with 3-0 Maxon and 3-0 nylon.

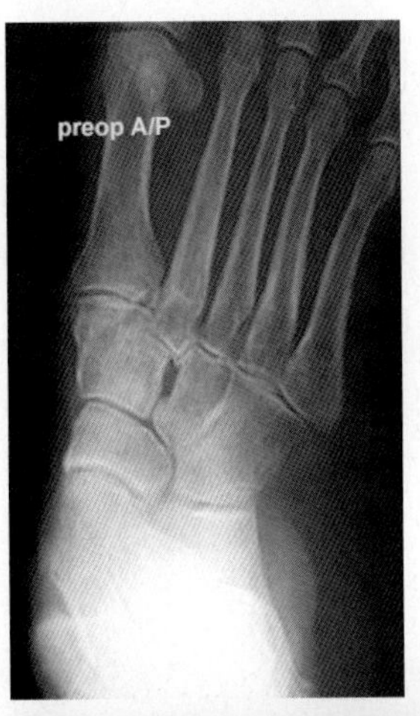

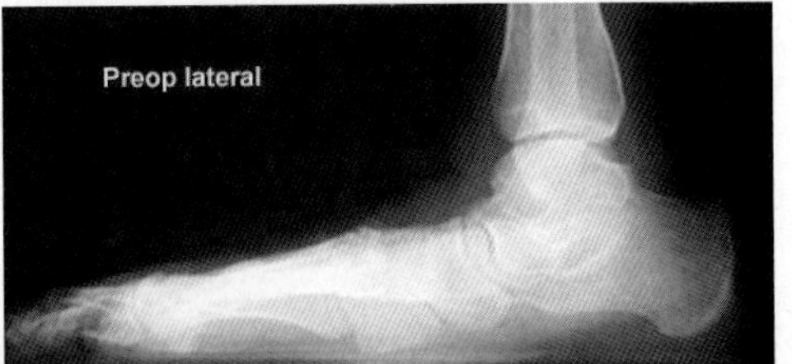

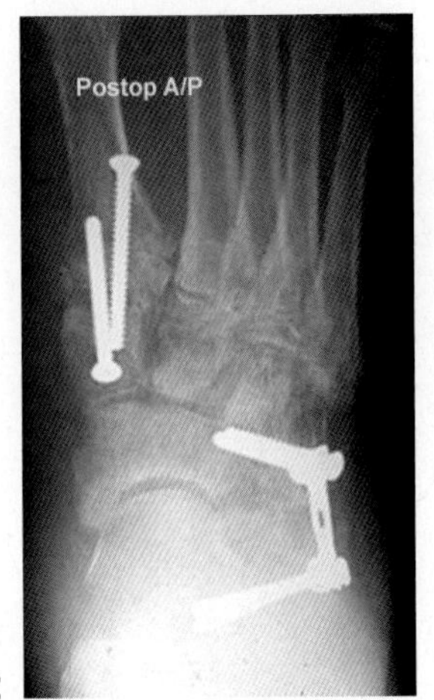

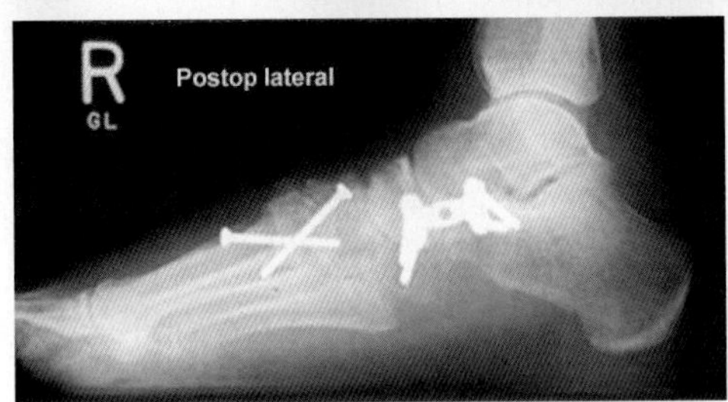

TECH FIG 4 • Preoperative AP (**A**) and lateral (**B**) radiographs. Postoperative AP (**C**) and lateral (**D**) radiographs after lateral column lengthening through the calcaneocuboid joint. (**A–D**: by permission from Bruce Sangeorzan, MD).

PEARLS AND PITFALLS

Physical examination	■ Examine the patient in the sitting position with the knee bent and the hindfoot reduced to evaluate Achilles tendon contracture and with the knee straight and the hindfoot reduced to evaluate gastrocnemius contracture. ■ Watch for the peroneal spastic flatfoot and evaluate appropriately for tarsal coalition. ■ Evaluate for ipsilateral ankle instability. ■ Assess the foot for fixed forefoot supination. Even when the hindfoot is supple and can be passively corrected, the forefoot may have compensatory supination that does not correct spontaneously. Lateral column lengthening may correct the hindfoot but could worsen the relative forefoot supination. An adjunctive medial column stabilization procedure to plantarflex the first ray may be necessary (Lapidus procedure or plantarflexion osteotomy of the medial cuneiform).
Approach	■ Evaluate and be prepared to treat any concomitant peroneal tendon pathology, such as splits or contracture.
Osteotomy	■ Take care not to place the osteotomy too far distal and destabilize the calcaneocuboid joint. ■ Take care not to place the osteotomy too far proximal and violate the middle or posterior facet of the subtalar joint. ■ If the calcaneocuboid joint is unstable, secure the joint with a 0.062 Kirschner wire before distracting the osteotomy. ■ Retract the peroneal tendons with a small Lambotte osteotome under the inferior edge of the calcaneus and watch carefully to avoid accidental laceration of the tendons by the oscillating saw. ■ Angle the fixation screw slightly plantar to avoid placing the screw in the subtalar joint (**FIG 5**).
Graft size	■ Graft is usually close to 10 mm. ■ Ensure that the allograft has been soaking for about 20 minutes to prevent graft fracture as you are cutting the block. ■ Place the small lamina spreader in the osteotomy and open and close the device to find the appropriate amount of correction.

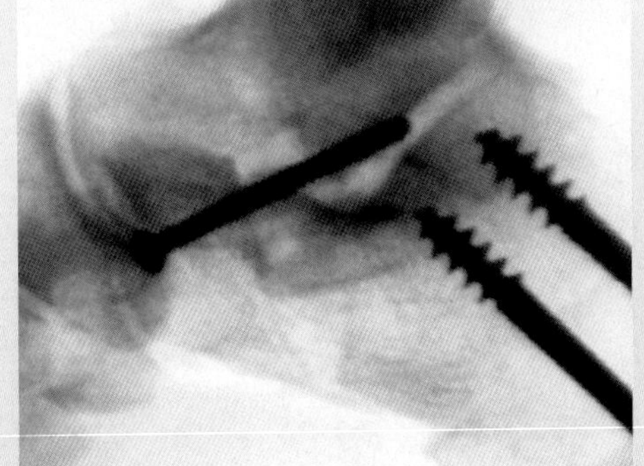

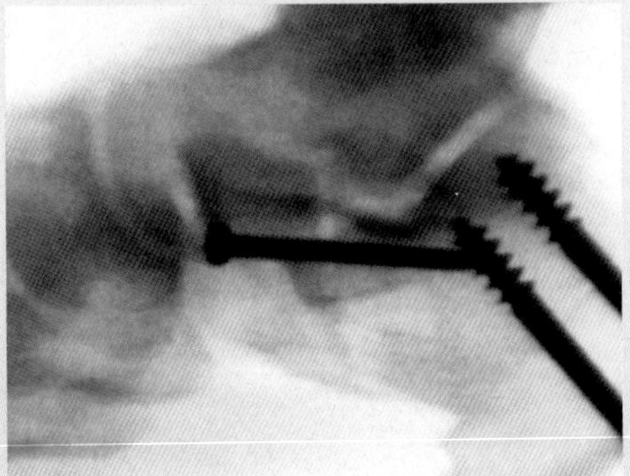

FIG 5 • **A.** Misplaced lateral column screw. **B.** Corrected position.

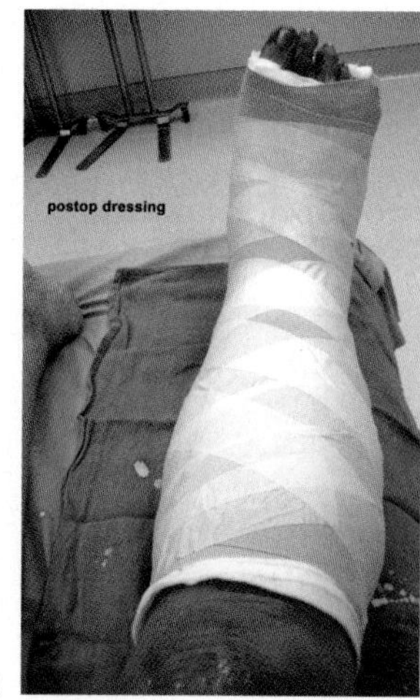

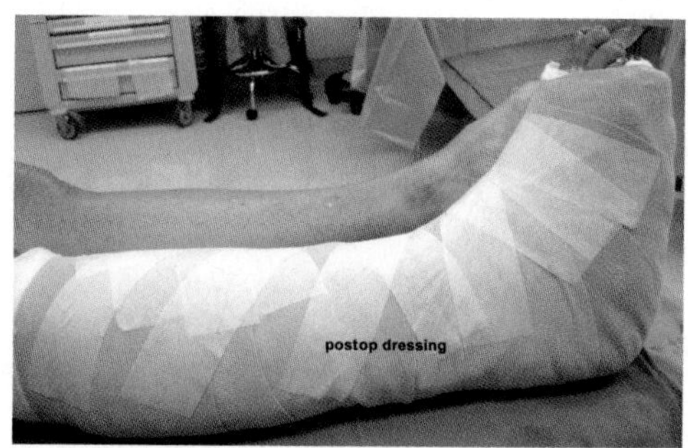

FIG 6 • Immobilization in a bulky Jones dressing and posterior splint dressing postoperatively.

POSTOPERATIVE CARE

- We typically immobilize our patients in a postoperative splint (**FIG 6**).
- At 2 weeks, we remove sutures, obtain simulated weight-bearing radiographs (AP, lateral, oblique) and the Harris view, and allow touch-down weight bearing in a short-leg cast.
- At 6 weeks the patient is transitioned from the cast into a fracture boot and from touch-down to partial weight bearing, with gradual progression to full weight bearing over the next 4 weeks.
- Our patients participate in a simple physical therapy protocol to assist with safe mobilization, modalities, and a protocol to strengthen the posterior tibial tendon reconstruction.
- In general patients can return to wearing shoes at 10 weeks postoperatively.

OUTCOMES

- The selection of autograft versus allograft for lateral column lengthening in the adult does not alter the capacity of the osteotomy to heal.
- A prospective, randomized study of 33 patients randomized to allograft versus autograft showed no difference in the union rate.[2]
- Calcaneocuboid joint arthritis has been proposed as a consequence of lateral column lengthening through the anterior process of the calcaneus.
- Mosier-LaClair et al[4] showed that 14% of their patients had evidence of calcaneocuboid joint arthritis at 5 years of follow-up; however, 50% had calcaneocuboid joint arthritis preoperatively.
- Lateral column overload may be more likely with a calcaneocuboid distraction arthrodesis than an Evans-type osteotomy (**FIG 7**).[6]

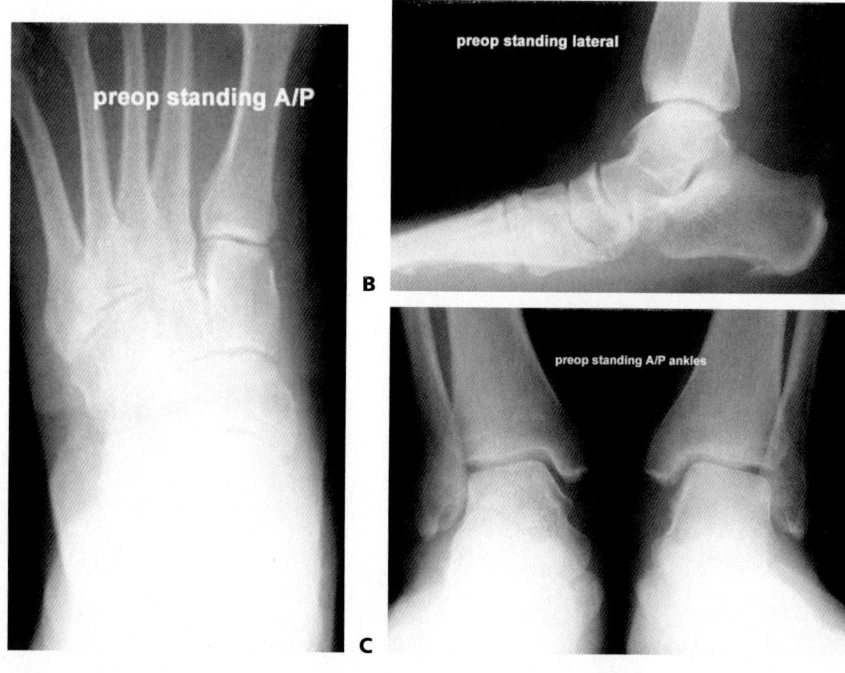

FIG 7 • **A–C.** Preoperative standing AP foot, lateral foot, and AP ankles. *(continued)*

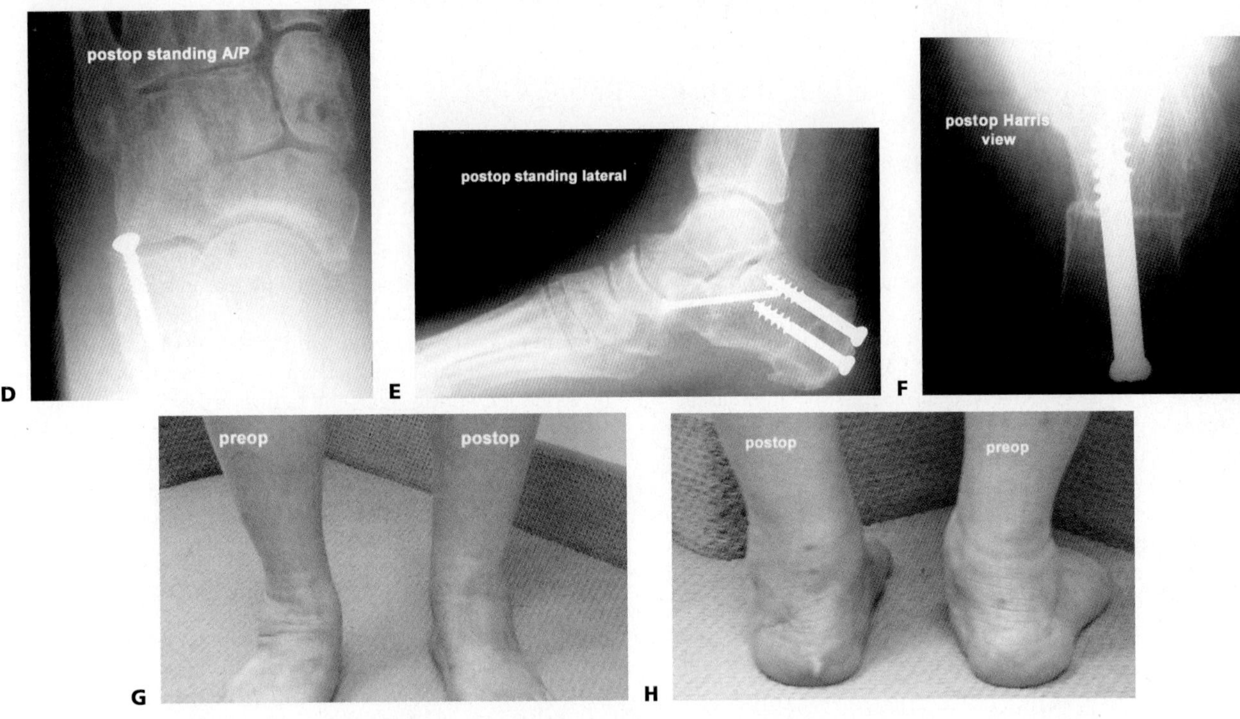

FIG 7 • *(continued)* **D–F.** Postoperative standing AP foot, lateral foot, and Harris view of the os calcis. **G.** Clinical photograph of the patient viewed from the front, comparing the unoperated side with posterior tibial tendon insufficiency and the corrected side. Note the corrected longitudinal height and forefoot abduction. **H.** Clinical photograph of the patient viewed from behind, comparing the unoperated side with posterior tibial tendon insufficiency and the corrected side. Note the corrected hindfoot valgus and the absence of a "too many toes" sign.

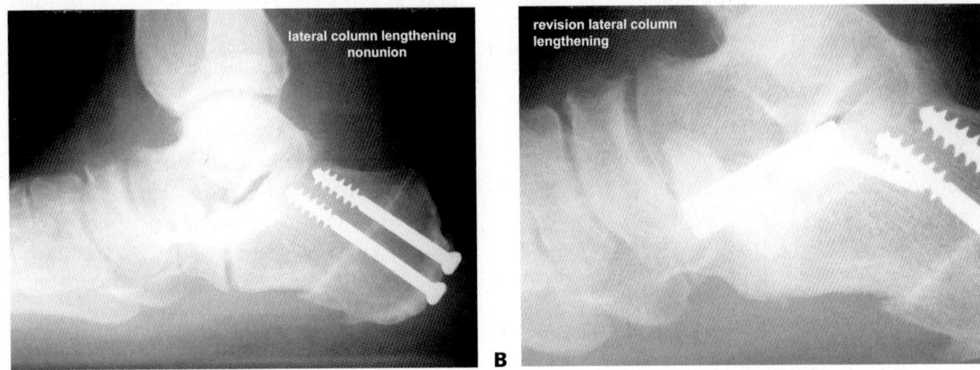

FIG 8 • **A.** Radiograph of late graft nonunion and hardware failure. **B.** Radiograph showing healed revision with plate fixation.

COMPLICATIONS

- Nonunion (**FIG 8**)
- Malunion
- Graft fracture
- Painful hardware
- Overcorrection
- Peroneal tendon irritation or injury
- Sural nerve irritation or injury

REFERENCES

1. Astion DJ, Deland JT, Otis JC, et al. Motion of the hindfoot after simulated arthrodesis. J Bone Joint Surg Am 1997;79A:241–246.
2. Dolan C, Henning J, Endres T, et al. Randomized prospective study comparing tri-cortical iliac crest autograft to allograft in the lateral column lengthening component for surgical correction of the adult acquired flatfoot deformity. Presented at the 73rd Annual Meeting of the American Academy of Orthopaedic Surgeons, Chicago, March 2006.
3. Hansen ST Jr., ed. Functional Reconstruction of the Foot and Ankle. Philadelphia: Lippincott Williams & Wilkins, 2000:198.
4. Mosier-LaClair S, Pomeroy G, Manoli A II. Intermediate follow-up on the double osteotomy and tendon transfer procedure for stage 2 posterior tibial tendon insufficiency. Foot Ankle Intl 2001;22: 283–291.
5. Mosier-LaClair S, Pomeroy G, Manoli A II. The difficult stage 2 adult acquired flatfoot deformity. Foot Ankle Clin 2001;6:95–119.
6. Tien TR, Parks BG, Guyton GP. Plantar pressures in the forefoot after lateral column lengthening: a cadaveric study comparing the Evans osteotomy and calcaneocuboid fusion. Foot Ankle Intl 2005; 26:520–525.

Chapter 48 Spring Ligament Reconstruction

Jonathan T. Deland

DEFINITION

- Spring ligament failure consists of lengthening or disruption of the spring ligament complex resulting in subluxation at the talonavicular joint.
- Spring ligament failure is commonly associated with considerable degeneration of the ligament. The ligament complex may have tears or large defects, or it may just be attenuated.
- Tears most commonly occur in the superomedial portion of the spring ligament complex, adjacent to the posterior tibial tendon, but can occur in the inferior portion as well.
- It is necessary to look at the alignment of the foot to determine how to treat failure in the spring ligament. If a flatfoot is present with increased heel valgus or abduction (or both) through the midfoot and there is a full tear of more than 30% of the ligament or severe attenuation, the risk of progression of deformity is high.

ANATOMY

- The spring ligament actually is a complex of ligaments composed primarily of a superomedial portion and an inferior portion. The deltoid ligament blends in with the superomedial portion.[1]
- The superomedial portion is medial to the posterior tibial tendon. It originates from the superomedial aspect of the sustentaculum tali and the anterior facet of the calcaneus to insert on the medial navicular adjacent to its articular surface (**FIG 1**).
- The inferior portion originates from the notch between the anterior and medial calcaneal facets. It inserts on the inferior surface of the midnavicular, just lateral to the insertion of the superomedial portion of the spring ligament (**FIG 2**).
- Because of location, failure of the superomedial portion should result in primarily medial migration of the talar head, whereas that of the inferior portion results in primarily plantar migration. Most commonly, the migration is both medial and plantar (**FIG 3**).

PATHOGENESIS

- Spring ligament failure is due most commonly to the repetitive stresses of a flatfoot causing increased strain on the medial ligaments of the foot.
- Failure most often occurs in the setting of a degenerated ligament, and it can be associated with an acute episode.
- Although spring ligament failure is associated with a preexisting flatfoot, it commonly results in progressive deformity of the foot at the talonavicular joint and hindfoot. Because the foot progresses out from under the talar head dorsally and laterally, the talar head migrates medially and plantarly compared with the rest of the foot.

NATURAL HISTORY

- Failure of the spring ligament complex most commonly occurs along with posterior tibial tendon insufficiency.[3]
- With or without tendon insufficiency, spring ligament failure places the patient at risk for progressive subluxation at the talonavicular joint. If subluxation is already present, progression of the subluxation is likely.[4]
- Progressive subluxation at the talonavicular joint eventually can cause enough deformity in the triple joint complex (ie, the talonavicular, calcaneocuboid, and subtalar joints) to result in lateral impingement and pain in the hindfoot, a collapsed foot.

PATIENT HISTORY AND PHYSICAL EXAMINATION

- Patients most commonly present with medial pain, which usually is associated with the posterior tibial tendon rather than the spring ligament, although isolated traumatic injuries to the spring ligament do occur. If enough deformity has occurred, pain occurs in the lateral hindfoot from impingement secondary to subluxation in the triple joint complex.

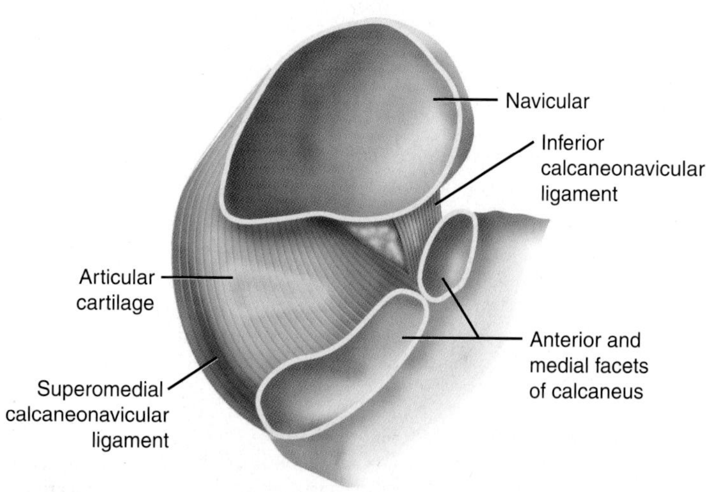

FIG 1 • Anatomy of the spring ligament complex (dorsal view with talar head removed). Note the location of the superomedial and inferomedial positions. The superomedial portion is medial to the posterior tibial tendon. It originates from the superomedial aspect of the sustentaculum tali and anterior facet of the calcaneus to insert on the medial navicular adjacent to its articular surface.

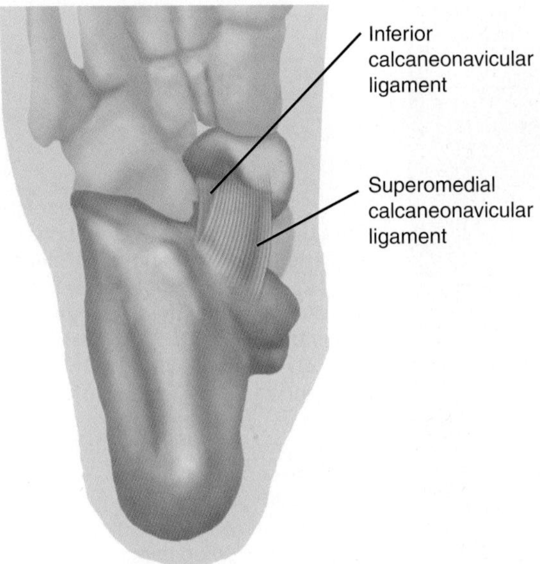

FIG 2 • Anatomy of the spring ligament complex seen from the plantar view. The inferior portion originates from the notch between the anterior and medial calcaneal facets. It inserts on the inferior surface of the midnavicular, just lateral to the insertion of the superomedial portion of the spring ligament.

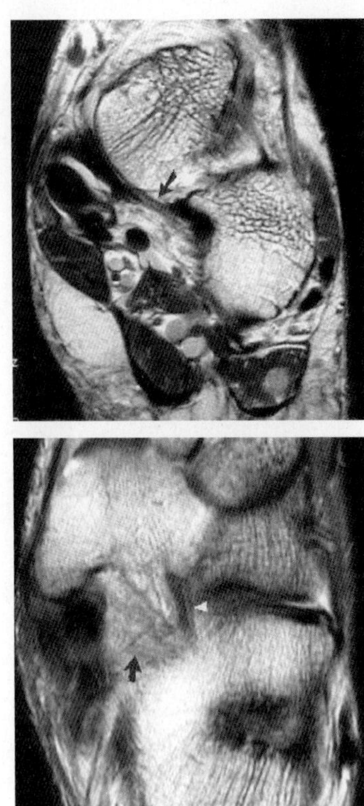

FIG 3 • Because of its location, failure of the superomedial portion should result in primarily medial migration of the talar head, whereas failure of the inferior portion results in primarily plantar migration. Most commonly, the migration is both medial and plantar. **A.** MRI scan with severe degeneration and attenuation (grade III/IV) of the superomedial portion of the spring ligament complex. **B.** MRI with a severely frayed and degenerated (grade IV/IV) plantar portion of the spring ligament complex.

- Depending on the presence and amount of deformity, the patient may or may not notice weakness or collapse in the arch. Most patients do notice some weakness.
- Physical examination should evaluate the posterior tibial tendon and alignment of the foot with the patient letting the arch sag fully when standing.
- The posterior tibial tendon should be palpated for tenderness. Inversion strength should be tested from an everted position to a plantarflexed and inverted position.
- Clinical alignment should be checked for midfoot abduction and height of the arch as noted on the frontal standing view. The degree of heel valgus is assessed from the posterior standing view.
- Physical examination may also include the following steps:
  - Palpate the medial talonavicular joint and posterior tibial tendon to evaluate swelling;. Acute and subacute tears.
  - Palpate the tendon versus the joint for tenderness. Tenderness on the tendon indicates tendon involvement and often masks tenderness from a tendon tear.
  - Evaluate range of motion. Compare the arc of motion (maximum eversion to maximum inversion) to the other foot. The arc of motion may be categorized as follows: full; some inversion present; motion only to neutral; or joint contracted in eversion. The joint must be mobile for tendon repair or reconstruction.
  - Evaluate inversion strength. Start with the foot in eversion and have the patient push against the examiner's hand to inversion and plantarflexion. For grades I through IV, tendon transfer may be required.

IMAGING

- The anteroposterior (AP) and lateral foot radiographs should be obtained standing with the patient told to let the arch sag. An AP standing radiograph of the ankle also should be performed to rule out valgus deformity at the ankle joint.
  - On the AP view of the foot, abduction at the talonavicular joint can be measured with the talonavicular uncoverage angle (ie, the amount of talar head not covered by the navicular; **FIG 4A**).
  - On the lateral view, plantar migration of the talar head in relation to the navicular can be checked (**FIG 4B**). The lateral talometatarsal angle, while a useful measurement, includes deformity at the naviculocuneiform and metatarsal-tarsal joints.
  - Radiographs are not diagnostic tools but are helpful in assessing deformity—as long as the patient is standing and the radiographic technique allows AP and lateral views with full weight bearing.
- An MRI scan visualizing the spring ligament complex can indicate the amount of degeneration or tear in the complex and is useful for diagnosis if it is of good quality and if it is read by an experienced examiner (see **FIG 3**).

DIFFERENTIAL DIAGNOSIS

- Degeneration or tear of the posterior tibial tendon without spring ligament failure
- Congenital flatfoot

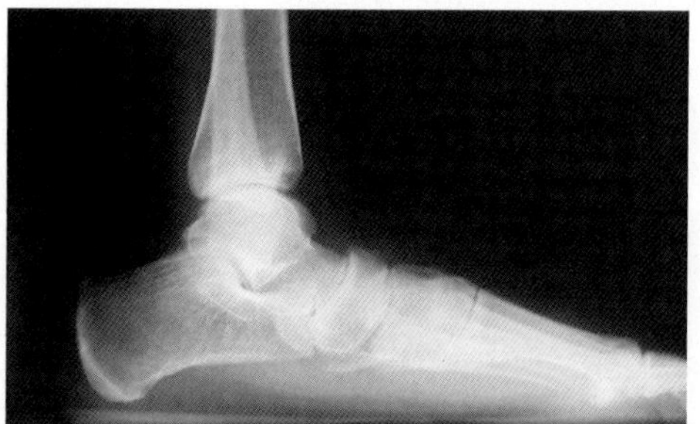

A

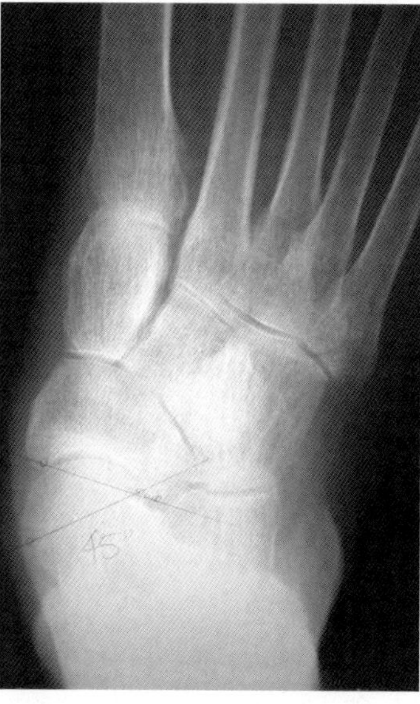

B

FIG 4 • The lateral and AP radiographic views of the foot should be obtained with the patient standing and told to let the arch sag. **A.** Standing lateral view of the foot showing a flat medial longitudinal arch with an increased talometatarsal angle on the lateral view. **B.** The AP view shows increased uncoverage of the medial talar head. These findings are characteristic–but not diagnostic–of a flatfoot associated with spring ligament pathology. Standing AP radiograph of the ankle also should be performed to rule out valgus deformity at the ankle joint.

NONOPERATIVE MANAGEMENT

- Nonoperative management is particularly appropriate for those patients for whom the tear and alignment are thought to have a low probability of progression. It also may be used for those patients who wish to delay surgery, but they must be informed of the risk of progression of deformity.
- Nonoperative management consists of support for the medial longitudinal arch with one of the following devices. (They do not at all guarantee stopping the progression of deformity.)
  - A removable boot is helpful for initial management. A medial longitudinal arch support inside the boot may be used.
  - A short, articulated ankle–foot orthosis is less cumbersome and allows ankle motion with a customized arch support.
  - A custom orthotic with a medial longitudinal arch support and medial heel wedge is the least cumbersome but also provides the least support.
  - A solid leather gauntlet or Arizona brace allows minimal motion. It is best for those patients with considerable deformity and limited function.
  - Patients receiving conservative care should be monitored for progression of flatfoot deformity.

SURGICAL MANAGEMENT

- Surgery is the best choice for patients with progression of flatfoot deformity associated with failure of the spring ligament complex or patients whose alignment and degree of injury to the spring ligament place them at high risk for progressive deformity.[4]
- Relative contradictions include medical conditions that adversely affect healing, such as diabetes, corticosteroid use, and neuropathy.
- Reconstruction of the spring ligament is not useful in those patients with rigid hindfoot deformity and is not necessary in those patients with small tears or good correction of ligament with bony procedures.

PREOPERATIVE PLANNING

- Standing clinical alignment and standing AP and lateral radiographs of the foot and ankle should be carefully reviewed to plan for correction of alignment as well as repair or reconstruction of the spring ligament.
- Surgeons should be prepared to deal with large tears or significant tissue loss in the spring ligament complex.
  - This may necessitate the use of tendon graft, possibly allograft tendon.
  - Possible Achilles contracture should be assessed.
  - Correction of the foot alignment should be considered an integral part of the procedure.
  - Remember that repair or reconstruction of the spring ligament has yet to be shown to correct bony malalignment and that a flatfoot deformity places strain on the spring complex.
  - Whether spring ligament reconstruction adds to alignment correction when bony procedures are being performed is debatable. In our experience, however, alignment correction is achieved by spring ligament reconstruction if osteotomies are performed at the same time and the foot is placed near the corrected position by the osteotomies.
  - Spring ligament reconstruction is the most logical choice for large tears and is performed along with bony realignment of deformity.[2,5,6]

POSITIONING

- The patient is placed in the supine position with a bolster under the greater trochanter so that the lower leg is neither internally or externally rotated. This allows good access to both sides of the foot.
- In this position, exposure of the spring ligament, posterior tibial tendon, and lateral hindfoot is possible.

APPROACH

- A medial incision is made from the tip of the medial malleolus to 2 cm distal to the navicular to inspect the posterior tibial tendon and expose the spring ligament complex by retracting the tendon.
- Lateral hindfoot incisions are used as necessary for calcaneal osteotomies.

PRIMARY SUPEROMEDIAL SPRING LIGAMENT REPAIR

- Primary repair rather than reconstruction is done when good tissue for repair is present and ends can be well apposed. Foot deformity is corrected at the same time.
- Figure 8 or horizontal mattress sutures are placed to appose both ends of the ligament with the foot in neutral position. Knots are placed to avoid impingement against the posterior tibial tendon (**TECH FIG 1**).
- If the ligament cannot be apposed with the foot in neutral or the tissue is attenuated, then reconstruction of the ligament is necessary for large tears. The reconstruction is performed together with osteotomies to correct bony alignment.

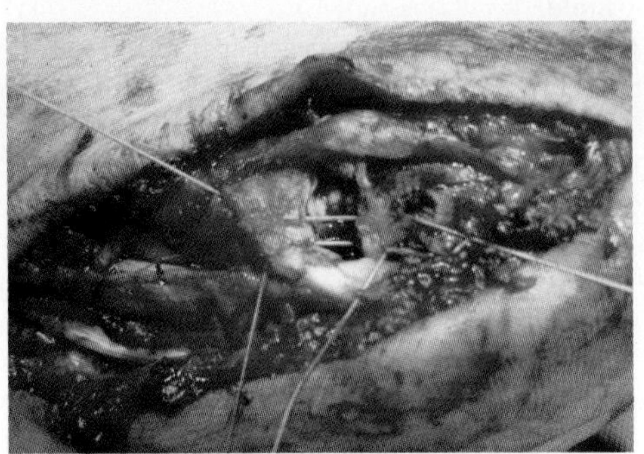

TECH FIG 1 • Operative photograph of repair of spring ligament. This repair was accompanied by a medial slide calcaneal osteotomy to address the deformity. Figure 8 or horizontal mattress sutures are placed to appose both ends with the foot in neutral position. Knots are placed to avoid impingement against the posterior tibial tendon.

SUPEROMEDIAL SPRING LIGAMENT RECONSTRUCTION

- Tendon graft is used to replace insufficient ligament tissue and block medial migration of the talar head.
- Achilles allograft is used most commonly, although peroneus longus can be used if both the longus and brevis are in good condition and overcorrection of bony realignment is avoided.
- Because the superomedial spring ligament blends in with the anterior deltoid ligament, which also can be attenuated, reconstruction of the anterior deltoid and superomedial spring ligaments is commonly performed together (**TECH FIG 2A**).
- Bone tunnels in the navicular and tibia are used to create a ligament path to support the medial talar head (**TECH FIG 2B**).
- The navicular tunnel is placed from dorsal to plantar/medial over a cannulated drill. The graft is to exit plantar medially and cross the medial talar head.
- A tibial tunnel beginning at the most inferior midportion of the medial malleolus tip is used.
  - The tibial tunnel exits laterally 5 to 9 cm above the ankle joint line.
  - A lateral longitudinal incision over the fibula is used to access the lateral tibia and fibula.

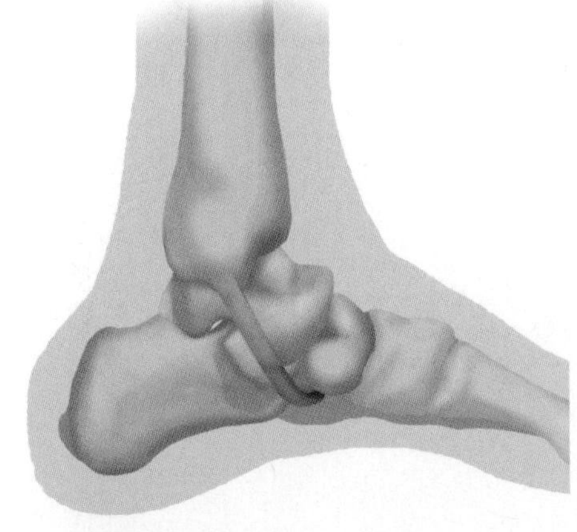

A

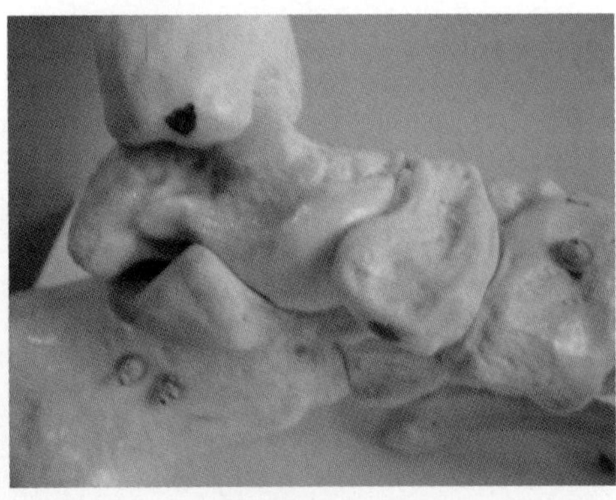

B

TECH FIG 2 • **A.** Diagram of superomedial spring ligament reconstruction. The repaired ligament crosses the medial aspect of the talar head to block medial migration of the head. An alternative to the tibial drill hole is a drill hole in the medial talar neck. Because the superomedial spring ligament blends in with the anterior deltoid ligament, which also can be attenuated, reconstruction of anterior deltoid and superomedial spring ligaments is commonly performed together. **B.** Exit hole of the graft at the inferior navicular and corresponding entrance hole into the tibia at the midportion of the tip of the medial malleolus. The navicular hole is drilled from dorsal to plantar and the tibial hole from the medial malleolus out the lateral tibia above the ankle. Bone tunnels in the navicular and tibia are used to create a ligament path to support the medial talar head.

- Given the size of the foot, the largest drill hole in the navicular is used, so a large tendon graft (6–9 mm) is possible.
- The graft is fixed at the navicular first and tensioned via the lateral ankle incision. The graft is tightened with the talonavicular joint in neutral to slight adduction.
- Fixation of the graft is via whipstitch using no. 2 nonabsorbable suture tied at each end, to a dorsal screw in the navicular and a lateral screw on the fibula.
  - With the navicular end tied down first, the foot is placed in neutral to slight adduction and the ligament graft tensioned and tied down laterally.
  - Alternative fixation with interference screws can be used, but the fixation may not be as strong with this technique in the tibia.
  - For large abduction deformities (ie, >30 degrees of talar head uncoverage), spring ligament reconstruction alone cannot be expected to hold correction and should, based on my experience, be used as a supplement to a lateral column lengthening procedure.
  - Lateral column lengthening—as minimal as possible—is done to place the talonavicular joint in neutral alignment.
  - The lateral column lengthening procedure should allow a minimum of 5 degrees of passive eversion to avoid excessive lateral tightness and should be tested in the operating room by everting the foot.
- An alternative to the tibial tunnel is a tunnel in the proximal talar neck with fixation using an interference screw.

INFERIOR SPRING LIGAMENT RECONSTRUCTION

- Tendon grafting also is used, but for deformity that is primarily plantar migration of the talar head.
- Graft is used to replace attenuated or degenerated tissue in combination with bony procedures to correct flatfoot deformity (TECH FIG 3A).
- Bone tunnels are used in the navicular and calcaneus (TECH FIG 3B).
  - The navicular tunnel is made from dorsal to plantar medial.
  - The calcaneal tunnel is drilled from underneath the distal medial and anterior facets and exits out the lateral calcaneus. The lateral exit point is exposed using the standard oblique incision for a posterior calcaneal osteotomy.
  - The graft is fixed first at the navicular, with the foot placed in 5 degrees of inversion with the calcaneus out of valgus (neutral). Calcaneal osteotomy is commonly performed and is fixed before the calcaneal drill hole is made and the graft is passed through.
  - Fixation of the graft is with nonabsorbable suture sewn in to the ends of the graft and tied down to screws in the dorsal navicular and lateral calcaneus. Alternative or supplemental fixation is done with interference screws.
  - The calcaneus cannot be left in valgus, or excessive strain on the graft will result.

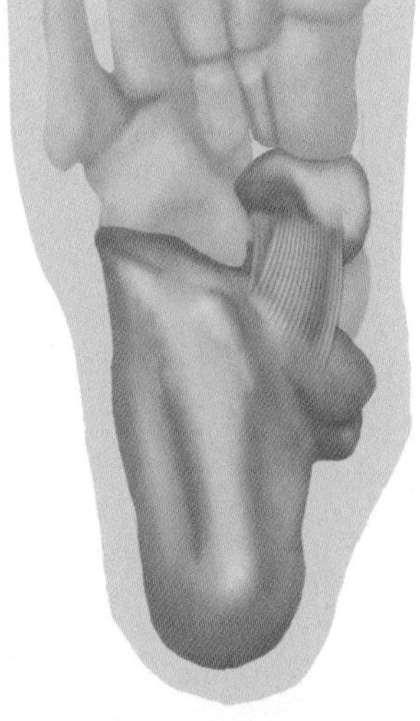

A

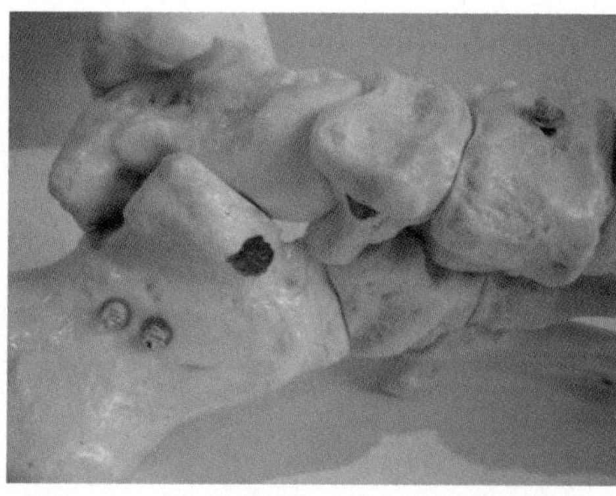

B

TECH FIG 3 • **A.** Diagram of plantar spring ligament reconstruction with the graft extending from the drill hole in the navicular to the calcaneus. Graft is used to replace attenuated or degenerated tissue in combination with bony procedures to correct flatfoot deformity. **B.** Navicular exit hole and calcaneal entrance for the graft. A drill hole is made dorsal (dorsal portion not shown) to plantar in the navicular and medial to lateral (not shown) in the calcaneus. Bone tunnels are used in the navicular and calcaneus.

COMBINED SUPEROMEDIAL AND PLANTAR SPRING LIGAMENT RECONSTRUCTION

- Combined superomedial and plantar spring ligament reconstruction is done for patients with considerable abduction of the talonavicular joint and plantar migration of the head.
- Two tendon grafts or a large tendon graft that is split at the plantar medial navicular tunnel is used (TECH FIG 4).
- The navicular tunnel is made as large as possible without fracturing the navicular to enable placement of large grafts. If allograft tendon is used, Achilles allograft with a bone block in the navicular tunnel is suggested (TECH FIG 5).
- The talonavicular joint is pinned in the corrected position (ie, 5 degrees of inversion and the calcaneus in neutral) after any bony procedures are fixed.
- The tendon grafts are then tensioned and fixed at the lateral calcaneus and fibula.
- Reconstruction with combined techniques is intended not to replace bony procedures but to supplement them when considerable tissue loss in the spring ligament complex is noted and correction of bony alignment has been gained at or near neutral position.
  - Commonly, a posterior osteotomy and, often, lateral column lengthening are performed.

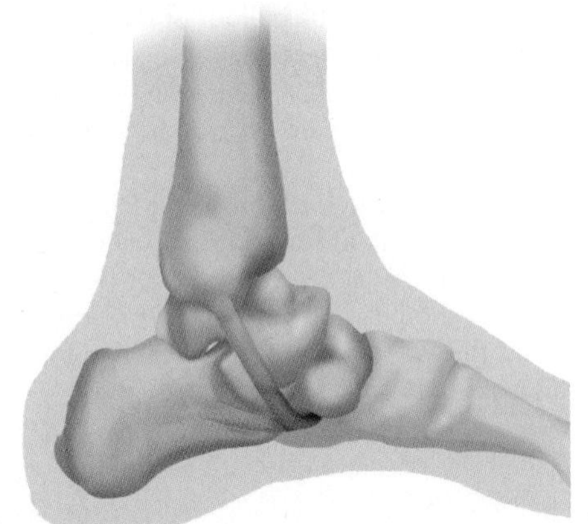
A

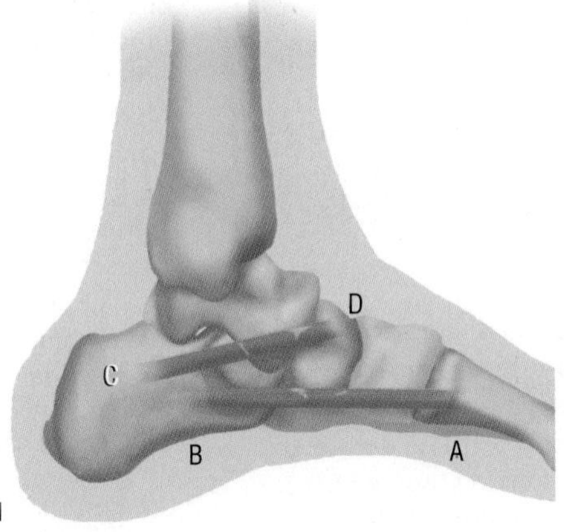

B1

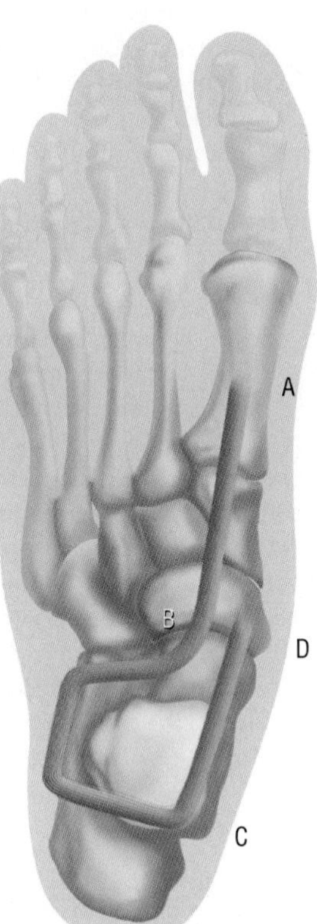

B2

TECH FIG 4 • A. Diagram of combined spring ligament complex reconstruction shows combined superomedial and plantar reconstruction. Two tendon grafts or a single large tendon graft that is split at the plantar medial navicular tunnel is used. **B.** Diagram of alternative combined spring ligament reconstruction using the peroneus longus left attached to first metatarsal base (shown) or free graft from the navicular plantar hole to the calcaneus and back to the navicular dorsal hole (not shown). Two tendon grafts or a large tendon graft that is split at the plantar medial navicular tunnel is used.

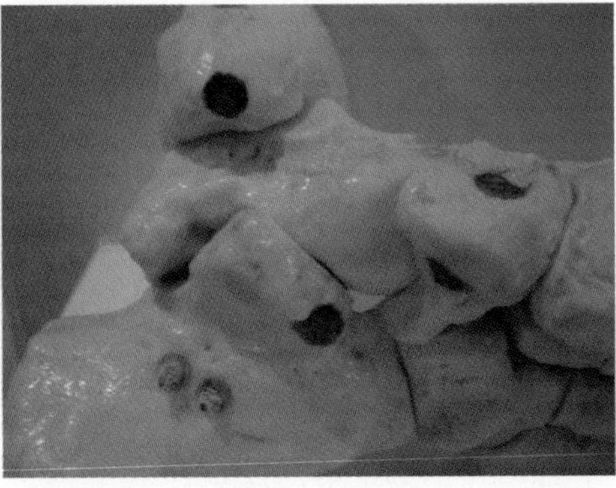

TECH FIG 5 • Drill holes for the combined spring ligament complex reconstruction with the graft exiting the plantar navicular and going into drill holes at the calcaneus. The navicular tunnel is as large as possible without fracturing the navicular, to enable placement of large grafts. If allograft tendon is used, Achilles allograft with a bone block in the navicular tunnel is suggested.

PEARLS AND PITFALLS

Do not expect soft tissue reconstruction to correct bony malalignment.	▪ The foot must be well aligned without excessive calcaneal valgus (≤ 5°) and without excessive abduction through the talonavicular joint (>30% uncoverage).
Avoid over- and undercorrection of deformity.	▪ Correct bony malalignment first. Then pin or hold the talonavicular joint in neutral position before tensioning the reconstruction.
Do not use lateral column lengthening, unless necessary.	▪ Bony procedures, while necessary to correct malalignment, have morbidity. Lateral column lengthening should not be used unless necessary, and overcorrection should be avoided.
Avoid weakening of tendon grafts.	▪ Fix bony procedures first to avoid crossing bony tunnels with screws, and use seizers to avoid multiple passages of the tendon grafts in tunnels.
Avoid unnecessary spring ligament reconstruction.	▪ Small tears do not necessitate spring ligament reconstruction.

POSTOPERATIVE CARE

- Touch-down weight bearing is allowed at 2 weeks and progressive weight bearing from 8 to 10 weeks.
- In reliable patients, a cast boot can be used instead of a cast beginning at 6 weeks.
- Full weight bearing without a boot is allowed at 12 to 16 weeks.
- Active inversion and eversion can be started at 6 weeks.

OUTCOMES

- Because spring ligament reconstructions are commonly combined with other procedures, it is difficult to define the contribution of these procedures to patient outcomes, and no reports have done so until recently.
- In our experience, spring ligament reconstruction does contribute to correction of deformity but only when most of the correction has been achieved through the bony procedures. I would use the superomedial spring ligament reconstruction for those feet with more of an abduction deformity and the plantar for those with more of a plantar sag deformity at the talonavicular joint. The superomedial may adequately correct combined deformity; if not, use the combined superomedial and spring ligament reconstruction.

COMPLICATIONS

- Failure of the graft can occur, particularly when a soft tissue procedure is used to try to correct large amounts of deformity without adequate bony correction of deformity.
- Failure of fixation of the graft. Interference screws are helpful, but the fit must be tight and tunnels must be made at somewhat of an angle to avoid straight pullout of the graft.
- Overcorrection with lateral weight bearing can occur, either with a medial slide osteotomy or, more commonly, if lateral column lengthening is used. Normal eversion motion should be maintained.
  - The heel should be in alignment with the lower leg (not in varus), and passive eversion into at least 5 degrees should be present after all the procedures are fixed.
  - The lateral column should not feel tight on range-of-motion testing in the operating room after the bony correction—eversion should be present.

REFERENCES

1. Davis WH, Sobel M, Deland JT, et al. The gross, histological and microvascular anatomy and biomechanical testing of the spring ligament complex. Foot Ankle Int 1996;17:95–102.
2. Deland JT. The adult acquired flatfoot and spring ligament complex, pathology and implications for treatment. Foot Ankle Clin 2001;6:129–135.
3. Deland JT, de Asla RJ, Sung I-H, et al. Posterior tibial tendon insufficiency: Which ligaments are involved? Foot Ankle Int 2005;26:427–435.
4. Deland JT, Page A, O'Malley MJ, et al. Posterior tibial tendon insufficiency. Results at different stages. HSS J 2006;2:157–160.
5. Hiller L, Pinney S. Surgical treatment of acquired adult flatfoot deformity: What is the state of practice among academic foot and ankle surgeons in 2002? Foot Ankle Int 2003;24:701–705.
6. Pinney SJ, Lin SS. Current concept review: acquired adult flatfoot deformity. Foot Ankle Int 2006;27:66–75.

Chapter 49

Calcaneonavicular Coalition Resection in the Adult Patient

Aaron T. Scott and H. Robert Tuten

DEFINITION

- A tarsal coalition is an abnormal fusion between two adjacent tarsal bones.
- Less than 2% of the general population is affected, and there appears to be no gender or racial predisposition.[2,6,10]
- Nearly 90% of all tarsal coalitions involve either the subtalar joint or the intervening space between the calcaneus and the navicular, with nearly an equal distribution between these two areas.[1]
- Although most calcaneonavicular coalitions are identified in children or adolescents, there does exist a subset of patients who become symptomatic in adulthood.

ANATOMY

- Unlike other tarsal coalitions, the calcaneonavicular coalition forms between two bones that normally do not articulate with each other.
- A calcaneonavicular coalition generally occurs between the anterior process of the calcaneus and the inferolateral aspect of the navicular.
- Histologically, these coalitions may be fibrous, cartilaginous, or osseous in nature, and may progress through these stages as the patient matures.

PATHOGENESIS

- Tarsal coalitions are most likely secondary to a failure of segmentation of the primitive mesenchyme.[2,3]
- In adolescents and young adults, the time at which the coalition becomes symptomatic appears to coincide with its ossification.[5]
- Although most coalitions are idiopathic, a dominant trait has been suggested.[10]

NATURAL HISTORY

- The natural history of a calcaneonavicular coalition is one of progressive disability.
- As the coalition ossifies in adolescence, the lack of subtalar range of motion may lead to hindfoot or midfoot pain, recurrent ankle sprains, and difficulty ambulating on uneven surfaces.
- In longstanding coalitions, the increased stresses imposed on the remaining mobile tarsal joints secondary to absent subtalar inversion and eversion may contribute to degenerative arthritic changes elsewhere in the foot.

PATIENT HISTORY AND PHYSICAL FINDINGS

- Symptomatic adults with calcaneonavicular coalitions generally present with hindfoot or midfoot pain, recurrent ankle sprains, or difficulty ambulating on uneven surfaces.
- In contrast to the often insidious onset of symptoms in adolescents with a calcaneonavicular coalition, onset in adults with this condition is abrupt and often coincides with a specific traumatic event, such as a severe ankle sprain.
- Other adults may simply present with a planovalgus foot deformity.
- Physical examination findings consistent with a calcaneonavicular coalition may include:
- Planovalgus foot deformity (rarely, a cavovarus deformity)
- Decreased or absent subtalar and transverse tarsal joint range of motion
- Tenderness in the region of the coalition
- Pain with inversion or eversion of the hindfoot
- Antalgic gait
- Instability secondary to multiple ankle sprains (as determined by anterior drawer testing)

IMAGING AND OTHER DIAGNOSTIC STUDIES

- Plain radiographs should be obtained in every patient suspected of having a tarsal coalition and should include AP, lateral, 45-degree oblique, and axial views of the foot.
- The 45-degree oblique view of the foot is the most useful plain radiograph for identifying a calcaneonavicular coalition. On this oblique view, the coalition may be seen as a discrete bony bridge between the calcaneus and the navicular, or this may simply be suggested by the presence of an extended, narrow beak of bone projecting from the anterior process of the calcaneus in the direction of the navicular (the "anteater sign"; **FIG 1A**).
- An axial view is important because it may aid in the identification of a talocalcaneal coalition.
- Computed tomographic scans should be obtained in all patients preoperatively to rule out a concomitant talocalcaneal coalition and to further evaluate for degenerative changes that may alter the surgical plan (**FIG 1B**).
- Magnetic resonance imaging may help identify a fibrous or cartilaginous coalition but is not necessary in the workup and treatment of most calcaneonavicular coalitions in adults.

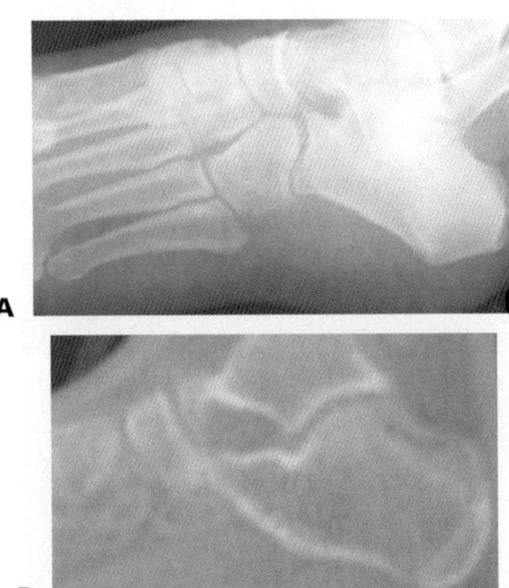

FIG 1 • **A.** A 45-degree oblique radiograph depicting a calcaneonavicular coalition (the "anteater sign"). **B.** Computed tomographic scan showing an isolated calcaneonavicular coalition.

DIFFERENTIAL DIAGNOSIS

- Talocalcaneal (subtalar) coalition
- Trauma or fracture of the hindfoot
- Arthritis (primary osteoarthrosis, posttraumatic arthritis, or inflammatory arthritis)
- Flatfoot secondary to posterior tibial tendon insufficiency
- Chronic ankle instability

NONOPERATIVE MANAGEMENT

- Initially, all patients with symptomatic calcaneonavicular coalition should be managed nonoperatively.
- Patients are first treated with nonsteroidal anti-inflammatory medications and custom orthotics that support the medial longitudinal arch.
- The UCBL brace is another orthotic option that acts to limit hindfoot motion.
- If patients fail this early conservative treatment, they are immobilized in a fiberglass short leg walking cast for 4 to 6 weeks.
- Symptomatic coalitions that are recalcitrant to casting in feet that display no degenerative changes may require surgical resection for relief of symptoms.

SURGICAL MANAGEMENT

- For patients who do not achieve relief with an adequate trial of nonoperative management, surgical intervention is warranted.

Preoperative Planning

- Plain radiographs, as well as computed tomographic or magnetic resonance imaging scans, are reviewed.
- All images are evaluated for additional pathology, including concomitant coalitions or degenerative arthritic changes that may alter the surgical treatment plan.

Positioning

- Thirty to 90 minutes before the incision is made, the patient is given an appropriate intravenous antibiotic.
- The patient is placed supine on the operating table, and a bump is placed under the ipsilateral sacrum to internally rotate the foot.
- A pneumatic tourniquet is placed around the upper thigh, and the extremity is prepped and draped in a standard, sterile fashion.

INCISION AND EXPOSURE

- After exsanguination with an Esmarch bandage and inflation of the tourniquet, a standard Ollier incision is created.
- This incision is centered directly over the dorsal aspect of the coalition and extends along a transverse Langer line plantarly to the peroneal tendon sheath and dorsally to the most lateral of the extensor digitorum longus tendons (**TECH FIG 1A**).
- Pre-emptive cauterization of any crossing vessels is performed.
- The sural cutaneous nerve and dorsal intermediate branch of the superficial peroneal nerve are identified and protected, as are the peroneal tendons.
- The extensor digitorum brevis muscle is visualized in the depths of the wound and subsequently elevated as a distally based flap using a scalpel and a Cobb elevator, with great care taken to preserve the overlying fascia, which will increase the suture-holding capacity of the flap (**TECH FIG 1B**).
- The elevated origin of the brevis is then grasped with a modified Mason-Allen stitch using 0-Vicryl (**TECH FIG 1C**).
- As the flap is retracted distally, the calcaneonavicular coalition is easily identified (**TECH FIG 1D**).

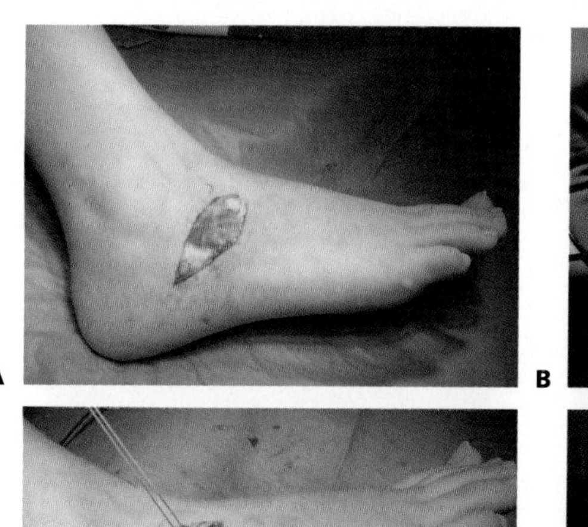

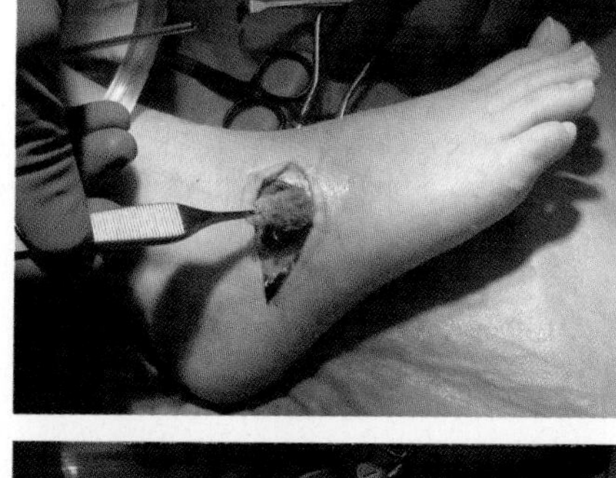

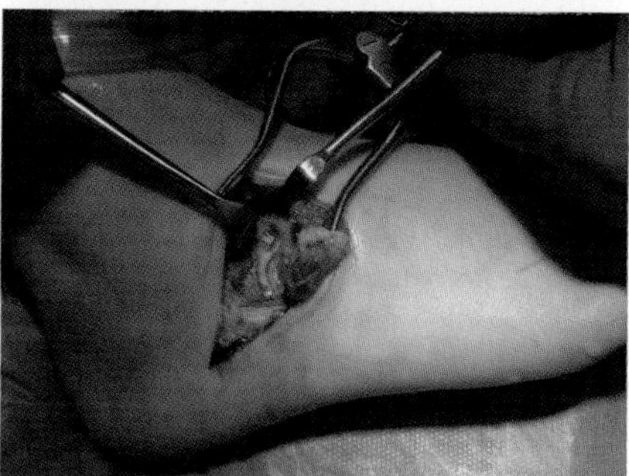

TECH FIG 1 • **A**. Incision. **B**. Elevation of the extensor digitorum brevis flap. **C.** Grasping of the extensor digitorum brevis with Vicryl suture. **D.** Flap retraction and visualization of calcaneonavicular coalition.

RESECTION OF CALCANEONAVICULAR COALITION WITH INTERPOSITION OF THE EXTENSOR DIGITORUM BREVIS

- After adequate visualization of the coalition, a straight osteotome is used to remove a 1-cm block to include the entire coalition.
- The osteotome cuts are made parallel to prevent the removal of a convergent, trapezoidal block of bone (**TECH FIG 2A**).
- Any remaining soft tissue within the resection site is cleared with a rongeur.
- The two limbs of the previously placed Vicryl suture attached to the extensor digitorum brevis flap are passed through the void created by coalition resection with the use of a free Keith needle (**TECH FIG 2B**).
- The tips of the Keith needles should pass just dorsal to the glabrous skin of the medial arch (**TECH FIG 2C**).
- The two limbs of the Vicryl suture are then tied over a soft dental bolster (no button; **TECH FIG 2D**).
- Alternatively, the raw bony surfaces of the resection site may be covered with bone wax, the void filled with gelfoam or autologous fat graft, and the brevis reattached to its origin.
- Radiographs are taken to confirm the adequacy of the resection (**TECH FIG 2E**).
- The wound is thoroughly irrigated, the tourniquet is released, and hemostasis is secured.
- Closure of the wound is performed using 2-0 Vicryl for the deep subcutaneous layer and 4-0 nylon horizontal mattress sutures for the skin (**TECH FIG 2F**).
- Finally, the wound is covered with a nonadherent dressing, sterile gauze, sterile cast padding, and a short leg fiberglass walking cast.

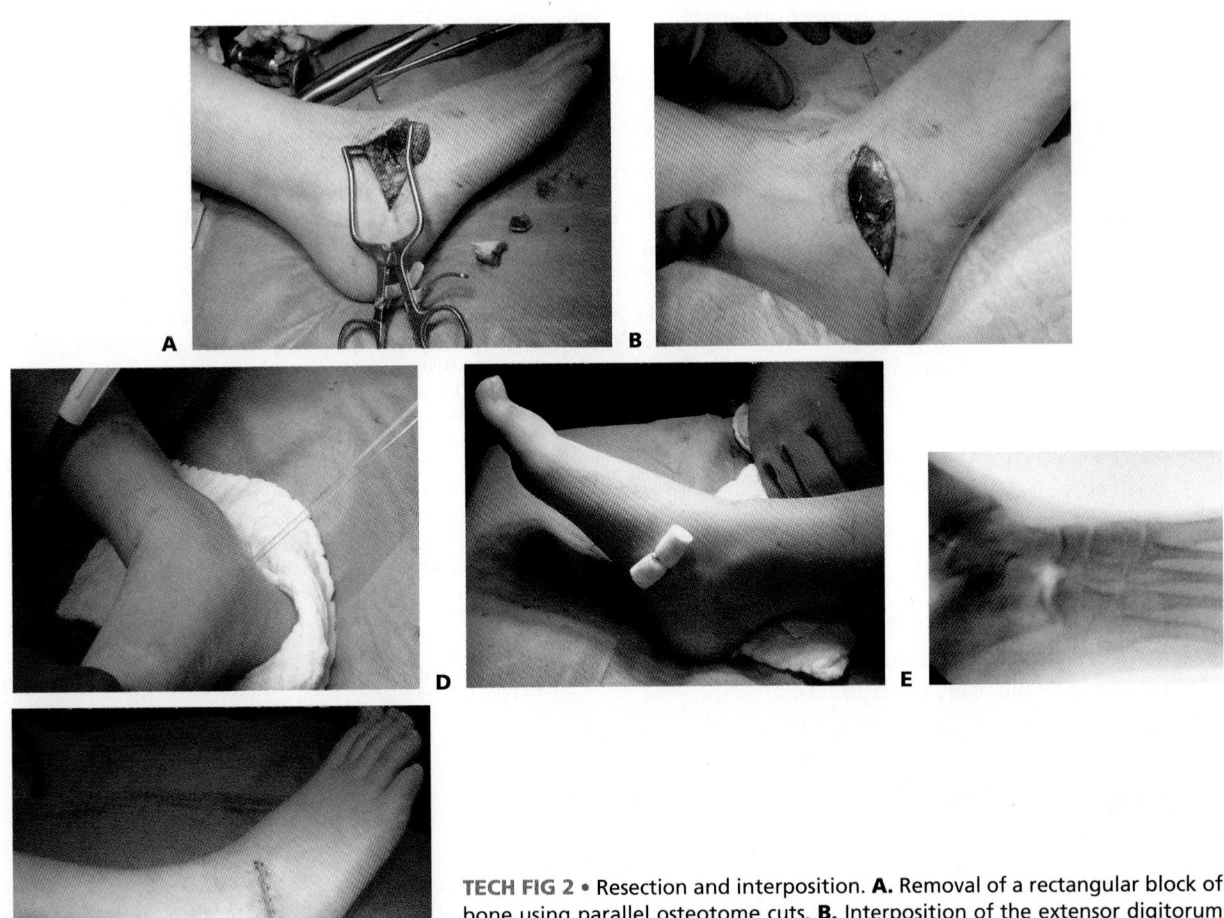

TECH FIG 2 • Resection and interposition. **A.** Removal of a rectangular block of bone using parallel osteotome cuts. **B.** Interposition of the extensor digitorum brevis flap into the void created by the resection. **C.** Passage of Keith needles through the skin of the medial arch. **D.** Flap sutures tied over soft dental bolster. **E.** Intraoperative radiographs to confirm the adequacy of the resection. **F.** Wound closure.

PEARLS AND PITFALLS

Preoperative workup	▪ Evaluate plain radiographs for the presence of significant degenerative changes, which would necessitate an appropriate arthrodesis. ▪ Review available computed tomographic or magnetic resonance imaging scans for the presence of any concomitant coalitions.
Coalition resection	▪ Osteotome cuts made in a parallel fashion will remove a rectangular block of bone rather than a convergent, trapezoidal segment, which may lead to recurrent pain secondary to an inadequate medial excision of the coalition.
Interpositional graft	▪ Preserve the fascia overlying the extensor digitorum brevis to increase the holding power of the Vicryl stitch.
Deformity correction	▪ Consider adding a lateral column lengthening procedure in the face of a significant pes planus.

POSTOPERATIVE CARE

- The patient is allowed to weight bear as tolerated in the cast on postoperative day 1.
- At 3 weeks, the patient returns to clinic for removal of the cast, wound sutures, and bolster stitch. At this point, the patient is placed in a walking boot.
- Following removal of the cast, physical therapy is initiated for ankle and hindfoot range-of-motion exercises.

OUTCOMES

- In the absence of significant degenerative changes that may necessitate an appropriate arthrodesis, resection of a calcaneonavicular coalition can be a successful procedure in symptomatic adults or adolescents.
- Cohen et al reviewed results of calcaneonavicular coalition resection in 12 adult patients. Subjective relief was attained in 10 patients and the average increase in total subtalar range of motion was 10 degrees.[1]
- In a group of 48 child and adolescent patients, Gonzalez and Kumar achieved 77% good to excellent results following calcaneonavicular coalition resection with interposition of the extensor digitorum brevis. The results did not deteriorate with time in those patients followed up for more than 10 years.[4]
- The importance of using an interpositional material has been reinforced in several publications.
- No recurrences of a calcaneonavicular coalition were noted by Moyes et al on oblique radiographs when an extensor digitorum brevis interposition was performed. However, in this same study, three of seven patients who underwent resection without interposition displayed radiographic evidence of a recurrence.[8]
- Swiontkowski et al used an interpositional material (fat or muscle) in 38 of 39 feet undergoing calcaneonavicular coalition resection and found no radiographic recurrences.[9]
- Mitchell and Gibson, on the other hand, found a recurrence of the coalition in nearly two thirds of their 41 patients who had undergone a simple coalition resection without interposition of the extensor digitorum brevis.[7]

COMPLICATIONS

- Superficial or deep infection
- Wound dehiscence[1]
- Recurrence of the coalition[7]
- Nerve damage
- Inadequate resection[3]
- Reflex sympathetic dystrophy[1]

REFERENCES

1. Cohen BE, Davis WH, Anderson RB. Success of calcaneonavicular coalition resection in the adult population. Foot Ankle Int 1996;17:569–572.
2. Cooperman DR, Janke BE, Gilmore A, et al. A three-dimensional study of calcaneonavicular tarsal coalitions. J Pediatr Orthop 2001;21:648–651.
3. Ehrlich MG, Elmer EB. Tarsal coalition. In: Jahss M, ed. Disorders of the Foot and Ankle, ed 2. Philadelphia: Saunders, 1991:921–938.
4. Gonzalez P, Kumar SJ. Calcaneonavicular coalition treated by resection and interposition of the extensor digitorum brevis muscle. J Bone Joint Surg Am 1990;72A:71–77.
5. Jayakumar S, Cowell HR. Rigid flatfoot. Clin Orthop Relat Res 1977;122:77–84.
6. Kulik SA, Clanton TO. Foot fellow's review: tarsal coalition. Foot Ankle Int 1996;17:286–296.
7. Mitchell GP, Gibson JMC. Excision of calcaneonavicular bar for painful spasmodic flatfoot. J Bone Joint Surg Br 1967;49B:281–287.
8. Moyes ST, Crawford EJP, Aichroth PM. The interposition of extensor digitorum brevis in the resection of calcaneonavicular bars. J Pediatr Orthop 1994;14:387–388.
9. Swiontkowski MF, Scranton PE, Hansen S. Tarsal coalitions: long-term results of surgical treatment. J Pediatr Orthop 1983;3:287–292.
10. Vincent KA. Tarsal coalition and painful flatfoot. J Am Acad Orthop Surg 1998;6:274–281.

Chapter 50 Isolated Subtalar Arthrodesis

Aaron T. Scott and Robert S. Adelaar

DEFINITION

- An isolated subtalar arthrodesis can be used in the treatment of a myriad of different hindfoot conditions, including primary arthrosis of the subtalar joint, posttraumatic arthritis secondary to a talar or complex calcaneal fracture, rheumatoid arthritis, and talocalcaneal coalition.
- Other indications include posterior tibial tendon insufficiency and any neuromuscular disorder presenting with instability of the subtalar joint.
- When the pathologic process resides solely in the talocalcaneal articulation, isolated subtalar arthrodesis is preferred over a triple arthrodesis for its preservation of hindfoot motion, its decreased potential for development of degenerative changes in neighboring joints, its relative simplicity, and its lower potential for pseudarthrosis of the talonavicular and calcaneocuboid joints.

ANATOMY

- The term *subtalar* refers to the articulation between the anterior, middle, and posterior facets of the inferior talus and the corresponding anterior, middle, and posterior facets located on the superior aspect of the calcaneus.
- The subtalar joint is a "plane type" synovial joint with a weak fibrous capsule supported by medial, lateral, and posterior talocalcaneal ligaments, as well as an interosseous talocalcaneal ligament.
- This important articulation provides for inversion and eversion of the hindfoot, which is critical for proper adaptation of the foot during ambulation on uneven terrain and for dissipation of heel strike forces.
- Isolated fusions of the subtalar joint have been shown to reduce talonavicular joint motion by 74% and calcaneocuboid joint motion by 44%.[1]

PATHOGENESIS

- Numerous causes of subtalar joint arthritis exist, including:
  - Primary osteoarthrosis: articular cartilage degeneration of unknown etiology
  - Secondary arthritis: caused by either traumatic articular cartilage damage or increased joint stresses following an arthrodesis of an adjacent joint
  - Inflammatory arthritis: autoimmune joint destruction (eg, rheumatoid arthritis, psoriatic arthritis)
- Other etiologies that may necessitate an isolated subtalar arthrodesis include:
  - Talocalcaneal coalition: abnormal fusion between the talus and calcaneus, most likely secondary to a failure of segmentation of the primitive mesenchyme
  - Instability or deformity secondary to muscular imbalance (eg, posterior tibial tendon insufficiency, Charcot-Marie-Tooth disease, poliomyelitis)

NATURAL HISTORY

- Depends on specific etiology
- In general, the various forms of subtalar arthritis are progressive in nature.
- Despite waxing and waning of symptoms, no spontaneous resolution of the pathologic process is noted.

PATIENT HISTORY AND PHYSICAL FINDINGS

- A problem-focused history should include direct questioning regarding the exact nature of the symptoms, specific location, duration and progression of symptoms, aggravating or alleviating factors, prior therapeutic interventions, and functional disability.
- Patients often complain of lateral ankle pain and difficulty ambulating on uneven terrain.
- The pain often gets better with rest and may be mitigated by wearing high-top shoes.
- Physical examination findings consistent with subtalar joint arthritis may include:
  - Hindfoot swelling
  - Tenderness within the sinus tarsi
  - Pain with inversion and eversion of the hindfoot
  - Limited range of motion of the subtalar joint
  - Antalgic gait
- To help localize the pathology to the subtalar joint complex, palpate and observe the sinus tarsi (the soft tissue depression just anterior and slightly distal to lateral malleolus) for swelling.
- Passively dorsiflex the ankle to neutral to lock the talus within the mortise. Descriptions of normal subtalar range of motion vary widely. Therefore, it is useful to describe the range as a fraction of the asymptomatic, contralateral side. Pain and decreased range of motion may be indicative of subtalar joint arthritis. Complete loss of range of motion is consistent with a tarsal coalition.

IMAGING AND OTHER DIAGNOSTIC STUDIES

- Plain radiographs should include standing AP, lateral, and oblique views of the foot, and standing AP, lateral, and mortise views of the ankle.
- Additional plain radiographs may include a Broden's view (lower extremity internally rotated 45 degrees; x-ray tube angled 10 to 40 degrees cephalad) to evaluate the posterior subtalar facet, and a Canale view (AP view of the foot in 15 degrees of pronation with tube angled 75 degrees from the horizontal) to evaluate the sinus tarsi.
- Radiographic findings consistent with a degenerative process include joint space narrowing, osteophytes, and subchondral cysts or sclerosis (**FIG 1**).

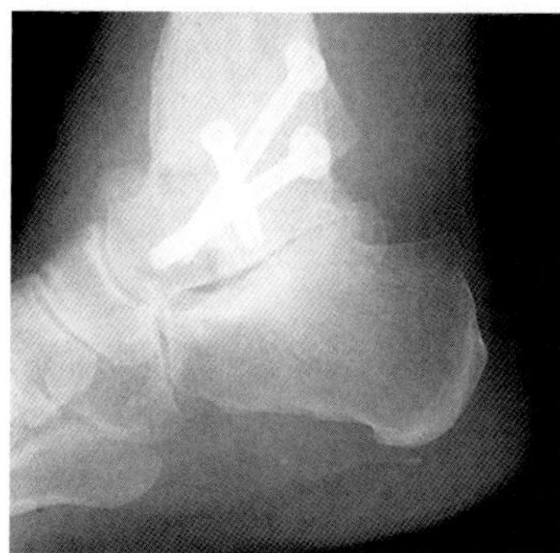

FIG 1 • Posttraumatic arthritis of the subtalar joint. Note the narrowing of the joint space, subchondral sclerosis, subchondral cysts, and osteophyte formation.

- Computed tomography and magnetic resonance imaging offer little additional information about the arthritic process involving the subtalar joint, but they may identify a previously undiagnosed tarsal coalition or concomitant soft tissue pathology.
- A diagnostic injection of a local anesthetic into the subtalar joint may help localize the patient's complaints, and if a corticosteroid is added to the injection, this procedure may provide significant short-term relief.

DIFFERENTIAL DIAGNOSIS

- Primary osteoarthrosis
- Posttraumatic arthritis
- Inflammatory arthritis
- Acute fracture
- Sinus tarsi syndrome
- Instability of the subtalar joint or subtalar sprain
- Fibrous or cartilaginous talocalcaneal coalition
- Subtalar loose body

NONOPERATIVE MANAGEMENT

- Subtalar joint arthritis is initially managed nonoperatively in all patients.
- Nonoperative management strategies may include:
  - Activity modification
  - Nonsteroidal anti-inflammatory medications
  - Intra-articular corticosteroid injection
  - Use of an ankle–foot orthosis or UCBL orthosis to limit hindfoot motion. Other options include an air stirrup or high-top boot.
  - Patellar tendon–bearing brace to unload the subtalar joint
- Conservative treatment may also be indicated in patients with significant peripheral vascular disease, active infection, inability to comply with the postoperative regimen, or a severe sensory neuropathy.

SURGICAL MANAGEMENT

- For patients who do not achieve relief with an adequate trial of nonoperative management, surgical intervention is warranted.

Preoperative Planning

- Plain radiographs are reviewed for deformity or malalignment, loose bodies, or retained hardware from a prior surgery.
- Computed tomographic or magnetic resonance imaging scans are reviewed, if available.

Positioning

- The patient is placed supine on the operative table, and the sole of the foot is aligned with the end of the bed to facilitate later screw insertion into the heel.
- A pneumatic tourniquet is placed around the upper thigh, and a soft bump is placed beneath the ipsilateral sacrum to internally rotate the operative extremity. Placement of the bump beneath the sacrum, rather than beneath the buttock, will prevent any undue pressure on the sciatic nerve.
- The fluoroscopy unit is brought in from the contralateral side of the bed.

Approach

- A tourniquet is elevated to a pressure of 100 mm Hg greater than the patient's systolic pressure.
- The incision begins approximately 1 cm below the tip of the lateral malleolus and progresses distally to a point just shy of the base of the fourth metatarsal (**FIG 2A**). Alternatively, a modified Ollier incision may be used.
- The subcutaneous tissue is incised in line with the skin incision, and preemptive hemostasis of any crossing vessels is performed using electrocautery.
- The origin of the extensor digitorum brevis muscle is identified and elevated along with the sinus tarsi fat pad as a distally based flap. A small cuff of tissue is preserved proximally for later reattachment of this flap (**FIG 2B,C**).
- At this point, the subtalar joint is well visualized.

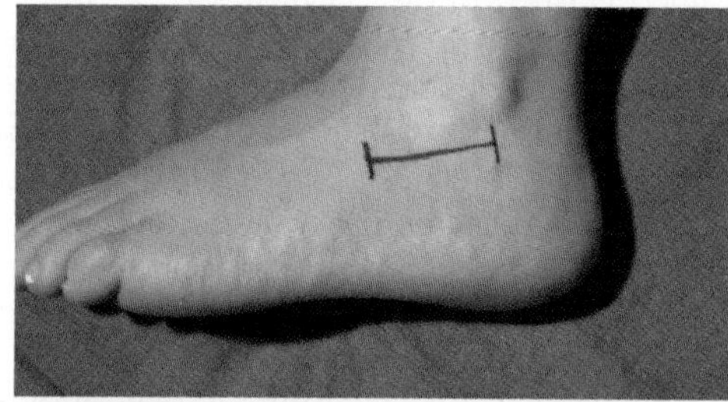

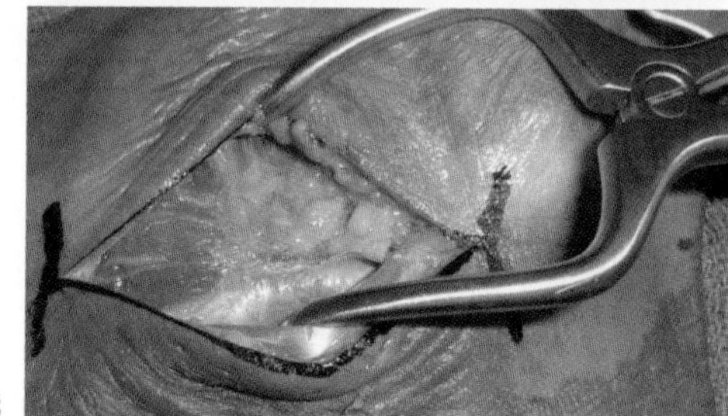

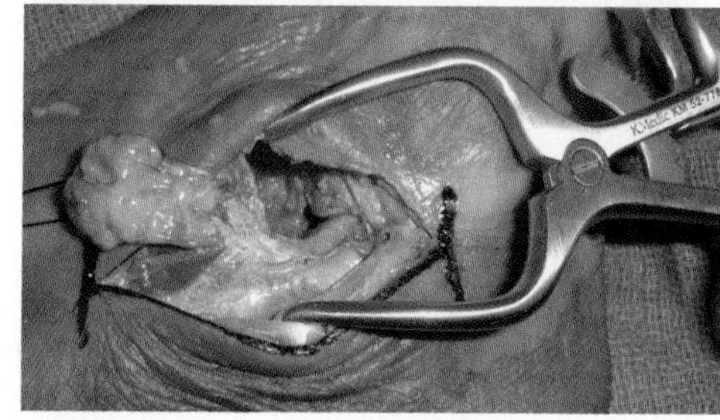

FIG 2 • Surgical approach. **A.** Incision. **B.** Exposure of the extensor digitorum brevis muscle, sinus tarsi fat pad, and peroneal tendons. **C.** Elevation of extensor digitorum brevis and sinus tarsi fat pad as a distally based flap.

PREPARATION OF THE ARTHRODESIS SITE

- After adequate visualization of the lateral aspect of the subtalar joint has been attained, any remaining fatty or ligamentous tissue is removed from the joint with a rongeur (TECH FIG 1A).
- Using a straight curette or chisel, the articular cartilage is removed from the lateral half of the inferior talus and superior aspect of the calcaneal facets (TECH FIG 1B). Note that the goal is to maintain the normal, curved contours of the articular facets.
- A lamina spreader is then inserted to allow access to the medial half of the joint, which is then cleared of its articular cartilage using a combination of straight and curved currettes (TECH FIG 1C).
- After complete removal of all articular cartilage, K-wire holes are created in the denuded inferior surface of the talus and the superior surface of the calcaneus to produce vascular channels that will aid in the fusion (TECH FIG 1D). These K-wire holes may be further augmented with larger holes created through the use of a 3-mm burr, and by feathering of the subchondral bone with a curved osteotome.
- Cancellous autograft obtained from the proximal tibia (see Techniques) is inserted into the subtalar joint, and the extensor digitorum brevis muscle is reattached to its site of origin to help seal the fusion site (TECH FIG 1E).

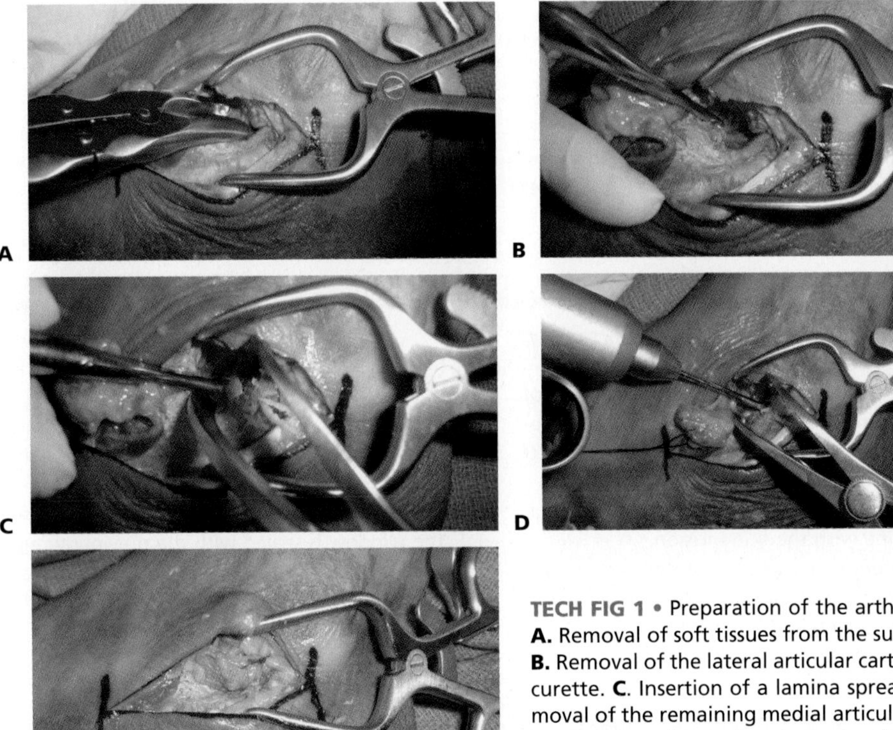

TECH FIG 1 • Preparation of the arthrodesis site. **A.** Removal of soft tissues from the subtalar joint. **B.** Removal of the lateral articular cartilage with a curette. **C.** Insertion of a lamina spreader and removal of the remaining medial articular cartilage. **D.** Creation of vascular channels with a K-wire. **E.** Reattachment of the extensor digitorum brevis to its origin after insertion of a tibial bone graft.

INSERTION OF HARDWARE

- At this point, the subtalar joint is positioned into 5 degrees of valgus.
- A 1-cm incision is created at the apex of the heel for insertion of a guide pin, which is subsequently driven through the posterior tuberosity, across the subtalar joint, and into the talar neck (TECH FIG 2A). This guide pin is placed fluoroscopically using axial (Harris) heel and lateral views.
- A second guide pin is placed through a 1-cm incision just medial to the anterior tibialis tendon into the dorsomedial aspect of the talar neck, across the subtalar joint, and into the posterior calcaneal tuberosity (TECH FIG 2B).
- The initial guide pin is occasionally overreamed proximally (not necessary with self-drilling, self-tapping screws), and a 6.5-mm partially threaded cancellous lag screw of an appropriate length is inserted after minimal use of the cannulated countersink. This procedure is repeated for the dorsomedial lag screw.
- Final fluoroscopic images are obtained to verify proper screw position (TECH FIG 2C).

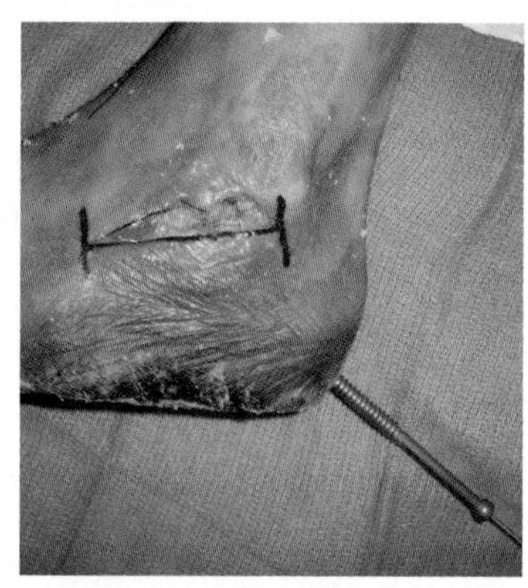

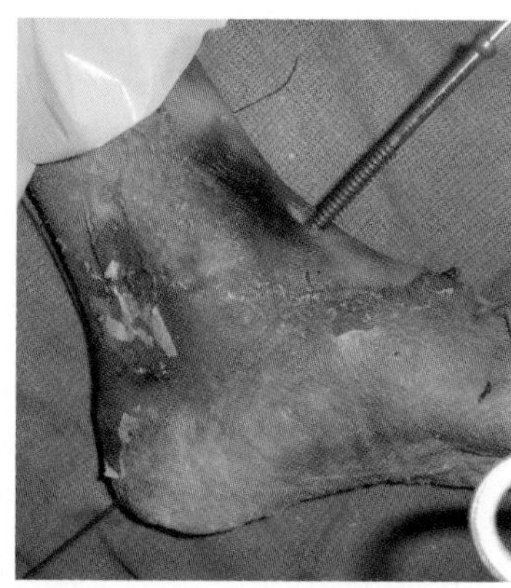

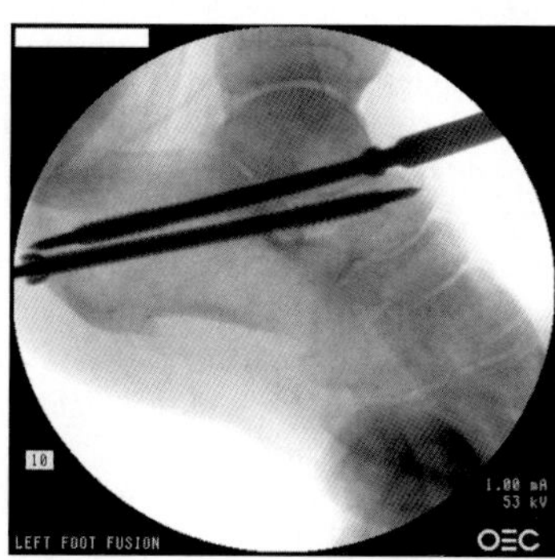

TECH FIG 2 • Internal fixation **A.** Placement of the first guide pin and screw from the apex of the calcaneal tuberosity. **B.** Placement of the second guide pin and screw from the dorsomedial aspect of the talar neck. **C.** Final fluoroscopic images.

WOUND CLOSURE

- The tourniquet is released and hemostasis is secured.
- The wound is then closed using 2-0 Vicryl for the subcuticular layer and 3-0 nylon horizontal mattress sutures for the skin.

HARVESTING OF TIBIAL BONE GRAFT

- An incision beginning 1 cm distal to the distal aspect of the tibial tubercle and 1 cm lateral to the anterior tibial crest is carried distally for a length of 4 cm (**TECH FIG 3A**).
- The fascia overlying the anterior compartment musculature is divided in line with the skin incision.
- Muscle and periosteum overlying the anterolateral face of the tibia is elevated using a periosteal elevator, thus exposing the anterolateral cortex (**TECH FIG 3B**).
- A 1 by 1–cm square (or elliptical) window is created in the center of the anterolateral face, and a curette is inserted into the window for removal of cancellous graft (**TECH FIG 3C,D**).
- After an adequate amount of cancellous graft is harvested, the window is sealed with the previously removed square plug of bone, and a layered closure of the fascia, subcutaneous tissue, and skin is performed.
- Time from graft harvest to insertion into the fusion site should be less than 30 minutes.

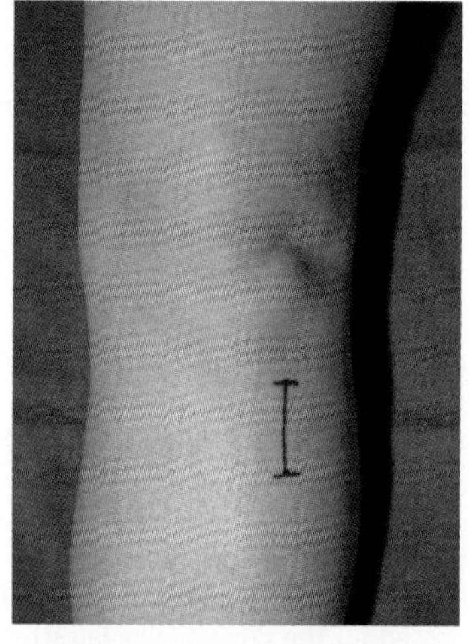

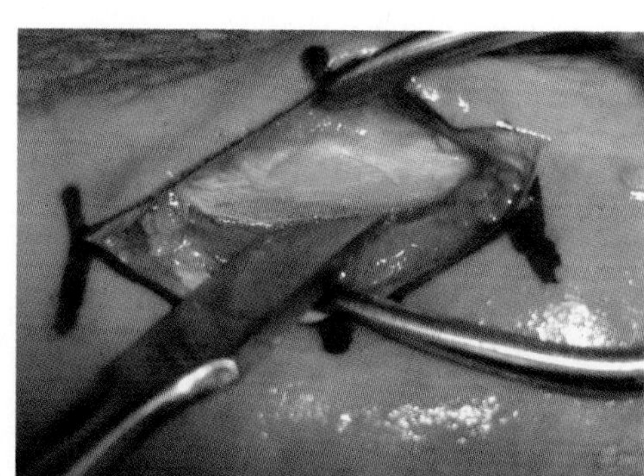

TECH FIG 3 • Harvesting of the tibial bone graft. **A.** Incision. **B.** Periosteal elevation along the anterolateral cortex. *(continued)*

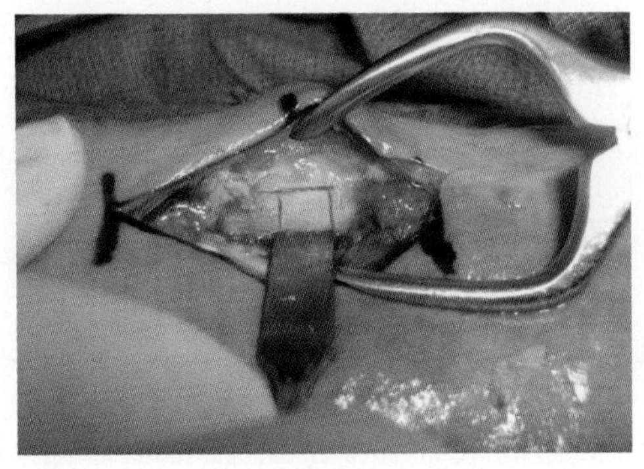

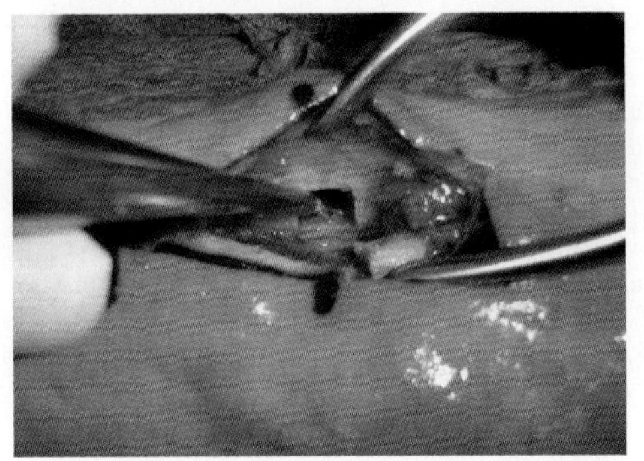

TECH FIG 3 • *(continued)* **C.** Creation of a 1 by 1–cm square window. **D.** Removal of the cancellous autograft with a curette.

PEARLS AND PITFALLS

Preparation of joint surfaces	■ Remove articular cartilage only. ■ Preservation of subchondral bone will provide structural support and will allow for better coaptation.[9] ■ Use of a K-wire to perforate the residual subchondral bone of the talus and calcaneus will allow communication between the marrow cavities and the arthrodesis site, and will aid in the fusion.
Positioning of arthrodesis	■ The arthrodesis is ideally placed in 5 degrees of valgus.[6] ■ Fusing the subtalar joint in varus will lock the transverse tarsal joint, leading to increased lateral forefoot pressures with weight bearing. [10] ■ Fusing the subtalar joint in excessive valgus can potentially lead to subfibular impingement.[10]
Internal fixation	■ Use of a partially threaded cancellous lag screw with a short threaded region will reduce the likelihood of any threads crossing the arthrodesis site. ■ Countersinking of the screw heads and avoidance of a screw head placed on the weight-bearing plantar surface of the calcaneus will reduce complaints related to the hardware.

POSTOPERATIVE CARE

- The extremity is placed in a well-padded, non–weight-bearing short leg plaster cast before the patient leaves the operating room.
- In the recovery room, the cast is widely split along its anterior surface to allow for immediate postoperative swelling.
- The patient is seen in clinic at 2 weeks postoperatively, at which point the initial cast and sutures are removed.
- A short leg fiberglass cast is applied and the patient is kept non–weight-bearing.
- At the 6-week mark, radiographs are obtained, and the patient is converted to a fiberglass short leg walking cast.
- If radiographic union is appreciated at the 12-week appointment, casting is discontinued and gentle range of motion of the foot and ankle is initiated. At this point, the patient is often placed in a CAM walker to ease the transition from the cast to normal shoe wear.

OUTCOMES

- At an average of nearly 5 years' follow-up, Mann et al reported a 93% satisfaction rate with isolated subtalar arthrodesis.[12]
- In another study by Mann and Baumgarten, subtalar joint fusion in 6 degrees of valgus resulted in the maintainence of approximately 50% of the transverse tarsal joint motion as compared with the unaffected, contralateral extremity. In this same study, minimal degenerative changes were noted at the talonavicular and calcaneocuboid joints, a finding that was not clinically significant.[11]
- In a retrospective study, Dahm and Kitaoka demonstrated a 96% union rate in 25 adult feet.[3]
- Similarly, Easley et al demonstrated a 96% subtalar fusion rate after excluding smokers, revision arthrodeses, fusions using a structural graft, and subtalar fusions performed in an extremity with a previously fused tibiotalar joint.[4]

COMPLICATIONS

- Infection[8]
- Nonunion[4,7,10]
- Malalignment
  - Varus leading to increased lateral column forefoot pressures[6,10]
  - Valgus leading to subfibular impingement[6,10]
- Symptomatic hardware[4]
- Superficial wound breakdown[2]
- Reflex sympathetic dystrophy[5]

REFERENCES

1. Astion DJ, Deland JT, Otis JC, Kenneally S. Motion of the hindfoot after simulated arthrodesis. J Bone Joint Surg Am 1997;79A:241–246.
2. Chandler JT, Bonar SK, Anderson RB, Davis WH. Results of in situ subtalar arthrodesis for late sequelae of calcaneus fractures. Foot Ankle Int 1999;20:18–24.
3. Dahm DL, Kitaoka HB. Subtalar arthrodesis with internal compression for posttraumatic arthritis. J Bone Joint Surg Br 1998;80B: 134–138.
4. Easley ME, Trnka H-J, Schon LC, Myerson MS. Isolated subtalar arthrodesis. J Bone Joint Surg Am 2000;82A:613–624.
5. Flemister AS, Infante AF, Sanders RW, Walling AK. Subtalar arthrodesis for complications of intra-articular calcaneal fractures. Foot Ankle Int 2000;21:392–399.
6. Kile TA, Bouchard M. Degenerative joint disease of the ankle and hindfoot. In: Thordarson DB, ed. Orthopaedic Surgery Essentials: Foot and Ankle. Philadelphia: Lippincott Williams & Wilkins, 2004: 195–220.
7. Kitaoka HB. Talocalcaneal (subtalar) arthrodesis. In: Kitaoka HB, ed. Master Techniques in Orthopaedic Surgery: The Foot and Ankle, ed 2. Philadelphia: Lippincott Williams & Wilkins, 2002:387–399.
8. Lin SS, Shereff MJ. Talocalcaneal arthrodesis: a moldable bone grafting technique. Foot Ankle Clin 1996;1:109–131.
9. Lippert FG, Hansen ST. Subtalar arthrodesis. In Lippert FG, Hansen ST, eds. Foot Ankle Disorders: Tricks of the Trade. New York: Thieme, 2003:133–139.
10. Mann RA. Arthrodesis of the foot and ankle. In: Coughlin MJ, Mann RA, eds. Surgery of the Foot and Ankle, ed 7. St Louis: Mosby, 1999: 651–699.
11. Mann RA, Baumgarten M. Subtalar fusion for isolated subtalar disorders: preliminary report. Clin Orthop Rel Res 1988;226:260–265.
12. Mann RA, Beaman DN, Horton GA. Isolated subtalar arthrodesis. Foot Ankle Int 1998;19:511–519.

Chapter 51

Surgical Management of Calcaneal Malunions

Michael P. Clare and Roy W. Sanders

DEFINITION

- A calcaneal malunion refers to residual bony malalignment and associated clinical sequelae resulting from inadequate treatment of a displaced intra-articular calcaneal fracture.

ANATOMY

- The calcaneus is an odd-shaped bone that supports full body weight and provides a lever arm through which the powerful gastrocnemius–soleus complex assists with forward propulsion during gait (**FIG 1**).
- The calcaneus also provides articulations for the subtalar and calcaneocuboid joints, and thus is integral to function of the triple joint complex of the hindfoot for normal ambulation and accommodation to uneven ground (**FIG 2**).
- The normal orientation of the calcaneus is reflected radiographically as calcaneal pitch, talocalcaneal height, and calcaneal length, which directly affect the three-dimensional alignment of the hindfoot and midfoot and indirectly affect ankle dorsiflexion (**FIG 3**).

PATHOGENESIS

- In a displaced intra-articular calcaneal fracture, there is typically not only intra-articular displacement of the posterior facet but also loss of calcaneal height, shortening and varus angulation of the calcaneal tuberosity, extension into the anterior process or calcaneocuboid joint, and expansion of the lateral calcaneal wall.
- Nonoperative treatment, or inadequate operative treatment, of a displaced intra-articular calcaneal fracture results in a calcaneal malunion, which affects function of the ankle, subtalar, and calcaneocuboid joints and leads to pain and disability.[4,15] Associated sequelae include:
  - Posttraumatic subtalar and calcaneocuboid arthritis due to residual articular incongruity[8,17]
  - Lateral subfibular impingement from residual lateral wall expansion and heel widening[8,16]
  - Peroneal tendon stenosis, tenosynovitis, or subluxation–dislocation as a result of adjacent bony prominence[2,5,12]
  - Anterior ankle impingement and loss of ankle dorsiflexion due to loss of calcaneal height, resulting in relative dorsiflexion of talus[3]
  - Hindfoot malalignment (typically varus) affecting gait pattern and shoe wear and potentially producing a leg-length discrepancy[13]

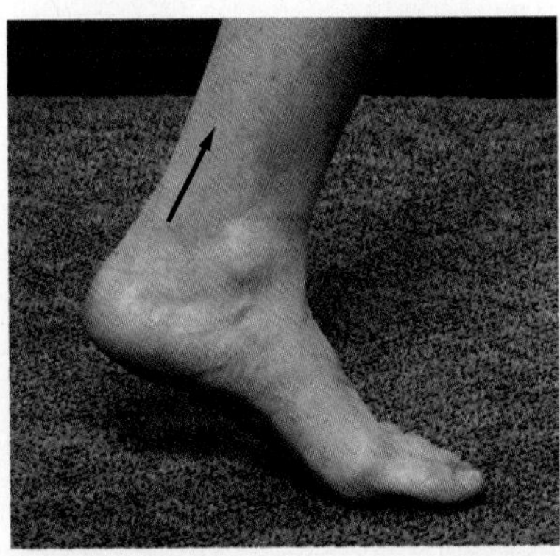

FIG 1 • The calcaneus serves as a lever arm for the powerful gastrocnemius–soleus complex.

NATURAL HISTORY

- Patients with displaced intra-articular calcaneal fractures that go on to malunion typically have a poor result, including pain with weight bearing, limitations in shoe wear, secondary gait alterations, and progressive posttraumatic subtalar arthritis.[6,11]

PATIENT HISTORY AND PHYSICAL FINDINGS

- History of prior calcaneal fracture (displaced intra-articular fracture) (the examiner should note the prior method of treatment, operative or nonoperative)
- Pain with weight bearing (standing or walking, particularly on uneven terrain)
- Thorough examination of the ankle and hindfoot should also include assessment of:
  - Skin and soft tissue envelope, including location of previous surgical incisions, overall mobility of lateral hindfoot skin, swelling, or any dystrophic changes where present
  - Neurovascular status (particularly the presence or absence of palpable pulses)
  - Hindfoot malalignment: excessive hindfoot varus or valgus relative to uninvolved limb represents malalignment
  - Subtalar range of motion: decreased subtalar range of motion may result from posttraumatic arthritis
  - Subtalar arthritis: tenderness to palpation suggests articular degeneration
  - Subfibular impingement, bony prominence, and tenderness suggest peroneal stenosis or tenosynovitis from residual lateral wall expansion. Peroneal tendons may actually be subluxed or dislocated in severe cases.

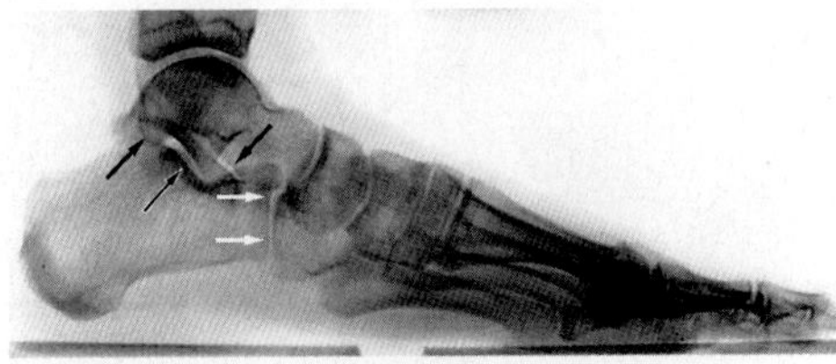

FIG 2 • Normal weight-bearing lateral radiograph demonstrating posterior and middle facets of subtalar joint (*black arrows*), and calcaneocuboid joint (*white arrows*).

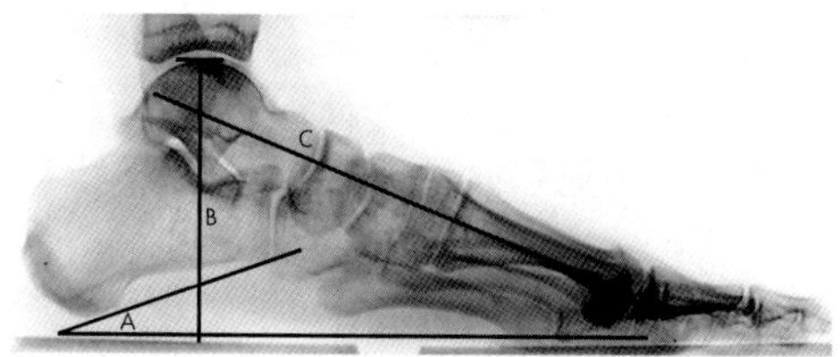

FIG 3 • Normal weight-bearing lateral radiograph; note downward orientation of talus. **A.** Calcaneal pitch angle. **B.** Talocalcaneal height. **C.** Talo–first metatarsal angle.

- Ankle range of motion: decreased dorsiflexion compared to uninvolved limb may indicate anterior impingement from relative dorsiflexion of talus and loss of calcaneal height.

IMAGING AND OTHER DIAGNOSTIC STUDIES

- Standard weight-bearing radiographs of the ankle and foot, in addition to a Harris axial view of the calcaneus, reveal the calcaneal malunion.
- The lateral view of the hindfoot demonstrates loss of calcaneal height and relative dorsiflexion of the talus (**FIG 4**).
- The mortise view of the ankle demonstrates residual lateral wall expansion and degenerative changes in the subtalar joint, as well as a fracture-dislocation variant fragment where present (**FIGS 5 AND 6**).
- The axial view shows residual shortening of the calcaneus, and any hindfoot malalignment where present (**FIG 7**).
- Once the diagnosis is established, a CT scan of the calcaneus, including axial, sagittal, and 30-degree semicoronal images, further delineates the extent of subtalar and calcaneocuboid arthritic change, hindfoot malalignment, lateral wall exostosis, and subfibular impingement, as well as any associated talar or other ankle joint pathology (**FIGS 8–10**).

DIFFERENTIAL DIAGNOSIS

- Posttraumatic subtalar arthritis (without malunion)
- Subtalar osteoarthritis

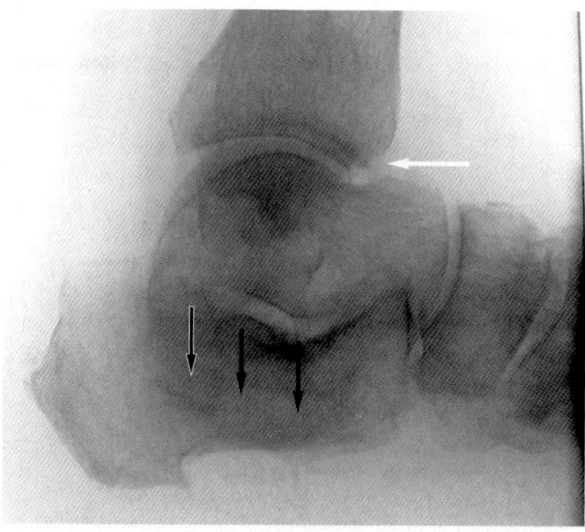

FIG 4 • Weight-bearing lateral radiograph of calcaneal malunion. Note loss of calcaneal height (*black arrows*), producing relative dorsiflexion of talus and anterior impingement at ankle joint (*white arrow*).

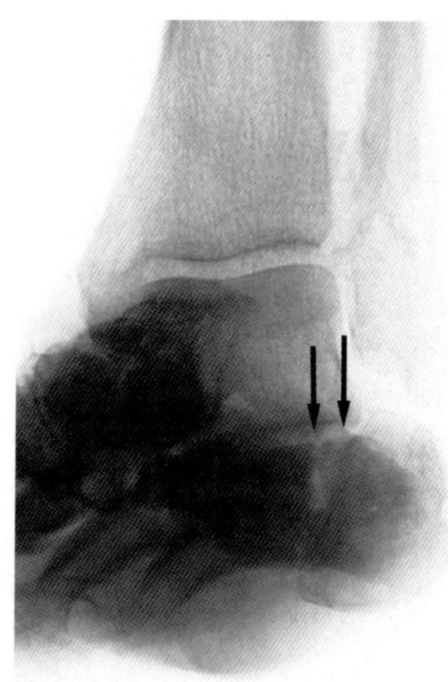

FIG 5 • Weight-bearing mortise radiograph of calcaneal malunion; note residual intra-articular step-off and associated degenerative changes (*black arrows*).

- Calcaneal fracture nonunion
- Lateral ankle instability or peroneal tendon pathology

NONOPERATIVE MANAGEMENT

- Nonoperative treatment options are limited but consist primarily of supportive modalities to lessen inflammation and painful motion through the hindfoot.
- A lace-up ankle brace, UCBL, ankle–foot orthosis, or Arizona-type brace may be beneficial in limiting painful subtalar motion and providing symptomatic relief. A prefabricated fracture boot may be used intermittently for episodes of arthritic flare-up.

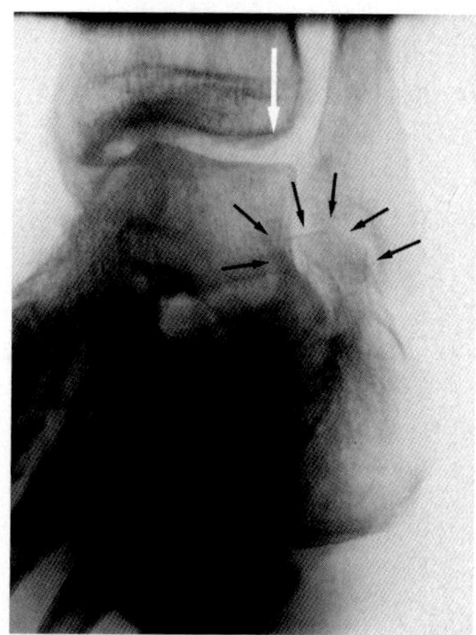

FIG 6 • Weight-bearing mortise radiograph of calcaneal malunion from fracture-dislocation variant pattern. Note residually dislocated posterolateral fragment wedged within talofibular joint (*black arrows*), and subtle varus tilt within ankle mortise (*white arrow*), suggesting incompetence of lateral ligamentous complex.

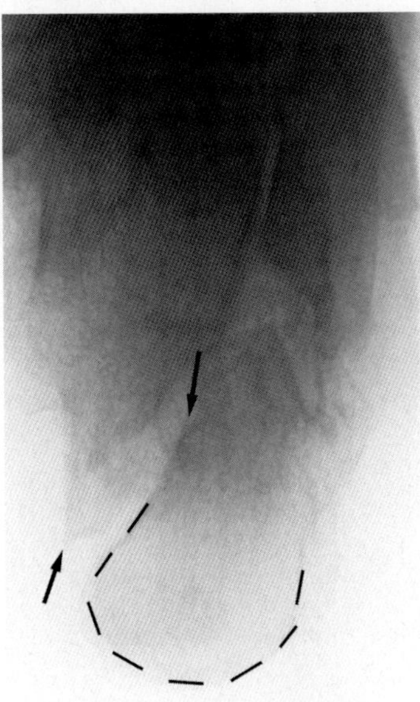

FIG 7 • Axial radiograph of calcaneal malunion. Note marked residual shortening (*black arrows*) and varus angulation of calcaneal tuberosity (*dashed lines*).

- Intermittent use of nonsteroidal anti-inflammatory medication can also be beneficial in disrupting the inflammatory cycle.
- Activity modification, such limited standing and walking, particularly on uneven terrain, may also lessen symptoms.

SURGICAL MANAGEMENT

- We use the Stephens-Sanders classification system and treatment protocol for calcaneal malunions, which is based on CT evaluation.[17] Type I malunions include a large lateral wall exostosis, with or without far lateral subtalar arthrosis. Type II malunions include a lateral wall exostosis and subtalar arthrosis involving the entire width of the joint. Type III malunions include a lateral wall exostosis, subtalar arthrosis, and malalignment of the calcaneal body resulting in significant hindfoot varus or valgus angulation (**FIG 11**).

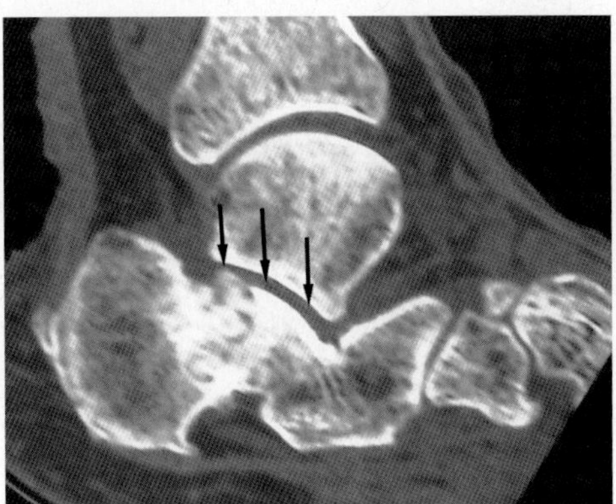

FIG 9 • Sagittal CT image demonstrating loss of calcaneal height (*black arrows*).

Preoperative Planning

- The calcaneal malunion is evaluated with plain radiographs and CT scan and classified according to the Stephens-Sanders classification.[17] Treatment is based strictly on malunion type:
  - Type I malunions are managed with a lateral wall exostectomy and a peroneal tenolysis.[2,5,12]
  - Type II malunions are managed with a lateral wall exostectomy, peroneal tenolysis, and a subtalar bone block arthrodesis, using the excised lateral wall as autograft.[10]
  - Type III malunions are managed with a lateral wall exostectomy, peroneal tenolysis, subtalar bone block arthrodesis, and a calcaneal osteotomy to correct hindfoot malalignment.[7]
- The procedure requires use of a radiolucent table and a standard C-arm.

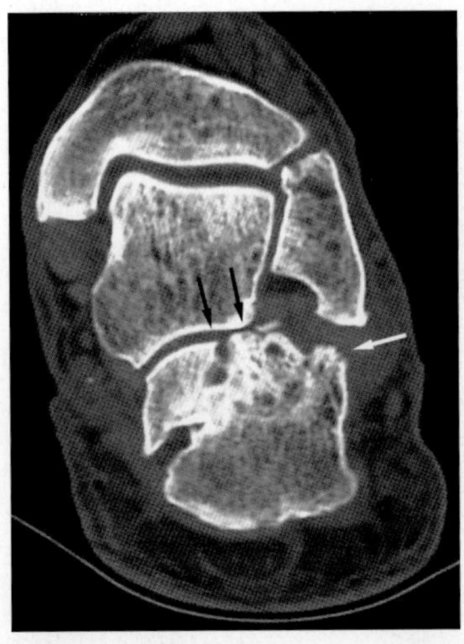

FIG 8 • Semicoronal CT image demonstrating subfibular impingement (*white arrow*) and posttraumatic arthritic changes in posterior facet (*black arrows*).

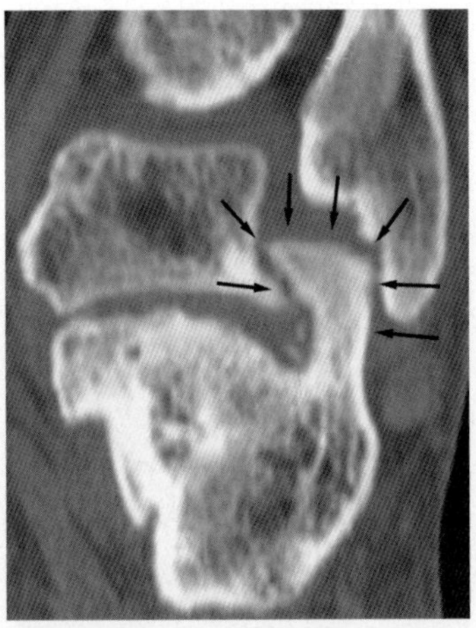

FIG 10 • Semicoronal CT image of calcaneal malunion from fracture-dislocation variant pattern (*black arrows*). This 25-year-old laborer had unfortunately been treated nonoperatively and rapidly developed posttraumatic arthritis.

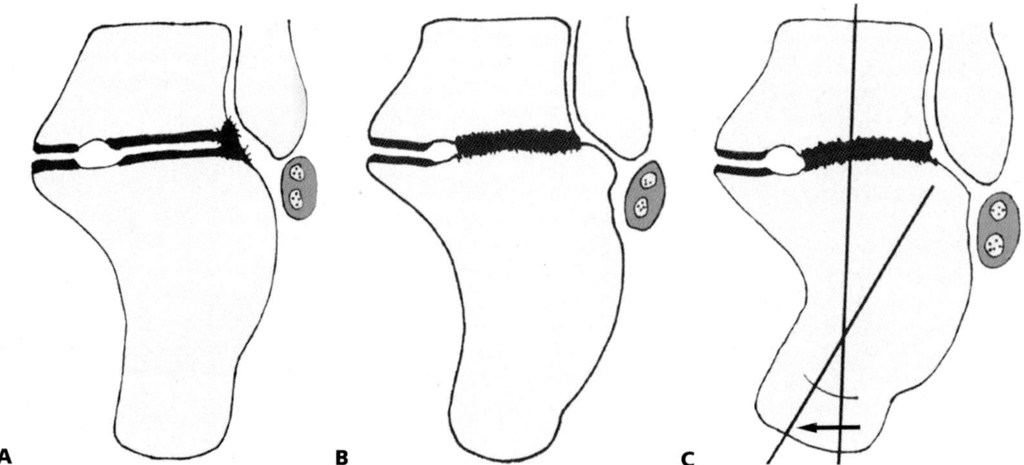

FIG 11 • Stephens-Sanders classification of calcaneal malunions. **A.** Type I malunion. **B.** Type II malunion. **C.** Type III malunion.

- A pneumatic thigh tourniquet is used. The procedure should be completed within 120 to 130 minutes of tourniquet time to minimize potential wound complications.

Positioning

- The patient is placed in the lateral decubitus position on a beanbag. The lower extremities are positioned in a scissor configuration such that the operative ("up") limb is flexed at the knee and angles toward the distal, posterior corner of the operating table, while the nonoperative ("down") limb is extended at the knee and lies away from the eventual surgical field. This facilitates intraoperative fluoroscopy without interference from the nonoperative limb. Padding is placed beneath the contralateral limb to protect the peroneal nerve, and an operating "platform" is created with blankets and foam padding to elevate the operative limb (**FIG 12**).
- Alternatively, the prone position may be used for bilateral procedures.

Approach

- We use the extensile lateral approach for surgical management of the calcaneal malunion, regardless of malunion type. The lateral calcaneal artery, typically a branch of the peroneal artery, supplies the majority of the full-thickness flap.[1] Thus, strict attention to detail with respect to placement of the incision and gentle handling of the soft tissues is of paramount importance.
- The planned extensile lateral approach is then outlined on the skin:
  - The incision begins about 2 cm proximal to the tip of the lateral malleolus, just lateral to the Achilles tendon and thus posterior to the sural nerve and the lateral calcaneal artery, and the vertical limb extends toward the plantar foot.
  - The horizontal limb is drawn along the junction of the skin of the lateral foot and heel pad; this skin demarcation can be identified by compressing the heel. We substitute a gentle curve where these two lines combine to form a right angle, primarily to avoid apical necrosis. The horizontal limb also includes a gentle anterior curve along the skin creases distally, ideally ending over the calcaneocuboid articulation (**FIG 13**).

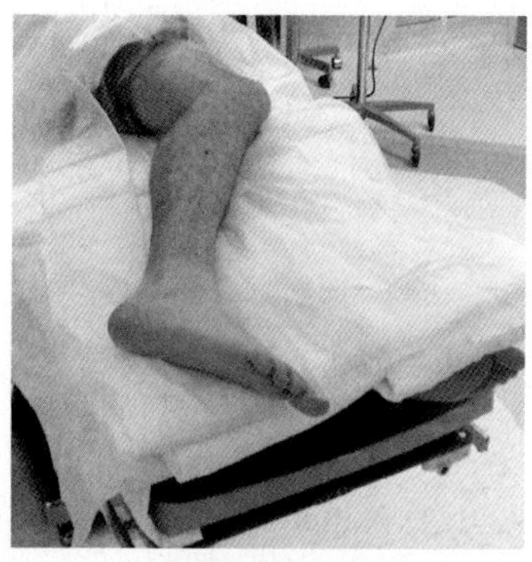

FIG 12 • Lateral decubitus position. Note scissor configuration of limbs to facilitate intraoperative fluoroscopy.

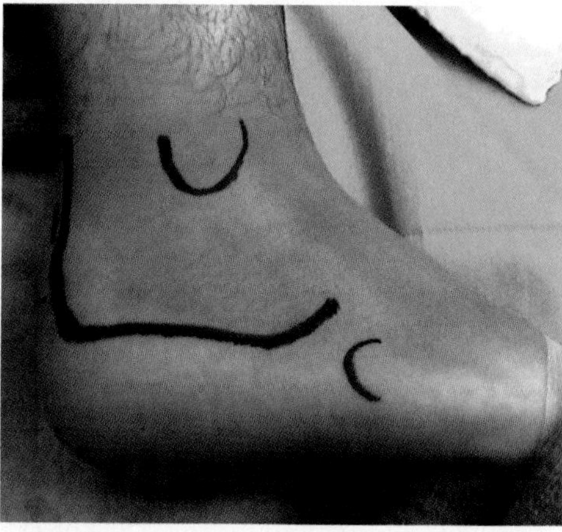

FIG 13 • Planned incision for extensile lateral approach.

EXTENSILE LATERAL APPROACH

- Place the limb on a sterile bolster and begin the incision at the proximal portion of the vertical limb. It becomes full thickness at the level of the calcaneal tuberosity—literally "straight to bone," while avoiding any beveling of the skin.[9] Again lessen scalpel pressure beyond the apical curve of the incision, and develop a layered incision along the horizontal limb of the incision.
- Raise a full-thickness, subperiosteal flap starting at the apex, specifically avoiding use of retractors until a considerable subperiosteal flap is developed, in order to prevent separation of the skin from the underlying subcutaneous tissue (**TECH FIG 1A**).
- Sharply release the calcaneofibular ligament from the lateral wall of the calcaneus, and release the adjacent peroneal tendons from the peroneal tubercle through the cartilaginous "pulley" to avoid iatrogenic injury (**TECH FIG 1B**).
- Use a periosteal elevator to gently mobilize the tendons along the distal portion of the incision, which then exposes the anterolateral calcaneus. Thus, the peroneal tendons and sural nerve are contained entirely within the flap, and devascularization of the lateral skin is minimized (**TECH FIG 1C**).
- Continue deep dissection to the sinus tarsi and anterior process region anteriorly, the calcaneocuboid joint distally, and the superior-most portion of the calcaneal tuberosity posteriorly.
- Place three 1.6-mm Kirschner wires for retraction of the subperiosteal flap: one into the fibula as the peroneal tendons are slightly subluxed anterior to the lateral malleolus; a second in the talar neck; and a third in the cuboid as the peroneal tendons are levered away from the anterolateral calcaneus with a periosteal elevator. Thus, each Kirschner wire retracts its respective portions of the peroneal tendons and full-thickness skin flap (**TECH FIG 1D**).

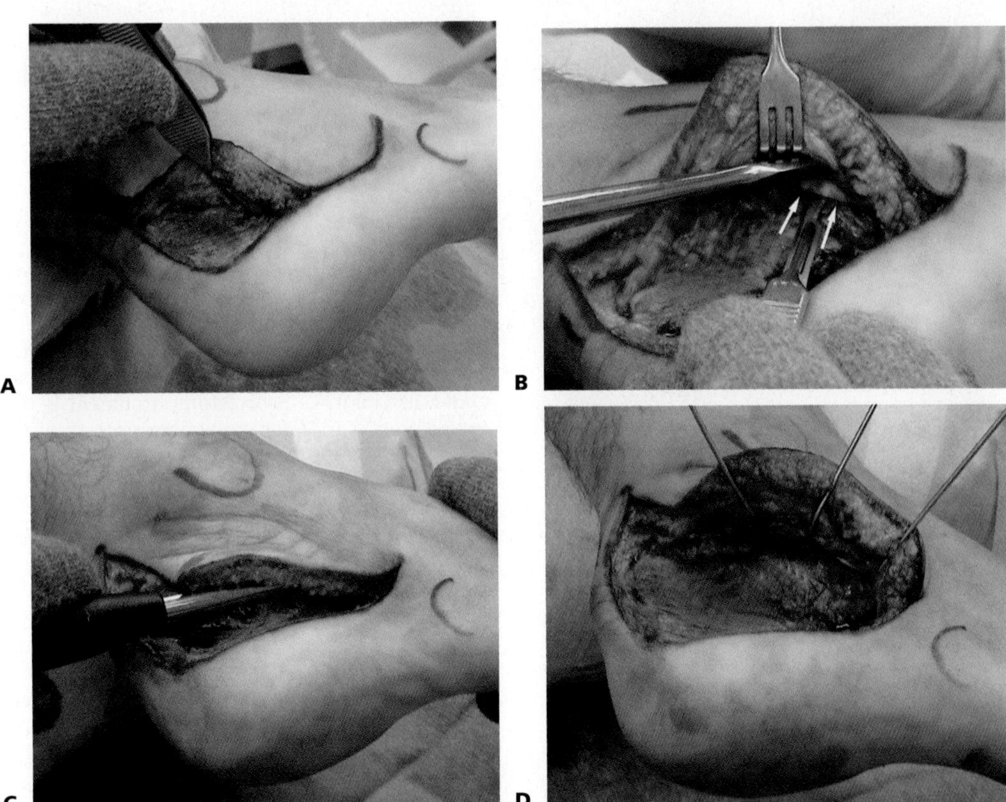

TECH FIG 1 • Extensile lateral approach. **A.** Note absence of retractors until a sizeable subperiosteal flap has been raised. **B.** Mobilization of peroneal tendons (*white arrows*). **C.** Gentle mobilization of flap along anterolateral wall of calcaneus. **D.** 1.6-mm Kirschner wire retractors.

LATERAL WALL EXOSTECTOMY

- A lateral wall exostectomy is completed for all three malunion types.
- Starting posteriorly, angle the A/O osteotomy saw blade slightly medially relative to the longitudinal axis of the calcaneus, preserving more bone plantarly and thereby providing decompression of the subfibular impingement (**TECH FIG 2A, B**).

- Take care throughout the exostectomy to avoid violation of the talofibular joint: place a small Bennett-type retractor at the level of the posterior facet (**TECH FIG 2B**).
- Continue the exostectomy to the level of the calcaneocuboid joint and complete it with an osteotome. Remove the fragment en bloc as a single fragment and preserve it in saline on the back table for later use as autograft (**TECH FIG 2C**).
- The width of the exostectomy fragment varies (about 10 to 15 mm) but is generally proportional to the extent of loss of calcaneal height and lateral wall expansion from the original injury, which reflects the amount of initial energy involved.

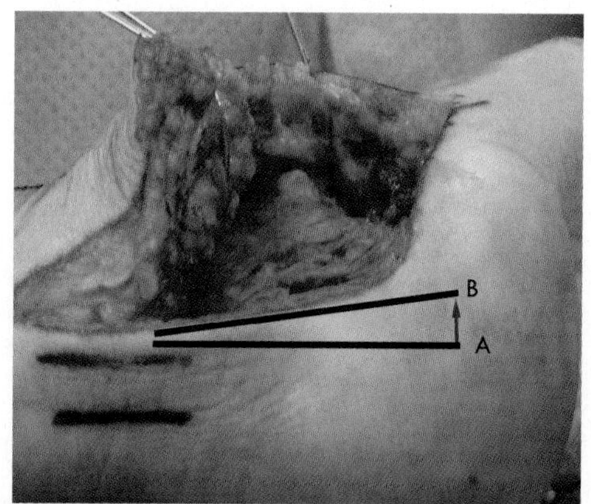

A

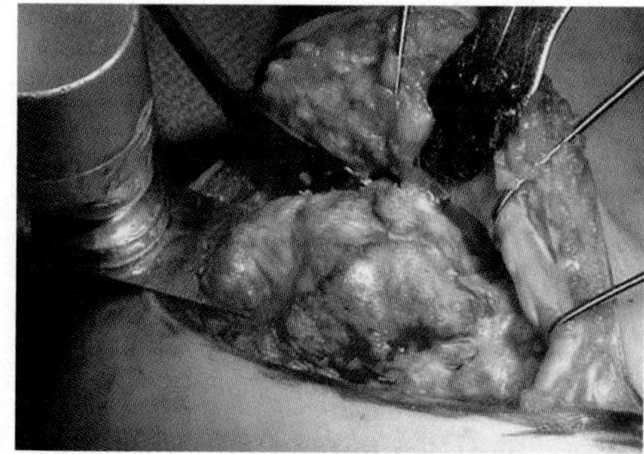

B

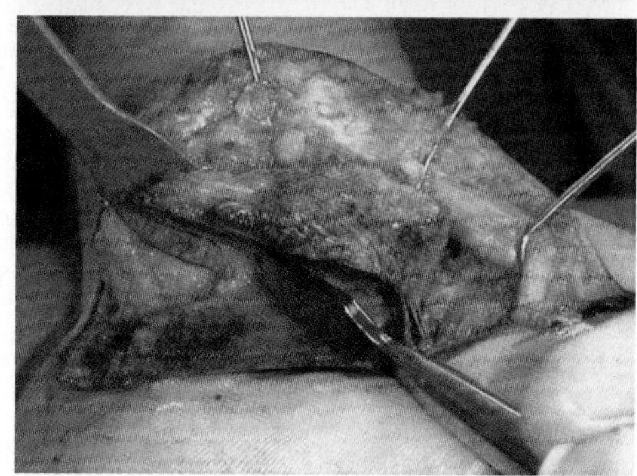

C

TECH FIG 2 • Lateral wall exostectomy. **A.** Intraoperative photo demonstrating vertical axis of limb (line A) and plane of lateral wall exostectomy (line B). **B.** Use of A/O osteotomy saw; note presence of small Bennett retractor protecting talofibular joint. **C.** Exostectomy fragment is removed en bloc for later use as autograft.

SUBTALAR BONE BLOCK ARTHRODESIS

- In patients with a type II or III malunion, gently mobilize the subtalar joint with a small osteotome, carefully identifying the plane of the posterior facet.
- Place a laminar spreader and meticulously débride the joint of any residual articular surface while preserving the underlying subchondral bone; we prefer to use a sharp periosteal elevator and pituitary rongeur.
- Irrigate the joint and make multiple perforations in the subchondral surface with a 2.5-mm drill bit to stimulate vascular ingrowth. Place highly concentrated platelet aspirate both within the joint and upon the previously resected lateral wall fragment.
- Place the lateral wall fragment within the subtalar joint as an autograft bone block; we prefer to place the laminar spreader posteriorly to facilitate bone block placement (**TECH FIG 3A**).
- Position the fragment such that the widest portion of the autograft is oriented posteromedially to avoid varus malalignment (**TECH FIG 3B**).
- Fill any remaining voids within the subtalar joint with supplemental allograft.
- With the subtalar joint held in neutral to slight valgus alignment, obtain definitive stabilization with two large (6.5 to 8.0 mm) partially threaded cannulated screws placed from posterior to anterior in diverging fashion: the more lateral screw is placed in the talar dome, while the more medial screw is placed in the talar neck.
- A third screw may be placed extending from the anterior process region into the talar neck and head, avoiding violation of the talonavicular articulation (**TECH FIG 4**).

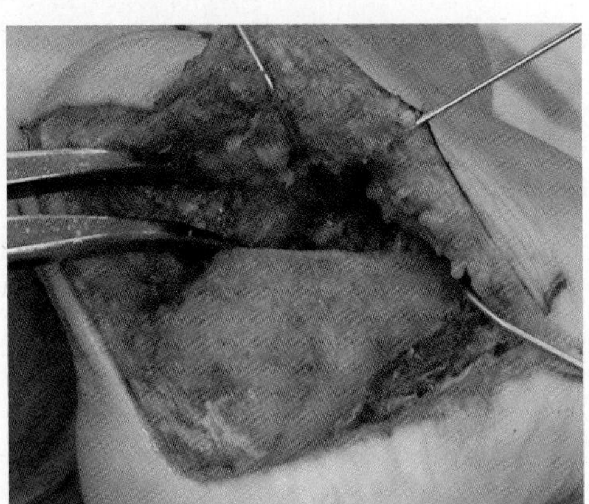

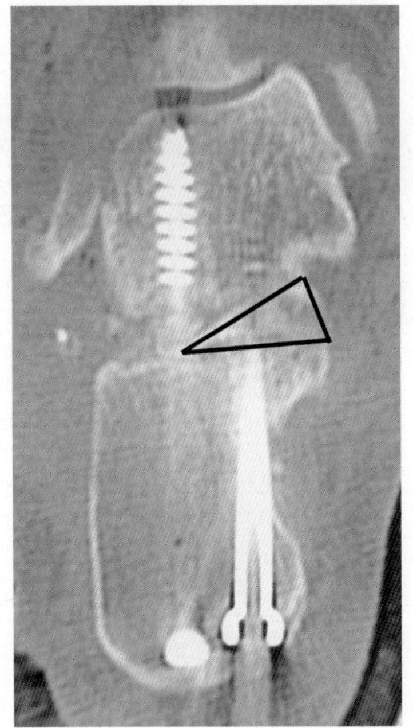

TECH FIG 3 • Placement of autograft bone block. **A.** Note position of laminar spreader within subtalar joint posteriorly. **B.** Postoperative semicoronal CT image demonstrating proper orientation of autograft bone block (*black triangle*), with widest portion placed posteromedially.

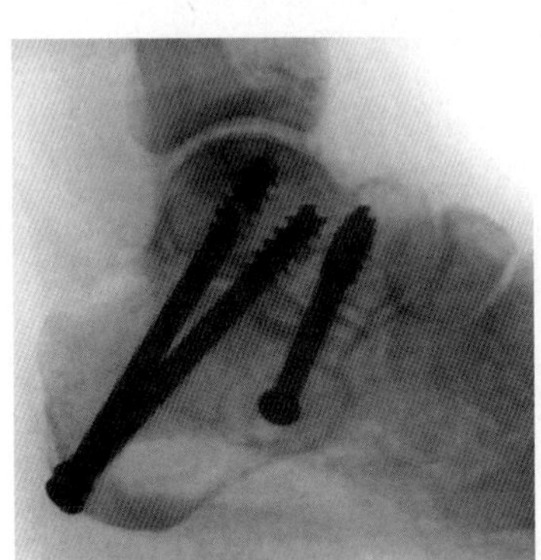

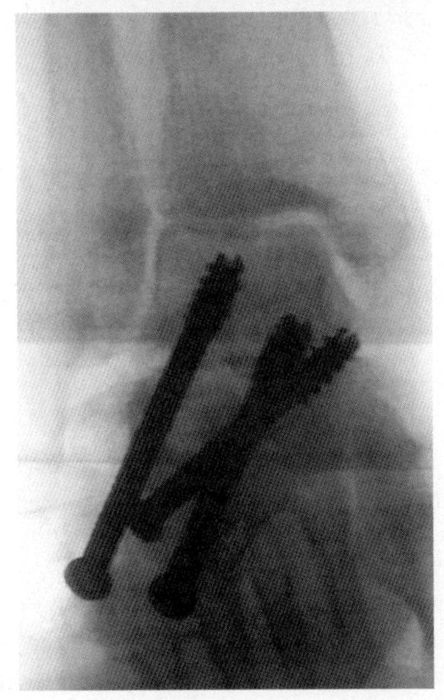

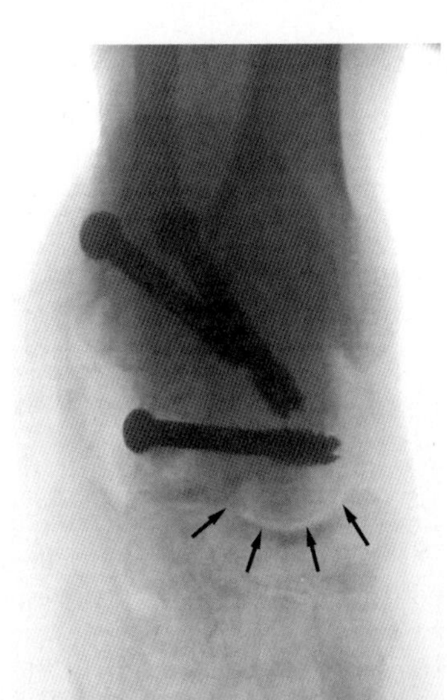

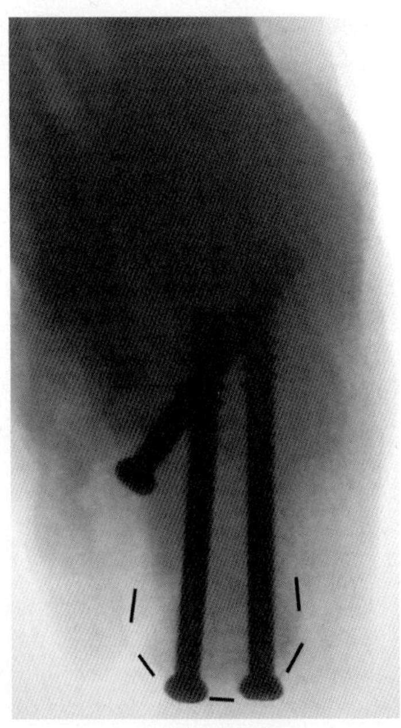

TECH FIG 4 • Definitive stabilization. **A.** Intraoperative fluoroscopic lateral view demonstrating diverging orientation of large cannulated screws posteriorly, and supplemental screw traversing middle facet. **B.** Intraoperative fluoroscopic mortise view; note slight medial angulation to avoid violation of talofibular joint. **C.** Intraoperative fluoroscopic anteroposterior view; note transverse orientation of anterior screw, avoiding violation of talonavicular joint (*black arrows*). **D.** Intraoperative fluoroscopic axial view; note neutral hindfoot alignment.

CALCANEAL OSTEOTOMY

- For patients with a type III malunion, angular malalignment in the calcaneal tuberosity is corrected before implant placement.
- A Dwyer-type closing wedge osteotomy is performed for those with varus malalignment (**TECH FIG 5**).
- A medial displacement calcaneal osteotomy is used for those with valgus malalignment (rare).
- Because the plane of the osteotomy is nearly parallel to the plane of the posterior facet, the osteotomy and subtalar joint are stabilized simultaneously as described above.

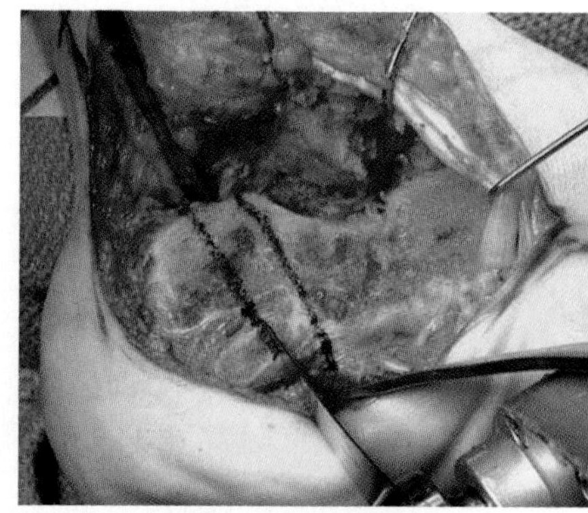

TECH FIG 5 • Calcaneal osteotomy. Dwyer closing wedge osteotomy for correction of varus malalignment in calcaneal tuberosity.

PERONEAL TENOLYSIS

- Remove the Kirschner wire retractors and incise the peroneal tendon sheath along the undersurface of the subperiosteal flap over a length of 2 to 3 cm. A peroneal tenolysis is then completed.
- Advance a Freer elevator within the tendon sheath to the level of the lateral malleolus proximally, thereby mobilizing the peroneal tendons.
- Assess the competence of the superior peroneal retinaculum (SPR) by gently levering the Freer elevator forward while observing the overlying skin. The presence of an endpoint indicates an intact retinaculum, but with an incompetent SPR the elevator will easily slide anterior to the lateral malleolus, with no demonstrable endpoint.
- Advance the Freer elevator within the tendon sheath distally to the cuboid tunnel.

SUPERIOR PERONEAL RETINACULUM REPAIR

- If the SPR is incompetent, make a separate 3-cm incision along the posterior border of the lateral malleolus, exposing the tendon sheath.
- With the peroneal tendons held reduced in the peroneal groove, use one or two suture anchors to secure the detached SPR to bone (**TECH FIG 6**).
- Reassess tendon stability using a Freer elevator in the same manner.

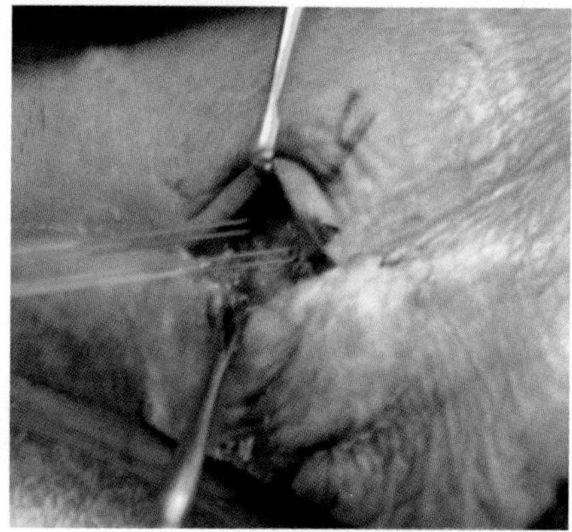

TECH FIG 6 • Superior peroneal retinaculum repair and suture imbrication of incompetent superior peroneal retinaculum.

CLOSURE

- Place a deep drain exiting proximally in line with the vertical limb of the incision.
- Place deep no. 0 absorbable sutures in interrupted, figure 8 fashion, beginning with the apex of the incision and progressing to the proximal and distal ends. The sutures are temporarily clamped until all sutures have been passed, then hand-tied sequentially, starting at the proximal and distal ends, and working toward the apex of the incision, so as to eliminate tension at the apex of the wound (**TECH FIG 7A**).
- Because of the lateral decompression from the exostectomy, the flap should close fairly easily with minimal tension (despite restoration of calcaneal height).
- Close the skin layer with 3-0 monofilament suture using the modified Allgöwer-Donati technique, again starting at the ends and working toward the apex (**TECH FIG 7B**).
- Deflate the tourniquet and place sterile dressings, followed by a bulky Jones dressing and Weber splint.

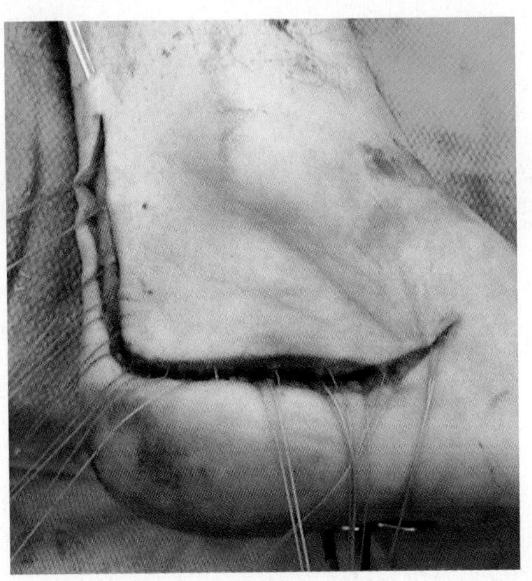

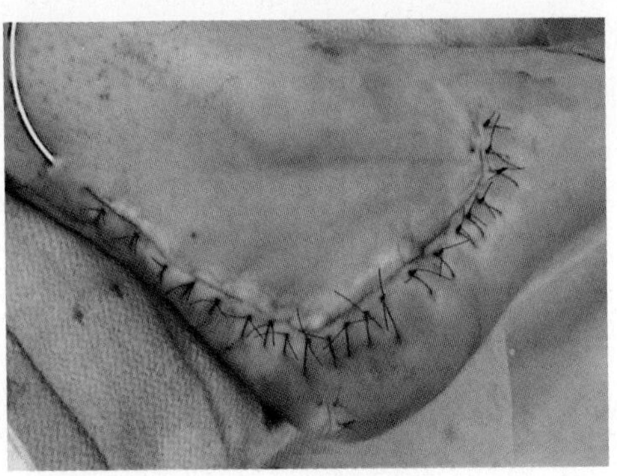

TECH FIG 7 • Flap closure. **A.** Deep absorbable sutures placed and temporarily clamped. **B.** Skin closure using modified Allgöwer-Donati technique.

PEARLS AND PITFALLS

Lateral wall exostectomy	■ Avoid violating the talofibular joint during lateral wall exostectomy. ■ Gently place a small Bennett-type retractor within the subtalar joint at the level of the posterior facet to protect the talofibular joint.
Placing autograft bone block	■ Use of an additional laminar spreader at the crucial angle of Gissane may facilitate graft placement. ■ Release of the deltoid ligament should be strictly avoided as this destabilizes the ankle joint. ■ The peripheral margin of the fragment may need to be shaped slightly to prevent overhang and prominence laterally.
Definitive stabilization	■ Avoid violating the talofibular joint by angling slightly medially during placement of guide pins (**FIG 14A**). ■ Fluoroscopic visualization of the ankle joint before screw placement is of paramount importance (**FIG 14B**).

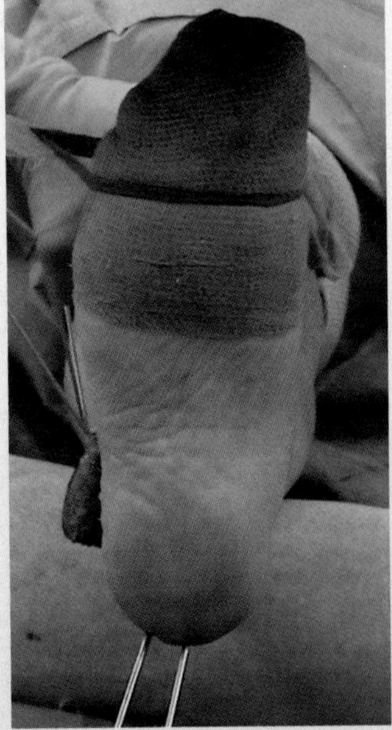

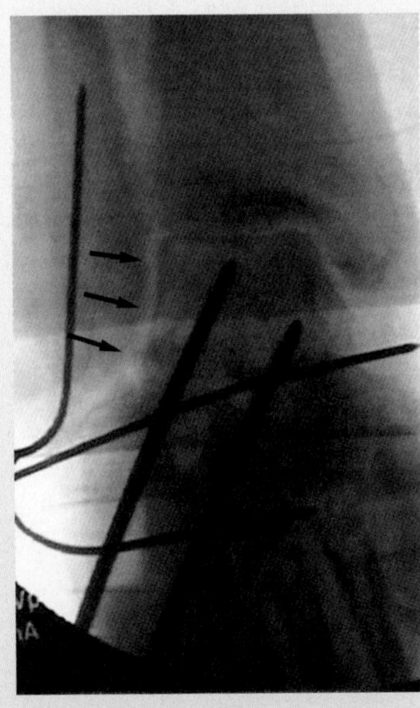

FIG 14 • Axial orientation of guide pins traversing posterior facet of subtalar joint. **A.** Intraoperative photo. **B.** Intraoperative fluoroscopic view. Note slight medial angulation to avoid violation of talofibular joint.

Fracture-dislocation variant patterns	▪ With fracture-dislocation variant patterns, the posterolateral fragment is typically wedged within the talofibular joint; this is often associated with secondary lateral ankle instability. ▪ Mobilize the subtalar joint before the lateral wall exostectomy and excise the prominent portion of the posterolateral fragment flush with the remaining posterior facet articular surface. ▪ At the conclusion of the procedure, the ankle joint should be stressed (varus force) under live fluoroscopy and lateral ligament reconstruction completed where necessary.

POSTOPERATIVE CARE

- For type I malunions, the patient is converted to a prefabricated fracture boot at 2 weeks postoperatively. Weight bearing and range-of-motion exercises are initiated once the incision has fully healed.
- For type II or type III malunions, the patient is converted to a short-leg non–weight-bearing cast at 2 to 3 weeks and again at 6 to 7 weeks postoperatively. Weight bearing is not permitted until 10 to 12 weeks postoperatively, at which point radiographic union is confirmed.
- The patient is then converted to a prefabricated fracture boot, and weight bearing is initiated. The patient is gradually transitioned to regular shoe wear and activity is advanced as tolerated thereafter.

OUTCOMES

- This is intended as a salvage procedure for pain relief and restoration of alignment.
- We recently reported our intermediate- to long-term results of this protocol[4]:
  - The initial arthrodesis union rate was 93%.
  - Ninety-three percent had neutral or slight valgus hindfoot alignment; 100% had plantigrade foot.
  - There was no statistical difference in outcome scores among the three malunion types.
  - Significantly greater restoration of talocalcaneal height was found among patients with type III malunions.

COMPLICATIONS

- Delayed wound healing, wound dehiscence, deep infection
- Arthrodesis delayed union or nonunion
- Postoperative ankle stiffness
- (Late) Lateral ankle ("sprain") pain from coronal plane stresses applied to ankle joint
- (Late) Compensatory ankle joint arthritis (theoretical)

REFERENCES

1. Borrelli J Jr, Lashgari C. Vascularity of the lateral calcaneal flap: a cadaveric injection study. J Orthop Trauma 1999;13:73–77.
2. Braly WG, Bishop JO, Tullos HS. Lateral decompression for malunited os calcis fractures. Foot Ankle 1985;6:90–96.
3. Carr JB, Hansen ST, Benirschke SK. Subtalar distraction bone block fusion for late complications of os calcis fractures. Foot Ankle 1988;9:81–86.
4. Clare MP, Lee WE III, Sanders RW. Intermediate to long-term results of a treatment protocol for calcaneal fracture malunions. J Bone Joint Surg Am 2005;87A:963–973.
5. Cotton FJ. Old os calcis fractures. Ann Surg 1921;74:294–303.
6. Crosby LA, Fitzgibbons T. Computerized tomography scanning of acute intra-articular fractures of the calcaneus. J Bone Joint Surg Am 1990;72A:852–859.
7. Dwyer FC. Osteotomy of the calcaneum for pes cavus. J Bone Joint Surg Br 1959;41B:80–86.
8. Gallie WE. Subastragalar arthrodesis in fractures of the os calcis. J Bone Joint Surg 1943;25:731–736.
9. Gould N. Lateral approach to the os calcis. Foot Ankle 1984;4:218–220.
10. Kalamchi A, Evans J. Posterior subtalar fusion. J Bone Joint Surg Br 1977;59B:287–289.
11. Kitaoka HB, Schaap EJ, Chao EY, et al. Displaced intra-articular fractures of the calcaneus treated non-operatively: clinical results and analysis of motion and ground-reaction and temporal forces. J Bone Joint Surg Am 1994;76A:1531–1540.
12. Magnuson PB. An operation for relief of disability in old fractures of the os calcis. JAMA 1923;80:1511–1513.
13. Myerson M, Quill GE. Late complications of fractures of the calcaneus. J Bone Joint Surg Am 1993;75A:331–341.
14. Radnay CS, Clare MP, Sanders RW. Subtalar fusion after displaced intra-articular calcaneal fractures: does initial operative treatment matter? J Bone Joint Surg Am 2009;91:541–546.
15. Sanders R, Fortin P, DiPasquale T, et al. Operative treatment in 120 displaced intraarticular calcaneal fractures: results using a prognostic computed tomography scan classification. Clin Orthop Relat Res 1993;290:87–95.
16. St C Isbister JF. Calcaneo-fibular abutment following crush fracture of the calcaneus. J Bone Joint Surg Br 1974;56B:274–278.
17. Stephens HM, Sanders R. Calcaneal malunions: results of a prognostic computed tomography classification system. Foot Ankle Int 1996;17:395–401.

Chapter 52

Calcaneal Osteotomy and Subtalar Arthrodesis for Calcaneal Malunions

Michael M. Romash

DEFINITION

- Malunited calcaneal fractures pose a complex reconstructive problem.
- The presenting symptoms are caused by posttraumatic subtalar and calcaneocuboid arthritis, fibulocalcaneal impingement that displaces the peroneal tendons, talotibial impingement due to the loss of normal talar inclination, and sural nerve entrapment.

ANATOMY

- As the calcaneus is exposed to axial loading, stress occurs obliquely across the tuberosity as the tuber is lateral to the axis of the tibia (**FIG 1**).
- Burdeaux[2] was unable to produce calcaneal fractures with the heel inverted and in the line of the tibia.
- The bone fails along this line. The tuberosity translates proximally, laterally, and anteriorly. The lateral posterior facet is driven plantarly into the calcaneus by the talus, causing a fracture at the angle of Gissane and either a tongue or joint depression pattern posteriorly. The lateral wall expands outward, further widening the heel (**FIG 2**).
- Calcaneal fractures have certain recurrent patterns.[7,8]
- There are four major fragments: the tuberosity, posterolateral facet, sustentaculum, and anterolateral fragments. The sustentacular fragment stays in anatomic position (**FIG 2**).

PATHOGENESIS

- When union occurs in this pathologic position, the lateral and proximal displacement of the tuberosity causes calcaneus–fibular impingement and displacement of the peroneal tendons.
- The disruption of the posterior facet causes posttraumatic subtalar arthritis.
- The loss of height of the heel results in the loss of the talar inclination angle and tibial talar impingement.
- Plantar subluxation of the navicular at the talonavicular joint may also occur (**FIG 3**).

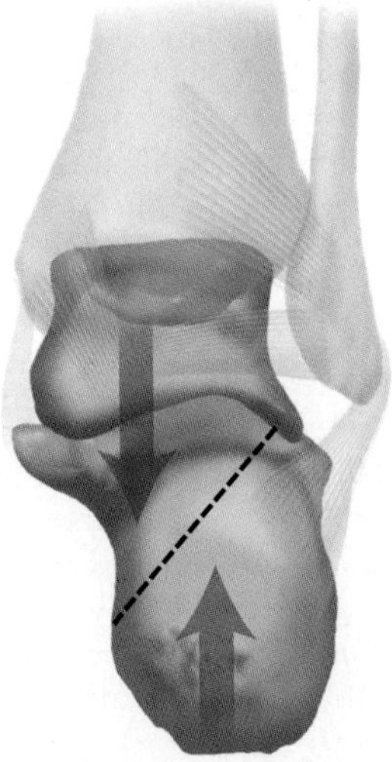

FIG 1 • Offset forces cause internal stress, which results in primary oblique fracture. (From Kitaoka H. Master Techniques of Orthopedic Surgery series: Foot and Ankle, 2nd ed. Philadelphia: Lippincott Williams & Wilkins, 2002, with permission.)

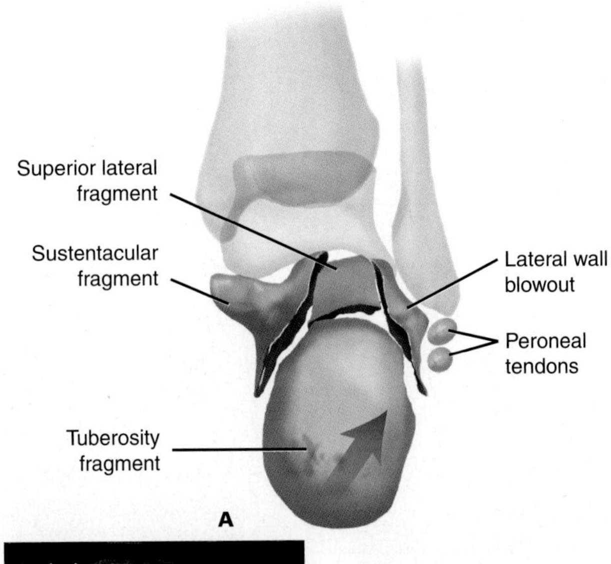

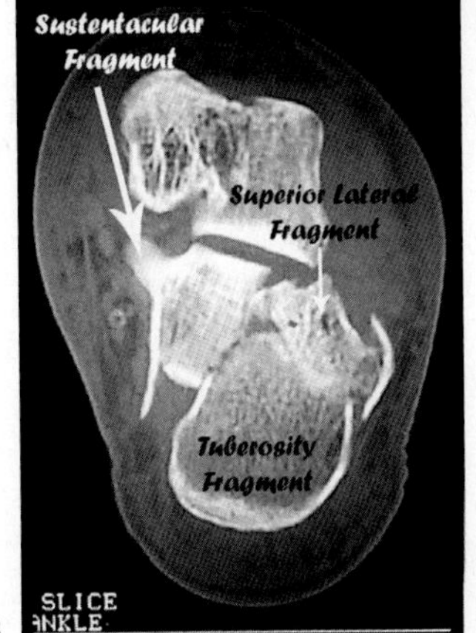

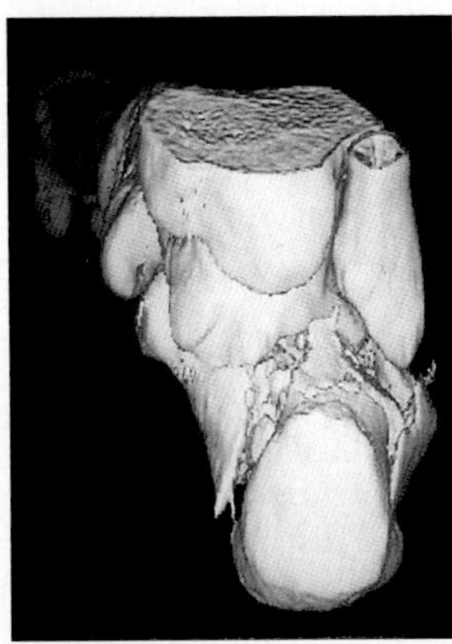

FIG 2 • **A.** Diagram of fracture demonstrating primary oblique fracture, lateral, and proximal displacement of tuberosity, impaction of posterior lateral facet, and expansion of lateral wall. **B.** CT scan of acute calcaneal fracture demonstrating the fracture and displacement. **C.** Three-dimensional volumetric reconstruction of acute fracture demonstrating the displacements. (From Kitaoka H. Master Techniques of Orthopedic Surgery series: Foot and Ankle, 2nd ed. Philadelphia: Lippincott Williams & Wilkins, 2002, with permission.)

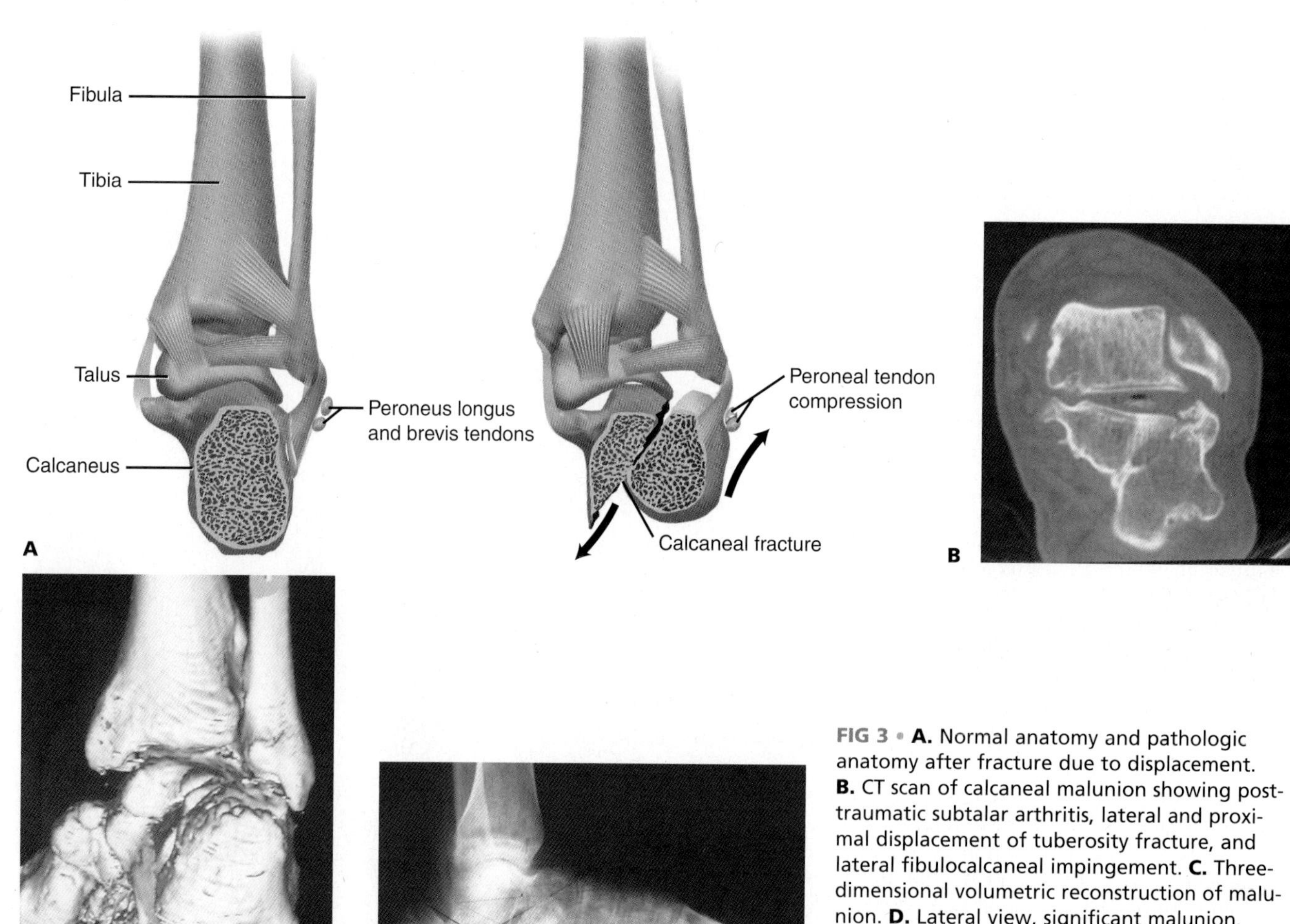

FIG 3 • **A.** Normal anatomy and pathologic anatomy after fracture due to displacement. **B.** CT scan of calcaneal malunion showing posttraumatic subtalar arthritis, lateral and proximal displacement of tuberosity fracture, and lateral fibulocalcaneal impingement. **C.** Three-dimensional volumetric reconstruction of malunion. **D.** Lateral view, significant malunion, reverse angle of Bohler, tibial calcaneal impingement. (**B** and **C** from Kitaoka H. Master Techniques of Orthopedic Surgery series: Foot and Ankle, 2nd ed. Philadelphia: Lippincott Williams & Wilkins, 2002, with permission.)

NATURAL HISTORY

- The anatomic disruption, posttraumatic arthritis, and impingement cause increasing pain with activity.
- The stiff malpositioned hindfoot will lead to arthritic changes at the talonavicular joint.
- Tibial talar impingement and loss of ankle dorsiflexion puts more stress on the transverse tarsal articulation, causing secondary arthritis there.
- The displacement of the peroneal tendons and peroneal impingement will eventually cause tendinosis or tear.

PATIENT HISTORY AND PHYSICAL FINDINGS

- There will be a history of a calcaneal fracture, which may have been treated by nonoperative or operative means. Not all patients will know that they have had a heel fracture.
- Symptoms include pain at the fibulocalcaneal junction and sinus tarsi. Hypoesthesia or dysesthesia in the sphere of the sural nerve may be present.
- Physical findings are the loss of the usual step-off or indentation just distal to the tip of the fibula, loss of subtalar motion, and some loss of dorsiflexion of the ankle.
- The examiner should look for hypoesthesia in the sphere of the sural nerve with a positive percussion or Tinel test.
- Methods for examining malunited calcaneal fractures include:
  - Examining for loss of "fibular sulcus." The physician should palpate the area just distal to the tip of the fibula of both ankles. With a calcaneal malunion, there will be no sulcus for the peroneal tendons. This is indicative of the lateral displacement of the tuberosity fragment and "blow out" of the lateral wall, causing fibulocalcaneal impingement.
  - Evaluating for hindfoot stiffness. The physician should examine the range of motion of the hindfoot, checking inversion and eversion. A malunion will have little if any motion, which may be painful. The stiffness is indicative of subtalar arthritis and scarring of the subtalar joint.

IMAGING AND OTHER DIAGNOSTIC STUDIES

- Radiographs show loss of the angle of Bohler, loss of talar inclination, and widening of the heel.
  - The primary fracture line is often identifiable on axial heel views and Broden views.

- CT scans show all of the above and give information about the internal architecture of the heel, confirming the deformity, impingements, and arthritis.

DIFFERENTIAL DIAGNOSIS

- Posttraumatic subtalar arthritis without deformity
- Peroneal tendon tear
- Sural neuritis
- Tarsal coalition

NONOPERATIVE MANAGEMENT

- Judicious use of nonsteroidal anti-inflammatories (NSAIDs) will diminish some of the symptoms, as will sparing use of steroid injections into the sinus tarsi.
- Bracing the foot and ankle as well as the use of heel cups or heel lifts may provide some relief.

SURGICAL MANAGEMENT

- This technique is capable of correcting height losses of up to 1.5 cm. Greater height loss will require augmentation with an interpositional bone block.
- The correction-limiting factor is the amount of bone available for transverse fixation as the fragments slide relative to each other. Moving the fixation anteriorly will give windows for fixation as less translation occurs in this portion of the calcaneus.
- Indications include malunited calcaneal fractures that exhibit the signs and symptoms of fibulocalcaneoperoneal impingement, posttraumatic subtalar arthritis, loss of the angle of Bohler (and talar inclination), widening of the heel, and tibial talar impingement. Not all of these need to be present.
- Joint depression fractures are better suited for correction by this procedure than tongue-type fractures.
- If painful arthritis is present at the calcaneocuboid joint, arthrodesis of this joint may be added to the procedure.
- Smoking, diabetes, and vascular impairment must be evaluated in each patient and certainly can be contraindications to the procedure.

Preoperative Planning

- Quality radiographs are essential.
- Radiographs include weight-bearing AP, lateral, axial heel, and Broden views of the affected foot.
- A weight-bearing lateral view of the unaffected foot will provide normal parameters for the patient and allow measurement of the deformity and the amount of correction desired.
- The AP view will show the calcaneocuboid joint, which may be involved.
- The lateral view will demonstrate the loss of height and loss of talar inclination and will demonstrate tibial talar impingement.
- The axial heel film will show the oblique primary fracture line and shift of the tuberosity.
- Broden views will show the subtalar joint and demonstrate fibular calcaneal impingement.
- A CT scan of the foot with axial, semicoronal, sagittal, and three-dimensional volumetric reconstructions is suggested.
- This study will confirm what is suggested by the plain films and provide a "blueprint" of the internal architecture of the calcaneus (**FIG 4**).

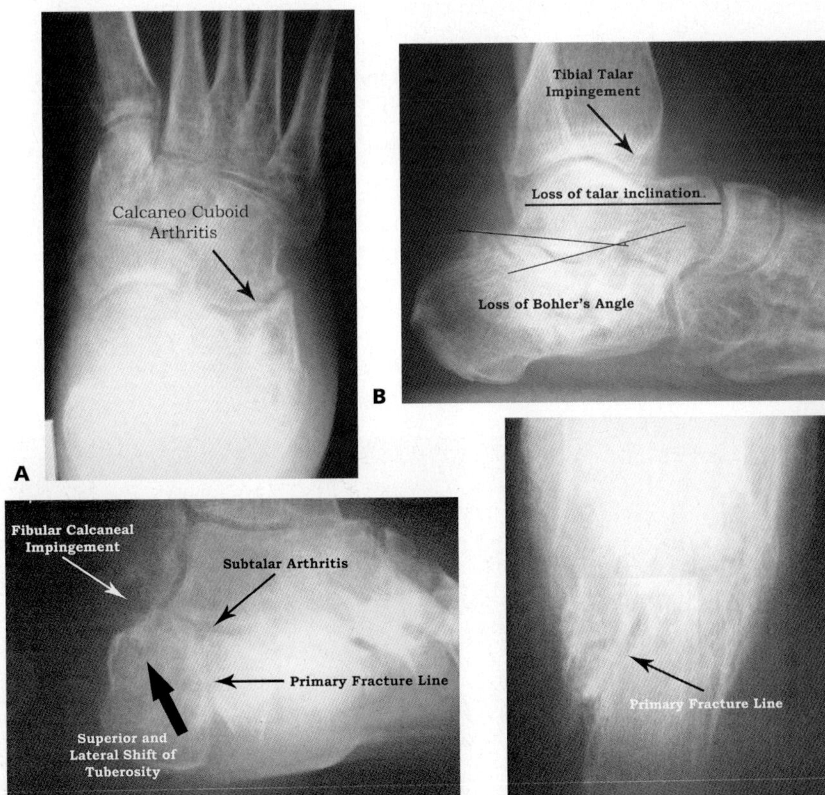

FIG 4 • **A.** AP radiograph of foot with calcaneal malunion affecting the calcaneocuboid joint. **B.** Lateral view of calcaneal malunion showing loss of angle of Bohler, loss of talar inclination, and anterior tibial talar impingement. **C.** Broden view of calcaneal malunion showing tuberosity translation, lateral impingement, and subtalar arthritis. **D.** Axial heel view of calcaneal malunion showing oblique primary fracture line, displacement of the tuberosity, and lateral impingement.

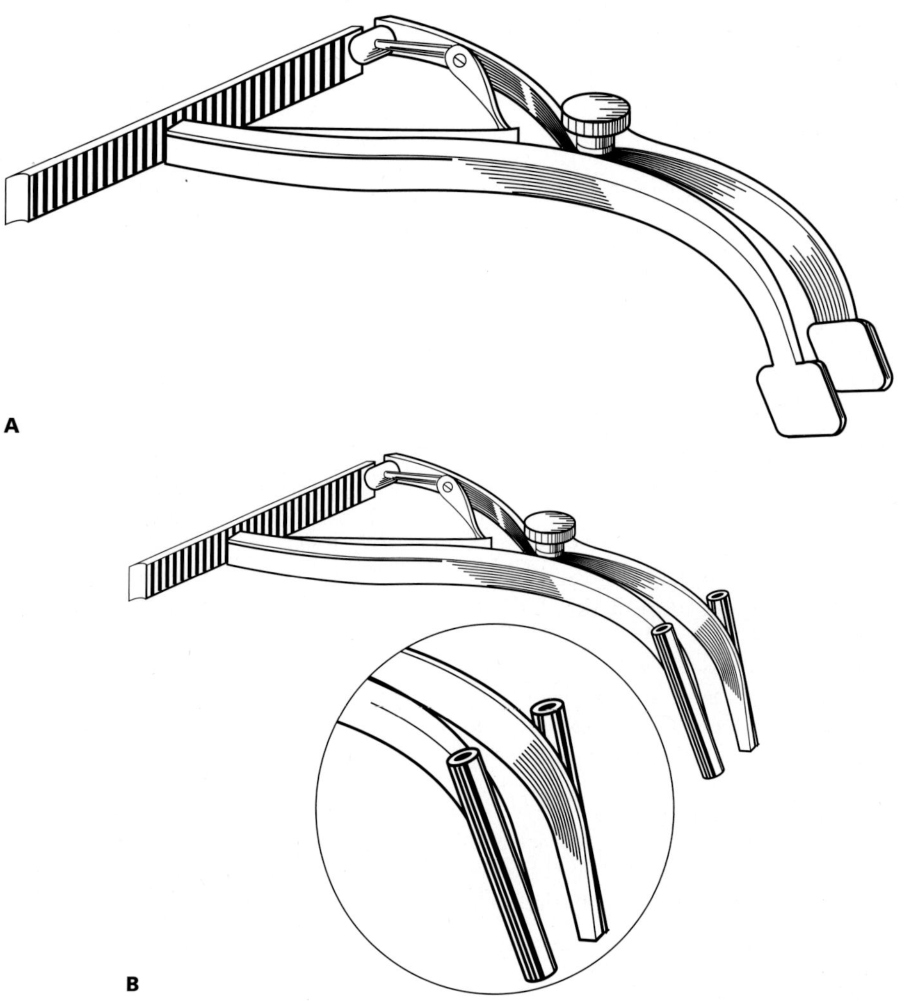

FIG 5 • **A.** Calcaneal spreaders. **B.** Steinmann pin calcaneal spreaders.

- Special instruments for the procedure are required:
  - 7.0-mm cannulated screws (we tend to use fully threaded screws)
  - Anterior cruciate ligament drill guide to assist in placement of the guidewire for the 7.0-mm cannulated screws
  - Baby Inge lamina spreaders, with and without serrations
  - "Calcaneal spreaders"—wide, flat-faced, and Steinmann pin fixation spreaders (**FIG 5**)
  - Smaller screws; 3.5-, 4.0-, or 4.5-mm cannulated screws for transverse fixation
  - A "power" osteotome is helpful.

Positioning

- The patient is positioned in lateral decubitus with the affected limb up. A tourniquet is applied to the thigh. The entire leg as well as the iliac crest is prepared and draped.

Approach

- A straight incision is made from just below the tip of the fibula, directed anteriorly in the line of the fourth–fifth ray interval past the calcaneocuboid joint. (Slight posterior elongation of the incision may be needed.)
- The area at the tip of the fibula is often congested due to the impingement, and the peroneal tendons will be displaced (**FIG 6**).

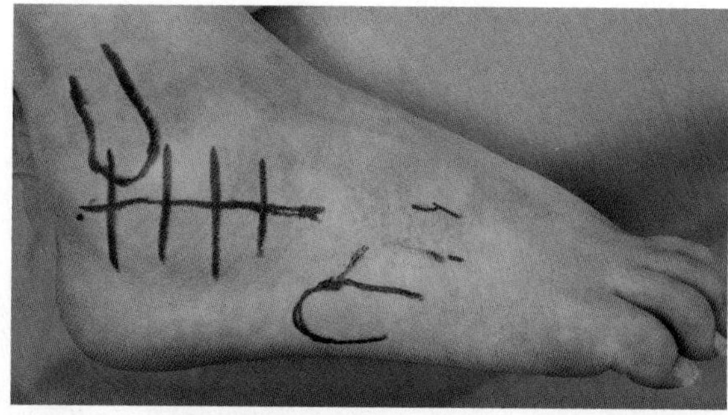

FIG 6 • Incision.

OBLIQUE CALCANEAL OSTEOTOMY WITH SUBTALAR ARTHRODESIS

- Enter the subtalar joint and mobilize it.
- Place a baby Inge lamina spreader in the sinus tarsi to distract the joint. Incise the scar and capsule including the fibulocalcaneal ligament laterally.
- Incise the posterior capsule and clear tissue from the posterior calcaneus up to the flexor hallucis longus tendon, which can be observed through the joint.
  - Do not incise the interosseous ligaments if possible, as these will help stabilize the sustentacular fragment to the talus (**TECH FIGS 1, 2**).
- The fracture line can usually be observed on the surface of the posterior facet of the calcaneus. Mark this line (**TECH FIG 3**).
- Decorticate the undersurface of the talus and the posterior facet of the calcaneus. Make sure that the fracture line is preserved or marked again.
- Under fluoroscopic control, drill a Steinmann pin from superior anterior lateral to inferior posterior medial in the plane of the primary fracture.
- Visualize this on the axial heel view, which may be obtained by having the C-arm in a horizontal plane or by externally rotating the leg to verify the pin placement (**TECH FIG 4**).
- I perform an osteotomy in the plane of the primary fracture, using the Steinmann pin as a guide. A saw is used to start the osteotomy, which may then be finished with osteotomes. This osteotomy exits the medial wall of the calcaneus posterior and inferior to the neurovascular bundle (**TECH FIG 5**).
- The most difficult part of the procedure then follows. This is shifting the tuberosity medially, plantarly, and slightly posterior.
- I first distract the fragments from each other by placing the calcaneal spreader, then lamina spreaders between the fragments to relax any soft tissue attachments.
  - The tuberosity may then be moved as far as possible easily, then "walked" further using small (quarter-inch to half-inch) curved osteotomes to lever the tuberosity down and the medial side up (**TECH FIG 6**).
- Steinmann pins may be inserted transversely into the medial fragment at the superior surface of the lateral fragment to act as "dead men" (carpentry term) to prevent loss of correction. On occasion a large Steinmann pin is

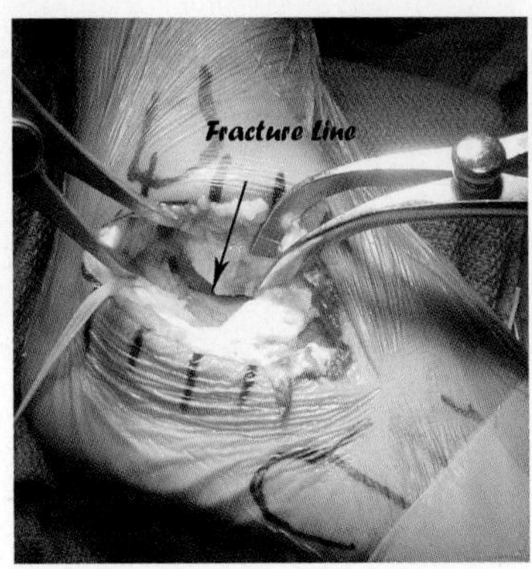

TECH FIG 2 • Subtalar joint opened; fracture can be observed.

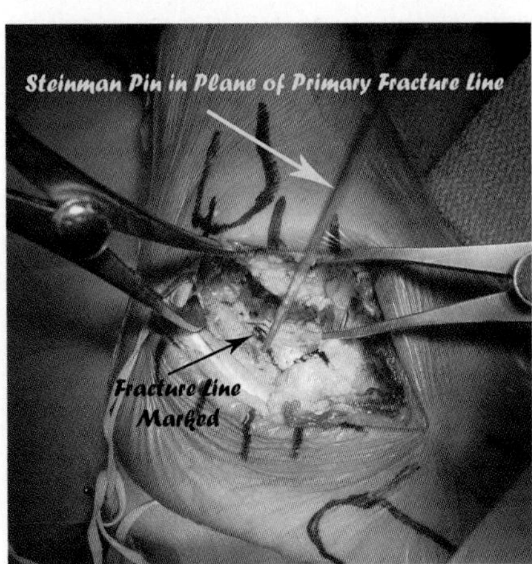

TECH FIG 3 • Fracture marked and Steinmann pin placed in plane of fracture.

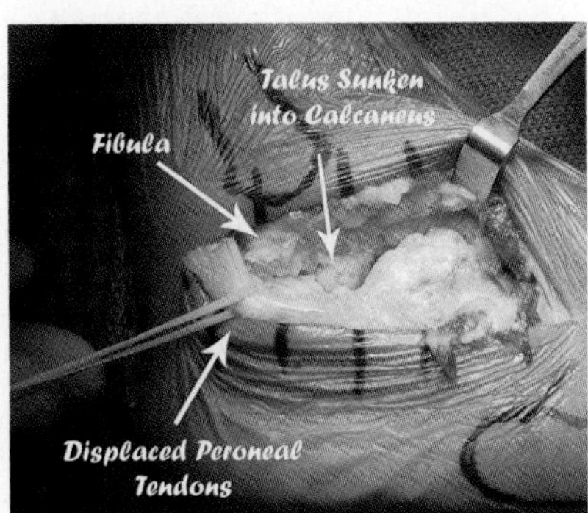

TECH FIG 1 • Peroneal tendons retracted, sinus tarsi and calcaneus exposed.

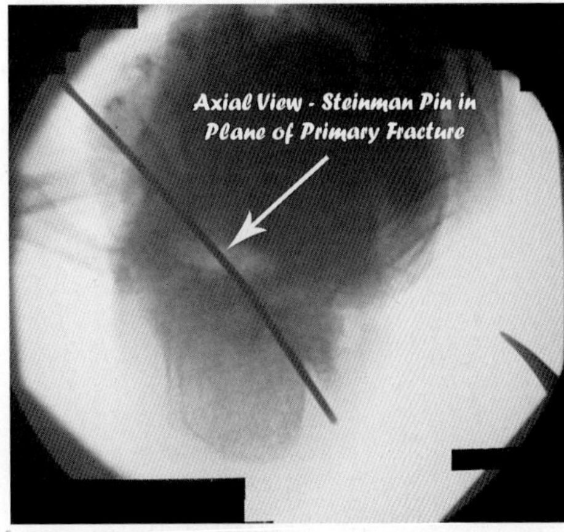

TECH FIG 4 • Intraoperative radiograph confirming Steinmann pin placement.

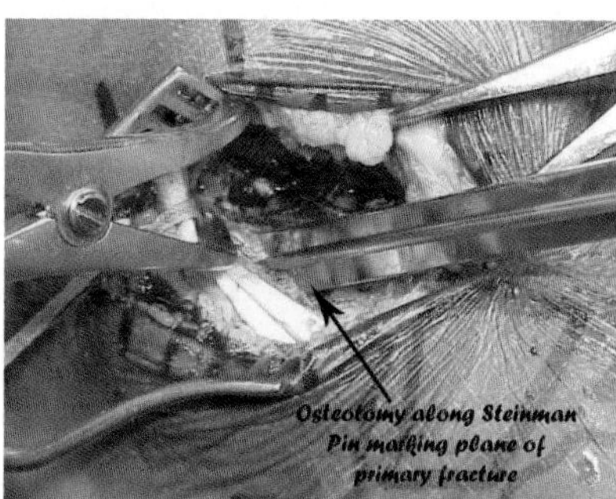

TECH FIG 5 • Osteotome being guided by Steinmann pin finishing osteotomy.

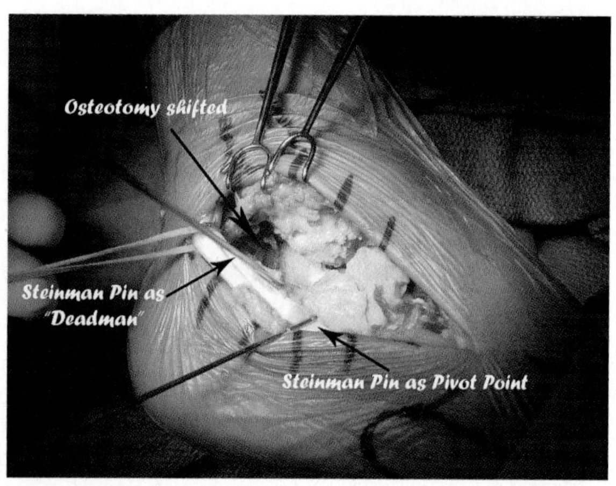

TECH FIG 7 • Steinmann pin in anterior calcaneus perpendicular to plane of osteotomy to act as pivot (this is optional), osteotomy displaced and held by Steinmann pin "dead man."

placed temporarily through the talus into the medial calcaneus to stabilize this fragment while the lateral tuberosity is being moved (TECH FIG 7).

- It is also helpful to plantarflex the ankle to relax the triceps surae, thus facilitating the plantar shift.
  - A smooth Steinmann pin may be placed across the anterior osteotomy to act as a pivot point to obtain more of a rotational correction (TECH FIG 7).
- I have had success with a Steinmann pin anchored calcaneal spreader placed from posteriorly, with one pin in the medial fragment and the second pin in the tuberosity.
  - Opening this spreader aids the shift, and twisting the instrument helps oppose the fragments (TECH FIG 8).
- Once the correction has been obtained, fixation from lateral to medial is obtained using the smaller cannulated screws in compression (TECH FIGS 9, 10).
- Use the anterior cruciate ligament drill guide to place a guide pin for the 7.0-mm cannulated screw. The entry point is the posterolateral tip of the tuberosity and the exit is through the medial aspect of the posterior facet, thus engaging fragments on both sides of the osteotomy (TECH FIGS 11, 12). Use the motion of the hindfoot complex to place the hindfoot in a neutral position. At this point in the procedure, the subtalar joint, talonavicular joint, and calcaneocuboid joint are mobile and height has been corrected. It is now possible to invert and evert the foot using the normal axis of motion of the hindfoot complex to a neutral position. (This is a crucial point of the procedure and differentiates it from interpositional bone block procedures where hindfoot position is dependent on the size and placement of the structural grafts.) Oppose the medial aspect of the subtalar joint to the talus and drive the guide pin into the talus. Stabilize the construct by a 7.0-mm screw in mild compression. Place a second screw if desired (TECH FIG 13).
- Check the ankle's range of motion. If a triceps surae contracture limits ankle dorsiflexion, remedy it by a percutaneous Achilles tendon lengthening.
- Harvest bone graft from the iliac crest. This may be cancellous or a corticocancellous block. Fit this graft into the empty space under the talus created by the displacement of the tuberosity with the depressed portion of the lateral posterior facet. Position this graft only to the lateral border of the talus. If a corticocancellous block is chosen, impact it into the space after properly shaping it. I have usually used cancellous bone. Allograft bone may also be used (TECH FIG 14). If a calcaneocuboid arthrodesis is needed, it is done now.
- Place a small drain if needed, and close the wounds in layers. Apply a well-padded short-leg cast. I place an AV impulse pump bladder under the cast. The cast is bivalved within 24 hours.

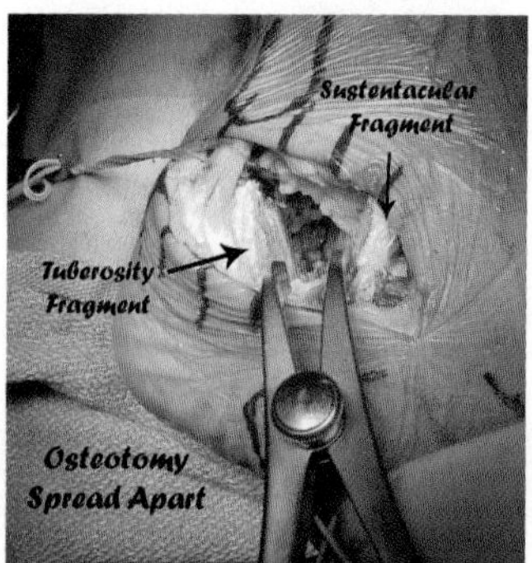

TECH FIG 6 • Osteotomy distracted by lamina spreaders.

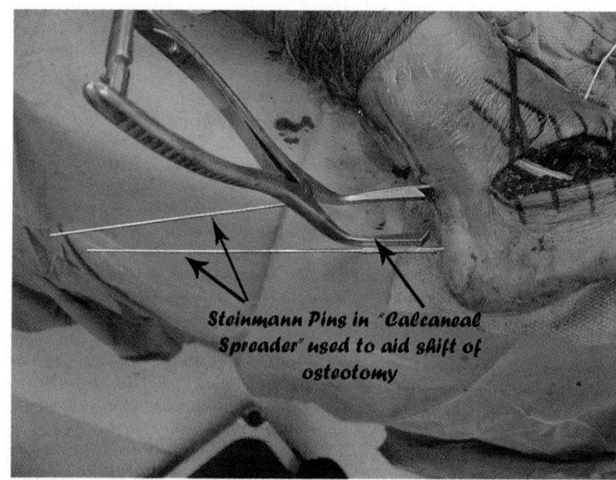

TECH FIG 8 • Calcaneal distractor applied to help displace and control osteotomy fragments.

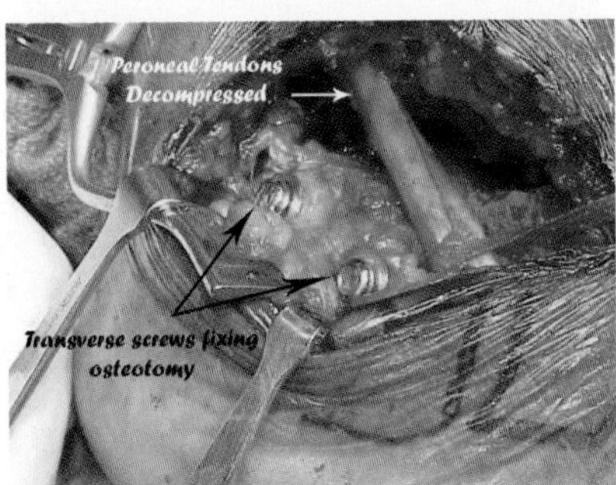

TECH FIG 9 • Transverse fixation with two cannulated compression screws.

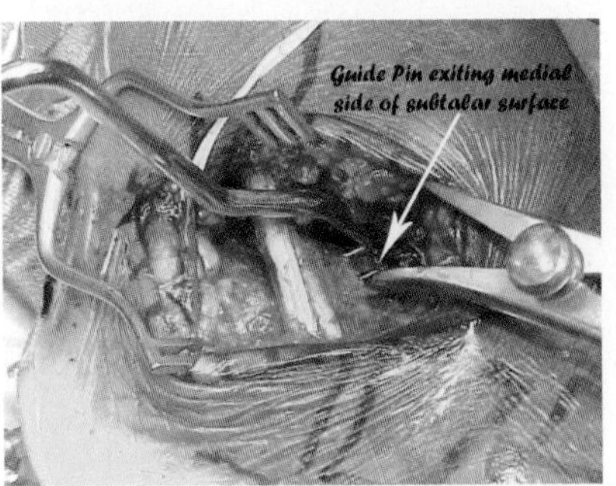

TECH FIG 12 • Tip of guidewire visible exiting sustentacular fragment. (From Kitaoka H. Master Techniques of Orthopedic Surgery series: Foot and Ankle, 2nd ed. Philadelphia: Lippincott Williams & Wilkins, 2002, with permission.)

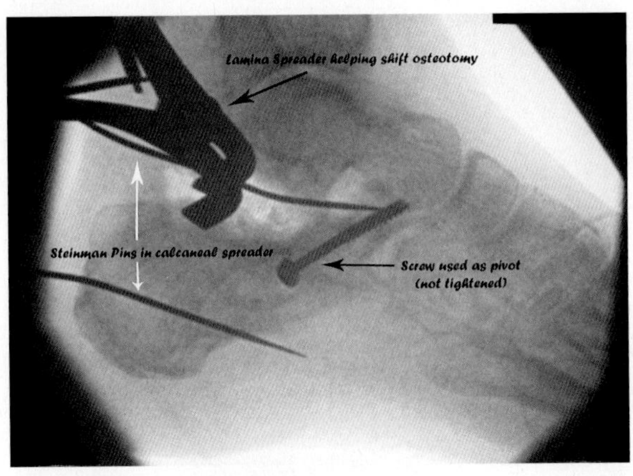

TECH FIG 10 • Intraoperative radiograph, transverse screw placed, distractor in place.

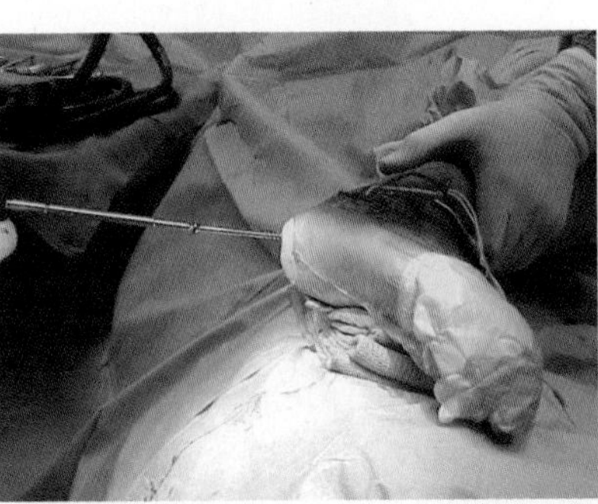

TECH FIG 13 • 7.0-mm screw being inserted. (From Kitaoka H. Master Techniques of Orthopedic Surgery series: Foot and Ankle, 2nd ed. Philadelphia: Lippincott Williams & Wilkins, 2002, with permission.)

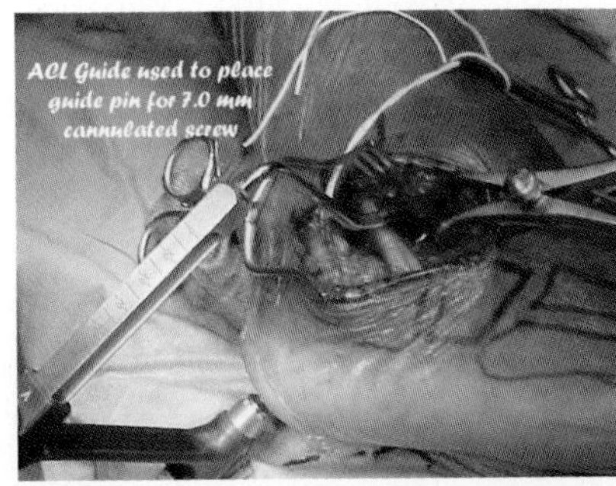

TECH FIG 11 • Anterior cruciate ligament drill guide used to place guidewire for 7.0-mm screw through tuberosity and sustentaculum.

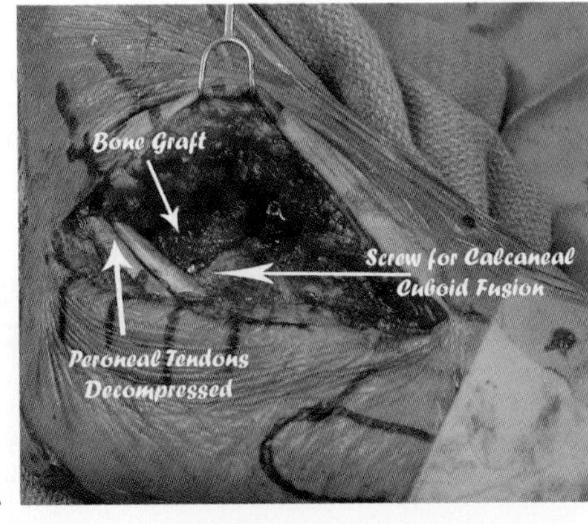

TECH FIG 14 • **A.** Final construct with bone graft in place. *(continued)*

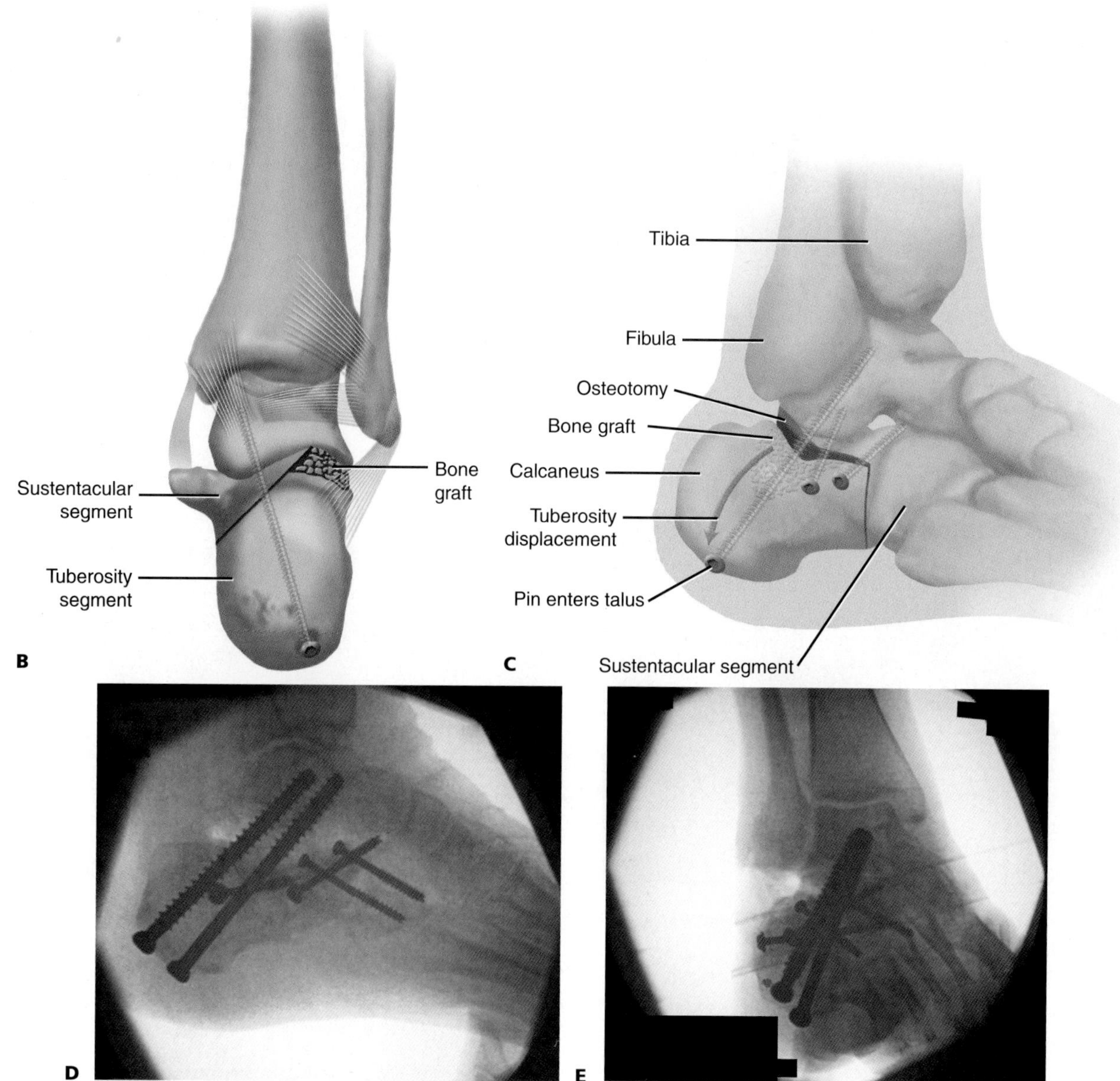

TECH FIG 14 • *(continued)* **B.** Diagram of final construct, axial view. **C.** Diagram of final construct, oblique view. **D.** Radiograph, lateral view, final construct (note calcaneocuboid joint arthrodesed in this case). **E.** Radiograph, Broden view, final construct. (From Kitaoka H. Master Techniques of Orthopedic Surgery series: Foot and Ankle, 2nd ed. Philadelphia: Lippincott Williams & Wilkins, 2002, with permission.)

EXTRA-ARTICULAR OBLIQUE OSTEOTOMY

- Hansen has described an extra-articular oblique osteotomy combined with subtalar arthrodesis. This is done in a similar fashion. The osteotomy does not follow the primary fracture line, but parallels it outside the joint. The obliquity of the osteotomy may be varied.

VERTICALLY ORIENTED OSTEOTOMY

- A vertically oriented osteotomy displaced directly plantarly has also been described. This increases the height of the heel and is aimed at correcting the talar inclination. This osteotomy may be shifted medially as well.

PEARLS AND PITFALLS

Mobilization and shift of the tuberosity	■ Ensure that the lateral ligaments and scar about the subtalar joint are released. Also make sure that the posterior capsule and scar are released. ■ Separate the osteotomy side to side with lamina spreaders to stretch the soft tissue preliminary to the plantar shift.

POSTOPERATIVE CARE

■ The drains are removed on the first postoperative day. The cast and bandages are changed on the third postoperative day. The patient is non–weight-bearing in a short-leg cast for 8 to 12 weeks until union is demonstrated.

■ The patient then progresses to weight bearing as tolerated. A removable fracture boot may be used.

■ Physical therapy is prescribed to gain ankle range of motion and calf strengthening.

OUTCOMES

■ The first cases were reported in 1993. We have continued to perform this procedure over the intervening years; about 45 procedures have been performed. The results have been reproducible. A 1.5-cm correction and increase of the Bohler angle of 25 degrees can be expected. There have been no osteotomy nonunions and one nonunion of the subtalar fusion in a smoker. There have been two patients treated by osteotomy alone (no subtalar arthrodesis) with satisfactory results.

COMPLICATIONS

■ Nonunions of the osteotomy or arthrodesis sites are possible but have not proven to be a problem. Malposition of the arthrodesis is possible, but attention to inversion–eversion before fixation of the calcaneal construct to the talus avoids this potential complication.

■ Inadequate correction can be avoided by proper selection of patients. The magnitude of the deformity should be within the limits of correction described above. The surgeon should have patience and be persistent in gaining correction, especially in the initial procedures undertaken. The correction is not achieved immediately, but gradually as tissues are freed and stretch.

■ Wound dehiscence due to skin tension after correction has not been a problem as the wound is anterior to the greatest correction. The skin is not stretched.

REFERENCES

1. Bradley SA, Davies AM. Computerized tomographic assessment of old calcaneal fractures. Br J Radiol 1990;63:926–933.
2. Burdeaux BD. Reduction of calcaneal fractures by the McReynolds medial approach technique and its experimental basis. Clin Orthop Relat Res 1983;177:87–103.
3. Carr JB, Hansen ST, Benirshke SK. Subtalar distraction bone block fusion for late complications of the os calcis fractures. Foot Ankle 1988;9:81–86.
4. Conn HR. The treatment of fractures of the os calcis. J Bone Joint Surg 1935;17:392.
5. Gallie WE. Substragalar arthrodesis in fractures of the os calcis. J Bone Joint Surg 1943;25:731–736.
6. Hansen ST Jr. Calcaneal osteotomy in multiple planes for correction of major posttraumatic deformity. In: Functional Reconstruction of the Foot and Ankle, pp. 380–383. Philadelphia: Lippincott Williams & Wilkins, 2000.
7. Leung K, Chan W, Shen W, et al. Operative treatment of intra articular fractures of the os calcis—the role of rigid internal fixation and primary bone grafting: preliminary results. J Trauma 1989;3:232–240.
8. Palmer I. The mechanism and treatment of fracture of the calcaneus: open reduction with the use of cancellous bone grafts. J Bone Joint Surg Am 1948;30A:2–8.
9. Romash MM. Reconstructive osteotomy of the calcaneus with subtalar arthrodesis for malunited calcaneal fractures. Master Techniques in Orthopedic Surgery series: The Foot and Ankle, 1st and 2nd eds. Philadelphia: Lippincott Williams & Wilkins.
10. Romash MM. Reconstructive osteotomy of the calcaneus with subtalar arthrodesis for malunited calcaneal fractures. Clin Orthop Relat Res 1993;228:157–167.

Chapter 53 Traditional Triple Arthrodesis

Mark E. Easley

DEFINITION

- Triple arthrodesis is a procedure performed to restore and maintain physiologic hindfoot alignment.
- It is typically reserved for:
  - Severe fixed deformity not amenable to joint-sparing procedures
  - Inflammatory arthropathy of the hindfoot

ANATOMY

- The hindfoot comprises the talus, calcaneus, navicular, and cuboid.
- Physiologic alignment is generally defined as a congruent talar–first metatarsal alignment in both the anteroposterior (AP) and lateral planes with weight bearing.
- The talar–calcaneal articulation is referred to as the subtalar joint.
- The combination of the talonavicular and calcaneocuboid articulations is known as the transverse tarsal joint.
- Multiple ligamentous static restraints support the hindfoot. In fact, in stance phase, the physiologically normal foot is balanced and plantigrade without any dynamic muscle forces acting on it.
- Physiologic hindfoot alignment is influenced by the ankle, midfoot, and forefoot.
- The hindfoot is a component of the ankle–hindfoot complex. To an extent, ankle malalignment can be compensated by the hindfoot.
- The foot is balanced when there is relatively even pressure distribution on the heel, first metatasal–sesamoid complex, and the fifth metatarsal (ie, a plantigrade foot).
- Physiologically normal hindfoot alignment can be distorted by ankle, midfoot, and forefoot deformity.
- While the ankle is primarily responsible for dorsiflexion and plantarflexion, the hindfoot has some capacity to compensate in the sagittal plane with ankle stiffness, as evidenced by residual dorsiflexion and plantarflexion following ankle arthrodesis.
- Ambulation
  - With transition from heel strike to stance phase, the hindfoot becomes accommodative to the surface it contacts by "unlocking" the hindfoot joints.
  - With push-off, the posterior tibial tendon (PTT) inverts the hindfoot, thereby locking the transverse tarsal joints and hindfoot.
    - This converts the foot's accommodative function to one of biomechanical advantage with creation of a rigid lever arm for the Achilles tendon.

PATHOGENESIS AND NATURAL HISTORY

- Hindfoot alignment is easily distorted by imbalance of its dynamic stabilizers, in particular the posterior tibial and peroneal tendons.
  - If the imbalance persists and becomes chronic, the hindfoot's static ligamentous restraints may weaken, creating a hindfoot deformity that ultimately may become fixed.
  - PTT dysfunction leads to a flatfoot deformity with attenuation of the medial static restraints (spring ligament complex, medial talonavicular capsule) and pes planovalgus (flatfoot) deformity.
  - Peroneal tendon dysfunction may lead to lateral ankle–hindfoot attenuation and a pes cavovarus (hindfoot varus) deformity.
- Posttraumatic or inflammatory arthritis may also create a stiff and painful hindfoot, with or without deformity.

PATIENT HISTORY AND PHYSICAL FINDINGS

- The patient typically describes aching in the hindfoot, particularly in the sinus tarsi area, with weight bearing.
- There may be a report of a progressive deformity.
- Stiffness and swelling are common complaints.
- It is important to elicit a history of an inflammatory arthropathy.
- A neurologic and vascular examination is required.
- The patient should be examined while standing and ambulating.
  - The deformity may not be obvious with the patient non–weight-bearing.
  - Typically the patient will walk with a limp.
  - A single limb heel rise for a patient with pes planovalgus deformity, if possible, will determine if the deformity is flexible and if the PTT is functional.
- With the patient seated, range of motion (ROM) is assessed.
  - Inversion and eversion are almost always restricted in patients being considered for triple arthrodesis.
  - The talus can be stabilized with a thumb on the talar neck to determine dorsiflexion and plantarflexion in the hindfoot.
  - Ankle ROM and stability also should be evaluated.
  - An equinus contracture may be present and is important when considering surgery. Achilles tendon lengthening may be required to reposition the hindfoot anatomically. Many hindfoot deformities result in Achilles tendon contractures.

IMAGING AND OTHER DIAGNOSTIC STUDIES

- Plain radiographs of the weight-bearing foot in the AP, lateral, and oblique views (**FIG 1**).
- Occasionally, contralateral foot radiographs are useful in understanding what is physiologically normal for an individual.
- I routinely obtain ipsilateral ankle radiographs as well.
- In severe deformity there may be a pre-existing talar tilt.
  - If this is the case, proper operative realignment of the hindfoot may be compromised by the more proximal deformity.
  - One needs to be aware of pre-existing talar tilt or ankle malalignment to ensure that the hindfoot deformity is corrected appropriately.
  - I will check the ankle alignment fluoroscopically while realigning the hindfoot in surgery.
- Rarely is computed tomography or magnetic resonance imaging necessary.

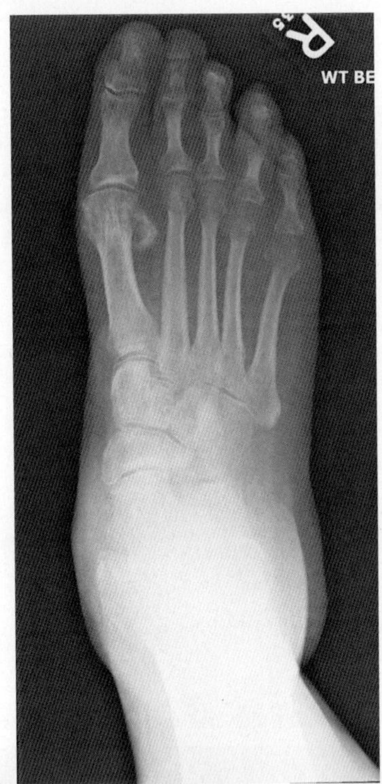

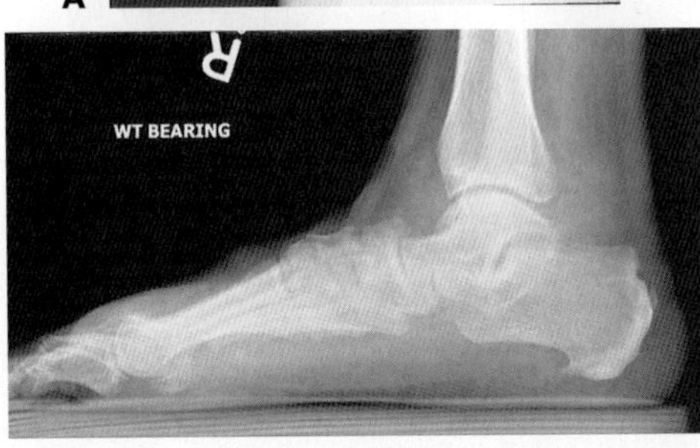

FIG 1 • AP and lateral weight-bearing radiographs of patient with posterior tibial tendon dysfunction, spring ligament rupture, and fixed hindfoot deformity. Note severe talonavicular sag visible in **B**.

NONOPERATIVE MANAGEMENT

- Activity modification
- Nonsteroidal anti-inflammatory agents
- Corticosteroid injection
- Bracing
  - Lace-up brace
  - Hinged or fixed ankle–foot orthosis

SURGICAL MANAGEMENT

- A spectrum of pathologies may warrant triple arthrodesis:
  - Stage III posterior tibial tendinopathy
  - Chronic peroneal tendinopathy
  - Posttraumatic hindfoot arthritis
  - Inflammatory arthritis
  - Charcot neuroarthropathy
  - Chronic spring ligament rupture
- If a joint-sparing procedure can be performed, it should be favored over triple arthrodesis.
- Selective hindfoot arthrodesis may also be considered.
- There has been a trend toward double arthrodesis in lieu of triple arthrodesis.
  - The concept is to preserve the accommodative effect of the calcaneocuboid joint when possible and only perform talonavicular and subtalar joint arthrodeses.
  - Isolated talonavicular joint arthrodesis restricts hindfoot motion by 90%.

Preoperative Planning

- The preoperative deformity needs to be assessed to determine what correction is warranted.
  - If there is a severe pes planovalgus deformity, consider a single medial approach double arthrodesis to eliminate the risk of lateral wound problems that may occur with a lateral approach in such deformity.
- Equinus contracture: It may be necessary to lengthen the Achilles tendon to correct the deformity.
- Equipment
  - Fluoroscopy unit to confirm reduction and hardware placement
  - Preferred screw (and plating or staple) system
  - Bone graft is not required but may be useful to fill any voids or gaps with deformity correction.

Positioning

- With a traditional triple arthrodesis, the patient is placed on the operating table in a modified lateral decubitus position ("sloppy lateral position"; **FIG 2**). This allows access to the lateral and medial hindfoot.
- The patient's torso is supported with a beanbag.
- An axillary roll is usually indicated.
- The contralateral hip is flexed slightly to make room for a stack of folded sheets on which the operative leg is placed.
  - The opposite leg must be padded if it contacts the beanbag.
- I routinely use a thigh tourniquet if I am considering an Achilles tendon lengthening.
  - If an Achilles tendon lengthening is unnecessary, a calf tourniquet is adequate.

Approach

- The traditional utilitarian lateral approach uses a 7- to 8-cm incision from the tip of the fibula toward the base of the fourth metatarsal.
- The traditional utilitarian dorsomedial approach uses a 7- to 8-cm incision from the anterior aspect of the anterior medial malleolus toward the dorsomedial base of the first metatarsal.
- If equinus contracture is present, I first perform an Achilles tendon lengthening.

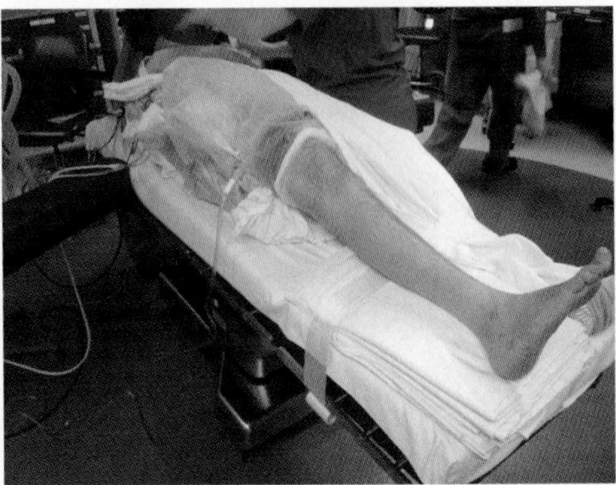

FIG 2 • The patient is placed on a beanbag in a modified lateral position that allows access to the medial and lateral foot. A stack of folded sheets is placed under foot to be operated.

LATERAL EXPOSURE

- Create a lateral longitudinal incision (TECH FIG 1A).
- Protect the sural nerve (TECH FIG 1B).
- Create the interval between the peroneal tendons and the extensor digitorum brevis (EDB) muscle.
- Elevate the EDB muscle with its fascia dorsally (TECH FIG 1C).
  - Avoid "shredding" the muscle and fascia, as it will be used as the deep layer closure at the completion of the surgery.
- Release the bifurcate (calcaneonavicular and calcaneocuboid) ligament that lies deep to the EDB muscle.
- Release the calcaneocuboid capsule also (TECH FIG 1D).

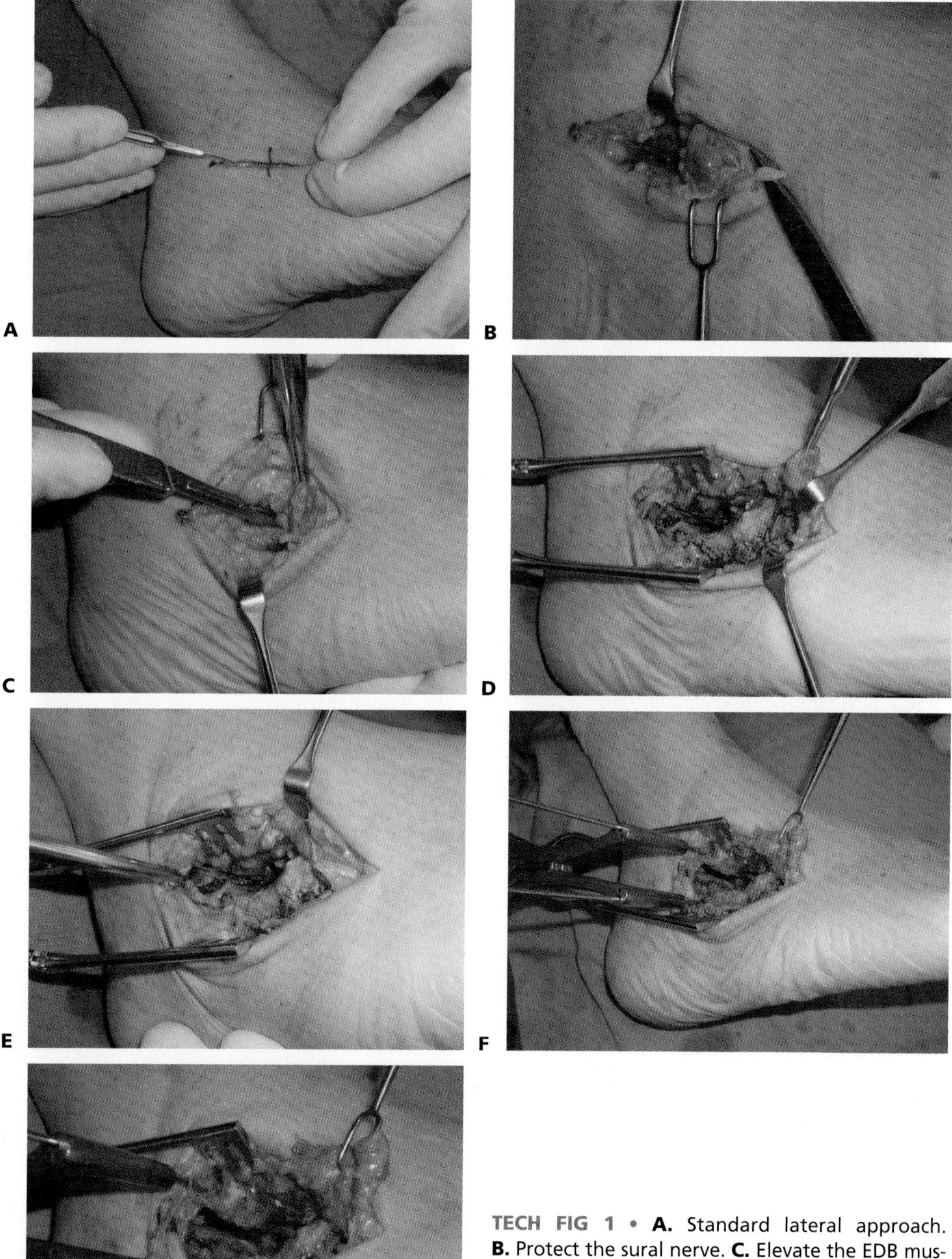

TECH FIG 1 • **A.** Standard lateral approach. **B.** Protect the sural nerve. **C.** Elevate the EDB muscle and fascia. **D.** Expose the subtalar joint. A blunt retractor may be placed deep to the calcaneofibular ligament. **E.** Identify the calcaneocuboid joint. In this patient with an inflammatory arthropathy, the joint is distorted. **F,G.** Subtalar joint exposed with a distraction device.

- Place a blunt retractor between the lateral subtalar joint and the calcaneofibular ligament (TECH FIG 1E).
- Use a distractor to expose the subtalar joint first (TECH FIG 1F,G) and then the calcaneocuboid joint.
- The lateral talonavicular joint may also be accessed through this approach.

SUBTALAR, CALCANEOCUBOID, AND LATERAL TALONAVICULAR JOINT PREPARATION

- The preparation is the same for all three joints.
- Remove residual articular cartilage with an sharp elevator or chisel (TECH FIG 2A).
- Preserve the native subchondral bone architecture.
- Drill or chisel ("feather") the subchondral bone to allow for vascular channels to form at the arthrodesis surfaces while maintaining subchondral bone architecture (TECH FIG 2B,C).
- For the subtalar joint, include not only the posterior facet but also the middle and anterior facets.
  - However, be careful to not disrupt the delicate vasculature on the undersurface of the talar neck, if possible.
- The calcaneocuboid joint is a "saddle" joint, so avoid simply driving a chisel directly across the joint surfaces as it may result in more than desired bone removal, particularly when correcting pes planovalgus (TECH FIG 2D,E).
- The lateral talonavicular joint is often difficult to reach from the medial approach, but the lateral exposure affords satisfactory access to prepare this aspect of the talonavicular joint (TECH FIG 2F,G).
- I irrigate the joint before drilling the subchondral bone. Drilling creates reamings that serve as bone graft, and I do not want to wash the reamings away.

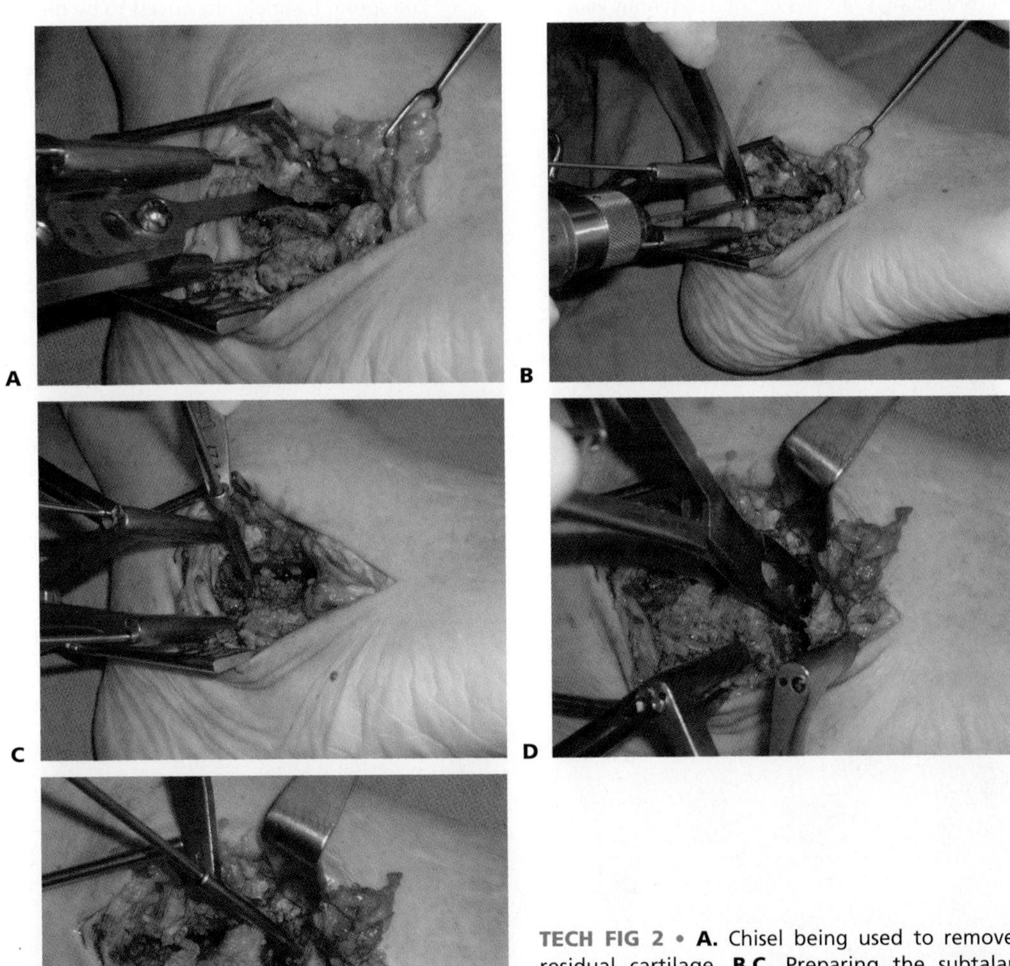

TECH FIG 2 • **A.** Chisel being used to remove residual cartilage. **B,C.** Preparing the subtalar joint. **B.** Drill being introduced. **C.** The reamings created will serve as bone graft. **D,E.** Preparing the calcaneocuboid joint. **D.** Chisel being used to remove residual cartilage. **E.** Drilling the subchondral bone to promote fusion and adding reamings that serve as bone graft. *(continued)*

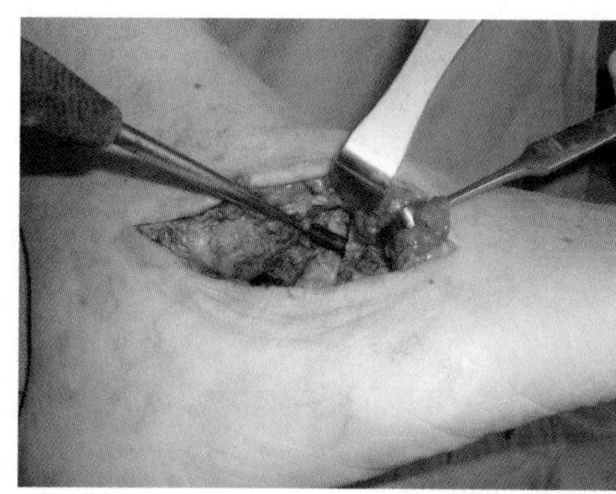
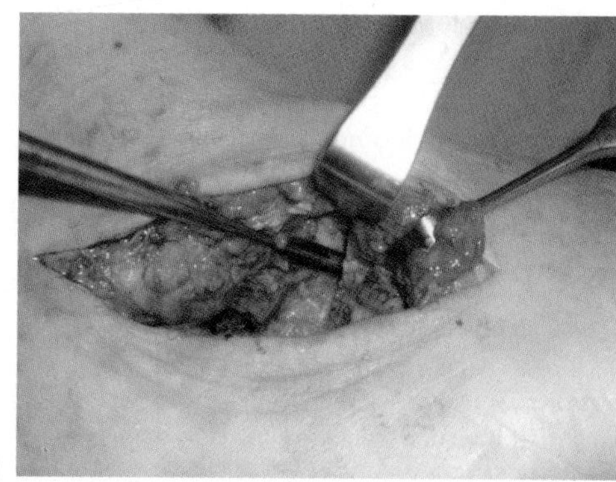

TECH FIG 2 • *(continued)* **F,G.** Exposure of the lateral talonavicular joint.

MEDIAL EXPOSURE

- Create a longitudinal incision (TECH FIG 3A).
- Cauterize connecting branches of the saphenous vein so the vein can be mobilized.
- Identify the tibialis anterior tendon and protect it throughout the procedure (TECH FIG 3B).
  - Typically fibers of the extensor retinaculum must be released to access the tibialis anterior tendon.
- Perform a longitudinal capsulotomy (TECH FIG 3C,D).
  - The spring ligament may need to be divided and the PTT tendon may need to be released from the navicular to improve access to the talonavicular joint.

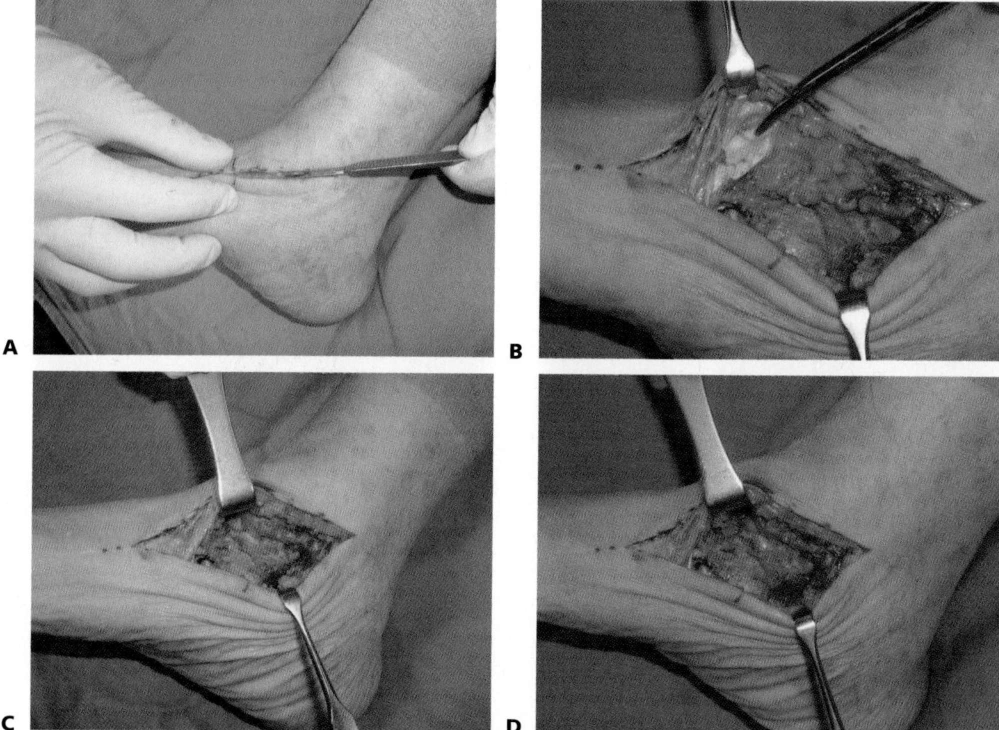

TECH FIG 3 • **A,B.** Medial approach to the talonavicular joint. **C.** Medial exposure after capsulotomy. **D.** Close-up demonstrating erosive changes in the talonavicular joint in a patient with an inflammatory arthropathy.

TALONAVICULAR JOINT PREPARATION

- Use a distractor to gain full exposure to the talonavicular joint (TECH FIG 4A,B).
  - In brittle bone, be careful when applying pressure to the navicular as it may fracture.
- Remove the residual articular cartilage from the talonavicular joint (TECH FIG 4C).
  - In pes planovalgus deformity, the talar head may be weak, so be careful not to gouge the talar head when attempting to delaminate the residual articular cartilage.
  - The lateral talar head should have already been prepared from the lateral approach.
  - Remove cartilage from the navicular.
- Penetrate the subchondral bone to promote fusion.
  - The talus is relatively easy to access with a small-diameter drill bit (TECH FIG 4D). Be careful using a chisel on the talar head as it may fracture.
  - The navicular can also be readily drilled.
  - I do not often use a burr to prepare subchondral bone for fusion, but on the navicular it is sometimes very effective, provided cold water or saline irrigation is used simultaneously to limit bone necrosis. However, this may wash away desirable reamings that could serve as bone graft.
  - As for the preparation of the other joint surfaces, I irrigate the talonavicular joint before drilling then try to maintain the reamings so they can be used as bone graft.

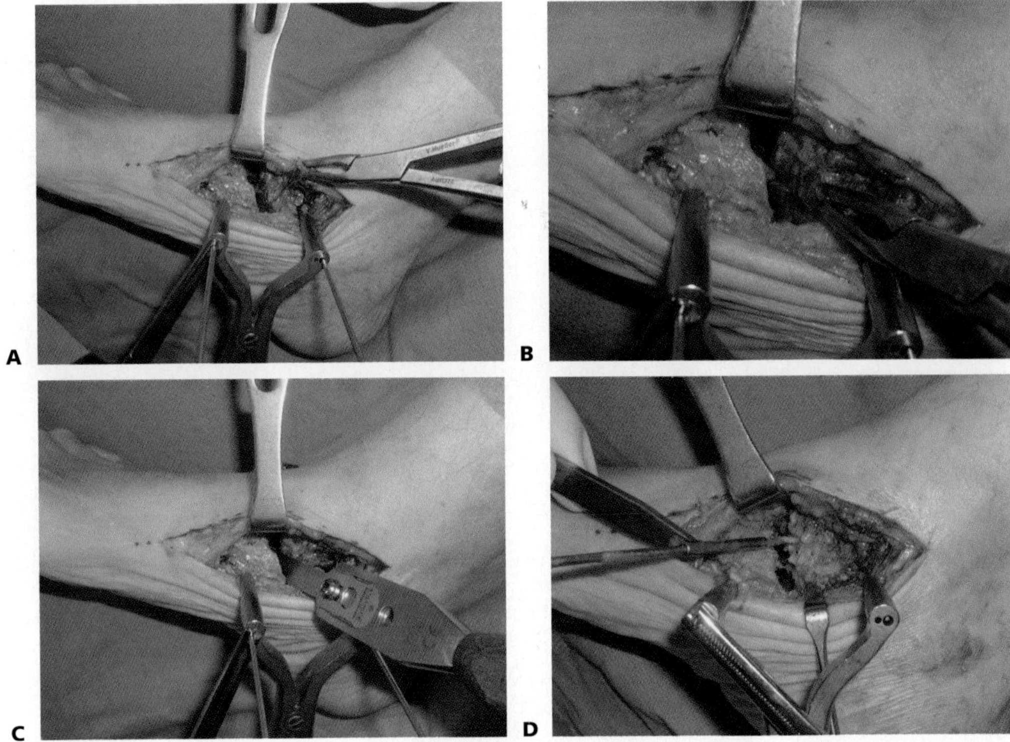

TECH FIG 4 • **A.** Talonavicular joint distracted. **B.** Dèbriding the joint with a rongeur. **C.** A chisel is used to remove residual articular cartilage. **D.** Drilling the subchondral bone to promote fusion.

HINDFOOT REDUCTION

- Place bone graft in the arthrodesis sites at this time, before the reduction is performed.
  - I routinely use bone graft to fill voids at the surfaces to be fused. While this is not mandatory, I believe that filling the voids enhances the body's ability to form bridging trabeculations.
- The calcaneus must be centered properly under the talus.
  - Through the lateral wound, the optimal relationship of the posterior facet can be assessed and controlled. (TECH FIG 5A,B).
  - Physiologically there is a gap between the anterolateral talus and the anterior calcaneal process, and this should be re-created.
  - In correcting severe pes planovalgus, I aim to overcorrect the calcaneus beneath the talus (TECH FIG 5C).
- Once the optimal subtalar relationship established, I provisionally pin the subtalar joint.
  - I use a guide pin for the intended cannulated screw and try to place the pin in the intended trajectory for the screw (TECH FIG 5D,E).

- Typically I have an assistant working with me, so I hold the reduction while the assistant places the guide pin from the calcaneal tuberosity into the talar body.
- The dual-incision approach affords the surgeon the ability to palpate the talonavicular and calcaneocuboid joint reductions simultaneously.
  - With the subtalar joint reduced, I then attempt to reduce the talonavicular joint to an anatomic position. I can palpate both sides of the talonavicular joint by having two incisions (**TECH FIG 5F**).
  - When correcting pes planovalgus deformity, I err on the side of overcorrection of the navicular on the talar head.
- Once I have the talonavicular joint reduced, I protect the tibialis anterior tendon and have my assistant drive two guide pins, appropriately spaced from one another, from the navicular into the talar head (**TECH FIG 5G**).
  - I attempt to place the screw from the most distal aspect of the navicular, even reaming the medial wall of the first cuneiform slightly, so the pin needs to be flush against the medial aspect of the first cuneiform.
- Finally, I provisionally pin the calcaneocuboid joint.
  - To create a relief area on the anterior process of the calcaneus for the screw insertion, I remove a small wedge of bone from the anterior process using a rongeur.
  - I routinely push up on the cuboid and down on the anterior process of the calcaneus to reduce the joint.
  - Despite the lateral approach, optimal longitudinal orientation of the guide pin across the calcaneocuboid joint is not possible.
    - I sometimes create a stab incision behind the peroneal tendons, dissect carefully deep to the sural nerve and tendons, creating a soft-tissue tunnel, insert a drill sleeve, and then deliver the guide pin safely to the anterior process of the talus.
  - The guide pin is driven across the joint.

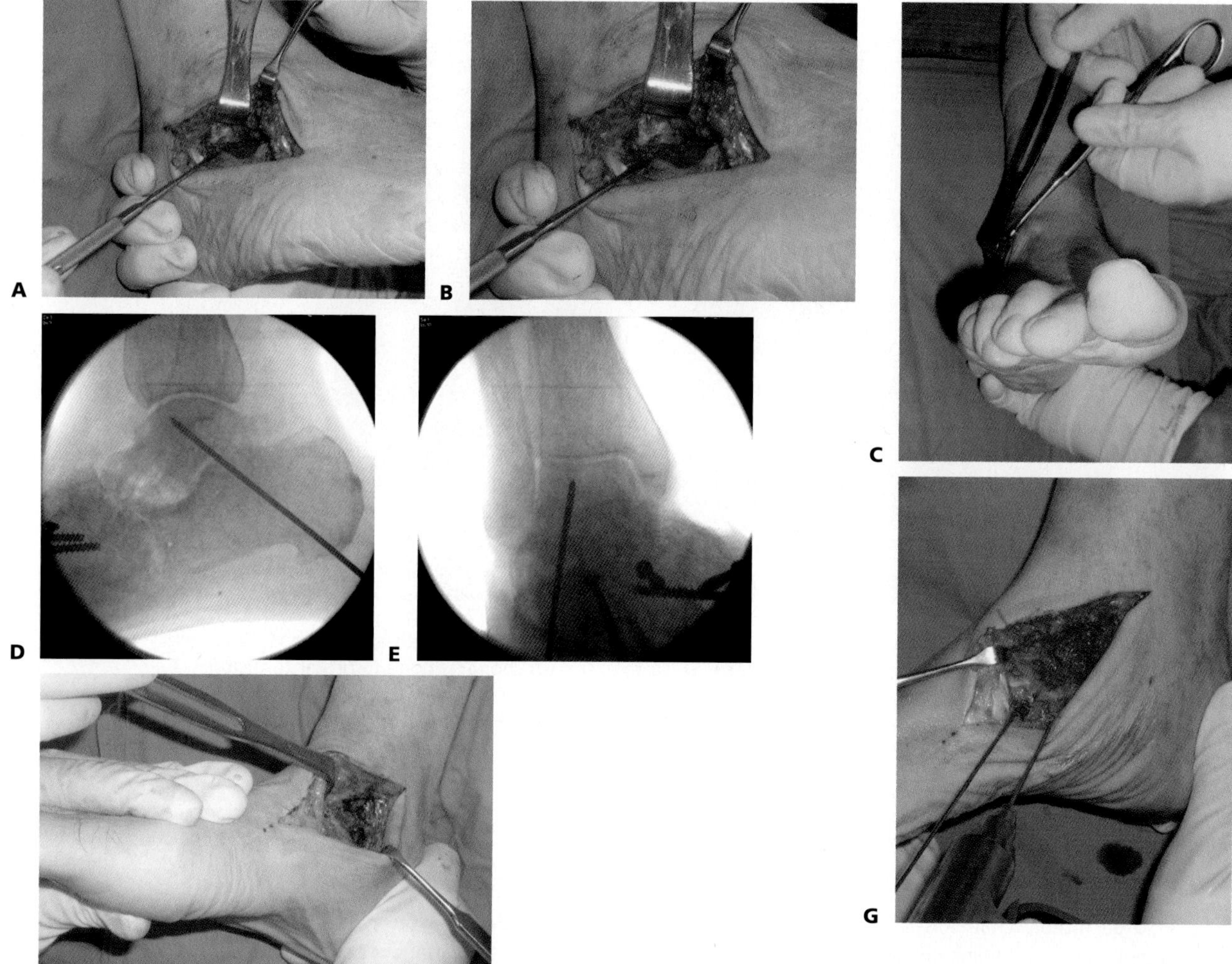

TECH FIG 5 • Reducing the hindfoot. **A,B.** Checking the subtalar joint reduction. **C.** The hindfoot is maintained in the corrected position. Lateral (**D**) and mortise (**E**) fluoroscopic views after a guide pin was placed across the reduced subtalar joint. **F.** Reduction of talonavicular joint. **G.** Guide pins placed across talonavicular joint.

HINDFOOT STABILIZATION

- The reduction and the position of the guide pins are checked fluoroscopically (TECH FIG 6A).
  - Adjustments are made as necessary.
  - At this stage, I also routinely check the ankle fluoroscopically to be sure there is no ankle deformity that may distort the true hindfoot alignment.
- I determine proper screws lengths and overdrill the guide pins, but only to the initial aspect of the second bone.
  - Most modern screws are self-drilling and self-tapping; however, particularly in the navicular, I prefer to predrill to diminish the risk of navicular fracture.
  - By not drilling the full length of the planned screw, purchase of the screw is typically improved.
- I first place the subtalar screw, as a compression screw (TECH FIG 6B,C).
- Next, I place the two talonavicular screws (TECH FIG 6D–F).
  - The first screw is a compression screw.
  - I use a positional screw for the second screw.
  - If greater talonavicular stability is needed, I create a small dorsal incision over the midfoot; protect the superficial peroneal nerve, extensor tendons, and the deep neurovascular bundle; and using a drill sleeve, place a guide pin from the centrolateral navicular into the talar body or sometimes through the inferior talar body and into the calcaneus. Over this I place a third talonavicular screw, either positional or compression, although with two screws medially further compression is generally not possible.
- For the calcaneocuboid joint, I protect the soft tissues and overdrill only the anterior calcaneal process. Then I insert a compression or positional screw across the calcaneocuboid joint (TECH FIG 6G,H).
  - If the joint is well reduced, I tend to use a positional screw; if the joint could stand to be compressed for better bony apposition, however, I place a compression screw.
  - As mentioned earlier, I push up on the cuboid and down on the anterior calcaneal process to maintain the reduction and to make sure the cuboid does not sag, occasionally leaving it prominent postoperatively. However, with an anatomic reduction, this is rarely an issue.
  - Occasionally, I add a lateral compression plate or staple across the calcaneocuboid joint to augment the fixation.
- I get final fluoroscopic confirmation of alignment, bony apposition at the arthrodesis sites, and hardware position (TECH FIG 6I,J).

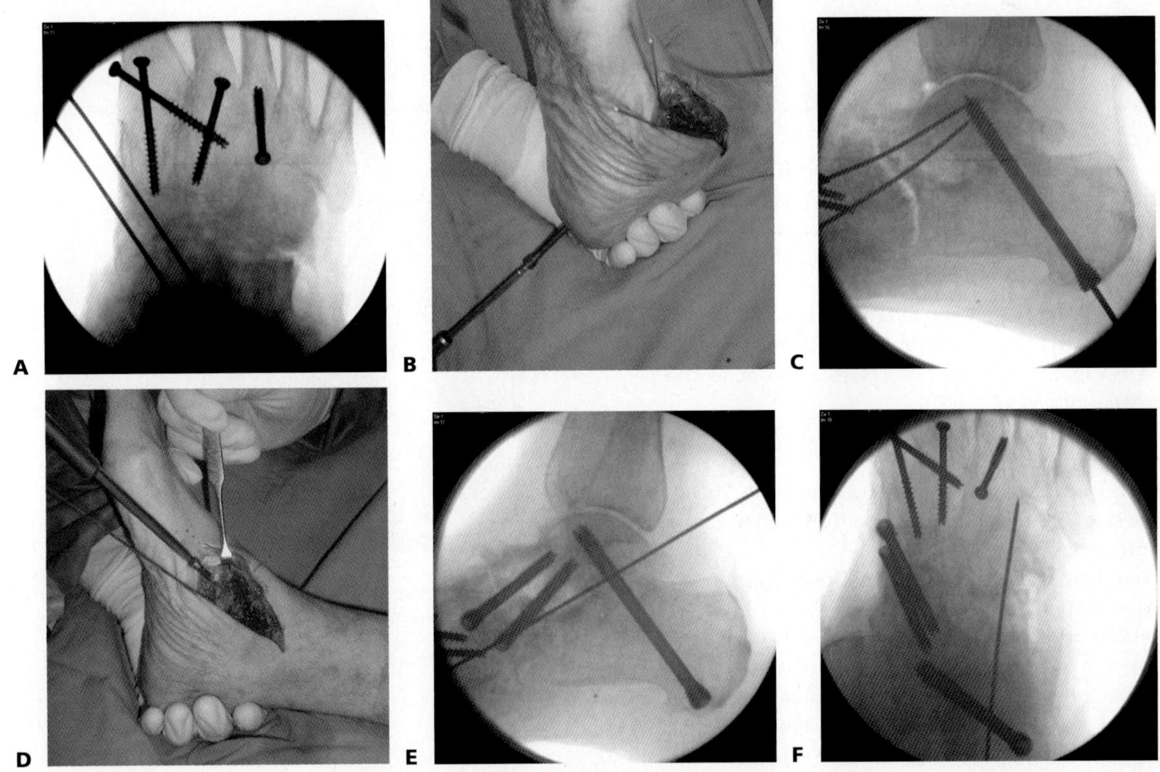

TECH FIG 6 • A. Fluoroscopic confirmation of the guide pins placed across the talonavicular joint (this patient had undergone prior midfoot arthrodesis). **B,C.** Clinical and fluoroscopic views of the subtalar screw in place. **D–F.** Clinical and fluoroscopic views of the talonavicular screws in place. One partially threaded compression screw is placed first, and one fully threaded positional screw is placed second. *(continued)*

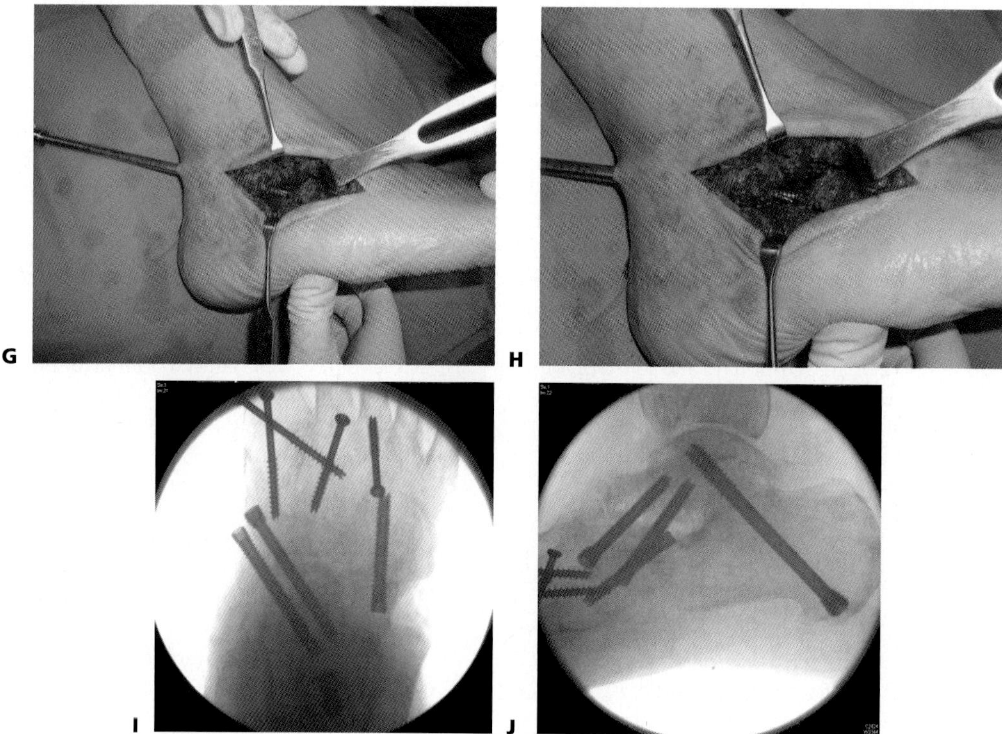

TECH FIG 6 • *(continued)* **G,H.** Calcaneocuboid screw. A separate stab incision is made with a carefully prepared soft tissue tunnel under the sural nerve and peroneal tendons. Note thumb pressure pushing up on the cuboid to maintain joint reduction and a more favorable position of the cuboid. **I,J.** Final AP and lateral fluoroscopic views confirming appropriate reduction, bony apposition at the arthrodesis sites, and proper hardware position.

CLOSURE

- I routinely pack bone graft at the "quadruple arthrodesis" site, where talus, calcaneus, navicular, and cuboid meet at the lateral aspect of the talonavicular joint (TECH FIG 7).
- Medially the capsule is reapproximated.
- Laterally the fascia overlying the EDB muscle can usually be reapproximated to soft tissues adjacent to the peroneal tendons.
- Any bone graft in the soft tissues is irrigated away, as it may interfere with wound healing.
- Next, the subcutaneous tissues are closed.
- The skin incisions are then reapproximated to tensionless closures.
- I routinely release the tourniquet prior to subcutaneous layer closure.
- I also routinely use a lateral drain.
- The stab incisions for screw placement are closed.
- Sterile dressings and a posterior or sugar-tong splint are placed over adequate padding, with the ankle in neutral position.

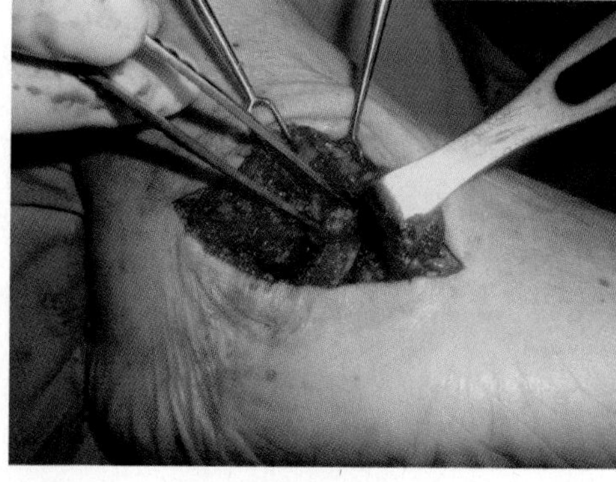

TECH FIG 7 • Bone grafting the confluence of all four hindfoot bones, at the "quadruple arthrodesis" site.

PEARLS AND PITFALLS

Achilles tendon	■ If an equinus contracture is not corrected, anatomic reduction will be difficult or impossible.
Severe pes planovalgus deformity	■ This is perhaps more safely corrected with a single incision medial approach double arthrodesis. A traditional dual-incision triple arthrodesis may lead to a lateral wound complication when correcting severe flatfoot deformity.
Ankle	■ In severe deformity, be sure to check the ankle preoperatively. With pre-existing ankle deformity, a triple arthrodesis is sure to fail.
Sequence of reduction	■ While the talonavicular joint may be reduced first, the most important correction of deformity, in my opinion, is the centering of the calcaneus anatomically under the talus.
Talonavicular joint preparation	■ If a traditional dual-incision triple arthrodesis is performed, use the lateral access to prepare the lateral talonavicular joint because it is difficult to reach the lateral talar head from the medial approach.

POSTOPERATIVE CARE

- I routinely keep patients overnight for pain control, nasal oxygen (which may improve wound healing), and limb elevation.
  - While I recognize that some of my colleagues perform this surgery as a pure outpatient procedure, I believe that one night (which still qualifies as an outpatient procedure) is in the patient's best interest after major hindfoot surgery.
- The patient wears a splint for 2 weeks.
- The patient returns to the clinic at 2 weeks for suture removal and short leg cast.
- The patient returns to the clinic at 6 weeks after surgery for radiographs out of cast and repeat casting.
- Touch-down weight bearing is the rule for a full 10 weeks.
- The patient returns to the clinic at 10 weeks and if repeat simulated weight-bearing radiographs suggest healing and no complications, he or she can be placed in a cam boot with gradual progression to full weight bearing by 12 to 14 weeks.
- The patient returns to the clinic at 14 to 16 weeks for full weight bearing radiographs (**FIG 3**), then gradual progression to full activities.

OUTCOMES

- Patients are generally improved with an appropriately performed triple arthrodesis.
- At intermediate to long-term follow-up, patients are functional in their activities of daily living but few are able to perform demanding recreational activities.
- With time, patients tend to develop adjacent joint arthritis, but it is unclear if this causes functional deficits.
- "Triple arthrodesis" performed through a single medial incision and including only the subtalar and talonavicular joints is gradually displacing the traditional triple arthrodesis. Results of this procedure are promising, but it is not clear if they are more favorable than those of the traditional triple arthrodesis.

COMPLICATIONS

- Nonunion
- Malunion
- Wound dehiscence
- Infection
- Sural neuralgia
- Prominent hardware
- Persistent pain despite appropriate management and satisfactory clincal and radiographic findings

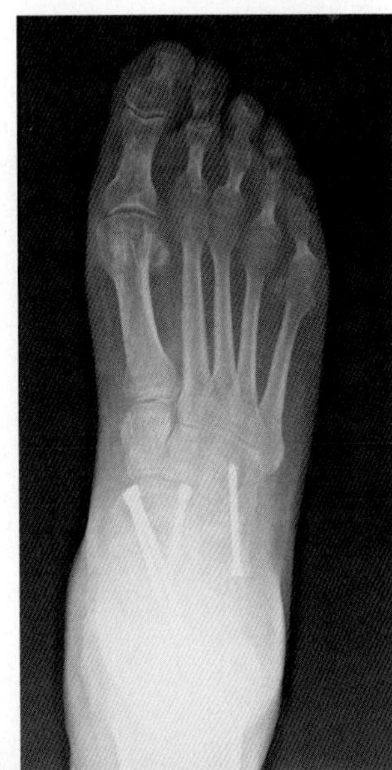

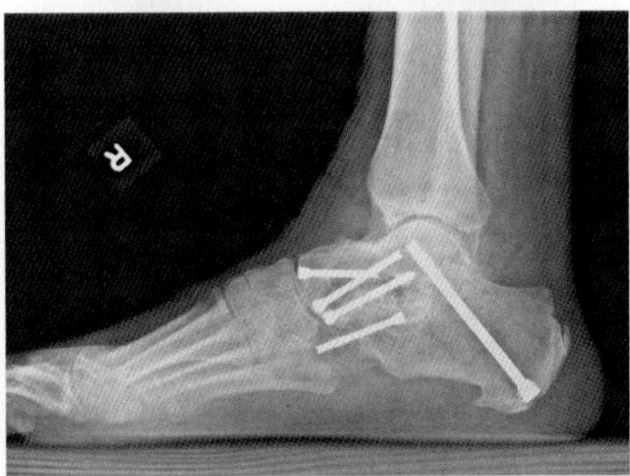

FIG 3 • Follow-up weight-bearing radiographs of the patient with fixed hindfoot deformity secondary to posterior tibial tendon dysfunction and spring ligament tear. Note the congruent alignment of the talar–first metatarsal axis in both the AP and lateral views.

REFERENCES

1. Bednarz PA, Monroe MT, Manoli A II. Triple arthrodesis in adults using rigid internal fixation: an assessment of outcome. Foot Ankle Int 1999;20:356–363.
2. Haritidis JH, Kirkos JM, Provellegios SM, Zachos AD. Long-term results of triple arthrodesis: 42 cases followed for 25 years. Foot Ankle Int 1994;15:548–551.
3. Knupp M, Skoog A, Törnkvist H, Ponzer S. Triple arthrodesis in rheumatoid arthritis. Foot Ankle Int 2008;29:293–297.
4. Pell RF IV, Myerson MS, Schon LC. Clinical outcome after primary triple arthrodesis. J Bone Joint Surg Am 2000;82A:47–57.
5. Rosenfeld PF, Budgen SA, Saxby TS. Triple arthrodesis: is bone grafting necessary? The results in 100 consecutive cases. J Bone Joint Surg Br 2005;87B:175–178.
6. Sangeorzan BJ, Smith D, Veith R, Hansen ST Jr. Triple arthrodesis using internal fixation in treatment of adult foot disorders. Clin Orthop Relat Res 1993;294:299–307.
7. Saltzman CL, Fehrle MJ, Cooper RR, et al. Triple arthrodesis: twenty-five and forty-four-year average follow-up of the same patients. J Bone Joint Surg Am 1999;81:1391–1402.
8. Smith RW, Shen W, Dewitt S, Reischl SF. Triple arthrodesis in adults with non-paralytic disease: a minimum ten-year follow-up study. J Bone Joint Surg Am 2004;86A:2707–2713.
9. Song SJ, Lee S, O'Malley MJ, et al. Deltoid ligament strain after correction of acquired flatfoot deformity by triple arthrodesis. Foot Ankle Int 2000;21:573–577.

Chapter 54

Single-Incision Medial Approach for Triple Arthrodesis

Clifford L. Jeng

DEFINITION

- Severe rigid planovalgus foot deformity may be a result of multiple underlying causes.
- In longstanding rigid hindfoot valgus deformities, the lateral skin and soft tissues may become severely contracted. In these cases, adequate correction of a severe valgus deformity may stretch and compromise the lateral soft tissues if a standard two-incision approach is used for triple arthrodesis.
- Previous surgical incisions, soft tissue injuries, or infections may further compromise wound healing if a lateral incision is used.
- A single-medial-approach triple arthrodesis technique offers adequate exposure of the subtalar, talonavicular, and calcaneocuboid joints for preparation without putting the lateral skin at risk.

ANATOMY

- The posterior and middle facets of the subtalar joint lie directly deep to the excised posterior tibial tendon (**FIG 1**).
- The flexor digitorum longus tendon and the posterior tibial neurovascular bundle lie just posterior and plantar to the subtalar joint. These must be protected with a retractor during joint preparation.
- The talonavicular joint is easily accessible through the extensile medial approach.
- The calcaneocuboid joint is directly lateral to the talonavicular joint across the foot. It can be adequately accessed through the extensile medial incision after the talonavicular joint is distracted with a lamina spreader (**FIG 2**).

PATHOGENESIS

- The medial longitudinal arch is supported by both static and dynamic anatomic structures.
- The static component includes the spring ligament (calcaneonavicular ligament), the plantar fascia, and the long plantar ligament.
- The dynamic component includes the posterior tibial tendon.
- In the adult acquired flatfoot, the spring ligament, plantar fascia, and long plantar ligament become attenuated and the posterior tibial tendon becomes dysfunctional. It is controversial whether the static or dynamic stabilizers fail first.
- In severe flatfoot patients, the peroneal tendons and the laterally shifted Achilles tendon overpower the dysfunctional posterior tibial tendon, forcing the subtalar joint into heel valgus.
- The transverse tarsal joints (talonavicular and calcaneocuboid joints) are abducted by the relative overpull of the peroneus brevis, causing lateral subluxation of the talonavicular joint and uncovering of the talar head.

NATURAL HISTORY

- Severe hindfoot valgus deformity, if left untreated, may lead to gradual attenuation of the deltoid ligament. Once this occurs, the tibiotalar joint becomes incongruent and tilts into valgus. This will eventually lead to ankle joint arthritis.
- The association of severe hindfoot valgus and valgus tilt of the ankle is difficult to treat and generally requires either (1) a pantalar arthrodesis or (2) ankle arthroplasty with an underlying triple arthrodesis.
- In my opinion, it is critical to intervene in these patients with severe hindfoot valgus before the deltoid ligament becomes incompetent in order to preserve the ankle joint.

PATIENT HISTORY AND PHYSICAL FINDINGS

- While a single-incision medial triple arthrodesis is feasible in most patients recommended for triple arthrodesis, we favor employing this technique in the most severe cases of hindfoot valgus or in high-risk patients.
- Risk factors exist that may predispose to severe pes planovalgus or may put the patient at risk for wound healing complications. Rheumatoid arthritis is a common cause of severe hindfoot valgus. Rheumatoid patients can sometimes present

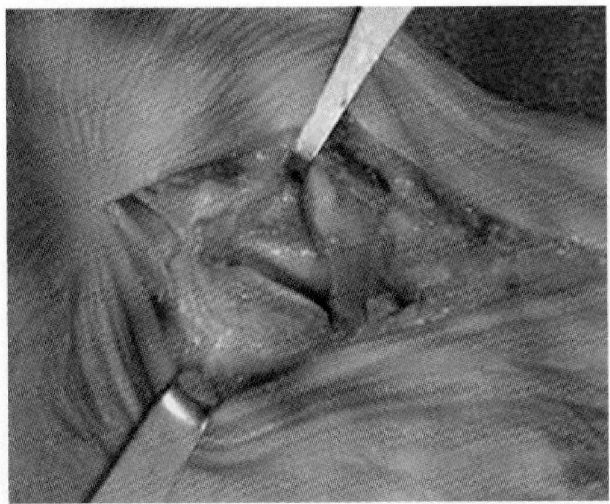

FIG 1 • The subtalar joint lies directly beneath the excised posterior tibial tendon.

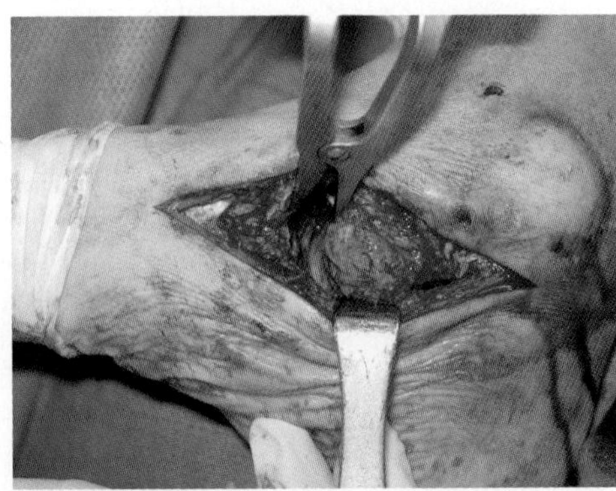

FIG 2 • View of the calcaneocuboid joint from the medial approach.

with greater than 30 degrees of valgus through the subtalar joint. Many of these patients will have gross subluxation of the posterior facet of the subtalar joint on radiographs.

- Likewise, diabetic patients with Charcot-like subtalar joint subluxation or dislocation may present with severe hindfoot valgus. These patients are at increased risk of wound healing complications, and in our opinion represent patients in whom a lateral sinus tarsi approach is not advised.
- Anyone with a history of previous soft tissue trauma laterally, open wounds, active infection, or recent surgical incisions that may compromise the ability of a lateral sinus tarsi incision to heal may benefit from a single-medial-incision technique.
- Examination should include the following:
  - Standing hindfoot alignment. The examiner should visually inspect the posterior heel alignment with respect to the tibia with the patient standing. Physiologic hindfoot valgus is usually 5 to 7 degrees. Significantly greater valgus may be pathologic. In patients with severe hindfoot valgus greater than 30 degrees, a lateral sinus tarsi incision may be difficult to heal once the heel is reduced.
  - Subtalar range of motion. The examiner should maximally invert and evert the heel to determine the range of motion with respect to the tibial axis. Normal subtalar range of motion is 5 degrees of eversion and 20 degrees of inversion. Most severe, longstanding pes planovalgus deformities will be rigid. If the hindfoot is flexible, the surgeon may consider osteotomies or lateral column lengthening to correct the malalignment.
  - Peroneal tendon contracture. With the heel maximally inverted, the examiner should palpate the peroneal tendons to determine how much they are contributing to valgus contracture. If the peroneal tendons are excessively tight, they will need to be released for the heel alignment to be corrected to neutral.
  - Contracture of the skin overlying the lateral hindfoot. The examiner should visually inspect the lateral skin to see whether it is loose or taut. If the lateral skin is tight before correcting the heel valgus, a sinus tarsi incision will be very difficult to close once the heel is neutral.

IMAGING AND OTHER DIAGNOSTIC STUDIES

- Standard weight-bearing radiographs of both the foot and ankle are critical in evaluating severe pes planovalgus deformities. The foot films will determine the amount of subluxation or dislocation of the subtalar and transverse tarsal joints that must be corrected. They can also determine whether there is deformity or bone loss that demands the addition of structural bone grafts. The ankle radiographs are required to confirm that the severe heel valgus is isolated to the hindfoot. Occasionally, severe valgus hindfoot deformity leads to increasing deltoid ligament incompetence, creating a valgus tilt of the talus within the ankle mortise. Deltoid ligament incompetence and valgus tilt of the ankle may necessitate surgical correction of the ankle as well should hindfoot realignment with triple arthrodesis fail to rebalance the tibiotalar joint (**FIG 3**).

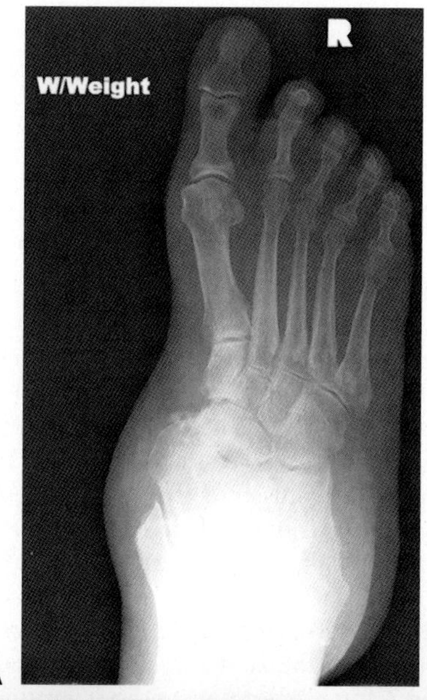

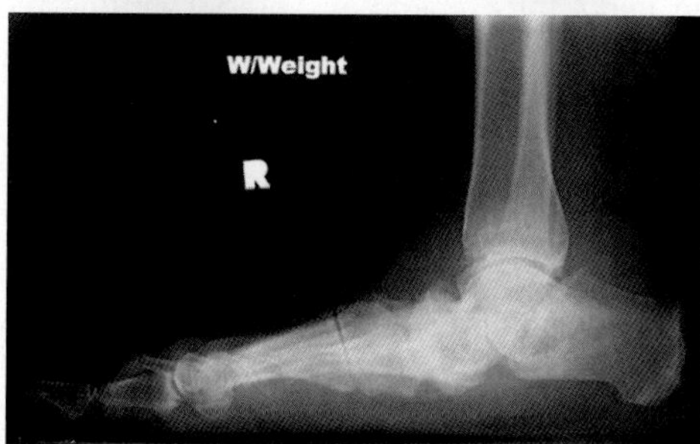

FIG 3 • Radiographs of a 56-year-old diabetic woman with severe pes planovalgus deformity and gross subluxation of the subtalar and transverse tarsal joints radiographically.

DIFFERENTIAL DIAGNOSIS

- The possible underlying causes of flatfoot in an adult include:
  - Posterior tibial tendon dysfunction
  - Inflammatory arthritis
  - Osteoarthritis
  - Calcaneus fracture
  - Navicular fracture
  - Spring ligament rupture
  - Lisfranc fracture-dislocation
  - Crush injury
  - Tarsal coalition
  - Accessory navicular
  - Charcot neuroarthropathy
  - Cerebral palsy
  - Poliomyelitis
  - Nerve injury
  - Longstanding idiopathic flatfoot

NONOPERATIVE MANAGEMENT

- In patients with longstanding pes planovalgus feet, the deformity is frequently fixed, meaning that the deformity cannot be actively or passively corrected. Orthotics and braces can only help by supporting the arch, unloading prominences, or immobilizing arthritic joints. Several over-the-counter braces are available commercially that may be effective in immobilizing and supporting the painful flatfoot. The gold standard is a custom-made relatively rigid lace-up ankle brace. In-shoe orthotics for rigid flatfeet should be custom-molded to accommodate the deformity and any prominences.

- Nonsteroidal anti-inflammatory medications may be helpful in alleviating arthritic pain or synovitis. Occasionally a cortisone shot may be beneficial to relieve an acutely painful joint.

SURGICAL MANAGEMENT

Positioning

- The patient is positioned supine on the operating table with a small bump beneath the contralateral hip. This places the operative foot nearly parallel to the table, which is critical because all of the exposure and preparation will be performed through the medial incision. A well-padded thigh tourniquet is placed on the proximal thigh.

Approach

- An extensile medial incision affords satisfactory exposure to the talonavicular and subtalar joints. With talonavicular joint distraction, the calcaneocuboid joint may also be accessed.

TECHNIQUES

RELEASE OF THE PERONEAL TENDON CONTRACTURE

- Make a 3-cm longitudinal incision posterolaterally about 10 cm above the level of the ankle joint. This incision is made directly over the peroneal tendons, immediately behind the posterior border of the fibula.
- Open the peroneal tendon sheath longitudinally in line with the skin incision.
- Use a hemostat to remove the peroneus longus and brevis tendons from their sheath. Transect each tendon completely and return them into the sheath (**TECH FIG 1**).
- Close the sheath and skin in layers.

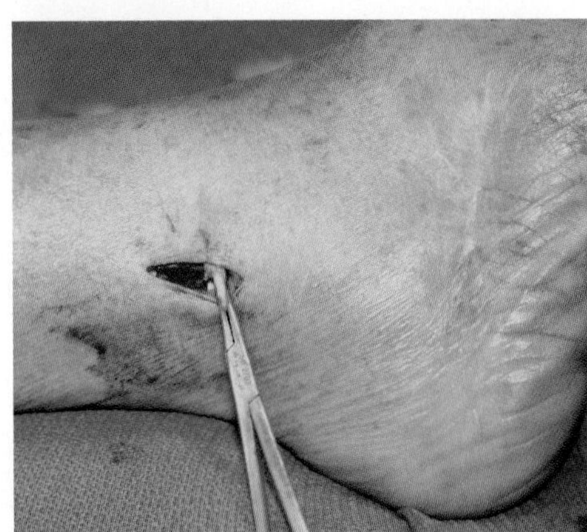

TECH FIG 1 • The peroneus longus and brevis contractures are released through a small incision well above the level of the ankle joint to avoid wound complications.

EXPOSURE AND PREPARATION OF SUBTALAR JOINT

- Make an extensile longitudinal incision medially from the tip of the medial malleolus to the tarsometatarsal joint level.
- Open the sheath of the posterior tibial tendon longitudinally in line with the skin incision.

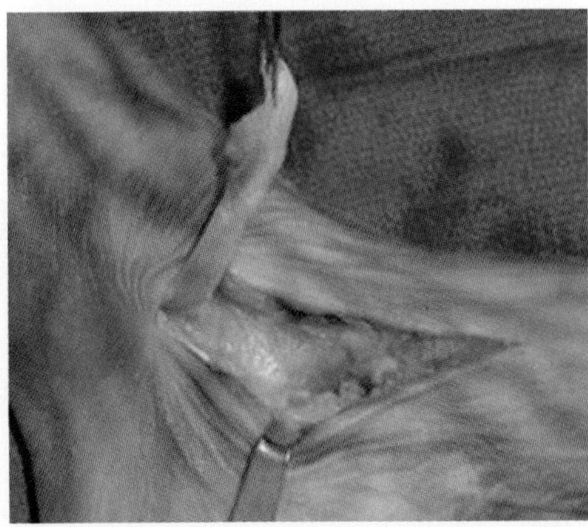

TECH FIG 2 • The posterior tibial tendon is detached from its insertion on the navicular and excised to expose the underlying subtalar joint.

- Completely release the posterior tibial tendon from its insertion onto the navicular. Use a Köcher clamp to pull out the tendon as far as possible, and excise the posterior tibial tendon proximally in the incision (**TECH FIG 2**).
- Using a retractor, pull the flexor digitorum longus tendon posteriorly. This will protect the posterior tibial neurovascular bundle behind it.
- Use a scalpel blade to localize the posterior and middle facets of the subtalar joint by probing deep to the excised posterior tibial tendon. Once the joint is identified, use an osteotome or elevator to release the joint capsule and ligaments (**TECH FIG 3**).
- Insert a lamina spreader between the talar neck and calcaneus and open it to expose the subtalar joint for preparation (**TECH FIG 4**).
- Using a combination of osteotomes and curettes, remove all remaining articular cartilage from the joint down to the subchondral plate.
- Use a curved osteotome to aggressively "feather" the articular surfaces of the posterior and middle facets of the subtalar joint, creating increased surface area for fusion and serving to provide local bone graft.

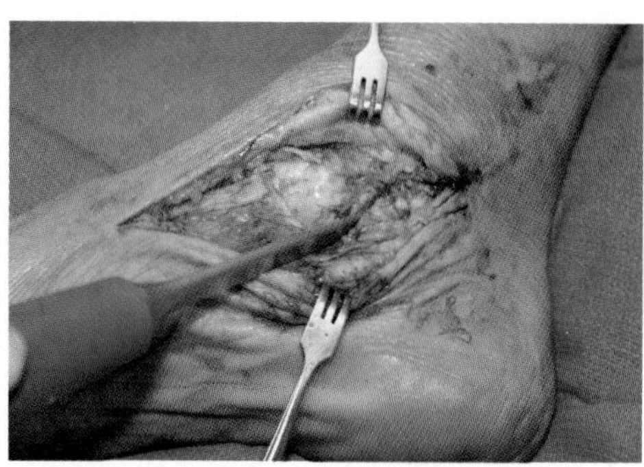

TECH FIG 3 • A scalpel or osteotome is used to identify the subtalar joint.

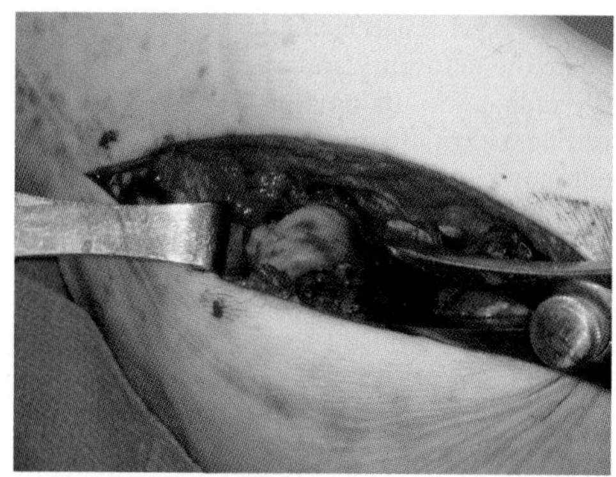

TECH FIG 4 • With a lamina spreader between the talar neck and the calcaneus, the middle and posterior facets of the subtalar joint are easily visualized.

EXPOSURE AND PREPARATION OF THE TALONAVICULAR JOINT

- Through the medial incision, the talonavicular joint is easily approached. Make a longitudinal capsulotomy in line with the skin incision over the talonavicular joint.
- Elevate the dorsal and plantar capsule off the joint to expose the articular surfaces.
- Insert an elevator across the talonavicular joint and use it to release the lateral capsule. This will permit distraction of the joint.
- Use a small lamina spreader to distract open the joint for preparation.
- Using curettes and osteotomes, remove the articular cartilage down to the subchondral plate.
- Use a curved osteotome to aggressively feather the articular surfaces of the talus and navicular.

EXPOSURE AND PREPARATION OF THE CALCANEOCUBOID JOINT

- Insert a large lamina spreader into the talonavicular joint and open it to gain access to the calcaneocuboid joint across the foot.
- Identify the calcaneocuboid joint using a scalpel or elevator. Check this position with intraoperative fluoroscopy.
- Use the elevator to open the joint. Pass a scalpel across the joint to release the lateral capsule and bifurcate ligaments (ligaments that bifurcate from the anterior process of the calcaneus and the cuboid and navicular). Be careful not to violate the lateral skin from inside to out as it will be placed on stretch with correction.
- Remove the articular cartilage with a combination of curettes and osteotomes down to subchondral bone.
- Aggressively feather the articular surfaces with a curved osteotome (TECH FIG 5).

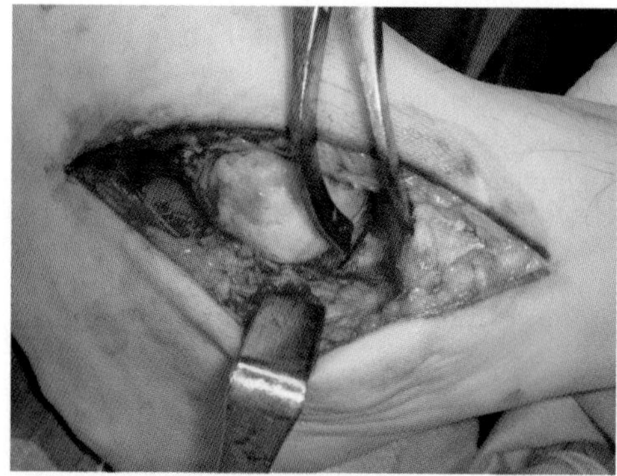

TECH FIG 5 • The calcaneocuboid joint is easily accessed across the foot after distracting open the talonavicular joint with a lamina spreader.

REDUCTION OF THE DEFORMITY AND INTERNAL FIXATION

- Based on the surgeon's preference, the talonavicular or subtalar joint is reduced and fixed first.
- Position the subtalar joint in 5 to 7 degrees of hindfoot valgus and fix it with a partially threaded 6.5-mm cannulated screw from the heel into the body of the talus. I also make sure that the calcaneus is translated fully under the talus; residual hindfoot valgus may look good on the operating table but will fail to do so once the patient bears weight.

- Reduce the transverse tarsal joints by adducting the transverse tarsal joints and pronating the forefoot. Fix the talonavicular joint with two parallel 4.5- to 5.0-mm cannulated screws from the navicular into the talar body.
- Fix the calcaneocuboid joint percutaneously. Insert the 4.5- or 5.0-mm cannulated screw dorsally on the cuboid and pass it retrograde into the tuberosity of the calcaneus (**TECH FIG 6**).

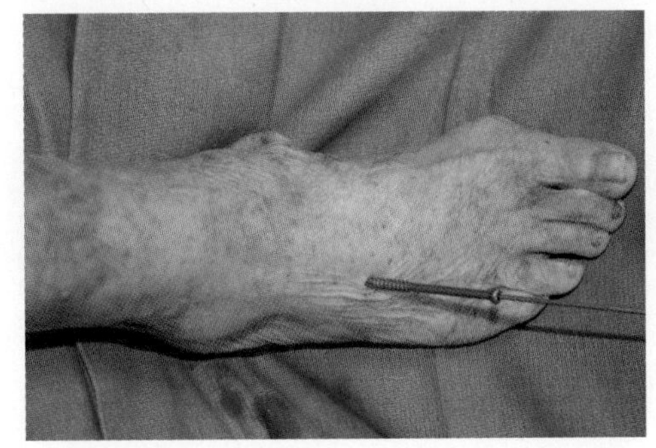

TECH FIG 6 • The calcaneocuboid joint is fixed percutaneously with a screw from distal to proximal.

PEARLS AND PITFALLS

Osteoporotic bone	▪ When spreading open the talonavicular joint to expose the calcaneocuboid joint, the lamina spreader may crush the talar head if the bone is soft. In these cases, prepare the calcaneocuboid joint first and leave the subchondral plate of the talonavicular joint intact to distract against. This will avoid crushing the talar head.
Incorrect identification of calcaneocuboid joint	▪ When approaching the calcaneocuboid joint from across the foot, confirm the position of the joint fluoroscopically before preparing it. The tarsometatarsal joint can be mistakenly entered from this approach.

POSTOPERATIVE CARE

- The patient is placed in a well-padded plaster splint until the incisions have healed. A cast or removable cam-boot is then used for immobilization until 12 weeks postoperatively. Patients are instructed to be strictly non–weight-bearing for the first 6 weeks; they then may progressively bear weight as tolerated. At 12 weeks, immobilization is discontinued and the patient is sent to physical therapy.

OUTCOMES

- Seventeen patients underwent single-medial-incision triple arthrodesis.
- All 17 demonstrated clinical improvement in alignment and pain relief.
- All talonavicular and subtalar joints healed (**FIG 4**).
- Radiographic correction was comparable to previous series describing traditional two-incision triple arthrodesis.
- In a cadaver study, 90% of the calcaneocuboid joint articular surface was able to be prepared successfully from the medial incision.

COMPLICATIONS

- Two of the 17 patients (12%) developed a nonunion of the calcaneocuboid joint. Neither of these was symptomatic.
- Three patients developed valgus ankle arthritis after successful triple arthrodesis. These were managed with total ankle replacement in two patients and ankle arthrodesis in one patient.

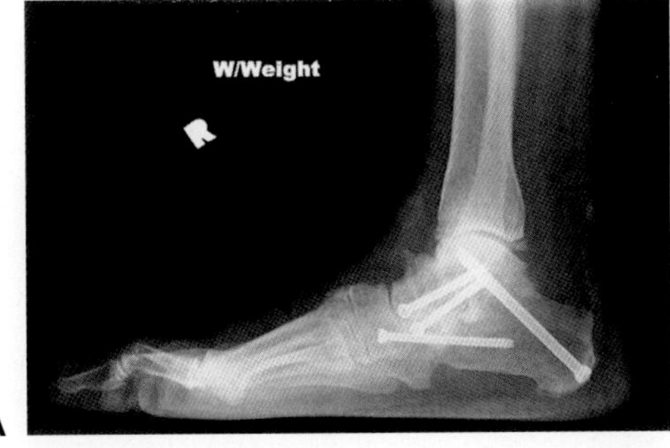

A

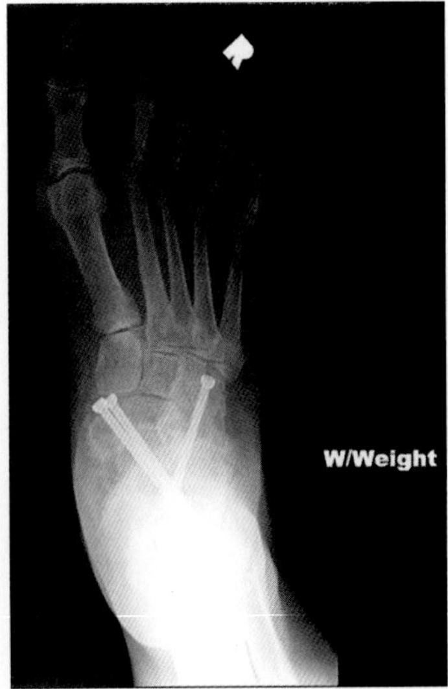

B

FIG 4 • After single-medial-incision triple arthrodesis, the patient shown in Figure 3 had excellent correction of her deformity without wound-healing complications.

REFERENCES

1. Brilhault J. Single medial approach to modified double arthrodesis in rigid flatfoot with lateral deficient skin. Foot Ankle Int 2009;30: 21–26.
2. Jackson WF, Tryfonidis M, Cooke PH, et al. Arthrodesis of the hindfoot for valgus deformity: an entirely medial approach. J Bone Joint Surg Br 2007;89B:925–927.
3. Jeng CL, Tankson CJ, Myerson MS. The single medial approach to triple arthrodesis: a cadaver study. Foot Ankle Int 2006;27: 1122–1125.
4. Jeng CL, Vora AM, Myerson MS. The medial approach to triple arthrodesis: indications and technique for management of rigid valgus deformities in high-risk patients. Foot Ankle Clin 2005;10: 515–521.
5. Knupp M, Schuh R, Stufkens SA, et al. Subtalar and talonavicular arthrodesis through a single medial approach for the correction of severe planovalgus deformity. J Bone Joint Surg Br 2009;91B: 612–615.
6. O'Malley MJ, Deland JT, Lee KT. Selective hindfoot arthrodesis for the treatment of adult acquired flatfoot deformity: an in vitro study. Foot Ankle Int 1995;16:411–417.
7. Sammarco VJ, Magur EG, Sammarco GJ, et al. Arthrodesis of the subtalar and talonavicular joints for correction of symptomatic hindfoot malalignment. Foot Ankle Int 2006;27:661–666.

Chapter 55 Comprehensive Correction of Cavovarus Foot Deformity

Michael Barnett, Arthur Manoli, Bruce J. Sangeorzan, Gregory C. Pomeroy, and Brian C. Toolan

SURGICAL MANAGEMENT

Preoperative Planning

- Imaging studies are reviewed.
- Physical examination should be done to test for rigidity or flexibility of the foot.
- Plain radiographs should be examined for arthritic changes, with triple arthrodesis reserved for severe, rigid deformity.[6]
- CT scanning can aid in determining arthritis when plain radiographs are unclear but suspicion is high.
- A tight Achilles tendon should be addressed during the same procedure (gastrocnemius recession, percutaneous, or open Achilles lengthening).
- Coleman block testing confirms forefoot-driven hindfoot varus or primary hindfoot varus.
- Concurrent problems, such as lateral ankle instability, should be addressed during the same procedure.

Positioning

- The patient is positioned supine on the table with the heel resting at the end of the bed (**FIG 1**).
- Thigh tourniquets are used and well padded.

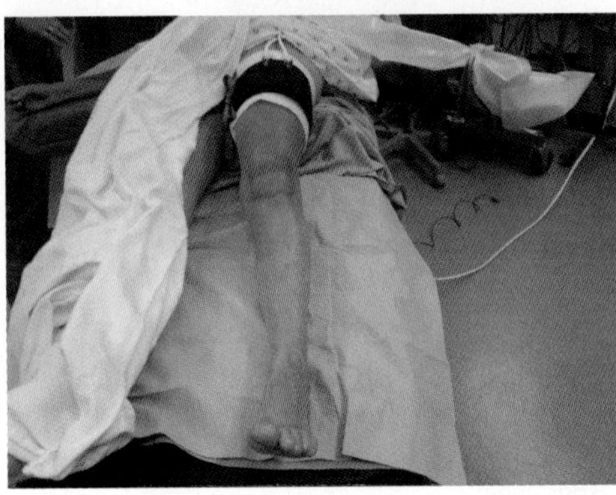

FIG 1 • Positioning for cavovarus reconstruction. The patient is supine with a bump under the ipsilateral hip. The foot is placed perpendicular to the floor to facilitate medial and lateral foot access.

- A bump is placed beneath the ipsilateral hip until the foot is perpendicular to the table to facilitate medial and lateral exposures if needed.
- The leg is prepared to the knee.

Approach

- Achilles tendon pathology is addressed first so this will minimize the deforming force on the heel when shifted.
- Either a lateral displacement or Dwyer-type osteotomy is performed, depending on the surgeon's preference, if rigid heel varus is present.
  - The lateral displacement osteotomy is used for most adult cases, as the Dwyer weakens the moment arm of the Achilles and often cannot achieve the desired correction.[7]
- Through the same incision, a peroneus longus to brevis transfer is done if appropriate.
- Attention is then turned toward the first metatarsal, where a dorsiflexion osteotomy of the first ray is performed until the first ray is out of plantarflexion.
  - This is the most common location needing osteotomy in our practice.
- For more severe cases, multiple metatarsal dorsiflexion osteotomies may be required in a similar fashion.[5]
- More advanced cases with extensive cavus through the midfoot and forefoot may require dorsal wedge osteotomies at more proximal levels, as described by multiple authors.[2,3]
- Adequate preoperative planning should alert the surgeon to the need for these more advanced procedures.
- A plantar fascia release is useful as an adjunct when midfoot flexion is severe and prevents adequate reduction of the forefoot after osteotomy.
  - This can also be done first in deformities associated with increased calcaneal pitch, where a proximal slide of the calcaneus is being done to lower the arch.
- A Jones procedure can be used to correct residual claw hallux with Girdlestone and Taylor hammer toe procedures for the lesser toes if required.
- Transfer of the tibialis posterior to the lateral cuneiform is a useful adjunct in cases of Charcot-Marie-Tooth associated with dorsiflexion weakness of the ankle.[4]

GASTROCNEMIUS RECESSION

TECHNIQUES

- Isolate the gastrocnemius fascia through a longitudinal incision just distal to the musculotendinous junction of the gastrocnemius on the medial side of the leg (**TECH FIG 1**).
- Identify the deep fascia of the leg and incise it in line with the incision, revealing the muscle and tendon structures beneath.
- The plantaris tendon will be visible along the medial border of the tendons and may be cut.
- Using blunt dissection, the separation of the deep soleus and the more superficial gastrocnemius can be recognized.
- The gastrocnemius fascia is easily isolated using a pediatric vaginal speculum, but various retraction techniques may be employed.
  - Retraction helps protect the sural nerve, which lies adjacent to the gastrocnemius at this level near the midline.
- Once isolated, cut the entire fascia transversely using tenotomy scissors.
- Fifteen to 20 degrees of increased ankle dorsiflexion with the knee extended can usually be obtained.
- Reapproximate the deep fascia using 3-0 absorbable sutures.

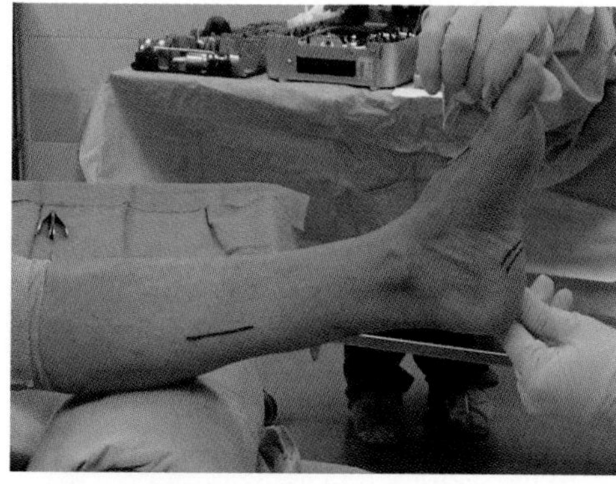

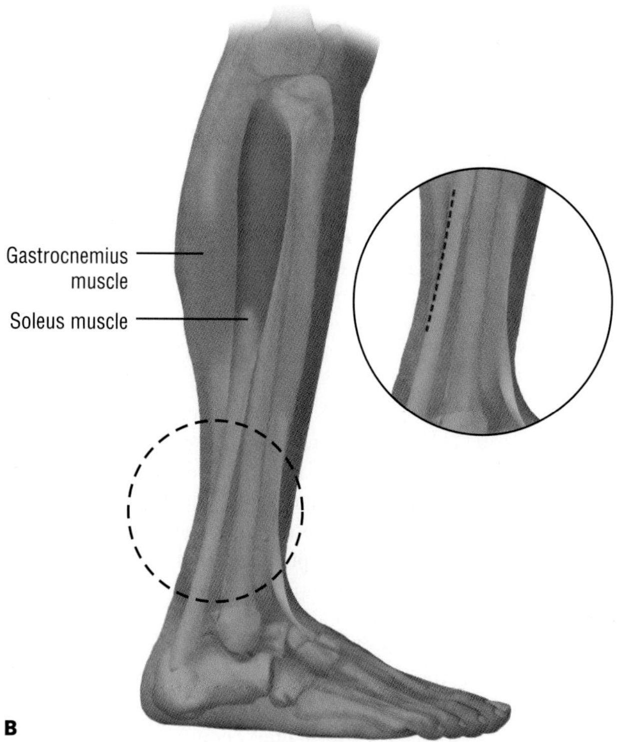

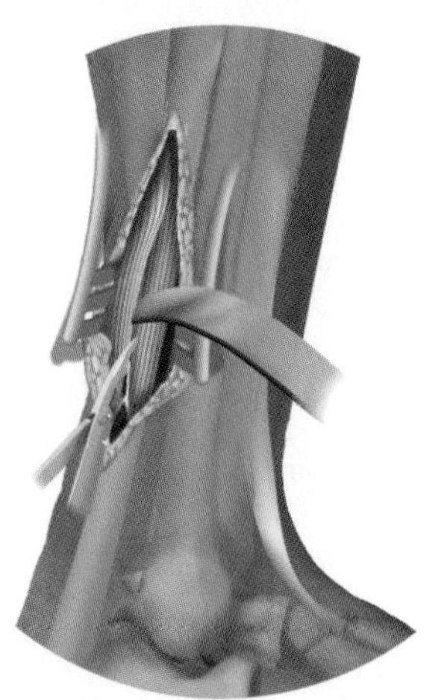

TECH FIG 1 • A. Location of incision along medial leg. **B.** Deep fascia has been incised, revealing division of gastrocnemius and soleus fascias. **C.** Gastrocnemius fascia is isolated and cut from medial to lateral using tenotomy scissors. This protects the overlying sural nerve and saphenous vein.

LATERAL DISPLACEMENT CALCANEAL OSTEOTOMY AND PERONEUS LONGUS TO BREVIS TRANSFER

- The incision to accomplish both of these procedures is made inferior to but parallel to the peroneus longus tendon (**TECH FIG 2**).
- Deepen the dissection from the original incision until the peroneal tendons are identified.
- Enter the sheaths for the length of the incision, making sure to preserve the superior peroneal retinaculum (SPR).
  - The SPR may be taken down directly off the posterior fibula and reattached with a suture anchor if tendon pathology exists such as tears or instability, such as in our example.
  - Otherwise, the tendons can be sutured together, preserving this structure.
- Remove a section of the peroneus longus with a knife.
- Reapproximate the longus and brevis tendons proximally and hold them together with figure 8-0 nonabsorbable suture, making sure the knot does not impinge below the SPR.
- Carry dissection inferior to the sural nerve, taking care to identify and protect it.
- Once the calcaneus is reached, carry the subperiosteal dissection inferior.
- Place small Hohmann retractors superior and anterior to the calcaneal tuberosity, protecting the insertion of the Achilles tendon and the origin of the plantar fascia, respectively.
- With soft tissues protected, use a sagittal saw to make the osteotomy perpendicular to the axis of the calcaneus.
- Shift the free tuberosity piece lateral until a physiologic valgus position of 5 degrees is obtained (usually 8 to 10 mm).
- Make a midline longitudinal incision just off the posterior plantar heel pad.
- Carry dissection straight through subcutaneous fat to bone.
- An assistant or Kirschner wire holds the heel shift in the corrected position while two 6.5-mm partially threaded cancellous screws are placed in lag fashion.
- The screws should be off the posterior weight-bearing surface of the heel and should not penetrate the subtalar joint.
- Use a rasp to smooth down the prominent lateral bone after the heel shift.

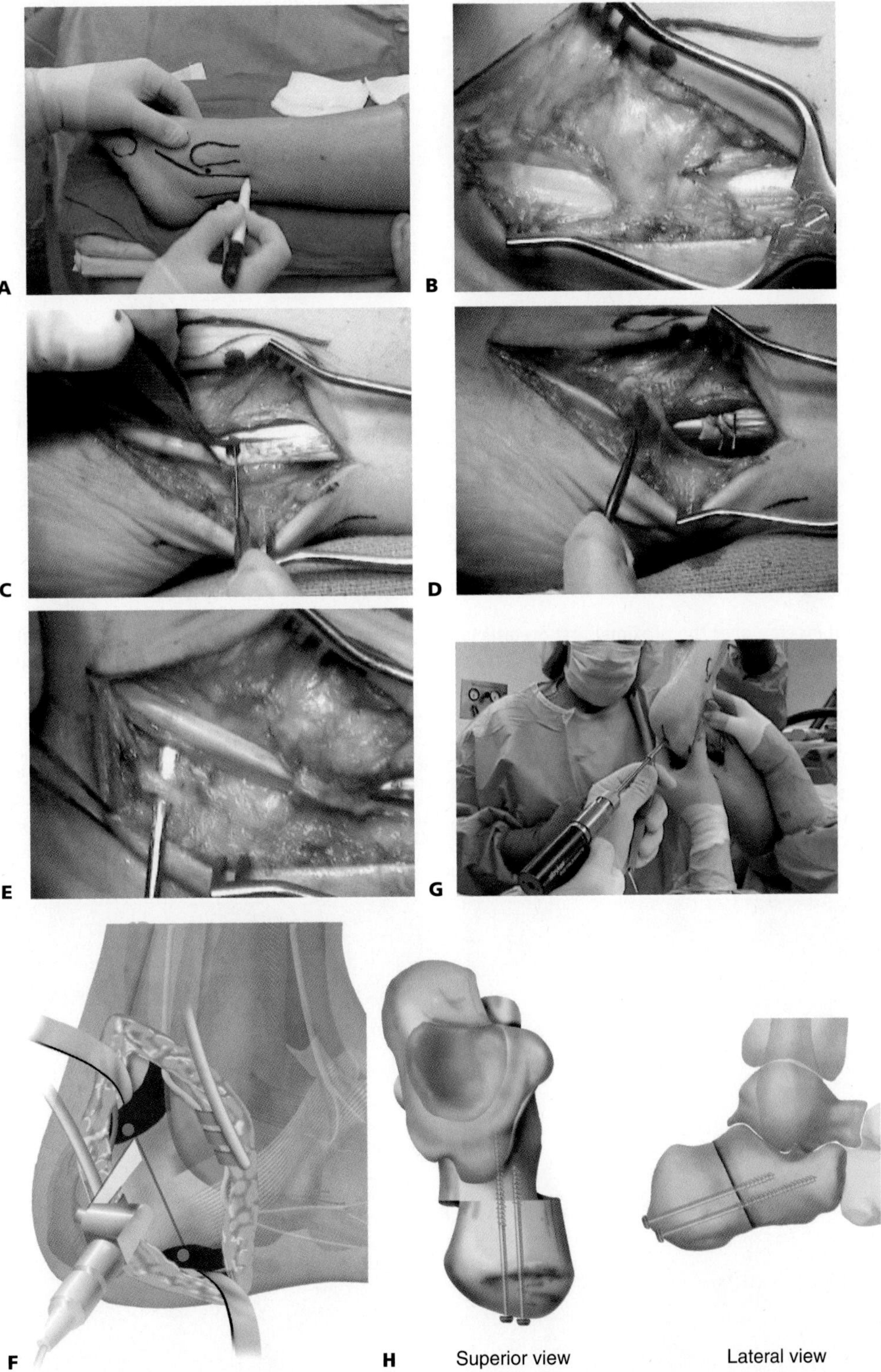

TECH FIG 2 • Lateral displacement calcaneal osteotomy and peroneus longus to brevis transfer. **A.** Lateral incision over hindfoot just posterior to peroneal tendons. **B.** Dissection carried down to the peroneal tendons, with the superior peroneal retinaculum still intact. **C.** With the superior peroneal retinaculum flap taken posterior, a section of the peroneus longus is removed. **D.** The peroneus longus has been sutured to the brevis, making sure the knot does not impinge under the superior peroneal retinaculum through range of motion of the tendon. **E.** Sural nerve is identified as dissection is carried inferior. **F.** A saw is used to cut across the calcaneus, perpendicular to its long axis, protecting the Achilles and plantar fascia. **G.** An assistant holds the lateral shift while two 6.5-mm partially threaded cancellous screws are placed across the osteotomy. **H.** Final screw positioning as seen from lateral and superior views.

DWYER LATERAL CLOSING-WEDGE CALCANEAL OSTEOTOMY

- Use the approach outlined above for the lateral sliding calcaneal osteotomy.
- Instead of a transverse cut with a shift, remove a wedge of bone, based laterally, using a sagittal saw (TECH FIG 3).
- The size of the wedge depends on the desired correction but should bring the heel to a physiologic valgus position.
- Once the bone is removed, dorsiflex the foot to close the wedge and proceed with fixation as described previously.[1]

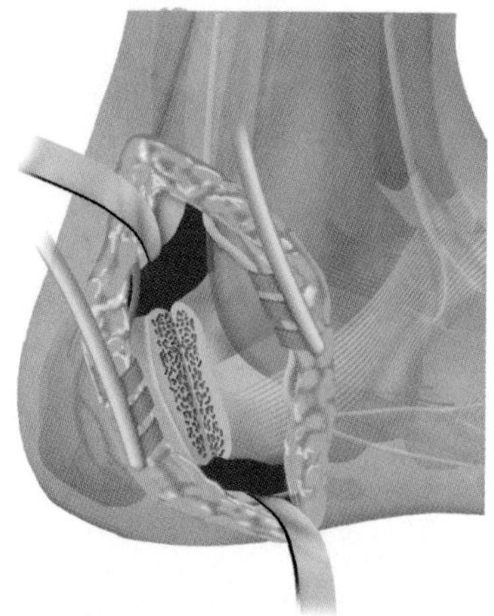

TECH FIG 3 • Dwyer calcaneal osteotomy. Instead of a straight cut through bone, a lateral-based wedge is removed.

FIRST METATARSAL DORSIFLEXION OSTEOTOMY

- Make a dorsal incision over the proximal first metatarsal and carry dissection down to the extensor tendons (TECH FIG 4).
  - Retract them lateral so dissection can be carried down to bone.
- Subperiosteal dissection allows exposure of the proximal metatarsal to the first tarsometatarsal joint.
- Mark a line transversely on the bone 1 cm from the joint for the bone cut.
- Place small Hohmann retractors around the bone to protect the soft tissues, and perform a dorsal closing-wedge osteotomy using a sagittal saw.
- The first cut is through 90% of the bone and perpendicular to the diaphysis.
- The second cut is 2 to 3 mm distal and angled back toward the plantar endpoint of the first cut.
- Complete the first cut and remove the bone wedge. Take enough bone to restore anatomic alignment of the talus

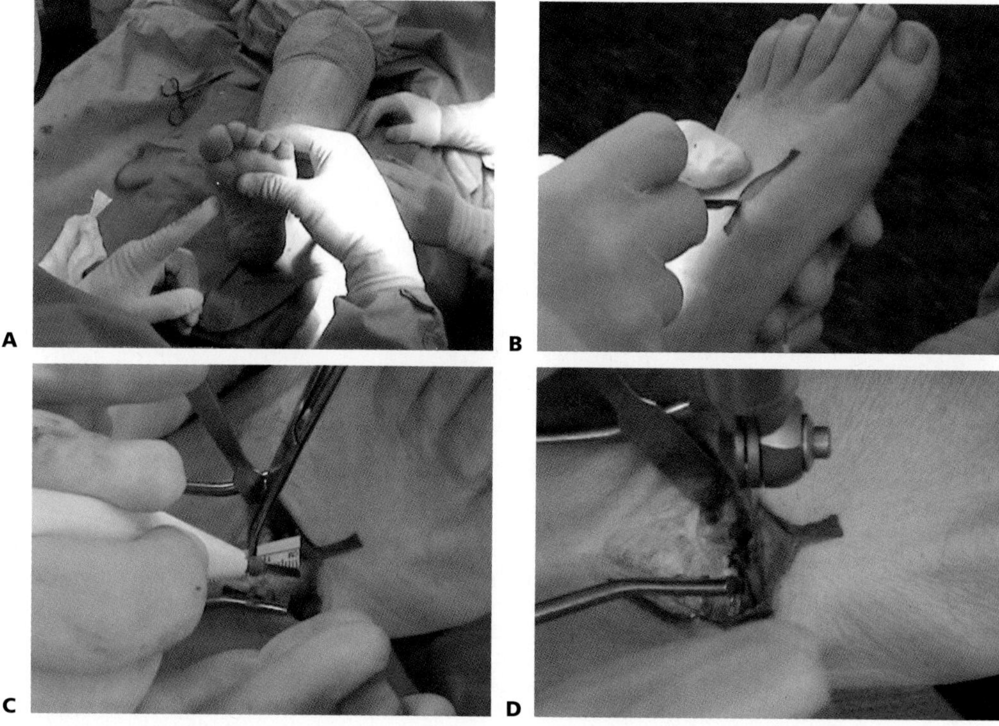

TECH FIG 4 • First metatarsal dorsiflexion osteotomy. **A.** Plantarflexed first ray. **B.** Incision over first metatarsal. **C.** Measuring 1 cm from first tarsometatarsal joint. **D.** A small dorsally based wedge is removed. *(continued)*

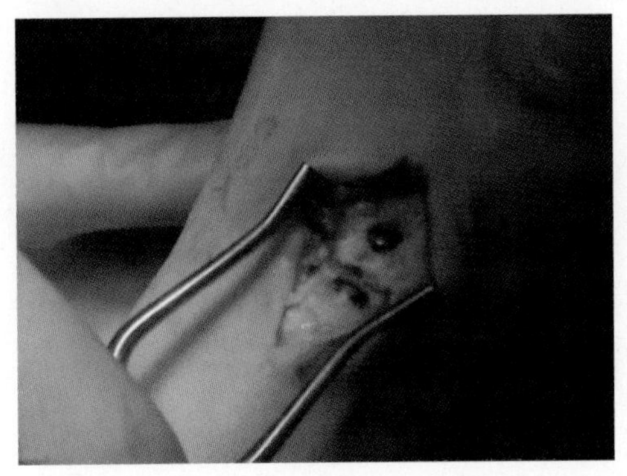

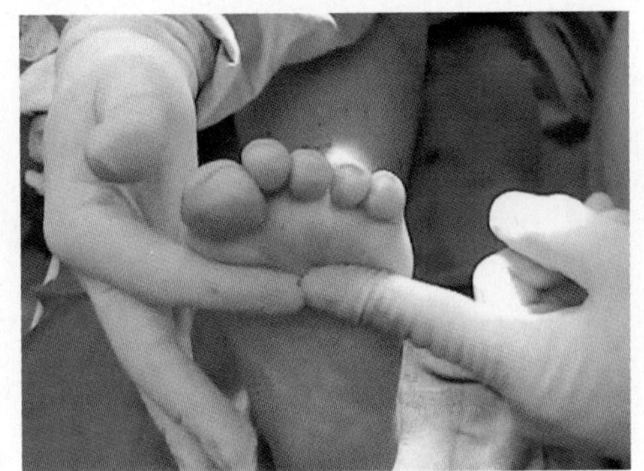

TECH FIG 4 • *(continued)* **E.** The wedge is closed and held with a screw recessed in the first metatarsal. **F.** Final first ray position.

and first metatarsal on the lateral radiograph (about 0 degrees).

- Use a small burr to make a shallow hole in the dorsal bone to recess the screw head.
- Reduce the first metatarsal and place a 3.5-mm lag screw from the burr hole across the osteotomy, taking care not to enter the first tarsometatarsal joint.

PARTIAL PLANTAR FASCIOTOMY

- Make an incision just distal and parallel to the plantar heel pad (**TECH FIG 5**).
- Dissection through subcutaneous fat exposes the plantar fascia.
- When the medial and lateral borders of the fascia are identified, partial or complete release may be undertaken.
- Begin transection 1 cm from the origin on the calcaneus and proceed medial to lateral.
- More severe deformities may require more of a release.

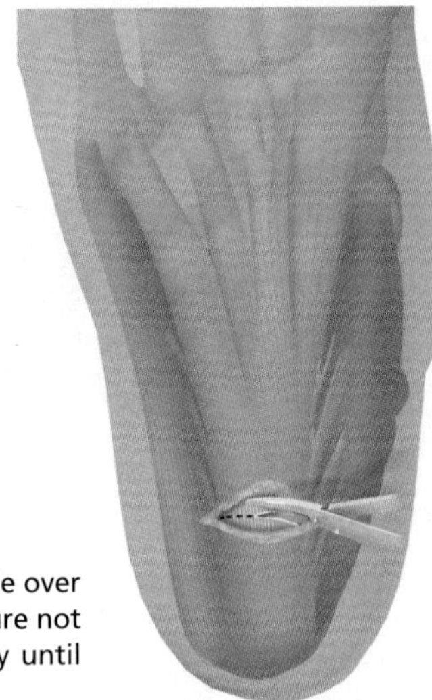

TECH FIG 5 • Partial plantar fasciotomy. Incision is made over medial hindfoot, off weight-bearing surface, making sure not to disturb nerves. The plantar fascia is cut transversely until desired correction is achieved.

JONES PROCEDURE

- The interphalangeal (IP) fusion of the great toe begins with a transverse incision over the IP joint dorsally (**TECH FIG 6**).
- Cut the extensor hallucis and make an arthrotomy in the joint, freeing up the collateral ligaments.
- Use curettes to remove the articular cartilage and use a 2-mm drill bit to fenestrate both sides of the joint.
- Place a Kirschner wire from proximal to distal through the distal phalanx and out the tip of the toe just under the nail, leaving minimal wire within the joint.
- Place the wire retrograde across the IP joint while holding it reduced.
- Make a transverse incision at the toe tip to allow drilling over the wire.
- Measure the length of screw so it does not penetrate the metatarsophalangeal joint.
- Place a 4.0-mm partially threaded cannulated screw over the wire for compression.
- Confirm the position on fluoroscopy and remove the wire.
- Center a dorsal midline incision over the first metatarsal neck.
- Identify the extensor hallucis longus and bring its distal end into the wound.
- Make 4.0-mm drill holes on the medial and lateral aspects of the metatarsal neck and connect them using a curette.
- Pass the tendon from lateral to medial through the hole and suture it back on to itself using nonabsorbable suture while holding the ankle in a neutral to slightly dorsiflexed position.

TECHNIQUES

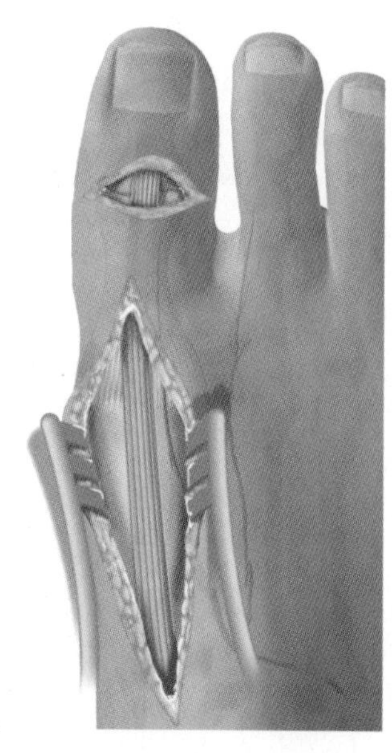

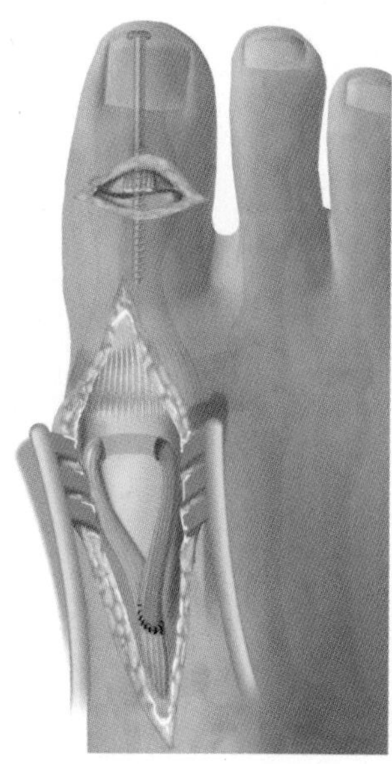

TECH FIG 6 • Jones procedure of first toe. **A.** Incision is made transversely over the interphalangeal joint to remove cartilage and harvest extensor hallucis longus tendon. **B.** Incision is made longitudinally over the first metatarsal, transferring the tendon to the neck, and a screw is placed across the interphalangeal joint in lag mode.

PEARLS AND PITFALLS

Preoperative assessment	▪ A neurologic workup is indicated if no identifiable neurologic cause for deformity is known, as a progressive muscle imbalance may cause recurrence.
Heel screw placement	▪ With a lateral heel shift, the tendency is to place screws too far lateral. ▪ The drill should be angled slightly medial to ensure entering the remaining calcaneus.
First metatarsal osteotomy	▪ The tendency is to take too little of a dorsal wedge, leaving the first metatarsal plantarflexed and making the patient susceptible to recurrence.
Plantar fascia release	▪ The medial calcaneal branch of the tibial nerve and the intrinsic musculature of the foot are at risk, so careful dissection is warranted.

POSTOPERATIVE CARE

- Posterior sugar-tong splinting is used immediately postoperatively with the ankle in neutral dorsiflexion.
- Skin staples are removed at 2 weeks.
- Patients are kept immobilized and non–weight-bearing for a total of 8 weeks, and weight bearing is begun when bony healing has occurred.

OUTCOMES

- Long-term studies of cavovarus correction in adults are lacking, likely given the varied presentation and multiple modes of treatment for the disorder.
- Early treatment while feet are flexible is advised to prevent more extensive procedures required for rigid deformities and complications from progressive arthrosis.

COMPLICATIONS

- Painful hardware
- Infection
- Recurrence of deformity
- Wound dehiscence
- Nonunion

REFERENCES

1. Dwyer FC. The present status of the problem of pes cavus. Clin Orthop Relat Res 1975;106:254–275.
2. Jahss MH. Tarsometatarsal truncated-wedge arthrodesis for pes cavus and equinovarus deformity of the fore part of the foot. J Bone Joint Surg Am 1980;62A:713–722.
3. Japas LM. Surgical treatment of pes cavus by tarsal V-osteotomy: preliminary report. J Bone Joint Surg Am 1968;50AL927–944.
4. McCluskey WP, Lovell WW, Cummings RJ. The cavovarus foot deformity: etiology and management. Clin Orthop Relat Res 1989; 247:27–37.
5. Sammarco GJ, Taylor R. Cavovarus foot treated with combined calcaneus and metatarsal osteotomies. Foot Ankle Int 2001;22:19–30.
6. Wetmore RS, Drennan JC. Long-term results of triple arthrodesis in Charcot-Marie-Tooth disease. J Bone Joint Surg Am 1989;71A: 417–422.
7. Younger AE, Hansen ST. Adult cavovarus foot. J Am Acad Orthop Surg 2005;13:302–315.

Chapter 56

Management of Equinocavovarus Foot Deformity

Wolfram Wenz and Thomas Dreher

DEFINITION

- Pes cavus is characterized by increased plantarflexion of the forefoot and midfoot in relation to the hindfoot. An isolated pes cavus is rare; it is commonly accompanied by other deformities of the foot. Therefore, pes cavus should be classified in different groups: pes cavovarus, pes equinocavus, pes calcaneocavus, and pes valgocavus (**FIG 1**). In many cases a combination of the first two types occurs, called the pes equinocavovarus.
- The equinocavovarus foot describes a mostly acquired foot deformity consisting of an increased arch of the foot (forefoot and midfoot equinus), a limited dorsiflexion of the ankle joint (hindfoot equinus), and a hindfoot varus. A concomitant forefoot and midfoot adductus, supinatus, or pronatus can occur, depending on the underlying pathology.
- "The cavovarus foot is one of the most perplexing and challenging of all foot deformities."[2]
- "The literature on pes cavus is extremely confusing."[15]

ANATOMY

- Equinus deformity of the ankle (limited dorsiflexion)
- Hindfoot in varus position (inversion of the calcaneus, flexible or rigid)

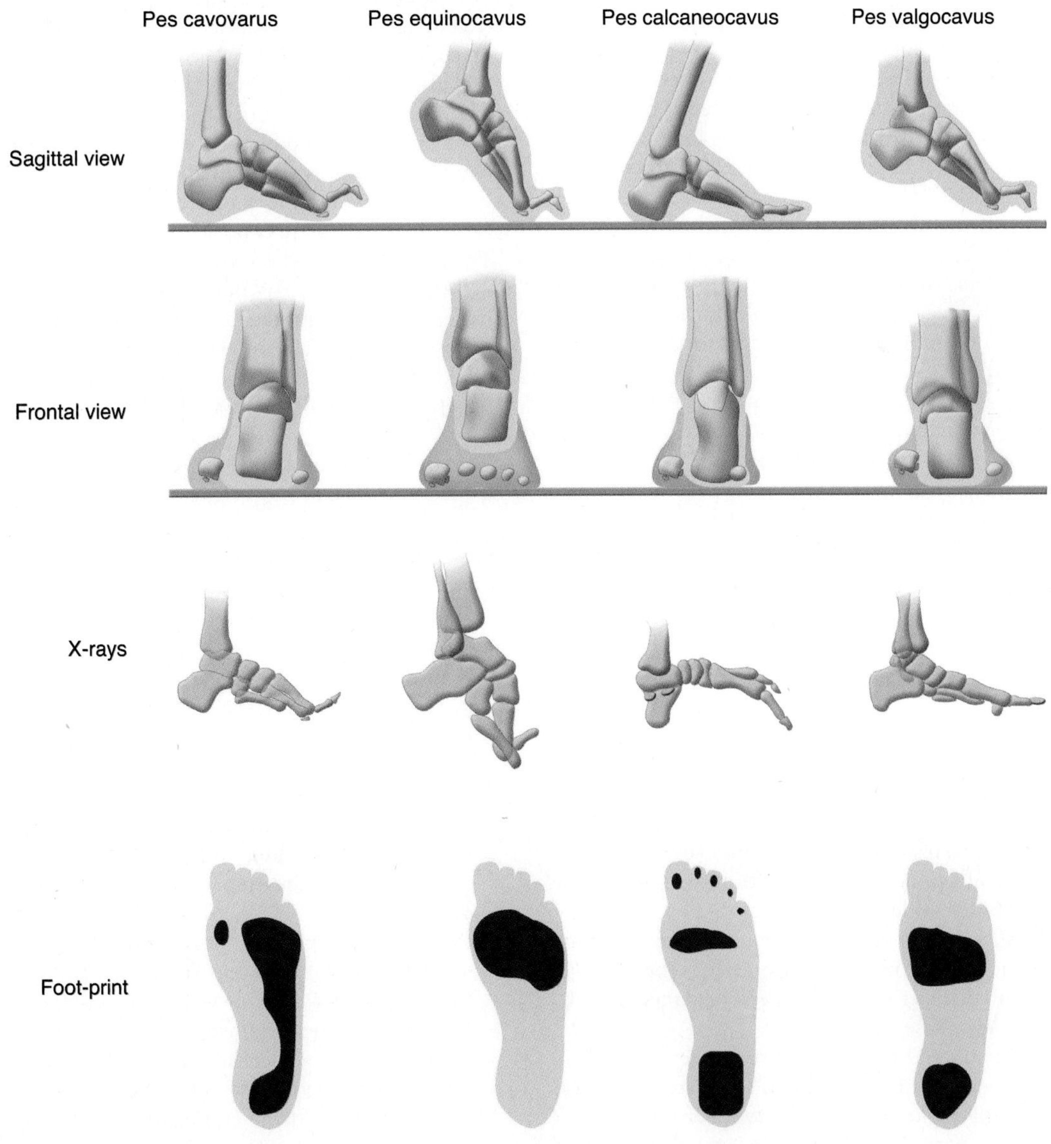

FIG 1 • Cavus foot deformities.

- External rotation of the talus and retraction of the lateral malleolus
- Medial dislocation of the navicular and the cuboid bone in the Chopart joint
- Cavus deformity medially (flexible or rigid)
- Plantarflexed position of the first metatarsal bone (flexible or rigid)
- Pronation and adduction of the forefoot (flexible or rigid)
- Claw toes, isolated to the hallux or involving all five toes (flexible or fixed)

PATHOGENESIS

- "...a story of repeated failure to comprehend the basic pathogenesis and mechanics of a deformity which remains a mystery to this day, comparable only to problems such as scoliosis."[6]
- There are various theories concerning the pathogenesis of pes equinocavovarus:
  - "There is little doubt that the condition is caused by a muscle imbalance, involving both the intrinsic and the extrinsic muscles of the foot."[15]
  - Weakness of the anterior tibial muscle (progressive plantarflexion of the first metatarsal bone) because of relative overactivity of the long peroneal muscle; the long toe extensors try to compensate the reduced dorsiflexion force of the anterior tibial muscle. This results in an overbalance of the extrinsic extensor muscles in comparison to the intrinsic extensor muscles. The toes are hyperextended in the metatarsophalangeal joints. At the same time the long toe flexors pull the end phalangeal bone into plantarflexion. Both mechanisms result in increased cavus (forefoot and midfoot equinus).
  - Weakness of the short peroneal muscle (peroneus brevis). Relative overactivity of the posterior tibial muscle forces the hindfoot into varus position. The force of the long toe flexors (increased flexion of the metatarsophalangeal joints) is antagonized by increased activity of the long peroneal muscle (peroneus longus) that also pulls the first metatarsal bone into plantarflexion. Because of its limited effects on the hindfoot, the peroneus longus cannot antagonize the overactivity of the posterior tibial muscle.

NATURAL HISTORY

- One functionally relevant consequence of the deformity is the limited ankle dorsiflexion. Its causes can be an isolated shortened Achilles tendon, which is rare. An acquired horizontal position of the talus resulting from hindfoot supination can cause a limited dorsiflexion. The cavus deformity itself may be responsible for limited ankle dorsiflexion.
- The limited ankle dorsiflexion in pes equinocavovarus may cause a genu recurvatum. Another consequence is toe walking with excessive load transfer to the metatarsophalangeal joints and a reduced stance phase of gait.
- Pronation in the subtalar joint is inhibited, potentially causing impingement between the medial malleolus and the talus, similar to the impingement in severe clubfoot deformity.
- Another consequence is the medialization of the navicular, which migrates toward the medial malleolus to cause additional bony impingement. Osteophytes often develop at the talar neck.
- In the case of a concomitant hindfoot equinus and subtalar joint compensation, the acquired varus stress in the subtalar joint frequently cannot be compensated by the ankle joint, leading to eventual varus talar tilt in the ankle mortise.

PATIENT HISTORY AND PHYSICAL FINDINGS

- A characteristic description of a patient with pes equinocavovarus can be found in the book by Tubby and Jones[22] for Charcot-Marie-Tooth (hereditary motor sensory neuropathy):
- "The patient was a healthy-looking country-woman, aged fifty-six years, practically free from any disability from this condition. The patient stated that when about seven years old she found that her ankles, especially the right, easily 'turned in', and that consequently she often suffered from sprains. She was unaware that there was anything unusual about her hands. The muscles of the rest of the upper extremity and of the shoulder girdle did not appear to be in any way affected. In the lower extremity deformity was more advanced and unequally developed on either side. On the right the foot was hollowed and inverted, and also somewhat dropped. The tendon of the tibialis anticus stood out as a taut cord. The toes and ankle joint could be freely moved in all directions except that of eversion, owing to complete paralysis of the peronei muscles. In addition to pes cavus there was some equinovarus. The other muscles of the lower extremity were capable of causing powerful movements. The knee jerks could not be obtained."
- "A man, aged thirty-one years, the third child of the above patient showed a marked club-foot on both sides, and the feet were inverted and dropped, but without any contracture of tendons. The power of dorsiflexion and of eversion was completely lost. The toes were in the characteristic position."

Dynamic Examination

- Problems during stance phase of the gait cycle
  - Initial contact with the toes (toe walking, hindfoot equinus, limited dorsiflexion)
  - Hyperextension of the knee (genu recurvatum, due to equinus) and proximal compensatory mechanisms
  - Overload of the lateral border of the foot (varus deformity)
  - Instability in loading response of the gait cycle
  - Main load on the first and fifth metatarsal head, in some cases with ulceration
  - Limited roll-off movement due to reduced dorsiflexion in mid-stance
  - Internal rotation moment due to rolling off over the lateral border of the foot and the forefoot
  - Missing load bearing of the toe tips due to claw toe deformity
- Problems during swing phase of the gait cycle
  - Drop foot (weak extensor muscles, primarily the anterior tibial muscle) with foot clearance problems; this is aggravated by hindfoot equinus
  - Compensatory mechanisms for drop foot (eg, increased knee or hip flexion, circumduction of the leg)
  - Equinus foot at the end of the swing phase, which leads to forefoot initial contact
  - Overactivity of the long toe extensors to compensate for decreased dorsiflexion force with consecutive claw toe deformity

Methods for Examining the Equinocavovarus Foot Deformity

- In stance: medial view. The examiner inspects the medial aspect of the foot, evaluating for elevated heel, increased medial arch, plantarflexion of the first metatarsal bone, and claw toe deformity of the first column of the foot.
- In stance: lateral view. The examiner inspects the lateral aspect of the foot, evaluating for posterior shift of the lateral malleolus, convexity of the lateral border of the foot, prominent basis of the fifth metatarsal bone, and prominent head of the talus on the lateral dorsum of the foot.
- In stance: dorsal view. The examiner inspects the posterior aspect of the foot, evaluating for varus deformity of the heel, elevation of the heel, prominent lateral malleolus, pronation of the forefoot, and "hello big toe" sign (normally, the hallux cannot be seen from posterior view, but in case of forefoot adduction it may be visible).
- In stance: plantar view. The examiner inspects the plantar aspect of the foot, evaluating for convex lateral border of the foot and prominent basis of the fifth metatarsal bone, increased weight bearing of the heads of the first and fifth metatarsal bones, increased skin wheal (in severe cases, the heads of all metatarsal bones are involved), and hindfoot equinus (lack of weight bearing on the heel).
- In stance: anterior view. The examiner inspects the ventral aspect of the foot, evaluating for lateral prominence of the talar head, convex lateral border of the foot, forefoot adduction, and clawing of the first through fifth toes.
- Coleman block.[3] With a block placed under the hindfoot and the second through fifth toes, the examiner tests the compensability of the hindfoot in fixed forefoot pronation and compensation of the plantarflexion of the first metatarsal bone.
- Silfverskiöld test.[18] Dorsiflexion is examined in knee flexion and knee extension. This test is important for detecting equinus deformity and differentiating between the involvement of gastrocnemius and soleus muscles.
- "Trying to assess actions of individual muscles is a trap for the unwary because muscle action is so much one of synergism and unassessable motive power that it becomes impossible to apportion with any accuracy the actions of single muscles."[6]

Problems Due to Footwear

- Ulcerations over the interphalangeal joints of the toes
- The food is broad and short (problems wearing regular shoes)
- Wearing out of the lateral border of the shoes or the forefoot, respectively

Further Problems

- Cosmetically disturbing
- Rapid fatigue
- Progressive deformities

IMAGING AND OTHER DIAGNOSTIC STUDIES

Conventional Radiographs

- Lateral view (standing) (**FIG 2A**)
  - Posterior shift of the lateral malleolus
  - The longitudinal axis of the talus is parallel to the axis of the calcaneus.
  - The calcaneus seems to be shortened due to varus position.
  - There is decreased distance between the navicular and the medial malleolus.
  - The calcaneocuboid joint is visible; it is normally obscured by the talonavicular joint.
  - The first metatarsal is plantarflexed and its head has a plantar prominence.
  - Claw toes
  - The posterior subtalar joint is projected horizontally.
  - Opened sinus tarsi ("sinus tarsi window")
- AP view (standing) (**FIG 2B**)
  - Longitudinal axes of the talus and calcaneus are parallel.
  - There is a medial shift of the talonavicular joint and in some cases the calcaneocuboid joint.
  - The first metatarsal seems to be shortened, due to its plantarflexed position.
  - There is overlapping of the metatarsal bones, especially the fourth and fifth.
- AP view of the ankle joint (standing) (**FIG 2C**)
  - Varus deformity of the ankle joint?
  - Hindfoot varus

Computed Tomography with 3D Reconstruction

- In severe cases CT imaging with 3D reconstruction may be needed (**FIG 2D**).

Dynamic Pedobarography

- An objective method to measure the pressure distribution pattern is the dynamic pedobarography EMED® examination.
- It is used to identify the imbalance of the major pressure points of the foot due to the deformity.
- A mildly involved footprint is shown in comparison with the typical pattern for a severe equinocavovarus foot (**FIG 2E**).

A
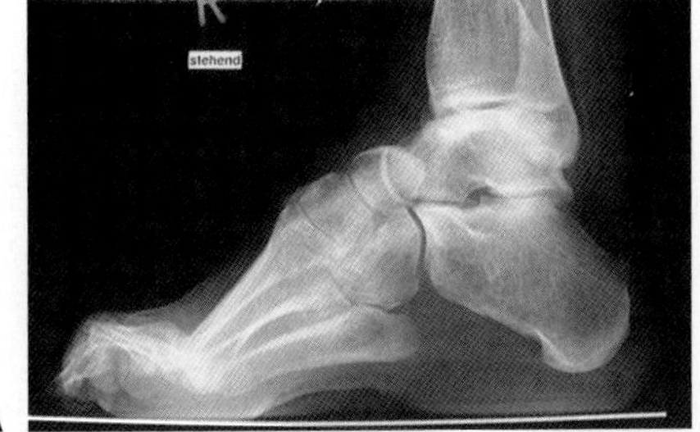

B
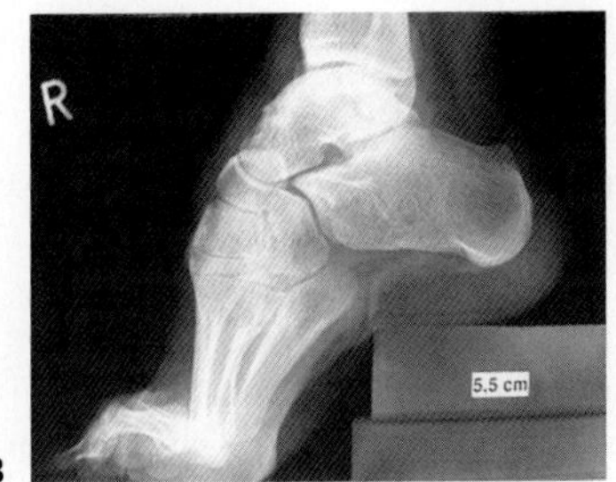

FIG 2 • Conventional radiograph. **A,B.** Lateral view with and without correction of the forefoot equinus. *(continued)*

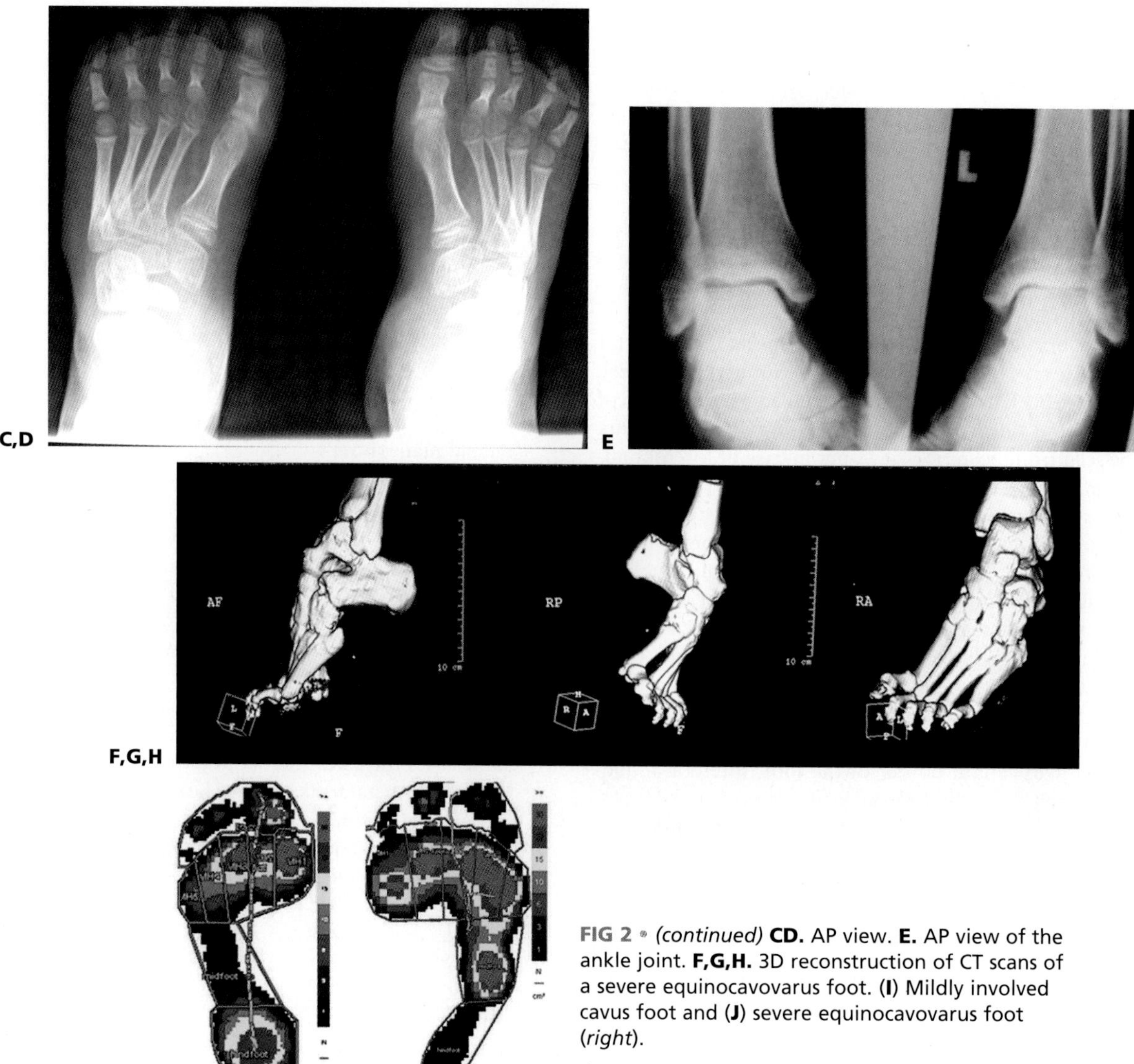

FIG 2 • *(continued)* **CD.** AP view. **E.** AP view of the ankle joint. **F,G,H.** 3D reconstruction of CT scans of a severe equinocavovarus foot. (**I**) Mildly involved cavus foot and (**J**) severe equinocavovarus foot (*right*).

3D Foot and Gait Analysis (Heidelberg Foot Model®)

- This objective and computer-assisted method records movements between single segments of the foot in all three planes (sagittal, frontal, transverse) during walking.
- The foot and shank are equipped at typical anatomic landmarks with 17 reflective markers (**FIG 3**).[16] Special cameras send and record reflected ultrared light while the patient walks over a defined distance.
- After processing by dedicated software, characteristic segment movements in all three planes can be visualized.

DIFFERENTIAL DIAGNOSIS

Pes equinocavovarus can occur in different primary diseases:

- Central nervous system
  - Progressive diseases
    - Increased muscle tone (eg, multiple sclerosis)
    - Reduced muscle tone (eg, tethered cord syndrome)
    - Diastematomyelia, syringomyelia, intraspinal tumor
  - Limited diseases
    - Increased muscle tone (cerebral palsy, traumatic brain injuries, stroke)
    - Reduced muscle tone (eg, spina bifida)
    - Lipoma, angioma
    - Encephalitis
- Peripheral nervous system
  - Progressive diseases
    - Hereditary sensory motor neuropathy (Charcot-Marie-Tooth disease)
    - Spinal muscular atrophy
    - Polyneuropathy
  - Limited diseases
    - Poliomyelitis
    - Arthrogryposis multiplex congenita
- Other causes
  - Compartment syndrome
  - Burn injuries
  - Inflammatory arthritides
  - Diabetic neuropathy

NONOPERATIVE MANAGEMENT

- "Nonsurgical management of cavus, cavovarus and calcaneocavus is uniformly unsuccessful in the long run."[20]

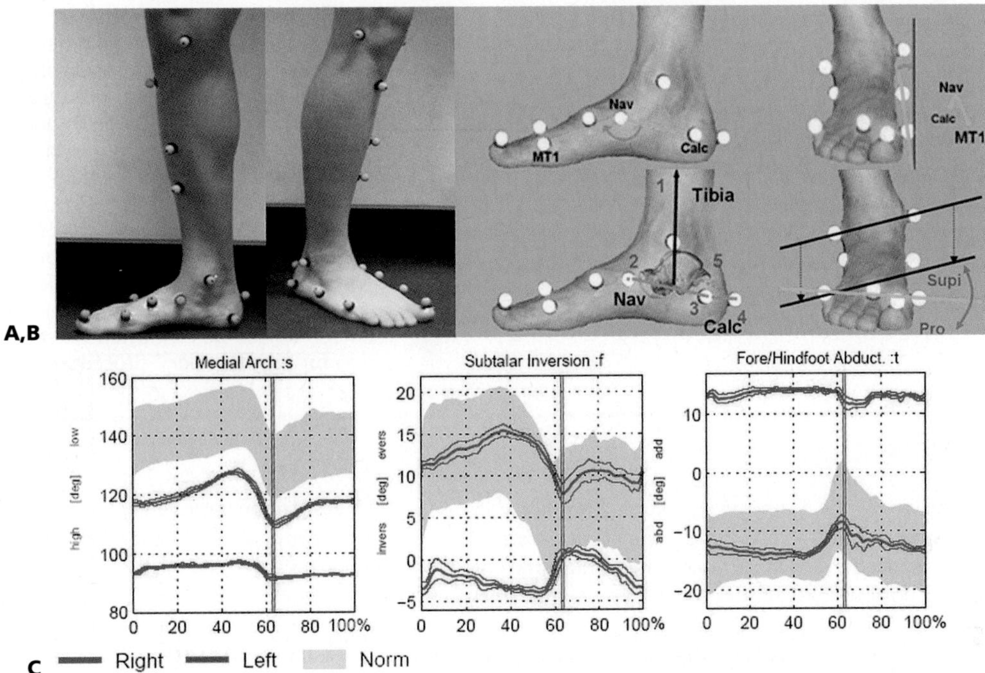

FIG 3 • Heidelberg foot motion measurement. **A.** Marker placement and angle calculation. **B.** Examples of motions in different planes for an equinocavovarus foot. **C.** *Left*: increased medial arch; *middle*: increased subtalar inversion; *right*: increased forefoot adduction.

- "Nonoperative measures generally do not stop progression or prevent deformity, therefore their role is extremely limited."[17]
- Nonoperative treatment can only compensate for the functional problems in pes equinocavovarus; it cannot stop its progression.
- Possible nonoperative treatment methods are:
  - Orthopaedic arch support (reduced head of the first metatarsal bone and smooth bedding)
  - Orthopaedic shoes

SURGICAL MANAGEMENT

Preoperative Planning

- "Muscle balance is the key to understanding the production of pes cavus."[12]
- "A foot will deform in the presence of a solid, well-performed triple arthrodesis when the foot is not in gross muscular balance....When definite muscular imbalance is evident, tendon transfer is mandatory."[10]
- Preoperative clinical examination, radiographs, EMED, dynamic foot analysis (instrumented foot gait analysis), and clinical examination (Silfverskiöld test[18]) under anesthesia represent optimal preoperative planning.

Positioning

- The patient is placed supine on the operating table. We routinely drape the iliac crest into the operative field when there may be a need for iliac crest bone harvest (**FIG 4**).

Approach

- The different approaches that we consider in equinocavovarus deformity correction are shown in **FIGURE 5**.
  - Dorsal incision for the modified Jones[4] procedure
  - Lateral–dorsal incision for the triple or Lambrinudi arthrodesis[14] or the Cole procedure[1] and the posterior tibial tendon transfer as well as the Russel-Hibbs procedure[8]
  - Ventral incision for the posterior tibial tendon transfer[19]
  - Distal medial shank incision for the open Achilles tendon lengthening, the posterior tibial tendon transfer, and, if needed, the intramuscular lengthening of the long toe flexors
  - Skin incision for the triple or Lambrinudi arthrodesis,[14] the Cole procedure,[1] and the posterior tibial tendon transfer; this incision can be connected with the previous one (distal medial shank) if needed
  - Skin incision for the Steindler procedure[19]

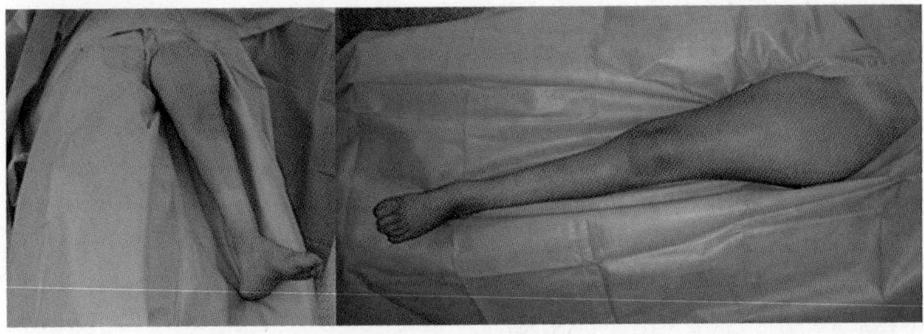

FIG 4 • Positioning in the operating room.

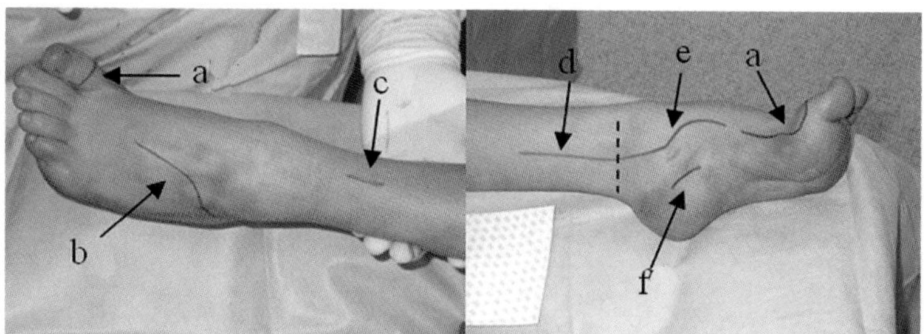

FIG 5 • Approaches for foot deformity correction. (*a*) Dorsal incision for the modified Jones[13] procedure. (*b*) Lateral/dorsal incision for the Triple/Lambrinudi arthrodesis[14] or the Cole procedure[1] and the posterior tibial tendon transfer as well as the Russel-Hibbs procedure.[8] (*c*) Ventral incision for the posterior tibial tendon transfer.[17] (*d*) Distal medial shank incision for the open Achilles tendon lengthening, the posterior tibial tendon transfer and, if needed, the intramuscular lengthening of the long toe flexors. (*e*) Skin incision for the Triple/Lambrinudi arthrodesis,[14] the Cole procedure,[1] and the posterior tibial tendon transfer; incision (*e*) and (*d*) can be connected if needed. (*f*) Skin incision for the Steindler[19] procedure.

TECHNIQUES

OVERVIEW

- The first step is the Steindler procedure.[19] In mildly involved cases it is possible to correct the cavus deformity with this procedure. In most cases, however, a total correction is not possible and this procedure is followed by bony correction of the cavus component.
- After the Steindler procedure, the tendon transfers are prepared (split posterior tibialis transfer,[19] modified Jones procedure[4]). **Important:** Tendon transfers and Achilles tendon lengthening are only prepared at this point; they are eventually secured with suture during the final stages of the reconstruction.
- Next, we correct the clawed hallux (modified Jones procedure[4]). **Important:** The tendon transfer of the extensor hallucis longus (EHL tendon) is sutured at the end of all procedures.
- Bony correction of the midfoot and hindfoot is performed next. Depending on the severity of deformity, an arthrodesis of the Chopart joint or triple arthrodesis may be required. In cases of dorsal impingement of the talus on the tibia with limited dorsiflexion or extreme hindfoot equinus, we recommend adding a modified Lambrinudi procedure.[14]
- In select cases an extra-articular correction of the cavus (Cole procedure[1]) and the hindfoot varus (Dwyer osteotomy[5]) are indicated.
- To correct hindfoot equinus, an intramuscular lengthening of the calf muscles or an open or percutaneous Achilles tendon lengthening is carried out. In cases of severe equinus tested in knee flexion and extension proximal or distal Achilles tendon lengthening (open or percutaneous) is considered. The choice of open or percutaneous lengthening depends on the surgeon's preference. A percutaneous TAL (tendo Achilles lengthening) is more prone to overcorrection, whereas with an open technique, tension can be more easily controlled. In mildly involved cases intramuscular calf muscle lengthening is done (eg, Baumann procedure[23]).
- After correction of the hindfoot and midfoot, we typically reassess the forefoot. In the case of shortened long toe flexors (masked on initial examination by the equinus deformity), an intramuscular lengthening of the long digitorum and hallucis flexor tendons (EDL and EHL tendons) can be done through the same approach used for the open Achilles tendon lengthening.
- When satisfactory correction of first metatarsal plantarflexion is not possible with the modified Jones procedure alone, we routinely add a first metatarsal dorsiflexion osteotomy.[11]
- The final step before wound closure is securing all tendon transfers. We do not routinely use bone anchors but instead suture tendons directly to target other tendons or soft tissues at the site of desired transfer (EHL, tibialis posterior) and the lengthened Achilles tendon slips.

STEINDLER PROCEDURE (TRANSECTION OF THE PLANTAR APONEUROSIS)

- While an important step in the correction of the equinocavovarus foot deformity, our experience is that it does not afford much correction if used in isolation. In our hands, this technique represents the first step in the treatment of pes equinocavovarus. It is a simple method for correcting flexible forefoot and midfoot cavus deformity.
- Make a slightly dorsal convex, 3- to 4-cm-long incision at the medial border of the foot directly above the origin of the plantar aponeurosis at the calcaneus (**TECH FIG 1**).
- Carefully divide the subcutaneous tissue and retract it with Langenbeck retractors. Expose the origin of the

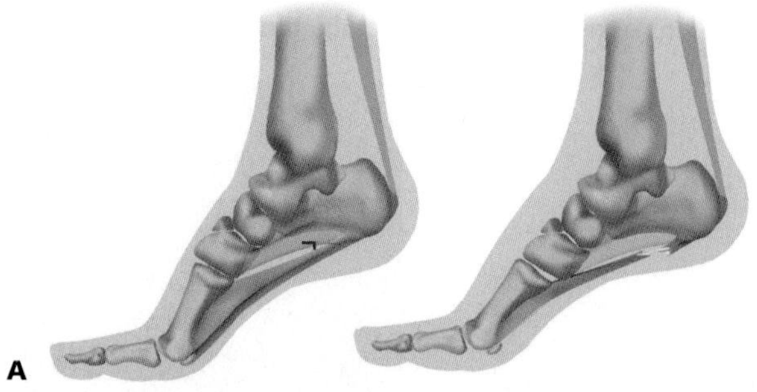

TECH FIG 1 • Steindler procedure. *(continued)*

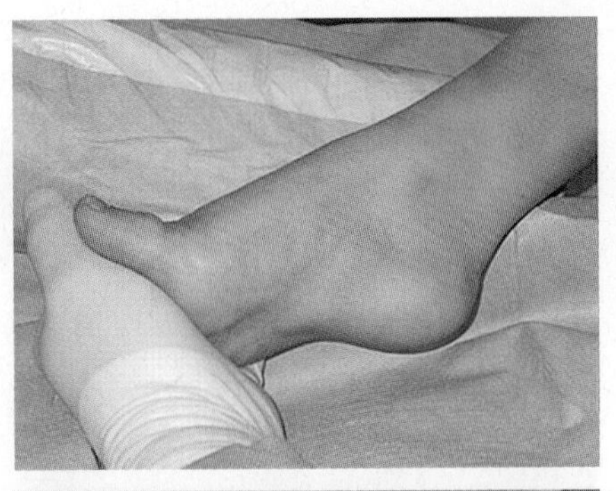
B

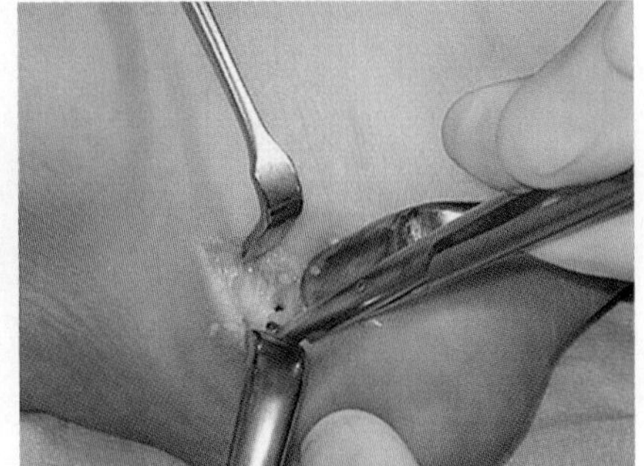
C

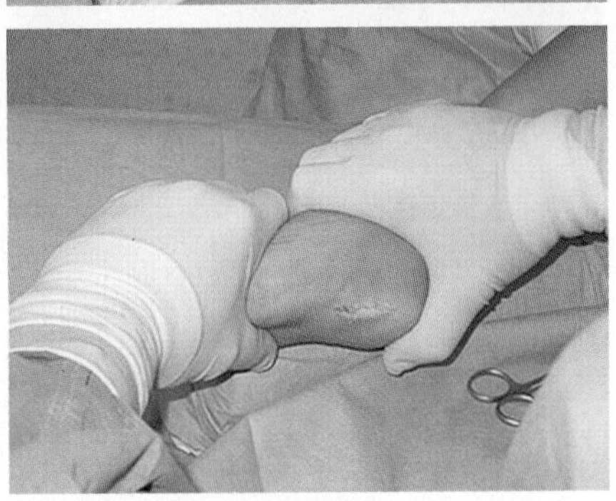
D

TECH FIG 1 • *(continued)*

plantar aponeurosis at the calcaneus as far proximally as possible. Sharply transect the aponeurosis as well as the origin of the short flexor digitorum muscle with the strong preparation scissors.

- It is important to stay directly at the bone and to feel for the peak of the scissors at the lateral border of the foot. After the transection, use a clamp to create the lengthening effect.

T-SPOTT (TOTAL SPLIT POSTERIOR TIBIAL TENDON TRANSFER, MODIFIED SPOTT)[19]

- The purpose of this technique is the augmentation of the attenuated ankle dorsiflexor muscles that are often compromised by longstanding hindfoot equinus deformity. Furthermore, it eliminates the function of the posterior tibial muscle on the hindfoot position.
- Make a 3- to 4-cm incision over the insertion of the posterior tibial tendon (PTT) at the navicular. After dividing the subcutaneous tissue, incise the flexor retinaculum and PTT sheath. Tension the tendon using an Overholt clamp and release it at its insertion point with the scalpel as distally as possible.
- Make another skin incision (3 cm) at the distal medial calf, three to four fingerbreadths proximally to the ankle, directly behind the posterior edge of the tibia.
- After dividing the subcutaneous tissue, incise the fascia and retract it with Langenbeck retractors. Identify and retract the tendon of the long toe flexor muscle (FHL tendon). Immediately deep to the FHL tendon, identify the PTT. Expose it with an Overholt clamp and pull it out (TECH FIG 2).
- Bisect the tendon and tag both halves with atraumatic 1-0 Vicryl sutures.
- Make a third skin incision 3 cm in length on the lateral side of the shank on the same height directly ventrally to the fibular bone. Beneath the subcutaneous tissue, incise and retract the fascia.

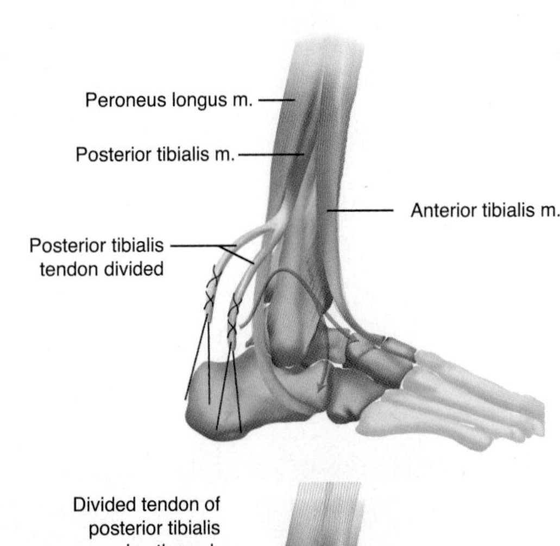

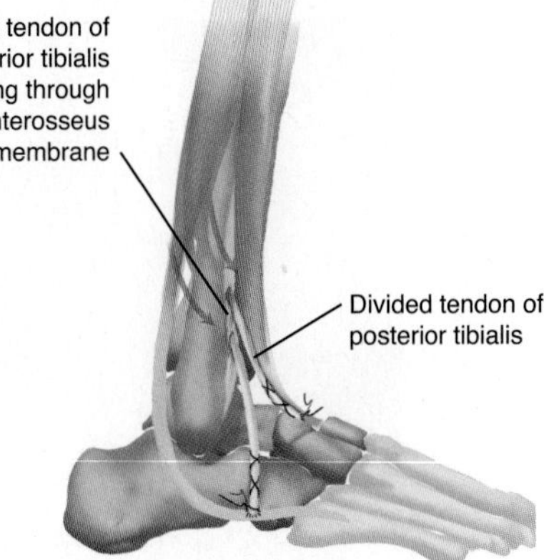

TECH FIG 2 • Total split posterior tibial tendon transfer. *(continued)* A

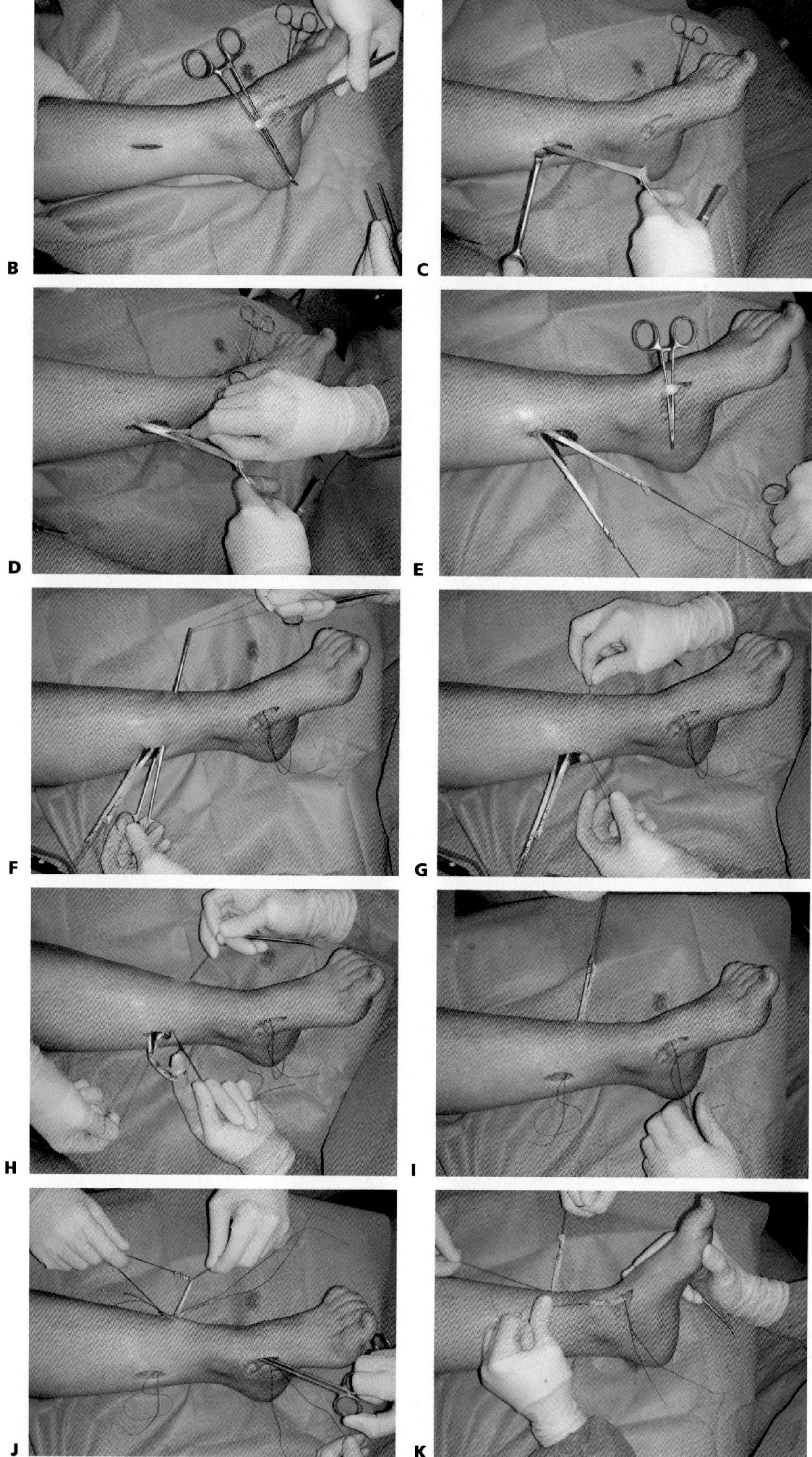

TECH FIG 2 • *(continued)*

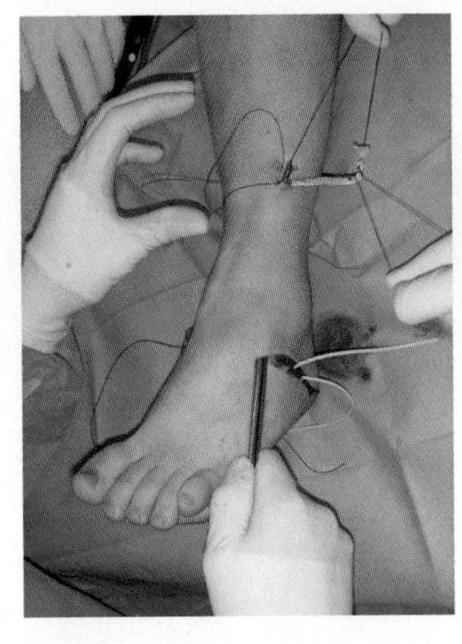
L

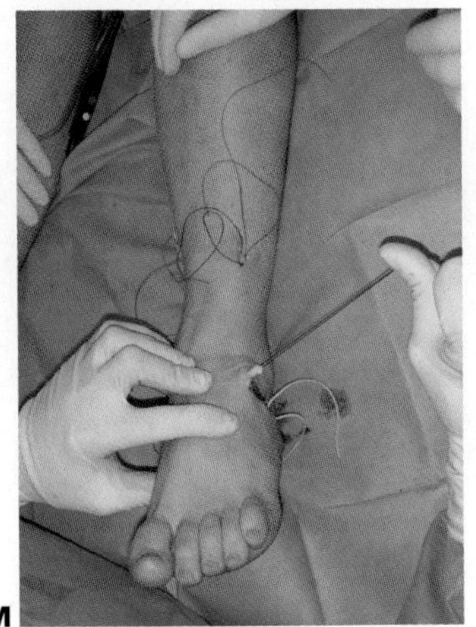
M

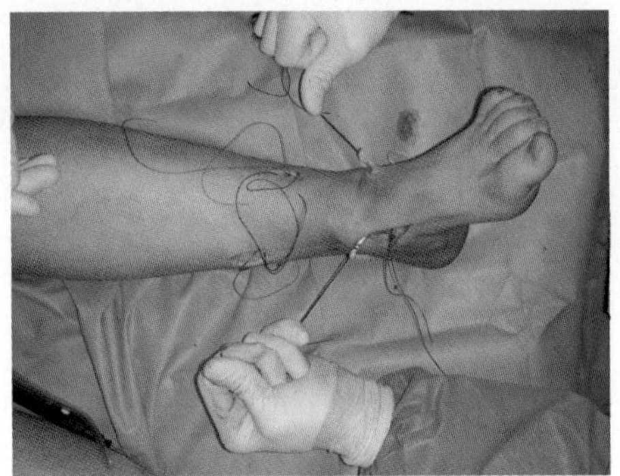
N

TECH FIG 2 • *(continued)*

- Perform the following preparation of the interosseous membrane with caution because of the superficial peroneal nerve. Carefully direct a narrow forceps through the interosseous membrane from the medial wound to lateral wounds.
- Grab a single thread with the forceps and pull it through the medial wound. Capture the tag sutures of the two halves of the PTT in the loop. Transfer the split PTT to the lateral wound by pulling the end of the single thread.
- To maintain the ability to pull back the transferred tendons, loop another single thread around the tendons.
- Expose the anterior tibial tendon by making a 2- to 3-cm skin incision. When planning this incision, take into consideration the possible need for an arthrodesis of the talonavicular joint. If it is needed, the incision should be in line with the previous incision made to expose the PTT.
- After dissecting the subcutaneous tissue, incise the sheath of the anterior tibial tendon and pass the forceps through its sheath to the extensor compartment, where the two halves of the PTT were transferred before.
- There, grab the tagged suture of one half and transfer it distally. For the transfer of the second half of the tendon, make an additional skin incision on the dorsal foot.
- Expose the tendons of the long toe extensors (EDL) and incise their sheath. The same technique is used for the distal transfer of the other half of the PTT. Perform any other concomitant procedures now, before securing the tendon transfers.
- At the end of the operation, suture the medial half of the PTT to the anterior tibial tendon and suture the lateral half to the peroneus brevis tendon, which is previously exposed.
- When tensioning the tendon transfers, we routinely position the ankle in neutral and avoid not only undercorrection but also overcorrection of the foot.
- After suturing the transfers, the foot should rest in the corrected position. Therefore, hindfoot equinus must be corrected before suturing the tendon transfers.

MODIFIED JONES PROCEDURE (ROBERT JONES, 1916)

- The purpose of the modified Jones procedure[4] is to eliminate the overactive EHL muscle and to correct the clawed hallux.

Exposure

- Make an S-shaped skin incision from the proximal first metatarsal to the first interphalangeal (IP) joint.
- After careful soft tissue dissection and protection of the dorsomedial sensory nerve to the hallux, tag the EHL tendon distally with a 0 Vicryl suture.
- Release the tendon as far distally as possible and perform an arthrotomy of the first IP joint (TECH FIG 3).

Hallux Interphalangeal Joint Arthrodesis

- We use a rongeur to remove cartilage at the hallux IP joint (TECH FIG 4A–C).
- We then place two crossing Kirschner wires (1.4 mm for children, 1.8 for adults) through the distal fragment, antegrade from proximal to distal.
- Using the wire driver on the distal aspect of the wires, retract the Kirschner wires from the IP joint arthrodesis site, reduce the IP joint, and advance the Kirschner wires retrograde across the IP arthrodesis site (TECH FIG 4D–F).
- Avoid excessive IP joint extension because it may lead to problems with shoe wear.
- Confirm proper toe rotation after placing the first wire, and then advance the second wire.
- We routinely use two Kirschner wires for fixation; however, the combination of one longitudinal screw and a derotational Kirschner wire is a reasonable alternative. We caution against using only a single screw since this fixation may prove rotationally unstable.

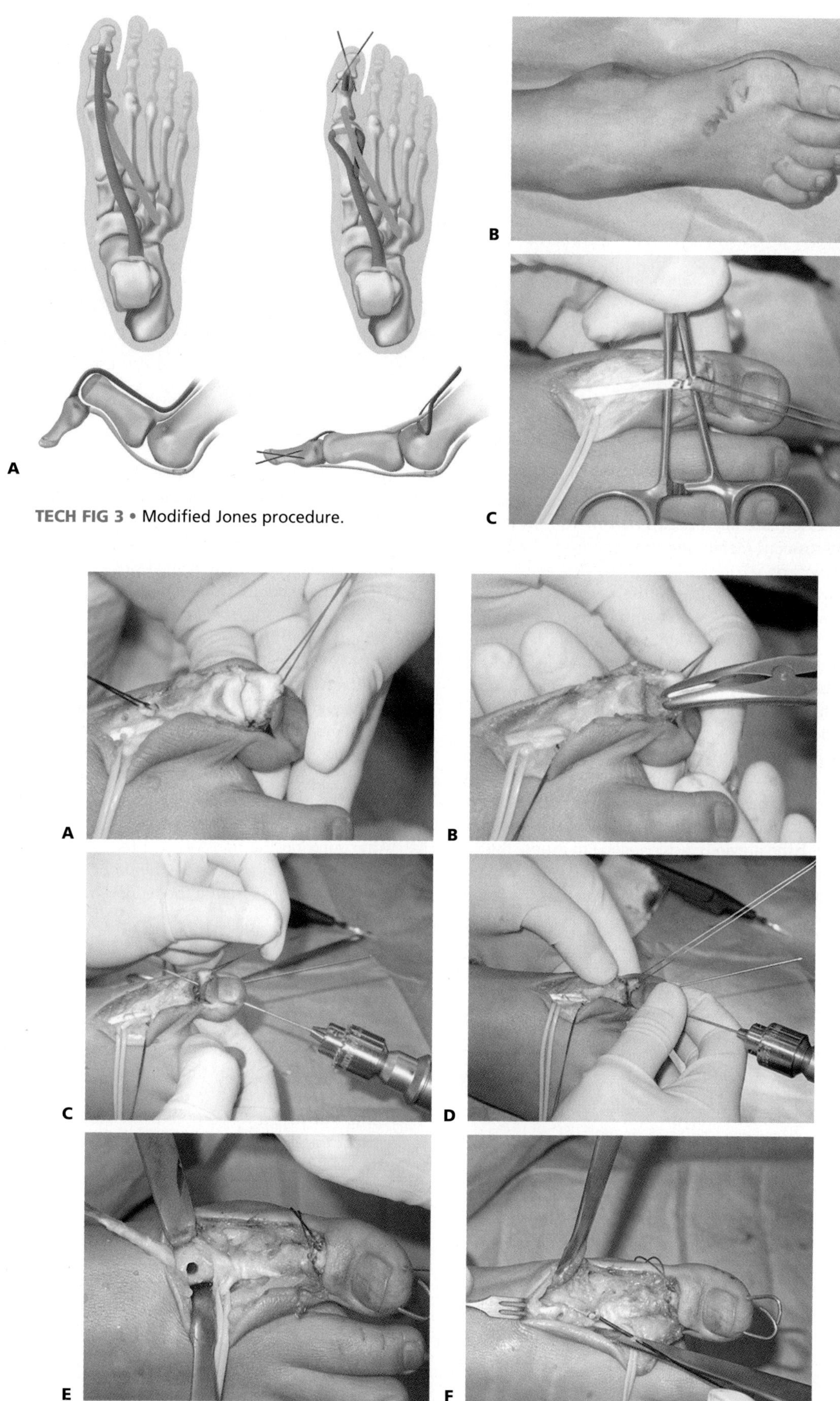

TECH FIG 3 • Modified Jones procedure.

TECH FIG 4 • Modified Jones procedure.

Extensor Hallucis Longus Tendon Transfer (With or Without Dorsiflexion Osteotomy of the First Metatarsal)

- Expose the first metatarsal to the proximal third of its shaft. If the plantarflexion of the first metatarsal bone cannot be corrected by soft tissue correction alone, a dorsiflexion osteotomy of the first metatarsal must be performed. (The technique will be described in greater detail later.)
- Extend the approach a few more centimeters proximally.
- Perform the dorsiflexion osteotomy with an oscillating saw, removing a dorsal wedge of bone in the proximal third of the metatarsal and leaving the plantar cortex intact.
- Secure it with Kirschner wires, a small dorsal plate, or a screw and tension band technique.
- For the EHL tendon transfer, use a periosteal elevator to expose the bone at the first metatarsal head–neck junction.
- Place two Hohmann retractors to protect the soft tissues and drill a hole centrally in the first metatarsal bone with sequentially larger-diameter drill bits: first 2.0 mm, then 2.7 mm, followed by 3.2 mm.
- Advance the tagged EHL tendon through the hole with a needle and suture it to itself with 1-0 Vicryl.
- If the hallux tends to plantarflex after the tendon transfer, the distal end of the transferred EHL tendon or its suture tags may be reattached to the periosteum of the distal phalanx as a tenodesis to avoid undesirable postoperative flexion of the first toe.

FUSION OF THE CHOPART JOINT, TRIPLE FUSION (HOKE, 1921[9]), LAMBRINUDI FUSION (LAMBRINUDI, 1927[7,14])

- Fixed hindfoot cavus deformity may warrant talonavicular and calcaneocuboid joint (Chopart joint) arthrodesis. However, when the deformity is isolated to a fixed, plantarflexed first ray, a dorsiflexion first metatarsal osteotomy may be adequate. Likewise, global cavus of the entire forefoot may be effectively treated with a dorsiflexion midfoot osteotomy (Cole procedure).
- In select cases of flexible hindfoot varus, a Dwyer lateral closing wedge calcaneal osteotomy (see below) may be performed in lieu of hindfoot arthrodesis.
- The lateral approach is performed with an S-shaped skin incision, beginning 2 cm distally and dorsally to the lateral malleolus, proceeding in an arch shape to the navicular, distally to the palpable talar head.
- Expose the sural nerve in the proximal wound edge with its accompanying vessels and retract it.
- The preparation leads to the peroneal tendon sheath and the origin of the extensor digitorum brevis muscle (EDB) at the anterior processes of the calcaneus.
- With an L-shaped incision, release the EDB. Using a concave chisel, detach its origin from the anterior processes of the calcaneus bone. Expose the calcaneocuboid joint by inserting a Vierstein retractor.
- Use an additional Vierstein retractor to expose the talonavicular joint.
- The hindfoot arthrodesis may be performed with preservation of the subchondral bone architecture or as a corrective wedge resection. If cavus was not corrected by the Steindler procedure, a dorsally based wedge must be taken from the Chopart joint.
- With extreme forefoot and midfoot adduction, the dorsal wedge resection may need to include an additional lateral-based wedge resection.
- The more conservative arthrodesis that maintains subchondral bone architecture of the joints is reserved for mild to moderate deformity. Remove the cartilage and penetrate the subchondral bone with a chisel or drill to promote fusion.
- If a wedge resection is required to correct the deformity, we prefer to use an oscillating saw.
- After the complete release of the Chopart joint, the cavus foot can be manually corrected and the navicular centered on the talar head.
- We routinely stabilize the reduced joints with Kirschner wires (two through the talonavicular joint, two through the calcaneocuboid joint). Alternatively, the fixation can be done with screws.
- If a satisfactory deformity correction is not possible by Chopart arthrodesis, especially with severe hindfoot varus, the hindfoot arthrodesis must be extended to the subtalar joint to complete the triple arthrodesis.
- In severe deformity, a laterally based wedge can be removed from the subtalar joint. Dorsal impingement of the talus on the tibia, in cases with limited ankle dorsiflexion or extreme hindfoot equinus, may warrant a modified Lambrinudi procedure.
- For both the triple arthrodesis and modified Lambrinudi procedure the sinus tarsi is freed from all soft tissue structures (interosseous ligaments and fat). The most important structure to be dissected is the interosseous ligament between the talus and calcaneus. To expose the subtalar joint, use a lamina spreader in the subtalar joint and place a Vierstein retractor below the apex of the lateral malleolus.
- Prepare the surfaces at the arthrodesis site with a concave chisel or with the oscillating saw, depending on the amount of correction needed.
- A severe hindfoot varus is corrected by removing a lateral-based wedge from the subtalar joint (**TECH FIG 5**). If a Lambrinudi fusion is needed, a dorsally based wedge is taken out of the subtalar joint.
- The determination of the osteotomy lines is important for the size of the remaining bone. The first osteotomy runs parallel to the ankle joint line and through the talar head. It should not take more than 50% of the talus head.
- The osteotomy ends dorsally in the posterior edge of the subtalar joint. The second osteotomy runs parallel to the

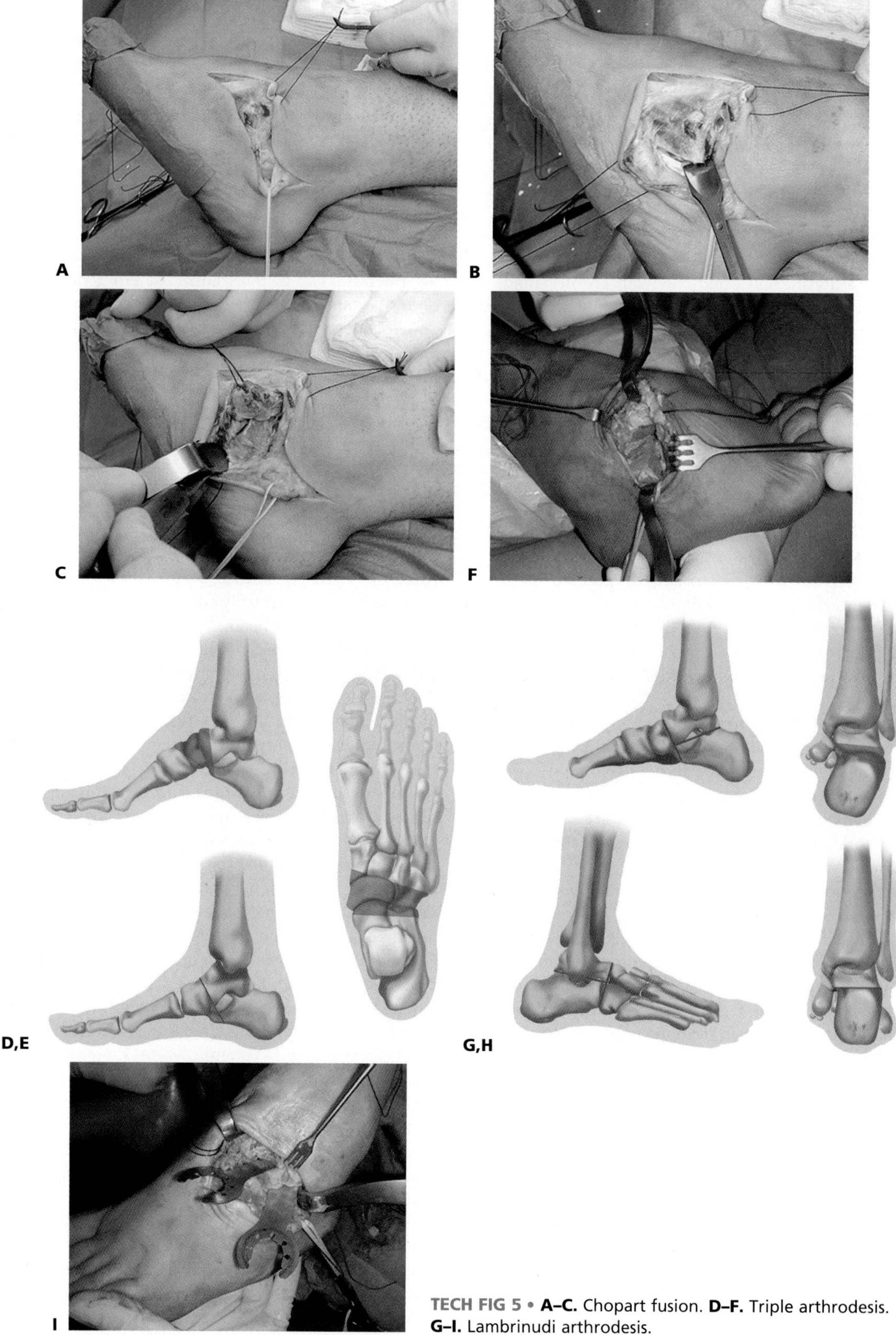

TECH FIG 5 • **A–C.** Chopart fusion. **D–F.** Triple arthrodesis. **G–I.** Lambrinudi arthrodesis.

subtalar joint line and through the calcaneal bone. Both osteotomies unite in the posterior edge of the subtalar joint, forming a dorsally based wedge with its apex in the posterior aspect of the subtalar joint.

- After resecting the cartilage or the bony wedge, assess the effect of correction by the reposition of the talocalcaneal and the Chopart joint. In addition to the correction of the cavus hindfoot varus components, it is very important that the foot can be repositioned in a plantigrade position.
- The osteosynthesis can be done with six Kirschner wires (2.2 to 2.5 mm, two for the talonavicular joint, two for the calcaneocuboid joint, and two for the subtalar joint). Alternatively, the fixation may be performed with screws or a locking plate.

COLE OSTEOTOMY[1]

- This procedure is used for bony correction of cavus deformity when the talonavicular and calcaneocuboid joints can be reduced. A dorsally based wedge is removed from the navicular–cuneiform joints and the cuboid.
- We perform this procedure through a lazy S-incision at the lateral midfoot. Expose the sural nerve in the subcutaneous tissue and retract it.
- Make an incision between the sheath of the peroneal tendons and the EDB to expose the cuboid. Perform the osteotomies with an oscillating saw or osteotome.
- The distal osteotomy should be driven exactly through the cuneiforms and the cuboid; the proximal osteotomy runs through the cuboid and navicular. At least 0.5 cm of bone must be preserved between the proximal osteotomy and the talonavicular joint.
- These osteotomies converge on the plantar aspect of the midfoot. Remove a dorsal-based bony wedge (TECH FIG 6).
- After the resection, the osteotomy can be closed and fixed with two to four Kirschner wires (talonavicular and calcaneocuboid joint, Chopart fusion). Alternatively, screws or locking plates can be used.

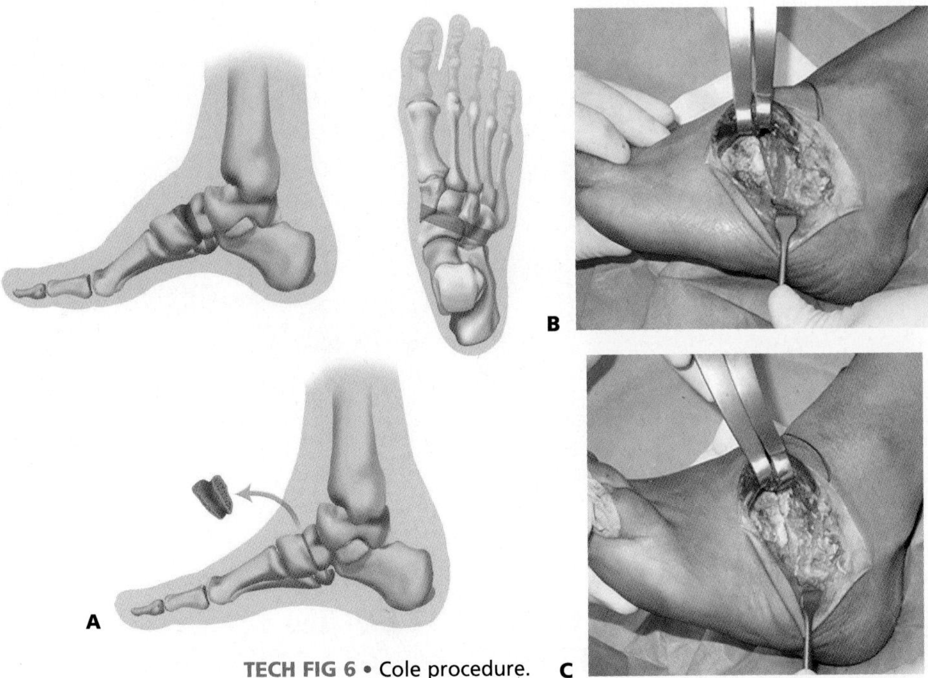

TECH FIG 6 • Cole procedure.

DWYER OSTEOTOMY[5]

- This procedure is used for bony correction of hindfoot varus deformity, when subtalar joint fusion is not indicated, the hindfoot cannot be completely reduced, and a correction of the hindfoot varus correction cannot be achieved by tendon transfer alone.
- Make a skin incision (about 5 cm) at the lateral border of the hindfoot above the peroneal tendons, vertical to the longitudinal axis of the calcaneus. Expose the sural nerve in the subcutaneous tissue and retract it.
- Expose the neck of the calcaneus subperiosteally by two Hohmann retractors.

- A laterally based bony wedge may be resected from the calcaneal neck with the oscillating bone saw if greater correction is required (TECH FIG 7).
- Avoid overpenetration of the medial calcaneal cortex with the saw blade, which may injure the medial neurovascular bundle.
- The osteotomy can be opened with a straight chisel. The osteotomy is then closed holding the hind foot into slight valgus position.
- Use two crossing Kirschner wires inserted from posterior for transfixion.

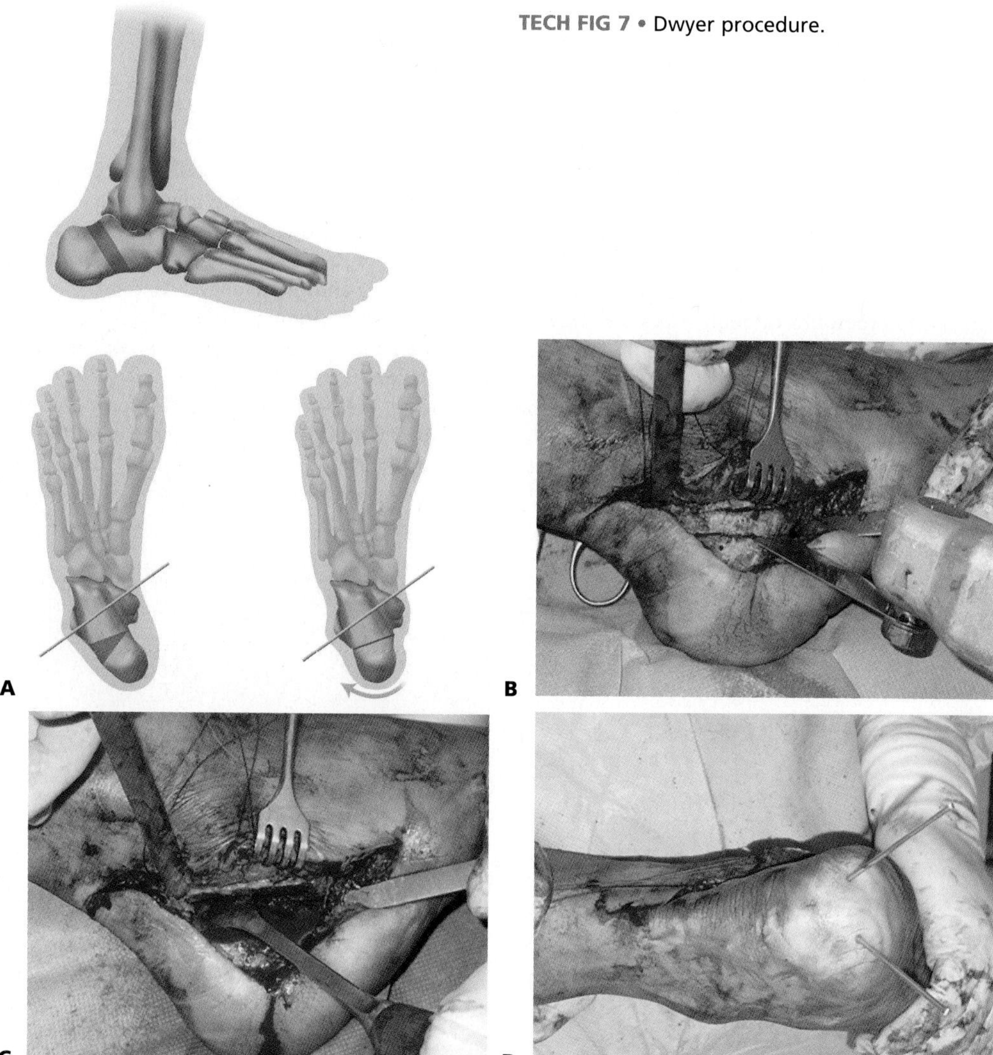

TECH FIG 7 • Dwyer procedure.

SOFT TISSUE CORRECTION OF HINDFOOT EQUINUS (BAUMANN PROCEDURE, ACHILLES TENDON LENGTHENING)

- Achilles tendon lengthening is done when both calf muscles are shortened and the equinus is severe and fixed. In case of a flexible and mild equinus, intramuscular recession (Baumann technique) is done.
- The approach for an open Achilles tendon lengthening is done though a 6- to 10-cm skin incision made at the medial distal calf, about 3 to 4 cm above the ankle joint, running proximally. The length of the skin incision varies with the amount of Achilles tendon lengthening needed for equinus correction.
- After identifying and retracting the saphenous nerve and vein, expose the fascia and incise and divide it proximally and distally. Beneath the fascia, identify the Achilles tendon and elevate it with two Langenbeck hooks, inserted under the tendon proximally and distally.
- Perform the Z-lengthening with a small scalpel over the entire tendon (TECH FIG 8A–C).
- In hindfoot varus deformity, we prefer to preserve the lateral half of the tendon distally. Do not dissect the underlying muscle tissue.
- Tag both tendon slips with 1-0 Vicryl sutures.
- The ankle joint can now be reduced to 10 to 20 degrees of dorsiflexion, so that both tendon slips slide apart.

With the ankle joint in neutral position, suture together both tendon slips with atraumatic 1-0 Vicryl suture.

- For the Baumann procedure, make a 4- to 5-cm skin incision in the medial aspect of the proximal third of the calf. Expose and incise the fascia after tagging it with two sutures.
- Open the interval between the gastrocnemius and the soleus muscle and insert two broad Langenbeck retractors.
- Perform an intramuscular recession of the aponeurosis of the gastrocnemius, soleus, or both (**TECH FIG 8D–F**), based on an intraoperative Silfverskiöld test.
- After recession, the ankle can be redressed. The aponeurosis will slide apart.

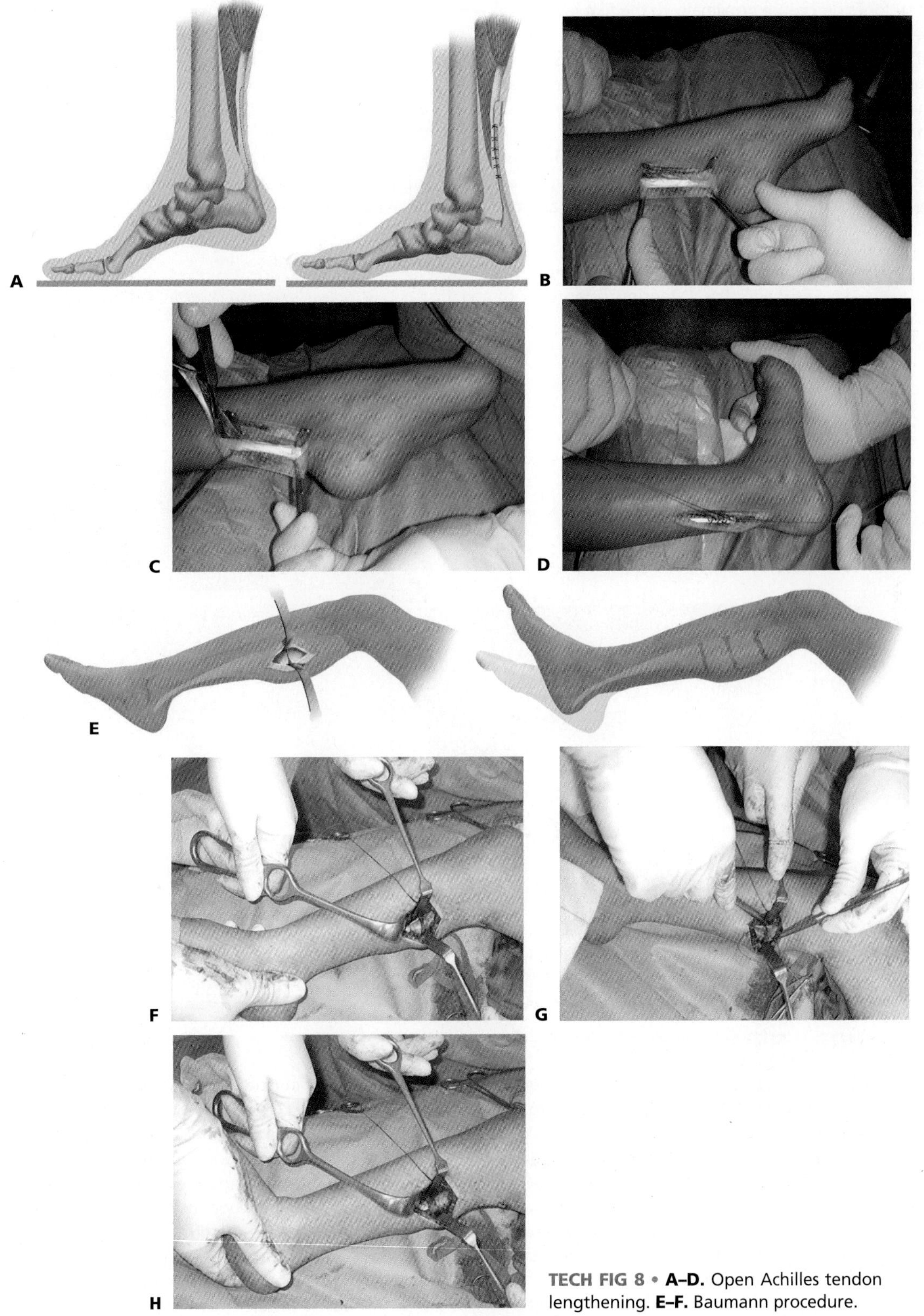

TECH FIG 8 • A–D. Open Achilles tendon lengthening. **E–F.** Baumann procedure.

DORSIFLEXION FIRST METATARSAL OSTEOTOMY (A.H. TUBBY, 1912[21])

- This procedure is one of the final steps in the surgical correction of pes equinocavovarus. It is warranted when fixed plantarflexion of the first metatarsal fails to correct with the modified Jones procedure alone.
- The approach is easily done by lengthening the incision for the Jones procedure proximally to the first metatarsal base.
- Sharply incise the periosteum over the dorsal first metatarsal lengthwise approaching the first tarsometatarsal joint, protecting the soft tissues with two Hohmann retractors.
- Perform the proximal limb of the osteotomy with an oscillating saw, vertical to the first metatarsal, about 0.5 cm distal to the first tarsometatarsal joint in adults and the growth plate in children. It is important to keep the plantar cortex intact to control rotation error.
- The distal osteotomy converges with the first osteotomy at the plantar cortex, creating a dorsal wedge (**TECH FIG 9A**).
- The width of the dorsal wedge is determined by the planned correction; in our experience, bone resection of 2 to 3 mm is appropriate.
- Close the osteotomy with plantar pressure on the head of the first metatarsal (**TECH FIG 9B**).
- We routinely secure the osteotomy with two crossing Kirschner wires (**TECH FIG 9C**). Alternatively, a dorsal locking plate or screw and tension band technique may be used to stabilize the osteotomy.

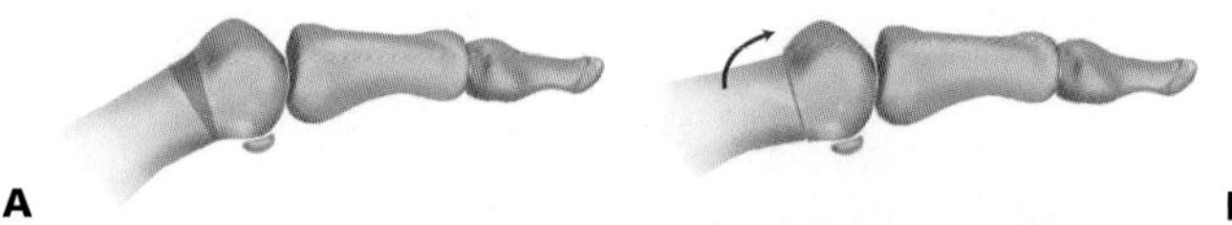

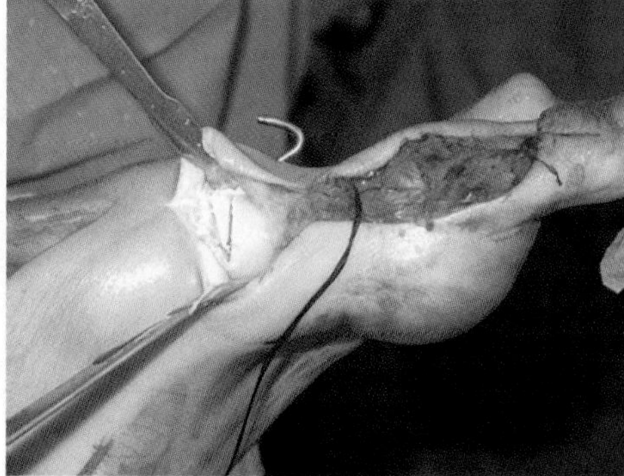

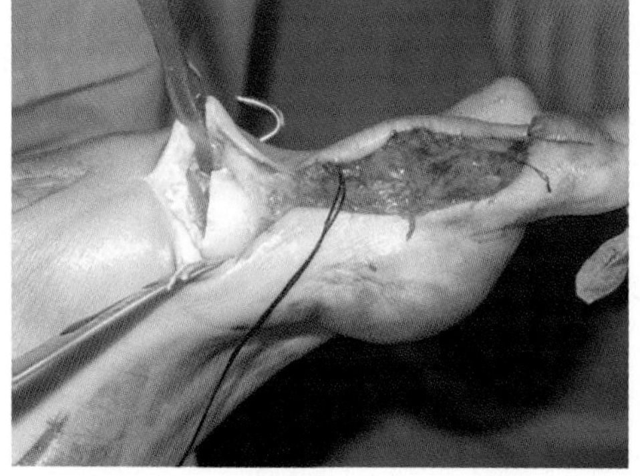

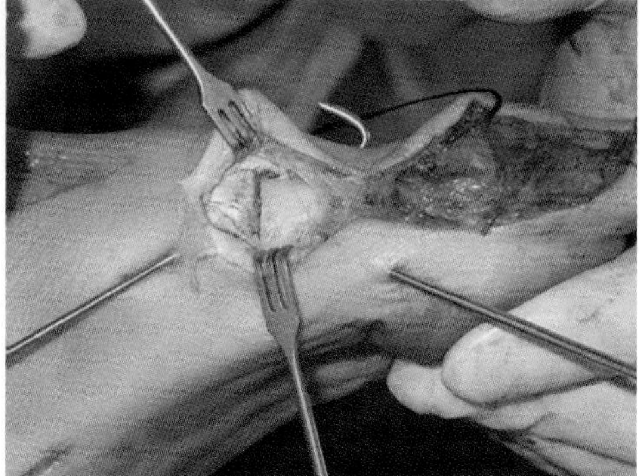

TECH FIG 9 • Extension osteotomy of the first metatarsal bone.

RUSSEL-HIBBS PROCEDURE (1919)[8]

- This procedure corrects claw toes secondary to overactivity of the extrinsic (long extensor and flexor digitorum muscles) relative to the intrinsic muscle groups.
- We use a convex lateral 4-cm incision over the fourth metatarsal. Identify and retract the superficial peroneal nerve.
- Expose the EDL tendons of the second through fourth toes and tag them together proximally and distally (**TECH FIG 10**) with atraumatic 1-0 Vicryl sutures.
- Cut the tendons between the two sutures.
- Dissect the EDB muscle carefully and expose the underlying bone.
- In children, the proximal endings of the tendons can be sutured to the periosteum. The foot should come into neutral position spontaneously after the suture.
- In adults a tendon anchor is secured to the underlying bone (intermediate cuneiform body), and the tendons are secured to the anchor. The distal part of the tagged tendons should also be sutured to periosteum or the anchor to create a distal tenodesis.

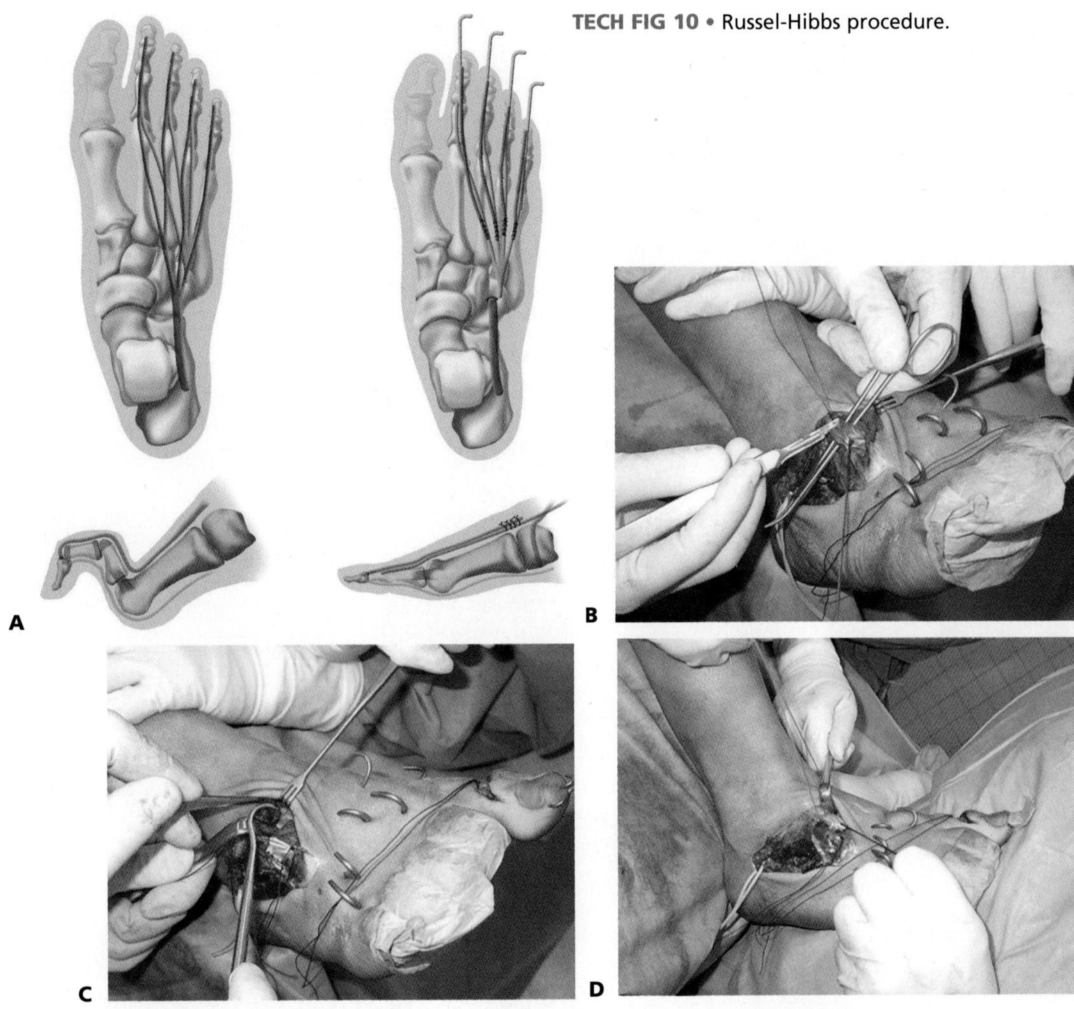

TECH FIG 10 • Russel-Hibbs procedure.

WOUND CLOSURE

- Tendon transfers and lengthened Achilles tendon are sutured with atraumatic 1-0 Vicryl. All wounds are closed in layers.
- At the calf the fascial incisions are sutured with 0 Vicryl.
- If removed, the anterior processes of the calcaneus are reattached with 1-0 Vicryl.
- Afterwards the subcutaneous tissue is closed (2-0 Vicryl).
- We routinely use a simple suture technique (and occasionally the Donati-Allgower technique) for skin closure on the foot (3-0 Ethilon), and we use an intracutaneous technique for skin closure on the calf.

PEARLS AND PITFALLS

Indications	■ A detailed clinical examination is the basis for the correct indication and a good outcome. Concomitant deformities should be considered when planning the treatment.
Order of procedures	■ Begin with soft tissue procedures before performing bony procedures. This may decrease the extent of bony wedge resection. Sutures of soft tissue procedures are done after the bony correction.
Joint fusion	■ Ensure that all cartilage is removed from the resection areas to avoid nonfusion.
Overcorrection	■ Avoid overcorrection; start with small wedges and extend the resection if needed.
Wound closure problems	■ In severe cases that demand significant correction, skin closure can be difficult. This should be considered before performing skin incisions. The problem often can be solved with S-shaped incisions.

POSTOPERATIVE CARE

- In the operating room, we apply a short-leg cast with the ankle in neutral ankle position and the hindfoot in slight eversion.
- On postoperative day 1, we routinely obtain a radiograph and change the plaster cast.
- With bony procedures, weight bearing is restricted for 6 weeks and 4 weeks for adults and children, respectively. At the subsequent follow-up, new radiographs are obtained, the Kirschner wires are removed, and a short-leg, weight-bearing plaster cast is applied for an additional 6 weeks and 4 weeks for adults and children, respectively.
- In contrast, without bony procedures, the weight-bearing plaster cast is applied immediately after the operation for 6 (adults) or 4 (children) weeks.
- The stitches are removed 14 days postoperatively, when we perform a routine cast change. After the removal of the final plaster cast, we advise our patients to use a brace for 6 months to a year, depending on the severity of deformity and correction required.

OUTCOMES

- References concerning long-term outcomes after complex foot reconstruction surgery in pes equinocavovarus are rare. Controlled outcome studies, based on clinical, radiographic, and functional data (3D foot analysis, EMED), are needed.

Case 1

- This 16-year-old patient with tethered cord syndrome and myelolysis suffered from a painful equinocavovarus foot on the right side with hindfoot varus and equinus, cavus

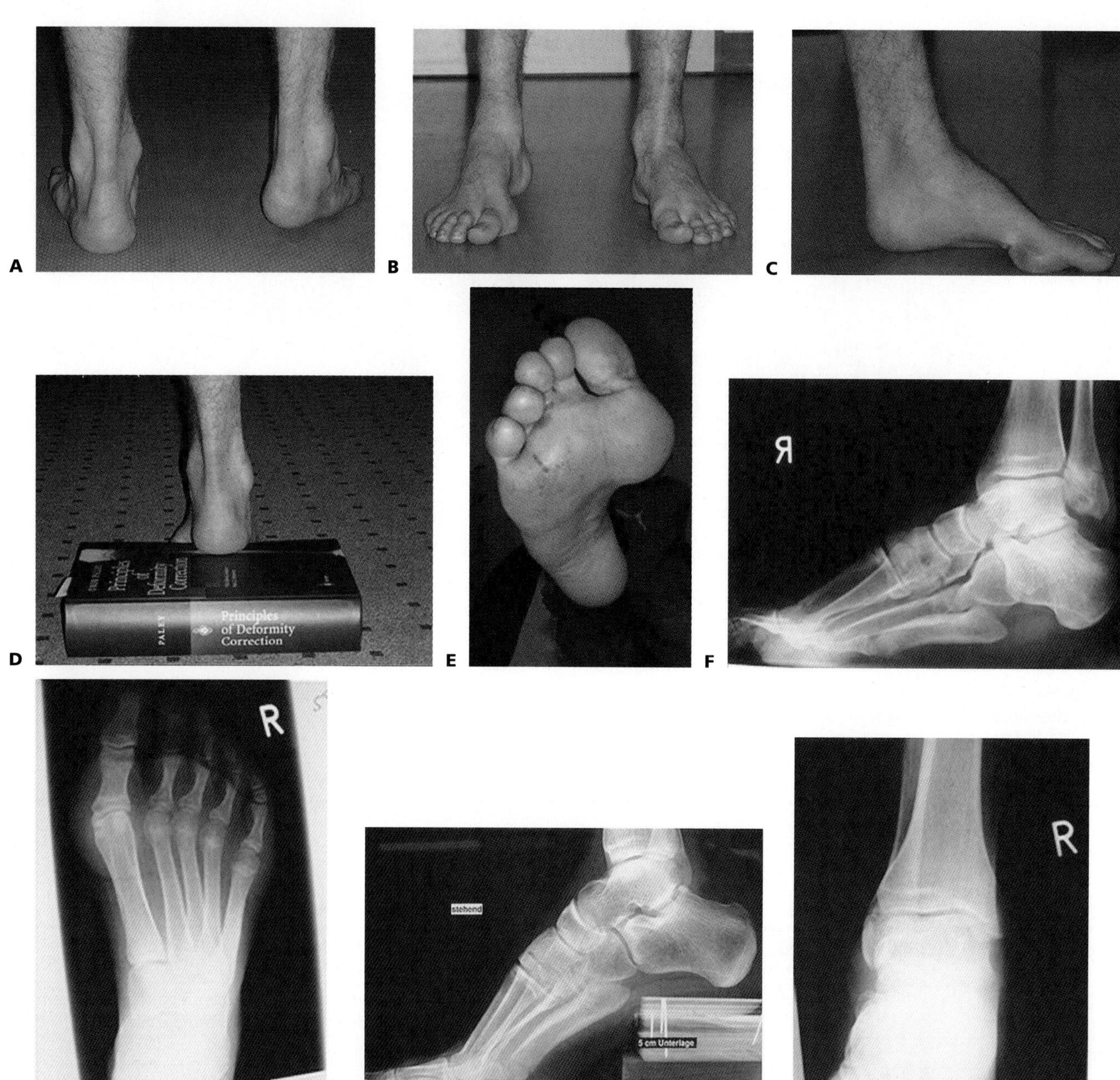

FIG 6 • **A–I.** Preoperative clinical and radiographic findings of a 16-year-old patient with tethered cord syndrome, myelolysis, and an equinocavovarus foot deformity on the right side. *(continued)*

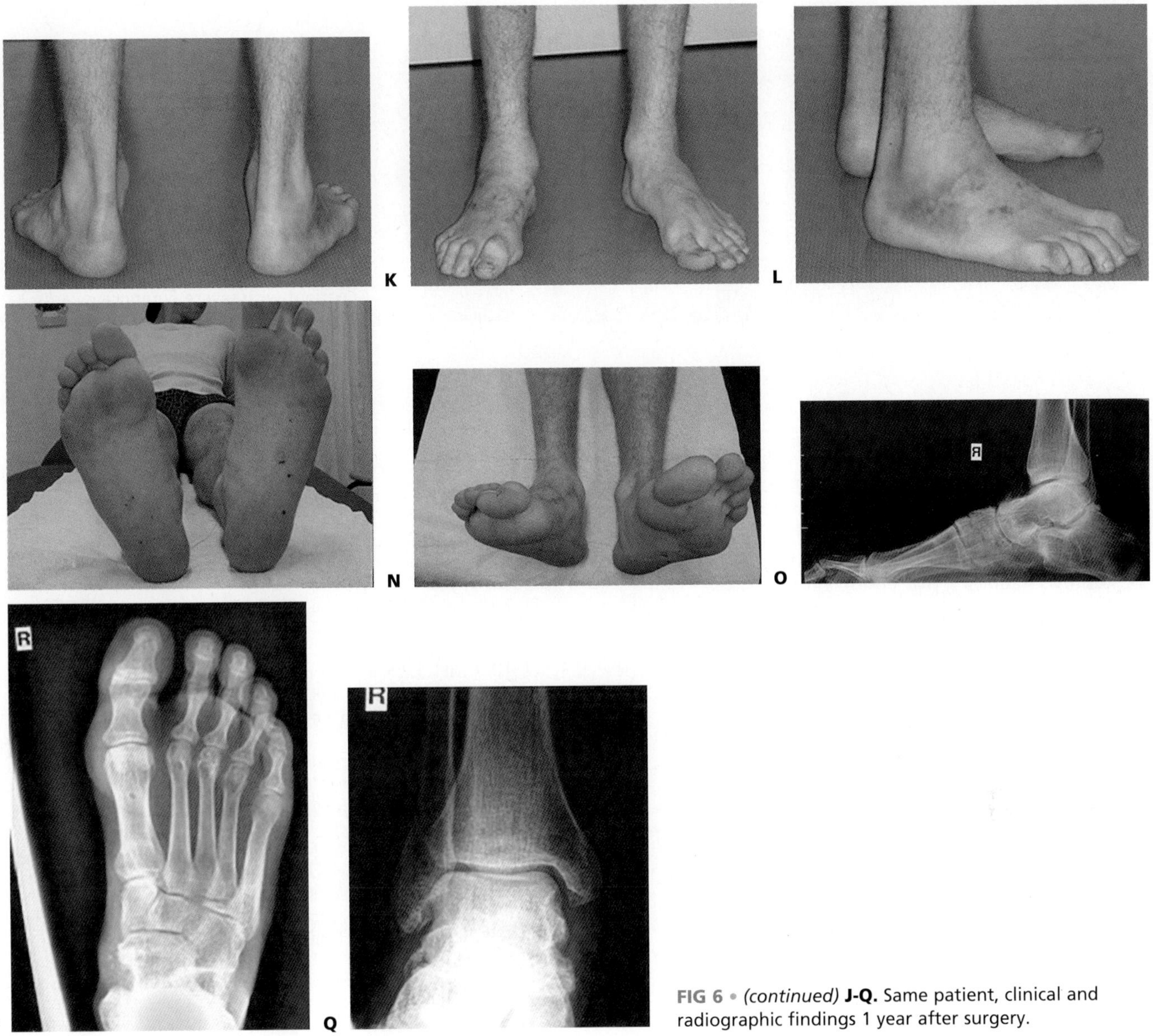

FIG 6 • *(continued)* **J-Q.** Same patient, clinical and radiographic findings 1 year after surgery.

deformity, plantarflexion of the first metatarsal, and claw toes (**FIG 6A–I**).

- He was treated with a Steindler procedure, a Jones procedure, a PTT transfer, a Chopart fusion, an Achilles tendon lengthening, and a dorsiflexion first metatarsal osteotomy. The postoperative results are shown in **FIGURE 6J–Q**.
- After his foot deformity correction he is now able to work as a roof tiler without functional limitations or pain.

Case 2

- A 32-year-old man with severe equinocavovarus had as his major problems combined forefoot and hindfoot equi-

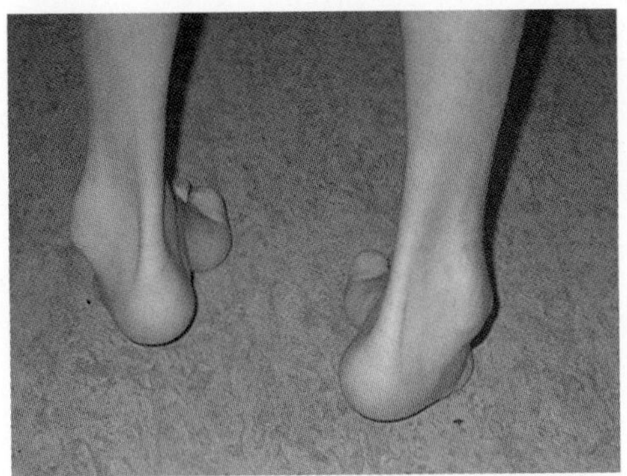

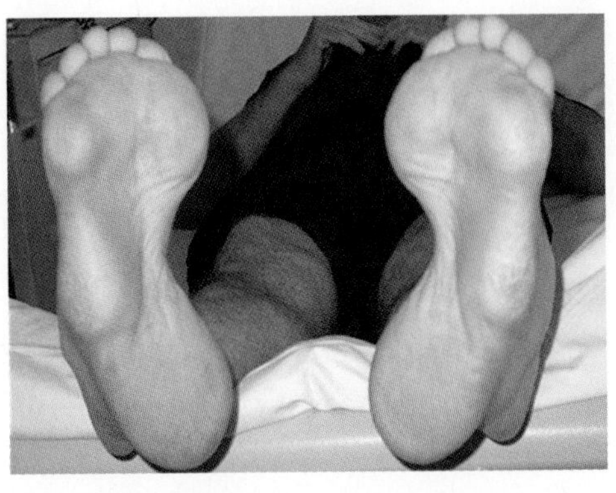

FIG 7 • Preoperative (**A, B**) and postoperative *(continued)*

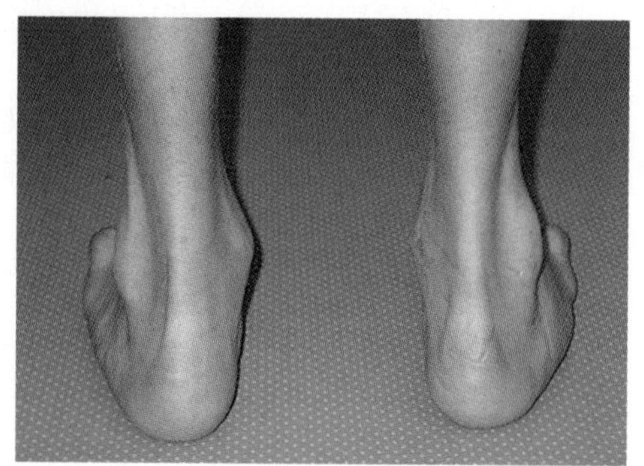

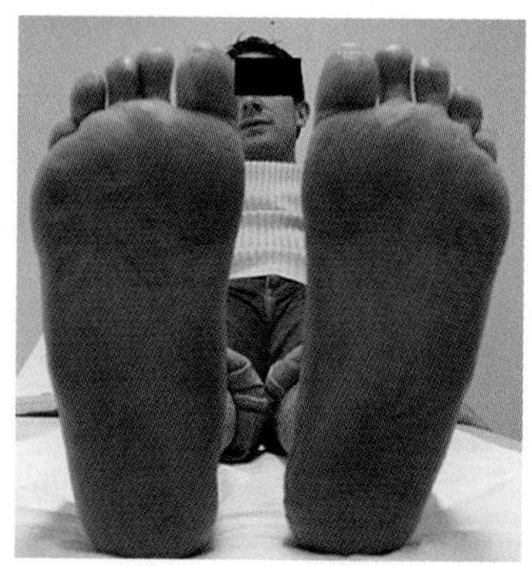

FIG 7 • *(continued)* **(C, D)** clinical and radiographic findings of a 32-year-old patient with severe equinocavovarus foot deformity bilaterally.

nus, hindfoot varus, a cavus component, and clawing of the toes.

- After Achilles tendon lengthening, a split PTT transfer, a Steindler procedure, a Chopart fusion, a dorsiflexion first metatarsal osteotomy, and a modified Jones procedure, a plantigrade functional foot was restored.
- **FIGURE 7A,B** shows preoperative findings and **FIGURE 7C,D** shows findings 1 year postoperatively.

COMPLICATIONS

- Infection
- Vessel or nerve bundle injury
- Nonunion
- Overcorrection (flatfoot, valgus foot, calcaneus foot)
- Undercorrection
- Recurrence
- Ulceration due to plaster casting
- Pin tract infection from the Kirschner wires

REFERENCES

1. Cole WH. The treatment of claw-foot. J Bone Joint Surg 1940; 22:895–908.
2. Coleman SS. Complex Foot Deformities in Children. Philadelphia: Lea and Febiger, 1983.
3. Coleman SS, Chesnut WJ. A simple test for hind-foot flexibility in the cavo-varus foot. Clin Orthop Relat Res 1977;123:60–62.
4. DePalma L, Colonna E, Travasi M. The modified Jones procedure for pes cavovarus with claw hallux. J Foot Ankle Surg 1997; 36:279–283.
5. Dwyer FC. Osteotomy of the calcaneum for pes cavus. J Bone Joint Surg Br 1959;41B:80–86.
6. Dwyer FC. The present status of the problem of pes cavus. Clin Orthop Relat Res 1975;106:254–275.
7. Hall JE, Calvert PT. Lambrinudi triple arthrodesis: a review with particular reference to the technique of operation. J Pediatr Orthop 1987;7:19–24.
8. Hibbs RA. An operation for "claw foot." JAMA 1919;73:1583–1585.
9. Hoke M. An operation for stabilizing paralytic feet. J Orthop Surg 1921;3:494.
10. Hsu JD, Hoffer MM. Posterior tibial tendon transfer anteriorly through the interosseous membrane. Clin Orthop Relat Res 1978; 131:202–204.
11. Imhäuser G. Treatment of severe concave clubfoot in neural muscular atrophy [in German]. Z Orthop Ihre Grenzgeb 1984;122: 827–834.
12. Jahss MH. Evaluation of the cavus foot for orthopedic treatment. Clin Orthop Relat Res 1983;181:52–63.
13. Jones R. An operation for paralytic calcaneo-cavus. Am J Orthop Surg 1908;5:371–376.
14. Lambrinudi C. New operation for drop foot. Br J Surg 1927;15:193.
15. Mann RA. Pes cavus. In: Mann RA, Coughlin MJ, eds. Surgery of the Foot and Ankle, Vol. 1, 6th ed. St. Louis, Baltimore, Berlin: Mosby, 1992:785–801.
16. Samilson RL, Dillon W. Cavus, cavovarus and calcaneocavus: an update. Clin Orthop Relat Res 1983;177:125–132.
17. Shapiro F, Bresnan MJ. Orthopaedic management of childhood neuromuscular disease, parts I–III. J Bone Joint Surg Am 1982;64A: 785–789, 64A:949–953, and 64A:1102–1107.
18. Simon J, Doederlein L, McIntosh AS, et al. The Heidelberg foot measurement method: development, description and assessment. Gait Posture 2006;23:411–424.
19. Steindler A. The treatment of pes cavus (hollow claw foot). Arch Surg 1921;2:325–337.
20. Thometz JG, Gould JS. Cavus deformity. In: Drennan JC, ed. The Child's Foot and Ankle. New York: Raven Press, 1992:343–353.
21. Tubby AH. Deformities Including Diseases of Bones and Joints, 2nd ed. London: Macmillan, 1912.
22. Tubby AH, Jones R. Modern Methods in the Surgery of the Paralysis. London: Macmillan, 1902.

Chapter 57

Plantar Fascia Release in Combination With Proximal and Distal Tarsal Tunnel Release

John S. Gould and Benedict F. DiGiovanni

DEFINITION

- Chronic plantar fasciitis with distal tarsal tunnel syndrome is an underrecognized disorder in which the patients with the typical enthesopathy of plantar fasciitis develop neurogenic symptoms and signs, becoming recalcitrant to the usual management of the initial condition.
- This chapter will concentrate on the most common type of distal tarsal tunnel syndrome: chronic plantar fasciitis associated with the involvement of the lateral plantar nerve and the first branch of the lateral plantar nerve.

ANATOMY

- Proximal or classic tarsal tunnel syndrome was first described by Koppell and Thompson in 1960. It was subsequently named by Keck and Lam in two independent reports in 1962.[8,10] Entrapment of the entire tibial nerve as it courses beneath the the flexor retinaculum behind the medial malleolus defines proximal tarsal tunnel syndrome (**FIG 1A**). The flexor retinaculum or laciniate ligament is formed by joining the deep and superficial aponeurosis of the leg, and it is closely attached to the sheaths of the posterior tibial, flexor digitorum longus, and flexor hallucis tendons.
- Distal tarsal tunnel syndrome, proposed by Heimkes et al in 1987,[6] results from irritation of one or more of the terminal branches of the tibial nerve. The three terminal branches are the medial plantar nerve, lateral plantar nerve, and medical calcaneal nerve.
  - The first branch of the lateral plantar nerve occurs just after the lateral plantar nerve branches from the posterior tibial nerve (**FIG 1B**). The first branch travels between the abductor hallucis muscle deep fascia and the medial fascia of the quadratus plantae muscle. It then changes direction and travels laterally in a horizontal plane between the quadratus plantae and the flexor digitorum brevis muscles, sending a sensory branch to the central heel pad, and terminates as motor branch to the abductor digiti quinti.
  - The lateral plantar nerve follows the same course initially, passing under the deep fascia of the abductor hallucis and the medial edge of the plantar fascia and over the quadratus plantae fascia, and then turns distally under the flexor digitorum brevus, emerging distally just under the plantar fascia to form the intermetatarsal nerves to the 4/5 interspace and contributing to the 3/4 intermetatarsal nerve as well.

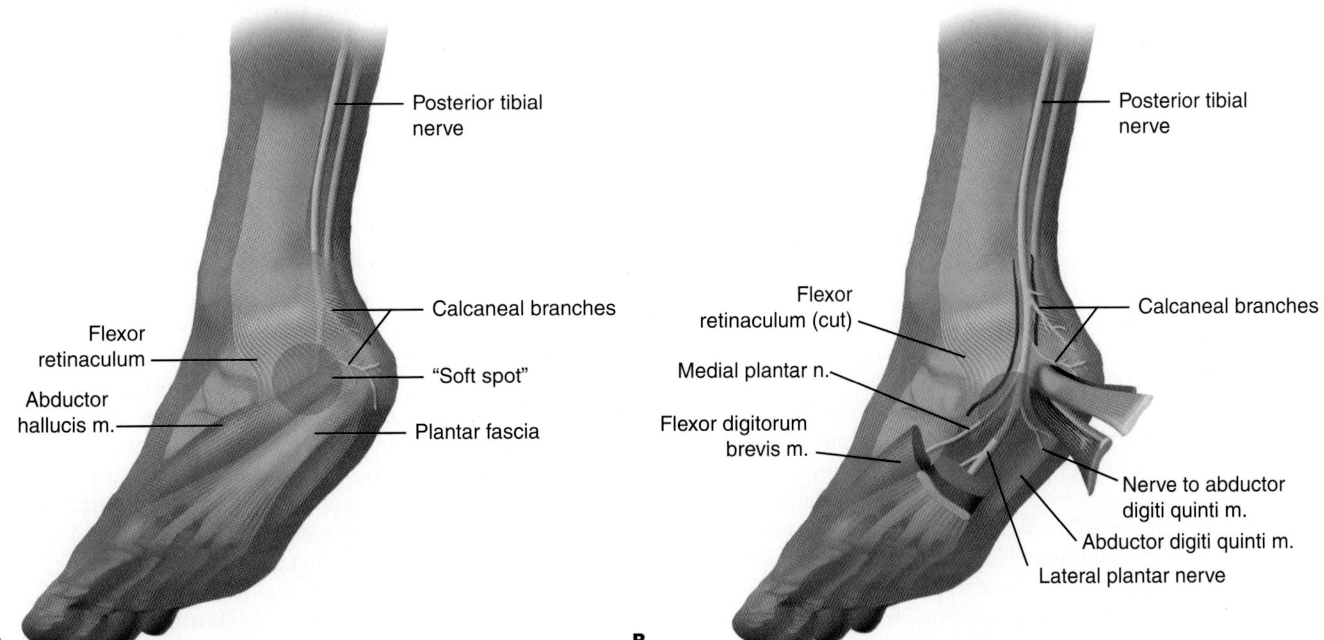

FIG 1 • **A.** The laciniate ligament, three branches of the tibial nerve, and the classic tarsal tunnel. **B.** Detailed anatomy of the tibial nerve and branches.

- The medial plantar nerve leaves the tibial nerve just proximal to or just under the abductor hallucis and travels under the abductor hallucis, innervating it and forming the intermetatarsal nerves to the 1/2, 2/3, and 3/4 interspaces. Both the medial and lateral plantar nerves provide innervation to the interossei and lubricals.

- The medial calcaneal nerves may be multiple and emerge from the tibial nerve proximal to the proximal (upper) edge of the abductor hallucis.
- The plantar fascia or aponeurosis arises from the os calcis and is composed of three segments—the central, medial, and lateral portions.
  - Clinically, the central portion is considered to be the plantar fascia and originates from the medial tuberosity of the os calcis and inserts into all five toes.
  - Extension of the toes and the metatarsophalangeal (MTP) joints tightens the plantar aponeurosis, elevates the longitudinal arch, and inverts the hindfoot. This mechanism, which is entirely passive and depends on bony and ligamentous stability, is referred to as the "windlass mechanism."

PATHOGENESIS

- Plantar fasciitis is thought to be a result of repetitive microtearing of the origin of the central band of the plantar aponeurosis.
  - This repetitive trauma results in inflammation and persistent pain, especially pain with the first steps in the morning or with the first steps after periods of inactivity.
- Chronic symptoms of plantar fasciitis develop in about 10% of patients with plantar heel pain.
  - We believe that these patients experience partial ruptures or attenuation of the plantar fascia, as suggested by clinical findings in which the medial border of the fascia becomes less distinct than the normal side when the ankle and toes are dorsiflexed.
  - A subset of these patients has chronic, disabling plantar heel pain with associated neurogenic symptoms of distal tarsal tunnel syndrome.

NATURAL HISTORY

- In 1986, Rondhuis and Huson[12] described compression of the first branch of the lateral plantar nerve and its association with heel pain.
- Baxter et al[1] further studied and reported on the priniciple of isolated compression of the first branch and its association with chronic plantar fasciitis.
- Further studies by Lau and Daniels[11] demonstrated that increased traction in the lateral plantar nerve and in its first branch is noted as the supporting structures of the longitudinal arch are selectively divided, including the plantar fascia, which could result in a "traction neuritis" of the nerves.
- Inflammatory conditions and local edema affect the nerve as it travels in the hindfoot. Entrapment, or *traction irritation,* of the lateral plantar nerve and its first branch is though to occur between the abductor hallucis muscle deep fascia, the medial border of the plantar fascia, and the medial caudal margin of the quadratus plantae muscle.
  - Electrodiagnostic evidence of compression of the first branch lateral plantar nerve and its association with chronic plantar fasciitis have been reported by Schon et al.[13]

PATIENT HISTORY AND PHYSICAL FINDINGS

- Patients with chronic proximal plantar fasciitis with distal tarsal tunnel syndrome have signs and symptoms typical of both plantar fasciitis and neuritis.
- We believe that chronic plantar heel pain that does not respond to a standard nonoperative protocol is the result of attenuated or significant partial plantar fascia rupture, in addition to some degree of neuritis or nerve entrapment.
- The patient population is diverse, with a wide age range and varied activity levels, and includes both nonathletes and elite competitive athletes. Occupations are also diverse, although many patients are employed in vocations that require prolonged standing or walking.

Plantar Fasciitis

- Plantar fasciitis symptoms are considered chronic when they persist for at least 9 months.
  - Typically, symptoms include plantar heel pain that is most severe with the first steps in the morning or with the first steps after prolonged sitting. This pain disappears relatively quickly after walking for a few moments and is relieved immediately upon non–weight-bearing. It does not become increasingly painful with increased walking or at rest.
- On physical examination, there is tenderness at the medial tubercle of the calcaneus, which correlates with the origin of the plantar fascia. This area of tenderness is focal and reproducible and is located at the plantar medial heel.
  - Most patients in the chronic state have evidence of attenuation of the plantar fascia and probable biomechanical incompetence.
  - This asymmetry between the two feet in terms of firmness of the plantar fascia is noted when recreating the windlass mechanism (ankle dorsiflexion and 1–5 MTP joint dorsiflexion) and palpating the plantar fascia medial border. This difference is thought to represent a significant chronic partial plantar fascia tear.
  - Significant attenuation of the plantar fascia was noted at preoperative evaluation in 15 of 22 patients in the series reported by DiGiovanni et al.[4]

Neuritis/Distal Tarsal Tunnel Syndrome

- Neuritic symptoms and signs may be subtle and not appreciated unless the examiner is aware of their potential presence and checks for their possible existence.
- Neuritic symptoms typically include reports of a long "afterburn" rather than instant relief of heel pain with non–weight-bearing after prolonged activity.
  - Patients may also describe radiation of pain in the posteromedial ankle, medial hindfoot, and distal plantar foot, often with numbness or burning and often worse with prolonged standing or when resting after prolonged activity.
  - Neuritis pain may radiate up the medial aspect of the leg, a condition known as the Valleix phenomenon.
  - Radiation of the neuritic pain may occur along the lateral aspect of the plantar heel, following the course of the lateral plantar nerve first branch.
  - In many cases, the patient will have difficulty describing the exact nature of the pain but may report diffuse tingling, burning, or numbness.

- The medial hindfoot tenderness is located over the abductor hallucis muscle at a position approximately 5 cm anterior to the posterior border of the heel at the intersection of the plantar and medial skin.
  - If one palpates the medial border of the heel, the examiner's digit will suddenly feel a "soft spot," which corresponds with the course of the lateral plantar nerve and its first branch as they pass from the ankle into the foot at the lower edge of the fascia of the abductor hallucis, an area that is associated with nerve entrapment or neuritis.
  - This is a separate area from the medial tubercle of the calcaneus tenderness associated with plantar fasciitis.
- In athletes (especially basketball players) or individuals whose occupations involve prolonged standing, enlargement or hypertrophy of the abductor hallucis muscle may be appreciated.
- Patients with such irritation of the tibial nerve and its branches may also be tender over the nerves in the arch, noted with the plantar fascia relaxed by passively plantarflexing the ankle and toes.
  - These patients have been diagnosed with so-called distal plantar fasciitis, an entitiy we doubt exists except with midsubstance ruptures of the plantar fascia.
  - These patients with tarsal tunnel syndrome may also have tenderness in the intermetatarsal spaces, suggesting intermetatarsal neuritis, Morton's neuroma, or a "double-crush" syndrome. This is usually not the case, however, as patients with primary pathology proximally in the distal tarsal tunnel and plantar fascia complain of heel, arch, and posteromedial ankle pain, while those with primary disease distally complain of metatarsal pain (metatarsalgia) and may incidentally also have tenderness over the nerves proximally.

IMAGING AND OTHER DIAGNOSTIC STUDIES

- Electrodiagnositic studies are usually performed before surgical intervention, with most aimed at ruling out associated pathology, such as radiculopathy and generalized peripheral neuropathy.
  - If diffuse peripheral neuropathy rather than localized nerve entrapment is suspected, screening for diabetes, thyroid dysfunction, or alcoholism may be indicated.
  - Lower extremity electrodiagnostic studies are known to be less reproducible than upper extremity studies and are also dependent on the expertise and skill of the electrodiagnostician in performing detailed foot and ankle studies. The studies should evaluate potential entrapment of both the lateral and medial plantar nerves.
  - Electromyelographic results for the abductor hallucis or abductor digiti quinti are more likely to be abnormal than are nerve conduction studies.
  - A positive result adds confirmation to the clinical diagnosis, but because the neuritic component is thought to be a traction neuropathy, as demonstrated by Lau and Daniels,[11] and is believed to be most evident in the dynamic situation, which is not usually tested, a negative result does not rule out the diagnosis. Accordingly, it is not uncommon to have negative electrodiagnostic studies despite signs and symptoms of neuritis.
- Serologic studies may be indicated to evaluate for possible inflammatory arthritis in patients with bilateral heel pain of simultaneous onset and similar severity.
- Weight-bearing foot radiographs are obtained to rule out such associated pathology as calcaneal stress fracture and hindfoot degenerative joint disease.
  - Patients with subtalar and sometimes ankle arthrosis or with tenosynovitis of the posterior tibial, flexor digitorum longus, and flexor hallucis may have sufficient swelling to irritate the tibial nerve.
  - A subset of patients with posterior tibial tendon dysfunction may also have tarsal tunnel symptoms.[9]
  - If there is a history of previous fracture or significant trauma, radiographs of both the ankle and foot should be otatined to rule out external sources of nerve compression such as exostosis.
- Computed tomography (CT) has a limited role but may be helpful if there is a prior history of trauma with posttraumatic changes to assess for bony exostosis and deformity.
- Technetium bone scans have a poor specificity and are rarely indicated.
- Magnetic resonance imaging (MRI) is sensitive for detecting frank fascial rupture and confirming proximal plantar fasciitis, but it is not indicated in most cases.
  - MRI can demonstrate occult pathology, such as a space-occupying lesion in the proximal or distal tarsal tunnel or a subtle calcaneal stress fracture.

DIFFERENTIAL DIAGNOSIS

- Diffuse peripheral neuropathy (diabetes mellitus, thyroid dysfunction, alcoholism)
- Lumbar radiculopathy
- Inflammatory arthritis
- Calcaneal stress fracture, hindfoot degenerative joint disease

NONOPERATIVE MANAGEMENT

- Initial nonoperative treatment includes relative rest, plantar fascia and Achilles tendon stretching exercises, ice, and nonsteroidal anti-inflammatory drugs.
- Physical therapy modalities that involve or promote heating of the tissues, such as whirlpool baths, hydroculator packs, diathermy, ultrasound, or phonophoresis, seem to irritate the neuritic symptoms and increase rather than decrease symptoms.
  - Iontophoresis, which diffuses steroid with electrolysis, is well tolerated and is worthwhile.
- Steroid injections into the plantar fascia or the nerve itself are discouraged.
  - Many patients present with a history of earlier episodes of plantar fasciitis that responded to steroid injections. These patients are now unresponsive to injection and have an obviously attenuated plantar fascia. This suggests an association of steroid injection with plantar fascia rupture and the ensuing chronicity.
- Inexpensive over-the-counter orthotics are prescribed to support the arch and cushion the heel. With chronicity, a semirigid, accommodative, custom orthotic is prescribed. These are cork based and triple layered and include a "nerve relief channel" made of viscoelastic polymer, which is placed along the path of the lateral plantar nerve beginning at the proximal abductor hallucis muscle belly and extending to the soft spot.

- If the patient has more symptoms in the central heal pad, which involves the first branch of the lateral plantar, the channel is carried more posteriorly and onto the plantar heel to include the painful central area.
- The same orthotic devices are used postoperatively if the patient requires surgery.

- Preliminary studies with extracorporeal shock wave lithotripsy (ESWL), of both low and high intensity, for chronic plantar fasciitis report a positive response, and the modality appears to be safe and effective.
  - For individuals with chronic plantar fasciitis and associated signs and symptoms of neuritis, however, ESWL was not as effective. The treatment has the potential to further aggravate the inflamed nerves and is therefore not recommended.
  - Controlled ESWL studies in which patients with neurogenic symptoms were excluded had better results. Additional investigations are needed to clarify these issues.

SURGICAL MANAGEMENT

- In the late 1980s and early 90s, Baxter and colleagues[1] reported on and popularized their surgical approach to painful heel syndrome in athletes with entrapment of the first branch of the lateral plantar nerve. This approach includes partial release of the plantar fascia combined with release of the first branch of the lateral plantar nerve and removal of a heel spur if present. The investigators have reported a high success rate, particularly in the athletic population.
  - More recent reports using this approach in a more general patient population have noted mixed results, however, with Davies et al[2] in 1999 reporting less than 50% of patients with complete satisfaction as a result of persistent symptoms.
- DiGiovanni and Gould and their colleagues[3,4] have devised and reported on a modified surgical approach based partially on the work of Baxter and colleagues. The approach is also based on the observation that patients with plantar fascia rupture and chronic pain who do not have neurogenic symptoms respond to a complete surgical release of the plantar fascia.
  - Patients who had the release described by Baxter and continued to be symptomatic responded to the complete release and neurolysis as described below.
  - The more-extensile approach is used to allow the release of all potential sources of entrapment of the tibial nerve and its branches, and thus allow for improved rates of complete resolution of pain and elimination of activity limitations.
  - This technique combines a complete plantar fascia release with a proximal and distal tarsal tunnel release, without bone spur removal.
- The philosophy behind a complete release rather than a partial release of the plantar fascia is as follows:
  - The literature does not provide information about the optimal amount of partial release to perform to allow for reproducible resolution of plantar heel pain. The amount is probably highly variable from patient to patient and depends on a number of factors, including the type of foot arch.
  - Patients with chronic heel pain commonly have evidence of attenuation of their plantar fascia and probably have pre-existing biomechanical incompetence. A further partial release in feet with pre-existing plantar fascia attenuation has not consistently led to resolution of plantar heel symptoms.
  - Complete release of the plantar fascia from the abductor hallucis to the abductor digiti quinti has consistently relieved the pain experienced after the first step in the morning or after recumbency.
- The nerve component of the pathology is also specifically addressed. In our experience, release of the plantar fascia alone in patients with chronic plantar fasciitis often leads to increased neuritic symptoms. Consequently, the nerve procedure is always performed in addition to the plantar fascia release.
  - Rather than an isolated release of the first branch of the lateral plantar nerve, a proximal (or classic) as well as a distal tarsal tunnel release is performed to address all potential sites of nerve entrapment.
  - Proximal tarsal tunnel syndrome may coexist distal and can be difficult to differentiate and isolate.
  - In addition, more than one branch of the terminal tibial nerve branches may be entrapped.

Preoperative Planning

- Good history taking, specifically to determine when and in which anatomic location symptoms occur, is essential. We cannot emphasize enough that the history will differentiate metatarsalgia, pure plantar fasciitis, radiculopathy, and neuropathy.
- A careful physical examination must be done as indicated previously.
- Electrodiagnostic testing is useful when the history and physical have not clearly ruled out neuropathy particularly or radiculopathy.
  - Tibial nerve entrapment may coexist with neuropathy, but the prognosis for a good result with this surgery is guarded, and we believe such a combination accounts for less than optimal results.

Positioning

- The patient is positioned supine without a bump under the hip, allowing the leg to externally rotate.
- Multiple folded surgical towels are placed under the foot to allow the surgeon to easily operate posteromedially and to allow room for the assistant to retract. The foot is positioned near the foot of the table, but not at the end, so the surgeon has the table on which to rest the forearms and not be forced to operate in midair.
- We operate from the seated position across the normal leg and use a rolling surgical stool so that we can move from facing the medial side to the plantar side.
  - When we move around to the plantar side, we ask the anesthetist to place the foot of the bed in Trendelenburg to improve access.

Approach

- We use a posteromedial and plantar approach to fully visualize the anatomy.
- The procedure is done with high thigh tourniquet control after exsanguination of the leg.
- Bipolar cautery is used for minimal tissue necrosis.
- Loupe magnification is always used, with a preference of 3.5 to 4.5 magnification.

COMPLETE RELEASE OF THE PLANTAR FASCIA AND TARSAL TUNNEL[5]

- The midpoint between the posterior border of the medial malleolus and the medial border of the Achilles tendon is marked. The medial edge of the heel is palpated beginning posteriorly and moving distally until the palpating finger feels the soft spot where the neurovascular bundle enters the foot, and this point is marked as well.
- The midpoint of the malleolar–tendon interval is marked proximally, and the incision extends plantarly and curves distally to cross the soft spot, continuing onto the plantar skin at the distal portion of the heel pad, and extending transversely about three quarters of the width of the heel skin (**TECH FIG 1A**).
- The entire skin incision is made following the skin marking.
- The proximal subcutaneous tissue is separated bluntly to identify the superficial vessels, and a double skin hook is placed on the far side of the surgeon and lifted away from the ankle.
- The surgeon easily spreads, cuts, and cauterizes superficial vessels and identifies the flexor retinaculum (laciniate ligament). This layer is divided directly over visible posterior tibial veins distally to the level of the abductor hallucis muscle. No attempt is made to isolate the tibial nerve (**TECH FIG 1B**).
- The superficial fascia of the abductor hallucis is divided sharply with a no. 15 surgical scalpel or no. 64 Beaver blade.
- The hooks are now moved distally to the plantar surface, and spreading and cutting is done with a long-handled tenotomy scissors down to the plantar fascia. Two sharp Senn retractors are now used, which gather the fat away from the fascia and improve visualization.
- A Meyerding retractor is placed at the distal extent of the incision to expose the fascia overlying the abductor digiti quinti fascia. The knife blade is used to sharply cut the plantar fascia from its lateral extent, at the edge of

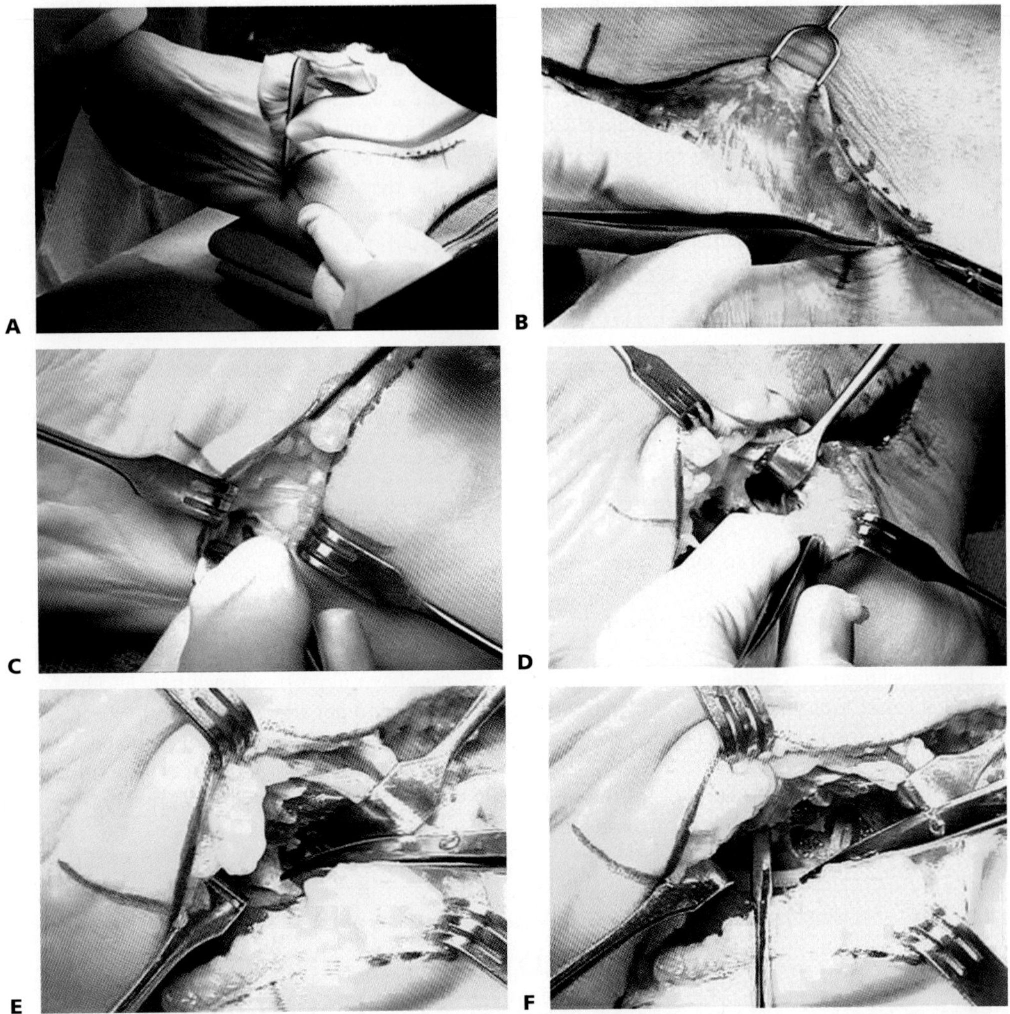

TECH FIG 1 • **A.** The skin incision for the complete release. **B.** Dividing the laciniate ligament. **C.** Dividing the entire plantar fascia. **D.** Dividing the deep fascia of the abductor hallucis. **E.** The abductor hallucis and flexor digitorum brevis interval. **F.** Lateral plantar nerve overlying the quadratus plantae fascia.

the abductor digiti quinti fascia medially to the abductor hallucis fascia, fully exposing the flexor digitorum brevis muscle (**TECH FIG 1C**).
  - The plantar fascia surface is actually convex and meets each of the abductor fascias more deeply or dorsally than at its midpoint.
- As right-handed surgeons, we release this deep fascia on the right foot from the laciniate ligament distally. On the left foot, we begin from the plantar fascia side. In either case, we now place a self-retaining retractor in the wound to allow the assistant to help with the next step (**TECH FIG 1D**).
- The blades of the tenotomy scissors are spread between the muscle of the abductor hallucis and its deep fascia to initiate its exposure. The Meyerding retractor is used to further tease the muscle off the fascia and enhance and complete its visualization.
- The fascia is divided under the muscle, exposing the neurovascular structures and the tarsal tunnel. We divide the deep fascia as far as we can see it and then expose the structure from the opposite side (either proximally and distally) and complete the release.
- The muscle of the flexor digitorum brevis is then retracted laterally, and the fine fascia overlying the neurovascular structures is divided.
- The interval between the abductor hallucis and the flexor brevis is then exposed. The self-retaining retractor is placed on the skin and subcutaneous fat at this interval. One Meyerding (or similar right-angle) retractor is placed under the abductor muscle, retracting it proximally. Another right-angle retracts the flexor digitorum brevis laterally (**TECH FIG 1E**).
- The posterior tibial artery and veins are easily seen. Parallel to them but slightly more anterior is the lateral plantar nerve, often with a little fat around it. The whiteness of the nerve and its striations make it obvious. The first branch is not specifically exposed but lies more posteriorly.
- The nerve is carefully teased from its surrounding tissues and gently retracted, and the underlying quadratus plantae fascia is observed.
  - A small vessel may obscure visualization of the nerve in some patients. In such cases, with the power of the bipolar cautery turned down, we carefully cauterize and cut it to provide the needed exposure.
  - The quadratus fascia is often a dense band over which the nerve is obviously tented. In other cases, the white bands of fascia are visible but less dense. They are cut sharply with the scissors to expose the muscle. The nerve now lies under no tension (**TECH FIG 1F**).
- With the confluence of the superficial and deep abductor fascias distally and the medial border of the plantar fascia, a dense band of fascia overlies the lateral plantar nerve, and with the dense band of the quadratus fascia below, it is easy to visualize a pincer effect on the nerve at this point with weight bearing and particularly when the plantar fascia is less taut.
- Closure is carried out after irrigation of the wound. The ankle subcutaneous is closed with 4-0 absorbable suture and the skin with 4-0 nonabsorbable suture. The glabrous plantar skin is closed with only 3-0 or 4-0 skin permanent suture, with no subcutaneous suture.
- A soft bulky dressing is applied and the tourniquet released. Sterility is not broken until the toes show good perfusion.

COMPLETE PLANTAR FASCIA AND TARSAL TUNNEL RELEASE FOR PRIOR INCOMPLETE AND FAILED RELEASES

- The same basic approach is used as just described but with several additions to the technique.
- The new incision begins proximal to the original one to start in normal tissue.
- The old incision is incorporated into the new, ensuring access to the soft spot.
- When the laciniate ligament is divided, the tibial nerve is exposed, and a vessel loop is placed around the nerve and a tie is placed on the loop as opposed to a hemostat to avoid any traction on the nerve.
- As the release proceeds, external neurolysis of the tibial nerve and of the medial and lateral plantar branches is carried out. The calcaneal nerves are identified and protected. The first branch of the lateral plantar nerve is identified.
- The muscle belly of the abductor hallucis is often divided with a cutting cautery with careful blunt dissection to protect the underlying critical structures. The muscle of the flexor digitorum brevis may also be partially or fully divided to get adequate exposure.
- If there is no evidence of damage to the nerves or marked wound scar or scar around the nerves, the wounds are closed as in the primary procedure.

COMPLETE PLANTAR FASCIA AND TARSAL TUNNEL RELEASE WHEN EXTENSIVE SCARRING OF THE NERVE IS PRESENT, WITH THE USE OF BARRIER WRAPPING OF THE NERVE

- The complete release as described above is performed.
- For nearly 20 years, we have used greater saphenous vein wrapping of scarred mixed nerves that must be preserved. More recently, we have used barrier wrapping with commercially available collagen tubes. Both techniques are described below.

Use of the Greater Saphenous Vein

- The greater saphenous vein is harvested with a longitudinal incision beginning in the midpoint between the crest of the tibia and its posteromedial margin. One usually has to harvest a length of vein three times the length of nerve to be wrapped.
  - At harvest, metal ligaclips are used for the branches, which are few in number in the distal vein. Double medium clips are used at either end of the vein, and one is left on the end of the harvested proximal vein to indicate the orientation of the vein.
- The vein is placed in lidocaine to relax the smooth muscle component. It is then dilated from distal to proximal either with mechanical dilators or hydrostatically with lidocaine inserted under pressure with a syringe, using a vein plastic adaptor fitted to the syringe.
- All metal clips are then removed and the vein divided longitudinally.
- The vein is then curled around the involved nerve in barber pole fashion with the venous intima adjacent to the nerve. The vein is wrapped without tension, and each end is attached to surrounding tissues so as not to have a closed loop at either end. The coils are attached to each other with two 7-0 Prolene sutures placed about 180 degrees apart (TECH FIG 2).
- The medial and lateral plantar nerves are wrapped separately.
  - The tibial nerve may be wrapped and then the surgeon may continue down one or the other of the branches.
  - The wrap of the other plantar nerve joins the initially wrapped portion.

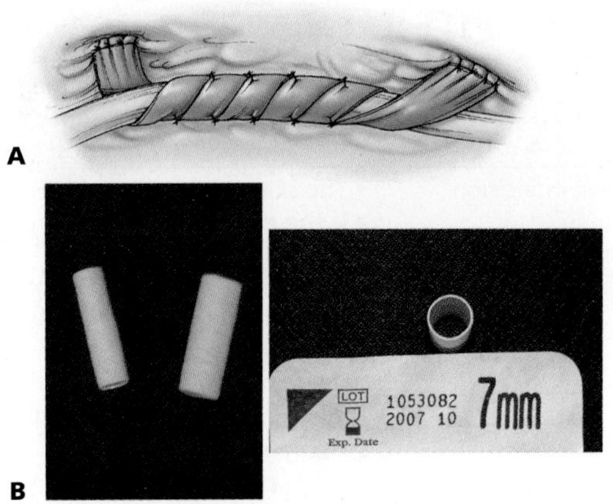

TECH FIG 2 • **A.** Vein wrapping. **B.** Bovine collagen longitudinally split tubes for wrapping.

  - The first branch of the lateral plantar may be initially wrapped with the lateral plantar and then allowed to travel independently distally.
  - The calcaneal branches are allowed to escape between the coils and must not be entrapped in the procedure.

Use of Commercial Collagen Tubes

- Use of the commercially available collagen tubes simplifies the process. The tubes come in diameters ranging from 2 to 10 mm and lengths of 2 to 4 cm. The tubes are provided longitudinally divided.
- The size to be used is determined by the surgeon's estimation of the needed diameter and lengths. Several lengths may be joined or a slightly long segment may be trimmed.
- The slit in the tube is closed, not too tightly, with a few interrupted 6-0 nylon sutures.

USE OF CONDUITS FOR NEUROMAS OF THE CALCANEAL BRANCHES

- A neuroma of a calcaneal branch is treated with either a vein or a collagen conduit.
- The neuroma is exposed and excised.
- A conduit of at least 2 cm should be used.
  - Collagen tubes of a proper diameter to loosely enclose the nerve are available, and the 4-cm lengths may be trimmed as needed.
  - When using a vein, the diameter must also be large enough to loosely accommodate the nerve, and the lumen diameter may need to be narrowed a bit so that it fits a little more closely around the nerve end.
- A nylon suture is placed through the end of the nerve, the needle is removed, and the two ends of the suture are grasped with a hemostat.
- A suture passer (Hewson) is placed through the conduit, and the nylon suture attached to the nerve is placed through the suture passer loop.
- The conduit is slid over the nerve, overlapping by 5 mm to 1 cm, and 8-0 sutures are used to attach the conduit lumen to the epineurium of the nerve. Typically, two sutures at 180 degrees are placed. The nylon suture used to draw the nerve into the conduit is removed (TECH FIG 3).
- The nerve and its "conduit to nowhere" is buried posteromedially, often into the retrocalcaneal space.

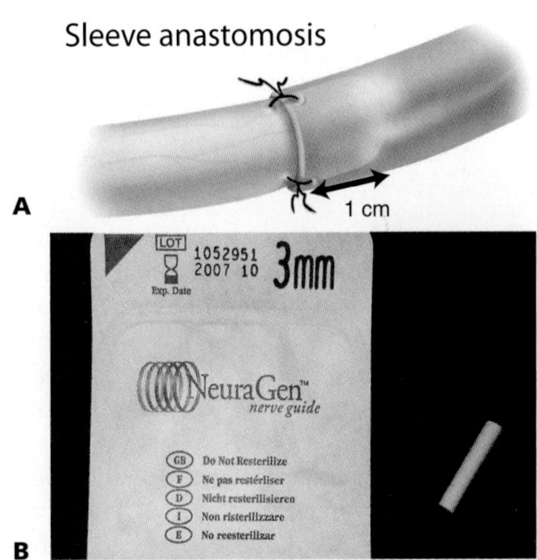

TECH FIG 3 • **A.** Vein conduits. **B.** Bovine collagen conduits for neuromas (or nerve guide for repairs).

PEARLS AND PITFALLS

Indications	■ It is essential that the patient's history is compatible with the diagnosis and that he or she is tender or has a Tinel sign at the soft spot. ■ If the history and physical examination do not correlate, look elsewhere for the diagnosis.
Accuracy of the skin incision	■ The skin incision must be accurate and the anatomy clearly seen. ■ If the entrance of the neurovascular bundle to the foot is not accurately located, the release will be unsuccessful. ■ If there is difficulty finding the nerve in the interval between the abductor and the flexor brevis, divide the muscle of the abductor hallucis and find the nerve more proximally and follow it through the interval. ■ If you are lost, find the nerve under the laciniate ligament (it is posterior to the vessels and more lateral), and follow it and the lateral plantar branch more distally to carry out a proper release.
Bleeding	■ Use of loupes and careful hemostasis will prevent bleeding, which prevents accurate visualization of the structures. ■ Postoperative bleeding will irritate the nerve and create more scarring, and can compromise the result. ■ Make sure the tourniquet is of proper size for the size of the thigh, and exsanguination must be right up to the tourniquet. This may necessitate the use of a sterile tourniquet, applied after draping. At times, with a very obese thigh, a calf tourniquet may be used. ■ We cannot emphasize enough the importance of excellent visualization of the anatomy.
Completeness of the release	■ All structures noted in the description must be fully released.

POSTOPERATIVE CARE

- The patient is placed in a soft bulky dressing at surgery, and crutches are used for non–weight-bearing. From immediately after the operation, motion of the foot and ankle is encouraged.
- Sutures are removed at 2 weeks, and a light dressing is applied. Gentle range-of-motion exercise of the ankle is re-emphasized to promote gliding of the nerve, but non–weight-bearing continues for 2 more weeks.
- At 4 weeks, the patient is allowed to bear weight using the custom orthotic described earlier.
  - The orthotic is used for at least 9 months and then may be phased out.
  - If the patient fails to comply, pain will be experienced, usually on the dorsum and lateral border of the foot, presumably from "arch strain." Most patients comply, without too much encouragement.

OUTCOMES

Primary Surgery

- DiGiovanni and Gould et al[3,4] reported an 82% rate of total satisfaction in primary surgery patients, with a marked decrease in pain to a level of no pain or mild, intermittent pain. This is a significant improvement over the less than 50% total satisfaction reported in most recent studies of limited plantar fascia release with a limited nerve release, or nerve release without plantar fascia release.
- The improved rate of total satisfaction is reflective of the lower rates of residual pain and activity limitations. Improved surgical results in primary surgery patients are thought to be due to the comprehensive surgical approach with the goal of addressing all potential sites of pathology—nerve and plantar fascia.
- Our unreported data from more than 100 cases followed for over 2 years indicate that patients take varying periods of time to reach a steady state or complete relief of all symptoms. This averaged about 18 months, and varied from 6 months to 2.5 years.[7]
- The surgical technique described here is highly recommended in patients with chronic plantar fasciitis and neuritic signs and symptoms, without prior surgery.

Revision Surgery

- Less predictable results have been reported for revision surgery. Although 73% of patients indicated they were better off than before surgery, total satisfaction was reported by only 27%, and 36% were dissatisfied with the procedure. There was a much higher incidence of residual pain and activity limitation.
- In revision situations, patients with evidence of inadequate prior distal tarsal tunnel release and those with persistent mechanical plantar fasciitis are most likely to have good resolution of their symptoms.
- Although the results for barrier wrapping and of the use of conduits for neuromas are less certain than those for the primary releases, they are still superior to results for other techniques reported to date. Data on the use of collagen conduits and wraps are being collected, with encouraging early outcomes.

COMPLICATIONS

- A low rate of complications, both intraoperatively and postoperatively, can be expected with this technique.
- Meticulous technique is needed to avoid potential complications, which include wound dehiscence, perineural scarring, and direct nerve injury. We recommend using bipolar electrocautery and surgical loupe magnification.
- Development of complex regional pain syndrome is possible postoperatively. Early diagnosis and aggressive treatment improves the prognosis.

REFERENCES

1. Baxter DE, Pfeffer GB, Thigpen M. Chronic heel pain: treatment rationale. Orthop Clin North Am 1989;20:563–569.
2. Davies MS, Weiss GA, Saxby TX. Plantar fasciitis: how successful is surgical intervention? Foot Ankle Int 1999;20:803–807.
3. DiGiovanni BF, Abuzzahab FS, Gould JS. Plantar fascia release with proximal and distal tarsal tunnel release: surgical approach to chronic, disabling plantar fasciitis with associated nerve pain. Tech Foot Ankle Surg 2003;2:254–261.
4. DiGiovanni BF, Rodriguez del Rio FA, Gould JS. Chronic, disabling heel pain with associated nerve pain: primary and revision surgery results. Podium presentation and abstract at the 17th Annual Summer Meeting of the American Orthopaedic Foot and Ankle Society, San Diego, July 2001.
5. Gould JS. Chronic plantar fasciitis. Am J Orthop 2003;32:11–13.
6. Heimkes B, Posel P, Stotz S, et al. The proximal and distal tarsal tunnel syndromes: an anatomic study. Int Orthop 1987;11:193–196.
7. Hollis M, Ferguson A, Gould JS, et al. American Sports Medicine Institute review of 104 feet (92 patients) following the complete plantar fascia and tarsal tunnel release between 1996–2000. Unpublished.
8. Keck C. The tarsal-tunnel syndrome. J Bone Joint Surg 1962;44A: 180–182.
9. Labib SA, Gould JS, Rodriguez del Rio FA, Lyman S. Heel pain triad: the combination of plantar fasciitis, posterior tibial tendon dysfunction, and tarsal tunnel syndrome. Foot Ankle Int 2002;23:212–220.
10. Lam SJS. A tarsal-tunnel syndrome. Lancet 1962;2:1354–1355.
11. Lau TC, Daniels TR. Effects of tarsal tunnel release and stabilization procedures on tibial nerve tension in a surgical created pes planus foot. Foot Ankle Int 1998;19:770–776.
12. Rondhuis JJ, Huson A. The first branch of the lateral plantar nerve and heel pain. Acta Morphol Meerl Scand 1986;24:269.
13. Schon LC, Glennon TC, Baxter DE. Heel pain syndrome: electrodiagnostic support for nerve entrapment. Foot Ankle 1993;14: 129–135.

Chapter 58 Endoscopic Plantar Fasciotomy

Steven L. Shapiro

DEFINITION

- Plantar fasciitis is the most common cause of heel pain in adults.
- The predominant symptom is pain in the plantar region of the foot when initiating walking.
- The cause is a degenerative tear of part of the fascial origin from the calcaneus, followed by a tendinopathy-type reaction.

ANATOMY

- The plantar fascia is a ligament with longitudinal fibers originating from the calcaneal tuberosity.
- The normal medial band is the thickest, measuring up to 3 mm.
- The central and lateral bands are 1 to 2 mm thick.[1]
- Distally, the plantar fascia divides into five slips, one for each toe.
- The plantar fascia provides support to the arch. As the toes extend during the stance phase of gait, the plantar fascia is tightened by a windlass mechanism, resulting in elevation of the longitudinal arch, inversion of the hindfoot, and external rotation of the leg.
- Endoscopically, the pertinent anatomy is the abductor hallucis muscle medially, then the plantar fascia. After fasciotomy, the flexor digitorum brevis comes into view as the medial intermuscular septum.

PATHOGENESIS

- Specimens of plantar fascia obtained during surgery reveal a spectrum of changes, ranging from degeneration of fibrous tissue to fibroblastic proliferation.
- The fascia is usually markedly thickened and gritty. These pathologic changes are more consistent with fasciosis (degenerative process) than fasciitis (inflammatory process), but fasciitis remains the accepted description in the literature.

NATURAL HISTORY

- The typical patient is an adult who complains of plantar heel pain aggravated by activity and relieved by rest.
- Start-up pain when initiating walking is common.
- Strain of the plantar fascia can result from prolonged standing, running, or jumping and activities that create repetitive stress on the plantar fascia. Excessive pronation is a common mechanical cause.
- The rigid cavus foot type can also predispose to plantar fasciitis.
- Obesity is present in up to 70% of patients.
- Plantar fasciitis is common among runners and ballet dancers.
- About 15% of cases are bilateral. Women are affected more than men.

PHYSICAL FINDINGS

- Localized tenderness over the plantar calcaneal tuberosity is the most common physical finding.
- Pain is usually medial, but occasionally lateral. Rarely, pain may be located distally; this condition is called distal plantar fasciitis. Frequently there is soft tissue swelling of the plantar medial heel.
- Careful comparison to the contralateral heel is useful in confirming tenderness typical for plantar fasciitis.

IMAGING AND OTHER DIAGNOSTIC STUDIES

- Radiographs are ordered routinely in patients with plantar heel pain.
- Plantar calcaneal spurs occur in up to 50% of patients but are not thought to cause heel pain; these are commonly associated with calcification in the origin of the flexor hallucis brevis, which is located proximal to the origin of the plantar fascia.
- Stress fractures, unicameral bone cysts, and giant cell tumors are usually identified with plain radiography.
- Three-phase technetium bone scans are rarely necessary but are positive in up to 95% of cases of plantar fasciitis.
- MRI can be used in questionable cases and elegantly demonstrates thickening of the plantar fascia and rules out soft tissue and bone tumors, subtalar arthritis, and stress fractures.
- Ultrasound is cost-effective and easily measures the thickness of the plantar fascia, documenting plantar fasciitis when thickness exceeds 3 mm.

DIFFERENTIAL DIAGNOSIS

- **Plantar fascia rupture:** Generally occurs acutely after vigorous physical activity. There may be visible ecchymosis in the arch. MRI or ultrasound confirms the diagnosis.
- **Tarsal tunnel syndrome:** Compression of the tibial nerve can cause numbness and pain in the heel, sole, or toes. Positive percussion and compression tests are elicited, and electromyography and nerve conduction studies are positive in 50% of cases.
- **Distal tarsal tunnel syndrome,** compression of the first branch of the lateral plantar nerve (Baxter's nerve), is often confused with plantar fasciitis and may be associated with plantar fasciitis. In fact, some surgeons recommend decompressing Baxter's nerve with every plantar fascia release. In our opinion, these two entities are separate, and with careful examination plantar fasciitis may be isolated and effectively treated with endoscopic plantar fascia release.
- **Stress fractures:** With a calcaneal stress fracture, tenderness is not localized to the plantar medial heel but instead is more diffusely present in the calcaneus, suggested by a calcaneal squeeze test. Plain films usually suggest a fracture line, but if there is any doubt, MRI clearly demonstrates stress

fractures and readily distinguishes plantar fasciitis from stress fracture.

- **Neoplasms:** Visualized on plain films at times. MRI is diagnostic. Pain is typically achy, constant, nocturnal, and even present without weight bearing and at rest.
- **Infection:** Pain is often constant. There may be swelling, redness, or fluctuance. Plain films, MRI, or a white blood cell-labeled scan can be diagnostic. Laboratory tests may show increased erythrocyte sedimentation rate, C-reactive protein, or white blood cells.
- **Painful heel pad syndrome:** Occurs most often in runners; thought to result from disruption of fibrous septa of the heel pad
- **Heel pad atrophy:** Occurs in the elderly, usually not characterized by morning pain, and a "central heel pain syndrome" with tenderness more plantar than in plantar fasciitis, directly under the bony prominence in the calcaneus
- **Inflammatory arthritis:** Usually bilateral and diffuse in nature. May be associated with positive RA, HLA, and B27 and an increased erythrocyte sedimentation rate.

NONOPERATIVE MANAGEMENT

- Conservative management includes rest, ice, nonsteroidal anti-inflammatories, plantar fascia and Achilles tendon stretching, plantar fascia-specific stretching protocols, silicone heel pads, prefabricated and custom orthoses, night splints, CAM walkers, casts, physical therapy, athletic shoes, judicious use of steroid injections, and shockwave therapy.
- Ninety-five percent of patients will respond to conservative management.
- Surgery is indicated after 6 to 12 months of conservative treatment.

SURGICAL MANAGEMENT

- Plantar fasciotomy is indicated in the few patients who fail to respond to conservative treatment.
- Although open techniques have yielded good results, endoscopic plantar fasciotomy (EPF) offers several important advantages:
  - Minimal soft tissue dissection
  - Excellent visualization of the plantar fascia
  - Precision in transecting only the medial third to half of the plantar fascia
  - Minimal postoperative pain with early return to full weight-bearing status
  - Earlier return to activities and work

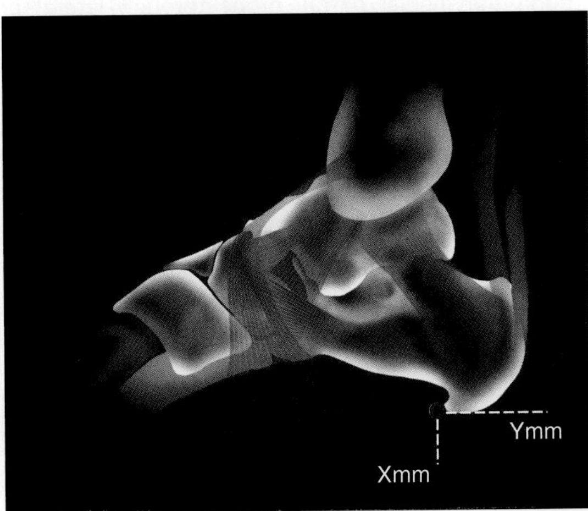

FIG 1 • Diagram of preoperative non–weight-bearing lateral radiograph showing appropriate measurements to identify the location of the medial portal incision.

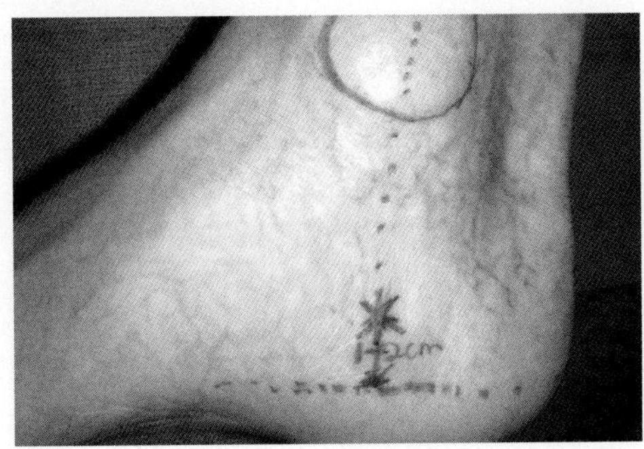

FIG 2 • A second method to determine the placement of the medial incision. The incision is made along a line that bisects the medial malleolus 1 to 2 cm superior to the junction of keratinized and nonkeratinized skin.

Preoperative Planning

- Non–weight-bearing lateral radiographs of the affected foot are performed (**FIG 1**).
- A point just anterior and inferior to the calcaneal tubercle is marked and measurements are made to the inferior and posterior skin lines.[2]
- These measurements are used to select the incision site (**FIG 2**).

Positioning and Anesthesia

- The patient is positioned supine with a bump under the ipsilateral hip of the affected side to limit external rotation of the limb.

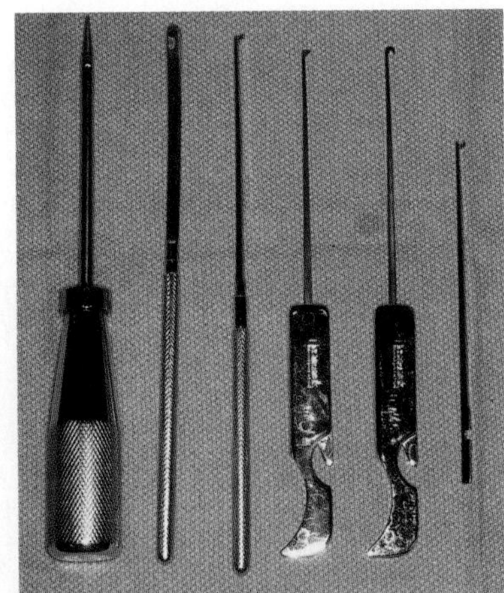

FIG 3 • Instratek Endotrac system for endoscopic plantar fasciotomy. From left to right: obturator with cannula, plantar fascia elevator, probe, disposable triangle knife with nondisposable handle, disposable hook knife with nondisposable handle, and disposable triangle knife without handle.

- The operative foot is then elevated on a foot prop with a tourniquet in place at the distal calf. The limb is prepared and draped in this position.
- We routinely order 1 g of cefazolin (Ancef) perioperatively.
- Anesthesia may be regional or general.
  - We prefer an ankle block or popliteal nerve block with intravenous sedation.
- The procedure is performed on an outpatient basis.

Equipment

- The equipment required includes the Instratek Endotrac System (Instratek, Houston, TX), which consists of a plantar fascia elevator, cannula and obturator, probe, nondisposable knife handles, and disposable hook and triangle knives (**FIG 3**).
- We use a 4-mm 30-degree short arthroscope.
- Several cotton-tipped applicators lightly fluffed with a Bovie scratch pad are needed.

TECHNIQUES

SET-UP

- The foot is prepared and draped on the foot prop and then exsanguinated with an Esmarch bandage.
- The tourniquet is inflated at the distal calf to 250 mm Hg.
- Make an 8-mm vertical incision just anterior and plantar to the medial tubercle of the calcaneus.
- Use the measurements from the non–weight-bearing lateral film as a guide.
- A good landmark is the medial malleolus.

IDENTIFYING THE PLANTAR FASCIA ENDOSCOPICALLY

- The incision can be placed on a line dropped from the midpoint of the medial malleolus or the junction of the middle and posterior thirds of the medial malleolus.
- Portal placement is critical to the success of the procedure.
- Deepen the incision with blunt tenotomy scissors.
- Place the plantar fascia elevator through the incision and sweep it from medial to lateral just plantar to the plantar fascia.
- Pass the obturator and cannula through this pathway and bring them out through a lateral incision overlying the tip of the obturator.
- Remove the obturator from the cannula and clear the cannula of fat with cotton-tipped applicators (**TECH FIG 1**). The cannula should be perpendicular to the long axis of the foot.
- Bring the 4-mm 30-degree scope into the medial portal.
- Visualize the abductor hallucis muscle medially, and then the plantar fascia. Pass the probe from the lateral portal and advance it medially to palpate the medial band of the plantar fascia (**TECH FIGS 2 AND 3**).

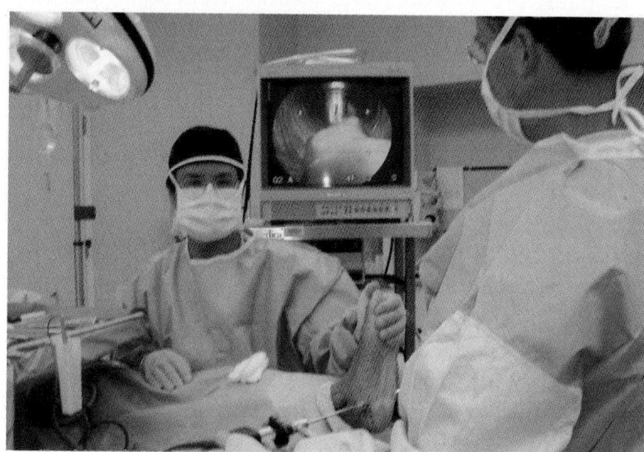

TECH FIG 2 • Intraoperative set-up with foot draped on foot prop, monitor on same side as foot, scope placed in cannula through the medial portal, probe through lateral portal. Plantar fascia is visualized on the monitor with the probe palpating the fascia.

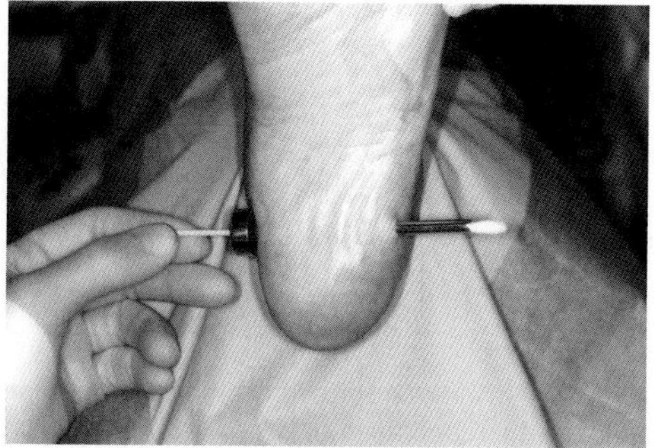

TECH FIG 1 • Clearing fat from cannula with fluffed cotton-tipped applicator to allow good visualization of the plantar fascia.

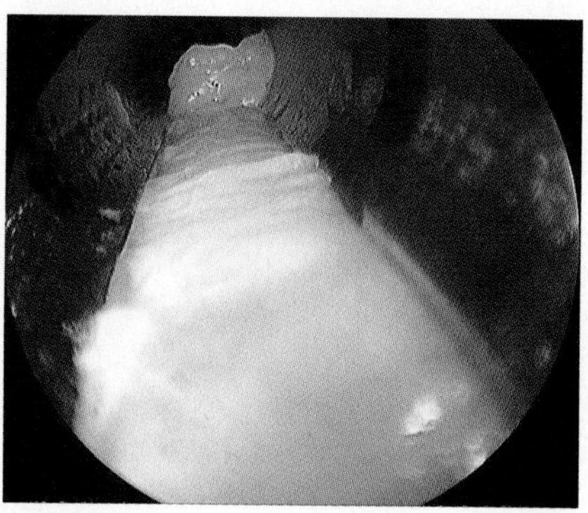

TECH FIG 3 • Plantar fascia before fasciotomy as seen through cannula.

PLANTAR FASCIA RELEASE

- Remove the probe and advance the triangle knife to the medial band.
- Dorsiflex the foot to place tension on the plantar fascia.
- With a controlled motion, pull the triangle knife across the medial band of the plantar fascia (**TECH FIG 4**).
  - Several passes are often necessary to completely divide this band.
- The flexor digitorum brevis muscle belly should be visible after the medial band is divided (**TECH FIG 5**). The fasciotomy is complete when the medial intermuscular septum is visualized.
- The amount of fascia divided is usually 14 mm, which can be measured off markings on the probe. The hook knife can be used to cut the fascia, but the triangle knife can be more easily manipulated with less likelihood of cutting into the muscle.

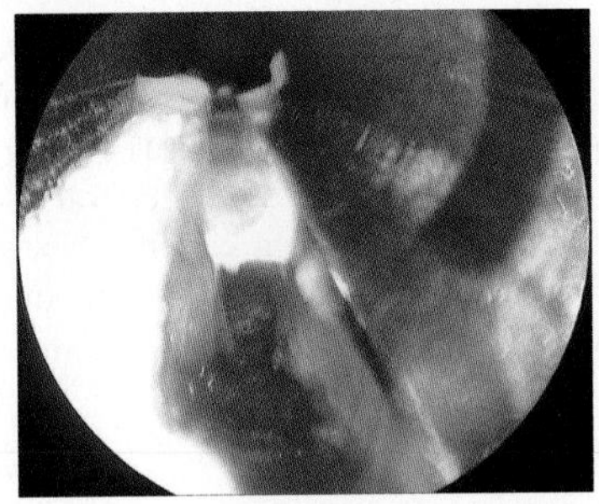

TECH FIG 4 • Endoscopic plantar fasciotomy performed with triangle knife as seen through cannula.

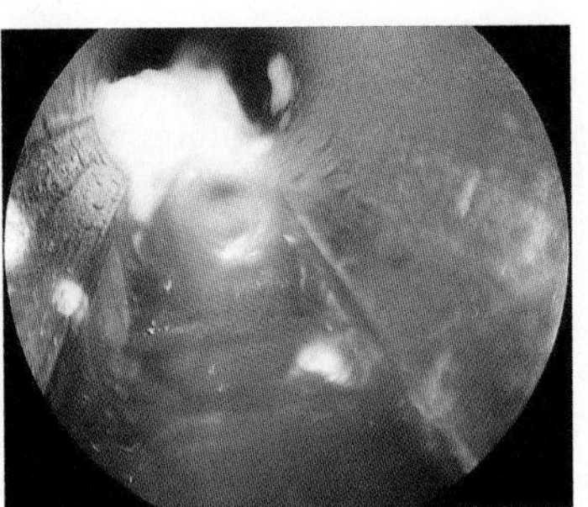

TECH FIG 5 • Flexor digitorum brevis muscle seen after endoscopic plantar fasciotomy. The central and lateral bands remain intact.

COMPLETION OF PROCEDURE

- After performing a partial fasciotomy, move the scope into the lateral portal to check if any bands of fascia remain uncut.
- The triangle knife can be passed through the medial portal to cut these bands.
- The two-portal system allows this versatility, which is lacking in the single-portal system.
- Irrigate the wound through the cannula.
- Reinsert the trocar and remove the trocar and cannula together.
- Close the incisions with 4-0 nylon.
- Apply a light dressing and posterior splint.
  - Make prints, a CD, or both of pre- and post-fasciotomy findings.

PEARLS AND PITFALLS

- Performing the procedure on a prep stand or prop and ensuring that the foot and ankle are stable is vital to the smooth operation of this procedure. U-shaped padded foot propping devices that attach to the side of the operating table are ideal. We also use the Lift-A-Limb foot prop, which cradles the limb and is an excellent device.
- The placement of the incision is critical. A point 1.5 to 2.0 cm superior to the junction of keratinized and nonkeratinized skin, on a plumb line from the midpoint of the medial malleolus, is ideal.
- Fluffed cotton-tipped applicators and a defogging liquid to apply to the tip of the scope allow good visualization.
- Maintaining tension on the plantar fascia while cutting is key. The triangle knife is usually more predictable than the hook knife. Staying in the center of cannula and not skiving are important elements of technique.
- Although it is possible for the surgeon to hold the scope in one hand and the knife in the other hand, it is usually easier to have the assistant hold the scope and dorsiflex the foot, while the surgeon makes precise and controlled cuts with both hands on the knife, if necessary.
- In some cases, the central band is incredibly thick and gritty. Several passes of the triangle knife may be needed. Using the hook knife as well in such cases may be helpful. Remember also to clearly see the complete separation of the plantar fascia with the flexor digitorum brevis muscle plainly visible. Failure of EPF is usually due to incomplete or inadequate division of the plantar fascia.
- Other causes of failure include portal placement that is too proximal. It is difficult to release the fascia so proximally, directly off the calcaneus.
- Finally, misdiagnosis may lead to a poor result. Carefully evaluate the patient before surgery to rule out other causes in the differential diagnosis (described in detail earlier).

POSTOPERATIVE CARE

- Ice and elevation are recommended for 48 to 72 hours postoperatively.
- Minimal postoperative pain medication is required.
- Sutures are removed at 1 week postoperatively and a CAM walker, weight bearing as tolerated, is used for 3 weeks to minimize the risk of lateral column pain.
- Most patients can resume normal activities at 6 weeks postoperatively and vigorous athletic activities at 12 weeks postoperatively.

OUTCOMES

- All published literature on EPF reports greater than 90% success, with shorter recovery times than traditional open surgery. Our experience mirrors the literature, with no infections or nerve damage and only four instances of lateral column pain in over 400 cases in the past 11 years.
- The success rate of EPF is significantly higher than extracorporeal shockwave treatment. In addition, EPF is reimbursed by all insurance companies, whereas shockwave procedures still have erratic insurance reimbursement.
- EPF is minimally invasive, with a simple, easy-to-learn surgical technique. The equipment is minimal and cost-effective.
- The incision is only 8 mm, compared to open procedures, where the incision is at least 4 cm and, with some more extensile approaches, as much as 10 cm.
- Surgeons with prior arthroscopic experience should find EPF to be a straightforward procedure to master. DVDs and technique guides are readily available through Instratek.
- Training courses with cadavers are also given through the Orthopaedic Learning Center or Instratek. After 10 cases, the surgeon should feel confident with this procedure. With experience, average surgery time should be 10 to 15 minutes.

COMPLICATIONS

- Lateral column pain and arch pain have been the most common complications, reported in up to 3% to 5% of cases.
- Immobilization in a CAM walker for 4 weeks and limiting the division of the plantar fascia to the medial and central bands should reduce this complication even further.
- The Instratek system has single and double lines etched into the cannula to guide the surgeon to limit the plantar fasciotomy to 14 mm. The probe also has 1-cm markings. The disposable knives can also be marked with a marking pen to 14 mm. Using the intermuscular septum as a guide for where to stop the fasciotomy is probably the best anatomic reference as to where the central band ends and the lateral band begins.
- Infection rates are extremely low with EPF. We have had just one superficial wound infection (a diabetic patient) in over 400 cases.
- Injury to the medial and lateral plantar nerves is discussed extensively but rarely reported. Cadaver studies reveal a reasonable safe zone as long as the incision is appropriate.
- One case of pseudoaneurysm of the lateral plantar artery has been reported and a case of a cuneiform stress fracture. With appropriate technique and postoperative immobilization these complications should be rare.

REFERENCES

1. Barrett SL, Day SV. Endoscopic plantar fasciotomy: preliminary studies with cadaveric specimen. J Foot Surg 1991;30:170–172.
2. Barrett SL, Day SV. Endoscopic plantar fasciotomy two portal endoscopic surgical techniques: clinical results of 65 procedures. J Foot Surg 2004;32:248–256.
3. Buchbinder R. Clinical practice: plantar fasciitis. N Engl J Med 2004;350:2159–2166.
4. Hofmeister EP, Elliott MJ, Juliano PJ. Endoscopic plantar fascia release: an anatomic study. Foot Ankle Int 1995;16:719–723.
5. Hogan KA, Weber D, Shereff M. Endoscopic plantar fascia release. Foot Ankle Int 2004;25:875–881.
6. Sabir N, Debirlenk S, Yagzi B, et al. Clinical utility of sonography in diagnosing plantar fasciitis. J Ultrasound Med 2005;24:1041–1048.
7. Saxena A. Uniportal endoscopic plantar fasciotomy: a prospective study on athletic patients. Foot Ankle Int 2004;25:882–889.

Chapter 59

Transection and Burial of Neuromas of the Foot and Ankle

Stuart D. Miller, Blake L. Ohlson, and Michael Scherb

DEFINITION

- Nerves in the peripheral limb are at risk for damage by direct contusion, by stretch injury, and by iatrogenic insult.
- Nerve pain can be severe and crippling.
- Sensory nerves are expendable in many cases and most patients adapt well to removal.
- The resected proximal end of a nerve will usually form a neuroma as new growth seeks to reconnect with the distal nerve; thus, attempts to bury the nerve into a safe haven are desirable.

ANATOMY

- There are five sensory nerves in the foot and ankle, but anatomic variability is common.
  - The tibial nerve splits into medial and lateral plantar nerves (this is mixed motor as well).
  - The saphenous nerve is an extension of the femoral nerve, found along the lesser saphenous vein.
  - The deep peroneal nerve lies along the anterior tibia with a neurovascular bundle, passes under the extensor retinaculum, and innervates the first web space. It has some muscle components to the flexor hallucis brevis muscle and some innervation to the sinus tarsi as well.
  - The superficial peroneal nerve, with the peroneal muscles, emerges from the peroneal retinaculum to innervate the dorsum of the foot. The terminal medial branch, the dorsomedial cutaneous nerve, is at risk with bunionectomy along the dorsomedial hallux.
  - The sural nerve runs superficial to the gastrocnemius muscle and then between the peroneals and the Achilles tendon to innervate the lateral foot and two toes.

PATHOGENESIS

- Nerve injuries are most commonly iatrogenic.
- Arthroscopic ankle lateral portal placement risks damage to the superficial peroneal nerve.
- Lisfranc fracture open reduction and internal fixation (ORIF) or second metatarsal–cuneiform arthrodesis procedures will challenge the superficial and deep peroneal nerves in the midfoot.
- Bunion procedures threaten the dorsomedial cutaneous nerve, a distal branch of the superficial peroneal nerve.
- Calcaneal ORIF and fifth metatarsal ORIF incisions risk damage to the sural nerve in the foot.
- Achilles tendon procedures and Haglund resections can damage the sural nerve and especially a posterior branch of that nerve.
- Ankle fracture ORIF risks damage to the saphenous nerve medially (**FIG 1**), and the superficial peroneal nerve runs a variable course in front of the fibula laterally.
- Nerves can be damaged in a stretch injury (**FIG 2**). The stretch usually involves a pathologic extreme of motion as might be seen with ankle fracture[5] or with ligament sprain.[4]

NATURAL HISTORY

- Neuromas can behave in a variety of ways, from a small benign bulb neuroma (**FIG 3**) to a massive accumulation of angry hypersensitive nerve endings.
- Stretch injuries can cause dysfunction resulting in decreased sensation, in hypersensitivity, or even in severe pain with independent nerve signal generators.
- Some nerve injuries will heal with a slow distal progression of symptoms.
- Most nerve injuries are unpredictable in their natural course.

PATIENT HISTORY AND PHYSICAL FINDINGS

- Examination of these nerve injuries requires understanding of natural anatomy.
- The nerves in the foot and ankle do not read the textbooks, and deviations from expected course are common.

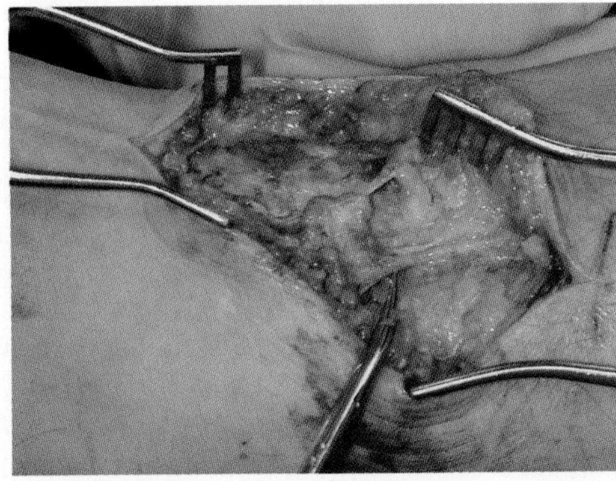

FIG 1 • Saphenous nerve neuroma at site of previous ankle fracture open reduction and internal fixation.

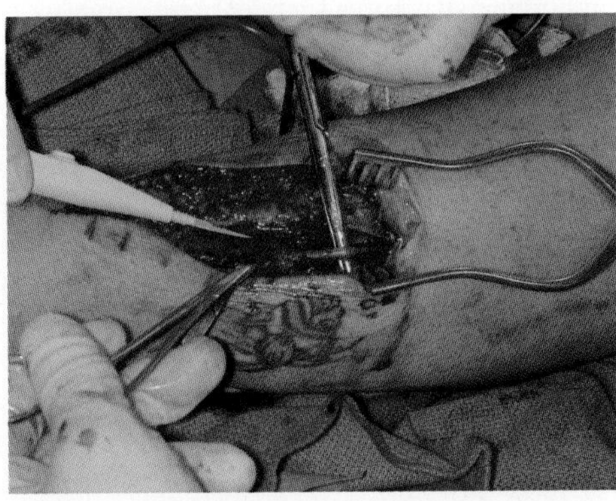

FIG 2 • Superior peroneal nerve adherent to muscle and fascia after severe stretch injury.

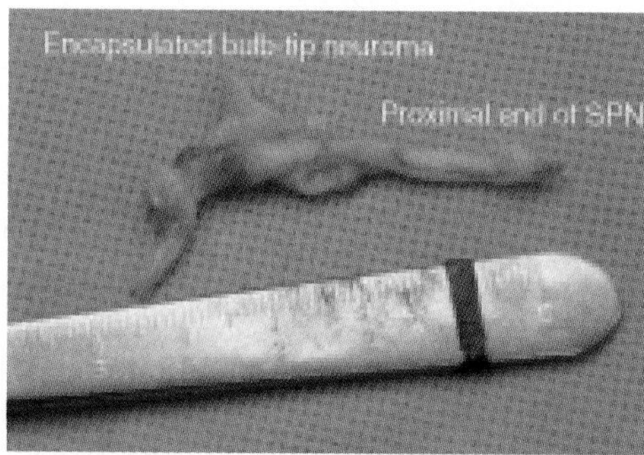

FIG 3 • Small nonpainful bulb neuroma from superior peroneal nerve buried in muscle.

- Nerves can suffer a stretch injury, especially the superficial peroneal nerve with severe ankle inversion due to sprain or fracture. The sural nerve can also be at risk with this injury.
- The saphenous nerve is especially at risk with contusion, as are all of the nerves, especially the deep peroneal nerve with a dorsal foot injury.
- Iatrogenic injury remains the most common form of nerve injury in the foot and ankle.
- Prior surgical intervention can result in confusing symptoms.
- Many nerve injuries are initially misdiagnosed. The nerve can often be suspected when the skin or subcutaneous tissues are hypersensitive (or hyposensitive) rather than the deep tissues.
- One of the best physical diagnostic findings is a nerve block using lidocaine hydrochloride (1% or 2%), Marcaine hydrochloride (0.5%), and a few drops of sodium bicarbonate solution in a mix. The bicarbonate acts to titrate the acidity of the local anesthetic and ease the burning pain of administration. The physician should return a few minutes after the injection to reexamine the patient rather than having him or her report on the effect of the injection at the next office visit.

IMAGING AND OTHER DIAGNOSTIC STUDIES

- Routine radiographs may provide evidence of mechanical imbalance, mechanical irritation (cyst or tumor), or osteophyte formation to suggest nerve entrapment.
- MRI helps to define any soft tissue irritation and helps to rule out impinging structures such as tumor or cyst. The MRI also helps the diagnostician by illuminating areas of inflammation. An exception is interdigital neuroma, for which MRI has proven less accurate.
- Electrodiagnostic studies can help differentiate between local and more proximal nerve pathology. Cervical spine or lumbosacral impingement as well as more generalized neuropathies can masquerade as local phenomena.
  - Electrodiagnostic studies are not helpful with interdigital neuroma or many small sensory nerves.
  - Electrodiagnostic studies should be performed in patients suspected of having tarsal tunnel syndrome. Sensory nerve conduction velocity may approach 90% sensitivity.

DIFFERENTIAL DIAGNOSIS

- Degenerative disc disease, disc herniation, radiculopathy
- Peripheral neuropathy
- Leprosy
- Diabetic neuropathy
- Peripheral vascular disease
- Tarsal tunnel syndrome
- Joint arthrosis or synovitis
- Tenosynovitis
- Giant cell tumor of the tendon sheath
- Intrinsic nerve damage, crush injury
- Rheumatoid arthritis
- Ganglion cyst
- Lipoma
- Neurilemmoma
- Abscess or infection
- Fracture
- Malalignment (varus or valgus foot or ankle)
- Plantar fasciitis

NONOPERATIVE MANAGEMENT

- Physical support to the limb
  - Observation often allows a nerve to regenerate, heal, and resume its normal sensitivity.
  - Periods of immobilization in a short-leg cast or walking boot may allow neuritic symptoms to subside, especially when traction causes pain.
  - Braces and splints can provide added stability and prevent recurrent stretching injuries, especially to the superficial and deep peroneal nerves.
  - Tarsal tunnel symptoms caused by mechanical imbalances—such as acquired pes planus secondary to posterior tendon dysfunction—may be alleviated with orthotic devices that restore foot balance.
- Multiple forms of pharmacologic intervention exist:
  - Nonsteroidal anti-inflammatories
  - Narcotics (caution must be exercised due to addiction potential, especially with chronic nerve pain)
  - Neuromodulators can help quiet nerve response.
    - Anticonvulsants such as pregabalin, gabapentin, or tricyclics often quiet nerve hypersensitivity.
    - Clonazepam and similar benzodiazepines may lessen nerve reactivity.
    - A variety of newer medications may be helpful; thus, referral to a pain management specialist often aids in complete patient care.
  - Lidoderm patches: Applied directly over the symptomatic area, lidocaine hydrochloride is released in a time-dependent manner through the skin.
  - Neuromodulators and local anesthetics and nonsteroidals in an absorbent gel for topical application; these creams can be found in compounding pharmacies.
  - Steroid injection, combined with local anesthetic, may serve a dual role as both therapeutic and diagnostic agent.
    - While sometimes useful, symptomatic relief is often temporary.
    - Injections should be limited to no more than two in a 1-year period.
    - Risks include skin discoloration, tendon rupture, atrophy of subcutaneous fat, and collateral ligament attenuation.
  - Ethanol injections: 4% ethanol in a Marcaine solution has been used for interdigital neuroma treatment.
    - The ethanol has been anecdotally useful for postincisional neuroma pain.

- The Morton neuroma protocol involves four injections a week apart, followed by three more injections similarly timed if partial improvement is noted.
- The benefit, besides avoiding at trip to the operating room, entails loss of nerve conduction without formation of postresection neuroma.

SURGICAL MANAGEMENT

- The decision to embark on surgical manipulation of persistent nerve pain often entails complex decision making. The resection of a nerve remains essentially a "one-way street," and careful discussion helps alleviate confusing results. Issues surrounding nerve ending regrowth and possible neuroma formation are dealt with easily later if they are understood preoperatively.
- Motor nerves can be sectioned but at a higher cost. The motor loss of the deep peroneal nerve branches is relatively well tolerated, while the posterior tibial nerve governs much more muscle activity in the foot. The posterior tibial nerve has been resected only in salvage procedures as a precursor to possible amputation if unsuccessful. Some surgeons continue to manage these problems with implantable nerve stimulators.

Preoperative Planning

- The preoperative planning includes patient education, careful patient evaluation, and decisions regarding the location of nerve burial. The final location of the proximal end of the nerve may be tender; thus, resection of the saphenous nerve just above the ankle in a patient who wears boots that may hit this level would be less desirable and a more proximal burial site would be advised.
- The best preoperative indicator of success remains the patient's response to a local anesthetic block. The surgeon should confirm the location of the nerve tenderness and further discuss postoperative expectations.
- Instrumentation is relatively simple. Appropriate retractors make the job easier, as does a small drill, a 2.5-mm and a 3.5-mm drill bit, and drill sleeves for creation of the bone hole.
- A tourniquet should be available but is often not used in order to better visualize the vessels accompanying the nerve. Under tourniquet, the vessel and the nerve can look very similar; thus, examination of the cross-section of the presumed nerve is essential at the time of surgery. Even the most experienced surgeons have been fooled by a vein impersonating the nerve: better to know at surgery than to be told by the pathologist the next day.
- If a patient had reflex sympathetic dystrophy or a complex regional pain syndrome involved with the leg, then consideration should be given to performing the surgery under epidural anesthesia. In theory, the diminution of painful stimulation may diminish the chance of triggering further hypersensitivity reactions.

Positioning

- Positioning depends on the location of the neuroma.
- The saphenous nerve is best explored with the patient supine and the leg externally rotated.
- The superficial and deep peroneal nerves are best approached with the patient positioned supine. A rolled towel placed beneath the ipsilateral hip may facilitate exposure.
- Sural nerve exposure often requires use of a rolled towel beneath the ipsilateral hip to provide better access to the nerve as it courses posteriorly. Currently, due to resection of the sural nerve very proximally in the leg, the patient is positioned in a semilateral decubitus position with the use of a beanbag.

Approach

- While each nerve dictates the appropriate surgical approach, a basic extensile exposure, following the line of the neurovascular structures, seems ideal.
- The incision is made with a scalpel and deeper dissection is usually performed with dissecting scissors. The variability of several nerves, especially the superficial peroneal nerve, warrants careful exposure and identification.
- The nerve can be fully exposed and separated from the vessels before resection and burial.
- If burying the nerve into bone, the surgeon should expose the area of bone to receive the nerve, incising the periosteum and drilling the appropriate hole.

TECHNIQUES

SURAL NERVE RESECTION AND BURIAL

- Regional or general anesthesia may be used.
- A local block is performed along the course of the nerve.
- A tourniquet may help with exposure, but the vein and branches are better identified without.
- The sural nerve, perhaps the easiest to find, has anecdotally proved difficult postoperatively with nerve regrowth. The current choice for burial is very proximal in the leg.
- The lesser saphenous vein serves as a key landmark in the posterior leg as it courses alongside the sural nerve. The nerve does not possess a lumen.
- Begin the incision just distal to the point of maximal tenderness and carry it proximally along the posterolateral ankle and posterior leg.
- Dissection usually proceeds distal to proximal (**TECH FIG 1**).

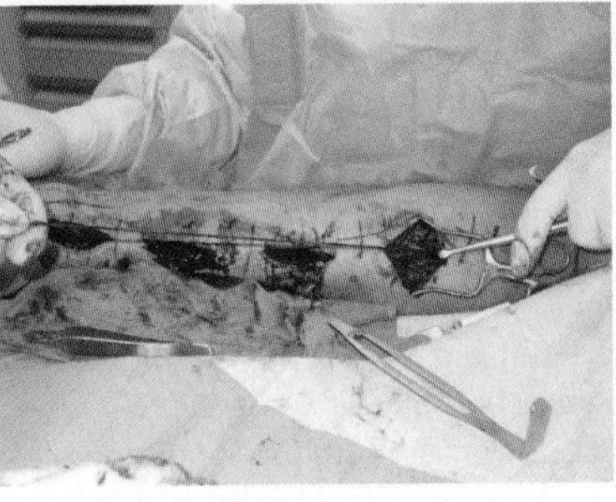

TECH FIG 1 • Progressive incisions made along the course of the sural nerve.

- Several skip incisions, usually three or four, can be made along the course of the nerve.
- These skip incisions can be avoided with one long incision, depending on the patient's preferences (**TECH FIG 2**).
- Identify the nerve proximally beneath the gastrocnemius fascia.
- Tension is placed on the proximal end of the nerve while it is sharply cut in an oblique fashion and allowed to retract into the surrounding tissues.

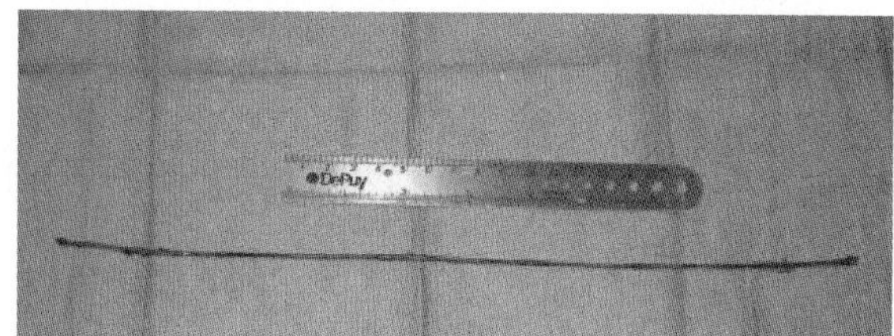

TECH FIG 2 • A long sural nerve harvest.

- The resected nerve is usually quite long (**TECH FIG 3**).
- Electrocautery may also be used on the distal fragments to prevent nerve regeneration via production of neurotrophic signals.
- Subcutaneous and skin sutures are usually bioresorbable to avoid any irritation in neuritic patients.

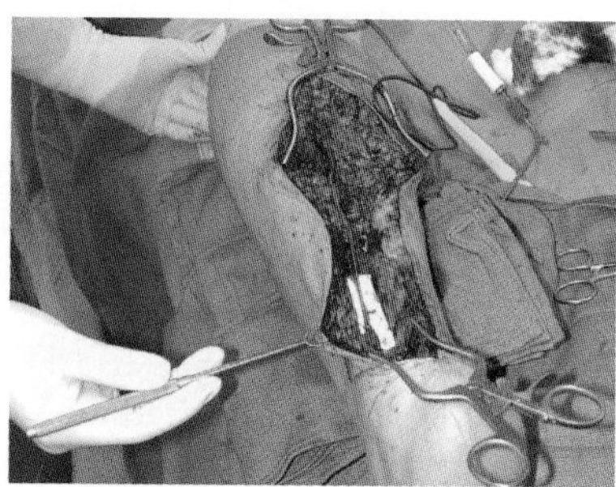

TECH FIG 3 • A long incision exposing the sural nerve with a neuroma at its end.

DEEP PERONEAL NERVE RESECTION AND BURIAL

- The deep peroneal nerve runs along the anterior border of the distal tibia; thus, the bone offers a fine burial site for the proximal nerve ending.
  - A straight anterolateral incision over the distal lateral border of the tibia works well; in cases of simultaneous superior peroneal nerve resection, a curved-S incision from this site more proximal and posterior allows an easy dual procedure.
- Incise the superficial retinaculum over the extensors in line with the incision and bluntly separate the muscles. The deep peroneal nerve usually lies between the extensor digitorum longus and the extensor hallucis longus muscles. Two large anterior tibial veins and the artery are close by the nerve; careful dissection avoids a messy field.
- Isolate and cut the nerve distally and cauterize the distal end.
- Bring the proximal nerve to a resting location over the tibia.
- The periosteum can be incised and drilled as above. Use a drill sleeve and round off or bevel the proximal edge of the hole to avoid a sharp edge for the nerve entry.
- Copiously irrigate the wound and then place the nerve into the distal tibial hole without tension.
- Allow the muscles to fall back over top the burial site. Repair the retinaculum if possible.
- Subcutaneous and skin sutures are bioabsorbable.

SUPERIOR PERONEAL NERVE RESECTION AND BURIAL

- Start with a longitudinal incision over the anterior compartment of the leg.
- Find the superficial peroneal nerve as it pierces the crural fascia about 10 to 12 cm proximal to the tip of the fibula.
  - The course is variable; the surgeon may need a more distal exposure to find the nerve and then trace it back proximally.
- Isolate the nerve and decide on the burial site in the fibula (**TECH FIG 4**) or into muscle (**TECH FIG 5**).
- The peroneal muscles can be split manually and the bone easily palpated.
  - The fibula can then be held in easy exposure with two small Hohmann retractors on each side of the bone.
  - The flat anteromedial wall of the fibula provides a fine resting place for the nerve.
  - Incise the periosteum longitudinally if it is thick enough to merit such action.

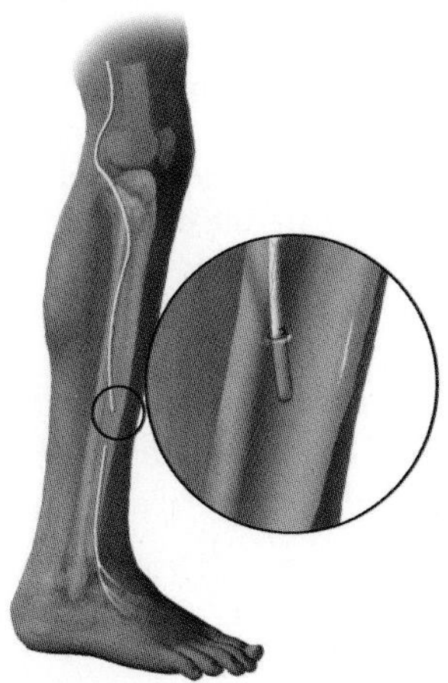

TECH FIG 4 • Diagram of burial of superior peroneal nerve into fibula bone.

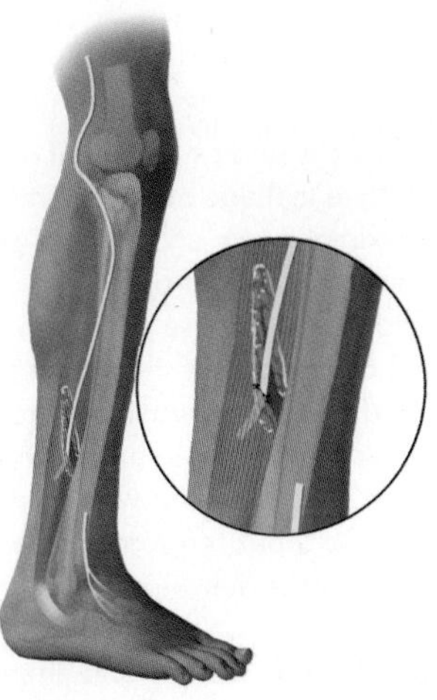

TECH FIG 5 • Diagram of burial of superior peroneal nerve into peroneal musculature.

- Cut the nerve sharply in the distal aspect of the dissection.
- Careful observation for a proximal split and a high medial superior peroneal nerve branch is important. If found, bury both branches or resect the nerve before the split.
  - Hold the distal portion of the nerve with a hemostat and cauterize it to prevent leakage of neurotrophic hormones.
- With a 3.5-mm drill bit, make a unicortical drill hole 3 to 4 cm proximal to the distal extent of the cut superior peroneal nerve to allow sufficient slack to bury the nerve without tension (TECH FIG 6). Carefully retract the nerve to prevent it from getting caught in the drill. Once the hole is made, angle the drill proximally to bevel the edge, allowing soft entry into the bone.
- Place the cut end of the proximal superior peroneal nerve into the hole after irrigation (TECH FIG 7).
- The nerve should have little tension on it and should be stable with ankle plantarflexion or dorsiflexion.

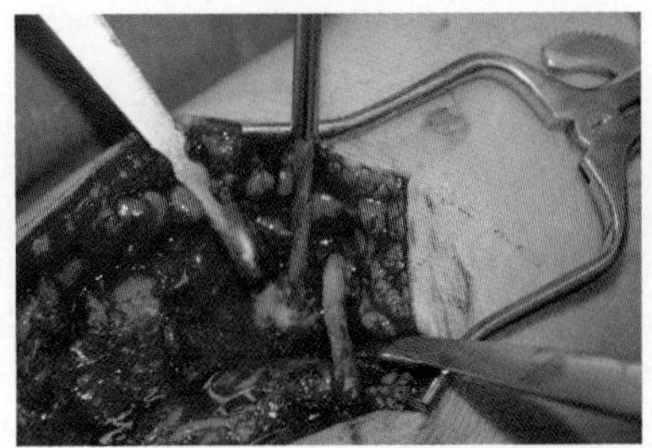

TECH FIG 6 • Drilling unicortical hole in fibula for transected superior peroneal nerve ending. (Note: drill guard removed for illustrative purposes.)

- The periosteum does not need to be sutured to the nerve epineurium to hold position.
- Gently remove the retractors, allowing the muscle to fall back over the fibula.
- Close the subcutaneous tissues with resorbable suture and close the skin with a resorbable suture as well, eliminating the need for suture removal.
- A splint is optional, depending on concomitant procedures and the amount of dissection.

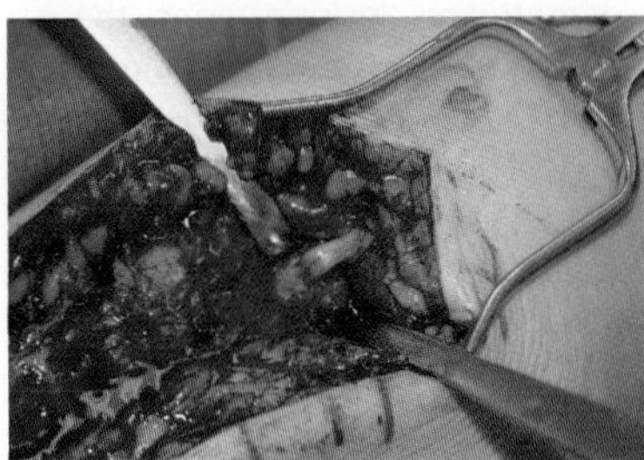

TECH FIG 7 • Final position of superior peroneal nerve into fibula hole.

DORSOMEDIAL CUTANEOUS NERVE

- This nerve is commonly damaged near the first metatarsal head in bunion surgery (TECH FIG 8). If a local block at the base of the metatarsal or cuneiform relieves the pain, then distal burial is a preferred solution.
- The incision often incorporates a prior incision over the dorsal metatarsal and is brought proximally over the cuneiform. Visualize the nerve and transect it as distally as possible; the surgeon need not find the distal neuroma if a proximal block relieved the pain. Cauterize the distal end and dissect the proximal end free.
- Using a 2.5-mm drill bit, drill a hole in the base of the first metatarsal or the medial cuneiform, whichever bone seems best anatomically for the nerve to inhabit. Bevel the hole proximally to allow a smooth gliding entrance for the nerve.
- Irrigate the wound and place the nerve into the hole; a tagging suture is usually unnecessary.
- Close the skin and subcutaneous tissues in a standard fashion with resorbable suture.

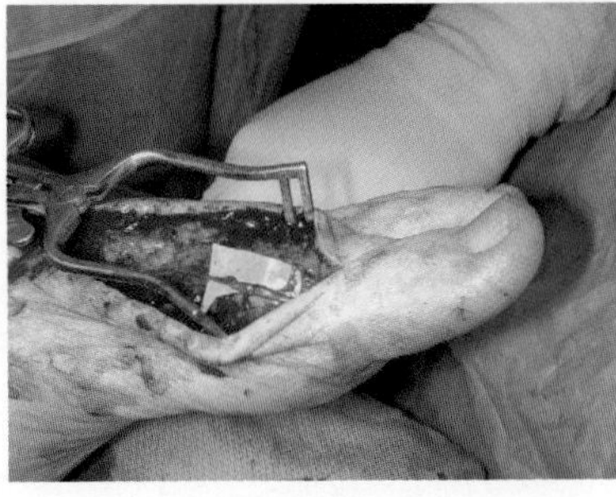

TECH FIG 8 • Neuroma of the dorsomedial cutaneous nerve.

SAPHENOUS NERVE RESECTION AND BURIAL

- Make a longitudinal incision over the lesser saphenous vein in the supramalleolar region of the medial ankle. The deep dissection should allow identification of the vein as well as the saphenous nerve. The nerve can be deceptively small here and has sometimes been found directly behind the vein. Take care to look for any branching (**TECH FIG 9**).
- Cut the nerve distally and cauterize all distal branches to limit postoperative leakage of any chemoattractants.
- Dissect the proximal nerve ending free and clear an appropriate spot on the medial tibia.
- Incise the periosteum and use a 2.5-mm or 3.5-mm drill bit (depending on the size of the nerve) to drill a unicortical hole. Tilt the drill bit proximally to round off the proximal edge and allow atraumatic nerve entry.
- Perform final irrigation of the wound. Place the nerve in the bone hole without tension. A suture from the periosteum to the epineurium is optional but rarely used any more.
- Close the subcutaneous tissues and then the skin with absorbable suture to limit any postsurgical irritation of the surgical site.

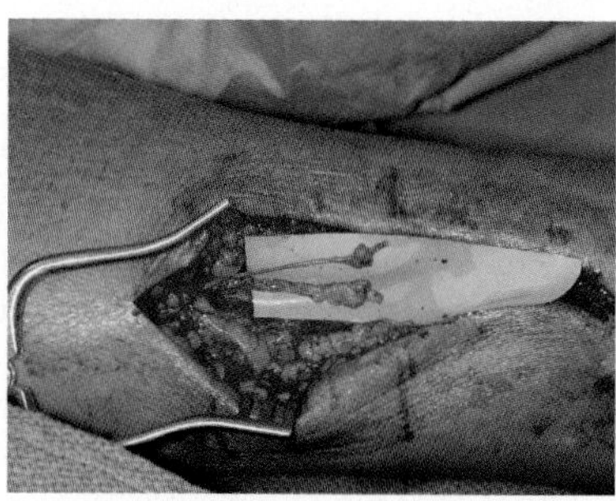

TECH FIG 9 • Saphenous nerve neuroma and small anterior branch.

MEDIAL PLANTAR NERVE

- Make a longitudinal incision along the course of the nerve on the plantar foot, attempting to avoid the heel and the ball, the primary weight-bearing areas.
- Gently carry the dissection through the subcutaneous tissues. The nerve lies just under the deep fascia. Take care to dissect the various branches to ensure adequate denervation (**TECH FIG 10**).
- Transect the nerve distally and bring it as far proximally in the midfoot as possible. Cut the nerve obliquely with an adequate length to allow burial into the deep musculature of the quadratus (**TECH FIG 11**).
- Close the subcutaneous tissues and skin with resorbable suture.

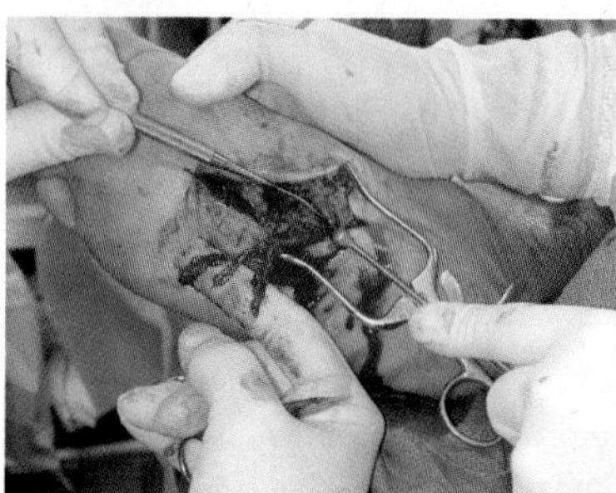

TECH FIG 10 • Dissection of the medial plantar nerve and branches.

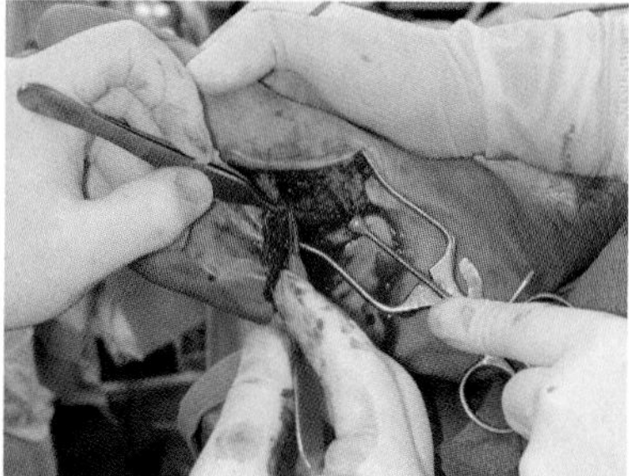

TECH FIG 11 • Transection of medial plantar nerve and burial deep into quadratus musculature.

TIBIAL NERVE

- Approach the tibial nerve in the supramalleolar space, similar to the tarsal tunnel incision. Resection of this nerve is for extreme salvage as a possible precursor to amputation.
- Resect the tibial nerve and branches, including possible high calcaneal branches, as distally as possible, cauterizing the distal ends to reduce chemoattractants.
- Obliquely resect the nerve proximally, leaving a length adequate for tension-free burial into the medial tibia.
- Using a 3.5- to 5.0-mm drill, acquire a burial site in the tibia. Bevel the unicortical hole proximally to allow an easy slide of the nerve into the tibia without a sharp edge.
- Close the subcutaneous tissues and skin with bioresorbable suture.

PEARLS AND PITFALLS

Indications	■ The nerve injury can be difficult to discern and may be associated with other pathology, which is usually addressed at the same surgical procedure.
Diagnosis	■ The nerve injury can be difficult to discern and may be associated with other pathology, which is usually addressed at the same surgical procedure.
Nerve resection level	■ The nerve should be cut above the level of multiple branching to simplify burial. The worry about obscure branches of other nerves providing innervation to the distal nerve remains.
Burial of nerve into bone hole	■ The surgeon should beware of an inadequate retraction and the mistake of wrapping the nerve in the drill bit; a tissue protector should be used when possible. ■ The foot, ankle, and knee are ranged while observing the nerve before closure. ■ A more proximal hole can always be drilled to eliminate tension on the nerve. ■ One case of fibular fracture occurred at the nerve burial hole. The patient did very well with conservative treatment.
Postoperative pain	■ Hypersensitivity often occurs in the early postoperative period as neighboring nerves react to the loss of a neighbor. ■ "Zingers" will often occur 1 to 3 weeks postoperatively and represent growth of the proximal nerve ending. These nerve pains will ease with time and are much better tolerated when the patient expects such a reaction to nerve resection.

POSTOPERATIVE CARE

- The postoperative rehabilitation must strike a balance between early return of motion and avoidance of mechanical trauma to the resected nerve.
- If the nerve is buried, immobilization time allows scarring into place.
- Many of these patients have some element of complex regional pain syndrome or reflex sympathetic dystrophy, so any stiffness will take a great deal of rehabilitation to recover full motion.
- The use of resorbable suture material seems especially prudent in these nerve patients, who are often hypersensitive after surgery.
- For simple neurectomy, the patient should have a soft compressive dressing with early range-of-motion exercises. Desensitization and nerve retraining should begin early.
- Most patients will have some degree of adjacent sensory nerve hypersensitivity; it can be better tolerated with advance warning.
- Many patients also get "zingers" starting at 7 to 14 days or so and lasting up to a month or so. These "electric" jolts of pain follow the resected nerve's distal sensory distribution and represent irritation of the cut proximal nerve ending. They usually begin to lessen in frequency and intensity after a week or so and gradually disappear. Again, discussion with the patient beforehand eliminates frantic office calls about the nerve growing back so quickly.
- For nerve resection and burial, the patient usually has a fairly high amount of pain simply from the mobilization of the muscle to allow nerve implantation. A well-padded splint similar to a Robert Jones dressing gives nice compression and stabilization for the initial 12- to 14-day postoperative period. After this time, a simple compressive wrapping will usually be sufficient and allows gradual recovery of range of motion.

OUTCOMES

- Chiodo and Miller[1] compared superior peroneal nerve resection and burial into muscle versus bone; the results favored burial into the fibula when possible.
  - Sixteen patients had burial into muscle, with improvement in the verbal analogue pain score (0 to 10) of 3.1 points and 46% relief of pain. Four required reoperation for neuroma.
  - Fifteen patients had burial into bone, with improvement in the pain score (0 to 10) of 5.4 points and 75% pain relief (statistically better than the muscle group).
- Dellon and Aszmann[2] reviewed 11 cases of superior peroneal nerve resection into anterior muscle with good or excellent results. They recommended compartment release as well.
- Miller[3] reviewed nine cases of dorsomedial cutaneous nerve resection and burial into the dorsal bones of the foot, with a verbal analogue scale improvement from 8.6 to 2.0 (on a 0-to-10 scale). All patients had relief of symptoms but most had a concurrent procedure to correct foot abnormality.

COMPLICATIONS

- Wound infection
- Neuroma
  - Neuroma can be expected to form at the end of a cut nerve as the nerve tries to reconnect with the distal end. Nerves can grow into:
  - Bulb neuroma: a small thickening on the end of the nerve; usually causes little pain (**FIG 4**)

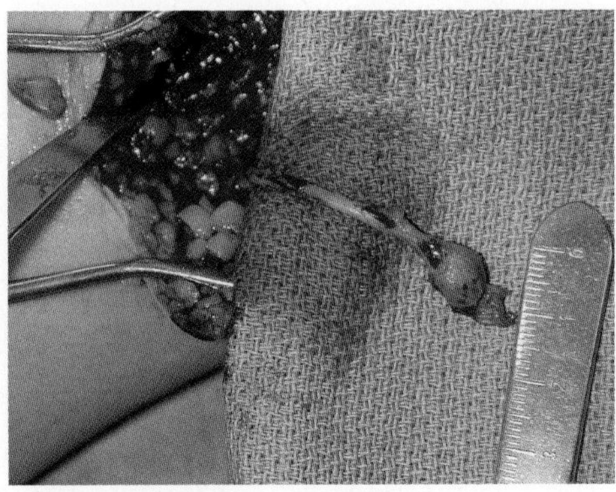

FIG 4 • Simple bulb neuroma after sural nerve resection.

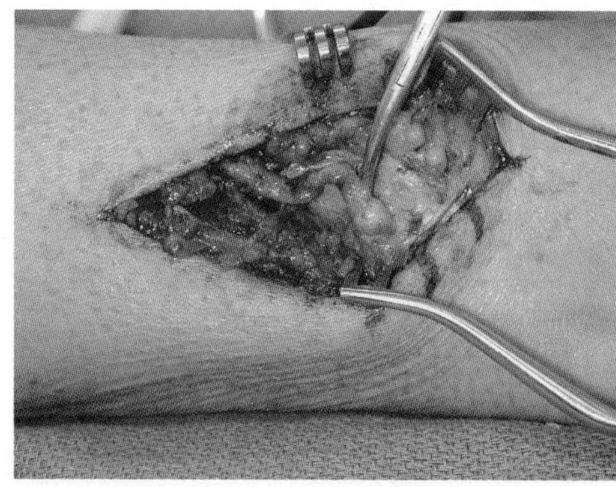

FIG 5 • Previous burial of superior peroneal nerve into bone with mild neuritis and small more proximal branch.

- Unorganized neuroma: a thick mass of nerve endings, usually with small very irritable extensions causing pain
- Nerve can regrow and reinnervate the distribution.
  - The speed of nerve regrowth should be 1 mm/day but can be faster.
  - Nerves can sprout new "rootlets" that will attempt to reinnervate the target area. Sometimes it may be difficult to determine whether a more proximal branch was missed at the prior surgery or if a new branch developed (**FIG 5**).
  - Adjacent nerves can sometimes provide an unexpected "feeder" innervation to the distal aspect of the resected nerve.
- Dysesthesias can be troublesome, with persistent pain in the distal nerve distribution.
- Denervation hyperesthesias can be horrible, with difficulty eradicating pain from nerve surgery.

REFERENCES

1. Chiodo CP, Miller SD. Surgical treatment of superficial peroneal neuromas. Foot Ankle Int 2004;25:689–694.
2. Dellon AL, Aszmann OC. Treatment of superficial and deep peroneal neuromas by resection and translocation of the nerves in the anterolateral compartment. Foot Ankle Int 1998;19:300–303.
3. Miller SD. Dorsomedial cutaneous nerve syndrome: treatment with nerve transection and burial into bone. Foot Ankle Int 2001;22:198–202.
4. O'Neill PJ, Parks BG, Walsh R, et al. Excursion and strain of superficial peroneal nerve strain during inversion ankle sprain. J Bone Joint Surg Am 2007;89A:979–986.
5. Redfern DJ, Sauve PS, Sakellariou A. Investigation of incidence of superficial peroneal nerve injury following ankle fracture. Foot Ankle Int 2003;24:771.
6. Schon, LC, Anderson, CD, Easley ME, et al. Surgical treatment of chronic lower extremity neuropathic pain. Clin Orthop Relat Res 2001;389:156–164.

Chapter 60 Barrier Procedures for Adhesive Neuralgia

Stuart D. Miller and Venus R. Rivera

DEFINITION

- Adhesive neuritis describes the pain from a nerve scarred to surrounding tissues. A common cause for such a condition in the lower extremity occurs after a tarsal tunnel release with subsequent scarring. While many nerves can be involved, the frequency of posterior tibial nerve involvement overwhelms that of other reported nerves and thus will be the primary focus of this chapter.

ANATOMY

- Adhesive neuritis can affect any nerve in the lower extremity. Lower extremity nerve anatomy involves the posterior tibial nerve, the superficial peroneal nerve, the sural nerve, the deep peroneal nerve, and the saphenous nerve, and distal branches of these nerves. The most common site of adhesive neuritis anecdotally seems to be the posterior tibial nerve, a continuation of the sciatic nerve, which courses along the medial leg in a discrete retinacular anatomic tunnel with the posterior tibial artery and vein. Around the medial malleolus, the nerve splits into the medial and lateral plantar nerves. The lancinate ligament obliquely crosses at this level and can cause tarsal tunnel compression. The calcaneal branches (usually one or two) split from the main nerve trunk or occasionally from the lateral plantar nerve alone and can be constricted in the medial soft tissues. More distally, the nerves run under the abductor hallucis muscle, which has a very thick lateral fascial covering. This fascia can be thickened and can become a major source of mechanical compression of the nerve.
- The superficial peroneal nerve runs in the anterolateral aspect of the leg, often in its own sheath, between the anterior intermuscular septum and lateral muscle compartment fascia. This nerve can be constricted at several points, but by far the most common area is above the level of the ankle joint, where it emerges from the deep fascia of the peroneal muscle. The nerve becomes subcutaneous distal to this region, usually splitting into two main branches. The nerve demonstrates a wide variation in its anatomic course in this region. Prior surgery or injury to this area can cause adhesive neuritis, from the posterior aspect of the fibula to the anterolateral portal for arthroscopy.
- The sural nerve can often be enveloped by scar tissue in the lateral aspect of the foot as a complication of surgery on the posterior calcaneus (Haglund deformity), on the calcaneus for fracture, for peroneal tendinitis, or for triple arthrodesis. The nerve also is at risk with surgery on the base of the fifth metatarsal as it drapes over the bone.
- The deep peroneal nerve lies along the anterolateral border of the tibia as it approaches the ankle between the extensor digitorum longus and the tibialis anterior muscles. This nerve has a muscle branch to the extensor digitorum brevis and may also send branches to the sinus tarsi before innervating the first web space distally. The deep peroneal nerve can become pinched at the anterior ankle retinaculum as well as scarred down over the dorsum of the foot at the cuneiforms. In addition to repetitive trauma, which can cause soft tissue inflammation and scar formation, the nerve is at risk from arthritic irritation and osteophyte formation, as well as from cyst encroachment.
- The saphenous nerve travels with the saphenous vein anteromedially. This superficial nerve is at risk with open reduction and internal fixation of the ankle joint and with any medial surgery, such as triple arthrodesis or arthroscopy.

PATHOGENESIS

- Adhesive neuritis may occur after insult to the nerve or neighboring tissues resulting in adhesion between the nerve and surrounding tissue. The local damage usually comes from mechanical irritation and scar, such as surgery or soft tissue damage. While any nerve can be affected, each nerve is at higher risk where it naturally rounds a bend or courses under a retinaculum. The scar tissue then prevents movement of the nerve along with normal range of motion of the foot or ankle, thus the designation adhesive neuritis.
- The most common cause of such a condition to the posterior tibial nerve would be after tarsal tunnel release. Other trauma, such as a severe contusion or stretch, surgery on adjacent tendons, or resection of tumor or cyst, can cause adhesions with healing.
- Other nerves, such as the superficial peroneal nerve, are at risk due to surgery as well, especially due to arthroscopic portals and after open reduction of lateral malleolus fracture. The saphenous nerve is at risk from open reduction of medial malleolus fractures as well. Sural nerves are at risk with open reduction of calcaneus fracture, with repair of the Achilles tendon, with triple arthrodesis, and with insertional Achilles tendinitis as well as resection of Haglund deformity.
- While the essential pathophysiology has yet to be defined, the end result is scar and fibrinous tissue adhering to the nerve epineurium. This scar can impede nerve conduction due to physical impingement. The infiltrative scarring can also directly affect nerve function and vascularity. The mechanical pull on the nerve can be irritating and limit conduction, particularly in extreme limb positions. The surgical guidance for simple nerve release versus epineurolysis has not been well delineated and remains at the surgeon's judgment.

NATURAL HISTORY

- The typical scenario of adhesive neuralgia is an initially good result after surgery with subsequent scarring and progressive nerve irritation. While a mild problem may ease with motion and tearing of the restricting tissues, the neuralgic pain often does not ease markedly with time, and often slowly worsens.
- After tarsal tunnel release, neuritis might be a recurrence of nerve pain 2 to 4 months after the original surgery. The pain

is often related to activity and foot position. Extremes of inversion or eversion put more mechanical strain on the posterior tibial nerve and strain the adhesions to the soft tissue, causing nerve pain. The nerve does seem to be at higher risk with more proximal nerve compression, such as a radiculopathy, represented by the term "double crush" syndrome.

PATIENT HISTORY AND PHYSICAL FINDINGS

- The patient with adhesive neuralgia will typically provide an event leading to the nerve issues. Prior surgery is a common trigger and the physician must determine whether the neuralgia is secondary to scarring or due to failure of the surgery to resolve the initial problem (ie, inadequate tarsal tunnel release). Prior medical history is essential; patients with diabetes or other metabolic insults to the nervous system should be fully evaluated and systemic neuropathy differentiated from local symptoms. The patient with any sciatica or symptoms extending proximally to the posterior thigh should be tested with electromyography and nerve conduction studies—not necessarily to diagnose the adhesive neuralgia as much as to rule out and possibly treat proximal causes of nerve pain.
- Physical examination must be taken in context of the extremity examination. A general leg examination sitting and standing is important, as varus or valgus angulation can cause many problems. Gait abnormalities may also be reflected in medial pain. A simple check for dorsal pedal pulses and toe capillary refill can find vascular insufficiency. Various joint issues such as synovitis or arthritis can contribute to nerve irritation, as could a palpable mass such as a ganglion cyst or neurilemmoma. Direct percussion can cause pain and pinpoint the location of impingement.
- Palpation of the posterior tibial nerve can often elicit pain at the area of the lancinate ligament and sometimes at the abductor fascia. Some surgeons have noted increased sensitivity of the nerve when the foot is passively placed in the dorsiflexed and everted position. Distal neural examination may map out a pattern of medial or lateral plantar nerve altered sensation or may demonstrate global peripheral neuropathy, sometimes with motor weakness. The irritation of the nerve to motion of the extremity is the hallmark of adhesive capsulitis and is a good prognostic sign for surgical intervention.

IMAGING AND OTHER DIAGNOSTIC STUDIES

- No radiologic studies are confirmatory for this condition. Indeed, most studies help in ruling out other causes for the pain.
- Plain radiographs are important to rule out other sources of lower extremity pain, such as fracture, severe malalignment, coalition, arthritis, or bone cysts.
- MRI may discern an underlying mechanical insult to the nerve, such as tendinitis, ganglion cyst, or tumor (**FIG 1**).
- Ultrasonography plays a similar role as MRI but involves a great deal of interpretation.
- An electromyelogram and nerve conduction studies help to rule out a systemic neuropathy or more proximal lumbosacral pathology.
  - The test may not always be confirmatory for significant tarsal tunnel nerve compression and often lacks the specificity for other peripheral nerves, but the exclusion of more proximal pathology is important.

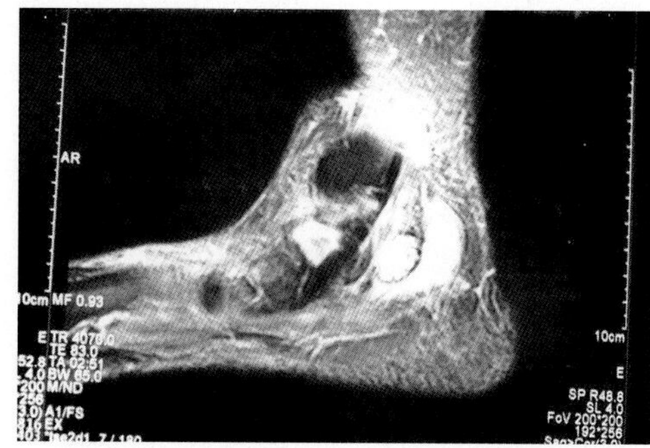

FIG 1 • MRI of cyst formation along the tibial nerve.

DIFFERENTIAL DIAGNOSIS

- Intrinsic nerve damage, crush injury
- Systemic neuropathy
- Diabetic neuropathy
- Leprosy
- Peripheral vascular disease
- Posterior tibial tendinitis
- Rheumatoid arthritis
- Ganglion cyst
- Lipoma
- Neurilemmoma
- Giant cell tumor of the tendon sheath
- Abscess or infection
- Spinal or nerve root pathology
- Fracture
- Malalignment (varus or valgus foot or ankle)
- Tarsal coalition
- Plantar fasciitis

NONOPERATIVE MANAGEMENT

- Tarsal tunnel syndrome, especially with adhesive neuritis, can often be mechanically exacerbated and a trial of immobilization is usually warranted. While a cast provides the best hold, a walker boot is much more practical, especially if some relief ensues. Many patients will begin walking postoperatively in a walker boot; thus, the investment can be worthwhile even if surgery later occurs.
- Pharmacologic management continues to develop, with anticonvulsants such as pregabalin or gabapentin augmenting the use of tricyclic antidepressants such as amitriptyline. Clonazepam and similar benzodiazepines also seem to help peripheral nerve irritation. Due to the complexity of these medications, referral to a pain management specialist often helps in patient care. Systemic anti-inflammatories can also help with pain control, especially when the nerve irritation is worsened by an arthritic or synovitic condition.
- Topical anesthetic creams can help with peripheral nerve irritation, especially with nerves close to the skin surface such as the sural or superficial peroneal nerves. Lidocaine can help either in a local pad or a gel. Other medications in a topical gel can be absorbed through the skin, such as ketamine or anti-inflammatories. Some patients respond well to capsaicin pepper cream, which raises the "background noise" about the nerve.

SURGICAL MANAGEMENT

Preoperative Planning

- The surgery should be respected as a revision nerve procedure, with attendant greater risk for intrinsic nerve damage, accompanying vessel damage, and time-consuming difficulty. A careful preoperative discussion regarding indications, risks, and expectations should be mandatory.
- Loupe or microscopic magnification can be very helpful. A 2.0× magnification has proven adequate for most cases.
- A microsurgical set of tools should be available, along with finer sutures, such as 8-0 nylon or Prolene, for repair of vascular structures. Sometimes a small branch will rip off the artery, and a simple suture of that resulting hole will control bleeding without arterial sacrifice. Documenting a good dorsal pedal pulse before surgery would greatly ease fears of vascular compromise to the foot. When in doubt (and especially when the dorsal pedal pulse is not palpable), a preoperative vascular consultation may prove fruitful.
- A set of bipolar forceps can ease some of the dissection difficulty.
- These procedures can be markedly variable in difficulty and duration. Some cases will "unzip" easily and allow easy nerve exposure while others may take several hours of meticulous dissection to uncover the nerve. Surgeons must allow adequate time to perform these operations, perhaps overbooking the time allotment to avoid rushing through a tough dissection.

Positioning

- Patients should be supine, perhaps on a bean bag positioner or a bump under the contralateral hip to allow easy access to the medial aspect of the foot. These surgical procedures can be long and appropriate padding to the bony prominences should be noted.
- A tourniquet is very helpful for control of vigorous bleeding, but its routine application is discouraged; we apply a tourniquet but rarely inflate the device. The dissection often proceeds more easily if the vessels remain full, thus being easily discerned against the nerve in a scar situation.
- A table that elevates and tilts is helpful for establishing a Trendelenburg position and lessening the blood flow to the limb.

Approach

- The surgical approach to the revision tarsal tunnel is usually along the same lines as the original incision with extension both proximally and distally. When in doubt, an extensile exposure seems ideal, following the line of neurovascular bundles. Often, the initial incision will cause difficulty with distal direction plantar as it included a plantar fascia release. For these occasions, especially when the bulk of symptoms are at the medial plantar nerve entrapment by the abductor fascia, the revision incision must curve anteriorly and at an angle to the original cut. The skin seems well vascularized here and sharp angles rarely have healing problems.
- The approach to the lesser peripheral nerves in the foot and leg usually follows anatomic guidelines. The superficial peroneal nerve can be compressed and adhesive to the peroneal muscle fascia at the supramalleolar level of the leg. The nerve here often runs in its own separate sheath and must be directly visualized to ensure complete release. Very little information has been presented regarding barrier procedures for these more purely sensory nerves.

REVISION NERVE RELEASE

- The revision nerve release remains the crucial and most difficult part of these procedures. The amount of scar tissue formation varies widely and dictates the pace of the surgery. Starting more proximally in "virgin" tissue seems wise as distal dissection proceeds more easily when the nerve and vessels have been identified. The initial skin incision should be superficial, especially distally when the nerve moves more medial and superficial by the lancinate ligament. Deep dissection with dissection scissors and simple blunt clearing of tissue allows the visualization of the fascia overlying the flexor digitorum longus tendon and then the tarsal tunnel. A band of yellow fat often marks the location of the tarsal tunnel under fascia.

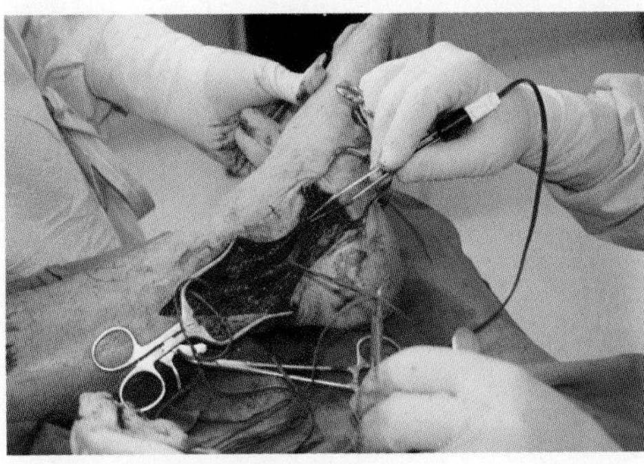

TECH FIG 1 • Dissection of the tarsal tunnel is facilitated by the bipolar forceps.

- Incise the fascia and isolate the nerve. Take care to cauterize small bleeding vessels; this is often made easier with use of the bipolar forceps (**TECH FIG 1**). The posterior tibial nerve will have a venous plexus around it, which can be stripped off with some bleeding. The larger vessels will send small branches by the nerve, and these may need cauterization or ligation depending on size.
- Separate the nerve from the artery and veins with care. Do not inflate the tourniquet unless severe bleeding occurs, as the vessels are more easily identified when full (**TECH FIG 2**). Persistent or vigorous bleeding can often be controlled with local pressure distally, but the tourniquet is sometimes needed to better dissect and cauterize the difficult venous plexus around the medial plantar nerve. Vessel loops aid with retraction of the vessels and for movement of the nerves without damage.
- The decision to perform epineurolysis depends on the clinical findings and on the dissected status of the nerve: grossly scarred nerves that then appear healthy after neurolysis probably do not warrant more extensive

incision of the epineurium, but no conclusive studies are available to help in this decision.

- The dissection must include the region above the ankle joint, and dissection proceeds distally beyond the abductor fascia. The abductor can be very thick and restrictive to the nerve (TECH FIG 3). The soft tissues should yield easily to a small hemostat sliding along the nerve, ensuring release.

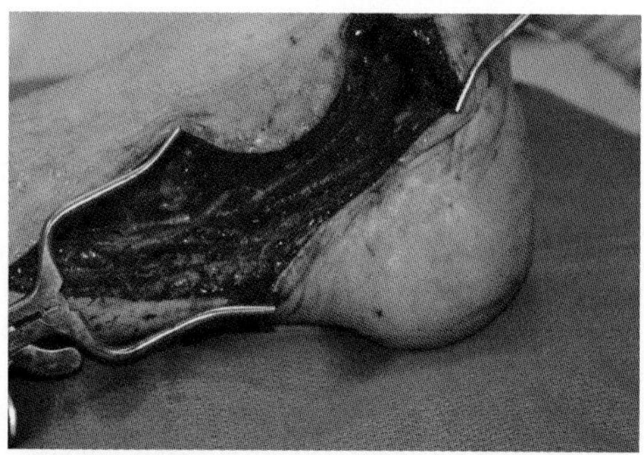

TECH FIG 2 • Wrapping with NeuraWrap. Note the intact vasculature, as the procedure is usually performed without inflation of the tourniquet.

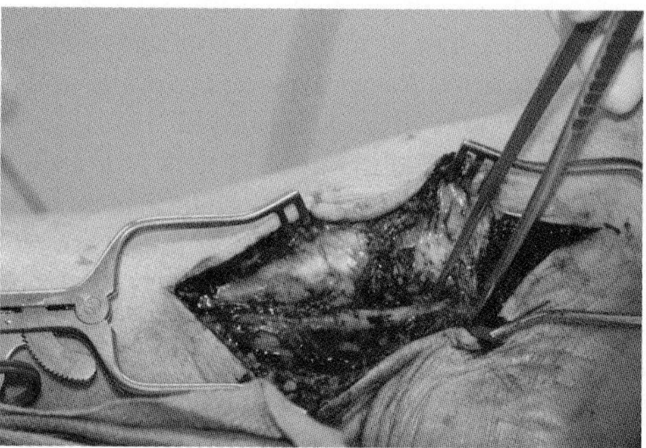

TECH FIG 3 • Typical scarring of the medial plantar nerve as it courses under the abductor fascia.

VEIN WRAP PROCEDURE

- The saphenous vein can be harvested by standard fashion (when in doubt, consult with cardiovascular surgical technicians, who harvest these veins daily), either by skip incisions or one long incision (TECH FIG 4).
- Tie off small side branch vessels to allow later expansion of the vessel.
- Once the maximal length is harvested, to the knee region, the vein is prepared.
- Mark the outer lining of the vessel with a marking pen (TECH FIG 5).
- Tie off the end of the nerve and any branches.
- Tie the vein ending around a bulb-tipped needle.
- Fill and then distend the vein with a Marcaine and saline solution (TECH FIG 6).
- Cut the vein longitudinally.

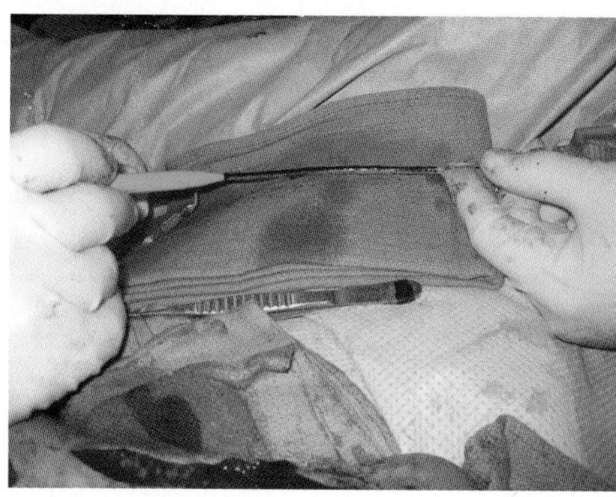

TECH FIG 5 • Labeling vein to later identify outside layer.

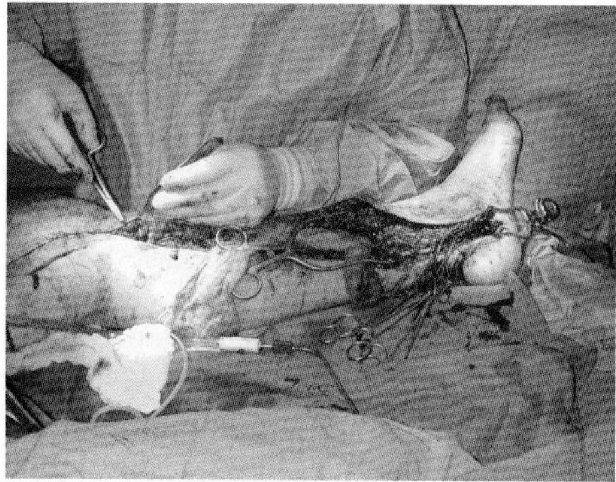

TECH FIG 4 • Extensive incision to see the tarsal tunnel and the saphenous vein dissection.

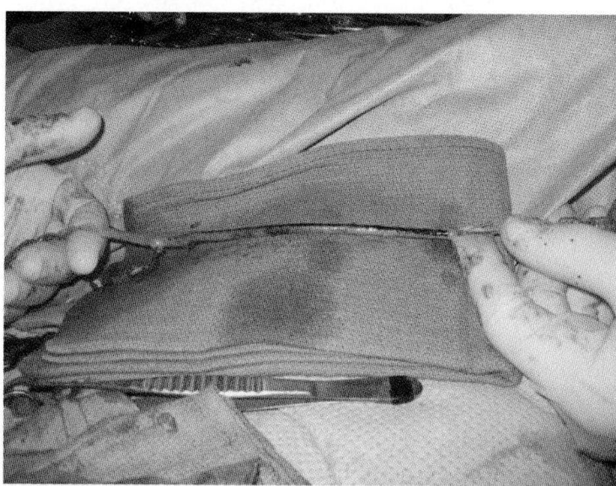

TECH FIG 6 • Distending saphenous vein graft with bupivacaine and saline.

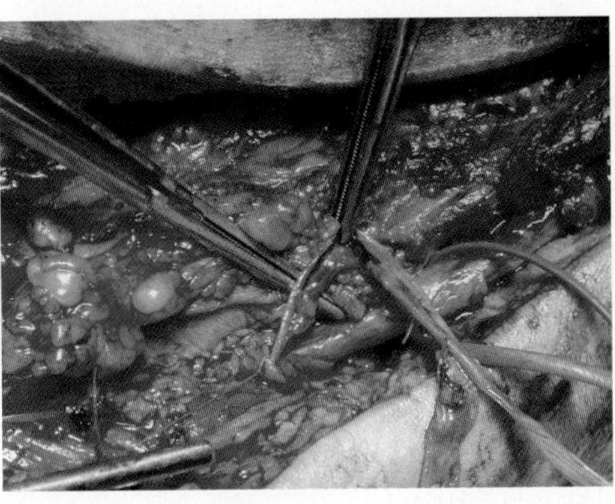

TECH FIG 7 • Vein being brought around the tibial nerve. Each throw is secured with 7-0 suture.

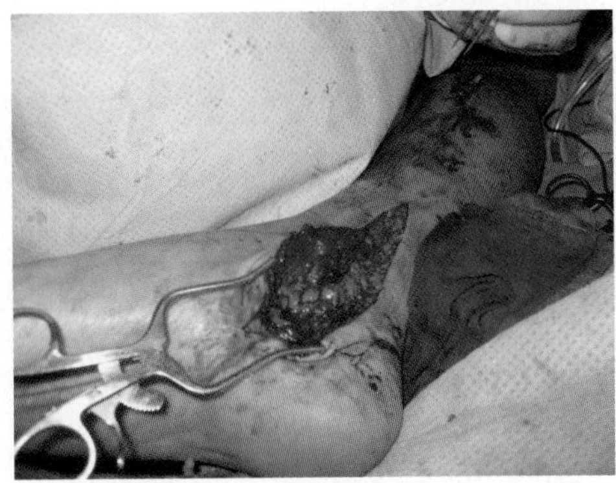

TECH FIG 8 • Vein wrapping in place.

- Begin wrapping the nerve with the vein, inner lumen to the nerve.
- Secure each turn with a simple suture of 7-0 Vicryl (**TECH FIG 7**).
- Once complete, put the foot and ankle through a full range of motion to ensure there is no binding (**TECH FIG 8**).
- Close the subcutaneous tissues with a 3-0 or 4-0 resorbable suture.
- Close the skin with 4-0 Monocryl suture.
- Place a bulky cotton wrap around the leg with a medial lateral U-splint and a posterior L-splint of plaster, covered with Coban or elastic wrapping.

NEURAWRAP APPLICATION PROCEDURE

- Once the nerve is exposed and free, the various sizes of NeuraWrap are selected. Each segment should be slightly larger than the portion of nerve being wrapped.
- The NeuraWrap sections should be soaked in saline for 5 minutes.
- Each section is simply wrapped around the nerve without tension. The material has a shape memory to be a tube (**TECH FIG 9**), and no suture is needed.
- Separate sections of NeuraWrap can be applied to each side branch.
- A branch can also be resected by cutting a small rectangular section of the NeuraWrap around the larger nerve to allow the branch to exit unimpeded.
- Most posterior tibial nerve segments require one or two 7 × 4-mm sections of NeuraWrap.
- Most medial or lateral plantar nerves require a 5 × 4-mm section of NeuraWrap (Tech Fig 2).
- Occasionally the calcaneal branch or the first branch of the lateral plantar nerve will be wrapped. These usually require a 3 × 4-mm section of NeuraWrap (**TECH FIG 10**, which shows the wrapping of patient seen in Tech Fig 3).

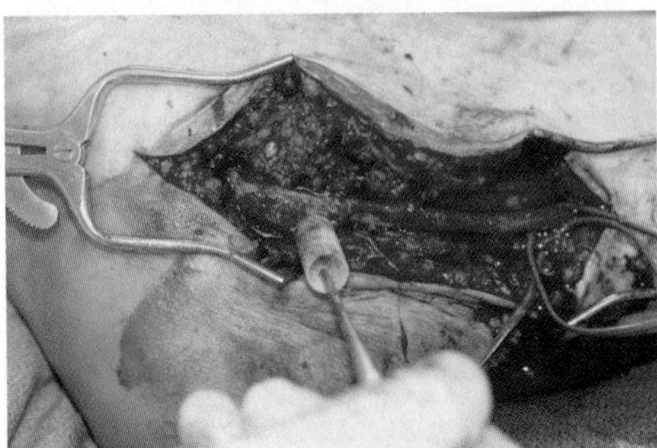

A

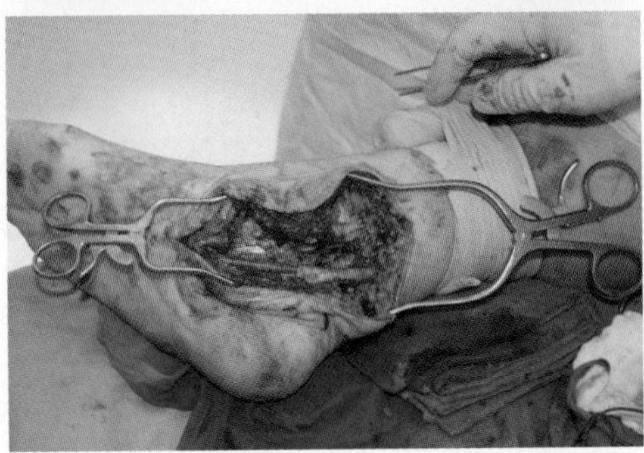

B

TECH FIG 9 • The NeuraWrap processed bovine collagen tube retains a convenient shape.

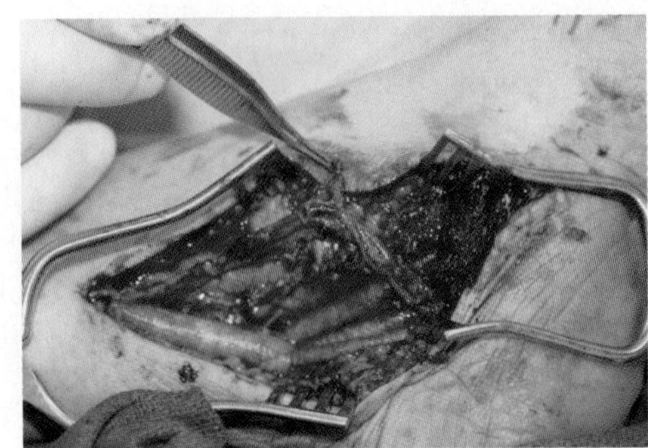

TECH FIG 10 • Release of the nerve with subsequent NeuraWrap placement. Note the large calcaneal branch.

- Once wrapping is complete, put the limb through a range of motion to ensure stability.
- Close the subcutaneous tissues carefully with resorbable suture and close the skin with resorbable suture when possible to avoid irritation in the postoperative period.
- Place a bulky cotton wrap around the leg with a medial lateral U-splint and a posterior L-splint of plaster, covered with Coban or elastic wrapping.

FETAL UMBILICAL VEIN WRAP OF TARSAL TUNNEL

- The use of fetal umbilical vein wrap for neuritis seems to have decreased with time. The procedure is similar to the above surgeries, with careful neurolysis (**TECH FIG 11**) followed by application of the vein wrap. This material is somewhat thicker than the saphenous vein but easier to apply because it can often be wrapped circumferentially rather than "barber-poled" with the labor-intensive wrap technique that the saphenous vein requires.
- Cut the fetal umbilical vein longitudinally (**TECH FIG 12**).
- Carefully wrap the material around the nerve (**TECH FIG 13**). The smaller side nerves may require a portal or hole cut in the nerve.
- The completed wrapping must glide easily with ankle motion (**TECH FIG 14**).
- In the case of postoperative infection, the material should be removed (**TECH FIG 15**), but the inflammatory reaction may leave a reasonable bed for the nerve.

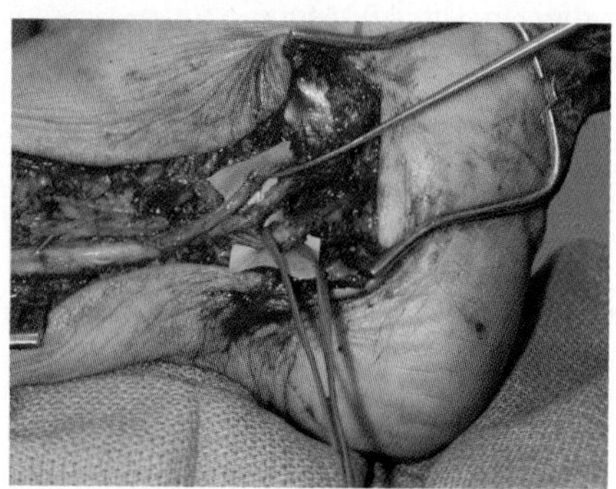

TECH FIG 11 • Tarsal tunnel released and ready for wrapping.

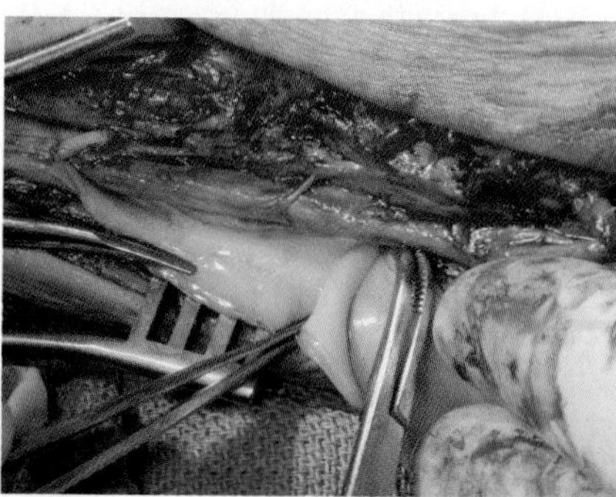

TECH FIG 13 • Placing the umbilical vein around the posterior tibial nerve.

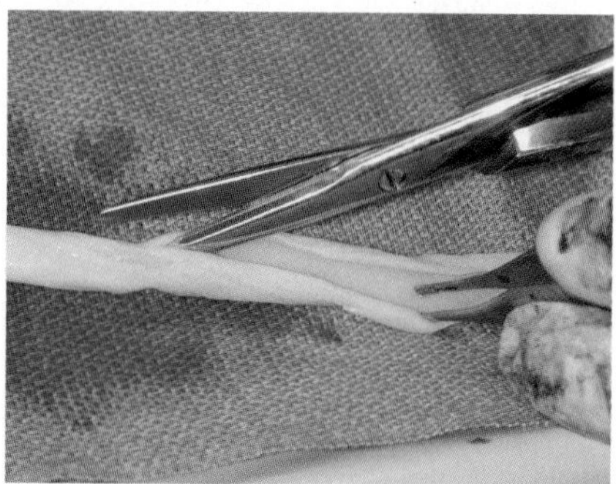

TECH FIG 12 • Cutting the fetal umbilical vein longitudinally.

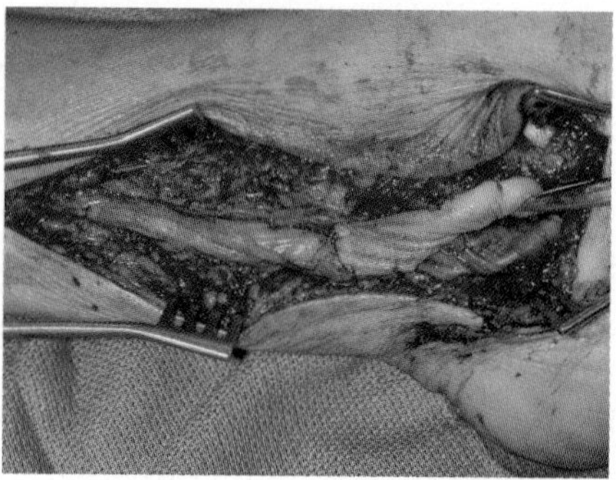

TECH FIG 14 • Finished umbilical wrap in place.

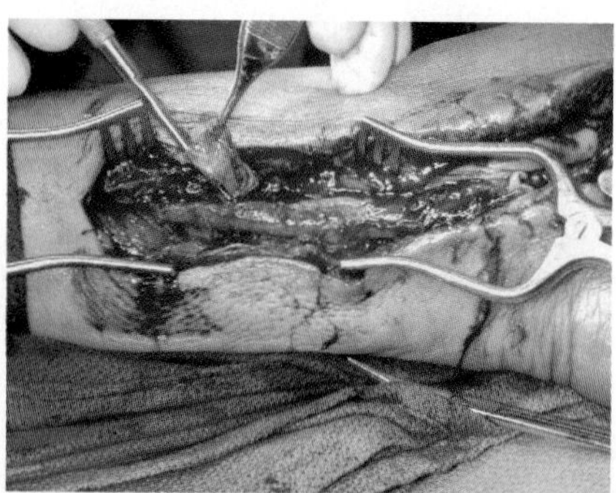

TECH FIG 15 • Infected graft removed at 3 weeks.

OTHER PERIPHERAL NERVE WRAP PROCEDURES TO MINIMIZE ADHESIVE CAPSULITIS

- The decision to wrap the superficial peroneal nerve, the deep peroneal nerve, the saphenous nerve, or the sural nerve must be made in light of reasonable results with neurotomy.
- The procedure would be similar to that for the posterior tibial nerve, with careful neurolysis and then wrapping with either autologous saphenous vein or NeuraWrap. The superficial peroneal nerve has been wrapped most often, with encouraging results.

PEARLS AND PITFALLS

Adequate preparation	▪ The surgeon needs a dedicated operating suite and staff for complicated surgery. The possibility of vascular damage requires microsurgical instruments and loupes (or microscope) available for repair (or availability of a vascular surgeon if desired). A tourniquet should be on the leg or a sterile one should be close by in case of excess bleeding with the complicated dissection.
Incomplete decompression	▪ Start more cephalad in virgin territory if possible to see the nerve more easily as well as to ensure adequate proximal decompression. Follow the nerve more proximally with finger exposure to confirm release. ▪ Distal release must be confirmed by easy passage of an instrument along the medial and lateral plantar nerves. We often take a piece of the abductor fascia out to prevent recurrent compression of the medial plantar nerve.
Residual neuritis	▪ This symptom is common; patience is warranted. Constricted nerves may take 3 to 6 months to recover, and some never do, but the prognostic guidelines remain muddy.
Unexpected tumor or cyst	▪ Most recurrent tarsal tunnel syndromes should be imaged preoperatively to rule out an extrinsic compression on the nerve. A large ganglion cyst should be completely resected, with care taken to find the stalk and source of the cyst. A neurilemmoma can often be carefully dissected, often with only minimal nerve loss.
Intractable damage to small nerve branches	▪ The sensory nerve branches, especially the calcaneal nerves, are often encased in severe scar. These may be sacrificed without many sequelae other than some heel numbness.

POSTOPERATIVE CARE

- Postoperative care depends on the extent of surgery performed and the risks of early motion on wound healing compared to the risks of stiffness.
- Most wounds are immobilized for 2 weeks to allow healing, and then a gentle range-of-motion protocol begins, often with formal physical therapy for desensitization as well.
- Weight bearing can begin at 2 weeks, progressing as tolerated.
- Physical therapy later can assist with motion, desensitization, and gait training.

OUTCOMES

- While outcome data can be difficult to interpret for initial tarsal tunnel release, the results of revision procedures can be even more confusing.
- The best study on revision tibial nerve release[5] found the best results when the initial distal release was inadequate.
- Easley and Schon[1] found significant improvement with peripheral nerve wrapping (scores improving from 8.5/10 to 5/10), especially with adhesive neuritis, which fared better than crush injury. They also found wrapping with fetal umbilical vein to be as effective as autologous saphenous vein. That study also included three superficial peroneal nerves and one deep peroneal nerve.
- The data on NeuraWrap are anecdotal at the time of this writing, although initial results have been very satisfying from two centers.

COMPLICATIONS

- The complications from revision nerve release and wrapping can be daunting, and careful preoperative discussion is essential. Most patients can expect some persistent nerve irritation for up to 6 months postoperatively, as some nerves are slow to recover (if they ever do). Sensory training can be very helpful in the postoperative period to recondition the limb.
- Infection can be devastating, especially with the extensive dissection required and the dysvascular material being applied. The senior author of this chapter treated one infected fetal umbilical graft (for revision tarsal tunnel) with a simple irrigation and débridement, leaving the graft in for 3 weeks. With a more formal removal and débridement at 3 weeks, the vein left an excellent bed of shiny tissue that healed uneventfully and with excellent results. Another surgeon left the vein in for months, with resulting inflammation and irritation and a less satisfactory outcome. Superficial wound infection can be treated with local and oral antibiotics, but deep infection must be treated aggressively.
- Vascular damage can often occur with the difficult dissection. Often, a small branch of the artery will be torn from the main posterior tibial artery. This problem can often be solved with one or two stitches of 8-0 or 9-0 suture, sealing the hole adequately. Preoperative evidence of a patent dorsal pedal pulse means that the posterior tibial artery may be able to be sacrificed, important knowledge in light of possible difficult repair.

■ Recurrent adhesive neuritis remains a difficult complication. Physical therapy, psychological counseling to deal with the stress of such an outcome, and possible revision procedures may offer some help to these patients.

REFERENCES

1. Easley ME, Schon LC. Peripheral nerve vein wrapping for intractable lower extremity pain. Foot Ankle Int 2000;21:492–500.
2. Kinoshita M, Okuda R, Morkikawa J, et al. The dorsiflexion-eversion test for diagnosis of tarsal tunnel syndrome. J Bone Joint Surg Am 2001;83A:1835–1839.
3. Schon LC, Anderson CD, Easley ME, et al. Surgical treatment of chronic lower extremity neuropathic pain. Clin Orthop Relat Res 2001;289:156–164.
4. Schon LC, Lam PW, Easley ME, et al. Complex salvage procedures for severe lower extremity nerve pain. Clin Orthop Relat Res 2001;391:171–180.
5. Skalley TC, Schon LC, Hinton RY, et al. Clinical results following revision tibial nerve release. Foot Ankle Int 1994;15:360–367.
6. Sotereanos DG, Giannakopoulos PN, Mitsionis GI, et al. Vein-graft wrapping for the treatment of recurrent compression of the median nerve. Microsurgery 1995;16:752–756.
7. Vartimidis SE, Vardakas DG, Goebel F, et al. Treatment of recurrent compressive neuropathy of peripheral nerves in the upper extremity with an autologous vein insulator. J Hand Surg Am 2001;26:296–302.
8. Xu J, Sotereanos DG, Moller AR, et al. Nerve wrapping with vein grafts in a rat model: a safe technique for the treatment of recurrent chronic compressive neuropathy. J Reconstr Microsurg 1998;14:323–330.

Chapter 61

Distraction Arthroplasty for Ankle Arthritis

Richard E. Gellman and Douglas N. Beaman

DEFINITION

- Ankle distraction arthroplasty is a new technique for the treatment of ankle arthritis in younger patients who wish to defer ankle arthrodesis or ankle replacement.
- Distraction arthroplasty is based on the hypothesis that healing of arthritic cartilage can occur when the joint is unloaded and subjected to intermittent intra-articular fluid pressure changes. Unloading is achieved with an Ilizarov external fixator, which is applied for 3 months to distract the joint.[9] During this time, it is essential that patients are weight bearing to provide the stimulus for fluid pressure changes. The flexibility of the fine wires used to construct the frame allows sufficient motion for this to occur.[9,10]
- In vitro and animal studies have shown that distraction with intermittent pressure change can reduce inflammation and normalize cartilage matrix turnover.[9] Clinical studies have demonstrated an increase in joint space and improvement in pain symptoms.[5,7,10]
- As this technique evolves, the optimal patient and arthritis stage and pattern for distraction arthroplasty will become better defined.

ANATOMY

- The anatomy of the arthritic ankle joint selected for ankle distraction arthroplasty should be carefully assessed. A well-aligned limb with a foot that is plantigrade to the long axis of the leg is essential to a good outcome in all distraction arthroplasty patients. Deformity can be present from articular wear or collapse, from bony deformity in the tibia or foot, and lastly from ligamentous laxity.
- The ideal arthritic pattern for ankle distraction treatment has uniform cartilage loss across the tibiotalar joint with no extra-articular bony malalignment or ligamentous laxity. Ankles with intra-articular collapse or uneven wear patterns can be treated successfully with ankle distraction only if extra-articular bony deformities and ligamentous laxity are addressed. The stage of ankle arthritis does not determine who is the ideal patient for distraction arthroplasty. If patients are able to maintain ankle range of motion, then satisfactory outcomes have been achieved even with advanced arthritic changes.
- Extra-articular deformities in the distal tibia will need to be corrected before or at the same time as the ankle distraction technique. The methods to correct angular deformity, acutely with osteotomy or gradually with an osteotomy followed by distraction osteogenesis, are not included in this chapter but have been well detailed in recent texts.[2,4,6]
- Deformities in the hindfoot and forefoot will also need to be corrected before or in conjunction with ankle distraction. This usually entails careful assessment of heel varus or valgus and compensatory forefoot deformities of forefoot valgus and varus. For most patients presenting with a primary complaint of ankle arthritis, it has been possible to acutely correct foot deformities at the same stage as ankle distraction arthroplasty. A calcaneal osteotomy or subtalar arthrodesis is performed to correct hindfoot deformity. A first metatarsal osteotomy or medial column arthrodesis is used to correct the forefoot.
- The presence of joint contractures will need to be carefully assessed. Ankle equinus is extremely common in ankle arthritis patients and clinically the most important feature limiting comfortable gait. It is essential to obtain 7 to 10 degrees of ankle dorsiflexion before or during ankle distraction arthroplasty to obtain a satisfactory outcome. Extra-articular contractures of the gastroc–soleus complex are less common and are readily treated with a percutaneous Achilles tendon lengthening during the frame application. Intra-articular contractures of the ankle can be corrected with the ankle distraction frame using universal hinges along the ankle joint axis and gradual correction of equinus simultaneous to ankle distraction. A more recent option is the use of Taylor Spatial struts to correct the equinus.
- Ligamentous stability will need to be assessed. Lateral ankle ligament instability is corrected before distraction. In general, medial deltoid ligament instability is addressed primarily by correcting planovalgus foot deformity or distal tibia valgus. The deltoid ligament can be tightened with nonabsorbable suture after a medial ankle arthrotomy to débride the joint, which is usually performed in these patients.

PATHOGENESIS

- Normal ankle articular cartilage is durable and resilient and distributes loads far in excess of single limb body weight. Articular cartilage has a highly organized structure consisting of chondrocytes and an extracellular matrix. The chondrocyte is responsible for synthesis and organization of the matrix molecules. The extracellular matrix consists of tissue fluid (water and cations); a collagen fibril meshwork, which provides form and tensile strength; and proteoglycans, which are responsible for stiffness and durability.
- Osteoarthritis in the ankle is the sequential change in the chondrocytes and matrix, resulting in the degradation of articular cartilage through the sequential loss of cartilage structure and chondrocyte number and metabolism.
  - Stage 1 osteoarthritis consists of matrix disruption with fibrillation, increasing water content and permeability, and changes in the matrix organization.
  - Stage 2 consists of a chondrocytic response with cellular proliferation, increased matrix turnover, and a repair response.
  - Stage 3 is the start of cartilage loss, with declining cellular response, bony changes, and progressive clinical symptoms.

NATURAL HISTORY

- Most patients have a history of trauma to the ankle, from an ankle or talus fracture or repetitive ankle sprains.

- The time between the initial trauma and presentation for ankle distraction is highly variable.
- Patients with ankle pilon fractures tend to be younger and usually develop the most rapid posttraumatic arthritis; therefore, they constitute the group to receive distraction arthroplasty closest to the time of their initial injury.

PATIENT HISTORY AND PHYSICAL FINDINGS

- Patient evaluation for ankle distraction arthroplasty includes a thorough history and physical examination.
- The optimal candidate is a compliant, motivated patient younger than 50 years of age who has posttraumatic arthritis or chronic ankle instability with arthritis, no previous history of ankle joint sepsis or ankylosis, no history of neuropathy, and an appropriate psychosocial support system to facilitate recovery and in-frame care.
- Clinically, patients must have pain primarily at the ankle joint along with documented arthritis on radiographs.
- Physical examination includes evaluation of ankle and foot range of motion.
  - Ankle motion (about 25 to 30 degrees), including dorsiflexion (5 to 10 degrees), is preferred for successful ankle distraction arthroplasty.
  - Subtalar arthrosis may affect the ability to achieve dorsiflexion, so both active and passive subtalar range of motion should be tested with the patient seated.
  - Hindfoot motion is not required but, if present, may improve the result of distraction arthroplasty.
  - Foot deformity such as cavovarus or flatfoot deformity is noted.
  - Ankle joint instability is assessed clinically and may be confirmed with ankle stress radiographs in addition to the radiographic evaluation of the deformity.
- Fluoroscopic evaluation is used to assess the arc of ankle motion. Hinge-type ankle motion, instead of the usual gliding tibiotalar motion, or loss of anterior ankle articular cartilage may be associated with less successful results.

IMAGING AND OTHER DIAGNOSTIC STUDIES

- Standard weight-bearing radiographs of the tibia, ankle, hindfoot, and foot provide sufficient information for the majority of ankle distraction candidates. CT scans, with or without reformations, are occasionally ordered for evaluation of complex deformity or to assist in defining focal wear patterns in the ankle joint.
- Standing full-length lower extremity AP and lateral radiographs from the hip to the ankle are obtained if there is deformity above the distal tibial region or a limb-length discrepancy. The long lateral view of the limb is made with the knee in full extension to assess tibial deformity, knee flexion contracture, or recurvatum from hyperlaxity. AP tibial radiographs are made with the patella facing forward. The x-ray beam is centered on the ankle to include the tibia. If a rotational deformity of the limb is present on clinical examination, an AP ankle radiograph is made in the foot-forward position to evaluate intra-articular wear or malalignment. Lateral ankle radiographs are made in the plane of the ankle malleoli.
- The hindfoot alignment view is a weight-bearing radiograph that enables observation of the tibia, ankle joint, and calcaneal tuberosity on a single view.[8] This view requires a specialized mounting box to angle the radiographic plate 20 degrees from the vertical plane.
- Another radiograph is the non–weight-bearing long axial view that visualizes the tibia, subtalar joint, and calcaneal tuberosity. A line drawn on the vertical axis of the midbody of the calcaneus should be parallel and about 1 cm lateral to the mid-diaphyseal line of the tibia. Valgus deformity and lateral translation indicate a pes planus deformity; varus angulation and medial translation indicate a cavovarus type of deformity.
- The weight-bearing AP foot radiograph is measured for the talo–first metatarsal angle, navicular coverage, and joint subluxation or arthritis. The lateral foot view is measured for the talo–first metatarsal angle, calcaneal pitch, and joint subluxation or arthritis.
- Comparison radiographs of the contralateral, asymptomatic limb should be obtained for preoperative planning.

DIFFERENTIAL DIAGNOSIS

- Arthritis associated with ankle pain is the indication for ankle distraction arthroplasty. As detailed previously, deformity evaluation and correction are needed before or in conjunction with ankle distraction.
- In patients with pain out of proportion to the degree of radiographic arthritis, the surgeon should assess for occult infection with joint aspiration for culture and a blood measurement of C-reactive protein.
- Any patients who are heavily narcotic-dependent or experience severe preoperative pain associated with early-stage arthritis are poor distraction candidates, as this technique is associated with the usual Ilizarov wire and pin site discomfort, especially in the foot.
  - These patients may not be able to perform intermittent partial weight bearing of 50 to 75 pounds in their frames and will not receive the intermittent joint pressure changes necessary for the distraction technique.

NONOPERATIVE MANAGEMENT

- Conservative treatment of ankle arthritis in younger patients is primarily activity modification.
- Running and jumping sports activities are discouraged; cycling, walking, and swimming are encouraged.
- Supportive braces, whether soft neoprene or rigid ankle–foot orthoses (AFOs), offer varying degrees of pain relief and can improve function.
- Anti-inflammatory medications, acetaminophen, and occasionally narcotics all have a role in alleviating mild to moderate arthritic symptoms.
- Homeopathic, naturopathic, or acupuncture remedies can all be used, but these are beyond our expertise for treatment recommendation in ankle arthritis.

SURGICAL MANAGEMENT

- All ankle distraction patients should be thoroughly counseled, including preoperative conversations with another patient who has undergone the procedure.

- Patient education is facilitated with a preoperative information packet reviewing external fixator and pin site care; this is given to the patient on his or her initial consultation.
- Pin and frame care is reviewed with the patient again after surgery.

Preoperative Planning

- Deformity analysis is conducted in the clinic from the radiographs.
- Previous scars or skin grafts are noted for their impact on planned approaches if joint débridement or tibial deformity correction is needed. The plan includes the need for possible fluoroscopic examination with the patient under anesthesia to assess joint tracking and fluoroscopic stress views to assess ankle joint stability.

Positioning

- The patient is positioned supine with a folded blanket under the ipsilateral hip to keep the patella facing upward.
- The entire leg to the upper thigh is draped free to allow placement of sterile bath blankets under the distal thigh and foot, leaving the posterior leg from the ankle to the knee free for ease of ring placement and positioning. This also allows optimal lateral fluoroscopic imaging during surgery.

Approach

- The ankle distraction procedure is an all-percutaneous surgery and therefore has no single surgical approach.
- Safe zones for wire and half-pin placement in the tibia and foot are detailed below (**FIG 1**). In addition, we do place sagittal half-pins in the tibia, just medial to the tibial crest.

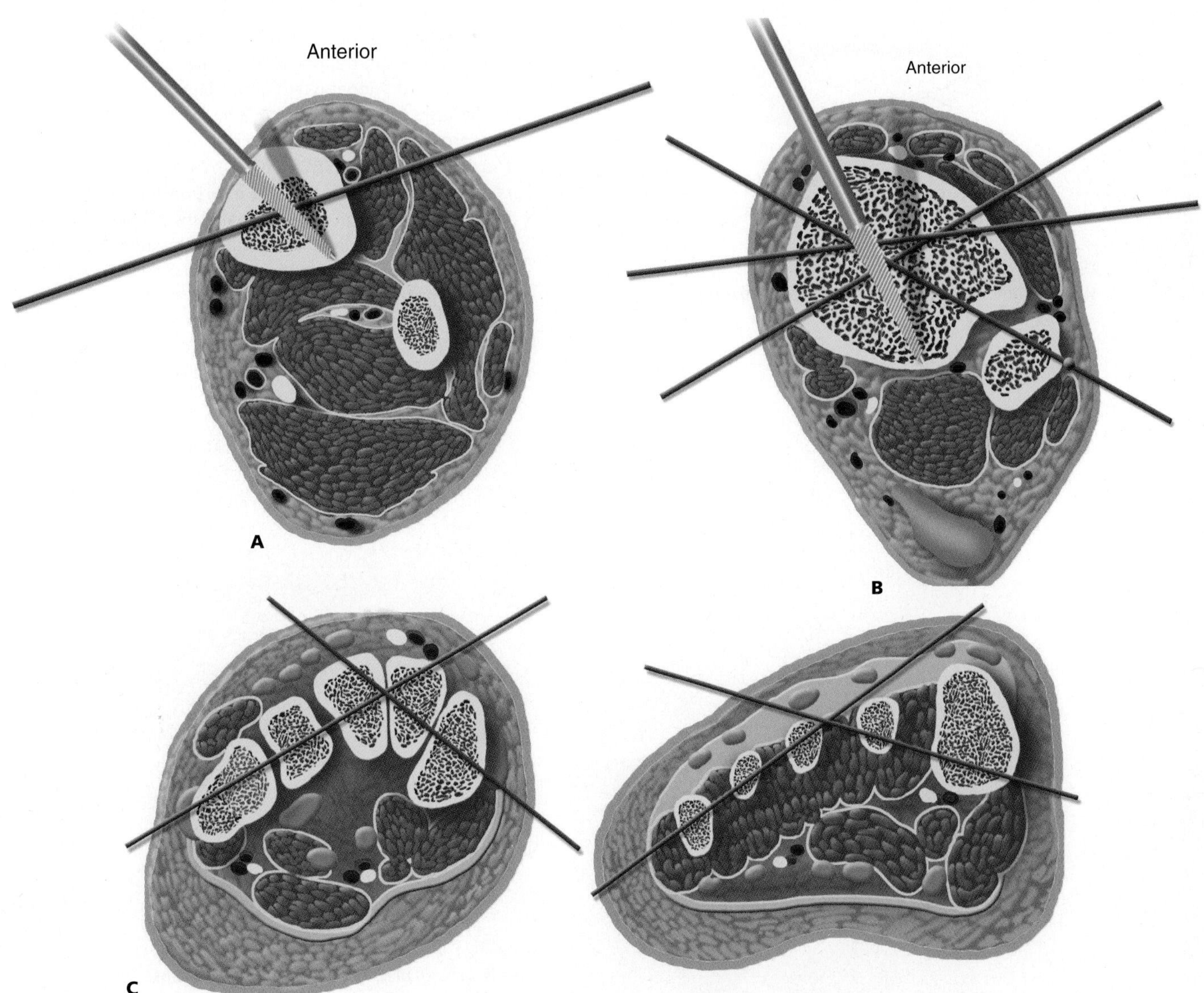

FIG 1 • Safe pin and wire placement for mid-tibia (**A**), distal tibia (**B**), and forefoot (**C**).

TIBIAL BASE FRAME APPLICATION

- Frame assembly for ankle distraction arthroplasty is similar with or without deformity correction.
- Assemble a two-ring tibial base frame. The two rings are separated by four 150- or 200-mm threaded rods, depending on the size of the patient (**TECH FIG 1**). We use Taylor Spatial rings for their strength and also the ability to use Taylor Spatial struts, as described below.

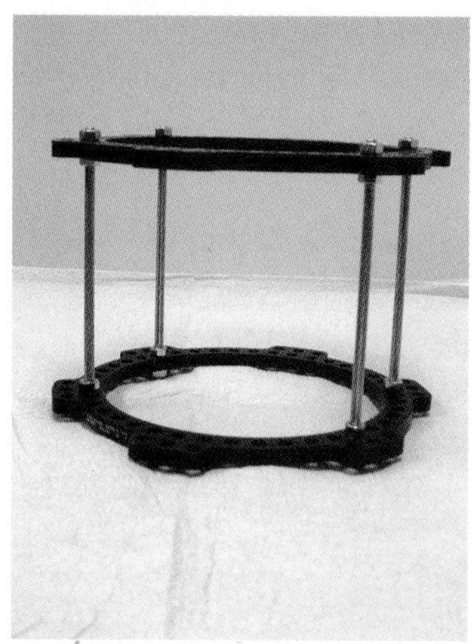

TECH FIG 1 • Tibial base frame. Two Taylor Spatial rings, usually 155 mm, are connected with four threaded rods.

- Pass the tibia base frame over the foot and place it proximal on the leg. For the distal ring, drive a transverse, smooth 1.8-mm reference wire through the tibia from medial to lateral, 5 cm proximal to the ankle joint.
- Connect the distal tibial ring to this wire orthogonal to the distal tibia with the limb centered within the ring to ensure soft tissue clearance between the limb and the rings, and tension the wire (**TECH FIG 2A,B**). A second wire may then be placed on the proximal ring and tensioned to secure the sagittal plane alignment (**TECH FIG 2C**).
- Six-millimeter half-pin fixation is now performed. Fix the proximal ring to the tibia with two 6.0-mm half-pins secured with connecting cubes or posts, one proximal and one distal to the ring in a multiplanar fashion; secure the most proximal half-pin to a two-hole connecting cube or post in the anteromedial to posterolateral plane, and secure the inferior half-pin to a two- or three-hole cube placed in the sagittal plane (**TECH FIG 3A**).
- Place two additional 6.0-mm half-pins and secure them to the distal tibial ring, also in a multiplanar orientation, one proximal and the other distal or both proximal to the distal tibial ring (**TECH FIG 3B**). Fluoroscopic imaging confirms appropriate half-pin insertion length. In general, the number of wire and half-pins placed increases as the patient's weight and neuropathy increases. Poor bone quality should be addressed with a greater number of wire fixation pins.

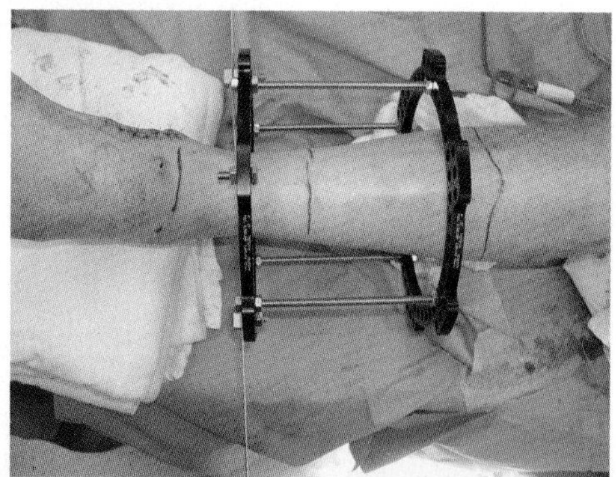

A

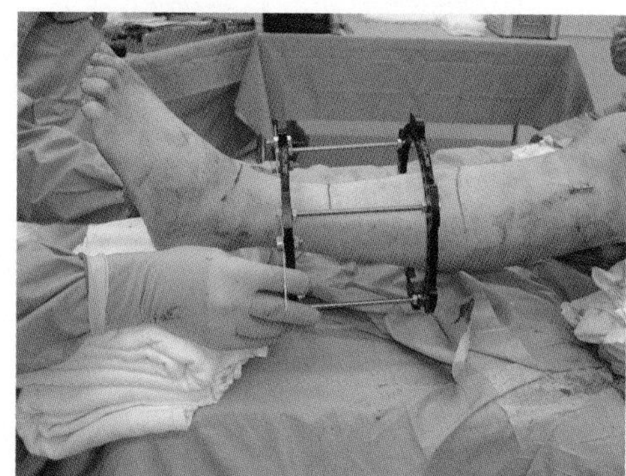

B

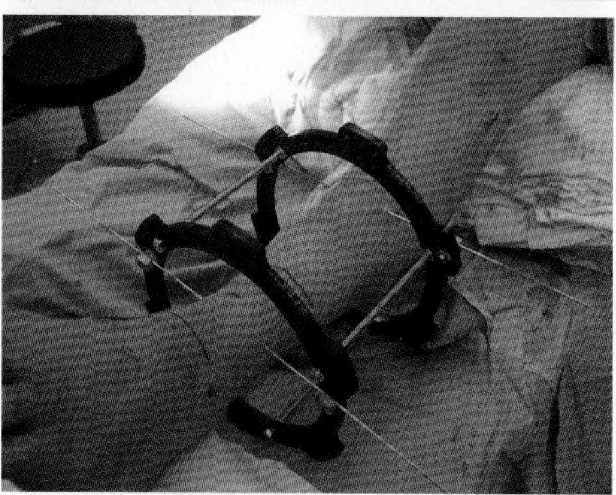

C

TECH FIG 2 • **A.** AP view of frame. The distal wire is placed first, 5 to 6 cm above the ankle joint. **B.** Lateral view. **C.** Tibial base frame. The proximal wire secures sagittal plane alignment. This wire may be removed in the office or later in the case once two half-pins are placed.

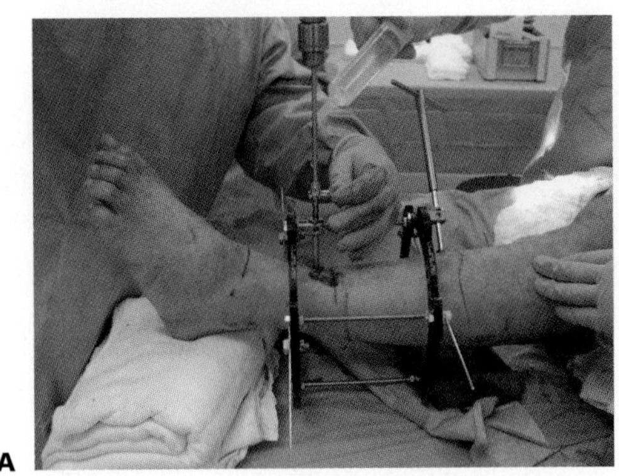

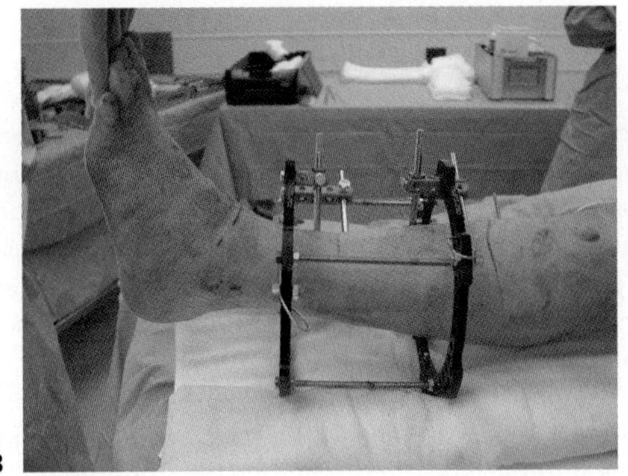

TECH FIG 3 • **A.** Half-pin fixation of tibia. **B.** Completed tibial base frame.

ANKLE HINGE PLACEMENT

- After applying the tibial base frame, place a smooth 1.8-mm wire temporarily from the tip of the lateral malleolus to the tip of the medial malleolus under fluoroscopic guidance. Cut the ends about 3 cm from the skin edges. This guidewire serves as a reference for hinge placement as it represents a good estimate of the coronal plane ankle joint axis (TECH FIG 4).
- Secure Ilizarov universal hinges to threaded rods, which are attached to the distal tibial ring, and align the hinges relative to the guidewire (TECH FIG 5A,B). Leave the threaded rods 1 to 2 cm long to allow for distraction. On the lateral fluoroscopic image, the universal hinges must align with the lateral talar process (TECH FIG 5C). If they do not, then move the hinges anterior or posterior until satisfactory position is achieved.
- After the hinges are properly positioned, remove the guidewire.

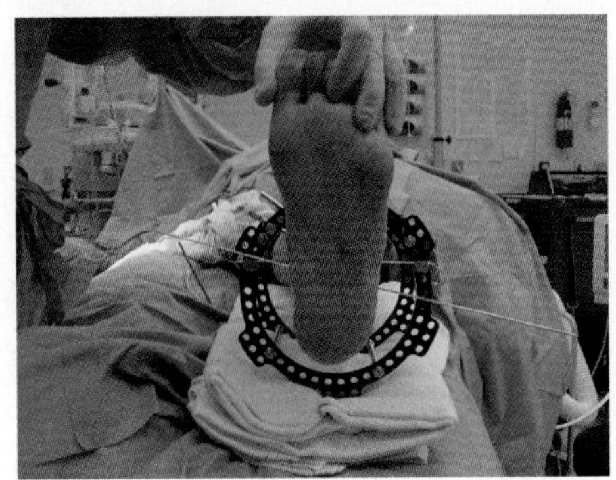

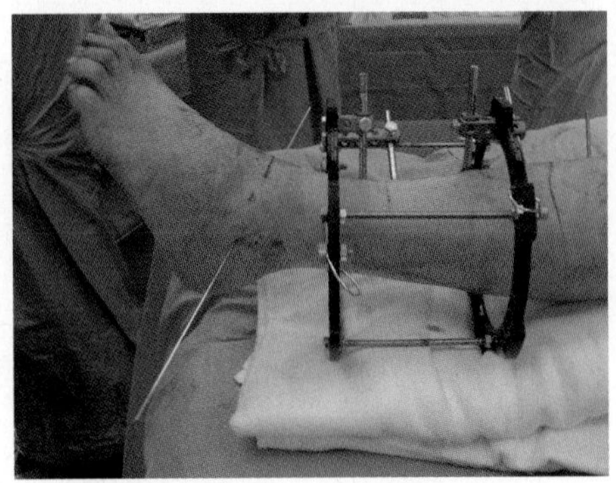

TECH FIG 4 • **A.** Ankle joint axis guidewire. AP view. This wire is placed with fluoroscopic guidance. **B.** Ankle joint axis guidewire, lateral view.

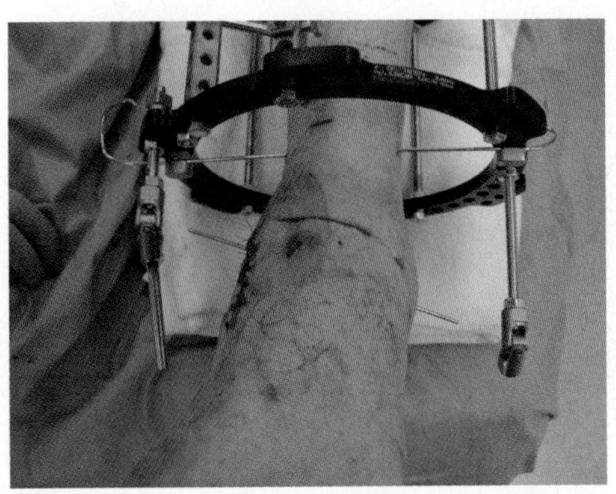

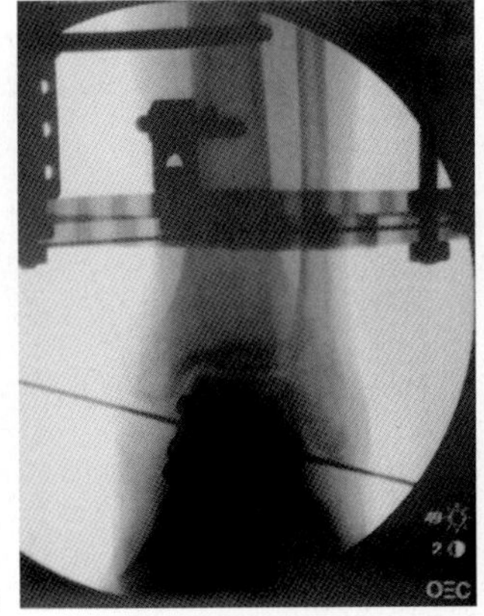

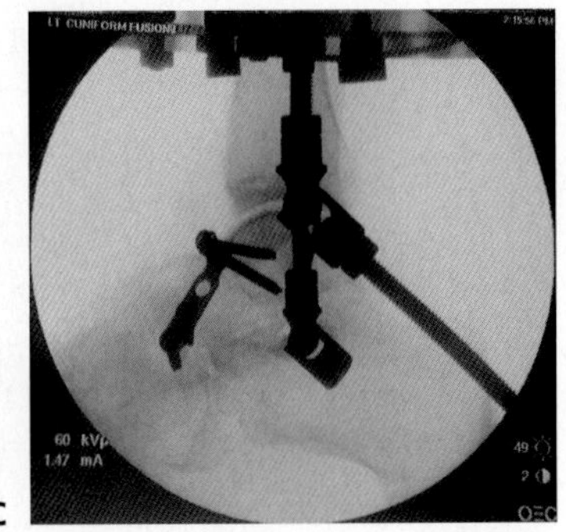

TECH FIG 5 • **A.** Clinical AP view of universal hinges mounted along joint axis. **B.** Fluoroscopic AP view. **C.** Fluoroscopic lateral view. The threaded rods of the hinges align with the lateral talar process and the center of the talar dome.

FOOT RING APPLICATION

- Center the foot in a foot ring and attach the hinges from the lower tibial ring to the foot ring. In most cases, the lateral hinge is placed directly on the ring, and a short threaded rod is used on the medial side (often a two-hole plate is needed off the foot ring to attach the medial hinge) (TECH FIG 6A,B). An assistant holds the foot ring in place during wire attachment (TECH FIG 6C).
- The foot ring is usually secured to the foot with five smooth 1.8-mm wires: one in the talar neck, two in the calcaneal tuberosity, and two in the forefoot. The weaker open section of the foot ring is enclosed with a half-ring placed parallel or at 90 degrees to the foot ring to prevent ring deformation (TECH FIG 6). An alternative method of enclosing the foot ring is the use of two oblique struts connected by a plate (TECH FIG 7).
- Place the first calcaneal wire from anteromedial to posterolateral, avoiding the neurovascular structures on the medial aspect of the hindfoot, and secure the foot ring to this wire parallel to the sole of the foot (TECH FIG 8). Place the first forefoot wire medial to lateral, engaging the first and second, and occasionally third, metatarsals. Tension these first two wires.
- Place the second calcaneal wire from distal-lateral to posteromedial. Then, place the second forefoot wire proximal to the fifth metatarsal head, engaging either the fifth, fourth, and third metatarsals or the fifth and first metatarsals (plantar to the second, third, and fourth metatarsals). Take care to avoid distorting the normal orientation of the metatarsals relative to one another (TECH FIG 9). At this point, the foot ring will move up and down in a constrained manner.
- Apply tension to the remaining calcaneal and forefoot wires.
- Place a 1.8-mm talar neck wire to avoid subtalar joint distraction. This wire is placed using fluoroscopic guidance. Often the attachment to this wire is performed on the inside of the foot ring to avoid the threaded rods of the universal hinges (TECH FIG 10A,B).
- Make a lateral and AP fluoroscopic check to ensure that normal ankle motion without joint subluxation is maintained after the foot ring has been applied (TECH FIG 10C,D).

A 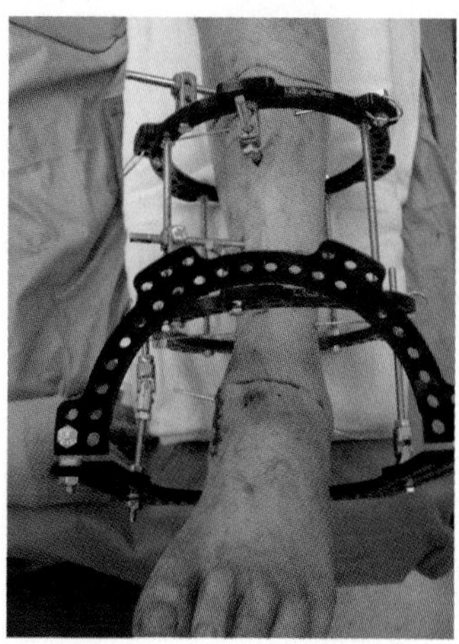

B 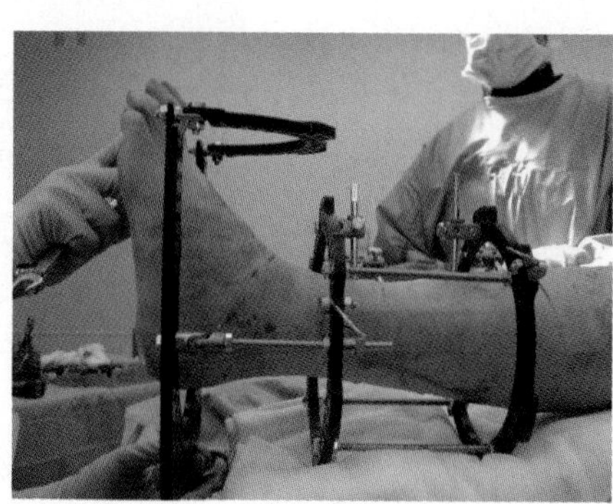

C 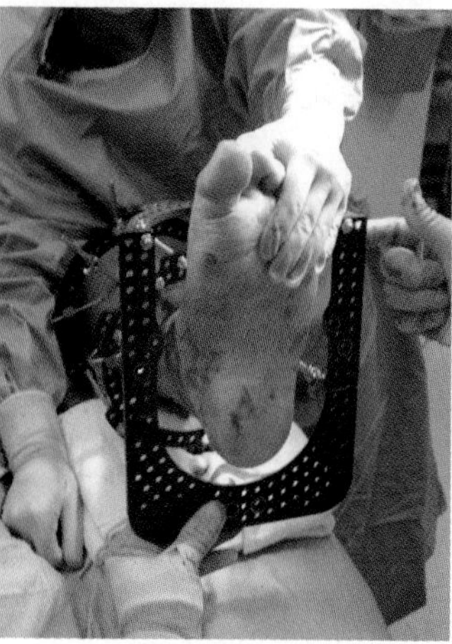

TECH FIG 6 • **A.** Foot ring is attached to the universal hinges. Lateral view. **B.** AP view. **C.** An assistant holds the foot with the ankle in neutral dorsiflexion before wire fixation is begun in the calcaneus.

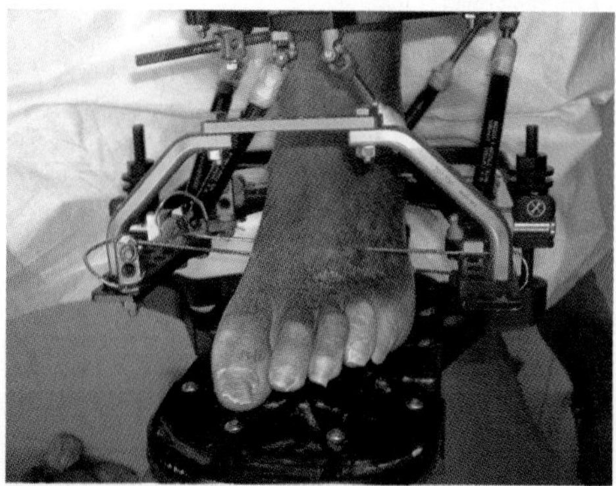

TECH FIG 7 • Oblique connecting struts are used to enclose the foot ring.

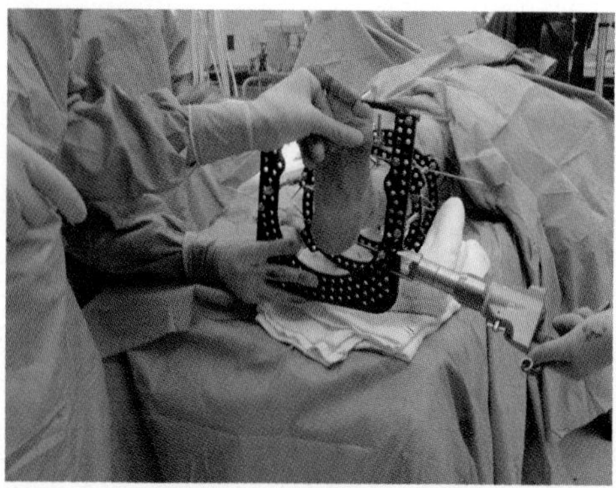

TECH FIG 8 • The calcaneal wire is tensioned first while an assistant holds the ankle in neutral and the footplate is parallel to the sole of the foot.

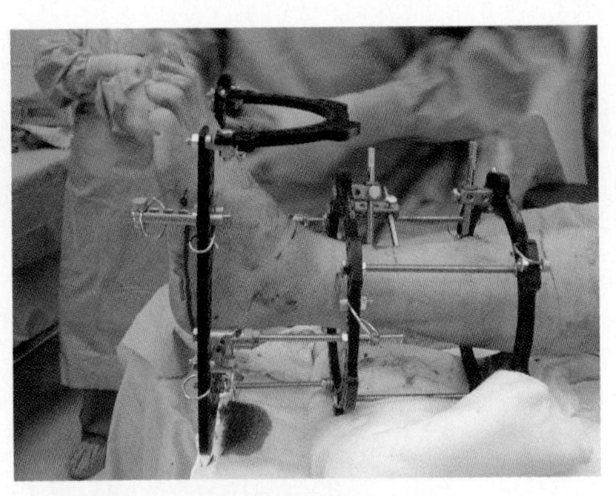
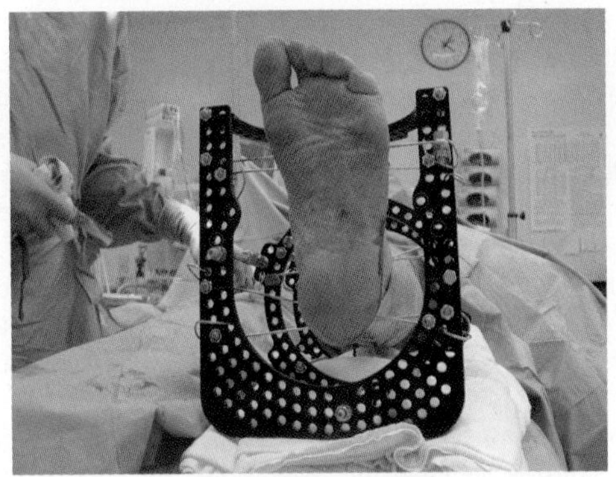

TECH FIG 9 • **A.** Foot fixation in place except for talar neck wire. Lateral view. **B.** Foot fixation in place; AP view from sole of foot.

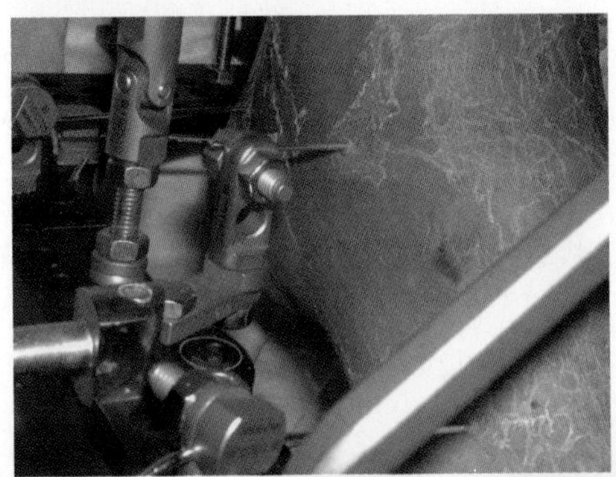
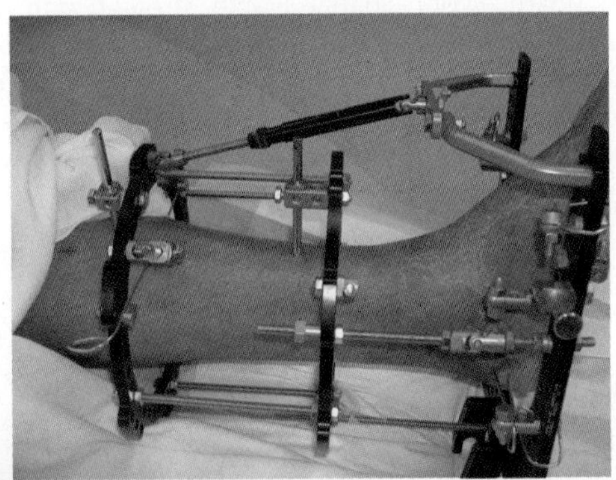
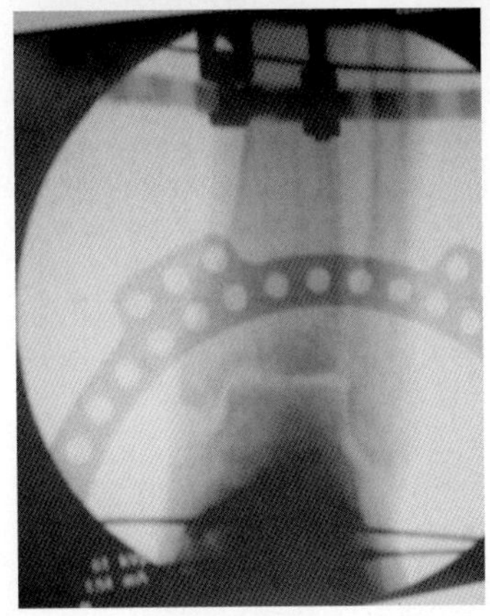
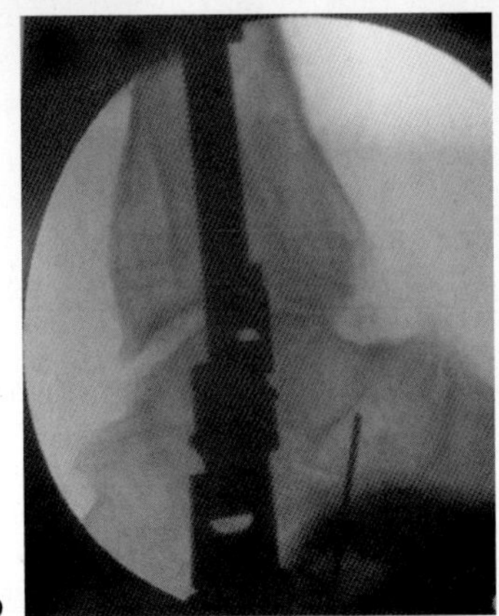

TECH FIG 10 • **A.** Talar neck wire. Attachment on the inside of the ring is often necessary. **B.** Completed ankle distraction frame with Taylor Spatial strut for anterior stability. **C,D.** AP and lateral fluoroscopic views to confirm concentric reduction before distraction. Note that the hinges align with the lateral talar process on the lateral view.

ANKLE DISTRACTION

- After applying the frame, acutely distract the ankle joint 3 to 5 mm from the preoperative position using the threaded rods attached to the universal hinges. This distraction usually is performed on the tibial ring attachment sites. Four-sided Ilizarov nuts facilitate counting the millimeters of distraction (TECH FIG 11).

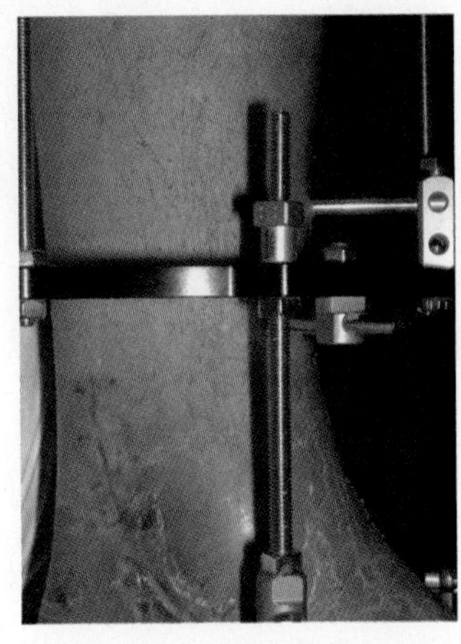

TECH FIG 11 • Four-sided nuts on the threaded rods allow for easy measurement of ankle distraction. Each 360-degree rotation equals 1 mm of movement along the threaded rod.

- Repeat fluoroscopic radiographs in neutral position, dorsiflexion, and plantarflexion to confirm satisfactory ankle distraction and motion without subluxation. If ankle distraction arthroplasty is done with either varus-to-valgus distal tibial or immediate equinus correction, minimize immediate ankle joint distraction to limit potential neurovascular compromise (**TECH FIG 12**).
- The ankle is held in neutral flexion by securing components (plates and threaded rods) from the distal tibial ring to the foot ring, which may be removed for range-of-motion exercises (**TECH FIG 13**).
- Alternatively, a frame strut (Fast Fix Taylor Spatial Frame Strut, Smith & Nephew Inc., Memphis, TN) may be secured from the proximal tibial ring to the foot ring, released to allow range of motion, and resecured with the foot held in neutral position (**TECH FIG 14A**).
- Two standard Taylor Spatial Frame struts (Smith & Nephew) placed anterior and posterior may be used for equinus correction. Take care to angle the posterior strut outward from the frame to prevent ankle joint subluxation, as shown in **TECH FIGURE 14B**.

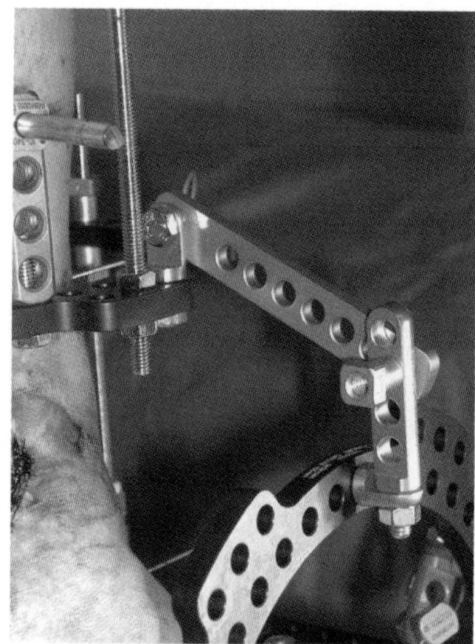

TECH FIG 13 • Anterior frame attachment with plates. This can be loosened by the patient to begin ankle range of motion.

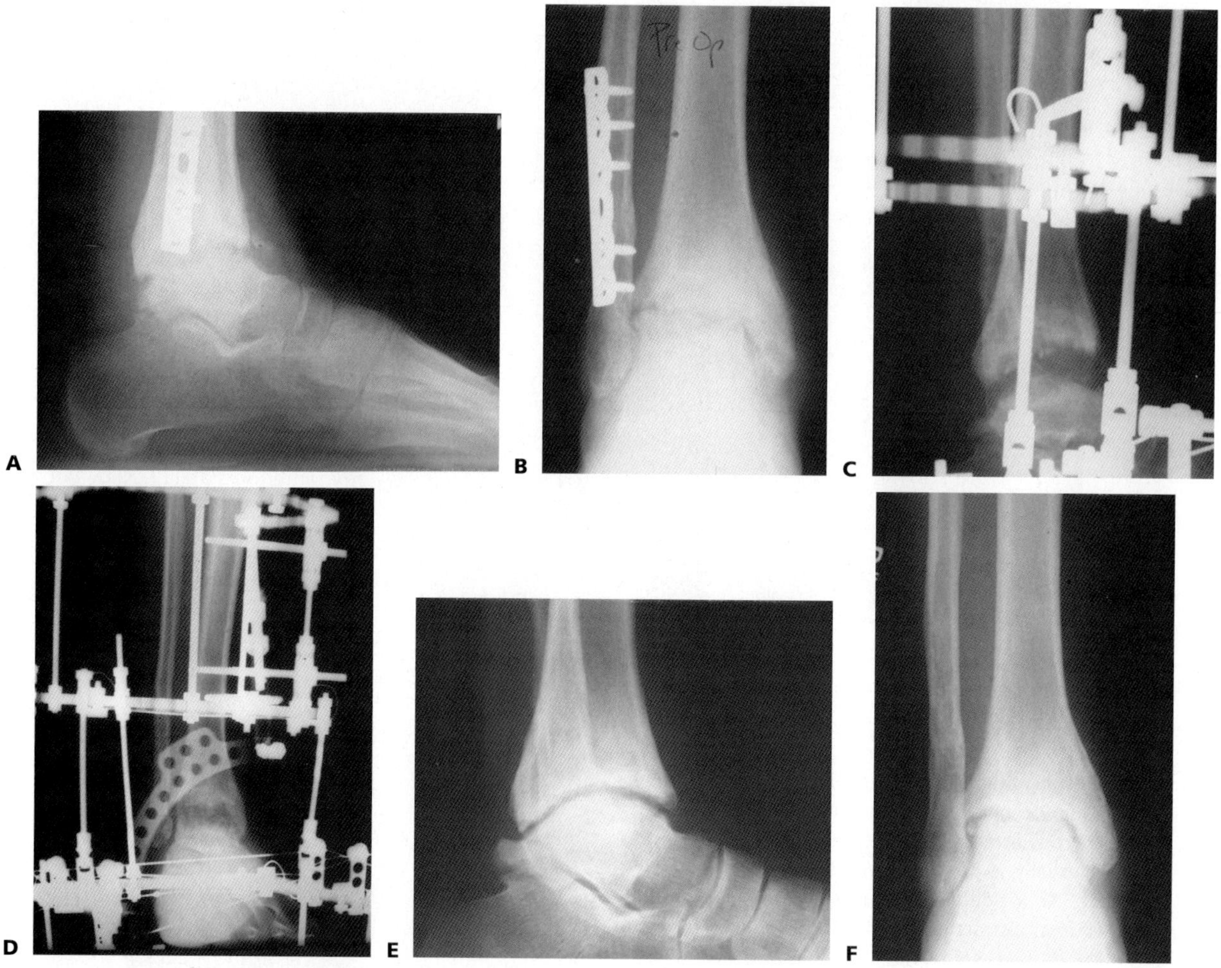

A B C D E F

TECH FIG 12 • A. Lateral radiograph of a 17-year-old boy who developed rapid posttraumatic ankle arthritis after an open ankle fracture. He required daily narcotics and anti-inflammatory medications. **B.** AP radiograph. **C,D.** Lateral and AP radiographs showing ankle distraction of 5 mm measured off the intact posterior tibiotalar joint. Bone loss anteriorly creates a greater distraction gap. **E,F.** Lateral and AP radiographs 18 months after surgery. The patient is an active college student. Pain is controlled with anti-inflammatory medications. Range of motion is 10 degrees dorsiflexion and 20 degrees plantarflexion.

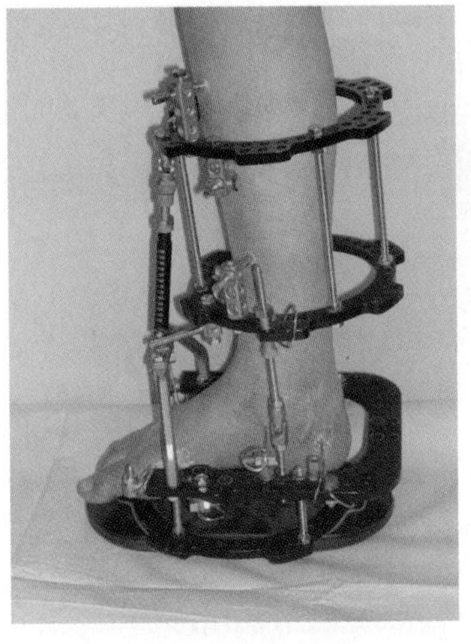

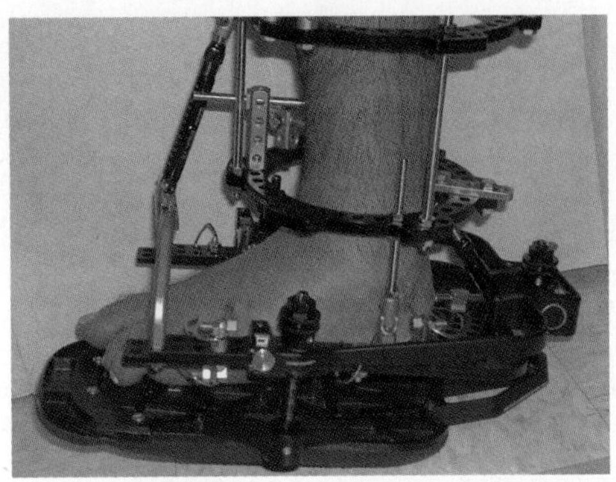

TECH FIG 14 • **A.** Taylor Spatial fast fix strut is used on the anterior frame to provide stability when locked and ankle range of motion when released. This simplifies the ability to range the ankle, since the patient does not need to carry around wrenches. **B.** Equinus correction ankle frame. Note the posterior angled "push" strut and anterior "pull" strut.

- An alternative to the use of universal hinges is to use Taylor Spatial struts for ankle distraction. There are numerous advantages to these struts. First, they allow safe, controlled ankle distraction that can be performed simultaneous to an equinus correction. Second, the struts control ankle subluxation since there is the ability to posterior translate the talus and foot during equinus correction. Third, they are very strong, which can be a factor in a heavy patient, where fatigue-related failure of the universal hinges can occur. And finally, although the struts increase the expense of the frame, they make attachment of the tibial ring to the footplate quick and easy, reducing the cost of operative time (**TECH FIG 15A**). The struts do not allow ankle motion; however, a conversion to universal hinges can be performed in the office if the surgeon wishes to start ankle motion before frame removal.

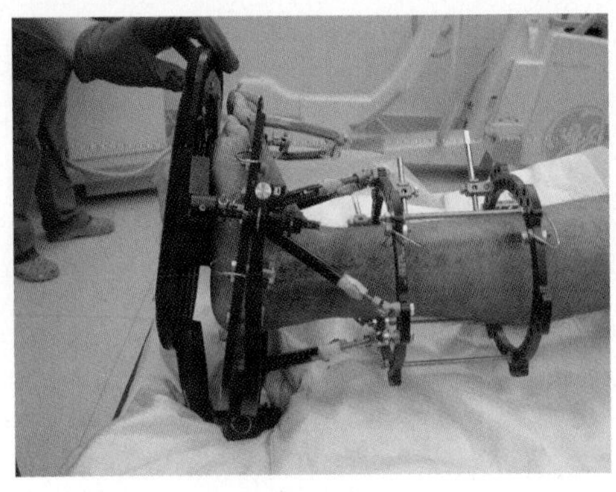

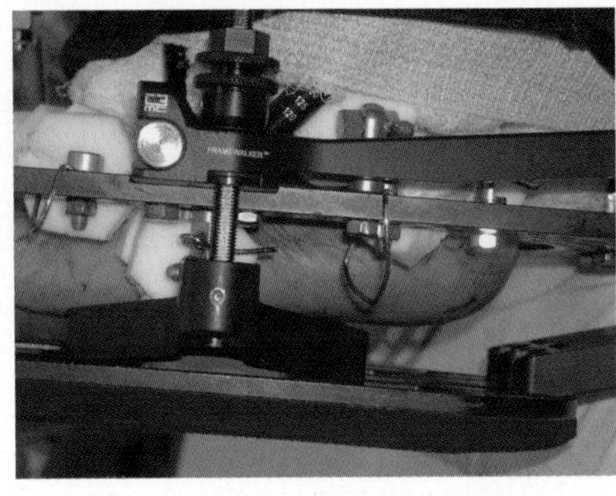

TECH FIG 15 • **A.** Taylor Spatial struts used to address rigid equinus contracture. The patient had failed open reduction and internal fixation of the ankle and syndesmosis with joint subluxation for 5 months. Frame was applied after revision surgery. The FrameWalker allows protected and more comfortable weight-bearing. **B.** Close-up view of FrameWalker attachment.

WOUND DRESSING

- Dress the wounds in routine fashion, and dress wires and half-pins with Ilizarov sponges stacked from the skin to the fixation attachment to provide soft tissue compression. During surgery or on the first postoperative day, a walking assembly (FrameWalker, Quantum Medical Concepts, Hood River, OR; www.quantummedicalconcepts.com) is attached to the foot ring to suspend the foot 1 to 2 cm from the floor (Tech Fig 15). This new device has improved patients' ability to comfortably bear weight due to some flex in the footplate device, and it also may decrease tibial half-pin loosening, which was occurring frequently with previous footplate designs. It also has design features that allow rapid adjustment to ensure a plantigrade foot position, and it easily snaps off and on for access to the sole of the foot for skin care.
- Place bulky roll (Kerlix, Kendall, Mansfield, MA) dressings between the rings and the limb, especially about the ankle and posterior leg and heel to limit swelling (**TECH FIG 16A**). Overwrap the rings with Ace bandages and an external fixator cover (Quantum Medical Concepts) for cleanliness and to protect the contralateral leg (as well as bed sheets and household furniture) from injury (**TECH FIG 16B**).

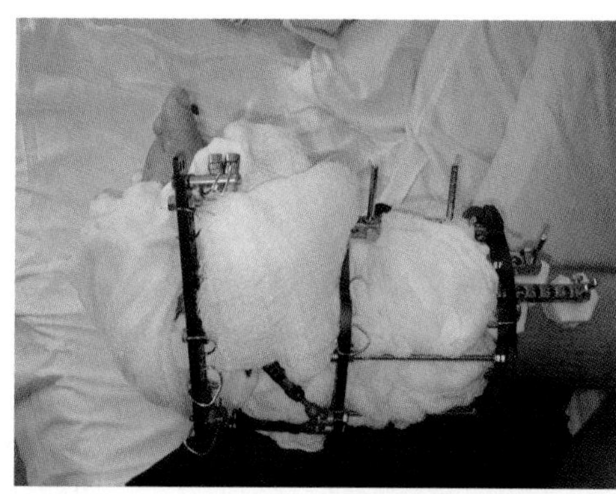

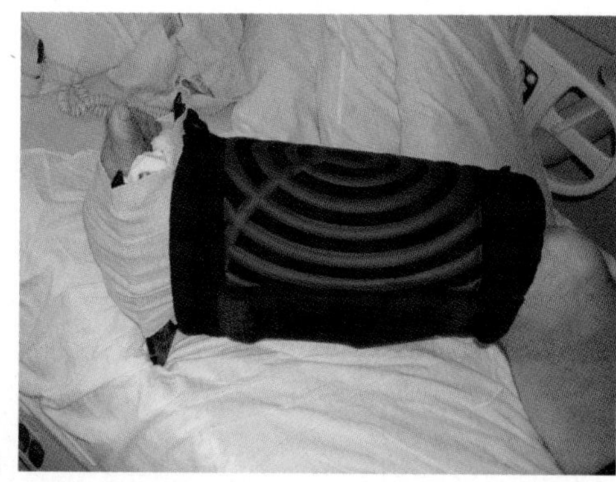

TECH FIG 16 • **A.** Postoperative dressings to absorb drainage and decrease swelling. **B.** Frame cover protects bedding and the other leg and helps keep the leg clean and dry.

PEARLS AND PITFALLS

Tibial base frame application	■ Ensure 5 cm of distance between the lower tibial ring and the ankle joint. Place at least four multiplanar half-pins, two off each tibia ring.
Hinge placement	■ Universal hinges must be aligned along the axis of the ankle joint and the tips of the malleoli on the fluoroscopic AP view and centered on the lateral talar process on the lateral view.
Foot ring application	■ Five-wire fixation in the foot for adequate stability. Add an axial calcaneal half-pin if a gradual equinus correction is necessary.
Ankle distraction	■ Acutely distract 3 to 5 mm, depending on the resistance of the joint capsule. Check fluoroscopic motion to ensure there is no joint subluxation.
Pin care	■ Daily shower once wounds are healed. Avoid cleaning with hydrogen peroxide; use normal saline or sterile water. Add oral cephalexin for pin infection.

POSTOPERATIVE CARE

- Postoperative dressings remain in place for 3 to 7 days. Pin care begins as an outpatient to avoid exposing pin sites in the inpatient setting. The contralateral leg is fitted with a shoe lift to balance the pelvis for gait.
- On the first postoperative day, the patient is advanced from bed to chair and physical therapy is begun for lower extremity function and gait. Partial weight bearing may begin on the first postoperative day and is progressed during the next 1 to 2 weeks, depending on the presence of other foot and distal tibia procedures. The patient is discharged from the hospital on the second or third postoperative day. Ankle range of motion is started 1 to 2 weeks after surgery, but this may be instituted later depending on individual circumstances.
- Pin care: The pin site sponges and dressings are removed and pin care is initiated 4 to 7 days after surgery. Normal saline or sterile water is used to remove significant accumulations of drainage around wire and half-pin sites. Hydrogen peroxide is avoided because it tends to irritate skin, and this can mimic an early pin infection.
- Two to 3 weeks after surgery, sutures are removed and the pin care may continue with a daily shower using antibacterial liquid soap and a thorough water rinse to the leg and fixator. The fixator and leg are dried with a clean towel and hair dryer (cool setting).
- The most common problem encountered with ring fixation is a localized wire or pin site infection. It is important to inspect all pin sites daily to assess for signs of infection or loosening, including localized redness, pain and tenderness, warmth, swelling (firm or fluctuant), and drainage from the pin or wire that may vary in color and odor. When early signs of pin site infection are noted, pin care is increased to twice daily, the pin site is wrapped with a gauze roll dressing, ankle range of motion is discontinued, and weight bearing and physical therapy are limited. If signs and symptoms of a pin site infection do not rapidly improve, oral antibiotics are prescribed (cephalexin or clindamycin) for 5 to 7 days. The pin site infection usually begins to resolve within 24 hours of starting oral antibiotic treatment. Recalcitrant pin site infection is treated with intravenous antibiotic therapy with or without pin removal.
- Physical therapy is started in the hospital and continued until after frame removal. Lower extremity motion, conditioning, and gait are emphasized. Non-impact activities, including swimming and pool therapy if available, are encouraged with the fixator in place.
- After adequate healing of an osteotomy, nonunion, Achilles lengthening, or ligament reconstruction, ankle range of motion can be initiated with attention to optimize dorsiflexion. Ankle range of motion is initially done for 30 minutes, three to five times per day, and then progressed as tolerated by the patient and pin sites.
- Follow-up evaluation: Weight-bearing AP, lateral, and oblique ankle radiographs are made at 1, 3, 6, and 9 weeks after frame application to confirm concentric ankle distraction and alignment. Distraction of about 4 to 5 mm greater than

preoperative ankle joint space is desired, and this usually is achieved intraoperatively and maintained during the postoperative course. With associated correction of equinus or varus deformity, immediate distraction is avoided, and gradual distraction (0.5 mm per day for 10 days, starting 3 to 10 days after surgery) is performed to limit potential tibial nerve injury. Weight-bearing radiographs are necessary to confirm, add, or delete distraction.

- Frame removal: The frame typically is removed 12 weeks after application under general anesthesia as outpatient surgery. This may be delayed until healing of a simultaneous osteotomy, nonunion correction, or malunion correction. After frame removal, soft dressings are applied and changed as needed for bleeding. A removable fracture walker boot is used for ambulation. Crutches or other assistive devices are used for the first several weeks after frame removal for comfort, but weight bearing as tolerated is allowed. Showers are resumed after the pin sites stop draining, usually within 3 days after frame removal.
- Care after frame removal: During the initial 6 to 8 weeks after frame removal, the patient gradually resumes regular footwear and full weight bearing without assistive devices. Maintaining ankle range of motion, especially dorsiflexion, may be facilitated with non-impact activities such as swimming, bicycling, and physical therapy. Prolonged weight bearing is avoided because this may delay recovery. A removable fracture walker boot, compression stocking, or light ankle brace may minimize discomfort and swelling. A stable level of function usually is not achieved until 6 to 12 months after frame removal.

OUTCOMES

- Ankle distraction arthroplasty is successful in 70% to 80% of patients in improving pain and function. Patient selection is critical, and success is more likely with motivated, compliant patients who have posttraumatic or instability-related ankle arthritis and retained preoperative ankle motion (5 to 10 degrees of dorsiflexion). Patients with minimal ankle motion and marked equinus contracture or severe arthritis localized to the anterior ankle are particularly susceptible to failure, and patients with previous septic ankle arthritis have suboptimal results.
- In an early study of ankle distraction for posttraumatic ankle arthritis with a hinged distraction apparatus, 13 (81%) of 16 cases had good results at 16 months of follow-up.[3] In 11 patients with posttraumatic arthritis, evaluation at 20 months after ankle distraction showed that all patients had less pain.[10] Persistent ankle swelling and crepitus have been noted after removal of the external fixator, but average function improved after 1 year after surgery.[9] In a more recent prospective study of 57 patients followed for an average of 2.8 years after ankle distraction, significant clinical improvement was noted in three fourths of the patients, improvement increased over time, and joint distraction had significantly better results than ankle joint débridement alone.[5] In a review by the same authors at a minimum of 7 years of follow-up, evaluation after ankle distraction for osteoarthritis showed that 16 (73%) of 22 patients had significant improvement of all clinical parameters and 6 (27%) patients had failed treatment.[7]
- Comparable results have been achieved when ankle distraction was used for arthritis in conjunction with osteotomy for deformity correction. In 11 patients with ankle arthritis associated with distal tibial deformity, treatment consisted of ankle joint distraction with the Ilizarov device, osteotomy, and range-of-motion exercises for 3 months.[1] Tibial deformity correction was gradual in three patients and acute in two patients, and all seven foot deformity corrections were done acutely. In 10 patients evaluated at an average of 18 months after surgery, 9 (90%) patients were very satisfied (3 patients) or satisfied (6 patients), 1 patient was not satisfied, and 9 patients stated that they would have the procedure again.[1] The average AAOS Foot and Ankle Outcome Score was 47 points (normal population average, 50 points). Dorsiflexion range directly correlated with AAOS score. It was concluded that deformity correction may augment the efficacy of distraction and that dorsiflexion may be an important factor in the success of the ankle distraction procedure.[1]
- A later study of 22 patients with longer follow-up (average 28 months) and a more detailed examination of ankle arthritic wear pattern showed that anterior joint involvement predominates in the patients with poor outcomes.[11] Of the patients without anterior wear, 83% had a successful outcome, compared to only 40% of patients with anterior wear.[11]

COMPLICATIONS

- The most common technical complications of ankle distraction arthroplasty are pin site inflammation or infection, wire or half-pin loosening, and frame hardware failure. Treatment for infection is usually oral antibiotics and checking to make sure the wire or half-pin is not loose. A loose wire can usually be retensioned in the office, whereas a loose half-pin can only be removed in the office. Frame modification is occasionally necessary if multiple half-pins become loose in the tibia early during the distraction period. Most broken hardware such as the universal hinges or threaded rods can be repaired in the office.
- The most significant complications of ankle distraction arthroplasty are failure to relieve pain and a loss of ankle motion. As a rule, swelling and stiffness do occur after ankle distraction as a result of the underlying arthritis. A period of increased pain and disability after ankle distraction may occur for 2 to 4 months after frame removal, occasionally persisting for up to 6 to 12 months. Physical therapy and non-impact activities are emphasized during this time, including swimming and bicycling. Patients should be counseled to wait a minimum of 12 months before judging the success or failure of ankle distraction arthroplasty.
- Direct neurovascular injury resulting from pin placement may occur despite operative caution because of posttraumatic distortion of the anatomy and scarring.
- Immediate correction of a distal tibial or foot deformity, especially with concomitant immediate ankle distraction, may be complicated by traction injury of the posterior tibial nerve and tarsal tunnel syndrome. Initial treatment includes restoration of deformity, if possible, and release of ankle distraction to decrease nerve tension. Correction and traction may be reapplied gradually. Prophylactic tarsal tunnel release may limit this complication, and careful postoperative monitoring to enable early recognition is important. Gradual deformity correction and ankle distraction may limit the risk of traction injury to the posterior tibial nerve.

REFERENCES

1. Beaman D, Domenigoni A. Distraction and deformity correction for ankle arthritis. Limb Lengthening and Reconstruction Society, 14th Annual Meeting, Toronto, 2004.
2. Beaman D, Gellman R, Trepman E. Ankle arthritis: deformity correction and distraction arthroplasty. In: Coughlin MJ, Mann RA, Saltzman CL. Surgery of the Foot and Ankle, 8th ed. St. Louis: Mosby, 2007.
3. Judet R, Judet T. The use of a hinge distraction apparatus after arthrolysis and arthroplasty. Rev Chir Orthop Reparatrice Appar Mot 1978; 64:353–365.
4. Kirienko A, Villa A, Calhoun JH. Ilizarov Technique for Complex Foot and Ankle Deformities. New York: Marcel Dekker, 2003.
5. Marijnissen AC, Van Roermund PM, Van Melkebeek J, et al. Clinical benefit of joint distraction in the treatment of severe osteoarthritis of the ankle: proof of concept in an open prospective study and in a randomized controlled study. Arthritis Rheum 2002; 46:2893–2902.
6. Paley D. Principles of Deformity Correction. New York: Springer Verlag, 2003.
7. Ploegmakers JJ, van Roermund PM, van Melkebeek J, et al. Prolonged clinical benefit from joint distraction in the treatment of ankle osteoarthritis. Osteoarthritis Cartilage 2005;13:582–588.
8. Saltzman CL, El-Khoury GY. The hindfoot alignment view. Foot Ankle Int 1995;16:572–576.
9. van Roermund PM, Lafeber FPJG. Joint distraction as treatment for ankle osteoarthritis. AAOS Instr Course Lect 1999;48:249–254.
10. van Valburg AA, van Roermund PM, Lammens J, et al. Can Ilizarov joint distraction delay the need for an arthrodesis of the ankle? J Bone Joint Surg Br 1995;77B:720–725.
11. Workman K, Gellman R, Beaman D. Ankle joint preservation arthroplasty. Inman Abbott Society Annual Meeting, San Francisco, 2007.

Chapter 62 Supramalleolar Osteotomy With Internal Fixation: Perspective 1

Emmanouil D. Stamatis

DEFINITION

- Ankle arthritis is characterized by loss of joint cartilage and joint narrowing.
- Primary ankle arthritis is relatively rare; most commonly, ankle arthritis is posttraumatic in origin. Inflammatory arthritides may also involve the ankle. While ankle arthrodesis and total ankle arthroplasty are accepted surgical treatments for advanced ankle arthritis, joint-preserving supramalleolar osteotomy is an attractive alternative in select patients with advanced ankle arthritis, particularly in ankle arthritis associated with malalignment.
- Supramalleolar osteotomy, whether opening or closing wedge, redistributes stresses on the ankle, transferring weight from an overloaded arthritic portion of the joint to a healthier aspect of the joint.[6,24,29] In theory, realignment also improves the biomechanics of the lower extremity[28] and may improve function and delay the progression of the degenerative process.

ANATOMY

- The ankle joint is the articulation formed by the mortise (tibial plafond–medial malleolus and the distal part of the fibula) and the talus.
- The ankle is a modified hinge joint with a slight oblique orientation in two planes: (a) posterior and lateral in the transverse plane and (b) lateral and downward in the coronal plane.
- This sagittal plane orientation affords about 6 degrees of rotation and 45 to 70 degrees in the flexion–extension motion arc.
- The tibiotalar joint functions as part of the ankle–subtalar joint complex during gait; portions of the medial and lateral collateral ligaments cross both the ankle and subtalar joints. The blood supply is provided by the anterior and posterior tibial arteries and the peroneal artery as well as their branches and anastomoses, forming a rich vascular ring.
- The distal tibial plafond is slightly valgus oriented, in the coronal plane, with respect to the tibial diaphysis, forming an angle called the tibial–angle surface (TAS) with a value of 93 degrees.[12]
- The same angle in the sagittal plane, with its apex posteriorly, is called the tibial–lateral surface (TLS), with a value of 80 degrees.[12]

PATHOGENESIS

- Idiopathic (primary) arthritis, or osteoarthrosis, is relatively rare in the ankle. The exact mechanism of cartilage degeneration and loss has not been clearly defined, although several theories have been proposed.
- Secondary arthritic involvement is mainly posttraumatic, occurring after intra-articular fractures, chondral or osteochondral injuries, and chronic instability.
- Other causes of ankle arthritis include peripheral neuropathy (neuroarthropathy) and various inflammatory disorders (such as rheumatoid arthritis, mixed connective tissue disorders, gout, and pseudogout), primary synovial disorders (pigmented villonodular synovitis), and septic arthritis, as well as seronegative arthritides associated with psoriasis, Reiter syndrome, and spondyloarthropathy.
- Distal tibial deformity may be a result of malunion of a distal tibial or pilon fracture, physeal disturbance from adjacent osteochondromata, physeal dysplasia, and so forth.

NATURAL HISTORY

- Untreated ankle arthritis typically progresses, with worsening pain that eventually interferes with daily activities. Gradually, ankle stiffness in addition to pain leads to a disturbance of physiologic heel-to-toe gait.
- Low-demand patients with isolated ankle arthritis may function surprisingly well because of the adaptive effect of the healthy subtalar and transverse talar joints. However, obesity, high-demand activity levels, and concomitant subtalar or transverse tarsal joint pathology typically contribute to the morbidity of ankle arthritis.
- To our knowledge there are no absolute numbers for tibiotalar angular alignment that predispose an ankle to the development of arthritis. Several authors have reported that angulation exceeding 10 degrees was compatible with long-term normal function and absence of pain in the ankle joint,[9,14] while biomechanical studies on cadavers have shown that there is a decrease of the contact surface area in the ankle joint of up to 40% in the presence of malalignment,[31,32] with the distal tibial deformities significantly altering total tibiotalar contact area, contact shape, and contact location.[31]

PATIENT HISTORY AND PHYSICAL FINDINGS

- A complete examination of the ankle and hindfoot joints should include the following:
  - Soft tissue condition: previous scars, callosities, ulcers, fistulas, and so forth
  - Vascular status: peripheral pulses, microcirculation (capillary refill), ankle–brachial index
  - Sensation: light touch and, if indicated, Semmes-Weinstein monofilament testing to rule out a peripheral neuropathy. A joint-preserving realignment supramalleolar osteotomy is feasible in select patients with peripheral neuropathy, but the potential for Charcot neuroarthropathy and failure of the procedure must be considered.
  - Stability: Anterior drawer test and inversion and eversion stress evaluation are performed to evaluate the integrity of the ankle and hindfoot ligaments. Realignment osteotomy with unstable or incompetent ankle or hindfoot ligaments may fail to improve function.
  - Motor strength: Manual motor testing of the major muscle groups is performed. Realignment in patients lacking

essential motor function at the ankle will improve function in stance phase but will typically necessitate bracing for effective gait.

- Alignment: The angle made by the Achilles and the vertical axis of the calcaneus is normally 5 to 7 degrees of valgus. Altered alignment to varus or increased valgus position indicates either abnormal tilt of the talus within the ankle mortise (eg, unicompartmental cartilage wear) or abnormality of the subtalar joint.
- Effusion testing: Elimination or fullness of the gutters indicates intra-articular fluid accumulation or hypertrophied capsular tissue.
- Normal ankle and hindfoot range of motion (ROM) in the sagittal plane is 20 degrees of dorsiflexion to 50 degrees of plantarflexion. Normal values of hindfoot motion are difficult to measure, since the motion is triplanar. A reasonable reference is 5 degrees of eversion and 20 degrees of inversion.
  - Isolated supramalleolar osteotomy for a stiff ankle rarely improves ROM; a stiff, diffusely arthritic and malaligned ankle may be best treated with realignment.
- Hindfoot stiffness must also be documented. In patients with malaligned ankles, the hindfoot compensates. For example, a varus ankle will generally be associated with a compensating hindfoot in excessive valgus. If the hindfoot has lost its flexibility due to longstanding compensation for ankle malalignment, then supramalleolar osteotomy may realign the tibiotalar joint but create hindfoot malalignment. With a flexible hindfoot, this is generally not a problem.

IMAGING AND OTHER DIAGNOSTIC STUDIES

- Weight-bearing AP, lateral, and mortise ankle and foot radiographs determine the extent of arthritic involvement, deformity, bone defects in the distal tibial plafond or talus, and the presence of arthritis in the adjacent hindfoot articulations. Radiographs may also suggest avascular necrosis (AVN) of the talus or distal tibia.
- With deformity, a minimum of full-length, weight-bearing AP and lateral tibial radiographs must be obtained. If more proximal deformity is suspected, then mechanical axis, full-length hip-to-ankle radiographs should be considered to accurately plan realignment. More comprehensive full-length weight-bearing radiographs are required to measure the TAS and TLS angles, the level of center of rotation of angulation (CORA) in case of existing deformity, and the preoperative leg-length discrepancy, since any substantial discrepancy may have an impact to the choice of osteotomy.
- Diagnostic injection. If there is uncertainty over whether the pain is originating from the ankle or hindfoot, selective injections may be of use in distinguishing the source of pain.

DIFFERENTIAL DIAGNOSIS

- Bone marrow edema
- Soft tissue pathology
- Distal tibial plafond or talar AVN
- Osteochondritis

NONOPERATIVE MANAGEMENT

- Nonoperative treatment of ankle arthritis includes pharmacologic agents, intra-articular corticosteroid injections, shoe wear modifications, and orthoses.
- Nonsteroidal anti-inflammatory agents (NSAIDs) are widely used and have proven efficacy in the management of arthritis, including ankle arthritis. In select patients with gastrointestinal irrigation, COX-2 inhibitors may offer a reasonable alternative to NSAIDs. Inflammatory arthritides are managed with immunosuppressive agents.
- Judicious use of intra-articular corticosteroid injections may temporize inflammation associated with intra-articular ankle pathology. Moreover, initial injections of the ankle or hindfoot may serve a diagnostic purpose to distinguish ankle from hindfoot pain. Indiscreet use of corticosteroid injections may have a deleterious effect on the residual joint cartilage as a result of the steroid, the anesthetic, or perhaps the accompanying preservative.
- Bracing to immobilize and support the arthritic ankle may provide some pain relief with weight bearing and ambulation. Specifically, polypropylene ankle–foot orthoses (AFOs), double-metal upright braces, and lace-up braces, combined with the use of a stiff-soled rocker-bottom shoe, may be of benefit. Bracing tibial and tibiotalar malalignment is challenging. With a flexible hindfoot, some axial realignment may be feasible, but correction is generally not possible at the focus of deformity.

SURGICAL MANAGEMENT

- We use the supramalleolar osteotomy for the following indications[25]:
  - Realignment of distal tibia fracture malunion without or with mild osteoarthritic changes of the ankle joint
  - Realignment of distal tibia malunion with mild to moderate osteoarthritic changes of the ankle joint
  - Ankle fusion malunion
  - Ankle arthritis with deformity secondary to intra-articular trauma or AVN of the distal tibia
  - Correction of valgus deformity associated with a ball-and-socket ankle joint configuration secondary to tarsal coalition
  - Tibiotalar osteoarthritis resulting from chronic lateral ankle instability or a cavovarus foot deformity
  - Restoration of a plantigrade foot position in ankle deformity resulting from Charcot neuroarthropathy, to create ankle and hindfoot alignment that may be safely braced
  - Correction of limb alignment in adolescents and young adults due to growth plate injury
  - Correction of lower limb alignment as staged planning for a total ankle replacement
- As a rule, we reserve supramalleolar osteotomy using internal fixation for mild to moderate angular deformities in the coronal or the sagittal plane. Severe angular deformities with concomitant translation of the distal segment or shortening are, in our opinion, better managed using external fixation and the principles of Ilizarov. Moreover, gradual correction of severe deformity with formation of a regenerate avoids large plates under a wound and typically thin soft tissues that would be under tension with acute correction using internal fixation.
- Comparing closing- and opening-wedge supramalleolar osteotomies: A closing-wedge osteotomy may result in limb shortening when compared to opening-wedge osteotomies. Conflicting reports exist regarding healing rates between the two methods. Studies suggest that closing-wedge osteotomies

exhibit delayed healing when compared to opening-wedge osteotomies,[28] but other reports demonstrate more rapid healing using a closing-wedge osteotomy.[24–26] One advantage of a closing-wedge osteotomy is that it does not necessitate incorporation of cancellous or structural interpositional graft. While an opening-wedge osteotomy may preserve limb length, resultant skin tension from acute correction may create problems with wound healing and potential vascular compromise if the vessels are put on sudden stretch. Gradual correction with external fixation may be a safer option in cases with severe deformity.

- In the absence of appreciable preoperative leg-length discrepancy, we recommend correcting distal tibial varus deformities with a medial opening-wedge osteotomy and valgus deformities with a medial closing-wedge osteotomy.

Preoperative Planning

- We routinely obtain bilateral, full-length weight-bearing radiographs of the tibia including the knee and ankle joints.
- We draw two lines on the preoperative radiographs: (a) the tibial mechanical axis (which for the tibia coincides with the anatomic axis) and (b) the distal tibial articular surface. On the AP view, the angle formed by these lines is the TAS angle (**FIG 1**). On the lateral view, these lines form the TLS angle.
- Ideally, we define the physiologic TAS and TLS angles for each patient using radiographs of the healthy contralateral limb. The goal of surgery is to realign the TAS and TLS to physiologic values and perhaps add a few degrees of (slight) overcorrection, to compensate for anticipated minor subsidence during healing of the osteotomy.
- The full-length weight-bearing radiographs serve to determine preoperative leg-length discrepancy, which may

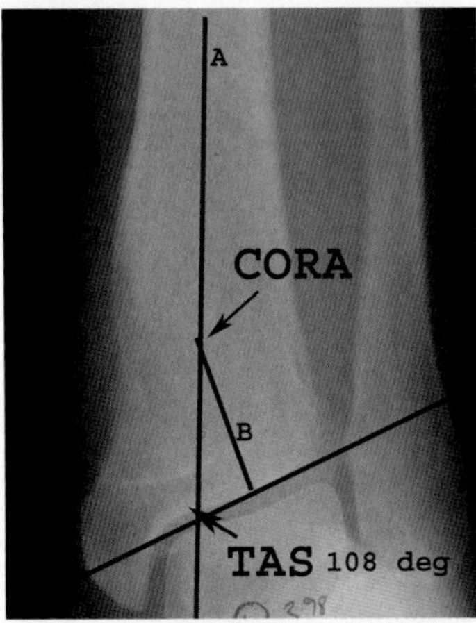

FIG 1 • Preoperative AP radiograph of a patient with severe valgus malalignment of the distal tibia, due to physeal disturbance from adjacent osteochondroma that was excised in a previous procedure. Note the location of center of rotation of angulation (CORA) at the intersection of two lines that represent the mechanical axes of the proximal (*line A*) and distal segments (*line B*). Line A, also representing the tibial mechanical axis (which in the case of the tibia coincides with the anatomic axis), and another line that is drawn to represent the distal tibial articular surface form the tibial–ankle surface (TAS) angle on the AP view with a magnitude of 108 degrees.

influence the choice between opening- and closing-wedge osteotomies.

- Determining the CORA of the deformity (Fig. 1): The CORA is the intersection of the two lines that define the deformity, lines that are drawn to represent the mechanical axes of the proximal (line A) and distal segments (line B).
- With isolated angular deformity, the CORA is at the apex of the deformity. When translation is also present, the CORA is located proximal to of the deformity.
- In very distal tibial deformities or ankle deformities with minor to moderate alterations of the TAS angle, the CORA is at the level of the ankle joint line.
- With distal tibial procurvatum deformity (malunion) or ankle fusion malunion in equinus, the CORA is the intersection of the tibial mechanical axis and a line representing the ankle's center of rotation. Typically, in such cases, the CORA is the level of the lateral process of the talus.
- Significance of the CORA: An osteotomy made at the level of the CORA, whether closing or opening, will predictably realign the ankle without translation of the distal segment and center of the ankle. If the osteotomy is not performed at the CORA, the center of the ankle will translate relative to the mechanical axis of the tibia, creating undesirable malalignment of the two segments and an unnecessary shift of loads to the ankle joint. To avoid secondary translational deformity when the osteotomy is intentionally made at a different level than the CORA, the distal segment must be translated relative to the proximal segment. These osteotomy rules apply irrespective of the method of fixation chosen.[19,20]
- The size of the opening-wedge or closing-wedge resection can be determined by drawing the desired correction angle on the preoperative radiographs and measuring the wedge size on a template, taking magnification into account.[1]
- The final step in preoperative planning is to determine the extent of compensation that is achieved by the subtalar joint before correction of the deformity. Deformities in the coronal plane are well compensated for by the subtalar joint, unless there is preoperative stiffness in the hindfoot.
- For example, a varus deformity of the tibia is compensated for by eversion of the subtalar joint. In cases of chronic deformity, this attempt to compensate and maintain the foot plantigrade may become fixed at the subtalar joint. Moreover, other adaptive changes may occur including the transverse tarsal joint or midfoot, creating a fixed forefoot deformity. These secondary fixed deformities may also require surgical correction after the ankle is realigned in order to create a functional, plantigrade foot.

Positioning

- The supramalleolar osteotomy is performed with the patient supine.
- A bump under the ipsilateral hip prevents the natural tendency of the lower extremity to fall into external rotation.

Approach

- The fibular osteotomy is performed first, using a small lateral incision, protecting the lateral branch of the superficial peroneal nerve.
- For the supramalleolar osteotomy, a medial skin incision is made and periosteal elevation is performed only to the extent needed to perform the osteotomy.

MEDIAL CLOSING-WEDGE SUPRAMALLEOLAR OSTEOTOMY

- Perform the fibular osteotomy first, using a small lateral incision. The osteotomy is oblique, located at the same level with the planned tibial cut. Some surgeons prefer to make the fibular osteotomy at a different level from the supramalleolar osteotomy.
- We do not routinely apply fixation to the fibular osteotomy, except in cases where it is felt that additional stability is required.
- When correcting tibial deformity, perform the osteotomy at the CORA (**TECH FIG 1**).
- In select cases, the supramalleolar osteotomy is not performed at the CORA. In some distal tibial deformities, the CORA may be located at the ankle joint, where the osteotomy is not feasible, and the translational component must be compensated. Also, in ankle deformity with only minor alterations of the TAS angle and when detrimental translation of the distal fragment is not a major concern, we generally perform the osteotomy 4 to 5 cm proximal to the medial malleolar tip.
- We routinely use Kirschner wires to define our proposed osteotomy; for an opening-wedge osteotomy we use a single Kirschner wire, but for the medial closing-wedge osteotomy, two Kirschner wires are required to define the tibial wedge resection. Under fluoroscopic guidance, insert the first Kirschner wire perpendicular to the mechanical axis and the second parallel to the ankle joint, intersecting the first Kirschner wire at the apex of the deformity. The size of the wedge has been determined during the preoperative planning, and the Kirschner wires are positioned 1 to 2 mm wider than the proposed osteotomy, so they can be left in place as a guide for the saw cuts. While the Kirschner wires define the osteotomy in one plane, the surgeon must also orient the saw blade perpendicular to the tibial shaft axis when performing the osteotomy. With the anterior and posterior soft tissue and neurovascular structures protected, we routinely use a broad oscillating saw, constantly irrigating the blade with cooled sterile saline or water to limit osteonecrosis. Ideally, a thin cortical bridge and periosteal sleeve on the opposite cortex will be preserved, to allow for a greenstick-like closure of the osteotomy that facilitates maintenance of alignment and enhances stability. However, when the osteotomy is intentionally performed at a level different than that of CORA, then the opposite cortex must be violated to allow the distal segment to be translated.

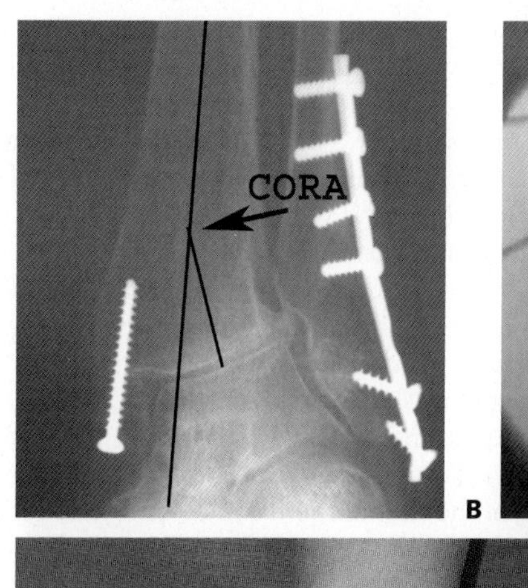

A

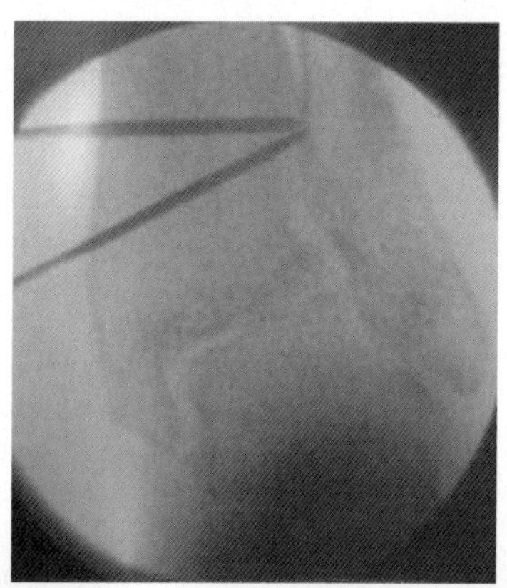

B

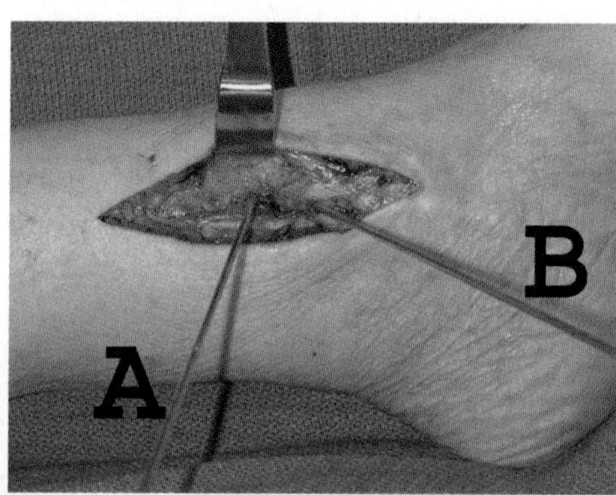

C

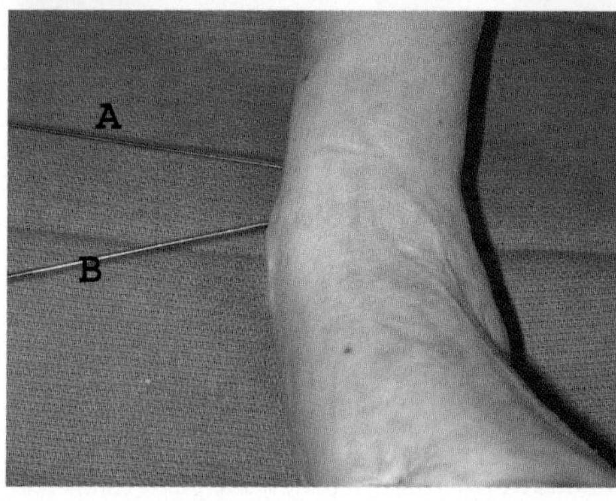

D

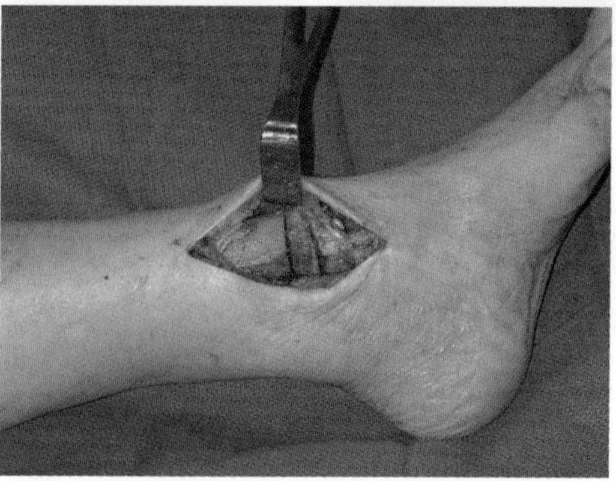

E

TECH FIG 1 • Medial closing-wedge supramalleolar osteotomy. **A.** Using a preoperative radiograph the center of rotation of angulation (CORA) is located at the intersection of two lines that represent the mechanical axes of the proximal and distal segments. **B.** Under fluoroscopy a Kirschner wire is inserted to the tibia perpendicular to the mechanical axis and a second Kirschner wire is inserted parallel to the ankle joint line intersecting the first wire, ideally at the apex of the deformity. **C, D.** Guide pin wires used to perform a closing medial wedge osteotomy. Pin A has been inserted to the tibia perpendicular to the mechanical axis and pin B has been inserted parallel to the ankle joint line, intersecting pin A at the apex of the deformity. **E.** The cut wedge. The pins have been used as a guide for the tibial cuts, while the size of the wedge has been determined during the preoperative planning. *(continued)*

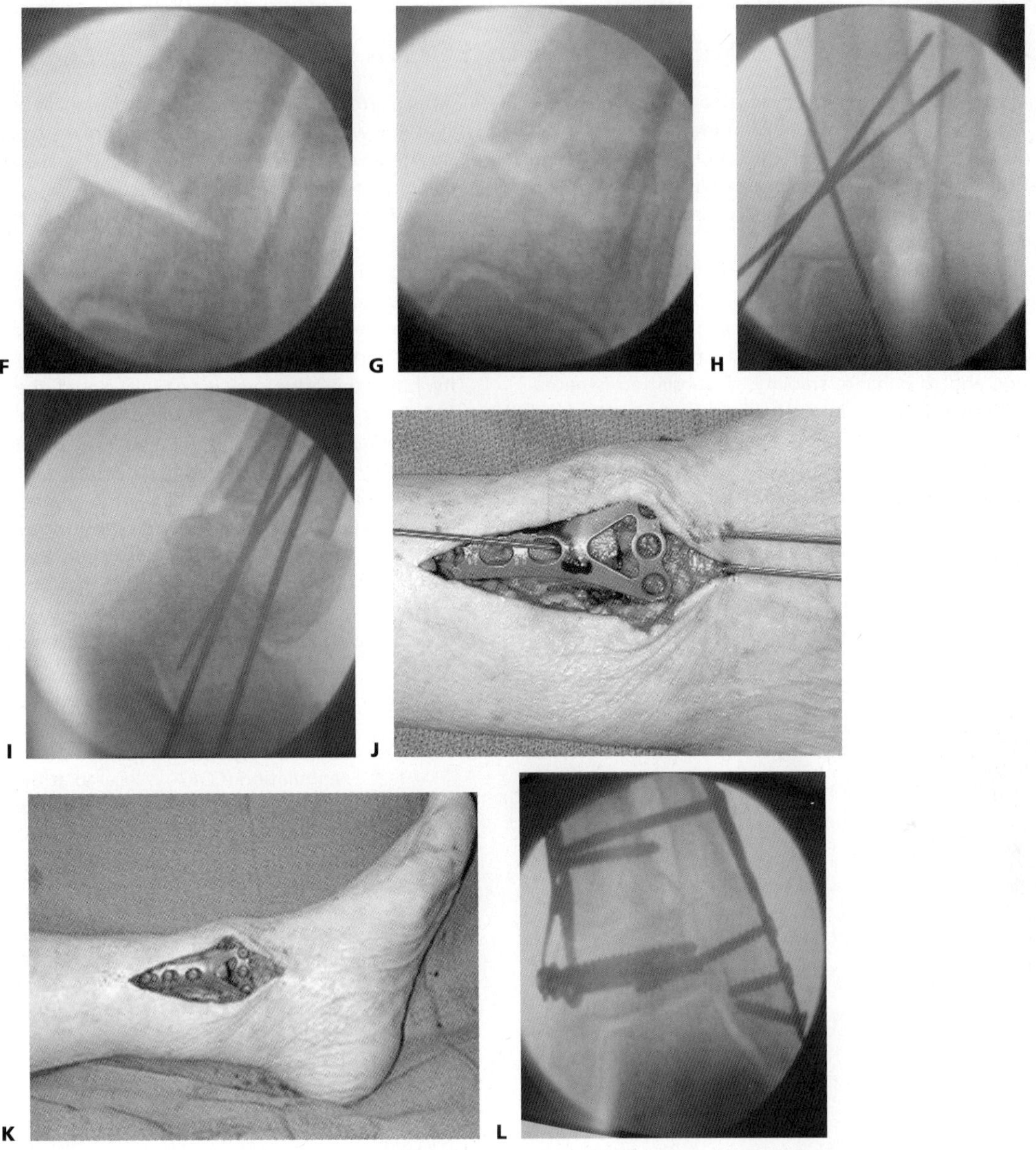

TECH FIG 1 • *(continued)* **F.** Fluoroscopic view of the resected wedge. **G.** Fluoroscopic view of the closed osteotomy. **H, I.** Fluoroscopic AP and lateral views of the provisionally fixed osteotomy with Kirschner wires. **J.** Photo of the applied periarticular plate. Note the excellent fit on the distal tibia. **K.** The applied periarticular plate after completion of fixation with three screws in the distal segment. **L.** Fluoroscopic view of the osteotomy after completion of fixation.

- After removing the resected wedge and performing appropriate translation of the distal segment, close the osteotomy and provisionally fix it with Kirschner wires. The provisional fixation may be guidewires for intended cannulated screws or it must be positioned so as not to interfere with the definitive fixation. Assess alignment of the tibia and ankle fluoroscopically, both in the AP and lateral planes.
- Several dedicated low-profile periarticular plating systems for the distal tibia are marketed, both locking and nonlocking. The majority of these plates were designed for the contours of the physiologic tibia. With a wedge resection the fit is typically acceptable but may not be perfect. Locking plates may provide optimal stability, but if the osteotomy is not fully closed, these may in fact delay or even hinder healing. Nonlocking plates, in our opinion, allow for a small amount of settling at the osteotomy with weight bearing, potentially facilitating healing. (If additional stability is required, then cannulated or solid screws may be used from the tip of the medial malleolus across the osteotomy. Alternatively, a second plate may be added anteriorly on the tibia to provide rotational control to the tibia; however, this requires greater soft tissue dissection.)
- We do not routinely apply fixation to the fibula, but if additional stability is required, then we apply a low-profile fibular plate.
- Final fluoroscopic images in the AP and lateral planes confirm proper alignment, apposition of the osteotomy, and position of hardware.

TECHNIQUES

MEDIAL OPENING-WEDGE SUPRAMALLEOLAR OSTEOTOMY

- Again, the osteotomy is ideally located at the level of the CORA (TECH FIG 2). If the CORA is located at the ankle joint level or if only minor correction is required and translation of the distal segment is of little concern, then we perform the osteotomy 4 to 5 cm proximal to the medial malleolar tip.
- We perform either a horizontal or slightly oblique (proximal medial to distal lateral) tibial osteotomy with a broad oscillating saw, preserving the opposite cortex and periosteal sleeve to serve as a fulcrum for the opening wedge and to enhance stability. If translation is necessary (the osteotomy is intentionally performed at a level different than that of CORA), then the opposite cortex is cut completely to allow the distal segment to move.
- Under fluoroscopy, gently distract the tibial osteotomy using a lamina spreader or alternative distraction system until desired correction is achieved.
- We routinely use contoured structural graft (generally the neck portion of a femoral head allograft) to fill the osteotomy.
- After correcting the deformity, provisionally fix the osteotomy with Kirschner wires in a manner that does not interfere with the definitive fixation. Assess the alignment using fluoroscopy, both in the AP and lateral planes.
- Several dedicated low-profile periarticular plating systems for the distal tibia are marketed, both locking and nonlocking. The majority of these plates were designed for the contours of the physiologic tibia. With an opening-wedge osteotomy the fit is typically acceptable but may not be perfect. Locking plates may provide optimal stability, but if the osteotomy is not fully closed, these may in fact delay or even hinder healing. Nonlocking plates, in our opinion, allow for a small amount of settling at the osteotomy with weight bearing, potentially facilitating incorporation of the interpositional graft. (If additional stability is required, then cannulated or solid screws may be used from the tip of the medial malleolus across the osteotomy. Alternatively, a second plate may be added anteriorly on the tibia to provide rotational control to the tibia; however, this requires greater soft tissue dissection.)

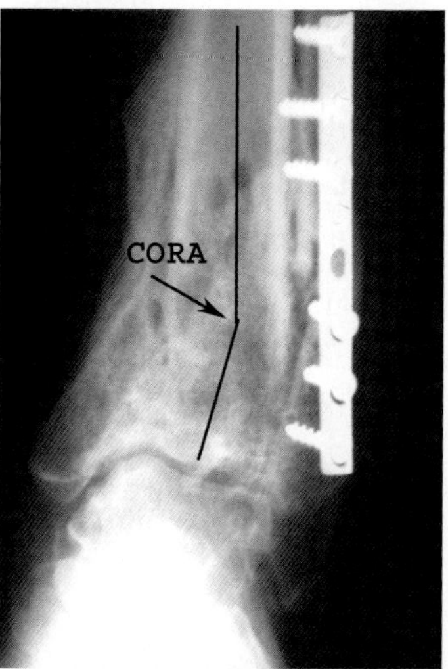

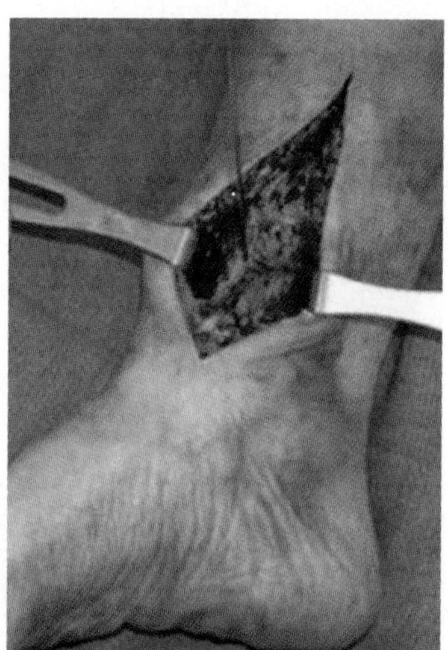

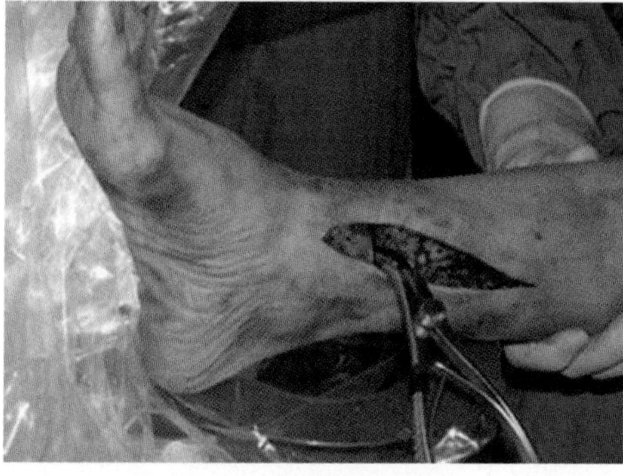

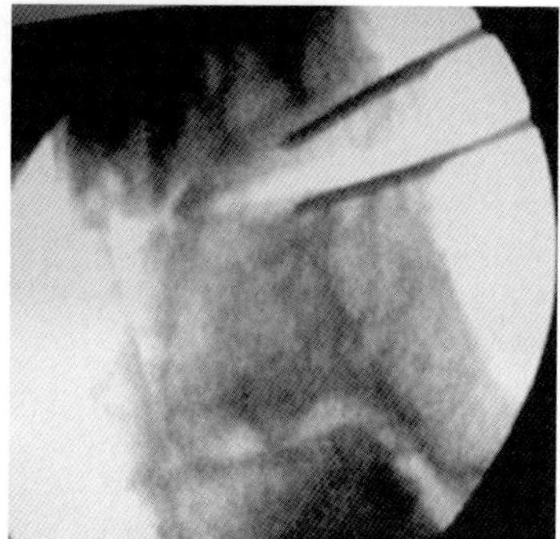

TECH FIG 2 • Medial opening-wedge supramalleolar osteotomy. **A.** Using a preoperative radiograph the center of rotation of angulation (CORA) is located at the intersection of two lines that represent the mechanical axes of the proximal and distal segments. **B.** Under fluoroscopy a Kirschner wire is used to mark the osteotomy site at the CORA level. **C, D.** Under fluoroscopy the tibial osteotomy is gently distracted using a lamina spreader until desired correction is achieved. (A, C, D: from Myerson MS. Reconstructive Foot and Ankle Surgery. Philadelphia: Elsevier; 205:254.

WOUND CLOSURE

- After completing the fixation, close the wound routinely in layers. With opening-wedge osteotomies, the skin tension is typically greater than before surgery, but with longitudinal incisions, this is rarely problematic. Use of a drain is at the discretion of the surgeon; we do not routinely use a drain.

PEARLS AND PITFALLS

Fixation	■ We recommend internal fixation for supramalleolar osteotomies in mild to moderate corrections. Complex and severe deformity may be best managed with external fixation and Ilizarov principles. Multiplanar correction with external fixation effectively manages angular and translational deformity and simultaneously compensates for potential loss of limb length. If there is no significant preoperative leg-length discrepancy, then all varus deformities are corrected using a medial opening-wedge osteotomy, while the valgus deformities are corrected with a medial closing-wedge osteotomy.
Exposure	■ Minimal periosteal elevation preserves vascularity at the osteotomy site.
Osteotomy level	■ A closing- or opening-wedge osteotomy at the level of the CORA will lead to complete realignment of the foot and ankle. If the osteotomy is made proximal or distal to the CORA, the distal segment and center of the ankle will translate relative to the mechanical axis of the tibia. When the osteotomy must be performed at a level different than the CORA, then the osteotomy must be completed on the lateral cortex and translated along with the angular correction. These osteotomy rules apply irrespective of the method of fixation chosen.
Fixation of the osteotomy	■ In our experience, medial plating is typically adequate for fixation of opening- or closing-wedge supramalleolar osteotomies. However, additional stability may be gained with (a) screws from the tip of the medial malleolus that cross the osteotomy or (b) supplemental anterior plating. No fixation is applied to the fibular osteotomy, except in cases where it is felt that additional stability is required.
Graft choice	■ The graft alternatives are to harvest it from the ipsilateral iliac crest or the proximal tibia or to use tricortical allograft. The two basic types of bone grafts are structural and cancellous. A structural bone graft is one that alters the shape during a reconstruction procedure by virtue of its size and dimension. The structural bone graft provides immediate mechanical support, with little likelihood of collapse even after the resorption that occurs during revascularization. Some structural integrity remains during the process of bone graft incorporation to allow the graft to withstand loads.
Locked vs. nonlocked plates	■ Locked plating affords optimal stability; however, if the plate is locked with suboptimal bony contact at the osteotomy site, then there may be a delay in osteotomy healing or incorporation of a structural graft. Nonlocked plating permits some settling during weight bearing that may promote healing of the osteotomy, provided stability is satisfactory.

POSTOPERATIVE CARE

- The procedure may be performed on an outpatient basis, but we routinely keep the patient overnight for monitoring and pain control (23-hour observation status).
- While rare, a tibial osteotomy, albeit distal to the lower leg muscles, could potentially create a compartment syndrome, and therefore overnight monitoring is prudent. All patients are discharged with a non–weight-bearing postoperative splint, are instructed to maintain elevation of the extremity, and are to return to the clinic 2 weeks after surgery for suture removal.
- At 2 weeks we routinely place the patient in a removable, prefabricated cam walker boot. If we have concern for the osteotomy stability or patient compliance, we obtain radiographs at this time to ensure satisfactory alignment and fixation, and place the patient into a short-leg non–weight-bearing cast.
- The patient returns at 6 weeks from surgery, at which time we routinely obtain simulated weight-bearing radiographs of the ankle. Depending on the stability of fixation and evidence for progression toward healing, we allow the patient to progressively advance weight bearing in the cam walker boot.
- Typically, with follow-up at 10 weeks from surgery, full weight bearing is permitted in the cam walker boot, with a rapid transition to a regular shoe, provided that weight-bearing radiographs of the ankle suggest satisfactory healing. Early ROM exercises without resistance are initiated early (at 2 weeks), when osteotomy fixation is deemed stable and if there is no concomitant procedure (eg, ligament reconstruction or tendon transfer) dictating adjustment of the rehabilitation protocol.

OUTCOMES

- Several studies have shown that the overall outcome of supramalleolar osteotomy is very good in terms of pain relief, correction of any existing mechanical malalignment, and the arresting of arthritic changes in the ankle joint.[6,24,28,29]
- The type of osteotomy (opening vs. closing wedge) does not influence the final outcome, even though a closing-wedge osteotomy may lead to leg-length discrepancy or decreased strength.[24]
- The type of osteotomy (opening vs. closing wedge) has no influence on the time of osseous healing.[24]

COMPLICATIONS

- Nonunion
- Delayed union
- Over- or undercorrection of the deformity
- Decreased postoperative ROM
- Failure to perform the osteotomy at the level of CORA, thus translating the distal fragment and center of the ankle away from the mechanical axis
- Failure to perform the appropriate translation of the distal segment, in cases where the osteotomy is intentionally performed at a different level than that of CORA (such as when the CORA is at the level or distal to the ankle joint), leading to mechanical axis shifting

Acknowledgment

I would like to thank my mentor Mark S. Myerson for his enlightening training, friendship, and help for the preparation of this chapter.

REFERENCES

1. Acevedo JI, Myerson MS. Reconstructive alternatives for ankle arthritis. Foot Ankle Clin 1999;4:409–430.
2. Becker AS, Myerson MS. The indications and technique of supramalleolar osteotomy. Foot Ankle Clin 2009;14:549–561.
3. Benthien RA, Myerson MS. Supramalleolar osteotomy for ankle deformity and arthritis. Foot Ankle Clin 2004;9:475–487.
4. Borrelli J Jr, Leduc S, Gregush R, et al. Tricortical bone grafts for treatment of malaligned tibias and fibulas. Clin Orthop Relat Res 2009;476:1056–1063.
5. Chao KH, Wu CC, Lee CH, et al. Corrective-elongation osteotomy without bone graft for old ankle fracture with residual diastasis. Foot Ankle Int 2004;25:123–127.
6. Graehl PM, Hersh MR, Heckman JD. Supramalleolar osteotomy for the treatment of symptomatic tibial malunion. J Orthop Trauma 1987;1:281–292.
7. Hintermann B, Knupp M, Barg A. Osteotomies of the distal tibia and hindfoot for ankle realignment [in German]. Orthopaede 2008;37:212–223.
8. Knupp M, Pagenstert G, Valderrabaro V, et al. Osteotomies in varus malalignment of the ankle [in German]. Oper Orthop Traumatol 2008;20:262–273.
9. Kristensen KD, Kiaer T, Blicher J. No arthrosis of the ankle 20 years after malaligned tibial-shaft fracture. Acta Orthop Scand 1989;60:208–209.
10. Lee KB, Cho YJ. Oblique supramalleolar opening wedge osteotomy without fibular osteotomy for varus deformity of the ankle. Foot Ankle Int 2009;30:565–567.
11. Lee HS, Wapner KL, Park SS, et al. Ligament reconstruction and calcaneal osteotomy for OA of the ankle. Foot Ankle Int 2009;30:475–480.
12. Mangone PG. Distal tibial osteotomies for the treatment of foot and ankle disorders. Foot Ankle Clin 2001;6:583.
13. Marti RK, Raaymakers EL, Nolte PA. Malunited ankle fractures. J Bone Joint Surg Br 1990;72B:709–713.
14. Merchant TC, Dietz FR. Long-term follow-up after fractures of the tibial and fibular shafts. J Bone Joint Surg Am 1989;71A:599–606.
15. Neumann HW, Lieske S, Schenk. Supramalleolar subtractive valgus osteotomy of the tibia in the management of ankle joint degeneration with varus deformity [in German]. Oper Orthop Traum 2007;19:511–526.
16. Pagenstert GI, Hintermann B, Barg A, et al. Realignment surgery as alternative treatment of varus and valgus ankle OA. Clin Orthop Rel Res 2007;462:156–168.
17. Pagenstert GI, Leumann A, Hintermann B, et al. Sports and recreation activity of varus and valgus ankle OA before and after realignment surgery. Foot Ankle Int 2008;29:985–993.
18. Pagenstert G, Knupp M, Valderrabano V, et al., Realignment surgery for valgus ankle OA. Oper Orthop Traum 2009;21:77–87.
19. Paley D. The correction of complex foot deformities using Ilizarov's distraction osteotomies. Clin Orthop Relat Res 1993;293:97–111.
20. Paley D, Herzenberg JE, Tetsworth K, et al. Deformity planning for frontal and sagittal plane corrective osteotomies. Orthop Clin North Am 1994;25:425–465.
21. Perena A, Myerson M. Surgical techniques for the reconstruction of malunited ankle fractures. Foot Ankle Clin 2008;13:737–751.
22. Rozbruch SR, Fragomen AT, Ilizarov S, et al. Correction of tibial deformity with use of the Ilizarov-Taylor spatial frame. J Bone Joint Surg Am 2006;88:156–174.
23. Sinha A, Sirikonda S, Giotakis N, et al. Fibular lengthening for malunited ankle fractures. Foot Ankle Int 2008;29:1136–1140.
24. Stamatis ED, Cooper PS, Myerson MS. Supramalleolar osteotomy for the treatment of distal tibial angular deformities and arthritis of the ankle joint. Foot Ankle Int 2003;24:754–764.
25. Stamatis ED, Myerson MS. Supramalleolar osteotomy: indications and technique. Foot Ankle Clin 2003;8:317–333.
26. Stamatis E, Myerson M. Supramalleolar osteotomy for the treatment of distal tibial angular deformities and arthritis of the ankle joint. Tech Foot Ankle Surg 2004;3:138–142.
27. Swords MP, Nemec S. Osteotomy for salvage of the arthritic ankle. Foot Ankle Clin 2007;12:1–13.
28. Takakura Y, Tanaka Y, Kumai T, et al. Low tibial osteotomy for osteoarthritis of the ankle: results of a new operation in 18 patients. J Bone Joint Surg Br 1995;77B:50–54.
29. Takakura Y, Takaoka T, Tanaka Y, et al. Results of opening-wedge osteotomy for the treatment of a post-traumatic varus deformity of the ankle. J Bone Joint Surg Am 1998;80A:213–218.
30. Tanaka Y, Takakura Y, Hayashi K, et al. Low tibial osteotomy for varus-type OA of the ankle. J Bone Joint Surg Br 2006;88B:909–913.
31. Tarr RR, Resnick CT, Wagner KS, et al. Changes in tibiotalar joint contact areas following experimentally induced tibial angular deformities. Clin Orthop Relat Res 1985;199:72–80.
32. Ting AJ, Tarr RR, Sarmiento A, et al. The role of subtalar motion and ankle contact pressure changes from angular deformities of the tibia. Foot Ankle 1987;7:290–299.
33. Weber D, Friederich NF, Müller W, et al. Lengthening osteotomy of the fibular for post-traumatic malunion: indications, technique and results. Int Orthop 1998;22:149–152.

Chapter 63

Supramalleolar Osteotomy With Internal Fixation: Perspective 2

Yasuhito Tanaka

DEFINITION

- Varus-type osteoarthritis is characterized by varus deformity combined with anterior opening of the articular surface at the distal end of the tibia.[1,2]
- It often develops bilaterally in middle-aged and elderly women.
- Low tibial osteotomy (LTO) was developed to treat varus-type osteoarthritis of the ankle. Cartilage defects can be repaired with fibrocartilage by resolving the stress concentration.

ANATOMY

- The distal joint surface of the tibia appears almost perpendicular to the anterior longitudinal axis of the tibia and slight anterior opening to the lateral longitudinal axis (**FIG 1**).

PATHOGENESIS

- The cause of varus-type osteoarthritis is not clear.
- Radiographic measurements showed varus tilt of the distal joint surface (Fig 1). It was thought that the varus tilt was caused by acquired changes, because the ankles of infants are in the valgus position.[3]
- Some biomechanical studies[4,10] showed that varus tilt of the distal joint surface of the tibia caused stress concentration on the medial side of the ankle (**FIG 2**). The stress moved to the lateral side after valgus osteotomy at a distal portion of the tibia.[8]

NATURAL HISTORY

- Osteophyte formation and sclerotic changes of subchondral bone initially appear in a medial gutter and an anteromedial corner of the ankle joint.
- Damage of articular cartilage gradually progresses from the medial side to the lateral side.
- Varus-type osteoarthritis of the ankle is classified into four stages (**FIG. 3**)[6,9]:
  - Stage 1: no joint space narrowing, but early sclerosis and osteophyte formation
  - Stage 2: narrowing of the joint space medially
  - Stage 3: obliteration of the joint space with subchondral bone contact medially
    - Stage 3a: obliteration of the joint space in the facet is limited to the medial malleolus
    - Stage 3b: obliteration of the joint space has advanced to the roof of the talar dome
  - Stage 4: obliteration of the entire joint space with complete bone contact

PATIENT HISTORY AND PHYSICAL FINDINGS

- The patient complains of ankle pain at the start of walking and after walking for a long distance.
- Pain on movement and swelling become significant as osteoarthritis progresses.
- A tender point is present at the medial joint space of the ankle.
- Motion of the ankle is retained until relatively advanced stages.

IMAGING AND OTHER DIAGNOSTIC STUDIES

- Weight-bearing AP and lateral radiographs should be taken to detect narrowing of the joint space.
- The angle between the tibial shaft and the distal joint surface of the tibia is measured on the AP view (TAS angle) and

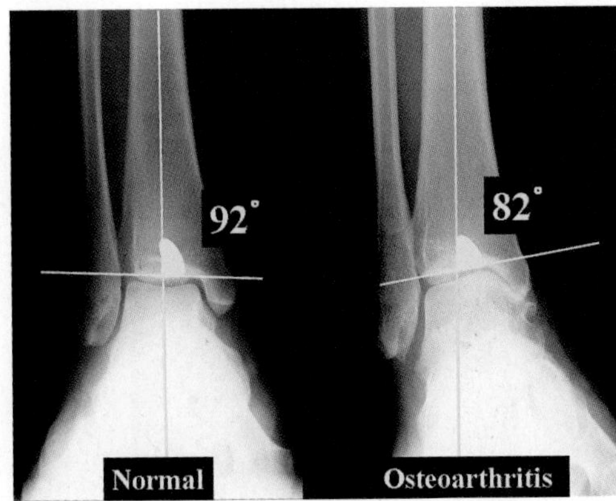

FIG 1 • Varus-type osteoarthritis is characterized by varus tilt of the distal joint surface.

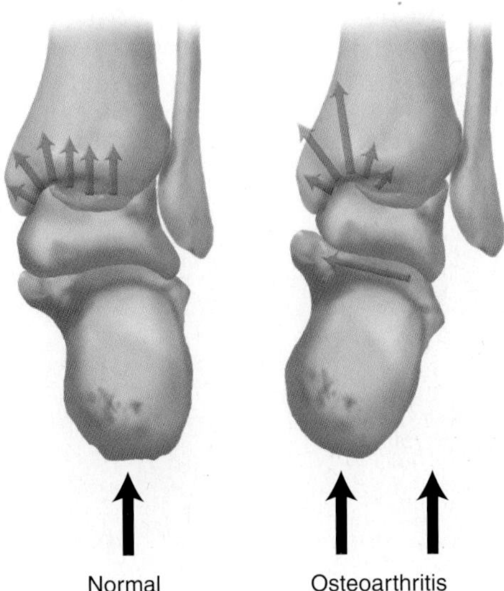

FIG 2 • Stress is distributed widely in a normal joint, but it is concentrated on the medial side of the ankle with varus-type osteoarthritis.

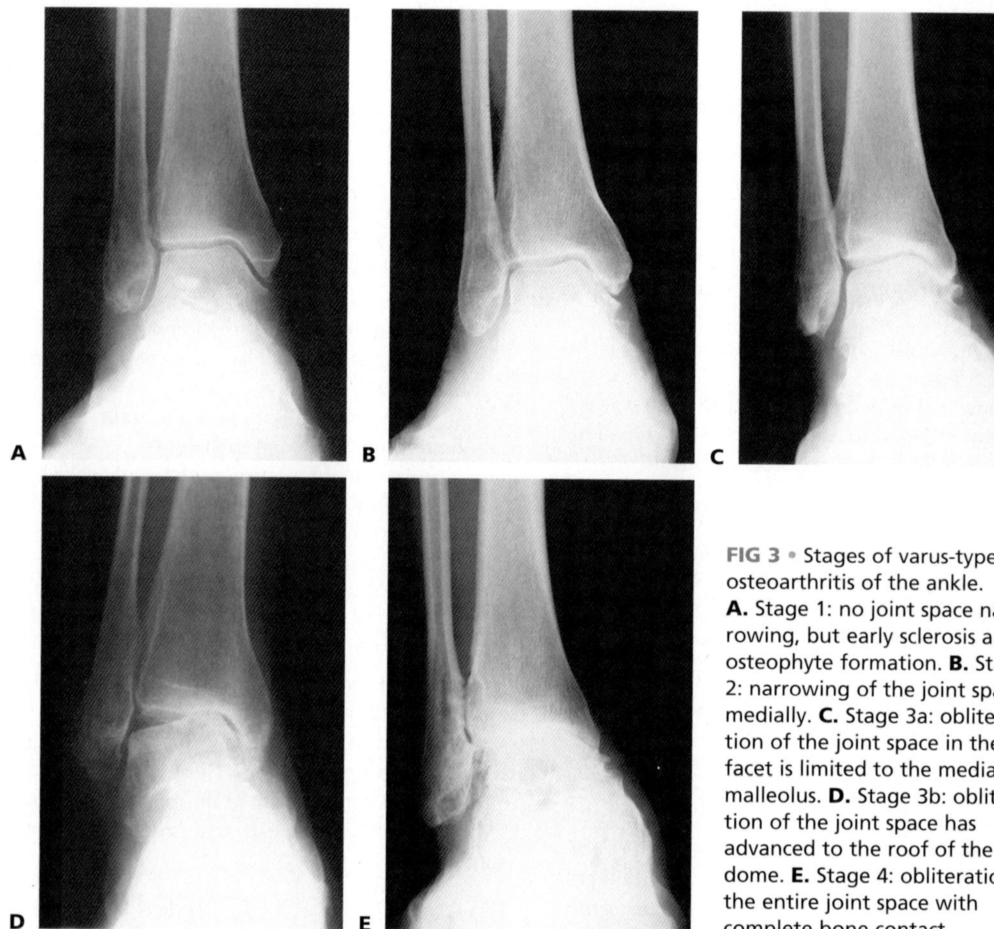

FIG 3 • Stages of varus-type osteoarthritis of the ankle. **A.** Stage 1: no joint space narrowing, but early sclerosis and osteophyte formation. **B.** Stage 2: narrowing of the joint space medially. **C.** Stage 3a: obliteration of the joint space in the facet is limited to the medial malleolus. **D.** Stage 3b: obliteration of the joint space has advanced to the roof of the talar dome. **E.** Stage 4: obliteration of the entire joint space with complete bone contact.

on the lateral view (TLS angle) (**FIG 4**).[1,2,5] Those angles represent the varus angle and the amount of anterior opening of the joint, respectively.

- Normal values are 88 to 90 degrees for the TAS angle and 80 to 81 degrees for the TLS angle.[1,2,5]
- The tibial axis is defined as the line between the midpoints of the tibial shaft at 8 cm and 13 cm above the tip of the medial malleolus.

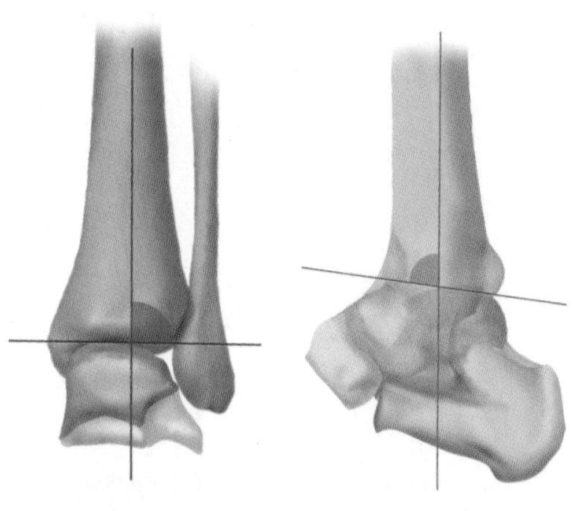

FIG 4 • The angle between the tibial shaft and the distal joint surface of the tibia on the AP view (TAS angle) and on the lateral view (TLS angle).

- Varus tilt of the talus has been observed in some ankles with osteoarthritis. The varus tilt angle is evaluated on a weight-bearing AP radiograph that shows the distal joint surface of the tibia and the upper surface of the talar dome (**FIG 5**).

DIFFERENTIAL DIAGNOSIS

- Posttraumatic osteoarthritis
- Rheumatoid arthritis
- Infectious arthritis
- Charcot joint
- Crystal-induced arthritis

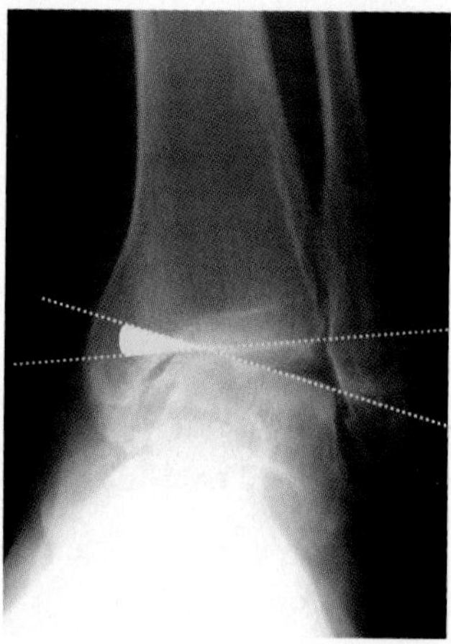

FIG 5 • Varus tilt angle on a weight-bearing AP view.

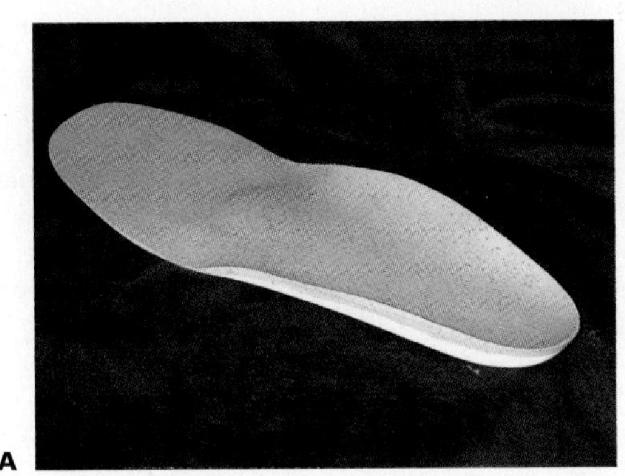

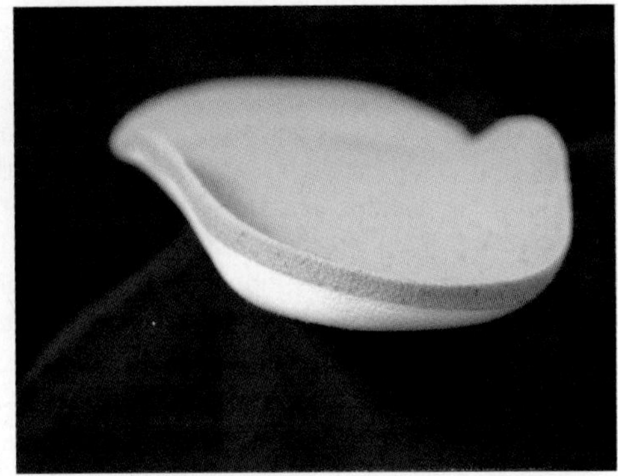

FIG 6 • A shoe insert with an outer wedge. **A.** Lateral view. **B.** Posterior view.

NONOPERATIVE MANAGEMENT

- Rest and avoidance of offending activity is recommended.
- Warming with hot packs and ultra microwave is effective.
- Nonsteroidal anti-inflammatories and an injection of hyaluronic acid are used for moderate and severe pain.
- A shoe insert with an outer wedge is very effective for osteoarthritis in stage 1 and stage 2 (**FIG 6**).

SURGICAL MANAGEMENT

- An anteromedial opening-wedge osteotomy to correct the varus and anterior opening of the distal joint surface should be planned (**FIG 7**). The open-wedge method of osteotomy is more effective than the closed-wedge method. The lateral closed-wedge method is difficult because of the presence of the fibula on the lateral side, and this method can weaken the peroneal muscles because it shortens the lateral side.
- LTO is very effective for patients with stage 2 or stage 3a, but clinical results for patients with stage 3b are unsatisfactory. There must be cartilage on the roof of the talar dome for this procedure to be indicated.
- If the varus tilt angle on the weight-bearing AP view is 5 degrees or less, good results can be obtained from osteotomy alone. However, no joint with a varus tilt angle exceeding 10 degrees can attain a normal joint space.[9]
- Although the indications for this procedure are very limited, LTO can provide relief of pain with retention of joint function.

Preoperative Planning

- In terms of the TAS angle, overcorrection has produced much better results than undercorrection, especially in cases of advanced osteoarthritis. Therefore, the ideal TAS angle is 96 to 98 degrees.
- With the TLS angle, overcorrection has been found to restrict dorsiflexion of the ankle. Consequently, the ideal TLS angle is 81 to 82 degrees.
- Preoperative drawing
  - The osteotomy site is set at 5 cm above the tip of the medial malleolus. The extent of correction is appropriate to the shape of the grafted bone.
  - The lengths of the outer and side margins of the wedge-shaped graft bone are measured during preoperative drawing for the osteotomy. The grafted bone is usually harvested from the iliac bone crest. The medial height of the graft usually ranges from 6 to 8 mm.

Positioning

- The operation is performed under general anesthesia or spinal anesthesia in a supine position using an air tourniquet.

Approach

- Usually two separate incisions are made, on the lateral side of the fibula and on the medial side of the tibia.

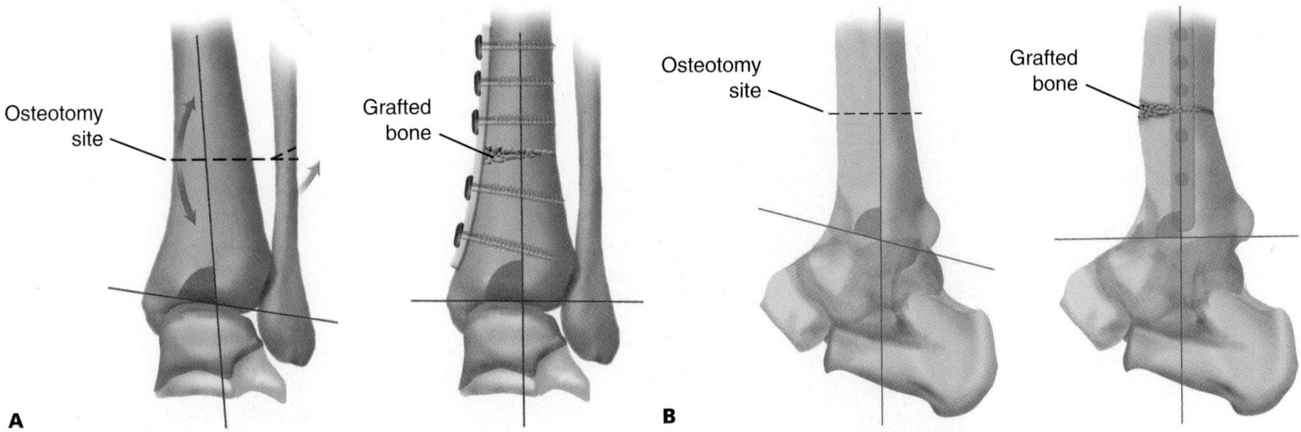

FIG 7 • Low tibial osteotomy. **A.** Anterior view. **B.** Lateral view.

FIBULAR OSTEOTOMY

- The fibular osteotomy is performed first. Make a 2-cm lateral longitudinal incision 7 cm proximal from the tip of the lateral malleolus. The tip of the lateral malleolus is detected using a needle percutaneously.
- Make an oblique cut on the fibula running from anteroproximal to posterodistal using a bone saw. When the tibia is corrected in the valgus direction, the hindfoot usually rotates laterally. This movement puts the osteotomy site in the appropriate position.
- If opening at the tibial osteotomy site is difficult, excise a 5-mm segment from the fibular osteotomy site.

TIBIAL OSTEOTOMY

- The tibial osteotomy is performed using an open-wedge technique.
- Make an 8-cm medial longitudinal incision beginning 5 cm proximal from the tip of the medial malleolus. The tip of the medial malleolus is detected using a needle percutaneously.
- The anterior surface of the distal part of the tibia is easily exposed, but retain as much of the periosteum as possible.
- Mark an osteotomy line using a chisel 5 cm proximal from the tip of the medial malleolus.
- Perform the osteotomy using a bone saw. Do not completely bisect the tibia. Retain several areas of cortex on the lateral side of the tibia. Open the osteotomy site carefully from the medial side using a chisel (**TECH FIG 1A,B**).
- Harvest grafted bone, the size of which has been decided during preoperative planning, from the iliac bone crest or a distal portion of the tibia.
- Form the grafted bone into a shape appropriate to an anteromedial opening-wedge osteotomy with reference to the drawing.
- Use the grafted bone to fill any open space at the osteotomy site (**TECH FIG 1C**).

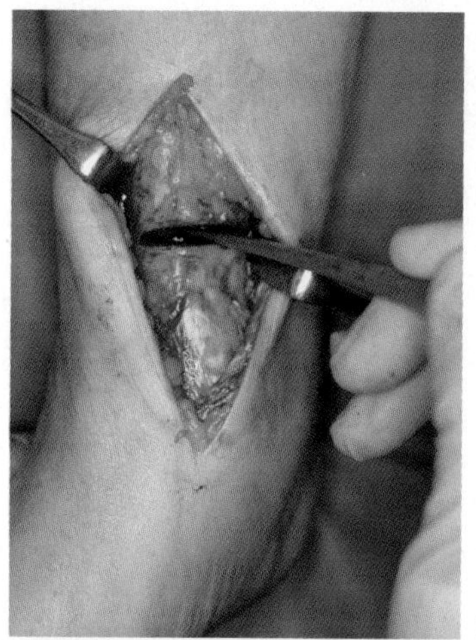

A

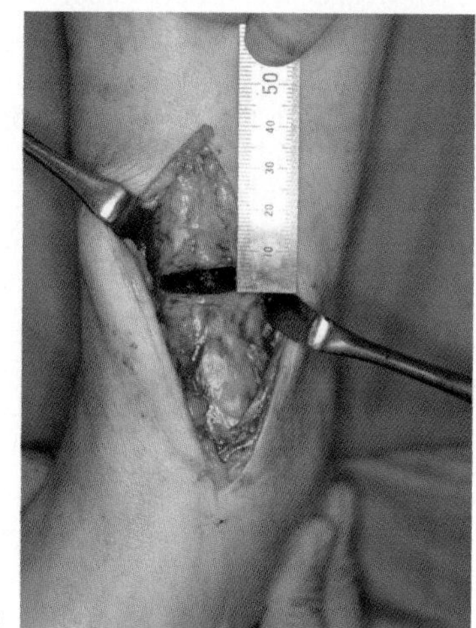

B

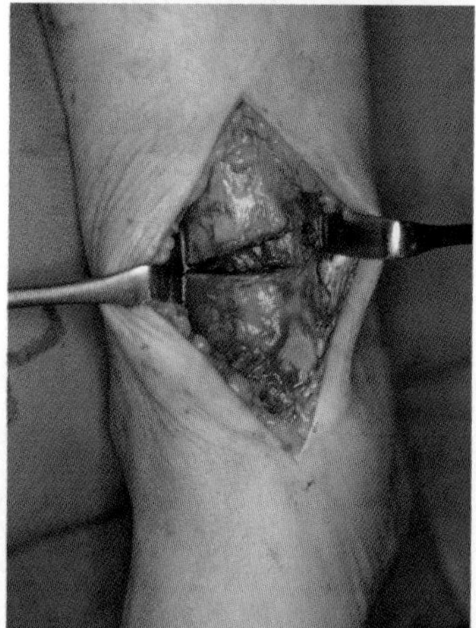

C

TECH FIG 1 • Tibial osteotomy. **A.** The osteotomy site is opened carefully. **B.** The size of the opening space is measured carefully. **C.** Open space is filled with bone graft.

FIXATION AT OSTEOTOMY SITE

- Fix the osteotomy site in the tibia using a four- or five-hole AO/ASIF Narrow Plate (Synthes), a six- or eight-hole Form Plate (Osteo), or a four- or six-hole Cloverleaf Plate (Stryker) (**TECH FIG 2**).
- Use cancellous screws for fixation at the distal end of the tibia to prevent fixing the distal talofibular joint.
- Fix the osteotomy site of the fibula using a screw or Kirschner wire.
- The compression mechanism of the screw holes on the plate sometimes causes loss of correction. If a plate has a compression mechanism, take extra care during the operation.

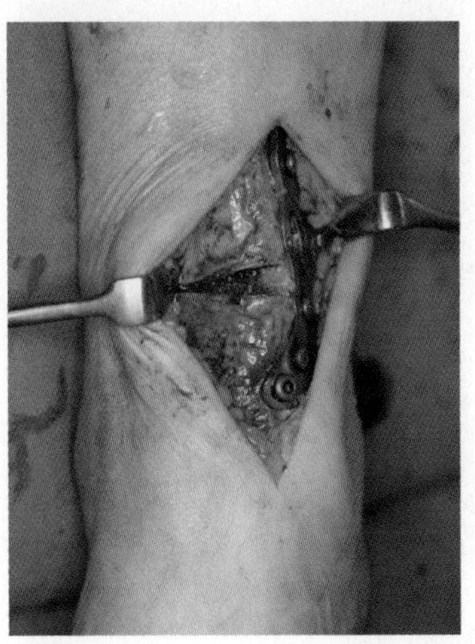

TECH FIG 2 • Plate fixation.

CLOSING

- Place a suction tube at the osteotomy site.
- Suture the subcutaneous fat tissue and close the skin.
- Apply a below-knee cast postoperatively.

PEARLS AND PITFALLS

Indication	■ LTO is indicated for stage 2 or 3A. ■ Retaining the cartilage of the roof of the talar dome is necessary to obtain good clinical results. ■ There is no indication for the ankle with more than 10 degrees of a weight-bearing talar tilt angle. ■ LTO cannot be expected to increase range of motion. It is indicated for the ankle that has at least 30 degrees of range of motion.
Fixation	■ If a plate has compression mechanism, take care to avoid loss of correction during fixation with screws.

POSTOPERATIVE CARE

- The leg is elevated with a pillow immediately postoperatively.
- The day after the operation, non–weight-bearing walking is allowed. Exercises for flexion and extension of the toes and knee are prescribed to prevent deep vein thrombosis and muscle weakness.
- A cast is used for 4 to 6 weeks. Touchdown with low–weight-bearing (5 kg) is allowed 2 weeks after the operation. Partial weight bearing (10 to 15 kg) is allowed 4 weeks postoperatively.
- After the cast is removed, a compression bandage is applied from the toes to the thigh to prevent edema. Active range-of-motion exercise of the ankle promotes repair of cartilage.
- The amount of weight bearing is increased gradually until full weight bearing on the ankle is allowed 2 months after the operation.

OUTCOMES

- The clinical results of 25 consecutive patients (26 feet) with varus-type osteoarthritis of the ankle who underwent LTO in our hospital were analyzed.[9] All were women aged 37 to 76 years (mean 54 years). Mean follow-up was 8 years 3 months.
- Patients reported marked relief of pain and exhibited significantly improved walking ability and activities of daily living. However, ankle movement did not improve postoperatively.
- The overall result was excellent in 4 ankles, good in 16 ankles, fair in 2 ankles, and poor in 4 ankles.
- Radiographic evaluation showed that the mean TAS angle was corrected from 83 degrees before surgery to 98 degrees at the follow-up examination; the mean TLS angle was corrected from 79 degrees before surgery to 85 degrees at the follow-up examination.
- In ankles that were radiographically classified as stage 2 or stage 3a, the lost joint space was restored. In contrast, only 2 of the 12 ankles that were classified as stage 3b exhibited restoration of the lost joint space. These findings indicate that LTO is indicated for stage 2 or 3a (**FIG 8**).

COMPLICATIONS

- Delayed union and nonunion are rare.
- Arthrodesis or total ankle arthroplasty as a salvage procedure should be selected for patients with poor results.

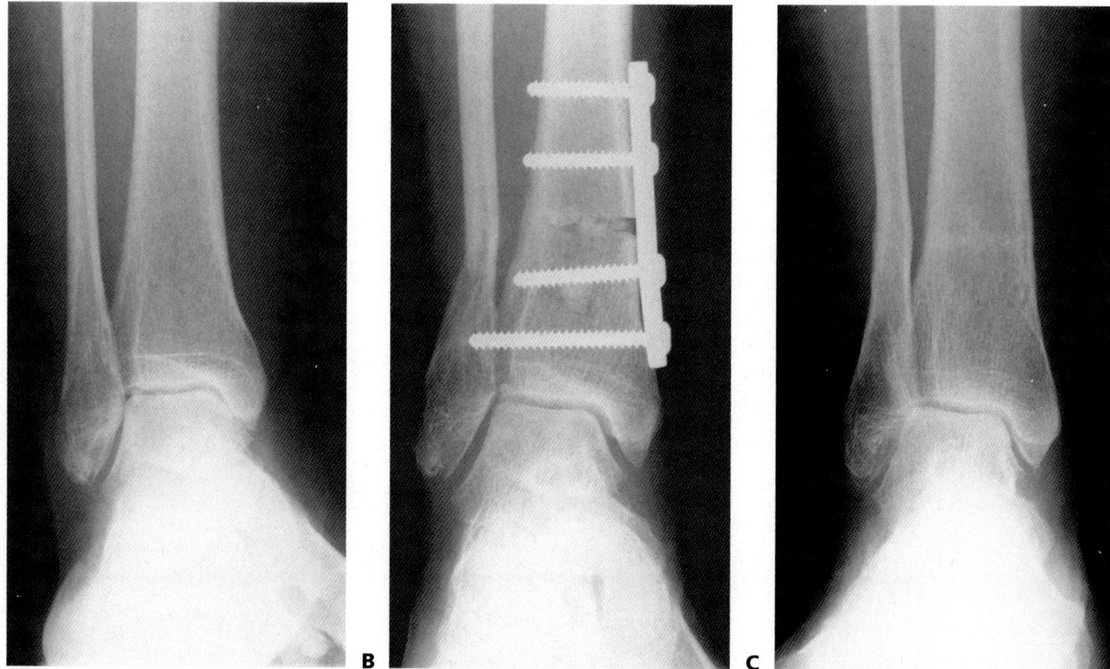

FIG 8 • A 44-year-old woman with stage 3a varus-type osteoarthritis. **A.** Preoperative obliteration of the joint space only at the tip of the medial malleolus. **B.** Immediate postoperative AP view. **C.** An excellent clinical result with no pain 11 years after the operation.

REFERENCES

1. Katsui T, Takakura Y, Kitada C, et al. Roentgenographic analysis for osteoarthrosis of the ankle. J Jpn Soc Surg Foot 1980;1:52–57.
2. Monji J. Roentgenological measurement of the shape of the osteoarthritic ankle. Nippon Seikeigeka Gakkai Zasshi 1980;54:791–802.
3. Nakai T, Takakura Y, Tanaka Y, et al. Morphologic changes of the ankle in children as assessed by radiography and arthrography. J Orthop Sci 2000;5:134–138.
4. Noguchi K. Biomechanical analysis for osteoarthritis of the ankle. Nippon Seikeigeka Gakkai Zasshi 1985;59:213–220.
5. Sugimoto K, Samoto N, Takakura Y, et al. Varus tilt of the tibial plafond as a factor in chronic ligament instability of the ankle. Foot Ankle Int 1997;18:402–405.
6. Takakura Y, Tanaka Y, Kumai T, et al. Low tibial osteotomy for osteoarthritis of the ankle. J Bone Joint Surg Br 1995;77B:50–54.
7. Takakura Y, Takaoka T, Tanaka Y, et al. Results of opening-wedge osteotomy for the treatment of a post-traumatic varus deformity of the ankle. J Bone Joint Surg Am 1998;80A:213–218.
8. Tanaka Y, Ohneda Y, Nakayama S, et al. Computer simulation of low tibial osteotomy using a three dimensional rigid body spring model. J Jpn Soc Surg Foot 1992;13:134–138.
9. Tanaka Y, Takakura Y, Hayashi K, et al. Low tibial osteotomy for varus-type osteoarthritis of the ankle. J Bone Joint Surg Br 2006;88B:909–913.
10. Unno M. An experimental stress analysis around the ankle after a low tibial osteotomy using two dimensional photoelasticity. J Nara Med Assoc 1984;36:524–546.

Chapter 64

Supramalleolar Osteotomy With Internal Fixation: Perspective 3

Markus Knupp and Beat Hintermann

DEFINITION

- A supramalleolar osteotomy is an osteotomy at the level of the distal tibia with or without osteotomy of the fibula.
- The correction is intended to normalize altered load distribution across the joint and may be indicated in cases of asymmetric osteoarthritis, malunited fractures of the distal tibial, and osteochondral lesions.

ANATOMY

- Trauma and neurologic disorders leading to varus and valgus alignment around the ankle joint predispose to asymmetric joint load. This causes cartilage wear, in particular in the presence of associated ligamentous instability and muscular imbalance (**FIG 1**).

PATHOGENESIS

- Various conditions, such as neurologic disorders, congenital and acquired foot deformities, posttraumatic malunions, and instability may be associated with malalignment of the ankle joint complex.

NATURAL HISTORY

- Malalignment of the hindfoot may result from bony deformity above or below the level of the ankle joint.
- Ligamentous instability or muscular imbalance may be a contributing or even an initiating factor in the natural history of malalignment around the ankle joint.

PATIENT HISTORY AND PHYSICAL FINDINGS

- A thorough medical history should be taken.
  - Systemic diseases, such as diabetes mellitus (Charcot arthropathy), rheumatoid arthritis, and neurovascular disorders need to be assessed carefully.

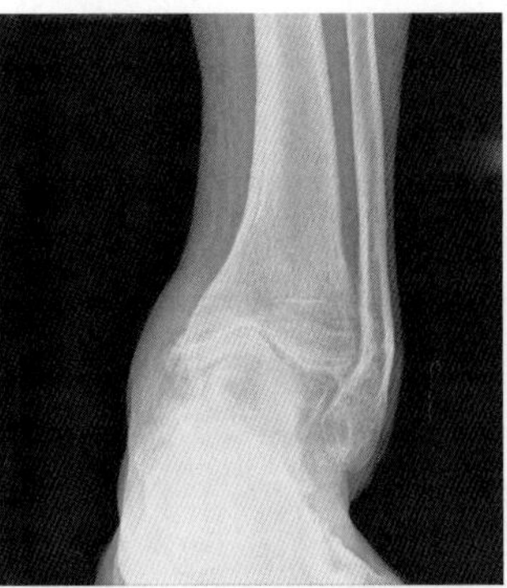

FIG 1 • Weight-bearing radiograph of a 65-year-old man with a posttraumatic varus deformity after a fracture of the distal tibia and fibula 26 years ago. The anteroposterior view shows the asymmetric osteoarthrosis of his tibiotalar joint due to the altered load distribution.

  - Tobacco use should be considered a relative contraindication to supramalleolar osteotomy.
  - Disorders that alter the bone quality and healing capacity (medication, osteoporosis, age) should be assessed carefully.
- Physical examination should include the following:
  - Drawer test and talar tilt test to assess ankle joint stability
  - Assessment of the inversion and eversion force to exclude peroneal tendon insufficiency
  - Subtalar range of motion
  - Coleman block test to exclude a forefoot driven hindfoot varus

IMAGING AND OTHER DIAGNOSTIC STUDIES

- Weight-bearing radiographs of the entire foot, the ankle, the tibial shaft (full-length radiographs) and the Saltzman hindfoot view are necessary to assess the nature and location of the deformity. Unless deformity at the level of the knee joint or the femur can be excluded clinically, whole lower-limb radiographs are obtained.
- Next to conventional radiography, computed tomography (CT) and magnetic resonance imaging are not routinely required. However, they could be of value when assessing osteochondral lesions and peroneal tendon disorders or evaluating the aspect of the ligament insufficiency.
- SPECT-CT has been found to be a valuable tool for the assessment and staging of osteoarthritis in asymmetric osteoarthritis of the ankle joint.

DIFFERENTIAL DIAGNOSIS

- Symmetric or end-stage osteoarthritis
- Muscular imbalance (eg, in neurologic disease)
- Forefoot-driven hindfoot deformities

NONOPERATIVE MANAGEMENT

- Asymptomatic, moderate malalignment usually is treated conservatively.
- Malalignment that is due to forces from the neighboring structures, such as plantarflexed first metatarsal or unbalanced muscle forces can be treated with physiotherapy or shoe wear modifications. Deforming forces, such as forefoot abnormalities or muscular imbalance, may require surgical procedures other than supramalleolar osteotomies.
- Recommendations for asymptomatic but severe malalignment, such as experienced by the patient in Fig 1, are controversial (surgical versus conservative). Because the deformity is likely to lead to excessive wear, surgery should be considered.
- An alternative surgical treatment is the calcaneal displacement osteotomy (medial or lateral). In my opinion, however, correction of malalignment is best performed at the level of the deformity.

SURGICAL MANAGEMENT

- Supramalleolar osteotomies are divided into opening and closing wedge osteotomies.
  - Valgus deformities are usually addressed with a medial closing wedge osteotomy.
  - Varus malalignment is corrected with a medial opening wedge osteotomy or a lateral closing wedge osteotomy.
- The decision between wedge removal laterally and wedge insertion is based on the amount of correction needed. In an extensive medial opening wedge osteotomy, the fibula may restrict the amount of correction possible, so deformities greater than 10 degrees are usually corrected through a lateral approach.

Preoperative Planning

- The most important aspect of the preoperative planning is the assessment of the origin of the deformity. Different entities need to be distinguished, and it is mandatory to separate the isolated frontal plane deformity of the hindfoot from complex deformities involving the transverse, sagittal, and coronal planes with or without muscular dysfunction and imbalanced ligamentous structures.
- To determine the size of the wedge that should be added or removed to restore anatomic alignment in the ankle, the tibiotalar angle should be measured.
  - On a standard anteroposterior image of the ankle joint, the tibiotalar angle is the angle between the tibial axis and the tibial joint surface. The wedge to be corrected can be measured out of the radiographs or calculated with the mathematical formula $\tan \theta = H/W$, where α is the angle to be corrected, H is the wedge height in millimeters, and W is the tibial width (**FIG 2**).
  - An overcorrection of 3 to 5 degrees is recommended by most authors for asymmetric osteoarthritis.
- Additional deviation (eg, rotational or translational deformities) must be taken into consideration during the planning of the osteotomy.

Positioning

- Positioning of the patient depends on the surgical approach:
  - Anterior approach: supine position
  - Lateral approach: lateral decubitus position or supine with a sandbag under the buttock of the affected limb
  - Medial approach: supine, ipsilateral knee in slight flexion with a sandbag under the calf

Approach

- An anterior, lateral, or medial approach can be chosen to correct the deformity. The choice depends on the nature of the deformity, the local soft tissue conditions, and previous approaches.

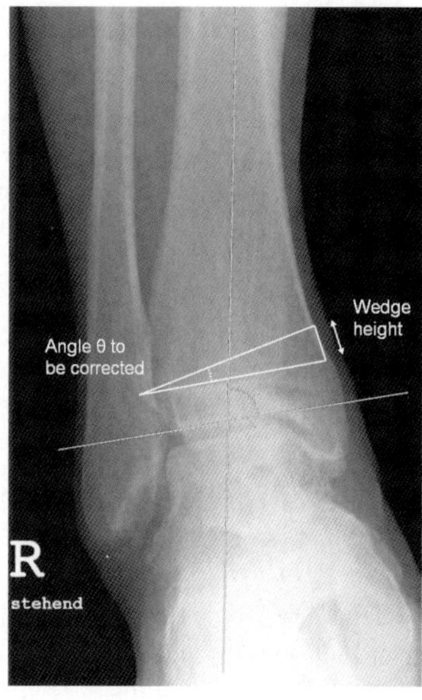

FIG 2 • Planning of the correction: measuring of the deformity and planning of the wedge to be inserted (lower line of the white triangle indicating the level of the osteotomy).

TECHNIQUES

LATERAL CLOSING WEDGE OSTEOTOMY TO CORRECT VALGUS

Details of Approach

- After exsanguination of the leg, a pneumatic tourniquet is inflated on the thigh.
- A 10-cm longitudinal slightly curved incision is made along the anterior margin of the distal fibula. If the incision needs to be extended distally, it is curved ventrally to end just distal to and anterior of the lateral malleolus (**TECH FIG 1**).
- The fibula and the tibia are then exposed laterally. To avoid devascularization of the bone, stripping of the periosteum is not performed.
- At the distal end of the incision, the anterior syndesmosis is exposed.
- The lateral branch of the sural nerve and the short saphenous vein run dorsal to the line of incision and are usually not seen during this procedure. Extended proximal dissection may require identification, exposure, and protection of the branches of the superficial peroneal nerve, however. Cauterization of some of the branches of the peroneal artery, which lie deep to the medial surface of the distal fibula, may be necessary.

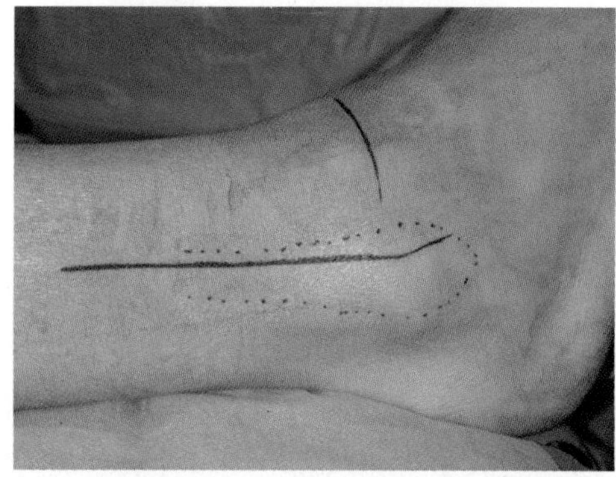

TECH FIG 1 • Lateral approach to the distal fibula and tibia.

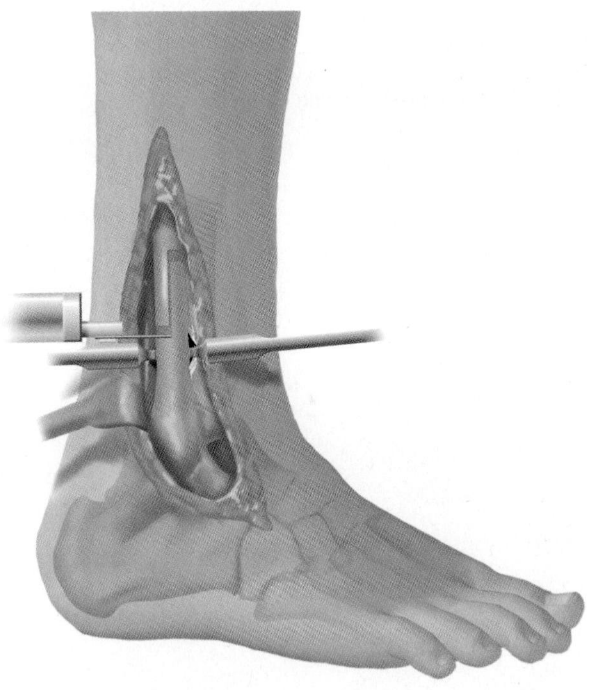

TECH FIG 2 • Drawing illustrating the Z-shaped osteotomy for shortening of the fibula.

Fibular Osteotomy

- In most cases in which a varus deformity is addressed with a lateral closing wedge osteotomy, the fibula needs to be shortened to preserve the congruency in the ankle joint. The shortening can be done by simple bone block removal or a Z-shaped osteotomy. I prefer the Z-shaped fibular osteotomy, which confers greater control of rotation and primary stability compared to a block resection for fibular shortening.
- The length of the Z-shaped fibular osteotomy is approximately 2 to 3 cm, starting distally at the level of the anterior syndesmosis.
- Kirschner wires can be placed as a reference at the level of the transverse cuts to confirm the location of the osteotomy fluoroscopically.
- The osteotomy is then carried out with an oscillating saw.
- After the fibula has been mobilized, bone blocks are resected on both ends of the Z based on the amount of the planned shortening (**TECH FIG 2**).
- To avoid interference from the dense syndesmotic ligaments when performing the Z-osteotomy, I routinely direct the proximal transverse cut anteriorly and the distal cut (which typically sits at the syndesmosis) posteriorly.

Lateral Closing Wedge Tibial Osteotomy

- To define the desired osteotomy, two Kirschner wires are drilled through the tibia, with the tips converging at the medial cortex, making sure that the angle between the K wires corresponds with the preoperative planning (see Tech Fig 2).
  - Unless the deformity is located proximal to the supramalleolar area, the wires are directed from proximal to the anterior syndesmosis to the medial physeal scar (**TECH FIG 3A**).
- After fluoroscopic verification of the location of the wires (**TECH FIG 3B**), the periosteum is incised only at the level of the planned osteotomy and carefully mobilized with a scalpel or periosteal elevator.
- The osteotomy is then performed using an oscillating saw cooled with saline or water irrigation to limit thermal injury to bone.
- Placing the K-wires accurately avoids cutting through the medial cortex; ideally, the medial cortex should serve as a hinge.
- Correction of the deformity must be performed at the center of rotation and angulation of the deformity to avoid relative translational malpositioning of the distal (ankle) and proximal (tibial shaft) fragments.
- The gap is then closed, and the osteotomy is secured with a plate. I prefer locking plates that afford optimal primary stability; however, it is imperative that the osteotomy is completely closed when employing locking plate technology (**TECH FIG 3C, D**).
- Prior to locking the plate both proximal and distal to the osteotomy, I use a tensioning device to optimally compress the osteotomy.
- I routinely close the periosteum over the osteotomy with 2-0 absorbable sutures.

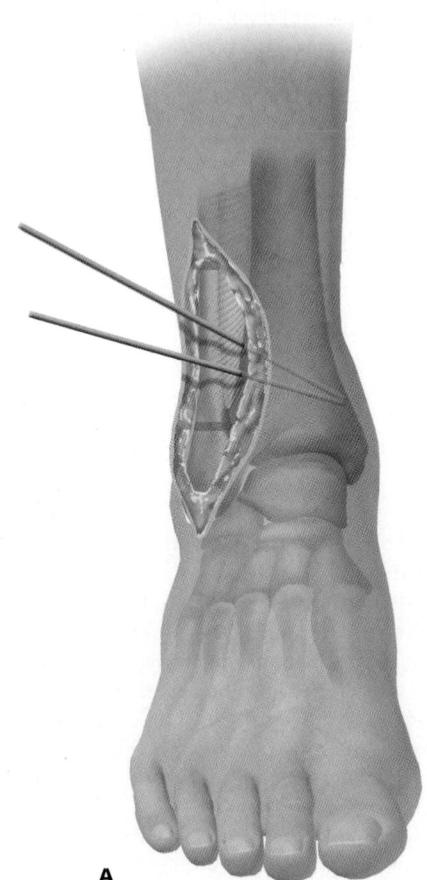

TECH FIG 3 • **A**. Placement of the K-wires for guidance of the osteotomy. *(continued)*

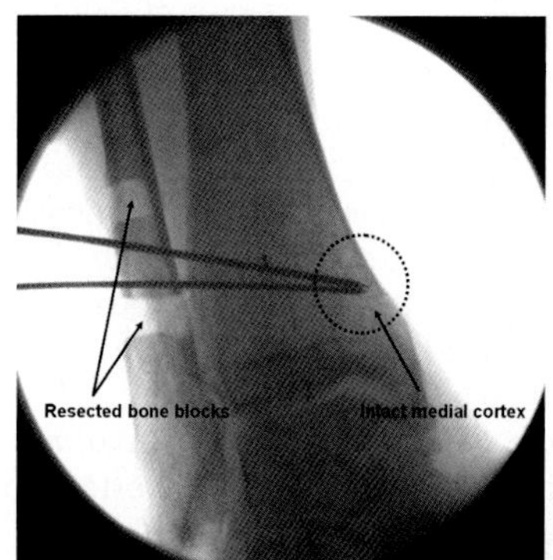

B

TECH FIG 3 • *(continued)* **B**. Intraoperative radiograph showing the guide-wires for the tibial osteotomy after the Z-shaped fibula osteotomy. Distal tibia/fibula before (**C**) and after (**D**) closure of the osteotomy. Note the shortening of the fibula.

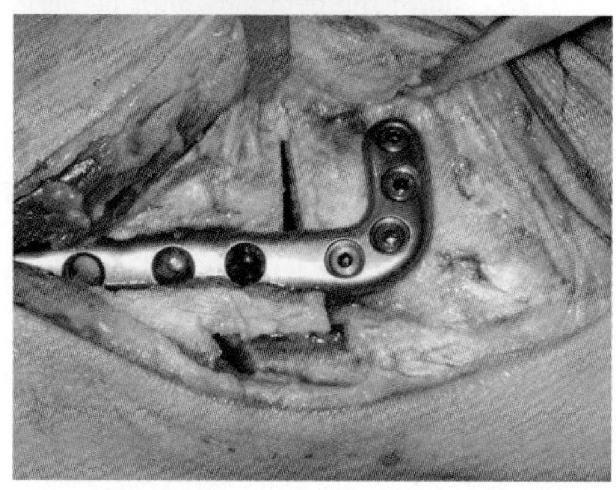

C

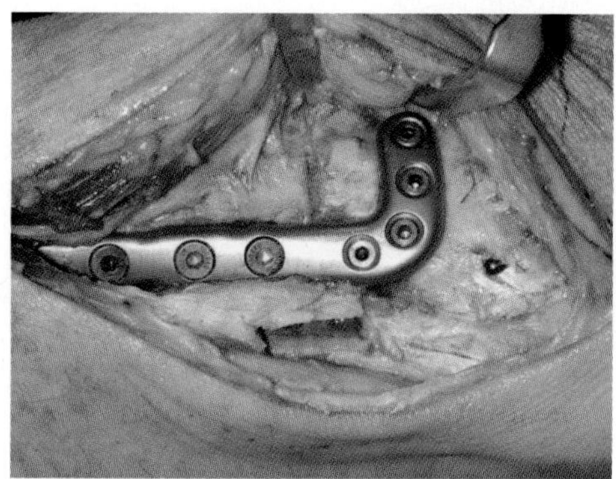

D

Optimizing Joint Congruity and Securing the Fibula

- Fluoroscopically, optimal tibiotalar joint congruity and fibular osteotomy reduction are determined.
- Once the joint is congruent, the fibula is secured with screws (in the longitudinal limb of the Z-osteotomy) or a one-third tubular plate (**TECH FIG 4**).
- The subcutaneous tissues and the skin are closed with interrupted sutures.

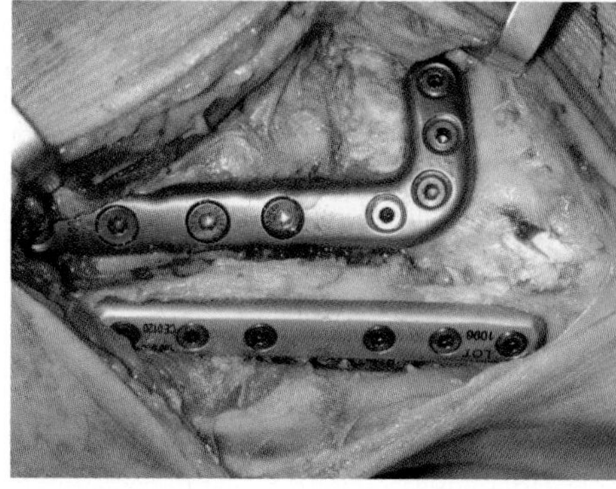

TECH FIG 4 • Fixation of the fibula with a plate.

MEDIAL OPEN WEDGE OSTEOTOMY FOR CORRECTION OF VARUS DEFORMITY

Anterior Approach

- The limb is exsanguinated and the thigh tourniquet is inflated.
- The anterior incision is made anteriorly over the distal tibia and ankle, immediately lateral to the tibial crest. The superficial peroneal nerve will cross the distal aspect of the incision and must be protected.
- The extensor retinaculum is then divided longitudinally to expose the extensor tendons. The approach uses the interval between the tibialis anterior and extensor hallucis longus tendons.
- A longitudinal incision in the extensor retinaculum is made between the anterior tibial tendon and the extensor hallucis longus tendon, starting 10 cm proximal to the joint, about midway between the malleoli (**TECH FIG 5**)
  - The anterior tibial tendon is retracted medially, and the tendon of the extensor hallucis longus is retracted laterally, if possible, without opening the tendon sheaths.
  - The deep neurovascular bundle (anterior tibial artery and deep peroneal nerve), located in the lateral aspect of the approach, must be identified and protected.
- The ankle joint is covered by an extensive fat pad that contains a venous plexus and requires partial cauterization.
- If tibiotalar joint debridement or exostectomy is required, I make an anterior capsulotomy at this time. If only a supramalleolar osteotomy is planned, however, there is no need to expose the joint.
- With all soft tissues and neurovascular structures protected, the anterior surface of the tibia can be exposed.

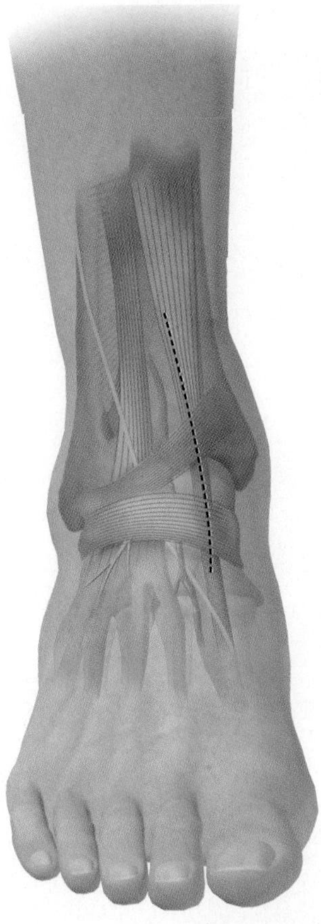

TECH FIG 5 • Anterior approach to the distal tibia with the interval between the extensor hallucis longus and the anterior tibial tendon and the neurovascular bundle lying lateral to it.

To promote healing of the osteotomy, periosteal stripping should be limited to the osteotomy site.

- The osteotomy is carried out as described below under Tibial Osteotomy.

Medial Approach

- The patient is positioned supine on the operating table; a bump placed under the contralateral hip may improve exposure.
- The limb is exsanguinated and the tourniquet is inflated.
- The great saphenous vein and the saphenous nerve usually lie anterior to the incision. A 10-cm longitudinal incision is made beginning over the medial malleolus and extending proximally over the distal tibia (**TECH FIG 6A**).

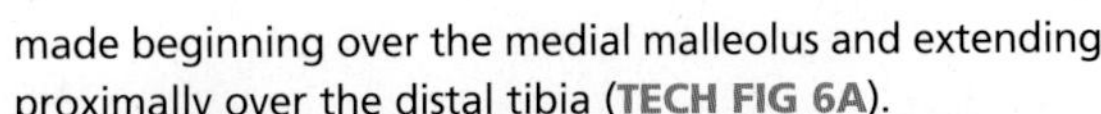

- The skin flaps are mobilized, with care taken not to damage the neurovascular bundle, which runs along the anterior border of the medial malleolus (**TECH FIG 6B**).
- The posterior tibial tendon, which lies immediately on the posterior aspect of the medial malleolus, must be identified and retracted posteriorly. It needs to be exposed, its sheath incised, and the tendon retracted posteriorly to visualize the dorsal surface of the distal tibia.

Tibial Osteotomy

- The tibia is exposed with minimal periosteal stripping (**TECH FIG 7A**).
- The plane of the osteotomy is determined under image intensification, and a K-wire is placed from the medial cortex into the physeal scar or, in case of a malunion, at the apex of the deformation (**TECH FIG 7B**).
- The periosteum is then incised at the level of the osteotomy and elevated off the bone using a scalpel or a periosteal elevator. The osteotomy must be planned carefully because placing it inaccurately may lead to relative translation of the distal and proximal fragments, malaligning the ankle joint under the tibial shaft axis.
- I recommend using a wide saw blade to create a congruent osteotomy (**TECH FIG 7C, D**).
  - Alternatively, a chisel or osteotome may be used instead of the oscillating saw to limit thermal injury to bone.
- The correction is based on preoperative planning.
- The gap can be filled with allograft (I use Tutoplast Spongiosa; Tutogen Medical GmbH, Neunkirchen, Germany) or autograft iliac crest bone (**TECH FIG 7E**).
- We typically secure the osteotomy with a medial locking plate, but plates with an integrated spacer (eg, Puddu plate; Arthrex, Naples, FL) can be used instead (**TECH FIG 7F**).

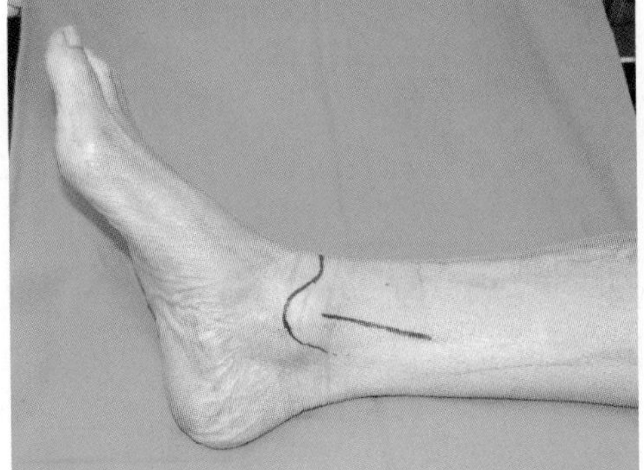

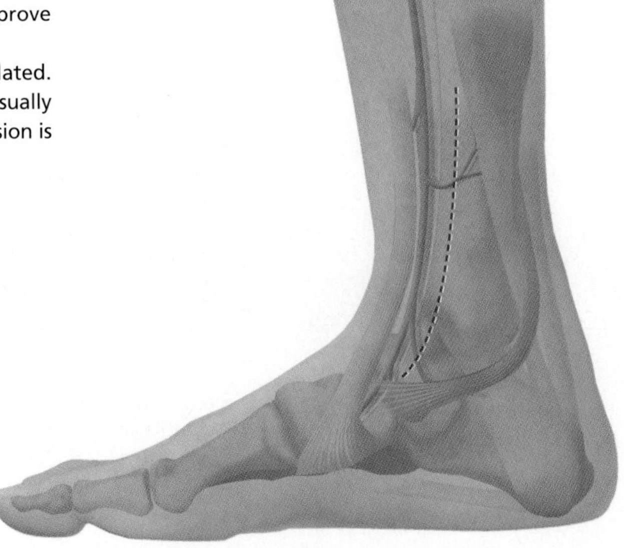

A B

TECH FIG 6 • **A, B.** Medial approach to the distal tibia.

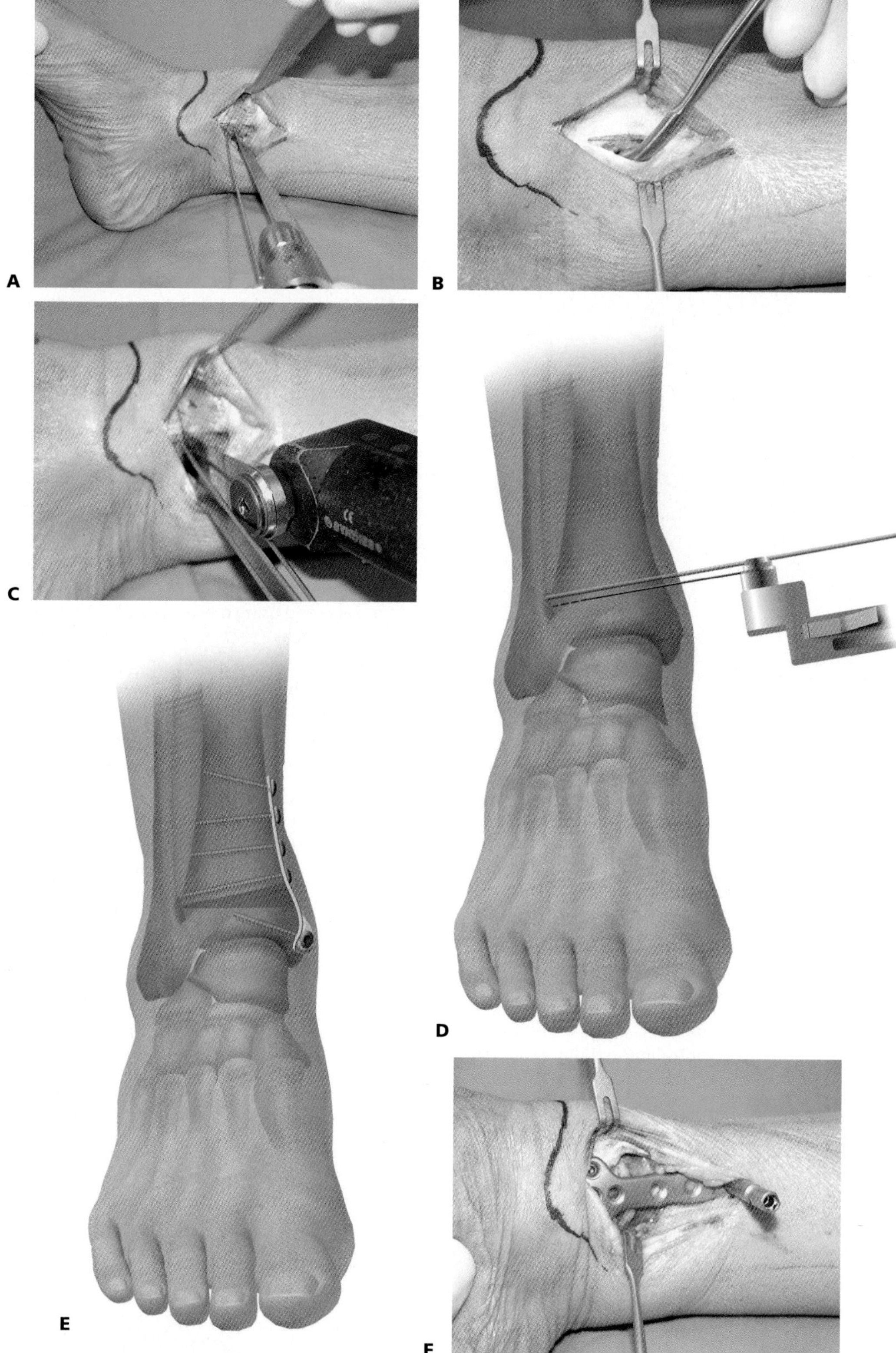

TECH FIG 7 • A. Intraoperative picture of the K-wire placement. **B.** Incision and careful stripping of the periosteum. **C.** Osteotomy of the tibia with an oscillating saw. **D.** Drawing of the saw cut for a medial opening wedge osteotomy. **E.** Fill the gap. **F.** Plate fixation of the osteotomy.

- Fixation of the osteotomy is as described for the lateral osteotomy (see earlier).
- The tendon sheath of the posterior tibial tendon is reapproximated with 2-0 absorbable sutures, and the subcutaneous tissues and the skin are closed with interrupted sutures. Do not overtighten the posterior tibial tendon sheath because it may create stenosing flexor tenosynovitis.
- Case results are shown in **TECH FIG 8**.

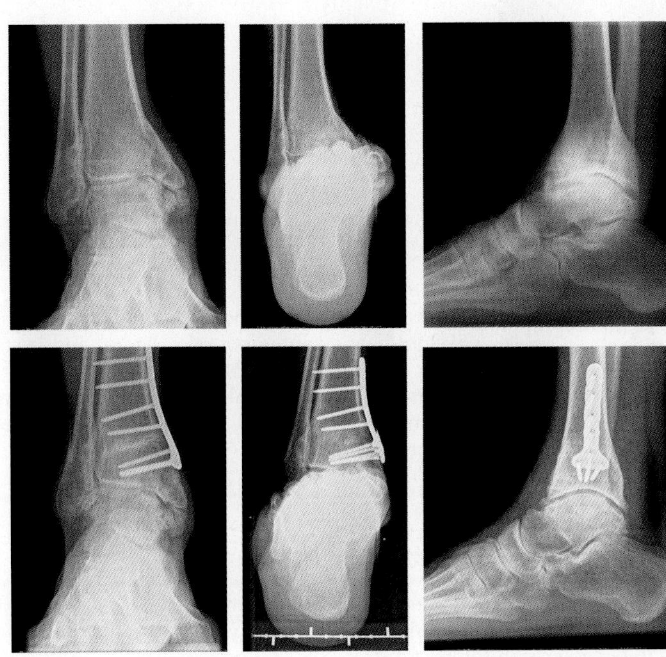

TECH FIG 8 • Pre- and postoperative radiographs (weight-bearing anteroposterior, lateral, and Saltzman views, respectively) of a 62-year-old male patient with varus osteoarthritis of his ankle joint. The postoperative images are made 1 year after a medial opening wedge osteotomy.

MEDIAL CLOSING WEDGE OSTEOTOMY FOR CORRECTING VALGUS MALALIGNMENT

- The technique essentially is the same as for the opening wedge osteotomy described in the previous section with removal of a bone wedge.
- K-wire placement is done according to the planned correction (**TECH FIG 9A**).
- The bone wedge is then removed (**TECH FIG 9B**) and the correction secured with a medial plate.
- A clinical example is shown in **TECH FIG 10**.

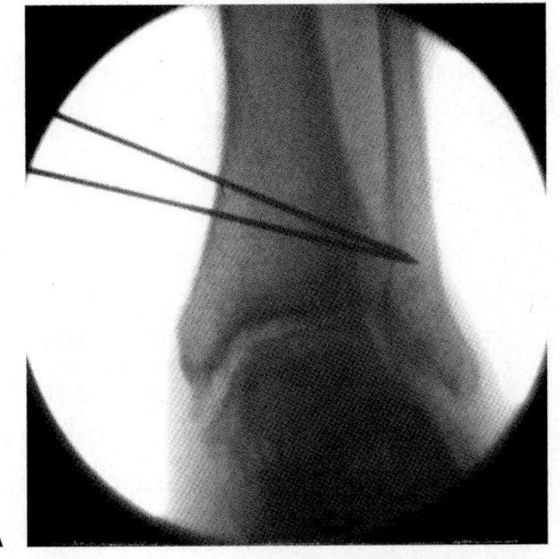

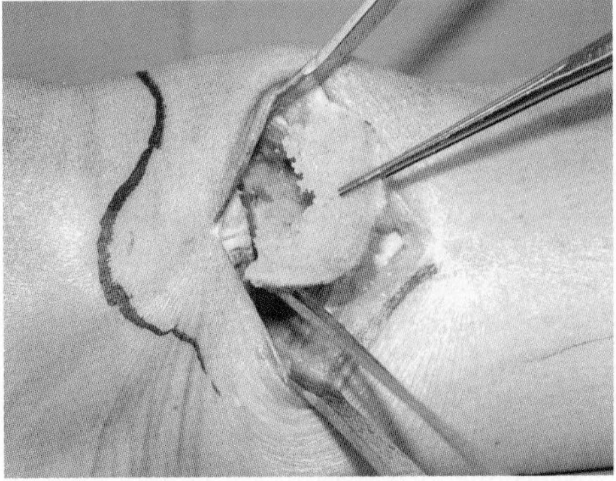

TECH FIG 9 • **A.** K-wire placement for a medial closing wedge osteotomy. **B.** Wedge removal in a medial closing osteotomy.

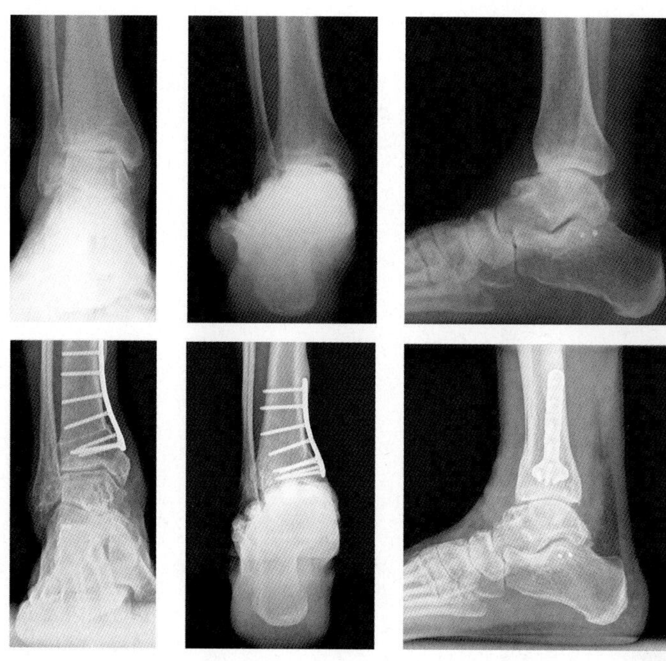

TECH FIG 10 • Pre- and postoperative radiographs (weight-bearing anteroposterior, lateral, and Saltzman views, respectively) of a 58-year-old male patient with valgus osteoarthritis of his ankle joint. The postoperative images are made 1 year after a medial closing wedge osteotomy.

PEARLS AND PITFALLS

Laceration of the posterior tibial tendon	▪ For lateral osteotomies in posttraumatic cases with extensive scarring on the posteromedial aspect of the ankle, it may be necessary to expose the tendon through a minimal incision to protect it.
Accidental cutting through the entire tibia	▪ This loss of the hinge mechanism of the far cortex introduces the risk for rotational or translational malpositioning and postoperative displacement of the osteotomy. ▪ Consider additional fixation with a second plate in a second plane.
Mobilization of the syndesmosis	▪ In select cases, the syndesmosis needs to be mobilized to maintain congruent tibiotalar joint alignment. I do this by releasing the anterior syndesmotic ligaments from the anterolateral distal tibia, immediately proximal to the ankle joint. The ligaments are released by removing Chaput's tubercle from the anterolateral distal tibia using an osteotome or chisel. Once the osteotomy is secured and the fibula is reduced to the desired position to create a congruent ankle joint, the syndesmosis is stabilized at its new resting tension by reattaching Chaput's tubercle with a screw and a washer or with transosseous sutures.
Loss of reduction of the osteotomy	▪ The risk can be lowered by the use of implants that provide angular stability and by leaving a hinge of bone and periosteum at the far cortex when performing the tibial osteotomy to achieve a controlled correction in the desired plane.

POSTOPERATIVE CARE

- The leg is elevated in the immediate postoperative period.
- A compressive dressing and splint are maintained for 2 days to diminish swelling.
- A short leg non–weight-bearing cast is used for 6 to 8 weeks.
- If radiologic evidence of consolidation is present after 6 weeks, partial weight bearing is allowed for 2 weeks, after which the patient advances gradually to full weight bearing.
- A rehabilitation program for strengthening, gait training, and range of motion is prescribed 8 weeks after surgery, with gradual return to full activities as tolerated.

OUTCOMES

- We have been observing our first series of 74 patients with a varus or valgus deformity of the ankle joint for 49 months (range of 24 to 146 months).
- For correction of a varus hindfoot malalignment, a medial opening wedge osteotomy was performed in 14 patients, and a combined lateral closing wedge osteotomy with a correction of the fibula in 13 patients.
- Valgus hindfeet were addressed with a medial closing wedge osteotomy in 42 cases and a lateral opening wedge in 5 cases.
- At the radiographic assessment after 6 months, all osteotomies showed complete consolidation. Pain reduction was found in all patients, which is similar to earlier reports. Improved radiographic osteoarthritis scores were noted in 75% of the patients. Additionally, patients exhibited a trend toward normalization of gait and function.

COMPLICATIONS

- Apart from perioperative complications such as delayed wound healing problems or infection, postoperative concerns include delayed union or nonunion of the osteotomy.

- Another potential complication is malunion, resulting from inaccurate alignment of the osteotomy at the time of surgery or postoperative loss of position.
- Intraoperative complications include nerve or tendon injury. We ensure that all adjacent neurovascular structures and tendons are identified and protected.

REFERENCES

1. Cheng Y-M, Huang P-J, Hong S-H, et al. Low tibial osteotomy for moderate ankle arthritis. Arch Orthop Trauma Surg 2001;121:355–358.
2. Hintermann B, Knupp M, Barg A. Osteotomies of the distal tibia and hindfoot for ankle realignment. Orthopade 2008;37:212–223.
3. Knupp M, Pagenstert GI, Barg A, et al. SPECT-CT compared with conventional imaging modalities for the assessment of the varus and valgus malaligned hindfoot. J Orthop Res 2009;27:1461–1466.
4. Knupp M, Pagenstert G, Valderrabano V, Hintermann B. Osteotomies in varus malalignment of the ankle. Oper Orthop Traumatol 2008;20:262–273.
5. Knupp M, Sufkens SAS, Pagenstert GI, et al. Supramalleolar osteotomy for tibiotalar varus malalignment. Tech Foot Ankle Surg 2009;8:17–23.
6. Pagenstert GI, Hintermann B, Barg A, et al. Realignment surgery as alternative treatment of varus and valgus ankle osteoarthritis. Clin Orthop Rel Res 2007;462:156–168.
7. Pagenstert GI, Knupp M, Valderrabano V, Hintermann B. Realignment surgery for valgus ankle osteoarthritis. Oper Orthop Traumatol 2009;21:77–87.
8. Stamatis ED, Cooper PS, Myerson MS. Supramalleolar osteotomy for the treatment of distal tibial angular deformities and arthritis of the ankle joint. Foot Ankle Int 2003;24:754–764.
9. Takakura Y, Takaoka T, Tanaka Y, et al. Results of opening-wedge osteotomy for the treatment of a post-traumatic varus deformity of the ankle. J Bone Joint Surg Am 1998;80A:213–218.

Chapter 65

Supramalleolar Osteotomy With External Fixation: Perspective 1

Austin T. Fragomen and S. Robert Rozbruch

DEFINITION

- Supramalleolar osteotomy (SMO) refers to an osteotomy of the distal tibia and fibula. Typically this is at the metaphyseal–diaphyseal junction, averaging 5 cm proximal to the ankle joint.
- The technique for SMO can vary greatly and includes both open and percutaneous approaches; use of a power saw, a Gigli saw, or an osteotome; use of internal fixation[3,26] or external fixation; and gradual or acute reduction of the bone.[1,2,6–8,10,14,19,27,29,30]
- The most common indication for SMO is malalignment of the distal tibia. Malalignment of the distal tibia and ankle is a common problem that is largely left untreated even in this era of modern orthopaedics. There is a general lack of interest in treating these deformities, which can be attributed to the deficiency of a safe and reliable method for correction.
- In our hands, correction of distal tibial and ankle deformities using a percutaneous osteotomy and a minimally invasive circular external fixator has yielded excellent and reproducible results with minimal complications.

ANATOMY

- Bony deformity
  - Common deformities that cause malalignment include distal tibial and ankle varus, valgus, apex anterior, apex posterior, malrotation, and shortening.
  - Typically, a patient has more than one of these deformities simultaneously.
- Tibial nerve
  - With longstanding varus or flexion (procurvatum) deformities of the distal tibia, the tibial nerve is often relatively shortened. An equinus contracture of the ankle joint will worsen the situation.
  - In these cases serious consideration needs to be given to the management of the nerve to prevent neurologic injury.
  - The two most common methods for avoiding injury are gradual correction of all deformities and tarsal tunnel release.
  - As long as one of these methods is employed, then the nerve should be protected.
- Poor skin
  - The condition of the skin around the operative site must be noted.
  - Many patients with posttraumatic deformities of the distal tibia have also sustained severe soft tissue injury. The skin is often matted down and adherent to the underlying bone. Skin grafts and free flaps are not uncommon and must be considered when choosing a correction technique.
  - Poor skin will often not tolerate large incisions. Wound dehiscence and even osteomyelitis are not uncommon in these circumstances. Internal fixation often will not fit underneath this skin and will often lead to wound breakdown and deep infection.
  - A minimally invasive technique relying on gradual correction is the ideal solution to avoiding further compromise of poor skin.
- Osteotomy level
  - Although the apex of the deformity (center of rotation and angulation [CORA])[16,17] often appears to be the obvious site for a corrective osteotomy, clinical factors must be weighed.
  - Often we make our osteotomy distal or proximal to the true CORA for a variety of reasons. The bone at the CORA is often very sclerotic and has suboptimal healing potential. An osteotomy through adjacent less sclerotic bone will result in more predictable and robust bone formation and a shorter time for consolidation.
  - Along the same lines, if there is a leg-length discrepancy (LLD), the surgeon must strongly consider whether the bone at the distal osteotomy site has the capacity to both heal and make good regenerate.
  - Often we will make a separate proximal tibial osteotomy for lengthening and use the SMO for deformity correction only.
- Percutaneous osteotomy
  - A thorough knowledge of the distal tibial anatomy is important before embarking on a percutaneous bone cut.
  - Judicious use of the C-arm fluoroscopy is needed to ensure that the osteotome has not passed beyond the far cortex of the bone and into the soft tissues.
  - With time this osteotomy can be done mostly by "feel" and repetition.
  - Pearls include making the incision medial to the tibialis anterior tendon and taking great care when the osteotome passes posteromedially.
  - We recommend rotating the foot internally to ensure the osteotomy is complete and to avoid stretching of the tibial nerve.
- Joint contracture
  - The surgeon must identify any coexisting joint contractures before planning the osteotomy.
  - Often there will be an equinus contracture of the ankle when there is a recurvatum deformity of the distal tibia.
  - Provisions need to be made for simultaneous correction of both the bony deformity and the capsular contracture.
  - When there is a longstanding varus deformity of the distal tibia, the subtalar joint will accommodate through hindfoot valgus. If this subtalar valgus is a fixed contracture, then further surgery will be needed to correct this second, more subtle deformity.

PATHOGENESIS

- A poorly aligned ankle joint experiences asymmetric forces on the articular cartilage that can lead to arthritis.
- We typically see two groups of patients with distal tibial malalignment: those with extra-articular deformity and those with intra-articular deformity.

- Patients with extra-articular malalignment have typically had a fracture of the distal tibial metaphysis that healed with deformity, yielding a malunion.
- If this deformity is corrected early, then the joint will not become arthritic and the prognosis is very good.
- If there is a delay in realignment, which is often the case, the patient will have developed posttraumatic ankle arthritis.
- The mechanism for the development of arthritis is the malalignment itself. The ankle joint was designed to function in its anatomic state. If the alignment of the joint is altered, there will be increased pressure in one area of the joint, and this leads to abnormal wear.
- For example, if a patient has a longstanding varus malunion of the distal tibia, the ankle joint will tend to wear out on the medial side, with relative sparing of the lateral joint surface.
- If the joint has asymmetric wear, SMO is still indicated. The goal is realignment of the distal tibia and even overcorrection to place more pressure on the more normal cartilage. This is the same concept as high tibial osteotomy, where the goal is to place the mechanical axis through the lateral compartment of the knee as opposed to through the middle of the knee. This overcorrection will unweight the damaged cartilage and reduce pain.
- The prognosis for patients with malalignment and joint arthritis is not as good as that for patients who did not present with arthritis.

PATIENT HISTORY AND PHYSICAL FINDINGS

History

- The surgeon should obtain information about the type of bony and soft tissue injury, surgical procedures performed, history of infection, and the use of antibiotics.
- High-energy injuries and open fractures are at a higher risk for infection.
- Information about back pain, perceived LLD, use of a shoe lift, and deformity should be elicited from the patient.
- The presence of deformity will often lead patients to report feeling increased pressure on the medial or lateral part of the foot with a valgus or varus deformity respectively.
- A short leg will often lead to complaints of low back pain and contralateral hip pain.
- If antibiotics are being used to manage an infected nonunion, an attempt should be made to discontinue these for 6 weeks before surgery to obtain reliable intraoperative culture samples. Discontinuation of antibiotics must be done with caution and careful observation, particularly in compromised patients like those with diabetes or on immunosuppressive medications.
- The current amount of pain, the use of narcotics, and the ability to walk with or without support should be noted.

Physical Examination

- The surgeon should look for deformity and LLD with the patient standing still and walking.
- Inability to bear weight suggests an unstable nonunion.
- The view from the back is helpful to identify a coronal plane deformity.
- LLD is evaluated by using blocks under the short leg and by examining the level of the iliac crests.
- The view from the side is helpful to observe sagittal plane deformity and equinus contracture. The combination of recurvatum deformity above the ankle and equinus contracture of the ankle will lead to a foot translated forward position, with an extension moment on the knee.
- The range of motion of the ankle, subtalar joint, forefoot, and toes should be recorded.
- Compensation for ankle deformity through the subtalar joint is an important factor. For varus deformity, the subtalar joint will slide into valgus. For valgus deformity, the subtalar joint will slide into varus. These compensatory deformities of the subtalar joint may become rigid and irreducible; this typically occurs with longstanding ankle deformity.
- If hindfoot deformity is present, it must be taken into account when correcting the ankle.
- The condition of the soft tissue envelope, especially previous surgical wounds and flaps, and neurovascular findings should be recorded. This includes the posterior tibial and dorsalis pedis pulses, foot sensation, and dorsiflexion and plantarflexion motor function of the ankle and toes.
  - Patients with poor pulses are sent for further vascular testing.
  - Many patients with Charcot joint destruction have apparently normal sensation to light touch.
- Rotational deformity is best assessed on clinical examination with the patient in the prone position.
  - The thigh–foot axis is used to assess rotational deformity of the tibia.
  - The rotational profile of the femur on examination is used to assess rotational deformity in the femur. CT scan can also be used for this purpose. CT scan cuts at the proximal femur, distal femur, proximal tibia, and distal tibia allow analysis of rotational deformity.[17,23]

IMAGING AND OTHER DIAGNOSTIC STUDIES

- Radiographs should include AP, lateral, and mortise views of the ankle, a Saltzman view of both feet (**FIG 1**), and a 51-inch bipedal erect leg radiograph including the hips to ankles with blocks under the short leg to level the pelvis.
- LLD and limb alignment can be measured from a standing bipedal 51-inch radiograph. The short leg is placed on blocks to level the pelvis, and the height of the blocks is recorded.[16,17] This can be performed with the patient using crutches if necessary.
- These radiographs yield crucial information about LLD, deformity, presence of hardware, arthritis, and bony union.
- A supine scanogram can also be used to measure length discrepancy, but this is not useful for alignment analysis.
- CT scan and MRI can be used for further evaluation as needed.
  - CT scan can provide more information about bony union.
  - MRI can be provide information about the condition of cartilage in the ankle and subtalar joints, and the presence of infection.
- Nuclear medicine studies can also be used, but we have not found them to be very helpful in this evaluation.
- Laboratory studies including white blood cell count, erythrocyte sedimentation rate, and C- reactive protein can help to diagnose the presence of infection.

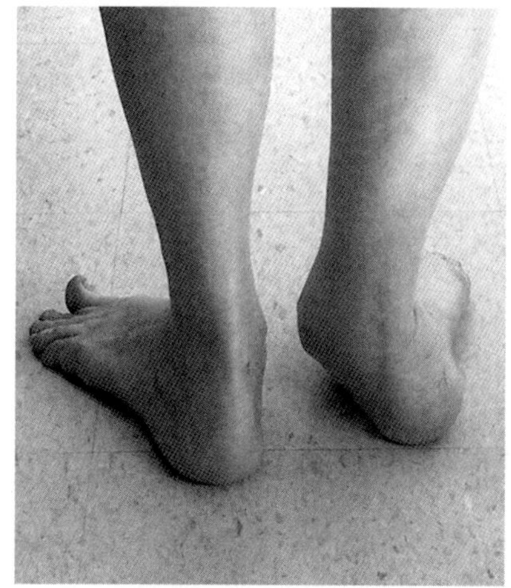

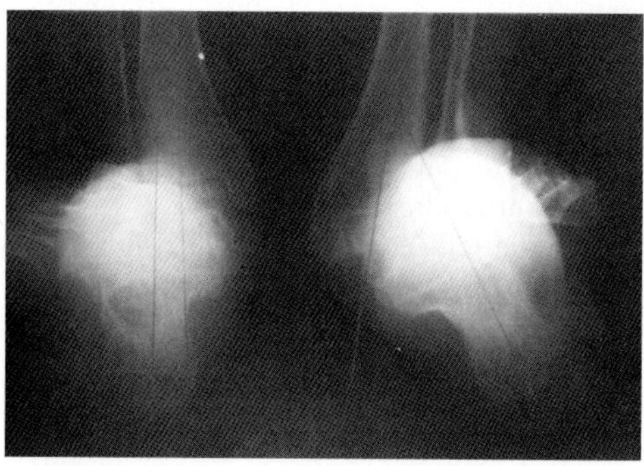

FIG 1 • Clinical photograph (**A**) of advanced hindfoot valgus and Saltzman (**B**) view of the same patient allowing for an objective measure of deformity severity.

- Selective lidocaine injections into the ankle and subtalar joints may help to diagnose the main source of pain.

DIFFERENTIAL DIAGNOSIS

- Ankle fusion malunion
- Joint contracture
- Joint deformity without distal tibial deformity (fixed or dynamic)

NONOPERATIVE MANAGEMENT

- Nonoperative management is not recommended because chronic deformity will lead to further ankle joint degeneration.
- Bracing is commonly employed to control pain associated with malalignment and arthritis.
- Some malalignment is accompanied by ankle ligamentous instability. For example, varus ankle deformity may lead to instability of the lateral ankle ligaments. Bracing will help provide stability but cannot correct the underlying bony deformity.
- Bone realignment will, however, reduce instability and obviate the need for bracing in most cases.

SURGICAL MANAGEMENT

Preoperative Planning

- The deformity is measured on AP radiographs (**FIG 2A**).
- The proximal tibial axis is represented with a mid-diaphyseal tibial line. The distal tibial axis is represented with a perpendicular line to the ankle joint drawn retrograde

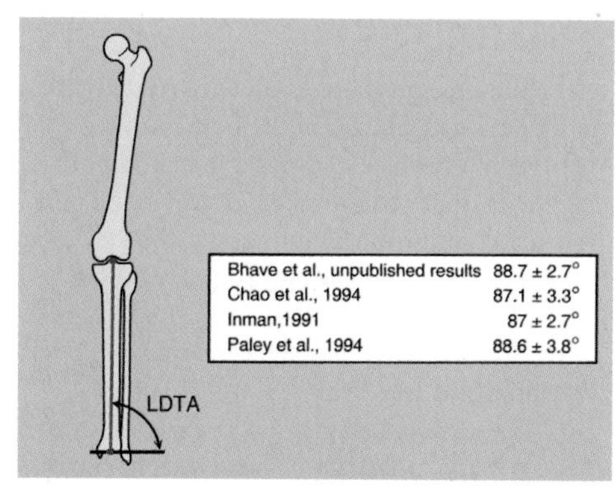

Bhave et al., unpublished results	88.7 ± 2.7°
Chao et al., 1994	87.1 ± 3.3°
Inman,1991	87 ± 2.7°
Paley et al., 1994	88.6 ± 3.8°

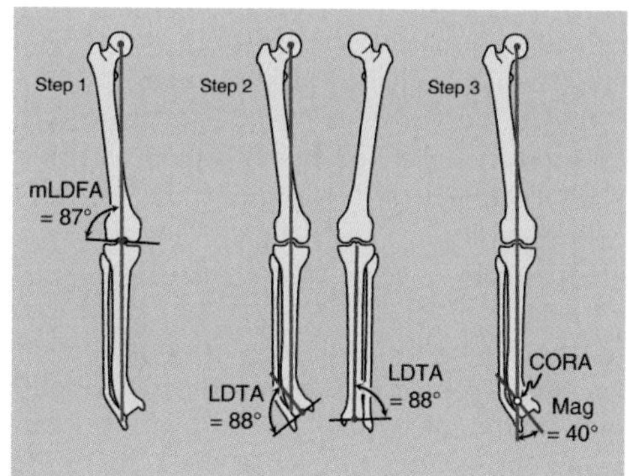

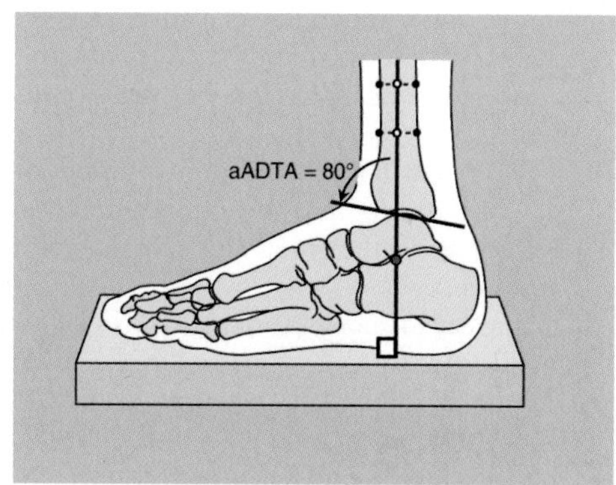

FIG 2 • **A.** Lateral distal tibial angle measurement and variations. **B.** How to find the center of rotation and angulation (CORA) of a distal tibial deformity, which will in turn help calculate the correct amount of translation needed at the osteotomy site. **C.** Normal anterior distal tibial angle. *(continued)*

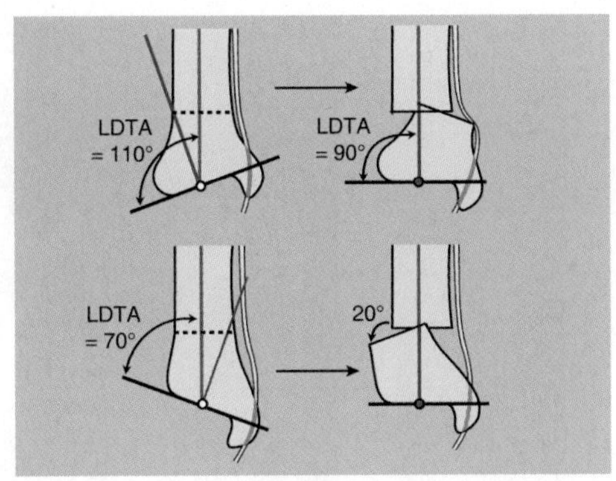

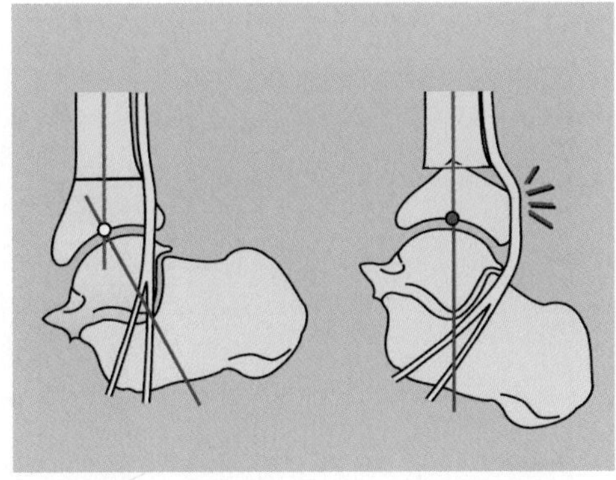

FIG 2 • *(continued)* **D.** Upper diagram demonstrates stretching of the tibial nerve with varus corrections. Valgus correction through the distal tibia does not stretch the same nerve (*lower diagram*). Both diagrams highlight proper translation needed to align the ankle under the tibia. This procurvatum deformity (**E**) results in symptomatic impingement of the talus on the anterior tibia with the ankle in the neutral position. Correction of this very distal procurvatum deformity with proper translation will stretch the tibial nerve significantly. One should consider gradual correction or tarsal tunnel release with an acute correction. (Reprinted with permission from Dror Paley. Principles of Deformity Correction. Springer-Verlag, 2003.)

(normal lateral distal tibial angle is 90 degrees). The intersection of these lines is the apex of deformity (**FIG 2B**).

- In the sagittal plane, the distal tibial axis is drawn 80 degrees to the lateral joint line (a normal anterior distal tibial angle is 80 degrees) (**FIG 2C**). The intersection of these lines is the apex of deformity.
- The rotational deformity is assessed from the tibiofemoral angle measured on physical examination. If the osteotomy is at the level of the CORA, no translation is needed. If the osteotomy is done at a level that is different from the CORA, then translation at the osteotomy site will be needed to fully correct the deformity (**FIG 2D,E**).[16,17]
- Either acute or gradual correction of a nonunion or malunion can be used.[20,21]
  - Acute correction can be performed in conjunction with all methods of fixation, including plates,[3,26] intramedullary nails, and external fixation frames.
  - Gradual correction requires the use of specialized frames.
- The personality of the problems helps guide the surgeon toward the best method. For example, a distal tibial malunion with 15 degrees of valgus deformity and 2 cm of shortening is best handled with an osteotomy to gradually correct the angular deformity and lengthen the bone with a specialized frame.
- The Ilizarov method allows gradual correction of all the components of deformity with distraction osteogenesis.
- One may choose to perform the deformity correction and lengthening at one level if bone regeneration potential is good (**FIG 3A,B**).
- Alternatively, one may choose to perform a double-level osteotomy: one level at the CORA[16] for deformity correction, and one level for lengthening in the proximal tibia metaphysis (**FIG 3C**).
- Gradual correction achieves lengthening and carries less risk of posterior tibial nerve stretch neuropraxia than if attempted with an acute correction.
- The use of plates and intramedullary nails requires an acute correction of angular and translational deformity. Acute corrections are particularly useful for modest deformity correction, mobile atrophic nonunions that are opened and bone grafted, and small bone defects that can be acutely shortened.
- The principal advantage of acute correction is earlier bone contact for healing and a simpler fixation construct.
- Acute corrections are generally better tolerated in the femur and humerus, and less well tolerated in the tibia and ankle, given the possible issues of neurovascular insult.
- Gradual correction with a specialized frame is useful for large deformity correction,[13,22,28] poor skin, associated limb lengthening, bone transport to treat segmental defects,[24] and stiff hypertrophic nonunion repair.[21]
- Gradual correction employs the principle of distraction osteogenesis, commonly referred to as the Ilizarov method.[9,15]
  - Bone and soft tissue are gradually distracted at a rate of about 1 mm per day in divided increments.
  - Bone growth in the distraction gap is called *regenerate.*
  - The interval between osteotomy and the start of lengthening is called the *latency phase* and is usually 7 to 10 days.
  - The correction and lengthening is called the *distraction phase.*
  - The *consolidation phase* is the time from the end of distraction until bony union.[9] This phase is most variable and is most affected by patient factors such as age and health.
- If the structure at risk is a nerve, such as the tibial nerve for an equinovarus deformity of the ankle, gradual correction may be the safer option. The correction can be planned so that the structure at risk is stretched slowly (**FIG 4**). If nerve symptoms do occur, the correction can be slowed or stopped. Neurolysis can be employed in select situations based on the response to gradual correction.[17]

Positioning

- The patient is given spinal-epidural anesthesia with intravenous sedation.
- The patient is then positioned supine on the operating table.

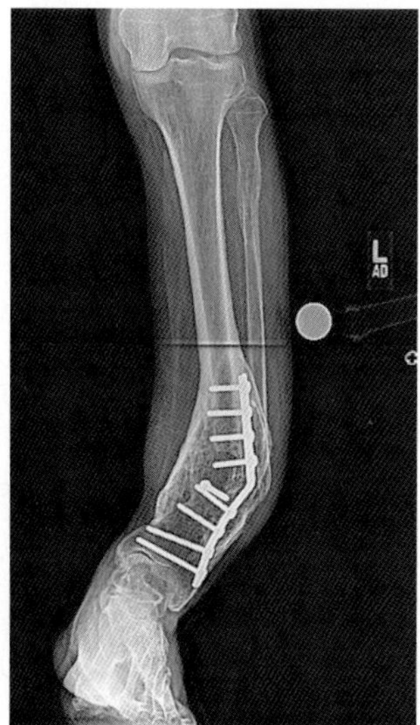

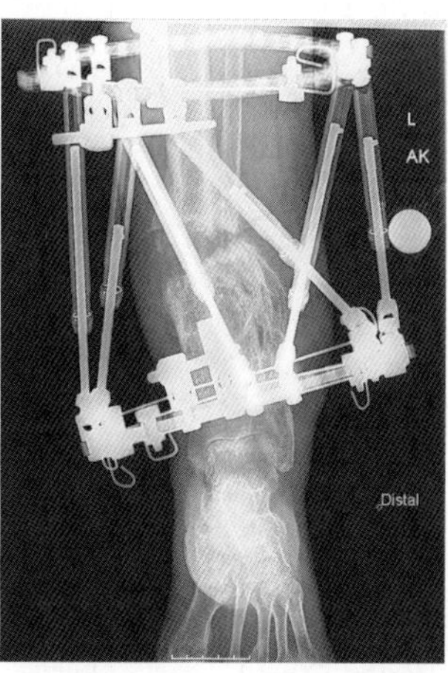

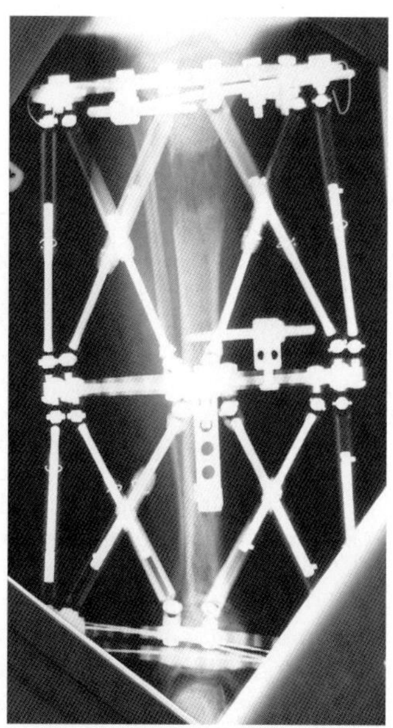

A B C

FIG 3 • A large distal varus deformity seen radiographically (**A**). Surgical reconstruction consisted of tibial osteotomy proximal to the center of rotation and angulation (CORA) (to avoid poor skin distal to the CORA). A gradual correction was employed with the Taylor Spatial Frame (**B**). Further translation may be performed by simply running a residual deformity correction to fine-tune the alignment. **C.** A supramalleolar osteotomy is accompanied by a proximal tibial osteotomy for lengthening. This technique allows lengthening to occur in a reliable location and brings more blood flow to the compromised distal tibia, which may accelerate the distal healing rate.

- A soft bump is placed under the ipsilateral buttock until the patella is facing upward.
- A well-padded pneumatic tourniquet is then placed around the thigh and set for 250 mm Hg.
- Two sterile bumps are during the frame application, one under the knee and the other under the heel. This will elevate the leg off the bed to accommodate the Ilizarov rings.

Approach

- The approach for the SMO will be anteromedial but can be altered somewhat depending on the skin condition about the ankle.
- The approach for the fibular osteotomy is direct lateral and at the same level as the tibial osteotomy.

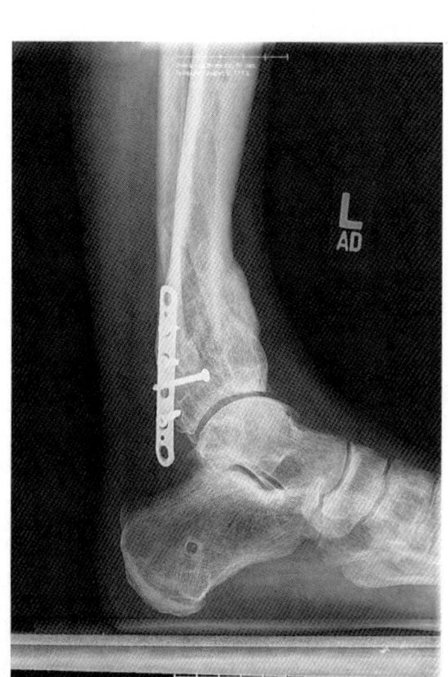

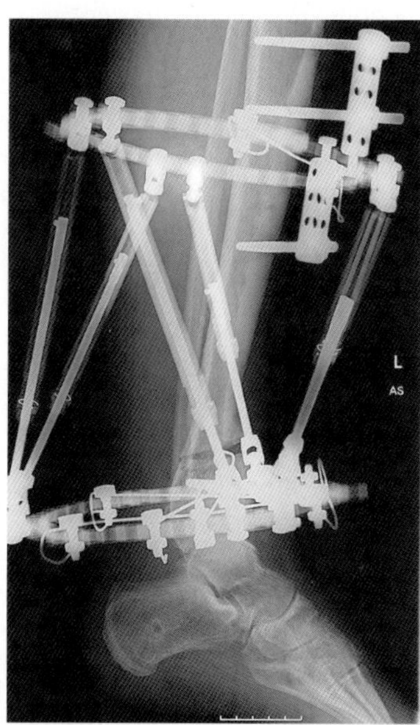

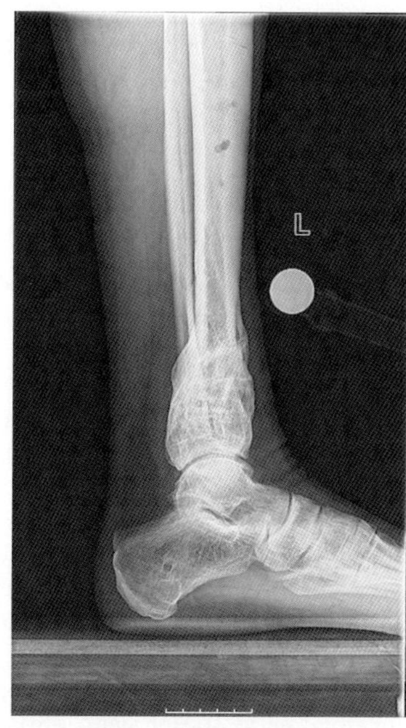

A B C

FIG 4 • A distal tibial malunion with a recurvatum deformity leaves the talus uncovered and often leads to equinus contracture of the ankle (**A**). Supramalleolar osteotomy with the Taylor Spatial Frame demonstrates an effective correction of alignment (**B,C**).

FIBULAR OSTEOTOMY

- Osteotomy of the fibula is usually performed with the use of a tourniquet at the beginning of the procedure before frame application. The leg is exsanguinated and the thigh tourniquet is inflated to 250 mm Hg.
- A small lateral exposure is a simple and safe way to approach the fibula. It is best to locate the osteotomy at or near the apex of deformity. Consider not performing the fibular cut at exactly the same level as the tibial cut to avoid formation of a synostosis.
- Cut the bone with an oscillating saw or an osteotome. Alternatively, the fibula can be fractured through the tibial osteotomy site.
- Once the tibial osteotomy is performed, keep the osteotome in the wound, redirect it posteriorly and laterally, toward the fibula, and advance it. This option works well when it is too risky to make a lateral incision.
- The shape of the osteotomy may be transverse or oblique.
  - When correcting valgus deformity gradually, a transverse osteotomy is performed. As the tibia is corrected, the fibula will be distracted and the gap will fill in with regenerate.
  - When correcting varus deformity, the fibula will need to be shortened.[8,14,22] This is accomplished with either fibula resection or an oblique osteotomy where the fragments can overlap.
- Do not close the fascia.
- Close the skin in layers.

FRAME APPLICATION: WIRE AND PIN CONFIGURATION

- Tensioned Kirschner wires and half-pins lend roughly the same stability to the frame.
- The proximal ring or ring block is secured with three or four points of fixation.
- When using the Taylor Spatial Frame one ring will suffice, as these rings are quite sturdy and deflection is minimal.
- Release the tourniquet before applying the external fixator.
- We typically use one 1.8-mm Kirschner wire as a reference wire from anterolateral to posteromedial (medial face wire) for purposes of mounting the ring. This wire is placed about 150 to 180 mm proximal to the ankle joint.
- Select the ring diameter according to the size of the leg. Ideally we leave 2 cm of space between the skin and the leg circumferentially.
- Secure the ring to the wire and tension the wire to 130 kg.
- Secure additional fixation with half-pins placed in slightly different planes.
- Make a pilot hole with a 4.8-mm drill bit through both cortices.
- 6-mm hydroxyapatite (HA)-coated pins are our first choice for adult patients.
- Use tall Rancho cubes to spread the fixation and achieve maximal stability.
- The distal tibial ring is usually secured with two or three 1.8-mm Kirschner wires (tensioned to 130 kg) and a half-pin.
- Place the reference wire in the tibia parallel to the ankle joint line and proximal to the ankle joint. Attach the ring proximal to the wire and tension the wire to 130 kg.
- Next, insert a fibula–tibia wire posterolateral to anteromedial to stabilize the syndesmosis and prevent fibula migration. The ring is oriented on the lateral radiograph to be perpendicular to the sagittal plane tibial anatomic axis (not parallel to the ankle joint line, as seen on the lateral view). A posteromedial to anterolateral wire can also be added.
- Finally, use an anteromedial (medial to the tibialis anterior tendon) to posterolateral 6-mm half-pin to add stability in the sagittal plane (**TECH FIG 1**).
- Fixation may be extended across the ankle to the foot if additional stability of the distal segment is needed.

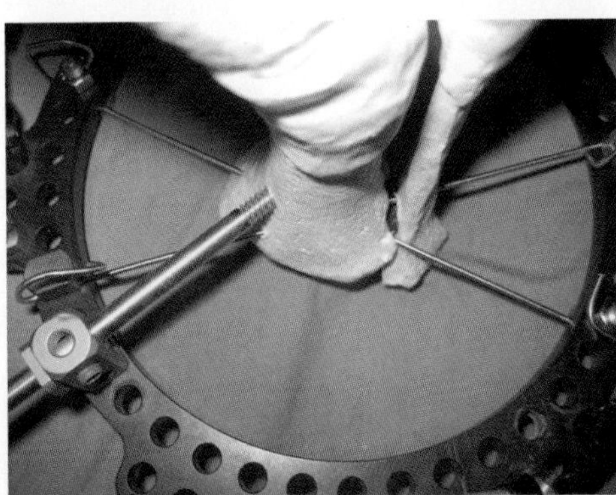

TECH FIG 1 • This sawbones model shows the typical fixation arrangement for the distal tibia with two tensioned wires and one half-pin.

TAYLOR SPATIAL FRAME

- The advantages of this frame over the classic Ilizarov frame are numerous. The application is easier and the fit on the leg is better when using the rings first method. Also, residual deformity at the lengthening and docking sites can be addressed by using the same frame to correct angulation and translation simultaneously in the coronal, sagittal, and axial planes without major frame modification. This minimizes angular deformity at the lengthening sites.[4,5]

- The rings have now been placed on either side of the deformity site and the anticipated lengthening site or sites. The rings have been placed independently to optimally fit the leg. This is called the *rings first method.*
- One ring is chosen as the reference ring for each level of movement, and this ring must be placed orthogonal (perpendicular) to the axis of the tibia.
- The "virtual hinge" around which the correction occurs is defined by the *origin* and the *corresponding point* (CP). The origin is a point chosen on the edge of one bone segment at the defect site. A CP on the other bone segment is chosen with the goal of reducing the CP to the origin.
- *Mounting parameters* define the location of the origin relative to the reference ring. Mounting parameters are defined by the spatial relationship between the center of the reference ring and the origin in the coronal, sagittal, and axial planes. This defines a virtual hinge around which the deformity correction will occur. Struts are used to connect the rings across the deformity.
- It is important to maintain enough distance between rings so that the struts can fit properly. In this frame, one is limited by the shortest length of strut.

Deformity Parameters

- Six deformity parameters describe the relationship between the proximal segment and the distal segment (the reference segment has the origin and the moving segment has the corresponding point) (**TECH FIG 2A,B**).
- Deformity parameters consist of an angulation and a translation in the coronal, sagittal, and axial planes.
  - In the coronal plane, the angulation is varus or valgus and the translation is medial or lateral.
  - In the sagittal plane, the angulation is apex anterior or apex posterior and the translation is anterior or posterior.
  - In the axial plane, the angulation is internal or external rotation, and the translation is short or long.

Mounting Parameters

- Since the Taylor frame enables correction around a virtual hinge, the surgeon must communicate its location (origin) to the computer program (**TECH FIG 2C**).
- A grid projected from the reference ring allows the surgeon to specify the location of the origin. The location of the origin relative to the center of the reference ring in the coronal, sagittal, and axial planes is recorded.[25]
- For example, the center of the reference ring may be 10 mm lateral, 25 mm posterior, and 35 mm distal to the origin.

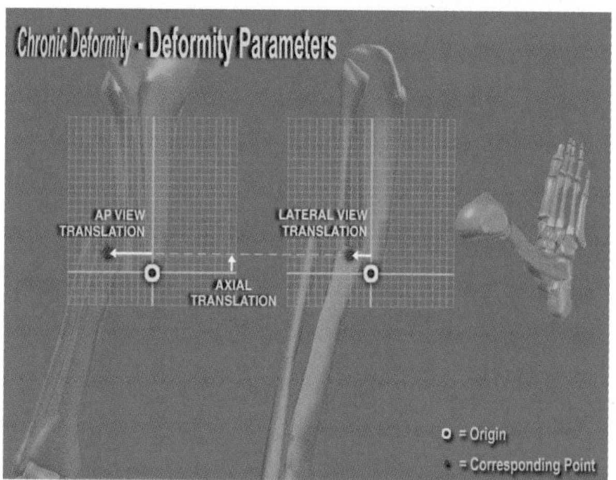

A

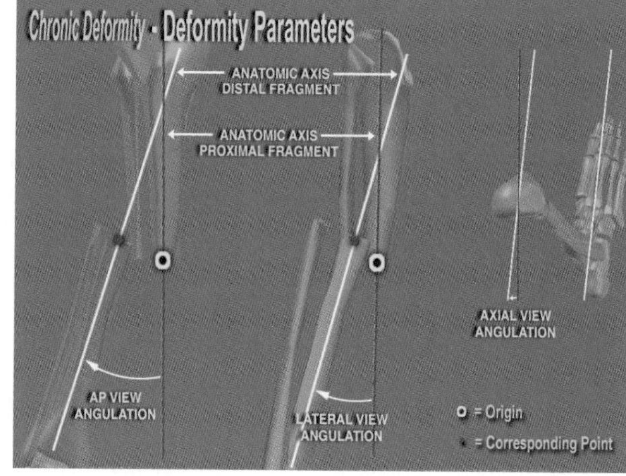

B

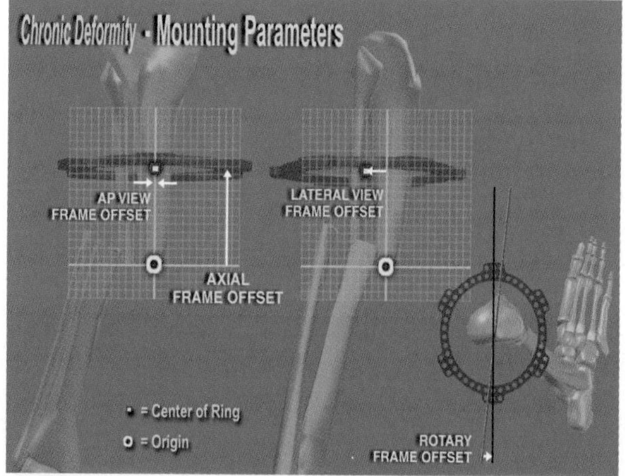

C

TECH FIG 2 • Taylor Spatial Frame concept and language. **A.** Measurement of translation deformity parameters. **B.** Measurement of angulation deformity parameters. **C.** Measurement of mounting parameters. *(continued)*

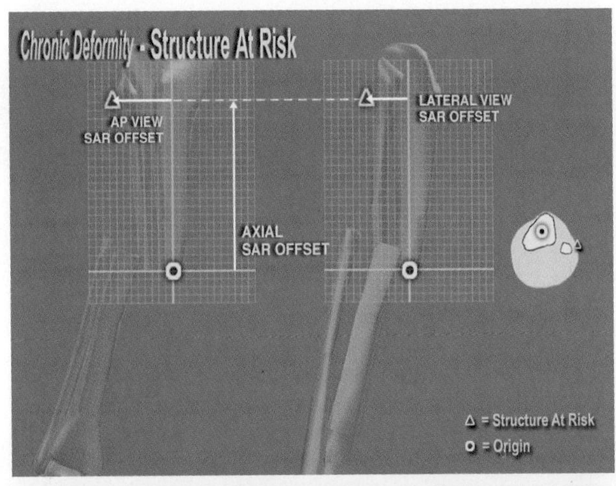

D

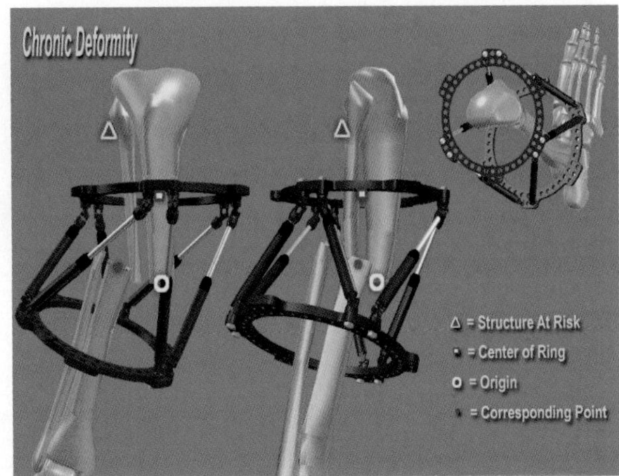

E

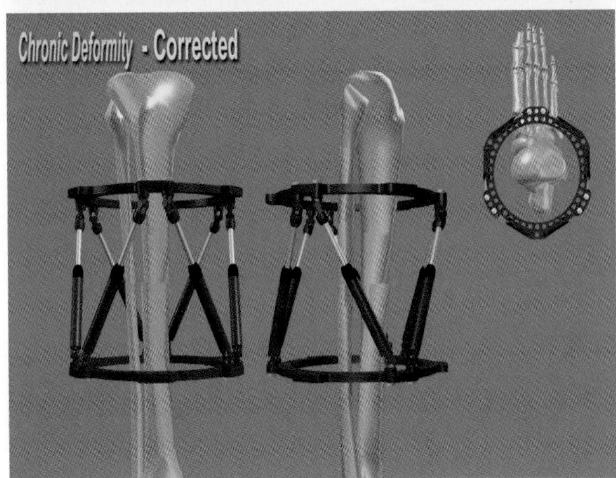

F

TECH FIG 2 • *(continued)* **D.** Structure at risk relative to origin. **E.** Before correction. **F.** After correction. (Reprinted with permission from Charles Taylor, MD.)

Structure at Risk

- The surgeon determines the speed of the correction by choosing a structure that he or she wants to move at a determined rate. Typically a structure in the concavity of the deformity is the structure at risk (SAR) (TECH FIG 2D–F).
- For example, if we are correcting a varus deformity, the SAR may be the medial cortex of the tibia or the posterior tibial nerve. If we are correcting a valgus, recurvatum deformity, the SAR will be the anterolateral surface of the tibia.
- We usually move the SAR at 1 mm per day,[25] although this can be varied.

SUPRAMALLEOLAR TIBIAL OSTEOTOMY

- After the frame has been mounted on the intact tibia, the tibial osteotomy is performed.
- Record the strut connections between the rings and then remove them.
- Perform the SMO through a 1-cm skin incision, medial to the tibialis anterior tendon and about 1 cm proximal to the distal tibial pins. This will typically place the osteotomy at the metaphyseal–diaphyseal junction about 5 cm proximal to the ankle joint.
- If the CORA is closer to the joint, then appropriate translation of the bone ends must be performed to prevent a translational deformity after correcting the angular deformity.
- The C-arm fluoroscope is positioned in the lateral position.
- Use a multiple drill hole osteotomy technique.
- Pass a 4.8-mm drill bit three times along the plane of the planned osteotomy line (TECH FIG 3A). Complete the SMO by passing the osteotome across the medial cortex and lateral cortex and through the bone center to crack the posterior cortex (TECH FIG 3B).
- Rotation of the osteotome and ultimately rotation of the rings completes the osteotomy. Alternatively, a Gigli saw technique can be used to perform the SMO.
- These are low-energy and low-heat techniques that will minimize bone and periosteal injury and optimize good regenerate bone formation. We believe that osteotomy with an oscillating saw will increase the risk of thermal necrosis to the bone.

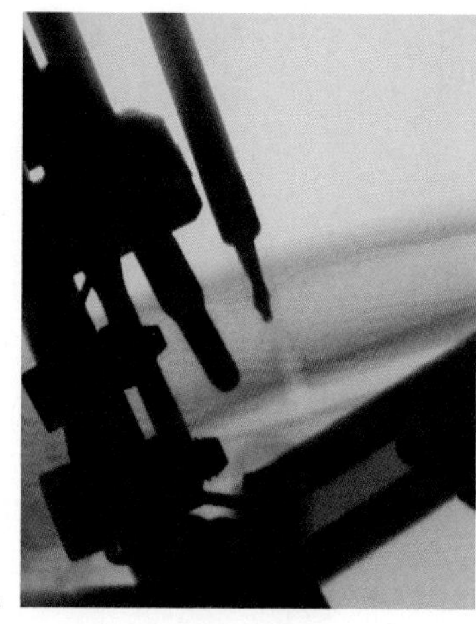

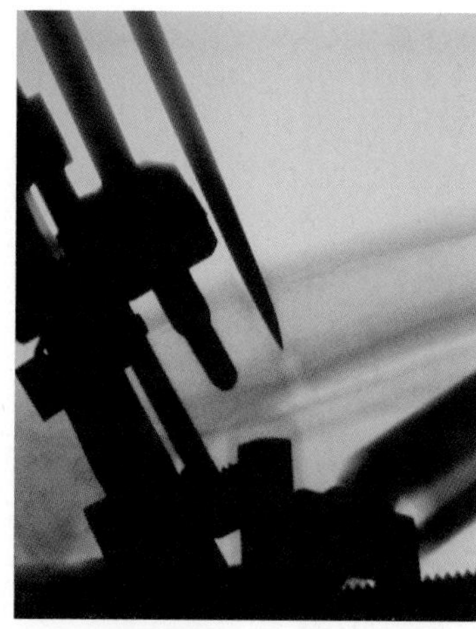

TECH FIG 3 • **A.** This intraoperative fluoroscopy film shows the 4.8-mm drill being passed in the plane of the planned osteotomy. **B.** A 7-mm osteotome is now being inserted along the same path as the drill holes.

FRAME EXTENSION ACROSS THE ANKLE

- If there is an ankle contracture, then a foot ring is placed, and gradual correction of the ankle deformity can be performed simultaneously.
- Hinges are placed along the axis of the ankle joint as is done in ankle distraction arthroplasty. A pulling rod can be placed anterior or a pushing rod posterior to motor the correction.

PROXIMAL TIBIAL OSTEOTOMY

- If there is shortening of the tibia, this can be addressed at the same time as the distal deformity correction.
- An osteotomy at the proximal tibia for lengthening can be done if the bone healing potential at the distal deformity site is not optimal.
- In general, the osteogenic potential of a sclerotic malunion of a distal tibial fracture is limited to deformity correction, and a bone lengthening of any significance should be done through a virgin site. In most cases that means going to the proximal tibia and carrying out an additional osteotomy for tibial lengthening.

EXAMPLE CASE (COURTESY OF MARK E. EASLEY)

- Fifty-five year old woman with a long-standing posttraumatic varus deformity and with a several year history of worsening symptoms (**TECH FIG 4A,B**).
  - Coronal plane deformity only
  - Symptomatic lateral foot overload along with ankle pain (**TECH FIG 4C**)
  - Failed nonoperative management
- Proximal ring block
  - Reference wire placed orthogonally to the tibia with fluoroscopic guidance (**TECH FIG 5A–C**)
    - Thin wire secured but not tensioned at this point (see **TECH FIG 5B,C**)
    - Note that wire is initially placed using power then fully positioned using a mallet (in theory, this will diminish postoperative pin problems)
  - A threaded rod extending proximally from the ring block may prove useful in determining the optimal ring position in relative to the tibial shaft axis (**TECH FIG 5D**)
  - Second thin wire placed at a different ankle than the first (**TECH FIG 5E**)
  - Half pins placed for further support (**TECH FIG 5F,G**)
    - Once half pins placed, thin wires tensioned (**TECH FIG 5H,I**)

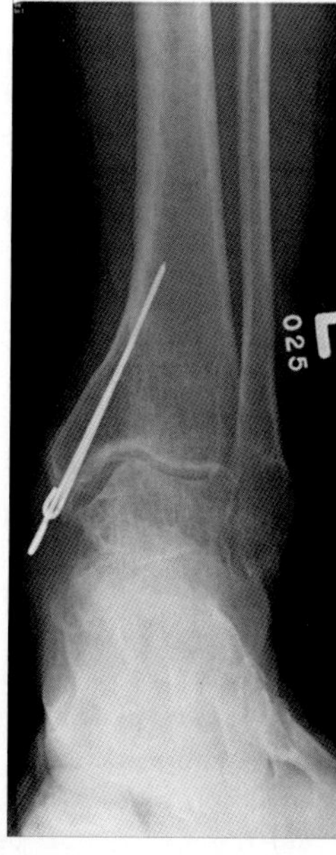

TECH FIG 4 • Preoperative weight-bearing ankle radiographs of 55-year-old woman with coronal plane varus ankle deformity. **A.** AP view. *(continued)*

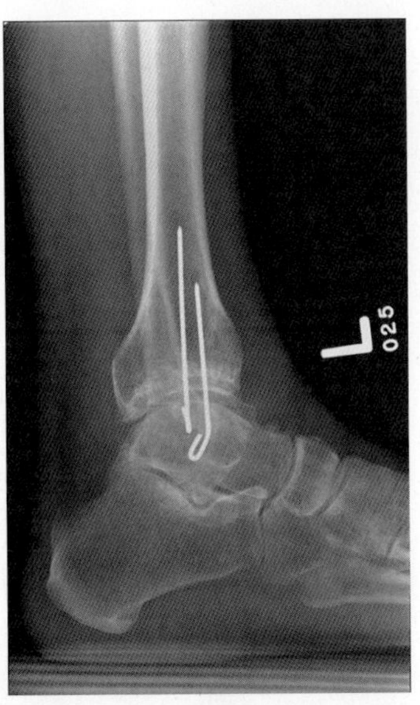

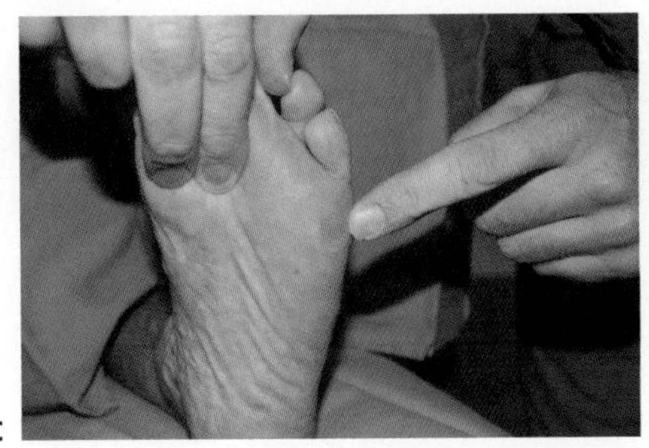

TECH FIG 4 • *(continued)* **B.** Lateral view. **C.** In addition to ankle pain, patient experiences lateral forefoot overload.

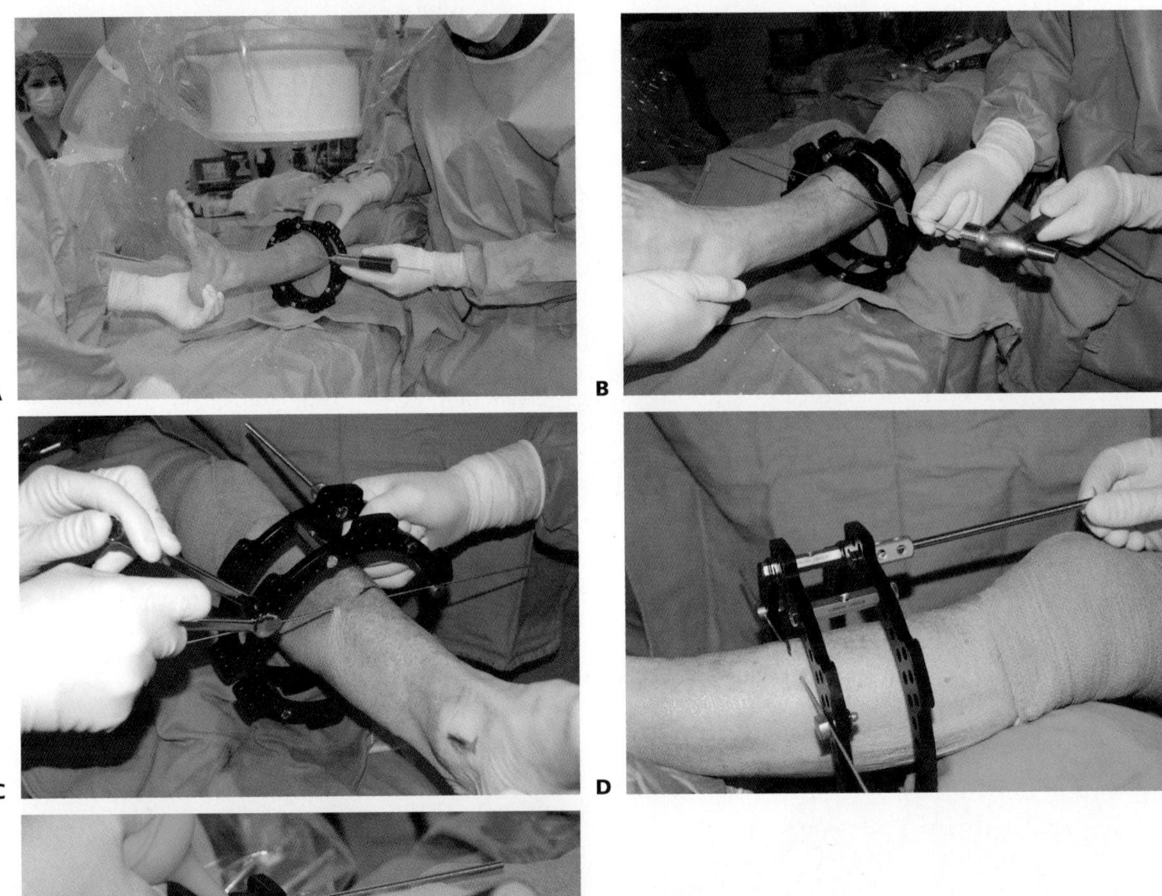

TECH FIG 5 • Proximal ring block. **A.** Reference wire placed under fluoroscopic guidance. **B.** Final position of wire achieved with a mallet to limit heat necrosis. **C.** Tightening the wire to the ring without tensioning at this point. **D.** A threaded rod may be temporarily placed on the proximal ring block to assist in sagittal plane position of the proximal ring block. **E.** Second thin wire being placed (note use of cold saline irrigation to limit heat necrosis). *(continued)*

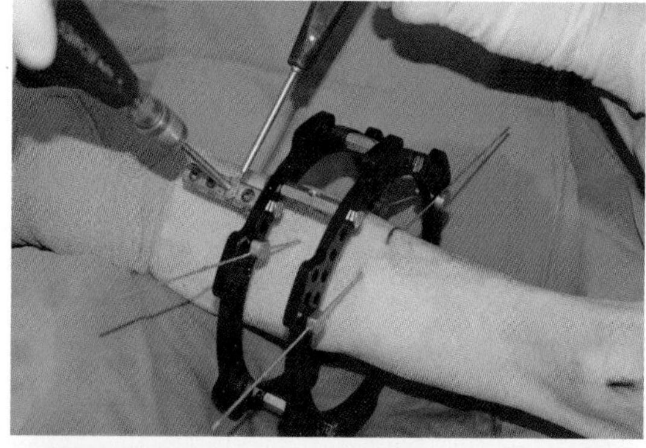

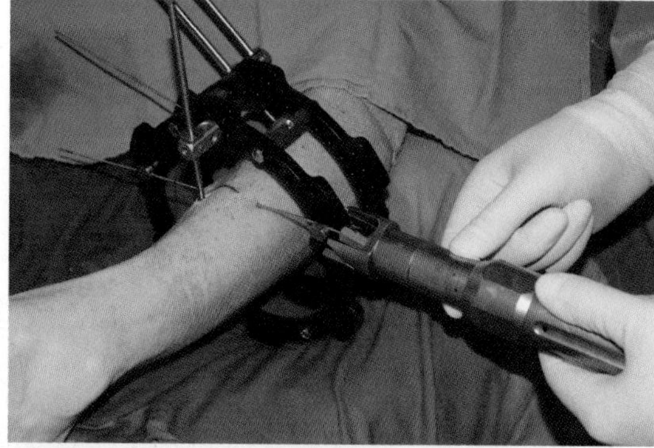

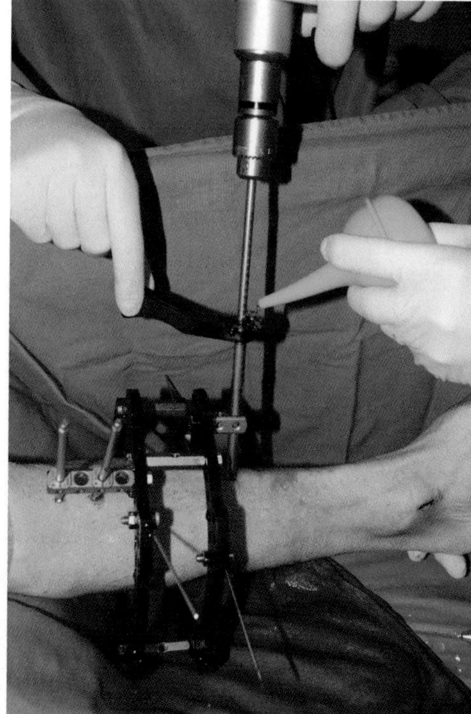

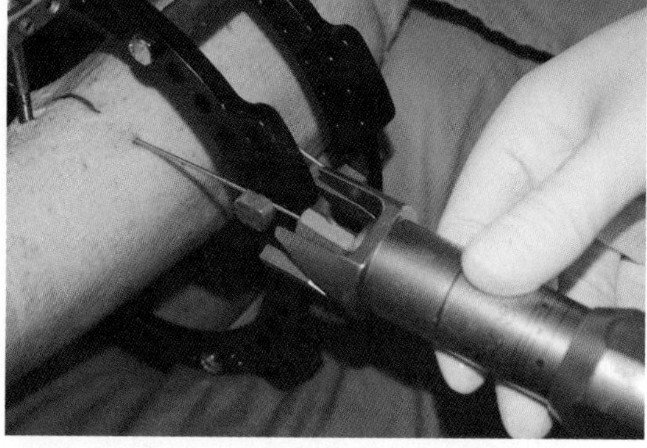

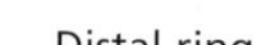

TECH FIG 5 • *(continued)* **F.** Half pins placed. **G.** Cold irrigation used to limit heat necrosis for half pins as well. **H,I.** Tensioning thin wires. **H.** Tensioning device on the proximal ring block. **I.** Close-up of tensioning device (note use of a "socket" in locations where the tensioning device cannot fully contact the ring).

  - Although this may not be in keeping with the Ilizarov principles, the half pins provide support to the ring while the thin wires are tensioned.
- If the tensioner cannot sit well on the frame, then a "socket" from the standard Ilizarov tray may be used to rest on the frame and still tension the thin wire.
- Distal ring
  - Reference wire placed orthogonally to the tibia and parallel to the tibial plafond in the coronal plane (coronal plane deformity only) (**TECH FIG 6A,B**)
  - First thin wire secured but not yet tensioned (**TECH FIG 6C**)

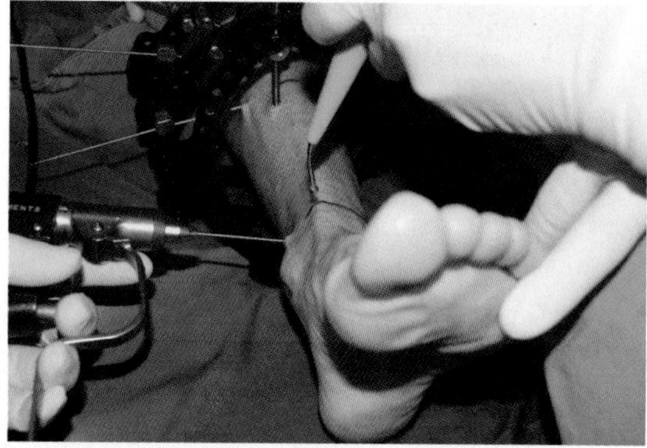

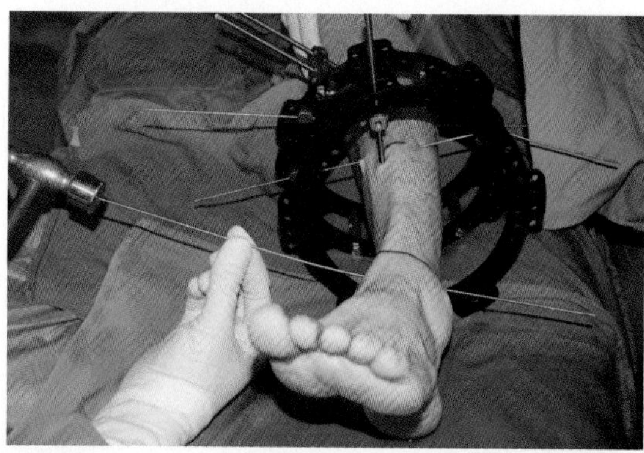

TECH FIG 6 • Reference pin for the distal ring. **A.** Pin place parallel to the tibial plafond (in this case in varus relative to the orthogonally placed proximal ring block. **B.** Final position achieved using a mallet. *(continued)*

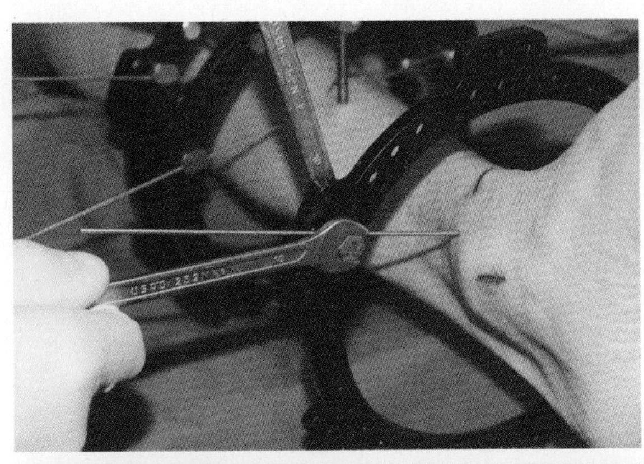

C

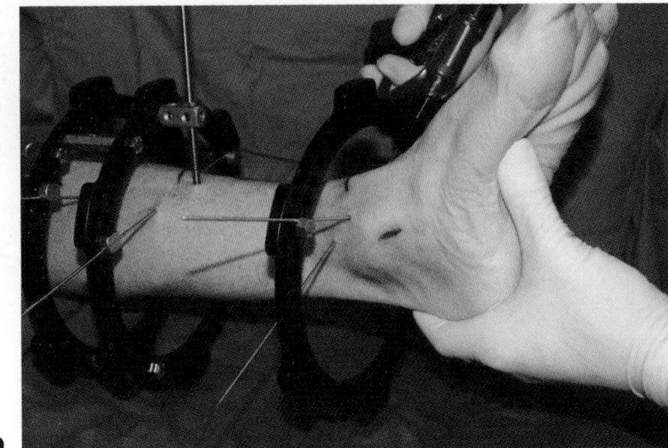

D

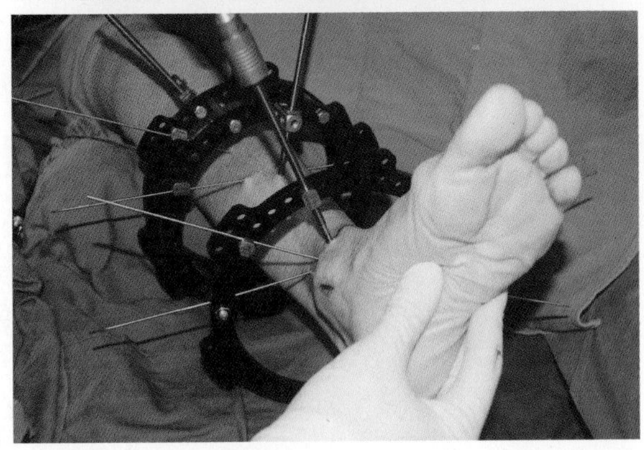

E

TECH FIG 6 • *(continued)* **C–E.** Securing the distal ring. **C.** Tightening the reference wire without tensioning. **D.** A second thin wire. **E.** Half pin added in a safe zone, after which the thin wires are tensioned.

   - Second thin wire placed and secured to the frame (TECH FIG 6D)
   - Half pin placed for further distal ring support (TECH FIG 6E)
   - Thin wires tensioned
- Connecting the struts
   - Struts are attached and each strut setting is recorded
      - This simplifies returning the tibia and fibula to their precorticotomy position after the corticotomy is performed
- Fibular osteotomy (TECH FIG 7)
   - Fibular osteotomy performed through small incision using a microsagittal saw to initiate the cut (the blade is cooled with cold saline) and completed with an osteotome
   - In this case, the fibular osteotomy is routinely performed slightly proximal to the tibial corticotomy for a supramalleolar osteotomy
   - It may have been prudent in this case to perform the oblique osteotomy in the opposite orientation
      - For correction of varus, the distal fibula would have been better contained under the proximal portion
- Supramalleolar tibial corticotomy
   - Minimally invasive approach with minimal periosteal stripping
   - Corticotomy predrilled
      - Larger diameter drill bit to create a defect in anterior cortex (TECH FIG 8A)
      - Smaller diameter drill bit to perform perforations in a single plane (TECH FIG 8B)

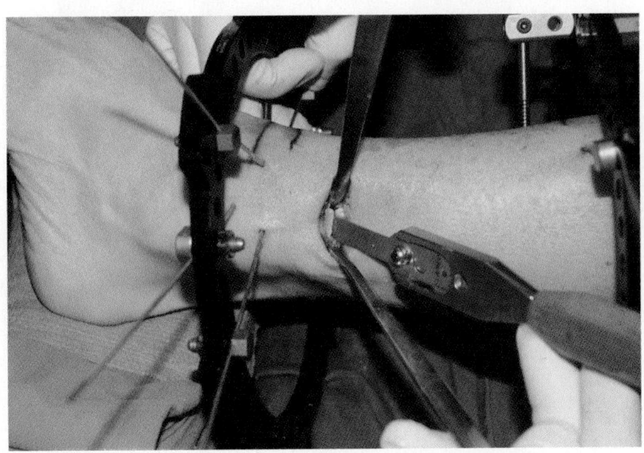

TECH FIG 7 • Fibular osteotomy.

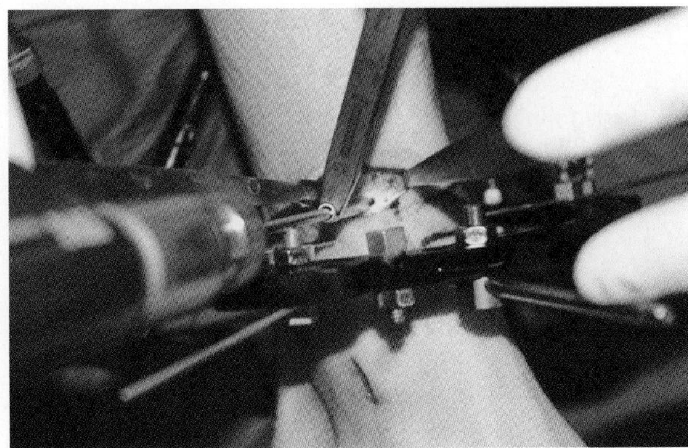

TECH FIG 8 • Tibial corticotomy. **A.** Limited incision through which a drill hole is made in the near cortex. *(continued)*

TECHNIQUES

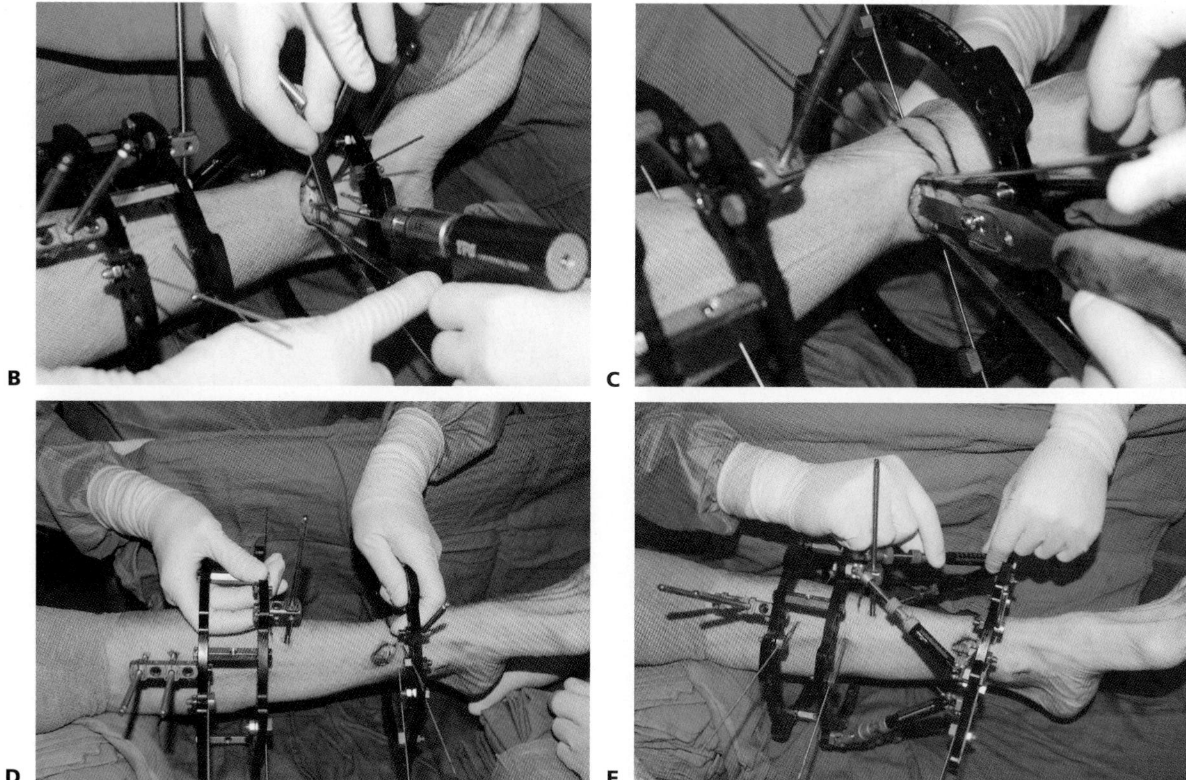

TECH FIG 8 • *(continued)* **B.** Through the initial cortical hole created, the remaining cortex at the same level is perforated with multiple small diameter drill holes. **C.** Corticotomy completed with a chisel (note the surrounding soft tissues are protected but minimal periosteal stripping is performed). **D.** Be sure the tibial corticotomy and fibular osteotomy are complete by rotating the distal and proximal rings in opposite directions. **E.** Secure the struts to connect the proximal and distal rings, spanning the corticotomy. We routinely place the struts prior to performing the corticotomy so that when the corticotomy is completed, we simply reset the struts at the same settings, thereby returning the tibia to its precorticotomy position.

  - Corticotomy completed using an osteotome (TECH FIG 8C)
- Confirming complete corticotomy
  - Once complete, two rings rotated in opposite directions to confirm that the corticotomy is complete (TECH FIG 8D)
- Reconnecting the struts to the precorticotomy position (TECH FIG 8E)
  - Struts are reconnected at the same settings that they were prior to the corticotomy, thereby re-positioning the osteotomy at the precorticotomy orientation
  - allows an appropriate gradual formation of the regenerate
- Early follow-up
  - In this case the single distal ring did not afford adequate stability (TECH FIG 9A,B)
    - This was inspite of several adjustments in the clinic
  - Repeat srugery to add a foot frame that afforded greater stability to the distal ring (block) (TECH FIG 9C,D)
    - In the face of ankle arthritis, slight distraction was added to the construct to distract the ankle.
- Gradual correction
  - Computer program utilized create a gradual correction of the coronal plane deformity (TECH FIG 10A,B)

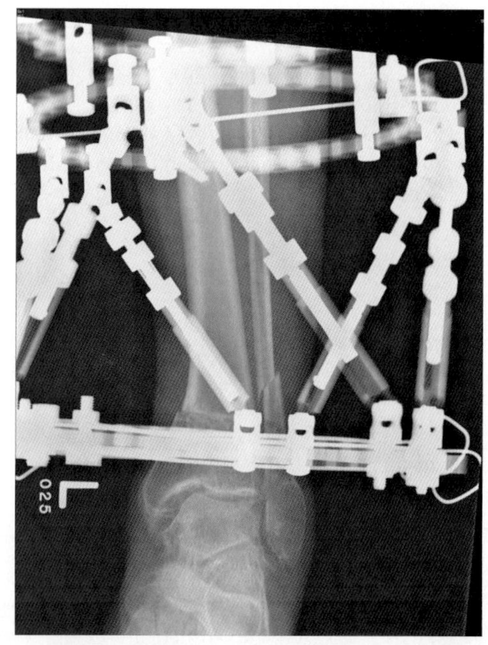

TECH FIG 9 • Early follow-up, in which the corticotomy is unstable despite several attempts at adjustments in the clinic using the Taylor Spatial Frame's dedicated computer software. **A.** AP view. *(continued)*

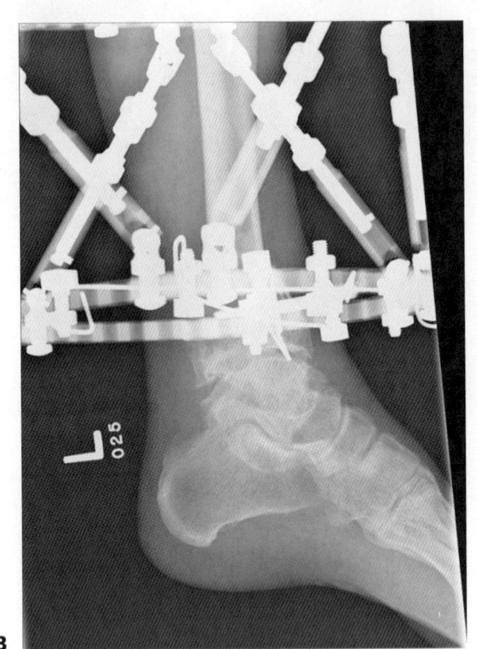

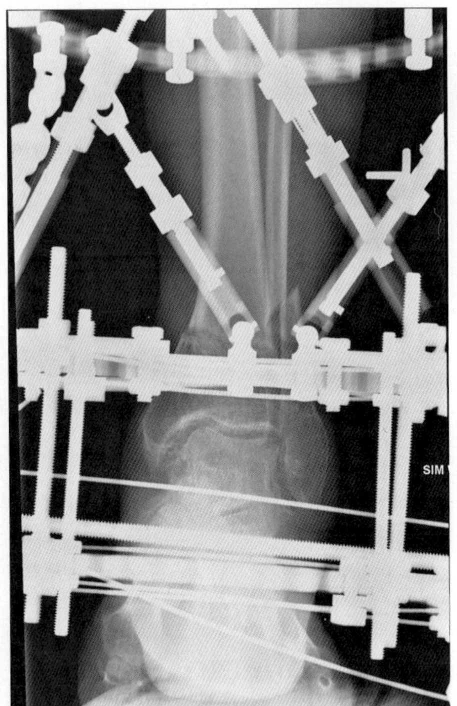

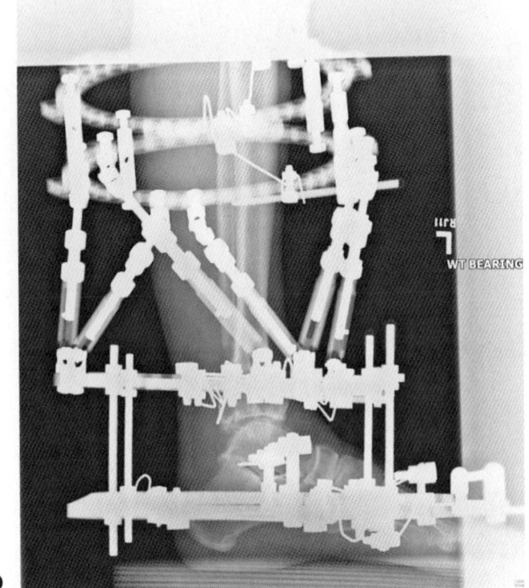

TECH FIG 9 • *(continued)* **B.** Lateral view demonstrates that the distal fragment is displacing anteriorly relative to the proximal fragment. **C,D.** Foot frame added to provide greater stability to the distal ring. **C.** AP view. **D.** Lateral view.

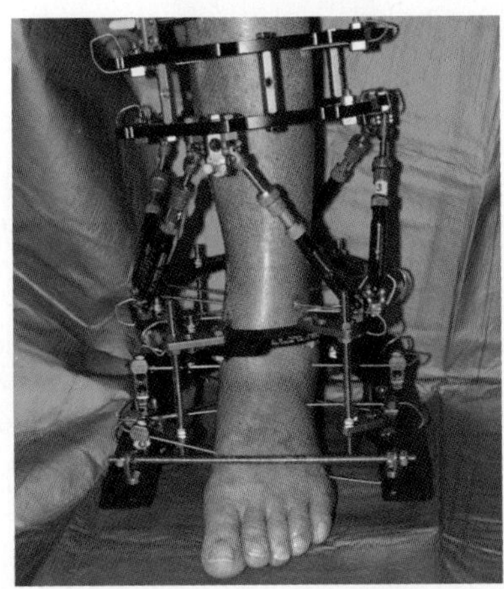

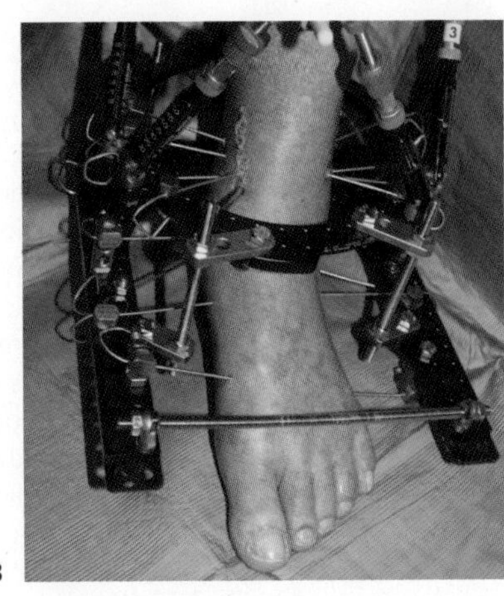

TECH FIG 10 • Further followup after foot frame added. **A,B.** Clinical view of frame now with the foot plate added to stabilize the distal ring. *(continued)*

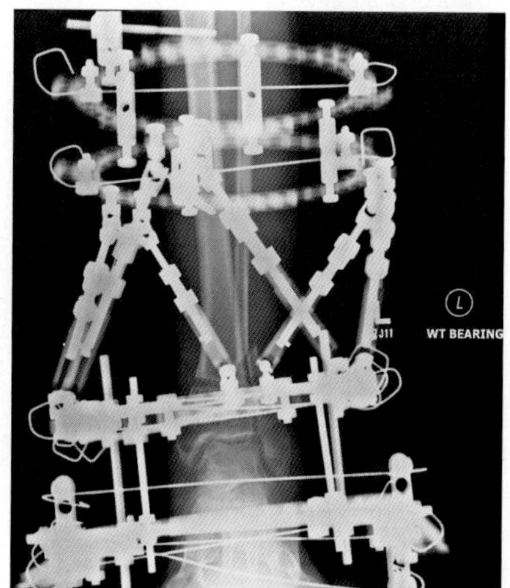

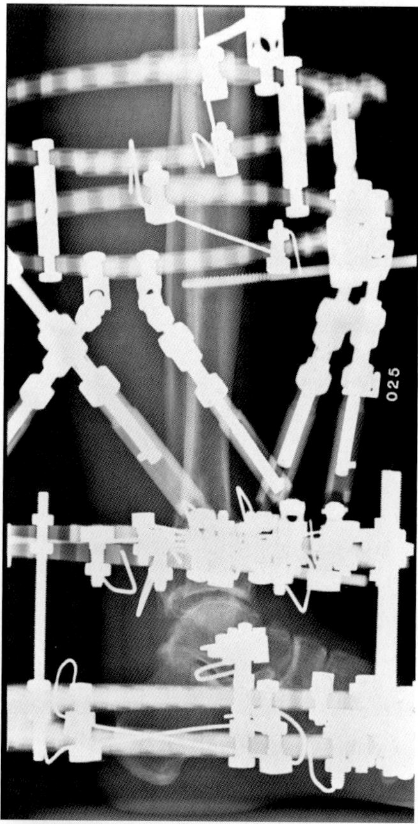

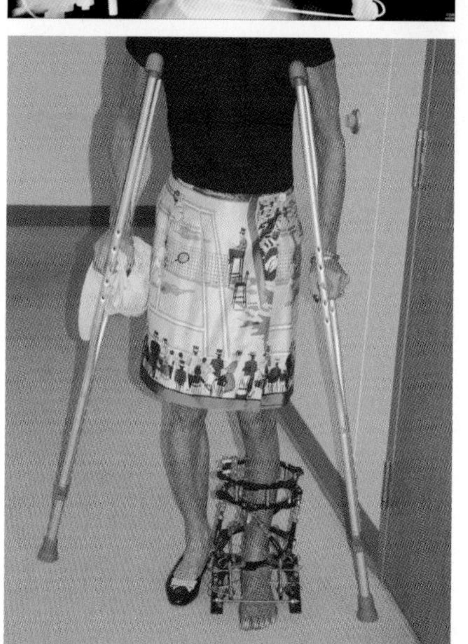

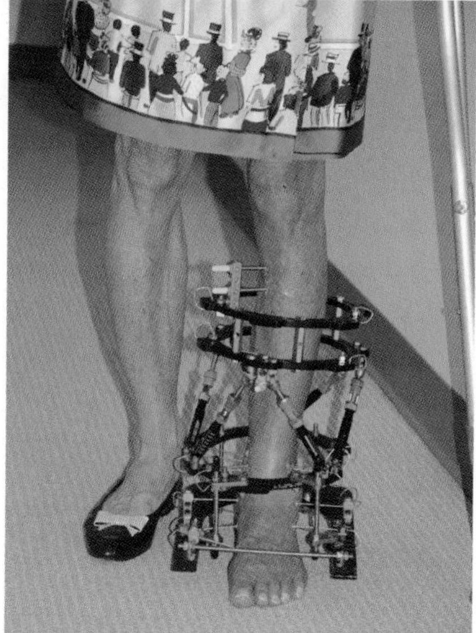

TECH FIG 10 • *(continued)* **C.** AP view (note the regenerate forming as the varus deformity is being gradually corrected). **D.** Lateral view. **E,F.** Patient can determine when the correction is adequate by weight-bearing on the foot as the deformity is being corrected. **E.** Patient weight-bearing with frame (crutches for balance, but patient able to fully bear weight). **F.** Close-up.

  - Radiographic follow-up to confirm that the correction is progressing appropriately with formation of a regenerate (**TECH FIG 10C,D**)
- Determining adequate correction
  - Although radiographs may be used and serve to confirm appropriate correction, simply having the patient stand on the foot as the correction nears completion allows the patient to report if the correction is adequate or if more adjustment is needed (**TECH FIG 10E,F**)
  - This is an advantage over internal fixation where full correction must be performed acutely at the index procedure
- Frame removal
  - Once the patient has achieved appropriate correction and has been weightbearing on the operated foot, follow-up radiographs dictate when the regenerate is consolidated allowing frame removal
- Further follow-up
  - Follow-up radiographs (**TECH FIG 11A,B**)
  - Improved lifestyle with less ankle pain

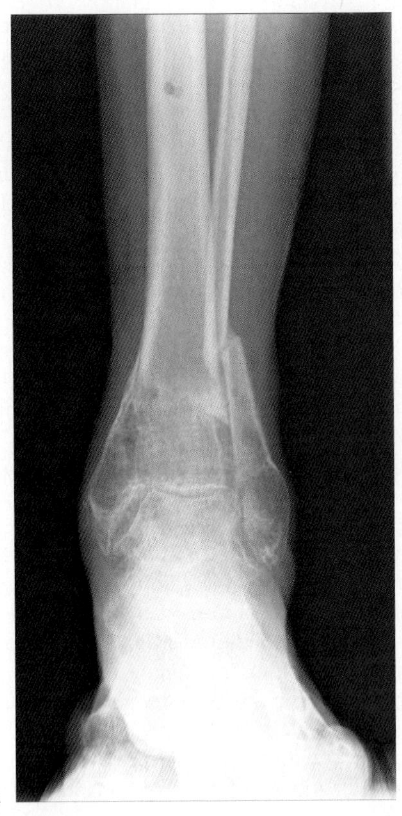

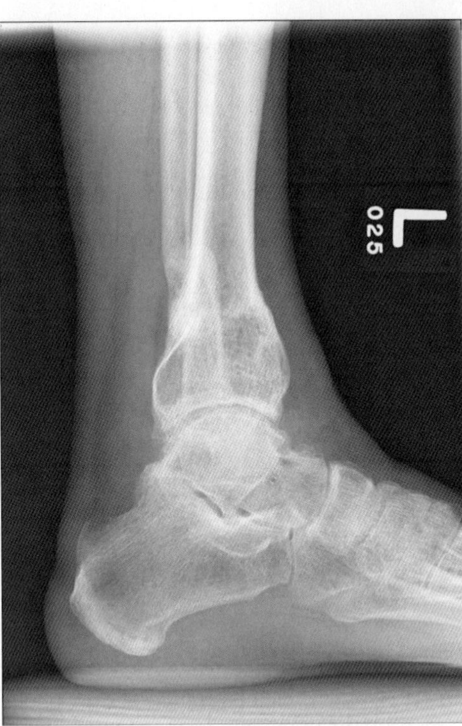

A B

TECH FIG 11 • Final correction after frame removal. **A.** AP view (note congruent alignment of tibial shaft axis and talus, with talus well centered under tibia). **B.** Lateral view also with talus well centered under tibia.

PEARLS AND PITFALLS

Space between the rings	▪ The rings should be about 150 mm apart to allow for use of medium Taylor Spatial Frame struts. Rings further apart will require long struts and will have less control over the bone. If the rings are too close, the shortest Taylor struts might not fit.
Osteotomy translation	▪ If the osteotomy site is not at the CORA, then the surgeon must translate the distal fragment to restore the mechanical axis.
Reference ring	▪ If the distal ring is mounted perfectly, it should be chosen as the reference ring. This is a distal reference system. ▪ Alternatively, the proximal ring can be the reference ring. This is less confusing, the proximal ring is easier to mount perpendicular to the tibia, and it is less likely to bend under stress.
LLD	▪ Best to correct through a separate proximal tibial osteotomy
Low-heat technique	▪ The success of this minimally invasive method relies on the ability to minimize injury to bone and soft tissue. Injury is most likely to occur during drilling and osteotomy. New drill bits are used for each case. Drill flutes are cleaned frequently when used in diaphyseal bone. Frequent pauses are included while drilling. No tourniquet is used during drilling.

POSTOPERATIVE CARE

General

- Patients are admitted to the hospital for 2 to 3 days.
- Nonsteroidal anti-inflammatory medications are avoided in all osteotomy patients for fear of adverse effects on bone formation.
- Patients receive intravenous antibiotics for 24 hours and are then switched to oral antibiotics.
- Patients are discharged on oral antibiotics for 10 days and oral pain medication.
- Patients return to the office 10 days postoperatively, when sutures are removed and they are educated on how to perform strut adjustments.
- Patients are seen every 2 weeks during this adjustment period, and then once monthly during the consolidation period.

Deformity Correction

- Correction of the deformity begins after a latency period of 7 to 10 days.
- The Web-based Smith & Nephew program is used to generate a daily schedule for strut adjustments that the patient will perform at home. The computer requires the input of basic information including the side, the deformity parameters, the size of the rings and length of struts used, the mounting parameters measured during frame application, and rate of daily adjustment.
- The structure at risk is selected and entered into the program to ensure the correct speed of gradual correction. For valgus-producing osteotomy the structures at risk are the medial soft tissues, as they are in the concavity of the correction and will be stretched the greatest distance.
- Using this information, a clear and simplified prescription is produced for the patient to follow every day. We prescribe that struts 1 and 2 be turned in the morning, struts 3 and 4 in the afternoon, and struts 5 and 6 in the evening for a total movement of 1 mm per day.[25]
- The duration of the adjustment phase depends on the amount of correction needed and is typically 14 to 28 days.
- The length of time in the frame is about 3 months.

Pain Management

- Transdermal wires and pins can be irritating, and we encourage patients to use appropriate oral pain medications. This is especially true during the adjustment period.
- Once the correction is complete, the frame is no longer moving, and the pain level decreases.
- Severe or atypical pain merits an evaluated for infection or deep vein thrombosis.

Pin Care

- The dressings are removed on the second postoperative day.
- Nurses teach proper daily pin care, consisting of a mixture of half normal saline and half hydrogen peroxide applied to the pin sites with sterile cotton swabs.
- Pins and wires are covered with dry gauze dressings at the skin.
- Patients are allowed to begin showering on the fourth postoperative day. They are instructed to wash the frame and pin sites with shower water daily.
- Antibacterial soap may be used as an adjuvant form of pin care.
- Problematic smooth wires can be removed in the office without anesthetic. This is commonly done after the distraction phase, or if a wire is painful and infected.

Rehabilitation

- Ilizarov stressed the importance of early physical conditioning in conjunction with the application of circular fixators. Early motion increases blood flow to the lower extremity, prevents joint stiffness, and shortens recovery time.[11]
- Physical therapy assists with ambulation with weight bearing as tolerated and range-of-motion exercises for the knee and ankle joints.
- Crutches are typically needed for the first 4 to 6 weeks after surgery.
- Occupational therapy provides a custom neutral foot splint to prevent the fall into equinus during sleep.
- Patients are encouraged to attend outpatient physical therapy where they continue with their rehabilitation programs.

Frame Removal

- The fixator is removed when the patient is walking without pain or the use of an assistive device and when callus is seen on three cortices around the osteotomy site. This is typically 3 to 4 months after the index surgery.
- We prefer to remove the frame in the operating room: the removal of HA-coated pins can be painful and is best done under sedation.
- We choose to curette all half-pin sites in an effort to keep pin tracts clean.
- Transfixion wire sites are not débrided unless there is concern over a specific site.
- At the time of frame removal, bony union and maturation of the regenerate may be evaluated with routine plain radiographs or a stress test under C-arm fluoroscopy.
- If there is a real concern about bony union, then the struts are removed and the rings are manually compressed and distracted, looking for motion at the osteotomy site.
- A lack of consolidation will require replacement of the struts and prolonging the time in the frame.
- Once the fixator is removed, patients are placed into a short-leg cast for 2 weeks. They are allowed 50% partial weight bearing for 2 weeks and then progress to full weight bearing thereafter, first in a cam walker boot and then in a regular shoe.

OUTCOMES

- Associated symptomatic arthritis may be addressed as well. Ankle distraction[11,31] or ankle fusion can be performed distal to the SMO with the addition of another level of treatment. In these cases the goal of realignment is to unload the area of diseased cartilage while trying to rebuild new cartilage and to ensure a well-aligned leg and foot in the setting of a fused ankle, respectively.
- The goal of PSMO is to correct the deformity in the coronal, sagittal, and axial planes. A lateral distal tibial angle of 90 degrees (Fig 2A) and an anterior distal tibial angle of 80 degrees are ideal (Fig 2C).[16,17]
- The use of the Ilizarov or Taylor Spatial Frame is particularly useful for a gradual correction of a simple or large oblique plane deformity.[4,5,21]
- At times the osteotomy is produced at a location other than the site of the malunion. For example, a malunion of the mid-distal third of the leg that is composed of varus and translation may have a CORA[16,17] or apex of deformity in the supramalleolar region. The SMO becomes a convenient way to correct this, since the supramalleolar bone is metaphyseal, is previously uninjured, and has better healing potential that the actual site of the malunion (**FIG 5**).
- Ankle fusion malunion can be corrected through a PSMO.[12,15,18,23,28] The osteotomy can be performed very distally, since wire penetration into the ankle joint is not a concern. One can correct all deformities effectively. If some lengthening is needed, it may be done through the same osteotomy or through an osteotomy in the proximal tibia.
- Tilt of the talus may develop with joint space narrowing on one side only of the ankle joint. In this situation, the SMO may be used to achieve a neutral talus relative to the axis of the tibia.[2,29,30] To achieve a talus position 90 degrees to the

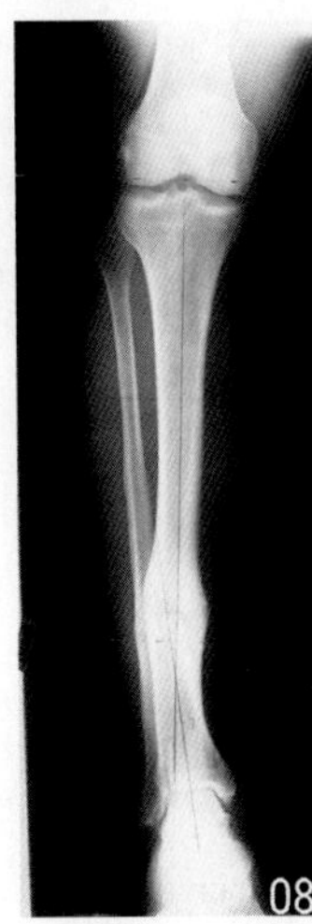

FIG 5 • Preoperative AP radiograph showing varus deformity at the mid-distal third of the tibia. The apex of the deformity is located in the supramalleolar region because of the lateral translation at the malunion site.

tibial axis the distal tibia must often be overcorrected. This can be combined with ankle distraction to stimulate cartilage regrowth.[11,23]

- In addition, internal rotation at the SMO can be used to compensate for some of the forefoot abduction.[2,27] Correction of a foot deformity above the ankle is very powerful, as a plantigrade foot can be obtained while avoiding more intricate and risky surgery to the feet in these complex cases.

COMPLICATIONS

Pin Infection

- Pin site infection is common when using external fixation.
- Pin infections manifest with erythema, increasing pain, and drainage around the pin or wire.
- The vast majority of these respond well to more aggressive local pin care and oral antibiotics.
- If the infection does not resolve quickly, then broader-spectrum antibiotics are added, or the pin or wire is removed.
- More advanced infections are treated with removal of the pin or wire and local bone débridement in the operating room, and intravenous antibiotics as needed.
- Loose pins and wires are removed and the pin sites are débrided even in the absence of infection.
- The use of HA-coated half-pins has decreased problems with pin loosening and infection.

Premature Consolidation

- Incomplete corticotomy can complicate SMO.
- A circumferential division of the tibial cortex may be ensured by rotating the proximal and distal rings in opposite directions and witnessing free motion at the corticotomy site.
- Other methods have been described, including acute distraction and angulation at the osteotomy site, but these techniques are more disruptive to the periosteum and not recommended.
- True premature consolidation of the osteotomy is rare in adult patients.
- Once the osteotomy is performed, there is a latency period of 7 to 10 days before correction is started. If the latency period is prolonged, the osteotomy site will consolidate prematurely.
- Similarly, if the correction is carried out too slowly, the osteotomy site may heal, preventing further correction.

Patient Related

- The success of any gradual correction system is based on the patient's ability to participate in his or her own care.
- Patients are responsible for performing their own strut adjustment three times a day at the outset of treatment.
- The Taylor Spatial Frame has simplified this process through color-coordination and a precise numbering system.
- Patients do make strut adjustment errors, but these mistakes are usually quickly acknowledged and remedied.
- Patients need to be seen frequently (every 10 to 14 days) during the adjustment period to avoid errors.

Nonunion

- Bony nonunion can complicate any osteotomy procedure.
- Causes may include inadequate fixation, lack of weight bearing, smoking and other causes of poor blood flow to the extremity, patient comorbidities, too rapid a correction, poor osteotomy technique, and an osteotomy through diaphyseal bone.
- Nonunions are treated aggressively with a variety of methods, including compression across the osteotomy site, percutaneous periosteal and endosteal stimulation, and additional points of fixation.
- Nonunions are rare when using the Taylor Spatial Frame technique. In fact, when there is impaired healing, this specialized frame is ideal for effective treatment.

Nerve Injury

- Direct injury to a nerve can occur during surgery from pin or wire insertion during the osteotomy.
- A more common mechanism is stretch injury during distraction. This is discussed above in the section on acute versus gradual correction.
- Gradual correction is much safer than acute correction and avoids stretching the nerves too rapidly.

Deep Vein Thrombosis

- Deep vein thrombosis is always a concern with any surgery of the lower extremity.
- Treatment is aimed at prevention. Patients are enrolled into early rehabilitation programs emphasizing immediate mobility to avoid venous stasis.
- There is no restriction to movement at the ankle, knee, or hip, and frame stability allows comfortable weight bearing early in the postoperative period.
- While in the hospital, patients receive subcutaneous low-molecular-weight heparin. After discharge, patients continue a 3-week course of subcutaneous low-molecular-weight heparin. Patients can then be switched to aspirin if they are still not walking well.
- With this regimen, we have not had any cases of deep vein thrombosis or pulmonary embolism.

Septic Arthritis

- This is a rare complication that needs to be recognized and treated quickly.

- The best way to avoid this is prevention. One must be careful not to insert the wires too close to the ankle joint capsule. In general, if the wires and pins are inserted proximal to the epiphyseal scar, there is little risk of an intra-articular wire.
- If ankle distraction is being performed simultaneously, then the talus wire is intra-articular and should be monitored.
- The surgeon should aspirate the joint immediately in the office and send cultures before giving any antibiotics.
- Septic arthritis is treated with removal of the infected intra-articular wire and open or arthroscopic joint lavage. The lavages are repeated until negative cultures are obtained.
- Appropriate systemic antibiotics are given once a culture has been taken.

Other

- Complications we have *not* experienced secondary to PSMO include necrotizing fasciitis, compartment syndrome, and osteomyelitis.

REFERENCES

1. Abraham E, Lubicky JP, Songer MN, et al. Supramalleolar osteotomy for ankle valgus in myelomeningocele. J Pediatr Orthop 1996;16:774–781.
2. Benthien RA, Myerson MS. Supramalleolar osteotomy for ankle deformity and arthritis. Foot Ankle Clin 2004;9:475–487.
3. Best A, Daniels TR. Supramalleolar tibial osteotomy secured with the Puddu plate. Orthopedics 2006;29:537–540.
4. Feldman DS, Shin SS, Madan S, et al. Correction of tibial malunion and nonunion with six-axis analysis deformity correction using the Taylor Spatial Frame. J Orthop Trauma 2003;17:549–554.
5. Fragomen A, Ilizarov S, Blyakher A, et al. Proximal tibial osteotomy for medial compartment osteoarthritis of the knee using the Taylor Spatial Frame. Techniques in Knee Surgery 2005;4:175–183.
6. Fraser RK, Menelaus MB. The management of tibial torsion in patients with spina bifida. J Bone Joint Surg Br 1993;75B:495–497.
7. Gessmann J, Seybold D, Baecker H, et al. Correction of supramalleolar deformities with the Taylor spatial frame. Z Orthop Unfall 2009;147:314–320.
8. Graehl PM, Hersh MR, Heckman JD. Supramalleolar osteotomy for the treatment of symptomatic tibial malunion. J Orthop Trauma 1987;1:281–292.
9. Ilizarov GA. Clinical application of the tension-stress effect for limb lengthening. Clin Orthop Relat Res 1990;250:8–26.
10. Inan M, Ferri-de Baros F, Chan G, et al. Correction of rotational deformity of the tibia in cerebral palsy by percutaneous supramalleolar osteotomy. J Bone Joint Surg Br 2005;87B:1411–1415.
11. Inda JI, Blyakher A, O'Malley MJ, et al. Distraction arthroplasty for the ankle using the Ilizarov frame. Tech Foot Ankle Surg 2003;2:249–253.
12. Katsenis D, Bhave A, Paley D, et al. Treatment of malunion and nonunion at the site of an ankle fusion with the Ilizarov apparatus. J Bone Joint Surg Am 2005;87A:302.
13. Mangone PG. Distal tibial osteotomies for the treatment of foot and ankle disorders. Foot Ankle Clin 2001;6:583–597.
14. Mendicino RW, Catanzariti AR, Reeves CL. Percutaneous supramalleolar osteotomy for distal tibial (near articular) ankle deformities. J Am Podiatr Med Assoc 2005;95:72–84.
15. Paley D. The correction of complex foot deformities using Ilizarov's distraction osteotomies. Clin Orthop Relat Res 1993;293:97–111.
16. Paley D, Herzenberg JE, Tetsworth K, et al. Deformity planning for frontal and sagittal plane corrective osteotomies. Orthop Clin North Am 1994;25:425–465.
17. Paley D. Principles of Deformity Correction. 1 ed. Berlin: Springer-Verlag, 2005.
18. Paley D, Lamm BM, Katsenis D, et al. Treatment of malunion and nonunion at the site of an ankle fusion with the Ilizarov apparatus: surgical technique. J Bone Joint Surg Am 2006;88A(suppl 1):119–134.
19. Pearce MS, Smith MA, Savidge GF. Supramalleolar tibial osteotomy for haemophilic arthropathy of the ankle. J Bone Joint Surg Br 1994;76B:947–950.
20. Pugh K, Rozbruch SR. Nonunions and malunions. In: Baumgaertner MR, Tornetta P, eds. Orthopaedic Knowledge Update Trauma 3. American Academy of Orthopaedic Surgeons, 2005:115–130.
21. Rozbruch SR, Helfet DL, Blyakher A. Distraction of hypertrophic nonunion of tibia with deformity using Ilizarov/Taylor Spatial Frame: report of two cases. Arch Orthop Trauma Surg 2002;122:295–298.
22. Rozbruch SR, Blyakher A, Haas SB, et al. Correction of large bilateral tibia vara with the Ilizarov method. J Knee Surg 2003;16:34–37.
23. Rozbruch SR. Post-traumatic reconstruction of the ankle using the Ilizarov method. J Hosp Special Surg 2005;1:68–88.
24. Rozbruch SR, Weitzman AM, Watson JT, et al. Simultaneous treatment of tibial bone and soft-tissue defects with the Ilizarov method. J Orthop Trauma 2006;20:197–205.
25. Rozbruch SR, Fragomen A, Ilizarov S. Correction of tibial deformity with use of the Ilizarov/ Taylor Spatial Frame. J Bone Joint Surg Am 2006;88A(suppl 4):156–174.
26. Selber P, Filho ER, Dallalana R, et al. Supramalleolar derotation osteotomy of the tibia, with T plate fixation: technique and results in patients with neuromuscular disease. J Bone Joint Surg Br 2004;86B:1170–1175.
27. Sen C, Kocaoglu M, Eralp L, et al. Correction of ankle and hindfoot deformities by supramalleolar osteotomy. Foot Ankle Int 2003;24:22–28.
28. Shtarker H, Volpin G, Stolero J, et al. Correction of combined angular and rotational deformities by the Ilizarov method. Clin Orthop Relat Res 2002;402:184–195.
29. Stamatis ED, Myerson MS. Supramalleolar osteotomy: indications and technique. Foot Ankle Clin 2003;8:317–333.
30. Stamatis ED, Cooper PS, Myerson MS. Supramalleolar osteotomy for the treatment of distal tibial angular deformities and arthritis of the ankle joint. Foot Ankle Int 2003;24:754–764.
31. Tellisi N, Fragomen AT, Kleinman D, et al. Joint preservation of the osteoarthritic ankle using distraction arthroplasty. Foot Ankle Int 2009;30:318–325.
32. Tellisi N, Ilizarov S, Fragomen A, et al. Humeral lengthening and deformity correction in Ollier's disease: distraction osteogenesis with a multiaxial correction frame. J Pediatr Orthop B 2008;17:152–157.

Chapter 66

Supramalleolar Osteotomy With External Fixation: Perspective 2

Bradley M. Lamm, Shine John, John E. Herzenberg, and Dror Paley

BACKGROUND

- Ankle arthrodesis remains the gold standard for ankle arthritis.
- Ankle arthrodesis is indicated for painful arthroses, instability, malalignment, and joint sepsis.
- Regardless of the method of arthrodesis, complications are not uncommon and include nonunion, malunion, infection, osteoarthrosis of contiguous joints, neurovascular injury, wound healing issues, and limb-length discrepancy.[6]
  - Rates of nonunion and other complications alone have been reported to be as high as 30% and 60%, respectively.
  - Malunion may be among the most consequential and detrimental complications because of its effect on functional outcome.
  - Sequelae of a malaligned ankle arthrodesis include subtalar degeneration, reduced foot flexibility, compensatory foot deformities, and pain with ambulation. Correction of malaligned ankle fusion is thus critical to preserve the functional mobility of neighboring joints.
- Revision of a malaligned ankle arthrodesis can be both technically demanding and traumatic to previously operated bone and soft tissue.
  - Preservation of compromised soft tissue structures, including the periosteum, is also a critical consideration when revising the failed ankle arthrodesis.
  - The amount of bone resection required to obtain apposition of viable bony surfaces can create an even greater limb-length discrepancy (larger than the expected 1 cm).
  - Malunion ankle deformities are typically multiplanar and therefore are not easily corrected acutely.
- The literature is sparse in regard to rates and management of the malpositioned ankle fusion. At our institution, we address these complex deformities through a minimally invasive osteotomy with gradual external fixation correction.
- In addition to presenting our technique and results, we will objectively define the optimal clinical and radiographic position for an ankle realignment arthrodesis.[7,10]

SURGICAL MANAGEMENT

- Our minimally invasive technique uses a four-incision percutaneous Gigli saw osteotomy with gradual external fixation correction of the ankle malunion.
- The subperiosteal Gigli saw osteotomy through a prior malaligned fusion site limits soft tissue compromise while optimizing soft tissue and bone healing.
- External fixation provides gradual accurate multiplanar (rotation, angulation, and translation) realignment, while simultaneously correcting limb length. In addition, obtaining proper alignment of an ankle fusion is paramount.

Positioning

- Under general anesthesia, the patient is positioned supine on the radiolucent table with an ipsilateral hip bump so as to place the foot in a foot-forward position.
- A nonsterile thigh tourniquet is placed, and sterile prep of the entire leg to the level of the tourniquet is performed.
- Under video fluoroscopy, a marking pen is used to indicate the desired level of the osteotomy on both the anteroposterior (AP) and lateral views. The thigh tourniquet is then inflated.

PERCUTANEOUS OSTEOTOMY

- The first incision is made transversely, just medial to the tibialis anterior tendon (**TECH FIG 1A–C**).
  - Subperiosteal dissection with a periosteal elevator is performed across the anterior tibia.
  - This subperiosteal dissection creates a subperiosteal tunnel that protects the tendons and neurovascular bundle along the anterior aspect of the ankle.
  - Along the desired level of the osteotomy, the periosteal elevator is then maneuvered in a rocking motion against the bone and across the entire anterior ankle to the lateral aspect of the ankle malunion.
- A vertical second incision is made where the skin is tented by the extension of the periosteal elevator, and the elevator is removed.
  - A no. 2 Ethibond suture is clasped with a curved tonsil hemostat and passed through the previously created subperiosteal tunnel from the medial incision to the lateral incision (**TECH FIG 1D**).
  - Once the suture is passed, the Gigli saw is tied to the suture and also pulled from medial to lateral through the same subperiosteal tunnel (**TECH FIG 1E**).
  - The position of the Gigli saw is then checked by image intensifier to ensure that the desired level of osteotomy has been properly maintained.
  - Through the lateral incision, the periosteal elevator is passed posterior subperiosteally to exit just on the posterolateral corner of the ankle malunion.
- A vertical third incision is made posterolaterally, where the elevator tents the skin (**TECH FIG 1F**).
  - The curved tonsil is then passed subperiosteally from the third incision to the second incision to clasp the Ethibond suture, and the suture with the

Gigli saw is passed through the third incision (TECH FIG 1G).
  - Again the elevator is extended from the third incision subperiosteally posterior to the ankle malunion deep to the flexor tendons to exit medially at the level just anterior to the posterior tibialis tendon (TECH FIG 1H).
- A transverse fourth incision is made where the elevator tents the medial skin.
  - From the fourth incision to the third incision, the curved tonsil is used to grasp the suture attached to the Gigli saw and pull them through the fourth incision.
  - The Gigli saw is now circumferentially around the ankle malunion (TECH FIG 1I).
  - Care must be taken during the passage of the Gigli saw to maintain the correct level of the planned osteotomy.
- The two Gigli saw handles are now attached, and, using a reciprocating motion, the ankle is cut from lateral to medial.
- To avoid injury to the medial skin, cutting is stopped just before the medial bone is exited, a periosteal elevator is placed between the fourth and first incisions crossing the Gigli saw, and then the cut is continued (TECH FIG 1J).
- When the cut is complete, the elevator will block further progression of the saw, thereby preventing medial soft tissue damage (TECH FIG 1K,L).
- The completion of the osteotomy is confirmed with the image intensifier.
- Then the Gigli saw is cut and removed (TECH FIG M,N).
- The tourniquet is deflated, and the incisions are closed.

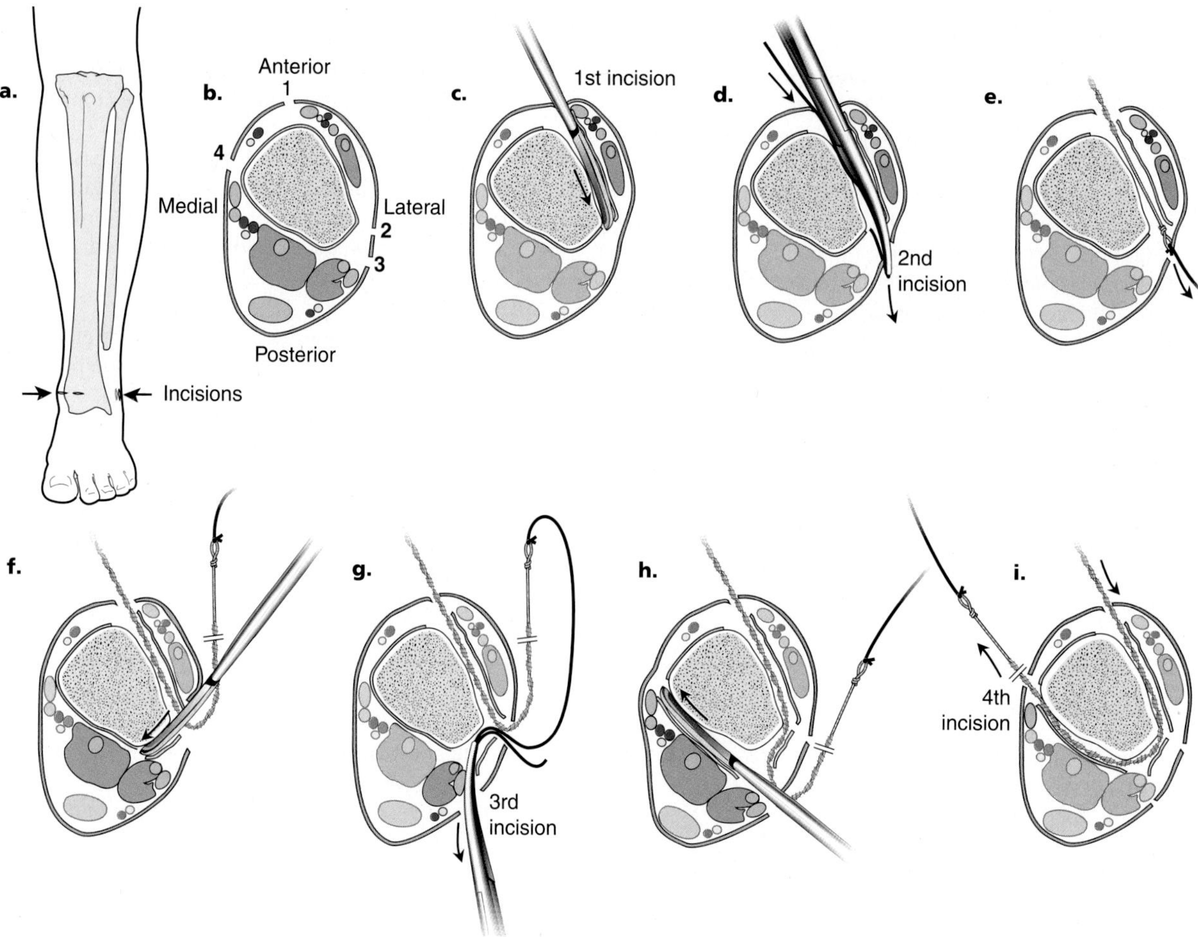

TECH FIG 1 • Percutaneous Gigli saw osteotomy of a malunited ankle arthrodesis. **A.** A Gigli saw can be passed percutaneously at the level of a previous ankle fusion. Four small incisions are used to pass the saw: two longitudinal medial and two transverse lateral incisions. **B.** Because of the square-shaped fusion mass, four incisions are used to safely pass the Gigli saw. The Gigli saw is passed subperiosteally starting anteromedial (*1*) and ending posteromedial (*4*). **C.** The medial longitudinal incision (*1*) is made just medial to the tibialis anterior tendon. Through the anterior medial incision, a periosteal elevator is passed subperiosteally across the anterior aspect of the fusion mass at the desired level. **D.** The second incision, which is transverse lateral (*2*), is made where the periosteal elevator tents the lateral skin. A suture is passed through the same subperiosteal tunnel from medial to lateral (the reverse can also be done). **E.** The suture with the attached Gigli saw is passed from medial to lateral anterior to the ankle fusion mass. **F.** Through the second incision, the lateral periosteum is elevated, and a third incision is made posterolateral (*3*). **G.** The suture and attached Gigli saw are passed through the third incision. **H.** The posterior periosteum is elevated. Care must be taken to avoid extra periosteal dissection. **I.** A fourth incision is made at the posterior medial corner of the ankle fusion mass. The suture and Gigli saw are passed around the malunited ankle fusion. Care must be taken to protect the peroneal tendons as the Gigli saw is being passed from the third to fourth incision. *(continued)*

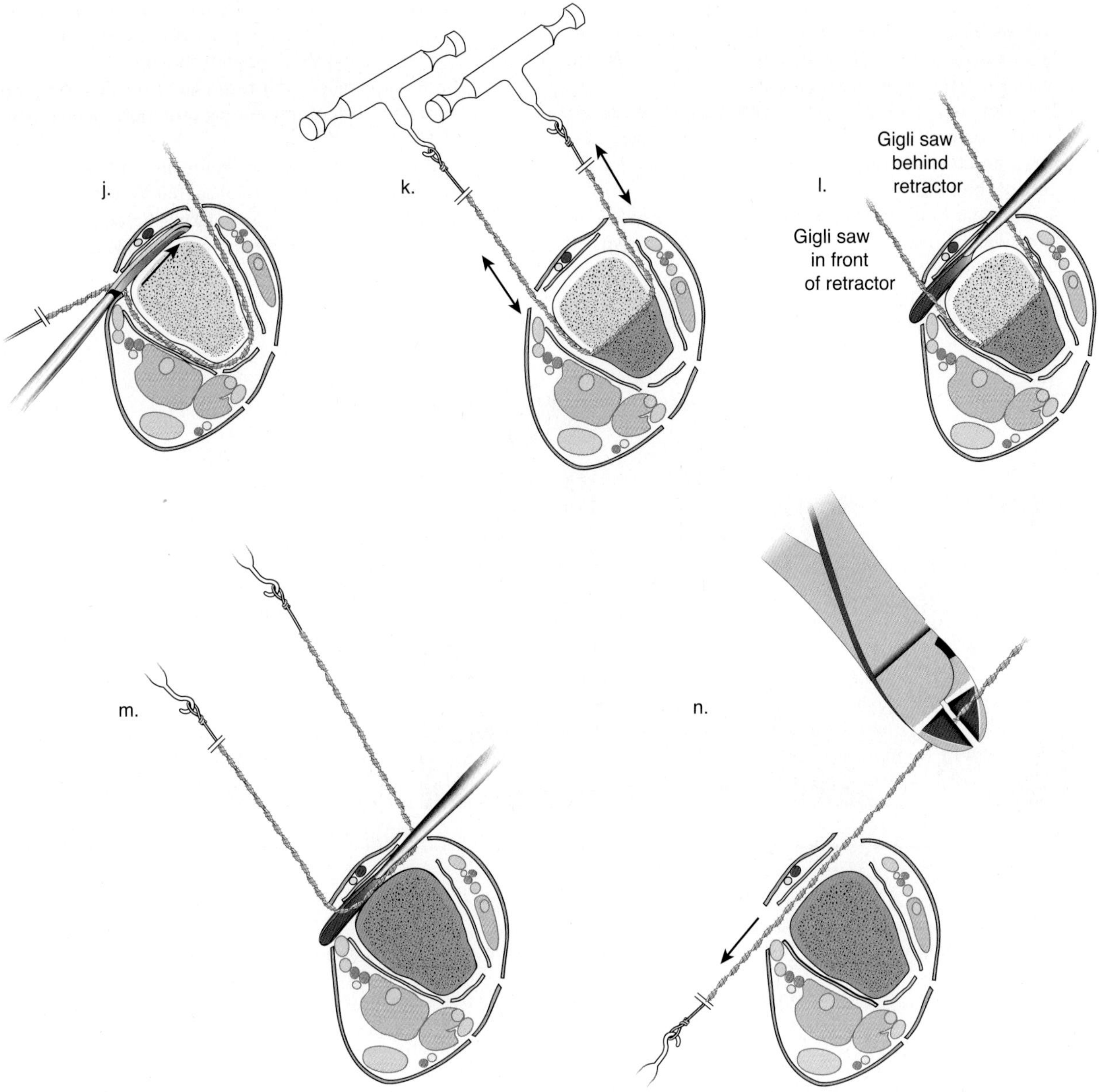

TECH FIG 1 • *(continued)* **J.** The medial periosteum is then elevated from the fourth incision to the first incision. **K.** The Gigli saw osteotomy is performed halfway through the fusion mass. **L.** The periosteal elevator is then inserted in the previously created tunnel, crossing the Gigli saw so as to protect the medial soft tissues. **M.** The osteotomy is completed. **N.** The Gigli saw is cut and removed. (Copyright 2008, Rubin Institute for Advanced Orthopedics, Sinai Hospital of Baltimore.)

EXTERNAL FIXATION APPLICATION

- The tourniquet is inflated only while passing the Gigli saw but is released before the fixator application.
- External fixation allows for gradual correction of deformity and lengthening, which can be accomplished by using the Ilizarov external fixator or the Taylor spatial frame (**TECH FIG 2**).
- The frame is built according to the deformity, with the proximal fixation block fixing the tibia and the distal fixation block fixing the talus, calcaneus, and foot.
- The goal is to achieve stable fixation proximal and distal to the osteotomy.
- Smooth wire (1.8 mm) or half-pin (6 mm) fixation is used per the surgeon's preference.
- The proximal ring is mounted perpendicular to the tibia in both the AP and lateral fluoroscopic views.
- The distal ring is mounted parallel to the plantar aspect of the foot. By using this mounting technique, at the end of correction, the foot and tibial rings will be parallel, confirming a plantigrade foot position.
- The proximal ring (full ring) is mounted on a lateral-to-medial smooth wire crossing the distal tibia perpendicular to the AP long axis of the tibia and tensioned.

- Then an anterior half-pin (6 mm) is inserted on this ring and two additional half-pins are inserted proximal or distal in a delta fashion. These half pins are placed perpendicular to the tibia in the sagittal plane.
- The foot ring is fixed in place with 1.8-mm tensioned smooth wires (two crossing calcaneal wires, two talar wires, and two forefoot wires) parallel to the plantar aspect of the foot.
- A foot board (an intraoperative rigid board that stimulates weight bearing) is used to ensure a plantigrade foot ring mounting.
- An oblique (posterolateral to anteromedial) talar wire and medial to lateral talar wires are placed for increased stability.
- Occasionally talar half-pins are used. Distraction of the subtalar joint is performed by rotating both talar wire fixation bolts using the Russian technique.
  - The Russian tensioning technique provides compression of the osteotomy site by pushing proximally on the talus.
  - Six struts are added between the distal tibial and foot rings to complete the Taylor spatial frame.
  - Computer planning on an Internet-based program is then performed, which generates a daily patient turn schedule.
  - Patients are followed biweekly during the gradual correction to ensure accurate final realignment.

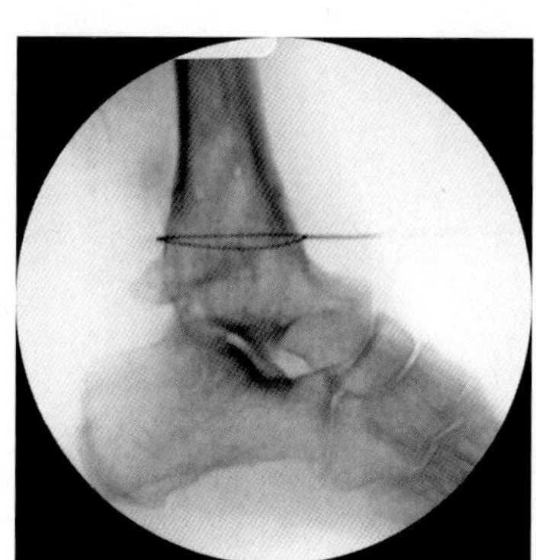
A

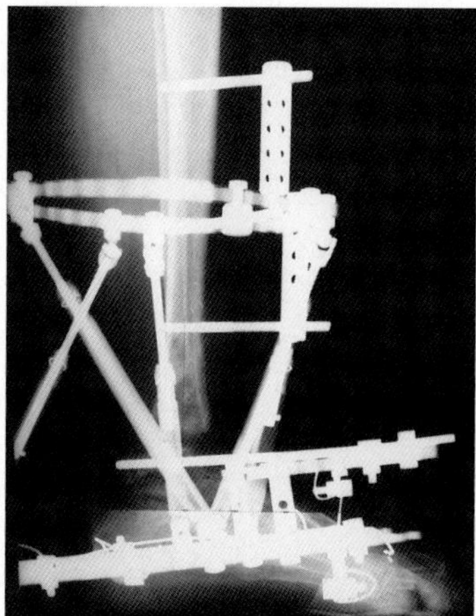
B

TECH FIG 2 • A. Lateral intraoperative radiographic view shows a malunion of the ankle (equinus of 15 degrees and the foot anteriorly translated) in an adult patient. The Gigli saw has been passed at the level of the ankle malunion. **B.** Lateral radiographic view showing opening posterior wedge of regenerate bone formation and posterior translation of the foot during distraction treatment with the Taylor spatial frame. (Copyright 2008, Rubin Institute for Advanced Orthopedics, Sinai Hospital of Baltimore.)

PEARLS AND PITFALLS

Optimal clinical and radiographic positions for ankle or tibiotalocalcaneal realignment arthrodesis[7,10]	■ In the sagittal plane, the foot is placed at a right angle to the limb (plantigrade angle, 90°) and the tibial mid-diaphyseal line coincides with the lateral process of the talus. ■ In the transverse plane, the foot is externally rotated to the limb so that the thigh–foot axis is 10° to 15° externally rotated. ■ In the axial plane, the calcaneal bisection line should be parallel or slightly valgus (0° to 2°) and coincide with the mid-diaphyseal line of the tibia. ■ The affected limb should be 1 cm shorter than the unaffected limb.

OUTCOMES

- The subperiosteal Gigli saw osteotomy through a prior malaligned fusion site limits soft tissue compromise while optimizing soft tissue and bone healing.
- External fixation provides gradual accurate multiplanar (rotation, angulation, and translation) realignment, while simultaneously correcting limb length.
  - In addition, obtaining proper alignment of an ankle fusion is paramount (**FIG 1**).
- Using this technique we have successfully realigned more than a dozen of these ankle malunions.

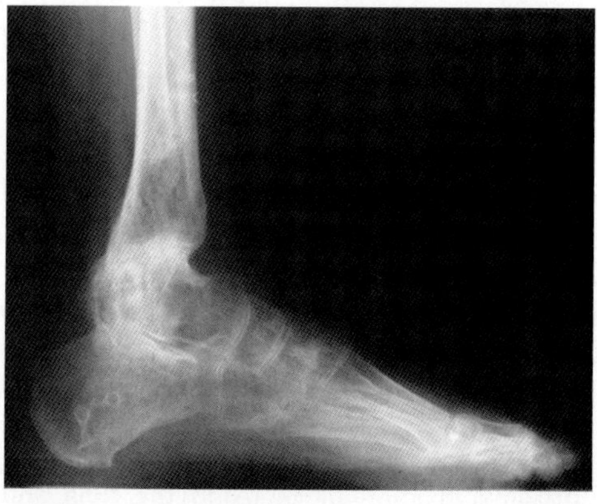

FIG 1 • Final weight-bearing AP radiographic view of the patient in Techniques Figure 2 shows full correction of the equinus deformity. (Copyright 2008, Rubin Institute for Advanced Orthopedics, Sinai Hospital of Baltimore.)

COMPLICATIONS

- Complications can occur (pin site infection, residual leg-length discrepancy, wound problems, premature or delayed consolidation, tarsal tunnel syndrome, and pin failure).

- A well-aligned ankle arthrodesis with a plantigrade foot was achieved in all patients using the described technique.
- Therefore, patients with a malunited ankle fusion, with or without a limb-length discrepancy, can be successfully treated with minimally invasive Gigli saw osteotomy and gradual external fixation correction.

ACKNOWLEDGMENTS

The authors thank Joy Marlowe, MA, for her excellent illustrative artwork, and Alvien Lee for his photographic expertise.

REFERENCES

1. Ahlberg A, Henricson AS. Late results of ankle fusion. Acta Orthop Scand 1981;52:103–105.
2. Ben Amor H, Kallel S, Karray S, et al. [Consequences of tibiotalar arthrodesis on the foot: a retrospective study of 36 cases with 8.5 years of follow-up]. Acta Orthop Belg 1999;65:48–56.
3. Frey C, Halikus NM, Vu-Rose T, Ebramzadeh E. A review of ankle arthrodesis: predisposing factors to nonunion. Foot Ankle Int 1994;15:581–584.
4. Jackson A, Glasgow M. Tarsal hypermobility after ankle fusion: fact or fiction? J Bone Joint Surg Br 1979;61B:470–473.
5. Johnson EW Jr, Boseker EH. Arthrodesis of the ankle. Arch Surg 1968;97:766–773.
6. Katsenis D, Bhave A, Paley D, Herzenberg JE. Treatment of malunion and nonunion at the site of an ankle fusion with the Ilizarov apparatus. J Bone Joint Surg Am 2005;87A:302–309.
7. Mendicino RW, Lamm BM, Catanzariti AR, et al. Realignment arthrodesis of the rearfoot and ankle: a comprehensive evaluation. J Am Podiatr Med Assoc 2005;95:60–71.
8. Moeckel BH, Patterson BM, Inglis AE, Sculco TP. Ankle arthrodesis: a comparison of internal and external fixation. Clin Orthop 1991;268: 78–83.
9. Ogilvie-Harris DJ, Lieberman L, Fitsialos D. Arthroscopically assisted arthrodesis for osteoarthrotic ankles. J Bone Joint Surg Am 1993;75A:1167–1174.
10. Paley D, Lamm BM, Katsenis D, et al. Treatment of malunion and nonunion at the site of an ankle fusion with the Ilizarov apparatus. J Bone Joint Surg Am 2006;88A:119–134.

Chapter 67 Total Ankle Shell Allograft Reconstruction

Michael E. Brage and Keri A. Reese

DEFINITION

- Articular defects of the tibiotalar joint, posttraumatic arthritis, and osteoarthritis can limit activity, make walking difficult, and lead to severe pain. Changes seen on radiographs include joint space narrowing, osteophytes, and subchondral bone sclerosis.
- Unlike the knee and hip, primary arthritis rarely affects the ankle. The most common causes of degenerative changes in the ankle are secondary to trauma and abnormal ankle mechanics. Posttraumatic arthritis is correlated to the severity of the fracture pattern and nonanatomic reduction of articular surfaces.[16]
- Osteoarthritis is described by degradation of the articular cartilage, subchondral sclerosis, and subchondral cyst and osteophyte formation. It is usually secondary to previous ankle fractures, talus fractures, or ligamentous instability.
- Rheumatoid or other inflammatory arthropathies and infection can cause significant ankle pain, deformities, and arthritis.
- Options for patients who fail to respond to conservative treatment for ankle arthrosis are tibiotalar arthrodesis, total ankle arthroplasty, and fresh ankle osteochondral shell allografts.[1,2,8,10,11,14] Tibiotalar osteochondral shell allografts are a reasonable alternative to tibiotalar arthrodesis and total ankle arthroplasty in young patients with posttraumatic ankle arthropathy.[8,11,14]

ANATOMY

- The ankle joint is complex, but its complexity may be simplified if the ankle is thought of as a single-axis joint in an oblique path from medial to lateral and oriented downward and backward. The main motion is dorsiflexion and plantarflexion, with some inversion and eversion of the tibiotalar joint.[3]
- The bones that make up the ankle joint are the tibia, fibula, and talus. The tibia plafond is concave anteroposteriorly and mediolaterally.
- The talus has no muscular or tendinous attachments and 60% of its surface is covered by articular cartilage.
- In addition to the bony support of the ankle, the medial and lateral ligamentous complexes provide stability to the ankle and hindfoot.

PATHOGENESIS

- The predominant collagen in articular cartilage is type II collagen. Articular cartilage has limited blood supply, cannot proliferate, and has little reparative potential.
- Type 1 injury to articular cartilage involves microscopic disruption of chondrocytes and the extracellular matrix, while type 2 injuries involve macroscopic damage to the surface. Since the subchondral bone is not involved, there is little inflammatory response and therefore poor healing of these injuries. Type 3 injuries also involve the subchondral bone and thus heal with a fibrocartilage, consisting mainly of type I collagen.[13]
- Ankle arthritis may cause loss of motion, pain, deformity, and instability.

NATURAL HISTORY

- Tibiotalar arthritis may result from trauma, inflammatory diseases, and osteoarthritis. Posttraumatic arthritis is the most common cause of ankle arthritis despite advances in open reduction and internal fixation of ankle and pilon fractures. Most likely, the tibiotalar chondral surfaces are injured and do not have the capacity to heal.
- Posttraumatic tibiotalar arthrosis often fails to respond to nonoperative management, and typically definitive surgical treatment has been ankle arthrodesis in a majority of patients and total ankle arthroplasty in select patients.[1,2,4,10,14]
- Ankle arthrodesis has been shown to alleviate pain in the arthritic ankle. However, loss of range of motion, functional limitation, and secondary progressive arthritis in the hindfoot and midfoot have been found in long-term follow-up studies on patients with isolated ankle arthrodesis.[2]
- Current total ankle prosthetic designs are a promising alternative to arthrodesis, but reportedly the patient's age has an adverse affect on the risk of failure and reoperation rate.[9,14,15]
- Osteochondral shell allografting, in which the tibial plafond and talar dome are replaced with a donor ankle matched for size, affords relief of pain, congruent articular surfaces, maintenance of bone stock, and preservation of surrounding joints. Recent improvements in surgical techniques and experience with allografts have improved short-term outcomes with this technique. Recent studies advocate the use of fresh osteochondral allografting as a alternative treatment for selected individuals with end-stage tibiotalar arthrosis.[8,11,17]

PATIENT HISTORY AND PHYSICAL FINDINGS

- A thorough history and physical examination of both lower extremities must be performed for any deformities or malalignment to identify multiple joint involvement, symmetric involvement, family history, and a history of trauma. The function and stability of the ligaments and tendons surrounding the ankle should be tested. This includes assessment for an equinus contracture or pes planus or pes cavus deformities. A neurovascular examination must also be performed before surgery.
- Physical examination methods include the following:
  - Anterior drawer test to evaluate the anterior talofibular ligament and ankle stability. The surgeon should look for a difference of 3 to 5 mm in the relationship between the lateral talus and the anterior aspect of the fibula.

- Inversion stress test to evaluate talar instability (somewhat difficult due to subtalar motion). Compared to the contralateral ankle, a difference of more than 15 degrees is significant.
- Equinus contracture assessment. A gastrocnemius recession or Achilles lengthening procedure may be required concomitantly if there is 5 degrees of equinus in the ankle.
- Range of motion: Normal total range of motion of the tibiotalar joint is from 20 degrees of dorsiflexion to 50 degrees of plantarflexion. Normal subtalar joint motion is about 20 degrees from maximal inversion to eversion.

- Contraindications for shell allograft ankle reconstruction are:
  - Diminished peripheral pulses
  - Varus or valgus malalignment of the tibiotalar joint of more than 10 degrees
  - Instability of the ankle joint

IMAGING AND OTHER DIAGNOSTIC STUDIES

- Weight-bearing radiographs of the ankle, including AP, lateral, and mortise views, are obtained (**FIG 1**).
- When indicated, AP stress radiographs may be obtained to confirm instability. Anterior translation between the talus and tibia of 3 to 5 mm greater than the contralateral ankle indicates instability.[3]
- Talar tilt on stress radiographs with the ankle internally rotated 30 degrees: A difference greater than 15 degrees compared to the contralateral ankle indicates instability.[3]

DIFFERENTIAL DIAGNOSIS

- Ankle instability or deformities
- Anterior or posterior impingement syndrome
- Osteochondritis dissecans lesions of talus or tibia
- Subtalar joint osteoarthritis
- Sinus tarsi syndrome

NONOPERATIVE MANAGEMENT

- Conservative treatment includes mechanical aids (such as ankle–foot orthoses [AFOs] and shoe modifications), anti-inflammatories, and intra-articular steroid injections.

SURGICAL MANAGEMENT

- For young healthy individuals who need alleviation of pain and retention of motion and function, osteochondral shell allografts represent an alternative to ankle arthrodesis and total ankle replacement.

Preoperative Planning

- Standard radiographs on the ankle are needed for preoperative planning. In our opinion, an external fixator or distraction device is useful during the operation. We routinely use the DePuy Agility ankle arthroplasty cutting block to increase the precision of cuts.
- Size-matched osteochondral allografts, based on radiographs, are procured from one of several regional tissue banks.

Positioning

- The patient is supine on a radiolucent operating table.

Approach

- A standard anterior approach to the ankle is used between the tibialis anterior and extensor hallucis longus tendons, while protecting the superficial peroneal nerve. The deep neurovascular bundle (deep peroneal nerve and anterior tibial and dorsalis pedis artery) is retracted laterally and dissection is carried through the joint capsule to expose the ankle.

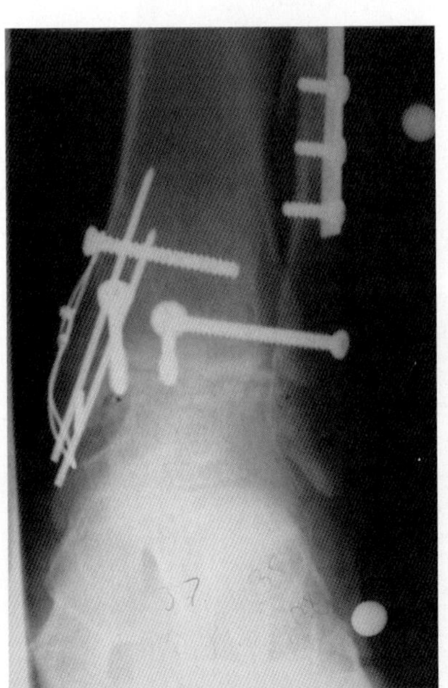

A

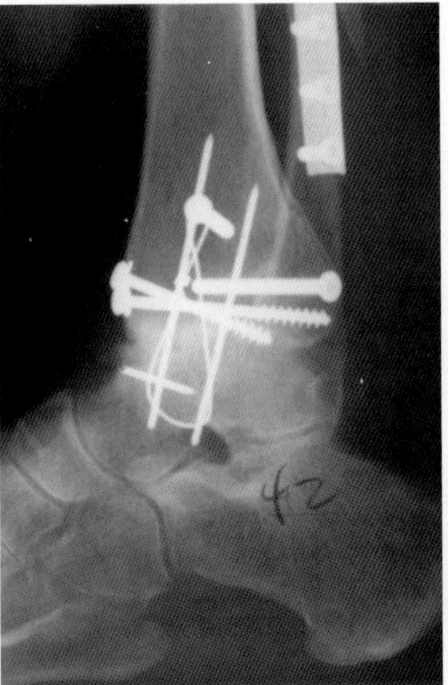

B

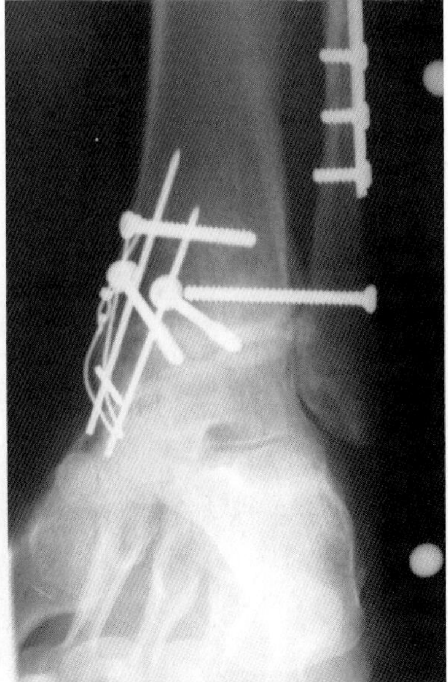

C

FIG 1 • **A.** Preoperative AP radiograph. **B.** Lateral view. **C.** Mortise view. (Courtesy of Dr. Michael Brage.)

DÉBRIDEMENT AND DISTRACTION OF THE ANKLE JOINT

- Through the anterior approach, excise synovitis and remove osteophytes using rongeurs and osteotomes. Next, apply an external fixator to distract the joint symmetrically about 1 cm (**TECH FIG 1**).

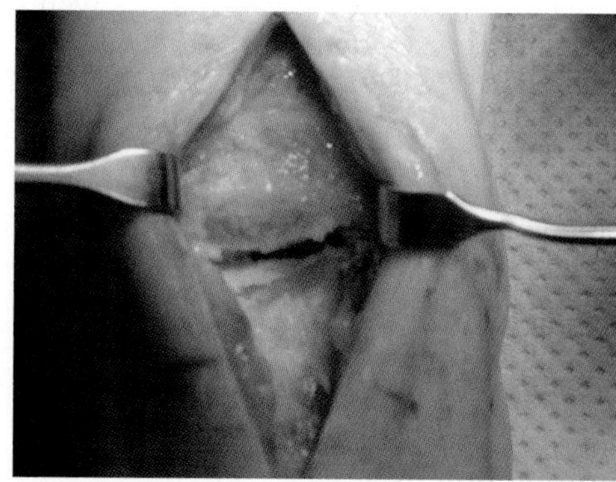

TECH FIG 1 • Débridement and distraction of the ankle joint. (Courtesy of Dr. Michael Brage.)

TIBIAL AND TALAR CUTS

- Although we always procure a complete ankle joint, careful inspection of the arthritic ankle may indicate that complete joint replacement may not be warranted. Occasionally, we perform only hemi-joint resurfacing, but with the disadvantage of loss of optimal articular congruency afforded by a complete or bipolar joint replacement. We determine the ideal Agility (DePuy, Warsaw, IN) cutting block by templating the ankle radiographs. Pin the corresponding Agility ankle arthroplasty cutting block into place over the anterior ankle (**TECH FIG 2A**). Confirm placement and size with intraoperative fluoroscopy (**TECH FIG 2B**).
- Using a blunt reciprocating saw, resect the tibial plafond and talar dome to a depth of about 7 to 10 mm.
- Remove an articular portion of the medial malleolus (about 3 to 4 mm) as well.
- Take extreme care as the posterior tibial neurovascular bundle is close to the posteromedial corner of the ankle joint.
- On the lateral aspect of the tibial cut, take care to avoid contract with the fibula to keep it fully preserved.

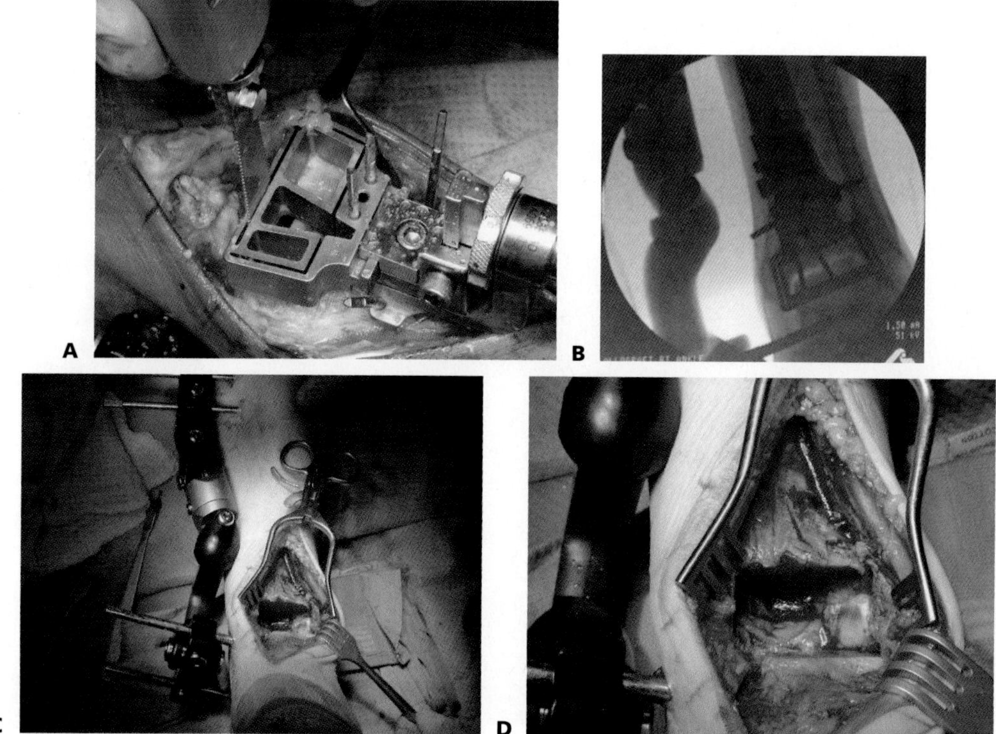

TECH FIG 2 • Tibial and talar cuts. **A.** Ankle arthroplasty jig is placed over tibia and pinned into place. **B.** Cutting jig size and placement are confirmed with fluoroscopy before cuts are made. (Courtesy of Dr. Michael Brage.)

ALLOGRAFT PREPARATION AND CUTS

- The Agility ankle cutting block for the tibial cut of the donor graft is one size larger than the block used on the recipient tibia. Pin the cutting block onto the graft using fluoroscopy and make the cut with an oscillating saw (TECH FIG 3A,B).
- Cut the talus graft free hand using an oscillating saw. The cut is made at the interface between the anterior neck and cartilage. We routinely lavage both the tibial and talar grafts to remove immunogenic marrow elements (TECH FIG 3C,D).

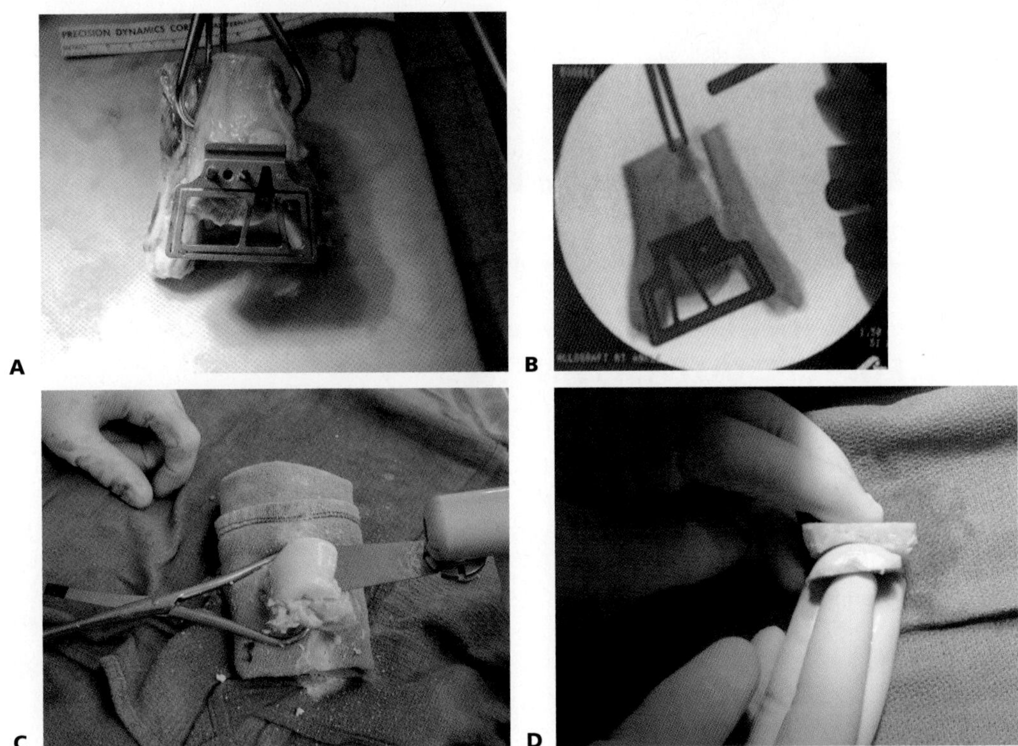

TECH FIG 3 • Allograft preparation and cuts. **A.** Cutting jig is pinned onto tibia. **B.** Size and position are confirmed with fluoroscopy. **C.** Talus allograft is cut free hand. **D.** Articulating tibial and talar allografts. (Courtesy of Dr. Michael Brage.)

PLACEMENT AND FIXATION OF THE GRAFTS

- With the ankle in plantarflexion, seat the grafts into the recipient mortise. We remove the external fixator and take the ankle through a range of motion to confirm graft and ankle stability.
- Imaging in the AP, mortise, and lateral planes confirms that the grafts have satisfactory apposition to the host bone and that the anatomy of the tibiotalar joint has been restored.
- Place two parallel 3.0-mm cannulated screws into each graft for fixation. Place them from the anterior portion of the tibial graft while aiming superiorly and posteriorly.
- Place two fixation screws on the anterior portion of the talar graft through the most anterior portion of the articular cartilage. Countersink these screws into subchondral bone (TECH FIG 4).

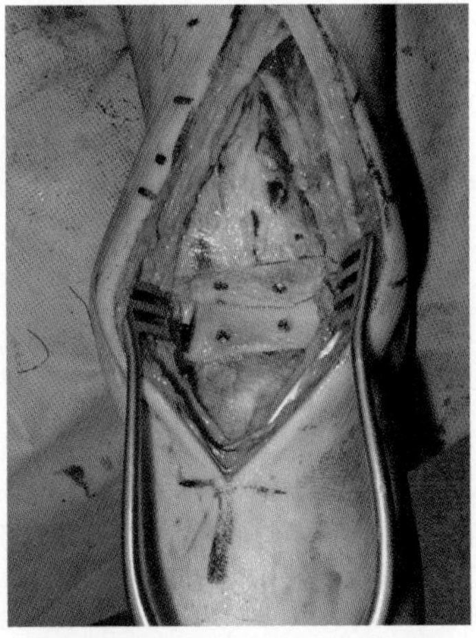

TECH FIG 4 • Placement and fixation of graft. **A.** Grafts are placed and fixed with two countersunk cannulated screws. *(continued)*

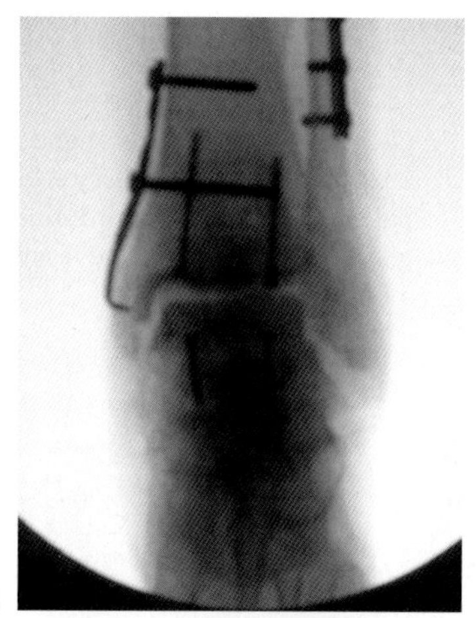

B

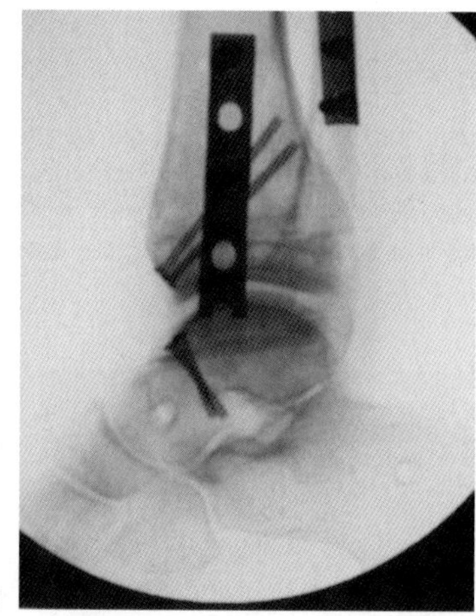

C

TECH FIG 4 • *(continued)* **B.** AP fluoroscopic view of grafts with fixation. **C.** Lateral fluoroscopic view. (Courtesy of Dr. Michael Brage.)

CLOSURE AND POSTOPERATIVE PLANS

- Perform copious irrigation and routine wound closure, and place the patient in a bulky cotton splint (**TECH FIG 5**).
- Range-of-motion exercises are started when the wound has sealed, typically at postoperative day 10. Patients are maintained non–weight-bearing for 3 months and then progressed to weight bearing as tolerated.

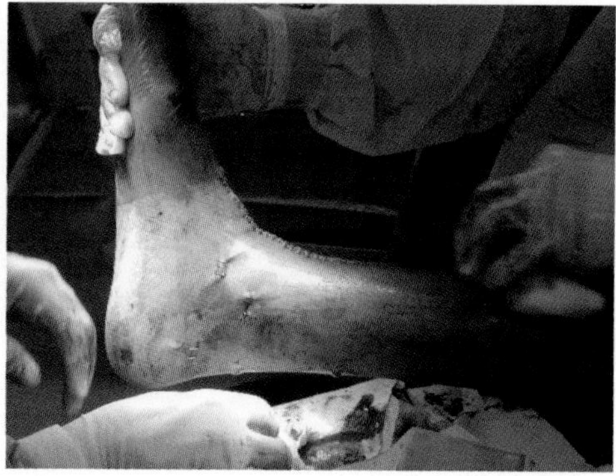

TECH FIG 5 • Wound is closed and range of motion is checked. (Courtesy of Dr. Michael Brage.)

PEARLS AND PITFALLS

Indications	■ Perform a complete history and physical examination. ■ Address associated pathology, such as an equinus contracture, pes planus, or pes cavus deformity.
Intraoperative fracture	■ Take care when making cuts to avoid fracture of the lateral or medial malleolus.
Graft preparation	■ Take care when preparing the allografts. ■ Use cutting guides to improve precision of cuts. Improper graft cuts may result in graft failure.
Neurovascular bundle	■ Avoid injury to the posterior tibial neurovascular bundle at the posteromedial corner of the ankle joint.

POSTOPERATIVE CARE

- Perioperative antibiotics and pain control are at the surgeon's discretion. The patient is placed in a bulky cotton splint with the ankle in neutral to slight dorsiflexion postoperatively.
- We routinely keep the operated extremity at touch-down weight bearing for 3 months.
- The patient begins range-of-motion exercises once the incision has healed (on roughly postoperative day 10).
- With satisfactory radiographs that suggest a progression toward graft incorporation, the patient may progress to weight bearing as tolerated after 3 months.

OUTCOMES

- Promising case series have reported on total ankle osteochondral shell allograft replacement of the tibiotalar joint as a

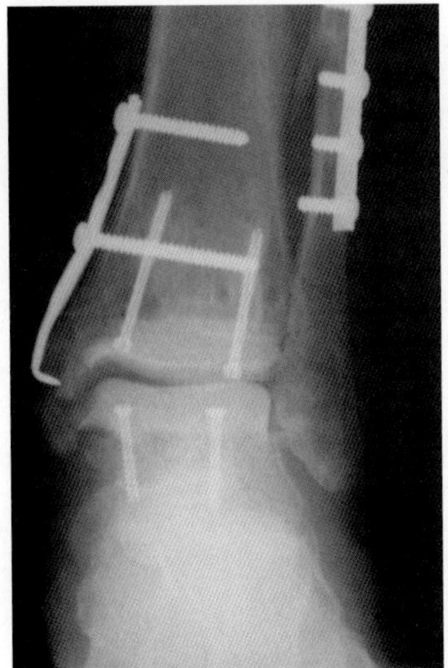

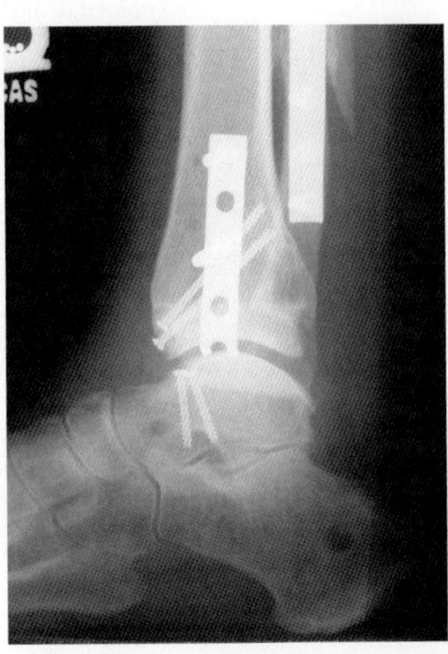

A B

FIG 2 • **A.** 4-month follow-up radiograph. **B.** Lateral view. (Courtesy of Dr. Michael Brage.)

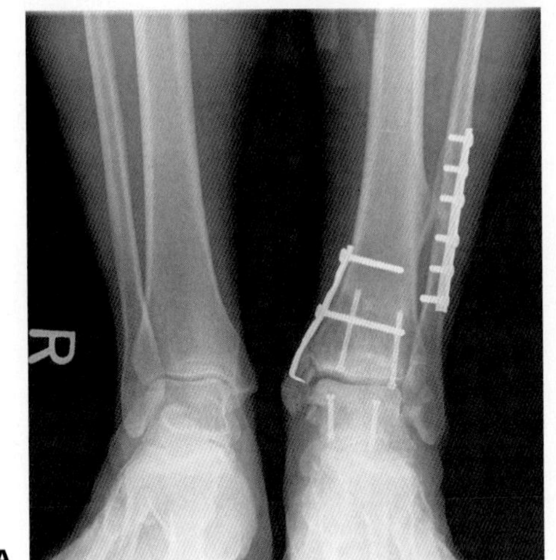

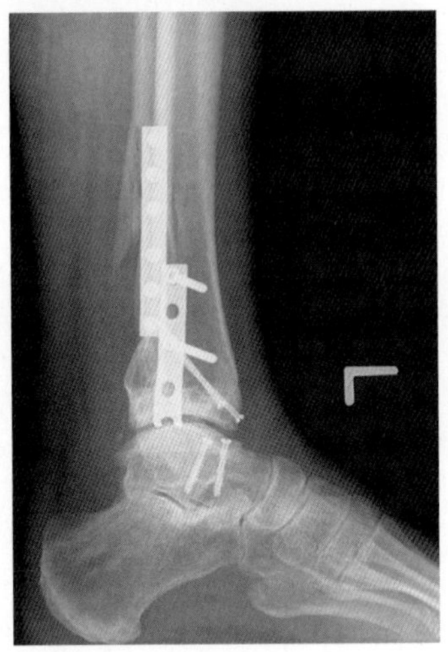

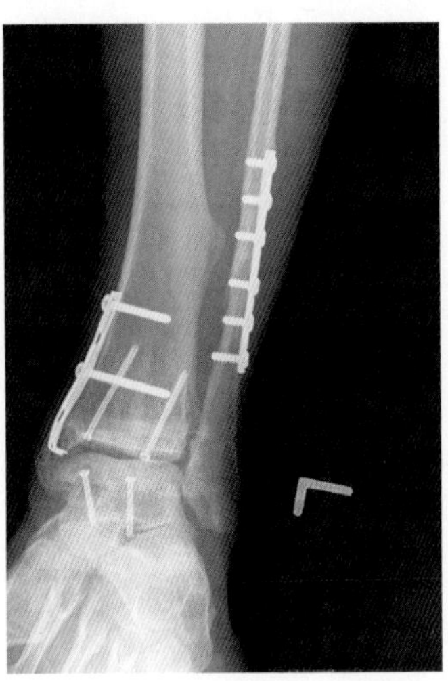

A B C

FIG 3 • **A.** Three-year follow-up radiograph, AP view. **B.** Lateral view. **C.** Mortise view. (Courtesy of Dr. Michael Brage.)

viable alternative for posttraumatic ankle arthritis in young patients (**FIGS 2 AND 3**).[8,11,17]

- The largest case series to date reports 6 out of 11 successful grafting procedures at a minimum follow-up of 24 months. Of the other five patients, three had revision allografting and one was revised to total ankle arthroplasty. The last patient did not have any further surgery.[11]
- Myerson reported that 14 of 29 fresh osteochondral shell allograft transplants had been revised to a repeat ankle transplant/arthrodesis. Six of the remaining 15 allografts were radiographic failures with progressive loss of joint space but did not require revision surgery. The remaining nine allografts (31%) were deemed a success. The authors concluded that patients with a lower body mass index, less angular deformity, and who refused arthrodesis did better. These authors did not use an external fixator during the procedure and did not use a cutting block one size bigger for the allograft as suggested in this article. Therefore their grafts may have been small/thin. Grafts should be at least 7 mm thick to prevent collapse.[7]
- Gross et al reported on nine patients treated with large fresh allografts of the talus to treat OCD lesions. Of the nine patients, six had successful procedures and remained in situ with a mean survival of 11 years. Three patients had fragmentation and collapse of the grafts and were converted to arthrodeses.[4]

COMPLICATIONS

- Intraoperative fracture
- Graft collapse
- Poor graft fixation
- Nonunion
- Need for additional débridement postoperatively

REFERENCES

1. Abidi NA, Gruen GS, Conti SF. Ankle arthrodesis: indications and techniques. J Am Acad Orthop Surg 2000;8:200–209.
2. Coester LM, Saltzman CL, Leupold J, et al. Long-term results following ankle arthrodesis for post-traumatic arthritis. J Bone Joint Surg 2001;83-A:219–228.

3. Coughlin MJ, Mann RA. Surgery of the Foot and Ankle. St. Louis, MO: Mosby, 1999.
4. Gross AE, Agnidis Z, Hutchison CR. Osteochondral defects of the talus treated with fresh osteochondral allograft transplantation. Foot Ankle Int 2001;22(5):385–391.
5. Haddad SL, Coetzee JC, Estok R, et al. Intermediate and long-term Outcomes of total ankle arthroplasty and ankle arthrodesis. A systematic review of the literature. J Bone Joint Surg 2007;89:1899–1905.
6. Hansen ST. Functional reconstruction of the foot and ankle. Philadelphia, PA: Lippincott Williams & Wilkins, 2000.
7. Jeng CL, Myerson MS. Fresh osteochondral total ankle allograft transplantation for the treatment of ankle arthritis. Foot Ankle Clin N Am 2008;13:539–547.
8. Kim CW, Jamali A, Tontz W, et al. Treatment of post-traumatic ankle arthrosis with bipolar tibiotalar osteochondral shell allografts. Foot Ankle Int 2002;23:1091–1102.
9. Kitaoka HB, Patzer GL, Ilstrup DM, et al. Survivorship analysis of the Mayo total ankle arthroplasty. J Bone Joint Surg 1994;76-A: 974–979.
10. Mann RA, Rongstad KM. Arthrodesis of the ankle: a critical analysis. Foot Ankle Int 1998;19:3–9.
11. Meehan R, McFarlin S, Bugbee W, et al. Fresh ankle osteochondral allograft transplantation for tibiotalar joint arthritis. Foot Ankle Int 2005;26:793–802.
12. Reider B. The Orthopaedic Physical Exam. Philadelphia, PA: Elsevier, 2005.
13. Richardson EG. Orthopaedic Knowledge Update: Foot and Ankle 3. Rosemont, IL: American Academy of Orthopaedic Surgeons, 2004.
14. Spirt AA, Assal M, Hansen ST. Complications and failure after total ankle arthroplasty. J Bone Joint Surg 2004;86-A:1172–1178.
15. SooHoo NF, Zingmond DS, Ko CY. Comparison of reoperation rates following ankle arthrodesis and total ankle arthrplasty. J Bone Joint Surg 2007;89:2143–2149.
16. Thomas RH, Daniels TR. Current concepts review ankle arthritis. J Bone Joint Surg 2003;85-A:923–936.
17. Tontz W, Bugbee W, Brage ME. Use of allografts in the management of ankle arthritis. Foot Ankle Clin N Am 2003;8:361–373.

Chapter 68 The STAR (Scandinavian Total Ankle Replacement) Total Ankle Arthroplasty

Mark E. Easley, James A. Nunley II, and James K. DeOrio

DEFINITION

- End-stage ankle arthritis failing to respond to nonoperative treatment

ANATOMY

- Ankle
  - Tibial plafond with medial malleolus
    - Articulations with dorsal and medial talus
    - In sagittal plane, slight posterior slope
    - In coronal plane, articular surface is 88 to 92 degrees relative to lateral tibial shaft axis.
  - Fibula
    - Articulation with lateral talus
    - Responsible for one sixth of axial load distribution of the ankle
  - Talus
    - 60% of surface area covered by articular cartilage
    - Dual radius of curvature
  - Distal tibiofibular syndesmosis
    - Anteroinferior tibiofibular ligament
    - Interosseous membrane
    - Posterior tibiofibular ligament
- Ankle functions as part of the ankle–hindfoot complex much like a mitered hinge.

PATHOGENESIS

- Posttraumatic arthrosis
  - Most common etiology
  - Intra-articular fracture
  - Ankle fracture-dislocation with malunion
  - Chronic ankle instability
- Primary osteoarthrosis
  - Relatively rare compared to hip and knee arthrosis
- Inflammatory arthropathy
  - Most commonly rheumatoid arthritis
- Other
  - Hemochromatosis
  - Pigmented villonodular synovitis
  - Charcot neuroarthropathy
  - Septic arthritis

NATURAL HISTORY

- Posttraumatic arthrosis
  - Malunion, chronic instability, intra-articular cartilage damage, or malalignment may lead to progressive articular cartilage wear.
  - Chronic lateral ankle instability may eventually be associated with:
    - Relative anterior subluxation of the talus
    - Varus tilt of the talus within the ankle mortise
    - Hindfoot varus position
- Primary osteoarthrosis of the ankle is rare and poorly understood.
- Inflammatory arthropathy
  - Progressive and proliferative synovial erosive changes failing to respond to medical management
  - May be associated with chronic posterior tibial tendinopathy and progressive valgus hindfoot deformity, eventual valgus tilt to the talus within the ankle mortise, potential lateral malleolar stress fracture, and compensatory forefoot varus

PATIENT HISTORY AND PHYSICAL FINDINGS

- Patient history
  - Often a history of ankle trauma
    - Ankle fracture, particularly intra-articular
    - Ankle fracture with malunion
    - Chronic ankle instability (recurrent ankle sprains)
  - Chronic anterior ankle pain, primarily with activity and weight bearing
  - Ankle stiffness, particularly with dorsiflexion
  - Ankle swelling
  - Progressively worsening activity level
- Physical findings
  - Limp
  - Patient externally rotates hip to externally rotate ankle to avoid painful push-off.
  - Painful and limited ankle range of motion (ROM), particularly limited dorsiflexion
  - Mild ankle edema
  - Potential associated foot deformity
    - Posttraumatic arthrosis secondary to chronic instability may be associated with varus ankle and hindfoot and compensatory forefoot varus.
    - Inflammatory arthritis may be associated with progressively worsening flatfoot deformity, valgus tilt to the ankle and hindfoot, and equinus.

IMAGING AND OTHER DIAGNOSTIC STUDIES

- Weight-bearing AP, lateral, and mortise views of the ankle (**FIG 1**)
- Weight-bearing AP, lateral, and oblique views of the foot, particularly with associated foot deformity
- With associated or suspected lower leg deformity, we routinely obtain weight-bearing AP and lateral tibia–fibula views.
- With deformity in the lower extremity, we routinely obtain weight-bearing mechanical axis (hip-to-ankle) views of both extremities.
- We typically evaluate complex or ill-defined ankle–hindfoot patterns of arthritis with or without deformity using CT of the ankle and hindfoot.

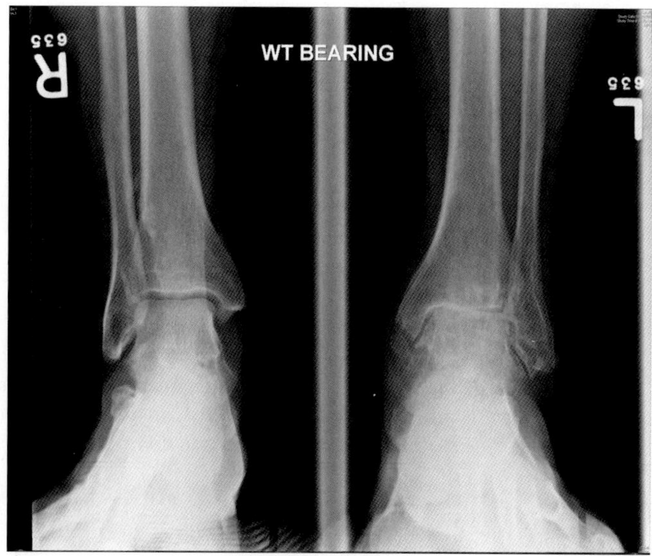

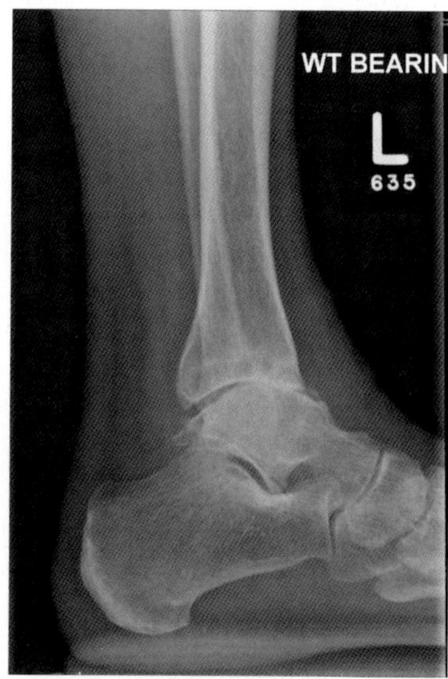

A B

FIG 1 • Weight-bearing ankle radiographs of a 60-year-old woman with end-stage posttraumatic left ankle arthritis. **A.** AP view (note slight varus talar tilt). **B.** Lateral view.

- If we suspect avascular necrosis of the talus or distal tibia, we obtain an MRI of the ankle.

DIFFERENTIAL DIAGNOSIS

- See the section on pathogenesis.

NONOPERATIVE MANAGEMENT

- Activity modification
- Bracing
  - Ankle–foot orthosis (AFO)
  - Double-upright brace attached to shoe
- Stiffer-soled shoe with a rocker-bottom modification
- Nonsteroidal anti-inflammatories or COX-2 inhibitors
- Medications for systemic inflammatory arthropathy
- Corticosteroid injection
- Viscosupplementation

SURGICAL MANAGEMENT

Preoperative Planning

- The surgeon must be sure the patient has satisfactory perfusion to support healing and is not neuropathic.
  - Noninvasive vascular studies and potential vascular surgery consultation should be obtained if necessary.
- The surgeon should inspect the ankle for prior scars or surgical approaches that need to be considered in planning the surgical approach for total ankle arthroplasty.
- The surgeon must understand the clinical and radiographic alignment of lower extremity, ankle, and foot.
  - The surgeon must be prepared to balance and realign the ankle. Occasionally, this necessitates corrective osteotomies of the distal tibia or foot, hindfoot arthrodesis, ligament releases or stabilization, or tendon transfers.
  - The surgeon should determine whether coronal-plane alignment is passively correctable; this provides some understanding of whether ligament releases will be required.
- Ankle ROM should be determined.
  - Ankle stiffness, particularly lack of dorsiflexion, needs to be corrected:
    - Anterior tibiotalar exostectomy
    - Posterior capsular release
    - Occasionally, tendo Achilles lengthening
- Instrumentation
  - These instruments facilitate total ankle arthroplasty:
    - Small oscillating saw to fine-tune cuts, resect prominences with precision, and easily morselize large bone fragments to be evacuated from the joint
    - A rasp for final preparation of cut bony surfaces
    - An angled curette, particularly to separate bone from the posterior capsule
    - A toothless lamina spreader to judiciously distract the ankle to improve exposure even after preparing the surfaces of the tibia and talus

Positioning

- The patient is positioned supine with the plantar aspect of the operated foot at the end of the operating table.
- The foot and ankle are well balanced, with toes directed to the ceiling.
- A bolster placed under the ipsilateral hip prevents undesired external rotation of the hip.
- We routinely use a thigh tourniquet and regional anesthesia.
  - A popliteal block provides adequate pain relief postoperatively, particularly if a regional catheter is used. Moreover, hip and knee flexion–extension is not forfeited, facilitating safe immediate postoperative mobilization.
  - However, using a thigh tourniquet with a popliteal block typically requires a supplemental femoral nerve block (patient forfeits knee extension) or general anesthesia.

Approach

- An anterior approach to the ankle is made, using the interval between the tibialis anterior (TA) tendon and the extensor hallucis longus (EHL) tendon.

APPROACH

- Make a longitudinal midline incision over the anterior ankle, starting about 10 cm proximal to the tibiotalar joint and 1 cm lateral to the tibial crest (TECH FIG 1).
- Continue the incision midline over the anterior ankle just distal to the talonavicular joint.
- At no point should direct tension be placed on the skin margins; we perform deep, full-thickness retraction as soon as possible to limit the risk of skin complications.
- Identify and protect the superficial peroneal nerve by retracting it laterally.
  - In our experience there is a consistent branch of the superficial peroneal nerve that crosses directly over or immediately proximal to the tibiotalar joint.
- We then expose the extensor retinaculum, identify the course of the EHL tendon, and sharply but carefully divide the retinaculum directly over the EHL tendon.
  - We always attempt to maintain the TA tendon in its dedicated sheath.
  - Preserving the retinaculum over the TA tendon:
    - This prevents bowstringing of the tendon and thereby reduces the stress on the anterior wound.
    - Should there be a wound dehiscence, then the TA is not directly exposed.
    - Preserving the retinaculum over the TA tendon is not always possible; some patients do not have a dedicated sheath for the TA.
- The interval between the TA and EHL tendon is used, with the TA and EHL tendons retracted medially and laterally, respectively.
- Identify and carefully retract the deep neurovascular bundle (anterior tibial–dorsalis pedis artery and deep peroneal nerve) laterally throughout the remainder of the procedure.
- Perform an anterior capsulotomy along with elevation of the tibial and dorsal talar periosteum to about 6 to 8 cm proximal to the tibial plafond and talonavicular joint, respectively.
- Elevate this separated capsule and periosteum medially and laterally to expose the ankle, to access the medial and lateral gutters, and to visualize the medial and lateral malleoli.
- Remove anterior tibial and talar osteophytes to facilitate exposure and avoid interference with the instrumentation.

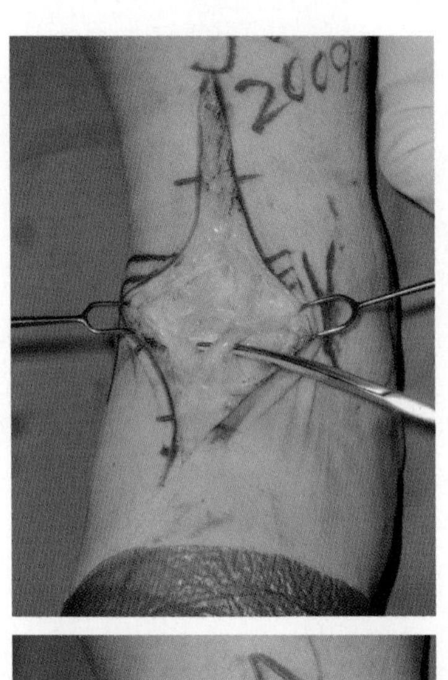
A

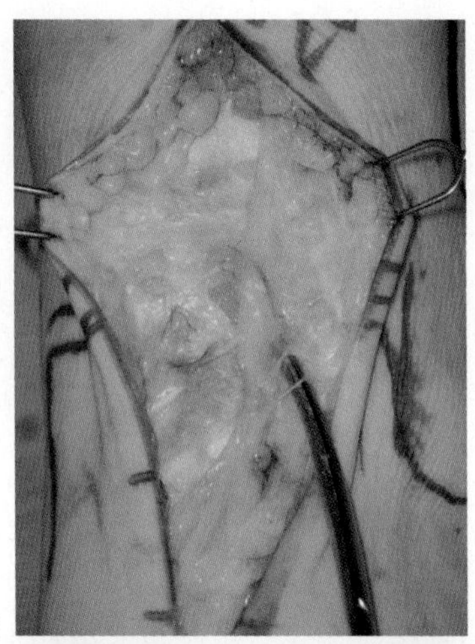
B

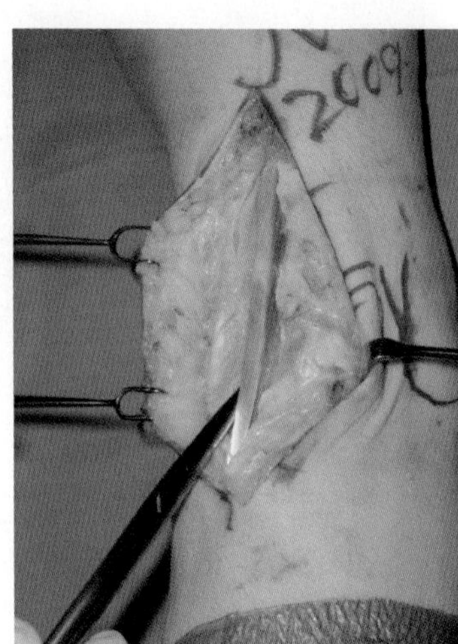
C

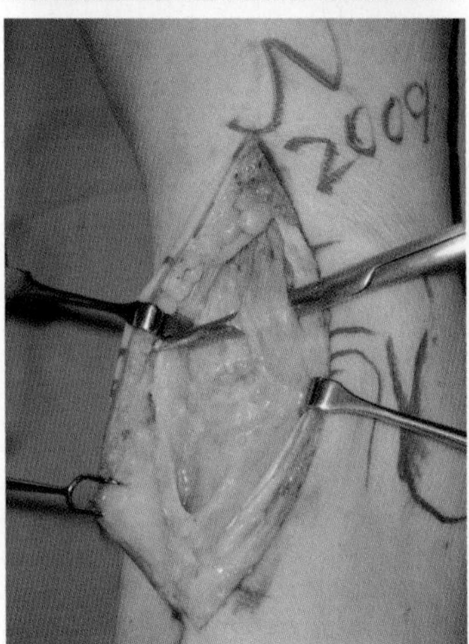
D

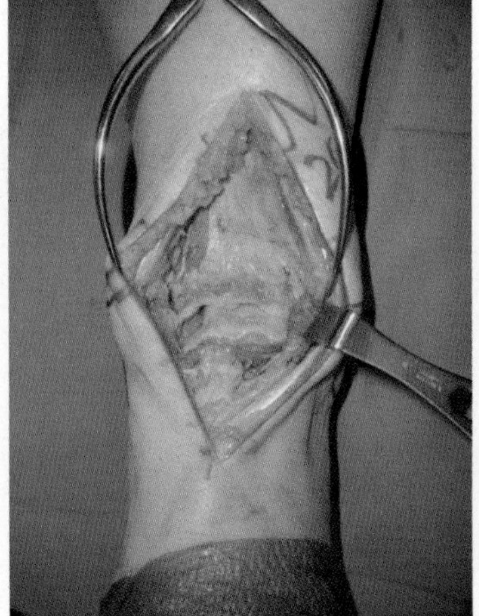
E

TECH FIG 1 • Anterior approach to the ankle. **A.** Approach. **B.** Close-up of superficial peroneal nerve. **C.** Division of extensor retinaculum directly over extensor hallucis longus tendon. **D.** Deep neurovascular bundle is identified and protected. **E.** After anterior capsulotomy, with ankle exposed.

TIBIAL PREPARATION

- An osteotome placed in the medial gutter serves as a reference for optimal rotation for the tibial preparation (TECH FIG 2).
- Place a pin in the proximal tibia via a 1-cm incision over the tibial tubercle.
  - When viewed in the AP plane, this pin is oriented parallel to the reference osteotome in the medial gutter.
  - When viewed in the lateral plane, the pin should be perpendicular to the tibial shaft axis if the physiologic 3 to 5 degrees of posterior slope to the tibial component is desired. We prefer to implant the tibial component perpendicular to the longitudinal tibial shaft axis (no posterior slope), aiming the pin slightly proximally. The external tibial alignment guide directs the initial tibial cut into 3 degrees of posterior slope; we aim to eliminate this slope.
- Suspend the external tibial alignment guide from the proximal pin. To further promote a perpendicular tibial preparation relative to the tibial shaft axis, we raise the proximal aspect of the external tibial alignment guide two to three fingerbreadths above the tibial spine before securing it to the proximal pin.
- Set the rotation of the cutting block for tibial preparation based on the reference osteotome set in the medial gutter. A dedicated T-guide temporarily attached to the distal aspect of the guide facilitates setting proper rotation. Lock the rotation of the distal block with the knob connecting the telescoping rods of the guide.
- While controlling rotation, set the proper length of the guide via the telescoping rods.
- Fine-tuning of the distal block's lateral-plane position is possible. We routinely separate the distal block of the

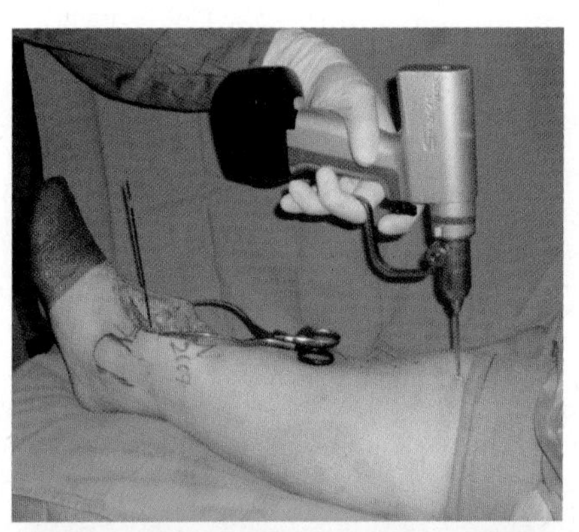

A

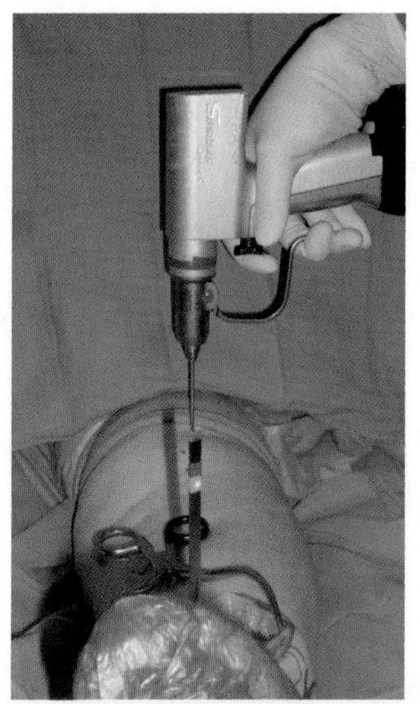

B

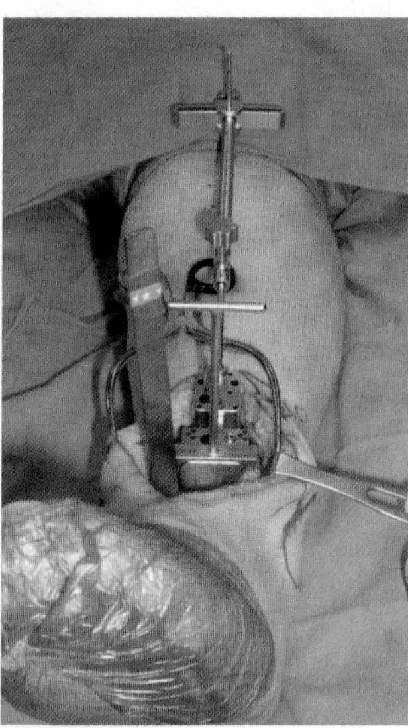

D

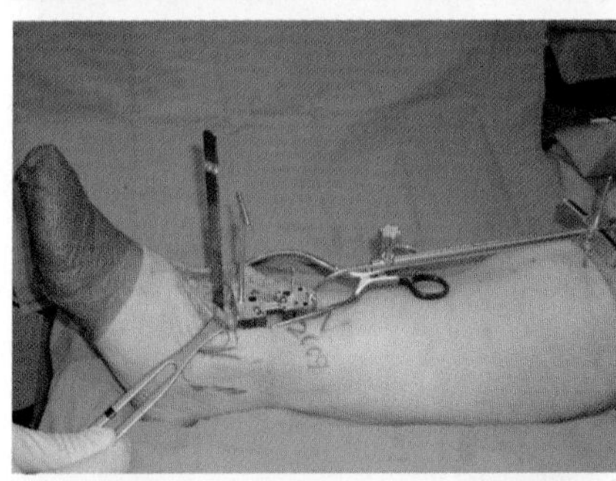

C

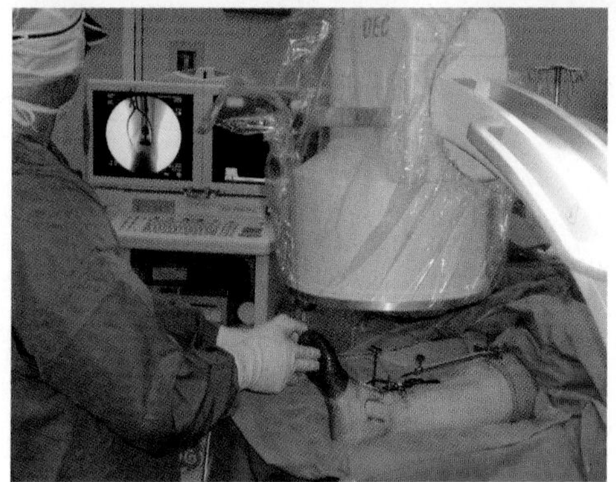

E

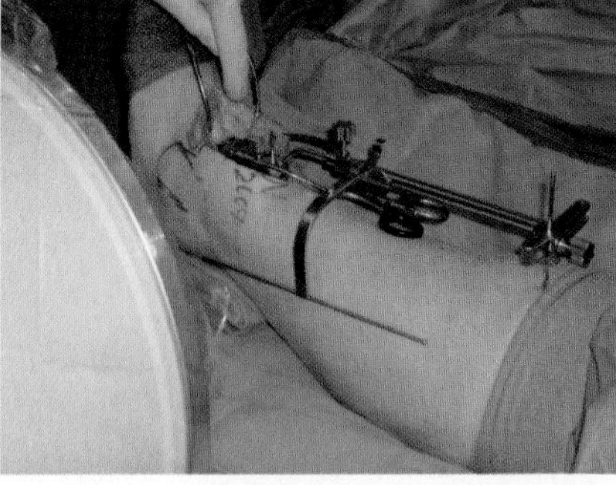

F

TECH FIG 2 • Positioning the external tibial alignment guide. **A, B.** Positioning the proximal pin relative to a reference osteotome placed in the medial gutter. **C, D.** Setting rotation of the distal cutting block of the guide relative to the medial gutter reference osteotome. **E, F.** Fluoroscopic confirmation of proper guide position in the AP and lateral planes.

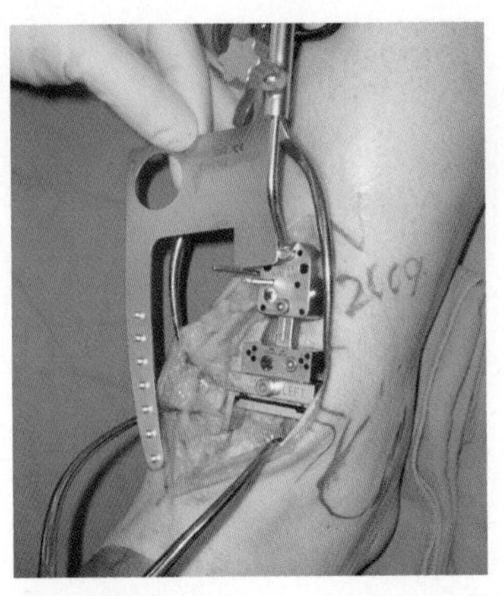

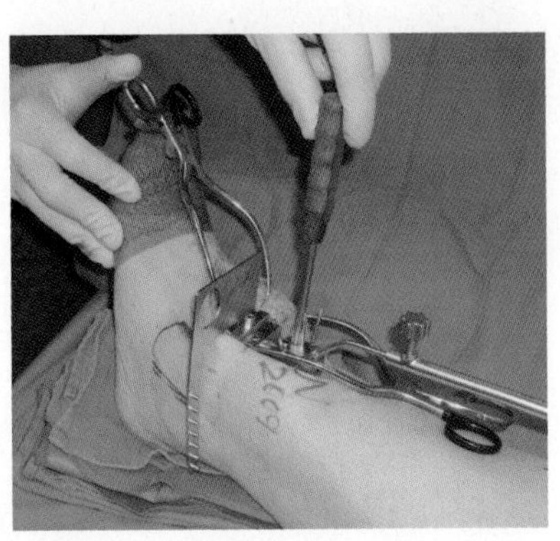

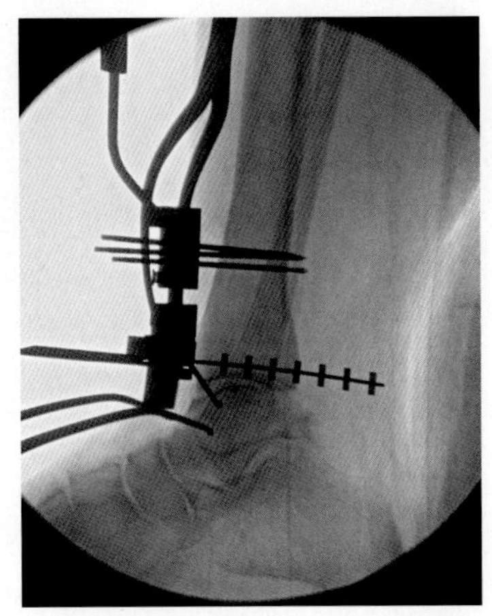

TECH FIG 3 • Determining tibial plafond resection level. **A.** Angel wing about to be inserted into capture guide attached to distal tibial cutting block. **B.** Angel wing in capture guide with height adjustment being made under fluoroscopy. **C.** Fluoroscopic image of angel wing confirming tibial resection level.

guide from the portion of the guide used to pin it to the tibia by at least 10 mm.

- If the initial position of the distal block is set at the apex of the plafond, the desired 5 mm of resection may be easily set and even greater resection is possible in a tighter ankle.
- We make sure that the block is positioned at the tibial plafond's apex, that it is properly rotated, and that we are able to fine-tune the block's proximal–distal position before pinning the guide to the tibia.
  - Multiple options exist to pin the guide to the tibia. We recommend using pins at different levels rather than pins in a single plane (risks creating a stress riser).
- Attach the cutting capture guide to the distal block, and insert an angel-wing resection guide in the capture guide. Use fluoroscopy in the lateral plane to determine the proper resection level for the tibial cut (TECH FIG 3).
- Adjust the cutting guide in the coronal plane to ensure that the malleoli are protected with tibial resection.
  - There is only a single capture guide size.
  - We routinely set the guide based on a pin placed loosely in the medial aspect of the capture guide.
  - We aim to position the guide so that the medial extent of tibial preparation is directly proximal from the transition of tibial plafond to medial malleolus.
  - Drive the pin used as a reference into the tibia through the medial aspect of the capture guide to protect the medial malleolus.
  - Similarly, place a lateral pin in the lateral aspect of the capture guide and advance it into the lateral gutter.
  - The capture guide has several options to place the lateral pin to accommodate any coronal plane dimension of the tibial plafond.
- With the soft tissues protected, particularly the deep neurovascular bundle, make the distal tibial cut with an oscillating saw through the horizontal portion of the capture guide. To complete the cut, use a reciprocating saw along the medial border of the capture guide, extending proximally from the medial gutter (TECH FIG 4).
- Remove the capture guide and evacuate the resected bone.
  - A toothless lamina spreader may be placed judiciously on the prepared tibial surface and dorsal talus to facilitate evacuation of bone from the posterior ankle.

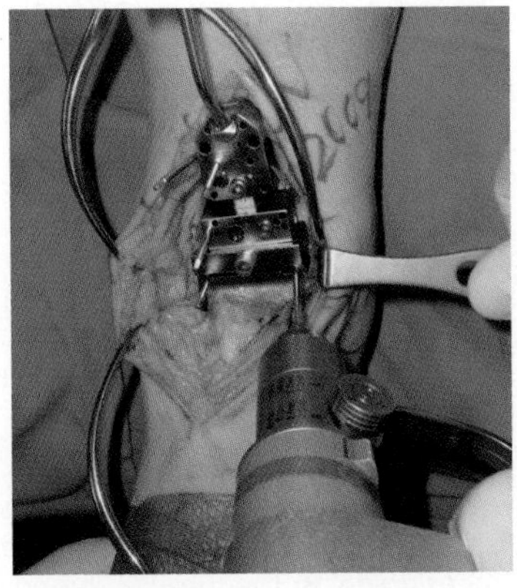

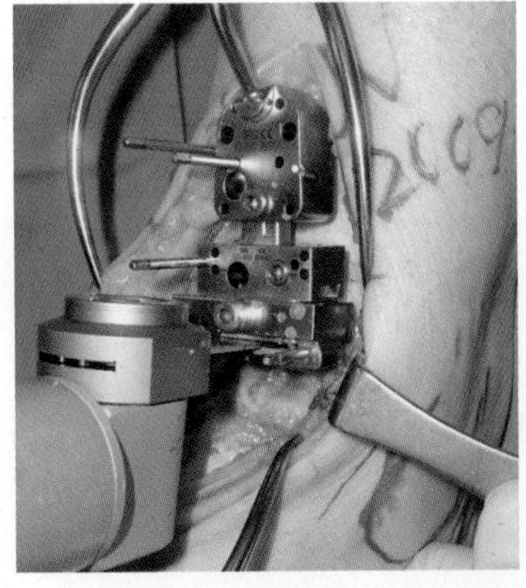

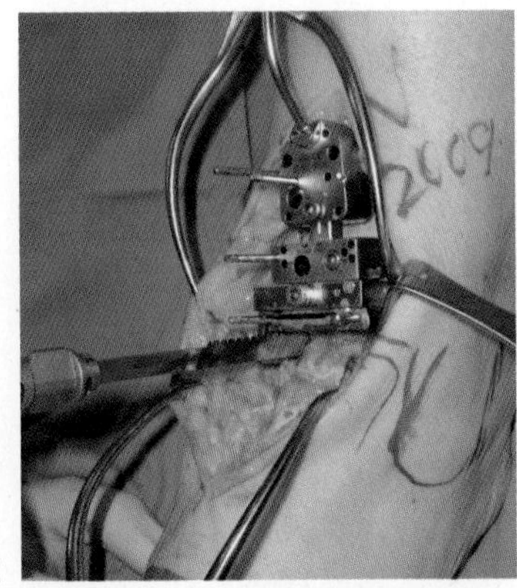

TECH FIG 4 • Initial tibial resection. **A.** After determining proper coronal placement of the tibial cutting block, the capture guide is pinned, with the pins used to protect the malleoli. **B.** Saw in the capture guide. **C.** Medial resection with a reciprocating saw to complete the initial tibial preparation. *(continued)*

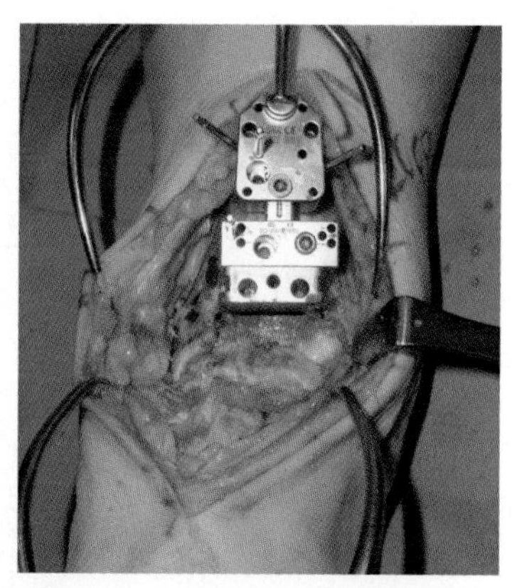
D

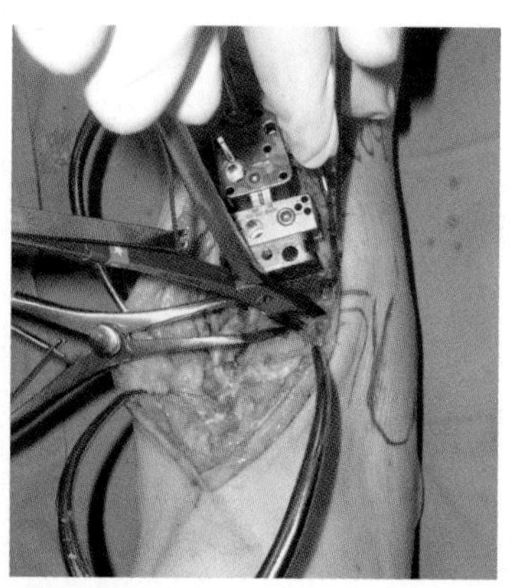
E

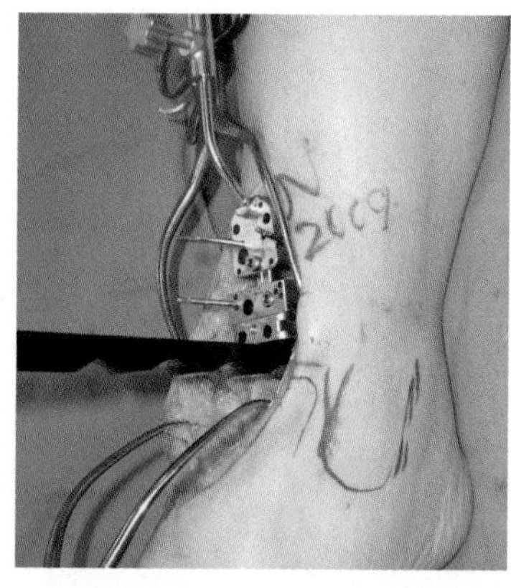
F

TECH FIG 4 • *(continued)* **D.** Tibial resection after removal of the capture guide (note that the cutting block was translated slightly medial for optimal positioning). **E.** Removal of the resected tibial bone (note the judicious use of a toothless lamina spreader to facilitate access to the posterior ankle). **F.** Confirming adequate tibial resection with plastic spacer (9 mm).

- We routinely use a small reciprocating saw to morselize the posterior fragments and a combination of curved curette and rongeur to retrieve the fragments that need to be separated from the posterior capsule.
  - The curette is used directly vertically in the ankle and never levered against a malleolus.
- We routinely perform a posterior capsular resection to optimize dorsiflexion.
- To ensure that the tibial resection is adequate, use the system's plastic spacer as a sizing guide. The 9-mm end of this sizing guide equals the combined height of the tibial component (3 mm) and the thinnest polyethylene component (6 mm).

TALAR PREPARATION

Initial Talar Preparation

- Residual articular cartilage must be removed from the dorsal talar dome so that the talar cutting guide may be properly balanced on the dorsal talus. We routinely use a thin oscillating saw to remove residual cartilage.
- Position the talar guide within the ankle joint and secure it to the distal block of the external alignment guide.
- We then hold the ankle in neutral dorsiflexion–-plantarflexion.
  - Excessive dorsiflexion risks talar preparation, leading to anterior translation and tilt of the talar implant. Moreover, an exaggerated notch will be created in the dorsal talar neck.
  - Excessive plantarflexion risks talar preparation, leading to posterior translation and tilt of the talar implant. In addition, too much posterior talus will be removed.
  - Excessive plantarflexion may be a result of fixed equinus. If the talus cannot be brought to a neutral position (confirm with an intraoperative radiograph), then consider a tendo Achilles lengthening rather than risk resecting too much of the posterior talus.
- With perfect contact of both the medial and lateral talar dome on the intra-articularly placed paddle of the talar cutting guide and a neutral sagittal plane alignment maintained, pin the talar guide.
- Place the angel-wing resection guide in the talar cutting guide and use lateral-plane fluoroscopy to confirm proper resection level and desired orientation for the guide.
- Place two more pins in the talar guide to protect the malleoli and further stabilize the guide.
- Make the initial talar cut using an oscillating saw, remove the guide, and evacuate the resected bone from the joint (TECH FIG 5).

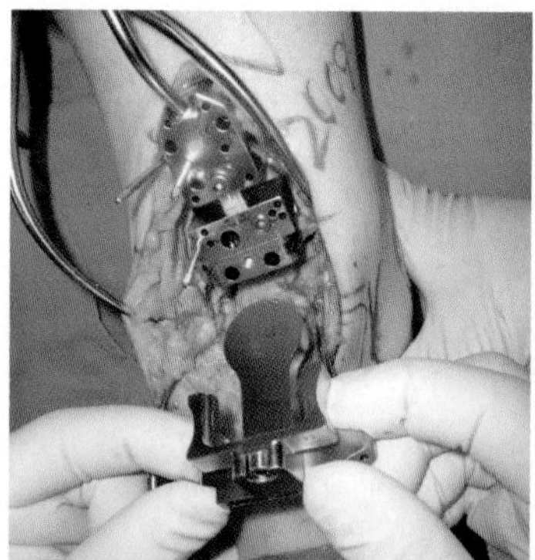
A

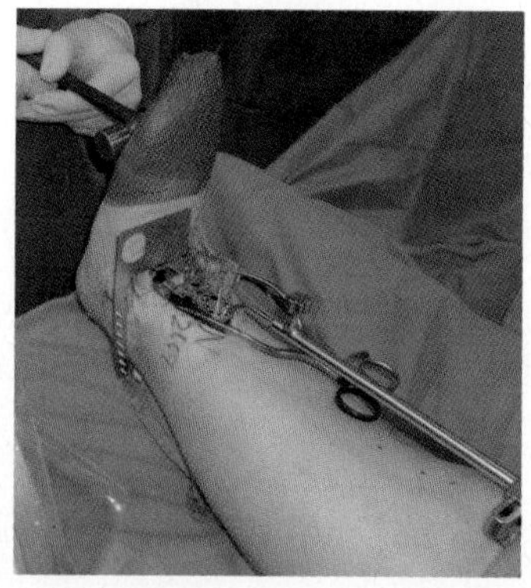
B

TECH FIG 5 • Talar resection. **A.** Talar resection guide to be suspended from the external tibial alignment guide. **B.** The surgeon should ensure proper talar alignment (patient had an equinus contracture, and gastrocnemius–soleus recession was required to obtain optimal talar position). *(continued)*

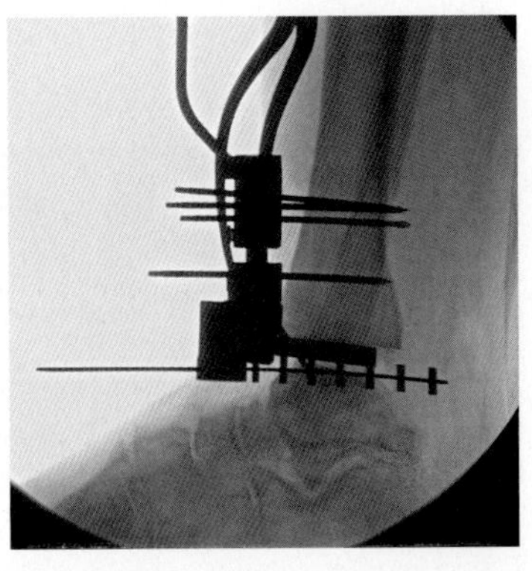

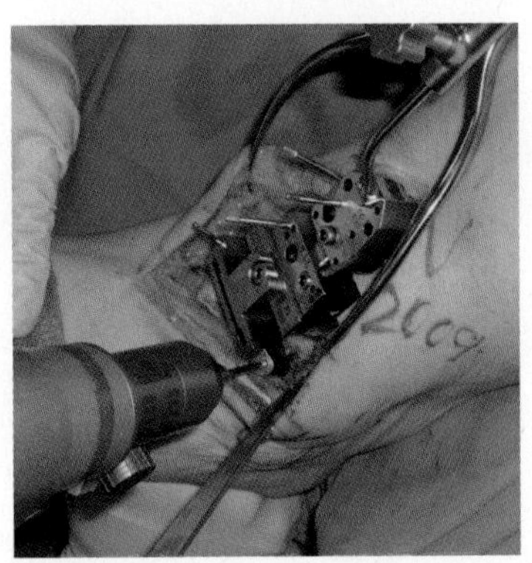

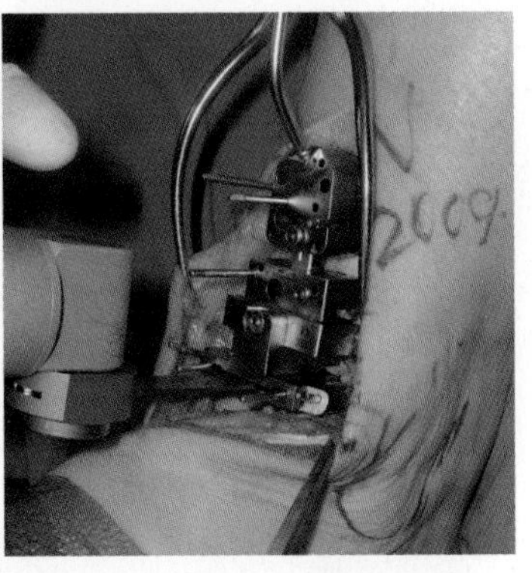

TECH FIG 5 • *(continued)* **C.** Intraoperative fluoroscopic view confirming resection level. Note the gap between intra-articular paddle of talar resection guide, suggesting some residual articular cartilage on talar dome and leaving talar resection too shallow. This prompted removal of residual talar cartilage to obtain optimal talar resection. **D.** Pinning the talar cutting guide. **E.** Talar resection with soft tissues protected.

- To ensure that a balanced resection was performed on the tibia and talus and that the resection levels are appropriate, use the plastic spacer–sizing guide–impactor and confirm proper alignment and resection levels on intraoperative fluoroscopy (TECH FIG 6).

Sizing the Talus and Positioning the 4-in-1 Talar Reference Guide ("Datum")

- Position a sizing guide on the dorsal prepared talar surface and properly rotate it with the second metatarsal. The proper sizing guide leaves 3 mm of medial and 3 mm of lateral bone (TECH FIG 7). Set the AP position of the sizing guide based on the resected surface; excessive bone should not be removed from the posterior talus. Mark the talar sizing guide on the prepared talar surface.
- Using the markings on the talus, position the 4-in-1 talar reference guide ("datum") on the prepared talar surface, with proper rotation, proper mediolateral-plane

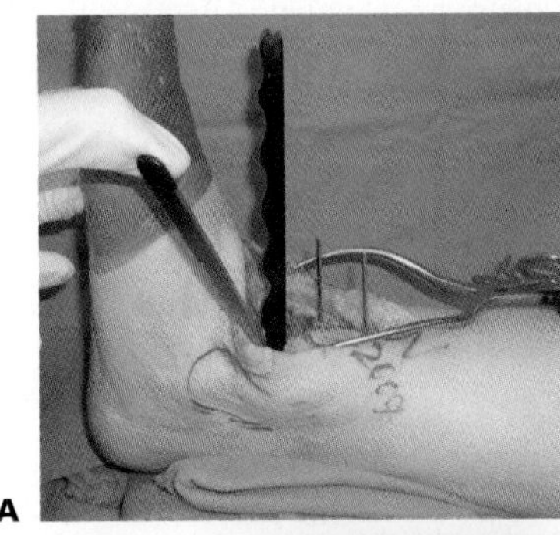

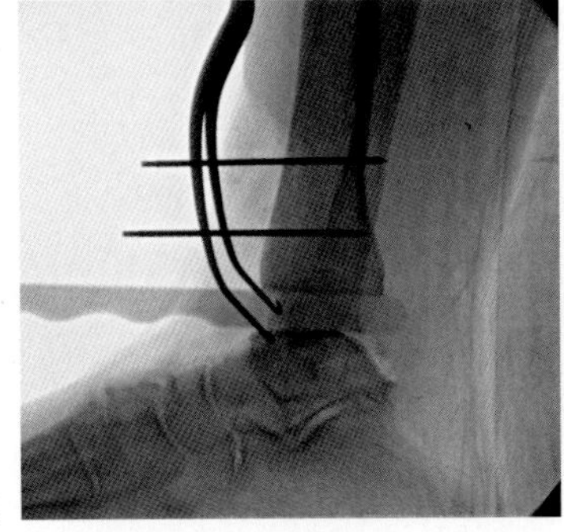

TECH FIG 6 • Confirming adequate and balanced gap. **A.** Plastic spacer confirms adequate resection (12-mm gap) **B.** Fluoroscopy confirms that the resections are balanced.

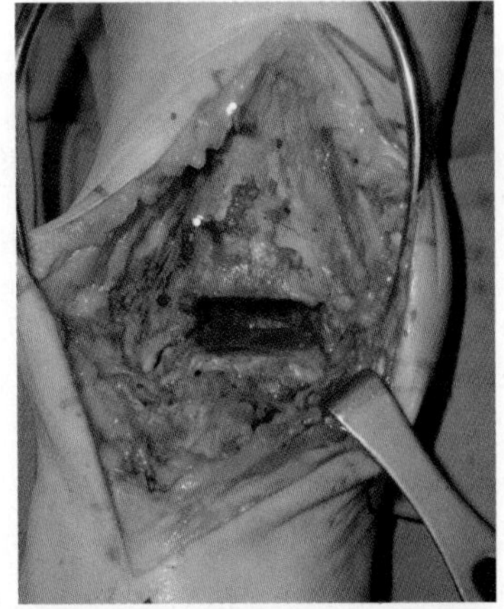

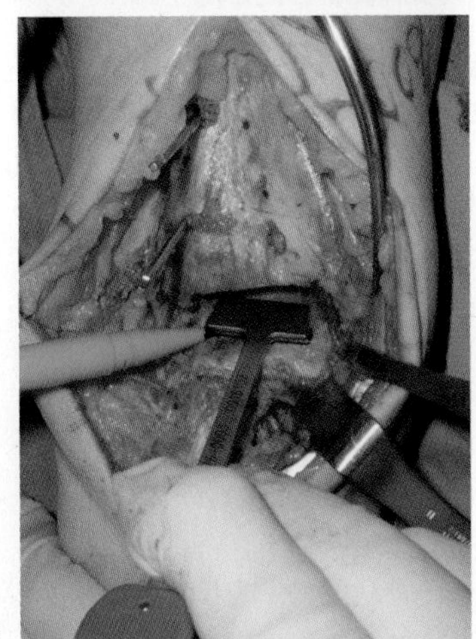

TECH FIG 7 • Talar sizing. **A.** Balanced resection. **B.** Talar sizing guide properly positioned (3 mm of residual talus on either side of sizing guide) on the prepared talar surface and properly rotated (oriented with second metatarsal axis). Note marking the talar surface to then place the talar reference guide.

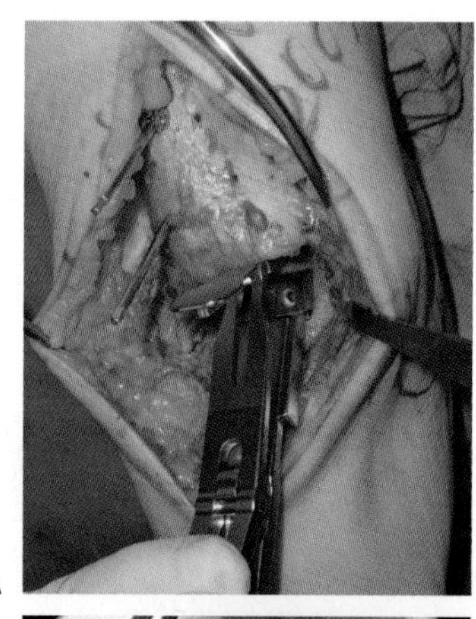
A

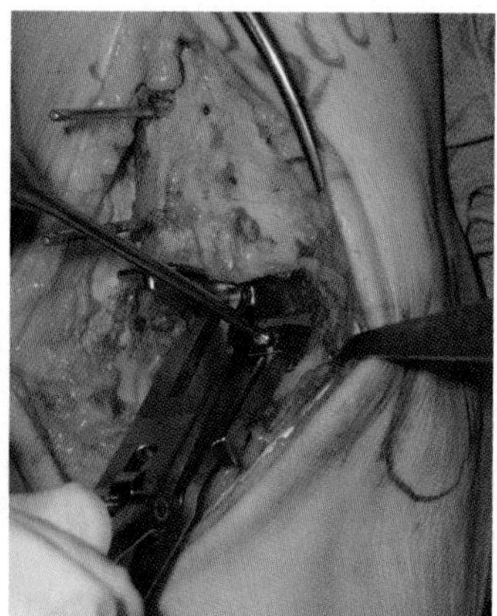
B

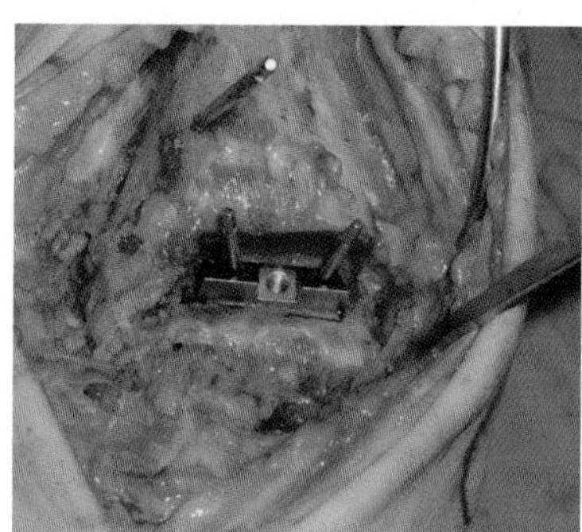
C

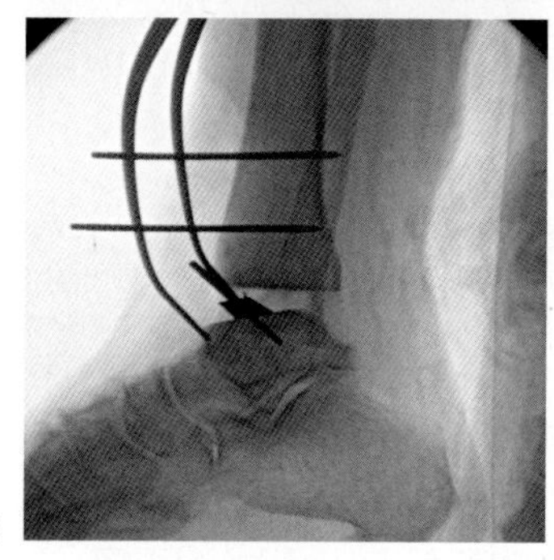
D

TECH FIG 8 • Positioning the 4-in-1 reference guide. **A.** Guide positioned on the prepared talar surface with the handle. **B.** Screw fixation of the 4-in-1 guide to the talus. **C.** 4-in-1 guide properly positioned with handle removed. **D.** Fluoroscopic confirmation of proper reference guide position.

position (3 mm of talus on either side of the guide), and a best estimate of proper anteroposterior position. Secure the 4-in-1 guide to the talus with dedicated pins (TECH FIG 8).

- Confirm proper position of the 4-in-1 guide with lateral fluoroscopy. Ideally, the center point of the undersurface of the guide rests directly over the lateral talar process. Another rough estimate of proper position is that the guide is centered under the tibia.
  - Full dorsiflexion of the talus is not possible due to impingement of the pins securing the guide to the talus.
- If this position cannot be confirmed, then the 4-in-1 talar guide must be repositioned and repinned.
  - This may be difficult, since typically only a subtle move of the guide is necessary, and securing a pin immediately adjacent to a previous pin position is possible but challenging.

COMPLETING THE TALAR PREPARATION AND IMPLANTING THE TALAR COMPONENT

Anteroposterior Talar Chamfer Cutting Guide

- Secure the anteroposterior talar chamfer cutting guide to the 4-in-1 talar reference guide and place an additional pin in the guide to stabilize it to the talus (TECH FIG 9).
- Cut the posterior talar chamfer using an oscillating saw in the posterior capture guide.
- Mill the anterior chamfer with the soft tissues and deep neurovascular bundle protected.
- Remove this guide, leaving the 4-in-1 guide in place.

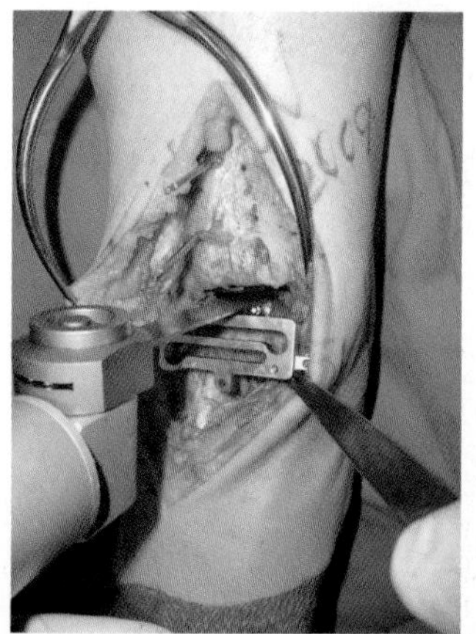
A

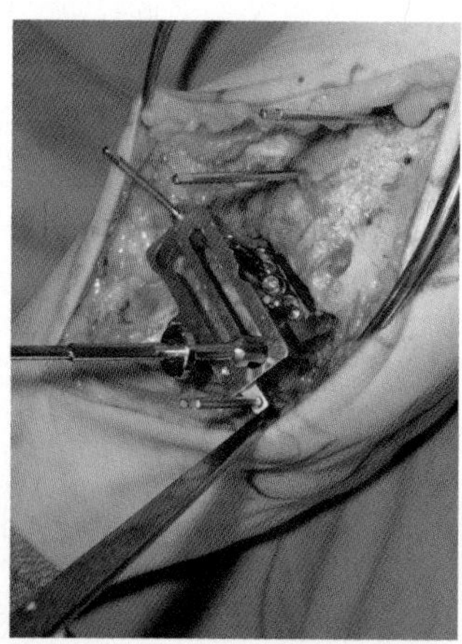
B

TECH FIG 9 • Anterior and posterior talar chamfer preparation. **A.** Pinning AP chamfer guide attached to 4-in-1 reference guide. **B.** Posterior chamfer resection. *(continued)*

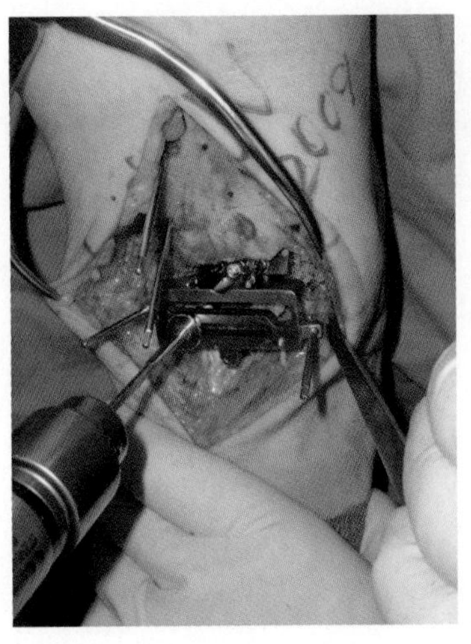

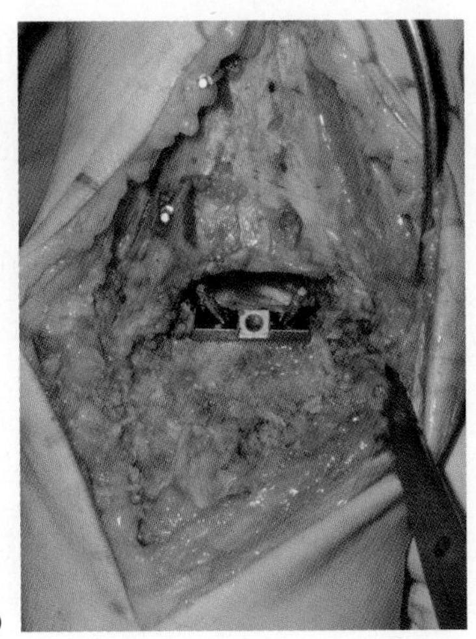

TECH FIG 9 • *(continued)* **C.** Anterior chamfer milling (additional pins were placed to support the guide in the talus). **D.** Talus with 4-in-1 reference guide in place and prepared AP chamfers.

Mediolateral Chamfer Cutting Guide

- Secure the mediolateral chamfer cutting guide to the 4-in-1 talar reference guide (TECH FIG 10).
  - Two additional smooth pins may be placed through this guide to further stabilize the guide to the talus.
- With the soft tissues and neurovascular structures protected, make the medial and lateral chamfer cuts with a reciprocal saw.
  - To accommodate the talar implant:
    - Medial cut is made to a depth of 10 mm.
    - Lateral cut is made to a depth of 15 mm.
- Remove the mediolateral chamfer and 4-in-1 reference guides.
- Evacuate the resected bone with:
  - A thin osteotome
  - A curved curette
  - A rongeur
- Inspect the prepared talus for any uneven surfaces or residual bony prominences, which may be removed judiciously with a small reciprocal saw and a rasp.

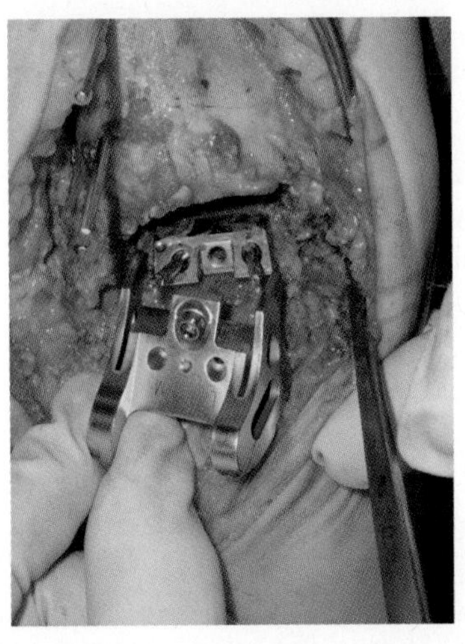

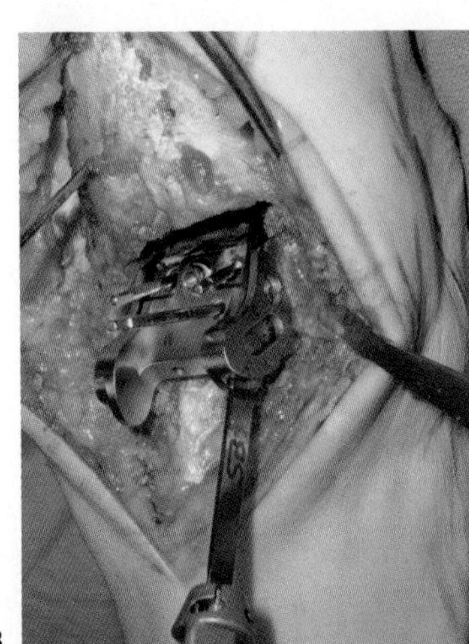

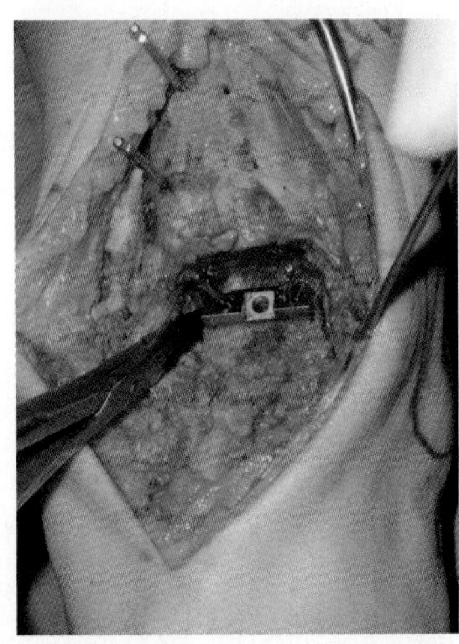

TECH FIG 10 • Mediolateral talar chamfer preparation. **A.** The mediolateral chamfer guide. **B.** Guide attached to the 4-in-1 reference guide and lateral chamfer being prepared with reciprocating saw (note protection of soft tissues with retractor). **C.** Talus after mediolateral chamfer resection and rongeur used to evacuate resected bone from medial gutter.

The "Window" Talar Trial

- Position the "window" talar trial on the prepared talus (TECH FIG 11).
- Often any incongruencies or prominences still need to be addressed to ensure that the guide rests completely flush on all prepared surfaces of the talus.
  - Since the guide is a "window," proper fit can be confirmed for the true implant that is resurfacing without any means of determining the actual bony contact between bone and implant.
- Pin the talar trial.

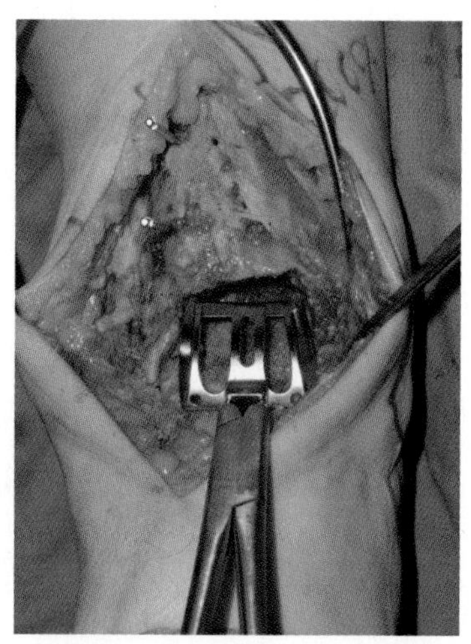

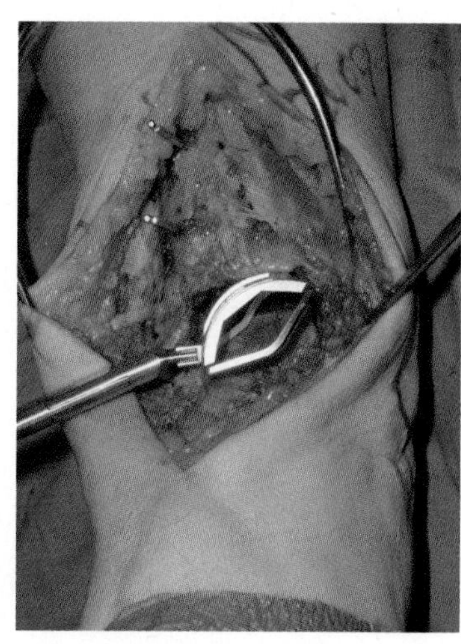

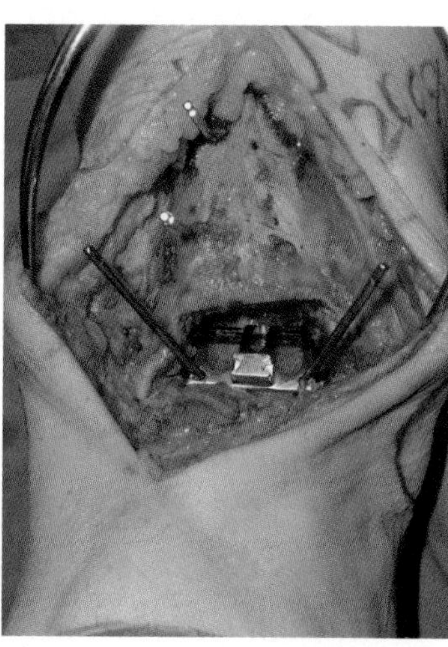

TECH FIG 11 • Trial talus ("window trial"). **A.** Lateral view of trial. **B.** AP view of trial. **C.** Trial pinned to talus; note congruent fit on all prepared surfaces.

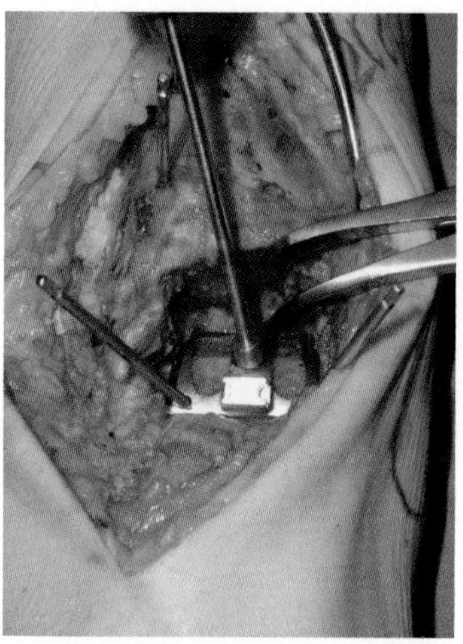

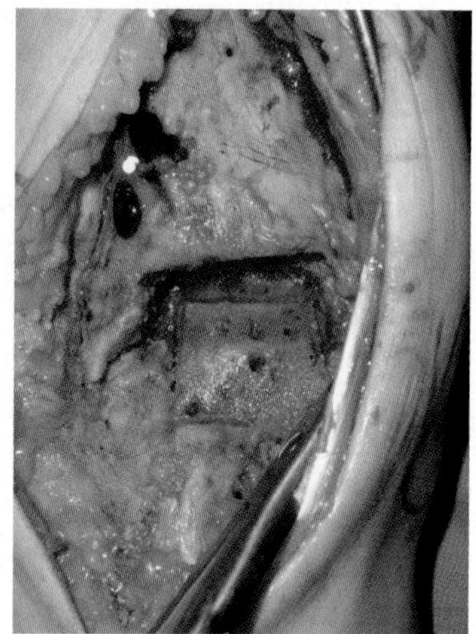

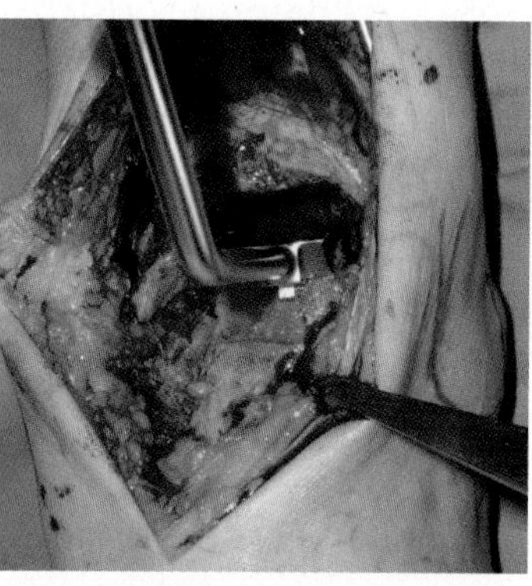

TECH FIG 12 • Preparing the fin slot for the talar stem. **A.** Using the router in the trial talus (note the judicious use of a toothless lamina spreader to afford greater support to the trial during talar stem preparation). **B.** Talus after removal of talar trial and fin slot preparation. **C.** Stem punch is used to complete preparation of fin slot.

- Use a router to create the slot in the talus to accommodate the talar implant's fin (TECH FIG 12).
- Use a stem punch to finish preparing the talar fin slot.

Implanting the Talar Component

- Orient the properly sized talar component with the longer side placed laterally (to articulate with the fibula) (TECH FIG 13).
- Gently tap the prosthesis posteriorly with the set's plastic impactor–spacer–sizer to rest in the optimal position over the fin slot.
- Use the talar dome impaction device to impact the talar component.
  - The anterior tibial cortex must be protected.
- We make sure that despite proper initial positioning the talar component does not tilt anteriorly, which it will tend to do given the limited access to the natural talus.
- Fully seat the talar component.

Final Preparation of the Tibial Plafond and Tibial Component Implantation

- Measure the AP dimensions of the tibia.
- Select the corresponding tibial component.
- If the mediolateral dimensions of the tibial plafond do not accommodate this component, then judiciously remove 1 or 2 more millimeters of medial bone to safely position the tibial trial.
- Also, all syndesmotic soft tissue impinging in the joint must be removed.
- The tibial trial should align with the center of the tibial shaft axis (TECH FIG 14).
  - It should not be tilted in varus or valgus.
  - It should not be lateral to the longitudinal center of the tibial shaft.

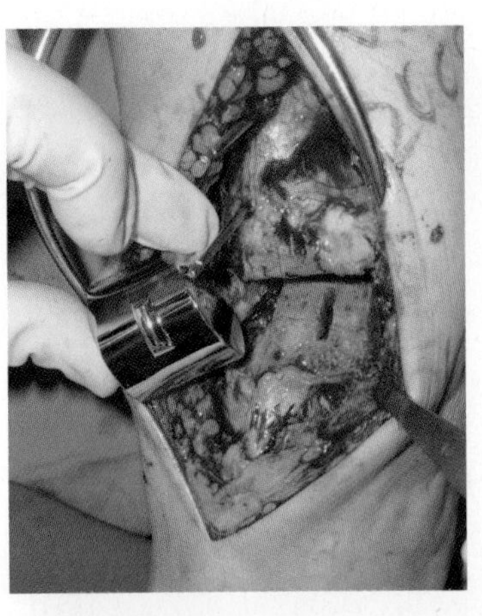
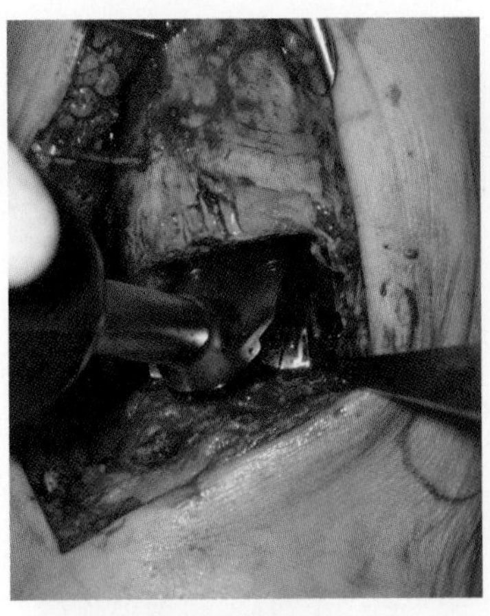

TECH FIG 13 • Inserting talar component. **A.** Talar component properly oriented. **B.** Impacting the talar component (note that the ankle is plantarflexed and the impactor is not contacting the anterior tibia).

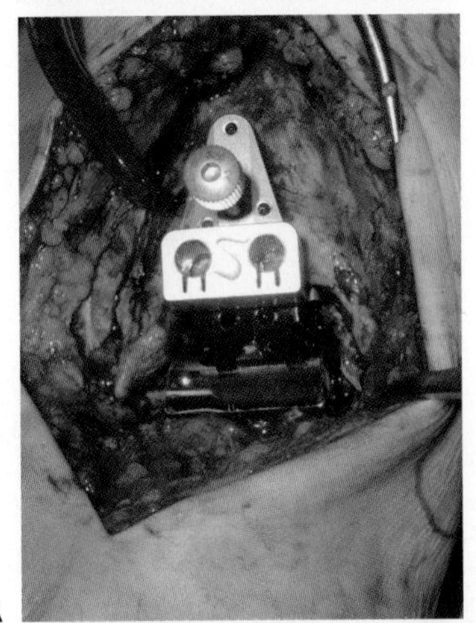
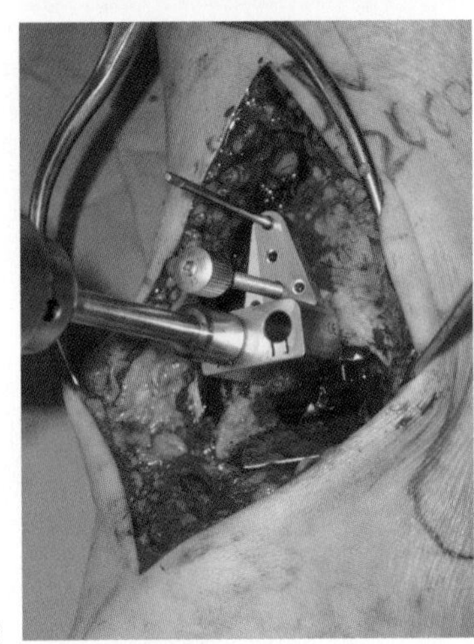
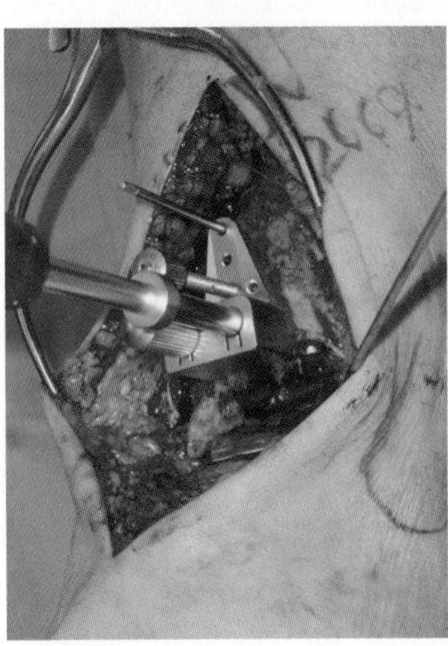
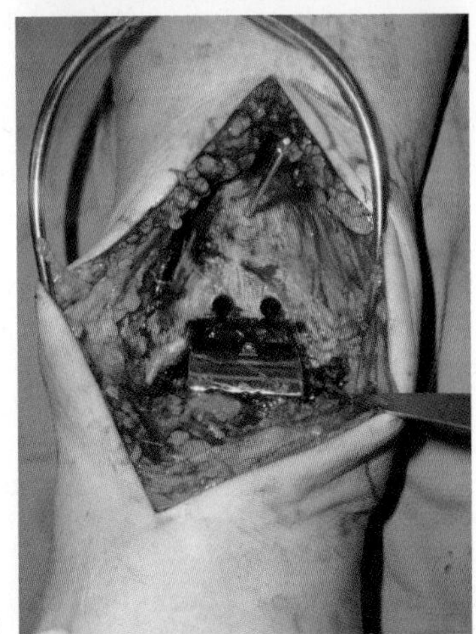

TECH FIG 14 • Final tibial preparation. **A.** Properly sized tibial trial in place, with trial polyethylene for support (we routinely obtain fluoroscopic confirmation in the lateral plane that the tibial trial is flush on the prepared tibial surface). **B.** Reaming the barrel holes. **C.** Using the dedicated chisel to complete the barrel hole preparation. **D.** Prepared tibia.

- After positioning the proper size of tibial component and confirming its position on intraoperative fluoroscopy, pin the tibial trial.
- Temporarily insert a trial polyethylene insert to maintain pressure on the tibial trial and therefore optimal bony apposition of the tibial trial base plate and prepared tibial surface.
- On intraoperative fluoroscopy, there should not be any posterior tibial tray lift-off from the prepared tibial surface and the tibial trial should be well aligned with the tibial shaft axis on the AP view.
- Prepare the barrel holes with the corresponding drill and chisel and remove the tibial trial and trial polyethylene. Leave the pin placed to secure the tibial trial as a reference.
- Irrigate the joint.
- Using the dedicated tibial impaction device, impact the tibial component almost fully (**TECH FIG 15**).
- Use the plastic spacer–sizer–impactor to advance the tibial component to its final position.
  - Again, use a trial polyethylene to afford further stability to the tibial trial as the final impaction is performed (**TECH FIG 16**).

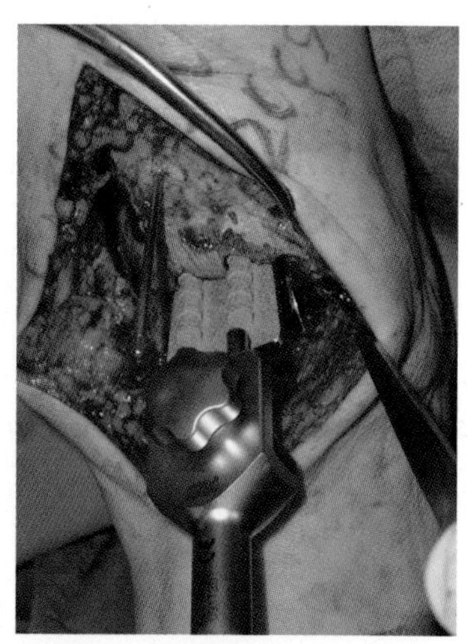
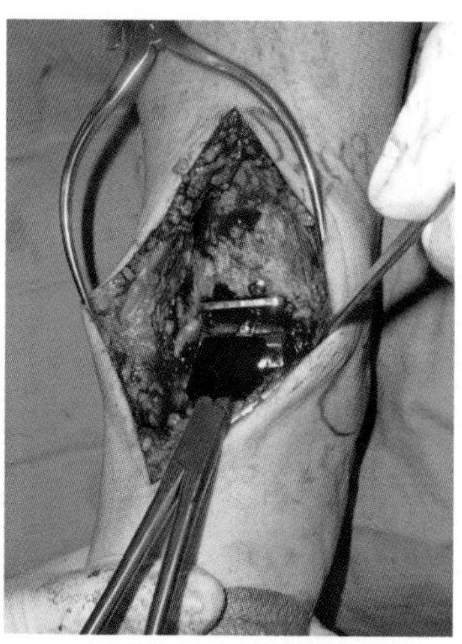
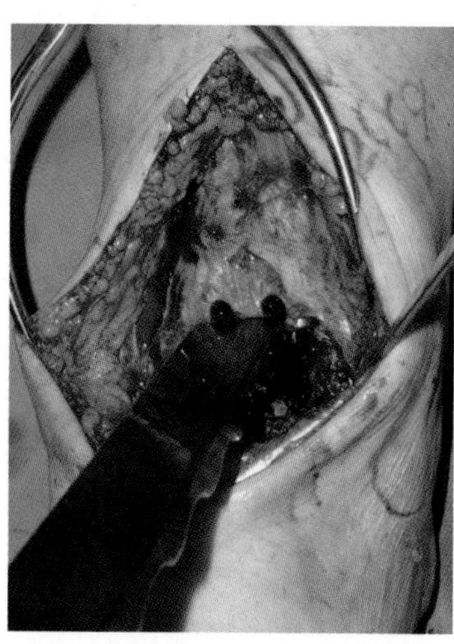

TECH FIG 15 • Tibial component insertion. **A.** Tibial component being advanced with insertion device. **B.** With tibial component nearly fully seated, trial polyethylene inserted to support posterior tibial component. **C.** Final impaction of tibial component.

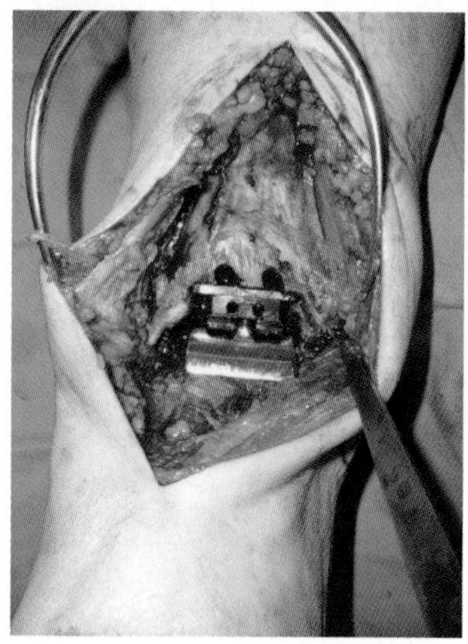
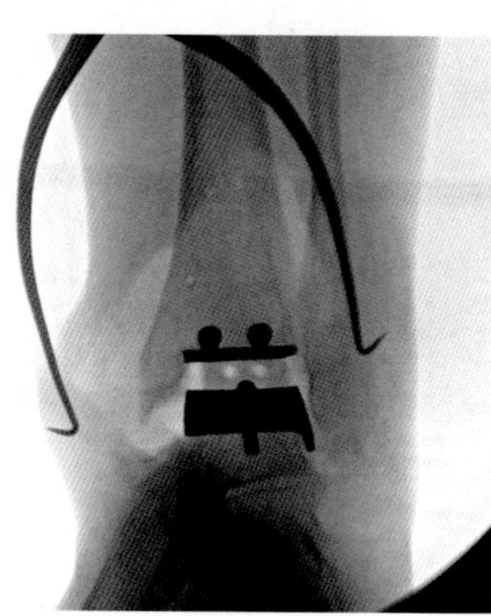

TECH FIG 16 • Trial polyethylene. **A.** Clinical view. **B.** Fluoroscopic view.

Final Polyethylene Implantation

- With the true tibial and talar components implanted, determine the optimal polyethylene size based on the trial polyethylenes (**TECH FIG 17**).
- With the ankle in neutral position, there should be virtually no lift-off at the two polyethylene–prosthesis interfaces when a varus or valgus stress is applied.
- ROM must allow dorsiflexion to at least 5 to 8 degrees, preferably more.
  - Occasionally, tendo Achilles lengthening is required. In these select situations we routinely perform a gastrocnemius–soleus recession.
- Contain the polyethylene meniscus under the tibial component during ROM (**TECH FIG 18**).

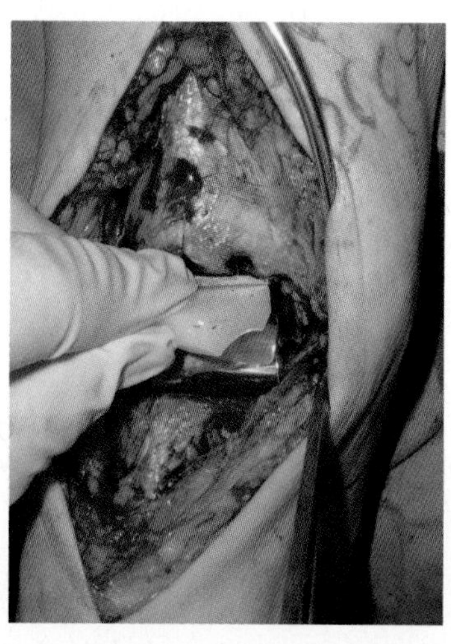

TECH FIG 17 • Insertion of final polyethylene. **A.** Manual insertion. *(continued)*

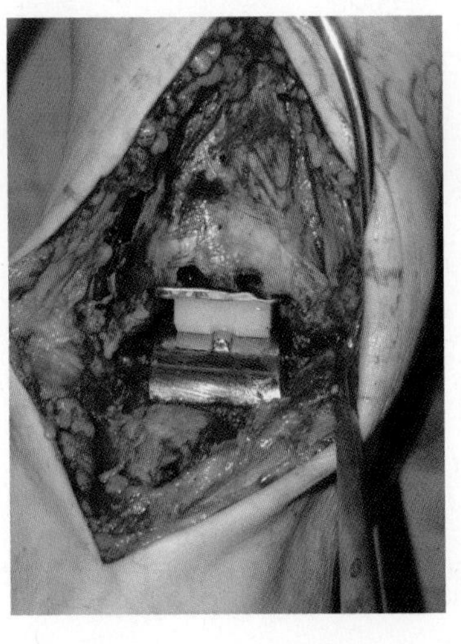

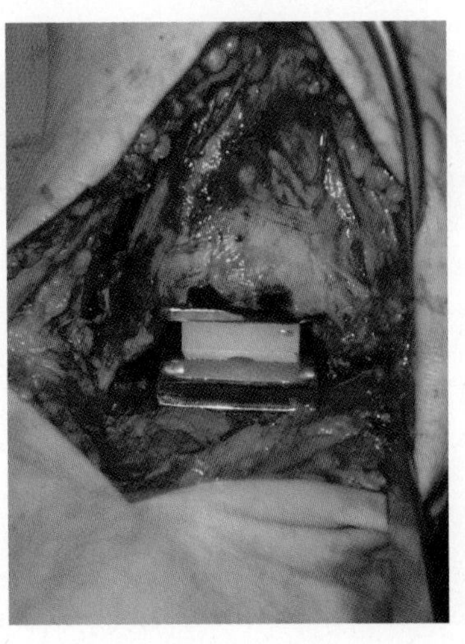

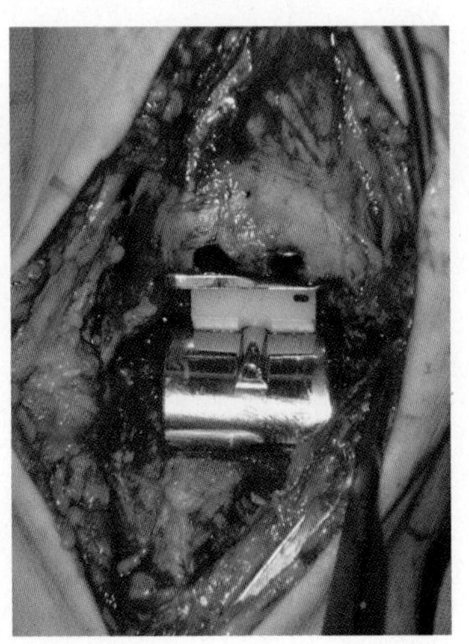

TECH FIG 17 • *(continued)* **B.** Polyethylene in place. **C.** Dorsiflexion. **D.** Plantarflexion.

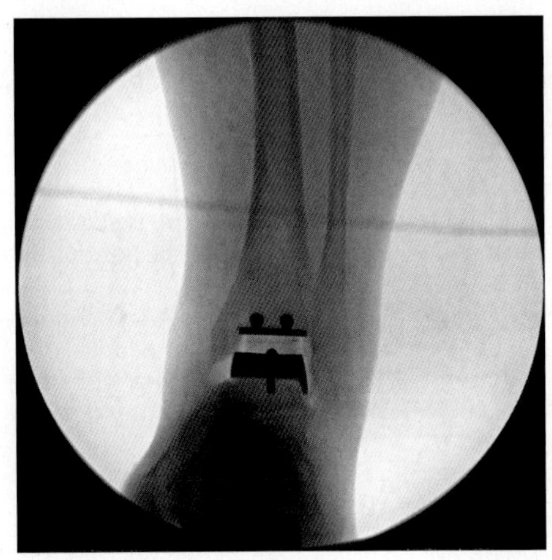

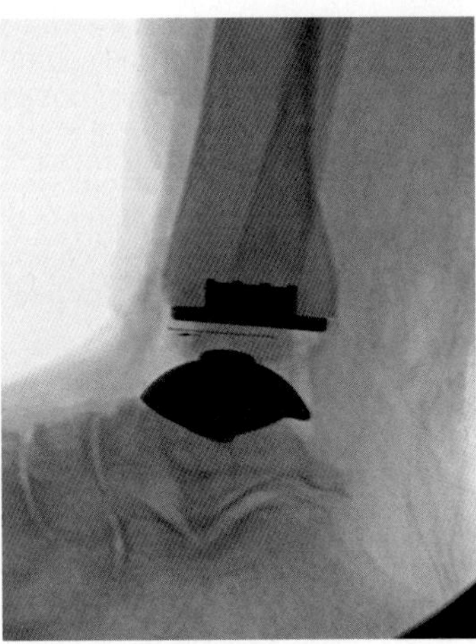

TECH FIG 18 • Final fluoroscopic views. **A.** AP. **B.** Lateral. The talus is proud posterior due to a relatively conservative initial talar cut. In our experience the component will settle (not subside) into a stable position.

CLOSURE AND CASTING

- Thoroughly irrigate the joint and implant with sterile saline.
- While protecting the prosthesis, fill the anterior barrel holes with bone graft from the resected bone (**TECH FIG 19**).
- Remove the pin from the proximal tibia.
- Reapproximate the capsule.
- We routinely use a drain.
- The tourniquet is released and meticulous hemostasis is obtained.
- Reapproximate the extensor retinaculum while protecting the deep and superficial peroneal nerves.
- Irrigate the subcutaneous layer with sterile saline and then reapproximate it.
- Reapproximate the skin to a tensionless closure.
- Place sterile dressings on the wounds, and apply adequate padding and a short-leg cast with the ankle in neutral position.

TECHNIQUES

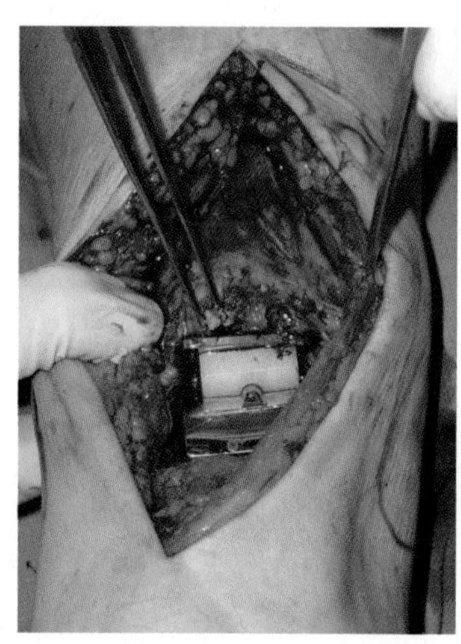

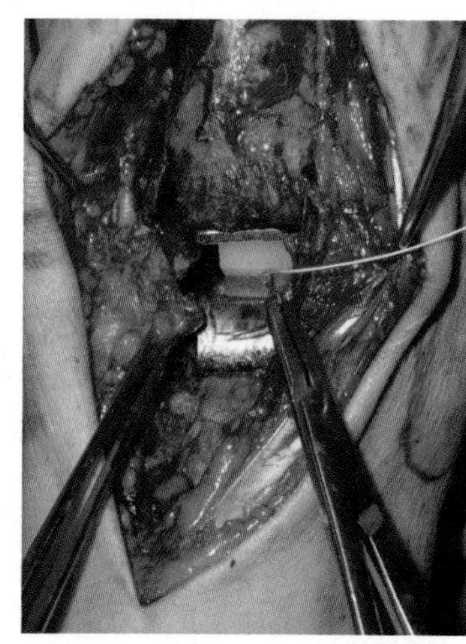

TECH FIG 19 • Bone grafting and closure. **A.** Bone grafting the anterior cortex at the barrel holes. **B.** Capsular closure.

PEARLS AND PITFALLS

Tibial preparation	▪ While traditionally up to 7 degrees of posterior slope was recommended, we favor 0 degrees of posterior slope. In our opinion, the mobile bearing will be more stable with a more uniform load distribution across the ankle.
Talar preparation	▪ Confirm fluoroscopically that the talus is in neutral dorsiflexion–plantarflexion in the sagittal plane so that the talar component will be in optimal position. If there is residual equinus despite anterior osteophyte removal, perform a tendo Achilles lengthening or gastrocnemius–soleus recession to position the talus correctly. ▪ Remove residual cartilage from the dome of the talus to ensure an adequate talar resection level. The distance between the cutting slot and paddle that rests on the talar dome is fixed. Therefore, if there is residual talar dome cartilage or a prominence that tilts the cutting guide, the initial talar cut will be less than desired or asymmetric.
Use of the 4-in-1 talar reference guide ("datum")	▪ Confirm its proper AP position with a lateral fluoroscopic view.
Impacting the talar component	▪ Because of the limited access to the ankle, the talar component tends to tilt anteriorly when impacted, even with optimal talar preparation. Be sure it is positioned properly in the sagittal plane over the talus (inserted posteriorly enough) before it is impacted. During impaction, carefully place a small osteotome under the anterior edge of the prosthesis to limit the anterior tilt.
Coronal plane position of the tibial component	▪ The tibial component must be centered under the tibial shaft axis. If performed judiciously, 1 to 2 more millimeters of medial tibial bone may be resected with a small reciprocating saw to translate the tibial component more medially, without compromising the medial malleolus.
Impacting the tibial component	▪ The tibial component is wider anteriorly than posteriorly. The medial malleolus must be carefully monitored during tibial component impaction. If the component begins to impinge on the medial malleolus, the reciprocating saw may be used to perform an anterior "relief" cut to relieve stress on the malleolus. With proper reaming of the barrels in the trial component, this is rarely an issue, but it may be encountered.

POSTOPERATIVE CARE

- Overnight stay
- Nasal oxygen while in the hospital
- Touch-down weight bearing on the cast is permitted, but elevation is encouraged as much as possible.
- The patient returns in 2 to 3 weeks for cast change and suture removal.
- The patient then returns at 6 weeks postoperatively for removal of cast and weight-bearing radiographs of the ankle.
- If there is no evidence of a stress fracture or failure of the procedure, then the patient can progress to a regular shoe and full weight bearing (**FIG 2**).

OUTCOMES

- While some recently reported outcomes are based on high-level evidence, results of total ankle arthroplasty (TAA) are almost uniformly derived from level IV evidence. Two recent investigations of the Scandinavian total ankle replacement are

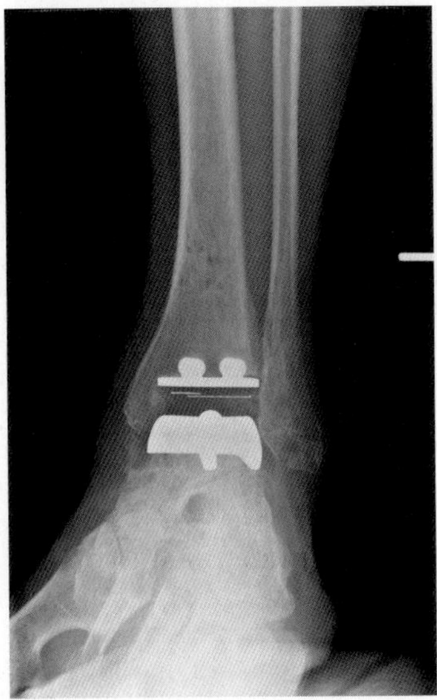

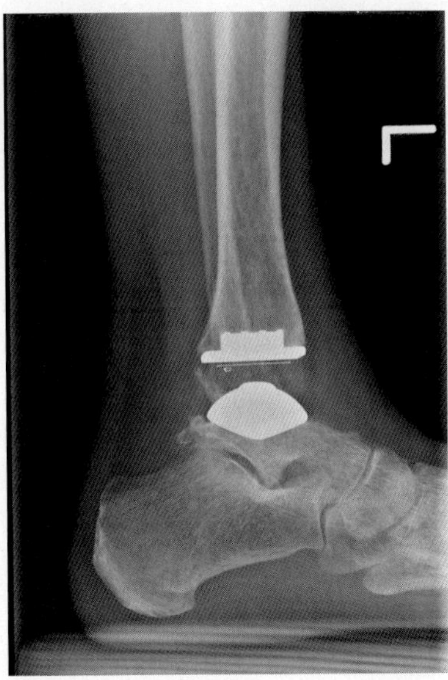

FIG 2 • Weight-bearing radiographs of same patient in Figure 1. **A.** AP view. **B.** Lateral view (note that talus has assumed anatomic position under tibial shaft axis).

level I[4] and level II[2], but with short- to intermediate-term follow-up only.

- Functional outcome using commonly used scoring systems for TAA (AOFAS,[1] Mazur, and NJOH [Buechel-Pappas]) suggest uniform improvement in all studies, with follow-up scores ranging from 70 to 90 points (maximum 100 points).
- Patient satisfaction rates for TAA exceed 90%, although follow-up for the patient satisfaction rating often does not exceed 5 years.
- Overall survivorship analysis for currently available implants, designating removal of a metal component or conversion to arthrodesis as the endpoint, ranges from about 90% to 95% at 5 to 6 years and 80% to 92% at 10 to 12 years.

COMPLICATIONS

- Infection (superficial or deep)
- Neuralgia (superficial or deep peroneal nerve; rarely tibial nerve)
- Delayed wound healing
- Wound dehiscence
- Persistent pain despite optimal orthopaedic examination and radiographic appearance of implants
- Osteolysis
- Subsidence
- Malleolar or distal tibial stress fracture
- Implant fracture (including polyethylene)

REFERENCES

1. Kofoed H. Scandinavian total ankle replacement (STAR). Clin Orthop Relat Res 2004;424:73–79.
2. Saltzman CL, Mann RA, Ahrens JE, et al. Prospective controlled trial of STAR total ankle replacement versus ankle fusion: initial results. Foot Ankle Int 2009;30:579–596.
3. Wood PL, Prem H, Sutton C. Total ankle replacement: medium-term results in 200 Scandinavian total ankle replacements. J Bone Joint Surg Br 2008;90B:605–609.
4. Wood PL, Sutton C, Mishra V, et al. A randomised, controlled trial of two mobile-bearing total ankle replacements. J Bone Joint Surg Br 2009;91B:69–74.

Chapter 69 The HINTEGRA Total Ankle Arthroplasty

Beat Hintermann and Alexej Barg

DEFINITION

- The HINTEGRA Total Ankle Prosthesis (Integra, Plainsboro, NJ) is an unconstrained, three-component system that provides inversion–eversion stability (**FIG 1**). Axial rotation and normal flexion–extension mobility are provided by a mobile bearing element.[3,6]
- The HINTEGRA ankle includes a metal tibial component, an ultrahigh-density polyethylene mobile bearing, and a metal talar component, all of which are available in six sizes. The metal components are manufactured of cobalt–chromium alloy with a porous coating of a 20% porosity. The porous coating is covered by titanium fluid and hydroxyapatite. The remaining metallic surfaces are highly polished.
- The tibial component employs a flat, 4-mm-thick loading plate with pyramidal peaks on the flat surface against the tibia and an anterior shield that allows for fixation by two screws through two oval holes. The anatomically sized flat surface allows for optimal contact with the subchondral bone, as well as optimal support of the cortical bone ring, providing a maximal load-transfer area. It also makes it possible to minimize bony resection to 2 to 3 mm of the subcortical bone. This fixation concept prevents any stress shielding from occurring.
- The talar component is conically shaped, with a smaller radius medially than laterally. It consists of a highly polished articular surface, and a medial and lateral surface. A 2.5-mm-high rim on the medial and lateral sides ensures stable position and anteroposterior translation of the polyethylene on the talar surface. The medial and lateral talar surfaces are covered by two wings that are anatomically sized and formed to the original articular, cartilage-covered surfaces. The inner, slightly curved surface of the wings allows for press-fit of the component to the bone. The anterior shield increases the bone support on weaker bone at the talar neck to increase stability in the sagittal plane and to prevent the adherence of scar tissue that might restrict motion. The current design, introduced in 2004, includes two pegs to facilitate the insertion of the talar component and to provide additional stability.

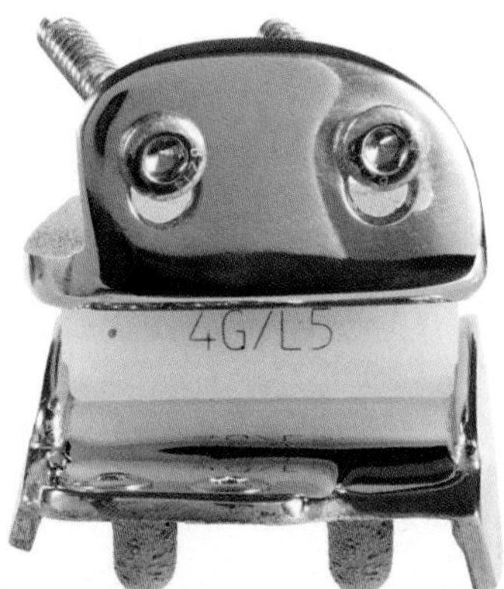

FIG 1 • The HINTEGRA ankle consists of three components.

- The high-density polyethylene mobile bearing (ultrahigh-molecular-weight polyethylene) consists of a flat surface on the tibial side and a concave surface that perfectly matches the talar surface. It has a minimum thickness of 5 mm but is also available for thicker sizes (6, 7, and 9 mm). The size of the bearing is determined by the talar size. As it fully covers the talar component, it ensures optimal stability against valgus–varus forces and minimal contact stress in both the primary and secondary articulating surfaces. The bearing is restrained by the compressive action of the collateral ligaments and adjacent tissues. Further, compressive muscle forces and gravitational loads across the joint hold the bearing against the metallic articulating surfaces. Thus, when properly positioned, dislocation of the bearing is unlikely.
- The HINTEGRA ankle provides 50 degrees of congruent contact flexion–extension and 50 degrees of congruent contact axial rotation, which provides congruent contact surfaces for normal load-bearing activities, even in the case of a distinct implantation error or pre-existing deformity. Limits of motion depend on natural soft tissue constraints: no mechanical prosthetic motion constraints are imposed for any ankle movement with this device.
- The HINTEGRA ankle uses all available bone surface for support. The anatomically shaped, flat tibial and talar components essentially resurface the tibia and talar dome, respectively, and the wings hemiprosthetically replace degenerate medial and lateral facets (a potential source of pain and impingement).

ANATOMY

- The superior extensor retinaculum is a thickening of the deep fascia above the ankle, running from tibia to fibula.
- It includes, from medially to laterally, the tendons of tibialis anterior, extensor hallucis longus, and extensor digitorum longus.
- The anterior neurovascular bundle lies roughly halfway between the malleoli; it can be found consistently between the extensor hallucis longus and extensor digitorum longus tendons.
- The neurovascular bundle contains the A. tibialis anterior and the deep peroneal nerve. The nerve supplies the extensor digitorum brevis and extensor hallucis brevis and a sensory space interdigital I–II.
- On the height of the talonavicular joint the medial branches of the superficial peroneal nerve cross from lateral to medial. It supplies the skin of the dorsum of the foot.

- On the posterior aspect of the ankle, the medial neurovascular bundle is located behind its posteromedial corner and the flexor hallucis longus tendon on its posterior aspect. The deltoid ligament is a multibanded complex with superficial and deep components.

PATHOGENESIS

- Primary osteoarthritis of the ankle joint is rare; degenerative disease of the ankle is more often seen after trauma and systemic diseases (eg, rheumatoid arthritis).
- Osteoarthritis of the ankle joint is often associated with malalignment, deformities, and instabilities of the foot, particularly in posttraumatic ankles.[5]

NATURAL HISTORY

- Development of osteoarthritis of the ankle joint can take years, particularly in posttraumatic ankles (eg, after fractures and sprains).
- Once it has become symptomatic, osteoarthritic changes usually progress, resulting in pain under loading and finally at rest.
- If associated with instability or muscular dysfunction, misalignment and deformity may occur.

PATIENT HISTORY AND PHYSICAL FINDINGS

- A careful history is taken to assess:
  - Previous trauma
  - Previous infections
  - Underlying diseases
  - Actual pain
  - Limitations in daily and sports activities
- While the patient is standing, a thorough clinical investigation of both lower extremities is done to assess:
  - Alignment
  - Deformities
  - Foot position
  - Muscular atrophy
- While the patient is sitting with free-hanging feet, the examiner assesses:
  - The extent to which a deformity is correctable
  - Preserved joint motion at the ankle and subtalar joints
  - Ligament stability of the ankle and subtalar joints with anterior drawer and tilt tests
  - Supination and eversion power (eg, function of posterior tibial and peroneus brevis muscles)

IMAGING AND OTHER DIAGNOSTIC STUDIES

- Plain weight-bearing radiographs, including AP views of the foot and ankle and a lateral view of the foot (**FIG 2**), are obtained to assess:
  - Extent of destruction of the tibiotalar joint (eg, tibia, talus, and fibula)
  - Status of neighboring joints (eg, associated degenerative disease)
  - Deformities of the foot and ankle complex (eg, heel alignment, foot arch, talonavicular alignment)
  - Tibiotalar malalignment (eg, varus, valgus, recurvatum, and antecurvatum)
  - Bony condition (eg, avascular necrosis, bony defects)
- A CT scan may be ordered for assessment of:
  - Destruction of joint surfaces and incongruency
  - Bony defects
  - Avascular necrosis
- Single-photon-emission computed tomography combined with computed tomography (SPECT-CT) with a superimposed bone scan (**FIG 3**) may be used to visualize:
  - Morphologic pathologies and associated activity process
  - Biologic bone pathologies and associated activity process
- MR imaging may be used to show:
  - Injuries to ligament structures
  - Morphologic changes of tendons
  - Avascular necrosis of bones (eg, talar body and tibial plafond)
- Gait analysis[7]

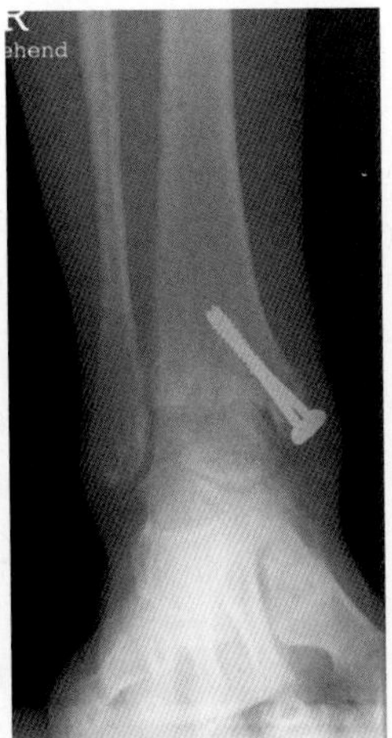

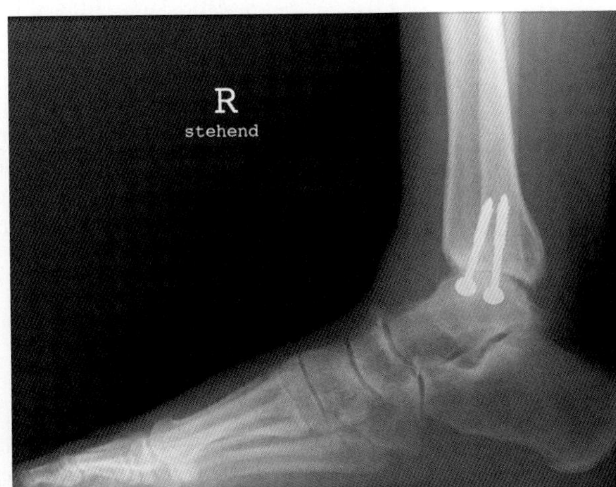

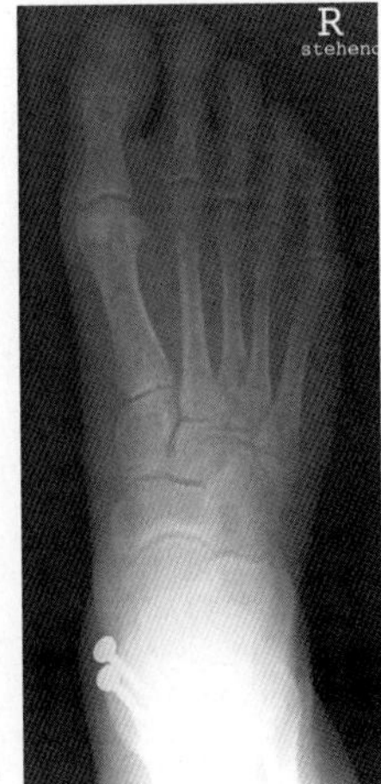

FIG 2 • Preoperative assessment includes weight-bearing standard radiographs as follows: (**A**) AP view of the ankle; (**B**) lateral view of the foot; (**C**) AP view of the foot.

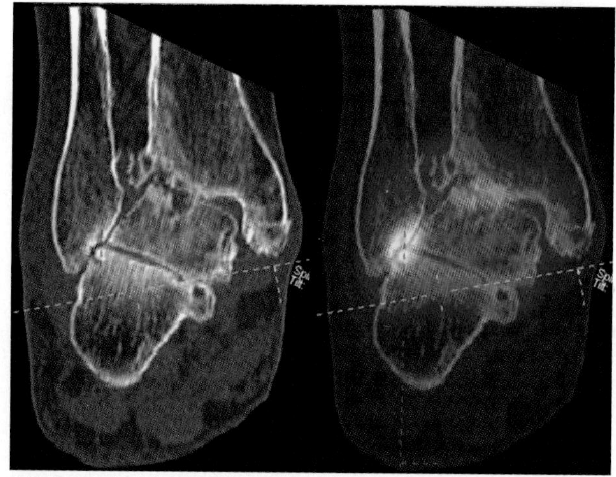

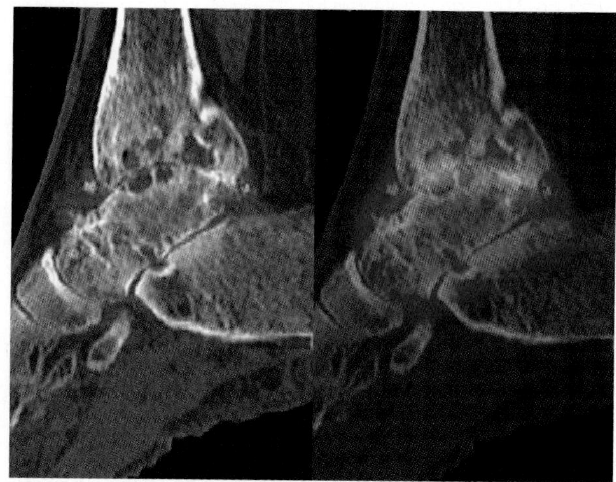

FIG 3 • Single photon emission computed tomography with combined computed tomography (SPECT-CT) in a patient with valgus deformity showing the pathologic process in the lateral tibiotalar and fibulotalar joints. **A.** AP view. **B.** Lateral view.

NONOPERATIVE MANAGEMENT

- Although nonoperative management is controversial, patients with less debilitating pain and dysfunction may be treated nonoperatively.
- Nonoperative treatment may consist of:
  - Shoe modifications to facilitate gait
  - Physiotherapy to decrease inflammatory response
  - Anti-inflammatory medicine for acute pain

SURGICAL MANAGEMENT

- Successful total ankle arthroplasty with an unconstrained three-component prosthesis demands thorough preoperative planning to address all associated pathologies.
- During surgery, the surgeon must continuously check whether these associated pathologies are sufficiently addressed. For instance:
  - Whether pre-existing deformity is sufficiently corrected
  - Whether the foot is properly aligned
  - Whether soft tissues are sufficiently balanced

Indications

- Primary osteoarthritis (eg, degenerative disease)
- Systemic arthritis (eg, rheumatoid arthritis)
- Posttraumatic osteoarthritis (if instability and malalignment are manageable)
- Secondary osteoarthritis (eg, infection, avascular necrosis) (if at least two thirds of the talar surface is preserved)
- Salvage for failed total ankle replacement (if bone stock is sufficient)
- Salvage for nonunion and malunion of ankle fusion (if bone stock is sufficient)
- Low demands for physical activities (hiking, swimming, biking, golfing)

Relative Indications

- Severe osteoporosis
- Immunosuppressive therapy
- Increased demands for physical activities (eg, jogging, tennis, downhill skiing)
- Bony avulsion fracture of medial malleolus (with or without fracture of the fibula–syndesmotic disruption)

Contraindications

- Infection
- Avascular necrosis of more than one third of the talus
- Unmanageable instability
- Unmanageable malalignment
- Neuromuscular disorder
- Neuroarthropathy (Charcot)
- Diabetic syndrome
- Suspected or documented metal allergy or intolerance
- Highest demands for physical activities (eg, contact sports, jumping)

Controversial Indications

- Diabetic syndrome without polyneuropathy
- Avascular necrosis of talus

Preoperative Planning

- All imaging studies are reviewed.
- Plain films should be reviewed to identify possible coexisting arthritis of adjacent joints as well as varus and valgus of the hindfoot and the longitudinal arch.
- Associated foot deformity, malalignment, and instability should be addressed concurrently.
- Examination under anesthesia should be accomplished to compare with the contralateral ankle.

Positioning

- The patient is positioned with the feet on the edge of the table.
- The ipsilateral back is lifted until a strictly upward position of the foot is obtained.
- A block is placed under the affected foot to facilitate fluoroscopy during surgery.
- The contralateral (nonaffected) leg is also draped if significant deformity is to be corrected.
- A tourniquet is applied on the ipsilateral thigh.

Approach

- An anterior longitudinal incision 10 to 12 cm long is made to expose the retinaculum.
- The retinaculum is dissected along the lateral border of the anterior tibial tendon, and the anterior aspect of the distal tibia is exposed.
- While the soft tissue mantle is dissected with the periosteum from the bone, attention is paid to the neurovascular bundle that lies behind the long extensor hallucis tendon.
- Capsulotomy and capsulectomy are done, and a self-retaining retractor is inserted to carefully keep the soft tissue mantle away (**FIG 4**).
- Osteophytes on the tibia are removed, particularly on the anterolateral aspect.
- Osteophytes on the talar neck and the anterior aspect of medial malleolus are also removed.
- The fibula usually cannot be fully visualized at this stage.

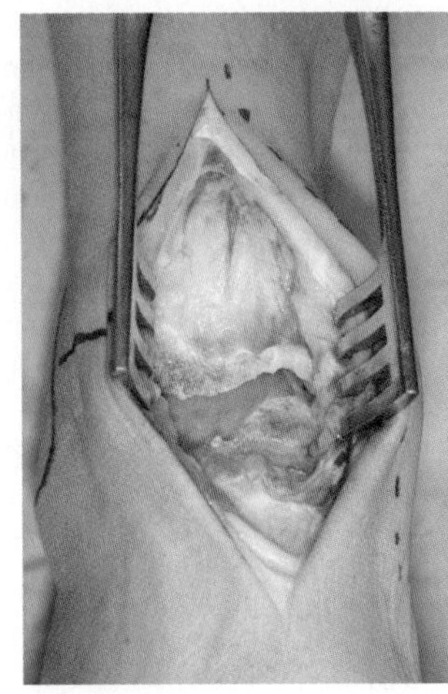

FIG 4 • The ankle joint is exposed through an anterior approach.

TIBIAL RESECTION

- Position the tibial cutting block with its alignment rod using the tibial tuberosity (eg the anterior cresta iliaca of pelvis in the case of leg deformity [**TECH FIG 1A**] as the proximal reference and the anterior border of the ankle (eg, the center of the resection block is supposed to be at intermediate line of the tibiotalar joint) as the distal reference.
- Make the final adjustment as follows:
  - Sagittal plane: Move the rod until a parallel position to the anterior border of the tibia has been achieved (**TECH FIG 1B**).
  - Frontal (coronal) plane: Frontal plane position is given by the position of the rod (eg there is a fixed

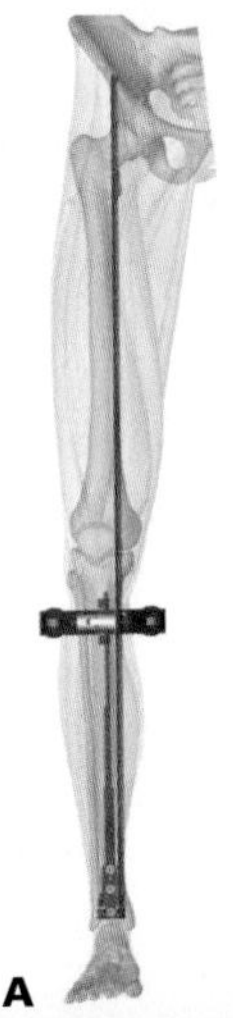

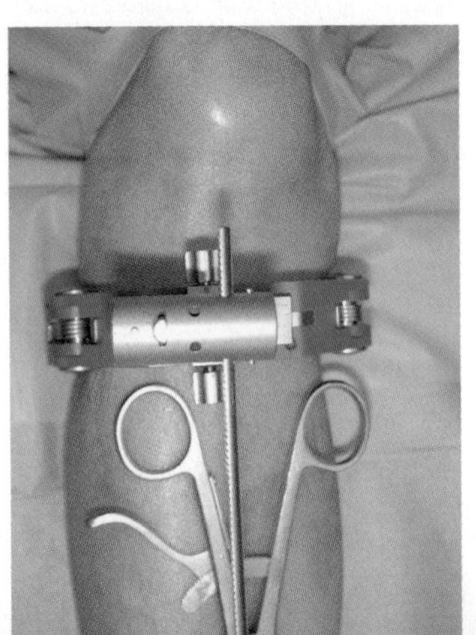

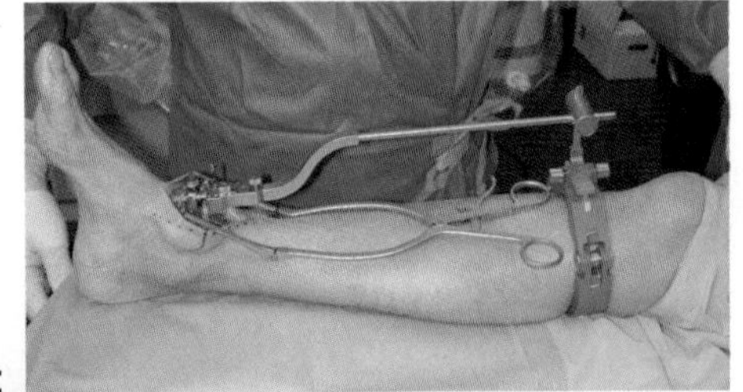

A B C

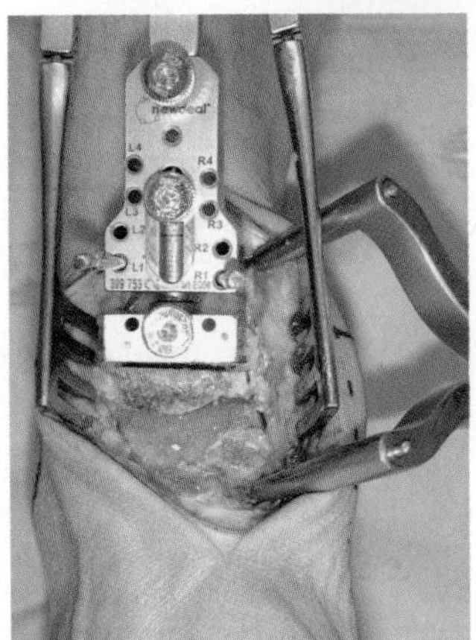

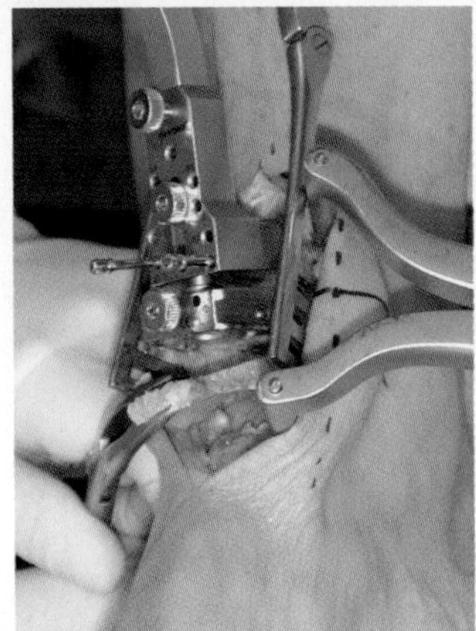

D E

TECH FIG 1 • Tibial resection. **A,B.** Tibial resection block is adjusted taking the tibial tuberosity or the anterior spina of iliac crest as the reference in the frontal plane, and (**C**) the anterior tibia in the sagittal plane. **D.** 2 to 3 mm of bone is removed, as measured at the apex of the tibial plafond. **E.** Bone is removed and resection is finalized at the lateral side, paying attention to not damaging the integrity of the fibula and at the medial side to get a sharp perpendicular cut along the medial malleolus.

90° angle between the resection surface and the rod). Once the rod is proximally centered to tibial tuberosity (TECH FIG 1C), two pins are used for fixation.

- Vertical adjustment: Move the tibial resection block proximally until the desired resection height is achieved. Usually resection of about 2 to 3 mm on the apex of the tibial plafond is desired. In varus ankles more tibial resection is usually needed, whereas in valgus ankles or in presence of high joint laxity, less bone resection is advised.
- Rotational adjustment: Rotate the tibial resection block to get a parallel position of its medial surface to the medial surface of the talus (eg, to avoid damaging the malleoli with the saw blade during resection).

- Slide the tibial cutting guide into the cutting block, creating a slot in which the saw blade will be guided. The width of the slot limits the excursion of the saw blade, thereby protecting the malleoli from hitting and fracturing.
- Once the tibial cut is made, a reciprocating saw might be used to finalize the cuts, particularly for the vertical cut on the medial side (TECH FIG 1D).
- Remove the remaining bone with a rongeur (TECH FIG 1E), including the posterior capsule.
- Use the measuring gauge to determine the size of the implant. In doubt (eg, if the anterior border of the tibia is projected onto the gauge between two markers), select the bigger size.

TALAR RESECTION

- Insert the talar resection block into the tibial cutting block.
- Move the resection block distally as much as possible to properly tension the collateral ligaments (TECH FIG 2A).
- Remove all distractors and spreaders before the foot is taken into neutral position (eg, with respect to dorsiflexion–plantarflexion and pronation–supination).
- Once the foot is in neutral position, fix the resection block with two pins (medially and laterally) (TECH FIG 2B,C).
- Resect the talar dome with the oscillating saw through the slot of the talar cutting block.
- Remove the tibial and talar resection block and again mount the distractor (Hintermann spreader) to distract the joint.
- Remove the posterior capsule completely until fat tissue and tendon structures are visible to achieve full dorsiflexion.
- Insert the 12-mm-thick spacer representing the thickness of the tibial and talar components and the thinnest 5-mm inlay into the created joint space (TECH FIG 2D). While the foot is held in neutral flexion position, this allows the surgeon to check:
  - Whether an appropriate amount of bone has been resected
  - Whether the achieved alignment is appropriate
  - Whether the medial and lateral stability are approximate
- If the spacer cannot be properly inserted into the joint space, and if there is no obvious contracture of the remaining posterior capsule present, additional bony resection might be considered. In most instances, such additional resection should be done on the tibial side. Reposition the tibial cutting block using the same fixation holes for the pins. Move the distal resection block proximally as desired, and make a new cut with the saw blade.
- If the alignment is not appropriate, and if an associated deformity of the foot itself (eg, varus, valgus heel) can be excluded, consider a corrective cut. In most instances, the resection should be done on the tibial side. Make the desired

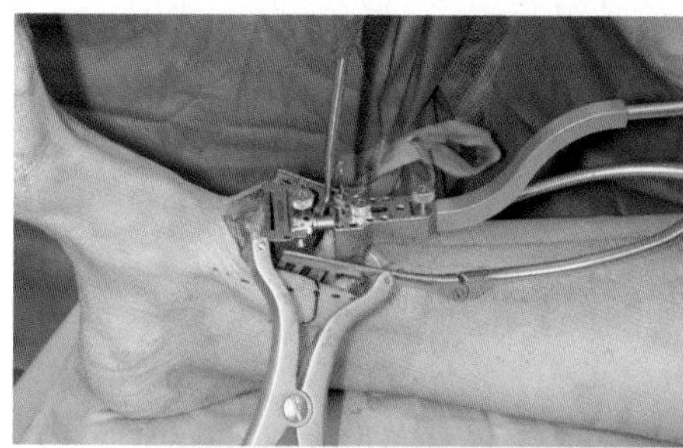

A

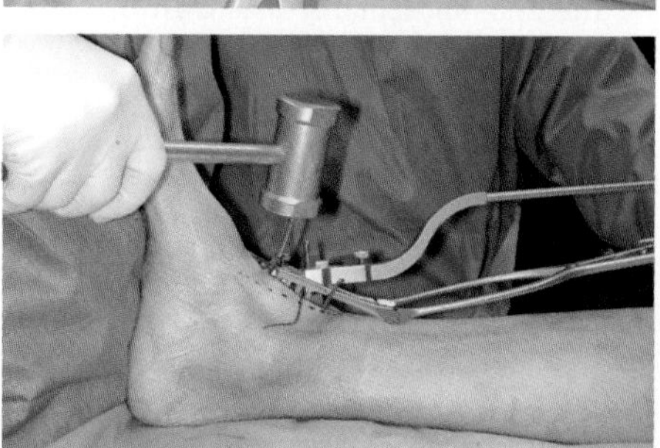

B

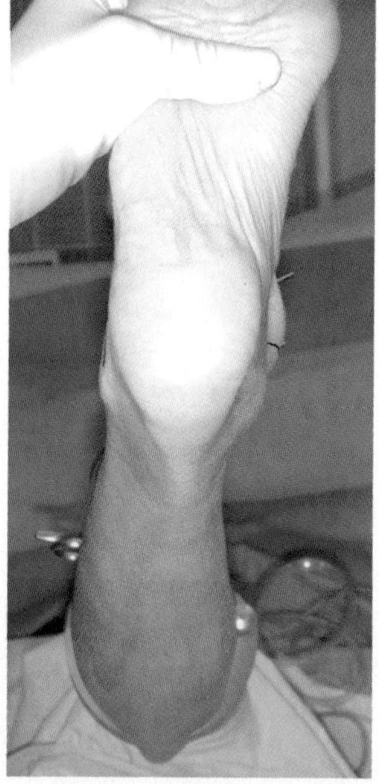

C

TECH FIG 2 • Talar resection. **A.** After insertion of talar resection block, the whole block is moved distally until collateral ligaments of ankle are fully tensioned. **B.** Talar resection block is fixed by pins to the talus while the foot is held in neutral position. **C.** Alignment of the hindfoot is carefully checked. *(continued)*

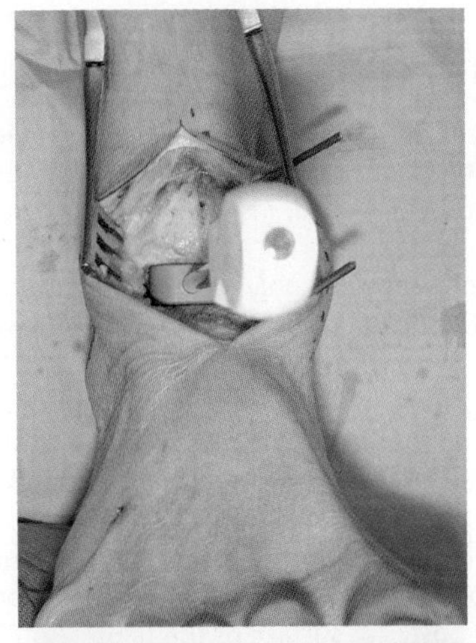

D

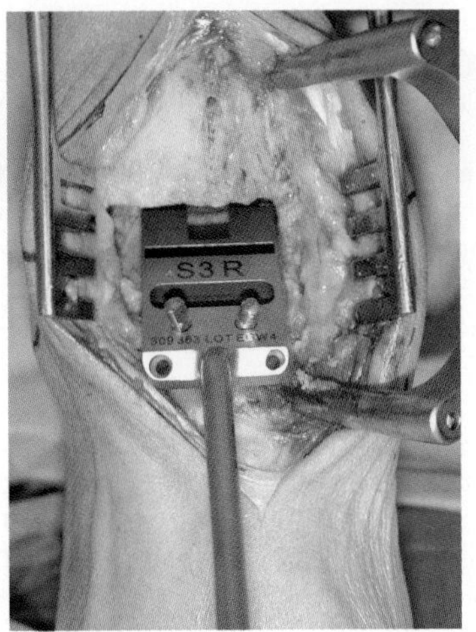

E

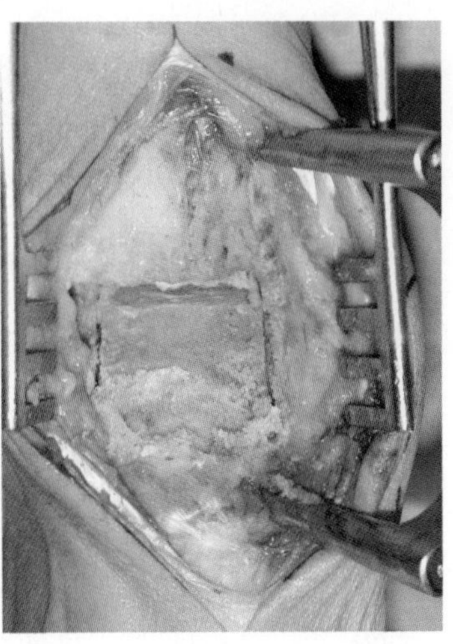

F

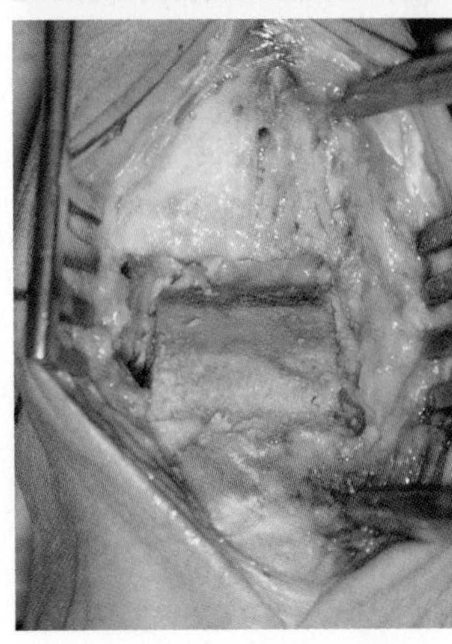

G

TECH FIG 2 • *(continued)* **D.** After the horizontal cut is made by the saw through the slot and the resection block is removed, the spacer is inserted to check alignment and stability of the ankle. **E.** Appropriate size of talar resection block is fitted to the bone using the medial border of the talus as the reference. **F.** After posterior, medial, lateral and anterior cuts are made, the block is removed. **G.** Bone stock of talus after careful debridement of the medial, lateral, and posterior compartment as well as complete resection of the posterior capsule of the ankle joint.

angular correction on the tibial resection block, and reposition the tibial cutting block using other fixation holes for the pins. Move the distal resection block proximally or distally so that an angular bony resection will result.

- If the ankle is not stable on both sides, consider using a thicker inlay. If the ankle is not stable on one side, consider a release of the contralateral ligaments or ligament reconstruction on the affected side. Ligament reconstruction is better done once the definitive implants have been inserted, and if there is still an obvious instability.
- Remove the spacer and mount the distractor (Hintermann spreader) using the same pins.
- Determine the size of the resected talar block as follows (TECH FIG 2E):
  - Use the medial side of the talus as the reference; position the resection block along the medial border of the talus so that 1 to 2 mm of bone will be removed from the medial side of the talus.
  - On the lateral side, the resection block is supposed to remove as little bone as possible on its posterior aspect; usually, more bone will need to be removed on the lateral aspect of the talus as there are osteophytes.
  - On the posterior side, the resection block is supposed to remove 2 to 3 mm of bone in addition to remaining cartilage; this is given by the distance of the posterior hooks of resection block that aim to be in strong contact with the posterior surface of talus.
  - The talar size should not exceed the previously determined tibial component by more than one size; if so, a smaller talar size must be selected.
- After selecting the appropriate size of talar cutting block, fix it with two or three short pins.
- Make posterior resection on the talus with an oscillating saw that is guided through the posterior slot of the talar cutting block.
- Make medial and lateral resections on the talus with a reciprocating saw that is guided along the talar cutting block. Make the cut as follows:
  - Medial side: 6 mm deep; the reference is the upper surface of the talus
  - Lateral side: 8 mm deep; the reference is the upper surface of the talus
- Make the anterior resection on the talus with a drill that is guided through the anterior slot of the talar cutting block.
- Remove the talar cutting block (TECH FIG 2F)
- On the medial and lateral sides, the cuts are finalized by using a chisel to make an almost horizontal cut along the base of the cuts previously made, thereby avoiding extended loss of bone stock and potential damage to the vascular supply of the talus.
- Clean the medial and lateral gutters using a rongeur.
- Remove the remaining bone and capsule of the posterior compartment (TECH FIG 2G).

TECHNIQUES

INSERTING TRIAL IMPLANTS AND FINALIZING CUTS

- Talar trial:
  - Insert the talar trial using the given impactor. The window on the posterior aspect of the trial allows the surgeon to check its proper fit to the posterior resection surface of the talus (TECH FIG 3A)
  - If proper position of the talus has been achieved, resect the anterior surface of the talus using a rongeur or the oscillating saw.
  - Fix the drill guide onto talar trial (TECH FIG 3B)
  - Make two drill holes with the provided 4.5-mm drill, and remove the trial (TECH FIG 3C).
- Tibial trial:
  - Use the tibial depth gauge to determine the size of tibial implant to be selected; insert it with the appropriate side (right/left) against the tibial surface, and hook the posterior edge on the posterior border of the tibia. The size to be selected can be taken from the scale on the depth gauge (TECH FIG 3D).
  - Remove the depth gauge and, if necessary, smooth the anterior border of tibia resection with an oscillating saw or rongeur according to the shape of indicated resection.
  - Insert the tibial trial. Try to get the tibial component in close contact with the medial malleolus and the anterior surface of tibia (TECH FIG 3E).
- Trial inlay: Insert the 5-mm inlay trial and remove the distractor (Hintermann spreader); if not enough soft tissue tension can be achieved, insert the 6-mm, 7-mm, or 9-mm trial.
- The use of fluoroscopy is highly recommended to check the position of implants while the foot is held in neutral position, particularly:
  - Appropriate length of the tibial component: its posterior border should be on line with the posterior aspect of the tibia so that the tibial surface is fully covered
  - Proper fit of the tibial component to the tibial surface
  - Proper fit of the posterior edge of the talar component to the posterior surface of the talus
  - Point of contact of the talar component to the tibial component. This contact point should be between 40% and 45% of the tibial component when the anterior border is taken as 0% and the posterior border as 100%, respectively. If the point of contact is too posterior, ligament balance will not be achieved.
- Carefully check the bony surfaces. Any cysts are removed with a curette, and filling with cancellous bone taken from the removed bony material is recommended. If there is sclerotic bone left on surface, drilling with a 2.0-mm drill is recommended.

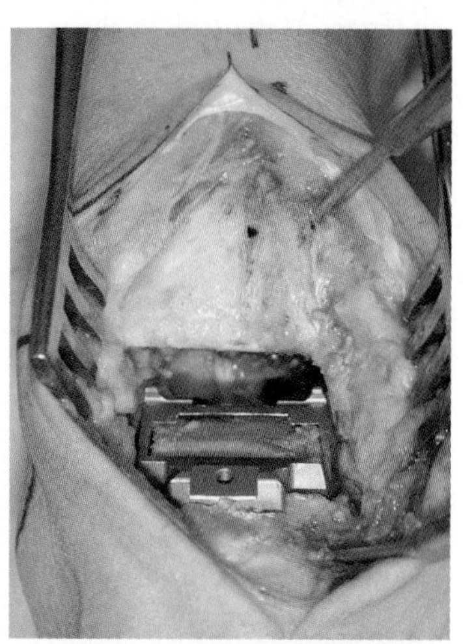
A

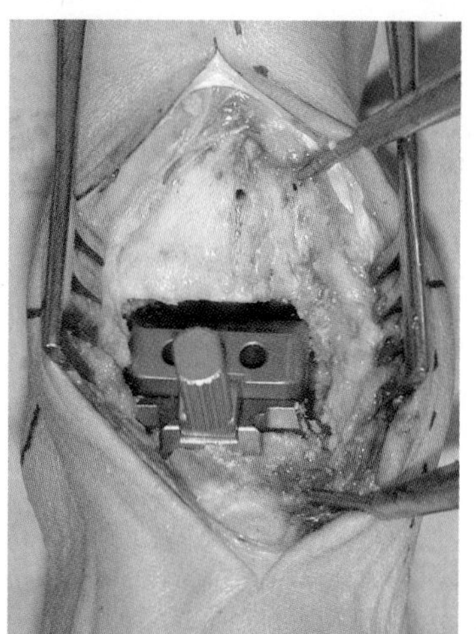
B

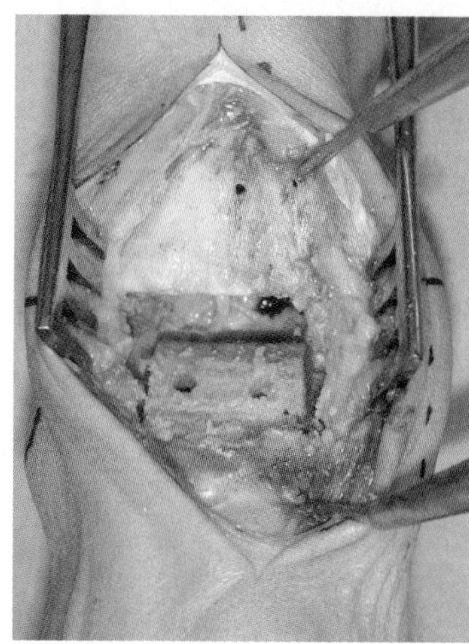
C

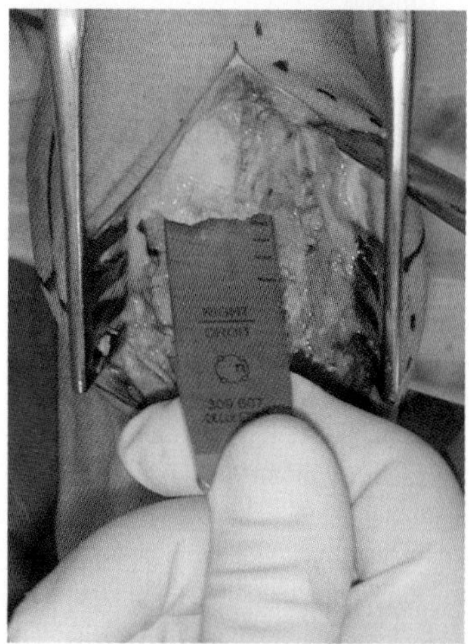
D

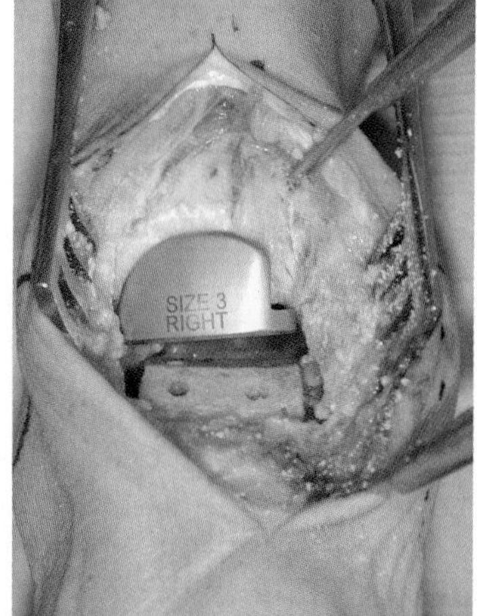

E

TECH FIG 3 • Trial implants. **A.** First, the trial implant of the talus is inserted, paying attention to obtain a proper fit to the posterior resection surface. **B.** After resection of anterior surface, the bloc is inserted and the holes for the pegs are drilled. **C.** The talar trial is removed. The resection surfaces of the talus and tibia are carefully checked for cyst formations. If present, they are meticulously removed. **D.** The tibial depth gauge is inserted and the size of tibial implant is determined. **E.** The tibial trial implant is inserted paying attention to get the tibial component in close contact with the medial malleolus and the anterior surface of tibia. If necessary, the anterolateral tibia has to be smoothed.

INSERTION OF IMPLANTS

- Insert the final implants, as previously selected, as follows:
  - Fill the talar component with bone matrix (ISOTIS) to get the cysts filled and then insert it such as the pegs can glide into the two drilled holes; use a hammer and impactor to obtain a proper fit of the component to the bone (**TECH FIG 4A**).
  - Insert the tibial component along the medial malleolus until proper fit to the anterior border of the tibia is achieved (**TECH FIG 4B**).
  - Insert the inlay (same size as the talar component). Remove the distractor (Hintermann spreader). Hammer and impactor might be used for appropriate fit to bone (**TECH FIG 4C**).
  - Check stability and motion clinically.
- While the foot is moved in dorsiflexion with the surgeon's maximal power, settling of the implant might be improved, and remaining soft tissue contracture on the posterior aspect of the ankle might be released (**TECH FIG 4D**).
- Screw fixation of the tibial component may be considered to achieve stability against rotational and translational forces during the osteointegration process; however, this is very seldom necessary as the proper fit and pyramidal peaks do provide sufficient primary stability.
- It is also highly recommended to check the position of the implants by fluoroscopy, as described for the trial implants (**TECH FIG 4E,F**). This also allows the surgeon to detect any remaining bony fragments or osteophytes that could be a potential source of pain or motion restriction.

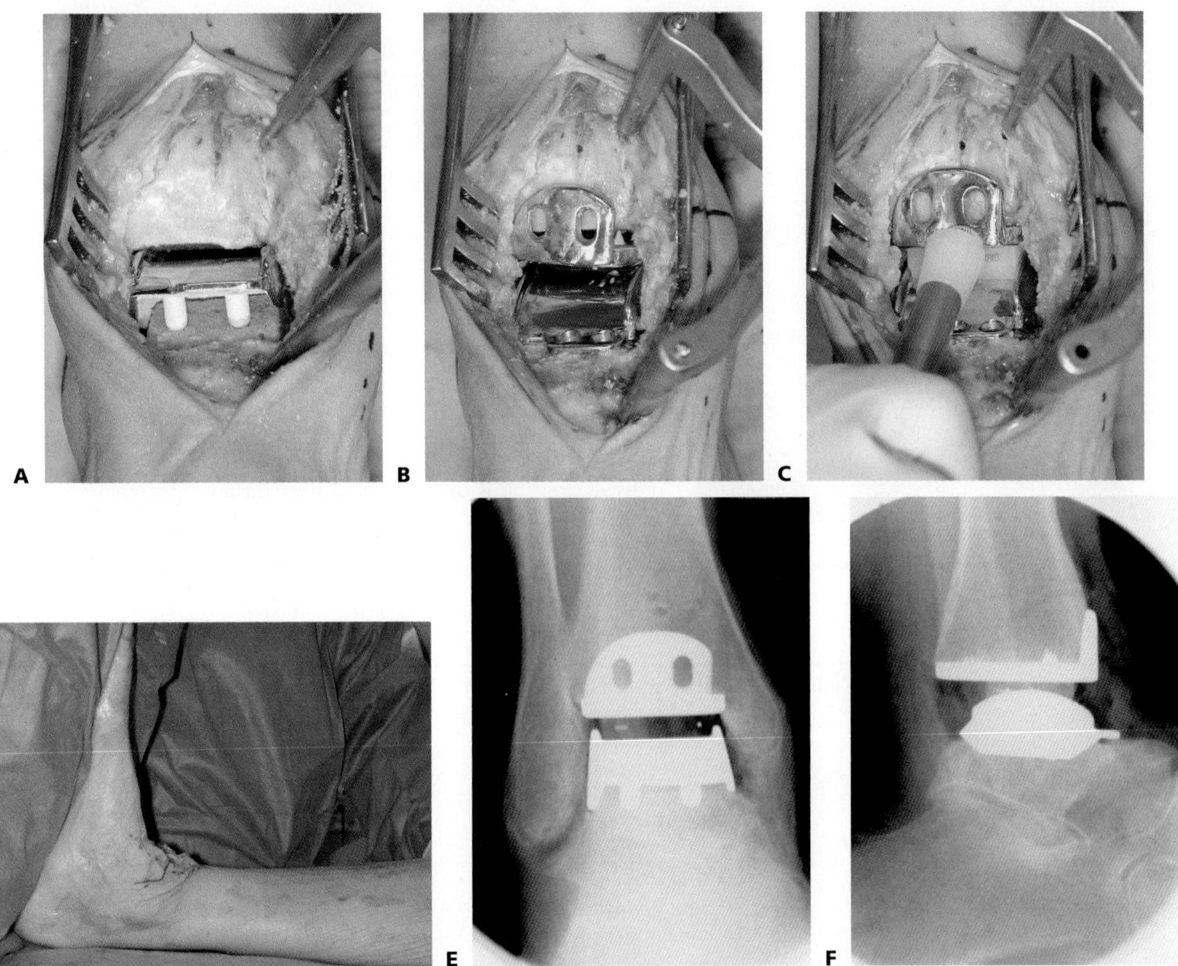

TECH FIG 4 • Insertion of definitive implants. **A.** The talar component is impacted first. **B.** After insertion of the tibial component and the polyethylene insert (**C**), the tibial component is impacted to obtain a proper fit to the tibial resection surface. **D.** The foot is moved in dorsiflexion with the surgeon's maximal power, thereby settling of the implant might be improved, and remaining soft tissue contracture on the posterior aspect of the ankle might be released. **E.** Final check of the position of the implants using fluoroscopy. On the AP view the surgeon checks the position of the implants for any misalignment that may cause edge load of the polyethylene insert, overall alignment in the frontal (coronal) plane, distraction of the ankle (gap between the fibula and talus), and medial and lateral gutters for any bone left that may cause bony impingement. **F.** On the lateral view the surgeon checks the position of the implants with regard to the bone surfaces (proper fit) and alignment of the implants with regard to contact area (usually, the apex of the talar component should meet the tibial component 3 to 5 mm anterior to its midpoint).

WOUND CLOSURE

- The wound is closed by suturing the tendon sheath and retinaculum (TECH FIG 5A) and the skin (TECH FIG 5B).
- Dress the wound, taking care to avoid any pressure to the skin (TECH FIG 5C).
- A splint is used to keep the foot in neutral position (TECH FIG 5D).

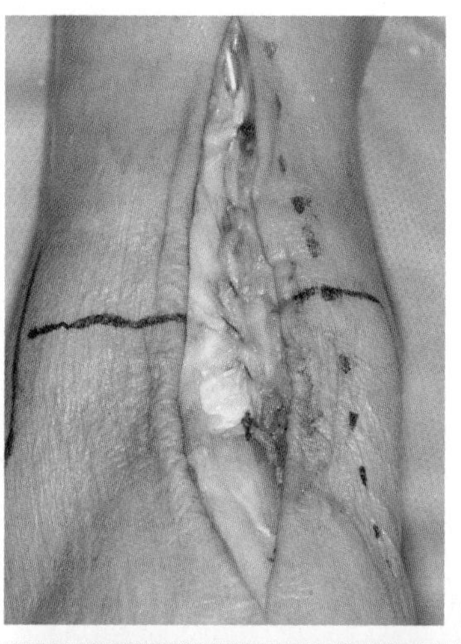
A

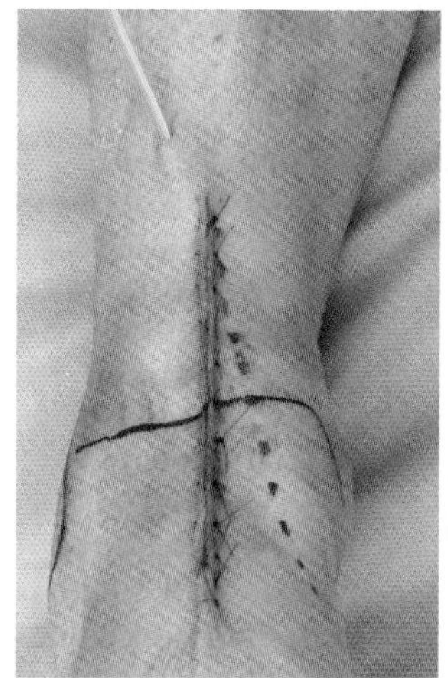
B

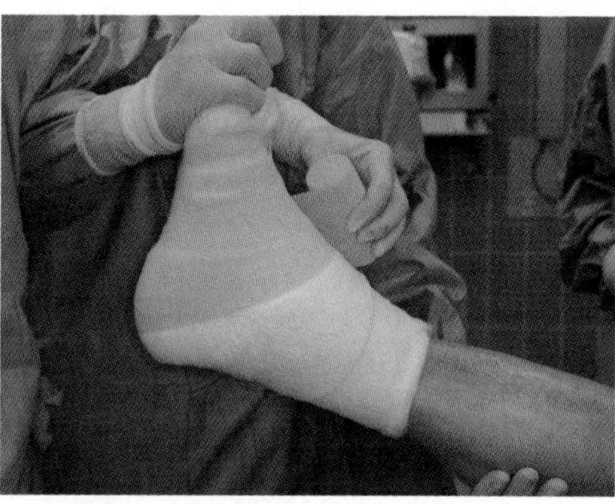
C

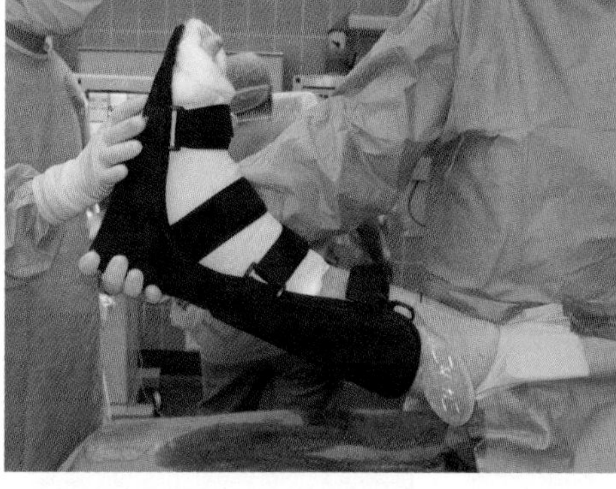
D

TECH FIG 5 • Wound closure and dressing. **A.** The extensor retinaculum is closed first. **B.** Then, the skin is closed by interrupted sutures. **C.** A compressive dressing is used to avoid swelling and hematoma formation. **D.** A splint is used to keep the foot in neutral position.

PEARLS AND PITFALLS

Malalignment or malunion above the ankle joint	■ Above the ankle joint: ■ Supramalleolar osteotomy ■ At the ankle joint: ■ Corrective tibial cut ■ Osteotomy of fibula or medial malleolus ■ Beneath the ankle joint: ■ Calcaneal osteotomy
Adjacent osteoarthrosis	■ Subtalar joint: ■ Subtalar arthrodesis ■ Talonavicular joint: ■ Talonavicular arthrodesis
Fixed deformity	■ Valgus deformity: ■ Triple arthrodesis ■ Medial sliding osteotomy of calcaneus ■ Varus deformity: ■ Release of medial ankle ligaments ■ Reconstruction of lateral ankle ligaments ■ Peroneus longus to brevis tendon transfer ■ Lateral sliding osteotomy of calcaneus ■ Dorsiflexion osteotomy of first ray

Ligamentous instability	▪ Lateral ankle ligaments: ▪ Lateral ligament reconstruction ▪ Medial ankle ligaments: ▪ Tibiotalar tilt of less than 10 degrees: medial ligament reconstruction ▪ Tibiotalar tilt of more than 10 degrees: ankle arthrodesis
Muscular dysfunction	▪ Peroneus brevis: ▪ Peroneus longus to brevis tendon transfer ▪ Tibialis posterior: ▪ Triple arthrodesis

POSTOPERATIVE CARE

- The dressing and splint are removed and changed after 2 days.
- When the wound is dry and proper, typically 2 to 4 days after surgery, the foot is placed in a stabilizing cast or walker that protects the ankle against eversion, inversion, and plantarflexion movements for 6 weeks.
- Active motion and lymphatic drainage may support recovery of soft tissues during the first 6 weeks. Overly aggressive motion during the first postoperative days, however, may lead to breakdown of soft tissues.
- Weight bearing is allowed as tolerated. Usually, full weight bearing is achieved after 1 week.
- In the case of additional osteotomies of the calcaneus, ligament reconstruction, or tendon transfer, cast immobilization for 6 weeks is advised.
- In the case of additional fusion of adjacent joints, cast immobilization for 8 weeks is advised.
- In the case of additional supramalleolar osteotomy, the patient should remain non–weight-bearing for 8 to 10 weeks.
- A rehabilitation program should be started for the foot and ankle after cast or walker removal, including stretching and strengthening of the triceps surae.[8]
- First clinical and radiologic follow-up is made at 6 weeks, to check the wound site and osteointegration and position of the implants.
- The patient should be advised to wear a compression stocking to avoid swelling for a further 4 to 6 months.

OUTCOMES

- Between May 2000 and December 2006, 574 primary total ankle arthroplasties were performed in 549 patients (272 women, 277 men; mean age 59.7 ± 12.6 years [range 19.8 to 90 years]; left side 277, right side 297, bilateral 26). The underlying diagnosis was posttraumatic osteoarthritis in 459 ankles, primary osteoarthritis in 40 ankles, and inflammatory arthritis in 63 ankles.
- The mean follow-up was 31.9 ± 19.7 months (range 12 to 82 months). The mean AOFAS improved from 42.1 ± 17.0 preoperatively to 78.1 ± 11.1 postoperatively, and the mean pain relief was from 6.8 ± 3.9 preoperatively to 2.9 ± 2.4 postoperatively. The mean plantarflexion at latest follow-up was 28.5 ± 10.2 degrees and the mean dorsiflexion was 6.4 ± 6.1 degrees. The satisfaction grade was excellent in 213 patients (38.8%), good in 238 patients (43.4%), and moderate in 87 patients (15.8%); only 11 patients (2.0%) were dissatisfied.
- Early complications included malleolar fractures intraoperatively, 11 patients; wound healing problems, 7 patients; infection, 4 patients; and polyethylene dislocation, 5 patients.
- Late complications included loosening of components, 24 patients (talar component, 22 patients, 7 of them with subsidence or migration; tibial component, 19 patients, none of them with subsidence or migration); polyethylene dislocation, 5 patients; polyethylene wear, 0; progressive loss of motion, 38 patients; chronic pain syndrome, 11 patients.
- Taking revision of a metallic implant or conversion into ankle arthrodesis as the endpoint, overall survivorship of both components at 6 years was 98.2% (97.9% for the talar component and 98.8% for the tibial component).
- Four ankles were revised to total ankle arthroplasty (component loosening, three; pain, one), and two ankles (component loosening and recurrent misalignment, one; pain, one) were revised to ankle arthrodesis.

COMPLICATIONS

- Intraoperative complications[1–4]
  - Malpositioning of prosthetic implant
  - Improper sizing of prosthetic implant
  - Fractures of malleoli
  - Tendon injuries
- Postoperative complications[1–4]
  - Wound healing problems
  - Infection
  - Swelling
  - Deep venous thrombosis
- Late complications[1–4]
  - Aseptic loosening
  - Subsidence
  - Polyethylene wear
  - Dislocation of polyethylene insert
  - Progressive loss of motion

REFERENCES

1. Haddad SL, Coetzee JC, Estok R, et al. Intermediate and long-term outcomes of total ankle arthroplasty and ankle arthrodesis: a systemic review of the literature. J Bone Joint Surg Am 2007;89A:1899–1905.
2. Henricson A, Skoog A, Carlsson A. The Swedish ankle arthroplasty register: an analysis of 531 arthroplasties between 1993 and 2005. Acta Orthop 2007;78:569–574.
3. Hintermann B, Valderrabano V, Dereymaeker G, et al. The HINTEGRA ankle: rationale and short-term results of 122 consecutive ankles. Clin Orthop Relat Res 2004;424:57–68.
4. SooHoo NF, Zingmond DS, Ko C. Comparison of reoperation rates following ankle arthrodesis and total ankle arthroplasty. J Bone Joint Surg Am 2007;89A:2143–2149.
5. Valderrabano V, Hintermann B, Horisberger M, et al. Ligamentous posttraumatic ankle osteoarthritis. Am J Sports Med 2006;34:612–620.
6. Valderrabano V, Hintermann B, Nigg BM, et al. Kinematic changes after fusion and total replacement of the ankle. Part 1: Range of motion. Part 2: Movement transfer. Part 3: Talar movement. Foot Ankle Int 2003;24:881–900.
7. Valderrabano V, Nigg BM, von Tscharner V, et al. Gait analysis in ankle osteoarthritis and total ankle replacement. Clin Biomech 2007;22:894–904.
8. Valderrabano V, Pagenstert G, Horisberger M, et al. Sports and recreation activity of ankle arthritis patients before and after total ankle replacement. Am J Sports Med 2006;34:993–999.

Chapter 70

The BOX Total Ankle Arthroplasty

Sandro Giannini, Matteo Romagnoli, Deianira Luciani, Fabio Catani, and Alberto Leardini

DEFINITION

- Severe erosions of the articular surfaces of the human ankle joint associated with arthritis drastically affect the normal interaction between muscles, bones, and ligaments and cause pain, joint instability, and disability.

SURGICAL MANAGEMENT

- Many surgeons maintain that arthrodesis is the surgical treatment of choice for these patients.[13]
- Arthrodesis has been associated with a high incidence of nonunion, secondary degenerative changes at adjacent joints, and postoperative infections.[3] Moreover, total loss of ankle motion often inhibits physiologic ambulation, particularly in patients with involvement of multiple lower extremity joints.[8] Patients who can walk with a fused ankle are generally inhibited in running and climbing.[3] These limitations of tibiotalar arthrodesis are prompting advances in total ankle arthroplasty (TAA).
- After encouraging early results of TAA, long-term clinical follow-up studies have been disappointing,[4,14,15,22] with poor results, especially in younger patients with isolated traumatic ankle arthritis. Recent clinical reports of TAA suggest only modest improvements in outcomes, outcomes that do not demonstrate the same success observed in comparable studies of total hip and knee arthroplasty.[2,5,11,12,25]
- However, several recent review papers[6,7,9,10,23,26] have demonstrated a renewed interest in TAA. Newer generations of TAA are again being touted as viable alternatives to ankle arthrodesis, although optimal restoration of physiologic tibiotalar motion and minimization of bone resection have not been achieved in any of the newer designs.
- Our extensive original research[16–21] has shown that physiologic mobility at the ankle involves rolling as well as sliding, guided by the preserved ankle joint's natural ligament apparatus.
- The BOX total ankle replacement is devised to reproduce physiologic mobility so that the ligaments continue to function normally (**FIG 1**).
- The unique three-component articulating geometry is designed to be compatible with the physiologic movement of isometric fibers within the calcaneofibular and tibiocalcaneal ankle ligaments. Sophisticated instruments have been developed to achieve accurate positioning of components relative to the ligament apparatus.[16,21]
- In our experience with the BOX prosthesis, physiologic motion and correct position are demonstrated by characteristic motion of the meniscal bearing on the tibial component, forward in dorsiflexion and backward in plantarflexion.[16,21]
- The BOX total ankle replacement is capable of restoring physiologic motion in the replaced joint with full congruence at the articulating surfaces over the entire motion arc. In our opinion, full congruence should result in minimum wear of the components, as preliminary results have indicated.[1]
- The technique, which uses instruments unique to the BOX prosthesis, involves removing a measured amount of bone from the talus (usually 4 mm) and minimal bone from the tibia (5 to 10 mm). A joint tensioning device is used so that ligament balance and tension are taken into account before the tibial cuts are made. The thickness of the meniscal implant is set via this device so that the appropriate amount of bone is resected. The amount of tension applied with this instrument represents the initial tension in the replaced joint.

Indications

- Patients with primary or posttraumatic tibiotalar arthrosis and preferably a low functional demand
- In general, patients over 50 years of age
- All patients with rheumatoid arthritis involving the tibiotalar joint
- Patients refusing arthrodesis, taking into account the following contraindications

Contraindications

- Severe morphologic defects of the ankle
- Significant osteoporosis or osteonecrosis, particularly affecting the talus
- Prior or active infections of the foot and ankle
- Vascular insufficiency or severe neurologic deficits (motor dysfunction, spasticity, neuropathy)

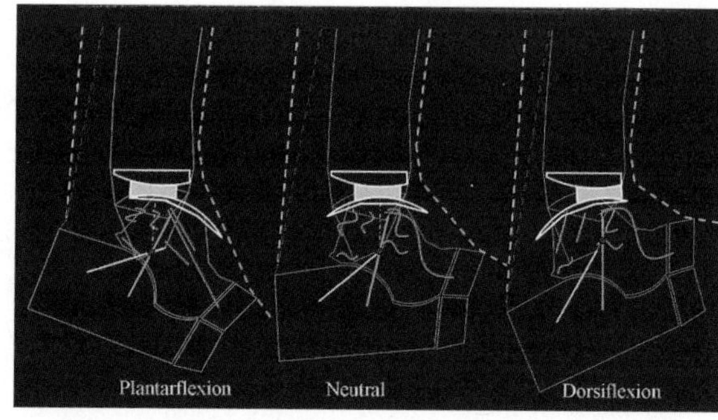

FIG 1 • The kinematics of the replaced ankle in the sagittal plane when guided by a computerized model of the four-bar linkage mechanism.[6,18,21] Arrangement of the two bone shapes (in *gray*), of the linkage (calcaneofibular in *yellow*, tibiocalcaneal in *green*) and other (slackened–tightened in *brick*) ligaments, muscle unit courses (*dashed lines*), and instantaneous center of rotation (at the crossing point between the linkage ligaments, *small circle in red*), corresponding joint contact line (*dash-dot in white*), of the metal (*empty white*) and meniscal (*gray* in between) components of the BOX Ankle, are all depicted at 20 degrees of plantarflexion (left), neutral (center), and 10 degrees of dorsiflexion (right). Details on the undersurface and fixation of the bone-anchored components are deliberately omitted because they are not relevant for this mechanism model.

- For our team, the following are contraindications only if they cannot be resolved before or during surgery (while performing TAA): capsuloligamentous instability that cannot be appropriately balanced; a foot deformity that cannot be corrected to a plantigrade position (ie, unstable platform on which to position the TAA); and severe ipsilateral hip and knee deformities or malalignment or previous arthrodesis at these joints.

Preoperative Planning

- Both AP and mediolateral ankle radiographs, taken with the patient in double leg support (fully weight bearing), are required to assess preoperative alignment and deformity of the tibiotalar joint.
- Radiographic magnification must be assessed, using a radiographic scaling technique or by comparing a measurement on the radiograph and the subject, such as foot length or ankle width. Radiographic templates are provided for the BOX prosthesis from 100% to 120% in 5% intervals to compensate for magnification discrepancies.
- The surgeon must assess the best fit of tibial and talar implants and the meniscal implant thickness. For the tibia component, the surgeon assesses the AP length at the level of resection and mediolateral fit between the malleoli. For the talar component, AP fit is assessed.
- We recommend that the tibial and talar implants are matched within one size up or down (eg, small tibia with medium talar or large tibia with medium talar, but preferably not small tibia with large talar). The meniscal implant corresponds with the size and color code of the talar implant.

Positioning

- The patient is positioned supine on the operating table.

Approach

- We routinely use a tourniquet in the upper third of the thigh after the foot and ankle have been exsanguinated with an Esmarch elastic wrap. The leg must be sterile up to the knee.
- An anterolateral skin incision 8 to 10 cm long is made, leaving one third distal and two thirds proximal to the joint line (**FIG 2A**).
- The subcutaneous tissue is dissected, identifying and protecting the superficial peroneal nerve. The superior and inferior extensor retinaculum is incised. The peroneus tertius tendon is identified and the incision is continued between this and the extensor digitorum communis tendons.
- A longitudinal capsulotomy is performed to expose the ankle joint (**FIG 2B**). The capsule and soft tissues are carefully elevated medially and laterally to the malleoli and retractors are inserted deep to the soft tissues and directly on the malleoli. Potentially harmful direct skin tension is avoided with deep retraction of the soft tissues.
- It is important to fully expose the medial and lateral aspects of the tibiotalar joint; all the fibrous tissue and osteophytes must be removed. Typically, soft tissue elevation is required on the distal anterior tibia, immediately proximal to the ankle joint, to permit satisfactory positioning of the tibial alignment guide. Distally, the incision and capsular–soft tissue elevation must be extended to identify the transition between the head and the neck of the talus, while protecting the deep neurovascular bundle.
- The ankle is positioned in maximum dorsiflexion and the most anterior borders of the articulating surfaces are marked, together with the central line mediolaterally. The latter is important for the correct later positioning of the tibial alignment mediolaterally to provide better support.

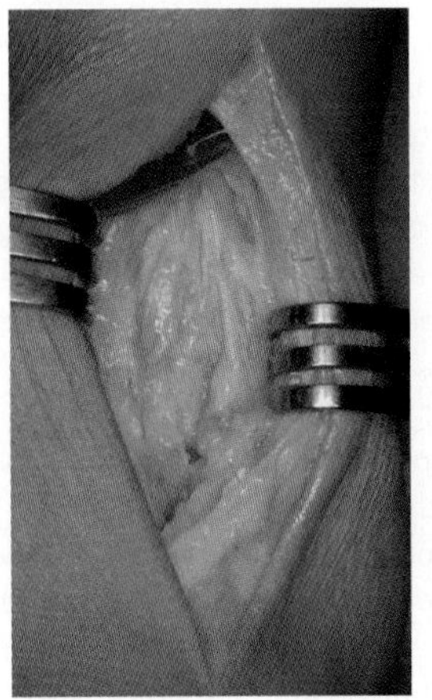

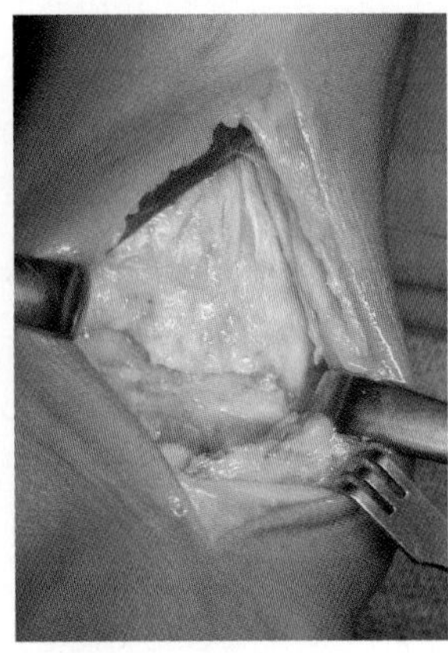

FIG 2 • **A.** An 8- to 10-cm anterolateral skin incision. **B.** Exposure of the ankle joint.

BOX IMPLANT

Initial Tibial Preparation

- Trim the anterior prominence and exostosis of the distal tibia using a chisel to gain access to the joint space (**TECH FIG 1**).
- Assemble the tibial alignment guide with proximal clamp and connector; tighten with the proximal screw. Insert the talar cutting block onto the tibial alignment guide and tighten with the frontal screw (**TECH FIG 2A**).
- With the button in the unlocked position and depressed, adjust the ratchet to the START position (Tech Fig 2A). Lock the ratchet to prevent it from moving out of position during positioning and sawing.
- Place the assembled guide onto the lower leg, inserting the posterior tongue of the talar cutting block into the joint space centered between the malleoli.

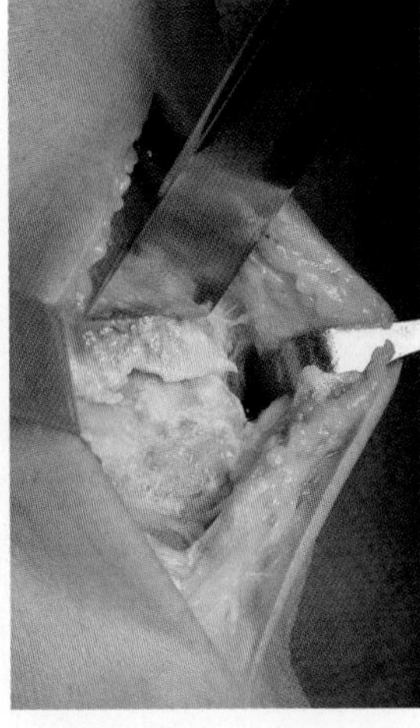

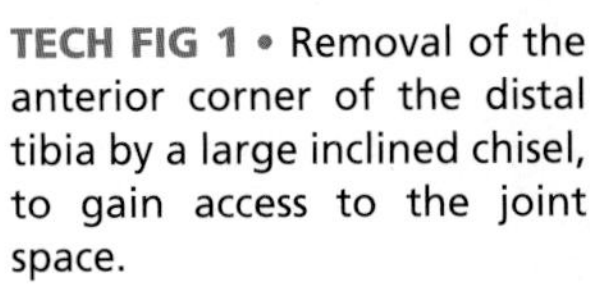

TECH FIG 1 • Removal of the anterior corner of the distal tibia by a large inclined chisel, to gain access to the joint space.

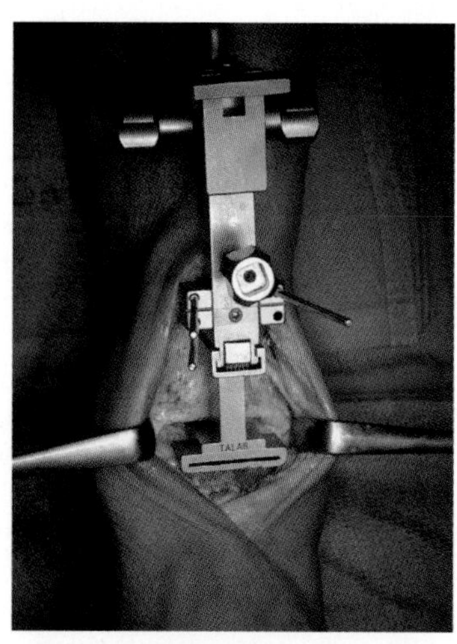

A

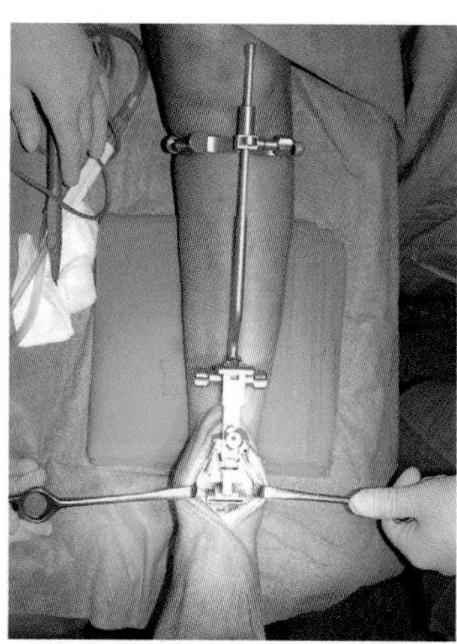

B

TECH FIG 2 • Placement of assembled guide for talar cut. **A.** Talar cutting block onto the tibia alignment guide, with the ratchet to the START position (same level of the central and lateral sulcus). **B.** Tibia alignment guide assembled onto the shank.

- Place the proximal clamp at the proximal tibial tuberosity (TECH FIG 2B).
- Fasten the spring around the proximal shank.
- Align the shaft of the tibial alignment guide parallel with the longitudinal axis of the tibia, in both anterior and lateral views, by adjusting the proximal clamp.
- Recheck that the tongue of the talar cutting block is centered between the malleoli and pin using two or three out of four diagonally opposite pin positions (pins converge toward the center of the tibial shaft).
- A common error is to align the shaft parallel to the front of the tibia rather than parallel to the longitudinal axis. This will result in an erroneous posterior inclination of the tibial component.

Horizontal Talar Cut

- Lock the position of the tongue as far as it will go into the joint space with the frontal screw.
- Ensure that the foot is in the neutral flexion position (0 degrees dorsiflexion and plantarflexion, 90 degrees between the tibia axis and the plantar aspect of the foot) and complete the horizontal talar cut.
- Remove the talar block, complete the cut, and remove the resected talar bone (TECH FIG 3).
- If the foot is in dorsiflexion or plantarflexion, a malrotation of the talar component will result, restricting final range of motion of the implanted prosthesis.

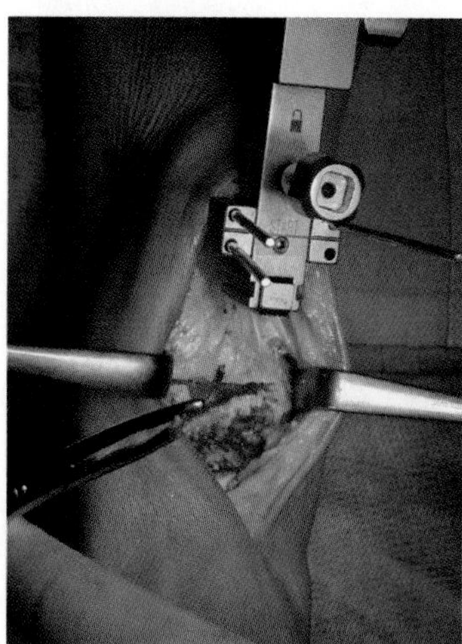

TECH FIG 3 • Removal of the talar bone stock.

Tibial Preparation

- Insert the selected size of tibial cutting block onto the tibial alignment guide (TECH FIG 4A) in neutral mediolateral adjustment (center of scale, TECH FIG 4B).
- Assess the central position of the block relative to the malleoli. If needed, adjust on the fine scale by moving the tibial cutting block forward (as if to remove it) until it is free to slide mediolaterally. Reinsert the block in the desired medial or lateral adjustment. Tighten with the frontal screw.
- Select the thinnest 5-mm tibial tensioner for minimum bone removal from the tibia (Tech Fig 4A). Slide the tensioner through the slot on the tibial cutting block, advancing the posterior tongue of the tensioner (most distal part of Tech Fig 4A) into the joint space.

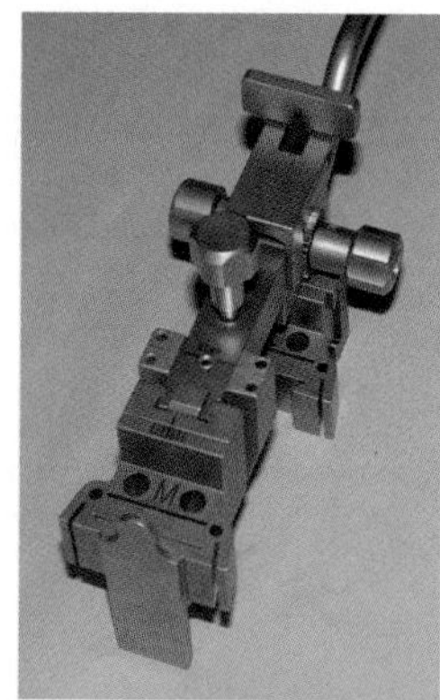

A

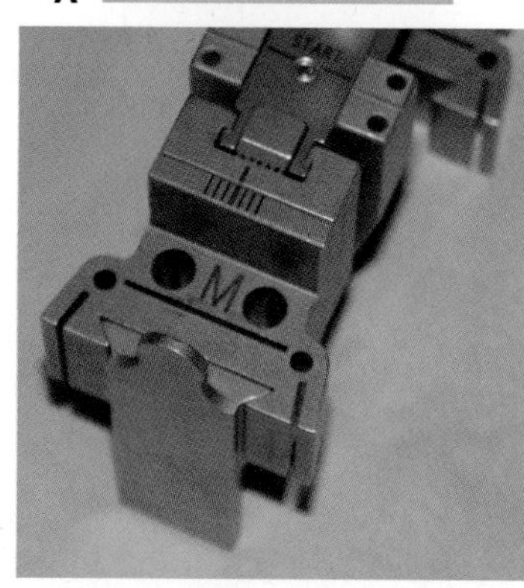

B

TECH FIG 4 • Details of the tibial cutting block.

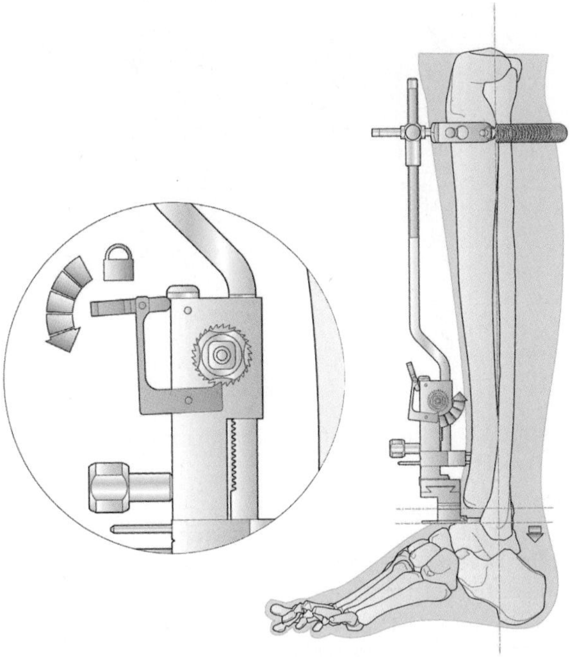

TECH FIG 5 • The ratchet applies tension to the joint via the tibial tensioner by turning the ratchet knob in a counterclockwise direction. At the end, the ratchet button is locked again. (Courtesy of Finsbury Orthopaedics Limited, Leatherhead, UK.)

- Assemble the knob tightener into the large blue handle and unlock the ratchet button (Tech Fig 4A).
- Insert the knob tightener into the ratchet knob and turn in a counterclockwise direction.
- The amount of tension applied will represent the tension in the replaced joint, provided the meniscal implant matches the tibial tensioner used (**TECH FIG 5**).
- If the selected position of the horizontal cut on the tibia is considered too distal (removing too little tibial bone), go back to the ratchet START position and insert the 6- or 7-mm tibial tensioner into the tibial cutting block and apply tension again.
- Lock the ratchet when the desired tension and level of tibial cut is reached.
- The position of the cuts on the tibia is now set, so that precisely the right amount of bone is resected to match the combined thickness of implant components.
- Tensioning the joint and using a meniscal implant as thin as possible are recommended to prevent excessive or unnecessary bone removal from the tibia.
- Complete the three tibial cuts without notching the malleoli with the saw blade.
- Drill the two 3.2-mm holes with the tibial corner drill up to the depth mark (S, M, or L), taking care not to drill too far.
- Select the appropriate 4.5-mm tibia drill (S, M, or L) to suit the tibial block used and drill the two 4.5-mm holes in the tibia through the tibial cutting block up to the depth stop.
- Remove the tibial cutting block by releasing the frontal screw and use the tibial corner gouge assembled in the large blue instrument handle to join the cuts in the two corners (**TECH FIG 6**).
- Fragment and remove the cut section of bone using a chisel (small 30 mm, medium 35 mm, large 40 mm long).
- Fragmenting thin sections of bone requires considerable care and patience because it is thicker posteriorly and retained by the posterior periosteum and capsule. Be careful to do so without leaning against the malleoli because this may result in their fracture.
- Before removing the tibial alignment guide, measure the AP length of the horizontal tibial cut with the tibial length gauge.
- The measurement indicates whether a small, medium, or large size of tibial implant is appropriate (small 30 mm, medium 35 mm, and large 40 mm).
- If in between sizes, size down to prevent overhang of the tibial component.
- If there is a need to increase the tibial implant size, select the next biggest tibia cutting block and increase the depth of the 4.5-mm holes using the next larger drill. Redrill the two 3.2-mm drill holes, recut the side cuts, and extend the top horizontal cut to meet the small holes. Remove the complete tibial cutting guide assembly.
- When increasing tibia implant size, be sure to increase the depth of the 4.5-mm holes; failure to increase the depth of the 4.5-mm holes may result in fracture of the posterior portion of the tibia.
- Use the tibial keyhole cutter assembled in the slide hammer to join the two 4.5-mm holes to the horizontal tibial

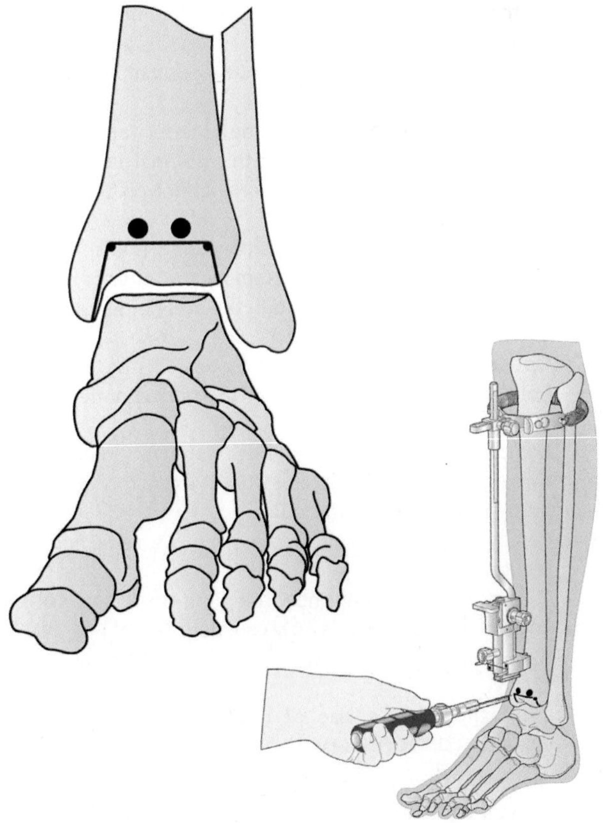

TECH FIG 6 • When the holes are drilled and the cuts are completed at the tibia (top left), the tibial corner gouge is used to join the three cuts in the two corners. (Courtesy of Finsbury Orthopaedics Limited, Leatherhead, UK.)

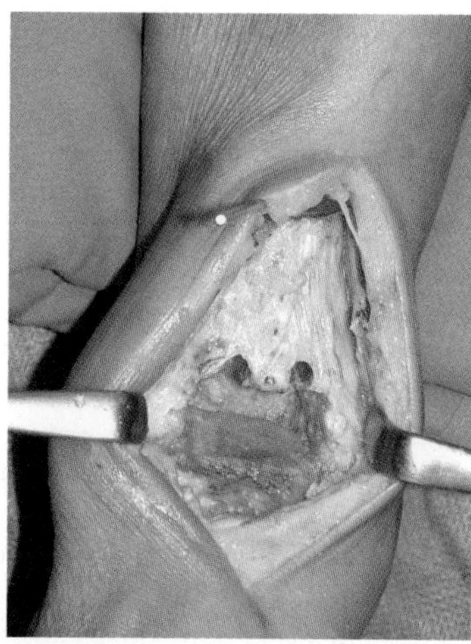

TECH FIG 7 • Completed tibial preparation.

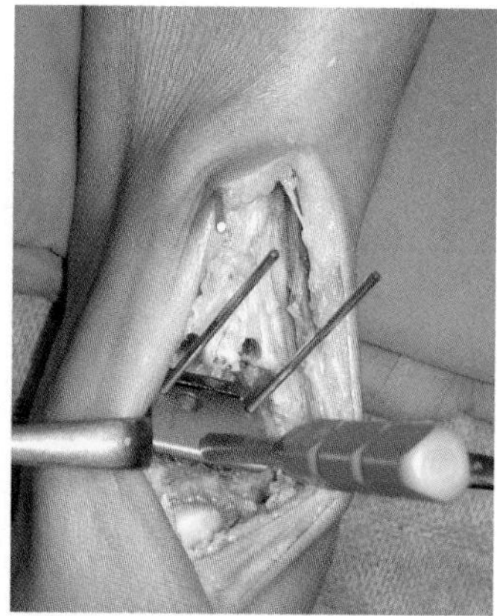

TECH FIG 8 • Placement of talar chamfer guide by the small blue handle in front.

cut. Care should be taken not to break out the holes by biasing the cutter proximally or distally.

- The tibial preparation is now complete (TECH FIG 7).

Completion of the Talar Preparation

- Select the appropriate size of talar chamfer guide and attach the small blue handle.
- Slide the guide onto the flat talar cut until the anterior chamfer abuts the front of the talus (TECH FIG 8).
- Using the appropriate-thickness flat spacer (blue, Tech Fig 9), assess the joint gap in neutral, maximum plantarflexion (TECH FIG 9A), and maximum dorsiflexion (TECH FIG 9B) positions.
- With the talar chamfer guide in the optimal AP position, the gaps will be equal.
- It is usually necessary to trim the anterior talus, moving the guide posteriorly to gain this optimal position because a good fit of the anterior chamfer on the talus is desired.
- Pin the guide in the final position using two short pins (pins converge centrally), and remove the anterior handle.
- Drill the two peg holes through the drill guide tube with the talar peg drill.
- Optionally, use the talar lever to distract the tibia and hold down the posterior part of the talar chamfer guide (TECH FIG 10A).
- Complete the posterior chamfer cut. Optionally, continue using the talar lever to hold down the posterior part of the talar chamfer guide.
- Remove the guide and complete the cut, removing the section of bone.
- The talar preparation is now complete (TECH FIG 10B).
- The tibial preparation is now complete (TECH FIG 11).

Trial Reduction

- Insert the selected size of talar trial using the talar impactor (TECH FIG 12).
- Insert the selected size of tibial trial using the tibial inserter (in the large blue handle) and the green profile spacer to keep the tibial trial hard up against the cut bone surface.
- A spacer one size thicker than the planned final meniscal implant is recommended (TECH FIG 13).
- Select the appropriate-sized meniscal trial matching the size of the talar trial used and the thickness of tibial tensioner used. Insert with the meniscal trial inserter–remover (TECH FIG 14).
- Assess the overall range of dorsiflexion–plantarflexion and joint function.
- The meniscal trial should traverse anterior to posterior on the tibial trial component by about 5 mm from maximum dorsiflexion to maximum plantarflexion.

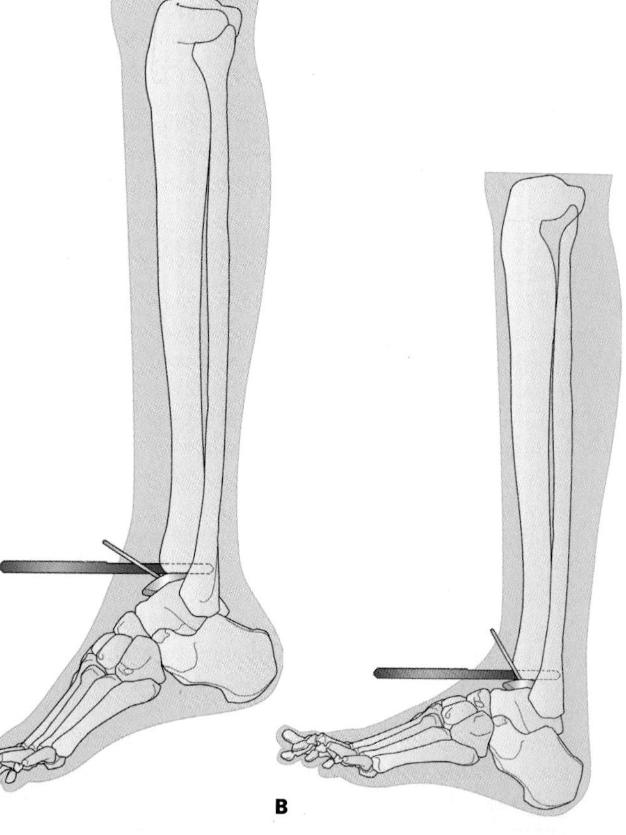

TECH FIG 9 • Joint gap by the blue flat spacer in maximum plantarflexion (**A**) and maximum dorsiflexion (**B**) positions. (Courtesy of Finsbury Orthopaedics Limited, Leatherhead, UK.)

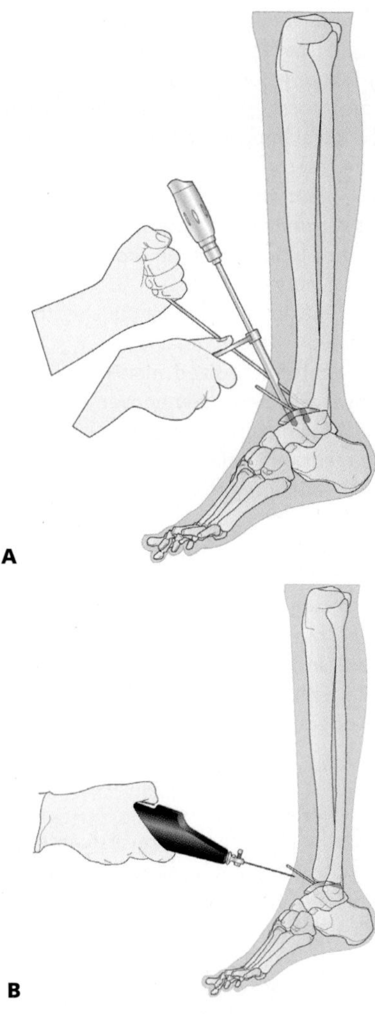

TECH FIG 10 • Final talar preparation. **A.** Drilling the anterior peg hole through the drill guide tube with the talar peg drill; the talar lever is used with the left hand to hold down the posterior part of the talar chamfer guide. **B.** The bone saw for the posterior chamfer cut. (Courtesy of Finsbury Orthopaedics Limited, Leatherhead, UK.)

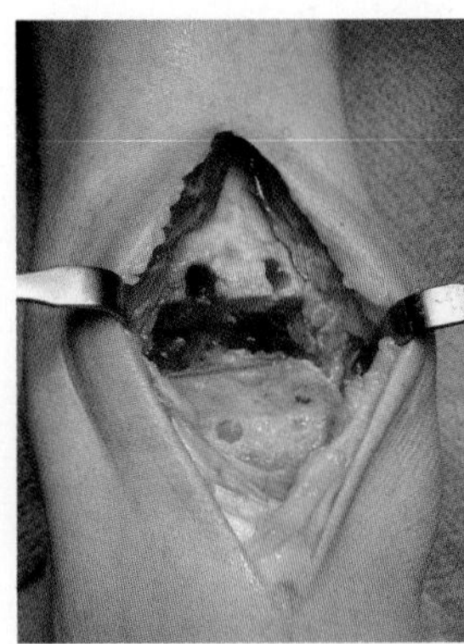

TECH FIG 11 • Completed tibial and talar preparation.

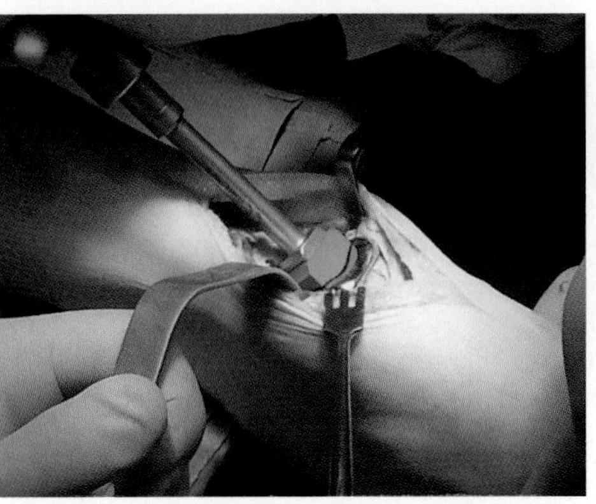

TECH FIG 12 • Insertion of the talar trial using the talar impactor.

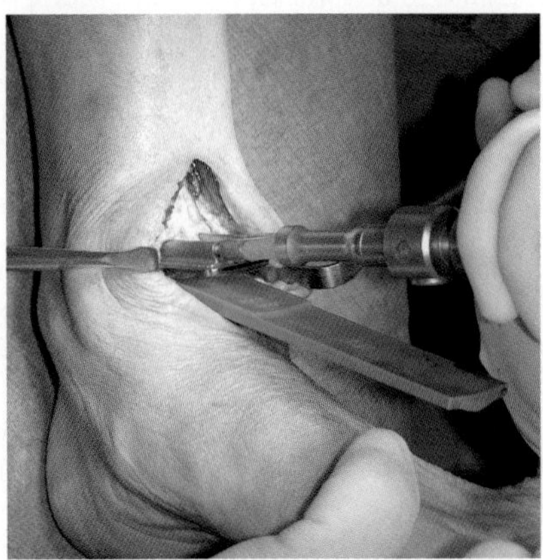

TECH FIG 13 • Insertion of the tibial trial using the tibial inserter and the green profile spacer.

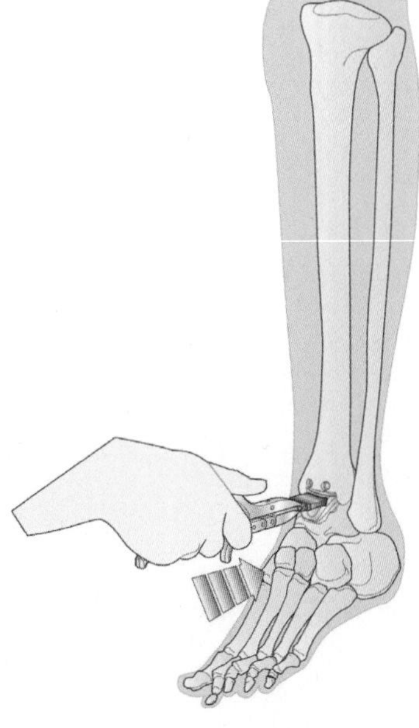

TECH FIG 14 • Insertion of the meniscal trial using the relevant inserter–remover. (Courtesy of Finsbury Orthopaedics Limited, Leatherhead, UK.)

- The meniscal trial should also remain in full contact with the two metal trials throughout flexion and the full range of internal–external rotation in the transverse plane.
- An intraoperative fluoroscopy or radiographic control should be considered to assess the AP position of both tibial and talar implants.
- If range of motion or stability is not satisfactory, it is possible to make a small adjustment in the tibial trial AP position or to try an alternative thickness of meniscal trial.
- Use the meniscal trial inserter–remover to remove the meniscal trial, as in Techniques Figure 14.
- Use the tibial trial remover attached to the slide hammer to remove the tibial trial (**TECH FIG 15A**) and the talar extractor aligned with the recesses in the anterior chamfer to remove the talar trial (**TECH FIG 15B**). Attaching the slide hammer is optional.
- Before attempting to move the tibial trial posteriorly, it is essential to increase the depth of the relevant two drill holes; failure to do this may result in fracture of the posterior portion of the tibia while inserting the tibial trial.

Final Implantation

- When selecting the implant components, ensure that the meniscal implant matches the talar implant size and color code.
- Both tibial and talar components are cementless.
- Clean the resected bone surfaces with a bone brush or pressurized lavage. Use suction to remove the debris and liquid. Dry thoroughly.
- Position the talar implant to engage the pegs with the drilled holes. Impact in line with the pegs using the talar impactor.
- Insert the tibial implant with the tibial inserter using the green profile spacer to avoid contact between the two highly polished metal components.
- The profile spacer also maintains optimal contact between the tibial implant and resected tibial surface during implant insertion.
- A spacer 1 mm thicker than the planned final meniscal implant is recommended. This is to avoid tibial component posterior tilting and to improve its primary fixation with a better press-fit.
- Impact the tibial implant until it matches the optimal position obtained with the tibial trial.
- Insert the appropriate-sized meniscal trial again using the meniscal trial inserter–remover to assess the final thickness of the meniscal implant.
- Insert the meniscal implant by hand with the two raised marker ball pads anterior and a single raised marker pad posterior.
- This is performed by pushing it with both thumbs. Considerable effort may be required. Usually this is expected to result in limited range of motion at the replaced joint, but this not the case for this TAA, because the meniscal implant sagittal shapes are designed to be compatible with the isometric motion of the ligaments and the operative technique allows this to be restored.[16,21]
- Assess the ankle range of dorsiflexion–plantarflexion and joint function.
- The meniscal implant should traverse anterior to posterior on the tibial implant by about 5 mm from maximum dorsiflexion (**TECH FIG 16A**) to maximum plantarflexion (**TECH FIG 16B**).

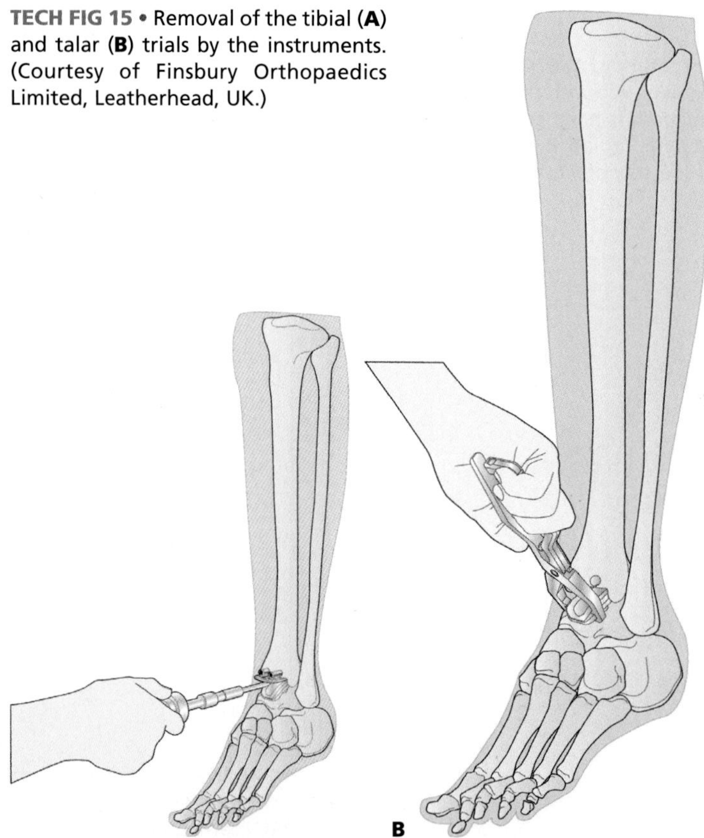

TECH FIG 15 • Removal of the tibial (**A**) and talar (**B**) trials by the instruments. (Courtesy of Finsbury Orthopaedics Limited, Leatherhead, UK.)

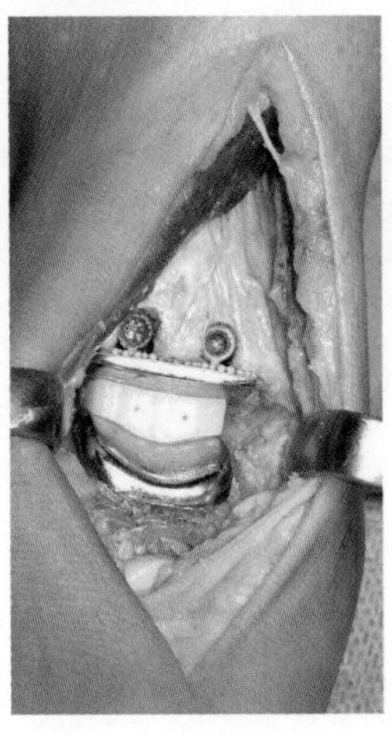

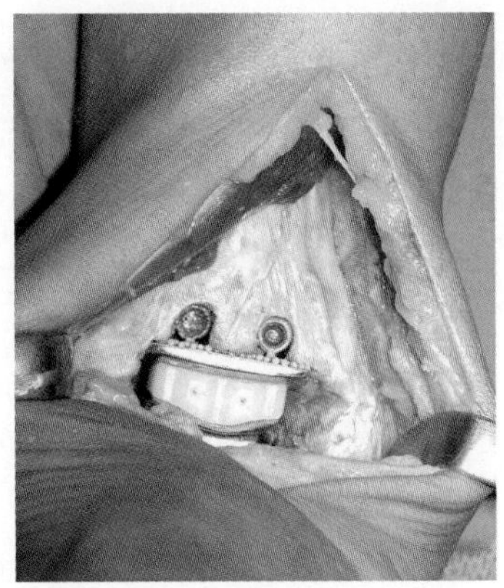

TECH FIG 16 • Final implantation and assessment of joint and meniscal mobility: maximum plantarflexion (**A**) and maximum dorsiflexion (**B**).

- The meniscal implant should also remain in full contact with the two metal components throughout flexion and the full range of internal–external rotation in the transverse plane.
- The only possible correcting actions at this stage are exchanging the meniscal implant thickness or inserting further the tibial implant (though the latter is critical because of the risk of posterior tibial fracture, as in the last paragraph of the previous section). In addition, if a limited range of dorsiflexion is observed and the replaced joint is stiff, a percutaneous Achilles tendon lengthening can be performed.

Closure

- Release the tourniquet and carefully cauterize any bleeding veins.
- Insert a drain and suture the anatomic planes.
- Closure of the extensor retinaculum is essential. The deep neurovascular bundle and superficial peroneal nerve must be protected. After closure, lateral and frontal radiographs are taken and the joint is cast in the neutral position.

ADDITIONAL TECHNIQUES

- Correction of forefoot deformity, particularly fixed forefoot varus
- Calcaneal osteotomy to correct hindfoot malalignment
- After final implantation, if the total ankle prosthesis does not provide at least 10 degrees of dorsiflexion, percutaneous Achilles tendon lengthening is performed by a laterally and medially based stab incisions of the tendon.
- Ligamentous reconstruction to treat the ankle instability, performed with a trial implant to ensure that proper ligamentous balance can be achieved with the final implant
- If widening of the mortise was present preoperatively, open reduction and internal fixation of the syndesmosis is performed by a syndesmotic screw.

PEARLS AND PITFALLS

Pearls	▪ Maintain proper indications. ▪ Address relative contraindications appropriately and TAA may still be favored over arthrodesis. ▪ With the ankle in maximum dorsiflexion and the most anterior borders of the tibial and talar articulating surfaces close together, mark both with a pen the central line mediolaterally. This procedure is performed for the correct positioning of the tibial alignment guide. ▪ Tensioning the joint by moving the tibial cutting block distally and using a meniscal implant as thin as possible implies that eventually the minimum bone removal from the tibia is performed; in other words, correct distraction of the joint prevents excessive or unnecessary bone removal from the tibia. ▪ If in between sizes, size down to prevent mediolateral and posterior overhang of the tibial component. ▪ It is usually necessary to trim the anterior talus, moving the guide posteriorly to gain this optimal position, to achieve an optimal fit of the anterior chamfer on the talus. ▪ A fluoroscopy or radiographic control should be considered to assess the correct AP position of both tibial and talar implants.

	■ A green spacer 1 mm thicker than the planned final meniscal implant is recommended during tibial implantation to force the component further against the bone; this avoids tibial component posterior tilting and improves primary fixation of the component with a better press-fit. ■ Perform necessary additional surgical procedures (ie, foot realignment and ligament rebalancing) to ensure optimal support and stability.
Pitfalls	■ A common error is to align the tibial alignment guide parallel to the front of the tibia rather than parallel to the longitudinal axis. This will result in an erroneous posterior inclination of the tibial component. ■ If the foot is in dorsiflexion or plantarflexion during the transverse talar cut, a malrotation of the talar component will occur, resulting in a likely restriction of the final range of motion at the replaced joint. ■ Avoid notching the malleoli with the saw blade during tibial bone preparation. ■ When increasing the size of the tibia implant during the intervention, failure to increase the depth of the 4.5-mm holes may result in fracture of the posterior portion of the tibia during impaction of the component. ■ Fragmenting thin sections of tibial bone resection requires considerable care and patience, particularly because it is thicker posteriorly and retained by the posterior periosteum.

POSTOPERATIVE CARE

■ Immediately after surgery a cast is placed for 2 weeks, and weight bearing is not allowed.

■ After 2 weeks a brace is placed and active and passive range of ankle motion is permitted. If the part of the wound not healed is small, motion is still permitted, but if it is large motion is not permitted until complete healing.

■ After 1 month full weight bearing with the brace is allowed.

■ After 2 months full weight bearing without the brace is allowed after bone ingrowth is suggested on follow-up radiographs. Rehabilitation is then recommended, particularly muscular reinforcement and proprioceptive exercises as well as functional restoration of walking patterns.

OUTCOMES

■ In an eight-center Italian clinical trial, 135 patients received implants between July 2003 and December 2006. Mean age was 60.7 years (range 31 to 80). The AOFAS clinical score systems and standard radiographic assessment were used to assess patient outcome, here reported only for the 90 patients with follow-up longer than 6 months.

■ Intraoperatively, the components maintained complete congruence at the two articulating surfaces of the meniscal bearing over the entire motion arc, associated with considerable anterior motion in dorsiflexion and posterior motion in plantarflexion of the meniscal bearing, as predicted by the previous mathematical models.

■ A mean of 10.1 degrees of dorsiflexion and 23.5 degrees of plantarflexion were measured immediately after implantation, for a mean additional range of motion of 18.6 degrees, which was maintained at follow-up.

■ Radiographs showed good alignment and no signs of progressive radiolucency or loosening.

■ The mean AOFAS score went from 37.0 before surgery to 64.7, 73.2, 78.4, and 85.9 respectively at 3-, 6-, 12-, and 18-month follow-ups.

■ One revision was performed 3 days after implantation because of a technical error; it was successful. Another revision in arthrodesis was performed at 19 months because of a wrong indication.

■ In the scoring system used, the function and range-of-motion sections scored better than any average previous total ankle result.[24] Pain scored similarly.

■ The satisfactory though preliminary observations from this novel design encourage continuation of the implantation, which has now been extended over a few European countries. Instrumented gait and three-dimensional fluoroscopic analyses are in progress to quantify functional progress.

COMPLICATIONS

■ The most common intraoperative complication is medial malleolus fracture. The medial malleolus should always be checked for fracture before wound closure. A medial malleolar fracture must be fixed with a screw, a medial buttress plate, or both.

■ Another intraoperative complication could be widening of the mortise, which is treated with open reduction and internal fixation of the syndesmosis (see above).

■ Less common complications include lateral malleolus fracture (managed with screw or Kirschner wire fixation), tendon laceration (treated with direct repair), or nerve or artery injury (treated with direct repair).

REFERENCES

1. Affatato S, Taddei P, Leardini A, et al. Wear behaviour in total ankle replacement: a comparison between an in vitro simulation and retrieved prostheses. Clin Biomech 2009;24:661–669.
2. Anderson T, Montgomery F, Carlsson A. Uncemented STAR total ankle prostheses: three to eight-year follow-up of fifty-one consecutive ankles. J Bone Joint Surg Am 2003;85A:1321–1329.
3. Bauer G, Kinzl L. Arthrodesis of the ankle joint. Orthopade 1996;25:158–165.
4. Bauer G, Eberhardt O, Rosenbaum D, et al. Total ankle replacement: review and critical analysis of the current status. Foot Ankle Surg 1996;2:119–126.
5. Buechel FF Sr, Buechel FF Jr, Pappas MJ. Ten-year evaluation of cementless Buechel-Pappas meniscal-bearing total ankle replacement. Foot Ankle Int 2003;24:462–472.
6. Chou LB, Coughlin MT, Hansen S Jr, et al. Osteoarthritis of the ankle: the role of arthroplasty. J Am Acad Orthop Surg 2008; 16:249–259.
7. Cracchiolo A III, DeOrio JK. Design features of current total ankle replacements: implants and instrumentation. J Am Acad Orthop Surg 2008;16:530–540.
8. Demetriades L, Strauss E, Gallina J. Osteoarthritis of the ankle. Clin Orthop Rel Res 1998;349:28–42.
9. Deorio JK, Easley ME. Total ankle arthroplasty. AAOS Instr Course Lect 2008;57:383–413.
10. Guyer AJ, Richardson G. Current concepts review: total ankle arthroplasty. Foot Ankle Int 2008;29:256–264.

11. Hintermann B, Valderrabano V, Dereymaeker G, et al. The HINTEGRA ankle: rationale and short-term results of 122 consecutive ankles. Clin Orthop Relat Res 2004;424:57–68.
12. Hurowitz EJ, Gould JS, Fleisig GS, et al. Outcome analysis of agility total ankle replacement with prior adjunctive procedures: two to six year follow-up. Foot Ankle Int 2007;28:308–312.
13. Katcherian DA. Treatment of ankle arthrosis. Clin Orthop Rel Res 1998;349:48–57.
14. Kitaoka HB, Patzer GL. Clinical results of the Mayo total ankle arthroplasty. J Bone Joint Surg Am 1996;78A:1658–1664.
15. Lachiewicz PF. Total ankle arthroplasty: indications, techniques, and results. Orthop Rev 1994;23:315–320.
16. Leardini A, Catani F, Giannini S, et al. Computer-assisted design of the sagittal shapes for a novel total ankle replacement. Med Biol Eng Comp 2001;39:168–175.
17. Leardini A, O'Connor JJ, Catani F, et al. Kinematics of the human ankle complex in passive flexion: a single degree of freedom system. J Biomech 1999;32:111–118.
18. Leardini A, O'Connor JJ, Catani F, et al. A geometric model of the human ankle joint. J Biomech 1999;32:585–591.
19. Leardini A, O'Connor JJ, Catani F, et al. The role of the passive structures in the mobility and stability of the human ankle joint: a literature review. Foot Ankle Int 2000;21:602–615.
20. Leardini A, O'Connor JJ. A model for lever-arm length calculation of the flexor and extensor muscles at the ankle. Gait Posture 2002; 15:220–229.
21. Leardini A, O'Connor JJ, Catani F, et al. Mobility of the human ankle and the design of total ankle replacement. Clin Orthop Relat Res 2004;424:39–46.
22. Rush J. Management of the rheumatoid ankle and hindfoot. Curr Orthop 1996;10:174–178.
23. Saltzman CL, McIff TE, Buckwalter JA, et al. Total ankle replacement revisited. J Orthop Sports Phys Ther 2000;30:56–67.
24. Stengel D, Bauwens K, Ekkernkamp A, et al. Efficacy of total ankle replacement with meniscal-bearing devices: a systematic review and meta-analysis. Arch Orthop Trauma Surg 2005;125:109–119.
25. Wood PL, Deakin S. Total ankle replacement: the results in 200 ankles. J Bone Joint Surg Br 2003;85B:334–341.
26. Younger A, Penner M, Wing K. Mobile-bearing total ankle arthroplasty. Foot Ankle Clin 2008;13:495–508.

Chapter 71 The Salto and Salto-Talaris Total Ankle Arthroplasty

Michel Bonnin, Brian Donley, Thierry Judet, and Jean-Alain Colombier

DEFINITION

- The Salto Total Ankle Prosthesis is a cementless resurfacing-type implant that is intended to restore near-normal joint kinematics. Fixation is achieved through bone ingrowth.
- The surgical technique is critical to a successful outcome, and some criteria are essential:
  - Tight fit of the components and extended contact area with bone to achieve good primary stability, which is a prerequisite for secondary biological fixation
  - Restoration of the mechanical axis of the ankle
  - Accurate restoration of the joint line (proper level and strict horizontal plane)
  - Preservation or restoration of the soft-tissue balance
  - Adequate soft tissue release to achieve good range of motion (ROM) intraoperatively

ANATOMY

The Mobile-Bearing Salto Prosthesis

- The Salto Total Ankle Prosthesis (Tornier SA, Saint- Ismier, France) was developed between 1994 and 1996 and has been used clinically since January 1997.
- Based on experience with the third-generation cementless meniscal-bearing designs, this system was designed to restore nearly normal kinematics of the ankle (**FIGS 1 AND 2**).
- A dedicated instrument system was developed to achieve optimal positioning of the components, and the design of the implant was optimized to better restore the natural anatomy and obtain an optimal primary fixation of the components while retaining a minimally invasive resurfacing concept.
- The tibial component accommodates the superior flat surface of the mobile bearing. Its smooth surface allows free translation and rotation of the mobile bearing. The 3-mm medial rim protects the polyethylene from impingement with the medial malleolus.
- The specific shape (segment of a cone of revolution) of the talar component replicates the anatomy of the talar dome. It is broader anteriorly than posteriorly, and the lateral condyle has a larger radius of curvature than the medial condyle. As a result, the axis of flexion and extension of the talar component, under the polyethylene, is aligned with the physiologic axis. The lateral aspect of the talus is resurfaced, allowing articulation with the lateral malleolus.
- The ultra-high-molecular-weight polyethylene (UHMWPE) insert articulates with the tibial component superiorly and with the talar component inferiorly. It maintains full congruency with the talar component in flexion and extension and accommodates as much as 4 degrees of varus and valgus in the coronal plane, thereby reducing the chance of polyethylene edge loading.
- The tibial component is available in three sizes and the talar component is available in four sizes. The mobile bearing is size-matched to the talar component in thicknesses from 4 to 8 mm.
- The mobile-bearing size must match the size of the talar component. The talar component must be equal to or one size less than the tibial component.

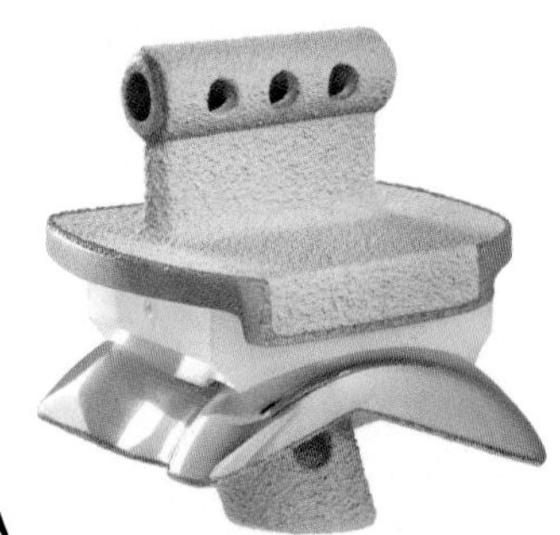

A

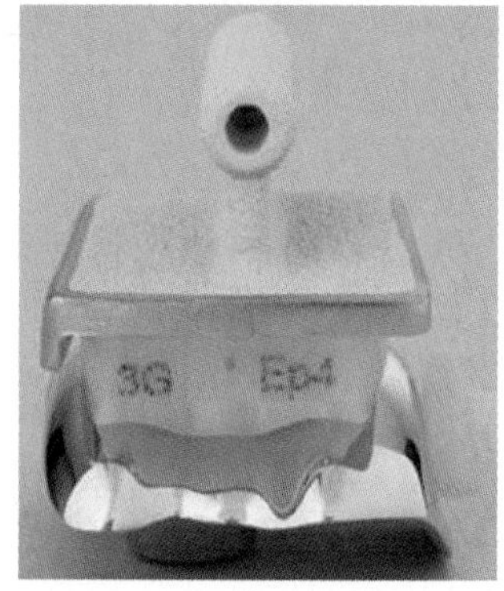

B

FIG 1 • **A.** An oblique view shows the Salto Total Ankle Prosthesis. **B.** An AP view shows the three main components and the malleolar component.

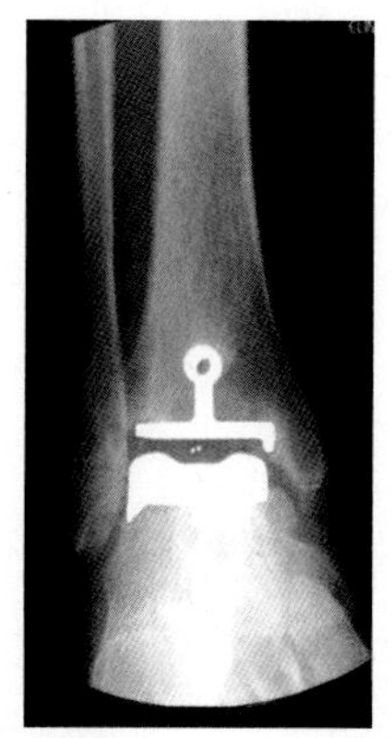

A

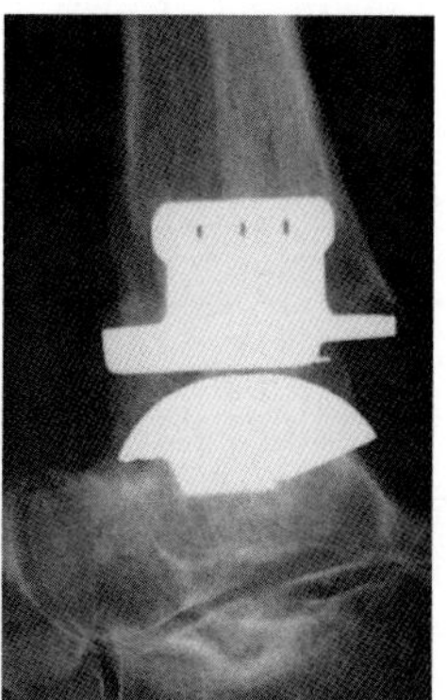

B

FIG 2 • AP (**A**) and lateral (**B**) radiographs show the Salto Total Ankle Prosthesis in situ.

Dr. Donley is a paid consultant for Tonnier, Inc., the company that makes the Salto Talaris Anatomic Ankle.

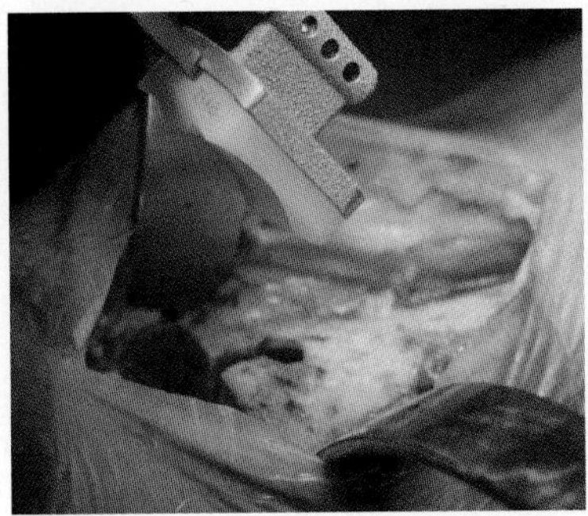

FIG 3 • The Salto-Talaris components and instrument system are the same as those of the Salto prosthesis, except that the tibial component is a fixed-bearing design.

- Primary fixation to the tibia is ensured by close match of the tibial component to the epiphysis, and enhanced by an AP keel and a tapered cylindrical plug.
- Stability of the talar component is provided by three bone cuts, and insertion of an 11-mm-diameter hollow fixation peg into the body of the talus.
- Secondary fixation is provided by bone ingrowth into a dual coating of hydroxyapatite applied to a 200-μm-thick layer of plasma-sprayed titanium.

The Fixed-Bearing Salto-Talaris Prosthesis

- Our experience with the Salto prosthesis has led us to revise our concept of mobility. As a matter of fact, owing to the anatomic design of the implant, the precision of the bone cuts, and the accuracy in component positioning, the need for and the potential problems associated with postoperative motion of the polyethylene bearing during flexion–extension movements have been almost completely eliminated. This has been confirmed in clinical studies based on standing dynamic views. On the other hand, intraoperative motion of the tibial component assembly is most helpful in allowing self-positioning of the bearing with respect to the talar component before the tibial keel preparation is completed.
- The Salto-Talaris components and instrument system are the same as those of the Salto prosthesis, except that the tibial component is a fixed-bearing design (**FIG 3**). The final position of the tibial component is fine-tuned at the end of the procedure to achieve perfect alignment with the talar component. In this manner the self-positioning feature of the mobile-bearing insert has been retained.

PATHOGENESIS

- In general, our indications for total ankle arthroplasty (TAA) are: end-stage ankle osteoarthritis (OA) or rheumatoid arthritis (RA).
- In OA, degeneration may be due to sequelae of trauma, chronic ankle instability, and rarely primary osteoarthritis.
- In our experience, RA occurs relatively infrequently in the ankle when compared to the hip or knee. However, there is no consensus on the actual rate of ankle joint involvement in RA patients, with figures ranging from 9% in the study by Vainio,[8] in which clinical criteria were used, to 40% in the study by Jakubowski et al,[6] which employed radiographic criteria.
- Occasionally, end-stage erosive or degenerative changes of the ankle may develop secondary to osteochondromatosis, pigmented villonodular synovitis, hemochromatosis, or osteochondritis dissecans.
- Ankle joint involvement in RA tends to occur late in the disease process, with symptoms not occurring until a mean disease duration of 17 to 19 years.
- Since the tibiotalar joint is rarely affected in isolation, treatment will need to be systemic and not only for the ankle.

NATURAL HISTORY

- Progressive tibiotalar arthritis typically is accompanied by progressive ankle stiffness. Loss of ankle ROM, particularly dorsiflexion, results from tibiotalar osteophytes and less resilience in the distal tibiofibular syndesmosis.
- Over time, the patient may develop an equinus gait with resultant Achilles tendon contracture, posterior capsular adhesions, and occasionally tibialis posterior adhesions.

PATIENT HISTORY AND PHYSICAL FINDINGS

Methods for Examining the Degenerative Ankle Joint

- Silfverskiold test
  - Passive ankle ROM with the patient supine and the knee flexed and extended
  - Physiologic ROM with this examination is 15 (dorsiflexion)/0/40 (plantarflexion).
  - An isolated gastrocnemius contracture is present when lack of dorsiflexion with the knee in extension is eliminated with knee flexion.
- Evaluation of ankle ROM with the patient standing and walking
- Visualizing the gait pattern. The patient may externally rotate the extremity, or female patients may be able to walk in high heels to mask the lack of ankle dorsiflexion.
- Hindfoot ROM
  - We use three grades of hindfoot motion: physiologic, diminished, or stiff. We favor total ankle arthroplasty (TAA) over ankle arthrodesis in patients with a stiff hindfoot.
- Hindfoot alignment with the patient standing or ambulating
  - Hindfoot malalignment (varus or greater than physiologic valgus) may be most pronounced with the patient walking.
- Hindfoot alignment with the patient supine
- We typically assess passive hindfoot motion to determine if the deformity can be reduced to a physiologic position. In our hands, this examination determines the type of hindfoot realignment that will be performed concomitant to TAA.
- Tibiotalar instability
  - The examiner successively assesses coronal plane and sagittal plane stability with varus–valgus stress and anterior drawer testing, respectively. In our hands, varus instability or fixed varus ankle requires careful ligament balancing.

IMAGING AND OTHER DIAGNOSTIC STUDIES

- In our preoperative assessment we not only determine the extent of deformity and instability at the ankle but also assess any concomitant ipsilateral lower extremity malalignment that may have a bearing on the outcome of TAA. We routinely obtain weight-bearing AP, mortise, and lateral radiographs of both ankles; radiographs of the uninvolved ankle typically provide some understanding of what is physiologic for the patient. Weight-bearing mechanical axis hip-to-ankle radiographs are required if there is associated deformity of the ipsilateral lower extremity.

- We recommend obtaining CT scans of the ankle and hindfoot, particularly to review coronal sections, to further evaluate tibial or talar bone loss or cysts not fully defined on plain radiographs.

DIFFERENTIAL DIAGNOSIS

- Septic arthritis
- Charcot neuroarthropathy

NONOPERATIVE MANAGEMENT

- We have had limited success with nonoperative management in active patients with end-stage ankle arthritis.
- Activity modification, rocker-bottom shoe modification, and bracing offer some relief.
- We reserve nonoperative management for low-demand patients who are poor surgical candidates.

SURGICAL MANAGEMENT

Total Ankle Arthroplasty Versus Ankle Arthrodesis

- In general, arthrodesis is favored over TAA because:
  - Lower risk of mechanical implant failure; no risk of implant wear
  - Lower risk of infection
  - Less chance of skin necrosis when the ankle has been previously operated on
  - In our hands, lower incidence of residual pain
- In general, TAA is favored over ankle arthrodesis because:
  - Less risk of developing adjacent (hindfoot) joint arthritis
  - In our hands, more favorable functional outcome
  - In our opinion, malunion or development of adjacent joint arthritis makes revision surgery more difficult after arthrodesis.

Preoperative Planning

- Preoperative evaluation of weight-bearing radiographs and CT scan to:
  - Choose the optimal implant size, with the use of available templates. This is important because an oversized prosthesis will alter the center of rotation, giving rise to pain and stiffness.
    - If the talus is particularly deformed, the template should be applied to the contralateral, unaffected ankle.
  - Determine the reference for establishing the ideal tibial resection level, taking into account the extent of wear in the tibial plafond
  - Analyze tibiotalar joint alignment relative to the tibial shaft axis. This allows differentiation between axial deviations:
    - Resulting from asymmetrical wear of the tibial plafond that may be corrected with tibial preparation.
    - Because of malunion that may require corrective osteotomy, simultaneous to or staged with TAA.
  - Analyze the residual talar body.
    - Asymmetry needs to be balanced in the talar preparation.
  - Evaluate the hindfoot.
    - A joint-sparing calcaneal osteotomy may be necessary to realign the hindfoot.
    - In the face of hindfoot arthritis or hindfoot instability, a subtalar or even triple arthrodesis may be warranted.

Positioning

- The patient is positioned supine on the operating table, with a pad under the ipsilateral hip to promote a neutral tibial and foot alignment with the foot pointing to the ceiling.
- The plantar aspect of the foot should be flush with the end of the table.
- Placing a rolled towel under the ankle facilitates subtle adjustments in ankle positioning.
- We routinely use a thigh tourniquet.
- In our experience, a pillow placed behind the knee allows the Achilles tendon to relax and may improve exposure.
- We recommend including the knee in the sterile field so that the limb can be positioned more freely and so that the patella and tibial tubercle may be used to confirm optimal alignment. The surgeon stands at the foot of the table, with the assistant at the lateral side of the operative leg.

Approach

- The tibiotalar joint is approached through an anterior midline incision starting 8 to 10 cm proximal to the joint line and extending to the midfoot.
- The soft tissues must be handled carefully, especially in patients being managed with systemic steroid treatment.
  - The surgeon should avoid undermining the skin.
  - The surgeon should maintain deep retraction only and avoid tension directly on the skin edges.
  - Extending the skin incision will further diminish skin tension.
- While we maintain meticulous hemostasis, we ligate vessels whenever possible and use electrocautery sparingly to diminish the risk of skin burns. We typically incise the crural fascia and extensor retinaculum along the lateral border of the tibialis anterior tendon, using the interval between the tibialis anterior and extensor hallucis longus tendons.
  - Whenever possible, the tibialis anterior tendon should remain protected in its individual sheath throughout the procedure (this also separates the tendon from the anterior incision during closure).
- Alternatively, the extensor retinaculum may be incised at the lateral border of the extensor hallucis longus tendon, using the interval between the extensor hallucis and extensor digitorum longus tendons. The tendons are retracted with angled retractors, and the deep neurovascular bundle (anterior tibial artery and deep peroneal nerve) is identified in the proximal wound and carefully reflected laterally.
- The periosteum and joint capsule are incised longitudinally. The medial and lateral flaps are elevated using a scalpel and an elevator to expose the tibiotalar joint to the anterior margins of the malleoli.
- To avoid direct tension on the skin margins, we use deep retractors, one at the proximal aspects of each malleolus.
- Anterior osteophytes are removed with an osteotome, and the talar facets are cleared with a rongeur.
- We then define the physiologic aspects of both malleoli, removing any osteophytes, ossifications, and loose bodies

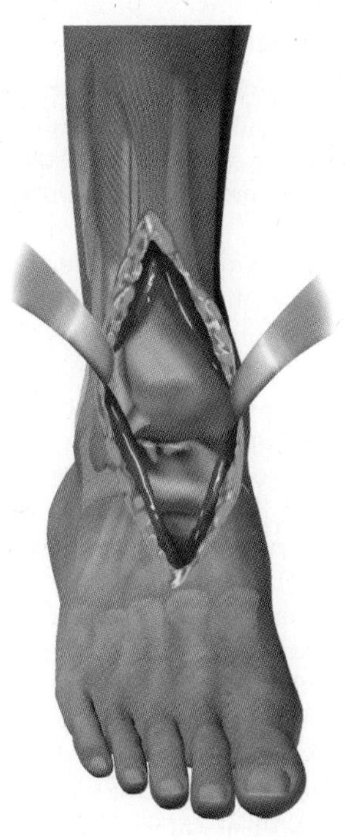

that obscure visualization of the medial and lateral ankle gutters, distort the natural anatomy, or impinge on the talus (**FIG 4**).

- Upon completion of these steps, the talus should be mobile and the medial and lateral gutters should be fully exposed.

FIG 4 • A lateral retractor is placed against the lateral malleolus and a medial retractor against the upper part of the medial malleolus. Anterior osteophytes are removed with an osteotome, and the talar facets are cleared with a rongeur.

TIBIAL RESECTION

- The goal is to restore a physiologic tibiocalcaneal axis. Ideally, implant position should produce a joint line at right angles to the mechanical tibial axis in the coronal plane and reproduce the physiologic 7-degree posterior slope in the sagittal plane.
- Align the extramedullary guide with the anterior tibial crest or a line joining the center of the knee and the midpoint of the distal tibial surface.
  - Proximally, secure the alignment guide to the anterior tibial tuberosity with a self-drilling pin, roughly perpendicular (in the sagittal plane) to the malleolar tips and distal medial tibial metaphysis in the sagittal plane (**TECH FIG 1**).
- We then perform five sequential adjustments.

Orientation in the Coronal Plane

- Provided there is anatomic or near-anatomic overall alignment of the lower extremity, the tibial cut should be horizontal and perpendicular to the tibial axis (**TECH FIG 2**).
- Perform resection using the extramedullary guide referencing off the anterior tibial border.
- A few degrees of coronal plane deviation proximal to the ankle or at the knee is readily compensated by realigning the proximal aspect of the external tibial alignment guide on the pin placed in the tibial tubercle. However, in our experience moderate to severe deformity proximal to the ankle should be corrected before TAA, typically in a staged fashion.

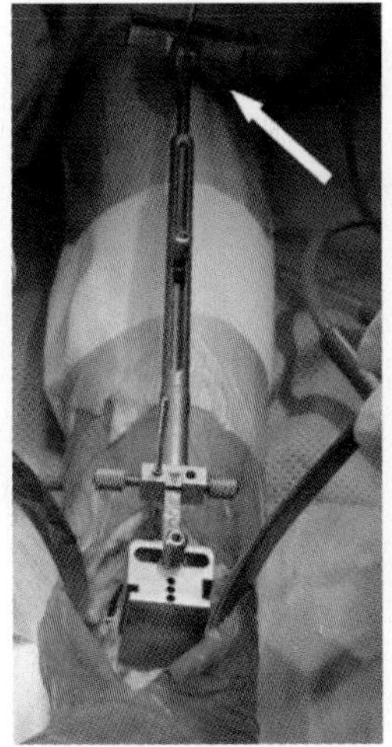

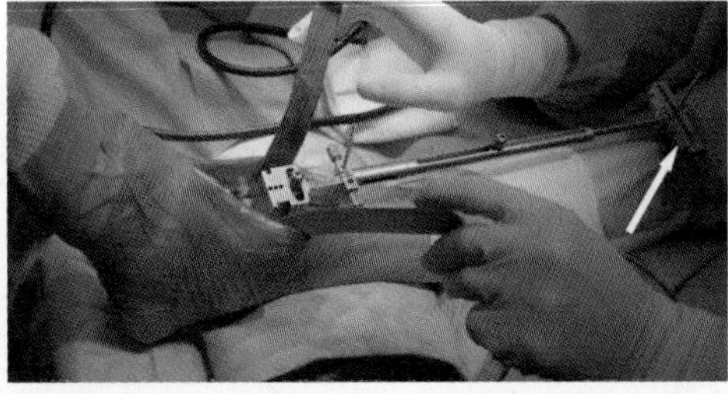

TECH FIG 1 • **A, B.** Left ankle. The extramedullary guide is aligned with the anterior tibial crest. It is attached with self-drilling pins at the anterior tibial tuberosity, roughly perpendicular (in the sagittal plane) to the malleolar tips, and then at the distal medial metaphysis of the tibia. Resection is performed using the extramedullary guide, referencing off the anterior tibial border. A few degrees of axial deviation of the knee joint in the coronal plane can be compensated for by using the proximal holes (*arrow*) to obtain a perfect adjustment and to perform a bone cut that will be almost horizontal.

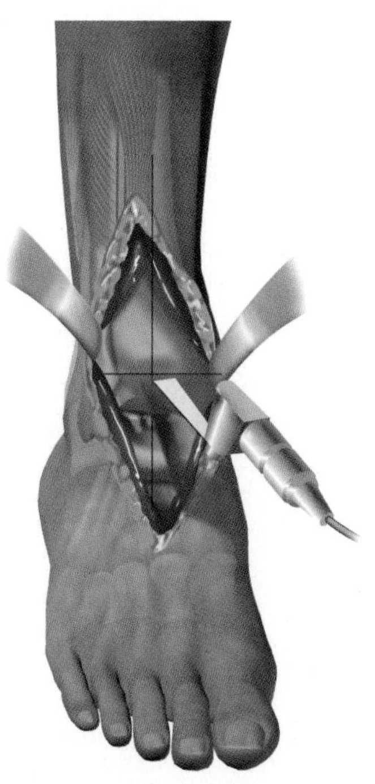

TECH FIG 2 • In the coronal plane, provided there is a good overall alignment of the lower extremity, the tibial cut should be horizontal and perpendicular to the tibial axis.

Orientation in the Sagittal Plane

- The external tibial alignment guide, when positioned parallel to the anterior tibial cortex, establishes a physiologic posterior slope of 7 degrees for the tibial cut.
- In our experience, to achieve correct angulation of the tibial cutting block, the extramedullary guide must rest on the tibia at both the proximal and distal ends.

Resection Level

- The goal is to restore an anatomic joint line level. When the subchondral architecture of the tibial plafond is intact, the amount of distal tibial resection should match the metal tibial base plate plus the polyethylene insert.
- We use the apex of the tibial plafond as the reference point for tibial resection. To expose this apex, we resect the anterior margin of the tibial plafond using an osteotome. With clinical inspection or fluoroscopic confirmation in the sagittal plane, the resection level is determined from this reference point (**TECH FIG 3**).
- For the Salto (three-part mobile-bearing) prosthesis, the tibial resection is 7 mm (3 mm for the thickness of the metal base plate plus 4 mm for the minimum thickness of the polyethylene).
- For the Salto-Talaris (two-part fixed-bearing) prosthesis, the minimum resection is 8 mm (3 mm for the thickness of the metal base plate plus 5 mm for the minimum thickness of the polyethylene). However, as a routine we resect 9 mm, which allows for downsizing of the polyethylene in the event that the joint is too tight.
- We modify the tibial cut based on the ligamentous tension in the ankle. In stiff ankles, we typically resect 2 mm more than the minimal resection; in ankles with instability, we generally resect 2 mm less than the minimal resection.
- Bone loss in the tibia may warrant adjusting the tibial cut to re-establish the proper joint line.

Orientation in Rotation

- Since both the tibial and initial talar cutting guides are suspended from the tibial alignment guide, thus linking the tibial and initial talar resection, proper rotational alignment is critical. Malrotation of the components may interfere with the implant's kinematics, create malleolar

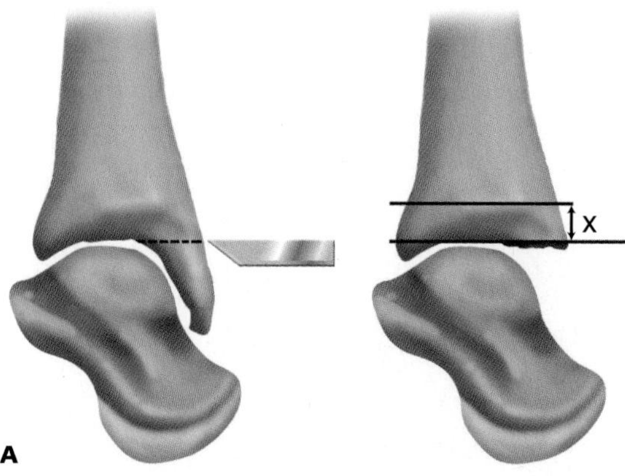

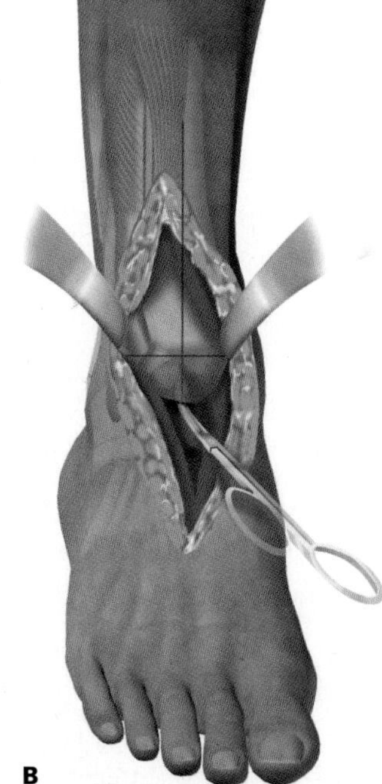

TECH FIG 3 • **A.** The goal with the Salto is to restore an anatomic joint line level. Then, in the absence of significant bone wear, the amount of bone resection on the tibia must fit exactly with the thickness of the tibial components (metal base plate plus polyethylene). **B.** The only reliable landmark is the plafond of the tibial pilon. The anterior margin of the tibial pilon is resected using an osteotome. This will provide direct exposure of the joint surface. From this reference level, the required cut is determined, aiming to remove as little bone as possible. *(continued)*

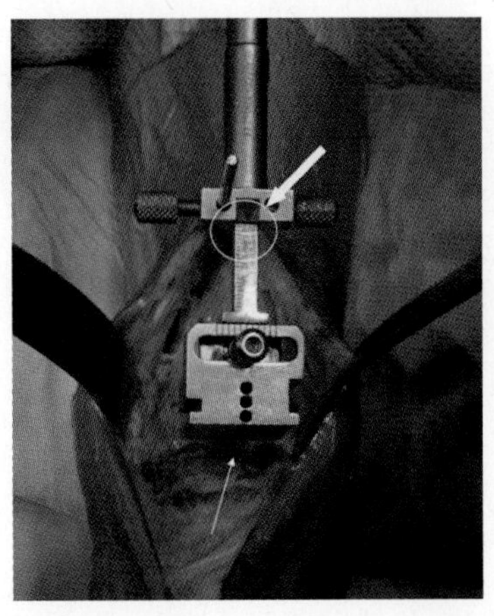
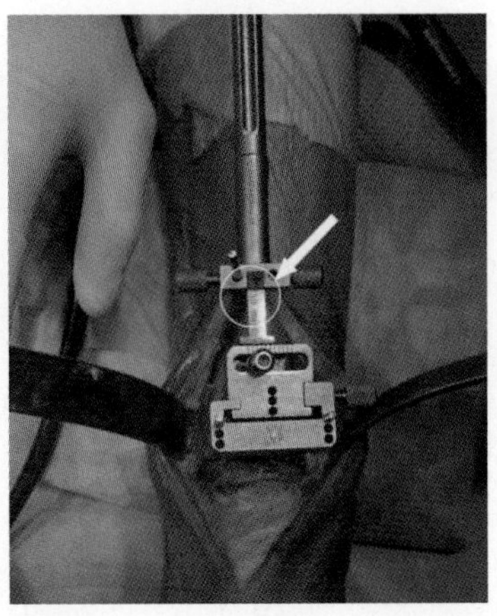

TECH FIG 3 • *(continued)* **C.** The guide is adjusted at the level of the tibial pilon (*small arrow*) and this level is observed on the scale on the tibial alignment jig (*large arrow and circle*). Left ankle. **D.** Then, from the initial reference position the guide is adjusted proximally from 7 to 9 mm according to the desired amount of resection (*arrow and circle*). Left ankle.

impingement, risk edge loading, and (particularly in the fixed-bearing Salto-Talaris) lead to increased constraint (**TECH FIG 4**).

- While the mobile-bearing Salto implant may compensate for a certain degree of malpositioning, edge loading or overhang of the polyethylene on the metal tibial tray may result. Therefore, every effort should be made to orient the implant on the center bisecting line of the talus in the coronal plane, the line that is parallel with the talus when it is taken through its motion arc. We rotate the cutting guide until it is centered on the line bisecting the space between the medial and lateral talar facets.
- Orienting the implant in line with the second metatarsal may be useful but introduces errors with associated midfoot or forefoot deformity.

Coronal Plane Positioning

- The final adjustment is to center the cutting block on the tibial plafond, often necessitating medial or lateral translation of the cutting block relative to the tibial alignment guide. The proper-size cutting block must be selected; the reference landmarks for sizing are the medial axilla and the lateral edge of the tibia.
  - Set the guide to avoid compromise of the malleoli. Secure pins within the cutting block at the level of resection to protect the malleoli from inadvertent saw blade excursion. (**TECH FIG 5A**).
- Bone resection
  - Before making the sagittal bone cuts (medial and lateral), drill holes through the appropriate-size cutting block and fully insert two short pins through the superior holes to protect the malleoli during resection. Before placing the protective pins, an AP radiograph may be obtained to confirm proper position and sizing of the cutting block in the coronal plane.
  - For a mobile-bearing Salto prosthesis, use the extramedullary guide to initially prepare for the tibial keel as it sets the rotational alignment of the tibial component.
  - When implanting a Salto-Talaris prosthesis, the rotational alignment is established using the trials and ranging the ankle to allow the tibial base and insert assembly to self-center with respect to the trial talar component.
  - The capture guide on the cutting block guides the saw blade.
  - The tibial resection must be completed through the posterior cortex of the distal tibia, without plunging the saw blade into the posterior soft tissues.
  - We typically use a saw blade of adequate length and limited excursion.
- Removing the resected bone
  - Remove the tibial cutting block but leave the external tibial alignment guide in position.
  - With a thin osteotome or small reciprocating saw, complete the two sagittal cuts through the predrilled holes created using the cutting block.
  - Remove the resected bone wafer.
  - The resected bone must be fully mobilized before attempting to extract it from the joint; abrupt mobilization of this bone may result in a fracture of

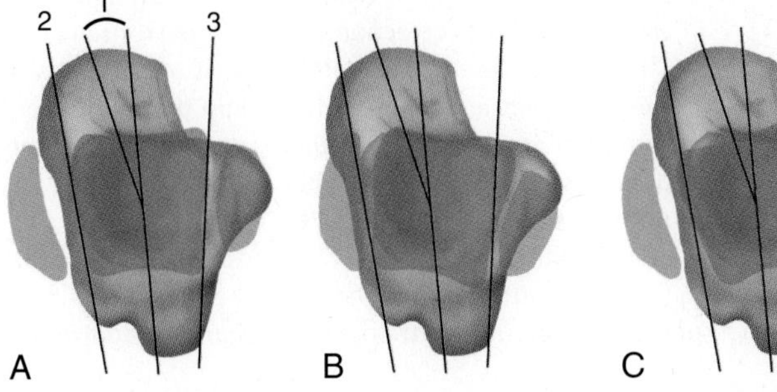

TECH FIG 4 • The rotational alignment is of critical importance even more so as the tibial and talar resections are linked. **A.** The talar component must be aligned with the axis of the talar dome (*1*) and is centered on the line bisecting the space between the medial and lateral talar facets (*2* and *3*). External (**B**) or internal (**C**) rotational malpositioning of the components will result in increased stress being placed on the fixation system, impingement with the malleoli and may interfere with the kinematics of the joint replacement.

the medial malleolus if the cut is not complete, especially in an ankle with an equinus contracture. The removal of the distal tibial resection is rarely done in one piece; usually piecemeal removal is required.

- Remove the anterior half. With the Salto and Salto-Talaris prostheses removal of the posterior portion may be delayed until after the posterior talar cut is completed (TECH FIG 5B).

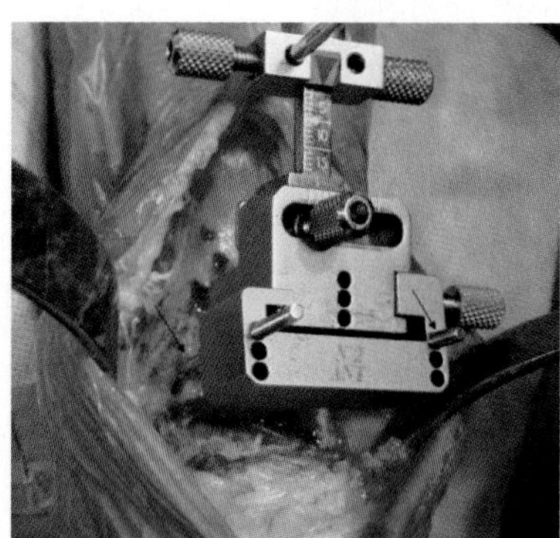

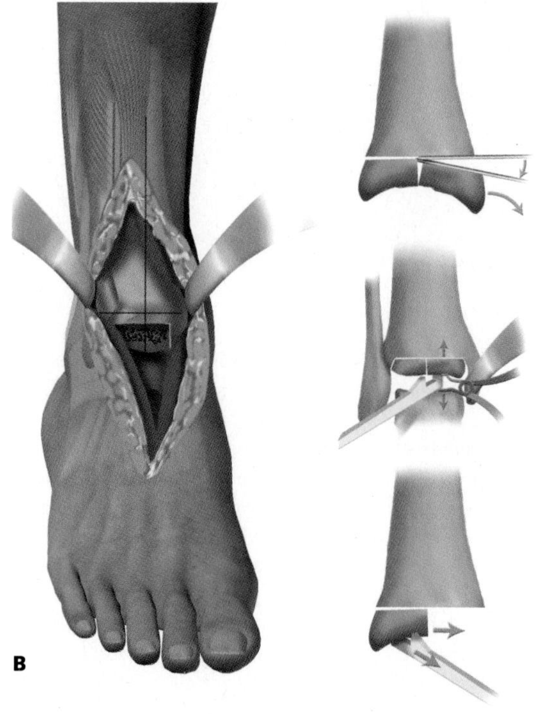

TECH FIG 5 • **A.** The instrument system provides accurate component positioning through adjustment of the resection level, translation, and rotation. Pins can be inserted in the medial and lateral holes of the guide to visualize the limits of the tibial cut with respect to the malleoli. Before the tibial cut is performed, holes are drilled through the appropriate-size cutting block, and two short pins are fully inserted through the superior holes to protect the malleoli during resection (*small arrows*). **B.** The removal of the distal tibial resection is rarely done in one piece; usually, piecemeal removal is required. The anterior half is removed, and then removal of the posterior portion can be delayed until after the posterior talar cut is completed.

TALAR PREPARATION

- Talar preparation requires that the ankle can be dorsiflexed to at least 90 degrees.
  - This angle is almost always obtained at this stage, since the removal of bone from the tibia (anterior part of tibial resection) will have created more space, even in a stiff ankle.
  - In the rare case that it is not achieved, then an Achilles tendon lengthening or gastrocnemius–soleus recession may need to be considered.
- Talar preparation comprises three cuts: posterior, anterior, and lateral. The native medial talar dome is left intact with this technique.

Posterior Talar Chamfer Cut

- To position the talar component properly on the prepared talar dome, the posterior talar cut must be inclined 20 degrees posteriorly.
- With the ankle maintained at 90 degrees of dorsiflexion and the hindfoot in physiologic valgus position, suspend the talar guide from the external tibial alignment guide and insert a pin into the talus (TECH FIG 6A).
  - This pin dictates the sagittal orientation of the talar component.
  - This reference pin must be placed with the ankle in a strictly neutral position between flexion and extension.
  - Excessive dorsiflexion will lead to anterior and flexed positioning of the talar component.
  - Excessive plantarflexion tilts the implant backward.
  - Secure the posterior chamfer talar cutting block on this reference pin.
  - Talar styli are available to determine the level for an anatomic resection that corresponds to the thickness of the talar component.
- In case of severe flattening of the talar dome, this resection level may need to be adjusted. The talar resection level depends on having satisfactory fixation of the implant in healthy bone while simultaneously trying to preserve as much talar bone stock as possible.
  - The posterior chamfer cut of the talus should be anatomic, parallel to the superior margin of the talar dome.
  - Asymmetric wear must be recognized and the posterior talar chamfer cut adjusted appropriately; shims are available to make such adjustments.
  - We do not recommend compensating extra-articular or hindfoot deformity by means of an asymmetric posterior talar chamfer cut; instead, simultaneous or staged hindfoot correction should be performed.
  - The talar guide orients the placement of four pins in the talus that are then used to guide the talar resection. Maintain the oscillating saw flush with the dorsal aspects of the pins while protecting the malleoli from injury (TECH FIG 6B).
- The residual tibial bone is relatively easy to extract at this point, along with the resected portion of talus. A lamina spreader without teeth, used judiciously, usually improves exposure.

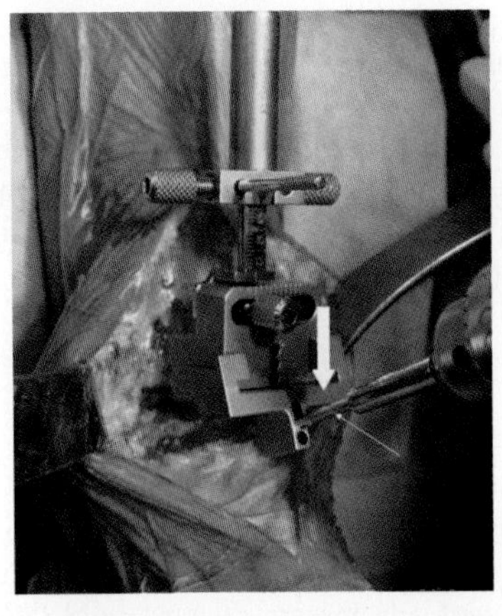

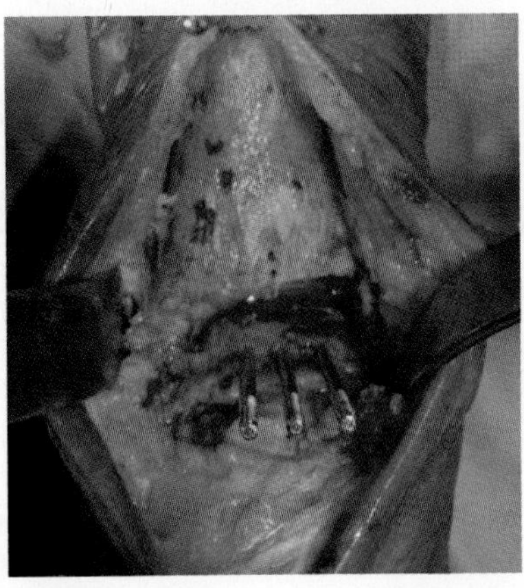

TECH FIG 6 • **A.** The talar pin setting guide (*large arrow*) is positioned on the distal end of the tibial guide. With the ankle positioned in neutral flexion, a pin is inserted through the hole into the talus (*small arrow*) (left ankle). **B.** The pin-guided resection is performed with an oscillating saw, taking care to keep the saw blade flat against the pin surface during resection.

Anterior Talar Chamfer Preparation

- Anterior talar preparation contributes to the correct AP and rotational positioning of the talar component.
- Perform the anterior chamfer cut with a milling device controlled by the anterior talar cutting guide, secured on the posterior resected surface (TECH FIG 7).
- Adequate anterior resection is essential to avoid an anterior talar position relative to the tibia, a situation that may lead to increased anterior contact stresses and potential edge loading.

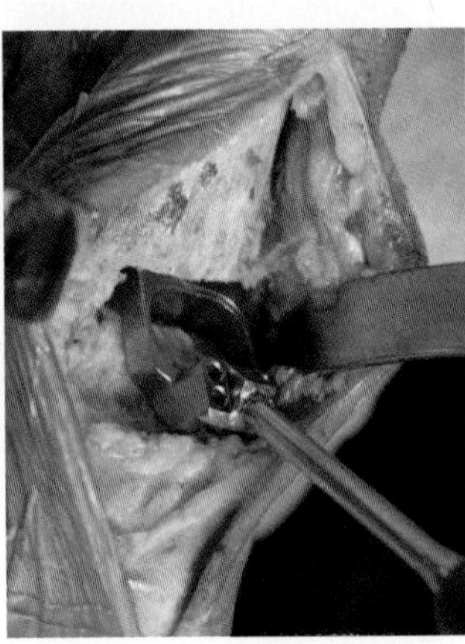

TECH FIG 7 • The anterior chamfer cut is performed with a end mill cutter controlled by the anterior talar cutting guide, which is positioned on the posterior resected surface.

  - In our experience, the threshold to deepen the anterior chamfer preparation should be low.
  - Removing anterior talar neck osteophytes allows the guide to be properly seated on the talus.
  - Appropriate anterior chamfer preparation is determined using the talar gauge.
  - With respect to rotation, the guide must be perfectly aligned with the axis of the talar body. The second metatarsal may be used as a reference provided there is no associated foot malalignment.

Lateral Chamfer and Talar Stem Preparation

- Proper positioning is essential.
  - In the sagittal plane, the guide should be positioned flush with the two previously resected surfaces, with no anterior overhang.
  - In the horizontal plane, rotation is determined with reference to the axis of the talar body.
  - In the coronal plane, correct mediolateral position is referenced from the lateral margin of the prepared talar dome.
  - Once correctly positioned, pin the cutting guide to the bone.
- First, prepare the talar stem recession using the bell saw. Then insert a dedicated metal peg into this prepared portion of talus to afford greater stability to the lateral talar chamfer cutting guide. Prepare the lateral chamfer using an oscillating or reciprocating saw.

INSERTION OF TRIAL COMPONENTS

- The appropriate-size talar trial is that which provides good coverage of the talus in the mediolateral plane, without medial overhang.
- The talar trial lacks the plasma spray coating and thus lacks the interference fit of the actual talar implant; therefore, the talar trial may appear loose. To determine optimal polyethylene thickness and ligament balance, the talar trial remains in situ during insertion of the tibial trials.
- Insertion of tibial trials
  - Salto mobile-bearing prosthesis
    - Insert the selected trial tibial component flush with the bone cut; this will serve as a drill guide for creation of the press-fit hole for the tapered cylindrical plug.
    - Insert the mobile bearing. Bearing thickness is crucial to the stability of the implant. A bearing of correct thickness will need to be pushed rather than slipped into the joint.
- Salto-Talaris fixed-bearing prosthesis
  - Push the trial tibial base and insert assembly into position; it is free to rotate relative to the tibia.
  - As the ankle is ranged from flexion to extension the tibial trial locates its ideal position and rotation with respect to the talus, unless the tibial trial has essentially the same dimensions as the prepared tibial surface.

TECHNIQUES

- When this automatic adjustment is obtained, the definitive position is determined.
- Perform preparation for the press-fit hole for the tapered cylindrical plug as described above for the Salto prosthesis.
- The use of a fixed or mobile bearing allows different sizes to be employed on the tibia and on the talus; when this option is being used, the choice of polyethylene size must be by the same size as the talar component.
- Range the joint and check stability. The implant should be stable in the coronal plane, without any residual laxity; dorsiflexion greater than 10 degrees should be readily obtained.

INSERTION OF THE DEFINITIVE COMPONENTS

- Insert the definitive components.
- The prosthesis must have sound initial stability, indicating appropriate ligament balance.
- Before impacting the components, any tibial or talar subchondral cysts or other bone defects may be filled with bone graft.
- Insert the talar component first.
- After inserting the tibial component, fill the anterior opening of the cortex with bone graft obtained from the bone cuts to prevent any ingress of joint fluid (**TECH FIG 8**), which may lead to osteolysis.

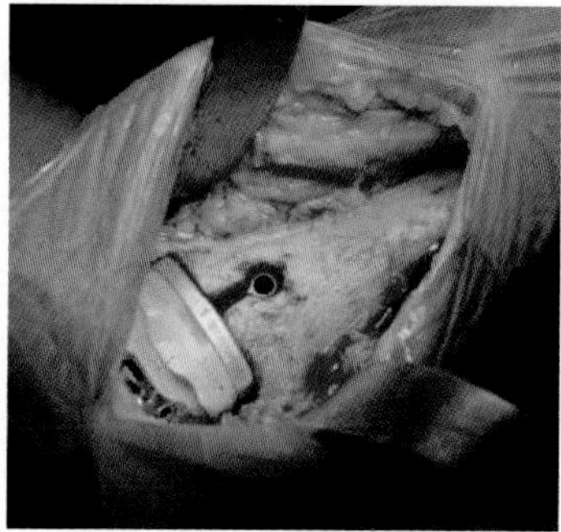

A

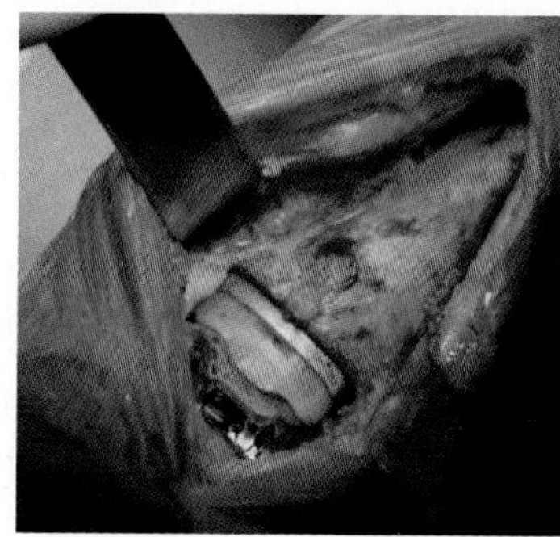

B

TECH FIG 8 • After insertion of the tibial component, the anterior opening of the cortex (**A**) is filled with bone graft obtained from the bone cuts to prevent any ingress of joint fluid (**B**).

CLOSURE

- Since the skin over the ankle is very delicate, closure must be meticulous.
- Close the wound over an intra-articular drain. Whenever possible, close the capsule with absorbable sutures.
- Suture the fascia and retinaculum. Isolate the toe extensor tendons and particularly the tibialis anterior tendon from the fascial suture line.
- Close the loose subcutaneous tissue and the skin with interrupted sutures.
- Apply a below-knee plaster cast with the ankle in maximum dorsiflexion.

PEARLS AND PITFALLS

Difficulties with trial components	Solution
Impossible to insert even the thinnest bearing	■ Tibial side will need to be re-resected.
Dorsiflexion unobtainable	1. Check the size and the positioning of the talar component. 2. Check that the posterior capsular structures and the medial and lateral talar margins have been adequately cleared. 3. Perform percutaneous lengthening of the Achilles tendon. 4. Re-resect the tibia.
Lateral residual laxity	1. Medial collateral ligament release, and use a thicker polyethylene component. 2. Consider lateral ligament reconstruction.
Absolute contraindications for TAA	■ Active infection ■ Poor anterior skin (multiple scars, previous graft) ■ Risk factors for skin necrosis ■ Major bone loss ■ Diffuse (as opposed to focal) osteonecrosis of the talus ■ Nonreconstructable ankle ligamentous instability

Relative contraindications for TAA	■ Eradicated tibiotalar infection ■ Previous medial or lateral surgical approaches to the ankle (TAA incision will be anterior and central) ■ Multiple prior surgeries to the ankle ■ High body mass index ■ High-demand patient (eg, construction work) ■ Unrealistic patient expectations

POSTOPERATIVE CARE

- The drain is removed the day after the operation.
- Once the swelling has subsided, a below-knee circular resin cast is applied.
- As a rule, weight bearing may be resumed once the resin cast has been applied.
- Patients who have undergone Achilles tendon lengthening will be non–weight-bearing for 3 weeks.
- Where there has been a malleolar fracture, the period of non–weight-bearing will be 45 days.
- The cast is removed after 45 days to prevent skin problems, and physiotherapy is commenced.

OUTCOMES

- Bonnin et al[4] reported the results of a consecutive series of their first 98 cases implanted between 1997 and 2000.
- With a mean 35 months of follow-up (range 24 to 57 months), they reported two failures requiring conversion to ankle arthrodesis.
- Reviewing the same consecutive series with a mean 6.4 years of follow-up (range 5 to 8.5), they reported five failures necessitating conversion into arthrodesis.[3]
- The mean AOFAS ankle–hindfoot score preoperatively was 32.3 (SD 10) and 83.1 (SD16) at last follow-up. The mean ankle range of motion measured on dynamic radiographs improved from 15.2 degrees preoperatively (SD 10) to 28.3 degrees at follow-up (SD 7).

COMPLICATIONS

- Technical difficulties in TAA may arise from a number of factors.

Failure to Re-establish the Physiologic Joint Line

- The final level of the implant joint line will depend upon the level of the tibial cut.
- The level is determined with reference to the preoperative radiographs. Depending on the status of the tibial plafond, the anatomy of the malleoli, and lateral talomalleolar congruency, four different patterns may be encountered (**FIG 5**):

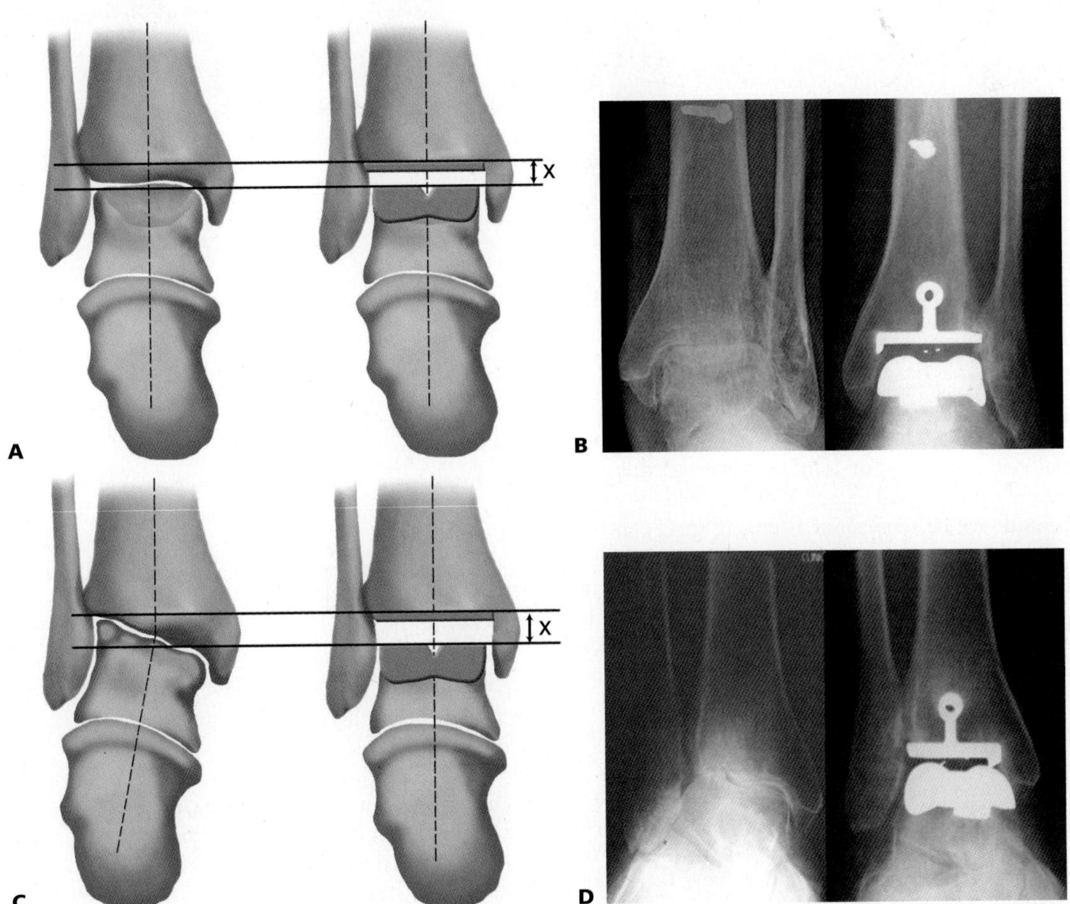

FIG 5 • **A, B.** Ankle mortise intact, no asymmetrical wear of the tibial pilon. **C, D.** Ankle mortise intact, tibial pilon asymmetrically worn. *(continued)*

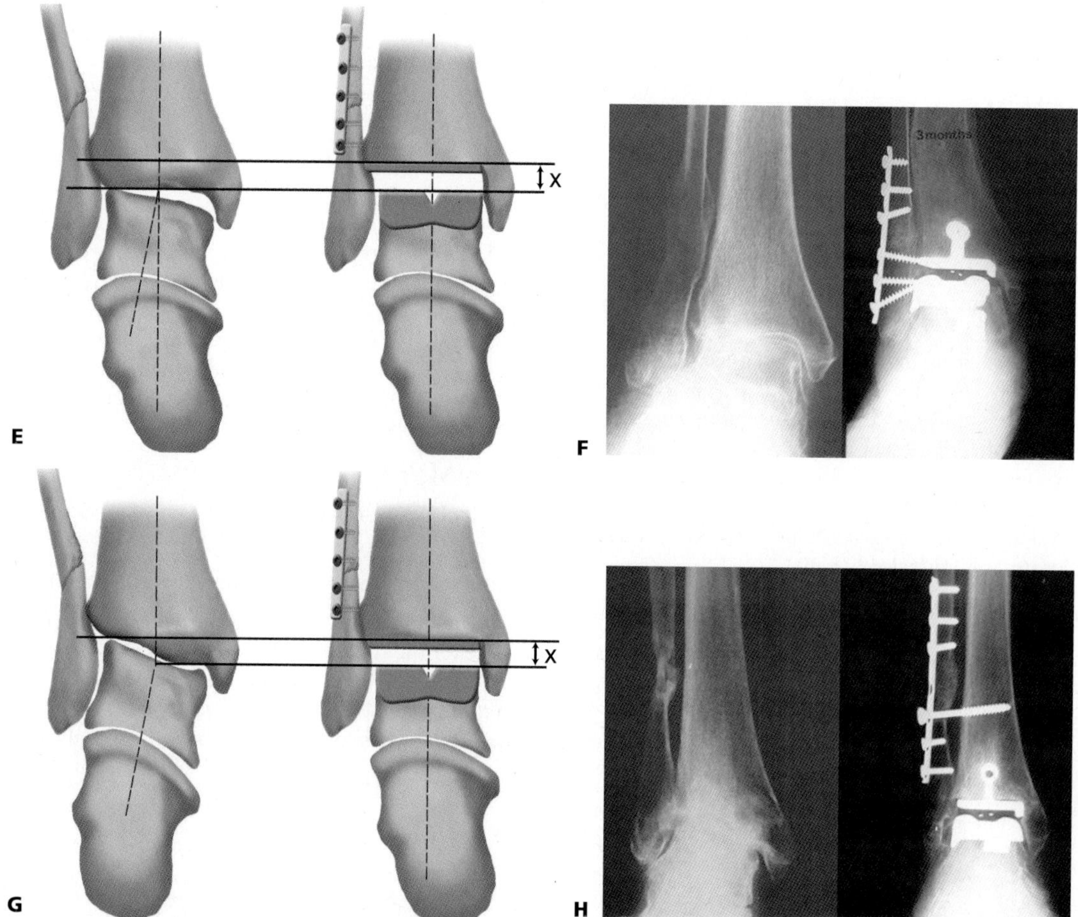

FIG 5 • *(continued)* **E, F.** Malleoli deformed, tibial pilon intact. **G, H.** Malleoli deformed, tibial pilon worn.

- The ankle mortise is intact, with symmetric wear of the tibial plafond. The procedure should be a simple resurfacing, with the metal tibial component and polyethylene thickness replacing exactly what is resected.
- The ankle mortise is intact, but the tibial plafond is asymmetrically worn. This pattern is seen in advanced RA, especially in the wake of long-term steroid therapy. In this case, a reasonable and balanced distal tibial resection level will need to be determined during preoperative planning.
- The malleoli are deformed, but the tibial plafond is intact. In our experience, this deformity involves the lateral malleolus. This pattern is seen in RA with severe hindfoot valgus that has resulted in a fatigue fracture of the fibula. In this case, the lateral malleolus will need to be managed with malleolar osteotomy and plating before TAA.
- The malleoli are deformed and the tibial plafond is worn or depressed. These cases will need to be managed with a combination of the principles discussed above: first, a normal ankle mortise pattern will have to be created, and then a resection level will need to be determined, taking into account the extent of loss of tibial bone stock.

Extra-articular Deformity

- The physiologic ankle joint line is perpendicular to the axis of the tibia, and the hindfoot axis is in slight (5 to 10 degrees) valgus in relation to the tibial axis. To promote long-term implant survival, physiologic alignment will need to be restored.
- Inserting a TAA prosthesis into a malaligned tibia or hindfoot is a recipe for early loosening and failure.
- Correction of deformities may be difficult in sequelae of trauma or RA. Preoperative evaluation should allow the determination of whether these deformities have an intra-articular or extra-articular origin.
- In our experience, most intra-articular deformities resulting from wear or laxity (including varus position caused by OA in chronic instability) can be corrected from within the joint with the prosthesis.
- In contrast, most extra-articular deformities cannot be corrected from within the joint with the prosthesis and must be treated independently with supramalleolar osteotomy, performed either staged or simultaneous to TAA (**FIG 6A**).
- In our opinion, hindfoot malalignment associated with arthritis must be corrected by doing a triple arthrodesis before TAA (**FIG 6B**).

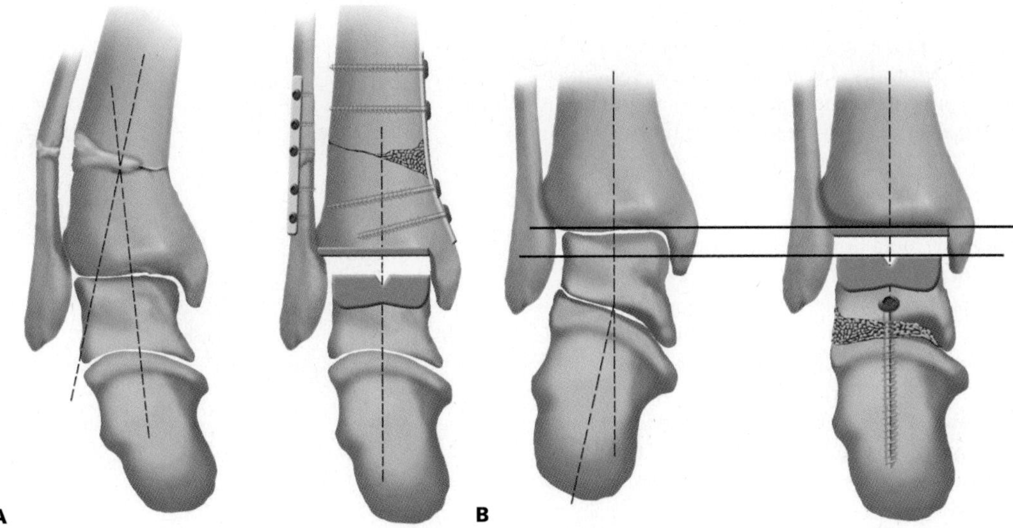

FIG 6 • **A.** In case of tibial malunion, a correction via a supramalleolar osteotomy must be associated with the ankle prosthesis. **B.** In case of hindfoot deformity, a correction via a subtalar or triple arthrodesis or calcaneal osteotomy must be done in association with the ankle prosthesis.

- We recommend performing staged triple arthrodesis and TAA to reduce the potential for skin problems and edema. In our hands, triple arthrodesis is usually done as a first-stage procedure 45 days before TAA, which avoids prolonged cast immobilization (**FIG 7**).
- We perform the triple arthrodesis by what would be an extension of the anterior approach to the ankle to prepare the talonavicular joint and a limited lateral–subfibular approach to the subtalar joint. We avoid dissection under the talar head to minimize the risk of necrosis of the talar body.

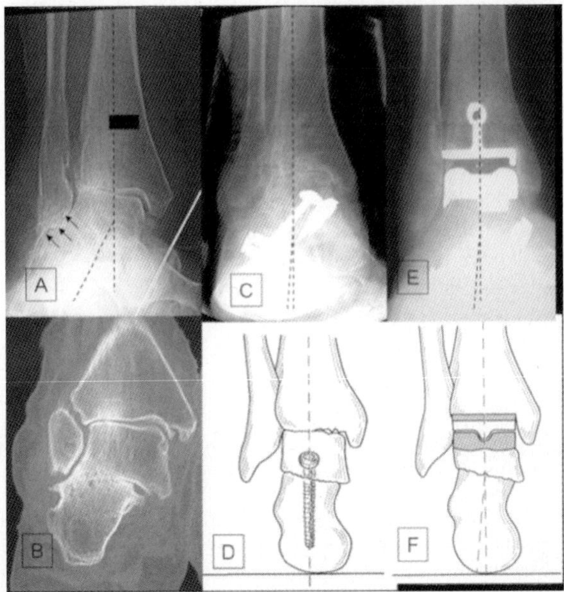

FIG 7 • Rheumatoid arthritis of the ankle, subtalar, and midtarsal joints, with valgus shift of the hindfoot causing a fatigue fracture of the lateral malleolus. A triple arthrodesis was done in association with lateral malleolus correction osteotomy. Forty-five days later, the total ankle prosthesis was implanted in a correctly aligned hindfoot. (From Bonnin M, Judet T, Colombier JA, et al. Mid-term results of the Salto total ankle prosthesis: report of 98 cases with minimum two years follow up. Clin Orthop Relat Res 2004;424:6–18.)

- Fixation is achieved using a talocalcaneal screw and two talonavicular and calcaneocuboid staples.
- The TAA prosthesis must be positioned on a properly aligned hindfoot.
  - In RA patients with a valgus deformity and severe lateral bone loss, bone grafting is the rule. Graft material is harvested from a local donor site (bone slices taken from the midtarsal joint, sometimes bone material taken from the proximal tibial metaphysis) and in some cases from the ipsilateral iliac crest in case of severe deformity.
- We stage the TAA 45 days after triple arthrodesis using the proximal extension of the same anterior approach. The talocalcaneal screw is removed.

Bone Loss

- Implant fixation requires sufficient tibial and talar bone stock and an intact ankle mortise.
- In RA patients or in posttraumatic OA, there may be major bone loss, and defects may have to be grafted. In particularly severe cases, TAA may be contraindicated.

Ankle Instability

- OA secondary to chronic lateral laxity is technically challenging because the persistence of lateral laxity may cause rapid deterioration of the prosthesis.
- In our experience, most cases can be balanced with TAA. We routinely restore the ankle's soft tissue balance with TAA and comprehensive soft tissue release on the concave side of the deformity.
  - Medial release in a varus deformity is challenging and involves the entire deltoid ligament, which is first released subperiosteally from its malleolar attachment and then detached from the talus. We have been satisfied with this balancing technique, which, in our hands, eliminates the need for the medial malleolar osteotomy technique to rebalance the deltoid ligament.

- With comprehensive and satisfactory medial release, we rarely need to perform a ligament reconstruction on the convex side of the deformity. Occasionally, however, for severe varus malalignment, we need to perform a lateralizing and valgus-producing calcaneal osteotomy to further realign the hindfoot.

Ankle Stiffness

- End-stage tibiotalar joint arthritis almost always leads to stiffness of the tibiotalar joint.
- Stiffness with equinus deformity requires sequential steps to regain dorsiflexion, beginning with excision of anterior ossifications, then freeing of talomalleolar adhesions, and finally posterior capsulectomy from within the joint.
  - The use of a lamina spreader greatly facilitates capsulectomy. However, great caution should be used to avoid avulsion of the medial malleolus and accidental penetration of the prepared tibial surface.
  - In particular, the surgeon must make sure that complete capsulectomy is performed at the posteromedial corner, flush with the tibialis posterior tendon.
  - Freeing up adhesions to this tendon is important as they may cause postoperative pain, particularly in patients who have previously undergone a procedure through a posteromedial approach.
  - In this case, tenolysis of the tibialis posterior tendon with opening of its retinaculum through a limited posteromedial approach may be useful. This approach makes posterior capsular release and even repair of associated fissures much easier.
- Lastly, contracture of the triceps surae and Achilles tendon is often responsible for a deficit of dorsiflexion. Therefore, lengthening should be considered whenever dorsiflexion is less than 10 degrees after insertion of the trials. Release of flexors may be achieved through either tendon lengthening or fasciotomy of the triceps surae.
- Achilles tendon lengthening
  - This simple procedure has little influence on the postoperative course, but it is associated with long-term persistence of posterior discomfort and sometimes with permanent loss of plantarflexion strength and range of motion.
  - Lengthening technique consists of making two or three percutaneous staged incisions with a fine scalpel; each incision should involve slightly more than half of the tendon.
  - The most distal incision may be performed on either side, depending on the fibers to be lengthened—laterally for a valgus deformity in order to preserve varus-oriented fibers, and medially for a varus hindfoot.
  - While making incisions, the ankle should be held in forced dorsiflexion with the trial components in place. Dorsiflexion suddenly increases as fibers slide over one another (**FIG 8**).
  - Fasciotomy of the triceps surae usually does not cause postoperative pain; it is performed through a limited midline posterior approach at the middle third of the leg. The sural vein is preserved.
  - The insertional fascia of the gastrocnemius is sectioned in a V-shaped fashion, and the underlying soleus fascia is sectioned in line with the muscle fibers. The postoperative course is the same as for Achilles tendon lengthening.

Anterior Translation of Talus

- Anterior translation of the talus must always be corrected to restore normal kinematics and avoid early wear due to overloading in a fixed-bearing prosthesis or due to overhanging of the polyethylene bearing in a mobile-bearing prosthesis (alignment between the polyethylene bearing and the talar component must be maintained at all times).
- Repositioning of the talar component requires complete soft tissue release (ie, talomalleolar compartment, posterior capsule) as well as correction of equinus deformity (if any) through Achilles tendon lengthening.
- Should these procedures prove ineffective, the talar component will have to be moved posteriorly, which means recutting the anterior chamfer.
- In our experience, the tibial component will have to be positioned as far anteriorly as possible beneath the distal tibia.

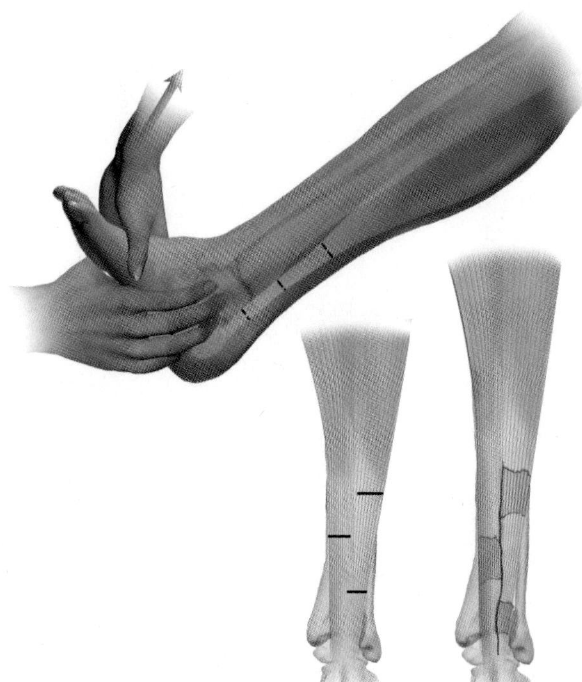

FIG 8 • Percutaneous lengthening of the Achilles tendon. Lengthening technique consists of making two or three percutaneous staged incisions with a fine scalpel; each incision should involve slightly more than half of the tendon.

REFERENCES

1. Bonnin M. La prothèse totale de cheville. Encycl Méd Chir (Editions scientifiques et médicales Elsevier Paris). Techniques Chirurgicales, Orthopédie Traumatologie, 44-903, 2002, 10p.
2. Bonnin M, Bouysset M, Tebib J, et al. Total ankle replacement in rheumatoid arthritis: treatment strategy. In: Bouysset Y, Tourné K, Tillmann M, eds. Rheumatoid Arthritis: Foot and Ankle. Paris: Springer Verlag, 2006.
3. Bonnin M, Judet T, Colombier JA, et al. Total Ankle Prosthesis: Five- to Eight-Year Results. Presented at the 22nd Annual Summer Meeting of the AOFAS, La Jolla, Calif., July 14–16, 2006.
4. Bonnin M, Judet T, Colombier JA, et al. Mid-term results of the Salto total ankle prosthesis: report of 98 cases with minimum two years follow up. Clin Orthop Relat Res 2004;424:6–18.
5. Bonnin M, Judet T, Siguier T, et al. Total ankle replacement: history, evolution of concepts, design and surgical technique. In: Bouysset Y, Tourné K, Tillmann M, eds. Rheumatoid Arthritis: Foot and Ankle. Paris: Springer Verlag, 2006.

6. Jakubowski S, Mohing W, Richter R. Operationen am rheumatischen Fuss. Therapiewoche 1970;20:762–768.
7. Judet T, Piriou P, Elis JB, et al. Total-endoprothese des oberen Sprunggelenkes. Konzepte und Indikationen der Saltoprothese. In: Imhoff AB, Zollinger-Jies H, eds. Fußchirurgie. Stuttgart, New York: Georg Thieme Verlag, 2003.
8. Vainio K. The rheumatoid foot: a clinical study with pathological and roentgenological comments. Ann Chir Gynaecol 1956;45(Suppl 1):1–12.
9. Weber M, Bonnin M, Colombier JA, et al. Erste Ergebnisse der Salto-Sprunggelenkendopprotheseseine fränzösische Multizenterstudie mit 115 Implantaten. Fuβ Sprunggelenk 2004;2:29–37.

Chapter 72

Mobility Total Ankle Arthroplasty

Pascal F. Rippstein, Mark E. Easley, and J. Chris Coetzee

DEFINITION

- Three-component, mobile-bearing total ankle arthroplasty system indicated for end-stage ankle arthritis failing to respond to nonoperative treatment

ANATOMY

- Ankle
  - Tibial plafond with medial malleolus
    - Articulations with dorsal and medial talus
    - In sagittal plane, slight posterior slope
    - In coronal plane, articular surface is 88 to 92 degrees relative to lateral tibial shaft axis.
  - Fibula
    - Articulation with lateral talus
    - Responsible for one sixth of axial load distribution of the ankle
  - Talus
    - 60% of surface area covered by articular cartilage
    - Dual radius of curvature
  - Distal tibiofibular syndesmosis
    - Anterior inferior tibiofibular ligament
    - Interosseous membrane
    - Posterior tibiofibular ligament
- Ankle functions as part of the ankle–hindfoot complex much like a mitered hinge.

PATHOGENESIS

- Post-traumatic arthrosis
  - Most common cause
  - Intra-articular fracture
  - Ankle fracture-dislocation with malunion
  - Chronic ankle instability
- Primary osteoarthrosis
  - Relatively rare compared to hip and knee arthrosis
- Inflammatory arthropathy
  - Most commonly rheumatoid arthritis
- Other
  - Hemochromatosis
  - Pigmented villonodular synovitis
  - Charcot neuroarthropathy
  - Septic arthritis

NATURAL HISTORY

- Post-traumatic arthrosis
  - Malunion, chronic instability, intra-articular cartilage damage, or malalignment may lead to progressive articular cartilage wear.
  - Chronic lateral ankle instability may eventually be associated with:
    - Relative anterior subluxation of the talus
    - Varus tilt of the talus within the ankle mortise
    - Hindfoot varus position
- Primary osteoarthrosis of the ankle rare and poorly understood.
- Inflammatory arthropathy
  - Progressive and proliferative synovial erosive changes failing to respond to medical management
  - May be associated with chronic posterior tibial tendinopathy and progressive valgus hindfoot deformity, eventual valgus tilt to the talus within the ankle mortise, potential lateral malleolar stress fracture, and compensatory forefoot varus

PATIENT HISTORY AND PHYSICAL FINDINGS

- History
  - Typically, history of trauma to the ankle
    - Intra-articular ankle fracture (bi- or tri-malleolar ankle fracture; tibial plafond [pilon] fracture)
    - Chronic ankle instability
  - Inflammatory arthropathy
  - Primary ankle arthritis
- Symptoms or complaints
  - Pain in anterior ankle with weight bearing and particularly with forced dorsiflexion
  - Often relieved by rest, but patient may have pain even at rest after vigorous activity or prolonged standing
  - Ankle swelling
  - Ankle stiffness
- Medications
  - If patient is taking anti-inflammatory agents, these will need to be stopped preoperatively to limit the risk of perioperative bleeding.
  - Rheumatoid medications may need to be stopped perioperatively to optimize wound healing and bone ingrowth into the prosthesis.
- Physical examination
  - Alignment
    - Ipsilateral limb alignment, not simply ankle alignment. The lower extremity should be examined from the hip to the foot. Optimal limb alignment is essential for longevity of the implant.
  - Ankle–foot alignment
    - The ankle functions as part of an ankle–subtalar joint complex.
    - The total ankle needs a solid, well-aligned platform on which to rest.
    - Hindfoot, midfoot, and even forefoot malalignment may need to be addressed as part of total ankle arthroplasty.
  - Range of motion (ROM)
    - Preoperative ankle ROM often dictates postoperative ROM. A stiff ankle before surgery may be a stiff ankle after surgery, despite total ankle arthroplasty. Dorsiflexion may be limited by anterior tibiotalar osteophytes, a tight Achilles tendon or posterior capsular contracture, or both.

The examination may identify a distinction between anterior impingement and a tight heel cord.

- Hindfoot ROM: Limitations in ROM of the hindfoot may place eccentric stresses on the implant.
- Soft tissues
  - An intact, relatively healthy soft tissue envelope surrounding the ankle is less likely to have soft tissue complications postoperatively, provided careful soft tissue handling is maintained.
  - Previous surgical scars must be considered. Either they can be incorporated into the surgical approach or the surgical approach may be modified to limit postoperative wound complications
  - Vascular status: Intact pulses and satisfactory refill must be confirmed; if not, a Doppler ultrasound, noninvasive vascular studies, or both must be performed before considering surgery.
  - Neurologic status: A peripheral neuropathy is a relative contraindication for total ankle arthroplasty, but in our opinion well-controlled diabetes without neuropathy is not. Established neuropathy and either existing or high risk of Charcot neuroarthropathy is a contraindication for total ankle arthroplasty.
  - Motor function: Intact motor function of the ankle and foot is essential to successful total ankle arthroplasty. In particular, lack of active dorsiflexion is a relative contraindication to total ankle arthroplasty. It is important to distinguish between anterior impingement or Achilles contracture or posterior capsular tightness versus lack of satisfactory tibialis anterior tendon function.

IMAGING AND OTHER DIAGNOSTIC STUDIES

- Weight-bearing AP, lateral, and mortise views of the ankle (**FIG 1A,B**)
- Weight-bearing AP, lateral, and oblique views of the foot, particularly with associated foot deformity
- We routinely obtain weight-bearing mechanical axis (hip-to-ankle) views of both extremities (**FIG 1C**).
- We typically evaluate complex or ill-defined ankle–hindfoot patterns of arthritis with or without deformity using CT of the ankle and hindfoot.
- If we suspect avascular necrosis of the talus or distal tibia, we obtain an MRI of the ankle.
- Electrodiagnostic studies are indicated with lack of active dorsiflexion that is not due simply to Achilles contracture, posterior capsular tightness, or anterior impingement.

DIFFERENTIAL DIAGNOSIS

- See the "Pathogenesis" section above.

NONOPERATIVE MANAGEMENT

- Activity modification
- Bracing
  - Ankle–foot orthosis
  - Double upright brace attached to shoe
- Stiffer-soled shoe with a rocker-bottom modification
- Nonsteroidal anti-inflammatories or COX-2 inhibitors
- Medications for systemic inflammatory arthropathy
- Corticosteroid injection
- Viscosupplementation

SURGICAL MANAGEMENT

Preoperative Planning

- The surgeon must be sure the patient has satisfactory perfusion to support healing and is not neuropathic.
  - Noninvasive vascular studies and potential vascular surgery consultation if necessary

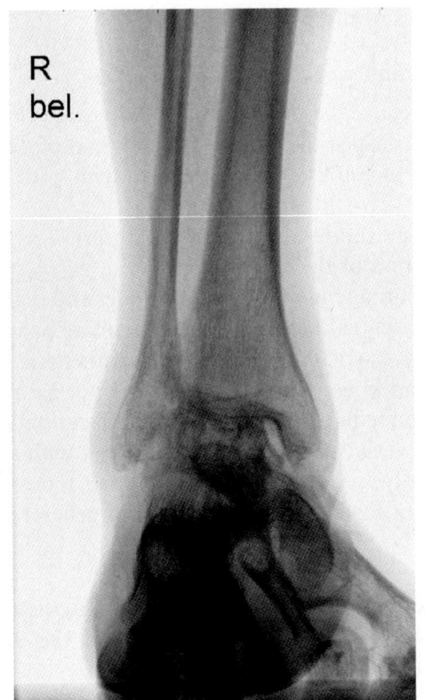

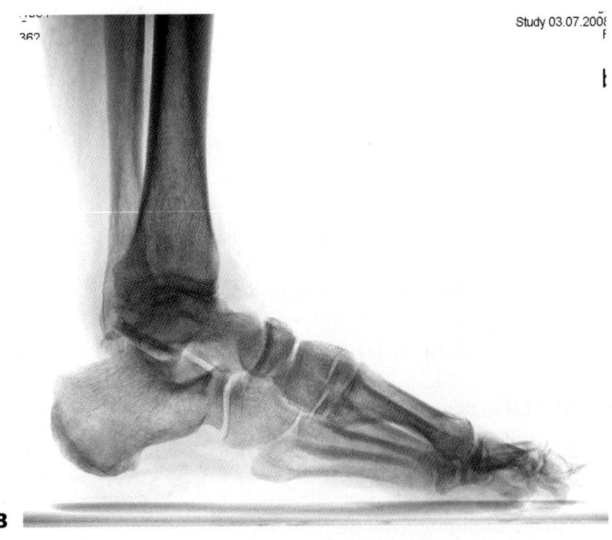

FIG 1 • Preoperative weight-bearing radiographs of a 75-year-old man with end-stage ankle arthritis. **A.** AP view of ankle. **B.** Lateral view of ankle. *(continued)*

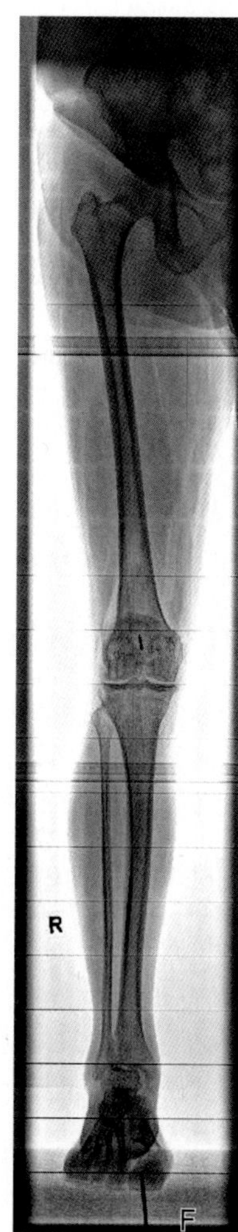

FIG 1 • *(continued)* **C.** Full-length mechanical axis views to rule out proximal malalignment.

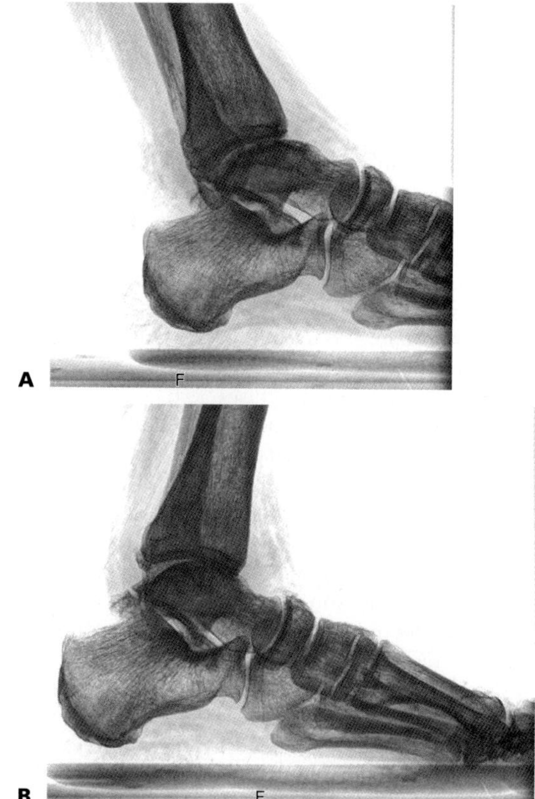

FIG 2 • Preoperative weight-bearing radiographs of same patient in Figure 1. **A.** Preoperative dorsiflexion. **B.** Preoperative plantarflexion.

- The surgeon must understand the clinical and radiographic alignment of the lower extremity, ankle, and foot.
  - The surgeon must be prepared to balance and realign the ankle. Occasionally, this necessitates corrective osteotomies of the distal tibia or foot, hindfoot arthrodesis, ligament releases or stabilization, and tendon transfers.
  - The surgeon should determine whether the coronal plane alignment is passively correctable; this provides some understanding as to whether ligament releases will be required.
- Ankle ROM is determined (**FIG 2A,B**).
  - Ankle stiffness, particularly lack of dorsiflexion, needs to be corrected:
    - Anterior tibiotalar exostectomy
    - Posterior capsular release
    - Occasionally, tendo Achilles lengthening
- Instrumentation
  - These instruments facilitate total ankle arthroplasty:
    - Small oscillating saw to fine-tune cuts, resect prominences with precision, and easily morselize large bone fragments to be evacuated from the joint
    - A rasp for final preparation of cut bony surfaces
    - An angled curette, particularly to separate bone from the posterior capsule
    - A toothless lamina spreader to judiciously distract the ankle to improve exposure even after preparing the surfaces of the tibia and talus

Positioning

- Supine
- Plantar aspect of operated foot at end of operating table
- Foot and ankle well balanced with toes directed to the ceiling
- A bolster under the ipsilateral hip prevents undesired external rotation of the hip.
- We routinely use a thigh tourniquet and regional anesthesia.
  - A popliteal block provides adequate pain relief postoperatively, particularly if a regional catheter is used. Moreover, hip and knee flexion–extension is not forfeited, facilitating safe immediate postoperative mobilization.
  - However, using a thigh tourniquet with a popliteal block typically requires a supplemental femoral nerve block (patient forfeits knee extension) or general anesthesia.

Approach

- Anterior approach to the ankle, using the interval between the tibialis anterior (TA) tendon and the extensor hallucis longus (EHL) tendon

APPROACH

- Make a longitudinal midline incision over the anterior ankle, starting about 10 cm proximal to the tibiotalar joint and 1 cm lateral to the tibial crest.
- Continue the incision midline over the anterior ankle just distal to the talonavicular joint.
- At no point should direct tension be placed on the skin margins; we perform deep, full-thickness retraction as soon as possible to limit the risk of skin complications.
- Identify and protect the superficial peroneal nerve by retracting it laterally.
  - In our experience there is a consistent branch of the superficial peroneal nerve that crosses directly over or immediately proximal to the tibiotalar joint.
- We then expose the extensor retinaculum, identify the course of the EHL tendon, and sharply but carefully divide the retinaculum directly over the EHL tendon.
  - We always attempt to maintain the TA tendon in its dedicated sheath.
  - Preserving the retinaculum over the TA tendon prevents bowstringing of the tendon and thereby reduces the stress on the anterior wound. Should there be a wound dehiscence, then the TA is not directly exposed. Preserving the retinaculum over the TA tendon is not always possible; some patients do not have a dedicated sheath for the TA.
- Use the interval between the TA and EHL tendon, with the TA and EHL tendons retracted medially and laterally, respectively (TECH FIG 1).
- Identify the deep neurovascular bundle (anterior tibial–dorsalis pedis artery and deep peroneal nerve) and carefully retract it laterally throughout the remainder of the procedure.
- Perform an anterior capsulotomy and elevate the tibial and dorsal talar periosteum to about 6 to 8 cm proximal to the tibial plafond and talonavicular joint, respectively.
- Elevate this separated capsule and periosteum medially and laterally to expose the ankle, access the medial and lateral gutters, and visualize the medial and lateral malleoli.
- Remove anterior tibial and talar osteophytes to facilitate exposure and avoid interference with the instrumentation.

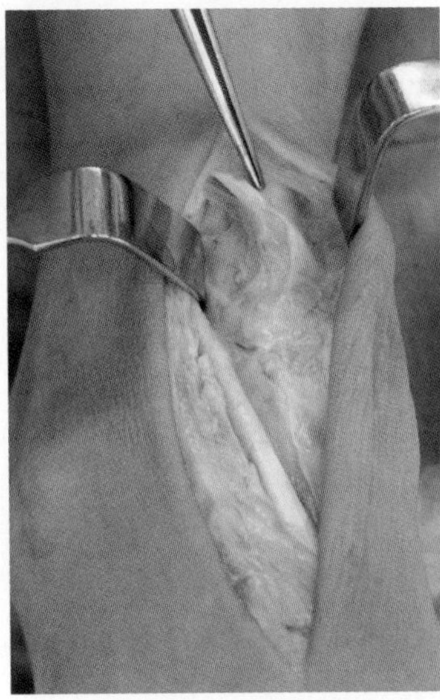

TECH FIG 1 • Anterior approach to the ankle.

EXTERNAL TIBIAL ALIGNMENT GUIDE

- Position the tibial alignment jig so that the clamp adjustment bar lies over the anterior crest of the tibia and the bar is parallel to the long axis of the tibia (TECH FIG 2A).
- The proximal end of the alignment jig is held in position by a 2.5-mm stabilizing pin.
- The adjustment tube on the yoke post and the extending tibial rod should be parallel to the tibia, or with deformity, aligned with the mechanical axis of the leg.
  - Adjust alignment to obtain proper positioning for the cutting block at the tibial plafond (TECH FIG 2B).
- Reference the tibial cutting block to the medial and lateral sides of the talus (TECH FIG 2C).
- Drill two 2.5-mm pins into the tibia through the guide holes to stabilize the tibial cutting block.
  - The configuration of the guide holes allows adjustment of the cutting block proximally or distally by increments of 2.5 mm to optimize the level of tibial resection.

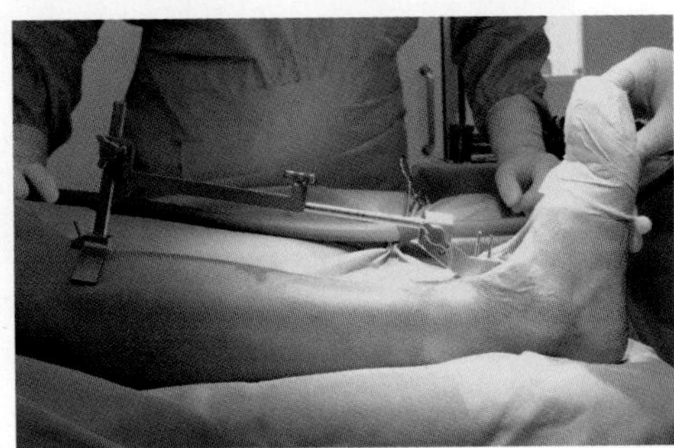

A

TECH FIG 2 • External tibial alignment guide parallel to the tibial shaft axis. **A.** Lateral view. *(continued)*

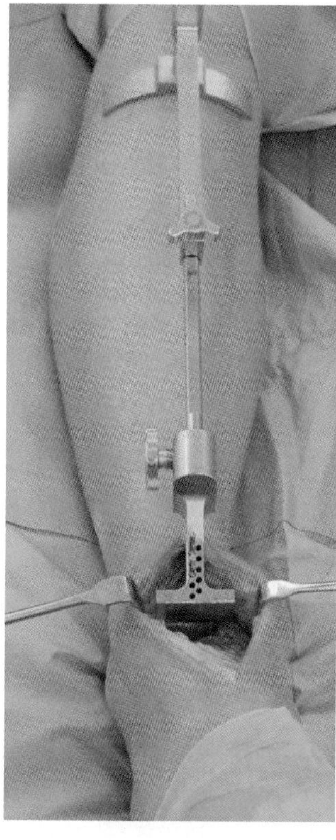

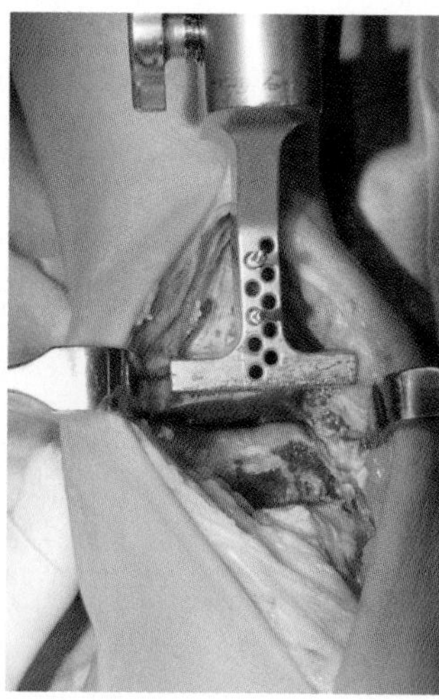

TECH FIG 2 • *(continued)* **B.** Anterior view. **C.** Initial tibial preparation, cutting block set for initial resection.

TIBIAL PREPARATION

Initial Tibial Resection

- The tibial resection is performed with an oscillating saw (TECH FIG 3A).
- With an asymmetric wear pattern in the tibial plafond, the resection may not be congruent but should be perpendicular to the tibial shaft axis or, with deformity, to the mechanical axis.
- In our experience, a stiff ankle warrants resection of 2 or 3 mm of distal tibia in excess of the resection needed to create sufficient room for the combined thickness of the implants.
- Do not attempt to remove the resected tibial bone until making a vertical tibial cut that is a vertical extension of the medial gutter of the ankle (TECH FIG 3B). This protects the medial malleolus from fracture.
- Do not lever on either malleolus while removing the resected bone because of the risk of fracture.
- Use the gap template to confirm and adequate tibial resection to accommodate the thickness of the tibial implant and thinnest mobile polyethylene bearing (TECH FIG 3C). If the guide does not fit in the space, further bone resection is required (TECH FIG 3D,E).

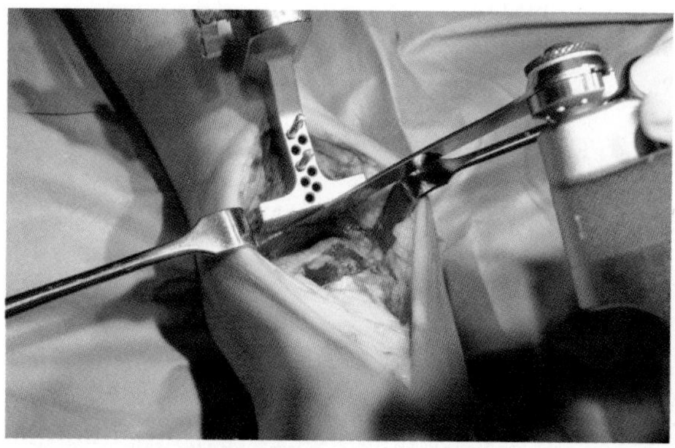

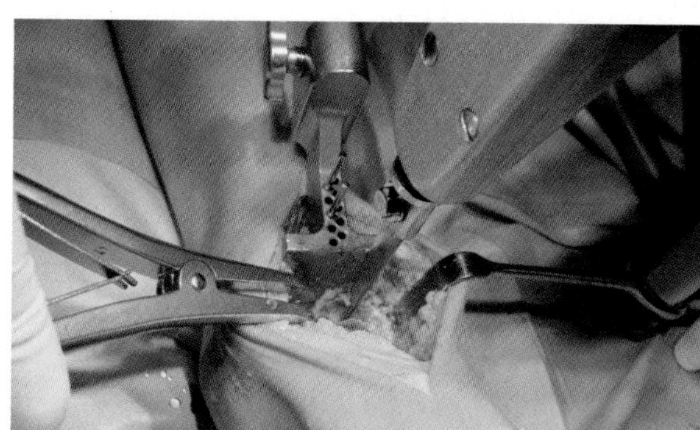

TECH FIG 3 • Initial tibial preparation. **A.** Oscillating saw. **B.** Vertical cut to complete initial tibial cut (protects medial malleolus from potential fracture). *(continued)*

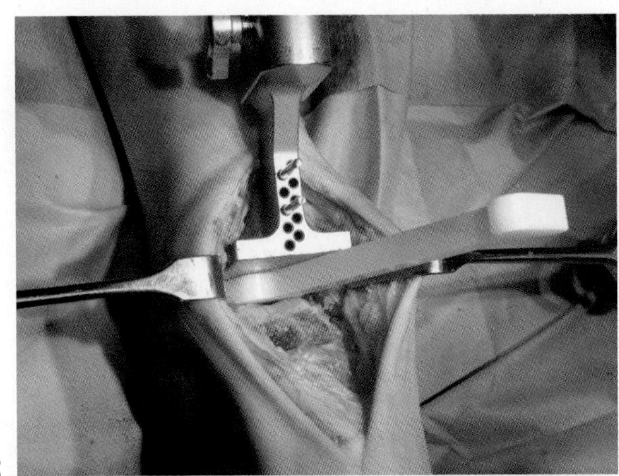

C

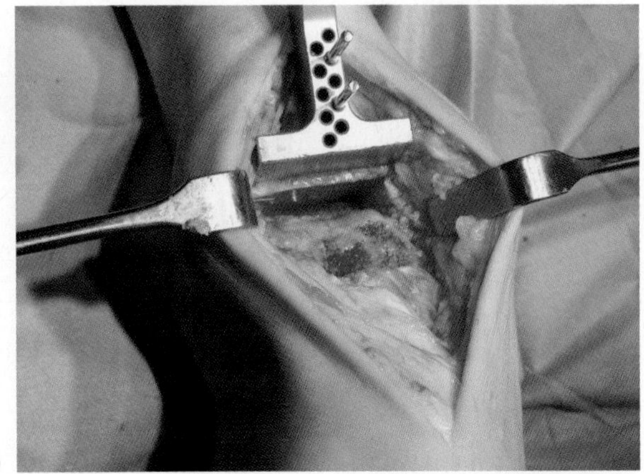

D

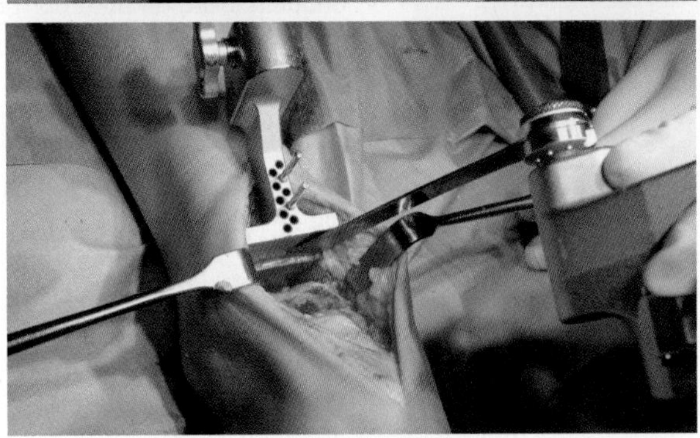

E

TECH FIG 3 • *(continued)* **C.** Gap template matches thickness of tibial base plate and the thinnest polyethylene bearing. **D.** Cutting block moved 2 mm more proximally on same pins to allow greater resection in same plane as initial cut. **E.** Repeat resection.

Tibial Sizing

- Use the tibial sizing gauge to determine the optimal tibial component size in the AP dimension (TECH FIG 4A).
  - The talar component may be of equal in size or smaller than the tibial component (TECH FIG 4B), but it cannot be larger than the tibial component (TECH FIG 4C).
  - Place the gauge on the prepared tibial surface and hook it on the posterior aspect of the tibia (TECH FIG 4D,E).
  - The proper component size is based on the markings on the upper surface of the gauge.
- Select the corresponding tibial profile guide to confirm that the size determined from the AP dimension is also appropriate in the medial-to-lateral dimension. If not, then downsizing is necessary.
- The tibial components are sized 1 through 6, with 1 being the smallest and 6 being the largest.
- Subsequent tibial cuts will be specific for the size of implant selected at this stage.

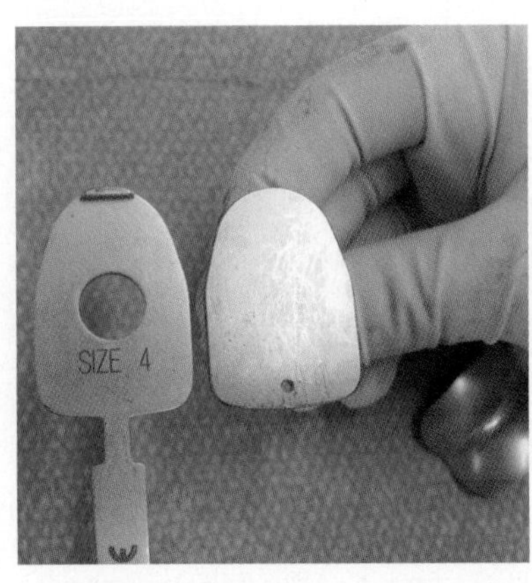

A

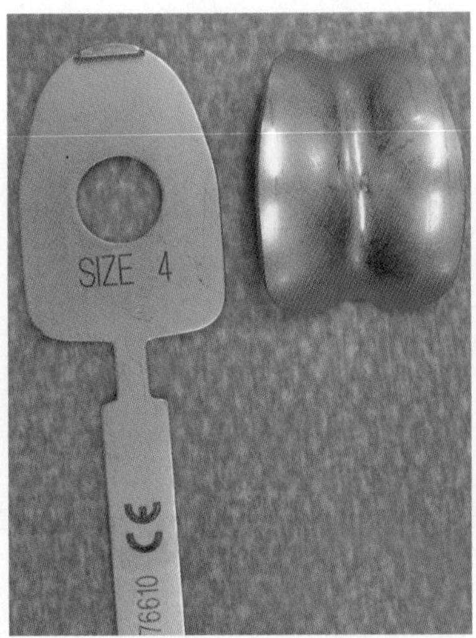

B

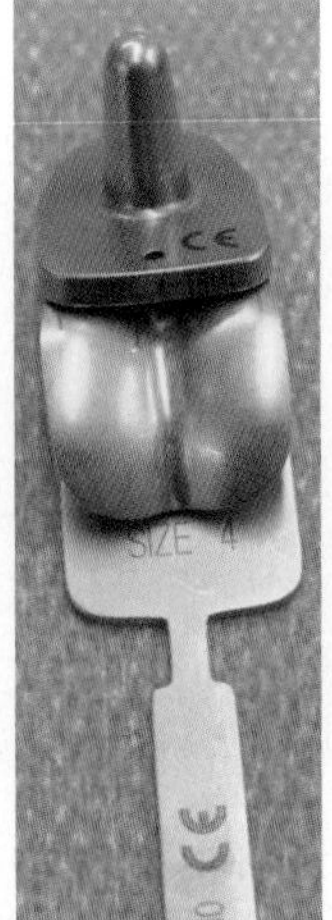

C

TECH FIG 4 • Tibial sizing. **A.** Tibial sizing gauge adjacent to corresponding tibial trial. **B.** Tibial sizing gauge next to talar trial. **C.** Corresponding tibial sizing gauge, tibial trial, and talar trial. *(continued)*

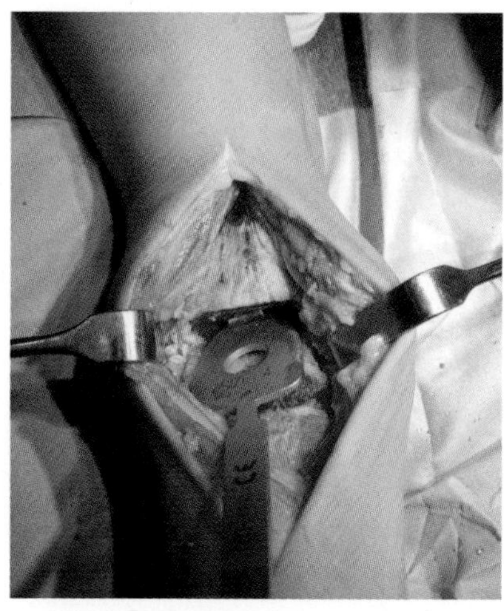

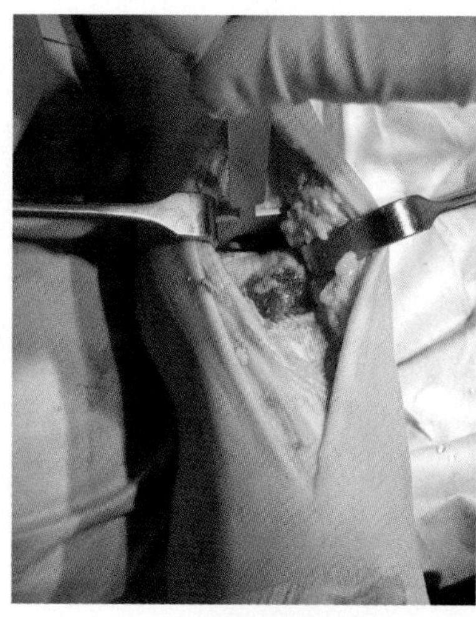

TECH FIG 4 • *(continued)* **D, E.** Tibial sizing using the tibial sizing gauge. **D.** Gauge being introduced to joint. **E.** Gauge hooked on posterior tibial cortex.

Tibial Window Resection

- Select the tibial template corresponding to the size determined from the guides used for sizing (**TECH FIG 5A**).
- Fit the tibial window cutting block to the tibial template and secure it with the system handle adapter.
- Place the assembly flush on the prepared tibial surface, with the tibial template flat against the resected plafond and the tibial window cutting block held firmly against the anterior tibia (**TECH FIG 5B**).
- The scissor distractor supports the tibial window cutting block–tibial template assembly.
- Use a 6-mm tibial drill to prepare the proximal aspect of the tibial window resection.
  - Drill to the depth stop.
  - Insert a tibial window peg to stabilize the tibial window cutting block.
  - Remove the system handle but leave the scissor distractor to further stabilize the tibial window cutting block–tibial template assembly.

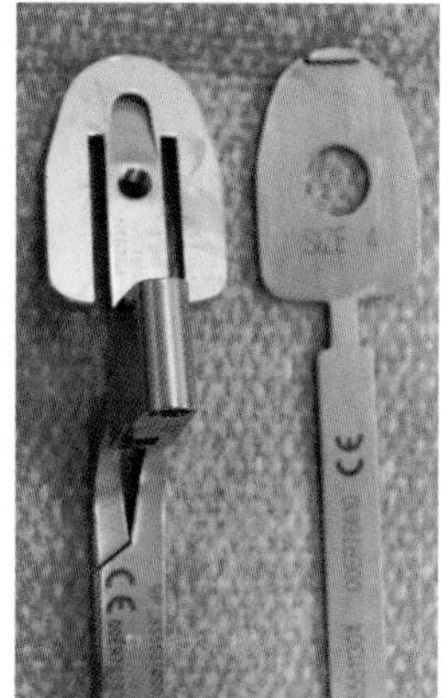

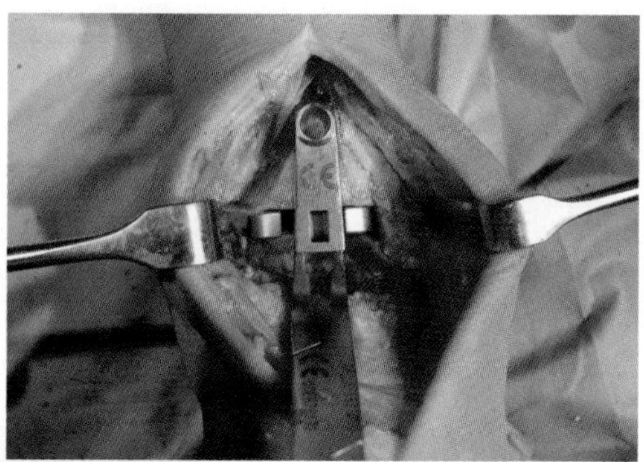

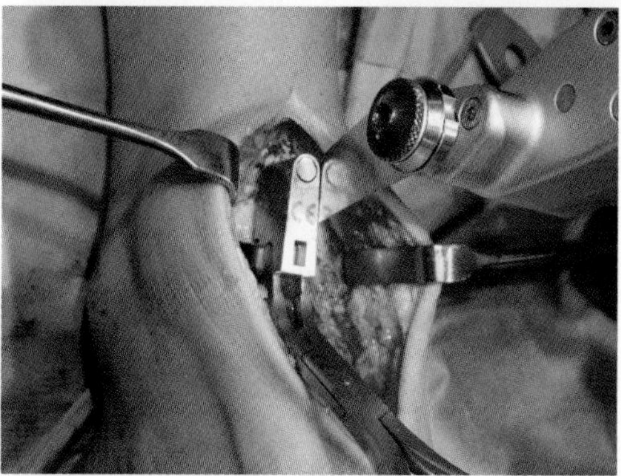

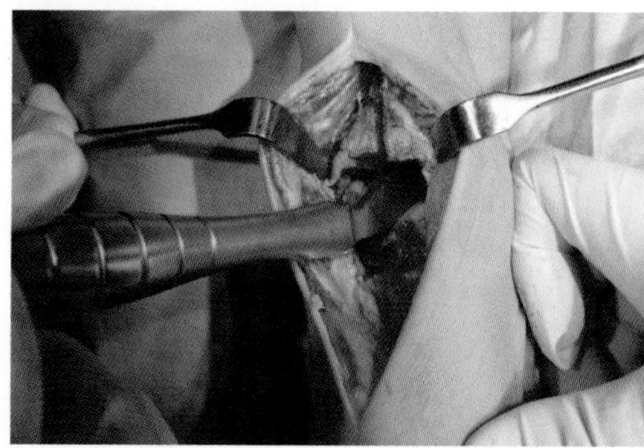

TECH FIG 5 • Tibial window preparation. **A.** Tibial window cutting block adjacent to its corresponding tibial template–sizing gauge. **B.** Tibial window cutting block assembled to the tibia template and placed flush against initial tibial prepared surface and flush with the anterior tibial cortex. **C.** After drilling proximal hole and placing a stabilizing post, the oscillating saw is used to cut the anterior tibial window. **D.** Tibial window extractor. *(continued)*

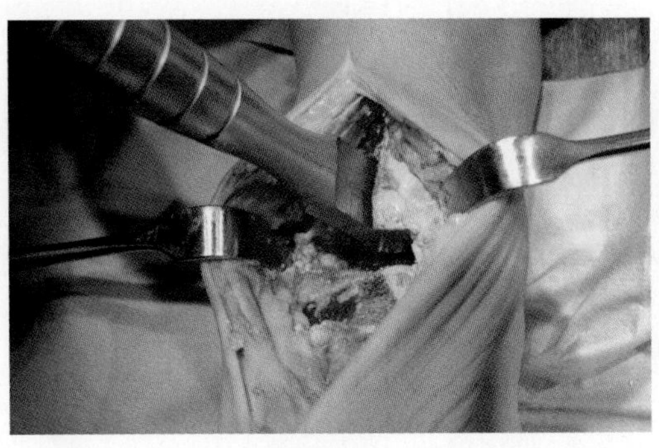

E

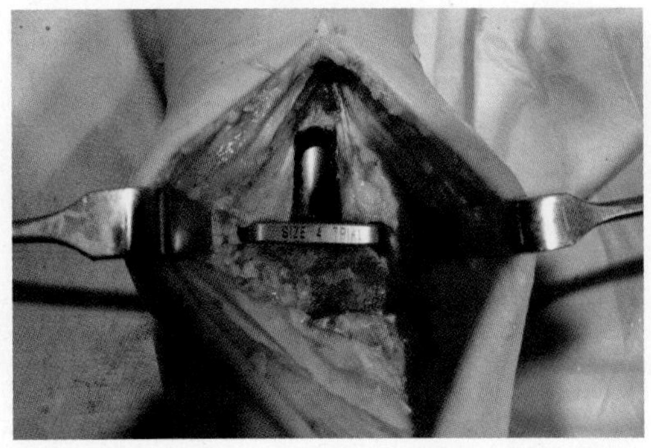

F

TECH FIG 5 • *(continued)* **E.** Tibial window impactor to finalize window preparation. **F.** Tibial trial confirming satisfactory window preparation.

- Immediately adjacent to the window cutting block, cut the medial and lateral sides of the window with an oscillating saw (**TECH FIG 5C**).
  - Mark the appropriate depth on the saw blade corresponding to the size of tibial component to be implanted.
- After preparing the tibial window sides, remove all instruments.
- Position the tibial window extractor on the distal tibial surface.
  - The appropriate mark on its upper surface must be positioned against the anterior tibial cortex.
- By carefully levering against the talus, force the cutting edge of the tibial window extractor into the firm subchondral bone of the distal tibia, thereby releasing the bony resection (**TECH FIG 5D**).
  - Retain this bone segment, as it is replaced after trimming at a later stage.
- Use the tibial window impactor to compact the most proximal cancellous bone in the tibial window to the required depth, indicated by the markings on the impactor (ie, size 1 through 6; **TECH FIG 5E**).
- Insert the tibial trial to be sure it fits appropriately and is perfectly centered over the talus (**TECH FIG 5F**).

TALAR PREPARATION

Superior Talar Flat Resection

- Assemble the tibial template used to make the tibial window resections with the tibial template post and the talar pin jig. The assembly is secured with the system handle adapter.
- There are four talar pin jigs: 5 mm, 7 mm, 9 mm, and 11 mm.
- Estimate the bearing insert thickness that is appropriately sized and avoids excessive dorsiflexion of the ankle.
- Place the tibial template, tibial post, and talar pin jig assembly in the resected tibial window (**TECH FIG 6A**). Use the system handle to hold this assembly in position.
- With the correct-thickness talar pin jig in place, hold the foot 90 degrees to the lower leg, and insert the first 2.5-mm pin through the talar guide (**TECH FIG 6B**). The foot must be held at 90 degrees relative to the lower leg; this is essential during talar drill pin insertion.
- Insert a second pin into one of the two other holes (**TECH FIG 6B**). Avoid the medial and lateral extremes of the talus.
- Remove all the instruments but leave the 2.5-mm talar drill pins, which should be parallel to the long axis of the talus (**TECH FIG 6C**).
- Slide the "standard" talar flat cutting block onto the 2.5-mm pins with the groove uppermost and on the left.
- Resect the superior flat of the talus (**TECH FIG 6D,E**). Keep the saw blade flush with the cutting block.

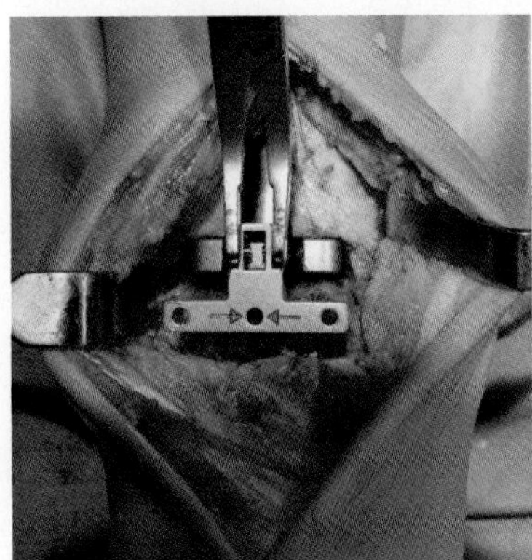

A

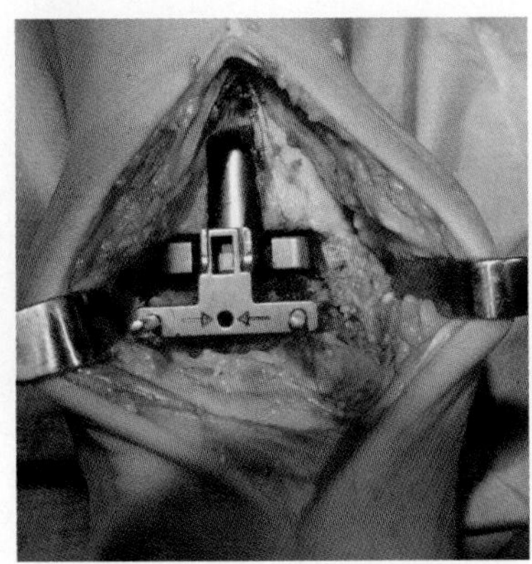

B

TECH FIG 6 • Initial talar preparation (superior talar flat cut). **A.** Tibial template, tibial post, and talar pin guide assembly in place. **B.** With ankle at neutral position, talus is pinned through the talar pin guide. *(continued)*

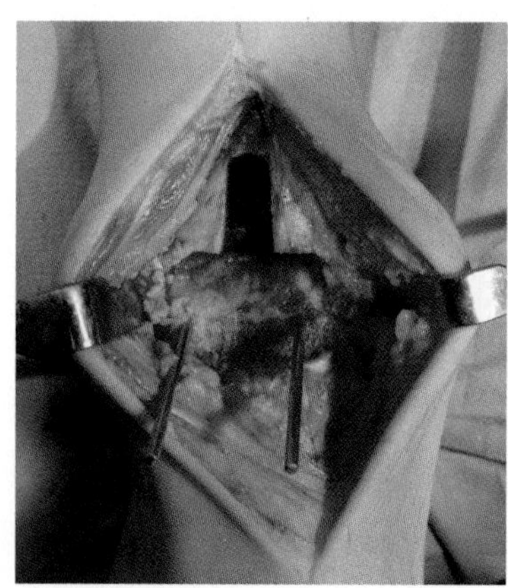
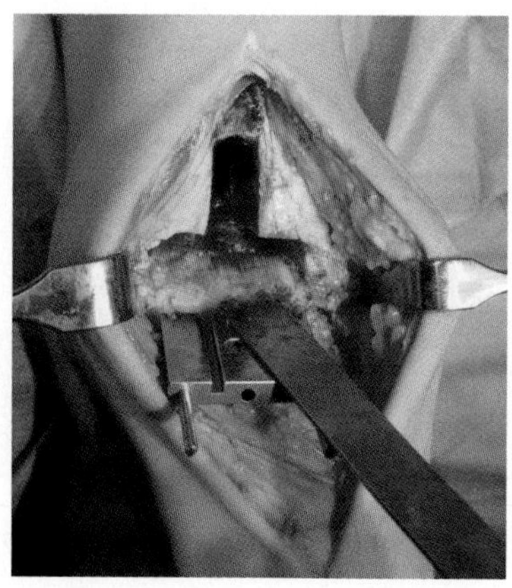
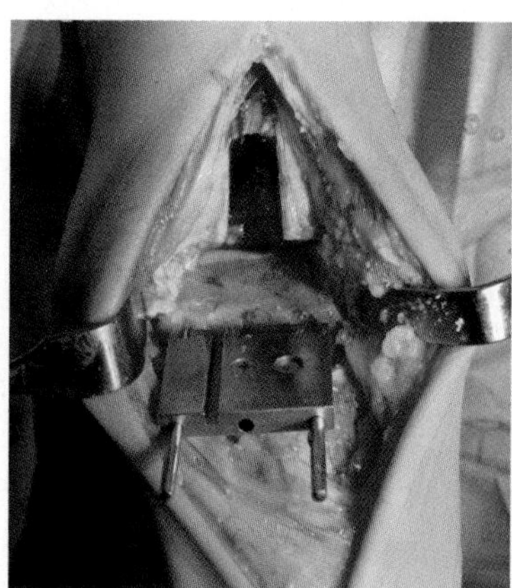

TECH FIG 6 • *(continued)* **C.** Talar pins in appropriate position. **D.** Oscillating saw for the superior talar flat cut. **E.** Initial talar preparation completed.

Transfer of Joint Center to Talus

- Assemble the talar center guide (**TECH FIG 7A,B**).
- Insert the tibial template into the resected tibial window with the 2.5-mm drill pins and the talar flat cutting block still in position (**TECH FIG 7C**).
- Align the foot into the neutral position and guide the locating runners on the talar center guide into the grooves in the tibial template superiorly and the groove in the talar flat cutting block inferiorly.
- Once the correct spacing is achieved, advance the talar center guide until the superior runners contact the end of the tibial template grooves. Use a center guide packing between the talar center guide and the tibial template if the space between the tibia and the talus is excessive.
- Advance the stop block until it meets the front of the talar flat cutting block and lock it into position using the locking screw.
- Plantarflex the ankle and remove the tibial template.
- Adjust the talar center guide on the talar flat cutting block so that the talar center guide's stop block contacts the top of the talar flat cutting block.
- The two bands marked on the talar center guide correspond to two ranges within the six available talar component sizes.
- The AP length of the talar flat must be at least equal to the bands for the smallest range of sizes marked on the talar center guide.
  - If the AP talar flat is less than the bands marked on the talar center guide, then more superior talar flat must be resected.
  - Use the "low" talar flat cutting block to remove more of the superior talus.
- At this point a decision must be made whether the optimal talar size falls in the size range 1–4 or 5–6. The anterior and posterior chamfer cuts are the same within these respective ranges but different as the size transitions from size 4 to 5.
- The size of the bearing insert component must match the size of the talar component.
- The size of the talar component and bearing insert must be smaller than or equal to that of the tibial component selected to prevent overhang of the bearing compared to the tibial plate.
- The sizes of subsequent cutting blocks used to further resect the talus are based on the talar size selection.
- Once the appropriate amount of talar flat cut has been confirmed, properly position the talar center guide against the talar flat cutting block and insert a 2.5-mm guide pin into the talus (**TECH FIG 7D**).

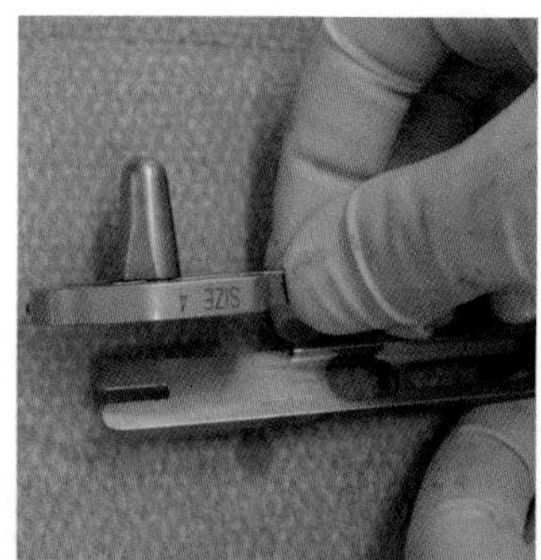
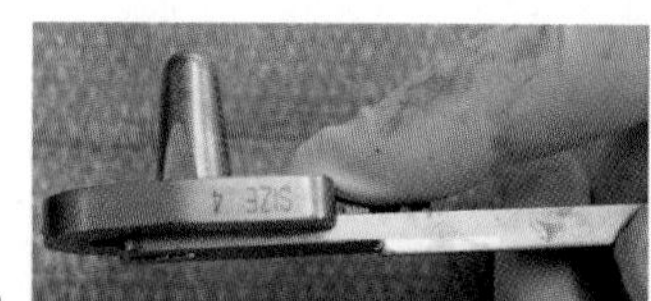
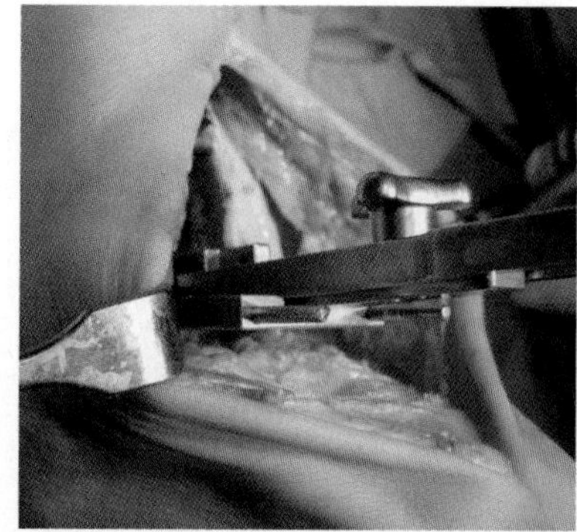

TECH FIG 7 • Transferring joint center to talus. **A, B.** Assembling the talar center guide. **C.** Advancing the talar center guide on the talar pin guide. *(continued)*

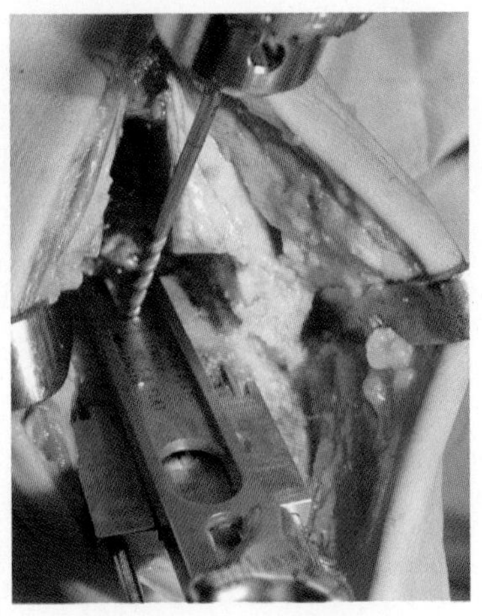

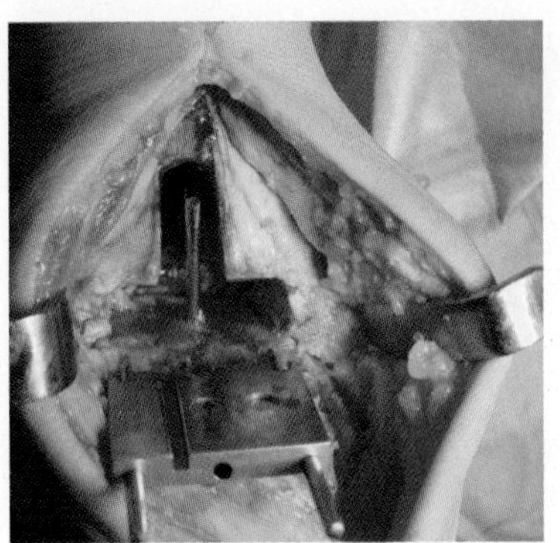

TECH FIG 7 • *(continued)* **D.** With the talar center guide appropriately positioned on the initial talar cut, the guide pin is drilled into the talus. **E.** Center pin position confirmed.

- The forked end of the talar center guide determines the position for the 2.5-mm pin.
- Insert the pin at about 60 degrees relative to the superior talar flat.

- This 2.5-mm pin identifies the AP center of the tibial component in relation to the talus.
  - Visually confirm that the 2.5-mm pin is in the AP center of the talus (TECH FIG 7E).
  - If the pin is not in the optimal position, repeat the transfer of the joint center and reposition the 2.5-mm guide pin in the exact AP center of the talus.

Anterior and Posterior Talar Flat Resection

- Remove the talar center guide but leave the 2.5-mm guide pin and the talar flat cutting block in position.
- Select the talar fin drill guide, either size 1–4 or size 5–6, to correspond to the size of talar component to be implanted, and attach it to the system handle.
- Guide the runner on the underside of the fin drill guide into the groove on the left side of the talar flat guide and advance the forked end along the resected talar flat cut until it abuts the 2.5-mm talar guide pin (TECH FIG 8A).
- Using the system handle to hold the fin drill guide in position, drill four holes into the talus using the 4.5-mm drill bit (TECH FIG 8B). Be sure to seat the drill fully against the talar fin guide so that the holes are created to the required depth.
- Remove the talar fin drill guide, the talar flat cutting block, and all 2.5-mm guide pins from within the joint space (TECH FIG 8C).

Trephine Guide

- Select the appropriate trephine guide (either size 1–4 [blue] or size 5–6 [green]) to correspond to the size of talar component to be implanted, and attach it to the system handle (TECH FIG 9A).
- The four posts in the trephine guide fit into the four drill holes made in the talus, and the guide is held in position using the system handle (TECH FIG 9B).
- Two posts are marked "A" for anterior and must be inserted into the anterior two holes in the talus.
- The other two posts are marked "P" for posterior and

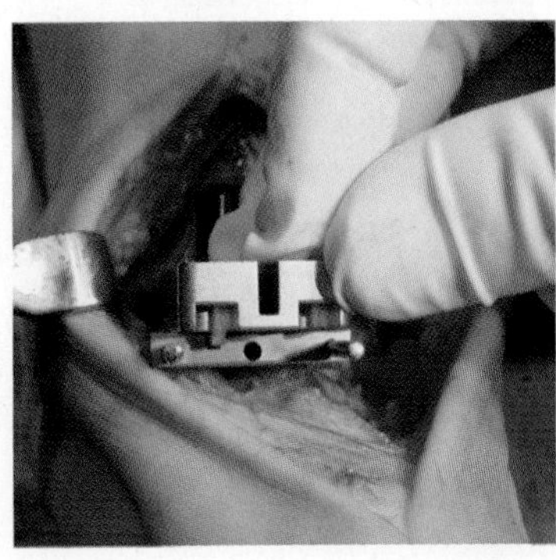

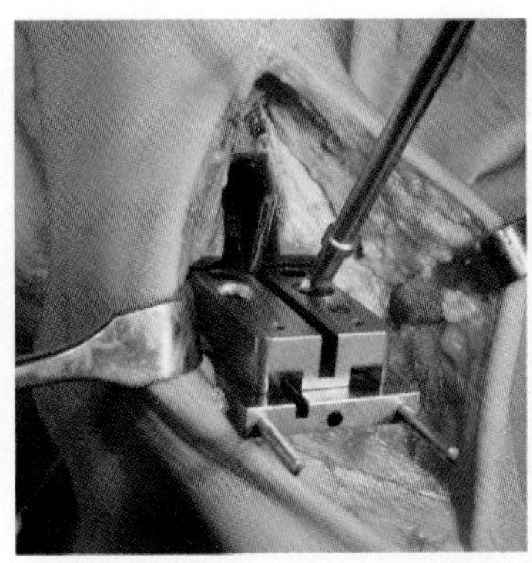

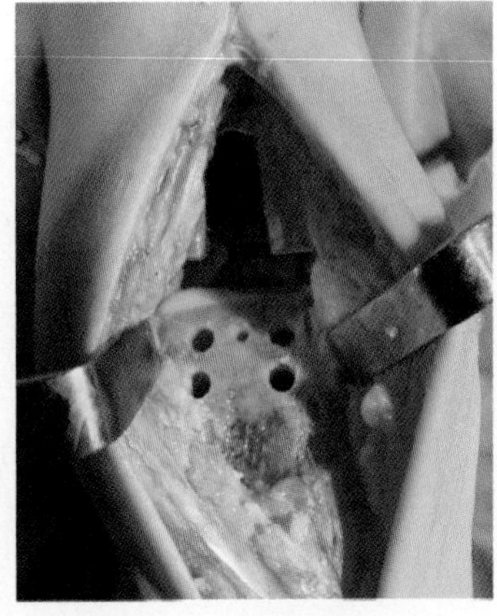

TECH FIG 8 • Talar fin drill guide. **A.** Guide positioned. **B.** Initial fin preparation. **C.** Initial talar fin preparation with talar fin drill guide removed.

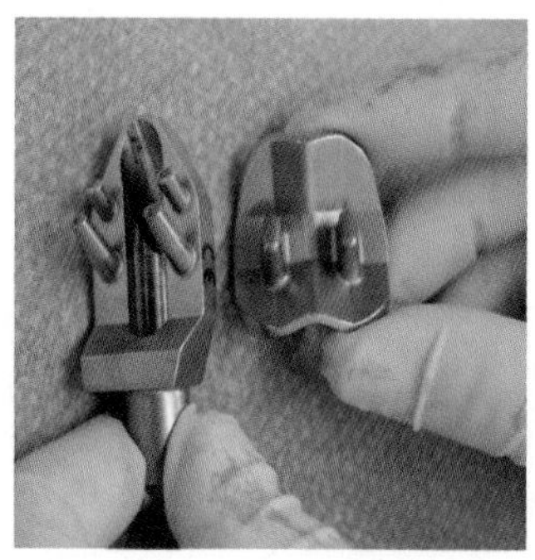

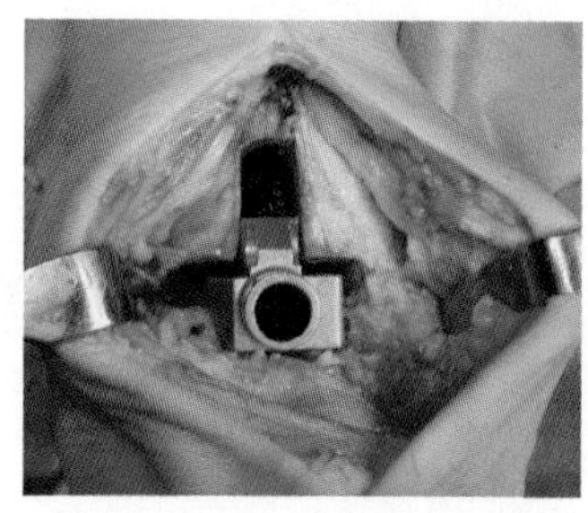

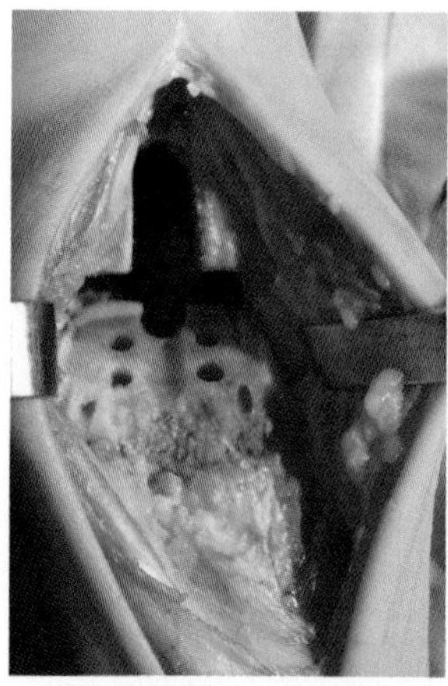

TECH FIG 9 • Talar trephine and posterior chamfer guides. **A.** Trephine guide adjacent to corresponding talar component. **B.** Trephine guide positioned on talus. **C.** After trephine preparation.

must be inserted into the posterior two holes in the talus.

- Trephine the superior and posterior talar sulcus using the specifically designed depth-stopped trephine.
- After the superior and posterior sulci have been trephined, remove the trephine guide (**TECH FIG 9C**).

Posterior Chamfer Preparation

- Select the appropriate posterior cutting block (either size 1–4 [blue] or size 5–6 [green]) to correspond to the size of talar component to be implanted, and attach it to the system handle.
- The two posts on the posterior cutting block are marked "A" for anterior. These posts must be inserted into the anterior holes in the talus.
- In the proper position, the tongue of the posterior cutting block will sit flush in the posterior sulcus that has just been trephined. The scissor distractors may be used to steady the cutting block.
- Resect the posterior talar flat and remove the posterior cutting block (**TECH FIG 10**).

Anterior Chamfer Preparation

- Select the appropriate anterior milling guide (either size 1–4 [blue] or size 5–6 [green]) to correspond to the size of talar component to be implanted, and attach it to the system handle (**TECH FIG 11A,B**).
- The two posts on the anterior milling guide are marked "P" for posterior; these posts must be inserted into the posterior holes in the talus.
- In the correct position the posterior face of the jig will be aligned with the resected posterior talar flat.
- The scissor distractors may be used to steady the jig.
- The talar anterior mill has a depth stop and is moved throughout the guide to prepare the anterior chamfer (**TECH FIG 11C**).
- The anterior milling guide restricts the mill from completely preparing the entire anterior chamfer.

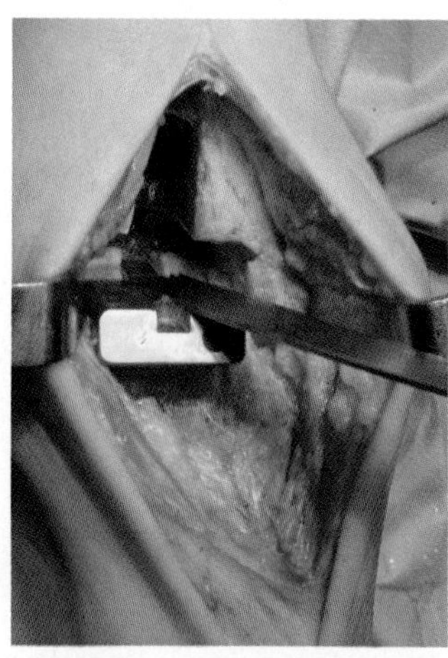

TECH FIG 10 • Posterior chamfer guide positioned and posterior chamfer cut being performed with an oscillating saw.

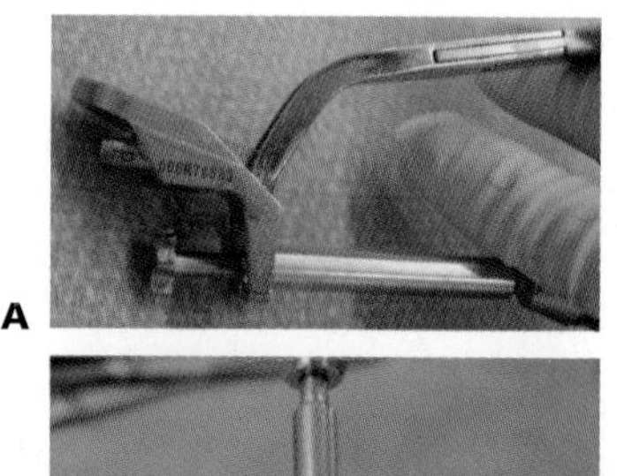

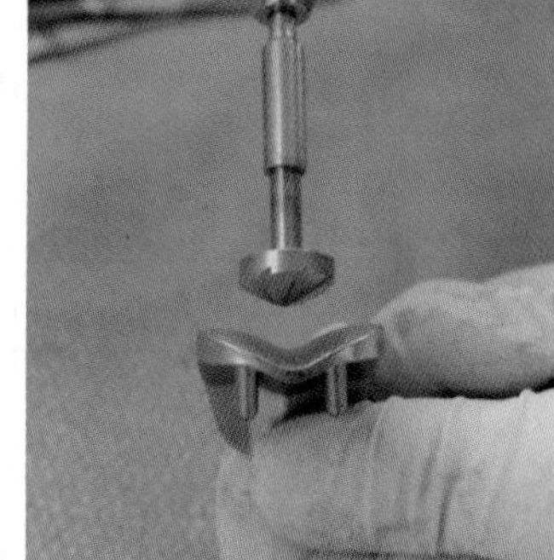

TECH FIG 11 • **A–C.** Anterior talar chamfer preparation. **A.** Anterior chamfer mill and guide. **B.** Depiction of the recess created by the mill for the talar component. *(continued)*

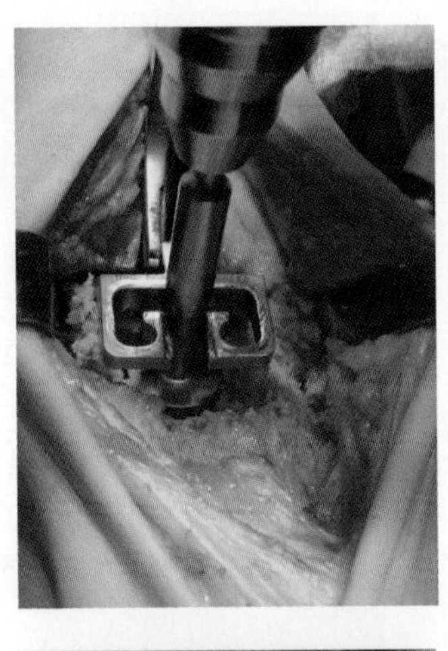
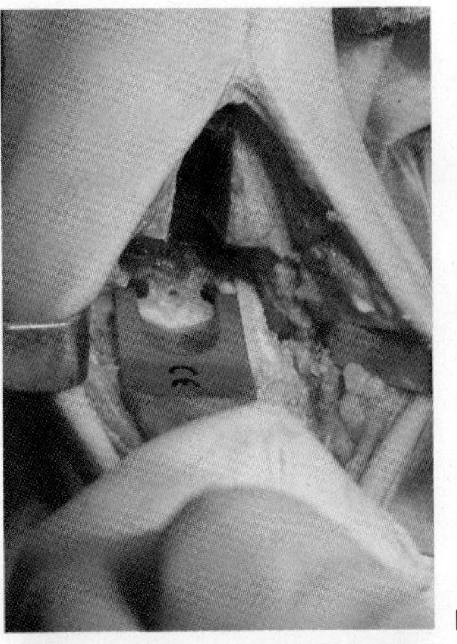
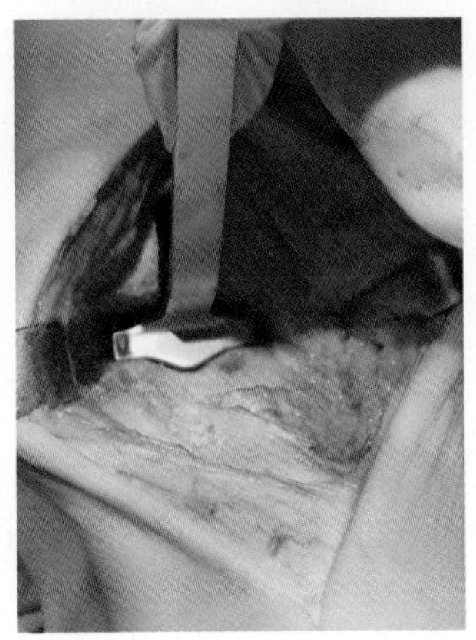
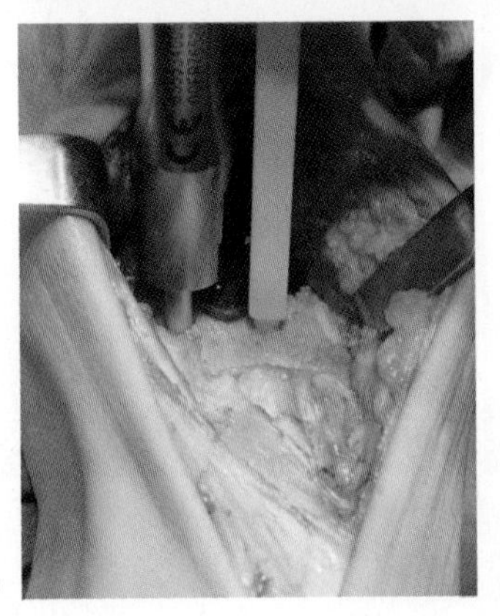
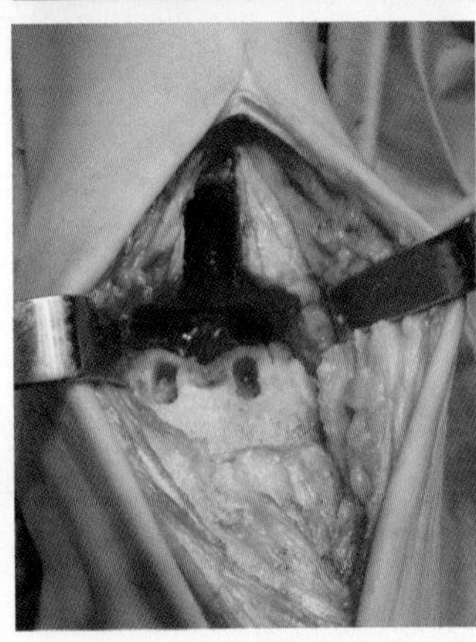

TECH FIG 11 • *(continued)* **C.** Talar milling for anterior chamfer preparation. **D–G.** Final talar preparation. **D.** Talar sulcus osteotome. **E.** Talar profile template to confirm adequate sulcus preparation. **F, G.** Completion of the talar fin slots.

- After removing the anterior milling guide, use a rongeur to remove residual anterior bony prominences.
- Finish the superior and posterior sulci by using the sulcus osteotome and the sulcus burr (**TECH FIG 11D**).
- The talar profile template confirms satisfactory preparation of the talus (**TECH FIG 11E**).
- Use the fin osteotome, the rongeur, or both to remove the small piece of bone between the anterior and posterior drill holes guided by the plastic fin angle guide (**TECH FIG 11F,G**).

TRIAL INSERTION

- There are six sizes of talar and tibial trials corresponding to the six available final component sizes.
- The size of talar implant must match or be smaller than the size of the tibial implant.
- Insert the proper talar trial, narrow aspect directed posteriorly. The tibial window serves as a convenient access for the talar impactor (**TECH FIG 12A**).
- Select the trial tibial component corresponding to the prepared tibial window and insert it straight anterior to posterior within the distal tibial window resection.
  - The curved aspect of the component is directed posteriorly.
  - The articular surface of the tibia component will be positioned about 85 degrees to the long axis of the leg.
  - The anterior aspect of the component should be flush with the anterior cortex of the tibia.
  - The posterior aspect of the component may overhang the rear of the tibia by 1 mm in the midpoint but should not do so near the malleoli as it may irritate the neurovascular bundle, tendons, or posterior soft tissues.
  - The medial and lateral dimensions of the tibial trial ideally should match the tibial resection. Most importantly it must cover all aspects of the polyethylene insert (**TECH FIG 12B**).
- The bearing insert is available in the six sizes, and there are five different thicknesses.
  - The six sizes of bearing insert trials are color-coded according to size (1, black; 2, brown; 3, purple; 4, yellow; 5, hot pink; 6, red).
  - The trial bearing insert's handle facilitates bearing removal without restricting trial joint motion or obstructing visualization of the resurfaced joint (**TECH FIG 12C**).
- Confirm proper alignment and trial component position fluoroscopically (**TECH FIG 12D–F**). Also confirm that there is no indication of stress fracture
- Confirm that the ankle is balanced and that ROM is adequate, particularly dorsiflexion beyond neutral (**TECH FIG 12G,H**).

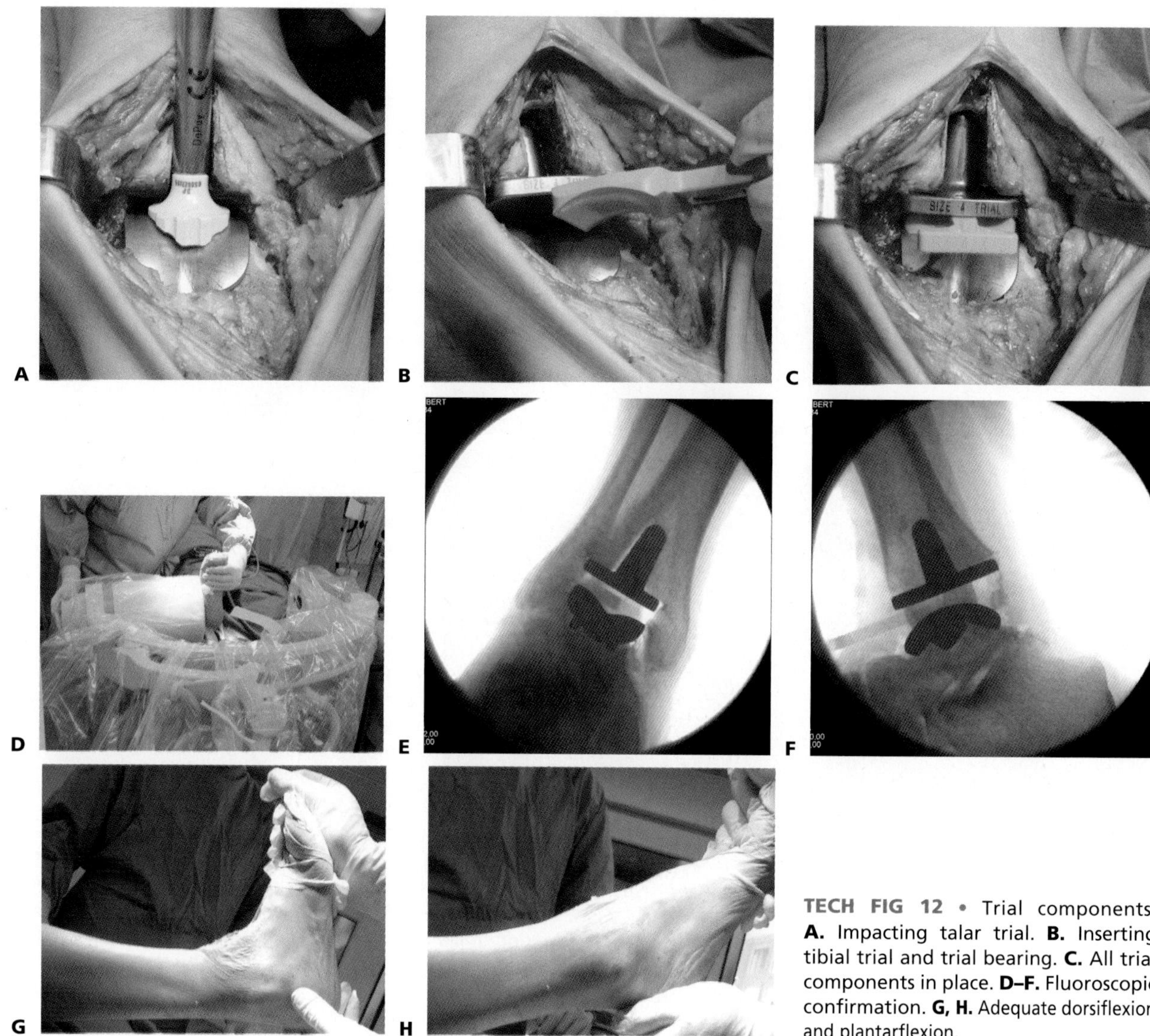

TECH FIG 12 • Trial components. **A.** Impacting talar trial. **B.** Inserting tibial trial and trial bearing. **C.** All trial components in place. **D–F.** Fluoroscopic confirmation. **G, H.** Adequate dorsiflexion and plantarflexion.

FINAL COMPONENT INSERTION

- The tibial and talar components are intended for uncemented use (**TECH FIG 13A**).
- Seat the talar component with the narrow aspect of the component directed posteriorly and the keel fins directed in line with the slots.
  - Use the component impactor, which can be positioned in the tibial window so that the posterior talus may be fully seated.
  - To avoid anterior tilt of the component, we routinely place an instrument under the anterior aspect of the component during initial impaction (**TECH FIG 13B**).
- Protect the articulating surface of the talar component with a trial insert bearing and insert the tibial component.
  - The curved aspect of the component is directed posteriorly.
  - Ensure that the implant is seated firmly on the prepared distal surface of the tibia (**TECH FIG 13C,D**).
- Check for any osteophytes that might impinge within the joint and trim if needed, taking care not to damage the polished articulating surfaces.
- Make the final decision about the thickness of the bearing, using trials as necessary.
- Insert the final polyethylene bearing (**TECH FIG 13E**).
- Trim and replace the resected bone in the tibial window, using slivers of bone in the saw cuts to enhance the stability of the "graft" (**TECH FIG 13F–I**).
- Be sure that motion is adequate, particularly dorsiflexion (**TECH FIG 13J–L**).
- Confirm proper alignment and implant position fluoroscopically. Also confirm that there is no indication of stress fracture.

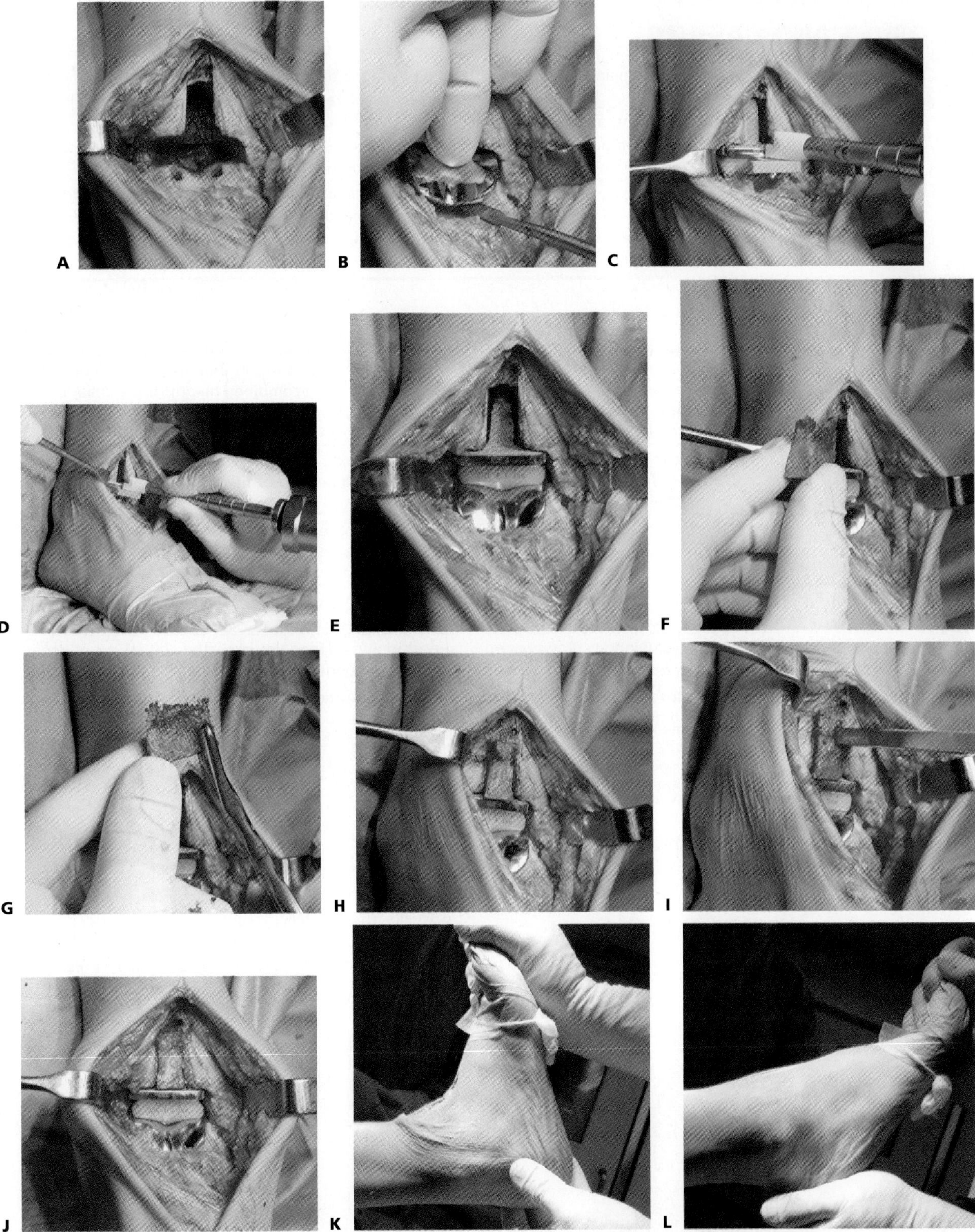

TECH FIG 13 • Final implants. **A.** Surfaces prepared for cementless implantation. **B.** The anterior lip of the talar component is supported during its initial insertion to keep it from tilting anteriorly. **C, D.** Tibial component insertion (note use of a bearing trial to support the tibial component during insertion and to protect the talar component). **E.** Final components in place, including mobile bearing. **F–L.** Final steps of implantation. **F.** Replacing anterior tibial cortical fragment that was removed to create tibial window. **G.** The cancellous portion must be carefully trimmed. **H–J.** Anterior cortex fragment in place and then impacted. **K, L.** Adequate motion confirmed.

TECHNIQUES

CLOSURE AND CASTING

- Thoroughly irrigate the joint and implant with sterile saline.
- While protecting the prosthesis, fill the anterior barrel holes with bone graft from the resected bone.
- The pin should have already been removed from the proximal tibia.
- Reapproximate the capsule.
- Use of a drain is by surgeon preference.
- Release the tourniquet and obtain meticulous hemostasis.
- Reapproximate the extensor retinaculum while protecting the deep and superficial peroneal nerves.
- Irrigate the subcutaneous layer with sterile saline and then reapproximate it.
- Reapproximate the skin to a tensionless closure.
- Place sterile dressings on the wounds, adequate padding, and a short-leg cast with the ankle in neutral position.

PEARLS AND PITFALLS

Tibial preparation	■ Use the gap template after the initial tibial resection to confirm that an adequate tibial resection has been completed. The gap template equals the combined height of the tibial base plate and the most narrow polyethylene bearing. If it does not fit, then more tibial resection is warranted.
Removing resected tibial bone	■ Be sure to make a vertical cut from the medial ankle gutter, all the way from anterior to posterior, before attempting to mobilize the resected portion of tibia. If it still has medial attachment, the medial malleolus may fracture.
Talar sizing	■ The talar preparation is in two ranges: sizes 1–4 have exactly the same talar preparation; sizes 5–6 have the same talar preparation. Therefore, a decision must be made between sizes 4 and 5 but not for sizes within a given range.
Tibial window preparation	■ Be sure to save the bone that is removed through the anterior tibial cortical window; it will be used to fill the defect at the conclusion of the surgery.
Impacting the talar component	■ The tibial window allows for optimal positioning of the talar impactor, so that it can impact directly vertically on the talar trial and final component.
Relative sizes of the tibial and talar components	■ The talus must be the same size as or smaller than the tibial component, and the polyethylene bearing must be smaller than the tibial base plate to avoid edge loading and impingement.
Final motion	■ If the ankle cannot be dorsiflexed beyond neutral with the components in place, consider a thinner polyethylene insert or a tendo Achilles lengthening versus gastrocnemius–soleus recession, or both.

POSTOPERATIVE CARE

- Overnight stay
- Nasal oxygen while in hospital
- Touch-down weight bearing on the cast is permitted, but elevation is encouraged as much as possible.
- Follow up in 2 to 3 weeks for suture removal and transition to a cam boot
- Weight bearing to tolerance starting at 3 weeks
- If the wound is stable, supervised therapy to reduce edema and optimize motion.
- At 6 weeks after surgery, weight-bearing radiographs of the ankle are obtained (**FIG 3**).
- If the wound is stable and radiographs suggest early bone ingrowth and no signs of stress fracture, weight bearing is

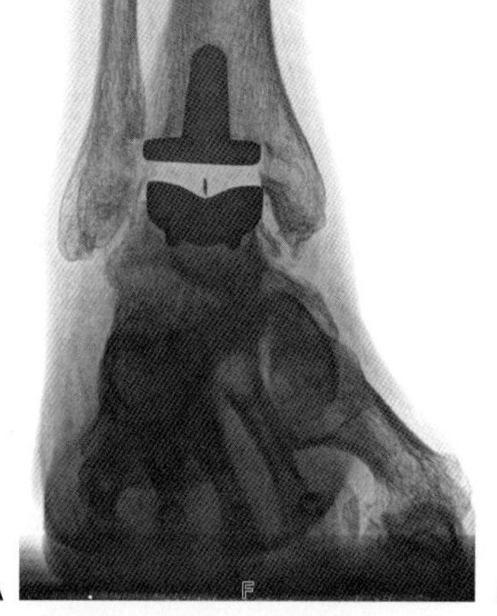

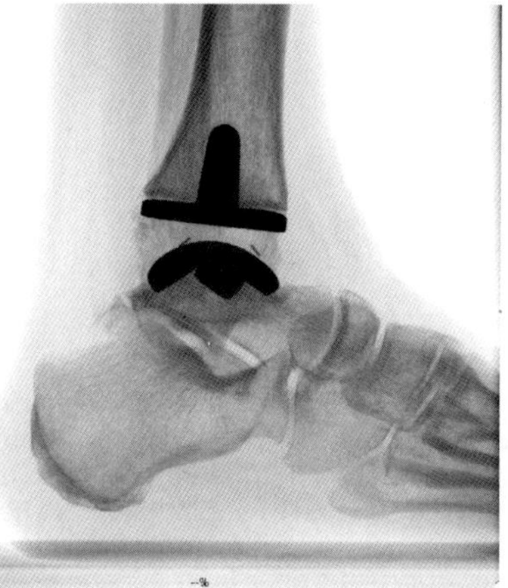

FIG 3 • Follow-up weight-bearing radiographs. **A.** AP view of ankle. **B.** Lateral view of ankle. *(continued)*

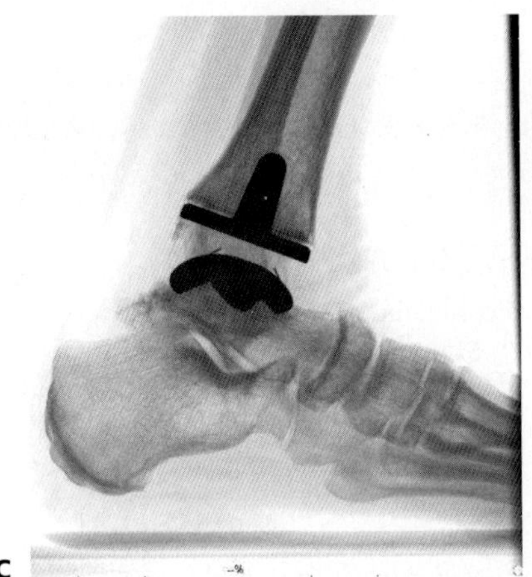

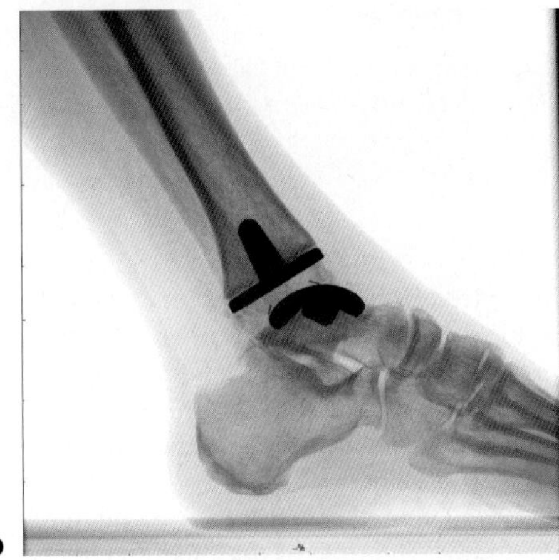

FIG 3 • *(continued)* **C.** Dorsiflexion. **D.** Plantarflexion.

gradually advanced and the patient is transitioned to a regular shoe.

- If there is no evidence of stress fracture or failure of the procedure, then the patient can progress to a regular shoe and full weight bearing.

OUTCOMES

- While some recently reported outcomes are based on high-level evidence, results of total ankle arthroplasty are almost uniformly derived from level IV evidence.
- Functional outcome using commonly used scoring systems for total ankle arthroplasty (AOFAS [Kofoed, Mazur] and NJOH [Buechel-Pappas]) suggest uniform improvement in all studies, with follow-up scores ranging from 70 to 90 points (maximum 100 points).
- Patient satisfaction rates for total ankle arthroplasty exceed 90%, although follow-up data for patient satisfaction often do not exceed 5 years.
- Overall survivorship analysis for currently available implants, designating removal of a metal component or conversion to arthrodesis as the endpoint, ranges from about 90% to 95% at 5 to 6 years and 80% to 92% at 10 to 12 years.
- At the time of this writing there are no published results available for the Mobility total ankle arthroplasty.

COMPLICATIONS

- Infection (superficial or deep)
- Neuralgia (superficial or deep peroneal nerve; rarely tibial nerve)
- Delayed wound healing
- Wound dehiscence
- Persistent pain despite optimal orthopaedic examination and radiographic appearance of implants
- Osteolysis
- Subsidence
- Medial malleolar stress fracture
- Implant fracture (including polyethylene)

REFERENCES

1. Gougoulias N, Khanna A, Maffulli N. How successful are current ankle replacements? A systematic review of the literature. Clin Orthop Relat Res 2010;468(1):199–208.
2. Haddad SL, Coetzee JC, Estok R, et al. Intermediate and long-term outcomes of total ankle arthroplasty and ankle arthrodesis: a systematic review of the literature. J Bone Joint Surg Am 2007;89A:1899–1905.
3. Stengel D, Bauwens K, Ekkernkamp A, et al. Efficacy of total ankle replacement with meniscal-bearing devices: a systematic review and meta-analysis. Arch Orthop Trauma Surg 2005;125:109–119.
4. Wood PL, Sutton C, Mishra V, et al. A randomised, controlled trial of two mobile-bearing total ankle replacements. J Bone Joint Surg Br 2009;91B:69–74.

Chapter 73 INBONE Total Ankle Arthroplasty

James K. DeOrio, Mark E. Easley, James A. Nunley II, and Mark A. Reiley

DEFINITION

- The INBONE™ (Wright Medical, Memphis, TN) total ankle system, like other total ankle systems, is indicated for end-stage ankle arthritis failing to respond to nonoperative intervention.
- In contrast to essentially all other total ankle systems, however, the INBONE™ total ankle system uses intramedullary rather than extramedullary referencing.
- While the intramedullary alignment guide passes through the plantar foot, calcaneus, talus, and tibia, it does so anterior to the posterior facet of the calcaneus and does not violate any articulations of the subtalar joint.
- To achieve reliable intramedullary alignment, the INBONE™ total ankle system uses a leg frame that is initially cumbersome, demands more pre-incision preparation, and requires greater fluoroscopy time than other total ankle systems. However, with experience this technique becomes manageable and allows the user to correct deformities prior to making bone cut.

ANATOMY

- Ankle
  - Tibial plafond with medial malleolus
    - Articulations with dorsal and medial talus
    - In sagittal plane, slight posterior slope
    - In coronal plane, articular surface is 88 to 92 degrees relative to lateral tibial shaft axis.
  - Fibula
    - Articulation with lateral talus
    - Responsible for one sixth of axial load distribution of the ankle
  - Talus
    - 60% of surface area covered by articular cartilage
    - Dual radius of curvature
  - Distal tibiofibular syndesmosis
    - Anterior inferior tibiofibular ligament
    - Interosseous membrane
    - Posterior tibiofibular ligament
- Ankle functions as part of the ankle–hindfoot complex much like a mitered hinge.

PATHOGENESIS

- Post-traumatic arthrosis
  - Most common cause
  - Intra-articular fracture
  - Ankle fracture-dislocation with malunion
  - Chronic ankle instability
- Primary osteoarthrosis
  - Relatively rare compared to hip and knee arthrosis
- Inflammatory arthropathy
  - Most commonly rheumatoid arthritis
- Other
  - Hemochromatosis
  - Pigmented villonodular synovitis
  - Charcot neuroarthropathy
  - Septic arthritis

NATURAL HISTORY

- Post-traumatic arthrosis
  - Malunion, chronic instability, intra-articular cartilage damage, or malalignment may lead to progressive articular cartilage wear.
  - Chronic lateral ankle instability may eventually be associated with:
    - Relative anterior subluxation of the talus
    - Varus tilt of the talus within the ankle mortise
    - Hindfoot varus position
- Primary osteoarthrosis of the ankle is rare and poorly understood.
- Inflammatory arthropathy
  - Progressive and proliferative synovial erosive changes failing to respond to medical management
  - May be associated with chronic posterior tibial tendinopathy and progressive valgus hindfoot deformity, eventual valgus tilt to the talus within the ankle mortise, potential lateral malleolar stress fracture, and compensatory forefoot varus

PATIENT HISTORY AND PHYSICAL FINDINGS

- Patient history
  - Often a history of ankle trauma
    - Ankle fracture, particularly intra-articular
    - Ankle fracture with malunion
    - Chronic ankle instability (recurrent ankle sprains)
  - Chronic anterior ankle pain, primarily with activity and weight bearing
  - Ankle stiffness, particularly with dorsiflexion
  - Ankle swelling
  - Progressively increased pain with activity
- Physical findings
  - Limp
  - Patient externally rotates hip to externally rotate ankle to avoid painful push-off.
  - Painful and limited ankle range of motion (ROM), particularly limited dorsiflexion
  - Mild ankle edema
  - Potential associated foot deformity
    - Post-traumatic arthrosis secondary to chronic instability may be associated with varus ankle and hindfoot and compensatory forefoot varus.
    - Inflammatory arthritis may be associated with progressively worsening flatfoot deformity, valgus tilt to the ankle and hindfoot, and equinus.

IMAGING AND OTHER DIAGNOSTIC STUDIES

- Weight-bearing AP with contralateral ankle included, lateral, and mortise views of the ankle

- Weight-bearing AP with contralateral foot included, lateral, and oblique views of the foot, particularly with associated foot deformity
- With associated or suspected lower leg deformity, we routinely obtain weight-bearing AP and lateral tibia–fibula views.
- With deformity in the lower extremity, we occasionally obtain weight-bearing mechanical axis (hip-to-ankle) views of both extremities.
- We occasionally evaluate complex or ill-defined ankle–hindfoot patterns of arthritis with or without deformity using CT of the ankle and hindfoot.
- If we suspect avascular necrosis of the talus or distal tibia, we obtain an MRI of the ankle.

DIFFERENTIAL DIAGNOSIS

- See the "Pathogenesis" section.

NONOPERATIVE MANAGEMENT

- Activity modification
- Bracing
  - Ankle–foot orthosis
  - Double upright brace attached to shoe
- Stiffer-soled shoe with a rocker-bottom modification
- Nonsteroidal anti-inflammatories or COX-2 inhibitors
- Medications for systemic inflammatory arthropathy
- Corticosteroid injection
- Viscosupplementation

SURGICAL MANAGEMENT

- In contrast to essentially all other total ankle systems, the INBONE™ total ankle system uses intramedullary rather than extramedullary referencing.
- While the intramedullary alignment guide passes through the plantar foot, calcaneus talus, and tibia, it does so anterior to the posterior facet of the calcaneus and does not violate any articulations of the subtalar joint.
- To achieve reliable intramedullary alignment, the INBONE™ total ankle system uses a leg frame that is initially cumbersome, demands more pre-incision preparation, and requires greater fluoroscopy time than other total ankle systems. However, with experience this technique becomes manageable and allows the user to correct deformities prior to making bone cut.
- In our opinion, the INBONE™ total ankle system is perhaps more stout than some other systems.
  - We have been able to correct coronal and sagittal plane deformities through the tibiotalar joint with appropriate soft tissue balancing and corrective osteotomies relying also on the durability of the implants, particularly the broad talar component and the tibial stem extensions to maintain correction.

Preoperative Planning

- The surgeon must be sure the patient has satisfactory perfusion to support healing and is not neuropathic.
  - Noninvasive vascular studies and potential vascular surgery consultation if necessary
- The surgeon must inspect the ankle for prior scars or surgical approaches that need to be considered in planning the surgical approach for total ankle arthroplasty.
- The surgeon must understand the clinical and radiographic alignment of the lower extremity, ankle, and foot.
  - The surgeon must be prepared to balance and realign the ankle. Occasionally, this necessitates corrective osteotomies of the distal tibia or foot, hindfoot arthrodesis, ligament releases or stabilization, and tendon transfers.
  - The surgeon should determine whether coronal plane alignment is passively correctable; this provides some understanding as to whether ligament releases will be required.
- Ankle ROM is determined.
  - Ankle stiffness, particularly lack of dorsiflexion, needs to be corrected.
    - Anterior tibiotalar exostectomy
    - Posterior capsular release
    - Occasionally, tendo Achilles lengthening
- Instrumentation
  - These instruments facilitate total ankle arthroplasty:
    - Small oscillating and reciprocating saws for fine cuts as well as larger oscillating saw for broad bone cuts. The smaller saws make it easier to resect prominences with precision, and easily morselize large bone fragments to be evacuated from the joint.
    - A rasp for final preparation of cut bony surfaces
    - A 90-degree angled curette, particularly to separate bone from the posterior capsule
    - A toothed lamina spreader to distract the joint and aid in realignment of preoperative ankle deformity. Since the INBONE™ prosthesis uses a monoblock cutting guide for tibial and talar resection, an intra-articular lamina spreader assists in limiting bone resection. A lamina spreader placed on the concave side of the joint also assists in realignment.
    - A toothless lamina spreader to judiciously distract the ankle to improve exposure even after preparing the surfaces of the tibia and talus
- Large fluoroscopic scanner
  - Fluoroscopy confirms proper alignment of the cutting guide to the ankle.
    - The leg holder maintains the leg in position relative to the alignment guides and reference drill.
  - With the leg holder, the large scanner is necessary to straddle the leg and leg holder.
  - Fluoroscopy through the operating table is necessary, so a little fluoroscopy unit is inadequate.
- Foot pedals to make adjustments to the table position
  - With the foot secured in the leg holder, subtle adjustments to the table's rotation confirm ideal alignment relative to the alignment guides.
- Subtle adjustments to the alignment guides relative to the ankle allow fine-tuning for the reference drill trajectory.

Positioning

- Supine
- Plantar aspect of operated foot at end of operating table
- Foot and ankle well balanced with toes directed to the ceiling
- A bolster under the ipsilateral hip prevents undesired external rotation of the hip.
- We routinely use a thigh tourniquet and regional anesthesia.
  - A popliteal block provides adequate pain relief postoperatively, particularly if a regional catheter is used. Moreover, hip and knee flexion–extension is not forfeited, facilitating safe immediate postoperative mobilization.
  - However, using a thigh tourniquet with a popliteal block typically requires a supplemental femoral nerve block (patient temporarily forfeits knee extension in the immediate postoperative period) or general anesthesia.

- The operative extremity needs adequate space for the INBONE™ leg holder. The surgeon should be sure the opposite extremity is not secured too close to the operative extremity.

Approach

- Anterior approach to the ankle, using the interval between the tibialis anterior (TA) tendon and the extensor hallucis longus (EHL) tendon

APPROACH

- Make a longitudinal midline incision over the anterior ankle, starting about 10 cm proximal to the tibiotalar joint and 1 cm lateral to the tibial crest.
- Continue the incision midline over the anterior ankle just distal to the talonavicular joint.
- At no point should direct tension be placed on the skin margins; we perform deep, full-thickness retraction as soon as possible to limit the risk of skin complications.
  - Identify and protect the superficial peroneal nerve by retracting it laterally.
  - In our experience there is a consistent branch of the superficial peroneal nerve that crosses directly over or immediately proximal to the tibiotalar joint.
- We then expose the extensor retinaculum, identify the course of the EHL tendon, and sharply but carefully divide the retinaculum directly over the EHL tendon.
  - We always attempt to maintain the TA tendon in its dedicated sheath if present.
  - Preserving the retinaculum over the TA tendon prevents bowstringing of the tendon and thereby reduces the stress on the anterior wound. Should there be a wound dehiscence, then the TA is not directly exposed.
  - However, preserving the retinaculum over the TA tendon is not always possible. Not infrequently only the retinaculum is present over the tendon and it will be free with the EHL tendon (**TECH FIG 1**).
- Use the interval between the TA and EHL tendons, with the TA and EHL tendons retracted medially and laterally, respectively.
- Identify the deep neurovascular bundle (anterior tibial–dorsalis pedis artery and deep peroneal nerve) and carefully retract it laterally throughout the remainder of the procedure.
- Perform an anterior capsulotomy and elevate the tibial and dorsal talar periosteum to about 6 to 8 cm proximal to the tibial plafond and talonavicular joint, respectively.
- Elevate this separated capsule and periosteum medially and laterally to expose the ankle, access the medial and lateral gutters, and visualize the medial and lateral malleoli.
- Remove anterior tibial and talar osteophytes to facilitate exposure and avoid interference with the instrumentation.

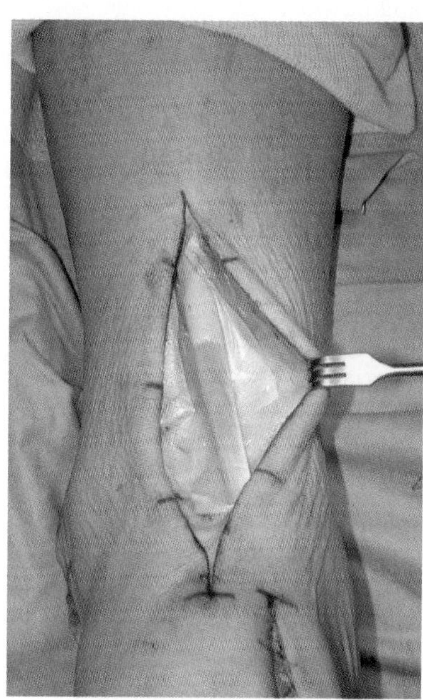

TECH FIG 1 • In this case there is no separate sheath for the tibialis anterior (TA) tendon. Nonetheless, the retinaculum was opened lateral to the tendon, and upon closure the TA will not be immediately up against the suture line.

TIBIOTALAR ALIGNMENT

- Before placing the lower leg in the INBONE™ foot and ankle holder, we optimize ankle soft tissue balance and alignment.
- Varus malalignment
  - We routinely perform a comprehensive medial release for moderate to severe varus malalignment.
  - The concept is similar to balancing the varus knee for total knee arthroplasty and was well described by Bonnin et al.[1] in their 2004 report of the Salto prosthesis.
  - We routinely subperiosteally raise a continuous soft tissue sleeve from the distal medial tibia to the medial talus.
  - There is no need to be aggressive on the medial talus, as this could compromise the deltoid branch of the posterior tibial artery that perfuses the medial talar dome.
  - The superficial deltoid (medial collateral) ligament is elevated but left intact proximally and attached distally. The release of these fibers is complete when the posterior tibial tendon can be visualized.
  - The deep deltoid (medial collateral) ligament may be peeled off the medial malleolus to balance the ankle appropriately. In severe varus deformity, the entire deep deltoid ligament must be released to achieve

tibiotalar balance (TECH FIG 2A). Overrelease is theoretically possible, but in our experience, with severe varus deformity, the ankle will not collapse into valgus even with a complete release.

- In our experience, with an appropriate medial release, optimal bony resection and metal component alignment, and proper sizing of the polyethylene, a lateral ligament reconstruction is seldom necessary. One exception is when there has been an avulsion fracture of the tip of the fibula: in that instance it is difficult to obtain any ability to rotate the ankle against the lateral tissue, and a Brostrom ligament reconstruction can be done at the beginning of the case (TECH FIG 2B–D). This marks a significant change from our initial practices in rebalancing the varus ankle.
- A lamina spreader placed in the medial tibiotalar joint maintains the correction.

- Valgus malalignment
  - Likewise, a valgus malalignment must be rebalanced.
  - However, in our experience, we rarely need to perform a ligament release.
  - Often, valgus malalignment is secondary to lateral ankle joint collapse and some medial (deltoid) ligament attenuation. This may involve a component of lateral ankle ligament instability as well.
    - While the latter portion of this statement seems counterintuitive, it has been our experience in treating many patients with end-stage ankle arthritis and valgus malalignment.
    - Moreover, lateral release in such situations may lead to paradoxical lateral instability!
  - We use a lateral lamina spreader to realign the ankle and regain functional tension in the medial ligaments (TECH FIG 2E,F).

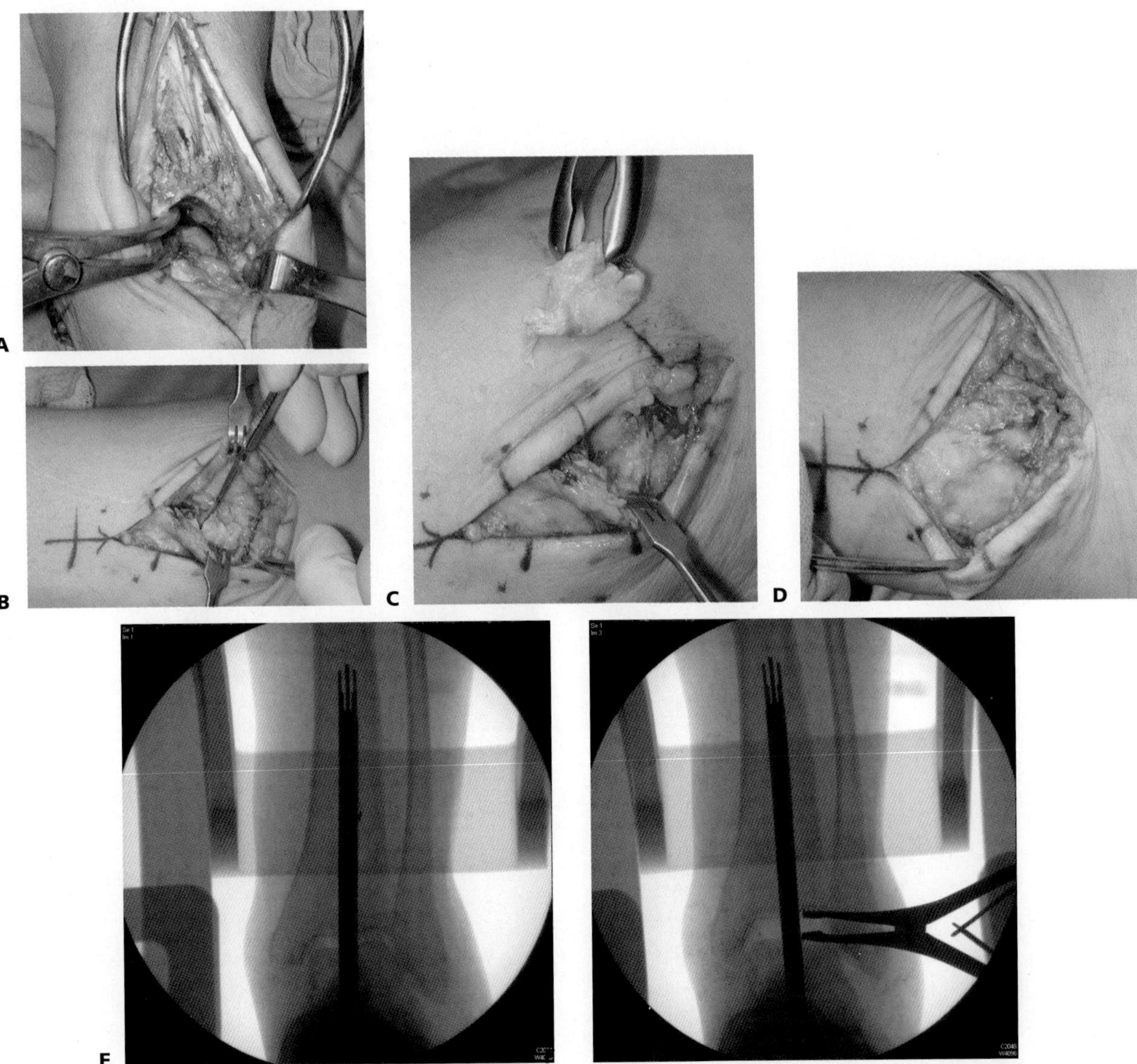

TECH FIG 2 • A. In this varus ankle a complete medial peel of the deltoid ligament has been performed and the ankle can be opened up with the lamina spreader. **B.** There was a large ossicle at the tip of the fibula representing an old avulsion fracture containing the anterior talofibular ligament. Hence, the bone was removed (**C**) and a Brostrom ligament reconstruction was performed (**D**). **E.** Valgus ankle with AP alignment guide properly rotated. However, the talus is not orthogonal to the guide or the tibia. **F.** In this view the lamina spreader has been placed laterally on the concave side, and now the talus is orthogonal to the tibia and the alignment guide.

INTRAMEDULLARY ALIGNMENT

- Be sure the foot and ankle frame is properly assembled and the alignment drill guide trajectory is calibrated. If unsure, you can assemble the cannula into the holder, put the drill in, and take a fluoroscopic view to make sure they coincide (**TECH FIG 3A**).
- The foot and lower leg are secured in the leg holder.
  - With correction of the preoperative deformity, we transfer the leg into the foot and ankle holder with the lamina spreader in place (**TECH FIG 3B**).
    - If the foot and ankle are secured first, it may be difficult to position the lamina spreader effectively.
  - Proper rotation
    - We use a small straight osteotome in the medial gutter as a reference. The foot is rotated until the osteotome is parallel with the leg holder foot plate.
  - Plantigrade foot
    - The heel must be flush with the foot plate of the guide.
    - If it is not, then the talar cut will have a posterior slope, removing an excessive amount of the talar body and increasing the risk of posterior talar component subsidence. Be sure all anterior tibiotalar osteophytes are removed. Perform a gastrocnemius release or tendo Achilles lengthening if necessary.
  - Coronal plane alignment
    - In the mediolateral plane, center the heel over the starting point for the reference drill.
    - We use the AP alignment guides to grossly set this alignment.
    - This position should also be in line with the tibial shaft axis so that minimal adjustments will be necessary.
    - Preoperative deformity complicates such preliminary alignment.
  - Sagittal plane alignment
    - We use the lateral alignment guides to grossly set this alignment.
    - The calf and Achilles rests need to be adjusted to optimize the lower leg's position relative to the foot (talus) (**TECH FIG 3C**).
  - In our experience, proper heel position, optimal tibial alignment, and ideal rotation may make the foot appear internally rotated relative to the lower leg.
  - Fluoroscopic confirmation of proper alignment
    - A large fluoroscopic scanner is needed (**TECH FIG 3D,E**).

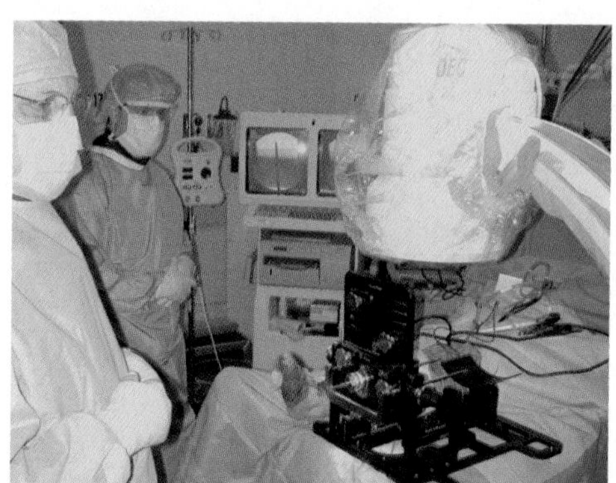
A

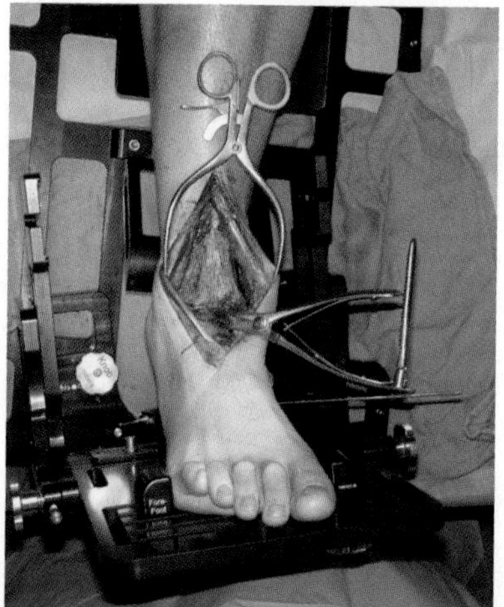
B

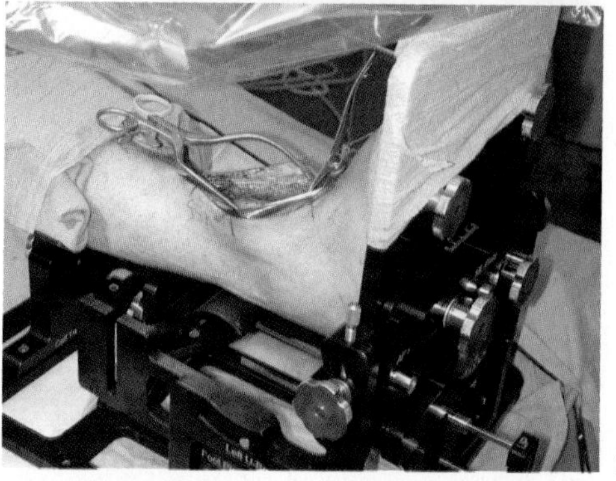
C

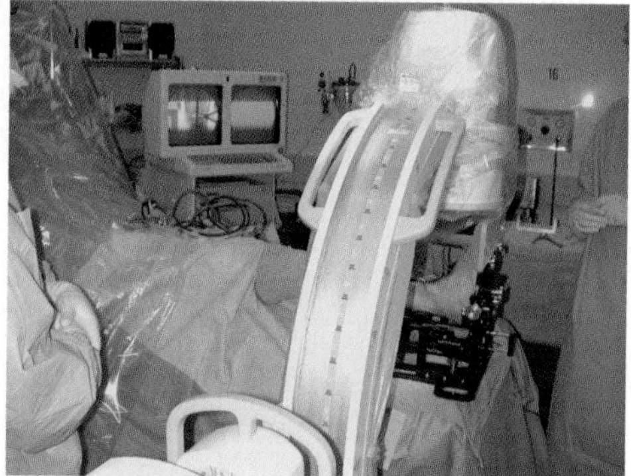
D

TECH FIG 3 • A. Fluoroscopic view being obtained of leg holder with cannula and drill in place to ensure correct assembly of leg holder. **B.** Gelpi retractor holding deep tissue aside with lamina spreader on concave medial side of varus ankle. **C.** Leg positioned in leg holder with Achilles and calf rests supporting leg. **D.** C-arm coming in to obtain AP view of ankle on ipsilateral side. *(continued)*

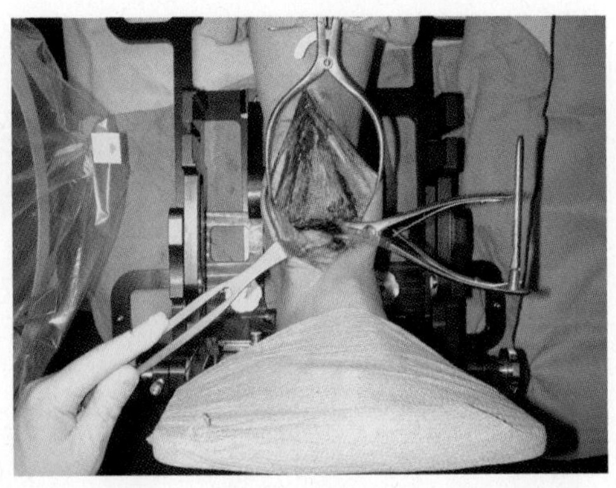

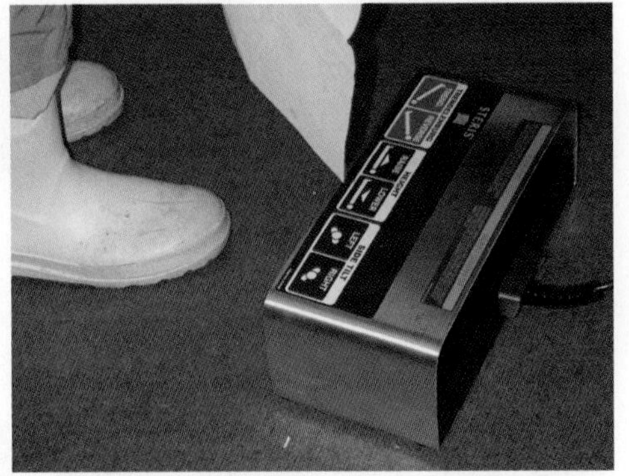

E **F**

TECH FIG 3 • *(continued)* **E.** Overhead view of lamina spreader in place and deep Gelpi retractor holding deep tissue apart. C-arm to the left is coming in for lateral view. **F.** Foot pedals are used to control tilting of the table to get the alignment sites exactly parallel to one another.

- Foot pedals to make adjustments to the table position (TECH FIG 3F)
  - With the foot secured in the leg holder, subtle adjustments to the table's rotation confirm ideal alignment relative to the alignment guides.
- Subtle adjustments to the alignment guides relative to the ankle to allow fine-tuning for the reference drill trajectory may be made with the foot pedal.
- Reference drill
  - Make a horizontally oriented 1-cm incision in the plantar foot, directly in the opening in the foot frame for passing the reference drill.
    - 1 cm allows for subtle adjustments to the medial and lateral position of the reference drill, even when its drill sleeve has been positioned on the plantar calcaneus.
    - The incision should not be more than a 5 mm deep, since otherwise it could injure the lateral plantar nerve.
  - Insert the drill guide to contact the plantar calcaneus.
    - Avoid holding the frame while inserting this guide as this could allow the drill to bend, achieving a different trajectory than the guide.
  - Secure the drill guide.
  - Advance the reference drill from calcaneus to tibia.
    - Since the trajectory may change when the drill hits the plantar medial calcaneus, we typically start the drill in reverse and "peck drill" (tap drill) to gradually penetrate the plantar calcaneal cortex without veering from the planned trajectory.
    - Once the plantar cortex is penetrated, the drill is run in forward.
  - Since drilling may shift the frame slightly, fluoroscopic confirmation of proper alignment must be re-established, after which proper alignment of the reference drill may be confirmed.
  - Advance the drill into the distal tibia, about 8 to 10 cm.
- Confirm appropriate reference drill position fluoroscopically in both the coronal and sagittal planes.

TIBIOTALAR JOINT PREPARATION

- Sizing
  - Approximate sizing for the component may be performed on preoperative radiographs of either the involved side or the uninvolved opposite ankle.
  - Position the cutting block in roughly the correct position by using the reference drill guide to estimate its position.
  - Fine-tune the cutting block using the reference drill guide under fluoroscopy.
    - In the AP plane we align the cutting guide with the reference drill guide (TECH FIG 4A).
    - In the lateral plane, we use saw blades through the cutting guide to determine the resection level (TECH FIG 4B).
    - The position of the cutting block should be finalized only if proper alignment has been confirmed fluoroscopically with the alignment guides.
    - It is important that the guide is centered medially and laterally and no more than 1 mm of bone is removed form the medial malleolus.
- Pinning the cutting block
  - Once proper position of the cutting block is established, the block is pinned, tibial pins first and talar pins next.
    - Occasionally the talar pins will skive and not engage the talus, particularly if a lamina spreader is being used to distract the joint or if the talar dome is sclerotic.
    - A toothless lamina spreader may be used to gently keep the talar pins in position as they are driven into the bone, but do this carefully because too much pressure may cause the pins to permanently bind in the cutting guide.
  - Two more pins are placed in the medial and lateral gutter.
    - Their mediolateral position is determined on the fluoroscopic image of the final cutting block position.
    - These pins protect the malleoli.
  - If a lamina spreader was used to distract the joint, it will interfere with the pin placement.

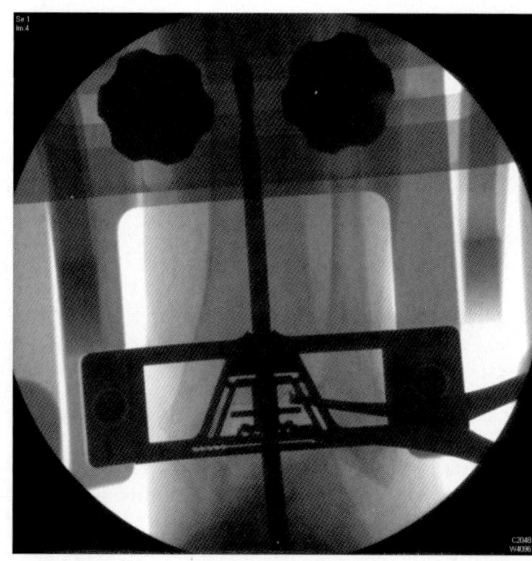

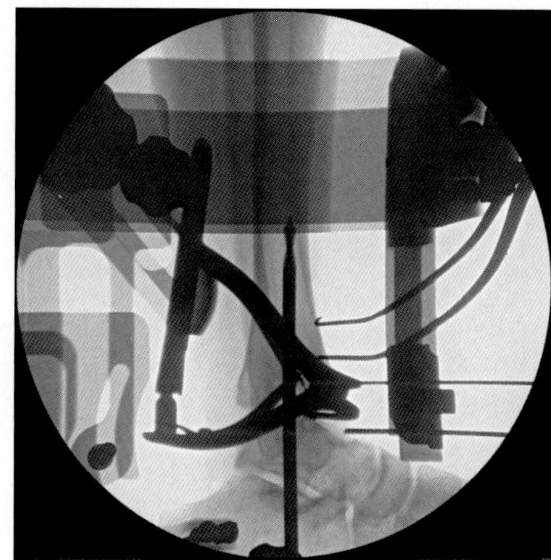

A B

TECH FIG 4 • **A.** The cutting guide has been placed over the ankle and centered on the drill. **B.** A lateral view of the cutting guides with the saw and "dummy" blade in place gives the surgeon the amount of bone resected on the top of the talus and the bottom of the tibia.

  - Try to keep it in place long enough to get enough pins in so that when the lamina spreader is removed, the correction is maintained.
- Withdraw the axial reference drill.
- Anti-rotation drill
  - The anti-rotation drill corresponding to the cutting block is used to drill the anti-rotation slot in the tibia (the sagittal prominence on the tibial base plate).
- Bone resection
  - With the soft tissues protected, make the tibial and talar cuts.
  - The bone resection should go all the way through the posterior cortex for each cut. It may not be possible on the initial pass, depending on the height of the cutting block and the particular saw used. After the initial cut, the cutting block can typically be lowered to complete the cuts, or the cuts can be freehand after the initial cuts. Obviously, avoid plunging the saw blade. Release the Achilles support to help prevent the flexor hallucis longus from being forced anteriorly and cut with the saw. Gently tapping the saw on the posterior cortex is usually possible to confirm that there is still cortex in place.
  - Once the posterior cortex has been penetrated for all cuts, the cutting guide and its pins can be removed.
- The resected bone is evacuated from the joint.
  - A toothless lamina spreader may be used to facilitate accessing the most posterior bone.
  - Avoid levering on the malleoli with the instruments, as they may break.
  - A rongeur and an angled curette are ideal to remove the bone.
  - A fine reciprocating saw may be necessary to morselize the resected bone to facilitate removing all of the bone. Avoid cutting into the prepared tibial and talar surfaces with this saw, and protect the malleoli.
- Tibial reaming
  - Secure the reamer tip to its shaft within the joint (TECH FIG 5). A toothless lamina spreader may be required to facilitate securing the reamer tip.
  - Advance the reamer. We typically use four segments for the stem extension; this requires reaming 55 mm into the tibia.
  - Extract the reamer tip from the joint. When the wrench is placed on the reamer tip, avoid activating the driver, as it will spin the reamer and the wrench, which then may fracture a malleolus. Keep your fingers off the trigger during this portion. With the wrench secured to the reamer tip and firmly held with one hand, set the driver for reverse and disengage the shaft from the tip, thereby protecting the malleoli. Extract the reamer tip from the joint and withdraw the reamer shaft from the plantar foot.
- Talar preparation
  - Secure the talar alignment guide sleeve to the plantar aspect of the foot plate.
  - Advance the talar positioning guide through this sleeve to the prepared talar surface.

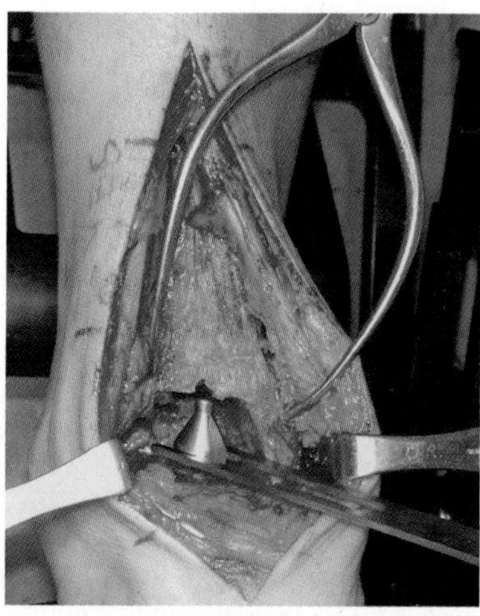

TECH FIG 5 • Reamer tip being assembled onto reamer to ream out distal tibia.

- Secure the talar pin guide to the positioning guide and place the talar pin. Check to see if the pin will be appropriately placed in the prepared talar surface; if not, then the talar pin guide affords multiple options for pin positioning. Alternatively, the pin may be placed in the "0" position and then the talar pin guide may be used over that initial pin to position a second, more appropriately positioned pin.
- We have also used the talar trial to determine optimal pin position. The talar trial may be positioned in the ideal mediolateral position and on the posterior cortex (TECH FIG 6A). The pin can then be placed through the talar trial and will then be in the ideal position. The talar trial is positioned on the talar pin and a lateral fluoroscopic view confirms that the talar component will be in the desired position.
- Optimally, the talar pin (which is the drill guide for the talar stem) is just posterior midpoint to the center of the calcaneal posterior facet. In the radiograph shown in Techniques Figure 6B, the component and talar pin are too far posterior. The talar trial and pin were moved anteriorly before drilling the talar stem hole. The new correct position is seen on the intraoperative films at the end of the case (TECH FIG 6C).
- This also determines which of the two stem sizes is to be used. The 10-mm stem can typically be attached to the talar component on the back table and the talar dome–stem combination may be inserted simultaneously. For the 14-mm stem, we typically place this stem first and then attach the talar dome separately.
- Remove the talar trial and ream the talar stem guide pin to either 10 mm or 14 mm (TECH FIG 6D).

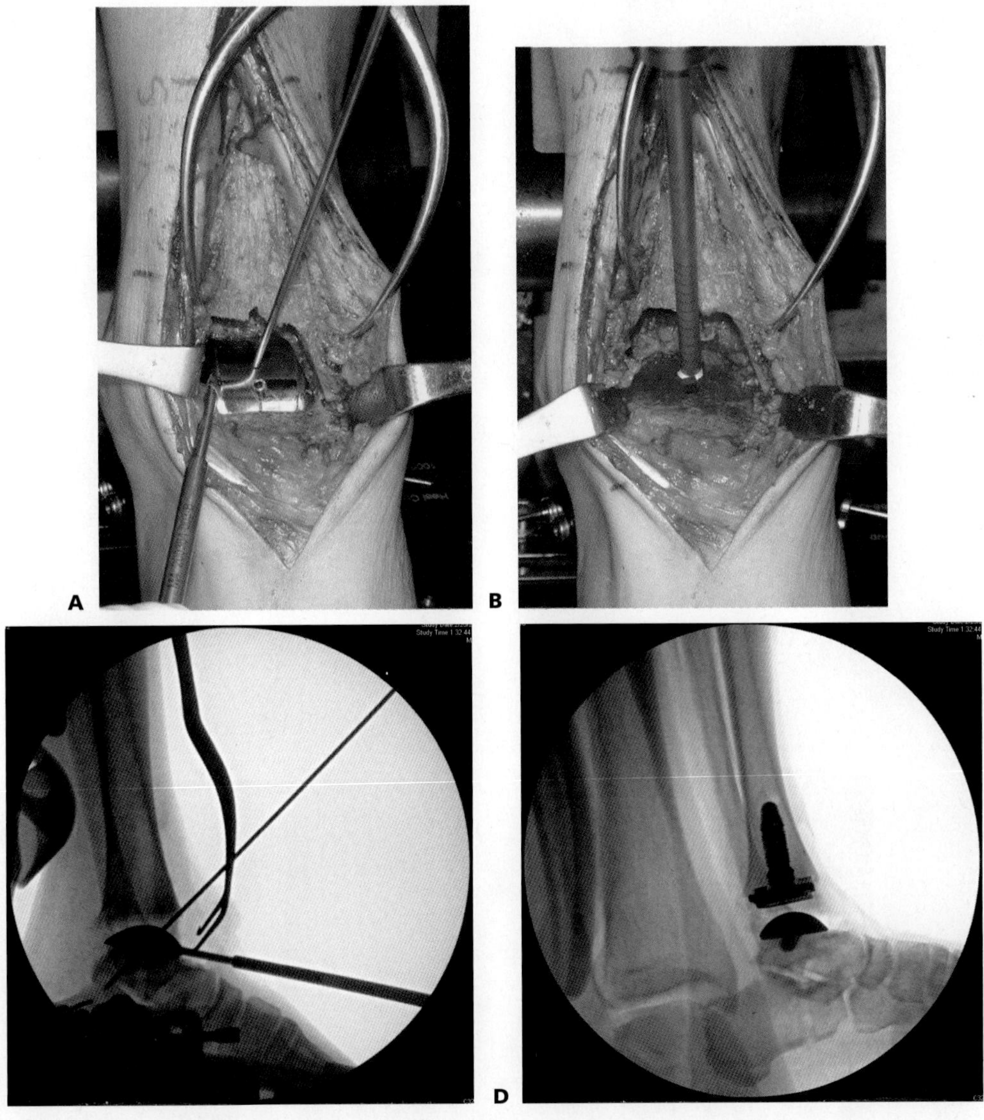

TECH FIG 6 • **A.** Talar component trial with hole and talar stem guide pin through it to determine position of stem. **B.** Cannulated drill being used over guide pin to create hole for stem. **C.** Lateral view of talar component with the talar stem guide through it. The guide and prosthesis are too far posterior and were brought forward. **D.** Final intraoperative lateral view showing that the prosthesis was moved forward and is in the correct position.

COMPONENT IMPLANTATION

- Assemble the tibial stem within the joint.
  - We routinely leave the ankle plantarflexed, assemble the first two segments of the tibial stem on the back table, and insert them into the reamed tibia with the corresponding wrench (TECH FIG 7A).
  - Return the ankle to the neutral position in which the tibia was reamed and introduce the "X-screw driver" from the plantar foot while the next tibial stem segment is positioned within the joint using the corresponding clip (TECH FIG 7B). A toothless lamina spreader to gently distract the joint may be needed to introduce the next segment.
  - Using the X-screw driver and while securing the wrench holding the other two segments in the tibia, secure the third segment to the stem (TECH FIG 7C). Be sure to hold the wrench that is stabilizing the two segments already in the tibia; if the third segment is advanced and secured and then turned, the wrench could impact the malleolus and break it.
  - Remove the X-screw driver and place the rod impactor from the plantar foot to advance the three-segment stem into the tibia (TECH FIG 7D). Obtaining a radiograph at this point can help ensure the correct angle of placement in this varus ankle (TECH FIG 7E). Be sure

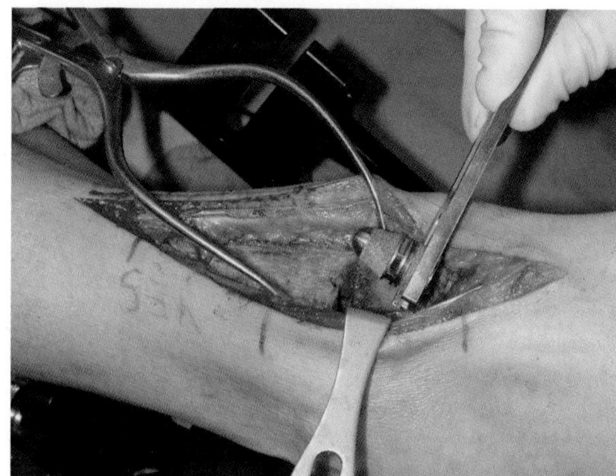
A

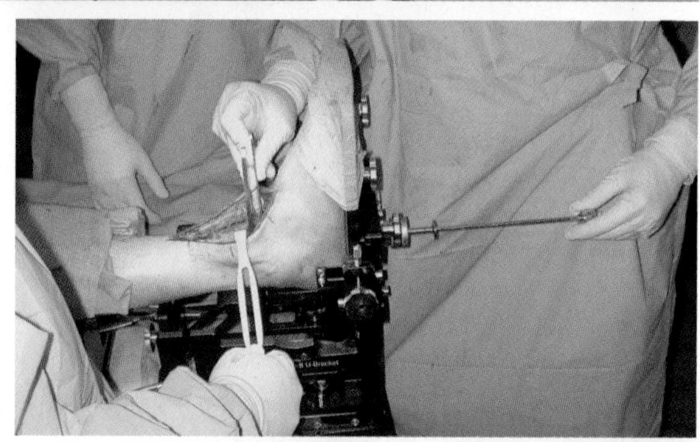
C

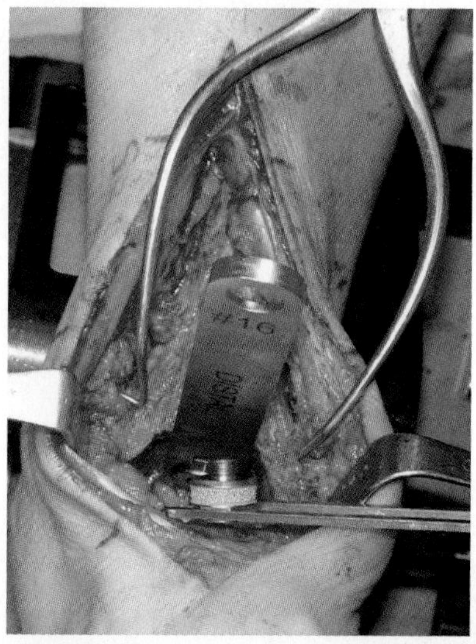

B

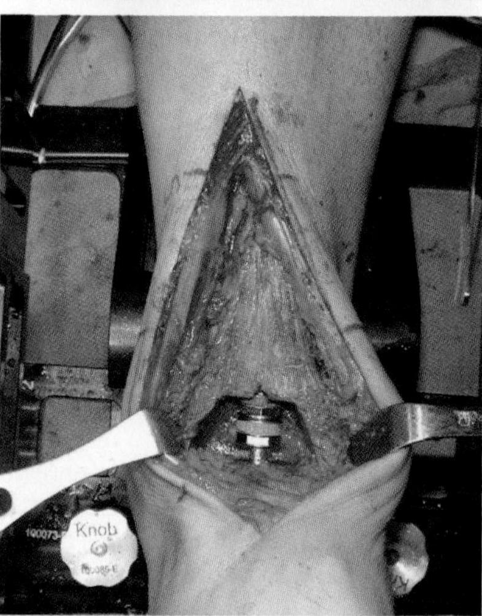

D

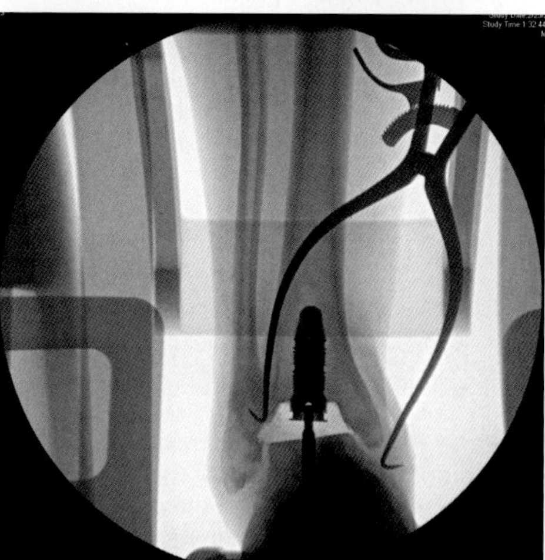
E

TECH FIG 7 • **A.** The foot is plantarflexed to allow insertion of the cone piece with one mid-stem cylinder attached. **B.** Wrench holding already inserted pieces in place while another mid-stem component is being inserted. **C.** X-screw driver being inserted into stem component to screw it in place. **D.** Stem components inserted waiting for wrench to be attached before tapping stem up into tibia **E.** AP view of stem just before wrench is attached and stem is pushed up into tibia.

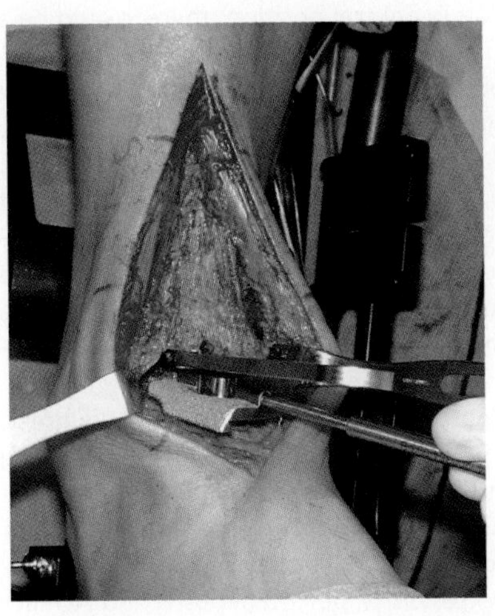

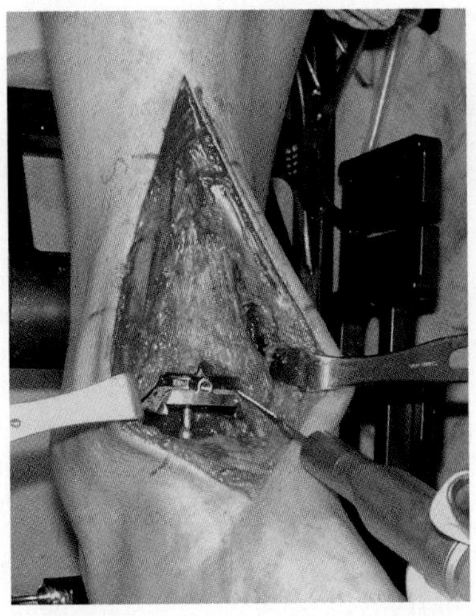

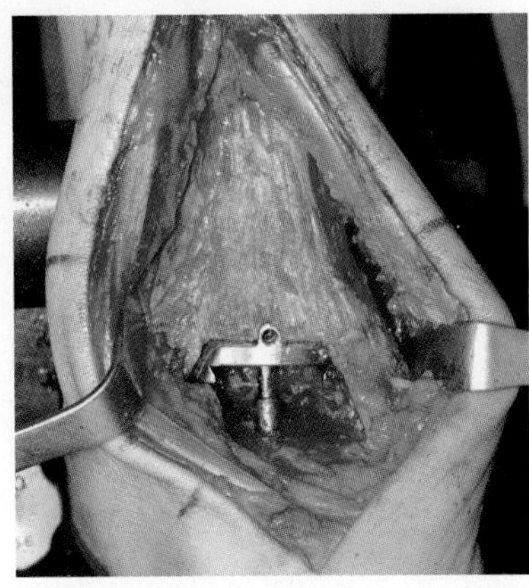

TECH FIG 8 • **A.** Base plate of tibial component being inserted onto base of stem. Note male Morse taper. **B.** Trimming away of bone using small reciprocating saw to ensure final fit. **C.** Base plate with stem being tapped up into tibia.

to attach the appropriate wrench to the third segment while impacting the stem to avoid having the stem advance too far into the tibia.

- Repeat the steps to attach the fourth segment to the third segment. Add additional segments as needed. We typically use four segments.
- The final segment is different from the others in that it houses the female portion of the Morse taper. It also has a small hole that indicates proper rotation. Be sure this segment is aligned and rotated properly. Then the entire stem is fully seated with its corresponding wrench using the rod impactor.

- Tibial base plate
  - Introduce the tibial base plate into the joint (TECH FIG 8A).
  - Withdraw the rod impactor from the stem slightly, allowing the tibial base plate to be positioned, and then use the rod impactor to secure the base plate to the stem. The tibial base plate is secured to the stem by means of a Morse taper (TECH FIG 8A).
  - Once the Morse taper is secured, remove the wrench on the stem and the composite base plate and stem combination is ready to be fully seated. Make sure there is enough room for the base plate, and trim out any bone on the sides, which could lead to a malleolus fracture (TECH FIG 8B).
  - During this step, rotation of the tibial component must be controlled. A narrow handle attaches to the anterior aspect of the base plate to control rotation as the tibial component is impacted. When the component is fully seated it should rest snugly in the mortise (TECH FIG 8C).
- Talar component
  - In our opinion, this is the most challenging step of the procedure, particularly if the joint was distracted to minimize bone resection or to correct deformity. In this situation, the joint space is quite tight by design, to achieve optimal soft tissue balance and ligament tension.
  - We routinely assemble a 10-mm stem to the talar dome component on the back table for the size 2 and 3 prosthesis, using the dedicated assembly device to secure the Morse taper.
  - Typically, a 14-mm stem is too long to be connected to the talar dome component before implantation. Therefore, we place the 14-mm talar stem first for size 4 and up if there is enough depth to the talus and seat it to the thin rib wrench that is flush with the prepared talar surface (TECH FIG 9). Since the Morse taper has not been secured, the rib wrench must remain under the 14-mm talar stem.
  - The joint must then be gently distracted with a lamina spreader, followed by insertion of the talar dome component. The toothless lamina spreader may need to go under the talar dome component to obtain the distraction, while the talar component is carefully forced posteriorly into position. A handle attached to the talar dome component facilitates driving the talar dome posteriorly. A protective plastic sleeve inserted onto the tibial base plate protects the talar dome from being scratched.

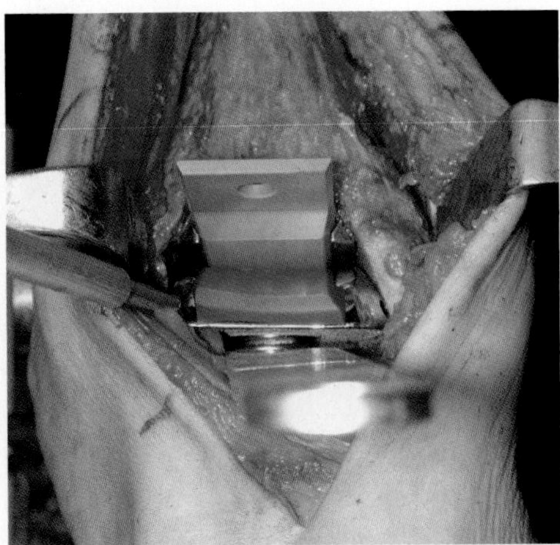

TECH FIG 9 • Fourteen-millimeter stem inserted first with rib wrench underneath and component impacted onto stem. Rib wrench prevents stem from being impacted before Morse tape is seated. Plastic trial protects talar dome surface.

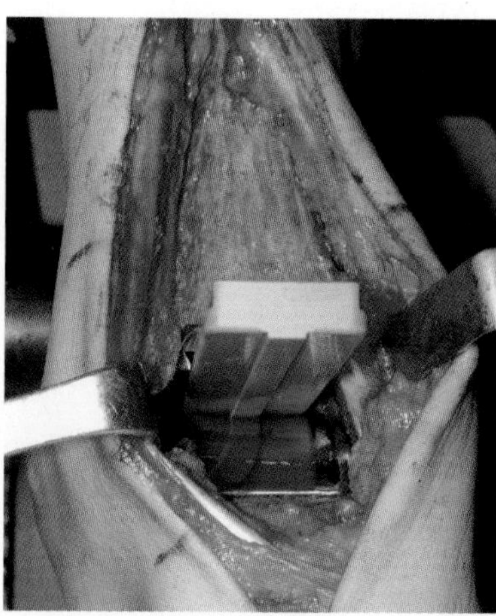

TECH FIG 10 • Trial in place to determine final thickness of final polyethylene component.

- Once the talar dome component seats on the stem, use the talar dome impactor to secure the Morse taper, with the rib wrench still between the talar dome component and the prepared talar surface.
- Remove the rib wrench and inspect the interface between talar dome and stem to ensure that the two talar components are securely attached. Use the impactor to fully seat the talar component.
- While impacting the talar component, use the handle that inserts into the talar dome to control subtle changes in rotation of the talar component.

- Polyethylene insertion
  - The polyethylene trials determine optimal polyethylene thickness (TECH FIG 10).
  - We routinely remove the leg from the leg holder and obtain AP and lateral fluoroscopic images at this stage to confirm proper position and balance of the components.
  - With the ankle in neutral position, there should be a balance with varus and valgus stress. If not, the polyethylene thickness may be inappropriate or, more likely, balance needs to be established. Typically, the medial joint (deltoid ligament) is too tight. Traditionally, we have performed a lateral ligament reconstruction (modified Brostrom or Brostrom-Evans); however, in our more recent experience, we have been successful in rebalancing the ankle with a deltoid ligament release (described above) and increasing the polyethylene thickness.
  - The ankle should dorsiflex to at least 5 degrees, preferably 10 degrees beyond neutral. If not, the polyethylene thickness may be too thick. If the polyethylene thickness is appropriate and the foot cannot be dorsiflexed to 90 degrees, consider a gastrocnemius recession or percutaneous tendo Achilles lengthening.
  - Using the dedicated polyethylene insertion device, insert the polyethylene (TECH FIG 11A). In our experience, the polyethylene will engage the tibial base plate's locking mechanism most effectively with the following maneuvers:
    - Have an assistant or co-surgeon distract the joint.
    - During the initial portion of the insertion, gently pull the insertion device into slight plantarflexion, thus driving the polyethylene into the tibial base plate's locking mechanism.
    - Once the polyethylene has cleared the superior dome of the talar component, ease off on the plantarflexion of the insertion device and have the assistant or co-surgeon compress the joint, thereby forcing the polyethylene into the locking mechanism.
    - Remove the insertion device and fully seat the polyethylene with the dedicated impactor. With that accomplished, the prosthesis should be fully seated (TECH FIG 11B).
- Obtain final AP and lateral fluoroscopic views of the valgus ankle (TECH FIG 12).

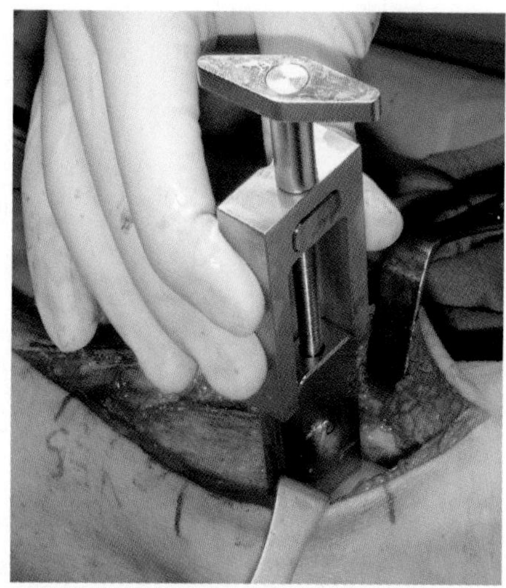

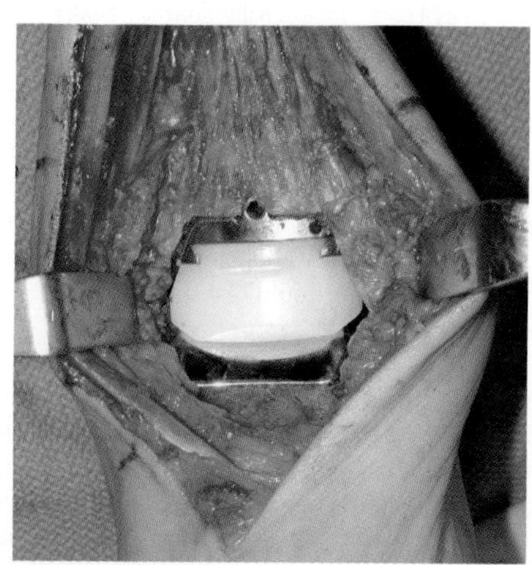

TECH FIG 11 • **A.** Polyethylene insertion device that screws down and pushes polyethylene onto tibial component tracks. **B.** Final component in position.

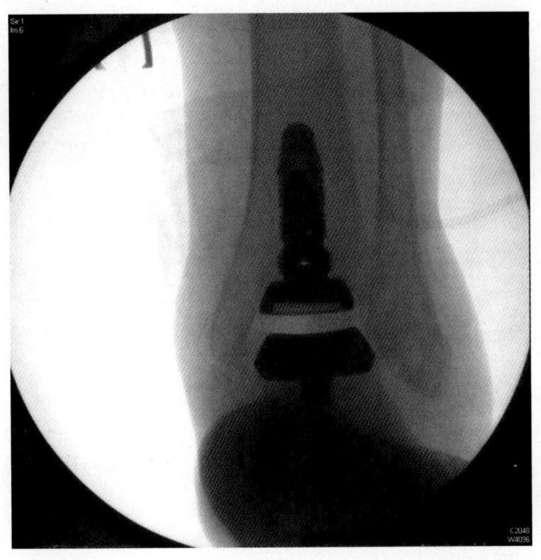

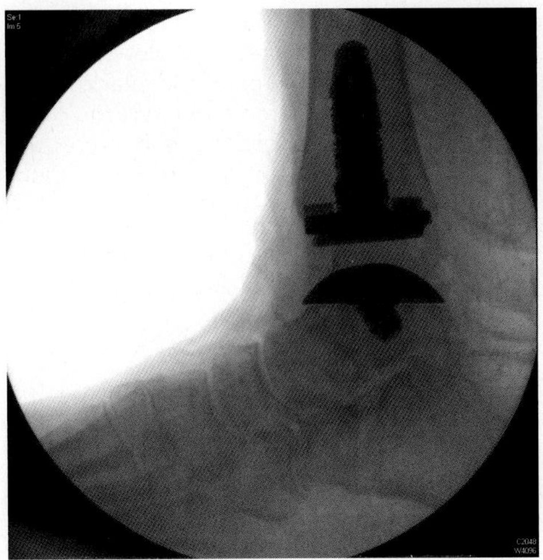

TECH FIG 12 • A, B. Final AP and lateral films taken in the operating room showing correction of initial valgus deformity.

CLOSURE

- Thoroughly irrigate the joint and implant with sterile saline.
- Reapproximate the capsule. We routinely use a drain.
- Release the tourniquet and obtain meticulous hemostasis.
- Reapproximate the extensor retinaculum while protecting the deep and superficial peroneal nerves.
- Irrigate the subcutaneous layer with sterile saline and then reapproximate it.
- Reapproximate the skin to a tensionless closure.
- Apply sterile dressings on the wounds, adequate padding, and a short-leg cast with the ankle in neutral position.

PEARLS AND PITFALLS

Equinus contracture	▪ Since the initial tibial and talar preparation is performed using a single monoblock cutting guide, an equinus contracture will lead to excessive and undesired resection from the posterior talus. Therefore, perform a tendo Achilles lengthening to get the talus in a neutral position before securing the leg in the leg holder. If the heel does not rest fully on the leg holder's foot plate with the toes touching the foot plate, there is equinus.
Rotation	▪ The foot and leg may be well positioned in the leg holder and fluoroscopy may suggest proper alignment, but the ankle may still be malrotated, leading to symmetric but malrotated tibial and talar preparation. Place a thin osteotome in the medial gutter of the tibiotalar joint to determine optimal rotation; the osteotome should be parallel to the side of the leg holder.
Varus ankle and valgus malalignment	▪ Balance the ankle before placing it into the leg holder. For varus perform the medial release; for valgus, the ankle is usually loose and simply needs the lamina spreader to realign the talus within the ankle mortise.
Place the ankle at the center of the fluoroscopic monitor.	▪ The ankle must be in the center of the monitor or alignment cannot be accurately determined. Therefore, first place the ankle in the center of the fluoroscopic beam, and then make adjustments. Note also that as adjustments are made to the operating table to optimize alignment, the ankle may "drift" from the center of the monitor and will need to be recentered in the fluoroscopic beam while alignment is being set.
Be sure alignment is proper before any reading is made off the fluoroscopy.	▪ Assessing the position of any instrument fluoroscopically demands that proper alignment has been confirmed first. For example, when positioning the cutting block relative to the reference drill, first check that alignment is perfect, and then assess the cutting block position.
Returning the ankle to neutral position while it is in the leg holder	▪ The stop on the side of the leg holder must be set before the ankle is plantarflexed with the frame or else it is difficult to return to the same neutral position.
Morse taper	▪ The tibial base plate and the talar dome components attach to their respective stems with Morse tapers; be sure these are fully secured before seating either composite (combination main component and stem) fully.

Insertion of talar component	■ May be difficult when joint distraction with lamina spreaders was used to minimize bone resection. However, judicious use of lamina spreaders is again possible to facilitate insertion of the talar component. When using a 10-mm talar stem, we typically have ample room to insert the combination talar dome and stem composite that was attached on the back table; however, we usually have to independently insert the 14-mm stem followed by the talar dome component, securing the Morse taper within the joint.

POSTOPERATIVE CARE

- Overnight stay
- Nasal oxygen while in hospital
- Touch-down weight bearing on the cast is permitted, but elevation is encouraged as much as possible.
- Follow up in 2 to 3 weeks for cast change and suture removal
- The patient returns 6 weeks after surgery for cast removal and weight-bearing radiographs of the ankle.

OUTCOMES

- While some recently reported outcomes are based on high-level evidence, results of total ankle arthroplasty are almost uniformly derived from level IV evidence.
- Functional outcome using commonly used scoring systems for total ankle arthroplasty (AOFAS [Kofoed, Mazur] and NJOH [Buechel-Pappas]) suggest uniform improvement in all studies, with follow-up scores ranging from 70 to 90 points (maximum 100 points).
- Patient satisfaction rates for total ankle arthroplasty exceed 90%, although follow-up data for patient satisfaction often do not exceed 5 years.
- Overall survivorship analysis for currently available implants, designating removal of a metal component or conversion to arthrodesis as the endpoint, ranges from about 90% to 95% at 5 to 6 years and 80% to 92% at 10 to 12 years.
- At the time of this writing there are no published results available for the INBONE™ total ankle arthroplasty.

COMPLICATIONS

- Infection (superficial or deep)
- Neuralgia (superficial or deep peroneal nerve; rarely tibial nerve)
- Delayed wound healing
- Wound dehiscence
- Persistent pain despite optimal orthopaedic examination and radiographic appearance of implants
- Osteolysis
- Subsidence
- Malleolar or distal tibial stress fracture
- Implant fracture (including polyethylene)

REFERENCES

1. Bonnin M, Judet T, Colombier JA, et al. Mid-term results of the Salto total ankle prosthesis: report of 98 cases with minimum two years follow up. Clin Orthop Relat Res 2004;424:6–18.
2. Gougoulias N, Khanna A, Maffulli N. How successful are current ankle replacements? A systematic review of the literature. Clin Orthop Relat Res 2010;468:199–208.
3. Haddad SL, Coetzee JC, Estok R, et al. Intermediate and long-term outcomes of total ankle arthroplasty and ankle arthrodesis: a systematic review of the literature. J Bone Joint Surg Am 2007;89A:1899–1905.

Chapter 74 TNK Total Ankle Arthroplasty

Yasuhito Tanaka and Yoshinori Takakura

DEFINITION

- Total ankle arthroplasty (TAA) is indicated for end stage osteoarthritis or rheumatoid arthritis.[2]
- The semi-constrained TNK ankle is a two-component total ankle implant (**FIG 1**).[10,11]
- It is made of alumina ceramic, and its interface with bone is coated with alumina beads. This prosthesis combines biocompatibility of alumina ceramics with a design that facilitates fixation to bone.

ANATOMY

- The physiologic alignment of the tibial plafond is nearly perpendicular to the anterior tibial shaft axis in the coronal plane and has a slight posterior slope relative to the lateral tibial longitudinal axis. To match this natural anatomy, the TNK ankle's tibial component is ideally implanted perpendicular to the anterior logitudinal axis of the tibia with a 10 degree posterior slope. The talar component is ideally set parallel to the ground or plantar aspect of the weight-bearing foot.

PATHOGENESIS

- Ankle osteoarthritis (OA) is most commonly posttraumatic in origin, often secondary to intra-articular fractures with cartilage injury and/or malunions of the tibial plafond.[1,6]
- Occasionally, severe pes planovalgus deformity, particularly that associated with stage IV posterior tibial tendon insufficiency, may result in a valgus-type ankle OA.[5]
- In our experience, a varus-type ankle OA may develop, typically characterized by varus deformity of the tibial plafond.[3,4]
- Advanced rheumatoid arthritis (RA) affects the ankle in 25% of patients.[8]
  - The talonavicular, subtalar, and calcaneocuboid joints are involved in 29%, 39%, and the calcaneocuboid joint in 25%, respectively.[7]

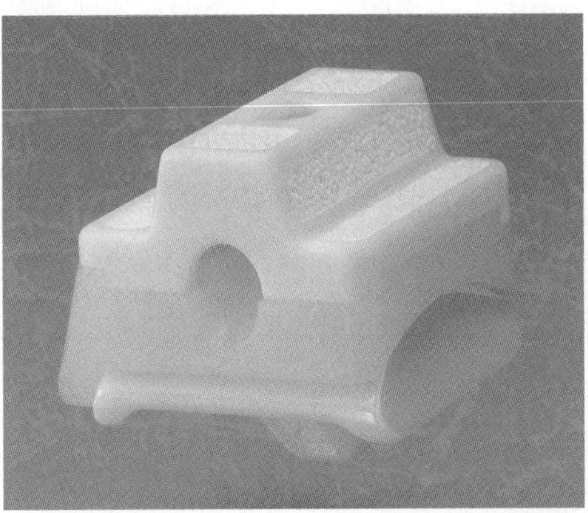

FIG 1 • The TNK ankle is a semiconstrained artificial joint made of alumina ceramic.

NATURAL HISTORY

- Irrespective of cause, OA is characterized by a gradual, progressive, and diffuse loss of articular cartilage with eventual complete eburnation down to subchondral bone on both sides of the joint. RA originates from an inflammatory process of the joint's synovial tissue.
  - We routinely use Larsen's grading scheme for evaluating the stage of RA.
  - TAA is indicated for Larsen's grades 3 and 4.
  - In our opinion, grade 5 (mutilans-type of RA) is contraindication for TAA.

PATIENT HISTORY AND PHYSICAL FINDINGS

- Osteoarthritis
  - Patients typically complain of ankle pain with weight-bearing, particularly start of pain in the first few steps and also with prolonged walking. With progressive OA, pain with ankle motion and ankle edema become more common. Ankle stiffness is associated with advanced stages of OA.
- Rheumatoid arthritis
  - Morning stiffness, symmetrical joint pain, and joint swelling in the hands, wrists, and feet are distinctive symptoms of RA.
  - In our experience, the ankle is usually not involved until advanced stages of RA.
  - Typically, patients complain of pain with ankle range of motion (ROM) and swelling.
  - Because RA may affect the talonavicular joint in isolation, ankle and talonvicular joint involvement must be distinguished. Careful examination of ankle and hindfoot palpation and stress usually allows differentiation between tibiotalar and talonavicular RA, but radiographic confirmation is often warranted.
- Advanced RA of the ankle associated with pes planovalgus often has concommittent posterior tibial tendon tendinopathy and spring ligament pathology.

IMAGING AND OTHER DIAGNOSTIC STUDIES

- Weight-bearing AP and lateral radiographs of the ankle determine the extent of arthritis and deformity at the ankle. Preoperatively, we determine the appropriate implant size using dedicated template for the TNK system.
  - Generally, we select the largest possible component to optimize the biomechanical advantage of maximum surface contact between implant and bone.
  - In complex cases, we utilize computer simulation to more accurately template the implants (**FIG 2**).
- Weight-bearing radiographs of the ipsilateral foot are important when ankle arthritis is associated with foot malalignment/deformity.

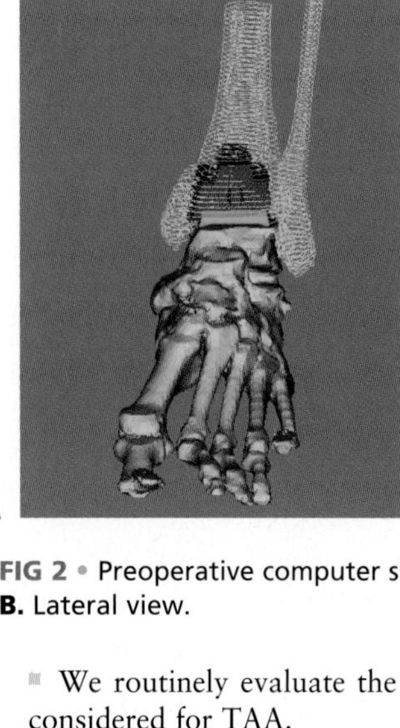

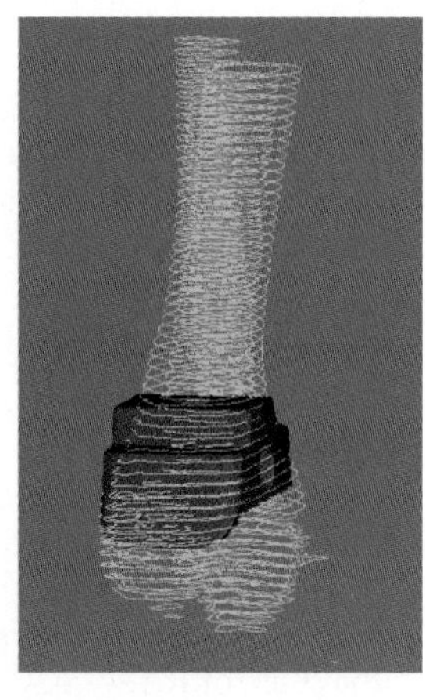

FIG 2 • Preoperative computer simulation. **A.** AP view. **B.** Lateral view.

- We routinely evaluate the hindfoot in any patient being considered for TAA.
- Occasionally, computed tomography (CT) is necessary to provide greater detail of potential subtalar pathology (**FIG 3**).
- As for laboratory tests, anticyclic citrullinated peptide (CCP) antibodies and galactose deficient IgG are useful to an early diagnosis.

NONOPERATIVE MANAGEMENT

- Osteoarthritis
  - Activity modification; bracing
  - Some patients benefit from heat treatments and ultrasound.
  - NSAIDs
  - Judicious use of corticosteroid injections
  - Viscosupplementation
- Rheumatoid arthritis
  - Anti-inflammatory medications
  - Systemic rheumatoid medical management through a rheumatologist
  - Bracing
  - Judicious use of corticosteroid injections

SURGICAL MANAGEMENT

- We favor TAA over tibiotalar arthrodesis for bilateral ankle arthritis and ankle arthritis associated with hindfoot stiffness/arthritis. In 1975, we developed a metal prototype of our TNK ankle.[9]
- In 1980, because of improvements in materials and operative procedures, we developed a TNK ankle made of alumina ceramic.[10] However, there were problems with the interface between bone and alumina ceramic, and the clinical results of the alumina ceramic TNK ankle were not satisfactory.

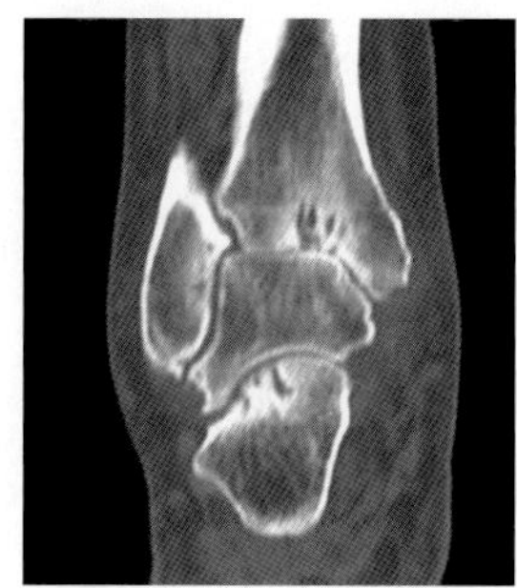

FIG 3 • CT is helpful for detecting subtalar lesions.

- In 1991, we developed a bead-coated alumina ceramic TNK ankle[11] and the current design has been modified from this version of the TNK implant.

Preoperative Planning

- Three sizes of the TNK prosthesis are available: small, medium, and large (**FIG 4**).
- We template for the TNK implant based on the preoperative weightbearing ankle radiographs, marking the proposed resection level. The planned resection line is 8 to 15 mm above the distal tibial surface, and has a 10 posterior slope.
- The antero-posterior dimension of the tibia plafond is measured to ensure optimal support for the tibial implant. While we favor noncemented implants, we rarely consider cement fixation for patients with osteopenic bone or bone defects that do not allow full support for the prosthesis with standard tibial and/or talar resections. In an effort to limit initial micromotion of the implant and to promote effective bone ingrowth, we routinely secure the prosthesis to bone with screw fixation.

Positioning

- Supine position
- Thigh tourniquet
- Bolster under the ipsilateral hip to prevent excessive external rotation of the operated extremity.

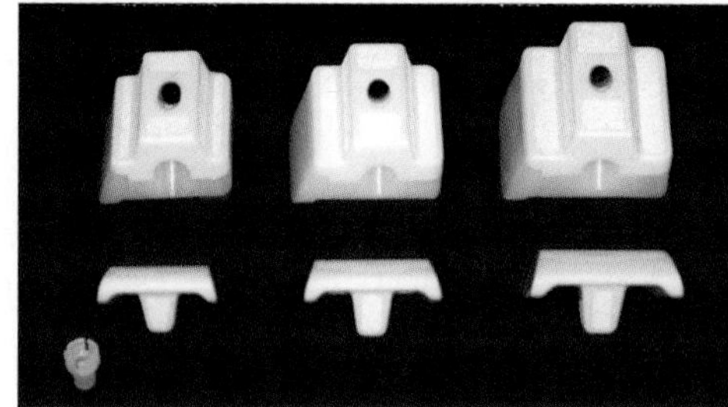

FIG 4 • Small, medium, and large sizes of the TNK ankle.

APPROACH

- A 10-cm longitudinal incision is centered over the anterior ankle. The extensor retinaculum is divided over the interval between the tibialis anterior and extensor hallucis longus tendons.
- The dorsalis pedis artery and the deep peroneal nerve are retracted to the lateral side.
- An anterior ankle capsulotomy is performed.
- In RA, a comprehensive synovectomy is performed, from the extensor tendon sheath(s) to the talonavicular joint.

TIBIAL PREPARATION

- Tibiotalar osteophytes are removed to expose the anterior joint. Based on preoperative templating and level of the tibial plafond, the tibial resection level is determined. The tibial cutting guide is positioned at the desired tibial resection level (TECH FIG 1A).
- The external tibial alignment guide attached to the cutting block is oriented in line with the tibial shaft axis and the center of the patella.
- Once properly oriented, the tibial cutting guide is secured to the tibia with a fixation pin and the distal tibial cut is performed with an oscillating saw advanced through the cutting block (TECH FIG 1B,C).
- Although we recommend 10 degrees of posterior slope, we caution that excessive posterior slope is detrimental.
- To maintain support for the prosthesis we avoid violating the posterior tibial cortex.
- The medial malleolar preparation is performed next.

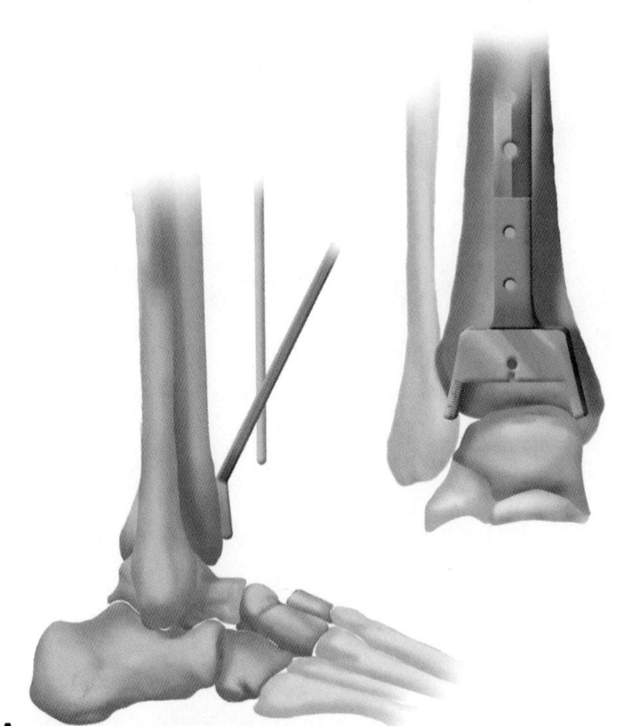

A

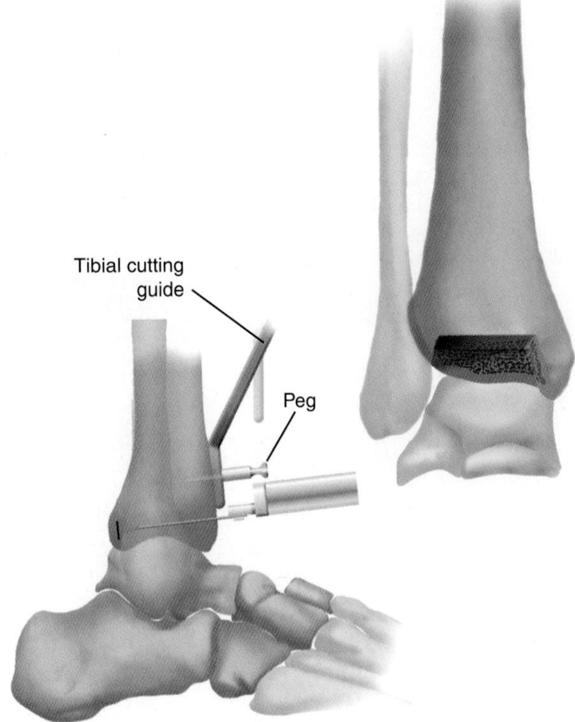

B

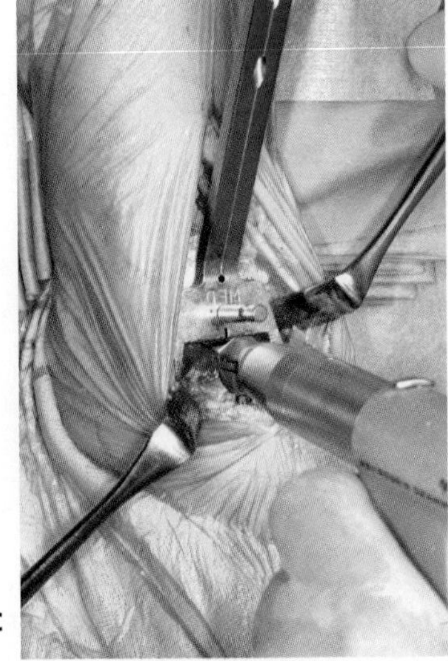

C

TECH FIG 1 • Osteotomy of the tibia. **A.** Tibial cutting guide and alignment bar. The alignment bar on the tibial cutting guide is adjusted to the center of the patella. **B.** Osteotomy is performed with 10 degrees of anterior opening. **C.** Osteotomy using a bone saw.

TALAR PREPARATION

- The superior surface of the talar cutting guide is brought into contact with the resected distal tibia, with traction applied to the ankle in approximately 10 degrees of plantar flexion.
- Proper alignment is confirmed using the external tibial alignment guide as was done prior to the tibial resection. The talar cutting is secured to the talus with a fixation pin.
- Using an oscillating saw, the superior surface of the talar dome is prepared using the talar cutting guide as a reference (TECH FIG 2A,B).
- A spacer is now inserted to confirm adequate and balanced bone resection (TECH FIG 2C).
- The mediolateral talar cutting guide is properly oriented to the talus and secured. Using an oscillating saw through the capture slots of the cutting guide, 2 mm are removed from the medial and lateral talar dome (TECH FIG 2D,E).
- Resection of more than 2 mm from either side of talus must be avoided by chosing the appropriate mediolateral cutting guide and orienting it properly; excessive resection may lead to talar component subsidence.
- Next, the appropriately sized talar peg cutting guide (TECH FIG 2F) is positioned on the prepared talar surface, and the tibial peg hole is created (TECH FIG 2G).

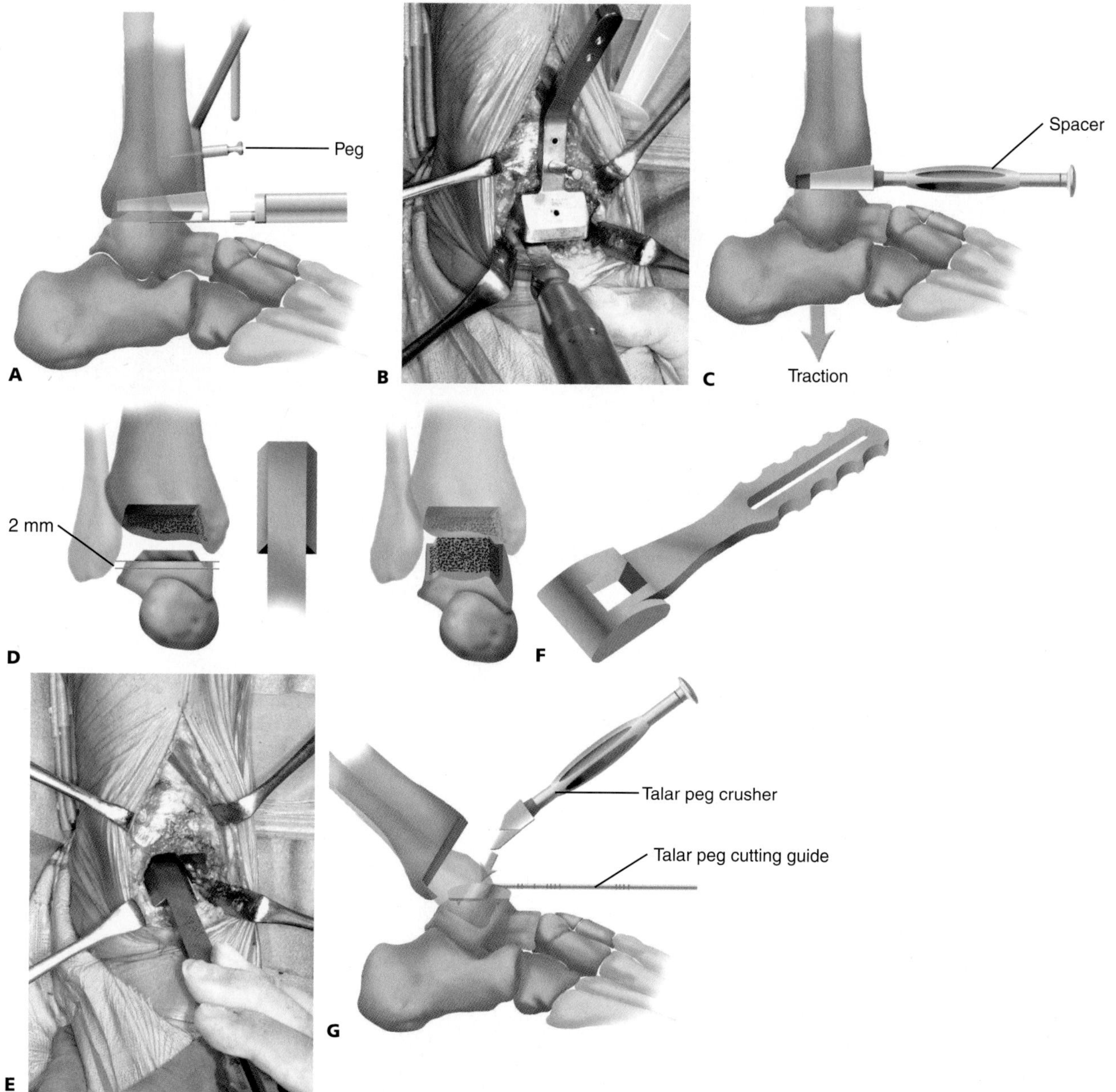

TECH FIG 2 • Osteotomy of the talus. **A.** Talar cutting guide. **B.** Osteotomy is performed parallel to a floor line. **C.** To confirm the osteotomy of the tibia and talus, a spacer is inserted under traction. **D.** The talar margin cutting guide. **E.** The talar margin is cut in a plantarflexion position of the ankle. **F.** The talar peg cutting guide. **G.** The talar peg crusher.

PREPARATION OF THE TIBIAL ANCHOR

- The talar trial corresponding to the component size is impacted with a talar impactor.
- The appropriately sized talar trial is positioned on the prepared talus and impacted.
- The tibial peg cutting guide is positioned on the anterior distal tibia (TECH FIG 3A).
  - The superior and medial aspects of the guide are aligned with the prepared tibial surface.
  - Once properly oriented with the prepared tibial surface and the talar trial, the tibial peg cutting guide is secured to the tibia (TECH FIG 3B, C).
- The tibial anchor is prepared along the inner surface of the guide.
  - We recommend preserving the posterior tibial cortex at the anchoring region mustbe left intact to prevent posterior tibial component migration (TECH FIG 3D).

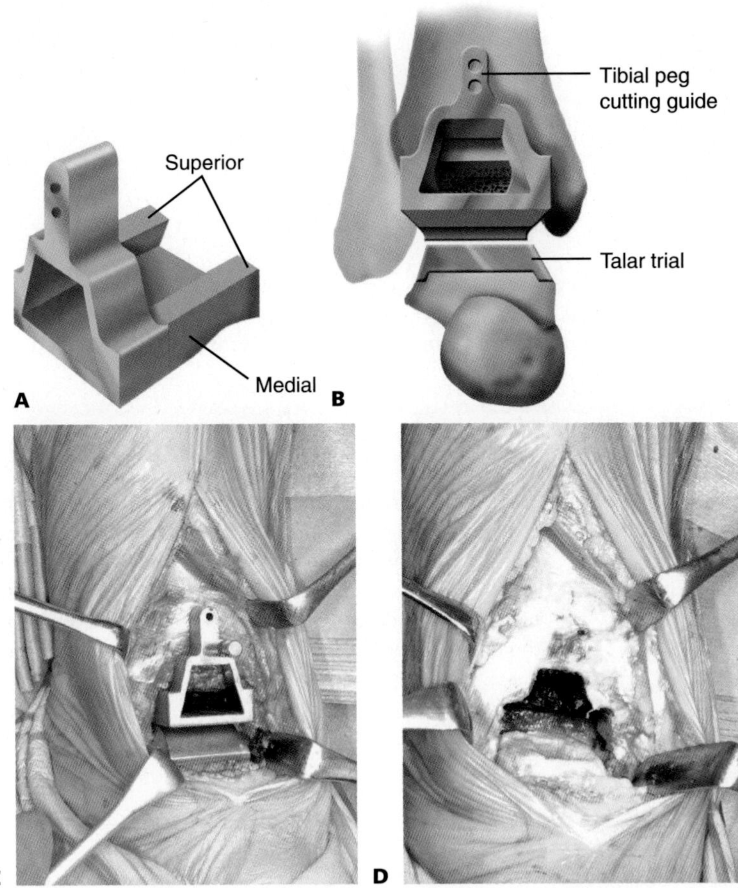

TECH FIG 3 • Osteotomy of tibial anchor region. **A.** The tibial peg cutting guide. **B.** The tibial peg cutting guide is inserted after placing the talar trial. **C.** Intraoperative view. **D.** Reaming is completed.

TRIAL AND SETTING

- The tibial trial is inserted
- Proper alignment and satisfactory ankle ROM are confirmed (TECH FIG 4A).
- Ideally, the tibial trial should be supported by both the anterior and posterior tibial cortices.
- Once optimal alignment and ROM are confirmed, the trial components are removed
- We favor applying bone marrow aspirate from the patient's iliac crest to the bone ingrowth surfaces of noncemented implants to to accelerate early bone ingrowth. (TECH FIG 4B).
- With the ankle held in plantarflexion, the final talar component is impacted using the dedicated talar impactor.
- Then, the tibial component is impacted with its specific impaction tool
- Via the screw hole in the tibial component, a 2.5-mm drill is advanced through the posterior tibial cortex.
  - A specially designed polyethylene sleeve is placed into the screw hole of the tibial component into which a 4.0-mm AO small fragment cancellous screw is inserted to secure the tibial component to the tibia (TECH FIG 4C, D).
- Any residual gapping between the bone and tibialcomponent should be filled with cancellous bone autograft.
- For patients with osteopenia, we routinely use bone cement for fixation of the components.

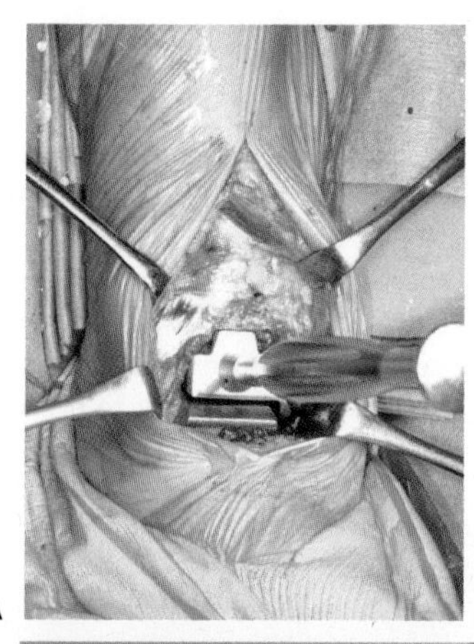

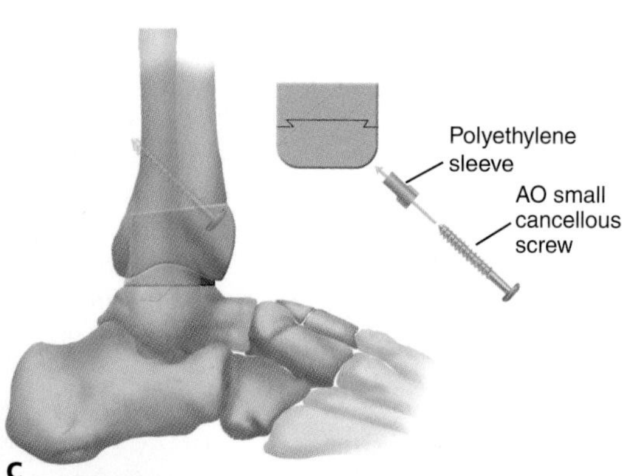

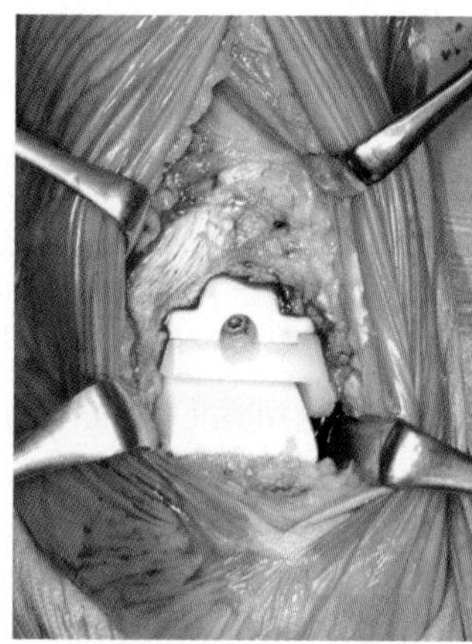

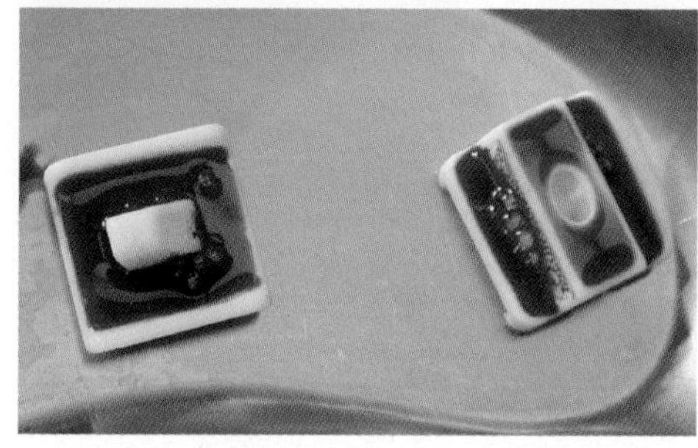

TECH FIG 4 • Trial and setting. **A.** The tibial trial is inserted. **B.** Bone marrow mounting. **C.** Screw fixation. **D.** Implantation is completed.

SUBTALAR ARTHRODESIS

- In patients with concomitant ankle and subtalar arthritis, we favor performing simultaneous TAA and subtalar arthrodesis (TECH FIG 5A, B).
- Through a 2.5-cm lateral incision over the sinus tarsi, the subtalar joint is exposed and residual articular cartilage is removed using a chisel and a curette.
- To facilitate fusion, a small diameter drill is used to penetrate the subchondral bone and increase the surface area of the subtalar joint.
- Through the anterior incision, anterior to the talar component, a standard AO cancellous screw is placed from the talar neck across the subtalar joint into the calcaneus.

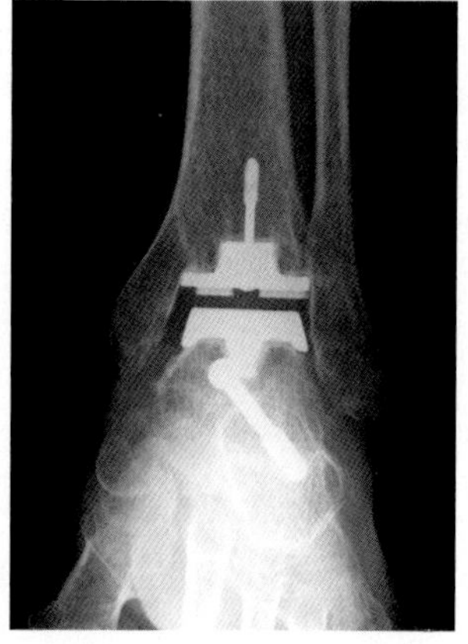

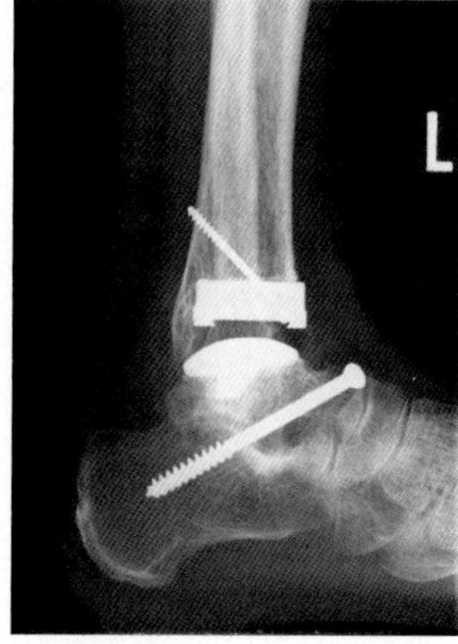

TECH FIG 5 • Subtalar arthrodesis. **A.** Postoperative AP view with subtalar arthrodesis using a single OA cancellous screw. **B.** Lateral view.

CLOSURE

- The wound(s) are thoroughly irrigated with sterile saline solution
- We routinely use a drain.
- The retinaculum and skin are reapproximated, taking care to protect the deep neurovascular bundle and superficial peroneal nerve.
- A short leg cast is applied with the ankle in a neutral position.

PEARLS AND PITFALLS

Contraindications to the TNK ankle	■ Patients planning high-impact, untreated osteoporosis, osteonecrosis of the talus, mutilans type of rheumatoid arthritis, and varus and valgus deformity of the ankle (>15 degrees); patients under the age 50 should only be considered if they have reasonable expectations and understand that they are very likely to require revision surgery in their lifetime.
Approach	■ The approach is anterior, but oriented toward the medial aspect of the ankle, because the TNK ankle does not have a fibular component. The deep peroneal nerve and the anterior tibial artery should be retracted to the lateral side.
Application of bone marrow aspirate to the bone ingrowth surfaces	■ The ideal timing to apply the bone marrow aspirate to the backside of the implants is when the marrow elements begin coagualting. Good timing of implantation is bone marrow just coagulating on the surface of the implant. In our opinion, this timing best promotes bone ingrowth.
Residual gap at the bone–prosthesis interface	■ We recommend filling this gap with autograft or even a thin cancellous wedge of bone from the patient's iliac crest.

POSTOPERATIVE CARE

- Patients with uncemented prostheses wear a cast for 3 weeks postoperatively, after which they gradually increase their active range of motion.
- During the first week, weight bearing is not allowed. In the following weeks, weight bearing to tolerance is permitted, with crutches. At 2 months postoperative, full weight bearing is initiated.
- Patients with cemented prostheses wear a cast for 2 weeks, and full weight bearing is allowed after the cast is removed.

OUTCOMES

- From 1991 to 2001, we performed 70 TNK TAAs in 62 patients (**FIG 5**).[10]
- Follow-up was possible for 67 ankles in 60 patients: 39 ankles in 36 patients with OA (osteoarthritis group), and 28 ankles in 24 patients with RA (rheumatoid arthritis group). Duration of follow-up ranged from 24 months to 134 months, with an average of 62 months.
- Cemented TAA was performed in three ankles with OA and 19 ankles with RA (**FIG 6**).
- Revision surgery was performed for three ankles in three patients: two ankles with collapse of the talus, and one infected ankle.
- Clinical evaluation was performed using our rating system,[9] in which the maximum score of 100 points is divided into 40 points for pain and 60 points for function. Satisfactory pain relief was obtained in majority of patients.

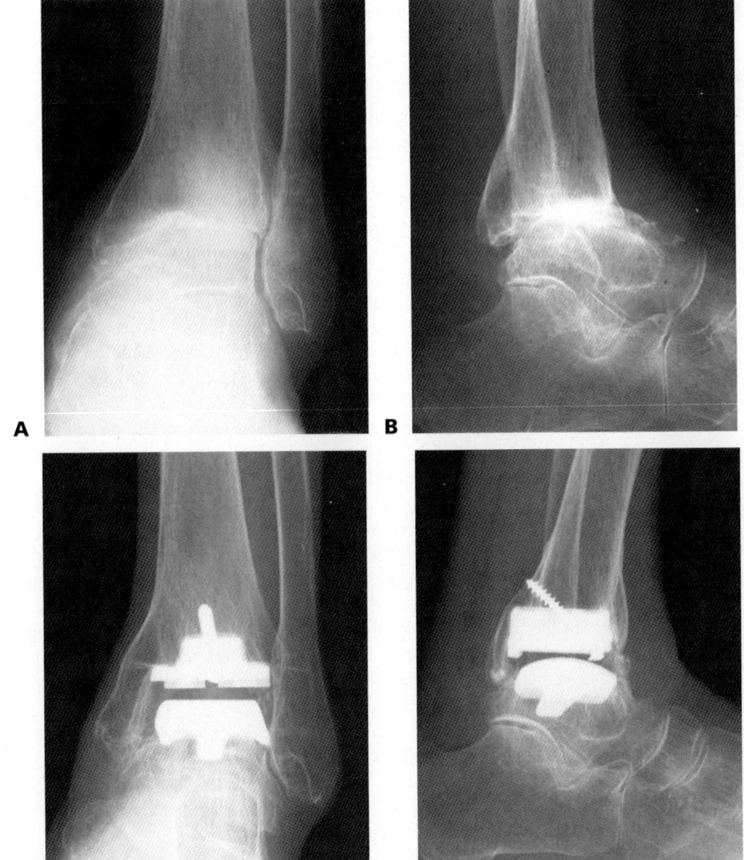

FIG 5 • The TNK ankle replacement for osteoarthritis of the ankle (noncemented replacement). **A.** Preoperative AP view. **B.** Preoperative lateral view. **C.** Postoperative AP view at 8 years. **D.** Postoperative lateral view.

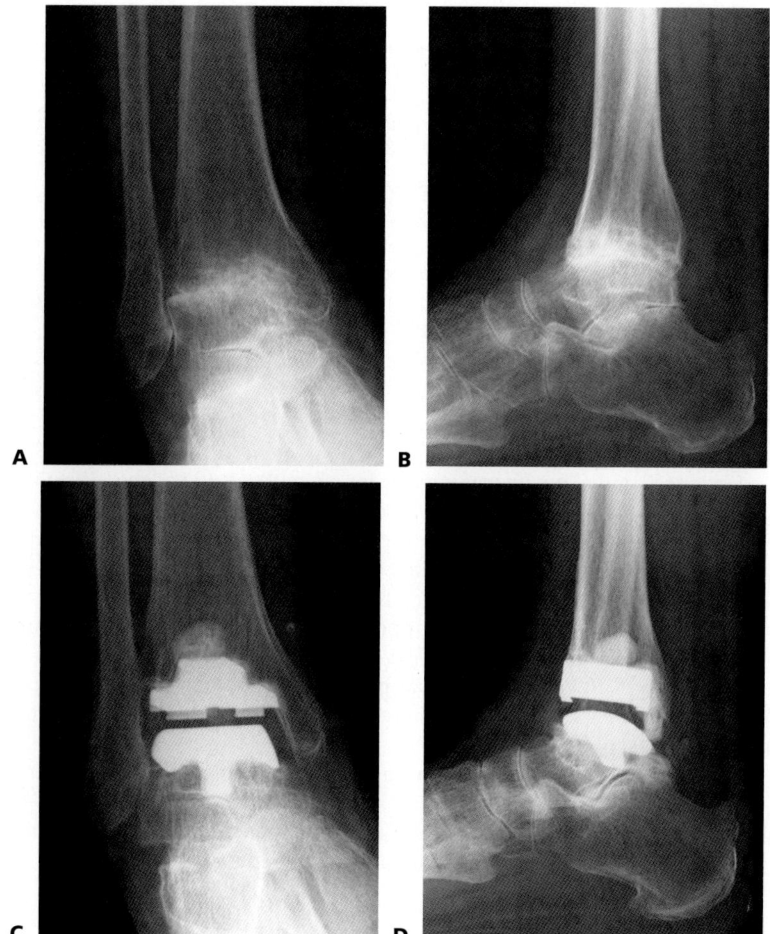

FIG 6 • The TNK ankle replacement for rheumatoid arthritis of the ankle (cemented replacement). **A.** Preoperative AP view. **B.** Preoperative lateral view. **C.** Postoperative AP view 2 years 6 months after the surgery. **D.** Postoperative lateral view.

- In the OA group, mean values of pain, function and total score improved from 14, 34, and 48 points preoperatively to 37, 49, and 86 points at last follow-up, respectively.
- In the RA group, the same mean values improved from 14, 31, and 35 points to 35, 39, and 74 points, respectively.
- Preoperative and postoperative mean ankle ROM was 28 and 33 degrees in the OA group and 22 and 22 degrees in the RA group, respectively.
- In the OA group, overall results were excellent in 24 ankles, good in 10 ankles, fair in 3 ankles, and poor in 2 ankles. In the RA group, overall results were excellent in 6 ankles, good in 12 ankles, fair in 7 ankles, and poor in 3 ankles.
- In the RA group, mean total scores (using our own ankle rating system) at the follow-up were 77 points for cemented fixation (18 ankles) and 71 points for cementless fixation (10 ankles).
- Radiography showed subsidence and loosening in four prostheses in the OA group (two tibial prostheses and two talar prostheses) and 17 prostheses in the RA group (six tibial prostheses and 11 talar prostheses).
- Although the results of the RA group were worse than those of the OA group, short- and medium-term results with bead-coated alumina ceramic prostheses were encouraging.

COMPLICATIONS

- Intraoperative fracture of the medial malleolus
- Superficial peroneal nerve palsy
- Wound edge necrosis
- Superficial infection
- Deep infection
- Loosening of the implant
- Subsidence of the implant

REFERENCES

1. Buckwalter JA, Saltzman CL. Ankle osteoarthritis: distinctive characteristics. AAOS Instr Course Lect 1999;48:233–241.
2. Easley ME, Vertullo CJ, Urban WC, et al. Total ankle arthroplasty. J Am Acad Orthop Surg 2002;10:157–167.
3. Katsui T, Takakura Y, Kitada C, et al. Roentgenographic analysis for osteoarthrosis of the ankle. J Jpn Soc Surg Foot 1980;1:52–57.
4. Monji J. Roentgenological measurement of the shape of the osteoarthritic ankle. Nippon Seikeigeka Gakkai Zasshi 1980;54:791–802.
5. Pomeroy GC, Pike RH, Beals TC, et al. Acquired flatfoot in adults due to dysfunction of the posterior tibial tendon. J Bone Joint Surg Am 1999;81A:1173–1182.
6. Saltzman CL, Salamon ML, Blanchard GM, et al. Epidemiology of ankle arthritis: report of a consecutive series of 639 patients from a tertiary orthopaedic center. Iowa Orthop J 2005;25:44–46.
7. Seltzer SE, Weissman BN, Adams DF, et al. Computed tomography of the hindfoot with rheumatoid arthritis. Arthritis Rheum 1985;28:1234–1242.
8. Spiegel TM, Spiegel JS. Rheumatoid arthritis in the foot and ankle: diagnosis, pathology, and treatment: the relationship between foot and ankle deformity and disease duration in 50 patients. Foot Ankle 1982;2:318–324.
9. Takakura Y. The total ankle prosthesis: experimental and clinical studies. J Nara Med Assoc 1977;25:582–598.
10. Takakura Y, Tanaka Y, Sugimoto K, et al. Ankle arthroplasty: a comparative study of cemented metal and uncemented ceramic prostheses. Clin Orthop Relat Res 1990;252:209–216.
11. Takakura Y, Tanaka Y, Kumai T, et al. Ankle arthroplasty using three generations of metal and ceramic prostheses. Clin Orthop Relat Res 2004;424:130–136.

Chapter 75

The Agility Total Ankle Arthroplasty

J. Chris Coetzee and Steven L. Haddad

DEFINITION

- The Agility ankle replacement is a fixed bearing device with a tibial base plate that requires a fusion between the distal tibia and fibula. This unique design feature allows a large surface area for bone ingrowth and also limits the likelihood of subsidence of the tibial component into the cancellous bone of the distal tibia.
- The tibial component is a porous-coated titanium implant designed to be positioned in 23 degrees of external rotation.
- It has an ultrahigh-molecular-weight polyethylene (UHMWPE) insert available in different thicknesses. The Agility LP uses a front-loading UHMWPE spacer, which makes insertion and revision simple.
- The talar component is a dome-shaped cobalt chrome alloy with a porous-coated undersurface. The Agility LP talar base plate covers the entire talar cut surface. The current design has six sizes and is a fixed bearing implant that is partially conforming (**FIG 1**).

ANATOMY

- The ankle joint is complex in that it involves four structures: the lower end and medial malleolus of the tibia and the lateral malleolus of the fibula and the trochlear surface of the talus (**FIG 2**).
- The ankle joint resembles a mortise-and-tenon joint as used in carpentry. The tibia and fibula must be bound together for the mortise to be stable. This is done by the syndesmosis, which consists of the anterior tibiofibular ligament, interosseous ligament, and posterior tibiofibular ligament. Instability of the mortise could lead to degenerative changes of the joint (**FIG 3**).
- The ankle acts mainly as a hinge joint, allowing plantarflexion and dorsiflexion. The ankle is strengthened on the medial side by the triangular deltoid ligament, which radiates from the medial malleolus to the sustentaculum tali of the calcaneus, the medial border of the plantar calcaneonavicular ("spring") ligament, the tuberosity of the navicular, and the neck of the talus.
- The lateral collateral ligament consists of the anterior and posterior tibiofibular ligaments and a calcaneofibular ligament.
- All these structures are essential for accurate function and stability of the joint.

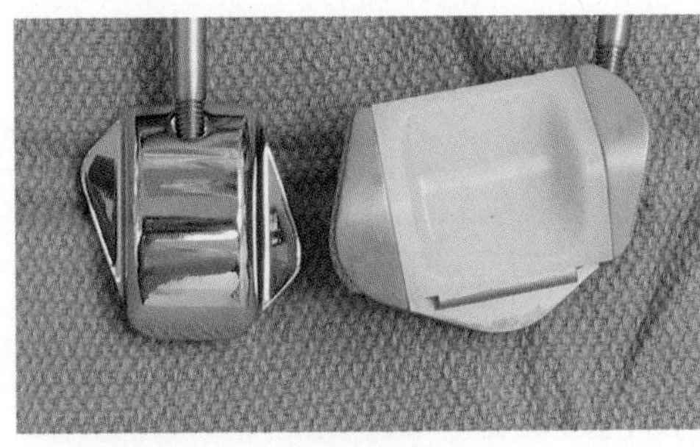

FIG 1 • The two-component design of the Agility ankle replacement with a fixed front-loading polyethylene bearing.

PATHOGENESIS

- The complexity of the ankle anatomy adds to the difficulty of successful ankle replacements.
- Most ankle arthritis is secondary to previous fractures. Intra-articular fractures are common, and especially pilon fractures have a high likelihood of resulting in degenerative changes.
- Syndesmosis injuries are notorious for causing ankle arthritis. One millimeter of translation of the talus in the mortis causes a 40% increase in force in the articular cartilage.[4]
- Collateral ankle ligament instabilities are also a major cause of ankle arthritis. Due to the close-packed nature of the ankle joint, any instability results in a significant increase in stress and force in the ankle.

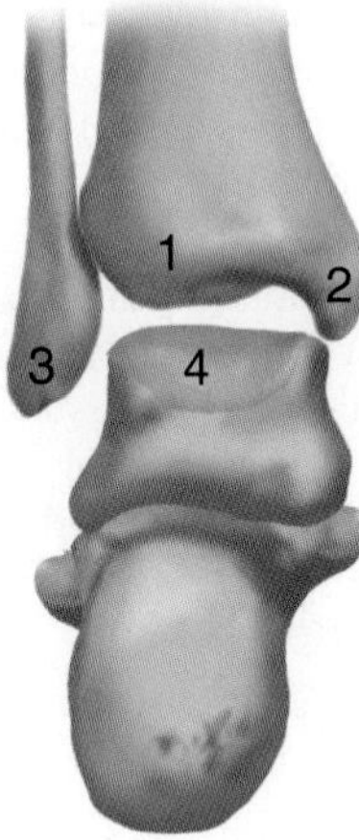

FIG 2 • Part of the complexity of ankle replacements stems from the fact that the ankle joint involves four "separate" entities: (1) the distal tibia, (2) the medial malleolus, (3) the lateral malleolus, and (4) the talus.

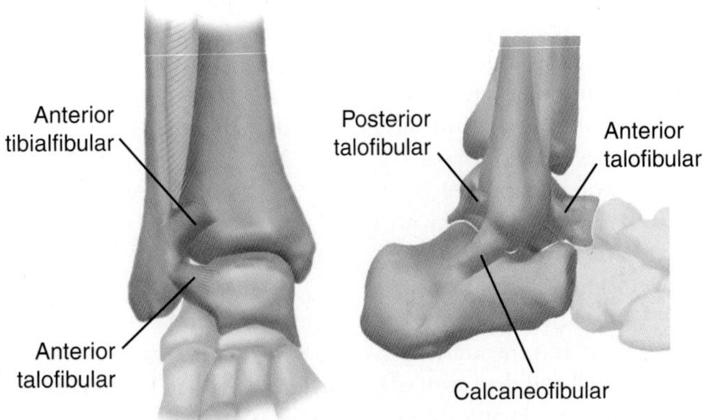

FIG 3 • Anterior and lateral views of the ankle show the multiple ligamentous structures involved in keeping the ankle and mortise stable.

- The most common is lateral instability. This is accentuated if there is a hindfoot varus deformity.
- The foot plays a major role in the pathogenesis of ankle arthritis, and also the outcome of ankle replacement surgery. A stable plantigrade foot is a prerequisite for a successful ankle replacement.
- Close attention should be paid to posterior tibial tendon insufficiencies, deltoid attenuation, gastrocnemius contracture, hindfoot varus, and forefoot supination in planning an ankle replacement. Any of these factors should be addressed before or at the time of the ankle replacement.
- At present a ligamentous instability of more than 20 degrees varus or valgus is felt to be a contraindication for a total ankle arthroplasty.

NATURAL HISTORY

- Degenerative change of the ankle occurs either after a fracture or after ligamentous instability. Only a few cases are truly idiopathic.[9]
- The postfracture group could be divided in two groups. The first comprises patients with severe soft tissue injury, high-energy injury, and multiple operated tibial pilon. These patients usually have a compromised, scarred soft tissue envelope, and the ankle has limited motion. Pain is due to the ankle arthritis but also the soft tissue problems, including scar and damaged lymphatic and venous outflow.
- The second group comprises patients with simple malleolar fractures, low-energy pilon with minimal soft tissue compromise. This group behaves more like the ligament instability or idiopathic group in that the soft tissues are friendly and the ankle range of motion is generally very well preserved.
- The instability group could have additional issues, including peroneal tendinosis or rupture as well as secondary subtalar arthritis or hindfoot varus.

PATIENT HISTORY AND PHYSICAL FINDINGS

- The history is usually very similar within the postfracture group. Depending on the severity and energy of the injury, as well as the accuracy of the reduction of the ankle mortise, the degenerative process will start early or many years after the incident.
- Patients in the ligamentous instability group usually present many years after multiple ankle sprains. The most common history is that of multiple ankle sprains while in school or college that were treated suboptimally. There is usually a history of ongoing instability and the need to use an ankle brace while playing sports in later years.
- Physical examination should include:
  - Range of motion of the ankle. Maximum plantarflexion and dorsiflexion are measured. At least 5 degrees of dorsiflexion is required for normal gait. As a general rule preoperative range of motion determines postoperative range of motion.
  - Gastrocnemius contracture. The examiner should lock the midfoot and then test passive dorsiflexion first with the knee extended and then with the knee flexed. With a gastrocnemius contracture dorsiflexion of the ankle is less with the knee extended. A gastrocnemius lengthening might need to be done.
  - Tibialis posterior tendon function. Evaluating the foot while the patient is standing and walking will show the triad of deformities: too many toes and loss of medial arch and hindfoot valgus. Grade 1 has no deformity but pain, swelling, and weakness. Grade 2 has weakness and correctable deformity. Grade 3 involves a rigid deformity.[5] Tibialis posterior tendon dysfunction is best treated before proceeding with ankle replacement surgery.

IMAGING AND OTHER DIAGNOSTIC STUDIES

- Weight-bearing AP, lateral, and oblique radiographs of the ankle are necessary. The lateral radiograph should include the entire foot to evaluate for midfoot and forefoot collapse.
- Obtaining weight bearing maximum plantarflexion and dorsiflexion radiographs of the ankle is the only reliable way to measure tibiotalar and midfoot motion.[2]
- Long-leg standing radiographs that include the knee and ankle will help to determine the axis of the leg and any alignment issues not shown on an ankle radiograph alone.
- CT scan and MRI could be helpful to determine the presence and size of bone cysts and avascular necrosis of the talus.

DIFFERENTIAL DIAGNOSIS

- Posttraumatic degenerative joint disease
- Degenerative joint disease secondary to ligamentous instability
- Rheumatoid or other seronegative arthritis
- Avascular necrosis
- Infection

NONOPERATIVE MANAGEMENT

- Medications
  - Nonsteroidal anti-inflammatories might give good medium-term relief.
  - Corticosteroids could be a valuable tool to delay total ankle replacement.
- Injections
  - Diagnostic
    - Invaluable; provides a way to determine if most of the pain is coming from the ankle joint
  - Palliative
    - Corticosteroids can give good anti-inflammatory and pain control over the short to medium term, but it is seldom, if ever, permanent pain relief.
- Footwear modifications
  - Wide, extra-depth, comfortable shoes with a low heel can help normalize the gait.
  - Heel wedges can compensate for a leg-length discrepancy or an equinus deformity.
  - Sole flares provide additional stability to the foot and ankle.
    - Medial heel flare provides stability for a valgus deformity of the hindfoot.
    - Lateral flare provides stability for a varus deformity of the hindfoot.
  - Rocker-bottom sole or a solid ankle cushioned heel (SACH) improves forward progression, reduces impact on the ankle at heel strike, and reduces the amount of plantarflexion required at gait.
- Orthotics: in-shoe[1,11]
  - Semirigid: vary from simple felt pads to custom-molded inserts
    - Accommodative inserts are best for rigid deformities. They can also support the medial arch and unload pressure areas. They can control an axial deformity to some degree.
    - Functional inserts are for flexible deformities. They support the foot and help maintain the axial alignment.

- Rigid orthotics
  - Give better control of axial deformity or misalignment and might help to control instability patterns to some degree
  - Unload pressure areas but might create new "hot spots"
  - The UCBL orthotic is a rigid polypropylene insert that aims to correct a flexible hindfoot deformity. It restricts painful hindfoot motion, supports the longitudinal arch, stabilizes the midfoot, and controls the forefoot.
- Laced-up ankle brace
  - Made from various materials (fabric, leather, plastic). It gives reasonable support and correction.
  - Limits motion to a variable degree (depending on the material)
  - Helps for swelling
  - Might simulate a fusion
- Ankle–foot orthosis (AFO)
  - Helps correct and maintain axial malalignment
  - Mimics an ankle fusion
  - Provides ankle stability
  - Might reduce pain but does not completely unload axial forces

SURGICAL MANAGEMENT

- It is of paramount importance to have a stable balanced foot before doing an ankle replacement. Any deviation from this tenet increases the likelihood of component malalignment and subsequent prosthetic failure.
- A concurrent tibialis posterior tendon dysfunction should be treated before the ankle replacement, especially if there are already secondary changes including hindfoot valgus, loss of the medial arch, or forefoot supination.
- Preoperative range of motion determines postoperative range of motion. On average there will be only a 5-degree increase in motion after a replacement.[2] Realistic expectations are therefore important.

Preoperative Planning

- The appropriate radiographs and other imaging studies should be available.
- If there is a significant ligamentous instability, one should plan to do a reconstruction at the time of the ankle replacement.
- Concurrent subtalar or talonavicular arthritis poses a challenge. If a diagnostic ankle joint injection relieved most of the pain, one should not fuse these joints. If it was necessary to inject these joints as well to get adequate pain relief, they should probably be fused at the time of the replacement.

Positioning

- The patient is placed supine on the table with a sand bag under the ipsilateral hip. It is easier to visualize the ankle if the foot is perpendicular to the bed (**FIG 4**). The operative extremity is placed on blankets to elevate the leg above the adjacent nonoperative extremity. This will allow easy visualization of the operative extremity on sagittal plane fluoroscopy.

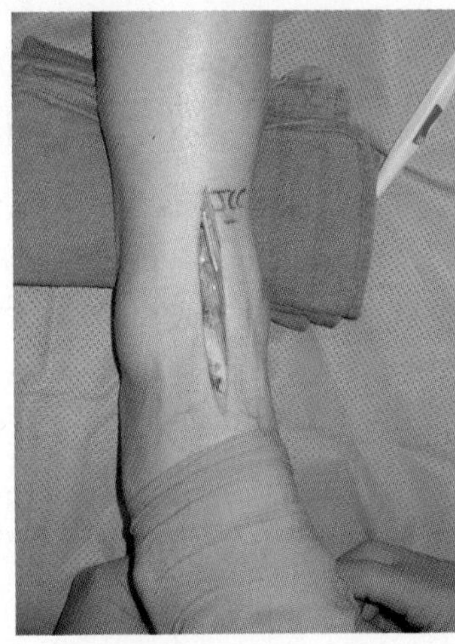

FIG 4 • The patient should be positioned with the foot close to the end of the bed. That makes it easier for the surgeon to visualize the joint without having to lean forward for an extended period. A sand bag is placed under the ipsilateral buttock to turn the foot perpendicular to the bed for equal access to the medial and lateral sides of the joint. The lower calf is supported to allow the ankle to hang free. That posteriorly translates the joint and also relaxes the posterior structures.

TECHNIQUES

EXPOSURE OF THE ANKLE

- Use an anterior approach between the extensor hallucis longus tendon and the tibialis anterior. Leave the sheath of the tibialis anterior tendon intact, and perform the dissection lateral to the tendon (**TECH FIG 1**).
- The medial branch of the superficial peroneal nerve is often found in the subcutaneous tissues in the distal half of the wound. It should be identified, protected, and retracted laterally.
- The deep neurovascular bundle is found deep to the extensor hallucis longus tendon. The medial malleolar arterial branches are coagulated or divided to free the neurovascular bundle so that it can be retracted laterally.
- Incise the ankle capsule longitudinally over the midpoint of the ankle; it may be necessary to excise the central portion of this capsule to gain good exposure. An

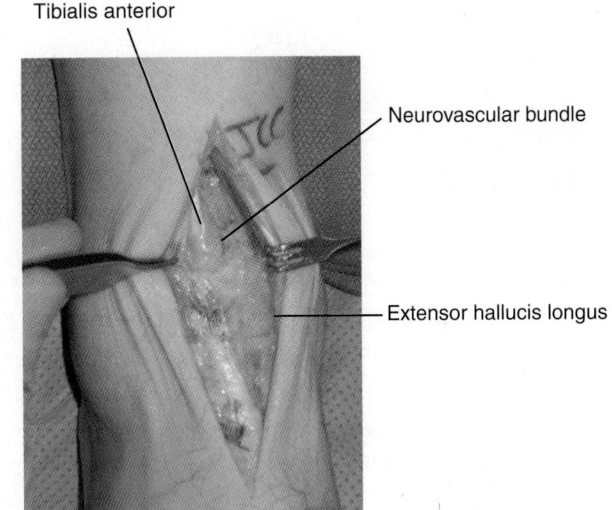

TECH FIG 1 • Anterior approach to the ankle between tibialis anterior and extensor hallucis longus.

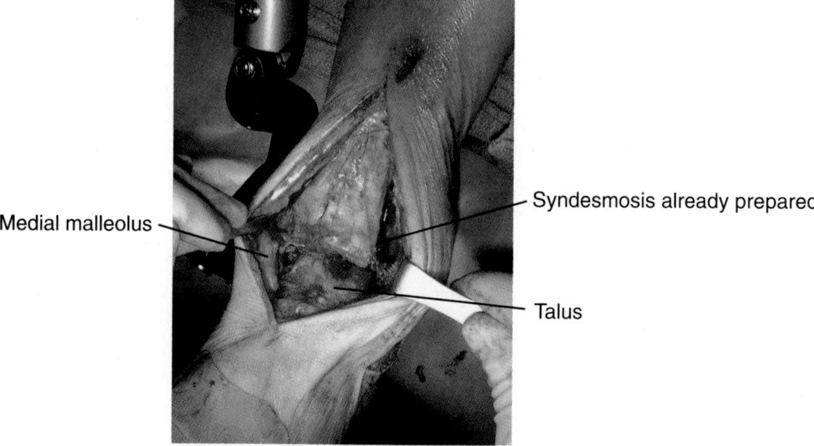

TECH FIG 2 • Adequate exposure is critical. This shows the medial malleolus, fibula, and syndesmosis. At this point the syndesmosis is already prepared for fusion by removing all the soft tissues and decorticating the apposing surfaces.

extensile exposure is required: the entire medial malleolus, syndesmosis, and lateral malleolus should be visible (TECH FIG 2).

- Remove the anterior osteophytes on the tibia with an osteotome to expose the extent of the depression in the tibial plafond.
- Also remove the osteophytes from the anterior aspect of the talus to allow the cutting block to be adequately placed (TECH FIG 3).
- Identify the medial and lateral sides of the talus. It is possible at this stage to assess whether soft tissue procedures are needed to realign the foot. Severe deformity is very difficult to correct, and deformity over 20 degrees may be regarded as a contraindication for ankle replacement with the Agility ankle. The lack of complete congruent contact between the dome of the talar component and the plafond of the tibial tray may encourage tilt of the prosthesis postoperatively.
- The syndesmosis is visualized and prepared for fusion using the same incision. Remove all the soft tissues and decorticate the apposing surfaces of the tibia and fibula over the distal 4 cm.

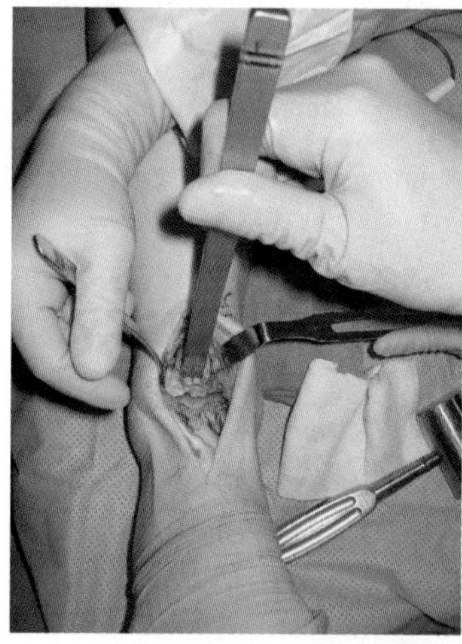
A

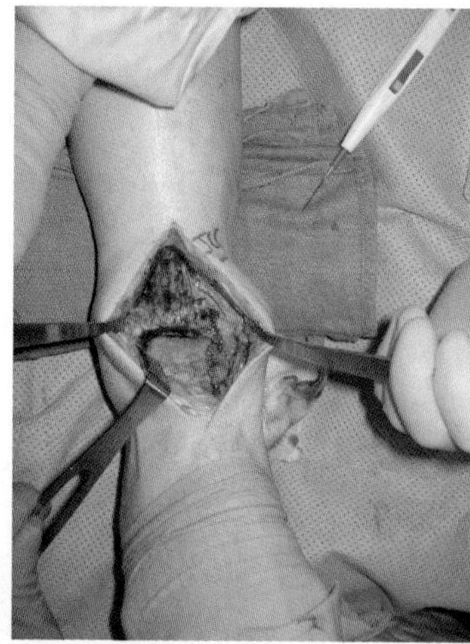
B

TECH FIG 3 • After adequate exposure of the ankle the anterior osteophytes are removed from the distal tibia and the talar neck. After the removal the entire joint should be visible. The neurovascular bundle is retracted laterally.

APPLICATION OF THE EXTERNAL FIXATION

- Apply the distractor with two pins in the foot and two in the tibia, all inserted from the medial side.
- The first pin goes into the talar neck. This pin is critical and should be parallel to the talar dome. For example, if the ankle is in valgus, the pin is inserted perpendicular to the axis of the deformity, which would be corrected as distraction is applied.
- With the dissection done first the actual placement of the talar pin can be verified under direct vision, which ensures accurate placement (TECH FIG 4).

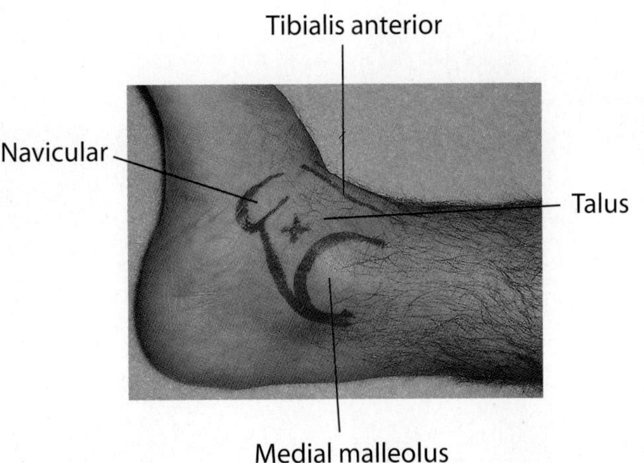

TECH FIG 4 • The talar pin placement is critical. It should be in the "soft spot" between the medial malleolus proximal, navicular distal, tibialis anterior tendon anterior, and tibialis posterior tendon posterior.

- Cancellous pins are used for the talus and calcaneus. Use the distractor guide to place the second pin through the calcaneus. Accurate placement of the first (talar) pin will ensure that the calcaneal pin is posterior and superior to the neurovascular bundle.
- This is followed by placing two proximal pins through the distractor guide into the tibia.
- Tighten all the distractor joints with the foot at 90 degrees to the tibial axis.
- Slowly distract the joint. There is no set distance for distraction, but the goal is to get close to the deltoid endpoint, where the deltoid is under tension. This is usually about 1 cm of distraction.
- If no distraction is possible due to scarring and ankylosis, use an osteotome to manually loosen the joint.
- Be careful not to overdistract. It could cause malleolar fractures, or "overstuffing" of the joint with limited range of motion.
- If distraction tilts the joint in varus or valgus, make adjustments to bring the ankle back to neutral before making the bone cuts.
- Use fluoroscopy liberally to ensure that the articular surfaces are parallel, joint space is restored, and the ankle is not in equinus (**TECH FIG 5**).

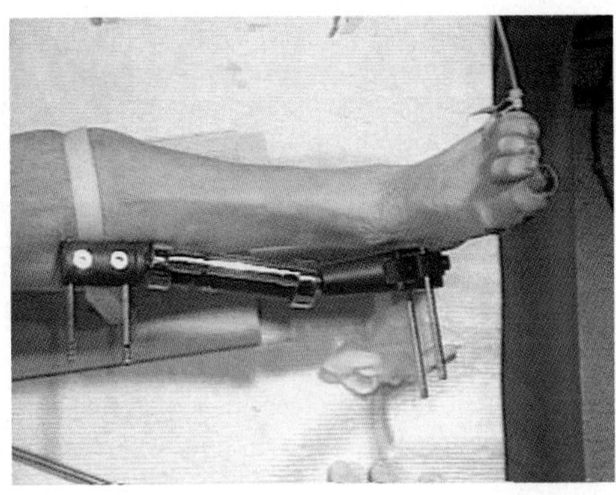

TECH FIG 5 • Proper placement of the distractor is critical to ensure correct bone cuts.

ALIGNMENT JIG AND CUTTING BLOCK

- Place the yoke of the tibial alignment jig on the leg so that the clamp adjustment bar lies over the anterior crest of the tibia.
- Center the proximal end of the ankle clamp alignment jig over the tibial tubercle and hold it in position by wrapping the ankle clamp spring around the leg. The adjustment tube on the yoke post and the extending tibial rod should be parallel to the tibia to give the correct angle for the cutting block at the ankle (**TECH FIG 6**).
- Turn the cutting block clamp fine-tuning screw to its halfway point. That will allow proximal and distal adjustment after securing the alignment guide to the tibia.
- Proper rotation of the cutting block is critical. With the jig parallel to the tibia, use the alignment stylus to

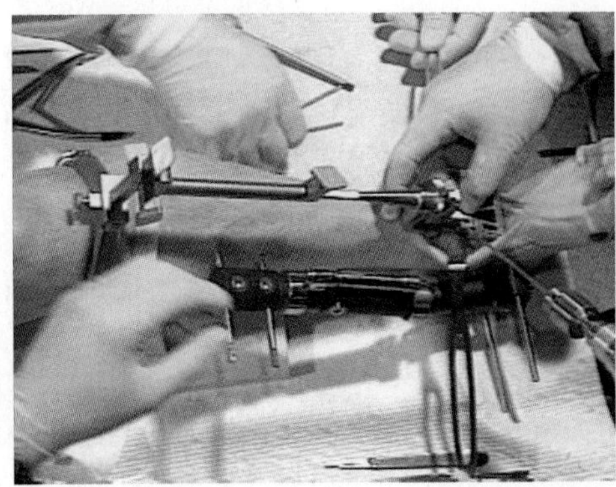

TECH FIG 6 • The yoke of the alignment jig should be centered over the tibial crest on an AP view and should be parallel to the tibia on a lateral view.

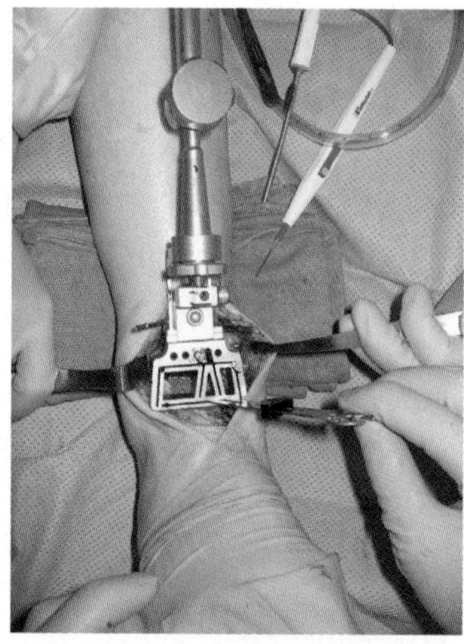

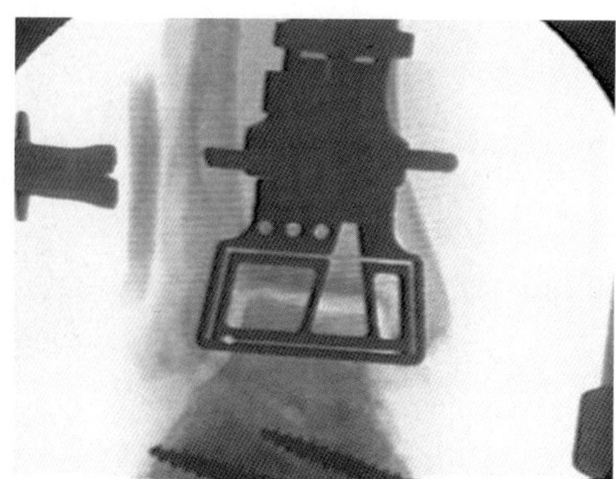

A B

TECH FIG 7 • The correct-size cutting block will remove equal bone from the tibia and talus, and about one third of the medial and lateral malleolus. At this point the alignment jig is secured to the tibia, but the cutting block can still be moved distal or proximal and lateral or medial. The correct position should be confirmed before securing the cutting block to the tibia.

ensure that the cutting block lines up with the second metatarsal. Then tighten the footpad assembly screw.

- Insert the correct-size cutting block into the alignment jig slot and roughly center it over the ankle joint. Secure the footpads to the tibia with the stabilizing pins.
- Center the cutting block over the ankle. Fluoroscopy is valuable. There is a notch on the lateral and medial wall of the cutting block to show the level of the joint. A lateral radiographic view can also be used to show that equal distances of the tibia and talus will be resected (**TECH FIG 7**).
- First insert the stabilizing pin on the proximal-medial aspect of the cutting block to ensure that the medial-lateral placement of the block will take equal bone from the medial and lateral malleolus (about one third of the width). With adequate placement of the cutting block, insert one or two more stabilizing pins.

BONE RESECTION

- Recheck the position of the ankle, especially in the sagittal plane, before making the saw cuts (**TECH FIG 8**).
- Perform the tibial, tibial keel, malleolar, and talar bone cuts using the respective slots in the cutting block. The tibial keel cut should go about half the depth of the tibia.
- Remove the cutting block and if necessary complete the corner cuts with a reciprocal saw.
- Remove the distal tibial bone, taking care not to rotate the fragments, as it can put excess pressure on the malleoli.
- This is followed by the talar fin cut. To allow placement of the burr guide, remove the distraction device to allow full plantarflexion of the ankle. Then place the burr guide centered on the cut surface of the talus, with the alignment jig parallel to the second metatarsal.
- Secure the burr guide to the talus with pins and prepare the keel. Remove the burr guide (**TECH FIG 9**).

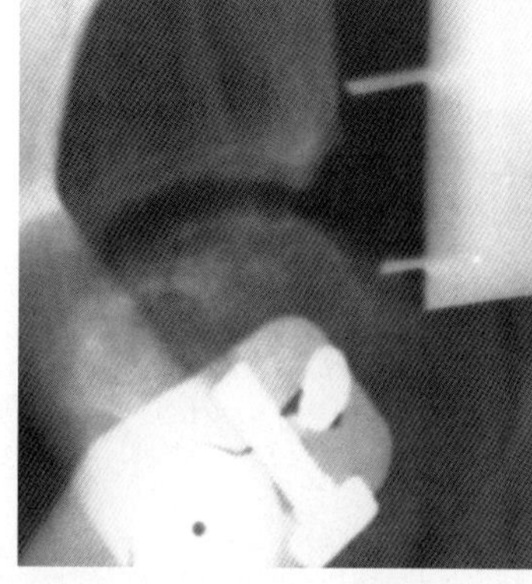

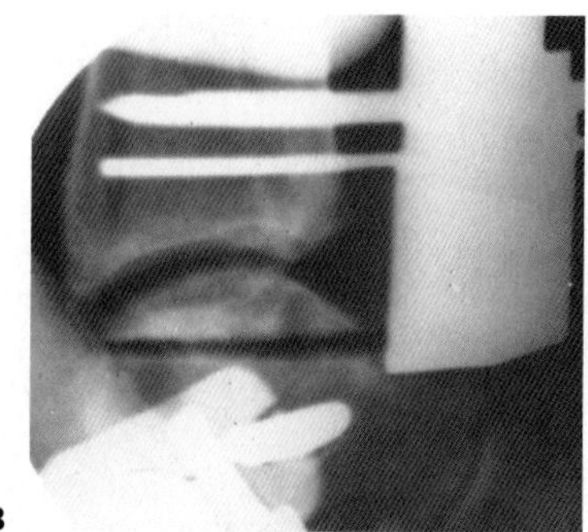

A B

TECH FIG 8 • A. The distractor is locked with the ankle in neutral. Note the distraction of the joint. Before securing the cutting block to the tibia, saw blades are used to verify that equal amounts of tibia and talus will be removed. **B.** The talar cut is complete and the tibia cut is being done.

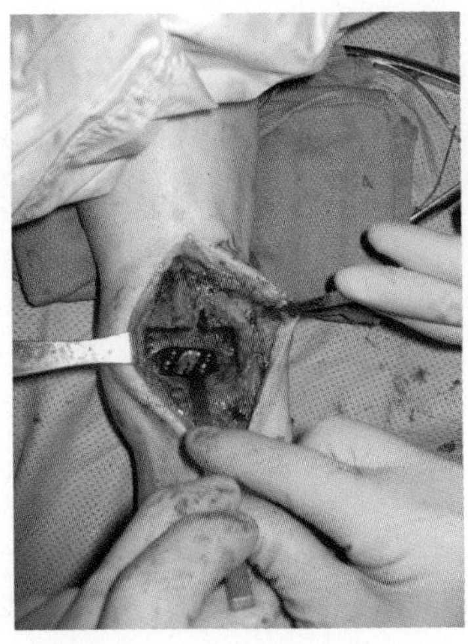

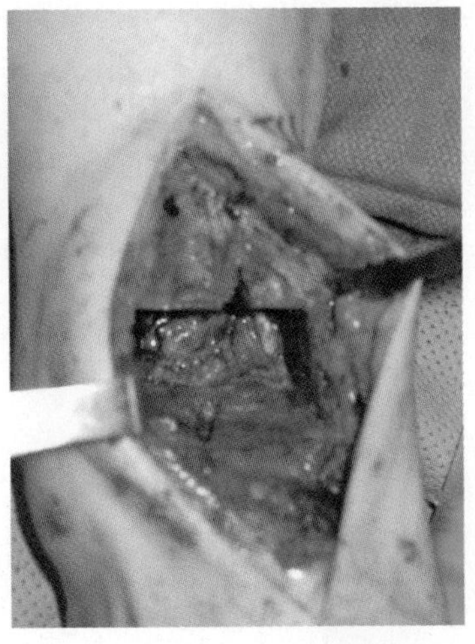

TECH FIG 9 • A. After removal of the bone from the tibia and malleoli, the burr guide for the talar keel cut is placed and secured. **B.** Final bone cuts, including the tibial and talar keel cuts. In the posterior-medial corner the tibialis posterior tendon is visible.

TIBIAL AND TALAR COMPONENT INSERTION

- Insert the trial components using the alignment handles. It might be helpful to gently spread the syndesmosis with a wide osteotome. The tibial component is inserted first, followed by the talus. A standard front-loading polyethylene component is then inserted into the tibial tray. It could be replaced with a +1 component if needed (**TECH FIG 10**).
- Test the range of motion and ankle ligament stability. If there is not at least 5 degrees dorsiflexion consider a gastrocnemius lengthening.
- Remove the trial components and thoroughly rinse the ankle to remove all debris. The final components are now inserted. The talar component insertion usually requires the foot to be in maximum plantarflexion (**TECH FIG 11**).

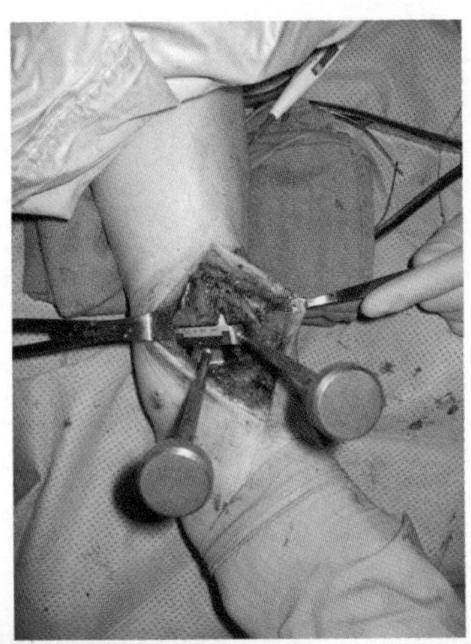

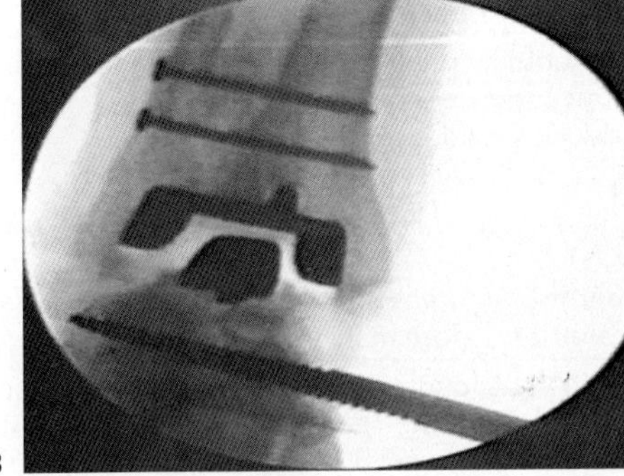

TECH FIG 10 • The trial components are inserted. The insertion handles should diverge about 23 degrees to confirm correct alignment of the two components. If it has not been done before, the distractor should be removed at this point and the ankle stability tested.

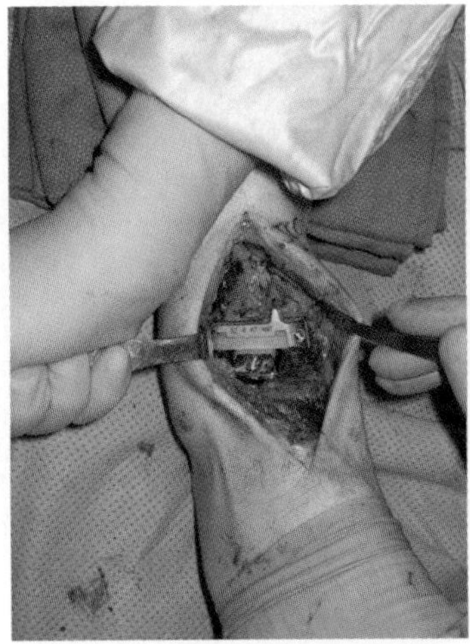

TECH FIG 11 • Final component placement.

SYNDESMOSIS FUSION

- Morselize the bone taken from the bone cuts in the tibia and talus and pack it in the syndesmosis.
- Place a three- or four-hole semitubular plate over the lateral aspect of the fibula through the anterior incision.
- Insert two screws percutaneously through the plate, fibula, and tibia to compress the syndesmosis. The distal screw should be about 1 cm proximal to the keel of the tibial component (**TECH FIG 12**).

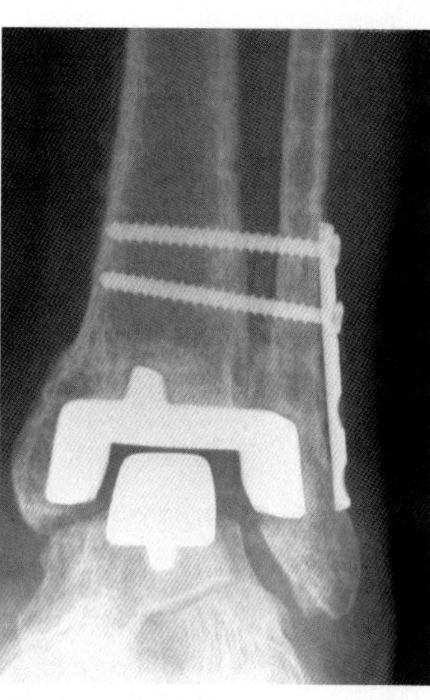

TECH FIG 12 • The syndesmosis is fused with a small plate on the fibula and two screws into the tibia. Bone taken from the bone cuts is morselized and packed into the syndesmosis.

PEARLS AND PITFALLS

Indications	■ A successful ankle requires a stable foot. Specifically look for and treat any muscle imbalances (ie, posterior tibial tendon dysfunction).
Varus or valgus malalignment	■ Preoperative varus is often due to chronic lateral ligament instability. ■ Valgus is often due to longstanding posterior tibial tendon dysfunction with secondary deltoid ligament instability. Ligamentous varus or valgus of more than 20 degrees may be a contraindication for an ankle replacement with the Agility ankle. ■ Bone erosion varus or valgus with no ligamentous instability is an acceptable indication.
Syndesmosis preparation	■ The entire syndesmosis should be débrided before attempting to spread the fibula from the tibia. ■ Failure to release the posterior tibiofibular ligament could result in a fibula fracture when spreading the syndesmosis or inserting the tibial component.
Ankle sizing	■ Take care to choose the correct ankle size. About one third of the medial and lateral malleolus should be removed. Overstuffing the joint will reduce the range of motion. ■ Too small a component will increase the risk of subsidence.
Distraction of the ankle	■ The talar pin should be parallel to the joint. ■ Lock the external fixator with the foot in 90 degrees. Locking the foot in plantarflexion will tilt the talar cut toward the subtalar joint. ■ Distract the ankle until the deltoid ligament is under tension. ■ Use fluoroscopy to confirm cutting block position before making bone cuts.
Malleolar fractures	■ Treat like any malleolar fracture. There is usually enough bone to insert one or two screws for fixation, or a tension band wire technique could be used. There are adequate amounts of bone from the bone cuts to graft the fracture site.

POSTOPERATIVE CARE

- The leg is placed in a short-leg posterior splint or leg walker with the ankle in neutral.
- The patient should be non–weight-bearing, or at most toe touch.
- The splint is removed at 2 weeks to remove the sutures.
- A leg walker is applied, and the patient can start with non–weight-bearing range of motion for 5 minutes three times a day.
- The patient continues to be non–weight-bearing for a further 4 weeks.
- At 6 weeks radiographs are obtained, and if there are adequate signs of syndesmosis healing the patient can progress to full weight bearing and start physical therapy to increase range of motion, proprioception, and strength.
- If soft tissue procedures were done to correct ligamentous imbalance, it is advisable to use a short-leg cast for the first 6 weeks.

OUTCOMES

- Alvine's series[6] has the longest follow-up (7 to 16 years) on the Agility ankle replacement.
- At a mean 9-year follow-up the revision rate was 11% (either a revision or a fusion).
- More than 90% of patients reported that they had decreased pain and were satisfied with the outcome of the surgery.
- Eighty-nine (76%) of the 117 ankles had some evidence of peri-implant radiolucency.
- Syndesmosis nonunion had a negative impact on the clinical and radiologic outcome.
- Deland et al[7] reported results at 3.5 years of follow-up on 38 patients. The American Orthopaedic Foot and Ankle Society (AOFAS) ankle–hindfoot scores increased from 33.6 preoperatively to 83.3 at final follow-up ($P < 0.001$).
- Postoperative Medical Outcomes Study Short Form-36 (SF-36) Physical Component Summary (PCS) and Mental Component Summary (MCS) scores averaged 49.5 and 56.1, respectively.
- Migration or subsidence of components was noted in 18 ankles. Overall, 37 of 38 patients were satisfied with the outcome of their surgery and would have the same procedure under similar circumstances.

COMPLICATIONS

- Hansen et al[10] reported on the complications on 306 consecutive ankle replacements.
- 28% underwent reoperations; the most common procedures were débridement of heterotopic bone, correction of axial malalignment, and component replacement. The below-the-knee amputation rate was 3.5%.
- Malleolar fractures happen in about 10% of cases. Further perioperative complications include tibial nerve injury, tendon injuries, and wound problems.[8]
- Late complications include syndesmosis nonunions in 6% to 26% of cases.[3]
- Infection
- Progressive varus or valgus deformities due to ligamentous imbalance
- Osteolysis, bone cysts, and subsidence

REFERENCES

1. Bono CM, Berberian WS. Orthotic devices: degenerative disorders of the foot and ankle. Foot Ankle Clin 2001;6:329–340.
2. Coetzee JC, Castro MD. Accurate measurement of ankle range of motion after total ankle arthroplasty. Clin Orthop Relat Res 2004;424:27–31.
3. Coetzee JC, Pomeroy GC, Watts JD, Barrow C. The use of autologous concentrated growth factors to promote syndesmosis fusion in the Agility total ankle replacement: a preliminary study. Foot Ankle Int 2005;26:840–846.
4. Gardner MJ, Demetrakopoulos D, Briggs SM, et al. Malreduction of the tibiofibular syndesmosis in ankle fractures. Foot Ankle Int 2006;27:788–792.
5. Johnson KA, Strom DE. Tibialis posterior tendon dysfunction. Clin Orthop Relat Res 1989;239:196–206.
6. Knecht SI, Estin M, Callaghan JJ, et al. The Agility total ankle arthroplasty: seven to sixteen-year follow-up. J Bone Joint Surg Am 2004;86A:1161–1171.
7. Kopp FJ, Patel MM, Deland JT, et al. Total ankle arthroplasty with the Agility prosthesis: clinical and radiographic evaluation. Foot Ankle Int 2006;27:97–103.
8. Myerson MS, Mroczek K. Perioperative complications of total ankle arthroplasty. Foot Ankle Int 2003;24:17–21.
9. Saltzman CL, Salamon ML, Blanchard GM, et al. Epidemiology of ankle arthritis: report of a consecutive series of 639 patients from a tertiary orthopaedic center. Iowa Orthop J 2005;25:44–46.
10. Spirt AA, Assal M, Hansen ST Jr. Complications and failure after total ankle arthroplasty. J Bone Joint Surg Am 2004;86A:1172–1178.
11. Wu WL, Rosenbaum D, Su FC. The effects of rocker sole and SACH heel on kinematics in gait. Med Engin Physics 2004;26:639–646.

Chapter 76 Revision Agility Total Ankle Arthroplasty

Steven L. Haddad

DEFINITION

- Revision of the Agility Ankle is required for a variety of circumstances. It may be necessary either relatively early after the index procedure, or delayed due to late mechanical failure.
- By definition, revision may be required around a stable arthroplasty (ie, correcting imbalance creating deformity in the prosthesis or repairing fractures around the prosthesis) or by implant removal and subsequent replacement of the prosthesis (whole or in part).

ANATOMY

- The anatomy of revision total ankle arthroplasty revolves around the specific mechanism of failure of the original prosthesis. Structures of concern include:
- Bone: the medial and lateral malleoli, the distal tibia, and the talus
- Ligaments: the anterior talofibular and calcaneofibular ligaments, the deltoid ligament, and the syndesmotic ligament complex
- Muscle and tendon: the Achilles tendon and the anterior tibial, extensor hallucis longus, extensor digitorum longus, peroneus longus and brevis, and posterior tibial tendons

PATHOGENESIS

- Malleoli: Failure of the malleoli may occur from fracture of these structures. Fracture can occur early (due to a technical complication sustained during the procedure) (**FIG 1A**) or late (from weakened bone architecture due to osteolytic cysts, or undue stresses applied to the malleoli from deformity or altered gait mechanics) (**FIG 1B**). Micro- or macromotion may occur through the prosthesis–bone interface at the fibula from lack of a syndesmotic fusion, creating the potential for lateral malleolar fracture.
- Distal tibia and talus: Failure is sustained through axial load applied to this portion of bone, compounded by the physiologic effects of the prosthesis. Osteolysis may occur from shed polyethylene particles, creating a macrophage reaction and autodestruction of bone. This weakened, cystic bone allows the prosthesis to subside through the resection margin, creating deformity and failure. In addition, compromise through lack of bone ingrowth into the sintered beads may create micromotion within the prosthesis–bone interface, creating further erosions and subsidence into the tibia or talus (**FIG 2A,B**).
- Lateral and medial ankle ligaments: Failure is sustained through ligaments that are often compromised before the surgical procedure (**FIG 3**). Often deformity exacerbates this problem, as chronic tension through weight bearing continues to attenuate the ligaments, creating further compromise.
- Extensor tendon complex (anterior tibial tendon, extensor hallucis longus, extensor digitorum longus): Issues involving the extensor complex revolve around scar tissue and anterior wound complication (**FIG 4A**), which as a baseline creates altered motion in the form of decreased plantarflexion (**FIG 4B**). In more advanced circumstances, wound coverage is required due to tendon exposure. Compromised blood supply to the anterior skin, multiple prior incisions in posttraumatic or reconstructive situations, and direct apposition of the tendon complex against the skin may all accelerate anterior incision failure.
- Infection: Early incision complication may provide a portal of entry for colonized bacteria, leading to superficial cellulitis or deep infection (**FIG 5A,B**). Early intervention in the form of parenteral antibiotics or operative débridement may allow salvage of the prosthesis. Deep infections involving the bone

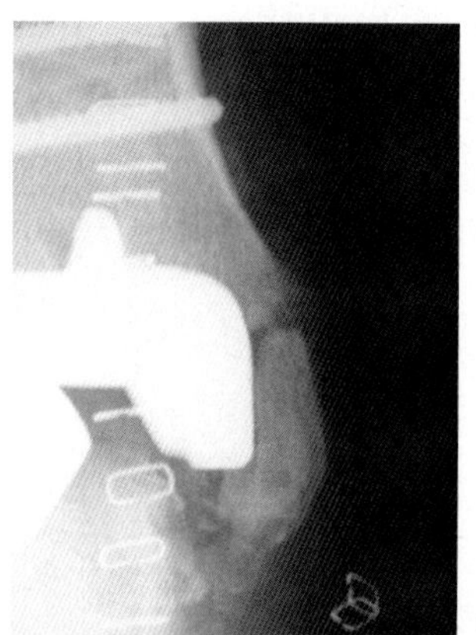
A

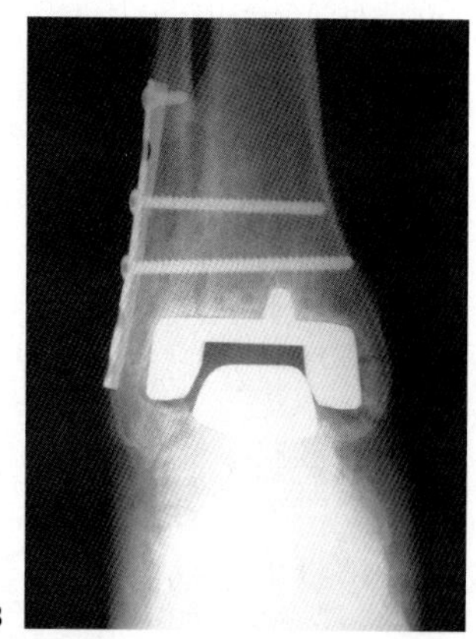
B

FIG 1 • Acute (**A**) and chronic (**B**) medial malleolus fractures. The former fractures occur due to an intraoperative technical error. The latter can occur from imbalance about the prosthesis with undue stresses.

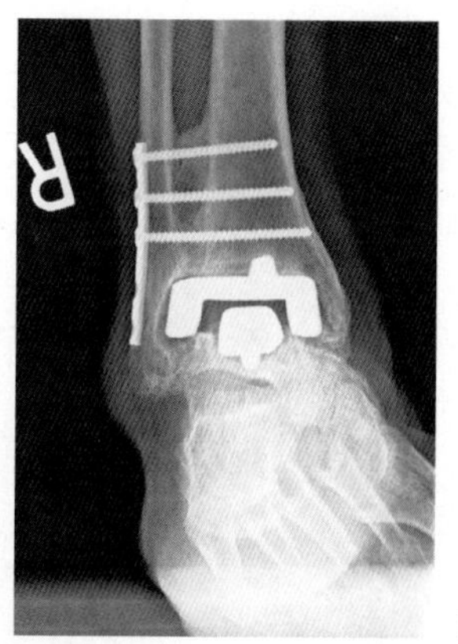

A

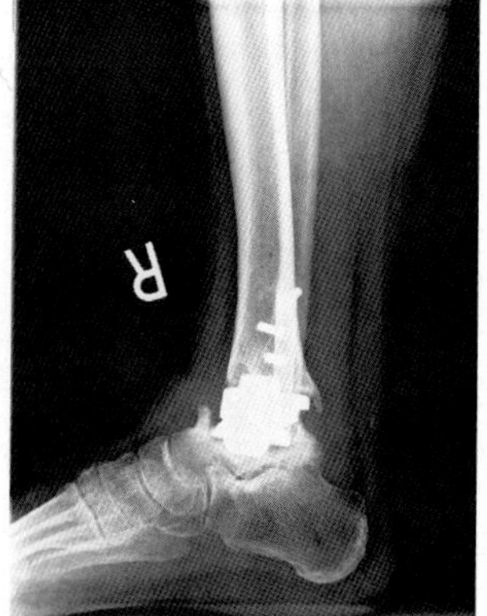

B

FIG 2 • AP (**A**) and lateral (**B**) radiographs of talar subsidence. Note the penetration of the talus into the nascent talus. Also note the osteolytic cyst in the distal tibia.

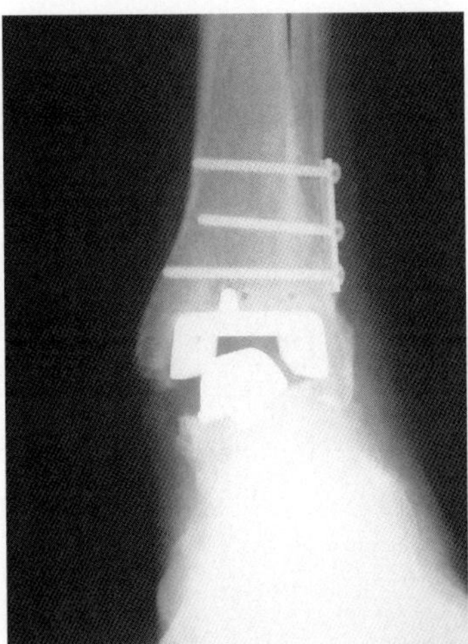

FIG 3 • Severe valgus after failure of the deltoid ligament. This is in combination with a structural foot deformity and hindfoot valgus.

(osteomyelitis) may result from direct extension from these superficial infections or may occur from bacteria seeded at the time of surgery, lying dormant for an undefined interval before presentation. Bacteria may cling to the prosthesis, creating a situation resistant to antibiotic intervention. They may form a glycocalyx, insulating themselves from both antibiotics and operative irrigation.

NATURAL HISTORY

- The natural history of all of the above-mentioned problems follows a course dependent on the index mechanism of failure.

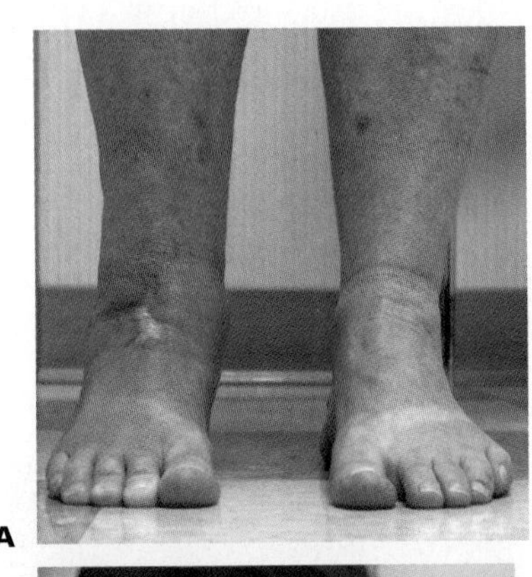

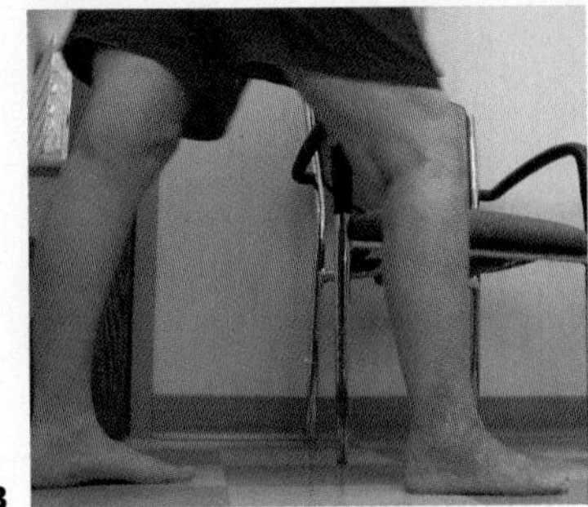

FIG 4 • Anterior wound complication (**A**) leads to excessive scar tissue, compromising the ability to plantarflex (**B**) the ankle.

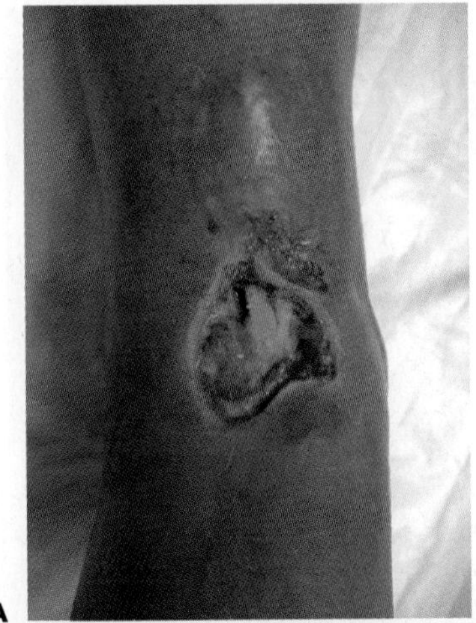

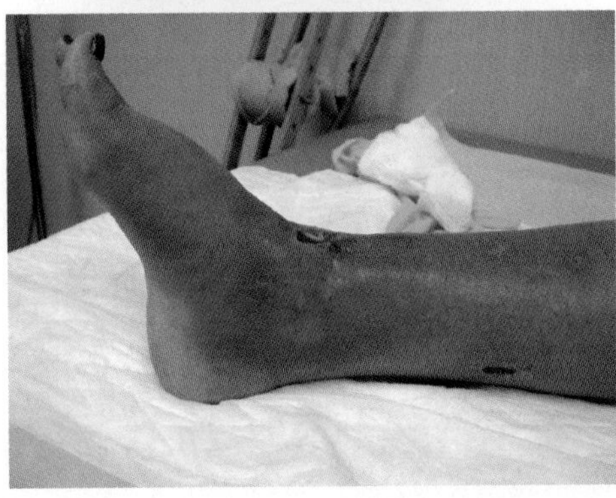

FIG 5 • Anterior wound complication has led to secondary deep infection and exposed tendons (**A**). The cellulitis is obvious (**B**), but the infection is deep.

- Malleolar fractures may occur early or late. In either case, resolution of the fracture is compromised by the limited bone available due to removal for implantation of the prosthesis. The natural history may thus progress to either successful union after repair, or nonunion. Nonunion may lead to a relative increased length of the malleoli and subsequently the ligaments, leading to deformity potential (**FIG 6**). Deformity, once present, prevents union.
- Ligament compromise follows a similar predictable course, with the endpoint being instability and subsequent deformity about the prosthesis. Lack of medial or lateral restraint allows edge-loading of the polyethylene, leading to osteolysis and implant subsidence.
- Incision compromise may begin as focal necrosis about the anterior wound. Blistering may be evident, or full-thickness necrosis. Necrosis presents as peri-incisional devascularized skin, which may be limited in extent or of greater breadth; either allows slough of the zone of injury. Full-thickness granulation tissue may develop, though it will be temporally slow. As such, scar tissue accumulates about the anterior tendon complex as motion must be restricted to provide the best healing environment. With exposed tendon, granulation tissue is less likely and plastic surgery involvement becomes a possibility.
- Infection may present in conjunction with wound compromise as cellulitis in the early postoperative period. Without attention, cellulitis may allow deep bacterial infestation, creating osteomyelitis or septic arthritis of the artificial joint. Salvage of

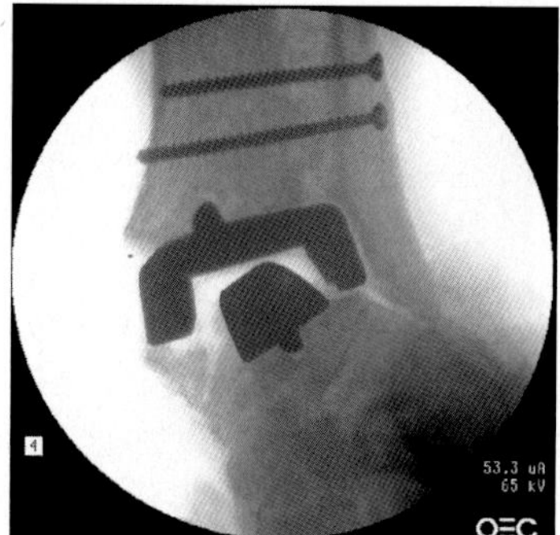

FIG 6 • Stressing the ankle in the operating room reveals significant medial bone compromise, leading to valgus deformity and medial instability.

the index prosthesis becomes less likely, as a glycocalyx may form about the polyethylene, shielding the bacteria from antibiotic penetration or irrigation.

- Malleolar fracture, ligament compromise, prosthesis subsidence, incision compromise, and infection will be discussed separately.

MALLEOLAR FRACTURE

PATIENT HISTORY AND PHYSICAL FINDINGS

- Evaluating the ankle for malleolar fracture should include the following:
  - Direct palpation to the medial or lateral malleoli, or pain with weight bearing medially or laterally. This is not the normal location of postoperative pain, so it creates clinical suspicion that fracture is present.
  - The examiner should look for increased swelling about the ankle joint after postsurgical resolution. The examiner should evaluate for deep vein thrombosis, but normally in combination with pain, one thinks of malleolar fracture.

IMAGING AND OTHER DIAGNOSTIC STUDIES

- Plain radiographs: Malleolar fractures may be subtle or obvious. Obvious fractures are visible at the level of the prosthesis, generally at the apex or superior corners of the prosthesis. In iatrogenic cases, the fractures occur at the level of the superior saw cut line on the tibia, where the sagittal saw violates the medial or lateral malleolus. Significant distraction via the uniplanar fixator upon osteoporotic bone may create avulsion fractures at the malleoli after saw cuts, where the thinned malleoli are subject to increased force per unit area. Subtle fractures are generally delayed in appearance and may involve periosteal reactions seen at the medial malleolus proximal to the prosthesis. This type of fracture occurs from an unbalanced prosthesis (**FIG 7A**) placing uneven load or compression about the malleoli (**FIG 7B**).
- Tc99 bone scans: This study is generally not helpful, as increased uptake is visible surrounding the prosthesis, making it difficult to discern a fracture from normal pooling.
- CT: This test is very helpful to evaluate both the presence and healing of malleolar fractures. CT scanning is not helpful during intraoperative occurrences but has value in delayed presentation, especially in subtle cases (**FIG 8**). Subtraction software minimizes interference from the prosthesis.

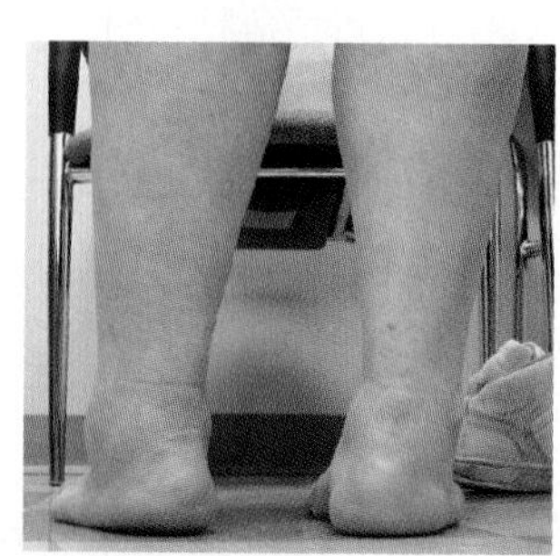
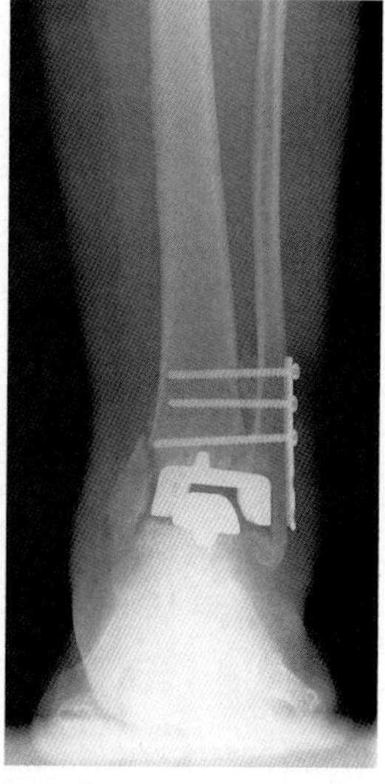

A B

FIG 7 • Hindfoot varus (**A**) places increased stress about the medial malleolus, which can create a delayed medial malleolus fracture. (**B**) Weight-bearing radiograph of the ankle demonstrates the most common pattern of late medial malleolus fracture: a vertical shear fracture pattern. Repetitive stress from the medial corner of the tibial implant creates the vertical fracture line that allows the prosthesis to shift into varus.

DIFFERENTIAL DIAGNOSIS

- Malleolar fracture
- Infection
- Deep venous thrombosis

NONOPERATIVE MANAGEMENT

- Conservative treatment for malleolar fractures involves cast immobilization until union is complete. Unlike malleolar fractures without ankle arthroplasty, immobilization is often extended beyond the standard 6 weeks, as the decreased surface area for healing due to the space-occupying prosthesis increases the likelihood of nonunion. If immobilization is terminated before complete union, refracture or separation of the fragments becomes likely, mandating surgical correction. A

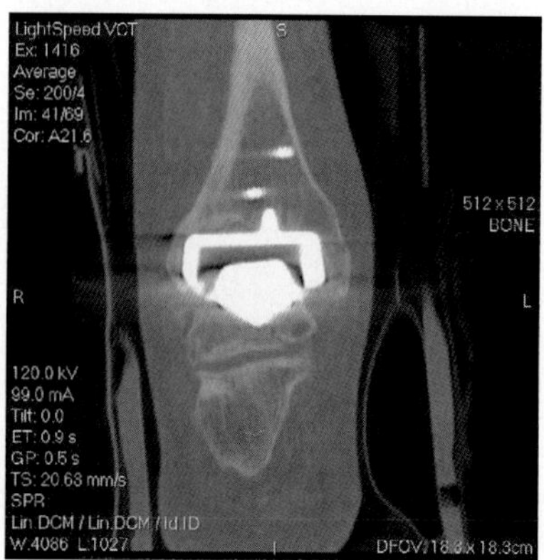

FIG 8 • CT scan of subtle medial malleolus fracture in a delayed presentation due to persistent hindfoot valgus.

CT scan is important to quantify union before discontinuing immobilization.

- Use of pulsed electromagnetic fields or ultrasound to stimulate union may enhance union.

SURGICAL MANAGEMENT

- Surgical repair of malleolar fractures is normally the treatment of choice after the fracture is recognized. As the rehabilitative goal of total ankle arthroplasty is early range of motion, prolonged immobilization to allow conservative union may lead to undue ankle stiffness, compromising patient satisfaction. Thus, upon visualization of a malleolar fracture (either acute or delayed), surgical repair is indicated.

Preoperative Planning

- In acute or iatrogenic situations, no preoperative planning is possible.
- In delayed or chronic situations, a CT scan is useful to evaluate the fracture pattern and determine screw placement. In addition, the CT scan may visualize partial union, allowing percutaneous fixation of the fracture fragments.

Positioning

- Positioning is supine for this procedure, with a bump under the ipsilateral hip of a diameter to rotate the knee, ankle, and foot to a neutral position (**FIG 9A**). Generally, blankets are used to elevate the involved extremity above the sagittal plane of the unaffected extremity (**FIG 9B**). This position improves the accuracy of sagittal imaging and prevents the need to lift or manipulate the involved extremity during the more tenuous portions of the surgical procedure.

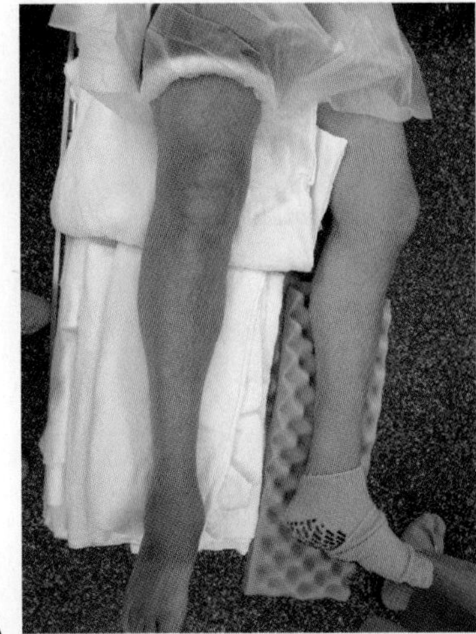

A

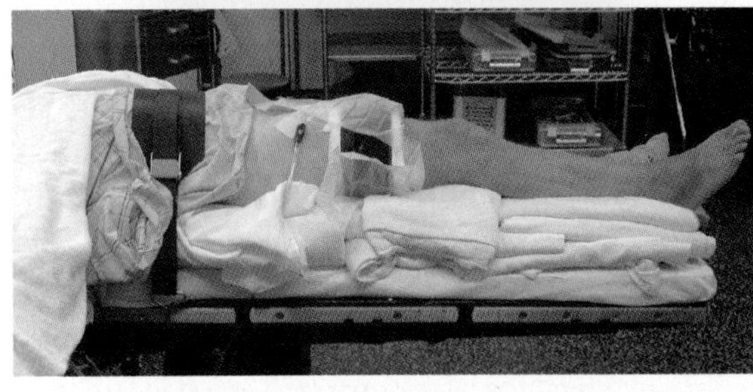

B

FIG 9 • AP positioning (**A**) reveals a knee placed in neutral alignment. Lateral (**B**) positioning on operating table. Note the rigid bump under the ipsilateral hip (rolled blankets) and the leg elevation on a firm surface of blankets.

Approach

- The surgical approach depends on whether the malleolar fracture is acute (noted intraoperatively) or chronic (occurs at a later date).
- The surgical approach for acute malleolar fractures is performed in the index procedure (ie, anterior approach for reduction and fixation of the medial malleolus fracture and lateral approach for the lateral malleolus fracture). The anterior approach allows evaluation of the fracture reduction, while screws are placed percutaneously medially. The lateral approach provides direct access for reduction and plate fixation.
- In chronic situations, the lateral approach is still used for lateral malleolar fractures. However, a medial approach is preferred for medial malleolar fractures, as direct visualization of the fracture fragments is critical, and often bone loss is present. The medial approach allows placement of either screws or plates, depending on the anatomy of the fragments.

TECHNIQUES

OPEN REPAIR OF THE ACUTE MEDIAL MALLEOLUS FRACTURE

- Reduce this fracture anatomically (**TECH FIG 1A**) during surgery and hold it with a reduction clamp.
- Place guidewires from the tip of the medial malleolus into the distal tibia (**TECH FIG 1B**). There is adequate room for one and possibly two guidewires despite the medial bone resection for the prosthesis.
- Perform screw fixation percutaneously with cannulated screws (**TECH FIG 1C**). Alternatively, if solid-core screws are preferred, drilling is done over the guidewire, followed by guidewire withdrawal and placement of the solid-core screws.

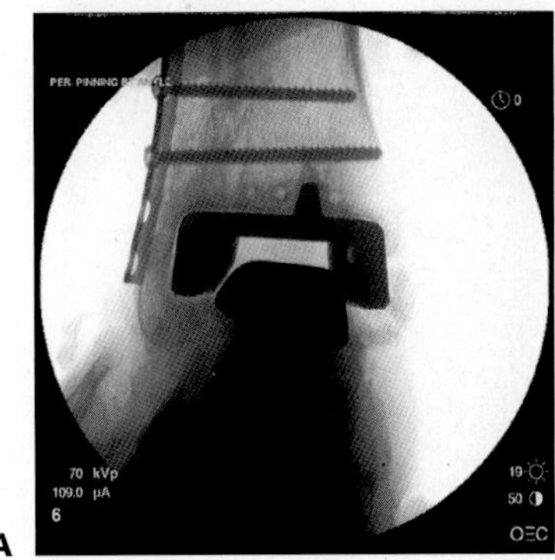

A

TECH FIG 1 • Stressing the ankle intraoperatively (**A**) reveals gapping at the medial malleolar fracture site. *(continued)*

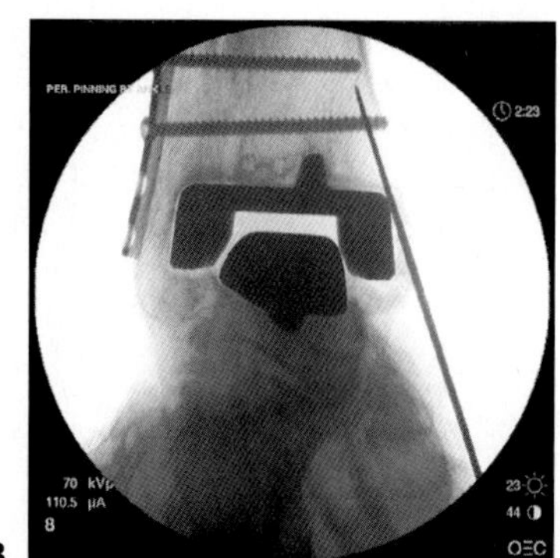

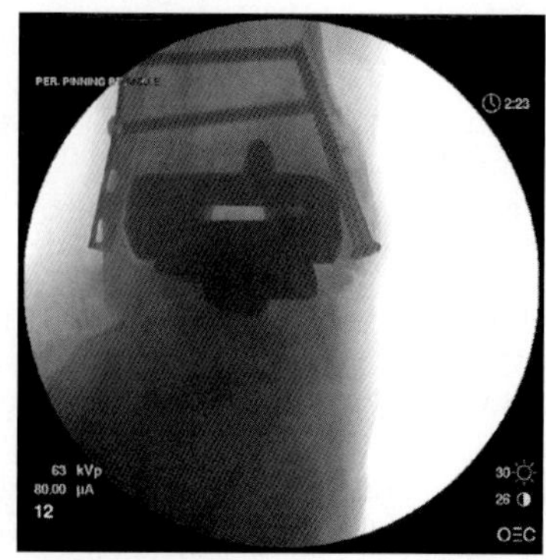

TECH FIG 1 • *(continued)* Two guidewires are placed across the fracture site (**B**) within the substance of the medial malleolar bone. Firm compression is achieved (**C**) across the fracture site.

OPEN REPAIR OF THE LATERAL MALLEOLUS FRACTURE

- Currently, standard fixation of the syndesmotic fusion is done percutaneously, after placing the plate against the distal fibula through the anterior approach (**TECH FIG 2A**).
- However, if a lateral malleolar fracture is sustained, extend the lateral approach as a standard lateral approach for this type of fracture pattern. Clean the fracture ends of debris (**TECH FIG 2B**).
- After direct exposure, reduce the fragments (**TECH FIG 2C,D**). Often the fracture is at the apex of the lateral portion of the prosthesis. Thus, it is difficult to provide standard lag-screw fixation.
- Prebend the plate to hook around the lateral malleolus tip (**TECH FIG 2E**).
- Apply the plate proximal to the fracture with three screws traversing the syndesmosis.
- Distal screw fixation generally allows placement of two screws, both cortical. The first, more proximal screw should be placed with lag technique. The second screw is placed intramedullary, at the tip, to provide stabilization.

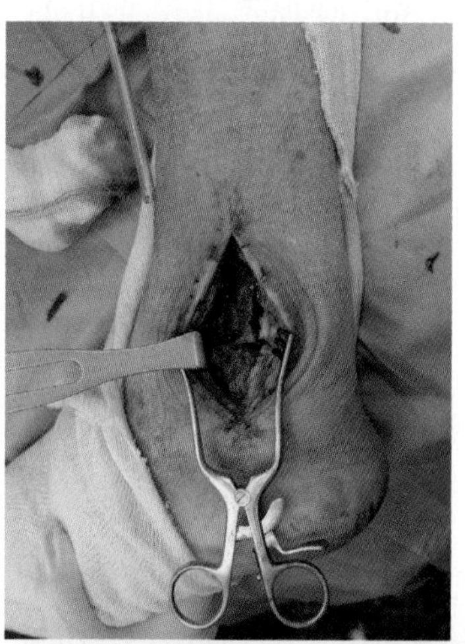

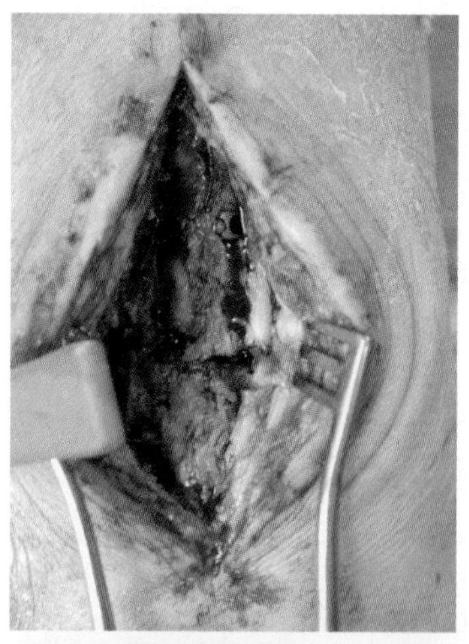

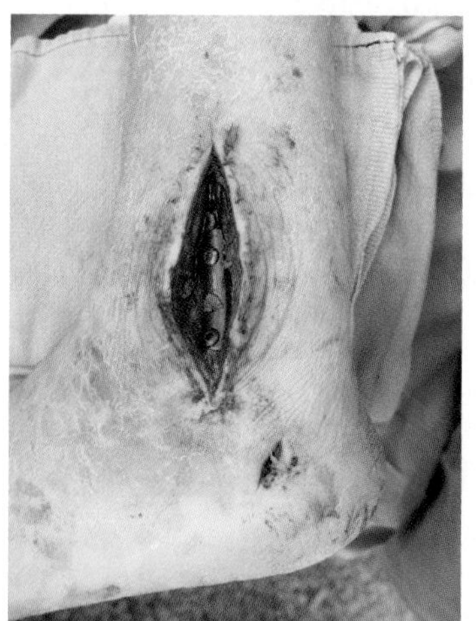

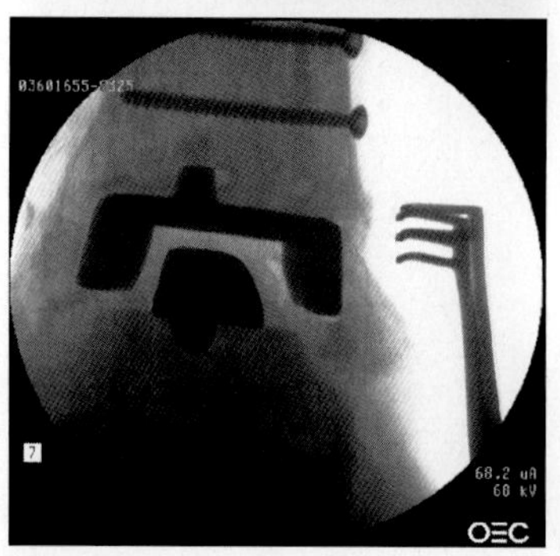

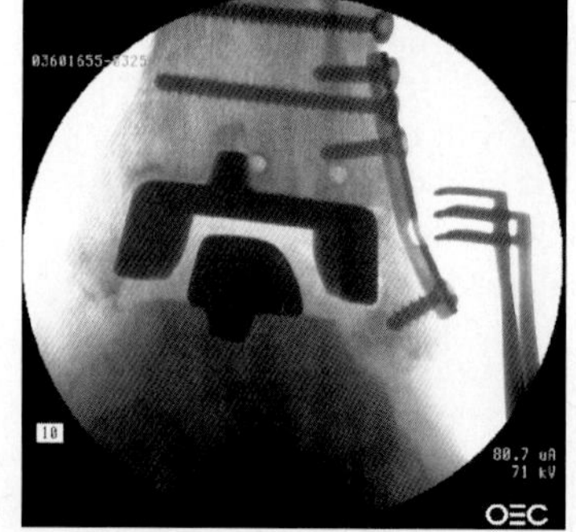

TECH FIG 2 • Lateral malleolus fracture. The lateral approach is chosen (**A**), and the fracture fragments are exposed and curetted (**B**). Intraoperative fluoroscopy demonstrates the fracture location (**C**) and reduction with plate fixation (**D**). Clinical photograph reveals contouring of plate (**E**) and screw fixation above and below the fracture to maintain stability.

REPAIR OF A LATE MEDIAL MALLEOLUS FRACTURE

- As mentioned above, a direct medial approach is used to provide better access to the fracture fragments while avoiding violation of the ankle prosthesis (**TECH FIG 3A**).
- Use a curette to remove all fibrous tissue present (**TECH FIG 3B**). This is a critical step, as good-quality vascular bone must be visualized on both sides of the fracture (**TECH FIG 3C**).
- It is critical to provide direct apposition of the fracture fragments to enhance the potential for union (**TECH FIG 3D,E**).
- Bone graft may be required to supplement any gaps present; it is generally taken from the calcaneus (**TECH FIG 3F–I**).
- Normally, axial fixation is preferred, as compression is achieved through standard medial malleolar fixation techniques. However, plate fixation may be used as a supplement after compression is achieved (**TECH FIG 3J–O**).

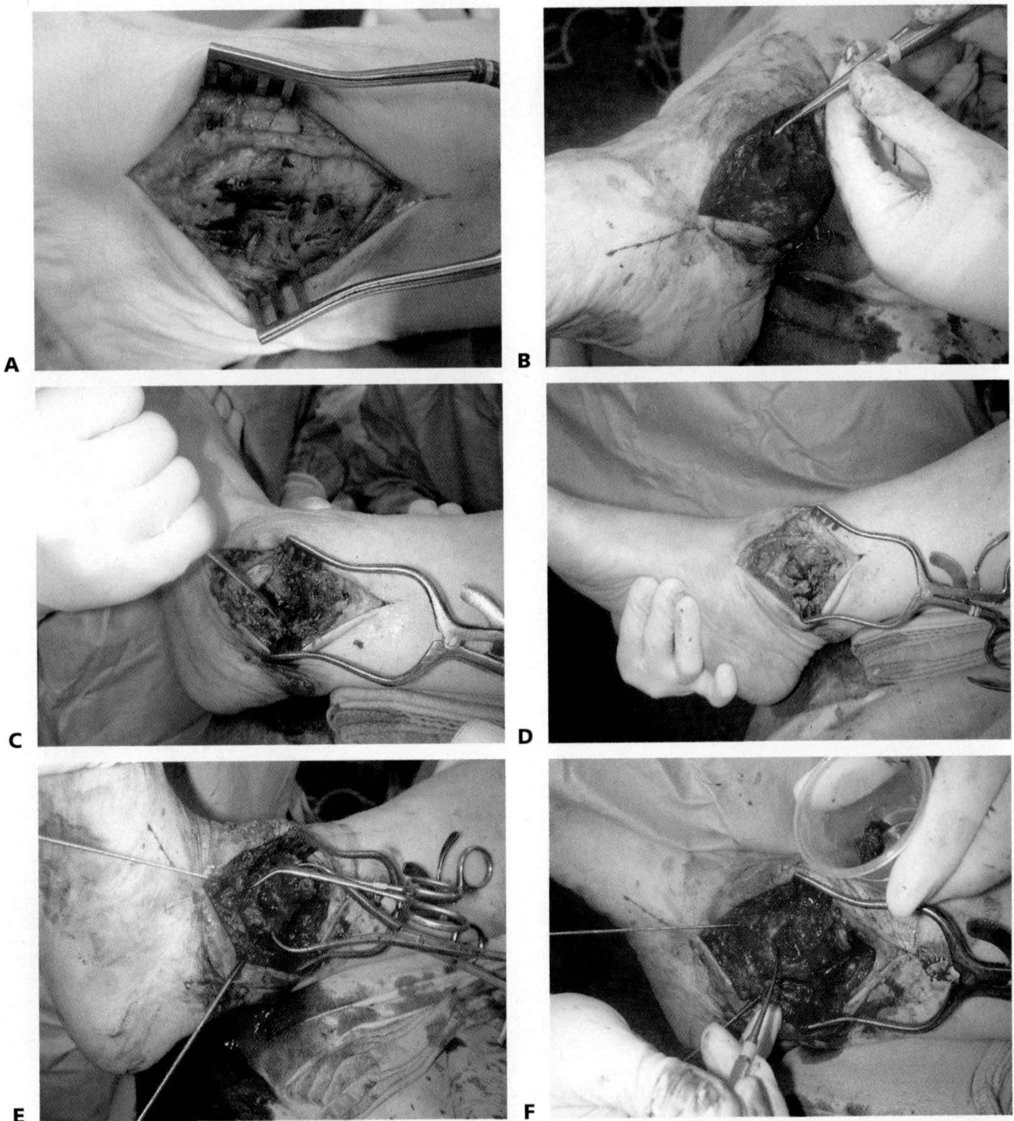

TECH FIG 3 • Late medial malleolus fracture. A direct medial approach is performed (**A**). Due to the delayed presentation and subsequent longevity of motion about the fracture site, significant bone erosion is present. The fracture site is curetted (**B**) and stressed (**C**) to check the stability of the prosthesis. The fracture is manually reduced (**D**) and clamped to maintain the reduction (**E**). The base of the fracture is packed with cancellous bone graft (**F**). *(continued)*

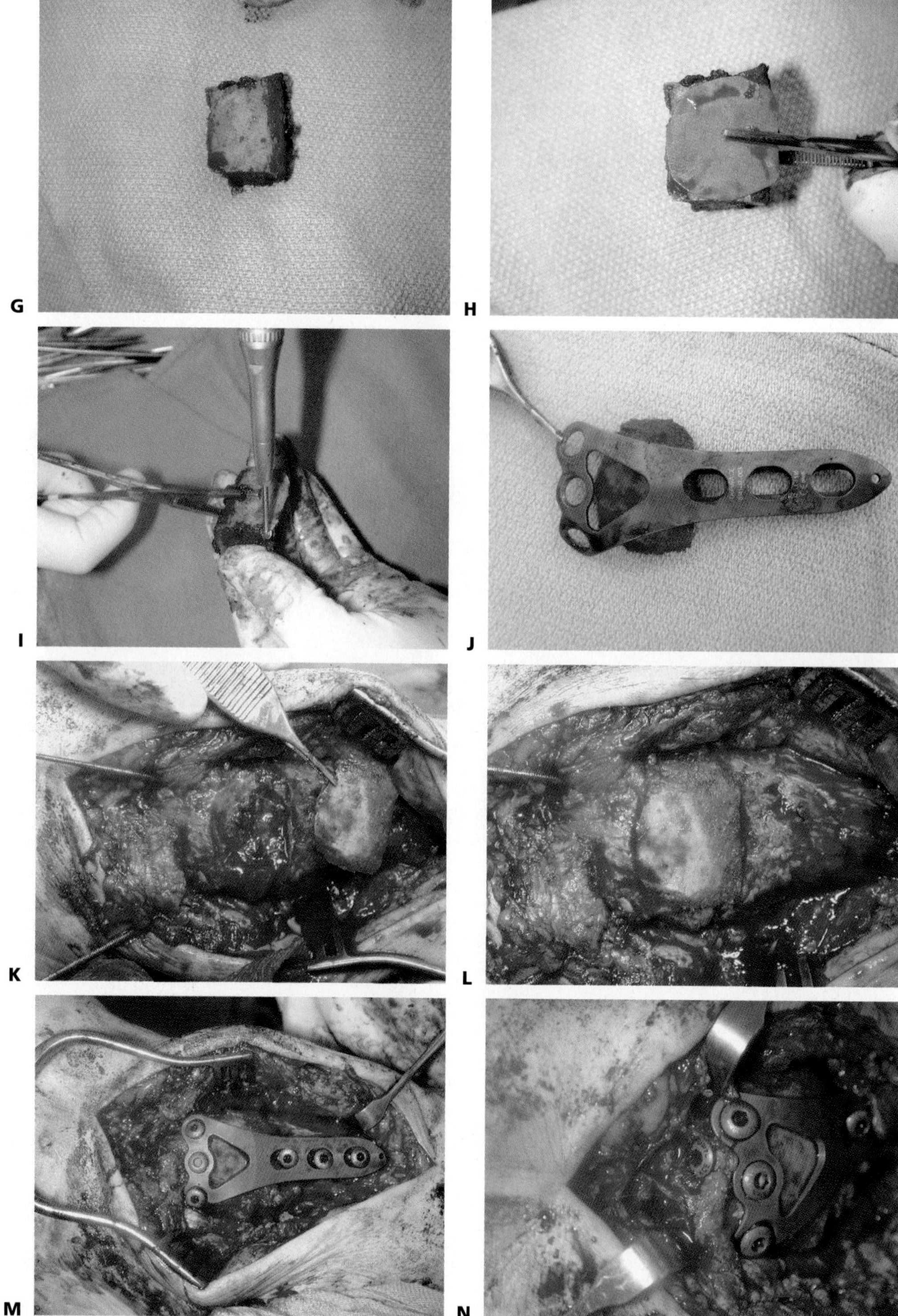

TECH FIG 3 • *(continued)* Tricortical graft is harvested (**G**), templated (**H**), and prepared (**I**) for a perfect fit in the cortical defect. A plate is contoured (**J**) and the bone graft inserted into the defect (**K,L**). The plate is applied (**M**) under compression (note eccentric placement of proximal screws). In addition, an axial screw (**N**) assists with this compression. *(continued)*

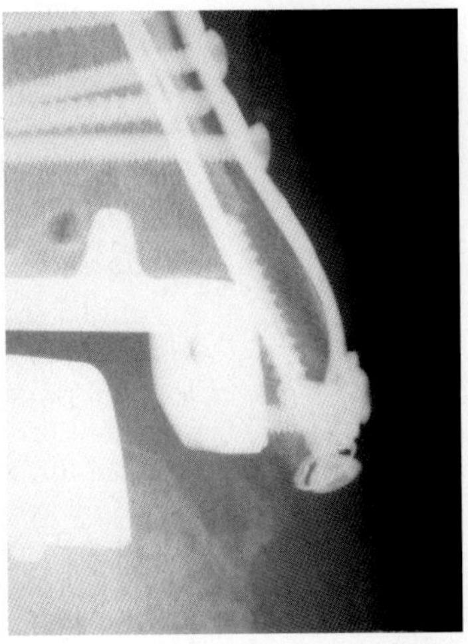

TECH FIG 3 • *(continued)* The fracture achieves successful union (**O**).

PEARLS AND PITFALLS

It is critical to assess for deformity if the medial or lateral malleolar fracture appears late.	■ If deformity is present, this must be corrected at the time of malleolar fracture. At a minimum, a calcaneal osteotomy is required. Additional procedures such as first-ray osteotomies may be used in supplement.

POSTOPERATIVE CARE

- Rigid internal fixation allows early motion, which is important after an ankle arthroplasty.
- After a brief period of immobilization (generally 10 days to 2 weeks), the patient is converted to a controlled-ankle-motion (CAM) boot.
- Range of motion is initiated at this time without weight bearing. Weight bearing is restricted until 6 weeks postoperatively, when union is generally present. It is extremely important not to allow an increase in activity or discontinuance of the CAM boot until union is complete. Nonunion of malleolar fractures in total ankle arthroplasty can severely compromise the result of the arthroplasty by creating intra-articular deformity and edge loading.

OUTCOMES

- Fracture fixation rarely results in nonunion. Without fixation, the risk of nonunion is high, compromising the arthroplasty through the potential for late deformity.

COMPLICATIONS

- Nonunion is the major potential complication.

LIGAMENT INSTABILITY

PATIENT HISTORY AND PHYSICAL FINDINGS

- Patients with ligament instability creating late malalignment of the prosthesis will develop increasing pain in the medial or lateral gutters around the prosthesis as the progressive tilt creates gutter impingement.
- Examination of the total ankle arthroplasty for ligament instability should include the following:
  - Medial–lateral stress radiographs. Medial and lateral stress is applied to the ankle, specifically looking for a soft endpoint or gross ligamentous laxity. This test will assist the examiner in determining the incompetence of the ligaments directly. Without a firm endpoint to stress, the ligaments are clearly compromised.
  - Thumb-to-forearm test, or hyperextension for the elbow: These basic tests examine for gross ligamentous laxity, often congenitally based. Patients with gross ligament laxity are at higher risk for failure of the prosthesis due to tilt, edge loading, and subsequent osteolysis.

IMAGING AND OTHER DIAGNOSTIC STUDIES

- Manual stress radiographs may assist the examiner in quantifying ligament laxity. Similar to the test mentioned above, stress is applied across the ankle joint while a mortise ankle radiograph is obtained. The examiner will specifically look for increased tilt of the talus upon the tibial tray.
- Weight-bearing AP and mortise radiographs may also be used to quantify ligament laxity, as the tilt of the prosthesis can be directly measured.
- Both radiographs must be interpreted with caution, for this tilt may be compounded by underlying foot deformities. Thus, these deformities must be corrected simultaneously, or any ligament reconstructive procedures will ultimately fail due to recurrent tension across the newly created ligament.

DIFFERENTIAL DIAGNOSIS

- Varus or valgus foot deformity
- Posterior tibial tendon insufficiency
- Peroneal tendon rupture

NONOPERATIVE MANAGEMENT

- Conservative care revolves around stabilizing the ankle with medial and lateral posts, often in the form of a lace-up brace, a U-shaped stirrup brace, a Ritchie-type brace, or an Arizona brace (**FIG 10**). All braces serve to limit varus or valgus thrust, and thus limit tilt.

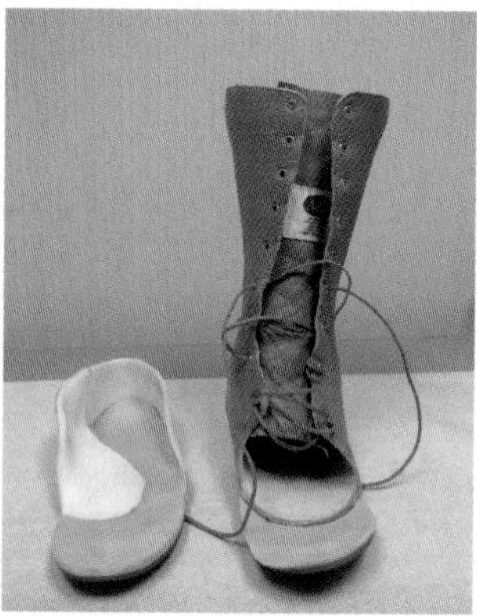

FIG 10 • Protective Arizona brace (*right*) offers a more secure option for stability over the UCBL orthotic (*left*).

SURGICAL MANAGEMENT

- Surgical ligament reconstruction is challenging due to the space occupied by the prosthesis. Thus, standard techniques need to be modified to accommodate the bone architecture provided by resection necessary for prosthesis implantation.

Preoperative Planning

- Patients with ligament incompetence are assessed for laxity via the stress radiographs mentioned above. The patient is assessed for hindfoot and forefoot deformities that may require simultaneous correction. Gross ligament laxity must be accounted for, as balance achieved through tightening one side of the ankle may create the opposite deformity from that corrected due to a lack of contralateral restraint. Finally, a diagnostic ultrasound may be used to assess the quality of the posterior tibial tendon and peroneal tendons, as an MRI will be compromised by the prosthesis.

Positioning

- Depending on the involved ligaments, the patient is positioned either laterally on the operating table for lateral ligament incompetence, or supine with a bump under the opposite hip for medial ligament incompetence.

Approach

- The approach parallels the standard anterior incision performed for ankle arthroplasty, maximizing the skin bridge to minimize wound complications. Exposure is carried proximal to the ankle joint a minimum of 5 cm and distal to the ankle joint a minimum of 6 cm. This generous incision allows access to reconstruct all aspects of the failed ligaments.

TECHNIQUES

DELTOID RECONSTRUCTION

- The patient is placed supine on the operating table, with a bump under the contralateral hip to externally rotate the involved extremity.
- The incision is medially based, extending from 1 cm proximal to the medial malleolus past the sustentaculum tali (**TECH FIG 4A**).
- Retract the posterior tibial tendon posteriorly, exposing the insertions of the deep and superficial components to the deltoid ligament (**TECH FIG 4B,C**).
- Using standard EndoButton technique, place drill holes at both insertions, exiting anterior to the fibula (**TECH FIG 4D–F**).

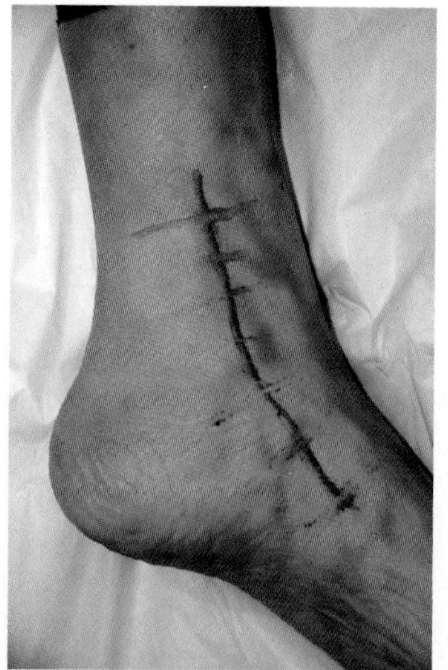

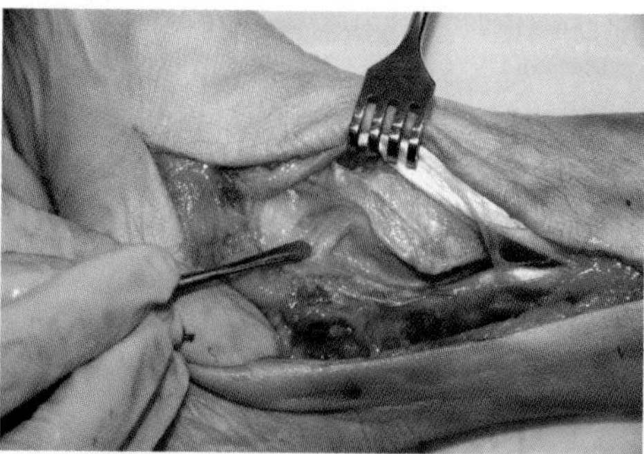

TECH FIG 4 • Deltoid reconstruction. Some photos are taken from cadaveric dissection during the development of the procedure; others are intraoperative photos taken during a reconstruction involving a stemmed talar component, calcaneal osteotomy, and Cotton osteotomy. The surgical approach is medial (**A**). After opening the posterior tibial tendon sheath and retracting the tendon anteriorly (**B**), the deep deltoid is visible. *(continued)*

- A cadaveric anterior tibial tendon is used for the reconstruction. Weave a Krackow suture stitch with no. 2 Ethibond through both ends of the tendon and anchor it to two separate EndoButtons with 1 cm of suture lead between the EndoButton and the tendon ends (**TECH FIG 4G**). The tendon is prestretched to minimize late plastic deformation of the tendon graft.
- Pass the ends through the drill holes and flip the buttons, providing secure fixation at both the superficial and deep insertions (**TECH FIG 4H–J**).
- Securely reproduce the ligament origin by placing a drill hole at the tip of the medial malleolus, directing the hole toward the anterior central tibia. This hole is placed obliquely to avoid the tibial component to the prosthesis (**TECH FIG 4K,L**).
- Double the tendon upon itself and thread it through this drill hole, with the looped end exiting the anterior tibia.
- Place a 4.5-mm drill hole proximal to the exit point of the looped tendon, 1 cm beyond the maximum stretch of the loop component of the tendon. By placing the drill hole 1 cm proximal to the extent of the loop, the ligament reconstruction will remain taut (**TECH FIG 4M**).
- Anchor the loop with a large-fragment screw and a spiked ligament washer (**TECH FIGS 4N–P**).

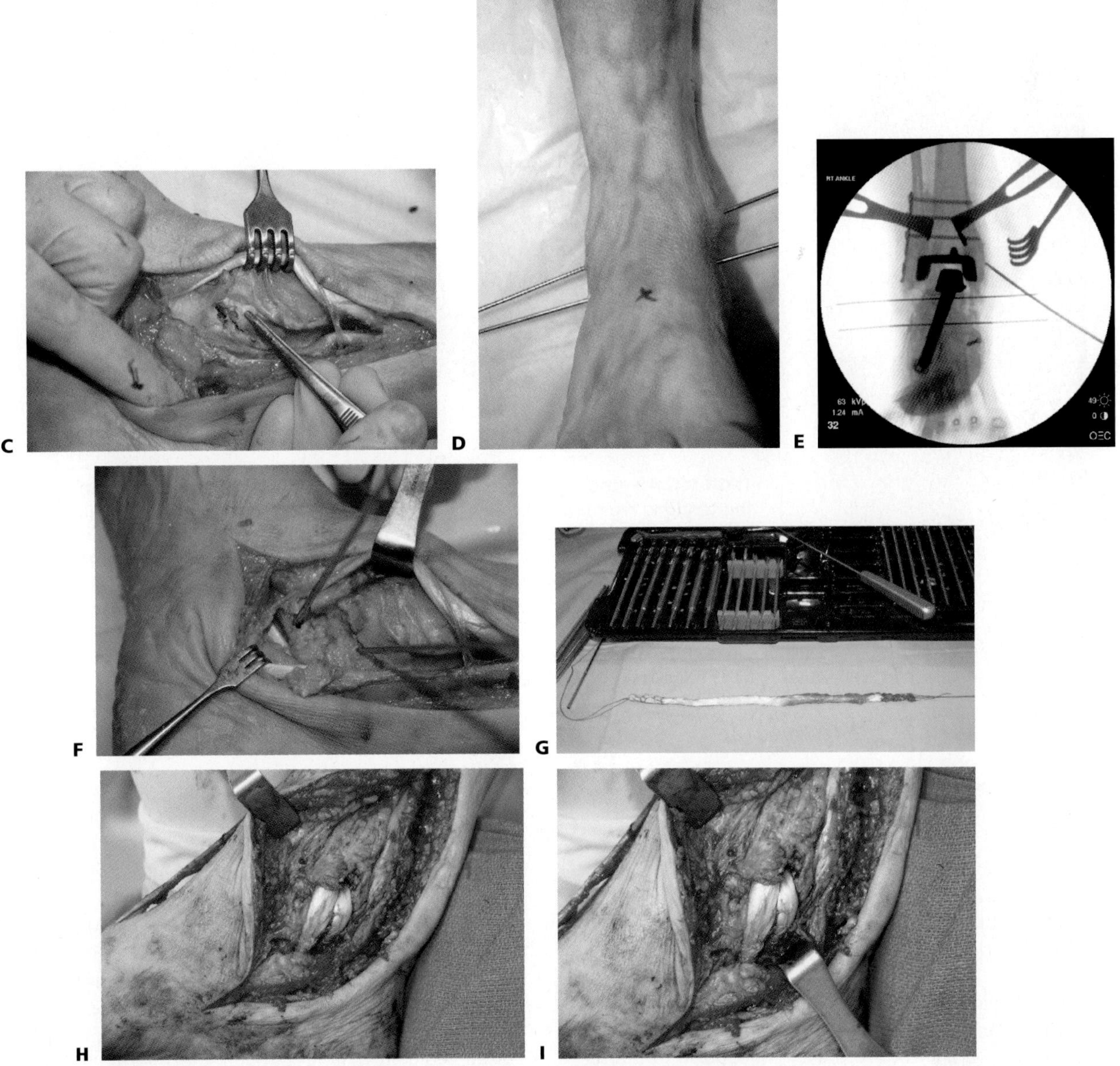

TECH FIG 4 • *(continued)* This ligament may be sectioned for lateral imbrications (**C**). Guidewires are passed for the EndoButton in a plane that emerges anterior to the fibula (**D**) and transtalar (**E**). The guidewires are placed at the insertion points of the native deep and superficial deltoid ligaments (**F**). The cadaveric tendon is prepared by placing Krackow suture weaves at both ends (**G**) and tensioned to minimize late plastic deformation. Each end of the graft is placed into the respective deep and superficial deltoid tunnel (**H,I**), held in place on the lateral side of the talus by the EndoButtons (**J**). *(continued)*

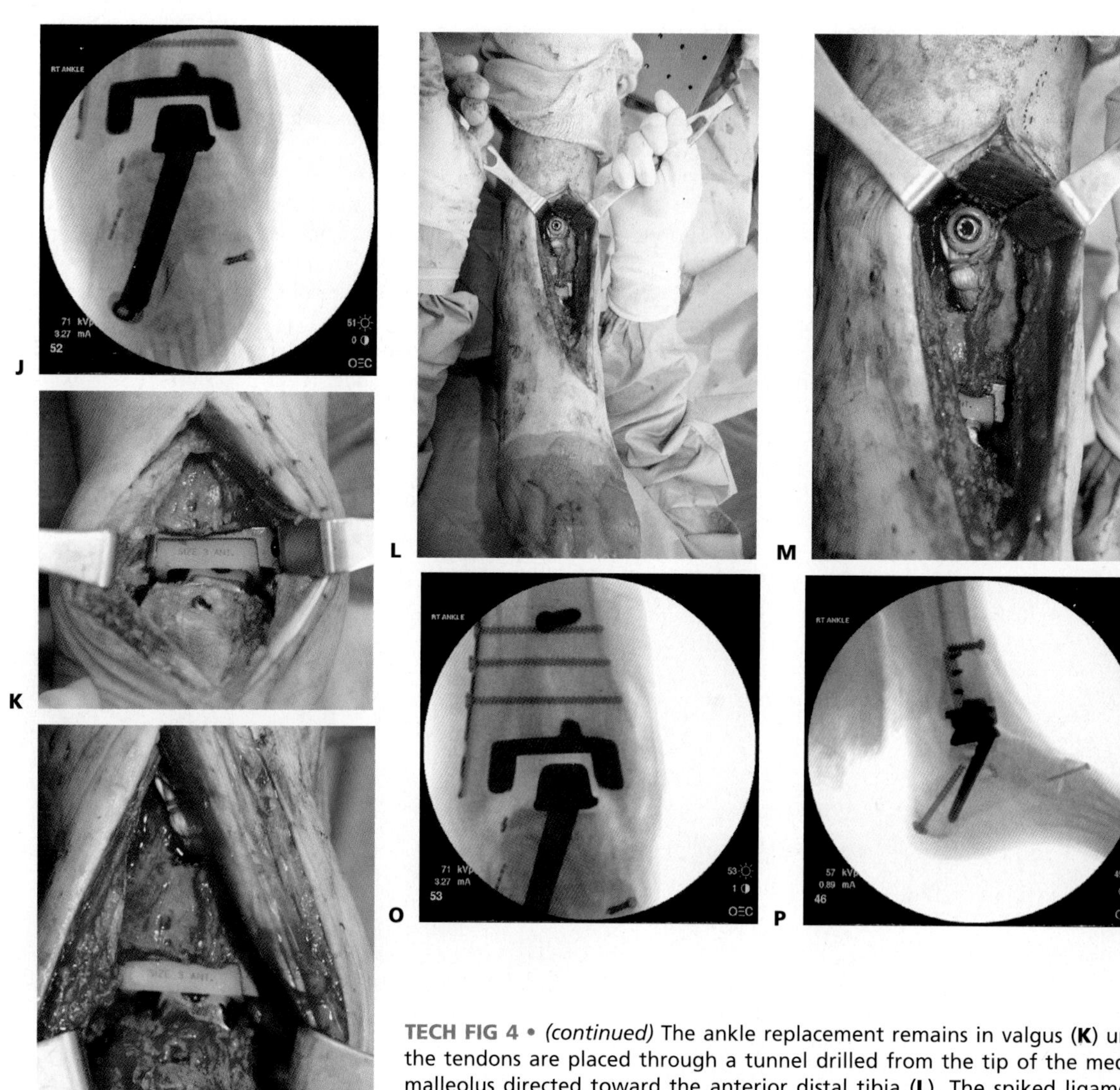

TECH FIG 4 • *(continued)* The ankle replacement remains in valgus (**K**) until the tendons are placed through a tunnel drilled from the tip of the medial malleolus directed toward the anterior distal tibia (**L**). The spiked ligament washer is placed proximal to the exit point of this tunnel to place the graft under maximal tension (**L**). The looped end of the graft is placed around the screw, and the ligament washer is tightened against it (**M**). The ankle is now aligned in neutral (**N**), and this position is confirmed under fluoroscopic imaging in the AP (**O**) and sagittal (**P**) planes. Note the position of the EndoButtons on the sagittal plane, anterior to the fibula and transtalar (**P**).

LATERAL LIGAMENT RECONSTRUCTION

- Unfortunately, a modified Brostrom procedure is not sufficient to stabilize the lateral ligaments in light of an ankle replacement. Thus, a similar cadaveric tendon transfer is performed to stabilize the deficient lateral ligaments.
- Use a cadaveric anterior tibial tendon, tubularizing the tendon and weaving a Krackow suture with no. 2 Ethibond on one end. Secure an EndoButton to this suture with a 1-cm gap between the end of the tendon and the EndoButton.
- Make a drill hole through the talar neck at the insertion of the anterior talofibular ligament, exiting anterior to the medial malleolus. The far cortex of the hole is smaller than the length of the EndoButton.
- If sufficient fibula is present distal to the lateral portion of the tibial tray, place 7.3-mm drill holes at the origins of the anterior talofibular ligament and calcaneofibular ligament. These holes meet in the central fibula.
- Place the allograft tendon through these holes, with the distal segment exiting through the inferior (calcaneofibular) hole.
- If there is not sufficient fibula at the tip, carry the plate for securing the syndesmotic fusion to the tip of the fibula, and place the cadaveric tendon deep to the plate.

Place a screw in the most distal hole of the plate to help stabilize the transferred tendon.

- In either case, place the hindfoot into eversion and make a 4.5-mm drill hole in the calcaneus, from lateral to medial, at the insertion of the calcaneofibular ligament.
- Place the cadaveric tendon under maximal tension, and use a knife to bisect the allograft proximal to the previously drilled hole.
- Place a 6.5-mm large-fragment screw with a large spiked ligament washer through the cadaveric tendon at the point of the previously placed incision. This screw is placed proximal to the previously drilled hole. Again, this technique will maximize tension on the transferred tendon.
- Insert the screw into the calcaneus, with the spiked washer completely engaging the tendon to provide rigid fixation.
- Place the peroneal tendons deep to this transferred tendon to prevent dislocation.
- If residual tendon is present, it may be doubled back over the lateral wall of the fibula and anchored to the bone to provide increased strength to the transfer.

PEARLS AND PITFALLS

Indications	▪ The surgeon must assess the patient for associated foot pathology (cavus with lateral ligament laxity, and flatfoot with deltoid ligament laxity). This must be addressed simultaneously in the form of osteotomies or arthrodeses, or the ligament repair will fail. ▪ The surgeon must assess the patient for generalized ligament laxity. Care must be taken not to overtighten the reconstruction, or the opposite deformity may occur.
Graft management	▪ The graft should be tubularized before performing the Krackow weave. This will increase the structural integrity of the cadaveric graft. ▪ The graft must be stretched to a minimum of 20 lbs of tension to prevent late stretch.
Tunnel placement	▪ The lateral (or medial, in lateral ligament reconstruction) portion of the tunnels (talar and calcaneal) must exit anterior to the fibula (or medial malleolus). Failure to achieve this placement will compromise flipping of the EndoButton and create malleolar impingement. ▪ The far cortical bridge of the tunnel must be a smaller diameter than the length of the EndoButton to ensure rigid fixation. ▪ Occasionally, a small incision is placed at the exit point of the EndoButton suture to assist with the flip. A hemostat can be used to assist with this maneuver.
Spiked ligament washer fixation	▪ Placing the spiked fixation beyond the maximum stretch of the proximal end of the cadaveric tendon is critical to maximizing tension on the ligament repair. The ligament must be tensioned to prevent late sag or recurrence.

POSTOPERATIVE CARE

- If the fixation is rigid and strong, the patient is placed in a cooling boot for 2 to 3 days and admitted to the hospital. This minimizes the risk of incision complications, but the patient must remain dormant with the leg elevated to prevent stretch on the newly reconstructed ligament.
- If the fixation has the potential for compromise, the patient is placed in a stirrup-type plaster splint in combination with a posterior mold splint. This construct will take tension off the ligament repair while simultaneously keeping the ankle flexed to neutral.
- The patient is changed to a cast at 5 to 7 days with windows placed in the cast for direct incision observation.
- Physical therapy is used at 6 weeks postoperatively to increase ankle range of motion. No inversion or eversion is attempted until 3 months postoperatively. The patient is in a CAM boot fully weight bearing at this time.
- The patient is placed in a lace-up brace at 12 weeks postoperatively. This brace may be discontinued at 4 months postoperatively.

OUTCOMES

- This technique is newly developed, so there are no long-term outcome studies at this time. A trial is under way.

COMPLICATIONS

- Wound infection, cellulitis, wound necrosis
- Nerve damage to superficial peroneal, deep peroneal, saphenous, sural, or tibial nerves
- Recurrence of deformity, tendon transfer failure
- Opposite deformity in cases of gross ligament laxity

PROSTHESIS SUBSIDENCE

PATIENT HISTORY AND PHYSICAL FINDINGS

- Patients with subsidence of the prosthesis have collapse and eventual impingement in the medial or lateral gutters. They often complain of increasing stiffness upon a prosthesis that was previously functioning well. This is rarely an acute phenomenon (unless fracture through an osteolytic cyst created the subsidence) and is often noticed as a part of a routine office visit. Pain follows the stiffness and is normally located deep, medial, and lateral to the prosthesis.
- The methods for examining the total ankle arthroplasty for subsidence include the following:
  - Standing flexibility (range of motion) of the ankle: The patient stands with the involved ankle anterior to the axis

of the body and the opposite ankle behind the body. To determine dorsiflexion, the knee is flexed forward as far anterior as possible (runner's stretch), and the angle between the foot and the tibia is measured. Plantarflexion is assessed by having the patient lean back on the involved extremity as far as possible while keeping the entire foot flat on the ground. The angle is then measured. This should be compared at each office visit and documented. Increasing stiffness is commonly seen with subsidence of the prosthesis. If this test is done routinely as a part of each office visit, accurate and reproducible values will allow measured changes in ankle flexibility.

- Direct palpation: The examiner must palpate deeply the medial and lateral gutters to elicit pain. In addition, the syndesmotic fusion is painful to palpation if a nonunion has led to tibial tray subsidence. Pain signifies increasing gutter impingement as the arthritic bone interacts due to loss of height. Pain in the syndesmotic region signifies a syndesmotic nonunion, which allows tibial tray subsidence (common in an undersized prosthesis).

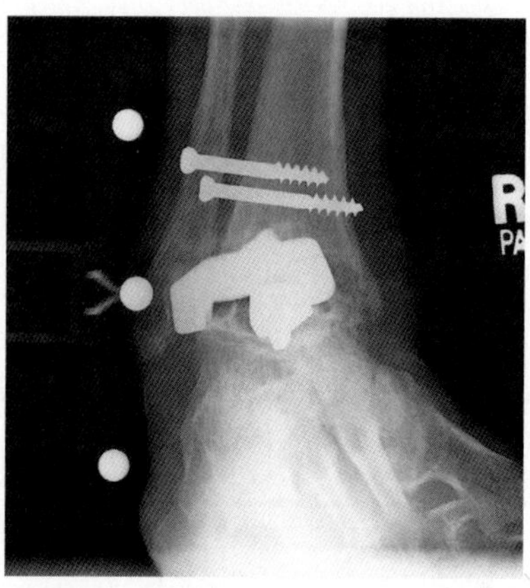

FIG 12 • Evaluation for tibiotalar tilt and lack of fibula coverage in the tibial tray on the AP radiograph. An assessment of deformity can guide the surgeon toward supplementary procedures done at revision surgery.

IMAGING AND OTHER DIAGNOSTIC STUDIES

- Standard radiographs include weight-bearing AP, lateral, and mortise views of the ankle. These radiographs reveal a tilt in the components if subsidence is not uniform. The lateral radiograph (**FIG 11**) is assessed for tibial tray subsidence (often at the anterior cortex of the tibia) and for talar subsidence (the talar fin may be penetrating the subtalar joint). The AP and mortise radiographs allow an assessment of measurable tilt and bone loss (**FIG 12**). Gutter impingement becomes obvious as contact between the talus and the mediolateral malleolus is visible.
- A CT scan is critical to assess penetration of the prosthesis into the subtalar joint (**FIG 13**). In addition, the nonunion of the syndesmotic fusion may be visualized, contributing to tibial tray subsidence. The surgeon can assess for an undersized prosthesis by examining the coverage of the tibial tray underlying the fibula. Lack of coverage by the fibula can lead to valgus subsidence of the tibial tray. The CT scan will reveal osteolytic cysts contributing to subsidence of the tibial tray or talar component, and potential fracture through these cysts. Finally, the CT can assess for ingrowth of the prosthesis and potential loosening. Subtraction software will assist in eliminating artifact due to the prosthesis.

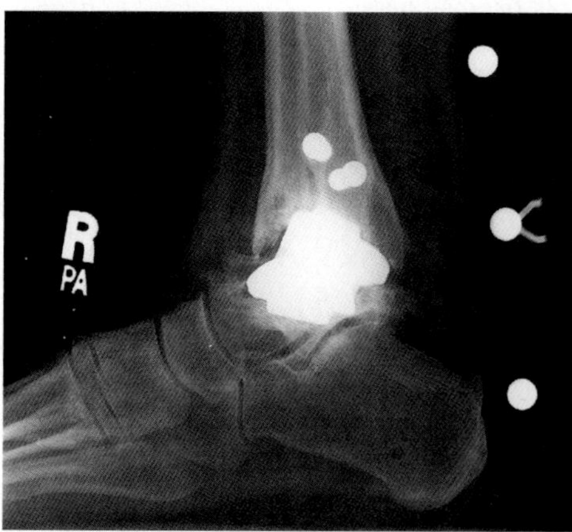

FIG 11 • Lateral radiograph of grossly subsided prosthesis. Note the lack of anterior coverage in the distal tibia and the subsequent anterior subsidence of the prosthesis. This preserved shelf of anterior bone can be used to re-establish the height of the tibial tray with a larger prosthesis offering better sagittal coverage. The lateral radiograph helps to assess talar subsidence, in particular looking for violation of the subtalar joint.

DIFFERENTIAL DIAGNOSIS

- Infection (osteolysis vs. osteomyelitis)
- Residual posttraumatic osteoarthritis in the medial or lateral gutters

NONOPERATIVE MANAGEMENT

- Nonoperative management involves bracing to prevent pain from arthritic or collapsed bone surfaces. In particular, a nonarticulating ankle–foot orthosis may limit pain.

SURGICAL MANAGEMENT

- The indications for surgical treatment of subsidence are three: pain, stiffness that is unacceptable to the patient, and prevention of substantial subsidence that will diminish bone stock to the point of preventing revision of the prosthesis in the future. Subsidence to this level may necessitate implant removal followed by arthrodesis of the ankle joint.

Preoperative Planning

- Assessment of the remaining bone stock after implant removal allows the surgeon to predict whether a custom prosthesis will need to be constructed to salvage the failed joint replacement. The most accurate way to make this assessment is a careful review of the CT scan.
- In addition, assessment for revision of the syndesmotic fusion may be made by CT scan. Underlying foot deformity that may have contributed to prosthesis subsidence is determined to allow planning for simultaneous flatfoot–cavovarus foot correction. The revised prosthesis must be placed upon a

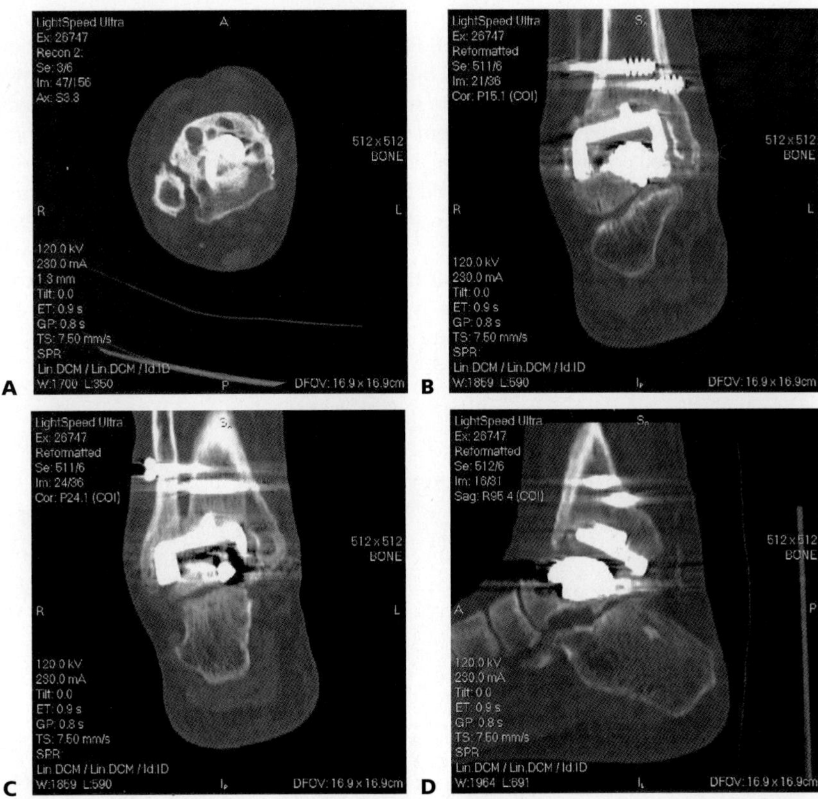

FIG 13 • CT scan of the ankle in the axial plane (**A**) reveals cystic changes to the distal tibia consistent with osteolysis. The coronal plane cuts (**B,C**) demonstrate the magnitude of subsidence and the syndesmotic nonunion. The sagittal cut (**D**) reveals the lack of penetration of the talar fin into the subtalar joint.

plantigrade foot to prevent uneven stresses leading to secondary failure.

- Infection is assessed via markers such as the white blood cell (WBC) count, erythrocyte sedimentation rate, and C-reactive protein. We have found limited value in a tagged-WBC scan, as the prosthesis itself may create an inflammatory foreign body reaction that mimics osteomyelitis on nuclear medicine scans.
- Bone stock and osteoporosis may be assessed via CT scan, plain radiographs, and a DEXA scan. If osteoporosis is present, a concerted effort to increase bone mass will assist in providing structural support to the prosthesis and should be performed before revision.

Positioning

- The patient is placed supine on the operating table.
- A bump is placed under the hip to rotate the extremity to neutral with respect to the knee.
- The lower leg is placed on multiple blankets to provide a firm working surface while simultaneously allowing shoot-through lateral radiographs to enhance the assessment of prosthesis coverage (anterior and posterior pillar).

Approach

- The surgical approach is anterior, following the initial incision done for the primary arthroplasty. The interval is the same as that mentioned above.

TALAR SUBSIDENCE

- Expose the talus by removing all associated scar tissue and necrosis. The fixator is applied to provide distraction and easy component access while providing stability (**TECH FIG 5A–D**).
- Remove the talar component. It is normally not ingrown and comes out simply after replacing the insertion rod and joysticking the component (**TECH FIG 5E,F**).
- Make saw cuts to restore the axis of the prosthesis to be perpendicular to the axis of the tibia (**TECH FIG 5G–I**). These cuts may use a standard (though larger) cutting block.
- There is often a rectangular void in the talus after component removal (**TECH FIG 5J,K**). Curette any fibrous tissue within that void, achieving healthy bleeding bone. There is normally a rim of excellent cortical bone in the nascent remaining talus, as the original Agility talar component does not conform to the entire talus after the initial cut.
- This rim of bone is advantageous, as the new Agility LP talar component does conform to the entire talus. As such, the talar component will sit on this rim, establishing the height of the nascent talus made with the original saw cut at the index procedure.

- The fin on the Agility LP will have no stability, due to the rectangular defect present in the central talus (TECH FIG 5L). One could consider bone grafting this defect, but I do not believe the bone graft will provide adequate stability in the short term, allowing the talar component to rotate or shift from the desired position after closure and rehabilitation. In addition, in the long term, it would be unusual for the bone graft to incite ingrowth into the Agility LP talar component.
- Thus, I use cement fixation for the talar fin. I fill the void present with polymethylmethacrylate while it is still softer and malleable. I then onlay the Agility LP talar component onto the talus, allowing it to sit on the rim of nascent bone while the fin conforms to the cement in the desired position (TECH FIG 5M–O). To do this, the tibial component must be in place so that appropriate rotation and mediolateral positioning can be determined. The remaining native talus provides some element of bone ingrowth into the prosthesis, while the cement interdigitates with the residual sintered beads on the talar component.
- I allow the cement to harden while I manually reduce the ankle joint, maintaining the correct position until the cement cures. The talus is now stable and ready to articulate (TECH FIG 5P–T).

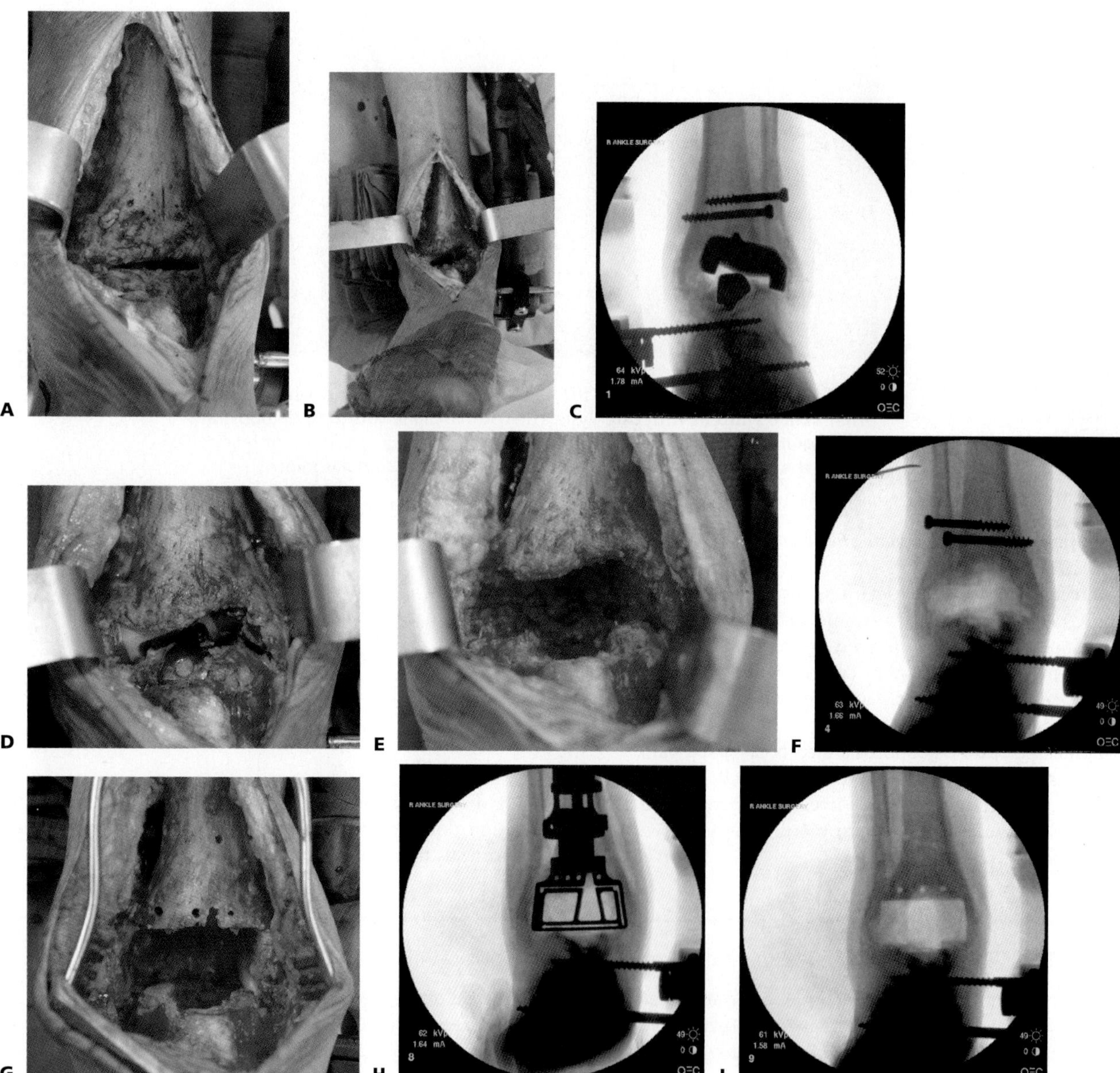

TECH FIG 5 • Operative management of severe subsidence of both the tibial and talar components via conversion of the primary replacement to an Agility LP component, with the addition of polymethylmethacrylate for stability. The anterior approach is reproduced, and no visible components are present due to the severe subsidence (**A**). The fixator is applied (**B**), allowing distraction and stabilization (**C**, reverse image). After distraction, the components become visible (**D**) and the magnitude of subsidence becomes obvious. After component removal (**E**), the bone defects are apparent (**F**) and the residual bone is truly appreciated. The saw cuts are made (**G**) after application of a large-sized cutting block (**H**), revealing a thinned but present medial malleolus (**I**). *(continued)*

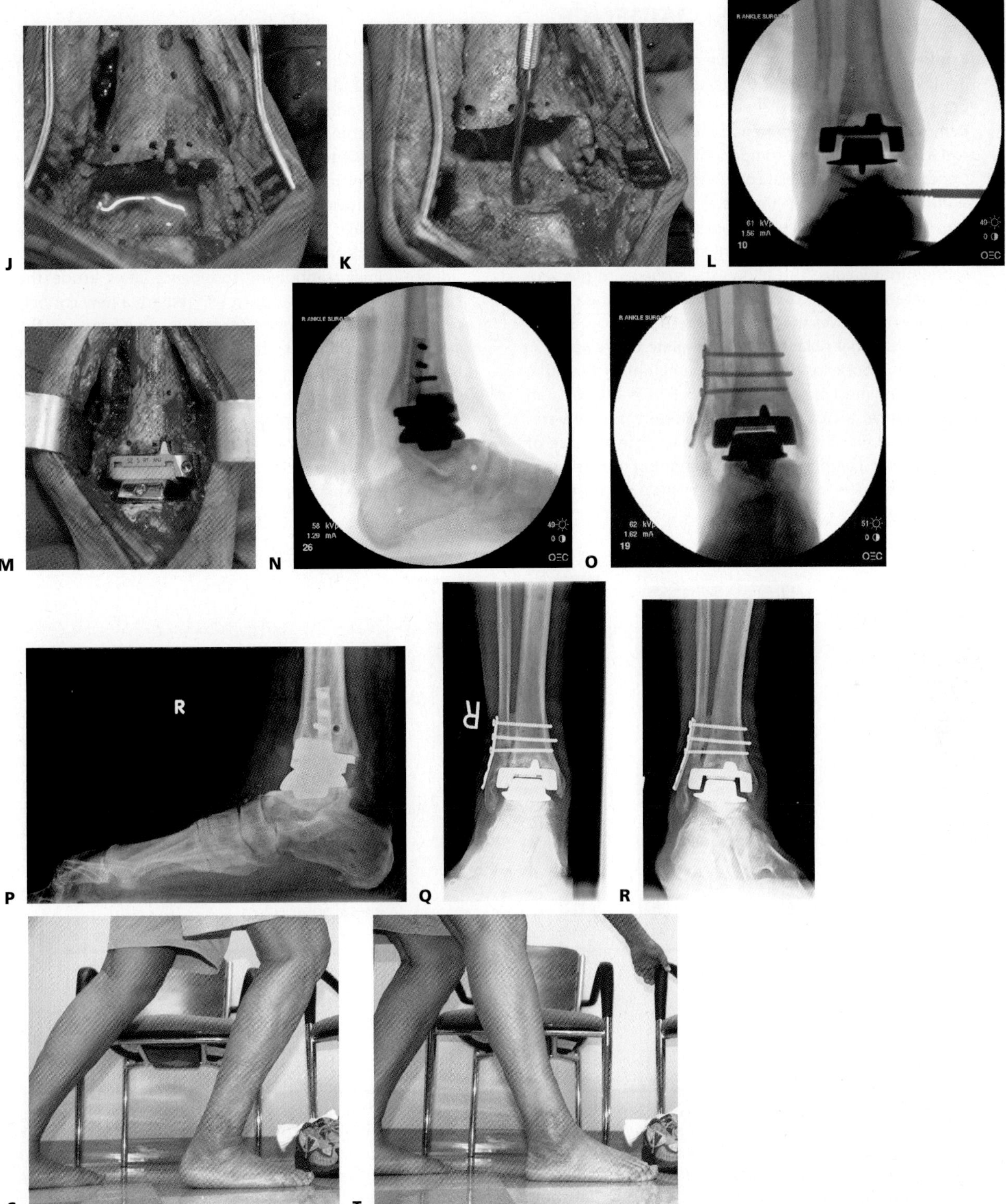

TECH FIG 5 • *(continued)* Clinical inspection demonstrates a preserved cortical rim in the tibia (**J**) and talus (**K**) with the central rectangular defect expected. The trial prosthesis confirms adequate rim support for the Agility LP (**L**), with restoration of height. The central defect is apparent and is filled with polymethylmethacrylate. The final components (**M**) are two sizes larger than the original. The syndesmosis has also been grafted, with fixation revised. The rim coverage is apparent on intraoperative fluoroscopy (**N,O**). At 1 year postoperatively (**P–R**) the prosthesis is stable and balanced, without laxity or tilt. The range of motion has been improved substantially by providing an appropriately articulating ankle replacement (**S,T**).

TIBIAL COMPONENT SUBSIDENCE

- Expose the tibia using the above-mentioned technique. Remove all associated scar tissue, and define the defects present.
- Remove the tibial component by replacing the insertion rod and joysticking the component.
- Generally, when the tibial component subsides, it creates significant bone loss in the distal tibia at the resection site. Often there is lack of appropriate fibula coverage on the tibial component, particularly those components that subside into valgus. This allows the surgeon to plan appropriate tibial tray coverage to ensure that the revised tibial tray will cover the fibula. In these instances, simply inserting a larger tibial tray will complete the revision.
- However, if bone loss is present, the height of the tibial component must be re-established (**TECH FIG 6A**). In this instance, a custom tibial component must be created (**TECH FIG 6B**). It is important to note the size of the original component when designing the revision component. The component itself may be based on standard mediolateral dimensions, simply adding height to the tibial tray. In this instance, it is important to use knowledge based on the size of the initial component in combination with calibrated radiographs (**TECH FIG 6C**) to determine the size (width) necessary to provide appropriate fibula coverage. This will lessen the risk of future tibial component subsidence.
- Unlike the talar component, which does not require a new cut in the talus due to the isolated central core subsidence, tibial component subsidence does erode the supportive bone, and as such will require a new cut perpendicular to the plane of the tibia. One may use the standard cutting blocks to make this cut, although custom cutting blocks can be manufactured.
- Once cuts are made, the revision component fits securely into its new space. Unlike revision of the talar component, polymethylmethacrylate is not necessary, as the new tibial component has the ability for ingrowth into the newly cut surfaces.

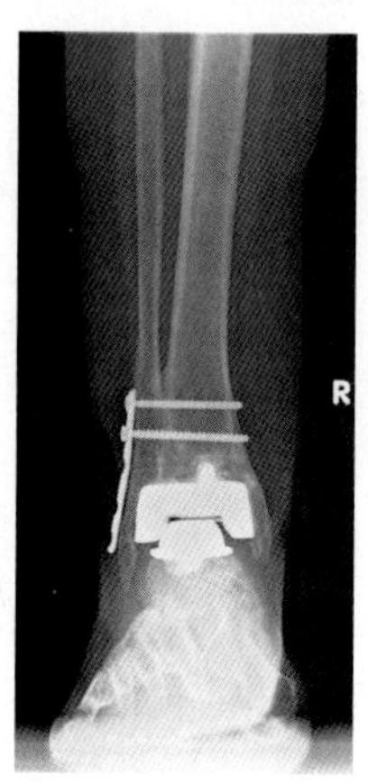

A

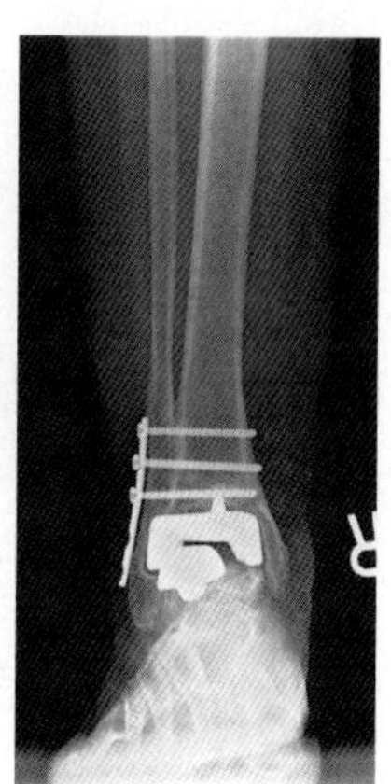

B

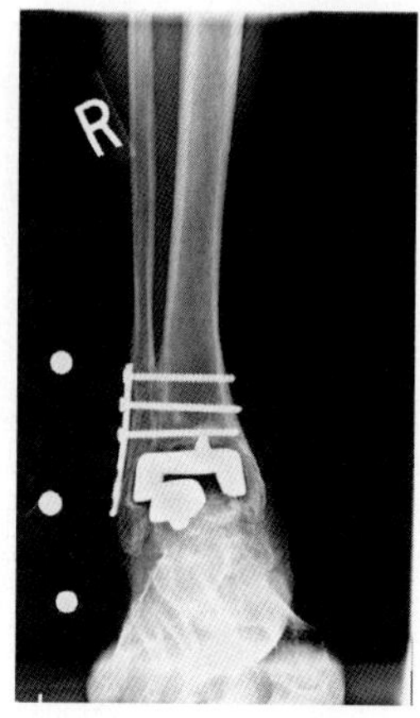

C

TECH FIG 6 • This patient had tibial tray subsidence leading to ligament laxity and a varus deformity (**A**). By revising the tibial component to a custom tray with increased height, ligamentotaxis is established and the varus deformity is eliminated (**B**). The use of calibrated radiographs (**C**) allows accurate size estimation for the revision components (note metal spheres).

PEARLS AND PITFALLS

Indications	■ The surgeon must carefully assess the patient preoperatively with plain radiographs as well as CT scans to estimate the residual bone present after removal of the subsided prosthesis. The CT will also document whether the talar fin has violated the subtalar joint. This may necessitate a subtalar fusion in conjunction with the revision. For tibial component subsidence, the surgeon must carefully assess syndesmotic fusion on the axial cuts. Revision of the syndesmotic fusion must be performed in conjunction with tibial tray revision in this instance.
Saw cuts	■ Use a large C-arm in the sagittal plane when making revised saw cuts. This will ensure that the cuts are perpendicular to the tibial–talar axis, avoiding a sloping of the components that will affect stability and flexibility. In addition, direct visualization in the sagittal plane will prevent violation of posterior neurovascular structures.
Fixation	■ Do not be afraid to use polymethylmethacrylate under these circumstances. This is essentially a hybrid revision. Some of the component remains in congruence for bone ingrowth, which will lessen the stress across the cement interface. Even in the tibial component revision, where a majority of the tray will be in contact with quality bone, I sometimes use cement at the fin to provide additional stability and allow early motion without worries of the component shifting.

POSTOPERATIVE CARE

- If the fixation is rigid and strong, the patient is placed in a cooling boot for 2 to 3 days and admitted to the hospital. This minimizes the risk of incision complications. We normally do not cast in the operating room under these circumstances, for preventing tension on the anterior surgical incision is the best method to avoid incision complications.
- The patient is changed to a cast at 5 to 7 days with windows placed in the cast for direct incision observation.
- Physical therapy is used at 2 weeks postoperatively to increase ankle range of motion, assuming the incisions have healed. Full weight bearing may be instituted before the standard 6-week interval if the patient had a previous successful fusion of the syndesmosis. If that is not the case, then weight bearing is restricted until the syndesmosis is fused.
- The patient may discontinue use of the CAM boot before 12 weeks if strength is appropriate and the syndesmosis is fused. Stability is enhanced if polymethylmethacrylate is used, and thus weight bearing without assistive devices is accelerated.

OUTCOMES

- These techniques are newly described, so there is no literature to support their use at this time. Anecdotal experience supports the techniques, however, with short-term outcomes (1 year) demonstrating substantial improvement at this time.

COMPLICATIONS

- Wound infection, cellulitis, wound necrosis
- Nerve damage to superficial peroneal, deep peroneal, saphenous, sural, or tibial nerves
- Subsidence of the newly placed components into poor-quality bone. This is a particular problem in patients with rheumatoid arthritis or other systemic conditions.

INFECTION

PATIENT HISTORY AND PHYSICAL FINDINGS

- The presentation of infection depends on the organisms involved. However, the common pathway is cellulitis, with or without a wound complication. Patients with joint infections often have fever and may have chills. Pain is often present about a previously painless prosthesis.

IMAGING AND OTHER DIAGNOSTIC STUDIES

- Plain radiographs may reveal a lucent line around the prosthesis, documenting lack of ingrowth. Cystic changes may be visualized in the bone surrounding the prosthesis.
- A CT scan is more specific for lucency about the prosthesis and poor ingrowth. In addition, the CT scan is more specific for bone cysts. Air or gas in the soft tissues is visible on CT scan. Contrast-enhanced CT scans can reveal a soft tissue abscess or a sinus tract communicating with an anterior wound complication.
- A nuclear medicine Tc scan combined with a tagged WBC scan may assist in differentiating infection from aseptic loosening of the components (**FIG 14**). The results should be interpreted with caution, however, for even in cases of aseptic loosening, inflammation around the prosthesis and foreign body reaction can create a false-positive WBC scan. Thus, this scan must be interpreted in combination with clinical and hematologic findings.

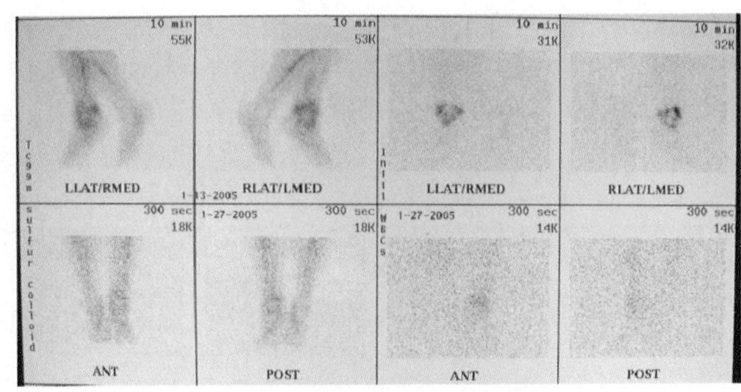

FIG 14 • A Tc99 scan is tagged with an indium (white blood cell) scan to increase the accuracy of the findings. The four images on the left are the Tc99 study done at 300 seconds and 10 minutes, and the equivalent temporal study using indium is on the right. This study suggests osteomyelitis, which was confirmed at débridement.

- Blood work must include a complete blood count with differential, an erythrocyte sedimentation rate, and C-reactive protein. Again, these results must be interpreted in combination with clinical and radiographic findings.

DIFFERENTIAL DIAGNOSIS

- Aseptic component loosening and subsidence

NONOPERATIVE MANAGEMENT

- Antibiotic management is the staple in treating infection but must be done in a thoughtful manner.
- Empiric therapy is appropriate only in cases of pure cellulitis without deep infection.
- If deep infection is suspected, débridement and deep cultures should be obtained before starting antibiotics. The exception to this rule would be circumstances where the patient's life is in danger (ie, the patient is septic and hemodynamically unstable).

SURGICAL MANAGEMENT

- The indications for surgery are the suspicion of a deep infection. If any suspicion is present, this is an indication for surgery.

Preoperative Planning

- The above-mentioned studies are all performed and interpreted.
- The incision is assessed for closure and the need for plastic surgery. If a wound complication is present, a preoperative assessment by a plastic surgeon is appropriate but not mandatory. If wound closure does not seem likely, the surgeon should plan on having a Wound VAC readily available for intraoperative application.

Positioning

- The patient is placed supine on the operating table.
- A bump is placed under the hip to rotate the extremity to neutral with respect to the knee.

- The lower leg is placed on multiple blankets to provide a firm working surface while simultaneously allowing shoot-through lateral radiographs to enhance the assessment of prosthesis coverage (anterior and posterior pillar).

Approach

- The surgical approach is anterior, following the initial incision done for the primary arthroplasty. The interval is the same as that mentioned above.

TECHNIQUES

IMPLANT REMOVAL

- Localize the implant through deep dissection. Follow any sinus tracts present to confirm direct communication with an infected incision.
- Remove the implant (all components) by applying the insertion rods and joysticking the components.
- Remove screws and plates about the syndesmotic fusion, as they are in direct communication with deep infection.
- Curette the bone surfaces and remove all necrotic tissues. Perform bone débridement. All residual tissue should be viable and demonstrate good vascularity. If a tourniquet is used, it should be released at this time.
- Perform irrigation with at least 6 liters of antibiotic-impregnated normal saline.
- Prepare the polymethylmethacrylate mixed with a heat-stable antibiotic (vancomycin, gentamicin). Often two bags are needed to manufacture enough cement to fill the void left by removing the prosthesis.
- Insert the cement into the newly created space while placing some distraction between the tibia and talus (**TECH FIG 7A**). This will maintain height by allowing the cement to fill the entire void. Ensure that the cement contacts the cut surfaces of the tibia and talus to maximize the local effect of the antibiotic and to provide enough stability to allow some weight bearing (**TECH FIG 7B,C**).
- Close the wound over a large suction drain, or, if this is not possible, apply a Wound VAC.

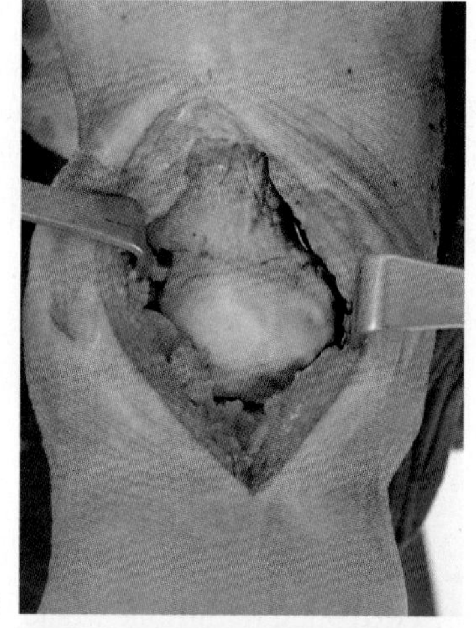
A

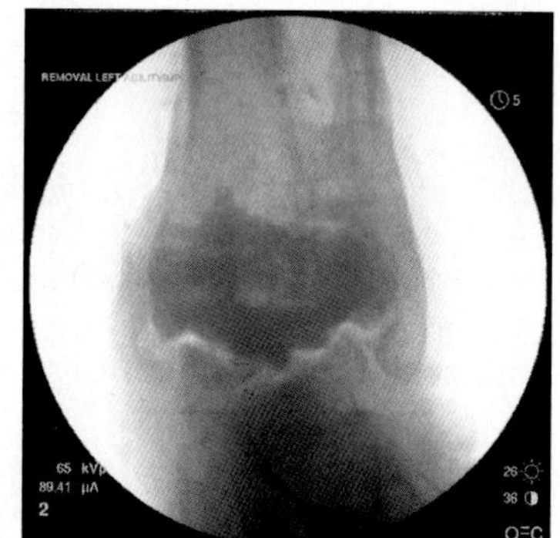

B

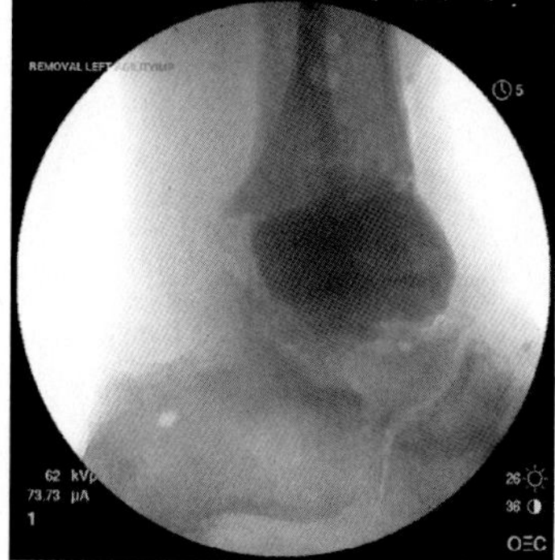

C

TECH FIG 7 • Implantation of an antibiotic-impregnated cement spacer (**A**) allows structural support and maintenance of height by providing complete fill in the AP (**B**) and sagittal (**C**) planes.

IMPLANT REINSERTION

- After 6 weeks of intravenous antibiotics and 6 weeks off of antibiotics (3 months total), hematologic tests are done to determine the potential for residual infection.
- The identical anterior approach is used.
- If bone loss was present, custom components are created based on both CT data and measured plain radiographs.
- Remove the spacer (**TECH FIG 8A**) and curette the bone of any defects or necrotic tissue.

- Make new bone cuts with a cutting block (**TECH FIG 8B**) to ensure that there is viable tibial and talar bone for ingrowth (**TECH FIG 8C**).
- Insert the prosthesis. If stability is in question, place polymethylmethacrylate on the fins of the tibia and talus before insertion (**TECH FIG 8D,E**). This limited application of cement allows bone ingrowth to the remaining prosthesis (the majority) while providing enough stability to allow early range of motion and weight bearing (**TECH FIG 8F–H**).

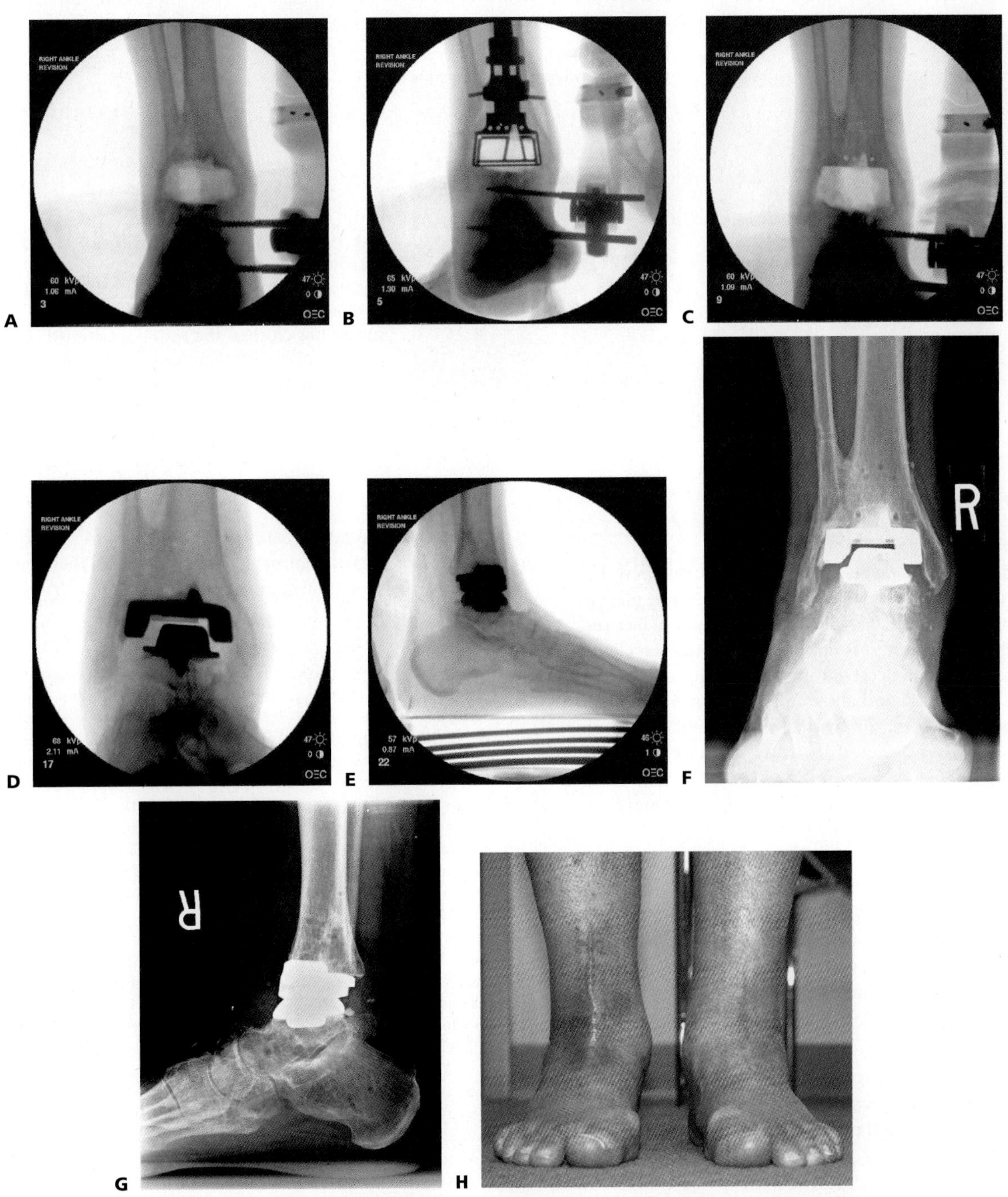

TECH FIG 8 • Revision after cement spacer. The spacer is first removed (**A**), followed by revision of the saw cuts (**B**). This allows a larger prosthesis seated against quality vascular bone (**C**). The prosthesis is balanced and stable (**D,E**). At 1 year postoperatively, there is no visible subsidence or cystic changes in the bone to suggest recurrent infection (**F,G**), and the incision demonstrates no compromise (**H**).

PEARLS AND PITFALLS

Indications	■ If there is any question of deep infection, obtain adequate deep cultures and biopsy specimens before starting antibiotics. Targeting specific organisms provides a better chance of eradicating infection than using broad-spectrum antibiotics.
Débridement	■ A generous débridement is critical to lowering the possibility of infection recurrence. This includes any posterior bone or abscesses deep to the posterior capsule.
Weight bearing	■ Caution should be used in patients wanting to bear weight on the cement spacer. This firm implant can cause additional bone destruction with full weight bearing, compromising revision surgery (**FIG 15A,B**).

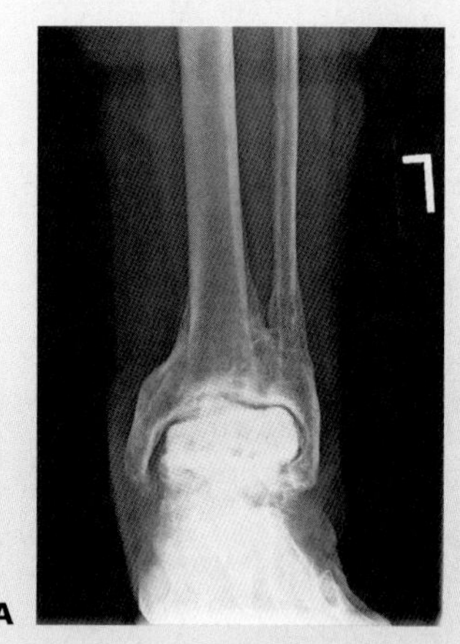

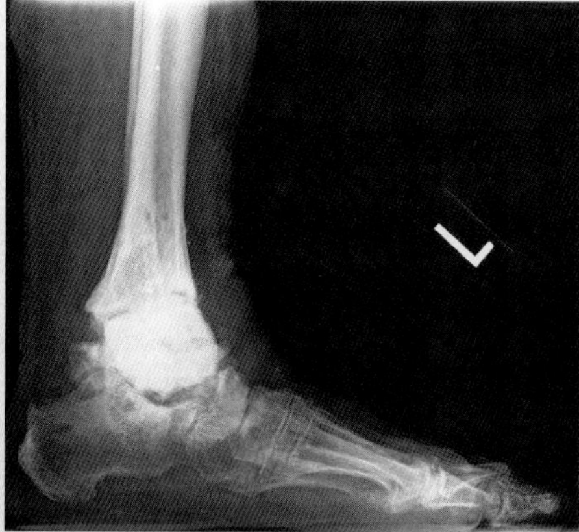

FIG 15 • This patient (seen in Tech Fig 8) decided to forgo revision surgery and continued to bear full weight on the cement spacer (**A**). After 1 year of repetitive impact, the spacer has crushed the residual talus (**B**). The patient, although symptom-free, can no longer contemplate revision total ankle arthroplasty and instead would have to undergo arthrodesis.

POSTOPERATIVE CARE

■ After the index débridement, further débridement may be required with gross infections. In addition, if necessary, plastic surgery is performed once Wound VAC application has resulted in a stagnant incision. It is important to obtain excellent soft tissue coverage (often necessitating a free flap) to improve resolution of the infection and allow implantation of the revision prosthesis. In this scenario, by the time revision surgery is performed, the flap has healed sufficiently to allow the anterior approach.

■ After revision surgery, the protocol is no different from that for subsidence.

OUTCOMES

■ These techniques are newly described, so there is no literature to support their use at this time. Anecdotal experience supports the techniques, however, with short-term outcomes (1 year) demonstrating substantial improvement.

COMPLICATIONS

■ Recurrent infection, osteomyelitis
■ Recurrent wound breakdown
■ Nerve damage to superficial peroneal, deep peroneal, saphenous, sural, or tibial nerves
■ Subsidence of the newly placed components into poor-quality bone. This is a particular problem in those with rheumatoid arthritis or other systemic conditions.

REFERENCES

1. Fevang BT, Lie SA, Havelin LI, et al. 257 ankle arthroplasties performed in Norway between 1994 and 2005. Acta Orthop 2007;78:575–583.
2. Haddad SL, Coetzee JC, Estok R, et al. Intermediate and long-term outcomes of total ankle arthroplasty and ankle arthrodesis: a systematic review of the literature. J Bone Joint Surg Am 2007;89A:1899–1905.
3. Hurowitz EJ, Gould JS, Fleisig GS, et al. Outcome analysis of agility total ankle replacement with prior adjunctive procedures: two to six year follow-up. Foot Ankle Int 2007;28:308–312.
4. Knecht SI, Estin M, Callaghan JJ, et al. The Agility total ankle arthroplasty: seven to sixteen-year follow-up. J Bone Joint Surg Am 2004;86A:1161–1171.
5. Kotnis R, Pasapula C, Anwar F, et al. The management of failed ankle replacement. J Bone Joint Surg Br 2006;88B:1039–1047.
6. Kurup HV, Taylor GR. Medial impingement after ankle replacement. Int Orthop 2008;32:243–246.
7. SooHoo NF, Zingmond DS, Ko CY. Comparison of reoperation rates following ankle arthrodesis and total ankle arthroplasty. J Bone Joint Surg Am 2007;89A:2143–2149.
8. Spirt AA, Assal M, Hansen ST Jr. Complications and failure after total ankle arthroplasty. J Bone Joint Surg Am 2004;86A:1172–1178.
9. Young J, May M, Haddad SL. Infected total ankle arthroplasty following a routine dental procedure. Foot Ankle Int 2009;30:252–256.

Chapter 77 Ankle Arthrodesis

Mark E. Easley

DEFINITION

- The procedure to fuse the tibiotalar joint for isolated end-stage tibiotalar arthrosis

ANATOMY

- Ankle
  - Tibial plafond with medial malleolus
    - Articulations with dorsal and medial talus
    - In sagittal plane, slight posterior slope
    - In coronal plane, articular surface is 88 to 92 degrees relative to lateral tibial shaft axis.
  - Fibula
    - Articulation with lateral talus
    - Responsible for one sixth of axial load distribution of the ankle
  - Talus
    - 60% of surface area covered by articular cartilage
    - Dual radius of curvature
  - Distal tibiofibular syndesmosis
    - Anterior inferior tibiofibular ligament
    - Interosseous membrane
    - Posterior tibiofibular ligament
- Ankle functions as part of the ankle–hindfoot complex much like a mitered hinge.

PATHOGENESIS

- Posttraumatic arthrosis
  - Most common cause
  - Intra-articular fracture
  - Ankle fracture-dislocation with malunion
  - Chronic ankle instability
- Primary osteoarthrosis
  - Relatively rare compared to hip and knee arthrosis
- Inflammatory arthropathy
  - Most commonly rheumatoid arthritis
- Other
  - Hemochromatosis
  - Pigmented villonodular synovitis
  - Charcot neuroarthropathy
  - Septic arthritis

NATURAL HISTORY

- Posttraumatic arthrosis
  - Malunion, chronic instability, intra-articular cartilage damage, or malalignment may lead to progressive articular cartilage wear.
  - Chronic lateral ankle instability may eventually be associated with:
    - Relative anterior subluxation of the talus
    - Varus tilt of the talus within the ankle mortise
    - Hindfoot varus position
- Primary osteoarthrosis of the ankle is rare and poorly understood.
- Inflammatory arthropathy
  - Progressive and proliferative synovial erosive changes failing to respond to medical management
  - May be associated with chronic posterior tibial tendinopathy and progressive valgus hindfoot deformity, eventual valgus tilt to the talus within the ankle mortise, potential lateral malleolar stress fracture, and compensatory forefoot varus

PATIENT HISTORY AND PHYSICAL FINDINGS

- History
  - Typically, history of trauma to the ankle
    - Intra-articular ankle fracture (bi- or tri-malleolar ankle fracture; tibial plafond [pilon] fracture)
    - Chronic ankle instability
  - Inflammatory arthropathy
  - Primary ankle arthritis
- Symptoms and complaints
  - Pain in anterior ankle with weight bearing and particularly with forced dorsiflexion
  - Often relieved by rest, but patient may have pain even at rest after vigorous activity or prolonged standing
  - Ankle swelling
  - Ankle stiffness
- Medications
  - If patient is taking anti-inflammatory agents, these will need to be stopped preoperatively to limit the risk of perioperative bleeding.
  - Rheumatoid medications; may need to be stopped perioperatively to optimize wound and bone healing
- Physical examination
  - Alignment
    - Ipsilateral limb alignment (not simply ankle alignment). The surgeon should examine the lower extremity from the hip to the foot. Optimal limb alignment is essential for the ankle arthrodesis to function well. Any ability for the lower limb to compensate for malalignment through the ankle is forfeited with ankle arthrodesis.
  - Ankle–foot alignment
    - The ankle functions as part of an ankle–subtalar joint complex.
    - Ankle fusion must be positioned on a sufficiently supportive and plantigrade foot.
    - Hindfoot, midfoot, and even forefoot malalignment may need to be addressed simultaneous to or staged with ankle arthrodesis.
  - Range of motion (ROM)
    - Ankle ROM is not critical since the ankle will be stiff following arthrodesis.

- Hindfoot ROM is essential for successful ankle arthrodesis. A stiff hindfoot and fused ankle allows very little accommodation and functions as a tibiotalocalcaneal or even pan-talar arthrodesis. Ankle arthritis associated with hindfoot stiffness, particularly if due to hindfoot arthritis, may be better treated with total ankle arthroplasty (TAA).
- Soft tissues
  - An intact, relatively healthy soft tissue envelope surrounding the ankle is less likely to have soft tissue complications postoperatively, provided careful soft tissue handling is maintained.
  - Previous surgical scars must be considered. Either they can be incorporated into the surgical approach or the surgical approach may be modified to limit postoperative wound complications.
  - Vascular status: Intact pulses and satisfactory refill must be confirmed; if not, a Doppler ultrasound or noninvasive vascular studies must be performed before considering surgery.
  - Neurologic status: A peripheral neuropathy is a relative contraindication for TAA; in our opinion, well-controlled diabetes without neuropathy is not. However, if there is any question about risks, then arthrodesis should be considered in lieu of arthroplasty for end-stage ankle arthritis. Established neuropathy and either existing or high risk of Charcot neuroarthropathy is a contraindication for TAA. Ankle arthrodesis or even tibiotalocalcaneal arthrodesis is favored over TAA for end-stage ankle arthritis associated with a dense peripheral neuropathy and risk of or existing Charcot neuroarthropathy.
  - Motor function: Intact motor function of the ankle and foot is essential to successful ankle arthrodesis. Lack of active dorsiflexion, plantarflexion, inversion, or eversion is a relative contraindication to ankle arthrodesis. Tibialis anterior function is still required to dorsiflex the foot at the transverse tarsal (talonavicular and calcaneocuboid) joints. Gastrocnemius–soleus function is needed to plantarflex the hindfoot. Posterior tibial and peroneal tendon function is necessary to maintain a dynamic balance of the foot under the ankle arthrodesis. Without these functioning muscle groups, a tibiotalocalcaneal or pan-talar arthrodesis or possibly a bridle tendon transfer may be warranted.

IMAGING AND OTHER DIAGNOSTIC STUDIES

- Weight-bearing AP, lateral, and mortise views of the ankle.
- Weight-bearing AP, lateral, and oblique views of the foot, particularly with associated foot deformity
- With associated or suspected lower leg deformity, we routinely obtain weight-bearing AP and lateral tibia–fibula views.
- With deformity in the lower extremity, we routinely obtain weight-bearing mechanical axis (hip-to-ankle) views of both extremities.
- We typically evaluate complex or ill-defined ankle–hindfoot patterns of arthritis with or without deformity using CT of the ankle and hindfoot.
- If we suspect avascular necrosis of the talus or distal tibia, we obtain an MRI of the ankle.

DIFFERENTIAL DIAGNOSIS

- See "Pathogenesis."

NONOPERATIVE MANAGEMENT

- Activity modification
- Bracing
  - Ankle–foot orthosis (AFO)
  - Double upright brace attached to shoe
- Stiffer-soled shoe with a rocker-bottom modification
- Nonsteroidal anti-inflammatories or COX-2 inhibitors
- Medications for systemic inflammatory arthropathy
- Corticosteroid injection
- Viscosupplementation

SURGICAL MANAGEMENT

- The trend is to perform ankle arthrodesis through an anterior approach with preservation of the malleoli.
  - Recently there have been favorable outcomes in conversion of ankle fusion to TAA.
    - While ankle arthrodesis is typically successful in relieving symptoms related to end-stage ankle arthritis, over time the hindfoot may develop compensatory degenerative changes (ie, adjacent joint arthritis).
  - If one or both of the malleoli are sacrificed, then this potential conversion is compromised.
  - The anterior approach is also used for the majority of TAA cases.

Preoperative Planning

- Vascular and neurologic examination
  - It is easy to focus on the patient's symptoms and radiographs demonstrating end-stage ankle arthritis.
  - Satisfactory circulation is essential to allow wound healing and fusion.
  - A neuropathy may warrant a more extensive ankle–hindfoot stabilization.
- Deformity correction
  - A sound preoperative plan facilitates effective intraoperative deformity correction.
- The surgeon should evaluate the contralateral extremity and ankle to have an understanding of what is physiologic for that patient.

Positioning

- Supine
- Plantar aspect of operated foot at end of operating table
- Foot and ankle well balanced, with toes directed to the ceiling
- A bolster under the ipsilateral hip prevents undesired external rotation of the hip.
- We routinely use a thigh tourniquet and regional anesthesia.
  - A popliteal block provides adequate pain relief postoperatively, particularly if a regional catheter is used. Moreover, hip and knee flexion–extension is not forfeited, facilitating safe immediate postoperative mobilization.
  - However, to use a thigh tourniquet with a popliteal block typically requires a supplemental femoral nerve block (patients temporarily forfeit knee extension postoperatively) or general anesthesia.

Approach

- Anterior approach to the ankle, using the interval between the tibialis anterior (TA) tendon and the extensor hallucis longus (EHL) tendon

APPROACH

- Make a longitudinal midline incision over the anterior ankle, starting about 10 cm proximal to the tibiotalar joint and 1 cm lateral to the tibial crest (**TECH FIG 1A**).
- Continue the incision midline over the anterior ankle just distal to the talonavicular joint.
- At no point should direct tension be placed on the skin margins; we perform deep, full-thickness retraction as soon as possible to limit the risk of skin complications.
- Identify and protect the superficial peroneal nerve by retracting it laterally.
  - In our experience there is a consistent branch of the superficial peroneal nerve that crosses directly over or immediately proximal to the tibiotalar joint.
- We then expose the extensor retinaculum, identify the course of the EHL tendon, and sharply but carefully divide the retinaculum directly over the EHL tendon (**TECH FIG 1B,C**).
  - We always attempt to maintain the TA tendon in its dedicated sheath.
  - Preserving the retinaculum over the TA tendon
    - Prevents bowstringing of the tendon and thereby reduces the stress on the anterior wound
    - Should there be a wound dehiscence, then the TA is not directly exposed.
  - Preserving the retinaculum over the TA tendon is not always possible; some patients do not have a dedicated sheath for the TA.
- Use the interval between the TA and EHL tendon, with the TA and EHL tendons retracted medially and laterally, respectively.
- Identify the deep neurovascular bundle (anterior tibial–dorsalis pedis artery and deep peroneal nerve) and carefully retract it laterally throughout the remainder of the procedure (**TECH FIG 1D**).
- Perform an anterior capsulotomy along with elevation of the tibial and dorsal talar periosteum to about 6 to 8 cm proximal to the tibial plafond and talonavicular joint, respectively (**TECH FIG 1E**).
- Elevate this separated capsule and periosteum medially and laterally to expose the ankle, access the medial and lateral gutters, and visualize the medial and lateral malleoli (**TECH FIG 1F,G**).
- Remove anterior tibial and talar osteophytes to facilitate exposure and avoid interference with the instrumentation (**TECH FIG 1H,I**).

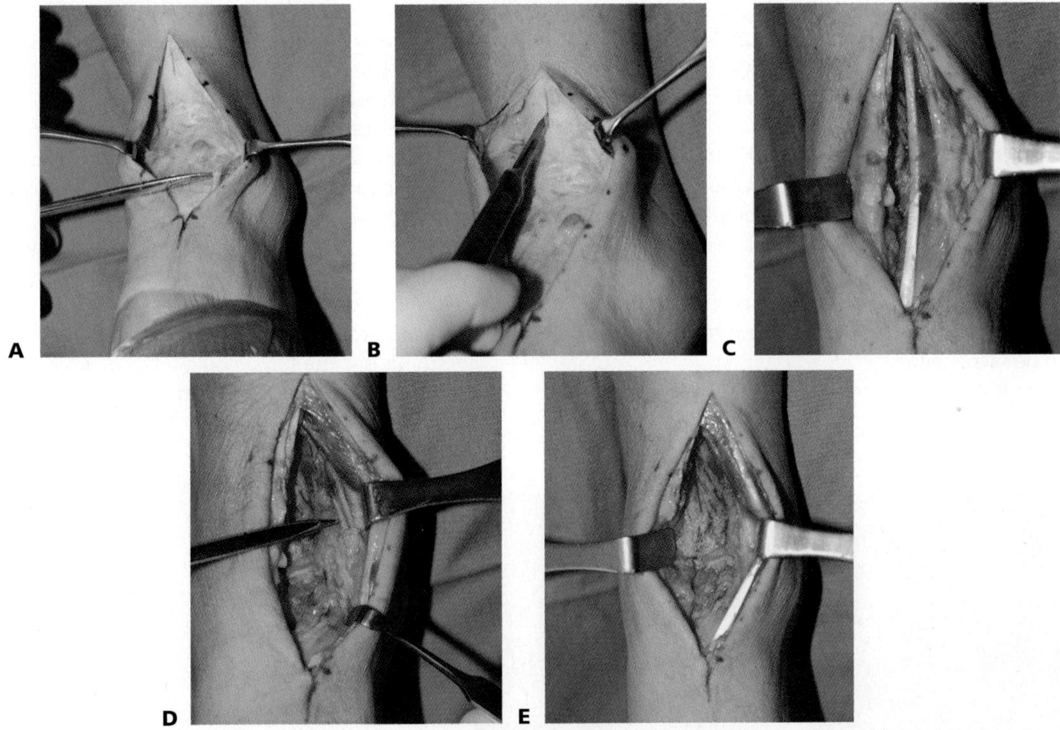

TECH FIG 1 • **A.** Anterior approach to ankle (note sural nerve). **B,C.** The extensor retinaculum is divided. **B.** Initiating the longitudinal incision in the retinaculum immediately superficial to the extensor hallucis longus (EHL) tendon. **C.** EHL tendon exposed. **D.** The deep neurovascular bundle must be identified and protected. **E.** Tibiotalar joint exposed after arthrotomy. *(continued)*

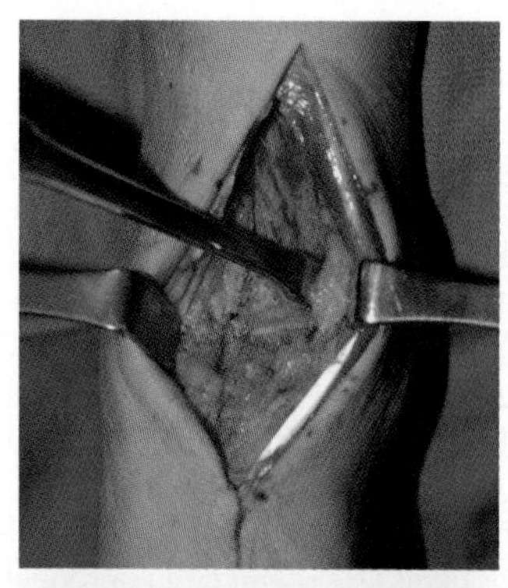

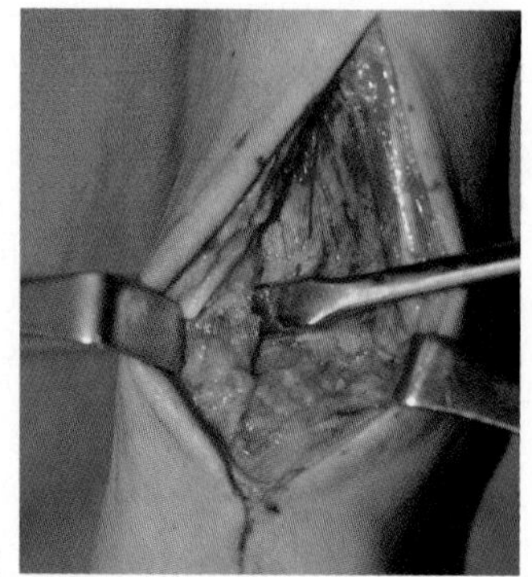

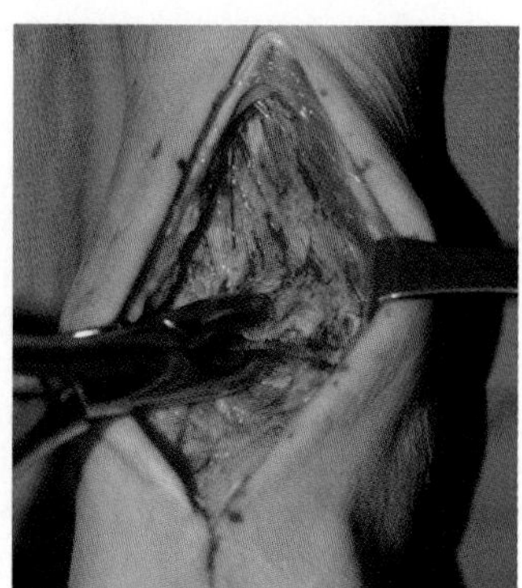

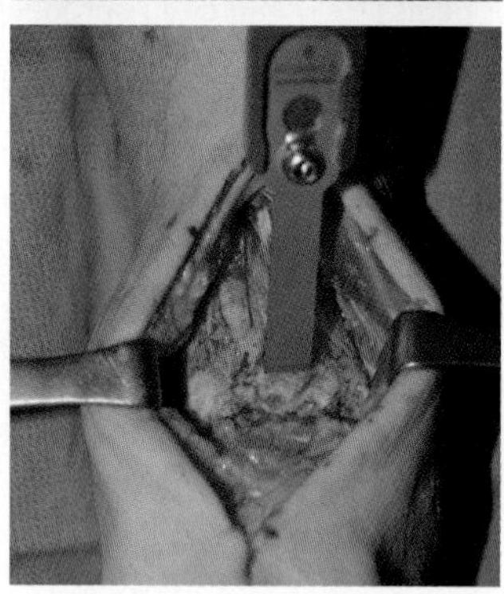

TECH FIG 1 • *(continued)* **F,G.** Exposure improved with capsular and periosteal elevation at the joint line. **F.** Laterally. **G.** Medially. **H,I.** Distal anterior tibial exostectomy. **H.** Rongeur. **I.** Chisel.

TIBIOTALAR JOINT PREPARATION

- I routinely use joint distraction (**TECH FIG 2A,B**).
- I prefer to maintain the subchondral bone architecture.
  - In preserving the essential anatomy of the talar dome and tibial plafond, I have the ability to adjust dorsiflexion–plantarflexion without compromising limb length or bony apposition at the arthrodesis site.
    - Flat cuts tend to forfeit limb length and the ability to adjust alignment without forfeiting optimal bony apposition.
  - Obviously, with deformity correction through the joint, some of the subchondral architecture may need to be sacrificed.
- I remove the residual cartilage with a sharp elevator or chisel (**TECH FIG 2A**).
- While preserving the subchondral architecture as best as possible I penetrate the subchondral bone with a drill bit, a narrow chisel, or both (**TECH FIG 2C–E**).
  - This increases surface area and promotes fusion.
- While careful to preserve the malleoli, I still prepare the tibiotalar joint gutters to further increase the surface area for fusion (**TECH FIG 2F,G**).
- Use of bone graft is at the surgeon's discretion.
  - I routinely use bone graft to fill any voids at the arthrodesis site.
  - Avoid excessive use of bone graft; the best chance for fusion is if the physiologic surfaces are appropriately prepared and well apposed.

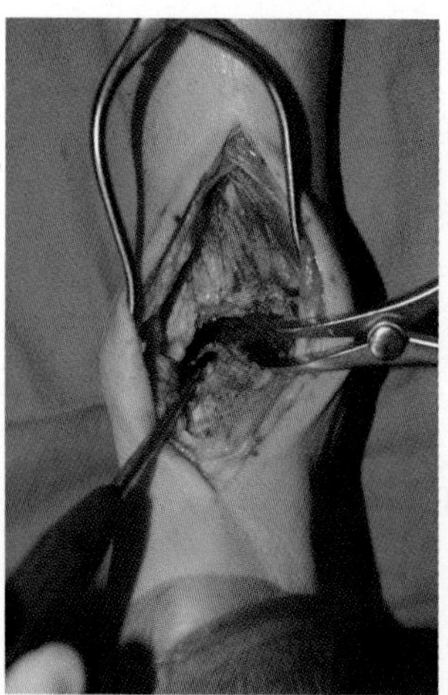

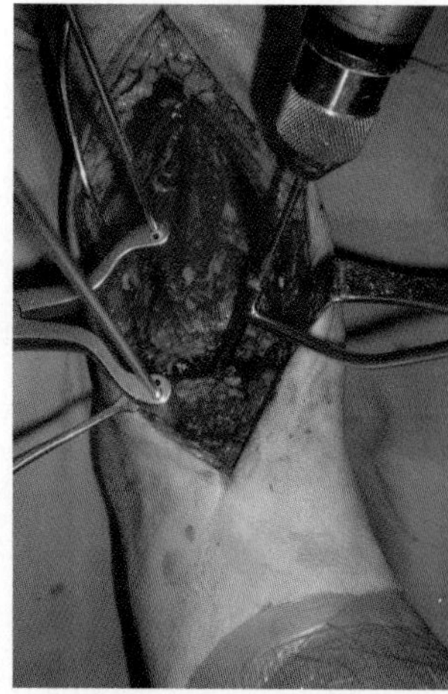

TECH FIG 2 • **A,B.** Tibiotalar joint preparation. **A.** Using a lamina spreader for distraction and a sharp elevator to delaminate residual cartilage. **B.** Alternatively, an invasive joint distractor may be used, here with drilling of the subchondral bone to promote healing. *(continued)*

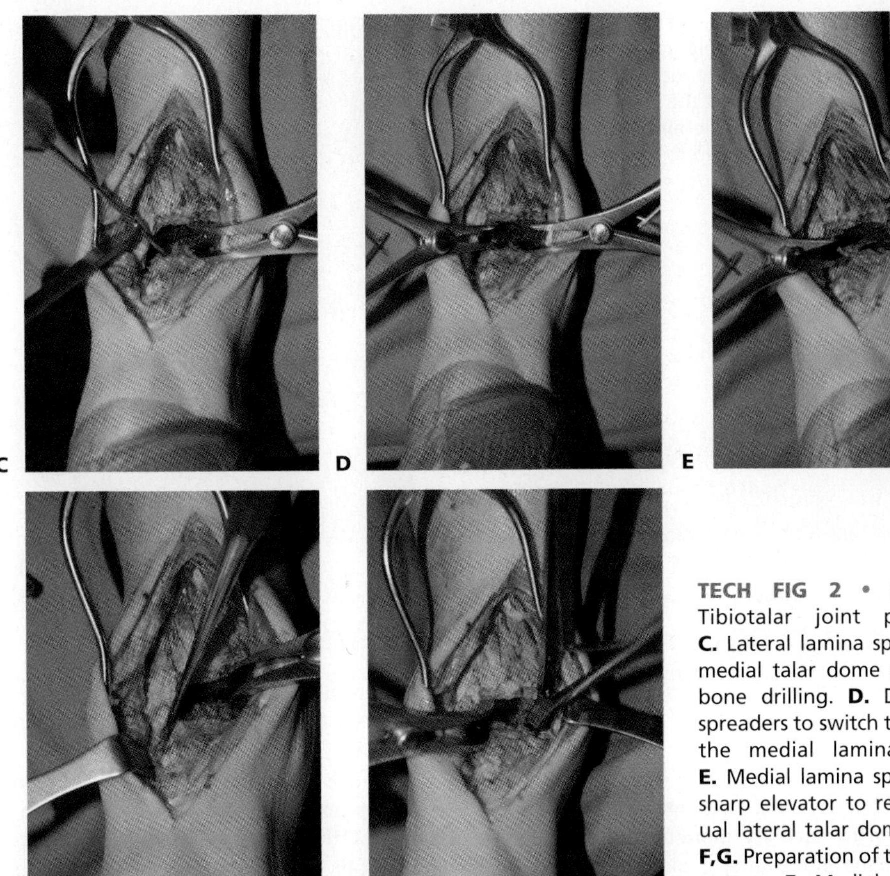

TECH FIG 2 • *(continued)* Tibiotalar joint preparation. **C.** Lateral lamina spreader with medial talar dome subchondral bone drilling. **D.** Dual lamina spreaders to switch to using only the medial lamina spreader. **E.** Medial lamina spreader with sharp elevator to remove residual lateral talar dome cartilage. **F,G.** Preparation of the tibiotalar gutters. **F.** Medial gutter with sharp elevator. **G.** Lateral gutter using a rongeur.

TIBIOTALAR JOINT REDUCTION

- For me, optimal tibiotalar joint alignment for arthrodesis is:
  - Neutral dorsiflexion–plantarflexion (**TECH FIG 3A**)
    - Many years ago, there was a tendency to fuse women's ankles in plantarflexion to facilitate wearing a heel. This is an idea that should be abandoned.
    - The tendency is to underestimate how much dorsiflexion is needed to get the ankle to neutral. Therefore, I typically dorsiflex the talus within the mortise just slightly more than what I think it may need. This usually results in neutral dorsiflexion–plantarflexion.
  - Slight hindfoot valgus
    - Balance the talus within the ankle mortise, but be sure that the hindfoot is in slight valgus.
    - If not, then contour the tibiotalar preparation to get the hindfoot in slight valgus.
    - A reasonable landmark is to have the lateral bony aspect of the calcaneus be in line with the fibula; if it is medial to the fibula, then a neutral to varus position is inappropriately set.
  - Rotation
    - Align the second metatarsal with the anterior tibial crest.
    - When the malleoli are preserved, rotation is often auto-adjusted.
    - External rotation is recommended by some authors, but I consider this only if the contralateral extremity dictates this position.
    - The goal is to avoid internal rotation.
  - Sagittal plane relationship of the talus to the tibia
    - Avoid anterior translation of the talus relative to the tibia. This places the ankle and foot at a biomechanical disadvantage.
    - With some deformity, it may be difficult to translate the talus posteriorly to a more physiologic position. In some cases, I have had to resect some of the posterior malleolus (through the joint from the anterior approach with joint distraction) to allow such posterior translation (**TECH FIG 3B**). Also, judiciously, the deltoid ligament may need to be partially released to allow posterior translation. Perform this cautiously, though, as some of the talar dome blood supply travels though the deltoid branch off the posterior tibial artery.
- I routinely obtain intraoperative fluoroscopic views in the AP and lateral planes to confirm appropriate alignment and bony apposition.

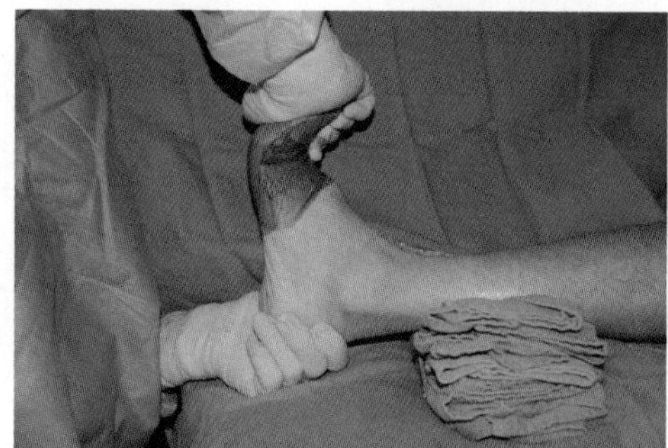

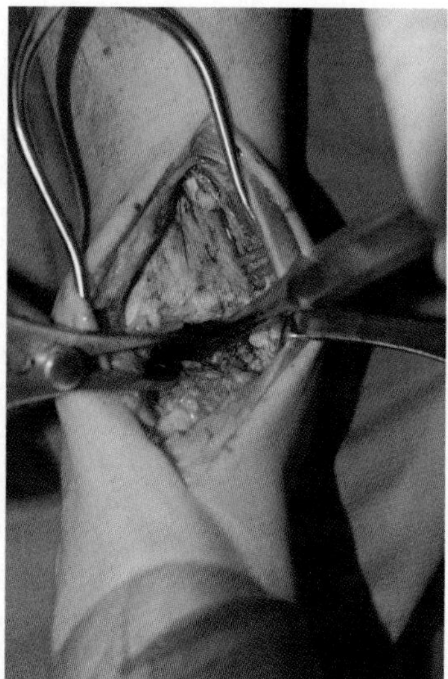

TECH FIG 3 • **A.** Tibiotalar joint reduction, with neutral dorsiflexion–plantarflexion, slight hindfoot valgus, and second metatarsal rotated to anterior tibial crest. **B.** If the talus fails to translate posteriorly in the ankle mortise, then the posterior malleolus may need to be weakened to allow the talus to reduce under the tibial axis.

INTERNAL FIXATION WITH ANTERIOR PLATING–SCREW FIXATION

- Internal fixation is contraindicated or less than optimal in the face of:
  - Infection
  - Osteopenic bone
- Traditionally, I performed screw fixation and added an anterior plate for further stability; more recently, I have switched to a technique where anterior plating is the primary technique, and I supplement with screws (other than those in the plate) only if I feel further stability is needed.
- Provisional fixation once optimal reduction is achieved
- Traditional screw fixation and supplemental anterior plate
- 55-year-old high-demand patient with anterior translation of the talus within the ankle mortise (TECH FIG 4A–C)
- Patient is positioned supine on the operating table with a bump under the ipsilateral hip to resist external rotation of the extremity.
- I typically use a medial screw first (TECH FIG 4D).
- Next, I place the posterior-to-anterior screw, the "home-run" screw.
  - With the newer anterior plating techniques that provide satisfactory stability, this screw has been largely abandoned; it is awkward to place and equally difficult to remove (TECH FIG 4E).

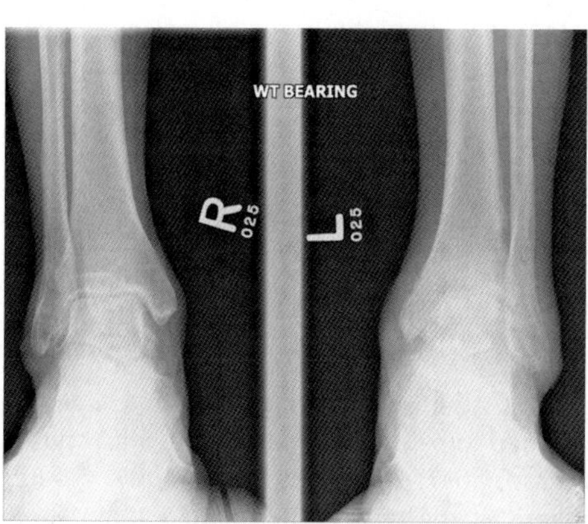

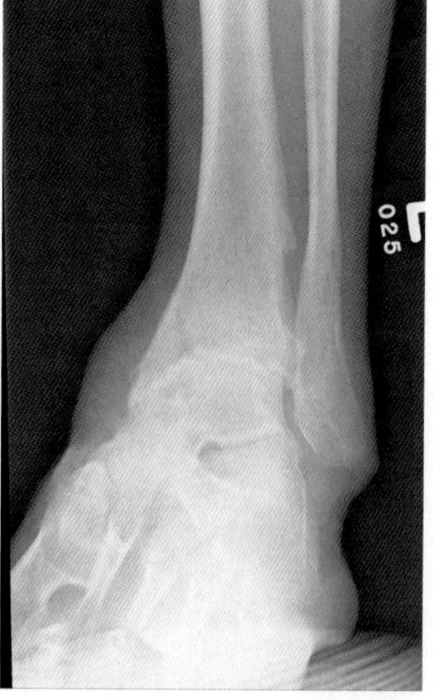

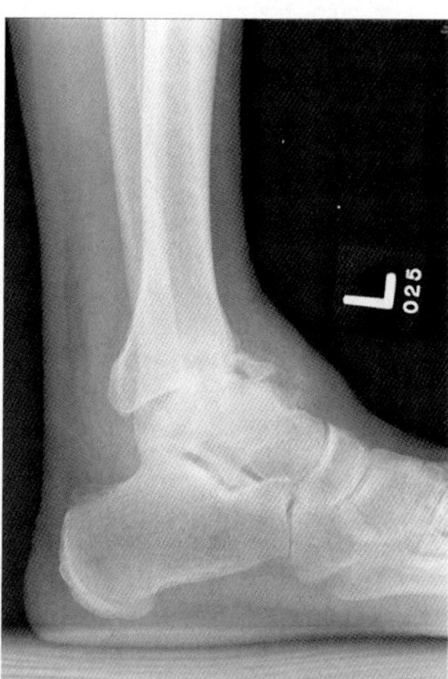

TECH FIG 4 • **A–C.** Fifty-five-year-old man with chronic instability and posttraumatic arthritis. **A.** AP view with comparison to contralateral ankle. **B.** Mortise view. **C.** Lateral view. There is considerable anterior translation of the talus from the ankle mortise. *(continued)*

- I add an anterolateral screw, one that is relatively vertical (TECH FIG 4F).
- Finally, I augment the fixation with an anterior plate. In this case a small fragment, non-locking plate was used (TECH FIG 4G–I).
  - In my experience, adding a supplemental anterior plate to an ankle arthrodesis construct adds considerable stability.
- Follow-up radiographs (TECH FIG 4J–N)
  - Patient returned to full activities, even playing doubles tennis.
  - He lacks some plantarflexion; time will tell what effect this will have on the hindfoot articulations that are attempting to compensate.
  - The talus is again in a physiologic relationship with the tibia, improving his biomechanics despite ankle arthrodesis.
- Plate fixation as the primary fixation
  - 33-year-old man with posttraumatic ankle arthritis and syndesmotic disruption (TECH FIG 5A–C)
  - Same joint preparation as described above
  - Provisional fixation with desired joint reduction
  - Plate locked to the dorsolateral talar neck with locking screws
  - Plate is precontoured based on average anterior ankle morphology.
  - Compression device is secured and compression is applied, thereby approximating the arthrodesis surfaces (TECH FIG 5D–F).

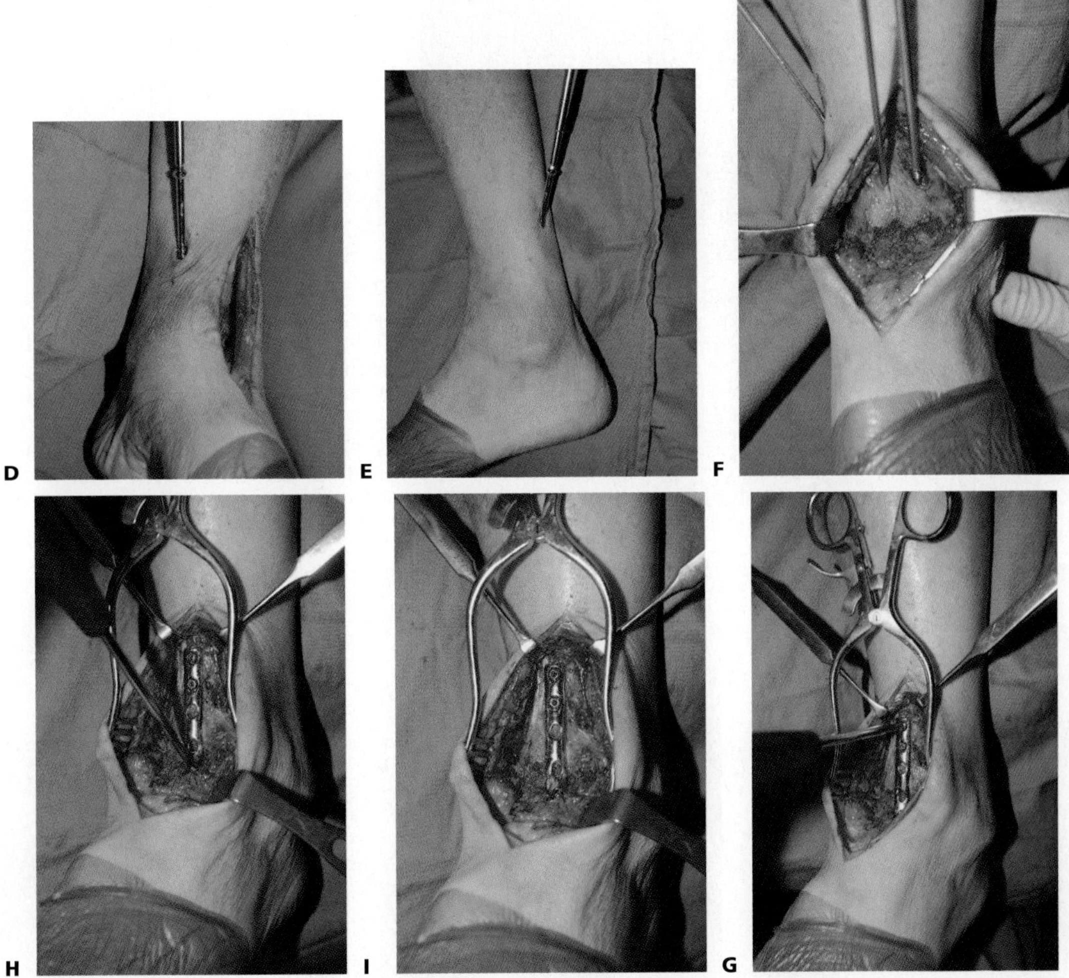

TECH FIG 4 • *(continued)* **D.** Medial screw placed first from the medial tibia to the talar dome, placed through a medial stab incision. **E.** Traditional posterior-to-anterior screw, placed via a posterolateral stab incision (care must be maintained to avoid injury to the sural nerve). **F.** Anterolateral screw placed through the anterior approach. Provisional fixation was placed adjacent to this screw. **G–I.** Anterior plating. **G.** Proximal screw fixation. **H.** Talar screw fixation. **I.** Final view of plate before closure. *(continued)*

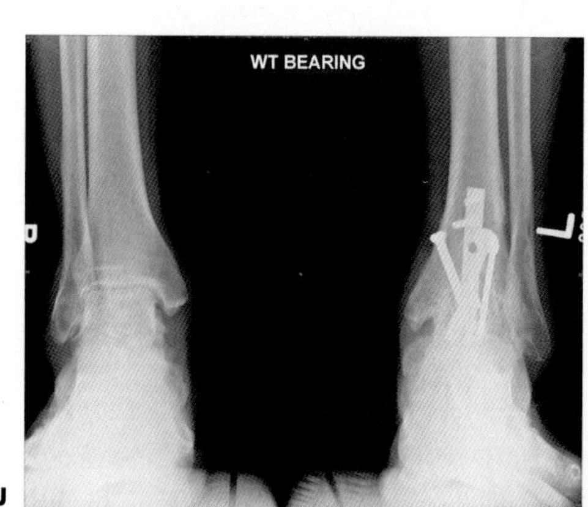

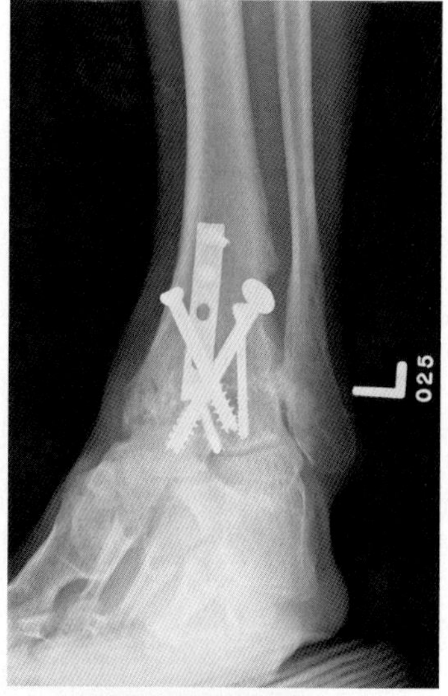

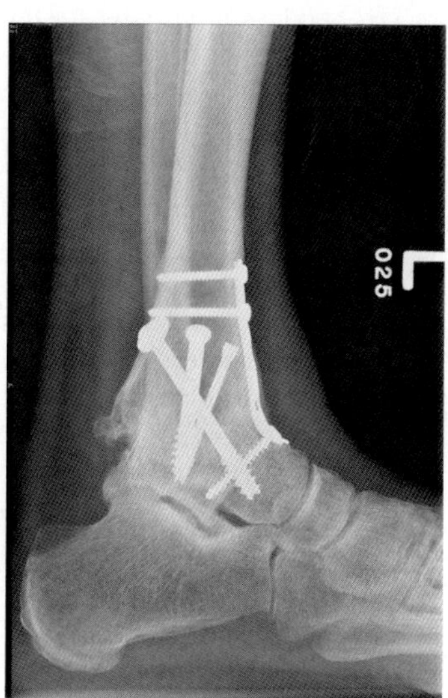

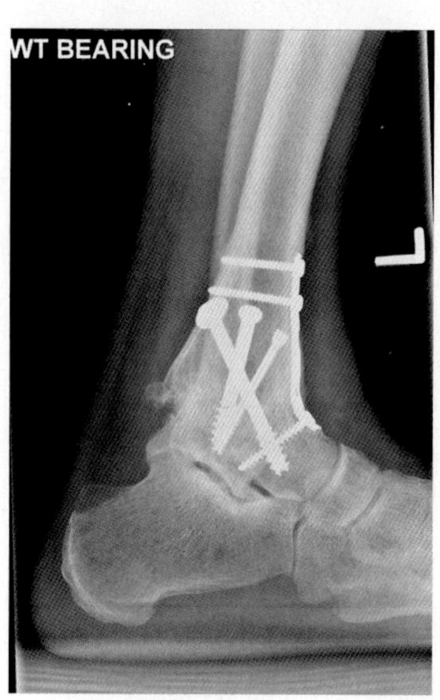

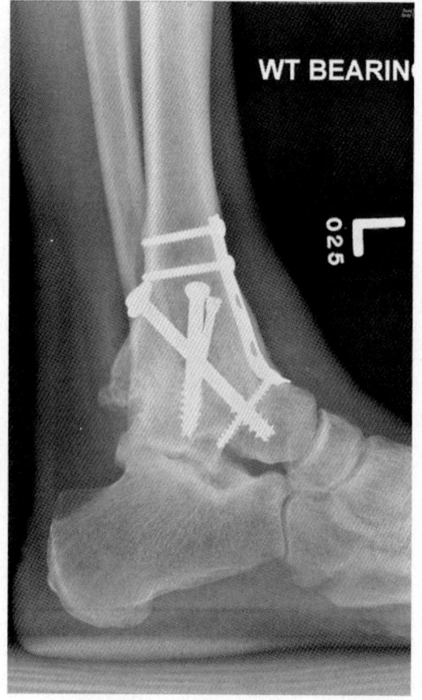

TECH FIG 4 • *(continued)* **J–N.** Postoperative weight-bearing radiographs of example patient with traditional screw fixation and supplemental anterior plate. **J.** AP radiograph. **K.** Mortise view. **L.** Lateral view (talus is reduced under tibial axis). **M.** Dorsiflexion view. **N.** Plantarflexion view. The patient lacks some hindfoot compensation for dorsiflexion and plantarflexion.

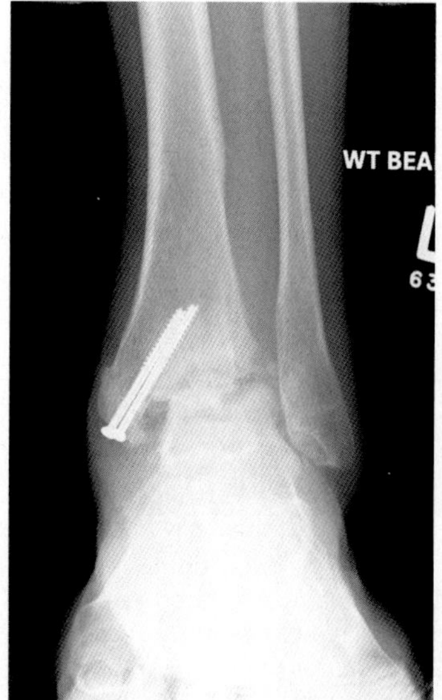

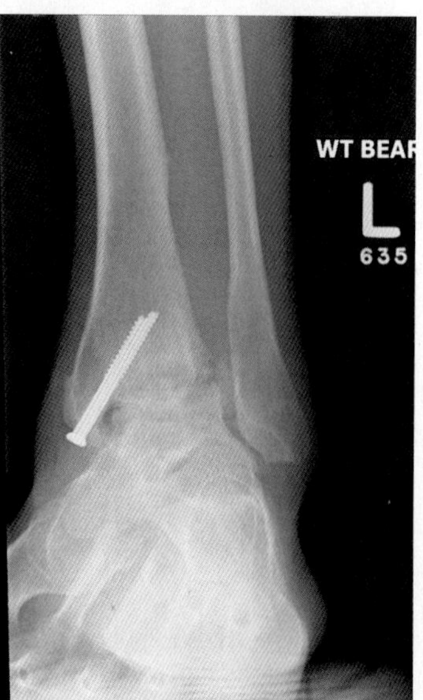

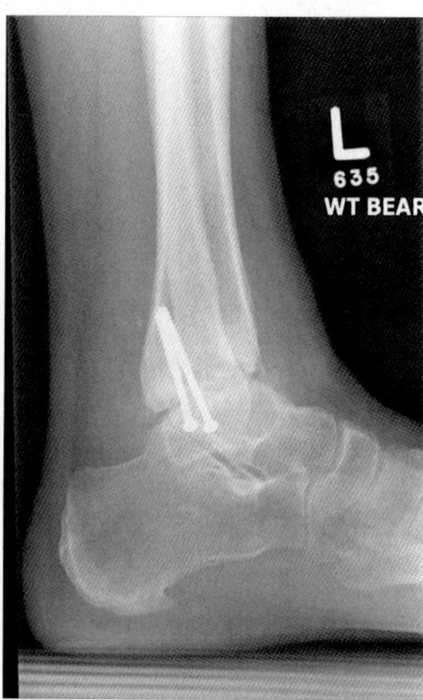

TECH FIG 5 • **A–C.** Preoperative radiographs of patient undergoing double anterior plating arthrodesis technique. **A,B.** AP and mortise views with end-stage ankle arthritis and chronic syndesmosis disruption. **C.** Lateral view. *(continued)*

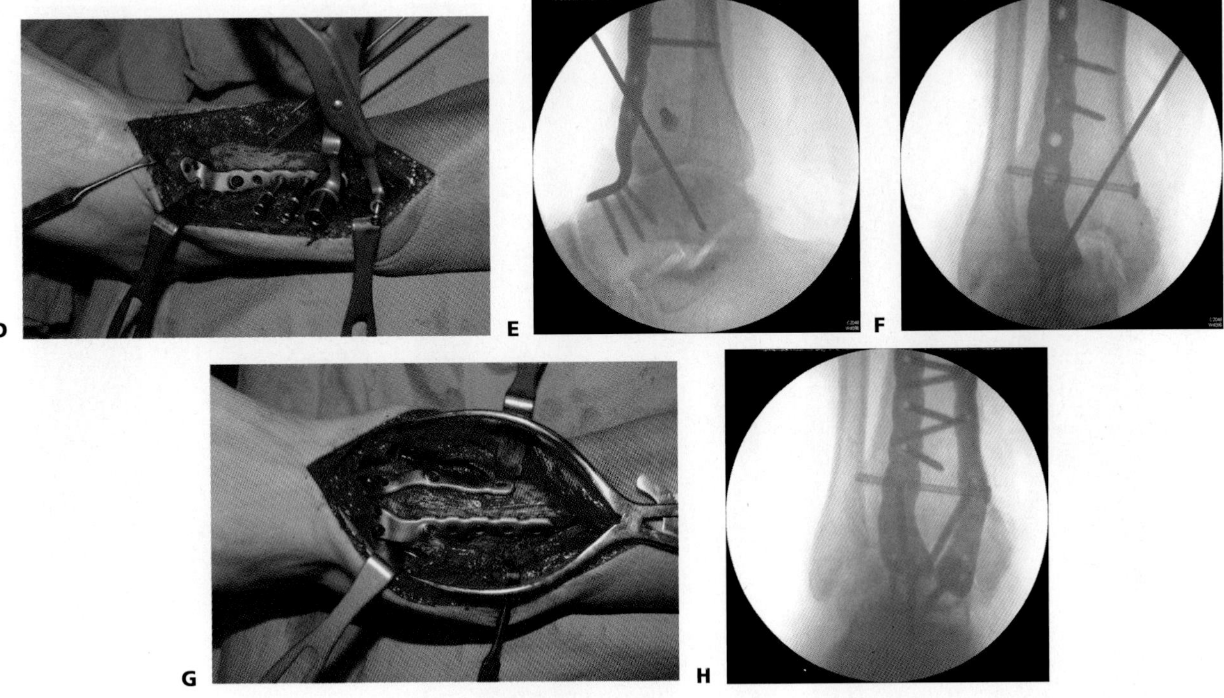

TECH FIG 5 • *(continued)* **D.** Lateral anterior plate applied and secured to talus and proximal compression device in place. **E,F.** Intraoperative fluoroscopic views of ankle of a different patient undergoing dual anterior plating, with provisional fixation and lateral plate in place. **E.** Lateral view. **F.** AP view. **G.** Example patient with both plates in place. **H.** Intraoperative fluoroscopic view of different patient with both plates in place.

  - While the locking plate creates axial compression, a mild but desirable valgus moment may be introduced since the lateral plate is being used for compression.
  - To obtain optimal compression, provisional fixation is removed before compression is applied but after the screws are locked into the talar neck and the compression device is secured proximally.
- After performing compression and securing the lateral plate in the tibia, the medial plate is applied (TECH FIG 5G,H).
  - Since compression has already been performed, this medial plate, which is also precontoured, serves to statically lock the arthrodesis.
- Each plate has a screw hole to allow non-locking screw fixation from the plate to the posterior talar body (TECH FIG 6A,B).
- Follow-up of case example (TECH FIG 6C–G)
- A supplemental screw may be added from the medial tibia to the talar body, but often this is unnecessary (TECH FIG 6H,I).

- Closure
  - I use a drain for 24 hours.
  - Standard wound closure
    - I routinely close the capsule, extensor retinaculum, subcutaneous layer, and skin (to a tensionless closure).
    - The deep neurovascular bundle, extensor tendons, and superficial peroneal nerve need to be protected during closure.
  - Sterile dressings on wound
  - Padding
  - Posterior–sugar-tong splint

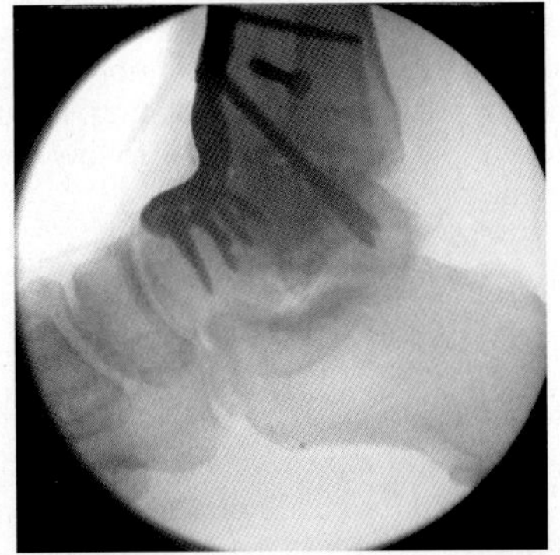

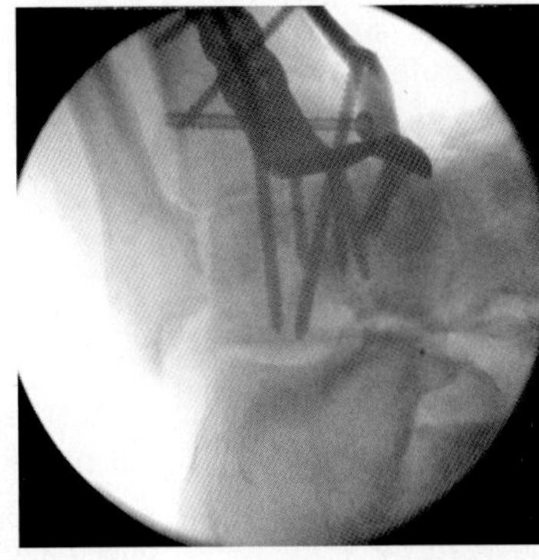

TECH FIG 6 • **A,B.** Intraoperative fluoroscopic views of two screws placed through the plate into the posterior talus for additional stability. **A.** Lateral view. **B.** Broden view to confirm that screws do not violate the subtalar joint. *(continued)*

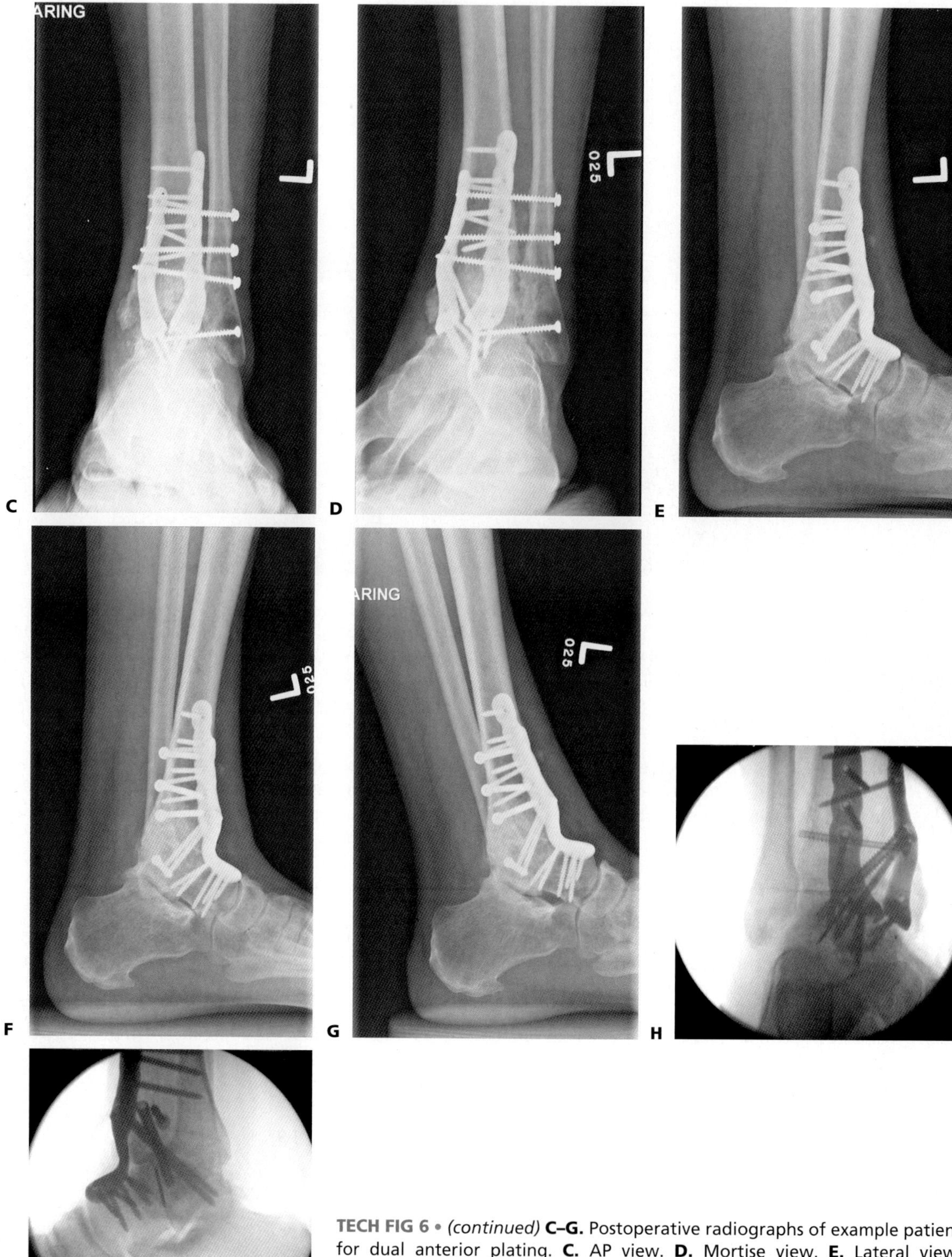

TECH FIG 6 • *(continued)* **C–G.** Postoperative radiographs of example patient for dual anterior plating. **C.** AP view. **D.** Mortise view. **E.** Lateral view. **F.** Dorsiflexion view. **G.** Plantarflexion view. **H, I.** Intraoperative fluoroscopic views of different patient with supplemental screw to anterior plating. **H.** AP view. **I.** Lateral view (note broken guide pin; it is important to follow the exact trajectory of the guide pin with cannulated screw systems).

EXTERNAL FIXATION

- Infection is not a contraindication for external fixation.
  - There will be no implant directly at the tibiotalar joint.
  - In some cases, I have performed a staged arthrodesis, with initial débridement and antibiotic bead placement. The external fixator may be placed at that initial procedure or at the definitive procedure when the antibiotic beads are removed and the joint is reduced and compressed with the external fixator.

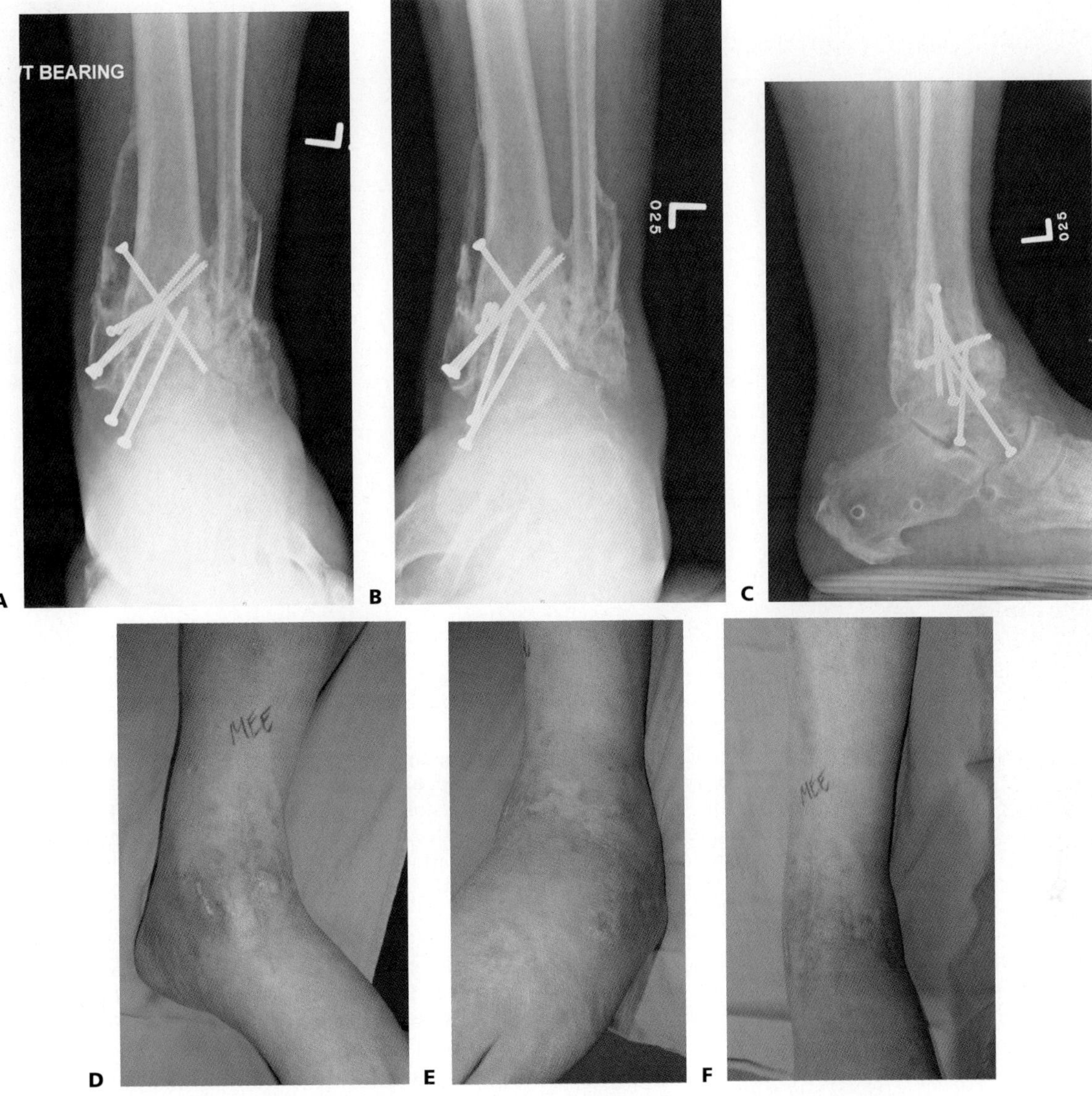

TECH FIG 7 • **A–C.** Preoperative radiographs of example patient for ankle arthrodesis with external fixation; patient has failed ankle arthrodesis with internal fixation. **A.** AP view. **B.** Mortise view. **C.** Lateral view. **D,E.** Poor skin condition. **D.** Medial ankle with prior anteromedial approach. **E.** Dorsolateral aspect with residual scarring. **F.** Patient positioned supine on the operating table. The external rotation malunion of the distal tibia creates excessive external rotation of the foot relative to the tibial axis.

- Forty-five-year-old patient with posttraumatic arthritis and deformity of the ankle, failing to respond to a prior attempt at ankle arthrodesis.
- Radiographs demonstrate nonunion and residual deformity (TECH FIG 7A–C).
  - Clinically, there are poor soft tissues anteriorly and a prior medial incision that will need to be incorporated into the surgical approach (TECH FIG 7D,E).
    - A standard anterior approach is too risky and, in my opinion, would leave an insufficient skin bridge to the prior incision.
- Supine on the operating table, again with a bolster under the ipsilateral hip to direct the ankle anteriorly
  - This patient also had a distal tibial external rotation malunion and an ankle nonunion with residual ankle external rotation (TECH FIG 7F).
- Hardware removal
- I used the prior incision and added another "mini-arthrotomy" incision laterally, thereby avoiding the unhealthy skin directly anteriorly over the ankle (TECH FIG 8A).
- I prepared the joint through the medial incision and used the lateral incision to provide joint distraction (TECH FIG 8B). I also switched the lamina spreader to the medial wound so that I could prepare the remainder of the joint via the lateral incision.
- From the preoperative radiographs it is obvious that there is distal tibial deformity and nonanatomic malleolar anatomy (TECH FIG 8C,D).
  - For this reason, the talus is not locked within the ankle mortise and rotation will need to be carefully controlled. However, this is more important with internal fixation; with external fixation such malrotation could still be corrected postoperatively with external fixator frame adjustment.

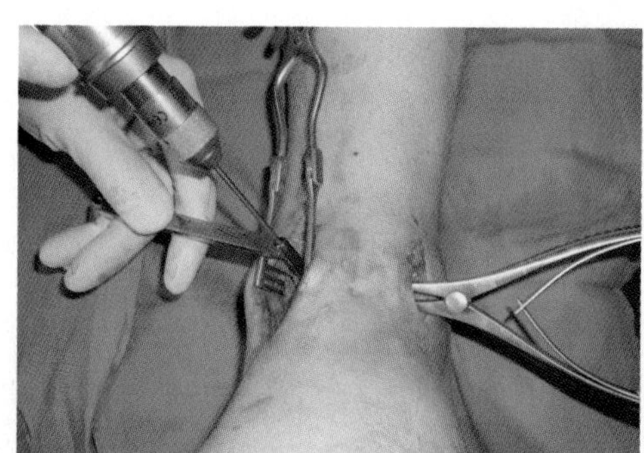

A

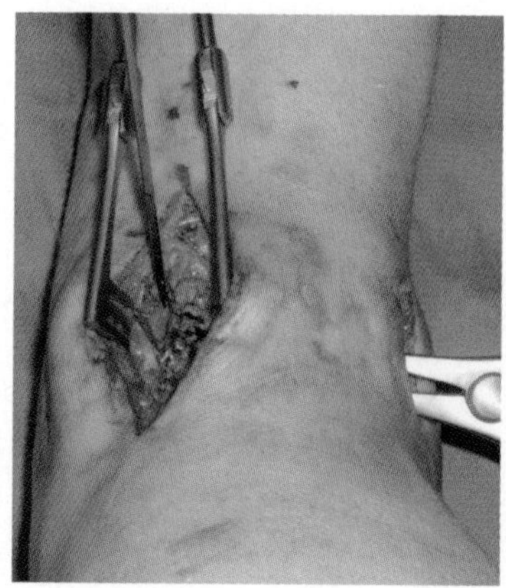

B

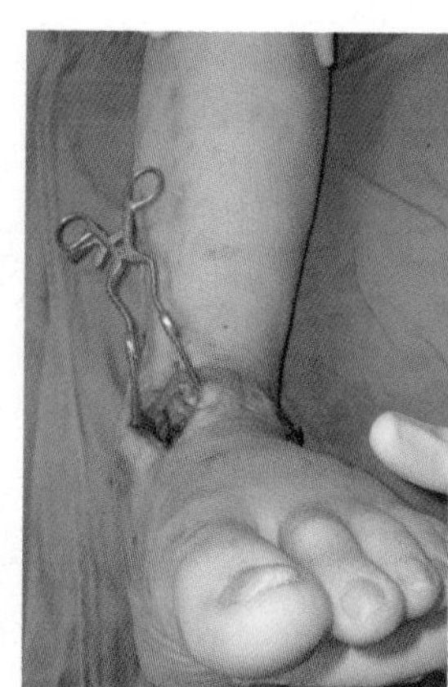

C

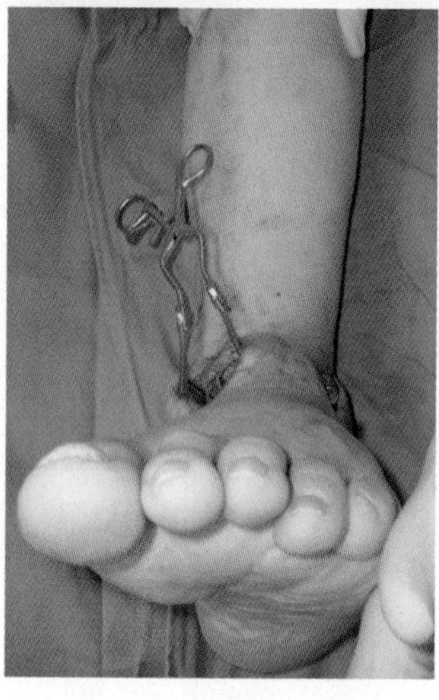

D

TECH FIG 8 • A. Modified "mini-open" arthrotomy approach to ankle arthrodesis. Previous medial incision used and a separate mini-lateral incision. Medial incision is being used for joint preparation while joint is being distracted by lamina spreader placed via lateral incision. Skin bridge between two wounds is adequate and previously compromised skin is not violated. **B.** Medial joint preparation. **C,D.** With distortion of the malleolar anatomy, the talus is not "locked" within the ankle mortise. **C.** Ankle tends to externally rotate. **D.** Ankle can be manually reduced to a physiologic position with the second metatarsal aligned to the anterior tibial shaft axis.

- Joint reduction
  - Neutral dorsiflexion–plantarflexion
  - Slight hindfoot valgus
  - Correct malrotation
    - Align second metatarsal with the anterior tibial crest.
- Provisionally pin the joint
  - I usually place two Steinmann pins axially. While this violates the subtalar joint, I do not believe that this has significant consequences in these patients with deformity, severe ankle arthritis, and compensatory hindfoot alignment.
- I routinely close the wounds at this point because once the external fixator is in place, suturing is particularly tedious.
  - However, if you prefer to delay the wound closure until the external fixator is in place, one or two struts can easily be reflected to allow adequate access to the wound or wounds.
- Proximal ring block (**TECH FIG 9A**)
  - I place the proximal ring block (I usually use two rings to create the "block") orthogonally to the tibia.
  - Initially, I stabilize the rings with two thin wires but do not tension them at this point.
  - I supplement the proximal ring block fixation with three half-pins (**TECH FIG 9B**).
  - Once the half-pins are secured, I tension the thin wires (**TECH FIG 9C**).
- Foot plate
- I suspend the foot plate ("horseshoe") from a transverse forefoot wire. This way I can control the foot's position within the foot plate (**TECH FIG 10A**).
- Once I am satisfied with the foot's position relative to the foot plate, I secure the hindfoot with two crossed thin wires, making sure the plantar surface of the foot is distal to the foot ring (**TECH FIG 10B**).
- I typically place a midfoot wire as well.
- Before tensioning the thin wires, I close the horseshoe-shaped foot plate anteriorly.
  - This can be done by adding a half-ring to the anterior foot plate, or I can have a double-decker foot plate and close the more proximal of the two foot plates (**TECH FIG 10C**).
  - Having two foot plate components affords less interference between the struts (that will connect the proximal ring block to the foot plate) and the thin wires to be passed through the foot from the foot plate.
- I then tension the thin wires in the foot (**TECH FIG 10D**).
- I also place one or two talar wires to provide greater support and to protect the subtalar joint (**TECH FIG 10E,F**).
  - These two wires either need to be built up from a single foot plate or connected to the proximal component of a two-ring foot plate set-up.

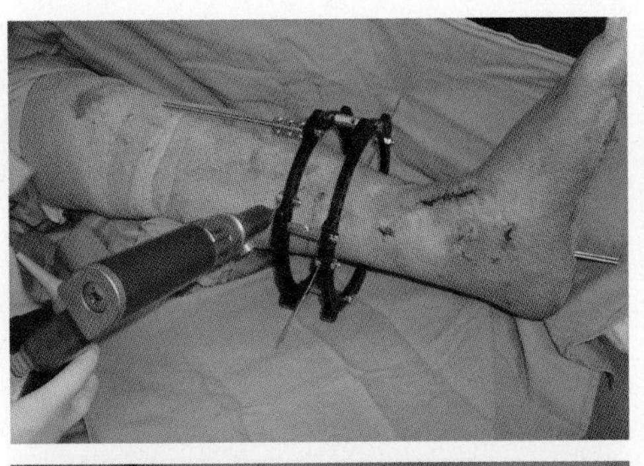

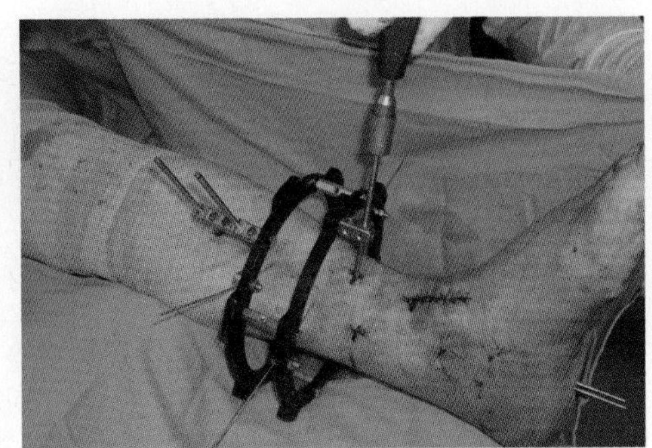

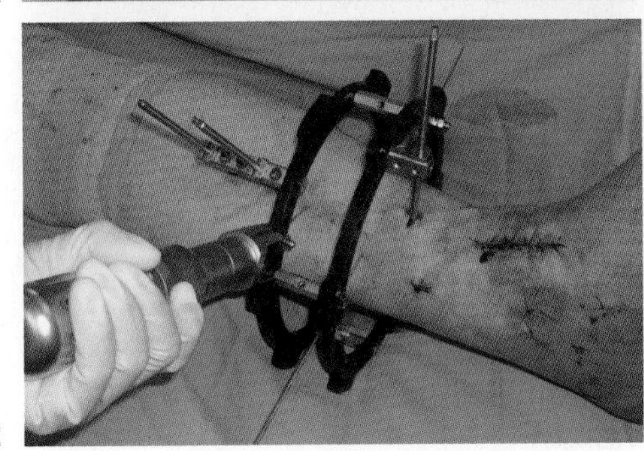

TECH FIG 9 • A. Building the proximal ring block, first with thin wires. Wounds were closed before applying external fixator. **B.** Half-pins added to stabilize the proximal ring block. **C.** Thin wires are tensioned within the proximal ring block.

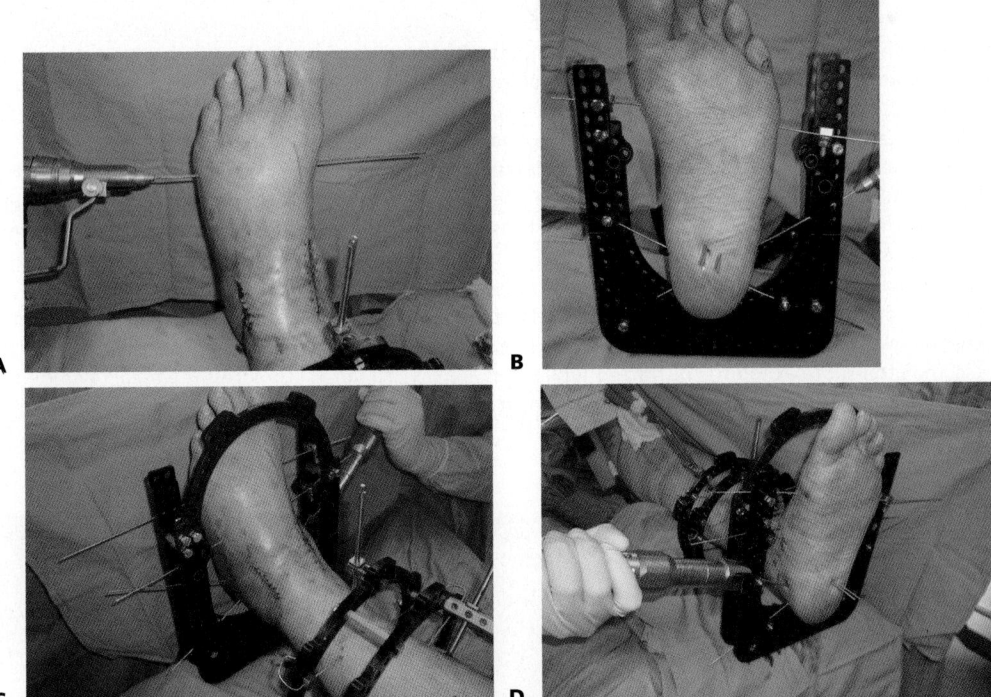

TECH FIG 10 • A. Forefoot wire placed to suspend the foot plate. **B.** Foot balanced within the foot plate. Foot plate suspended from forefoot wire and calcaneal wires being passed to stabilize the hindfoot. **C.** Tensioning the thin wires in the foot. The ring has been closed on the foot frame so that tension in all wires can be effectively maintained. **D.** In this case, two rings were used for the foot plate portion of the frame. Closing the top ring allows the foot frame to be closed even without placing a half-ring on the anterior portion of the "horseshoe." *(continued)*

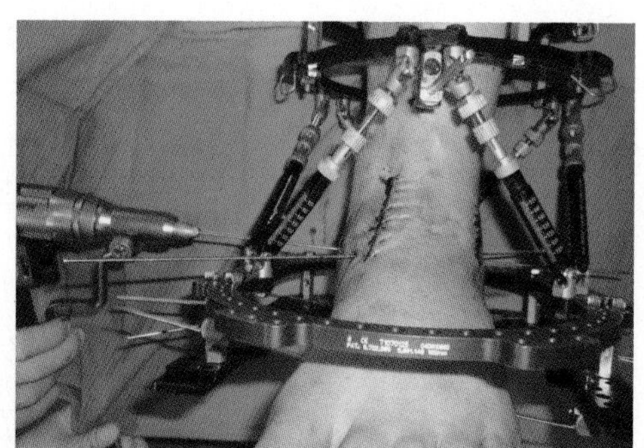
E

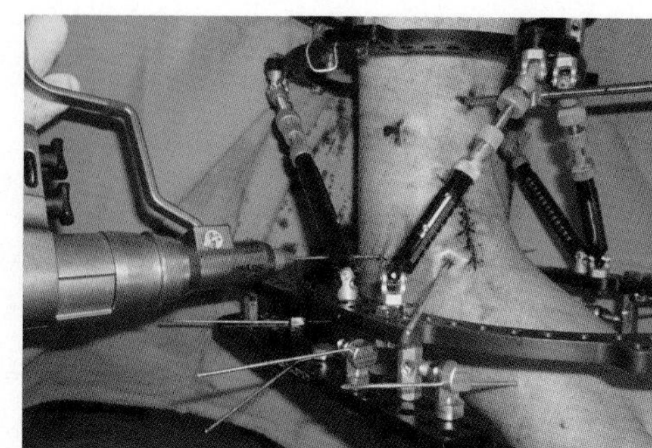
F

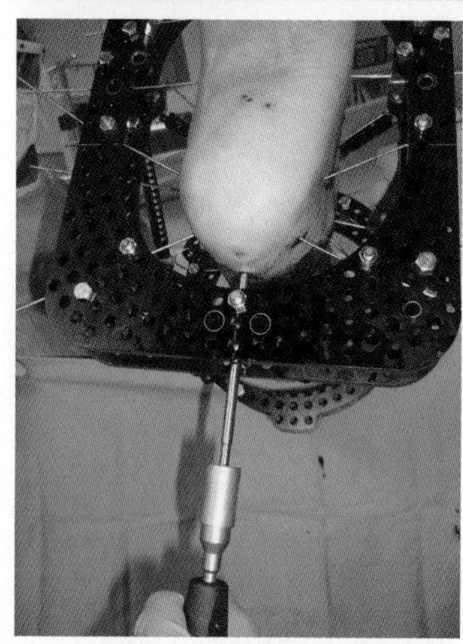
G

TECH FIG 10 • *(continued)* **E,F.** Two talar wires are passed. Without talar wires compression would be placed not only on the tibiotalar joint but also on the subtalar joint. **G.** Calcaneal half-pin for added foot frame stability.

- This is also essential to protect the subtalar joint from compression. If fixation from the foot plate to the foot is limited to the forefoot, midfoot, and calcaneus and no fixation is added to the talus, then axial compression will not be isolated to the tibiotalar joint but will also include the subtalar joint (with potential detrimental effects to the subtalar joint cartilage and motion). A perhaps more sophisticated (but not more complicated) construction of the foot plate is to distract between the two components of the foot plate, so that the subtalar joint is distracted while the tibiotalar joint is compressed. Although unproven, this may have a protective effect on the subtalar joint.
- I routinely add a calcaneal half-pin for added foot plate stability (TECH FIG 10G).
- Connect the proximal ring block and foot plate by struts and apply tibiotalar compression (TECH FIG 11A).
  - I make subtle adjustments at this point, which sometimes warrants removing one or both of the provisional fixation pins (TECH FIG 11B).
  - If the alignment is optimal, then I can leave one provisional pin in place (provided it is truly axial) to act as a rail as I compress the tibial talar joint with the external fixator.

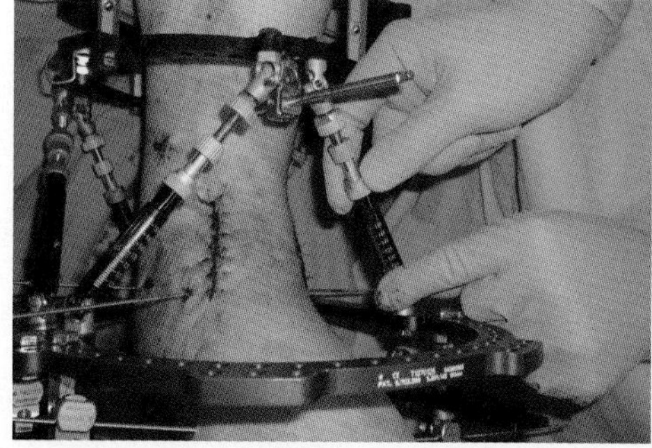
A

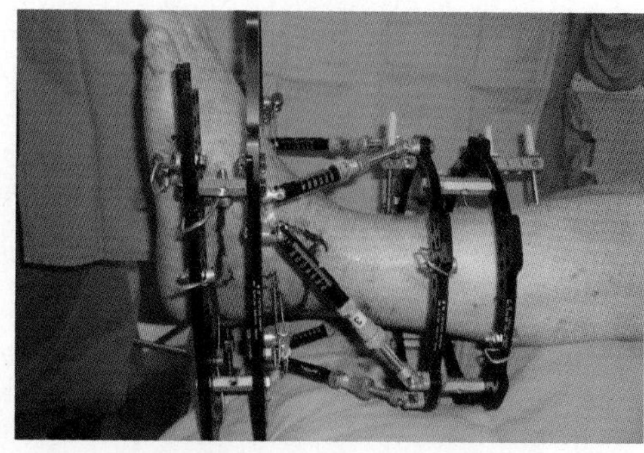
B

TECH FIG 11 • **A.** Adding struts to be used for compression between the proximal ring block and the foot frame. **B.** Proper position of the foot and leg within the external fixator. Ankle with neutral dorsiflexion–plantarflexion and plantar foot is distal to most distal ring–plate. The provisional fixation was removed for compression. *(continued)*

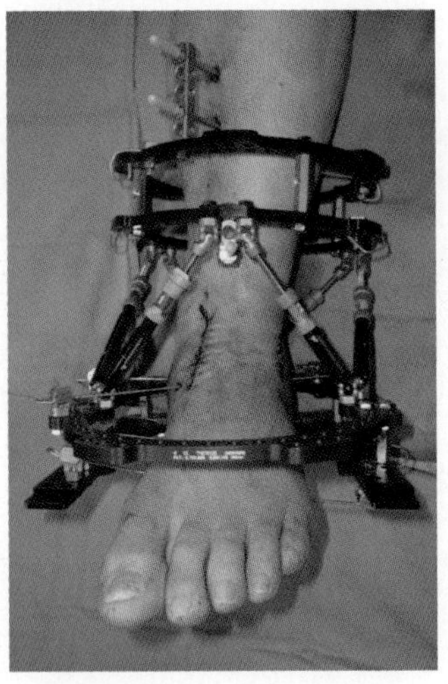

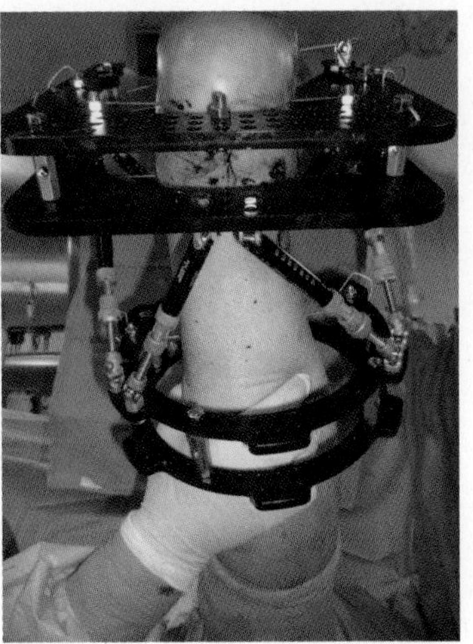

C D

TECH FIG 11 • *(continued)* **C,D.** Physiologic hindfoot valgus, with varus avoided. **C.** AP view. **D.** Posteroanterior view.

- If no translation, angulation, or rotation is required, which is often the case if the initial reduction was appropriate, then simply tightening the struts uniformly leads to satisfactory axial compression (**TECH FIG 11C,D**).
- If adjustments need to be made, the computer program may be used to run an effective correction at this time. However, on the operating table, the struts may simply be loosened, a gross manual adjustment can be made (with the provisional fixation removed), and the struts again secured. Then, uniform tightening of all struts can be performed.
- Final fluoroscopic views in the AP and lateral planes are sometimes difficult to interpret with an external fixator in place, but with subtle rotation of the limb, appropriate alignment and bony apposition can be confirmed.
- Final check to be sure that all bolts and connections are stable
- Sterile dressings on the wound
- Sterile dressings on the wires and half-pins
  - Pin irritation typically occurs because of skin motion or tension about the half-pins or thin wires.
  - I routinely place thick dressings around the thin wires and half-pins, creating moderate pressure from the dressing on the skin immediately adjacent to the half-pin or wire and thereby stabilizing the skin.
  - Prefabricated bolsters are also available to stabilize the skin around the pins.
- Final follow-up for external fixation case example (**TECH FIG 12**)
  - Alignment restored
  - Fusion apparent despite distorted distal tibial alignment

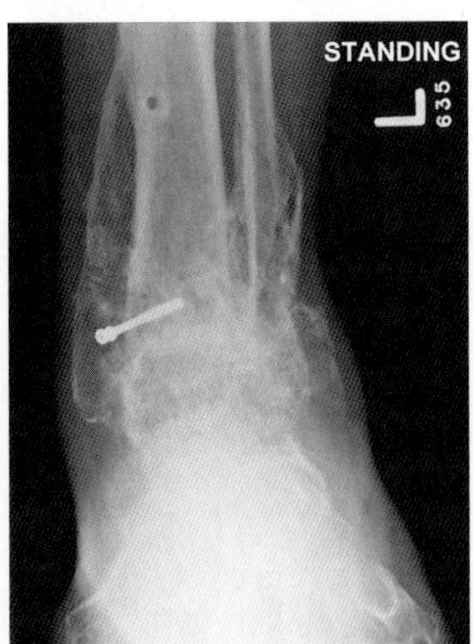

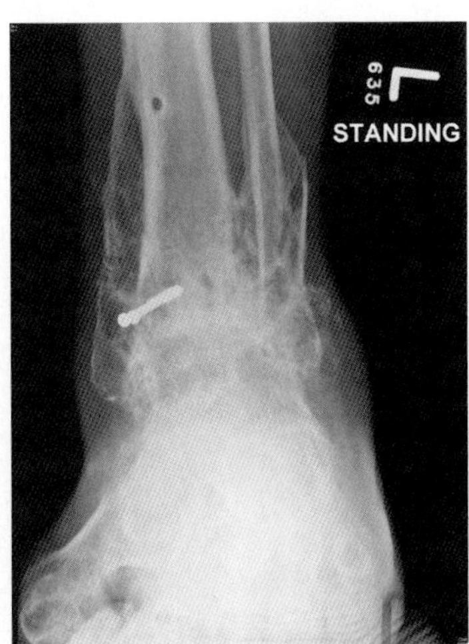

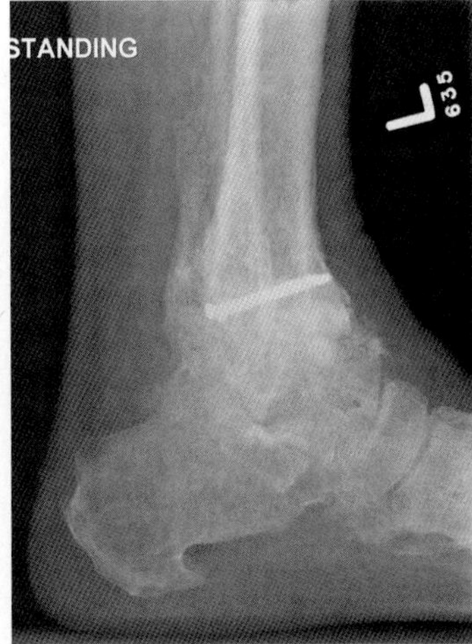

A B C

TECH FIG 12 • Follow-up radiographs suggesting successful revision ankle arthrodesis using external fixation. **A.** AP view. **B.** Mortise view. **C.** Lateral view.

PEARLS AND PITFALLS

Position of arthrodesis	▪ Avoid varus and internal rotation. Optimal position is neutral dorsiflexion–plantarflexion, slight hindfoot valgus, and the second metatarsal aligned with the anterior tibial crest.
Prior or active infection	▪ Internal fixation for ankle arthrodesis is probably contraindicated; however, arthrodesis is still possible with external fixation.
Joint preparation	▪ Internal and external fixation may stabilize the joint, but satisfactory joint preparation for arthrodesis is essential for fusion to occur.
Preservation of subchondral bone architecture	▪ If possible, maintain the subchondral bone architecture. This allows adjustments in dorsiflexion–plantarflexion position without forfeiting bony apposition at the arthrodesis site before fixation.
Potential advantages of internal fixation over external fixation	▪ No need for pin care; perhaps less intimidating to the patient
Potential advantages of external fixation over internal fixation	▪ Further compression and adjustments at the arthrodesis site are possible postoperatively; perhaps earlier weight bearing.

POSTOPERATIVE CARE

- With advances in anesthesia, ankle arthrodesis may be performed on an outpatient basis.
- However, we typically keep these patients at least overnight for pain control, nasal oxygen (which may have some positive effect on anterior wound healing), and prophylactic intravenous antibiotics.
- Follow-up in 10 to 14 days
  - Internal fixation
    - Suture removal
    - Short-leg, touch-down weight-bearing cast
  - External fixation
    - Suture removal
    - Radiographs to assess bony apposition at the arthrodesis site and alignment. If a subtle adjustment needs to be made, it is done at this time, typically with the computer program.
    - We routinely add more compression to the arthrodesis site at this and subsequent visits. Simple axial compression does not require use of the computer program; instead, uniform tightening of all struts creates axial compression at the arthrodesis site. This is a major advantage of external fixation over internal fixation. With internal fixation, bony apposition at the arthrodesis site cannot be altered after the index procedure.
    - The patient is instructed how to perform pin care. We do not usually have the patient perform pin care in the first 10 to 14 days in order to protect the wound. My routine pin care includes once-a-day pin cleaning with a sponge moistened with a 50–50 mixture of sterile saline and hydrogen peroxide. I instruct the patients to "shoeshine" the pins with the sponge so that the debris is removed at the pin–skin interface. If a pin is irritated, then we recommend placing an antibiotic ointment at that pin's interface with the skin and to continue to stabilize that particular pin with dressings that stabilize the skin adjacent to the pin. Oral antibiotics may be required in some situations.
    - We have the orthotist create a tread for the foot plate. Once the wounds have healed adequately and edema is controlled, the tread can be added and weight bearing through the external fixator is possible, another potential advantage of external over internal fixation.
- Follow-up at about 6 weeks
  - Internal fixation
    - Ankle radiographs
    - If healing is progressing well, the patient is progressed to a cam boot.
    - If more healing is necessary, a short-leg cast is continued.
    - Weight bearing may be progressively increased if healing is progressing, but we typically restrict the patient from full weight bearing until 10 weeks (longer if healing is delayed).
  - External fixation
    - Radiographs
    - We routinely add more axial compression.
    - Pin care is reinforced.
    - Weight bearing is encouraged with the tread on the foot plate.
- Follow-up at 10 to 12 weeks and beyond
  - Internal fixation
    - Radiographs
    - If healing is suggested, then the patient can progress to full weight bearing, first in the cam boot and then transitioning to a regular shoe by 12 to 14 weeks. If healing is delayed, then this protocol is delayed.
  - External fixation
    - Radiographs
    - More axial compression is added.
    - If healing is suggested radiographically, then the surgeon should plan for external fixator removal between 12 and 16 weeks.
    - If healing is delayed, more axial compression is added and follow-up is set for 3 to 4 more weeks. External fixator removal is delayed until healing is suggested.
    - Frame removal may be performed in the office, but removal of half-pins may be particularly uncomfortable for the patient (especially if hydroxyapatite-coated pins are used).
    - A short operating room procedure should be considered for frame removal with the patient under anesthesia.
    - We routine add a short-leg walking cast for an additional 2 to 4 weeks, then transition to a cam boot and regular shoe.

OUTCOMES

- The literature suggests favorable outcomes of ankle arthrodesis, with good relief of ankle pain and high rates of patient satisfaction (mostly level IV retrospective studies without standardized foot and ankle outcome measures).

- At intermediate follow-up, good to excellent results have been reported in 66% to 90% of patients (mostly level IV retrospective studies without standardized foot and ankle outcome measures).
- In long-term follow-up, a considerable number of patients with ankle arthrodesis develop adjacent joint (subtalar and, to a lesser degree, transverse tarsal joint) arthrosis.
- Although most patients with arthrodesis report satisfactory pain relief, functional outcome, particularly gait analysis, is not physiologic.

COMPLICATIONS

- Both internal and external fixation
  - Infection
  - Wound dehiscence or delayed wound healing
  - Nonunion
  - Malunion
  - Late development of subtalar (and, to a lesser degree, transverse tarsal joint) arthritis (adjacent joint arthritis)
- Internal fixation
  - Prominent hardware
  - Residual gapping at tibiotalar arthrodesis site that cannot be compressed postoperatively
- External fixation
  - Pin tract infection

REFERENCES

1. Agel J, Coetzee JC, Sangeorzan BJ, et al. Functional limitations of patients with end-stage ankle arthrosis. Foot Ankle Int 2005;26:537–539.
2. Anderson T, Montgomery F, Besjakov J, et al. Arthrodesis of the ankle for non-inflammatory conditions—healing and reliability of outcome measurements. Foot Ankle Int 2002;23:390–393.
3. Coester LM, Saltzman CL, Leupold J, et al. Long-term results following ankle arthrodesis for post-traumatic arthritis. J Bone Joint Surg Am 2001;83A:219–228.
4. Colman AB, Pomeroy GC. Transfibular ankle arthrodesis with rigid internal fixation: an assessment of outcome. Foot Ankle Int 2007;28: 303–307.
5. Easley ME, Montijo HE, Wilson JB, et al. Revision tibiotalar arthrodesis. J Bone Joint Surg Am 2008;90A:1212–1223.
6. Eylon S, Porat S, Bor N, et al. Outcome of Ilizarov ankle arthrodesis. Foot Ankle Int 2007;28:873–879.
7. Fuchs S, Sandmann C, Skwara A, et al. Quality of life 20 years after arthrodesis of the ankle: a study of adjacent joints. J Bone Joint Surg Br 2003;85:994–998.
8. Glazebrook M, Daniels T, Younger A, et al. Comparison of health-related quality of life between patients with end-stage ankle and hip arthrosis. J Bone Joint Surg Am 2008;90:499–505.
9. Greisberg J, Assal M, Flueckiger G, et al. Takedown of ankle fusion and conversion to total ankle replacement. Clin Orthop Relat Res 2004;424:80–88.
10. Haddad SL, Coetzee JC, Estok R, et al. Intermediate and long-term outcomes of total ankle arthroplasty and ankle arthrodesis: a systematic review of the literature. J Bone Joint Surg Am 2007;89A: 1899–1905.
11. Hintermann B, Barg A, Knupp M, et al. Conversion of painful ankle arthrodesis to total ankle arthroplasty. J Bone Joint Surg Am 2009;91A:850–858.
12. Holt ES, Hansen ST, Mayo KA, et al. Ankle arthrodesis using internal screw fixation. Clin Orthop Relat Res 1991;268:21–28.
13. Johnson EE, Weltmer J, Lian GJ, et al. Ilizarov ankle arthrodesis. Clin Orthop Relat Res 1992;280:160–169.
14. King HA, Watkins TB Jr, Samuelson KM. Analysis of foot position in ankle arthrodesis and its influence on gait. Foot Ankle 1980;1:44–49.
15. Kovoor CC, Padmanabhan V, Bhaskar D, et al. Ankle fusion for bone loss around the ankle joint using the Ilizarov technique. J Bone Joint Surg Br 2009;91B:361–366.
16. Mann RA, Rongstad KM. Arthrodesis of the ankle: a critical analysis. Foot Ankle Int 1998;19:3–9.
17. Monroe MT, Beals TC, Manoli A II. Clinical outcome of arthrodesis of the ankle using rigid internal fixation with cancellous screws. Foot Ankle Int 1999;20:227–231.
18. Muir DC, Amendola A, Saltzman CL. Long-term outcome of ankle arthrodesis. Foot Ankle Clin 2002;7:703–708.
19. Myerson MS, Quill G. Ankle arthrodesis: a comparison of an arthroscopic and an open method of treatment. Clin Orthop Relat Res 1991;268:84–95.
20. Nielsen KK, Linde F, Jensen NC. The outcome of arthroscopic and open surgery ankle arthrodesis: a comparative retrospective study on 107 patients. Foot Ankle Surg 2008;14:153–157.
21. Ogut T, Glisson RR, Chuckpaiwong B, et al. External ring fixation versus screw fixation for ankle arthrodesis: a biomechanical comparison. Foot Ankle Int 2009;30:353–360.
22. Plaass C, Knupp M, Barg A, et al. Anterior double plating for rigid fixation of isolated tibiotalar arthrodesis. Foot Ankle Int 2009;30: 631–639.
23. Salem KH, Kinzl L, Schmelz A. Ankle arthrodesis using Ilizarov ring fixators: a review of 22 cases. Foot Ankle Int 2006;27:764–770.
24. Saltzman CL, Mann RA, Ahrens JE, et al. Prospective controlled trial of STAR total ankle replacement versus ankle fusion: initial results. Foot Ankle Int 2009;30:579–596.
25. Sealey RJ, Myerson MS, Molloy A, et al. Sagittal plane motion of the hindfoot following ankle arthrodesis: a prospective analysis. Foot Ankle Int 2009;30:187–196.
26. SooHoo NF, Zingmond DS, Ko CY. Comparison of reoperation rates following ankle arthrodesis and total ankle arthroplasty. J Bone Joint Surg Am 2007;89:2143–2149.
27. Takakura Y, Tanaka Y, Sugimoto K, et al. Long-term results of arthrodesis for osteoarthritis of the ankle. Clin Orthop Relat Res 1999;361:178–185.
28. Thomas R, Daniels TR, Parker K. Gait analysis and functional outcomes following ankle arthrodesis for isolated ankle arthritis. J Bone Joint Surg Am 2006;88:526–535.
29. Thomas RH, Daniels TR. Ankle arthritis. J Bone Joint Surg Am 2003;85A:923–936.
30. Trouillier H, Hansel L, Schaff P, et al. Long-term results after ankle arthrodesis: clinical, radiological, gait analytical aspects. Foot Ankle Int 2002;23:1081–1090.
31. White AA III. A precision posterior ankle fusion. Clin Orthop Relat Res 1974;98:239–250.

Chapter 78 Transfibular Approach for Ankle Arthrodesis

Alex J. Kline and Dane K. Wukich

DEFINITION

- Ankle arthrodesis is performed for treatment of end-stage ankle arthritis, refractory to nonsurgical management. While ankle arthroplasty has become an increasingly popular procedure, arthrodesis remains an accepted surgical treatment for end-stage arthritis.
- Over 40 different techniques of ankle arthrodesis have been described in the literature.
- A traditional method of ankle arthrodesis is the transfibular approach, which uses a distal fibular osteotomy, allowing for optimal visualization of the joint surface, and provides a source of autogenous bone graft for fusion.

ANATOMY

- The ankle is a highly constrained hinge-type joint between the tibial plafond, the distal fibula, and the dome of the talus. Compressive forces across the ankle joint approach five times the body's weight at heel rise.
- The ankle is subjected to more weight-bearing force per square centimeter than any other joint. The articular cartilage of the ankle is relatively thin (1 to 2 mm) and the contact area is only one third of the hip or knee.
- The ankle joint is responsible for the majority of dorsiflexion and plantarflexion of the ankle–hindfoot complex.

PATHOGENESIS

- End-stage arthritis of the ankle results from progressive loss of the articular cartilage between the tibial plafond and the talar dome, resulting in inflammation, osteophyte formation, progressive loss of ankle motion, and increasing ankle pain with motion or weight bearing.
- Tibiotalar arthritis may be (1) posttraumatic arthritis (following ankle fracture, pilon fracture, talus fracture), (2) arthritis secondary to chronic ankle ligament instability, (3) primary arthritis, (4) one of a number of inflammatory arthritides (rheumatoid arthritis, gout or pseudogout, and mixed connective tissue disorders), (5) neuropathic arthrosis, or (6) postinfectious arthritis.

NATURAL HISTORY

- Most commonly, ankle arthritis is posttraumatic in origin, either from direct injury to the ankle's articular cartilage or due to chronic ligament instability.
- Primary ankle arthritis is relatively rare when compared to primary arthritis of the hip and knee.
- In general, once the cascade of cartilage degeneration is initiated, it will continue to progress, albeit at a variable rate.

PATIENT HISTORY AND PHYSICAL FINDINGS

- A careful history is obtained from the patient, including the cause of posttraumatic arthritis. Evaluation of posttraumatic arthritis should determine if there was a history of open fracture-dislocation and infection; evaluation of an inflammatory arthritis includes reviewing the patient's medications, particularly immunosuppressive medications. Diabetic neuroarthropathy may also be responsible for ankle arthritis.
- Social history includes the patient's age, occupation (and associated functional demands), and degree of functional limitation due to the arthritic ankle. Social history should also include tobacco use. Moreover, any concerns for the patient being incapable of maintaining a protected weight-bearing status postoperatively should be identified, including any restrictions to upper extremity function.
- Prior surgery, particularly to the arthritic ankle, is documented. When available, the surgeon should review prior operative reports. The most common symptom of ankle arthritis is anterior ankle pain that is increased with weight bearing and relieved by unloading the ankle joint, causing the patient to limp. Patients often report ankle stiffness and difficulty walking up inclines, which exacerbates their symptoms. Patients also notice that their foot is "turning out." Painless ankle arthritis may be indicative of a peripheral neuropathy, typically diabetic neuroarthropathy.
- While the ankle is not responsible for inversion and eversion, the surgeon should document any difficulties the patient may have walking on uneven terrain. This may indicate that there is associated hindfoot arthritis.
- Physical evaluation should include:
  - Evaluation of ankle and hindfoot alignment. The patient should be weight bearing. The examiner should inspect the position of the patient's foot and ankle, noting particularly any varus–valgus deformities. This is typically best accomplished from a posterior perspective, looking at the lower leg and heel. The lateral perspective may identify equinus. A careful understanding of weight-bearing preoperative alignment or malalignment allows for optimal intraoperative correction, which is done with the patient supine and non–weight-bearing.
  - Ankle range of motion. Passive and active range of motion of the ankle should be assessed and documented. This is best determined actively with the patient standing or passively with the patient seated. The patient with ankle arthritis typically experiences pain with ankle range of motion. Normal ankle range of motion is about 20 degrees of dorsiflexion and 50 degrees of plantarflexion. Limited dorsiflexion is most common, due to anterior ankle impingement or equinus contracture. It is often difficult to isolate ankle range of motion since the ankle functions in concert with the hindfoot, which also allows some dorsiflexion and plantarflexion, mostly through the transverse tarsal joint.
  - Hindfoot motion. Hindfoot motion is tested by grasping the hindfoot with one hand while the other hand passively inverts and everts the subtalar joint. The talar neck may be supported with one finger to ensure that hindfoot motion is

being tested in isolation. With isolated ankle arthritis, hindfoot range of motion is typically minimally symptomatic. Normal hindfoot motion is about 20 degrees of inversion and 10 degrees of eversion. Dorsiflexion and plantarflexion through the hindfoot is about 15 degrees for each. Ankle arthrodesis increases stresses in the hindfoot. With preexisting hindfoot arthritis and stiffness, symptoms may persist despite successful ankle arthrodesis.

- Vascular examination. Dorsalis pedis and posterior tibial pulses should be palpated and compared to the contralateral side. Capillary refill to the toes is also documented. Any asymmetry in pulses should prompt a further evaluation, including ankle–brachial indices and noninvasive vascular studies. Any reconstructive procedure for the foot and ankle requires satisfactory circulation. It is easy to recommend ankle arthrodesis based on the ankle's radiographic appearance but lose sight of the vascular status.
- Soft tissue envelope. The physiologically normal ankle affords little soft tissue reserves and is at risk for wound complications. Previous surgical scars or scars from soft tissue trauma about the ankle may increase the risk of reoperation on the ankle. Careful documentation of previous surgical scars is mandatory. The surgical approach must be carefully planned, particularly when there are prior surgical incisions or prior soft tissue trauma. In posttraumatic arthritis, open reduction and internal fixation of the fibula may have been performed, affording an ideal access to the ankle through the same incision for transfibular ankle arthrodesis.
- Gait. A limp is typically present, and as a compensatory mechanism, the patient often externally rotates the hip to avoid anterior impingement at the ankle. Gait analysis permits further understanding of the patient's hindfoot–ankle alignment and should be taken into consideration in planning ankle arthrodesis. External rotation occurs at the hip as a compensatory mechanism; a dramatic external rotation deformity at the ankle is rarely present.
- Edema, erythema, warmth, and draining sinus. A history of open fracture or postoperative infection after prior surgery should prompt comprehensive evaluation for septic arthritis and osteomyelitis.

IMAGING AND OTHER DIAGNOSTIC STUDIES

- Weight-bearing AP, mortise–oblique, and lateral radiographs of the ankle and foot are obtained to determine alignment, extent of arthritis, and retained hardware. Non–weight-bearing radiographs do not provide accurate determination of alignment and joint space narrowing. Occasionally, weight-bearing mechanical axis views of the tibia or even the entire lower extremity are necessary to accurately determine malalignment. This is particularly important for patients with ankle or tibial malunion or knee deformity. A more comprehensive radiographic evaluation may indicate that malalignment may not be corrected at the ankle alone and that more proximal realignment is required.
- Should radiographs suggest avascular necrosis of the talus or distal tibia, MRI may confirm avascular necrosis. CT provides greater detail of radiographic findings—in particular, large bony defects, such as subchondral cysts and suspected adjacent hindfoot arthritis.
- A history of open ankle fracture-dislocation, infection, or greater-than-anticipated erythema, edema, and warmth with greater-than-expected radiographic erosive changes should prompt a workup for septic arthritis or osteomyelitis so that implants are not placed in the face of infection. Laboratory tests should include a white blood cell count with differential, erythrocyte sedimentation rate, and C-reactive protein. The arthritic joint should be aspirated if possible for cell count, organism analysis, and cultures. MRI may identify effusion, abscess, or bone concerning for osteomyelitis; CT scan may reveal a sequestrum. The combination of a technetium bone scan and tagged WBC study tends to afford a high positive predictive value when infection is suspected. If an infection is still suspected despite a negative workup, then the surgical plan should start with obtaining a deep bone specimen to be evaluated for immediate frozen section and tissue sent for culture. Patients with asymmetric or weak pulses should undergo further diagnostic workup, including ankle–brachial indices or noninvasive vascular studies.
- Diabetic patients with suspected diabetic neuroarthropathy may not be candidates for isolated ankle arthrodesis and may be better served with tibiotalocalcaneal arthrodesis. However, well-controlled diabetic patients may be appropriate for isolated ankle arthrodesis. As for any orthopaedic procedure, these patients' blood glucose levels need to be optimized perioperatively.

DIFFERENTIAL DIAGNOSIS

- Osteoarthritis
- Posttraumatic arthritis
- Rheumatoid arthritis
- Inflammatory arthritides
- Postinfectious arthritis
- Osteonecrosis
- Idiopathic
- Congenital
- Neuroarthropathy

NONOPERATIVE MANAGEMENT

- Nonsteroidal anti-inflammatory agents (NSAIDs) are the mainstay of pharmacologic management of the arthritic ankle. With approval from the patient's primary care physician, COX-2 inhibitors can be considered if NSAIDs fail to relieve symptoms.
- Intra-articular corticosteroid injections may be judiciously used to help control flares of symptoms. We recommend administering these at no more than 3-month intervals.
- Shoe modifications, including the use of a stiff-soled rocker-bottom sole and solid ankle cushion heel (SACH), help some patients with mild to moderate arthritis. In patients with more advanced disease, bracing that further limits the degree of ankle motion may be required. These include a custom-molded ankle–foot orthosis (AFO), a rigid leather lace-up brace, or a double-upright bar brace.

SURGICAL MANAGEMENT

- The primary indication for ankle arthrodesis is the development of painful arthritis of the ankle joint that leads to progressive functional limitation. In such cases, the failure of nonoperative treatment is an indication for ankle arthrodesis.

Preoperative Planning

- Before planning an ankle arthrodesis, the adjacent joints must be carefully assessed. Concomitant moderate to severe arthritic changes in the adjacent joints (subtalar and transverse tarsal joints) are a relative contraindication to isolated fusion of the ankle joint. It is not unusual to see radiographic evidence of arthritis in the adjacent joints. In carefully selected patients, total ankle replacement in combination with hindfoot arthrodesis may afford a functional advantage over simultaneous ankle–hindfoot arthrodesis.
- Examination of the entire lower extremity should be performed to identify any proximal malalignment (internal rotation, external rotation, varus, valgus, and shortening) that needs to be corrected, either concomitant to ankle arthrodesis or in a staged fashion.
- As for any reconstructive procedure, patients should be medically optimized preoperatively. For example, diabetics must have their blood glucose levels normalized, and we recommend that smokers cease smoking 4 weeks before and 8 weeks after surgery. Infected wounds, septic arthritis, or osteomyelitis must be managed properly before internal fixation or bone graft is placed for ankle arthrodesis. It may be necessary to perform a preliminary irrigation and débridement and antibiotic bead placement to clear the infection, followed by a staged ankle arthrodesis.

Positioning

- The patient is placed supine on the operating table with a large bump underneath the ipsilateral hip to facilitate exposure. We routinely use a thigh tourniquet.

Approach

- For the transfibular approach, we make an incision over the posterior half of the fibula, starting about 8 to 10 cm proximal to the tip of the fibula, extending along the fibular shaft to the tip of the fibula, then curving anteriorly and distally over the sinus tarsi another 6 to 8 cm toward the base of the fourth metatarsal (**FIG 1**).

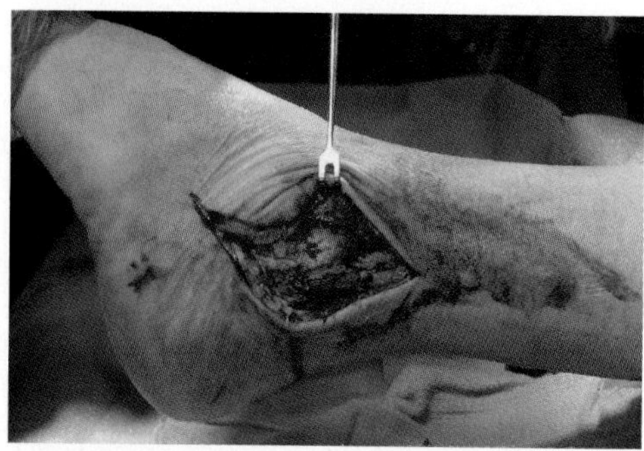

FIG 1 • Lateral transfibular approach to the fibula.

- The approach uses the internervous plane between the sural nerve posteriorly and the superficial peroneal nerve anteriorly.
- When performing the dissection at the level of the fibula, we create full-thickness flaps and perform a subperiosteal dissection to minimize soft tissue tension. At the proximal extent of the wound, the superficial peroneal nerve is protected; posteriorly the peroneal tendons and sural nerve are protected. We strip a minimal amount of fibular periosteum, with the majority being anterior using a periosteal elevator. We attempt to preserve a posterior hinge of fibular periosteum.
- The anterior syndesmotic ligaments, the anterior talofibular ligament, and the calcaneofibular ligament are fully exposed. An anterolateral ankle capsulotomy is performed and the anterior joint capsule and anterior distal tibial periosteum are elevated to expose the anterior tibiotalar articulation. Care is taken to avoid overzealous stripping over the talar neck in order to prevent devascularization of the talus.

TECHNIQUES

TRANSFIBULAR APPROACH FOR ANKLE ARTHRODESIS

- We perform a fibular osteotomy about 3 to 5 cm proximal to the level of the ankle joint. We prefer making an oblique osteotomy, from proximal lateral to distal medial. The cut edge is beveled to avoid creating a bony prominence. Alternatively, we make a transverse osteotomy 6 to 8 cm proximal to the ankle. We use a microsagittal saw to create the osteotomy while protecting the soft tissues. The anterior syndesmotic ligaments, the anterior talofibular ligament, and the calcaneofibular ligament are then transected, allowing the distal fibula to hinge on the intact posterior soft tissues and allowing some vascularity to remain intact. Using the microsagittal saw in the sagittal plane, the medial third of the fibula is removed, morselized, and saved as bone graft. Traditionally, the entire distal fibula was resected and used as bone graft. However, current practice favors leaving the malleoli, particularly because there has been some reported success in takedowns of ankle fusions and conversion to total ankle arthroplasty; future conversion to ankle replacement is not possible when the distal fibula is removed (**TECH FIG 1A**).
- At the distal tibia, elevate the anterior joint capsule and periosteum further, and remove impinging osteophytes that may block reduction. Posteriorly, use a periosteal elevator to elevate the soft tissues from the lateral and posterior aspect of the tibia and from the posterior talus.
- Once the soft tissues are released, retractors can be safely placed anteriorly and posteriorly about the distal tibia to protect the soft tissues and neurovascular structures. We typically use a joint distractor or laminar spreader to fully expose the tibial plafond and dome of the talus (**TECH FIG 1B**). Occasionally, we perform a limited medial arthrotomy to expose the medial gutter of the ankle joint.
- Tibial plafond and talar dome preparation may be performed with transverse flat cuts, a chevron pattern, or maintenance of the residual tibiotalar subchondral anatomy. We prefer maintaining the physiologic subchondral architecture to (1) maximize surface contact area, (2) maintain limb length, and (3) allow for subtle adjustments to tibiotalar arthrodesis without sacrificing contact area. We remove the residual articular cartilage

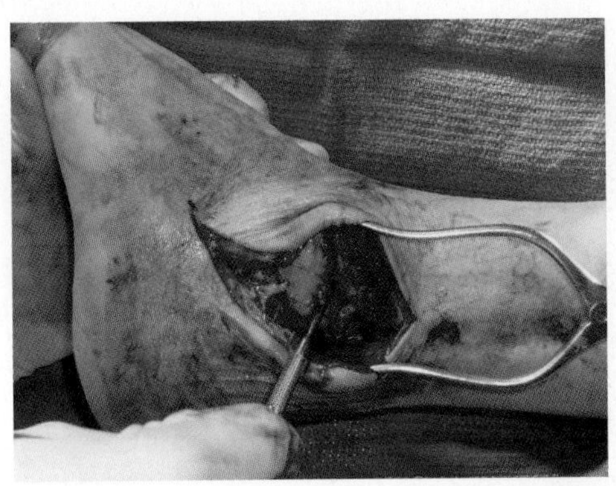

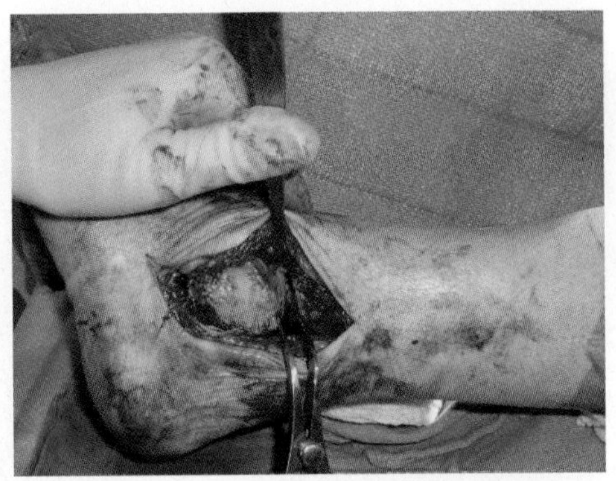

TECH FIG 1 • A. The fibula has been osteotomized proximal to the ankle joint and the dental Freer elevator is in the ankle joint. **B.** Lamina spreader is used to distract the joint.

with a sharp elevator, osteotomes, curettes, and a high-speed burr. The burr should be used with some cold sterile water or saline irrigation to minimize osteonecrosis. Once all cartilage has been removed, a small-diameter drill is used to penetrate the subchondral bone; alternatively, a narrow chisel may be used to "feather" the surfaces. Penetration of the subchondral bone by either method increases blood inflow to the arthrodesis site and increases surface area for fusion. Without disrupting the structure of the talar subchondral bone, the medial and lateral gutters should be denuded of residual articular cartilage. The accessory anteromedial arthrotomy affords access to the medial gutter that may not be feasible from the lateral approach. Based on the surgeon's preference, bone graft may be added directly to the arthrodesis site. We position the ankle and hindfoot in neutral dorsiflexion and plantarflexion, rotation to align the tibial shaft with the second metatarsal, and the hindfoot in slight (5 degrees) of valgus. The goal is to place the talar body directly under the tibial shaft axis. Often, this requires a few millimeters of posterior and medial talar translation in the ankle mortise. To accomplish the medial translation, we typically remove some of the medial malleolus, without disrupting the medial malleolar architecture. If cannulated screws are used for fixation, the guide pins are typically used for provisional fixation. We verify the position of the tibiotalar joint fluoroscopically using intraoperative C-image intensification. Multiple methods for insertion of the arthrodesis screws have been described, to include parallel and crossed screw techniques. In general, cross screws are more rigid than parallel screws, and three screws provide better compression and better resistance to torque than two screws.

- We routinely use cannulated screws for fixation of the tibiotalar arthrodesis. 6.5-mm, 7.3-mm, 7.5-mm, and 8.0-mm cannulated screw systems are available, and a variety of patterns for arthrodesis have been described. After manually positioning the tibiotalar joint in optimal position for arthrodesis, we typically place one guidewire from the lateral aspect of the base of the talus, aiming proximally and posteriorly through the body of the talus and laterally toward the medial tibial cortex. Alternatively, the initial guidewire may be placed from the medial tibia to the lateral talar dome. A second guidewire is inserted from the lateral tibia into the medial talus (**TECH FIG 2**). A final screw

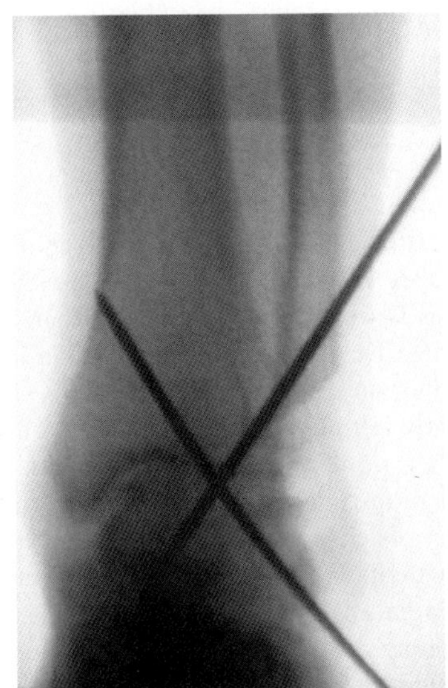

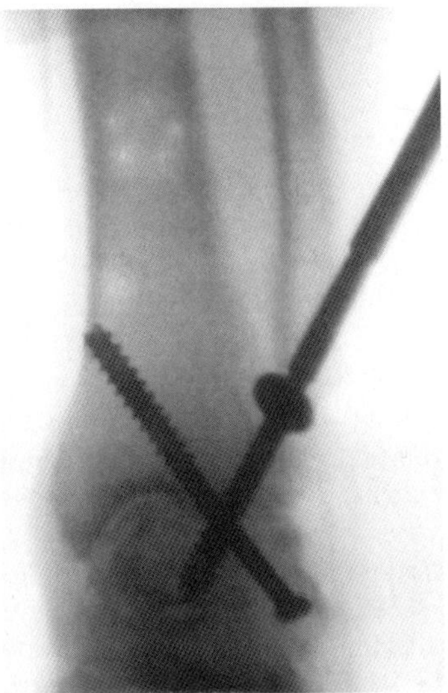

TECH FIG 2 • A. Two guide pins for the cannulated screws are inserted. **B.** The screws are inserted.

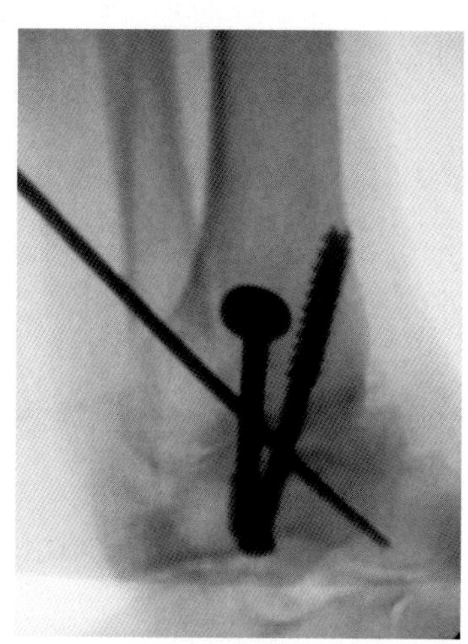

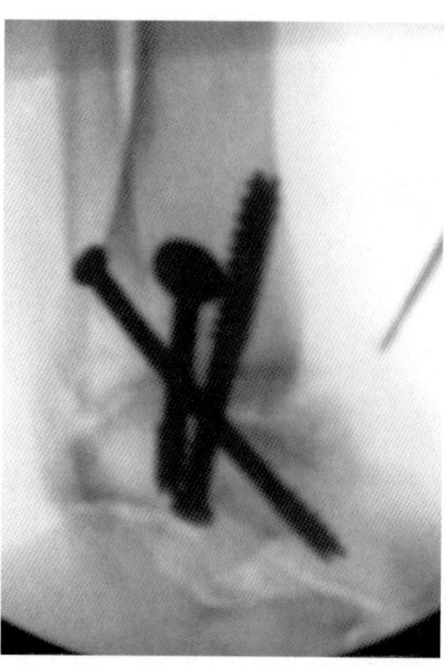

TECH FIG 3 • A. The guide pin for the "home run" screw is placed. **B.** The "home run" screw is inserted.

("home run screw") is inserted from the posterior malleolus into the neck of the talus (**TECH FIG 3**). We recommend using intraoperative fluoroscopy to confirm appropriate alignment, bony contact at the arthrodesis site, and satisfactory guidewire position and length. Three partially threaded cancellous screws are inserted over the guidewires, making sure that all threads cross the joint, to ensure compression. However, if one or two compression screws are supplemented with a fully threaded positional screw, the construct will be stable as well.

- Pack the morselized bone graft obtained from the excised section of the fibula anteriorly, laterally, and posteriorly at the arthrodesis site. The residual fibula is then repositioned as an onlay strut graft on the lateral aspect of the tibiotalar arthrodesis and secured with one screw from the distal fibula to the talus and a second more proximally from the fibula to the talus.

PEARLS AND PITFALLS

- Denuding cartilage from the medial malleolus and resecting some of the medial malleolus allows for slight medial translation and improved positioning of the talar body under the tibial plafond. A small accessory medial arthrotomy facilitates access to the medial gutter. Do not penetrate the subtalar joint with the screws.
- Varus and excessive valgus ankle and hindfoot position should be avoided.
- Equinus must be avoided; this is a particular risk if there is associated cavus or relative forefoot plantarflexion.
- The rate of nonunion for ankle arthrodesis is 10%.
- When transecting the anterior syndesmotic ligaments, avoid injuring the peroneal artery that lies directly posterior to the interosseous membrane.
- Resect the medial third of the fibula, morselize it to use as a bone graft, and use the residual fibula as a strut graft with a cancellous surface to heal to the tibiotalar arthrodesis.

POSTOPERATIVE CARE

- We routinely use a bulky Jones dressing with a plaster splint postoperatively. This is changed to a short-leg non–weight-bearing cast at the initial postoperative visit (usually in 7 to 10 days). Patients are kept non–weight-bearing for a total of 6 weeks, followed by a period of 6 weeks in which weight bearing is gradually progressed in a short-leg walking cast or cam walker boot. Weight bearing is then advanced in the cam boot and regular shoe over the subsequent few weeks.
- The use of a drain postoperatively is left to the discretion of the surgeon. Sutures are typically removed at 3 weeks. We typically observe radiographic evidence of tibiotalar fusion between 3 to 6 months.

OUTCOMES

- Reported rates of successful ankle fusion by any technique range from 60% to 100%. A recent study of transfibular approach ankle arthrodesis with screw fixation in 40 patients showed a fusion rate of 95%. Delayed unions were seen in four patients and nonunions in two patients. The mean AOFAS scores improved significantly in this patient population, and all patients except one said they would have the surgery again.
- Long-term follow-up demonstrates that two thirds to three quarters of patients are completely satisfied with minimal reservation. About 90% of patients would undergo ankle fusion again. Calf atrophy and adjacent joint hindfoot arthritis are universal findings during long-term follow-up. Eighty percent of patients demonstrate a gait abnormality.

COMPLICATIONS

- The incidence of wound complications and infections with ankle arthrodesis is roughly the same as in other elective foot and ankle cases. They can generally be managed with local débridement and antibiotics.
- Delayed union and nonunion occur relatively infrequently after ankle fusion, with a nonunion rate of about 10%. Infection must be ruled out as the cause for nonunion. Aseptic tibiotalar nonunion may be successfully managed with removal of hardware, repeat preparation of the arthrodesis site, bone grafting, and more rigid fixation. In osteopenic bone or where there is substantial bone loss at the arthrodesis site, a tibiotalocalcaneal arthrodesis may be warranted and external fixation may need to be considered.[4,5] Other potential complications of ankle arthrodesis include malunion, symptomatic hardware, reflex sympathetic dystrophy (complex regional pain syndrome), the development of symptomatic arthritis in adjacent joints, deep venous thrombosis, pulmonary embolism, and late stress fracture.

REFERENCES

1. Abidi NA, Gruen GS, Conti SF. Ankle arthrodesis: indications and techniques. J Am Acad Orthop Surg 2000;8:200–209.
2. Coester LM, Saltzman CL, Leupold J, et al. Long-term results following ankle arthrodesis for post-traumatic arthritis. J Bone Joint Surg Am 2001;83A:219–228.
3. Fuchs S, Sandmann C, Skwara A, et al. Quality of life 20 years after arthrodesis of the ankle: a study of adjacent joints. J Bone Joint Surg Br 2003;85B:994–998.
4. Haddad SL, Coetzee JC, Estok R, et al. Intermediate and long-term outcomes of total ankle arthroplasty and ankle arthrodesis. A systematic review of the literature. J Bone Joint Surg Am 2007; 89A: 1899–1905.
5. Levine SE, Myerson MS, Lucas P, et al. Salvage of pseudoarthrosis after tibiotalar arthrodesis. Foot Ankle Int 1997;18:580–585.
6. Thomas R, Daniels TR, Parker K. Gait analysis and functional outcomes following ankle arthrodesis for isolated ankle arthritis. J Bone Joint Surg Am 2006;88A:526–535.
7. Thordarson DB. Fusion in posttraumatic foot and ankle reconstruction. J Am Acad Orthop Surg 2004;12:322–333.
8. Wapner KL. Transfibular ankle fusion technique. Techniques Foot Ankle Surg 2002;1:17–23.

Chapter 79 The Miniarthrotomy Technique for Ankle Arthrodesis

Emmanouil D. Stamatis

DEFINITION

- Ankle arthritis is characterized by loss of joint cartilage and joint space narrowing.
- The etiology of ankle arthritis may be primary osteoarthritis, inflammatory arthritides, or posttraumatic, with posttraumatic being most common. Depending on the etiology, there may be a spectrum of concomitant findings, ranging from bone sclerosis and hypertrophy to osteopenia or absorption. Likewise, varying degrees of deformity and severity are observed, with and without inflammatory synovial proliferation.

ANATOMY

- The ankle joint is the articulation formed by the mortise (tibial plafond–medial malleolus and the distal part of the fibula) and the talus.
- The ankle is a modified hinge joint obliquely oriented in two planes (posteriorly and laterally in the transverse plane of the leg and laterally and downward in the coronal plane).
- The unique orientation of the physiologically normal ankle allows not only sagittal plane motion (approximately combined dorsiflexion and plantarflexion of 45 to 70 degrees) but also rotation (6 degrees) in addition to the movement in the sagittal plane.
- The ankle functions in concert with the subtalar joint as the ankle–subtalar joint complex, which is coupled by the medial collateral, lateral collateral, and tibiofibular ligaments to allow free movement of the ankle joint, stability, and cooperation with the subtalar joint during gait.
- The blood supply is provided by the anterior and posterior tibial arteries, the peroneal artery, and their branches and anastomoses, which form a rich vascular network.

PATHOGENESIS

- Idiopathic (primary) arthritis is better characterized by the term *osteoarthrosis* since it is not an inflammatory process. The exact mechanism of cartilage degeneration and loss has not been clearly defined. Secondary ankle arthritis is mainly posttraumatic, occuring after intra-articular fractures, chondral or osteochondral injuries, and chronic instability.
- Neuropathic arthritis is usually associated with diabetes mellitus, alcoholism, spinal cord injuries, peripheral nerve injuries, hereditary sensorimotor neuropathy, and proprioceptive nervous system injuries, or, more rarely, with congenital indifference to pain, tabes dorsalis, and leprosy.
- Other causes of ankle arthritis include the following:
  - Systemic inflammatory processes (rheumatoid arthritis, mixed connective tissue disorders, gout, and pseudogout)
  - Primary synovial disorders (pigmented villonodular synovitis)
  - Septic arthritis
  - Seronagative arthritides (associated with psoriasis, Reiter syndrome, and spondyloarthropathy)

NATURAL HISTORY

- The natural history of ankle arthritis is gradual progression of diffuse joint cartilage degeneration or erosion, osteophyte formation, and loss of joint space in the tibiotalar joint.
- In some cases, cartilage wear is not symmetric and deformity accompanies this arthritic process; this is particularly true of arthritis secondary to chronic ankle ligament instability and malunion.
- Body weight, level of activities, and concomitant subtalar or transverse tarsal joint pathology contribute to the morbidity of the disease. Patients with relatively low demands and isolated ankle arthritic involvement may function surprisingly well because of the adaptive effect of the healthy subtalar and transverse talar joints.

PATIENT HISTORY AND PHYSICAL FINDINGS

- Patients with end-stage ankle arthritis complain of severe ankle pain interfering with activities of daily living and typically note and demonstrate an obvious limp. Patients often report that their "foot is turning out" when walking; typically, this is a compensatory hip external rotation that relieves painful heel-to-toe gait. Recent literature suggests that ankle arthritis is as debilitating as hip arthritis.
- A complete examination of the ankle and hindfoot joints should include the following:
  - Soft tissue condition, including previous scars, callosities, ulcers, fistulas, and so forth. Elimination or fullness of the gutters indicates intra-articular fluid accumulation, or hypertrophied capsular tissue.
  - Vascular status, including peripheral pulses, microcirculation (capillary refill), ankle–brachial index
  - Sensation. Light touch is always tested to rule out peripheral neuropathy.
  - Stability. Anterior drawer and and inversion and eversion stress tests are performed to evaluate the integrity of the lateral collateral ligaments.
  - Motor strength: Manual motor test of the major muscular groups is performed.
  - Range of motion (ROM) of the ankle and hindfoot articulations. Loss of ankle extension may be the result of significant tibiotalar arthrosis, abutment of large anterior tibiotalar osteophytes, Achilles tendon contracture, or a combination of these. Loss of flexion may be related to significant tibiotalar arthrosis or subtalar pathology. Loss of hindfoot motion is the result of subtalar pathology (arthritis, fibrosis).

- Assessment of preoperative ankle, lower leg, and hindfoot alignment is important to understand what corrections must be considered in the ankle arthrodesis.

IMAGING AND OTHER DIAGNOSTIC STUDIES

- Plain weight-bearing radiographs—including anteroposterior (AP), lateral, and mortise views of the ankle joint—determine the extent of arthritis, deformity, bone defects in the distal tibial plafond or talus, potential avascular necrosis (AVN) in either the talar body or the distal tibia, and concomitant hindfoot arthritis.
  - The lateral and mortise ankle radiographs provide limited views of the hindfoot articulations; if foot arthritis or deformity is suggested, weight-bearing foot radiographs should be obtained (**FIG 1**).
  - Full-length weight-bearing bilateral radiographs are important in patients with suspected limb malalignment proximal to the ankle.
  - Weight-bearing radiographs of the foot are needed when the ankle arthritis is associated with pes cavus or pes planus or suspected concomitant hindfoot arthritis.

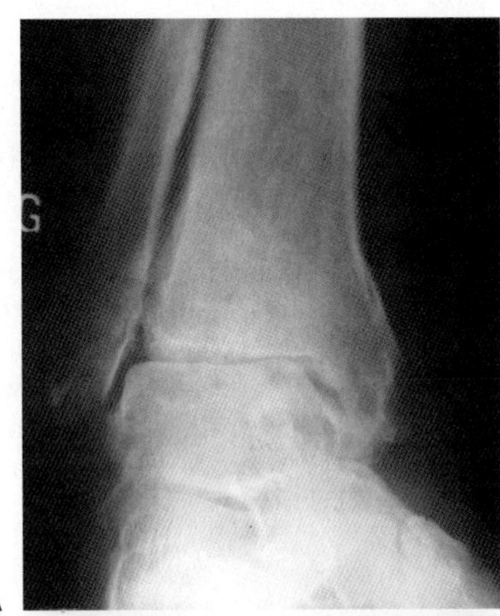

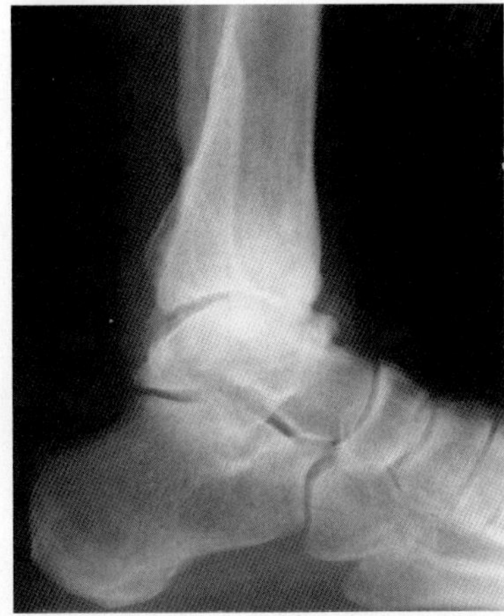

FIG 1 • AP and lateral weight-bearing radiographs of an arthritic ankle joint. Note the joint space narrowing with varus tilt of the talus (**A**), the anterior subluxation of the talus (**B**), and the presence of osteophytes (especially apparent in **B**).

- Computed tomogram provides detail of tibiotalar cysts and suspected hindfoot arthritis. Whereas large cysts in the tibia, talus, or both do not present a contraindication to the miniarthrotomy arthrodesis procedure, we recommend that these large defects be filled with autograft or allograft.
- If AVN is suggested by radiographs, magnetic resonance imaging typically is helpful in confirming the diagnosis and the extent. AVN also is not a contraindication to the miniarthrotomy procedure, but preoperative patient education is imperative since the nonunion rate is higher with AVN than without AVN.
- Combination three-phase technetium bone scan and and indium-labeled white blood cell scan are useful in ruling out or confirming suspected osteomyelitis.

DIFFERENTIAL DIAGNOSIS

- Bone marrow edema
- Soft tissue pathology
- Distal tibial plafond or talar AVN
- Osteochondritis

NONOPERATIVE MANAGEMENT

- Nonoperative treatment of ankle arthritis includes pharmacologic agents, intra-articular corticosteroid injections, shoe wear modifications, and orthoses.
- Nonsteroidal anti-inflammatory agents (NSAIDs) are widely used to provide pain relief, and other agents, such as gold, antimalarials, and immunosuppressives, are prescribed by rheumatologists to treat various inflammatory disorders.
- Intra-articular corticosteroid injections should be used judiciously since their repeated use accelerates the need for surgical treatment.
- High-top shoes restricting ankle motion or stiff-soled shoes with a rocker sole may be beneficial for pain relief.
- Polypropylene ankle–foot orthoses, with or without hinges, and orthoses with double metal upright bars and calf sleeves hold the joint still and limit the amount of pain.

SURGICAL MANAGEMENT

- Originally, the miniarthrotomy technique for ankle arthrodesis was described for use in arthritic ankles without deformity, bone defects, or AVN of talar dome or distal tibia.[5,8]
- With evolution of the technique, the indications for this procedure expanded to include end-stage ankle arthritis associated with the following[9]:
  - Marked joint space narrowoing
  - Severe ankle pain interfering with daily activities and walking ability
  - Failure of conservative treatment, including NSAIDs, intra-articular steroid injections, physical therapy, and use of ankle–foot orthoses
  - Absence of mechanical malalignment proximal to the ankle
  - A moderately deformed ankle joint with varus or valgus under 10 degrees
  - Less than 25% posterior or anterior subluxation
  - AVN of the talus involving less than 25% of its articular surface
  - Articular surface cavitations smaller than 1 × 2 cm
  - Intact sensation (absence of neuroarthropathy)

Preoperative Planning

- All imaging studies are reviewed.
- The ankle and adjacent hindfoot joints are evaluated for ROM and alignment.
- We typically perform diagnostic injections of the hindfoot articulations if symptomatic hindfoot arthritis is masked by the ankle arthritis. (Ankle arthrodesis in the face of hindfoot arthritis and stiffness will leave the patient with persistent symptoms.) Manual motor testing of the major muscular groups about the foot and ankle is important to identify weakness that may leave the patient with hindfoot imbalance despite successful ankle arthrodesis.
- Neuropathy, vascular insufficiency, venous stasis disease, or skin compromise at the ankle may warrant further evaluation or treatment before ankle arthrodesis. The advantage to the miniarthrotomy technique is minimal soft tissue and periosteal disruption, so it lends itself well to patients with some of these conditions.

Positioning

- The patient is positioned supine on the operating table. A support under the ipsilateral buttock allows balanced visualization to both sides of the ankle joint since the natural tendency of the lower extremity is to fall in external rotation.
- It is important to drape the leg well above the knee so that the patella may be used as a reference point for the aligning the ankle arthrodesis.
- We do not routinely use a tourniquet; this allows us to confirm that bleeding surfaces for fusion have been created.

TECHNIQUES

EXPOSURE AND VISUALIZATION OF THE JOINT

- Two 2.5-cm incisions are made, one anteromedial and one anterolateral, in approximately the same positions as arthroscopic portals created for standard ankle arthroscopy.
- The first incision is made just medial to the anterior tibial tendon, and the second immediately lateral to the peroneus tertius tendon (TECH FIG 1A).
- The medial incision is deepened through the subcutaneous tissues, avoiding inadvertent injury to the saphenous vein and nerve (TECH FIG 1B).
- The ankle retinaculum is identified and incised along the same line with the skin incision, and the anterior tibial tendon is retracted to identify the joint capsule.
- Sharp dissection or a rongeur is used to remove the hypertrophied capsular tissue from the anterior aspect of the joint, further improving the working space and visualization.
- A hemostat is driven through the medial incision, across the anterior aspect of the ankle joint, toward the lateral side to confirm the predetermined position of the lateral incision (TECH FIG 1C).
- The lateral incision is deepened through the subcutaneous tissues with careful subcutaneous dissection to avoid injury to the lateral branch of the superficial peroneal nerve (TECH FIG 1D).
- Again the ankle retinaculum is identified and incised along the same line with the skin incision, and the peroneus tertius tendon is retracted to identify the joint capsule.
- After removal of the hypertrophied capsular tissue from both the medial and the anterolateral aspects of the joint, resection of most osteophytes from the anterior tibia with flexible chisels further improves visualization.
- Any visible cartilage of the anterior ankle joint is resected with curettes of various sizes and shapes and a set of small rongeurs (TECH FIG 1E,F).

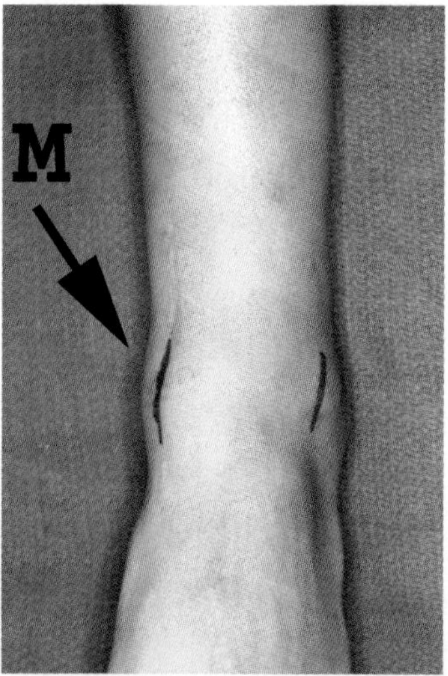

A

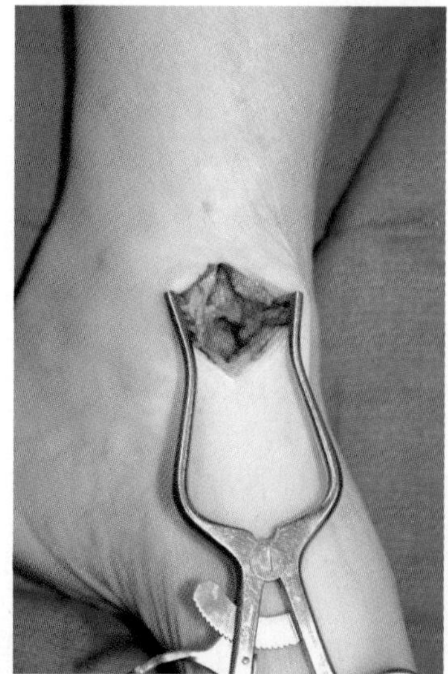
B

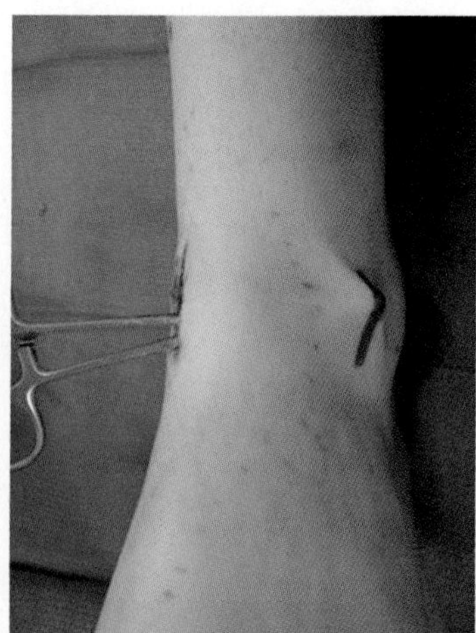
C

TECH FIG 1 • Incision and exposure. **A.** Incisions used for the miniarthrotomy technique for ankle arthrodesis. The medial incision is indicated (*M*). **B.** Exposure of the medial side of the joint. **C.** A hemostat is driven through the medial incision, across the anterior aspect of the ankle joint, and toward the lateral side, thus confirming the predetermined position of the lateral incision. *(continued)*

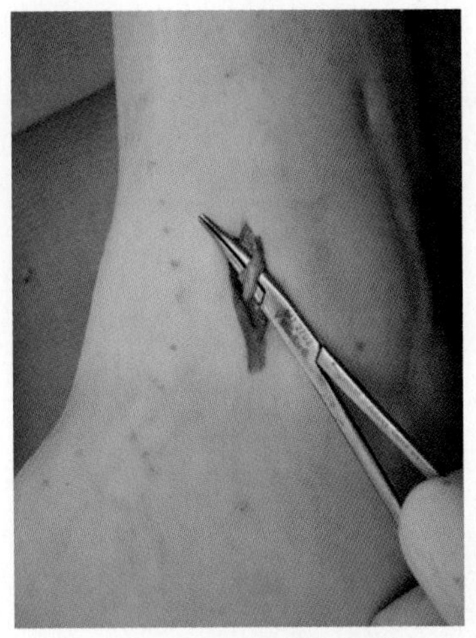

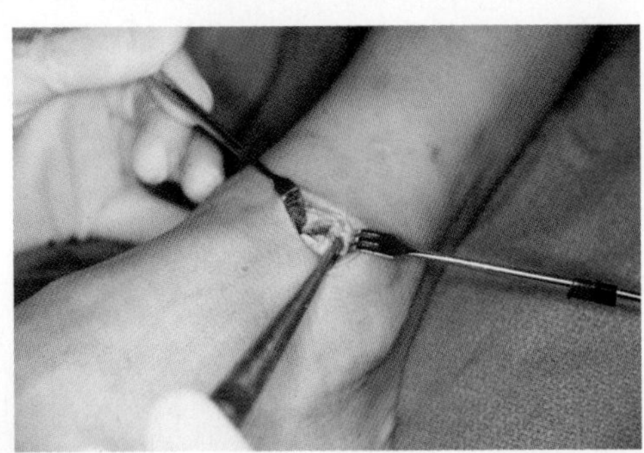

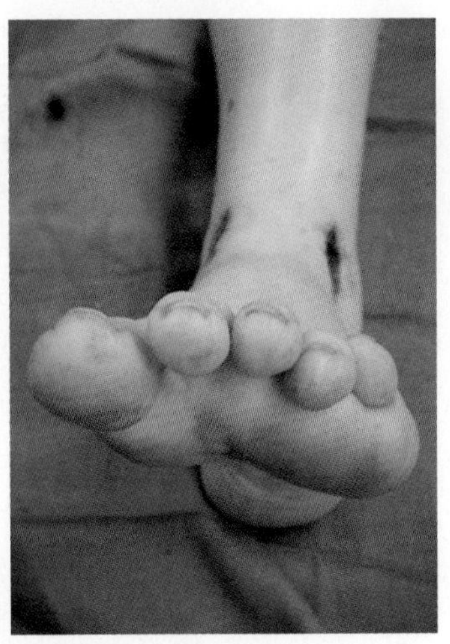

TECH FIG 1 • *(continued)* **D.** Identification and protection of the lateral branch of the superficial peroneal nerve during deepening of the lateral incision through the subcutaneous tissues. **E.** Any visible cartilage of the anterior ankle joint is resected with curettes of various sizes and shapes and a set of small rongeurs. **F.** Appearance of the ankle after completion of the exposure.

PREPARATION OF THE ARTICULAR SURFACES

- A small lamina spreader is inserted into either the medial or the lateral joint space, and further débridement is performed through the contralateral incision (TECH FIG 2A).
- This process is alternated between medial and lateral incisions (TECH FIG 2B).
- With the joint distracted, various instruments (rongeurs, curettes, and chisels) are used to débride any remnants of cartilage, synovial tissue, loose bodies, and sclerotic subchondral bone.
- The joint must be irrigated frequently to visualize the cancellous bone surfaces and to confirm uniform bleeding.
- Small bone wedges may be resected to obtain the ideal joint position, particularly when moderate deformity is present.

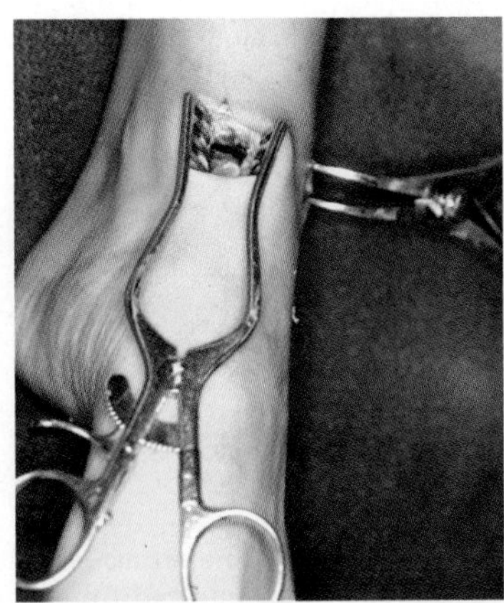

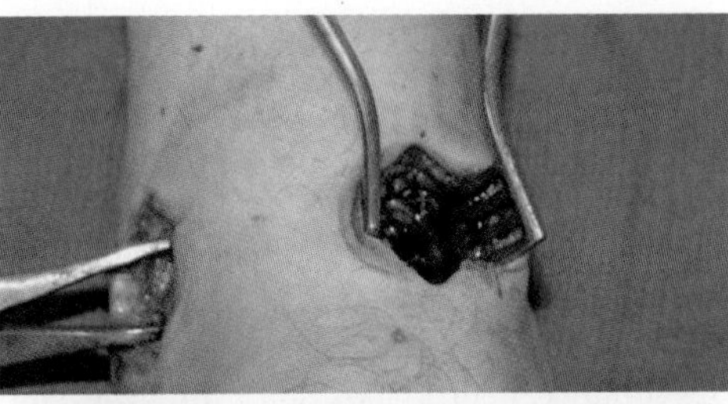

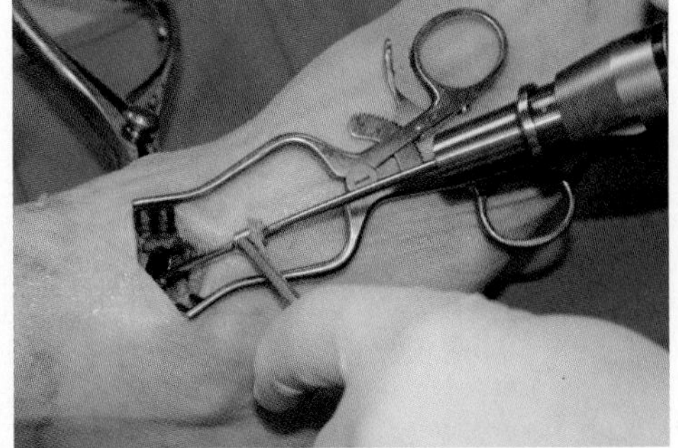

TECH FIG 2 • Preparation of the articular surfaces. **A.** A small lamina spreader is inserted into the lateral joint space, and further débridement is performed through the medial incision. **B.** The position of the instruments has been alternated. **C.** Any dense sclerotic subchondral bone of the distal tibia is drilled with a 2.5-mm drill bit to enhance revascularization. *(continued)*

- Any remaining cartilage on the lateral articular surfaces of the talus and of the articular surfaces of the malleoli is then meticulously removed.
- Any dense sclerotic subchondral bone can be drilled with a 2.5-mm drill bit to enhance revascularization (**TECH FIG 2C**). The use of a drill bit is preferable to use of a Kirschner wire, which is more likely to create osteonecrosis at the drill sites (**TECH FIG 2D,E**).
- Through the miniarthrotomies, the posterior 25% of the tibiotalar joint is not always accessed and therefore not prepared. In my experience, properly preparing the anterior 75% of the joint is sufficient to achieving union rates that equal or even exceed those of other ankle techniques for ankle arthrodesis.
- Cancellous allograft chips are used to fill in any defects.

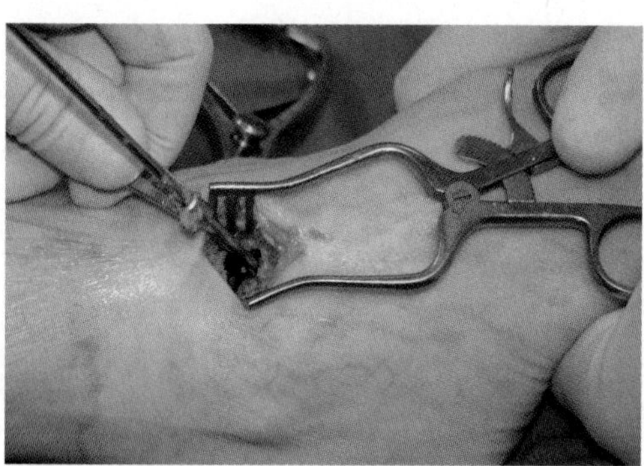

D

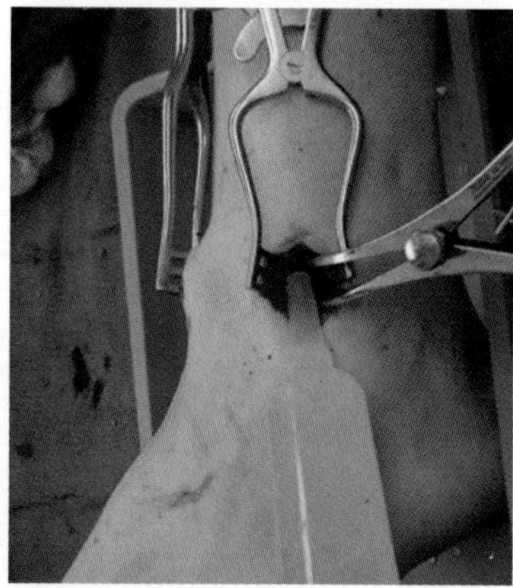

E

TECH FIG 2 • *(continued)* **D.** Drilling of the talus. **E.** The joint must be irrigated frequently to allow visualization of the cancellous bone surfaces and confirmation of uniform bleeding.

POSITION OF THE ARTHRODESIS SITE AND SCREW PLACEMENT

- Although the optimal position for an ankle arthrodesis has been debated, there is a consensus that the ankle should be in neutral position in the sagittal plane, with minimal valgus (up to 5 degrees) and external rotation symmetric with the contralateral uninvolved side (usually no more than 5 to 10 degrees).[1]
  - I generally set rotation by aligning the anterior tibial crest with the second metatarsal, when the foot is in a subtalar neutral position; with the miniarthrotomy technique, the ankle anatomy is left relatively undisturbed, and excessive malrotation is rarely possible.
- Most important is to avoid varus and internal rotation, both of which are poorly tolerated.
- I prefer to provisionally fix the ankle with three guide pins from a cannulated, self-tapping screw system.
- The first pin is inserted from the posterolateral aspect of the tibia in an anteromedial direction into the talar head. The guide pin is inserted immediately lateral to the Achilles tendon, approximately 3 cm proximal to the ankle joint. If there is some difficulty in maintaining the ankle position while inserting this first pin, the second pin can be placed first to lock the talus into the ankle mortise (**TECH FIG 3A**).
- The second pin is inserted from the anteromedial aspect of the tibia directly above the medial malleolus distally and anteriorly toward the sinus tarsi.
- The third guide pin is inserted from the lateral aspect of the joint anterior to the fibula and directed toward the medial talar neck. Occasionally, there is not enough space to insert the pin if there is no flare of the distal lat-

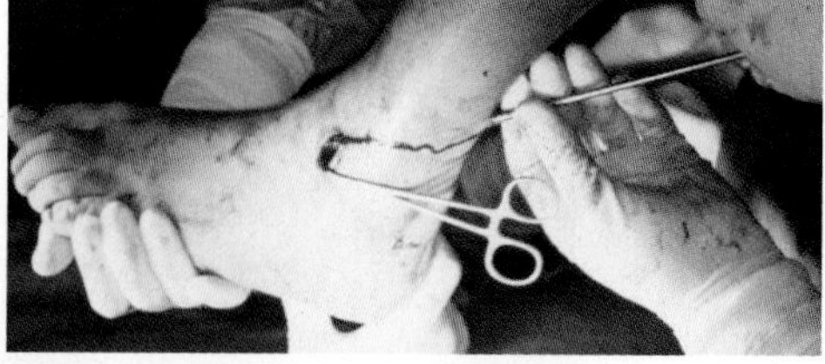

A

TECH FIG 3 • Position of the arthrodesis site and screw placement. **A.** The first pin is inserted from the posterolateral aspect of the tibia in an anteromedial direction into the talar head. The guide pin is inserted immediately adjacent to the Achilles tendon, approximately 3 cm proximal to the ankle joint. *(continued)*

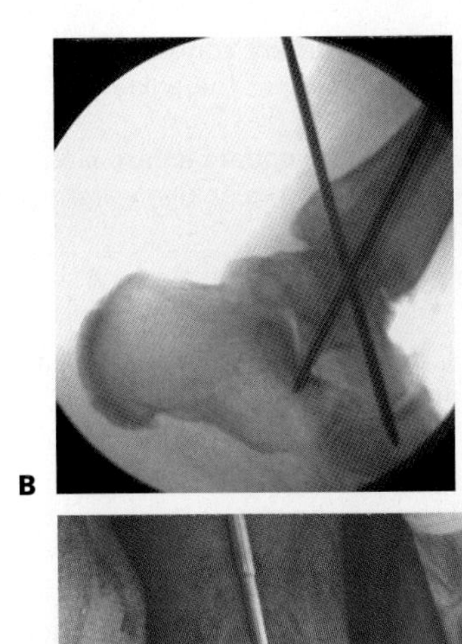
B

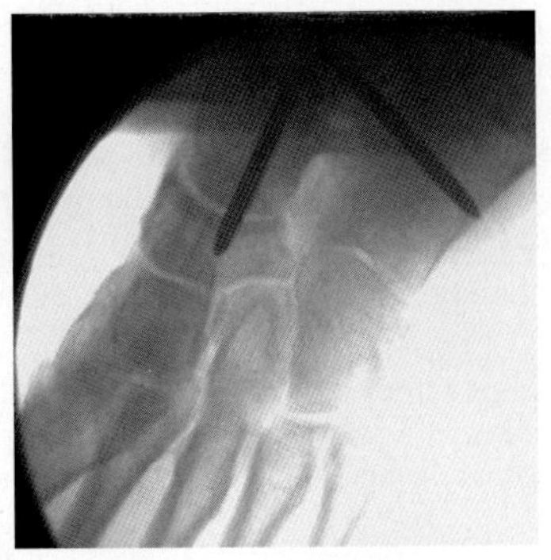
C

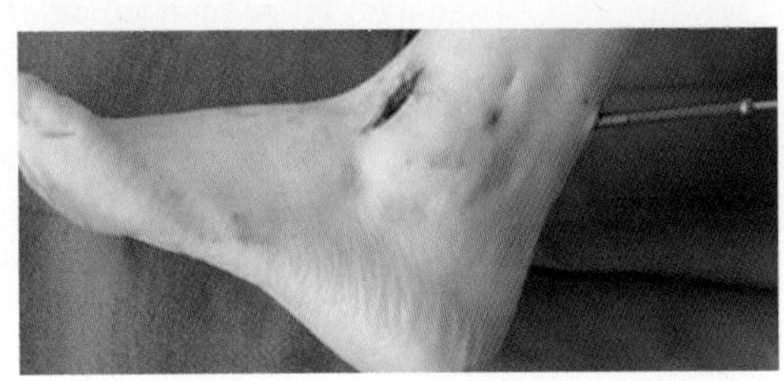
D

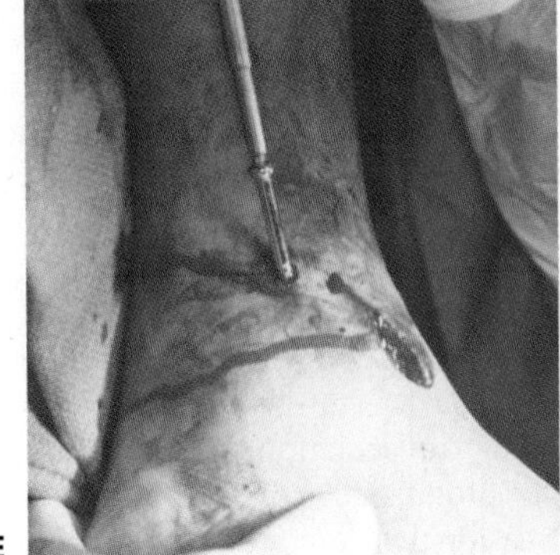
E

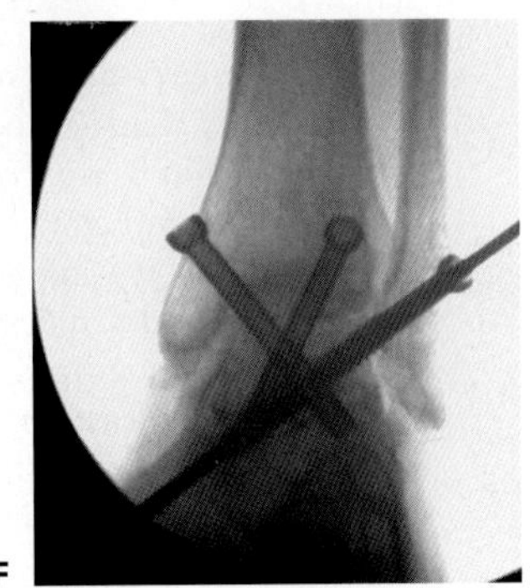
F

TECH FIG 3 • *(continued)* **B,C.** The positions of the first two guide pins are checked under fluoroscopy, and retrieval to appropriate length is performed when necessary. **D.** The first screw is inserted. **E.** The second screw is inserted just above the medial malleolus. **F.** The positions of the screws are checked under fluoroscopy.

eral tibia. In this case, the pin is inserted through the fibula into the talus.

- The positions of the guide pins and satisfactory tibiotalar apposition are then checked under fluoroscopy, and appropriate length 6.5-mm partially threaded cancellous screws are then inserted (**TECH FIG 3B–E**).
- Because the screws are not introduced parallel to each other, eccentric loading of the arthrodesis site may occur as the first one is inserted. This can be avoided by alternately tightening each screw until compression is obtained.
- After screw insertion, I check the stability of the construct. If there is residual motion in the arthrodesis, I retighten or reposition the screws.
- Final fluoroscopic views in the AP, mortise, and lateral planes confirm proper bony apposition, alignment, and screw position (**TECH FIG 3F**).
- With satisfactory stability, I place bone graft at the anterior tibiotalar arthrodesis.
- After closure of the retinaculum, the residual capsule, subcutanenous tissue, and skin are closed in routine fashion. I do not use a drain.

PEARLS AND PITFALLS

Screw insertion	■ The screw length inserted from the medial malleolus should be carefully checked because of the screw's proximity to the subtalar joint. ■ The screw inserted from the posterolateral tibia is critical because it obtains the best purchase in the talus and is in the plane of the most direct line of compression across the joint. ■ Because the screws are not introduced parallel to each other, eccentric loading of the arthrodesis site may occur as the first one is inserted. This can be avoided by alternately tightening each screw until compression is obtained.
Position of the arthrodesis site	■ I aim for neutral position in the sagittal plane, minimal valgus (up to 5 degrees), and external rotation symmetric with the contralateral physiologically normal ankle (no more than 5 to 10 degrees).
Preparation of the articular surfaces	■ A high-speed burr and smooth K-wires tend to create localized osteonecrosis that may delay healing. Moreover, the slurry created with a burr may predispose to symptomatic anterior joint synovitis. ■ The joint must be irrigated frequently to visualize the cancellous bone surfaces and confirm uniform bleeding. ■ Any dense sclerotic subchondral bone can be drilled with a 2.5-mm drill bit to enhance revascularization. ■ It is important to position the lamina spreader correctly to avoid tilting the talus from the neutral position.

Associated foot deformity	■ While not common with minimal ankle deformity, associated foot deformity may warrant concomitant osteotomies. Also, if a midfoot or forefoot deformity compromises optimal positioning of the ankle arthrodesis, adjunctive osteotomies of the foot may be warranted. ■ Alternatively, if a slight modification of the position for ankle arthrodesis may accommodate an associated fixed midfoot or forefoot deformity, such as equinus, it may be preferable to position the ankle in slight dorsiflexion to allow for a plantigrade foot position.
Pre-existing hardware	■ When using the miniarthrotomy technique, leave pre-existing hardware in place unless it interferes with insertion of the arthrodesis screws.
Joint preparation	■ The miniarthrotomy technique does not afford access to the posterior 25% of the tibiotalar Preparation of only the anterior 75% of the joint leads to fusion rates equal to those of other techniques of ankle arthrodesis in my experience and that of others.

POSTOPERATIVE CARE

- A bulky cotton dressing is applied with a medial to lateral coaptation-type splint and posterior mold of plaster.
- Radiographs are obtained at 2, 6, and 10 weeks to evaluate healing, maintenance of alignment and bony apposition, and screw position (**FIG 2**).
- If the operation was performed under regional ankle block, the patient is discharged the same day. The patient is given oral narcotics, NSAIDs, and oral antibiotics (at the surgeon's discretion).

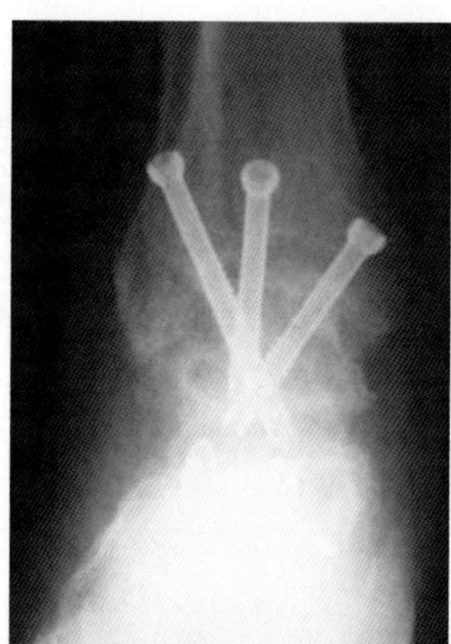

A

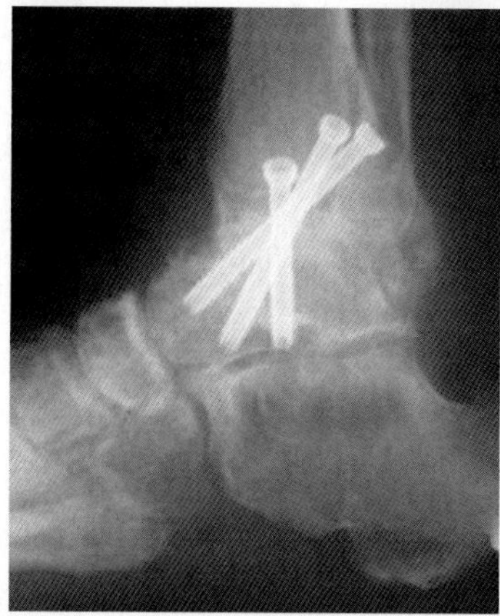

B

FIG 2 • AP and lateral postoperative radiographs are evaluated to ensure the desired alignment of the arthrodesis and check the screw position.

- At 2 weeks after surgery, the postoperative bulky cotton dressing is changed to a below-the-knee cast, and only touch-down weight bearing is permitted for 6 weeks or until early radiographic and clinical signs of healing are noted.
- Typically, we initiate progressive weight bearing in a cam boot at 6 weeks, unless a delay in healing is suggested on postoperative radiographs. With delayed union, we keep the patient in a short leg cast and on partial weight-bearing status. Once healing is confirmed (bridging trabeculation at the arthrodesis site), the patient is rapidly progressed from the cam walker boot to a regular shoe. Occasionally, transient use of a rocker-bottom shoe modification allows a more comfortable transition to normal gait.

OUTCOMES

- With appropriate indications and surgical technique, fusion rates for ankle arthrodesis in general are 90%.
- Clinical results and fusion rates of the miniarthrotomy arthrodesis technique are comparable to results with open and arthroscopic procedures.[3,4,6,7]
- Postoperative radiographs have demonstrated a fusion of the anterior three quarters of the joint as a result of inadequate visualization and débridement of the most posterior portion of the ankle joint. In our experience, lack of bony fusion across the posterior ankle is not a problem.

COMPLICATIONS

- Inadvertent laceration of the saphenous nerve and vein or the lateral branch of the superficial peroneal nerve
- Nonunion (limited incidence using the miniarthrotomy technique)
- Inadvertent penetration of the screws into the subtalar joint
- Infection
- Malposition of the ankle
- Symptomatic prominence of the screw heads

Acknowledgment

I would like to thank my mentor Mark S. Myerson for his enlightening training, friendship, and help for the preparation of this chapter.

REFERENCES

1. Buck P, Morrey BF, Chao EY. The optimum position of arthrodesis of the ankle: a gait study of the knee and ankle. J Bone Joint Surg Am 1987;69A:1052–1062.
2. Coester LM, Saltzman CL, Leupold J, et al. Long-term results following ankle arthrodesis for post-traumatic arthritis. J Bone Joint Surg Am 2001;83A:219.

3. Coughlin MJ, Mann RA. Arthrodesis of the foot and ankle. In: Myerson MS, ed. Surgery of the Foot and Ankle, ed 7. St Louis: Mosby, 1999:651–699.
4. Dent CM, Patil M, Fairclough JA. Arthroscopic ankle arthrodesis. J Bone Joint Surg Br 1993;75B:830–832.
5. Miller SD, Paremain GP, Myerson MS. The miniarthrotomy technique of ankle arthrodesis: a cadaver study of operative vascular compromise and early clinical results. Orthopedics 1996;19: 425–430.
6. Myerson MS, Quill G. Ankle arthrodesis: a comparison of an arthroscopic and an open method of treatment. Clin Orthop 1991;268:84–95.
7. Ogilvie-Harris DJ, Lieberman I, Fitsialos D. Arthroscopically assisted arthrodesis for osteoarthrotic ankles. J Bone Joint Surg Am 1993;75A:1167–1174.
8. Paremain GD, Miller SD, Myerson MS. Ankle arthrodesis: results after the miniarthrotomy technique. Foot Ankle Int 1996;17:247–252.
9. Stamatis E, Myerson M. The miniarthrotomy technique for ankle arthrodesis. Tech Foot Ankle Surg 2002;1:8–16.

Chapter 80

Arthroscopic Ankle Arthrodesis

James P. Tasto

DEFINITION

- Arthritis of the ankle can evolve from multiple causes, including, but not limited to, osteoarthritis, rheumatoid arthritis, and posttraumatic conditions. As the condition progresses, it generally leads to increased pain, gait abnormalities, and diminished function.
- Surgical remedies are employed when conservative measures fail; they consist of the time-honored tibiotalar arthrodesis as well as total ankle replacement.[2–4,9,19,21,28]
- We will be discussing and illustrating the technique of arthroscopic ankle arthrodesis (AAA).[7,12,17,23]

ANATOMY

- The ankle joint is composed of the tibiotalar and fibulotalar articulations, with the fibula bearing about one fifth of the weight-bearing stress across the ankle joint (**FIG 1**).

PATHOGENESIS

- As with any condition, when articular cartilage is destroyed, either by systemic or local disease, the progression of arthritis may be unpredictably slow or rapid. If malalignment is an accompanying factor, the progression and pain are usually more pronounced.

NATURAL HISTORY

- Once the breakdown of the articular surface has begun, it will progress at a rate that is not always predictable. Radiographic changes will not always reflect the degree of pain that the patient presents with. Some patients will come to surgery early while others may languish for decades without needing surgical intervention.

PATIENT HISTORY AND PHYSICAL FINDINGS

- Generally the patient will complain of pain with weight bearing, usually lateral more than medial. Generally it localizes anteriorly in a band from the lateral to the medial side of the ankle. There may be associated swelling and occasional night pain. The symptoms may in part be relieved by nonsteroidal anti-inflammatories (NSAIDs), acetaminophen, crutches, bracing, and activity modification. When other joints are involved, such as the knee and the hip, the discomfort in these areas may overshadow the ankle symptomatology.
- The patient will generally walk with an antalgic gait, and if there is any leg-length discrepancy, there may be a short-leg component to it. Gait will generally improve with the assistance of crutches or a cane.
- Stability is assessed with talar tilt and anterior drawer tests.
- Standing evaluation is critical in determining the feasibility of arthroscopic technique versus open as well as necessary osteotomies.
- Range of motion will be restricted in all planes, and pain will be elicited at the extremes of range of motion.
- Loss of dorsiflexion with plantarflexion contracture needs to be addressed at surgery.
- Careful isolation of ankle joint motion during the examination is critical so as not to confuse it with pathologic changes in the subtalar or midtarsal joints.
- There will usually be associated swelling about the ankle joint. Synovial hypertrophy, osteophytes, and generalized enlargement of the ankle will present rather than a frank effusion, which could indicate a systemic component.

IMAGING AND OTHER DIAGNOSTIC STUDIES

- Standing AP, lateral, and mortise radiographs are necessary to determine the extent of arthritis, alignment, presence of osteophytes, and the presence or absence of avascular necrosis of the talus (**FIG 2**). Minor degrees of malalignment may be corrected up to 7 degrees, varus being the most important element to reverse to neutral.
- MRI scans may be helpful if avascular necrosis is suspected.
- CT may be indicated if bone loss needs to be addressed.

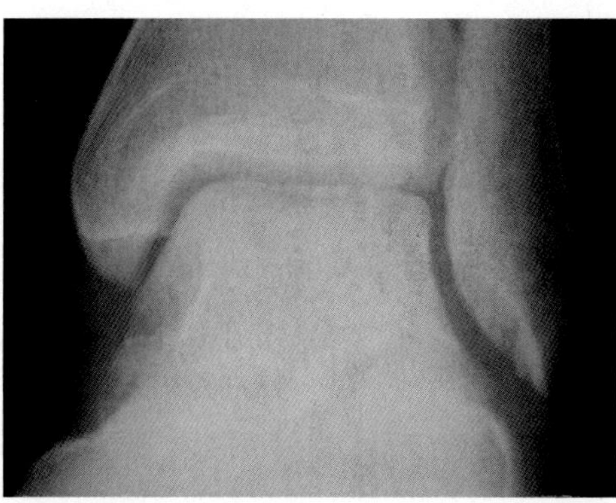

FIG 1 • Mortise view of right ankle.

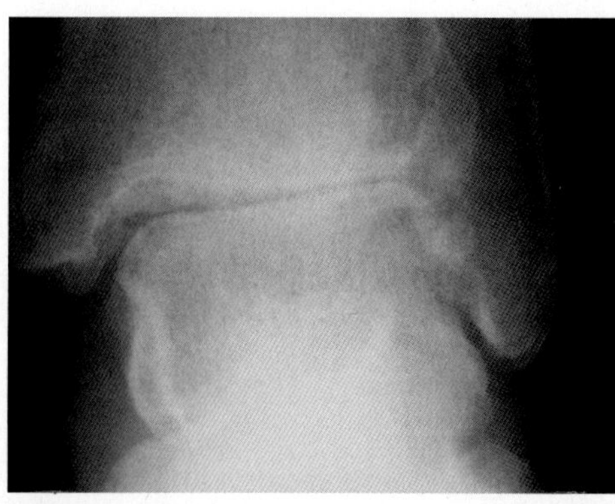

FIG 2 • Standing AP radiograph showing degenerative arthritis of the ankle.

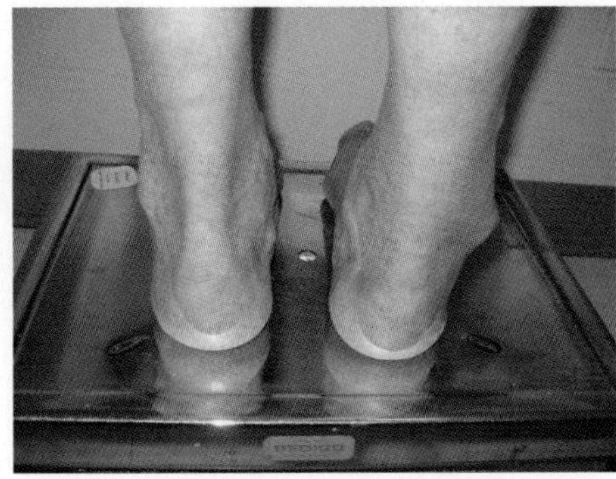

FIG 3 • Posterior view of varus malalignment, right ankle.

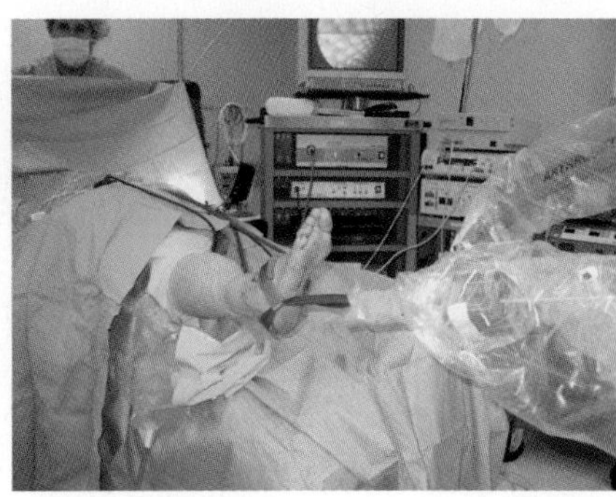

FIG 4 • Sterile traction device with tensionometer applied to right ankle.

- Should there be questions on the circulatory status, a vascular workup may be necessary.

DIFFERENTIAL DIAGNOSIS

- Infection
- Charcot joint
- Pseudogout and gout
- Osteochondral lesions of the talus
- Impingement
- Inflammatory synovitis

NONOPERATIVE MANAGEMENT

- As with most arthritic conditions, a wide variety of nonoperative measures can be employed. Medication in the form of NSAIDs, acetaminophen, and glucosamine sulfate can be used with careful monitoring for side effects. Bracing with simple soft tissue supports or a custom-made ankle–foot orthosis (AFO) can be effective. Cortisone injections, if used sparingly, can offer short-term pain relief. Off-label hyaluronic acid injections have been used with some reported success.

SURGICAL MANAGEMENT

- When patients fail to respond to conservative care, a number of procedures can be undertaken for isolated end-stage ankle arthritis. The time-honored procedure is an open ankle arthrodesis, but over the past 15 years some surgeons have come to prefer AAA.
- Total ankle arthroplasty has been popularized recently and has the obvious advantage of motion preservation at the cost of a more challenging technical procedure and a higher complication rate.[16]
- AAA will be discussed in detail in the following section.

Preoperative Planning

- We cannot overstress the need for a thorough evaluation of alignment before AAA is undertaken (**FIG 3**). The films must be done in a standing position and compared to the opposite side. Often patients will present with outside films showing a pseudo-varus deformity, but when a weight-bearing film is taken, the alignment is satisfactory.
- All medical conditions must be addressed. Vascular status needs to be examined as well as the skin condition. Patients

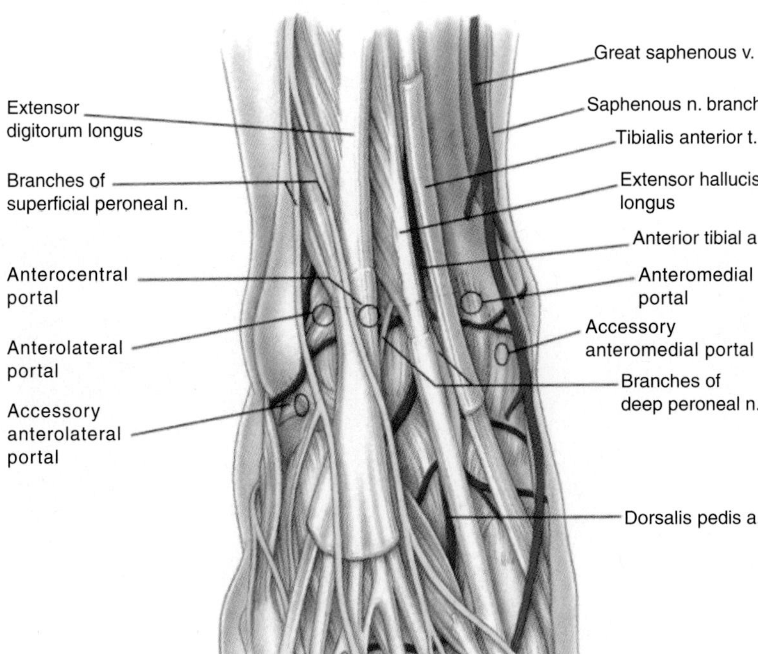

FIG 5 • Standard and accessory anterior portals for ankle arthroscopy.

need to stop smoking 3 months before the operative procedure and must stay off NSAIDs 5 days before and 3 months after the surgery.

- Perioperative antibiotics are used as well as postoperative deep venous thrombosis prophylaxis in high-risk patients.

Positioning

- The patient is placed in a supine position.
- The use of a leg holder and tourniquet allows the extremity to be placed in a neutral position so that both the anteromedial and anterolateral aspects of the ankle can be easily accessed.
- The foot of the table is dropped about 30 degrees.
- The ankle is placed in a sterile traction device using a tensionometer controlling traction to about 25 pounds (**FIG 4**).

Approach

- The approach that will be described is that of an AAA.
- Generally a two-portal technique can be used with anteromedial and anterolateral portals, and on occasion accessory portals located anterolateral, anteromedial, or posterolateral for additional flow or drainage (**FIGS 5 AND 6**).

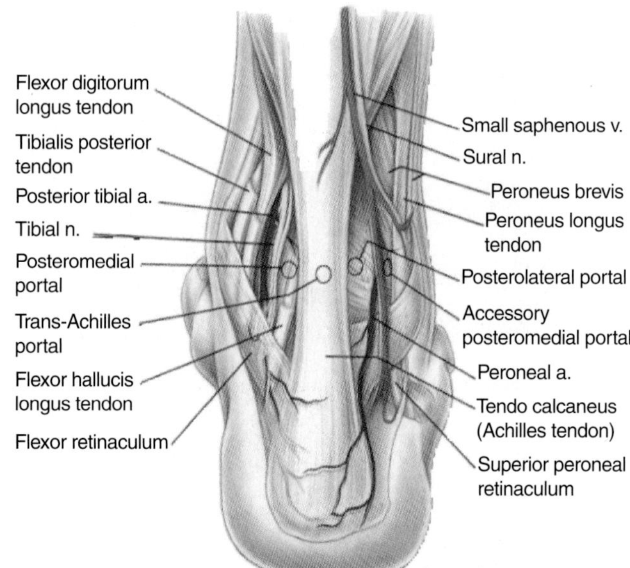

FIG 6 • Standard and accessory posterior portals for ankle arthroscopy.

TECHNIQUES

TRACTION AND EXPOSURE

- Delineate anatomic landmarks with a marking pencil (**TECH FIG 1**).
- Apply a traction device after thoroughly preparing and draping the ankle.
- Apply traction to about 25 pounds (**TECH FIG 2**).
- Countertraction is effective with the use of a tourniquet and leg holder.
- Dorsiflexion and plantarflexion are facilitated by the design of the traction strap.
- Instill 8 cc of normal saline into the ankle joint.
- Using a "nick and spread" technique, create the anteromedial portal with a no. 11 blade.
- Use a hemostat to bluntly dissect down to the capsule.
- Introduce a 2.7-mm wide-angled and small joint arthroscope through the anteromedial portal (**TECH FIG 3**).

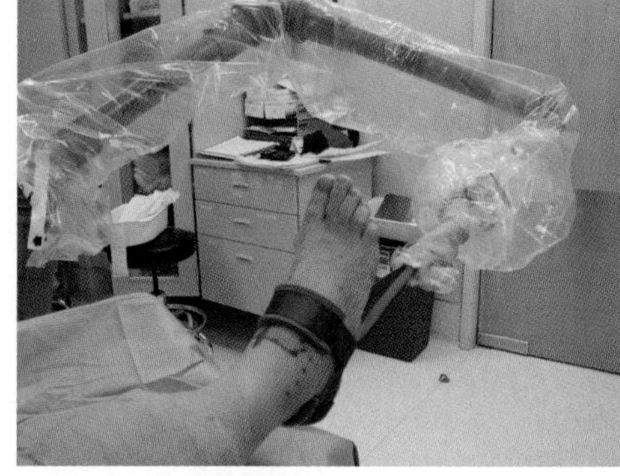

TECH FIG 2 • Soft tissue traction device for the ankle with 25 pounds of traction applied.

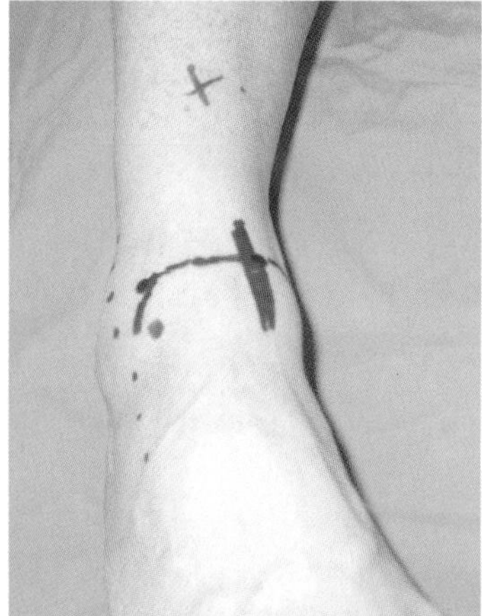

TECH FIG 1 • Anatomic landmarks consisting of the superficial peroneal nerve and anterior tibial tendon, right ankle.

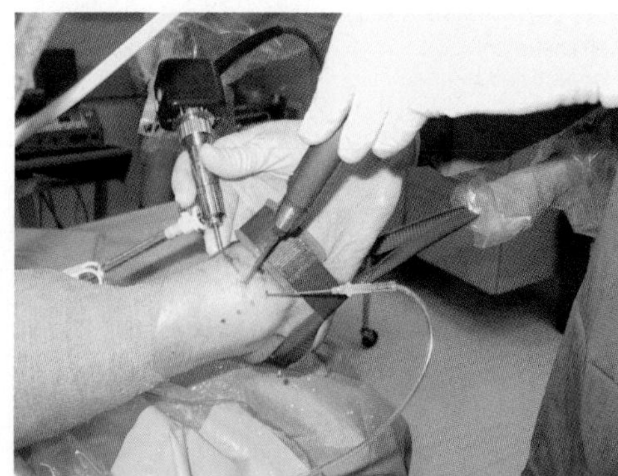

TECH FIG 3 • A camera and small arthroscope are introduced through the anteromedial portal, the shaver is introduced through the anterolateral portal, and drainage is introduced through an accessory inferior anterolateral portal, right ankle.

- Establish drainage through the anterolateral portal.
- Use a pump to control pressure at about 30 mm Hg.
- Take care, as with any infusion technique, to avoid excessive pressure and fluid extravasation.
- Anterior osteophytes may impede entry and visualization in the joint (TECH FIG 4).
  - Osteophytes can be removed anteriorly to create a space for visualization and performance of the arthrodesis.

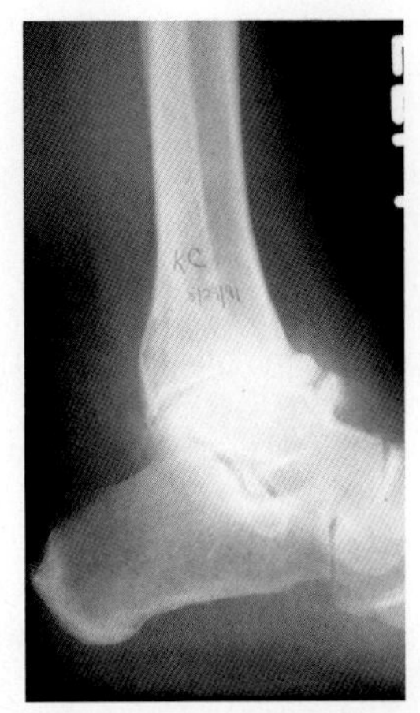

TECH FIG 4 • Lateral radiograph of an ankle with prominent tibial and talar osteophytes that need to be resected for access to the ankle joint during arthroscopy.

ARTHRODESIS

- Perform a synovectomy with a 3.5-mm resection blade (TECH FIG 5A).
- Use a soft tissue motorized blade and a burr to remove the articular cartilage.
- 1 to 2 mm of subchondral bone is generally removed with the burr (TECH FIG 5B).
- Spinal curettes can be used to débride the medial and lateral gutters as well as the posterior tibial plafond and posterior talus (TECH FIG 5C).
- A radiofrequency device can be used for débridement in some areas where access is limited.
- During débridement, maintaining the normal architecture of the tibiotalar joint is imperative.
- Medial and lateral gutters need to be débrided thoroughly, removing 1 to 2 mm of subchondral bone as well (TECH FIG 5D).
- Débriding the gutters allows for coaptation of the tibiotalar surfaces (TECH FIG 5E).
- Multiple spot welds placed on the tibiotalar surfaces will allow increased vascularity (TECH FIG 5F).
- Release the tourniquet and visualize the vascularity of both surfaces (TECH FIG 5G).
- Further débridement may be necessary if diminished vascularity is encountered in any one particular area.

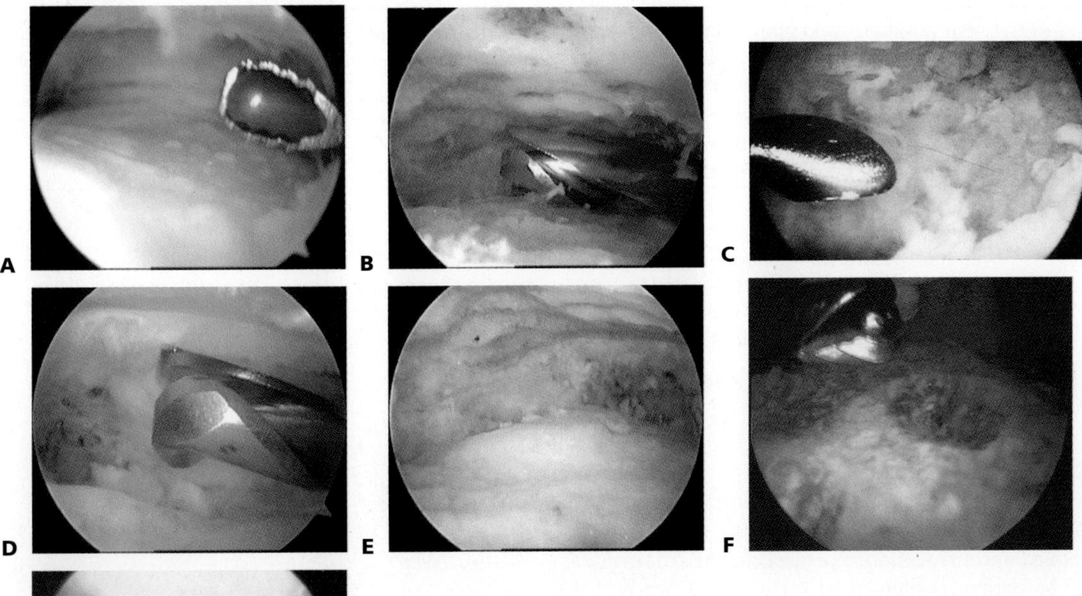

TECH FIG 5 • **A.** A soft tissue resection blade is being used to perform a synovectomy in the ankle joint. **B.** 1 to 2 mm of subchondral bone is removed with a burr and spot welds are created. **C.** A spinal curette is used to débride the medial gutter of the ankle. **D.** A burr is used to remove subchondral bone. **E.** Tibial–talar surfaces are prepared, as well as the gutters, for coaptation of the surfaces. **F.** A spot weld vascular access channel is created in the talus. **G.** After release of the tourniquet, vascularity of the tibial–talar surface is assessed.

STABILIZATION, FIXATION, AND CLOSURE

- Hold the ankle in the acceptable corrected neutral position and insert guidewires.
- Use two 7.3-mm AO cannulated cancellous screws to stabilize the tibiotalar joint.
- Place screws parallel and obliquely from the medial tibia into the lateral talus (**TECH FIG 6**).
- Perform fixation under fluoroscopic control to avoid any potential encroachment on the subtalar joint.
- Apply compression alternately to each screw.
- Check the final position both clinically and under fluoroscopy.
- Close the arthroscopic portals with Steri-Strips and close the operative site for screw insertion with 3-0 nylon sutures.
- Apply a local anesthetic and incorporate the leg into a bulky dressing and a bivalve cast.

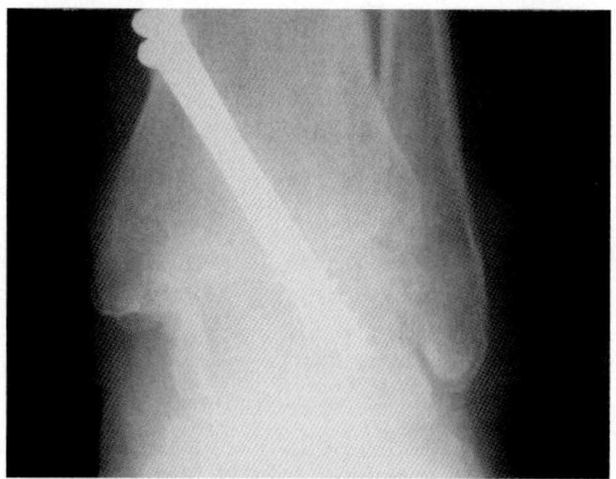

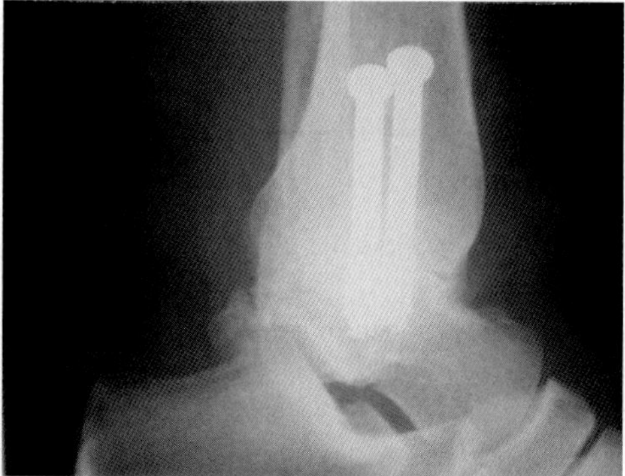

TECH FIG 6 • **A.** AP radiographs showing two parallel oblique screws used for fixation of the arthroscopic fusion. **B.** Lateral radiographs showing two parallel oblique screws fixing the ankle fusion.

PEARLS AND PITFALLS

Indications	■ If possible, avoid operating on smokers and patients with Charcot joints and avascular necrosis of the talus. ■ Carefully explain to the patient what the associated stiffness and lack of motion of the ankle will involve. ■ Avoid noncompliant patients.
Arthroscopic procedure	■ Use careful fluid management to avoid extravasation and compartment syndrome. ■ Do not exceed 25 to 30 pounds of traction. ■ Have the appropriate small joint arthroscopy system available.
Surgical technique	■ Early removal of the anterior osteophytes will aid in visualization. ■ Do not remove excessive amounts of subchondral bone. ■ Spot weld technique will increase the vascular access. ■ Medial and lateral gutters need to be débrided for better coaptation. ■ Guide pins need to be checked carefully under fluoroscopy. ■ Avoid violating the subtalar joint with screws.

POSTOPERATIVE CARE

- Patients are placed in a bulky dressing with a bivalve cast in the operating room. Circulatory checks are done in the recovery room and 24 hours postoperatively.
- The cast is removed and the wounds are inspected at 7 days postoperatively. The patient is then fitted for an AFO brace (**FIG 7**).
- The patient is allowed touch weight bearing the first few days after surgery, with progressive weight bearing, and may attain a full weight-bearing status as soon as tolerated.
- Generally the patient will use crutches for 2 to 3 weeks. Full weight bearing is encouraged.
- The patient is allowed to remove the AFO for bathing and range-of-motion exercises. Range of motion and weight bearing

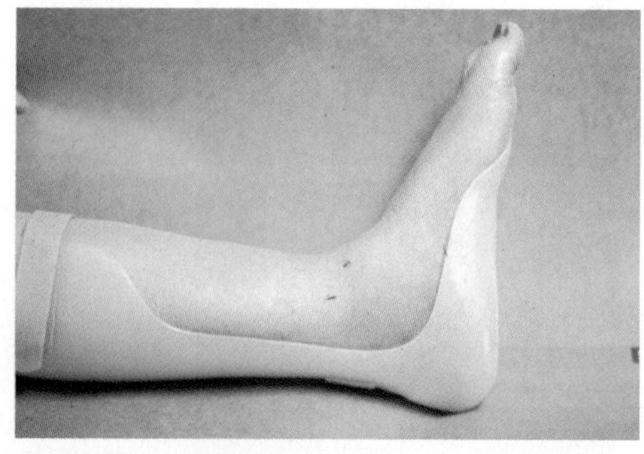

FIG 7 • An AFO brace is used for immobilization, postoperative week 1.

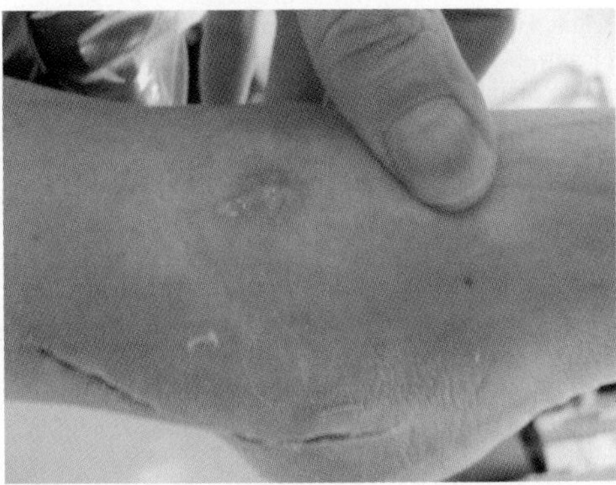

FIG 8 • Synovial fistula after ankle arthroscopy.

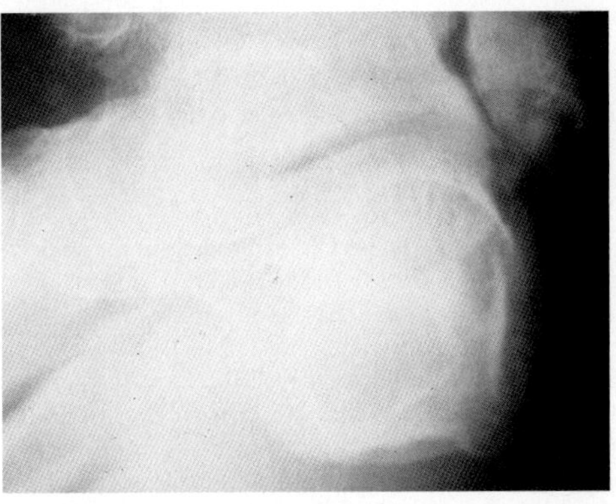

FIG 10 • AP radiograph in 40 degrees of internal rotation, showing fibular–talar and fibular–calcaneal impingement.

reduce stress deprivation. The patient is allowed to remove the AFO and walk with normal shoe wear when radiographic union has taken place, there is no motion at the screw sites, and the patient is essentially pain-free.

OUTCOMES

- Fusion rates for AAA are generally in the range of 90% to 95%.[10,15,27,30]
- There is definitely less pain after the arthroscopic procedure than with the open procedure.
- The operation is generally done as an outpatient procedure.
- Alignment is thought to be easier to obtain because of the maintenance of the normal architecture and geometry of the tibiotalar joint.

COMPLICATIONS

- The complication rate from ankle arthroscopy has been reported to be about 9%.[1,5,6,8,11,13,14,18,20,24–26]
- Infection
- Synovial fistula (**FIG 8**)
- Delayed union (**FIG 9**)
- Nonunion
- Charcot joint

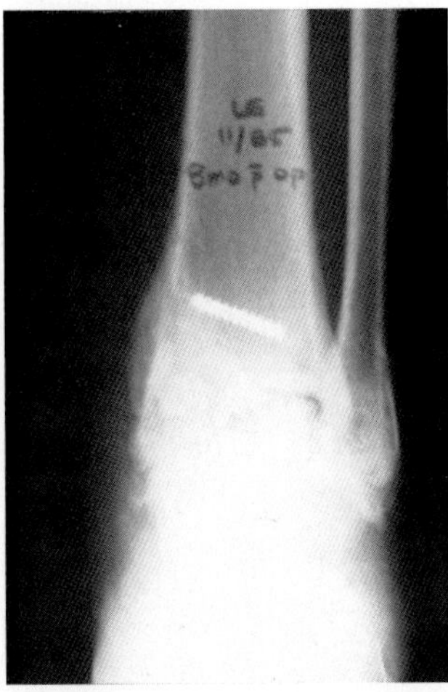

FIG 9 • AP radiographs showing delayed union–nonunion of open ankle arthrodesis.

- Secondary degenerative changes, subtalar and midfoot
- Equinus or dorsiflexion malposition
- Residual varus malalignment
- Fibular–talar and fibular–calcaneal impingement (**FIG 10**)
- Neurapraxia and nerve injuries
- Vascular injuries
- Skeletal traction complications (**FIG 11**)
- Screw encroachment in subtalar joint (**FIG 12**)

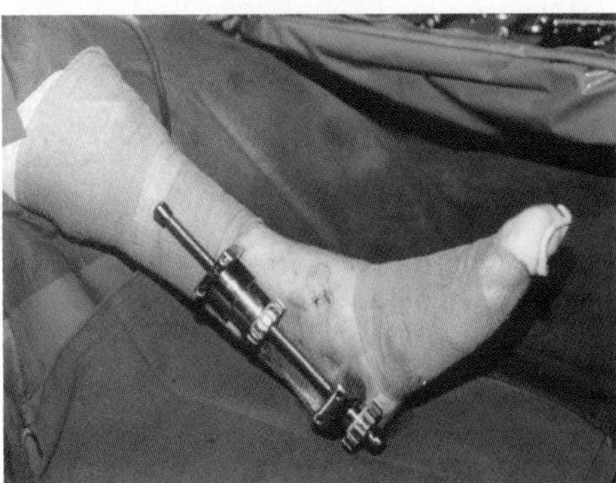

FIG 11 • Skeletal traction device previously used for ankle arthroscopy.

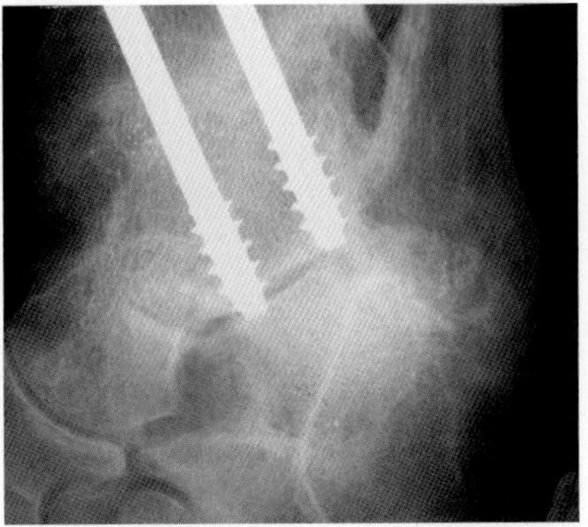

FIG 12 • Screw encroachment on the subtalar joint as seen with a 40-degree internal rotation and plantarflexion view.

REFERENCES

1. Alvarez RG, Barbour TM, Perkins TD. Tibiocalcaneal arthrodesis for nonbraceable neuropathic ankle deformity. Foot Ankle Int 1994; 15:354–359.
2. Boobbyer GN. The long-term results of ankle arthrodesis. Acta Orthop Scand 1981;52:107–110.
3. Braly WG, Baker JK, Tullos HS. Arthrodesis of the ankle with lateral plating. Foot Ankle Int 1994;15:649–653.
4. Chen YJ, Huang TJ, Shih HN, et al. Ankle arthrodesis with cross screw fixation. Acta Orthop Scand 1996;67:473–478.
5. Cobb TK, Gabrielsen TA, Campbell DC II, et al. Cigarette smoking and nonunion after ankle arthrodesis. Foot Ankle Int 1994; 15:64–67.
6. Collman DR, Kaas MH, Schuberth JM. Arthroscopic ankle arthrodesis: factors influencing union in 39 consecutive patients. Foot Ankle Int 2006;27:1079–1085.
7. Corso SJ, Zimmer TJ. Technique and clinical evaluation of arthroscopic ankle arthrodesis. Arthroscopy 1995;11:585–590.
8. Crosby LA, Yee TC, Formanek TS, et al. Complications following arthroscopic ankle arthrodesis. Foot Ankle Int 1996;17:340–342.
9. Dohm M, Purdy BA, Benjamin J. Primary union of ankle arthrodesis: review of a single institution/multiple surgeon experience. Foot Ankle Int 1994;15:293–296.
10. Ferkel RD, Hewitt M. Long-term results of arthroscopic ankle arthrodesis. Foot Ankle Int 2005;26:275–280.
11. Frey C, Halikus NM, Vu-Rose T, et al. A review of ankle arthrodesis: predisposing factors to nonunion. Foot Ankle Int 1994;15:581–584.
12. Glick JM, Morgan CD, Myerson MS, et al. Ankle arthrodesis using an arthroscopic method. Arthroscopy 1996;12:428–434.
13. Hagen RJ. Ankle arthrodesis, problems and pitfalls. Clin Orthop Relat Res 1986;202:152–162.
14. Helm R. The results of ankle arthrodesis. J Bone Joint Surg Br 1990; 71B:141–143.
15. Jerosch J. Arthroscopic in situ arthrodesis of the upper ankle. Orthopade 2005;34:1198–1208.
16. Jerosch J, Fayaz H, Senyurt H. Ankle arthrodesis versus ankle replacement—a comparison. Orthopade 2006;35:495–505.
17. Jerosch J, Steinbeck J, Schroder M, et al. Arthroscopically assisted arthrodesis of the ankle joint. Arch Orthop Trauma Surg 1996; 115:182–189.
18. Lynch AF, Bourne RB, Rorabeck CH. The long-term results of ankle arthrodesis. J Bone Joint Surg Br 1988;70B:113–116.
19. Mann RA, Van Manen JW, Wapner K, et al. Ankle fusion. Clin Orthop Relat Res 1991;268:49–55.
20. Moran CG, Pinder IM, Smith SR. Ankle arthrodesis in rheumatoid arthritis. Acta Orthop Scand 1991;62:538–543.
21. Morgan CD, Henke JA, Bailey RW, et al. Long-term results of tibiotalar arthrodesis. J Bone Joint Surg Am 1985;67A:546–550.
22. Muir DC, Amendola A, Saltzman CL. Long-term outcome of ankle arthrodesis. Foot Ankle Clin 2002;7:703–708.
23. Myerson MS, Quill G. Ankle arthrodesis. Clin Orthop Relat Res 1991;268:84–95.
24. Papa J, Myerson M, Girard P. Salvage, with arthrodesis, in intractable diabetic neuropathic arthropathy of the foot and ankle. J Bone Joint Surg Am 1993;75A:1056–1066.
25. Saltzman C, Lightfoot A, Amendola A. PEMF as treatment for delayed healing of foot and ankle arthrodesis. Foot Ankle Int 2004; 25:771–773.
26. Shibata T, Tada K, Hashizume C. The results of arthrodesis of the ankle for leprotic neuroarthropathy. J Bone Joint Surg Am 1990; 72A:749–756.
27. Stone JW. Arthroscopic ankle arthrodesis. Foot Ankle Clin 2006; 11:361–368.
28. Stranks GJ, Cecil T, Jeffery IT. Anterior ankle arthrodesis with cross-screw fixation. J Bone Joint Surg Br 1994;76B:943–946.
29. Turan I, Wredmark T, Fellander-Tsae L. Arthroscopic ankle arthrodesis in rheumatoid arthritis. Clin Orthop Relat Res 1995; 320:110–114.
30. Winson IG, Robinson DE, Allen PE. Arthroscopic ankle arthrodesis. J Bone Joint Surg Br 2005;87B:343–347.

Chapter 81 Tibiotalocalcaneal Arthrodesis Using a Medullary Nail

George E. Quill, Jr., and Stuart D. Miller

DEFINITION

- Tibiotalocalcaneal arthrodesis is the surgical procedure to simultaneously fuse the ankle and the subtalar joints.
- In cases of posttraumatic, neuropathic, or avascular talar body bone loss, tibiocalcaneal arthrodesis may be indicated. The term *pan-talar arthrodesis* refers to the surgical procedure to fuse all bones that articulate with the talus: the distal tibia, calcaneus, navicular, and cuboid. In essence, this is a combined ankle and triple arthrodesis.
- In our opinion, the term *medullary* refers to the inner marrow cavity of a long bone and the word *intramedullary* is a redundant, less useful term.
- The goal of tibiotalocalcaneal arthrodesis is to create a pain-free ankle and hindfoot that are biomechanically stable and fused in functional position.
- In our hands, tibiotalocalcaneal arthrodesis is a salvage operation performed for severe ankle and hindfoot deformity, bone loss, and pain.

ANATOMY

- Tibiotalocalcaneal arthrodesis aims to recreate physiologic ankle and hindfoot alignment with a plantigrade foot position (the foot is at a 90-degree angle to the long axis of the tibia) and about 5 to 7 degrees of hindfoot valgus.
- In general, rotation of the foot relative to the longitudinal axis of the tibia in the coronal plane is congruent with the anterior tibia—that is, the second ray of the foot is usually in line with the anteromedial crest of the tibia.
- Hindfoot position influences forefoot position. With long-standing ankle and hindfoot deformity, forefoot pronation, supination, adduction, and abduction may be affected. Proper positioning of a tibiotalocalcaneal arthrodesis must take forefoot position into account. Ideally, in stance phase the foot has near-equal pressure distribution under the heel and first and fifth metatarsal heads.

NATURAL HISTORY

- Severe ankle and hindfoot deformities and pathologic processes result in disabling pathomechanics and, when left untreated, often confine patients to cumbersome brace use, limited ambulation with assistive devices, or a wheelchair.
- Tibiotalocalcaneal arthrodesis is a major reconstructive process usually applied to otherwise disabling conditions.
  - Gellman et al.[2] noted that the dorsiflexion and plantarflexion deficits after ankle fusion compared to the nonfused contralateral ankle were 51% and 70%, respectively. Surprisingly, for tibiotalocalcaneal arthrodesis, dorsiflexion and plantarflexion deficits were 53% and 71%, respectively.
  - This same study concluded, however, that inversion and eversion were 40% less after tibiotalocalcaneal fusion than after tibiotalar fusion alone.

PATIENT HISTORY AND PHYSICAL FINDINGS

- The patient being considered for tibiotalocalcaneal arthrodesis with a medullary nail presents with a myriad of orthopaedic pathology affecting gait, weight bearing, and ability to earn a living.
- This patient may present with limited mobility, an equinus posture associated with genu recurvatum, and transverse plane deformity ranging from severe varus and instability of the hindfoot through profound valgus and ulceration over the medial structures (**FIG 1**).
- The neuromuscular or neuropathic patient may present with ulceration, intrinsic muscle loss, and multiple fractures in various stages of healing.
- The posttraumatic patient often has a compromised soft tissue envelope, previously placed hardware, and already medullary canal sclerosis that must be considered in preoperative planning (**FIG 2**). Evaluation must include gait and

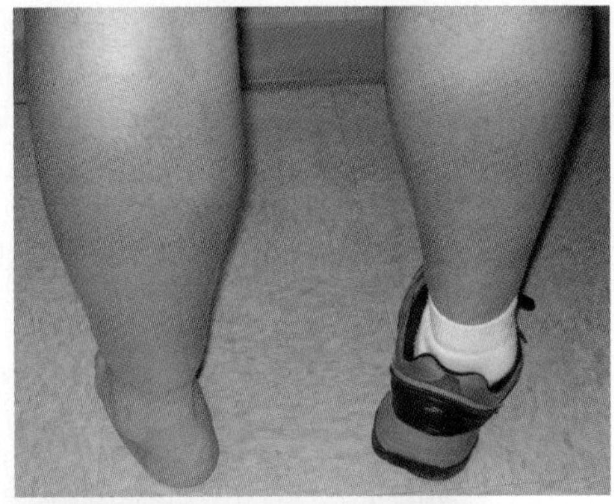

A

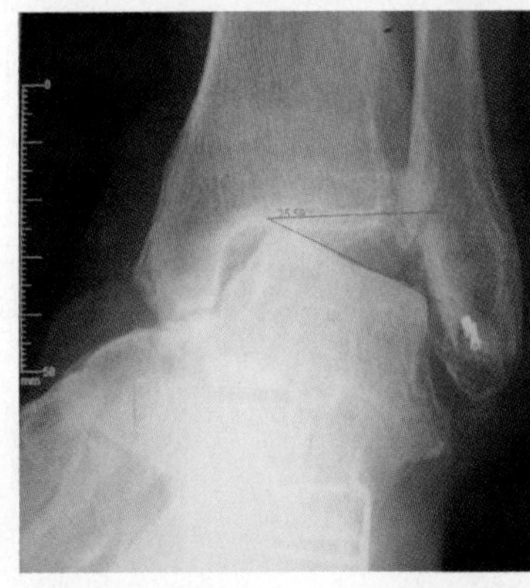

B

FIG 1 • Weight-bearing clinical photograph (**A**) and weight-bearing AP radiograph (**B**) of a 53-year-old laborer with persistent ankle and hindfoot varus instability after prior attempt at calcaneal osteotomy and lateral ligament reconstruction.

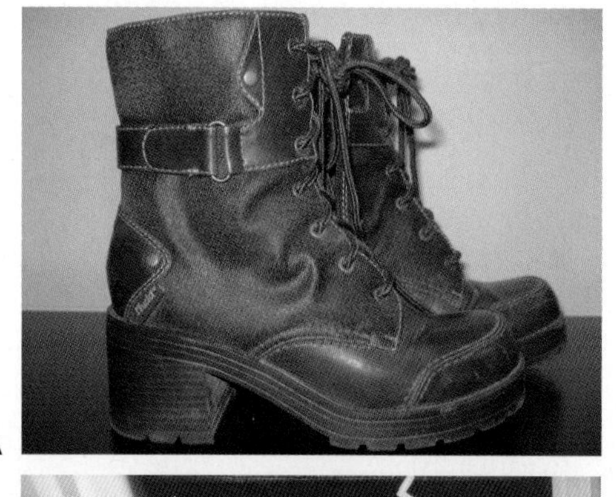

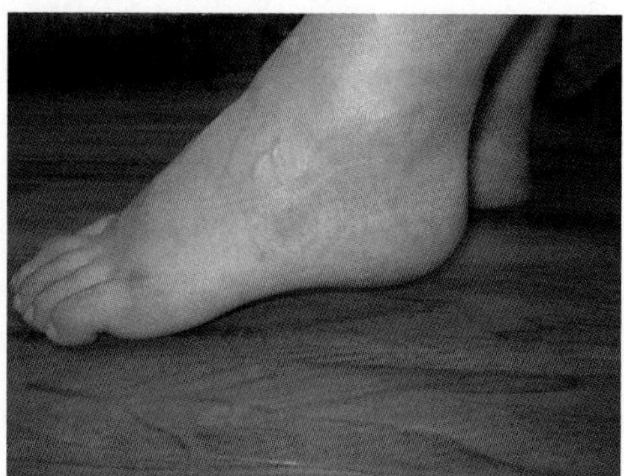

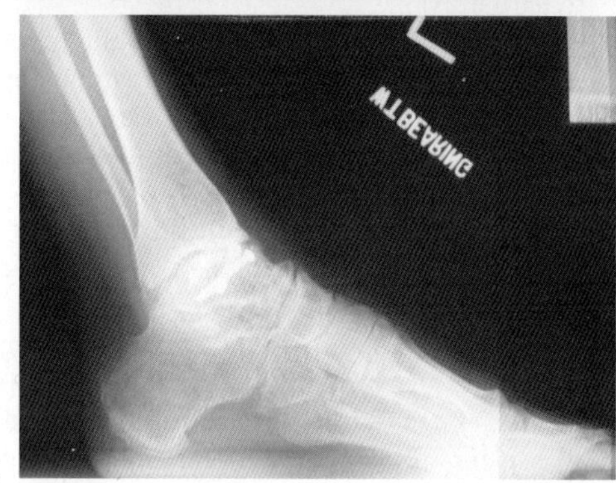

FIG 2 • **A.** Reportedly the only pair of high-heeled, high-topped boots that this 42-year-old woman was comfortable wearing 2 years after sustaining bilateral talus fractures malunited in equinus. **B.** Clinical appearance of this woman's foot in maximal passive left ankle dorsiflexion. **C.** Weight-bearing lateral radiograph of same woman. Note plantarflexion talus fracture malunion and posttraumatic osteoarthritis after open reduction and internal fixation.

weight-bearing posture, assessment of the soft tissue envelope, and a thorough neuromuscular examination.

IMAGING AND OTHER DIAGNOSTIC STUDIES

- We routinely obtain three weight-bearing radiographs of the ankle and foot. As many of these patients have deformity, we often obtain additional long-cassette radiographs of the ankle or even mechanical axis views of the lower leg from the hip to the foot.
- Posttraumatic and osteoarthritis
- Radiographs may reveal joint space narrowing, osteophyte formation, and subchondral sclerosis and cysts, all characteristic of osteoarthritis. Posttraumatic deformity and retained hardware may be identified and must be considered in preoperative planning (**FIG 3**).

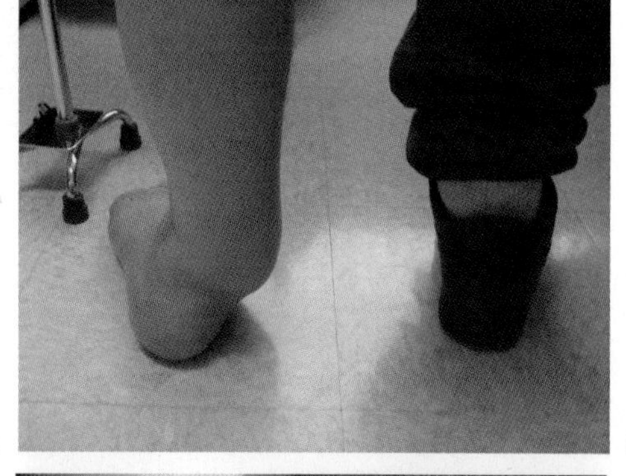

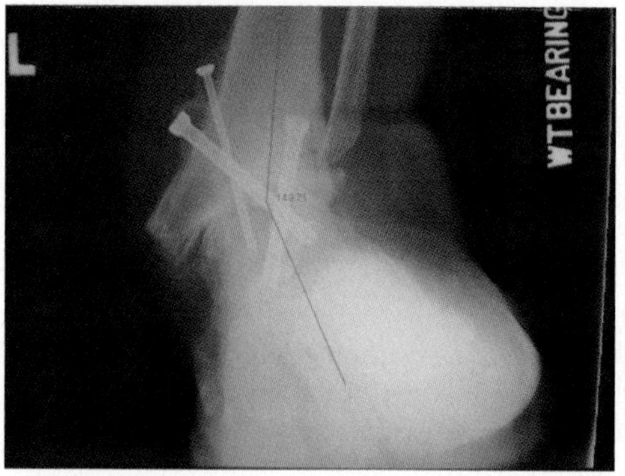

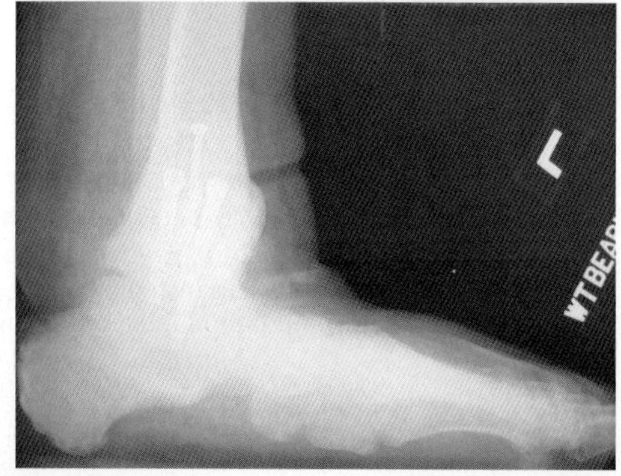

FIG 3 • Preoperative weight-bearing clinical appearance (**A**), AP radiograph (**B**), and lateral radiograph (**C**) of an obese 69-year-old man after valgus nonunion of attempted tibiotalar arthrodesis.

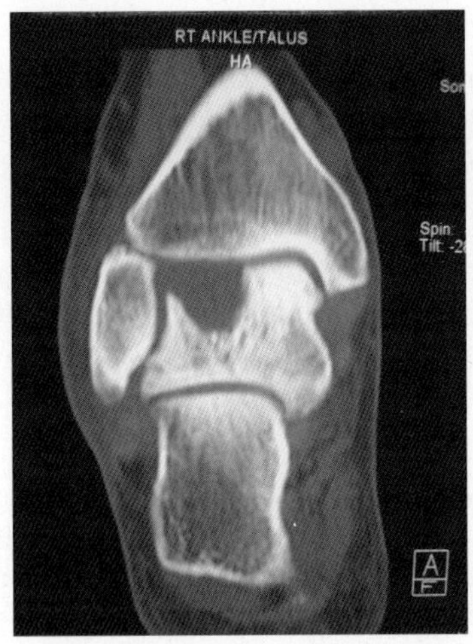

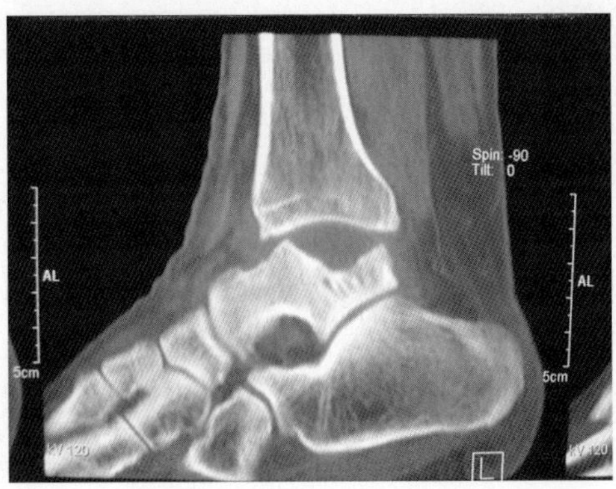

FIG 4 • Coronal (**A**) and lateral (**B**) CT images of a 48-year-old man with massive osteochondral talar insufficiency.

- Rheumatoid arthritis and other inflammatory arthritides
  - Radiographs typically identify periarticular erosions and osteopenia.
- Neuropathic arthrosis or Charcot neuroarthropathy
  - In our experience, this presentation is radiographically characterized by numerous fractures or microfractures in various stages of healing, hypertrophic new bone formation, and loss of normal weight-bearing architecture.
  - Bone resorption may be seen, along with vascular calcification and joint subluxation or dislocation.
- Plain tomography or CT may further define deformity, arthritis, bone loss, and prior malunion or nonunion (**FIG 4**).
  - We have not found three-dimensional CT reconstructions helpful in the routine setting.
  - CT is also useful in assessing progression toward union following tibiotalocalcaneal arthrodesis.
- MRI may complement CT by evaluating for fluid in and around the joints, bone marrow edema, talar vascularity, infection, and periarticular tendon and ligament pathology (**FIG 5**).
- Technetium-99 bone scans may be useful in the evaluation of osteonecrosis after talus fracture, arthritic involvement of one or several joints, stress fracture, or neoplasm.
- Indium-labeled white blood cell scans can be helpful in the diagnosis of osteomyelitis or septic arthritis.

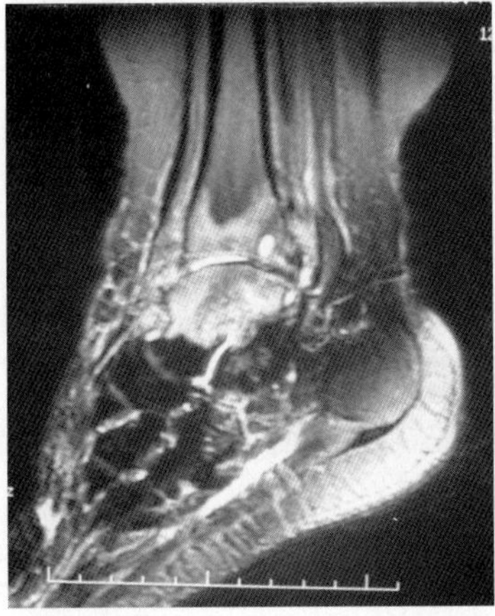

FIG 5 • MRI demonstrating extensive bone involvement of the talus.

DIFFERENTIAL DIAGNOSIS

- Primary and secondary osteoarthrosis, including posttraumatic osteoarthritis
- Rheumatoid arthritis and other inflammatory arthritides (gout, pseudogout, pigmented villonodular synovitis, septic arthritis, psoriatic arthritis, spondyloarthropathy, Reiter syndrome)
- Neuropathic arthropathy (diabetes mellitus, spinal cord injury, hereditary sensory and motor neuropathy, syringomyelia, congenital indifference to pain, alcoholism, peripheral nerve disease, tabes dorsalis, and leprosy)
- Infectious arthritis (sepsis, open trauma, or previous surgical procedure for fixation of fractures)
- Arthritis and joint subluxation resulting from generalized ligamentous laxity, mixed connective disease, posterior tibial tendinopathy, spring ligament insufficiency

NONOPERATIVE MANAGEMENT

- Selective (diagnostic) injection of local anesthetic may help locate the exact anatomic source of the patient's pain.
- Tibiotalar arthritis may be associated with a stiff, painful subtalar joint that has a relatively normal radiographic appearance.
- The injection of 5 to 10 mL of 1% lidocaine into the subtalar joint can clarify whether the pain may not be isolated to the ankle but in fact be generated in both the ankle and subtalar joints.
- This has important implications when considering isolated tibiotalar versus tibiotalocalcaneal arthrodesis. We do not routinely incorporate the subtalar joint into the arthrodesis when performing an ankle arthrodesis. In select cases of end-stage ankle arthritis associated with severe deformity and talar bone loss, we consider including an otherwise normal asymptomatic subtalar joint in the fusion mass achieved for tibiotalocalcaneal fusion. Alternatively, an injection carefully placed in the peroneal tenosynovial sheath may prove that pain may be related to the tendons rather than the joint.
- While often challenging for the patient with deformity, we recommend bracing for the patient with prohibitive medical illness or a dysvascular extremity, particularly for the patient with a non-fixed, passively correctible deformity. A custom

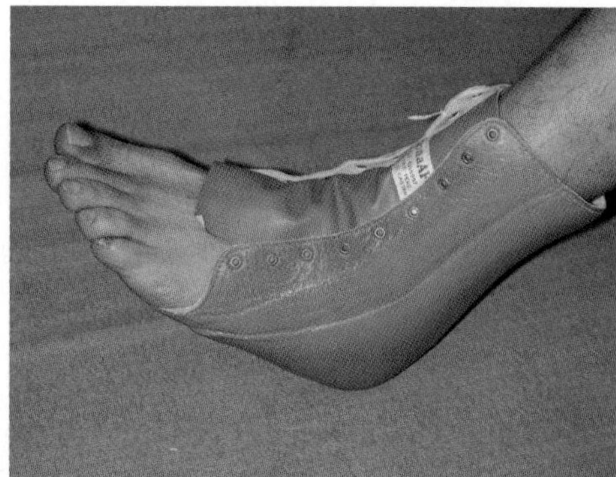

FIG 6 • Molded ankle–foot orthosis can provide stability and serve as an alternative to operative intervention.

polypropylene ankle–foot orthosis (AFO) or a supramalleolar AFO with Velcro closures may be considered as an alternative to tibiotalocalcaneal arthrodesis in poor surgical candidates (**FIG 6**).

- For the neuropathic patient in whom bracing can achieve a relatively plantigrade posture for the hindfoot and ankle, we prescribe a double-metal-upright AFO attached to an Oxford shoe that includes Plastazote liners (total contact inserts).
- In our experience, polypropylene in-shoe braces lead to ulceration in these patients with complex deformity.
- In severe deformity, a Charcot retention orthotic walker (CROW) may prove effective.
- While we favor tibiotalocalcaneal arthrodesis for patients with posttraumatic arthritis and deformity, we have had some success in relieving pain and improving function with a patellar tendon bearing brace for poor surgical candidates.

SURGICAL MANAGEMENT

Indications and Contraindications

- Indications for tibiotalocalcaneal arthrodesis
  - Sequelae of degenerative, posttraumatic, or inflammatory arthritis
  - Avascular necrosis of the talus
  - Severe instability or paralytic ankle and hindfoot weakness
  - Neuropathic arthropathy
  - Failed ankle arthroplasty with subtalar intrusion
  - Failed ankle arthrodesis with insufficient talar body
  - Severe deformity of talipes equinovarus
  - Neuromuscular disease
  - Skeletal defects after tumor resection
  - Pseudarthrosis
  - Flail ankle
- Absolute contraindications for tibiotalocalcaneal arthrodesis with internal fixation
  - Dysvascular extremity
  - Active infection
- Relative contraindication to tibiotalocalcaneal arthrodesis with closed nailing techniques
  - Severe, fixed deformity that precludes a colinear reduction of the tibia, talus, and calcaneus for rod placement

Preoperative Planning

- We glean essential information for preoperative planning from a thorough history and physical examination of the soft tissue envelope, vascular status, degree of deformity, and assessment of the entire limb and contralateral limb.
- We review all imaging studies, including longstanding radiographs of the lower extremity. Many of these patients have comorbidities, so we ensure that medical clearance is obtained.
- The availability of implant and instruments is ascertained and arrangements for perioperative care are confirmed.

Positioning

- The patient with severe preoperative valgus deformity is positioned supine on a radiolucent operating table with a well-padded bump under the ipsilateral buttock to rotate the involved extremity internally (**FIG 7A**). Another pad can be placed under the heel to facilitate cross-table fluoroscopic imaging.
- Alternatively and preferably, the patient with neutral to varus deformity is positioned in the lateral position with the affected extremity up (**FIG 7B**).
- We pad bony prominences and use an axillary roll in the recumbent axilla.
- The patient is usually fastened to the table with a beanbag and chest brace devices, and pneumatic tourniquet control at the level of the thigh is used.
- Parenteral, prophylactic antibiotics are administered before the tourniquet is inflated.

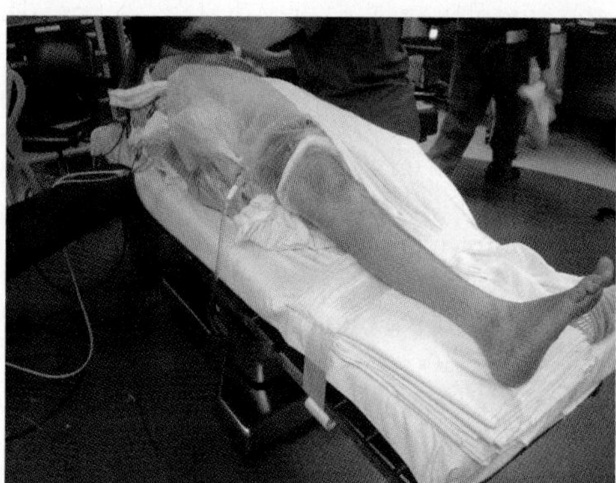

A

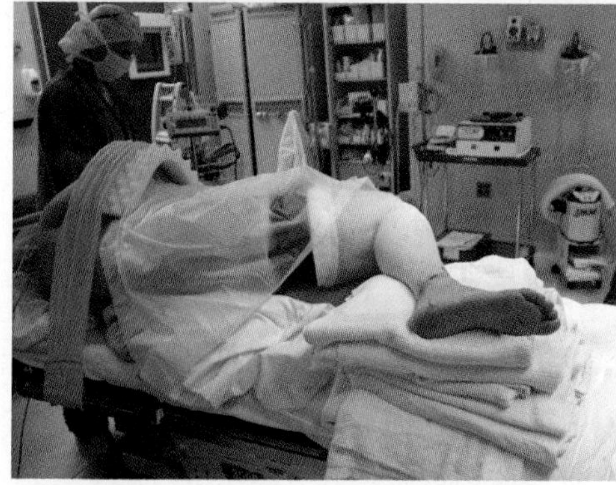

B

FIG 7 • **A.** Patient is positioned on a beanbag in a modified lateral position that allows access to the medial and lateral foot. Note stack of folded sheets under foot to be operated. **B.** Lateral position on blankets to level the leg with the pelvis; this position still allows for external hip rotation to see the medial ankle joint.

INCISION

- For the patient with severe preoperative valgus, we make a longitudinally oriented incision over the medial malleolus starting just at the supramalleolar level and carried 2 to 3 cm distal to the tip of the medial malleolus.
  - This allows a subperiosteal approach to the ankle and the removal of medially based closing-wedge osteotomies of diseased tibiotalar bone and cartilage to correct the preoperative valgus deformity.
- We identify and protect the medial neurovascular structures during this approach.
- For all patients other than those who present with severe preoperative valgus, we routinely use a lateral transfibular approach through a longitudinal incision over the distal fibula carried onto the sinus tarsi, curving slightly anteriorly as one extends beyond the distal end of the fibula.
  - This approach affords wide access to both the ankle and subtalar joints and eliminates the possibility of the lateral malleolus rubbing in normal shoe wear postoperatively, and the fibula serves as a source of abundant cancellous and corticocancellous bone graft material during the case (**TECH FIG 1**).
  - Fibular ostectomy should be especially considered at the time of hindfoot fusion if there is significant varus deformity or loss of tibial length relative to the fibula.
  - Resect the distal fibula in a beveled fashion with a microsagittal saw no more than 3 cm proximal to the level of the tibiotalar joint to preserve the distal tibiofibular syndesmosis and thereby minimize postoperative discomfort caused by distal tibiofibular movement and crepitus.
- *We would like to clarify that the transfibular approach with or without fibulectomy is reserved for patients with severe deformity who are not candidates, nor will ever be candidates, for future ankle fusion takedown and conversion to total ankle arthroplasty (TAA). For patients who may be considered for future TAA, every attempt should be made to preserve anatomy, especially the fibula—that is, the arthrodesis should be performed via an anterior or posterior approach.*

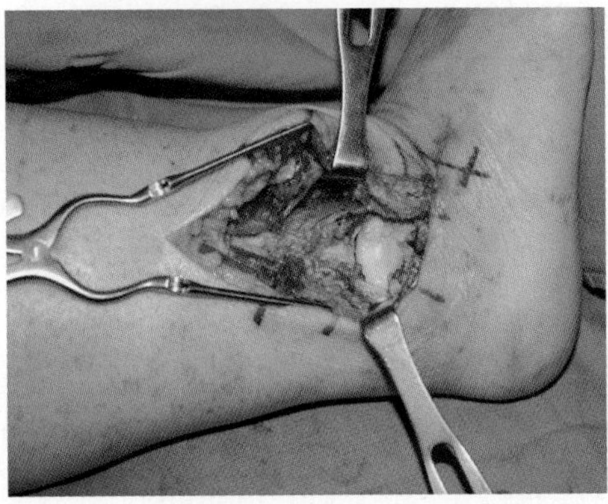

TECH FIG 1 • Lateral approach to the tibiotalar and subtalar joint after distal fibulectomy.

ANKLE ARTHROTOMY

- We use a lateral ankle arthrotomy with the incision carried over the sinus tarsi and subtalar joint to correct any deformity that may be present across the tibiotalar and subtalar joints and to prepare the joint surfaces by removing what is left of the diseased articular cartilage (**TECH FIG 2**).
- Small wedges of bone may be removed to obtain the appropriate plantigrade postoperative posture for the foot and ankle.
- These arthrotomies also leave space for insertion of bone graft as needed.
- Often combined medial and lateral arthrotomies are needed to achieve the appropriate plantigrade posture of the foot and to remove medial malleolar prominence.
- In the case of the ankle with preoperative valgus deformity, we use a medial approach to the tibiotalar joint in combination with a limited lateral exposure to decorticate and decancellate the subtalar joint via a separate lateral incision over the sinus tarsi.

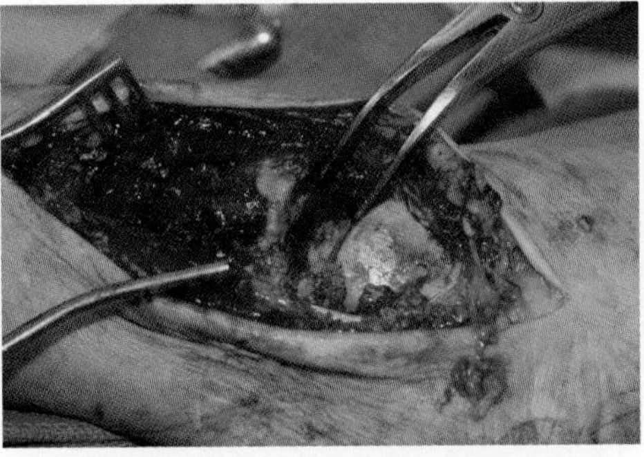

TECH FIG 2 • The lateral arthrotomy, with removal of fibula, allows easy access to the ankle joint as well as extending to the subtalar joint.

TECHNIQUES

PLANTAR INCISION FOR GUIDEWIRE INSERTION AND REAMING

- As is true with all other medullary fixation procedures, the starting point for insertion of the guidewire and subsequent medullary rod is critical to the success of the case.
- The correct starting point is midway between the tips of the medial and lateral malleoli, anterior to the subcalcaneal heel pad, and about 2.5 cm posterior to the transverse tarsal joints, in line with the longitudinal axis of the tibia (TECH FIG 3A).
  - Make a 2-cm, longitudinally oriented plantar incision just anterior to the weight-bearing subcalcaneal heel pad.
  - After the incision is carried through dermis sharply, blunt dissection only is taken down to the plantar fascia, which is split longitudinally.
  - The intrinsic muscles can be swept aside and the neurovascular bundle protected and retracted with the intrinsic flexors.
  - Place a smooth Steinmann pin or a guidewire, over which is passed a cannulated drill to provide access to the talus and tibial medullary canal after calcaneal corticotomy (TECH FIG 3B).
- Confirm optimal insertion of the cannulated drill, which passes sequentially through the inferior cortex of the calcaneus, the calcaneal body, the subtalar joint, the talar body, across the ankle, and finally into the distal tibial canal, using intraoperative fluoroscopic views in both the AP and lateral planes.
- After removing the cannulated drill, pass a bulb-tipped guidewire through the calcaneus and talus into the distal tibial medullary canal.
- Pass a series of progressively larger, flexible reamers over the guidewire, and use them to enlarge the tibiotalocalcaneal canal.
- We recommend that the final reamer diameter is a full 0.5 to 1 mm larger than the anticipated implant's diameter.
  - In our experience, overreaming avoids the risk of intraoperative and postoperative fracture at the proximal tip of the rod without compromising the construct's stability.
- Overzealous reaming in osteopenic bone may result in an intraoperative tibial fracture that then warrants using a longer medullary nail for spanning the fracture. When in doubt, check the reamer position with the fluoroscope.
- We are aware of several articles reporting fractures of the tibia at the proximal portion of the medullary nail when the nail is left at the relatively sclerotic distal tibial diametaphyseal isthmus.
- When closing the plantar wound, use simple interrupted or horizontal mattress sutures for a flat rather than inverted skin edge closure.

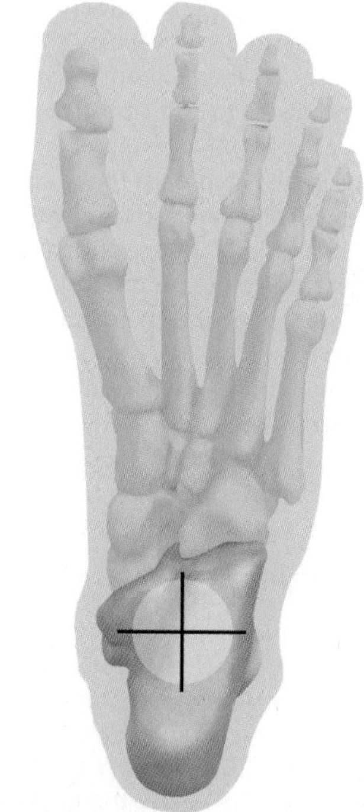

A

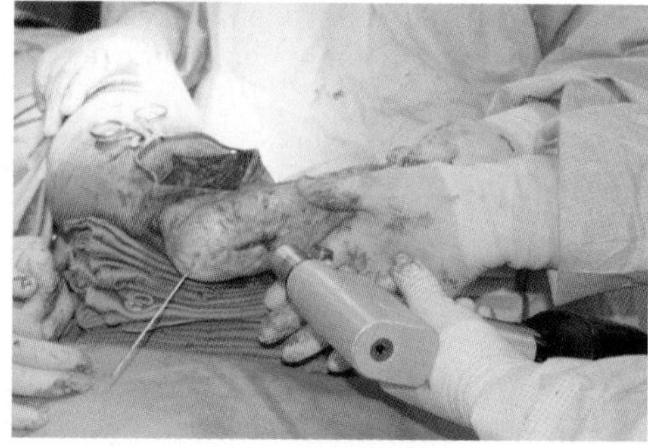

B

TECH FIG 3 • **A.** Desired starting point for the guide pin and medullary nail. With deformity, establishing this starting point's relationship to the talus and tibia may require some manipulation of the subtalar and ankle joints, but it is generally attainable. **B.** The guidewire should align with the tibial shaft.

NAIL SELECTION

- In most cases a nail length of 15 to 18 cm suffices for tibiotalocalcaneal arthrodesis with the proximal extent of the nail in metaphyseal bone, distal to the diametaphyseal isthmus, where the risk of tibia fracture is greatest.
- Nail diameter is dictated by the size of the native tibia.
  - In most cases, a 10-mm-diameter nail affords satisfactory stability to allow progression toward fusion.
  - While we acknowledge that an increase in nail diameter affords greater strength to the construct, we caution that aggressive overreaming of the cortex to place a larger-diameter nail may compromise the cortex, leading to a stress fracture.

- In profoundly neuropathic patients, we have used a long tibiotalocalcaneal nail that bypasses the distal tibial isthmus by a length equal to at least three times the diameter of the tibial canal measured at the level of the isthmus. A longer nail generally reduces the possibility of a distal tibial stress fracture, albeit by requiring more reaming of the tibia.

NAIL PLACEMENT ACROSS THE ARTHRODESIS SITE

- We find that locking the nail to its targeting arm, with each of two drill bits inserted through the drill guides and the two proximal-most screw holes in the nail before the nail and its targeting arm are tightened, ensures optimal alignment before placement.
- The medullary nail is attached to its alignment and targeting guide. As it is inserted in retrograde fashion at plantar foot, it is slightly internally rotated so that when the locking screws are passed from lateral to medial they will pass into the tibia without impingement upon the distal fibula (TECH FIG 4A).
- During insertion, the distal aspect of the nail should be countersunk at least 5 mm cephalad to the plantar surface of the os calcis or at least countersunk the same distance that the surgeon anticipates achieving axial compression across the ankle and subtalar fusion sites. Be sure not to leave the nail prominent on the plantar aspect of the foot (TECH FIG 4B).

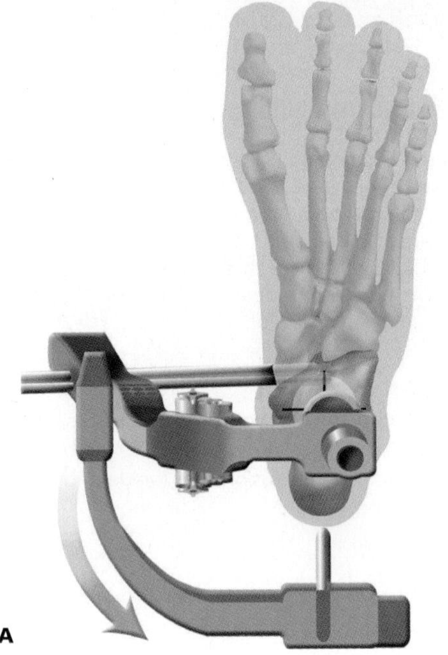
A

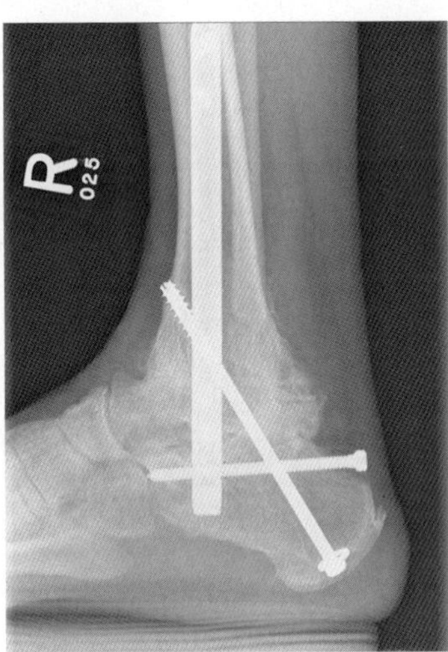

B

TECH FIG 4 • **A.** In our experience, internally rotating the nail and the guide slightly, posterior to anterior screws placed through the guide and the nail, tend to align optimally with the calcaneus. **B.** Follow-up radiograph demonstrating that the nail is slightly countersunk to avoid being prominent on the plantar surface of the foot. A nail that is slightly proud rarely creates a problem since that portion of the calcaneus is not weight bearing; in fact, it may afford some further support with the end of the nail engaged in the calcaneal cortex.

SCREW PLACEMENT IN THE INTRAMEDULLARY NAIL

- When determining the final position for the nail, we simultaneously estimate the position of locking holes in the nail relative to the distal tibia, the talar body, and the calcaneal body.
- It is preferable but not necessary to fill all the locking holes.
- Nail failure is likely to occur in the heavyset or neuropathic patient if locking holes are left open at the level of either the ankle or subtalar fusion site. Early reports of nail failure at the subtalar joint often noted failure to fuse the subtalar joint.
- An advantage of modern nail design includes placement of locking screws at various angles to one another.
- The position of the nail for the proximal screws into the tibia will dictate the final rotation; thus, the guide for the posteroanterior screw may be applied and used to check (including fluoroscopy) the later position for the posteroanterior screw in the calcaneus as well as the talar screws (TECH FIG 5A).
- A posterior-to-anterior calcaneal locking screw increases the torsional rigidity of the nail construct by at least 40% and improves purchase of the calcaneal bone exponentially when compared to simply locking in one plane relative to the long axis of the nail (TECH FIG 5B).
- Further manual compression and impaction can be done across the arthrodesis sites before the proximal interlocking screws are inserted. Some nails use an extramedullary compression device, while others use compression of the heel against the tibial screws.
- Some medullary rods include an inline compression device that can provide up to 15 mm of compression across the ankle and subtalar fusion sites (TECH FIG 5C).

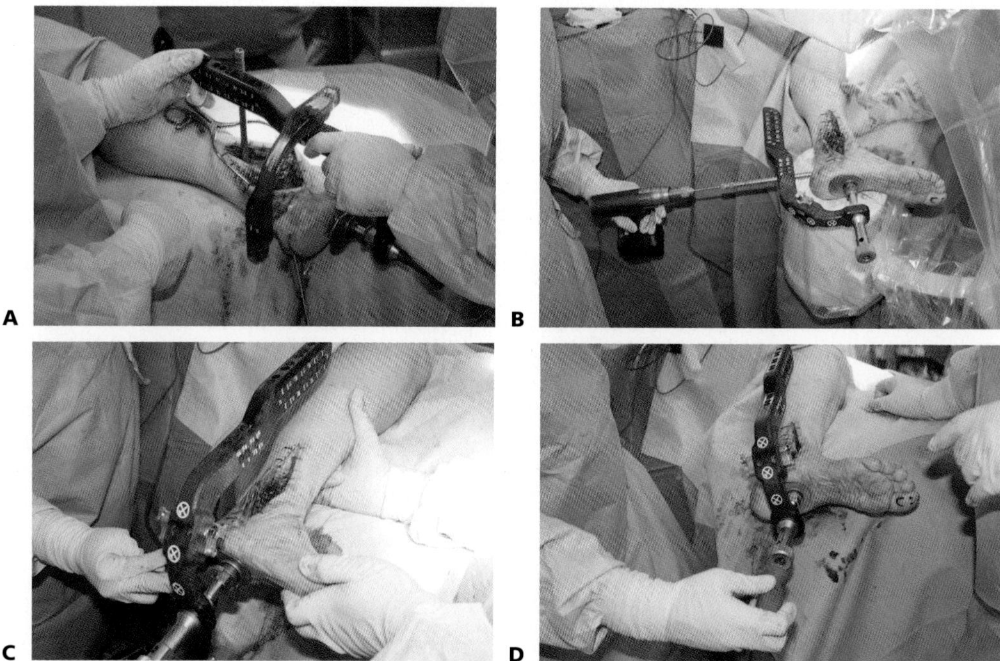

TECH FIG 5 • **A.** The alignment guide provides a quick check of overall positioning before drilling the proximal tibial screws. The surgeon should make sure the posteroanterior screw will be hitting the posterior calcaneus at an appropriate height. **B.** The posteroanterior screw is predrilled and measured via the C-arm to discern the length, usually just posterior to the calcaneal cuboid joint. **C.** A wrench is used to tighten the bolt compressing the heel plate toward the tibial screws; this intramedullary compression force is then held with distal screws through talus and calcaneus. **D.** Intraoperative view of screwdriver advancing the talar screw 7 mm proximally to augment ankle compression.

- Some nails also provide for compression of the talar screw proximally toward the tibial screws, further compressing the ankle joint 7 mm (TECH FIG 5D).
- Do not remove this compression until the rod is locked both in the talus and the calcaneus so that the benefits of compression across both fusion sites (ankle and subtalar) can be achieved.

END CAP INSERTION

- While some surgeons consider the end cap optional, we routinely secure it to the distal end of the nail after removal of the targeting arm. It restricts medullary bleeding, limits heterotopic calcification, and protects the threads of the nail should extraction be needed later.
- Permanent radiographs may be obtained in the operating room, both with AP and lateral projection, to ascertain appropriate alignment, position, and fixation.

BONE GRAFTING

- Autogenous or allograft bone grafting is done to improve healing rates.
- Medullary reamings can be mixed with a fibular autograft and inserted at the tibiotalar and subtalar fusion sites even before placement of the nail.
- After insertion of the nail, place bone graft anterior, lateral, and posterior to the fusion sites.
- For large defects, such as removal of ankle prostheses, a femoral head allograft may be cut to fit the large defect, and then the nail can be placed directly through the allograft (TECH FIG 6A–D).
- Because of the bleeding, cancellous surfaces of bone achieved at surgery, and the large amounts of bone graft employed, closed suction drainage is recommended.
- Some surgeons and investigators advocate internal or external electrical bone stimulators for improving healing rates in neuropathic, multiply operated patients or smokers.
- We have also used bone stimulation for patients with pre-existing avascular necrosis at the arthrodesis site.

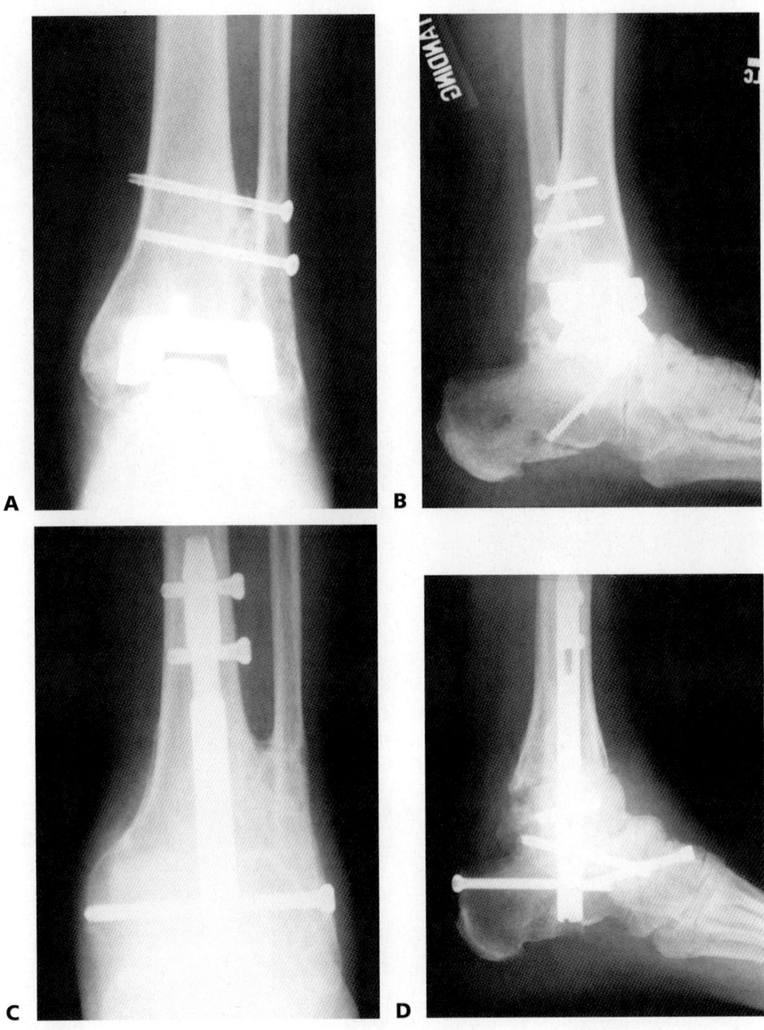

TECH FIG 6 • **A, B.** Preoperative AP and lateral views of failing Agility total ankle prosthesis. **C, D.** Postoperative AP and lateral views after placement of femoral head allograft (soaked in concentrated bone marrow aspirate) demonstrate the excellent stability of an intramedullary device in a complicated revision situation.

WOUND CLOSURE

- Take care to approximate the tissues in the ankle region. A layered closure is preferable.
- Apply a sterile, nonadherent dressing with adequate padding from the tips of the toes to just below the knee.
- This dressing includes a posterior plaster splint with the ankle and foot at neutral position and a gentle compressive wrap over padding.

EXAMPLE CASE

- The patient is a 58-year-old man with posttraumatic talar avascular necrosis who failed brace wear.
- Preoperative radiographs are shown in **TECHNIQUE FIGURE 7A–C**. The patient had pain from tibiotalar arthritis due to talar dome collapse. With increasing talar collapse, the foot gradually migrated anterior to the tibia, a biomechanically unfavorable position.
- Postoperative radiographs are shown in **TECHNIQUE FIGURE 7D,E**. Tibiotalocalcaneal arthrodesis with a medullary nail was performed. The anatomic relationship of the foot to the tibia has been re-established. The nail is not proud on the plantar foot. Despite the relatively large diameter of the nail, a supplemental cannulated screw can be placed adjacent to the nail from the calcaneus to the anterior tibia to provide further support to the construct. Also, a large buttress (much like the flying buttress on a French cathedral) was placed on the posterior tibia and dorsal calcaneus to increase the surface area for fusion.

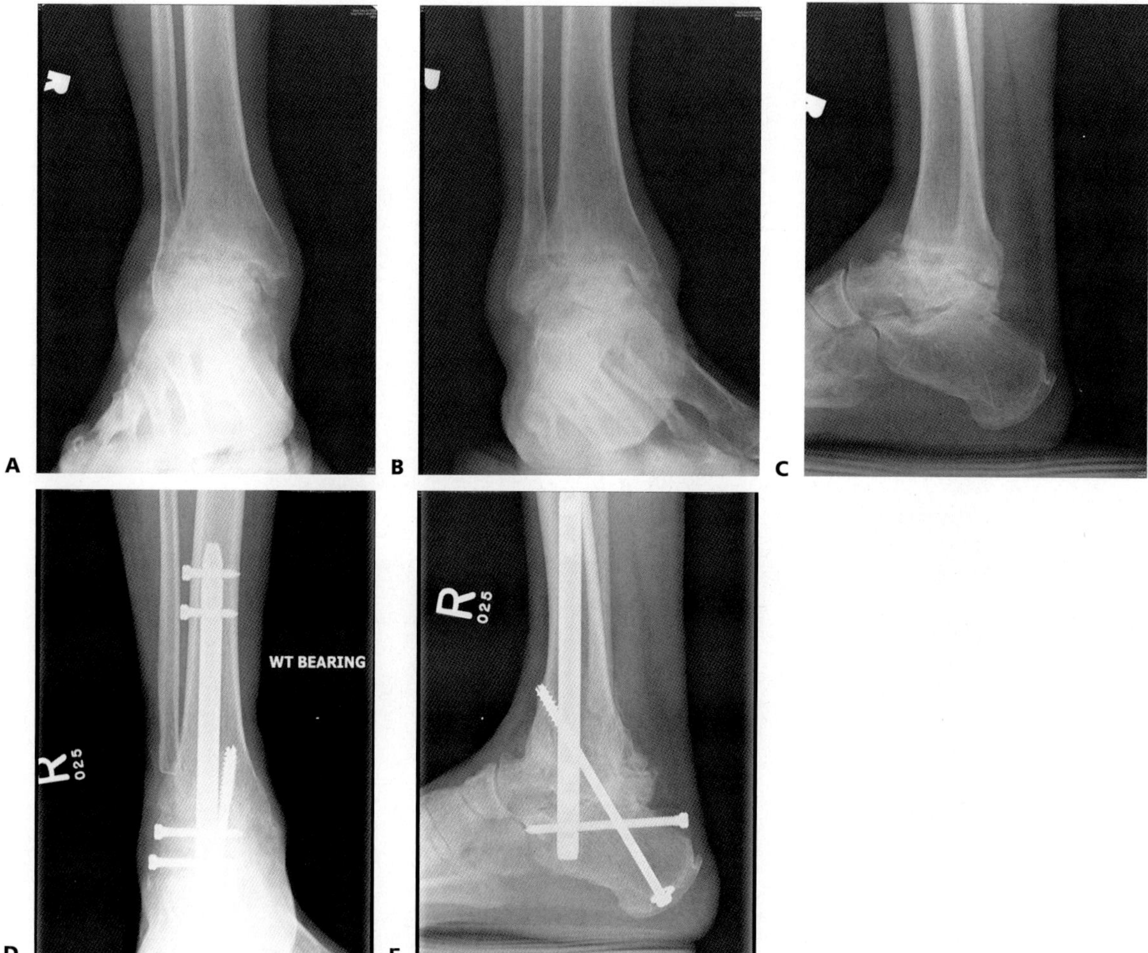

TECH FIG 7 • Preoperative weight-bearing ankle radiographs with avascular necrosis of the talar dome and some degree of anterior translation of the talus relative to the tibial axis. **A.** AP view. **B.** Mortise view. **C.** Lateral view. **D, E.** Postoperative weight-bearing ankle radiographs of the same patient after tibiotalocalcaneal arthrodesis. Fusion appears to have been successful based on the bridging trabeculation at the arthrodesis sites. In our experience, the increased surface area afforded by the bone graft to the prepared posterior tibia and dorsal calcaneus increases the chance of fusion. Note that the physiologic relationship of talus to tibial shaft axis has been re-established. Despite the nail's relatively large diameter, a supplemental cannulated screw could be passed adjacent to the nail to provide greater stability to the construct. **D.** AP view. **E.** Lateral view.

PEARLS AND PITFALLS

- The most important goal of tibiotalocalcaneal arthrodesis with medullary nail fixation is achieving satisfactory pain-free union of the ankle and hindfoot with the foot in optimal plantigrade posture.
- In our experience, radiographic and clinical assessment on the operating table before completion of the case is most important in achieving plantigrade posture.
- Intraoperative pearls include the need for appropriate positioning so that full access to the entire lower extremity is obtained.
  - We recommend that the patient with limited internal and external hip rotation should be positioned in slightly less than extreme lateral position to facilitate access to the medial malleolar side of the ankle and optimize AP imaging with a C-arm fluoroscope.
- The optimal insertion point for the nail is immediately lateral to the plantar calcaneus' midpoint and in line with the longitudinal tibial axis.
- Nail and targeting arm
  - Be sure that the targeting arm is rigidly coupled to the nail. Rigid coupling of the nail to its targeting arm in the appropriate position and alignment will save the surgeon a lot of effort and frustration in locking the nail proximally.
- Medullary nailing for tibiotalocalcaneal arthrodesis in the face of open ulcers or wounds is not absolutely contraindicated, but ulcers or wounds should be clean, non-cellulitic, and granulating before medullary nail fixation is considered.
- Rotational alignment of the tibiotalocalcaneal arthrodesis: Satisfactory rotational alignment is most readily achieved by comparison to the contralateral uninvolved limb and by preserving the natural concave–convex relationship of the tibiotalar and subtalar fusion sites at the time of removal of diseased cartilage and subchondral bone.

- Performing tibiotalocalcaneal arthrodesis with limited assistance: A holding pin from the calcaneus to the posterior tibia can help hold alignment during the reaming process (**FIG 8**).

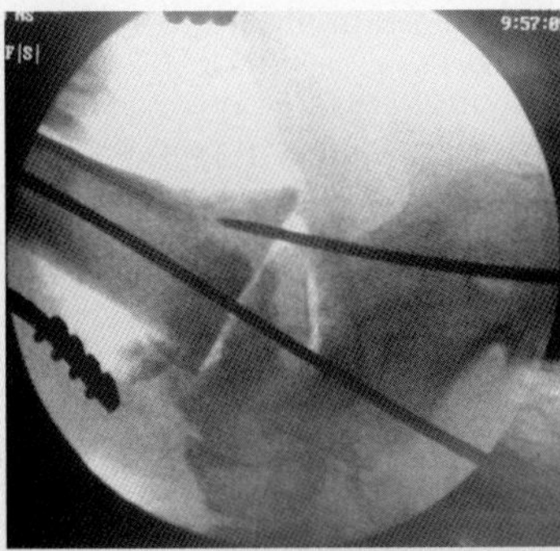

FIG 8 • A holding pin from the calcaneus to the posterior tibia can help hold position when reaming and placing the nail, as long as the pin remains out of the reamer's path.

POSTOPERATIVE CARE

- Most patients undergoing tibiotalocalcaneal arthrodesis with medullary nail fixation can be discharged the day after surgery with oral analgesics and after having received 24 hours of parenteral antibiotics.
- The typical case will require non–weight-bearing protection in a short-leg splint or cast for 6 weeks, followed by 4 to 6 weeks of weight bearing to tolerance in a short-leg walking cast.
- At 10 to 12 weeks postoperatively the patient is fitted with a removable fracture orthosis equipped with a rocker sole to ease the transition to weight bearing in more normal shoe wear by 12 to 16 weeks postoperatively.
- Less than half of the patients fused in the appropriate plantigrade posture with otherwise normal neuromuscular function will have a noticeable limp by 6 to 12 months postoperatively.
- Those requiring shoe wear modification are often best treated with a rocker-bottom sole or a cushioned heel to make up for the rigidity of the fused joints.
- Heel lifts can be employed to equalize limb lengths to within 10 to 15 mm, the side undergoing tibiotalocalcaneal fusion desirably being the short one to allow for toe clearance during the swing phase of gait.
- The vast majority of our patients are ambulatory postoperatively in a non-custom, off-the-shelf shoe.
- Rod removal has been required in less than 1% of Dr. Quill's operative series.

COMPLICATIONS

- We have not encountered plantar wound healing problems in any patient when the procedure is done as described above.
- Damage to the medial and lateral plantar nerves can be avoided by following the technique mentioned above and by dissecting with nothing sharper than a large key elevator deep to the dermis on the plantar aspect of the foot.
    - A three-quarter-inch key elevator can be used to bluntly spread the fibers of the plantar fascia and the intrinsic flexor muscles in line with the incision and to sweep soft tissues medially and laterally before inserting the guidewire through the sole of the foot.
- Complications of medullary nail fixation for ankle and hindfoot fusion include those germane to any orthopaedic procedure, such as infection, medical illness, and anesthetic perioperative complication, as well as hardware prominence.
- The complications unique to medullary nail fixation for tibiotalocalcaneal arthrodesis include delayed union, nonunion, and malunion and can be minimized by adhering to the technique described.
- The proximal dissection for screw fixation may encounter the superficial peroneal nerve and the distal dissection may expose the sural nerve; care must to be taken to avoid damage. In cases in which the medial malleolus is removed, the tibial nerve can be exposed to injury very easily.

OUTCOMES

- Medullary nail advantages over traditional fixation for arthrodesis of the ankle and hindfoot include the fact that a medullary nail is a load-sharing device that is especially indicated for the osteopenic or neuroarthropathic patient.
- Dr. Quill's personal clinical series includes a 93% union rate in an average of 12.2 weeks postoperatively (range 10 to 20 weeks).
    - Delayed nonunions have occurred in neuropathic patients, but most are asymptomatic.
    - Mean improvement in the AOFAS clinical scores for this series of patients has been 52 points.
    - Nail-related problems include the removal of 17 of 932 locking screws removed for fracture or local irritation.
    - There have been two fractured nails, both of which were in the face of severe persistent valgus and subtalar nonunion in neuropathic, obese patients.
    - One tibial fracture was sustained intraoperatively in an osteopenic rheumatoid patient. It was incomplete and healed during routine casting.
- Excellent early stability and rigid early fixation are achieved and maintained, providing for less perioperative morbidity and discomfort and shorter casting.
- The medullary nail ensures position and alignment from the immediate postoperative time frame, and the patients often require less activity restriction postoperatively.
- Medullary nail fixation for tibiotalocalcaneal arthrodesis has filled a particular niche in treating patients with severe deformities, disabilities, and bone loss who otherwise would have been severely disabled or would have needed to undergo limb amputation.

REFERENCES

1. Adams JC. Arthrodesis of the ankle joint: experiences with the transfibular approach. J Bone Joint Surg Br 1948;30B:506–511.
2. Gellman H, Lenahan M, Halikis N, et al. Selective tarsal arthrodesis, an *in vitro* analysis of the effect on foot motion. Foot Ankle 1987;8; 127–133.
3. Hefti FL, Baumann JU, Morscher EW. Ankle joint fusion: determination of optimal position by gait analysis. Arch Orthop Trauma Surg 1980;96:187.
4. Iwata H, Yasuhra N, Kawashima K, et al. Arthrodesis of the ankle joint with rheumatoid arthrodesis: experiences with the transfibular approach. Clin Orthop Relat Res 1980;153:189.
5. Kile TA, Donnelly RE, Gehrke JC, et al. Tibiocalcaneal arthrodesis with an intramedullary device. Foot Ankle Int 1994;15:669–673.
6. Papa J, Myerson M, Girard P. Salvage, with arthrodesis, in intractable diabetic neuropathic arthropathy of the foot and ankle. J Bone Joint Surg Am 1993;75A:1056–1066.
7. Papa JA, Myerson MS. Pantalar and tibiotalocalcaneal arthrodesis for posttraumatic osteoarthrosis of the ankle and hindfoot. J Bone Joint Surg Am 1992;74A:1042–1049.
8. Quill GE. An approach to the management of ankle arthritis. In Myerson M, ed. Foot and Ankle Disorders. Philadelphia: WB Saunders, 2000:1059–1084.
9. Quill GE. Tibiotalocalcaneal and pantalar arthrodesis. Foot Ankle Clin 1991;1:199–210.
10. Quill GE. Pantalar arthritis. In: Nunnelly JA, Pfeffer GB, Sanders RW, et al., eds: Advanced Reconstruction Foot and Ankle. Rosemont, IL: American Orthopaedic Foot and Ankle Society and American Academy of Orthopaedic Surgeons, 2004:209–213.
11. Quill GE. Tibiotalocalcaneal arthrodesis. Techniques Orthop 1996; 11:269–273.
12. Stewart MJ, Morrey BF. Arthrodesis of the diabetic neuropathic ankle. Clin Orthop Relat Res 1990;253:209–211.

Chapter 82

Tibiotalocalcaneal Arthrodesis Using Lateral Blade Plate Fixation

Christopher P. Chiodo and Catherine E. Johnson

DEFINITION

- Tibiotalocalcaneal arthritis is formally defined as the loss of cartilage from both the tibiotalar (ankle) and the talocalcaneal (subtalar) joints.
- Tibiotalocalcaneal arthritis can cause significant disability in terms of pain and limitation of function. Nonoperative treatment options are limited, as in most instances they only partially relieve pain and usually cannot correct deformity.
- The goal of tibiotalocalcaneal arthrodesis is to produce a stable, plantigrade, pain-free foot and ankle.
- Achieving stable fixation can be challenging in osteopenic bone. Blade plate fixation of the tibiotalocalcaneal joint has been shown in biomechanical studies to have higher initial and final stiffness.

ANATOMY

- The ankle joint comprises the talus as it articulates with the tibial plafond. The body of the talus is saddle-shaped dorsally and fits congruently within the mortise created by the distal tibia and fibula. In addition, the talus and the tibial plafond are narrower posteriorly to accommodate rotation with ankle dorsiflexion and plantarflexion.
- The subtalar joint comprises the talus and the calcaneus as they articulate through anterior, middle, and posterior facets.
- The talus is divided into head, body, and neck. Roughly 70% of the bone is covered with cartilage, and there are no muscular or tendinous attachments. The main blood supply of the talar body enters retrograde through the neck of the talus, which makes the body prone to avascular necrosis in the case of displaced talar neck fractures.
- The lateral aspect of the foot is innervated by the superficial peroneal and sural nerves. The superficial peroneal nerve typically exits the crural fascia 10 to 12 cm proximal to the tip of the lateral malleolus. The nerve then courses anteriorly to give sensation to the dorsal aspect of the foot.
- The sural nerve has contributions from branches of both the tibial and common peroneal nerves. It courses lateral to the Achilles tendon and is found about 1 cm distal to the tip of the fibula at the level of the ankle.

PATHOGENESIS

- Arthritis of the tibiotalar and subtalar joints has multiple causes, including primary osteoarthritis, trauma, neuroarthropathy, infection, avascular necrosis, inflammatory arthritis, and failed surgery.
- Patients typically complain of diffuse ankle pain and cannot differentiate tibiotalar from subtalar symptoms. Although it is preferable to fuse only one joint to retain an adjacent motion segment, such isolated fusion in the setting of residual arthrosis can result in persistent pain.
- In posttraumatic cases, failure to restore articular congruency can result in increased contact stresses, with resultant cartilage wear and the development of arthritis.

NATURAL HISTORY

- Hindfoot arthritis is usually a progressive disorder, although the rate of progression can vary. However, arthritis due to malalignment, trauma, and avascular necrosis of the talus can progress relatively rapidly.
- Nonoperative treatment of hindfoot arthritis in an ankle–foot orthosis (AFO) likely does not prevent or slow progression of the disease, but merely decreases symptoms.[3]
- Failed surgery can be quite debilitating and frequently needs expedited treatment.

PATIENT HISTORY AND PHYSICAL FINDINGS

- Physical examination should include:
  - Gait. The surgeon should watch the patient walking both toward and away from him or her and should clinically determine whether gait is normal or antalgic on both sides. The examiner should look for any assistive devices. Patients with painful arthritis will have an antalgic gait on that side. The patient may require the use of a cane or a walker.
  - Hindfoot alignment. The hindfoot is examined from behind. The surgeon should determine whether the hindfoot is in varus or valgus. Patients can have both varus and valgus malalignment.
  - Tibiotalar range of motion. Active and passive sagittal plane motion is assessed. Normal ankle motion is about 50 degrees of plantarflexion and 10 to 20 degrees of dorsiflexion. Tibiotalar motion is usually significantly decreased compared to the unaffected side.
  - Subtalar range of motion. Active and passive coronal plane motion is assessed. Normal subtalar motion is about 10 to 20 degrees of inversion and 5 to 10 degrees of eversion. Subtalar motion is usually significantly decreased compared to the unaffected side.
- Past medical history may be significant for antecedent ankle or hindfoot trauma, talar osteonecrosis, diabetes, neuroarthropathy, osteochondral defect, or recurrent ankle instability.
- Past surgical history may include previous ankle or hindfoot surgery, including open reduction and internal fixation, total ankle arthroplasty, and previous arthrodesis.
- Patients usually complain of pain and instability with weight bearing. Selective anesthetic injections into the ankle or subtalar joints can help to determine which joints are symptomatic.
- Upon examination, hindfoot swelling and tenderness are usually evident. Most patients have decreased passive range of motion in both joints. Malalignment is also often present.

IMAGING AND OTHER DIAGNOSTIC STUDIES

- Weight-bearing plain radiographs including AP, lateral, and mortise views of the ankle and AP, lateral, and oblique views of the foot are standard.

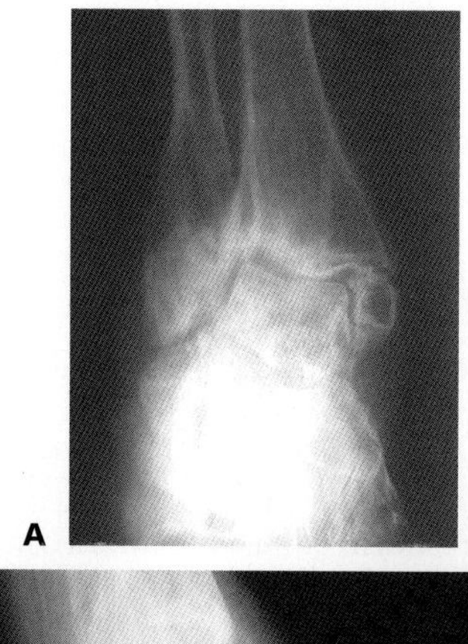

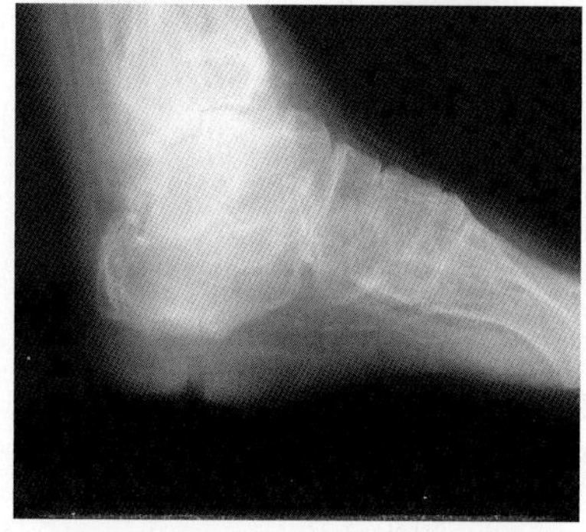

FIG 1 • Preoperative AP (**A**) and lateral (**B**) radiographs of the ankle.

- A weight-bearing lateral should be performed to assess talo–calcaneal and talo–first metatarsal angles (**FIG 1**).
- CT is often helpful preoperatively to assess bony anatomy, alignment, and articular integrity in greater detail.

DIFFERENTIAL DIAGNOSIS

- Talar avascular necrosis
- Talar osteochondral injury
- Isolated ankle arthritis
- Isolated subtalar arthritis
- Ankle instability
- Foreign body

NONOPERATIVE MANAGEMENT

- Nonoperative treatment is aimed primarily at alleviating symptoms rather than correcting deformity. The patient is placed in a robust brace such as an ankle–foot arthrosis (AFO) or Arizona brace in an attempt to provide support and limit motion.
- Bracing may not always be possible depending on the severity of the deformity. In addition, bracing typically does not prevent progression of disease.

SURGICAL MANAGEMENT

- Surgical management is generally indicated when nonoperative modalities have failed to provide adequate relief or are impractical (eg, a non-braceable deformity).
- Tibiotalocalcaneal fusion is indicated in patients with arthritis in both the tibiotalar and subtalar joints. The goal of surgical intervention is to obtain a stable, plantigrade, and pain-free foot and ankle.
- Blade plate fixation can be used primarily or in instances when the surgeon feels that intramedullary rod fixation is contraindicated. The latter may include poor bone stock or advanced osteopenia, a distal tibia deformity greater than 10 degrees, or significant loss of calcaneal height.[10]
- The main two contraindications to this procedure are (1) the presence of active infection and (2) destruction of calcaneal bone stock to the extent that purchase with the blade is compromised. In these instances, the use of a small wire ring fixator should be considered.

Preoperative Planning

- A full patient assessment is made before the operation. Smokers should be counseled with regard to smoking cessation because in this population, a 14-fold increase in the nonunion rate has been documented.[4]
- If active infection is suspected, an appropriate workup should be performed. This may include laboratory studies, MRI with contrast, and nuclear imaging. If there is still uncertainty despite these tests, a bone biopsy or joint aspirate may be necessary.
- Disease-modifying antirheumatic drugs (DMARDs) should be held preoperatively, typically for 2 weeks or a period determined in conjunction with a rheumatologist.
- Patients with significant comorbidities such as diabetes, cardiovascular disease, and nephropathy should be medically optimized by their primary care doctor before surgical intervention.

Positioning

- The patient is placed supine on the operating table with a bump under the ipsilateral buttock to maintain the foot in neutral or slightly rotated medially.
- The extremity is prepared and draped, including the iliac crest if structural autograft is desired. An alternative bone graft harvest site is the proximal tibia. A thigh tourniquet is used (**FIG 2**).

Approach

- Traditionally, an extensile lateral approach to the ankle and subtalar joints is used, although a posterior approach has also been described.[8]
- A 15- to 20-cm curvilinear incision is made through the skin centered over the fibula shaft proximally, then curving toward the base of the fourth metatarsal distally.

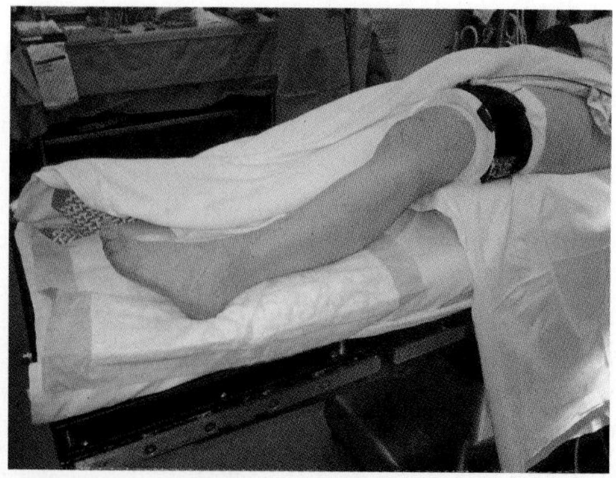

FIG 2 • Preoperative positioning of the patient.

- With deep dissection, care is taken to avoid injury to the superficial peroneal nerve, which exits the fascia about 12 cm proximal to the fibular tip. Distally, the surgeon must take care to avoid injury to the sural nerve along its course lateral to the fifth metatarsal (**FIG 3**).
- Distally, the extensor digitorum brevis is elevated to expose the subtalar joint.
- In some instances, a medial (longitudinal) incision may be necessary. These include (1) to remove medial bony prominences and debris and (2) to assist in resection of medial bone when advanced varus deformity precludes reduction of the foot to neutral.

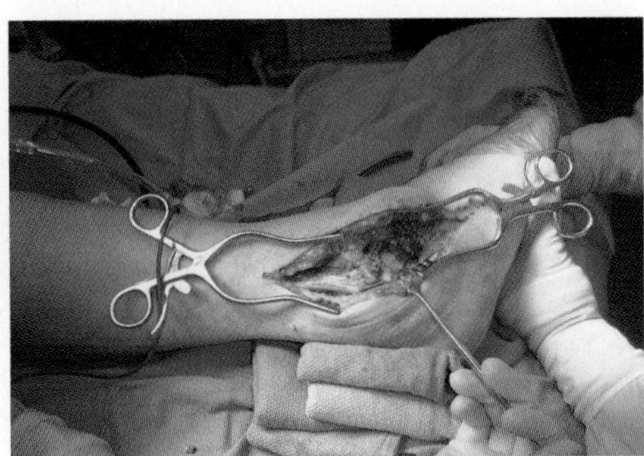

FIG 3 • The ankle and subtalar joints are approached through an extensile curvilinear incision.

OSTEOTOMY OF THE FIBULA AND PREPARATION OF THE TIBIOTALAR JOINT

- Make an osteotomy of the fibula about 6 to 10 cm proximal to the tip of the lateral malleolus (**TECH FIG 1**). Resect the distal section of the fibula. If desired, this can be morselized for bone graft. Retract the peroneal tendons posteriorly and protect them.
- Enter the ankle joint sharply and fully expose it by releasing the lateral ligaments and anterior and posterior capsule.
- Distract the joint using a lamina spreader.
- Remove any remaining cartilage with a curette.
- After removing the cartilage, prepare the joint surface with flexible chisels or a small, low-speed burr. If using a burr, use copious irrigation to avoid thermal necrosis. Burr holes should be just through the subchondral bone and separated by about 3 mm on all sides to avoid weakening or fracture of the cortex.

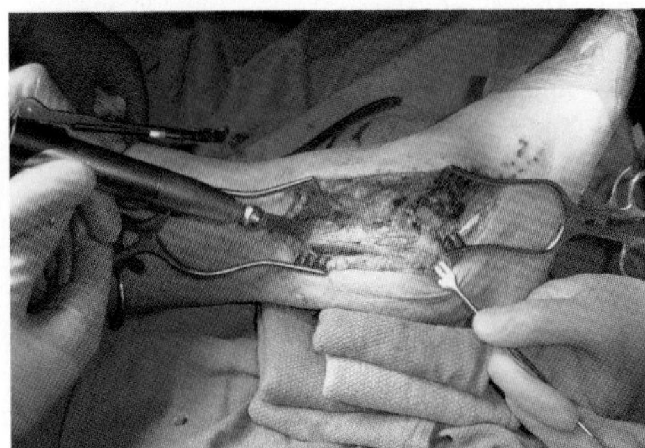

TECH FIG 1 • An osteotomy of the fibula is performed about 6 to 10 cm proximal to the tip of the bone.

PREPARATION OF THE SUBTALAR JOINT

- Enter the subtalar joint sharply with release of the lateral ligaments, capsule, and the talocalcaneal intraosseous ligament.
- Maintain distraction of the joint using a lamina spreader.
- Curette the remaining cartilage off the joint surface and prepare the subchondral bone with flexible chisels or a burr as described above.
- If there is significant bone loss or fragmentation of the talus, the tibia may have to be fused directly to the talus. In this case, the calcaneal articular processes will need to be removed with an osteotome to create a flat surface that will lie flush with the tibial plafond.
- Bone graft can be packed into the subtalar and ankle joints. If there is a large bony deficit with substantial loss of limb length, structural graft in the form of iliac crest autograft or femoral head allograft can be used to restore height.

INSERTION OF THE BLADE PLATE

- After preparing the joint surfaces, insert a 90- or 95-degree fixed-angle blade plate for fixation. The use of both an adolescent blade plate and a humeral blade plate has been described. The length of the blade is typically 40 mm. The side plate can range from five to eight holes based on the size of the patient and the surgeon's preference.
- Ensure that the hindfoot is positioned in neutral to 5 degrees of valgus and the ankle is in neutral dorsiflexion and plantarflexion. External rotation should

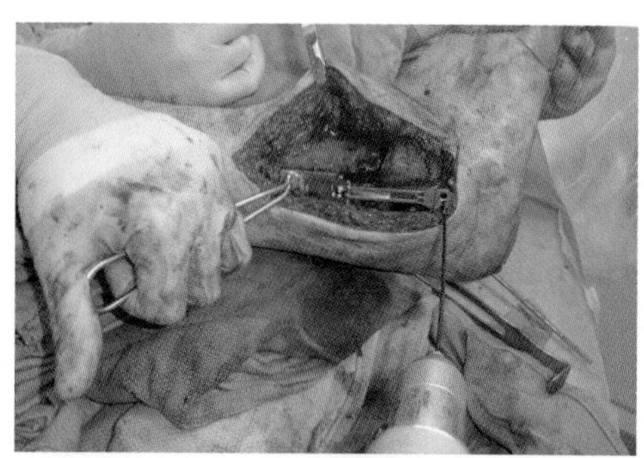

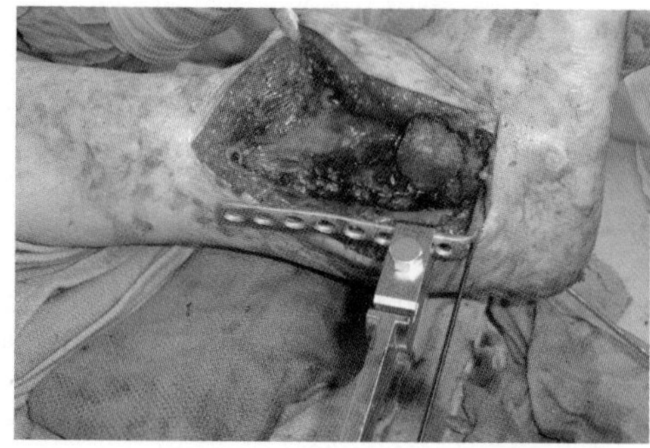

TECH FIG 2 • **A.** A 2.0-mm guidewire is inserted through the drill guide into the calcaneus. **B.** The blade plate is inserted over the guidewire using the insertion handle.

approximate that of the contralateral extremity, usually 5 to 10 degrees.

- The ankle and subtalar joints must be held rigidly during insertion of the blade plate. Provisional fixation can be obtained with guidewires or a Schanz pin.
- Use a 2.0-mm guidewire to facilitate insertion of the blade plate. The guidewire should be inserted such that 5 to 10 mm of calcaneal bone will remain plantar to the blade. Place the guidewire through the middle hole of the blade plate drill guide (TECH FIG 2A). The lateral calcaneal cortex may then be further prepared for blade insertion by predrilling with a 4.5-mm drill bit (through appropriate holes in the drill guide).
- Remove the drill guide and insert the blade plate over the guidewire using the inserter–extractor handle (TECH FIG 2B). Impact the blade until it is flush with the lateral cortex of the tibia. Rotational control is best achieved by using a slotted hammer.
- Contour the plate to the lateral aspect of the tibia and fill the screw holes sequentially. Use 4.5-mm cortical screws proximally and 6.5 mm cancellous screws distally.
- A single 6.5-mm or 7.3-mm cortical screw can be used to augment the blade plate fixation. Place the screw under fluoroscopic guidance from the calcaneal tuberosity into the anterior tibial cortex at roughly a 60-degree angle.

CLOSURE

- Given the large amount of bleeding cancellous bone exposed during the procedure, a meticulous layered closure should be performed. Further steps that will aid in the prevention of a postoperative hematoma include releasing the tourniquet and assessing hemostasis before closure, the use of drains, and the use of a compression dressing.

PEARLS AND PITFALLS

Pearl: Use a proximal guidewire to maintain sagittal plane alignment.	■ Once the blade engages the calcaneus, the position of the plate proximally cannot be changed. To avoid sagittal plane malalignment (ie, the plate coming off the tibial anteriorly or posteriorly), consider using another guidewire through the most proximal hole of the plate as the blade plate construct is inserted (**FIG 4**).

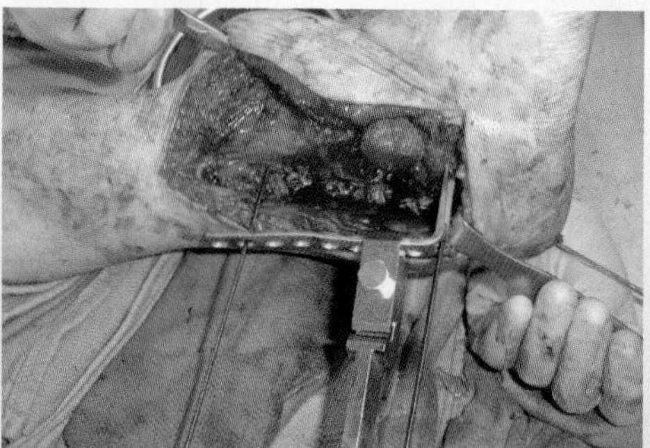

FIG 4 • Sagittal plane malalignment can be avoided using a proximal guidewire.

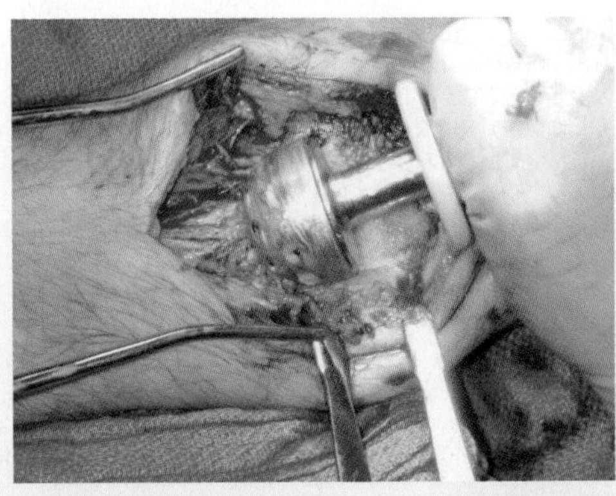

FIG 5 • The fibula can be morselized for bone graft using an acetabular reamer.

Pearl: Use the resected fibula for autogenous bone graft.	■ The distal fibula can be readily morselized into autogenous bone graft using a small acetabular reamer before resection[12] (**FIG 5**).
Pitfall: Tendency of hindfoot to fall into valgus	■ As the plate is screwed down to the tibia, there is a tendency for the hindfoot to be pulled into valgus given the normal contour of the lateral tibia. To avoid this, the blade plate should be carefully contoured before insertion. Resecting a groove for the plate in the most distal portion of the tibia using a chisel or burr may also be helpful.
Pitfall: Tendency of hindfoot to fall into varus	■ Failure to contour the blade plate when necessary can sometimes push the hindfoot into varus. Incorporating a small lateral "bow" distally will avert this.
Pitfall: Blade plate inserted too lateral	■ If the blade plate does not lie flush with the lateral calcaneus, the blade plate may be prominent, causing potential difficulties with wound closure and healing.
Pitfall: Dorsiflexion malunion with talectomy	■ In cases of talectomy, the foot must be aligned with the leg, as alignment of the distal tibia to the posterior calcaneal facet can result in a dorsiflexion malunion. The fused surfaces should be contoured accordingly.

POSTOPERATIVE CARE

- Postoperatively, patients are placed in a splint and admitted for 24 hours of intravenous antibiotics.
- After 10 to 14 days, patients return to the office for evaluation of the wound and suture removal. At this visit patients are placed in a non–weight-bearing short-leg cast.
- Patients remain non–weight-bearing in a short-leg cast for 6 to 12 weeks, based on radiographic healing.
- Thereafter, patients are transitioned to a short-leg walking cast or boot and progressive weight bearing is begun.
- The fusion is protected until sufficient clinical and radiographic healing is obtained (**FIG 6**). A CT scan may be needed to assess the adequacy of the fusion.

OUTCOMES

- A successful outcome is usually the norm for tibiotalocalcaneal fusion.
- Most studies report combined results of different approaches to fusion. In studies examining the use of blade plate fixation exclusively, the reported fusion rates have ranged from 90% to 100%.[2,8,10]

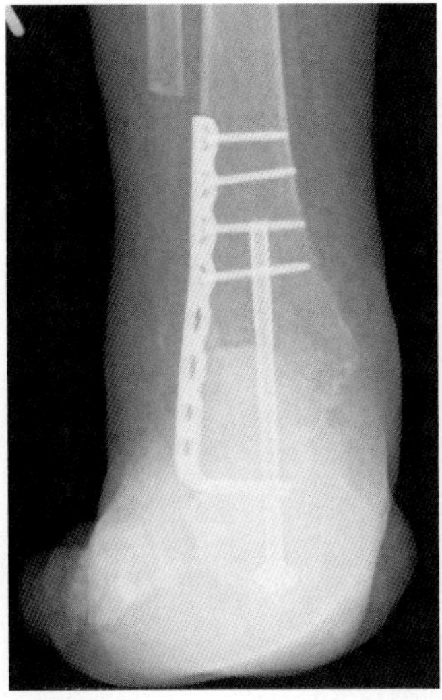

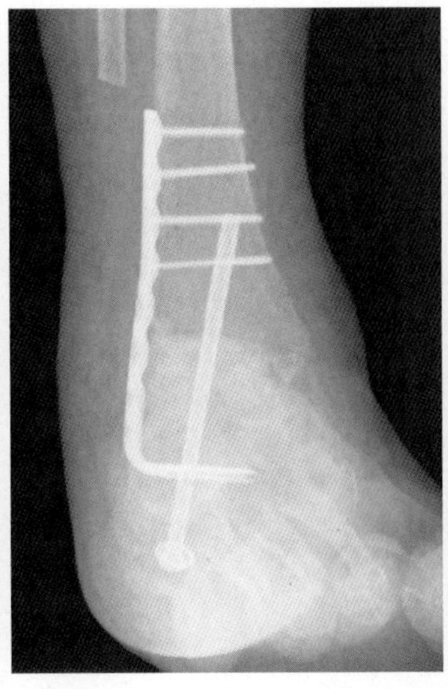

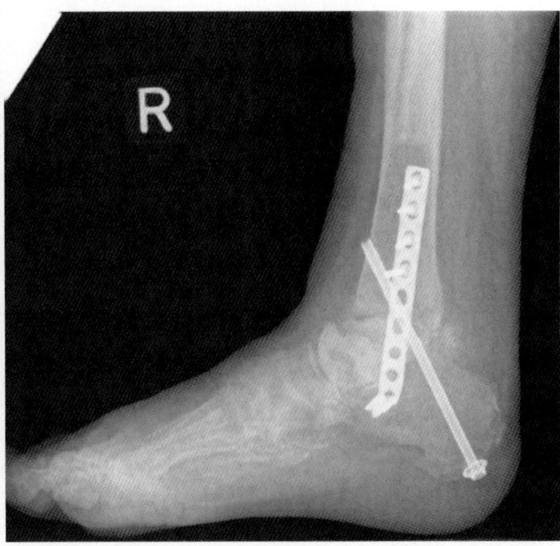

FIG 6 • Postoperative radiographs showing healing. In this case, the talus was "replaced" with a carefully contoured femoral head allograft.

COMPLICATIONS

- Overall complication rates for tibiotalocalcaneal fusion have been as high as 50% in some series.[3,5] The most common complications include nonunion, malunion, infection, and neuroma.
- In patients undergoing tibiotalocalcaneal fusion (regardless of fixation technique) the nonunion rate ranges from 0% to 40%. This is most common when there is avascular necrosis of the talus. In this patient population, the nonunion rate has been as high as 89%.[5] Nonunion rates are also significantly higher in smokers and patients with neuroarthropathy (33% to 75%).[4,5]
- Superficial and deep wound infection can be minimized through the use of appropriate perioperative antibiotics, meticulous soft tissue handling, a layered wound closure, avoidance of hematoma formation, and postoperative elevation.
- Peripheral neuroma of either the sural or superficial peroneal nerves can be minimized by careful incision placement and gentle retraction and soft tissue handling. In patients with neuroarthropathy, there is usually decreased if not absent distal sensation. In these patients, peripheral nerve injury is usually clinically insignificant.

REFERENCES

1. Alvarez RG, Barbour TM, Perkins TD. Tibiotalocalcaneal arthrodesis for nonbraceable neuropathic ankle deformity. Foot Ankle Int 1994;15:354–359.
2. Chiodo CP, Acevedo JI, Sammarco VJ, et al. Intramedullary rod fixation compared with blade-plate-and-screw fixation for tibiocalcaneal arthrodesis: a biomechanical investigation. J Bone Joint Surg Am 2003;85A:2425–2428.
3. Chou LB, Mann RA, Yaszay B, et al. Tibiocalcaneal arthrodesis. Foot Ankle Int 2000;21:804–808.
4. Cobb TK, Gabrielsen TA, Campbell II DC, et al. Cigarette smoking and nonunion after ankle arthrodesis. Foot Ankle Int 1994;15: 64–67.
5. Cooper PS. Complications of ankle and tibiotalocalcaneal arthrodesis. Clin Orthop Relat Res 2001;391:33–44.
6. Crosby LA, Yee TC, Formanek TS, et al. Complications following arthroscopic ankle arthrodesis. Foot Ankle Int 1996;17:340–342.
7. Frey C, Halikus NM, Vu-Rose T, et al. A review of ankle arthrodesis: predisposing factors to nonunion. Foot Ankle Int 1994;15: 581–584.
8. Hanson TW, Cracchiolo A III. The use of a 95-degree blade plate and a posterior approach to achieve tibiotalocalcaneal arthrodesis. Foot Ankle Int 2002;23:704–710.
9. Morrey BF, Wiedeman GP. Complications and long-term results of ankle arthrodesis following trauma. J Bone Joint Surg Am 1980;62A: 777–784.
10. Myerson MS, Alvarez RG, Lam PWC. Tibiocalcaneal arthrodesis for the management of severe ankle and hindfoot deformities. Foot Ankle Int 2000;21:643–644.
11. Papa JA, Myerson MS. Pantalar and tibiotalar calcaneal arthrodesis for post-traumatic osteoarthritis of the ankle and hindfoot. J Bone Joint Surg Am 1992;74A:1042–1049.
12. Raikin SM, Myerson MS. A technique for harvesting bone graft for arthrodesis about the ankle. Foot Ankle Int 2000;21:778–779.

Chapter **83**

Tibiocalcaneal Arthrodesis Using Blade Plate Fixation

Richard Alvarez, Delan Gaines, and Mark E. Easley

DEFINITION

- Because of the increased life expectancy of diabetic patients, neuropathic arthropathy is becoming a more prevalent problem.
- Resulting severe ankle and hindfoot deformities frequently are non-braceable. Bearing weight on such deformities can result in abnormal ipsilateral stresses on the knee, leg, ankle, hindfoot, and forefoot, causing ligament laxity, stress fractures, and recurrent ulcerations leading to cellulitis, abscess, and osteomyelitis (**FIG 1**).
- Before the 1990s, efforts in the reconstruction of these deformities often resulted in a below-knee amputation.
- Reconstructive efforts have included pan-talar and tibiotalocalcaneal fusions. These required an intact talus, adequate vascularity, and no infection. The prevailing feeling was that a fusion through a Charcot joint was impossible. After 1990, new techniques evolved, starting with blade plate fusions and soon followed by rods and Ilizarov techniques. All are important methods of solving these complicated problems.
- Each has its place in treating severe hindfoot and ankle deformity; however, the blade plate offers immediate deformity correction, rigid fixation, and skin closure in patients with talar fragmentation, avascular necrosis, or resorption.
- An additional problem for which the blade plate can be helpful is simultaneous tibiotalar and subtalar traumatic arthritis, frequently caused by talar fractures and untreated varus or valgus adult-acquired hindfoot problems.

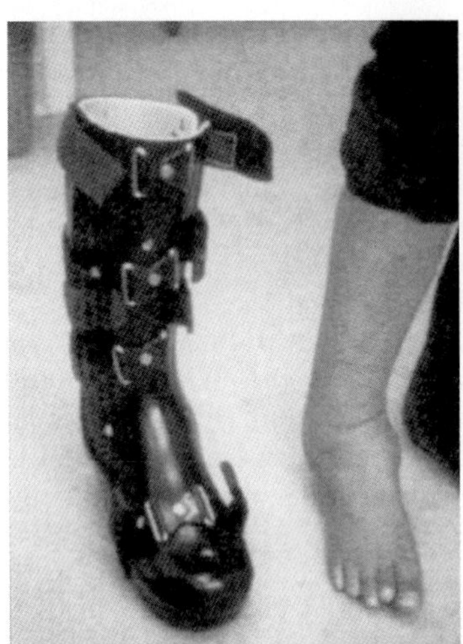

A

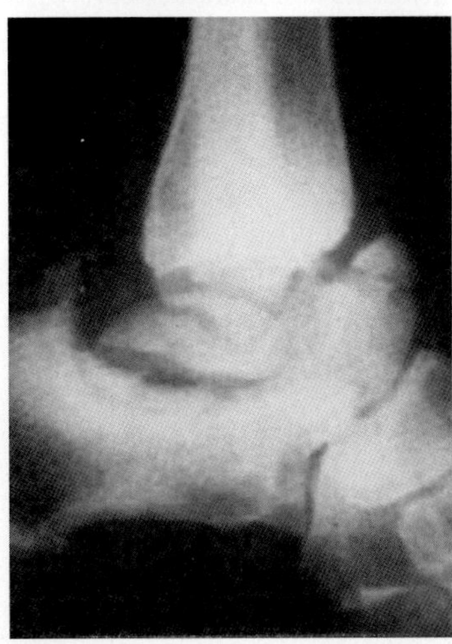

B

FIG 1 • **A.** Unbraceable Charcot ankle and hindfoot deformity, even with a Charcot retention orthotic walker (CROW). **B.** Lateral radiograph of Charcot neuroarthropathy of the ankle.

PATHOGENESIS

- Most commonly, the severe ankle and hindfoot deformity with talar fragmentation and resorption is seen in diabetic neuropathy. Other causes of Charcot arthropathy include tabes dorsalis, Hansen disease, syringomyelia, alcoholic neuropathy, Charcot-Marie-Tooth disease, lumbar radiculopathy, peripheral nerve lesions, Riley-Day syndrome, renal dialysis, congenital insensitivity to pain, and intra-articular steroid injections. Similar changes on radiographs can be seen in inflammatory arthritis, and in posttraumatic arthritis with talar avascular necrosis (**FIG 2**).
- Although the exact mechanism of neuropathic arthropathy is unknown, the presence of peripheral neuropathy (autonomic, sensory, and motor) is required.
- The sympathetic nerves supply the small vessels, sweat glands, sebaceous glands, and the erector pilae muscles of the hair follicles. The deficit of autonomic nervous system nerves results in the dry, flaky, warm skin with decreased skin appendages. However, more importantly, the loss of vasomotor tone produces a dramatic increase in the peripheral circulation, with the same effect as a surgical sympathectomy: warmth, vasodilation, and increased blood flow through the involved extremity.
- In the past, medical teaching was that complete anesthesia of the feet and/or legs had to be present for the Charcot joint and ulcerations to occur. However, patients frequently retain some sensation. Sensory neuropathy includes both skin sensations (eg, touch, pain, pressure) and proprioception. Decreased proprioception results in balance and gait difficulties that potentially result in injury from falls or missed steps. These injuries can include wounds, ligament injuries, and fractures. Because of the decreased sensation, injuries can be perceived as minor by patient, doctor, and podiatrist. However, for the diabetic patient, in the face of continued pain and swelling, a Charcot joint should be considered.
- Motor neuropathy involves weakness of extrinsic and intrinsic muscles of the leg and foot. The relative disproportionally stronger plantarflexors of the ankle (greater cross-sectional area than anterior muscles) inevitably lead to a tight heel cord. Abnormal stresses of a tight heel cord predispose the foot both to neuropathic ulcers, specifically under the interphalangeal

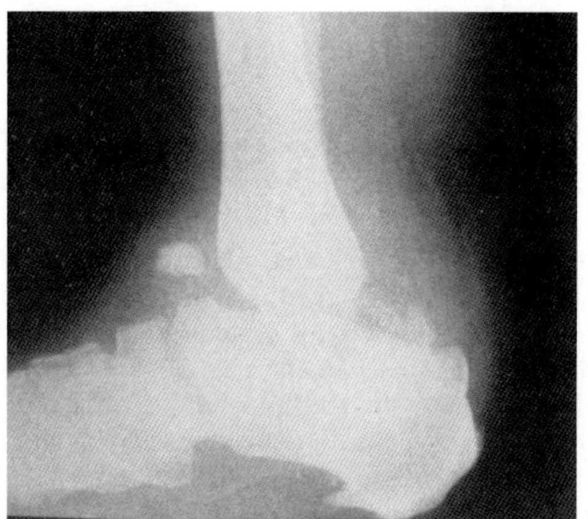

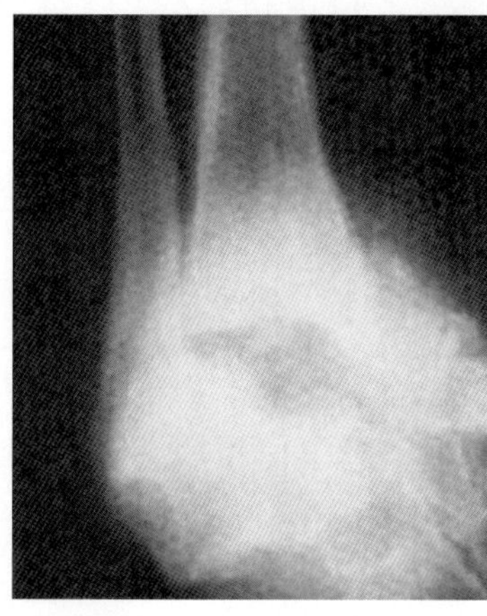

FIG 2 • **A**. Second example of lateral radiograph of Charcot neuroarthropathy of the ankle. **B**. AP radiograph of Charcot neuroarthropathy of the ankle.

joint of the great toe, first metatarsal head, and fifth metatarsal heads, and to tarsometatarsal, Chopart, or hindfoot collapse.

- In the hindfoot, the tight heel cord is also responsible for increased stress on the talus, by not allowing normal rotation of the tibia over the talus. The tibia, instead of rotating over the talus, crushes down into the talar body, fragmenting the talus by the so-called nutcracker effect. This devastating deformity is usually not braceable and often includes a large ulcer at the tip of the medial malleolus (**FIG 3**).

NATURAL HISTORY

- Eichenholtz described three stages of development for the Charcot joint, and to this Shibata added the stage 0.
  - Stage 0 (Shibata): Clinical signs of pain or swelling similar to what is seen in ankle and midfoot sprains. An overuse-type syndrome or minor fracture may preclude stage I. The presence of calcified vessels on a radiograph should arouse suspicion.
  - Stage I: In this "fragmentation" stage, clinically the joint appears hot, red, and swollen. Fragmentation, dissolution, or dislocation can appear on radiographs.
  - Stage II: The "coalescence" stage begins the reparative process with reduction of clinical signs. There may be residual inflammation, but without the severe warmth and edema. New bone formation appears on radiographs.
  - Stage III: In the "consolidation" stage the joint usually heals enlarged and deformed. Skin temperature and edema eventually decrease to normal. Radiographs show sclerotic bone formation with smoothing of fracture fragments, and fibrous ankylosis. The fixed deformity is usually associated with bony prominences. In the hindfoot, the patient may walk on the medial malleolus.

PATIENT HISTORY AND PHYSICAL FINDINGS

- Most cases of neuropathic arthropathy occur in patients with type 2 diabetes mellitus. Typically, the patients are obese, and many do not realize they have diabetes mellitus. Ten percent of these newly diagnosed patients will already have peripheral vascular disease, cardiovascular disease, cerebrovascular disease, and retinopathy. Many who are aware of their diabetes maintain poor control of their glucose level due to lack of information or lack of compliance.
- The diabetic with peripheral neuropathy typically has dry, flaky, hairless skin distally. The extremity may exhibit swelling, redness, and warmth. Patients complain of dysesthesia (eg, stinging, burning, cramping) rather than anesthesia. Stage 0 patients may complain of sprain-type pain and deep joint or deep bone pain, with or without a clear history of injury. Early, there may be little if any swelling. Later, as stage I approaches, swelling occurs. As the peripheral motor neuropathy progresses, Achilles contracture occurs. The appearance of a high arch in the foot actually may represent intrinsic muscle wasting. Early on before collapse occurs, the foot appearance is similar to that seen in Charcot-Marie-Tooth disease. Pulses in the extremity are usually present (**FIG 4**).

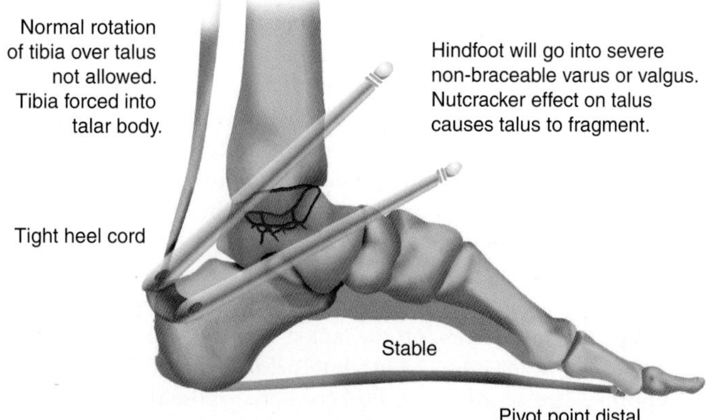

FIG 3 • "Nutcracker effect" theorized to lead to talar fragmentation in Charcot neuroarthropathy.

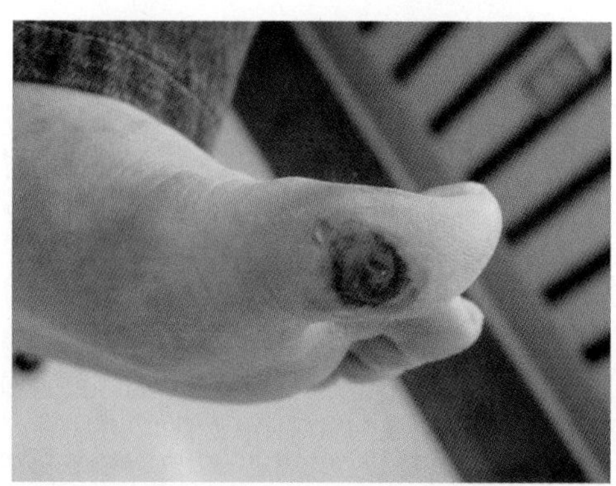

FIG 4 • Clinical picture of a diabetic foot ulcer.

- The examiner must rule out infection, especially in a patient with ulceration where deep infection (ie, abscess or osteomyelitis) must be considered. When in doubt, the physician should look at the patient: patients with osteomyelitis look and feel sick. Typically, if a Charcot extremity is elevated above the patient's heart, there is a decrease in redness and swelling after about 10 to 15 minutes (Brodsky test) compared with the infected extremity, which will remain unchanged. If there is no break in skin integrity, infection is unlikely.
- The physical examination should include:
  - A comprehensive neurologic evaluation using Semmes-Weinstein monofilament test, which indicates protective sensation
  - A vascular examination: Palpating pulses may be challenging with deformity. The threshold should be low to use a Doppler ultrasound or obtain noninvasive vascular studies.
  - Skin condition examination: The skin should be in satisfactory condition, to allow deformity correction. Even with complete or partial talectomy, correcting severe valgus deformity via lateral approach is risky. If the skin is suspect in valgus deformity and the heel is realigned, then skin perfusion may be compromised.

IMAGING AND OTHER DIAGNOSTIC STUDIES

- Radiographs showing calcified vessels may be an early warning of impending neuropathic problems. In fact, the surgeon must beware of a routine ankle fracture that has undergone an open reduction and internal fixation if calcified vessels are present on the radiograph. Often, the fracture falls apart and metal breaks with early range of motion and weight bearing. It is best to treat these two to three times longer with non-weight bearing and immobilization (**FIG 5**).
- Often, Charcot joints are confused with infection. Monitoring systemic clinical and laboratory markers of infection is important. However, a bone biopsy with a large-bore needle under fluoroscopy can quickly rule out osteomyelitis.

DIFFERENTIAL DIAGNOSIS

- Posttraumatic arthritis
- Inflammatory arthritides
- Charcot neuroarthropathy

NONOPERATIVE MANAGEMENT

- Goals of treatment are to achieve the third stage of bony healing, with as little resultant deformity as possible, and to minimize and treat soft tissue breakdown and ulcerations.

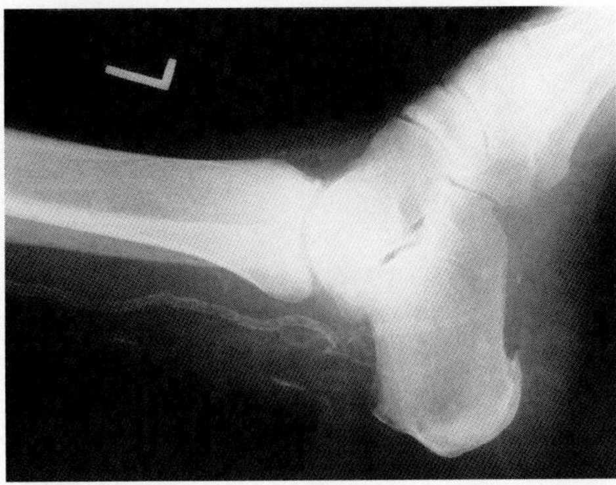

FIG 5 • Calcified vessels commonly seen radiographically in diabetics.

- A high index of suspicion is necessary to initiate treatment while the patient is still in stage 0. Patient compliance may be an issue. Risk factors for noncompliance include age, obesity, poor proprioception, and debilitation.
- The Charcot joint should be immobilized and elevated to reduce swelling. No weight bearing should be allowed until swelling and redness are resolved. The gold standard is total-contact casting (TCC) that should be changed weekly until stage III is reached. A Charcot rehabilitation orthotic walker (CROW) can be used once the limb is in stage II. At stage III, a custom ankle–foot orthosis (AFO) accommodates the resultant deformity.
- However, if the deformity is great, it may not be braceable. The brace may cause more soft tissue breakdown. Surgery becomes necessary to make the extremity braceable. The amount of talar body fragmentation and resorption with ensuing varus or valgus varies. Ulceration at the tip of the medial malleolus or lateral malleolus warrants a trial of nonoperative CROW bracing or TCC. Ideally, if wound healing can be accomplished and maintained, nonoperative management can be continued for the hindfoot. This most likely will be a CROW or molded solid ankle bivalved open AFO and a rocker shoe. However, most of these deformities are so severe that salvage surgery becomes necessary in an effort to save the extremity.

SURGICAL MANAGEMENT

- The surgical goal of correcting the alignment to make the foot and leg braceable can be achieved with a fibrous union, although bony union is preferable.
- There are four indications:
  - Non-braceable deformity
  - Chronic ulceration secondary to pressure from deformity not responding to bracing
  - Adequate circulation (usually not a problem)
  - Alternative to amputation

Preoperative Planning

- Patients must commit to 5 to 8 months of non–weight-bearing and must understand that complications can occur, such as incomplete healing, infection, hardware failure, and loss of correction. Amputation must be accepted as a possible consequence of failure of the procedure. Medical clearance should be obtained from the patient's internist or diabetologist. Emphasis should be that the patient must have strict control of blood glucose both preoperatively and in the postoperative healing period. Nutrition is, therefore, important.
- If there is a question of adequate circulation, even if pulses are present, a toe-level Doppler index or transcutaneous oxygen index at the first web space should be obtained; a reading greater than 0.45 predicts a 96% healing rate. Successful revascularization by a vascular surgeon may be necessary to reach the appropriate pressure.
- The presence of an ulcer is not a contradiction to this salvage as long as it is clean. If there is a question of infection, joint aspiration and talar biopsy should be acquired before proceeding.
- Absolute contraindications to hindfoot salvage include a patient who smokes, a patient who cannot comply with postoperative recommendations, or the presence of a deep abscess or osteomyelitis. A good indicator of patient compliance can be obtained during preoperative immobilization in a non–weight-bearing cast or CROW.

Positioning

- The patient is placed in the lateral decubitus position with operative side up. Imaging should be checked to ensure the ability to obtain AP and lateral views of the ankle and an axial view of the hindfoot.
- The skin is prepared with tincture of iodine and alcohol solution, as Betadine paint prevents Tegaderm from sticking and effectively marking the skin incision.
- The extremity is draped above the knee. The surgeon must make sure that the anterior superior iliac spine can be palpated through the drapes.
- Ulcers are covered with Tegaderm to isolate them from the rest of the surgical field (**FIG 6**).

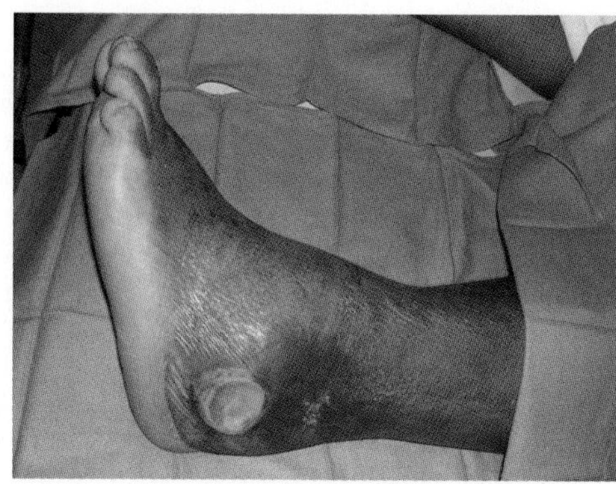

FIG 6 • Ulceration over the lateral malleolus in a neuropathic patient.

TECHNIQUES

INCISION

- Make a curvilinear incision over the distal 14 cm of the fibula and extend the incision over the lateral calcaneus, curving anterior.
- Try to incorporate previous incisions when possible if they are less than 2 years old.
- Developing a full-thickness soft tissue flap and retracting with skin hooks are particularly important in this patient population.
  - In patients with neuropathy, sacrificing the sural nerve as it crosses the field helps avoid excessive dissection and skin retraction.
  - A longer incision can be made to reduce skin retraction forces.
- Strip only the amount of periosteum needed to expose bone for cuts and fixation (**TECH FIG 1**).

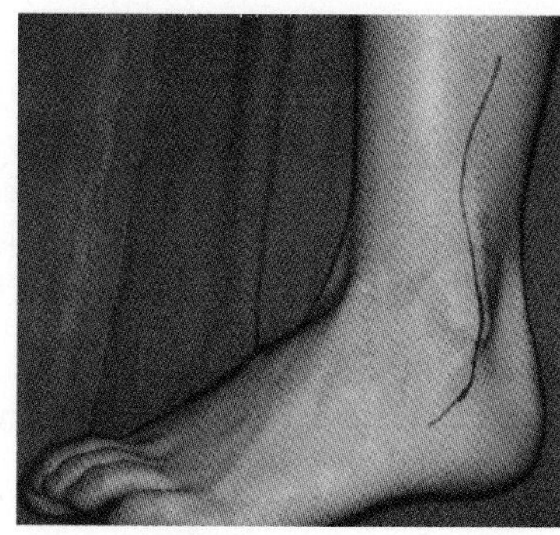

TECH FIG 1 • Our preferred lateral approach to the ankle and subtalar joints.

BONY EXCISION

- Once the fibula is exposed, the distal 10 to 14 cm of fibula may be excised using an oscillating saw. The fibula will serve as autograft. Take care to avoid damaging the perforating peroneal or anterior tibial arteries during the dissection.
- Excise the remaining talar body fragments. Preserve the remaining talar head and neck (**TECH FIG 2**).

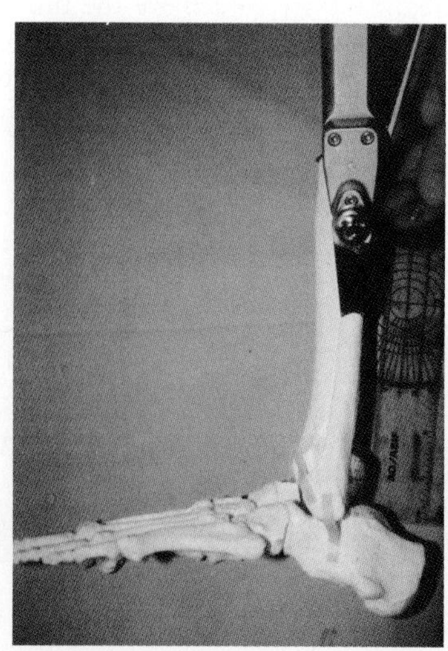

TECH FIG 2 • Sawbones model demonstrating routine fibular resection.

BONE GRAFT PREPARATION

- If the fibula is associated with any ulcerations, autograft from other sites or allograft can be used.
- Use a bone mill to morselize the fibula to 4-mm pieces.
  - If necessary, the autograft harvested from the fibula can be mixed with 4-mm cancellous chips.
- Combine the autograft and allograft combination with tobramycin (400 mg) and vancomycin (500 mg) powder.
- The antibiotic bone graft mixture is to be packed between the bony surfaces and to the anterior, posterior, medial, and lateral aspects of the tibia and calcaneus to facilitate an extra-articular fusion in addition to the intra-articular fusion.
- Tobramycin and vancomycin levels are not drawn as they do not reach systemic therapeutic levels (**TECH FIG 3**).

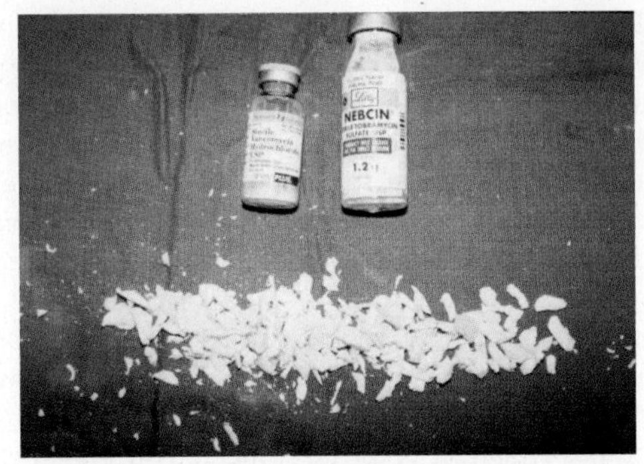

TECH FIG 3 • Our routine allograft bone for tibiocalcaneal arthrodesis. Note the addition of antibiotic powder to the graft (we typically use vancomycin and tobramycin).

PREPARING ARTICULAR SURFACES

- Drennen's principles for fusing neuropathic joints
  - Remove all cartilage and debris.
  - Remove all sclerotic bone down to bleeding, well-vascularized bone.
  - Fashion congruent surfaces for apposition.
  - Rigid fixation
  - Complete débridement of all synovial and scar tissue
- Cut the distal tibial surface flat with an oscillating saw and contour it with a large burr. Take care to maintain as much length as possible. The medial malleolus can be denuded of articular cartilage with a curette and a burr (**TECH FIG 4**).
- The anterior tibia will sit against the remaining talar neck and head. It can be slightly flattened with a saw or burr. Denude the calcaneus articular surfaces of cartilage, maintaining as much subchondral bone as possible. The posterior facet may need slight flattening so the tibia will sit stable on the calcaneus with the anterior tibia resting against the talar neck.
- Drill surfaces with a 3.2-mm bit to make holes in the subchondral bone of the calcaneus, the neck of the talus, the anterior tibia, and the pilon to provide channels for revascularization. Surfaces should be stable but not necessarily flat, as gaps can be filled with bone graft.

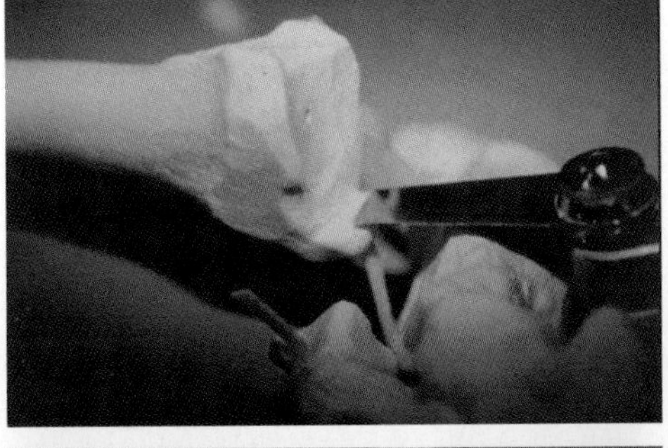

A

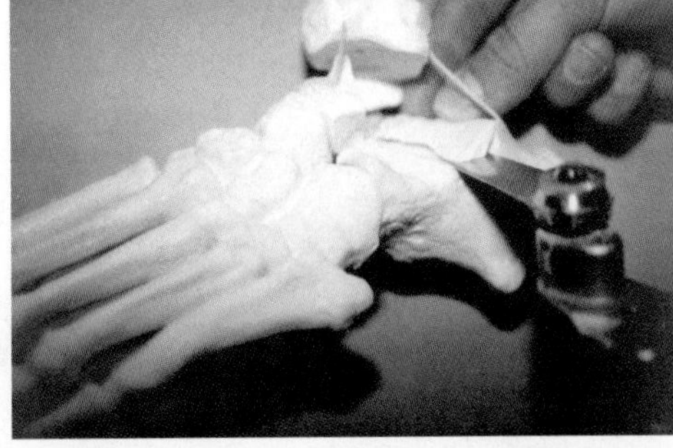

B

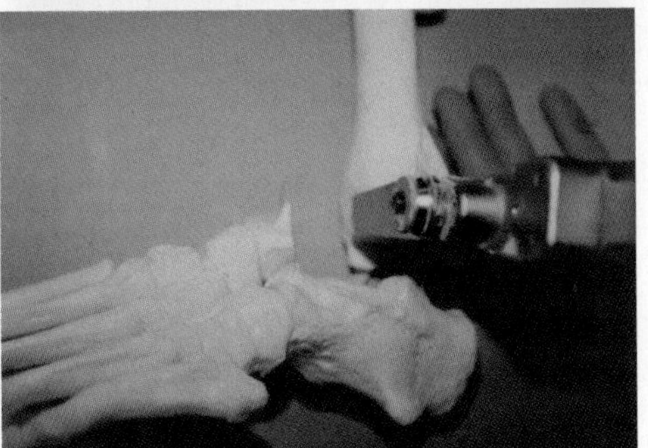

C

TECH FIG 4 • Sawbones model demonstrating preparation of the arthrodesis site. **A.** Tibial plafond preparation, including medial malleolus. **B.** Calcaneal preparation. **C.** Preparation of the anterior tibia to include an arthrodesis to residual talar head and neck.

STABILIZATION

- The deformity should be reduced so that the tibia sits flat on the calcaneus and the talar neck is flush to the anterior tibia. The foot should be plantigrade, at 90 degrees with respect to the leg and aligned with respect to the anterior superior iliac spine, anterior tibia tubercle, and second toe. The hindfoot should be placed in 5 degrees of valgus, with 5 to 10 degrees of external rotation of the foot.
- Use AO guide pins to hold the reduction. Place one 2.8-mm guide pin from the anterior distal tibial metaphysis into the posterior calcaneus. Place one 2.8-mm guide pin from the posterolateral distal tibial metaphysis into the talar head and neck. This pin may be advanced into the navicular if more purchase is needed. The pins serve as guides for 7.3-mm AO screws once the plate is fixed.
- Preparing for placement of the pediatric AO condylar blade plate
  - Place a pediatric blade plate laterally on the calcaneus near the posterior facet in line with the tibia. To do this, select the entry point for the blade plate at the junction of the lower and middle thirds of the calcaneus, at least 1 cm above the plantar cortex of the calcaneus.
  - Although rarely needed, the plate can be contoured to the lateral tibia with the table plate bender.
  - The 95-degree-angled pediatric condylar blade plate (PCBP) has a blade with a T profile.
  - The plate portion has varying lengths depending on the length needed to span. We have selected the five-hole plate with a 40-mm blade to traverse the width of the calcaneus. A longer plate may be necessary in fusions where the talus body is preserved (ankle and subtalar fusions) (TECH FIG 5A).
- Hold the alignment of the tibia on the calcaneus and the anterior tibia on the neck of the talus with the 2.8-mm guide pins for the cannulated 6.5- or 7.3-mm screws. Select an area at the lateral calcaneus at the junction of the middle and distal thirds, no less than 1 cm above the plantar cortex of the calcaneus and in line with the lateral tibia shaft. It is important that the plantar cortex of the calcaneus remain intact.
- Before the angled blade plate can be inserted into bone, a channel must be precut with the T profile seating chisel for the PCBP.
  - To do this, slide the base of the condylar blade guide (this subtends an angle of 85 degrees for the 95-degree angle of the PCBP) in the slot above the triple drill guide. Place this so that the 85-degree-angled plate guide portion of the condylar blade guide aligns with the tibia and the three-hole drill guide sets at the lateral calcaneus preselected entry point for the blade.
  - Drill three holes with the 4.5-mm drill bit no more than 1 cm deep.
  - Use a router or rongeur to convert the drill holes into a slit.
  - To receive the shoulder of the PCBP, bevel the slit hole proximally a few millimeters. This prevents shattering of the lateral calcaneal cortex.
- To cut the channel into the calcaneus, slide the seating chisel into the slot of the seating chisel guide with the adjustable flap to go proximally and the T profile

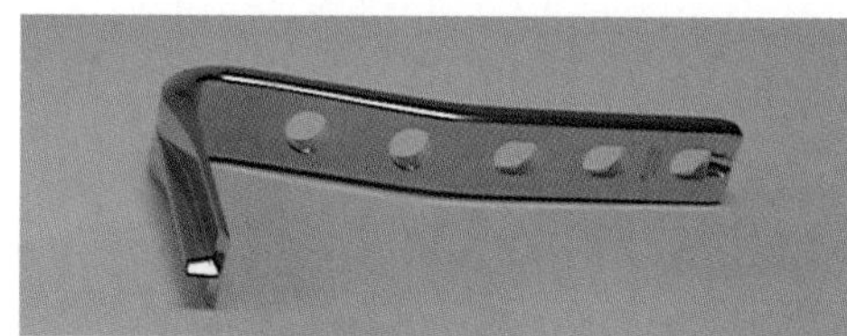
A

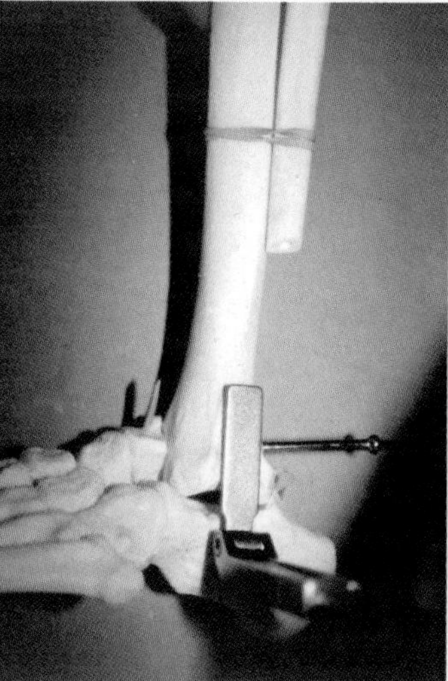
B

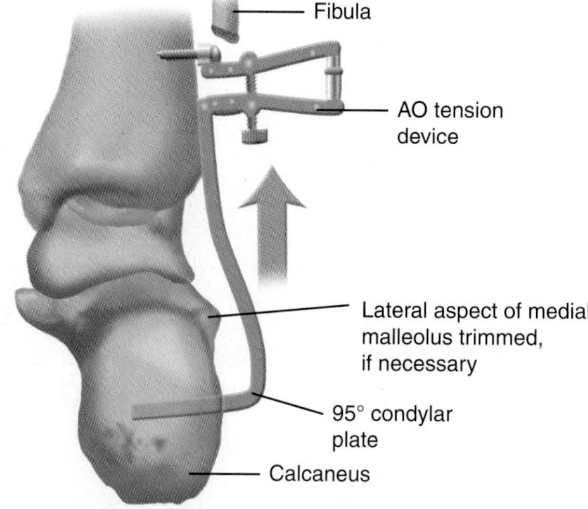

C

TECH FIG 5 • **A.** Typical fixed-angle blade plate used for tibiocalcaneal arthrodesis. **B.** Chisel used to create slot in calcaneus to insert blade plate. **C.** Compression device for the laterally applied blade plate. *(continued)*

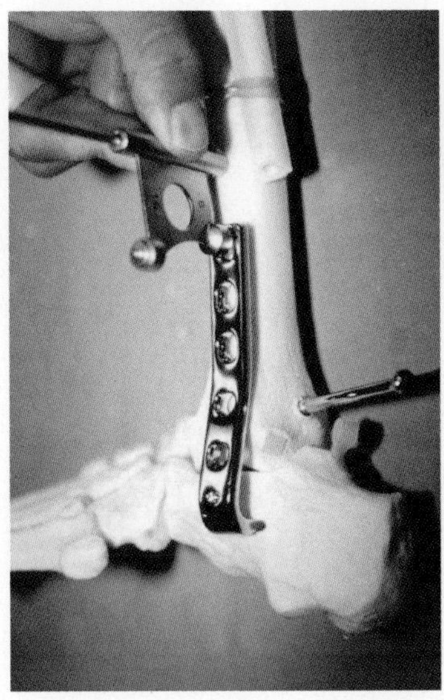

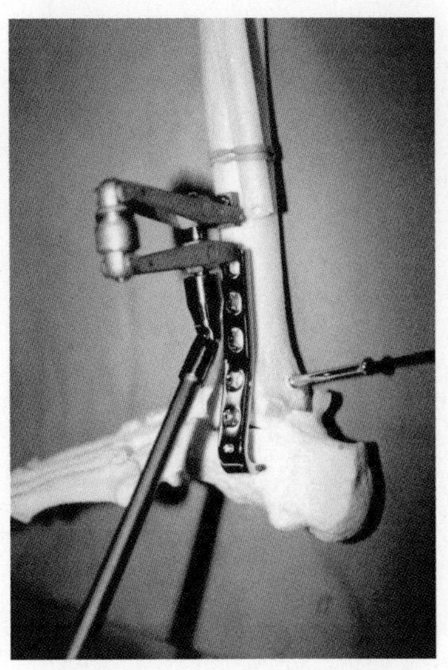

TECH FIG 5 • *(continued)* **D, E.** Compression device. **D.** Initial alignment guide for the compression device. **E.** Compression device in place.

distally toward the plantar calcaneus. The angle between the flap and the body of the seating chisel guide may be set with a triangular guide on the PCBP and maintained by tightening the screw with a screwdriver (TECH FIG 5B).

- This angle should be 85 degrees for the 95-degree PCBP (remember, this subtends an angle of 95 degrees with the tibia shaft). Now align the flap with the tibia and the chisel in the slot. The flap should align flat with the lateral tibia and the chisel handle 90 degrees to the lateral wall of the calcaneus (TECH FIG 5C).
- Hammer the chisel several centimeters and withdraw until the medial cortex is penetrated.
  - Using the plate holder, insert the PCBP into the precut channel to within 5 mm.
  - Remove the plate holder and use the impactor to drive and seat the plate into the bone.
- At this point, bone graft can be added to fill voids between the tibia and calcaneus and the anterior tibia and neck of the talus.
- Fix the articulated tension device to the tibia shaft and apply axial tension to mid-green.
  - Avoid overcompression with the tension device so that the calcaneus is not pulled into too much valgus. Compression can also be achieved with the plate's dynamic compression holes.
  - Fix the plate to the tibia with 4.5-mm cortical screws (6.5-mm cancellous screws may be needed in the distal tibia depending on screw purchase).
  - Use the previously placed 2.8-mm guide pins for placing 6.5- or 7.3-mm screws for the anterior tibia into the neck and head of the talus (navicular for more purchase).
  - A screw is placed from the anterior tibia into the talar calcaneus for a more rigid construct (TECH FIG 5D,E).

FIXATION

- Finally, use the guide pins to place a 6.5- or 7.3-mm cannulated cancellous screw from the posterior tibia into the head of the talus to increase rigid fixation and further control rotation and from the anterior tibia into the tuberosity of the calcaneus (TECH FIG 6).

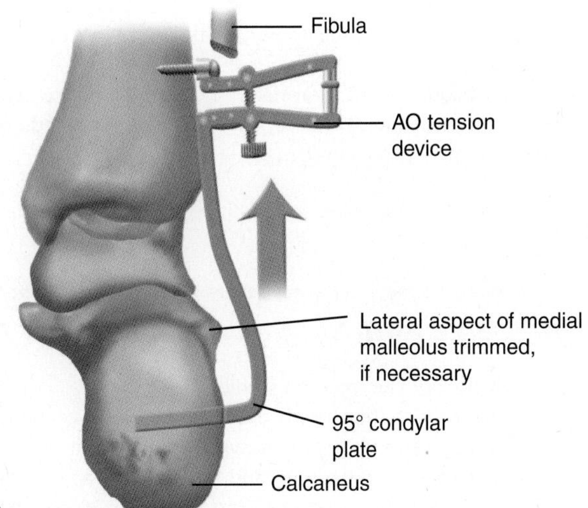

TECH FIG 6 • **A.** Blade plate and screw fixation construct for tibiocalcaneal arthrodesis. *(continued)*

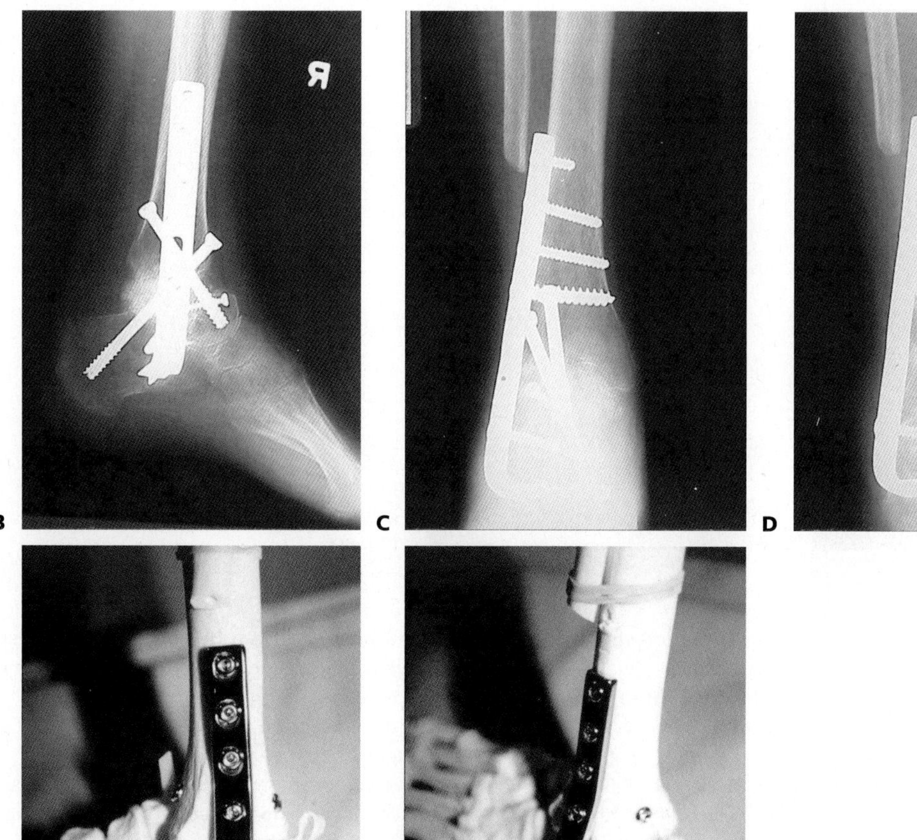

TECH FIG 6 • *(continued)* **B–D.** Postoperative radiographs of tibiocalcaneal arthrodesis. **B.** Lateral view. **C.** AP view. **D.** Mortise view. **E, F.** Sawbones model with blade plate in optimal position.

CLOSURE

- Close the wound in layers with 2-0 and 3-0 absorbable sutures.
- The skin may be closed loosely with 4-0 nylon or skin staples.
- If skin closure is tight, peroneal tendons may be excised to facilitate closure. However, with a curvilinear incision this will rarely be needed.
- The wound is dressed with Adaptic soaked in Betadine solution followed by fluff gauze and a well-padded cast applied from the tips of the toes to the tibial tubercle.

TIBIOCALCANEAL ARTHRODESIS (COURTESY OF MARK E. EASLEY, MD)

- Patient history and imaging studies
  - 60-year-old patient with avascular necrosis of talus and a 2-year history of pain with weight bearing
  - Walks with a severe limp and has failed bracing, including patellar-tendon bearing brace (TECH FIG 7A)
- Imaging studies
  - Initial review of AP and lateral radiographs suggests that talar anatomy is relatively well preserved; however, closer inspection of AP radiograph demonstrates some potential lucency/irregularity in

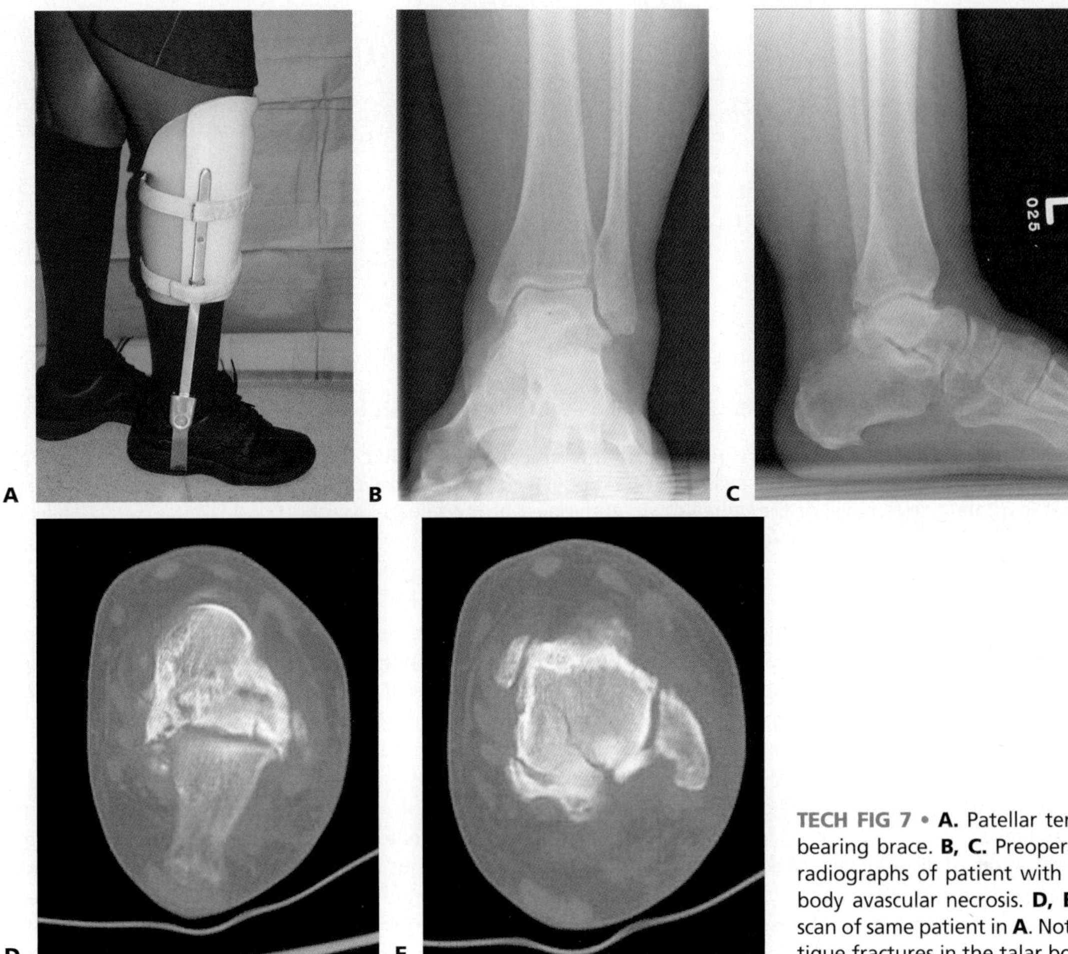

TECH FIG 7 • **A.** Patellar tendon bearing brace. **B, C.** Preoperative radiographs of patient with talar body avascular necrosis. **D, E.** CT scan of same patient in **A**. Note fatigue fractures in the talar body.

talar body, and lateral radiograph reveals some talar body collapse and subtalar incongruity (TECH FIG 7B,C).
    - CT scan shows fatigue fractures through avascular talar body (TECH FIG 7D,E).
- Positioning and surgical approach
    - Patient in lateral decubitus position, supported with a beanbag
    - Lateral transfibular approach
    - Fibula may be sacrificed and used as a bone graft in these patients since they are generally not candidates for total ankle arthroplasty, so fibular preservation is not critical.
    - Exposure of lateral ankle and subtalar joints. Note the fragmentation of the inferior surface of the talar body (TECH FIG 8).
- Extraction of residual talar body
    - It is always a difficult decision to extract a talar body, especially when the anatomy is relatively well preserved, at least on initial inspection.
    - However, this talar body was completely avascular. Note the unhealthy appearance of the talar body (TECH FIG 9A).
    - The talar body is extracted from the joint, in this case using a chisel. Note the fracture in the medial aspect of the talus that was revealed when the avascular lateral portion of talus is removed (TECH FIG 9B,C).
- Tibial, talar head, and calcaneal preparation
    - In addition to comprehensive removal of residual tibial plafond cartilage and penetration of the subchondral bone:
        - Prepare the anterior distal tibia to promote healing of the viable talar head to the distal anterior tibia (TECH FIG 10A).
        - Likewise, the talar neck must be prepared to promote fusion to the tibia.

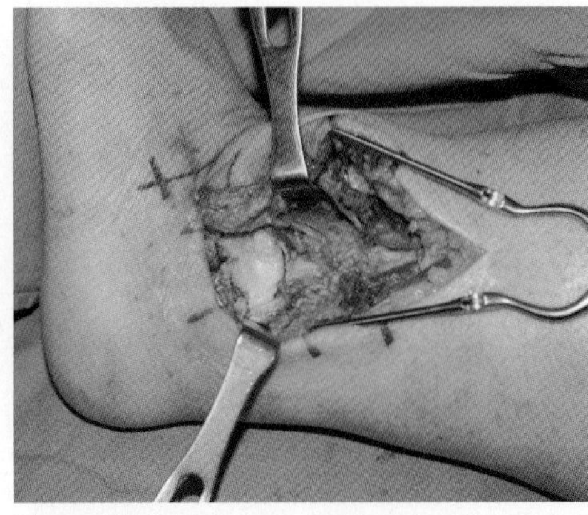

TECH FIG 8 • Lateral approach to ankle and subtalar joint after distal fibular resection.

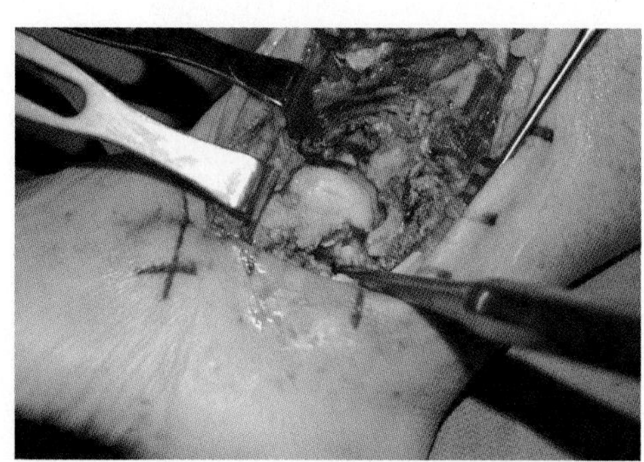

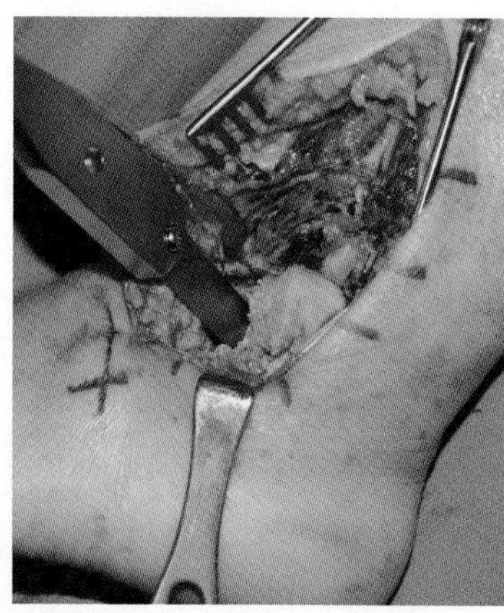

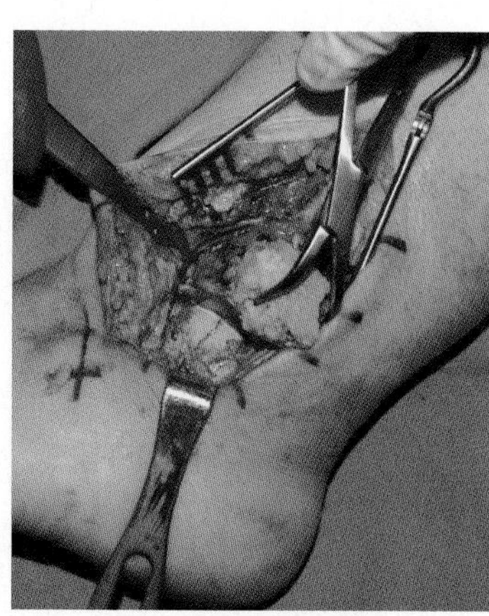

TECH FIG 9 • A. Avascular necrosis of the talar body. Note the unhealthy bone that is easily excavated from the inferolateral aspect of the talar body. **B, C.** Removal of the avascular talar body. **B.** Use of a chisel. **C.** Note the fatigue fracture in the medial talar dome that is visible with removal of the unhealthy lateral aspect of the talus.

  - In our experience, a medial malleolar osteotomy is necessary to allow the tibia to collapse to the calcaneal posterior facet. Even if structural autograft or allograft is introduced, then some of the medial malleolus should be scalloped out to allow better positioning of the allograft (TECH FIG 10B).
  - Finally, the posterior facet of the calcaneus must also be prepared.
  - Some degree of distal tibial and dorsal calcaneal contouring is necessary to optimize the match of these two noncongruent surfaces. Morselized fibular bone graft and cancellous allograft chips serve to fill any voids, but some contact between the tibia and the calcaneus or between the tibia, structural graft, and calcaneus is necessary.
- Initial positioning and provisional fixation
  - Alignment
    - Neutral dorsiflexion–plantarflexion, with a plantigrade foot
    - Slight heel valgus. If slight (physiologic) heel valgus is to be achieved and the lateral blade plate is compressed, then we recommend initially setting the heel in neutral position so that when compression is applied, the heel then aligns into slight valgus. If the heel is initially set in physiologic valgus and compression is placed on the lateral plate, then excessive heel valgus will result.
    - Rotation. Ideally, rotation is equal to that of the contralateral extremity. Internal rotation must be avoided, but likewise, excessive external rotation is not well tolerated. Since the extremity will tend to be slightly shorter than the contralateral leg, aligning the second ray of the foot with the anterior tibial crest is appropriate and allows for adequate clearance with a heel-to-toe gait.
    - Sagittal plane position. We ensure that the talar head and neck contacts the prepared anterior distal tibia. A foot forwardness position must be avoided; the majority of the calcaneus and all of the calcaneal tuberosity should be posterior to the tibia. Otherwise, the foot will be too anterior, necessitating that the patient vault over the foot to ambulate, which creates considerable mechanical disadvantage.

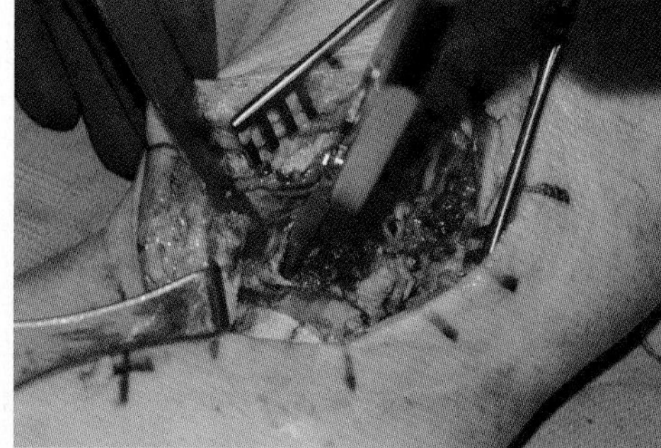

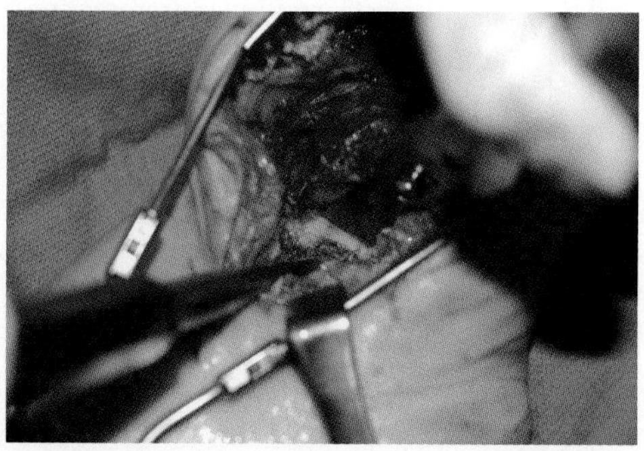

TECH FIG 10 • A. Preparation of the anterior distal tibia to promote fusion between the distal tibia and the head and neck of the residual talus. **B.** Partial resection of the medial malleolus to facilitate bony apposition of the tibia and calcaneus and potentially improve the position of a structural graft if it were used.

- Provisional fixation
  - Once this alignment is achieved, the construct should be provisionally pinned. Often a guide pin from the calcaneus to the anterior tibia that will then serve as the trajectory for one of the permanent screws is ideal. Also, an axial pin from the plantar calcaneus into the tibia is effective; however, it may interfere with the blade of the blade plate.
- Fluoroscopic confirmation
  - Be sure the position is confirmed in all planes and that bony contact is satisfactory at the arthrodesis site or sites.
- Bone graft
  - At this point, before permanent fixation and compression, we routinely add bone graft to fill any voids at the arthrodesis site.

- Permanent fixation
  - Positioning the blade plate
    - Since the blade plate is a fixed-angle device, we routinely place it backwards on the lateral tibia and calcaneus (**TECH FIG 11A–C**).
    - There is often a ridge of bone on the lateral tibia at the former incisura; this bone needs to be resected.
    - Occasionally a small relief area needs to be created in the calcaneus for the blade to sit flush on the lateral calcaneus.
    - We attempt to preserve the peroneal tendons so that they still function on the midfoot, but if they interfere, then they may be transected without appreciation of functional deficit in tibiocalcaneal arthrodesis.
  - Provisionally pin the blade to the lateral tibia and talus.
    - Place the pins so that the blade is optimally positioned on the tibia and calcaneus and so that the blade can easily be removed, turned to the correct orientation, and impacted.
    - Obtain fluoroscopic confirmation that the blade will be in the optimal position, both in the lateral and AP planes (**TECH FIG 11D,E**).
  - Reverse the blade and impact it on the calcaneus, using the pins to guide the blade into the optimal position.
  - Once fully seated, remove the guide pins and apply compression.
    - If the heel was set in neutral to begin, then the heel will end up in physiologic valgus.

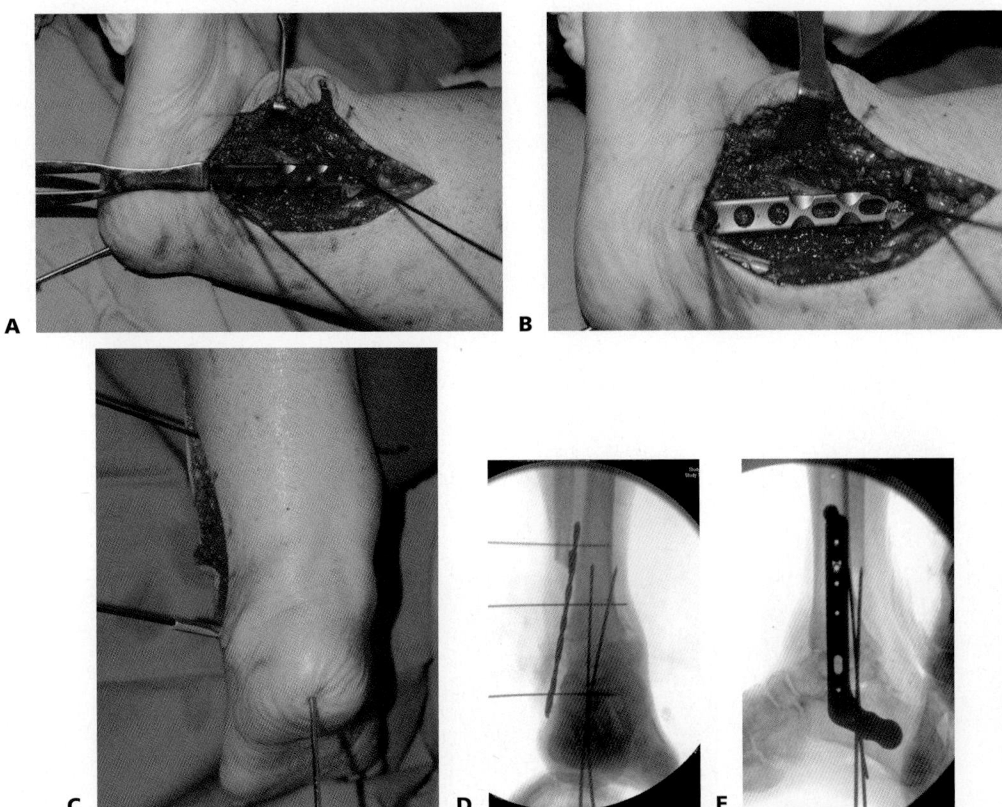

TECH FIG 11 • A–C. Fixed-angle blade plate placed backwards on the lateral tibia and talus to determine optimal position. **A.** Lateral view with perspective. Note the blade plate is placed backward to assess how well the plate fits, and note the guidewires to then guide the blade plate when it is turned around and impacted. **D, E.** Fluoroscopic views of an appropriately placed lateral tibiotalocalcaneal arthrodesis plate. This device has a locking mechanism to create a fixed-angle construct without a blade. **D.** AP view. Note appropriate contour of plate on lateral tibia and calcaneus. **E.** Lateral view. Note congruency of plate on lateral tibia and calcaneus. *(continued)*

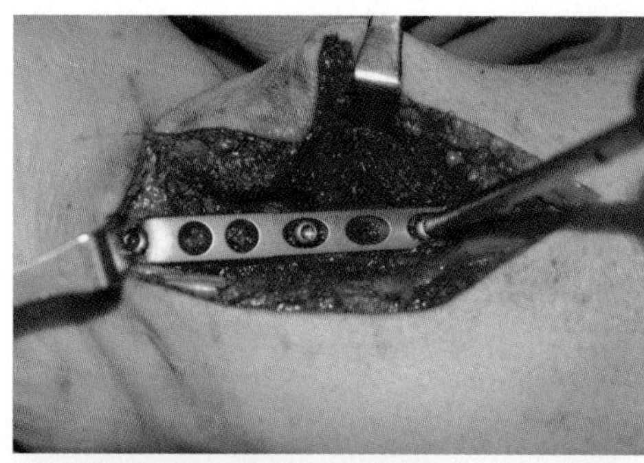

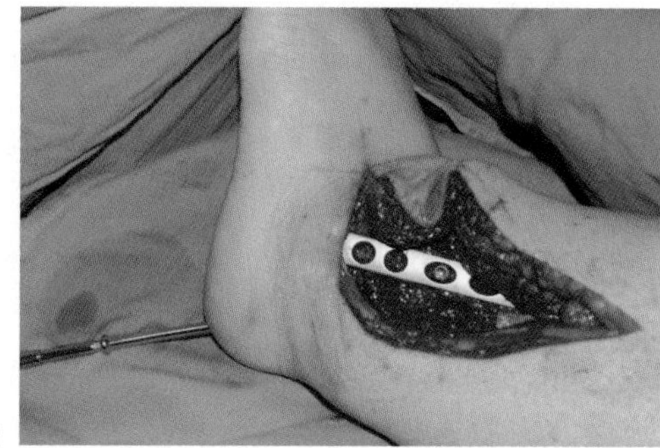

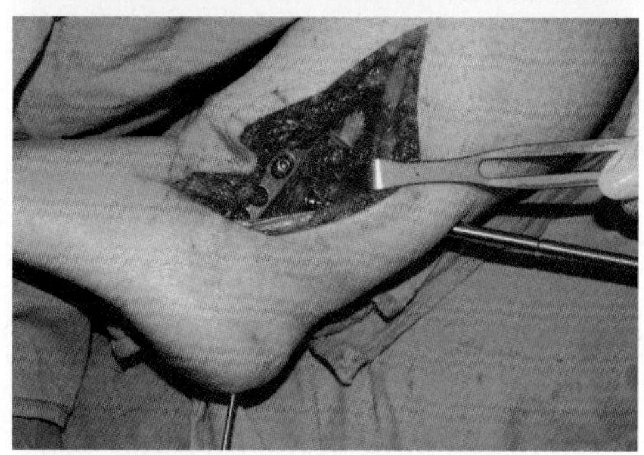

TECH FIG 11 • *(continued)* **F.** Lateral blade plate is impacted into lateral calcaneus, after compression is applied, with several proximal screws securing plate to lateral tibia. **G, H.** Supplemental fixation with cannulated screws. **G.** First screw from the calcaneal tuberosity to anterior tibia. **H.** Second screw from posterior tibia into talar head and neck to compress talar head and neck to prepared anterior distal tibial surface.

- Secure the plate to the tibia with several cortical or locking screws, depending on the implant used (TECH FIG 11F).
- We routinely augment the blade plate fixation with two screws.
  - One screw is directed from the plantar calcaneal tuberosity to the anterior tibia (TECH FIG 11G).
  - The second screw, from the posterior tibia to the center of the talar head, lags the talar head to the prepared anterior distal tibial surface (TECH FIG 11H). An AP view of the foot confirms that the guide pin is in the center of the talar head.
- Obtain fluoroscopic confirmation of the construct in the AP, mortise, and lateral planes.
  - Bone graft on the posterior tibia and calcaneus. In our opinion, one key to successful fusion is raising an osteoperiosteal flap on the posterior distal tibia and dorsal calcaneus and densely packing bone graft chips along the posterior construct, essentially creating a "flying buttress" effect.
- Follow-up (3 years)
  - Patient is ambulating comfortably without an assistive device; only a slight limp is appreciable.
  - She was issued a brace with a small lift but does not routinely wear it.
  - She is far more functional than preoperatively.
  - Radiographs demonstrate solid ankle and hindfoot fusion with near-physiologic alignment (TECH FIG 12).

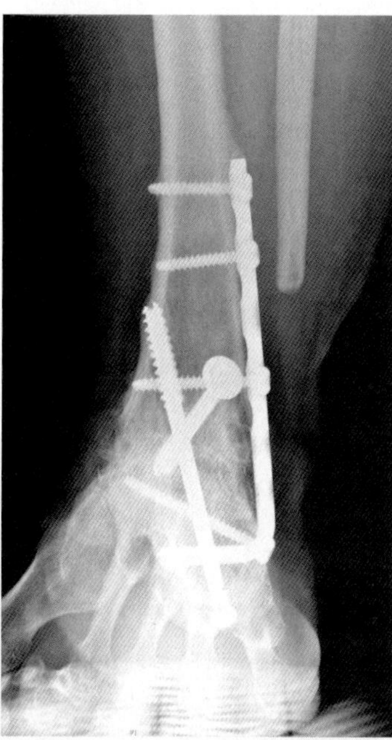

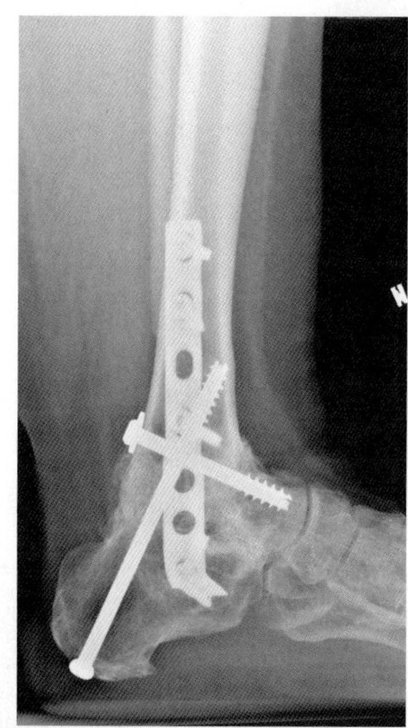

TECH FIG 12 • Final follow-up radiographs 3 years after procedure. **A.** AP view. **B.** Lateral view.

PEARLS AND PITFALLS

Arthrodesis of residual talar head and neck to the anterior distal tibia	▪ This will stabilize the construct and creates a more physiologic transition from fused hindfoot to supple midfoot.
Initial position with heel in neutral varus–valgus position	▪ If the heel is positioned in physiologic valgus before compression is applied through the blade plate, then excessive valgus will result.
Bone graft the posterior tibia and dorsal calcaneus	▪ Create an osteoperiosteal flap on the posterior distal tibia and dorsal calcaneus to densely pack bone graft that should incorporate to create a "flying buttress" of bone that greatly increases the surface area of the arthrodesis.
Avoid anterior translation of the foot relative to the tibia	▪ Be sure the foot is properly positioned under the tibia; if not, the lower extremity will be at a mechanical disadvantage.

POSTOPERATIVE CARE

- Intravenous antibiotics are continued for 2 to 3 days or until the patient is discharged.
- The cast should be changed first at 24 to 48 hours, then at 2- to 4-week intervals until the wound has healed.
- A CROW is used after this for non–weight-bearing immobilization for 4 to 6 months and weight bearing for 3 to 4 additional months and swelling has subsided.
  - Using a CROW instead of cast changes postoperatively allows patients to bathe around 2 to 4 weeks postoperatively.
  - Once the fusion is well healed, the patient may be changed to a bivalved AFO with a rocker sole.
- Weight bearing is started around the fourth to fifth month after there is radiographic evidence of healing of the fusion.
  - Starting at 25 pounds, weight is increased by 25 pounds at 1- to 2-week intervals.
  - Once 75% of the patient's weight is reached, full weight bearing is allowed in the CROW.
- Limb-length discrepancy can be corrected using a buildup for the rocker sole.
- A solid ankle cushion heel (SACH) can be added to dampen heel stride and simulate plantar fixation.
- The patient should be braced for life in a bivalved AFO that fits in a shoe.

OUTCOMES

- Fusion occurs in 93% of cases at an average of 16 weeks (range 12 to 18). Preoperative ulcerations heal after the precipitating deformity has been corrected.
- Tibial stress fractures occurring at the proximal end of the blade plate (the reason for bracing for life) can be prevented by placing the patient in a bivalved AFO. The anterior shell of the AFO prevents the moment or progression force of the tibia over the foot, thus reducing the chance of fracture.

REFERENCES

1. Alvarez RG. Chapter 12. Neuropathic joint: guidelines for treatment of great toe, midfoot, and hindfoot deformities. In: Pfeffer G, Frey C, eds. Current Practice in Foot and Ankle Surgery, Vol. 2. New York: McGraw-Hill, 1994:257–290.
2. Alvarez RG, Barbour TK, Perkins TD. Tibiocalcaneal arthrodesis for non-braceable neuropathic ankle deformity. Foot Ankle 1994;15: 354–359.
3. Alvarez RG, Trevino SG. Chapter 11. Treatment of the Charcot foot and ankle. In: Kelikian AS, ed. Operative Treatment of the Foot and Ankle. Stamford, CT: Appleton and Lange, 1999:147–177.
4. Brodsky JW. In: Coughlin MJ, Mann RA. Surgery of the Foot and Ankle, 7th ed. St. Louis: Mosby; 1999:895–969.
5. Brown MJ, Asbury AK. Diabetic neuropathy. Ann Neurol 1948;15: 2–12.
6. Cooper PS. Aplication of external fixators for management of Charcot deformities of the foot and ankle. Foot Ankle Clin 2002;7: 207–254.
7. Herbst SA. External fixation of Charcot arthropathy. Foot Ankle Clin 2004;9:595–609.
8. Johnson JE, Rudzki JR, Janisse E, et al. Hindfoot containment orthosis for management of bone and soft tissue defects of the heel. Foot Ankle Int 2005;26:198–203.
9. Logerfo FW, Coffman JD. Vascular and microvascular disease of the foot in diabetes. N Engl J Med 1984;311:1615–1618.
10. Orendurff MS, Sangeorzan B, Rohr E, et al. Ankle equinus has limited impact upon peak forefoot pressure during walking. Read at the Annual Meeting of the American Orthopaedic Foot and Ankle Society, July 14–17, 2005, Boston, MA.
11. Saltzman CL, Rashid R, Hayes A, et al. 4.5-gram monofilament sensation beneath both first metatarsal heads indicates protective foot sensation in diabetic patients. J Bone Joint Surg Am 2004;86A: 717–723.
12. Saltzman CL, Zimmerman MB, Holsworth RL, et al. Effect of initial weight-bearing in a total contact cast on healing of diabetic foot ulcers. J Bone Joint Surg Am 2004;86A:2714–2719.
13. Schon LC, Easley ME, Weinfeld SB. Charcot neuroarthropathy of the foot and ankle. Clin Orthop Relat Res 1998;349:116–131.
14. Texhammar R, Colton C. Angled Blade Plates and Instruments: AO/ASIF Instruments and Implants, 2nd ed. New York: Springer-Verlag, 1994:152–176.
15. Wagner FW. Transcutaneous Doppler ultrasound in the prediction of healing and the selection of surgical level for dysvascular lesions of the toes and forefoot. Clin Orthop Relat Res 1979;142: 110–114.
16. Wagner FW. The dysvascular foot. A system for diagnosis and treatment. Foot Ankle 1981;2:64–122.

Chapter 84 Treatment of Bone Loss, Avascular Necrosis, and Infection of the Talus With Circular Tensioned Wire Fixators

James J. Hutson Jr., Robert Rochman, and Oladapo Alade

DEFINITION

- Talus fractures are high-energy fractures that can have traumatic bone loss, avascular necrosis (AVN), and infected nonunion as the outcome of the injury.[1,3,16,23]
  - Acute talar bone loss and subsequent AVN and infection will present a cascade of hindfoot reconstruction problems (**FIG 1**).
  - Excision of the talus causes 3 to 4 cm of leg-length discrepancy (**FIG 2**). This defect can be reconstructed with internal fixation and bone grafting to maintain leg length.[17]
  - Traumatic loss of the talus or AVN is also treated with tibial calcaneal arthrodesis using internal fixation without reconstruction of leg length.[4,12,15,19]
  - Replacement of the traumatic extrusion of the talus has had a high level of infection in case studies.[6,16]
  - In recent case series, there has been success in reimplanting extruded talar body fractures without a high incidence of infection.[2,8,20]
  - If there is severe comminution of the talus, contamination from extrusion, infection, or a compromised soft tissue envelope, massive bone grafting and internal fixation would have a high risk of failure and infection. Half-pin fixators with a calcaneal tibial Steinmann pin have had a poor rate of arthrodesis.[18]
- Circular fixation provides an alternative to amputation in these complex cases.[5,10,11,22]
  - Because the pins and wires used in circular fixation are not in the zone of injury, a carefully débrided arthrodesis site can be compressed to achieve arthrodesis without foreign body internal fixation.
  - Wounds can heal by secondary intention over many weeks and the foot can be salvaged.
  - For patients with appropriate physiology, a proximal leg lengthening can be added to the reconstruction to equalize leg length.
  - The reconstructed extremity requires shoe modifications to improve gait.
  - With a well-aligned tibial calcaneal arthrodesis, the patient may participate in an active life without the problems and expense of a below-knee prosthesis.

ANATOMY

- The talus has precarious blood supply because approximately two thirds of the surface area is covered by articular cartilage.
- The ankle articulation, talar navicular joint and the three facets of the subtalar joint leave limited areas on the neck of the talus and inferior surface for penetration of blood vessels into the dense bone of the talus.
- The talus has no muscular attachments and is surrounded by the joint capsules of the multiple joints and a thin layer of soft tissue with bypassing tendons, vessels, and nerves.
- Open fracture dislocations of the talus are high energy injuries that cause disruption of the blood supply by dislocation, ejection of fragments, and fracture through the neck of the talus. This causes avascular necrosis of the body or entire talus, which is susceptible to infection (see Fig 1).

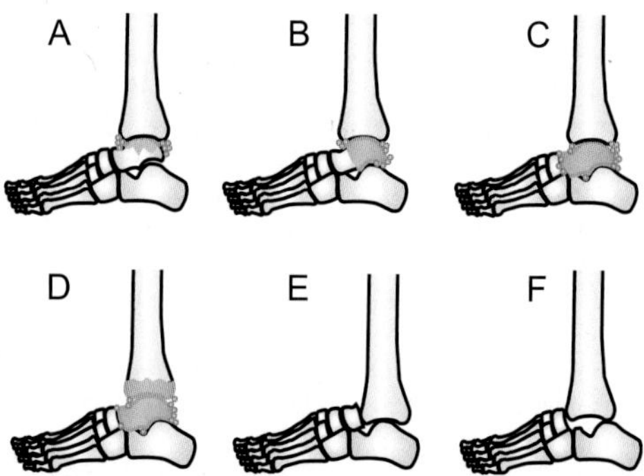

FIG 1 • The extent of bone loss and infection will determine the reconstruction. **A.** Extensive infection of the talar dome compromising tibial talar arthrodesis. **B.** Complete necrosis of the talar body. **C.** Necrosis of the entire talus. **D.** Necrosis of the plafond and talus. **E.** Traumatic ejection or crushing of the talar body. **F.** Traumatic ejection or crushing of the talus.

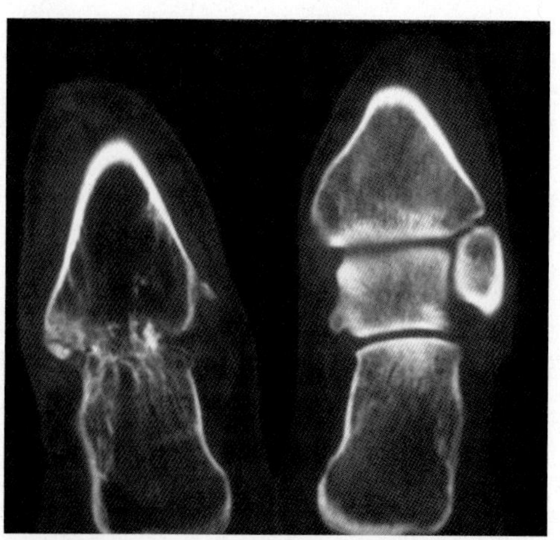

FIG 2 • CT scan of tibial calcaneal arthrodesis. The excision of the talus creates a 3- to 4-cm bone defect.

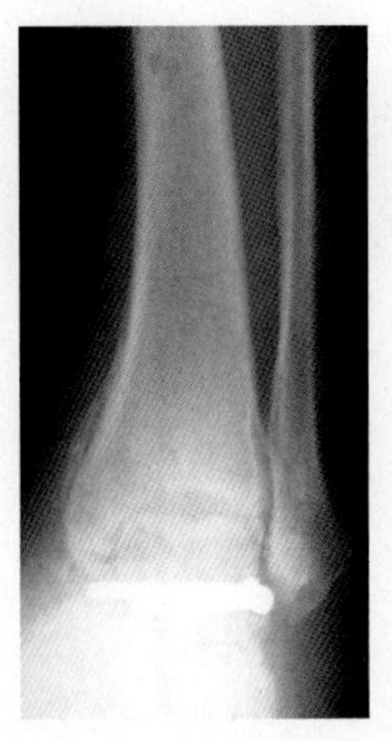
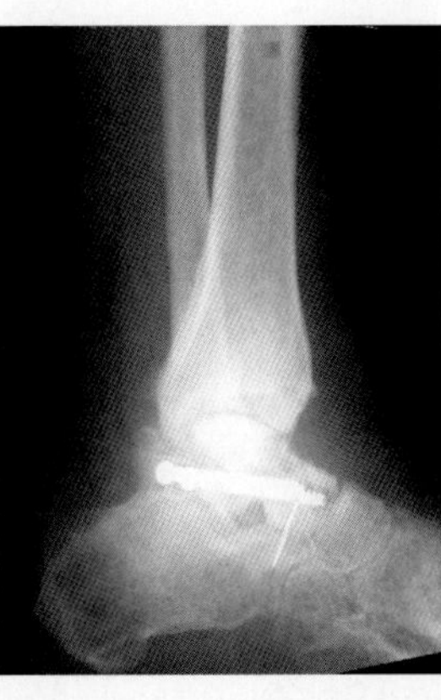

FIG 3 • **A,B.** Anterior and lateral x-ray of ankle with infected nonunion of talus. The ankle had a draining sinus. The talar body is avascular and the talar head has bone lysis around the two fixation screws. The plafond has erosion and destruction of the cartilage. There is reactive bone on the medial malleolus compatible with infection.

PATHOGENESIS

- High-energy ankle trauma
- Postoperative infection of open reduction and internal fixation of talus fractures
- Postoperative infection of ankle arthrodesis and ankle replacement

PATIENT HISTORY AND PHYSICAL FINDINGS

- Painful ankle with swelling and local inflammation
- Ankylosis of the hindfoot and ankle
- Shortening of the extremity
- A draining sinus indicates a deep infection.

IMAGING AND OTHER DIAGNOSTIC STUDIES

- An ankle series of radiographs will reveal the extent of the bone loss, the extent of AVN, and the location of internal fixation hardware in the talus and plafond (**FIG 3**).
- There may be local bone erosion of the talus, plafond, and malleoli from the chronic infection in the joint.
- A white blood cell count, erythrocyte sedimentation rate, and C-reactive protein study are screening tests that will indicate the possibility of a deep infection.
- Aspiration of the ankle joint under fluoroscopic guidance is indicated if there is suspicion of an infection.
- CT scanning will define the fragmentation of the talus and may reveal erosions of the plafond and malleoli compatible with infection.
- MRI will have diffuse signals caused by the fracture and inflammation that will provide little useful data in making the diagnosis.

DIFFERENTIAL DIAGNOSIS

- Charcot joint

NONOPERATIVE MANAGEMENT

- The patient may use a cane and ankle brace to improve gait.
- There will be chronic pain with AVN of the talus, infection, or traumatic ejection of the talus.
- There is no conservative treatment for an infected nonunion of the talus.
- Treatment with oral or intravenous antibiotics will only suppress the infection.

SURGICAL MANAGEMENT

Preoperative Planning

- Infection of the talus is treated with aggressive débridement.
- Oral antibiotics should be discontinued 2 weeks before the débridement to obtain accurate cultures.
- If there is infection and drainage that requires emergent débridement, the patient is taken to surgery and deep cultures are obtained before starting intravenous antibiotics.
- It is essential to identify the infecting organism.
  - Mycobacterium, yeast, and aerobic organisms may be the source of an infection, and cultures should be obtained.
  - The organisms cultured in our series include methicillin-resistant *Staphylococcus aureus*, *Enterobacter cloacae*, *Escherichia coli*, *Staphylococcus aureus*, streptococcus (nonhemolytic), *Alcaligenes xylosoxidans*, and *Pseudomonas aeruginosa*.

DÉBRIDEMENT OF INFECTION

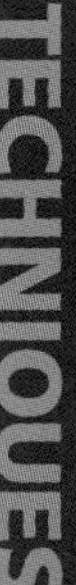

- Use an anterior medial approach located medial to the anterior tibial tendon to explore the talus (**TECH FIG 1A**).
- Before making the incision, elevate the leg for 3 minutes to drain blood from the extremity.
- Do not use an elastic compression bandage when there is a deep infection.
- Use a tourniquet during the initial excision of bone. Without a tourniquet, the field would be flooded with blood, obscuring the appearance of the infected bone.
- Carefully explore the infected talus.
- The necrotic bone will have a discolored avascular consistency.
  - Necrotic bone tends to have a brittle consistency compared to viable bone.
- Excise the bone in small fragments, carefully observing for vascularity and the transition from necrotic infected bone to viable bone.
- The preoperative radiographic evaluation may not clearly identify the extent of infection.
  - The talar head may be necrotic without the appearance of AVN on the radiograph.

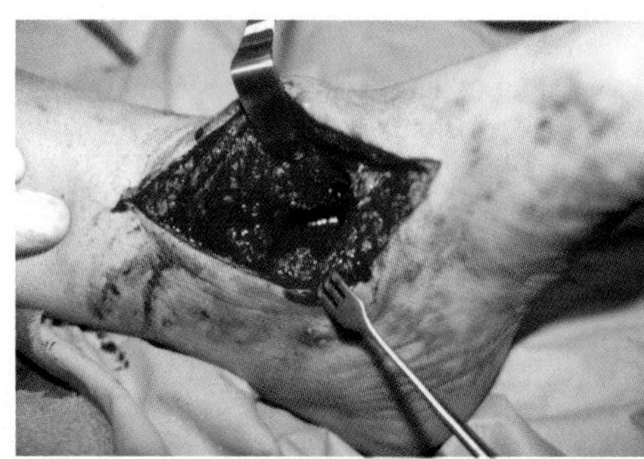
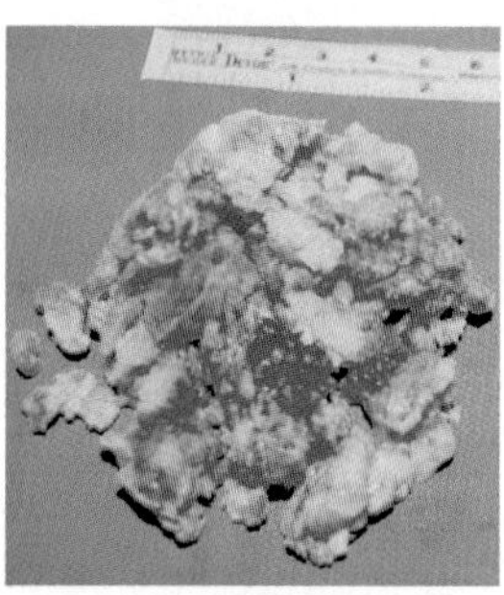
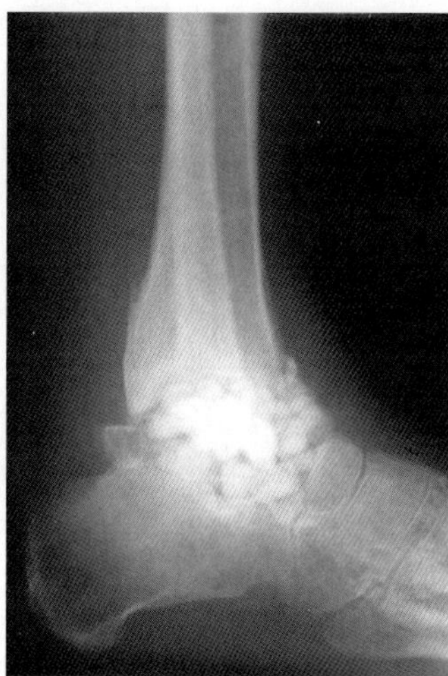

TECH FIG 1 • **A.** Anteromedial approach with excision of the entire talus. **B.** The talus is excised in small fragments using a 1/4-inch osteotome and pituitary rongeurs. This allows the entire talus to be removed without an extensive exposure. The bone is removed by working through the infected talus until the joint margins are cleared of all bone and cartilage. **C.** Debridement of the talus and distal plafond created a 5-cm bone gap. Antibiotic beads are placed in the ankle debridement.

- Remove all hardware as the talus is débrided.
- Take cultures from an area clearly involved with purulence.
- The infection and necrotic bone may be limited to the body of the talus, or the infection may have spread to the head of the talus, requiring excision of the entire talus (TECH FIG 1B).
- There may be a posteromedial section of the talus that is viable bone, but it is not large enough to be used for a pantalar arthrodesis.
- Once all necrotic bone is removed, lavage the joint with low-pressure saline and deflate the tourniquet.[7]
- Viable bone will have punctate bleeding.
  - If the margin of the bone resection does not bleed, excise the bone until bleeding is encountered.
  - This may lead to excision of the talar head.
- The tibial plafond can have invasion of infection and require removal of the joint surface and metaphysis for several centimeters (TECH FIG 1C).

Antibiotic Beads

- Antibiotic beads are manufactured on the back table.
  - The beads should have a small diameter (7 mm) to allow complete filling of the irregular volume created by the excision at the necrotic bone.
  - 2.4 grams of tobramycin powder is dry mixed with 1.0 gram of vancomycin and crushed with the rounded end of a Cobb elevator until there is a fine powder.
  - The antibiotics are dry mixed with 20 grams of methylmethacrylate cement before adding the liquid monomer.
- Using this large amount of antibiotics causes the cement to mix poorly, and it must be mashed into a paste before making the beads.
  - The cement is rolled into long 1-cm cylinders and cut into small pieces, which will form small-diameter beads.
  - The beads are formed and placed on a number 2 nylon suture that has had the heavy needle straightened.
  - Fifteen to 20 minutes of drying time is needed for the beads.
  - Once the beads have cooled, they are carefully packed into the wound to fill all of the space created by the talus excision (TECH FIG 1C).
  - The beads can be divided into two strings.
  - A half string usually fills the defect.
- The remaining beads are placed in a sterile container for repeat débridement if needed.

Wound Closure

- Close the wound with 2-0 nylon.
- Because of the thorough débridement, the wound can be closed primarily.
- Copious postoperative hemorrhage will drain through the single-layer closure.
- If the wound is left open, the edges will retract and a large open wound will develop that will take weeks to months to heal by secondary intention.
- If the infection was virulent, the patient is returned to surgery 24 to 48 hours later for a repeat débridement and bead exchange.
- The fibula is not excised at this time.
- With beads filling the defect and the fibula intact, the extremity is placed in a splint or fracture boot.

Postoperative Care

- Broad-spectrum antibiotics that cover methicillin-resistant *S. aureus* and gram-negative rods are administered until the cultures have identified the infecting organism.
- The extremity and surgical wound are examined daily.
- If the wound does not rapidly improve, a second débridement is indicated.
- After a week of intravenous antibiotics, the ankle is ready for tibial calcaneal arthrodesis.
- Extending the intravenous antibiotic course for 2 to 3 weeks and further observation may be indicated if the condition of the extremity requires further time to be ready for surgery.

TIBIAL CALCANEAL ARTHRODESIS

- Technically, the most difficult aspect of the surgery is fitting the concave surface of the plafond to the asymmetric surface to the posterior facet of the calcaneus, anterior calcaneus, and neck of the talus or the navicular (**TECH FIG 2A**).
- Cut the bone away in small shavings, with multiple trial fittings until the plafond fits securely into the calcaneus and talus or navicular.
- Approach the plafond and calcaneus from the lateral and medial sides of the ankle.

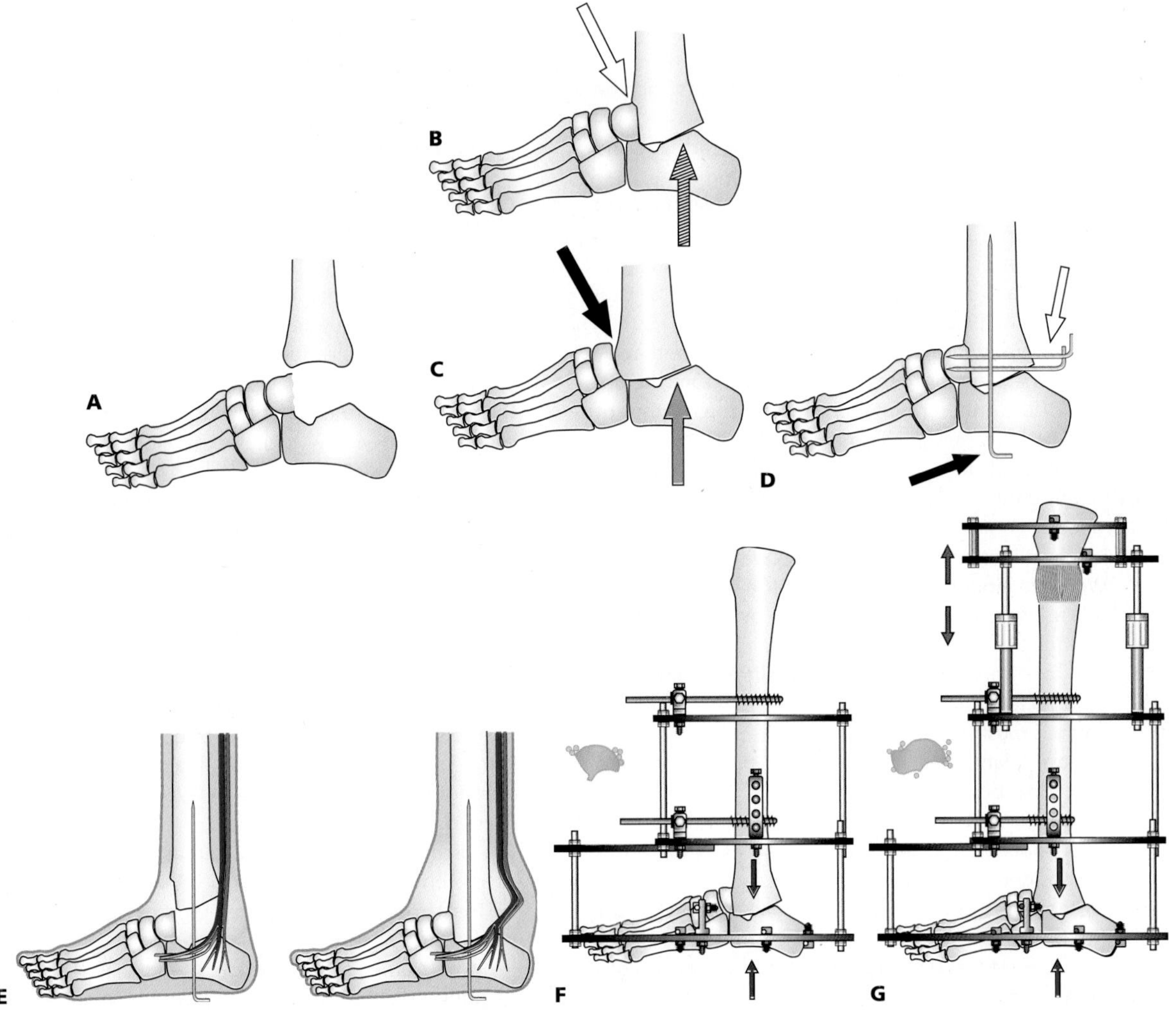

TECH FIG 2 • A. Fitting the incongruent surfaces of the tibial plafond to the calcaneus and talar neck or navicular requires craftsmanship. The osteotomy cuts are made with small cuttings until a stable compression surface is created. **B.** The anterior plafond is cut to align with the talar neck when the talar head is viable (*white arrow*). The posterior plafond osteotomy requires an oblique osteotomy to fit the posterior facet of the calcaneus (*striated arrow*). **C.** The anterior prominence of the tibial plafond is not removed when the talar head has been excised (*black arrow*). The anterior cortex is prepared to bleeding bone. The bone resection of the posterior plafond is shaped to fit the posterior facet (*gray arrow*). The resection of the posterior plafond is less because the tibia is located anteriorly with the talar head excised. The anterior process of the calcaneus is leveled to allow the tibia to compress onto the calcaneus. **D.** An inferior-to-superior Steinmann pin is placed to align the calcaneus with the tibial shaft after the arthrodesis osteotomies have been completed (*black arrow*). One or two Steinmann pins are placed from posterolateral through the plafond into the head of the talus to improve stability of the fixation if the talar head is preserved in the reconstruction. **E.** Acute shortening causes the soft tissues to bulge in the horizontal plane. After the calcaneal tibial pin is in place, the wounds can be closed with the extremity distracted. The tibia is compressed to the calcaneus after closure. Shortening causes distortion of the blood vessels crossing the ankle. Vascular flow must be carefully monitored after shortening. **F.** Monofocal tibial calcaneal talar head arthrodesis circular fixator. The frame consists of a double-ring fixation block and a foot fixation ring. The fixator is used to compress the arthrodesis. This illustration represents reconstruction of a talus with a viable talar head. **G.** Bifocal tibial calcaneal navicular arthrodesis circular fixator. The frame incorporates a proximal 5/8-full ring block and corticotomy to combine proximal lengthening with distal compression. The illustration depicts reconstruction after complete excision of the talus.

- Retention of the lateral malleolus is of no benefit.
- Excise the lateral malleolus through a lateral excision and perform an osteotomy 5 to 6 cm proximal with an oblique cut superior lateral to inferior medial.
- Carefully elevate the fascia overlying the lateral malleolus from the surface.
  - This fascia provides a deep closure of the lateral tissues after completion of the osteotomy.
- The lateral approach exposes the posterior facet of the calcaneus, lateral calcaneus, and anterior process.
  - Do not extend the vertical excision past the level of the peroneal tendons to prevent injury to the sural nerve.
- The anterior medial approach exposes the navicular, talar neck, and medial facets of the calcaneus.
- Evaluate the plafond and posterior facets of the calcaneus.
  - If the posterior facet is intact, excise the cartilage and expose the subchondral bone to bleeding bone.
- Débride the medial facet of cartilage and level the facet with the middle and anterior calcaneus.
- Cut the posterior plafond at an angle to match the posterior facet and remove the cartilage from the central plafond (**TECH FIG 2B,C**).
- If the talar neck is viable, cut the anterior plafond away to match the plane of the talar neck and flatten the underside of the anterior plafond to match the contour of the middle and anterior calcaneus (Tech Fig 2B).
- Cut away small amounts of bone from the tibia and calcaneus until there is a good fit between the tibia and calcaneus.
- Assess the alignment of the calcaneus with the tibia.
  - With the tibia compressed onto the calcaneus, the sole of the foot and heel should be in a foot-flat position.
  - The foot should be rotated straight forward or in slight external rotation.
  - Equinus must be avoided.
  - Neutral plantarflexion and slight dorsiflexion are functional positions.
  - It the arthrodesis is in equinus, the patient must wear shoes with a heel wedge to accommodate this malposition.
- The osteotomies of the tibia plafond and calcaneus must be fitted so that when the tibia is compressed onto the calcaneus, the fit of the osteotomy forces corrects alignment of the foot.
  - If the osteotomies are not correct, the compression applied by the circular fixation will malalign the arthrodesis.
- The bone cuts of the anterior plafond are modified if the talar head has been excised because of infection (Tech Fig 2C).
- Denude the navicular of cartilage to bleeding bone.
- Shape the bone contour of the anterior plafond to match the navicular concave surface.
- Flatten the anterior inferior plafond to fit the anterior calcaneus.
- The tibia is located in an anterior position toward the midfoot compared to the arthrodesis position if the talar head is present.
- Because of this anterior position, the osteotomy of the posterior plafond may require less bone resection.
  - Always align the plafond over the calcaneus and slowly cut away bone until there is a good fit of the bone surfaces.
- After completing the osteotomies, copiously lavage the operative field with low-pressure bulb irrigation to remove debris before closure.
  - The use of high-pressure pulsed irrigation destroys the exposed trabecular bone.[7]
- Deflate the tourniquet and examine the bone surfaces for punctate bleeding.
- If there is no bleeding, further bone resection is needed until viable bone is observed.
- Compress the calcaneus and align it manually, and drill a smooth Steinmann pin through the plantar surface into the tibial shaft (**TECH FIG 2D**).
  - This pin will guide the calcaneus to the correct position during compression with the circular fixator later during the technique.
- Close the medial and lateral incisions with a deep layer of absorbable suture and the skin with vertical nylon mattress sutures.
- The sutures may need to be in place for 3 to 4 weeks before there is adequate wound healing.
  - Never use staples for the skin closure.
- The shortening of the calcaneus onto the tibia will cause the soft tissues to expand in the horizontal plane (compression of a cylinder causes expansion of the diameter of the cylinder) (**TECH FIG 2E**).
- To facilitate closure, distract the calcaneus on the Steinmann pin and close the wounds with the foot out to length.
  - The amount of edema and fibrosis of the soft tissue will affect the ability to acutely shorten the arthrodesis.[9,14]
  - If there is severe edema and fibrosis, an acute shortening may not be possible, and a delayed shortening may be required to compress the arthrodesis.
  - The surgeon will gauge the effect of the shortening.
- If the calcaneus is compressed against the plafond and the foot becomes cyanotic, a delayed shortening will be needed for the reconstruction.
- The circular fixator is constructed as a monofocal frame or as a bifocal frame (**TECH FIG 2F,G**).
  - The circular rings are sized to provide 2 cm of soft tissue clearance.
  - Most frames are constructed with 160- or 180-mm rings.
- If the patient is a candidate for proximal distraction osteogenesis, the frame is assembled with a proximal 5/8-full ring block, a midtibial double ring fixation block, and a foot fixation block.
- If the patient has poor physiology for lengthening (end-stage diabetes, tobacco abuse, ischemic vascular disease, steroid dependency, or psychosis), the frame is assembled as a monofocal frame with a two-ring tibial fixation block and a foot fixation block.
- Carefully assess the ability of the patient to undergo distraction histogenesis.
- If there is failure of the arthrodesis, the salvage is a below-knee amputation.
- If a proximal corticotomy has been done on a patient with poor physiology, the below-knee level of salvage could be lost.

PROXIMAL LENGTHENING

- The proximal and midtibial ring blocks are assembled as a unit.
  - The proximal ring block is constructed with a 5/8 or 2/3 ring connected to a full ring with three 3.0-cm hexagonal sockets (**TECH FIG 3A**).
  - The midtibial ring block is constructed with two rings connected with four 120- or 150-mm threaded rods (**TECH FIG 3B,C**).
  - The proximal and midtibial ring blocks are connected with four 40-mm distraction telescopic rods (clickers).
  - A horizontal reference olive wire is placed 15 mm below the tibial plateau with a 3-degree varus alignment.
- The varus of the reference wire aligns the frame with the axis of the tibia shaft (**TECH FIG 3D**).
  - The frame is aligned and centered on the tibia with adequate soft tissue clearance (**TECH FIG 3E**).
  - Observe the posterior gastrocsoleus muscle to ensure proper clearance.
- Tension the horizontal reference wire to 110 kg.
- The center of the frame should align with the tibial shaft.
  - If the alignment is not axial, washers can be placed under the lateral or medial reference wire to correct the alignment.
- During this phase of the procedure, an assistant must support the distal leg and foot to prevent distorted positions, which could injure the soft tissues.
  - A towel block under the heel also prevents displacement.
- Align the distal tibial ring block with the tibia and place a 5-mm half-pin in the AP plane. Secure it with a universal Rancho cube on the distal ring (**TECH FIG 3F**).
  - The universal cube allows the ring to be aligned on the lateral view in an orthogonal position.
- Alternatively, a transverse olive wire may be used to align the distal fixation block (**TECH FIG 3C**).
- Once the frame is aligned, place a second AP 5-mm half-pin on the midtibial fixation block.
- Place a medial half-pin between the rings aligned 90 degrees to the two AP pins.
  - Place a second medial pin for large patients.
- Further stabilize the proximal 5/8-full ring block with a medial face olive wire on the inferior face of the full ring, and place a smooth wire though the fibula head, exiting the anteromedial tibial plateau.
- Connect the footplate to the midtibial fixation block with two threaded rods placed in the posteromedial and posterolateral ring (**TECH FIG 3G**).
  - The rods should have about 50 mm of excess length.
- Place a horizontal reference wire in the tuberosity of the calcaneus from lateral to medial.
- Compress the foot on the Steinmann pin until the calcaneus is in alignment with the tibia.

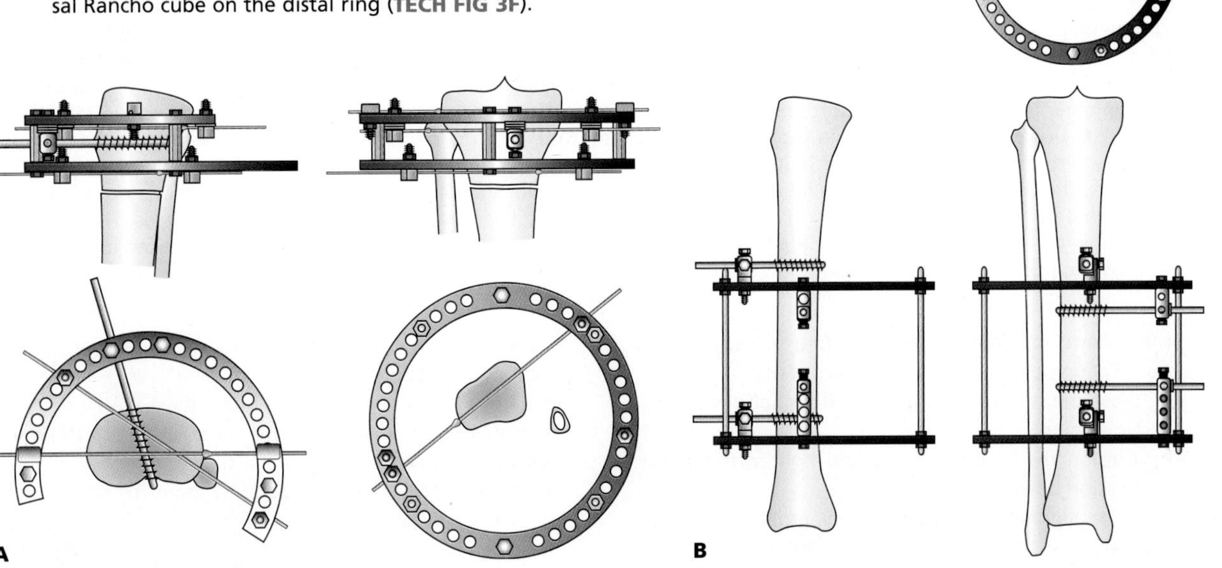

TECH FIG 3 • A. The 5/8-full ring proximal fixation block. The 5/8 ring is connected to the full ring by three 3-cm hexagonal sockets. The horizontal reference wire is 15 mm below the joint in 3 degrees of varus. A smooth wire is placed into the fibula head. If the fibula head is not fixated, the fibula will be dragged down the leg with lengthening. A medial face wire is placed on the inferior surface of the full ring. A 5-mm half-pin is placed anteromedial after completion of the corticotomy. The 5/8 ring is rotated to the lateral side to allow placement of the fibula head wire. **B.** The tibial shaft double-ring fixation block is aligned orthogonally on the tibia with two AP 5-mm half-pins mounted on universal Rancho cubes. The Rancho cube mountings allow the fixation block to be aligned orthogonally. One or two medial pins are added once the fixation block is aligned. The distal ring is located about 6 cm superior to the arthrodesis. *(continued)*

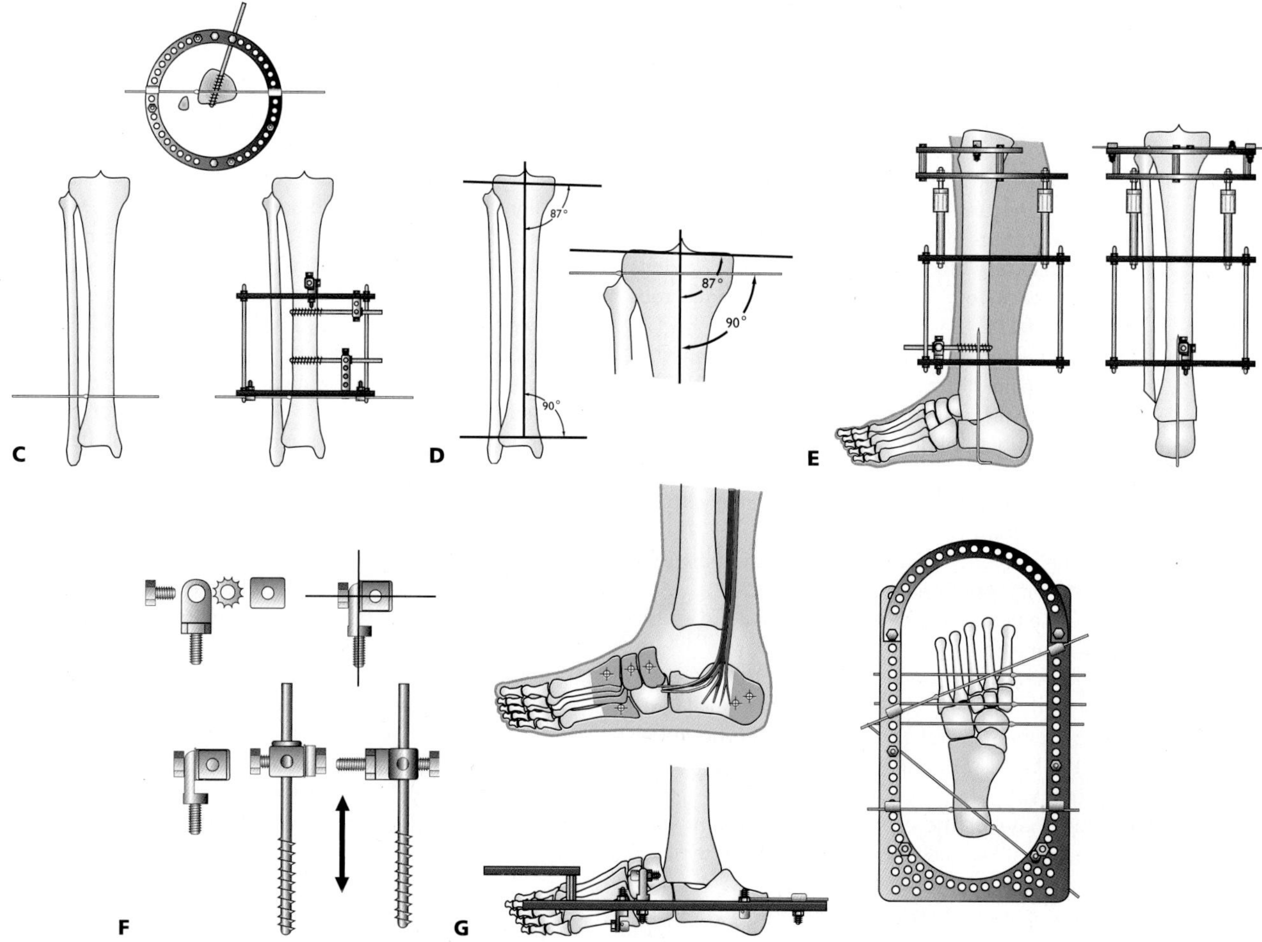

TECH FIG 3 • *(continued)* **C.** An alternative method to align the stable base is to place a horizontal reference above the plafond. The wire should be placed posterior on the shaft to avoid the anterior tibial artery. The distal wire is located about 6 cm proximal to the arthrodesis. **D.** The joint surface of the plateau forms a varus 87-degree angle with the shaft. A horizontal reference wire placed 90 degrees to the shaft will be slightly closer to the medial plateau compared to the lateral. **E.** The proximal 5/8 ring block and the tibial shaft double-ring block are connected by 40-mm distraction rods. The frame is aligned on the proximal reference wire followed by a 5-mm half-pin placed on the distal ring. Manipulating these two fixation points aligns the frame orthogonally on the tibia. The rings must have soft tissue clearance at the posterior gastrocnemius muscle and anterior ankle soft tissue prominence. **F.** Universal Rancho cube pin fixation. Three-axis adjustment of the pin alignment allows the frame to be aligned orthogonally with the tibia. Rancho cubes bolted directly to the ring fix the ring in the alignment of the half-pin. If the half-pin is not perfect, the ring block will be malaligned. **G.** The foot fixation block is constructed with a long footplate closed on the anterior open end with a half-ring. The ring extends above the toes to keep bed linen from irritating the toes. The surgeon should avoid wires that could penetrate the posterior tibial or plantar nerve. Two opposed olive wires are placed in the calcaneus and two opposed olive wires are placed in the forefoot.

- Manipulate the foot on the footplate to control rotational alignment and align the arthrodesis.
  - Close the footplate anteriorly with a half-ring before tensioning.
  - Tension the wire to 100 kg and tighten the slotted fixation bolts.
  - If the alignment is not satisfactory, repeat the process.
- Connect two threaded rods to the anterior foot plate with threaded rods using extension plates from the stable base.
- Stabilize the forefoot with opposed olive wires through the cuneiform row and metatarsal bases.
- Place a second wire from the posteromedial calcaneal tuberosity to the anterolateral calcaneal wall on the superior side of the foot plate.
- Assess the vascularity of the foot with the foot in the acutely shortened position.
  - There should be brisk capillary refill.
- Use a Doppler device to verify pulsatile flow in the dorsalis pedis and posterior tibial artery.
  - If the vascular flow is good, maintain the foot in the acute shortened position.
  - If the foot is cyanotic and no pulses are detected with the Doppler, slowly distract the foot by lengthening the threaded rods between the tibial fixation block and the foot ring.
  - Once pulsatile flow is detected, lock the threaded rod position in place.
- This position will create a gap between the tibia and calcaneus.

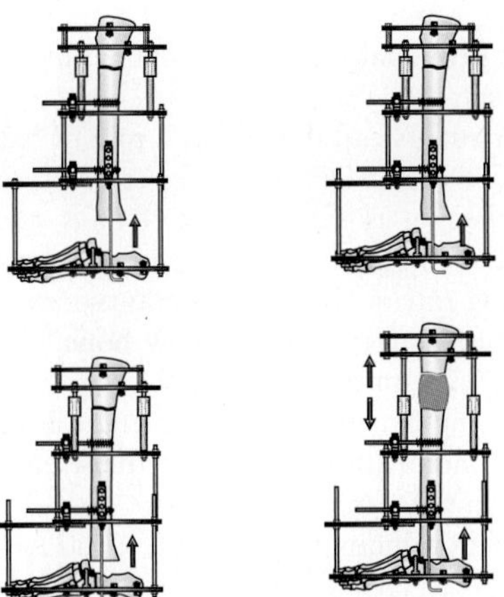

TECH FIG 4 • The technique of delayed shortening. The foot fixation block is compressed at a rate of 1 mm four times a day until the tibial calcaneal arthrodesis is compressed. The calcaneal tibial Steinmann pin aligns the foot during the compression. The proximal tibia is lengthened to equalize leg lengths.

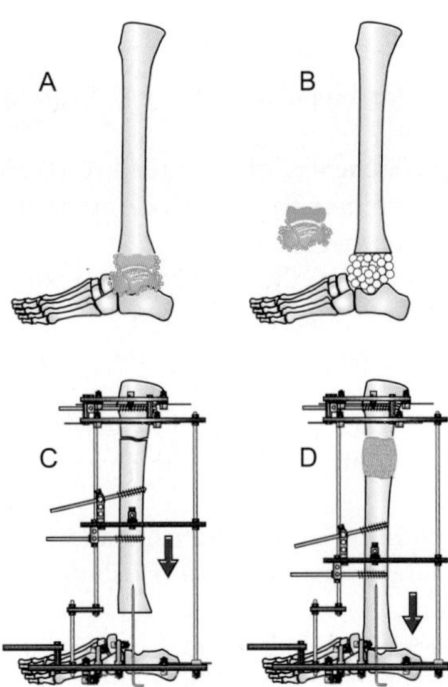

TECH FIG 5 • The technique of intercalary transport to arthrodesis. **A.** Infection of plafond and talus. **B.** Excision with bone gap greater than 5 cm. **C.** Ilizarov frame maintaining leg length before transport. **D.** Intercalary transport to docking. A revision of the docking site will improve alignment. A spatial frame could also be used in this configuration. Large defects can also be closed with an acute shortening of 3 cm combined with an intercalary transport to close the gap. The circular fixator is converted to a lengthening frame to equalize the leg length.

  - A delayed shortening is used to close this gap slowly over several days (TECH FIG 4).
  - The gap is closed at a rate of 1 mm four times a day until the arthrodesis is compressed.
- If the distal tibia plafond has extensive bone loss creating a bone deficit greater than 5 cm, the tibial calcaneal arthrodesis can be accomplished with an intercalary transport (TECH FIG 5).
- Reinflate the tourniquet and complete a corticotomy using an osteotome or a Gigli saw.
- After the corticotomy, place a 5-mm half-pin on the medial side of the tibial tubercle from anterior to posterior.
- The Steinmann pin is maintained for 6 weeks after surgery, which stabilizes the arthrodesis site.
- Place two more Steinmann pins from the posteromedial plafond into the talar head or navicular after compressing the arthrodesis (Tech Fig 2D).
  - These pins stabilize motion between the talar head and tibia, increasing arthrodesis between these structures.

TECHNIQUES WITHOUT LENGTHENING

- Apply a stable base to the distal tibia (Tech Fig 3B).
- Place two AP half-pins on universal Rancho cubes and align the ring block orthogonally.
- The distal ring is located about 6 cm above the arthrodesis site.
  - The ring is further stabilized with one or two 5-mm half-pins placed into the medial tibia.
  - An alternative method is to place a horizontal reference wire 6 cm above the ankle and align the double-ring fixation on the wire and place two AP pins and a medial face half-pin on the ring block (Tech Fig 3C).
- In patients with osteopenia, the entire fixation block can be fixated to the tibia with four olive wires placed in safe corridors.
- Complete the arthrodesis of the tibia to the calcaneus as described in the prior section.

PEARLS AND PITFALLS

The arthrodesis must be in a plantar-neutral position. A fusion with the foot in equinus will severely compromise the functional outcome.

POSTOPERATIVE CARE

- The foot is observed for blood flow every 4 hours for the first 2 postoperative days.
  - If the foot becomes ischemic, the threaded rods connecting the foot frame to the tibia fixation block are lengthened until the blood flow improves.
  - A delayed shortening is then carried out until the arthrodesis is compressed (**FIG 4**).
  - The patient is encouraged to mobilize the forefoot and toes and knee.
  - Toe loops on rubber bands are placed on a wire scaffold to prevent toe flexion contractures by the physical therapy service.
  - There will be significant bloody drainage and the bulky dressing placed in surgery may need to be changed on the first postoperative day.
  - Open wounds are treated with normal saline wet-to-dry dressings until closure by secondary intention.
  - Vacuum dressings are an alternative to wet-to-dry dressings.
  - The sutures are left in place for at least 2 weeks.
  - Many patients will require 3 to 4 weeks of suture closure before it is possible to remove the sutures.
- Intravenous antibiotics are administered for 2 days in patients without infections.
  - If the wounds are complex, the intravenous antibiotics will be continued for 7 days.
  - Patients with infected talus nonunions will be treated for additional weeks using intravenous antibiotics appropriate for the infecting organism.
  - There is debate on whether the antibiotics need to be given for an additional week or continued for a total of 6 weeks during the treatment course.
- The dressing sponges are removed 2 weeks after surgery and the pin sites are cleaned daily.
- Once the surgical wounds are healed, the leg is washed in the shower with soap and water, removing all dried secretions from the pins and wires.
  - Hydrogen peroxide 3% solution is used only occasionally to clean crust that cannot be removed with soap and water.
  - Cephalexin, trimethoprim–sulfamethoxazole (Septra DS), and ciprofloxacin are used if needed to control local pin or wire skin infections.
- Some patients will need only occasional use of antibiotics while others will require constant oral antibiotic coverage while the circular fixator is on the leg.
- Rarely, a more aggressive pin or wire infection will develop.
  - The infecting organism is most commonly methicillin-resistant *S. aureus*.
  - A 1-week course of intravenous vancomycin will be needed to control the wire infection.
  - If this is not successful, the wire is removed.
- The plantar and talar neck and navicular Steinmann pins are removed in the clinic 6 weeks after surgery.
  - The patient is started on partial weight bearing, increasing to 50% weight over the following month.
  - A shower sandal is placed over the toes when walking.
  - The sandal is elevated with a full sole elevation to equalize the leg lengths and the sole is cut down on the band saw as the lengthening progresses.
  - Most patients cannot tolerate full weight with wires in their foot.
- Lengthening proximally is at a rate of 0.25 mm (one quarter-turn) twice a day.
  - Younger patients can distract at a rate of 0.25 mm every 8 hours.
  - The lengthening is started 3 to 4 days postoperatively after the patient's pain has improved from the surgery.
  - The starting rate is always 0.25 mm twice a day.
    - If the patient forms robust new bone, this can be increased to 0.25 mm every 8 hours.
  - The leg is lengthened until the leg length is equal (Fig 4).
  - Given the choice, most patients request equal leg length rather than on to 2 cm of shortening.
  - The distraction index is between 1.5 and 2.0 months per centimeter.
  - For a patient with tibial bone loss, the lengthening required can exceed 5 cm, resulting in 10 or more months in the circular fixator.
  - Some patients will heal the arthrodesis before the lengthening is mature.
  - The foot frame can be removed before the proximal transport is mature.
- The tibial calcaneal arthrodesis requires 6 months for union.
  - The footplate is compressed 1 or 2 mm at each clinic visit to maintain compression over the course of treatment.
  - The fixator is removed under anesthesia.
  - A short-leg walking cast is applied and the patient walks with partial weight bearing.
  - The patient continues partial-weight gait until there is defined bone healing at the tibial calcaneal arthrodesis and the proximal bone transport has a well-developed medial, lateral, and posterior cortex.
  - Often patients will return to the clinic stating that they have advanced to full weight bearing around the house walking in the frame.
  - To increase the force transmitted across the transport, the frame is neutralized before frame removal.
  - This is accomplished by loosening the distraction clickers and allowing the distraction force to become neutral.
  - The rods are bolted in this neutral position and the patient is observed for several weeks to see if the cortex of the regenerate is strong enough to prevent collapse.
  - The fixator is removed under general anesthesia.
  - The leg is casted for 2 weeks after frame removal.
  - The radiograph out of plaster in the office with the Ilizarov fixator removed is analyzed for healing of the transport bone and arthrodesis.
  - A fracture walking boot with a rocker-bottom sole is applied.
  - The patient walks 50% weight bearing for 4 weeks.
  - The patient advances to full weight bearing with a cane and gradually increases his or her activity over the following year.
  - Activity is limited to walking on flat surfaces and light stress on the extremity.
  - The force applied to the leg is gradually increased with mature healing of the bone transport and arthrodesis observed at 1 year after fixator removal (Fig 4C,D).
  - The patient self-selects walking and training shoes that have cushioned heels with a rounded radius heel.
  - Patients who do not have proximal bone transport to equalize leg length have full sole elevations of 3 to 5 cm added to their walking shoes (shoe prosthesis) with a rocker sole.

- If the patient has mild valgus or varus foot alignment, an orthotic is prescribed that improves their foot loading when standing and walking.
- Long-term follow-up reveals osteophyte development at the talar navicular joint, which is associated with arthritic pain.

OUTCOMES

- The average AOFAS foot and ankle score was 65 for the 11 patients in our case series.[13]
  - Patients lose the ability to participate in sports and work as laborers.
  - The work status is reduced to light or sedentary work.
  - They can still ride motorcycles and drive cars.
  - Patients are aware of the asymmetry of their legs from atrophy of the muscles motorizing the foot and ankle.
  - When queried, no patient to date has considered having an amputation.
  - The long-term follow-up will probably reveal progression of midfoot arthritis.

COMPLICATIONS

- Failure of the bone transport to mature is a major complication.
  - The distraction index is between 1.5 and 2.0 months per centimeter of lengthening.
  - Bone growth is stimulated by weight bearing, so during the treatment course, the patient is encouraged to place 50% partial weight on the extremity.
  - An Exogen Bone Stimulator (Smith-Nephew) can be used once the distraction is completed.
  - Bone grafting of the distraction can also stimulate maturation if poor bone formation is observed.
- If deformation of the transport occurs after frame removal, this problem can be treated by several methods.
  - If there is less than 5 degrees of angulation, the patient is treated with a knee brace and non–weight-bearing for 6 weeks.
  - If greater deformity is observed, a second circular fixator is applied with angular correction and further time in the frame is indicated.
  - An alternative is to place a locked plate spanning the transport on the medial or lateral tibial shaft (Fig 4D).
  - An intramedullary nail can also be used for bone transport with poor bone formation.
  - The pin and wire tracks must be free of infection to use internal fixation after external fixation.
  - The patients walk 50% partial weight with crutches until healing of the transport.
- Failure to achieve arthrodesis is directly related to the physiologic status of the patient.
  - Patients with rheumatoid arthritis who are using steroids chronically are prone to nonunion of their tibial calcaneal arthrodesis.
  - If union has not occurred by 6 months of frame time, further time in the frame will not alter the outcome.
  - If the patient is not on steroids and is in good health, a revision arthrodesis is attempted.
  - Patients with rheumatoid arthritis are placed in a cast and encouraged to walk.
  - The mobile nonunion forms a pseudo-joint similar to fascial arthroplasty that allows them to walk independently (**FIG 5**).
  - We have observed four patients who have maintained this pseudo-joint for years and are able to participate in activities of daily living.

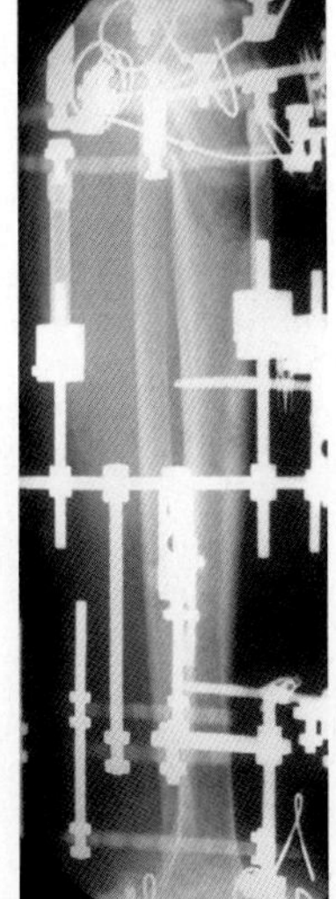
A
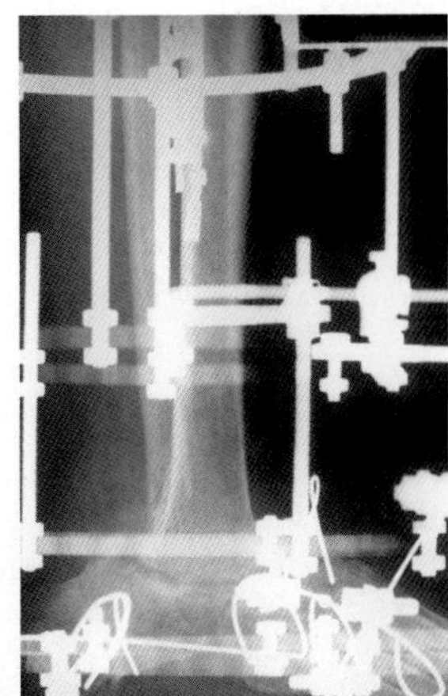
B
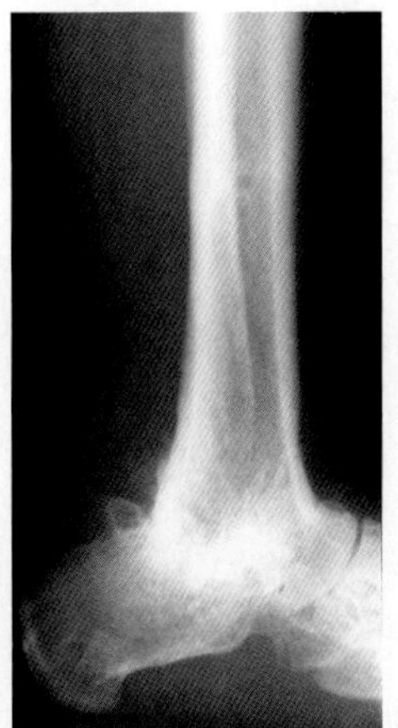
C
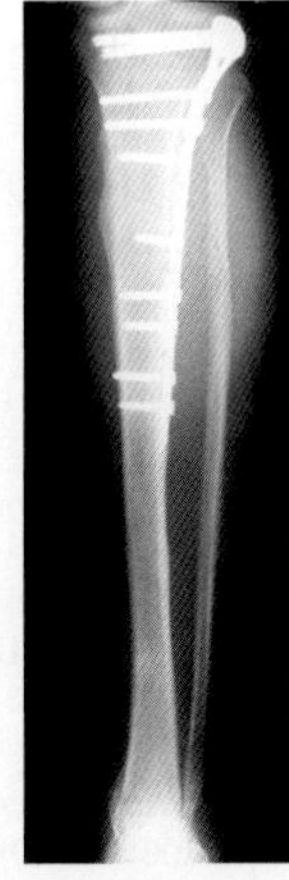
D

FIG 4 • **A.** Lateral x-ray of bifocal external fixator. The proximal tibia has been lengthened between the 5/8-full ring block and the double ring block on the mid tibia. **B.** Lateral x-ray of the tibia calcaneal arthrodesis with compression between the mid tibia and the foot plate. The foot is in plantar neutral alignment. **C.** Mature tibia1 calcaneal arthrodesis with the plafond fused to the calcaneus and navicular. **D.** AP x-ray with axial alignment of arthrodesis. The patient had a valgus deformity after frame removal of the transport. The tibia was realigned with a lateral locked plate.

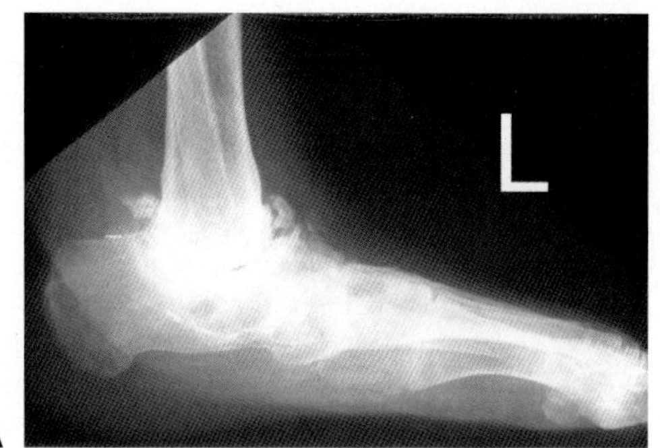

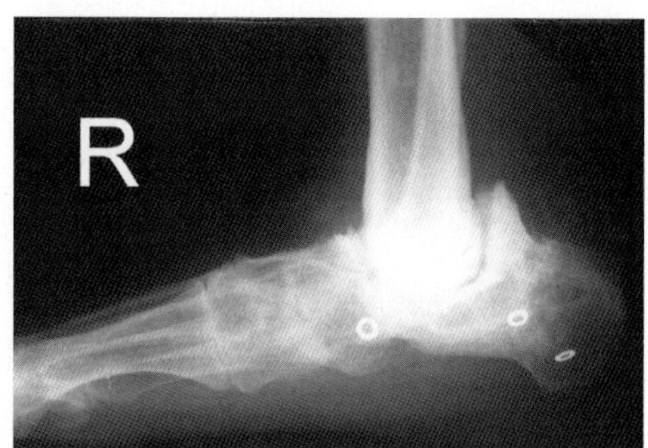

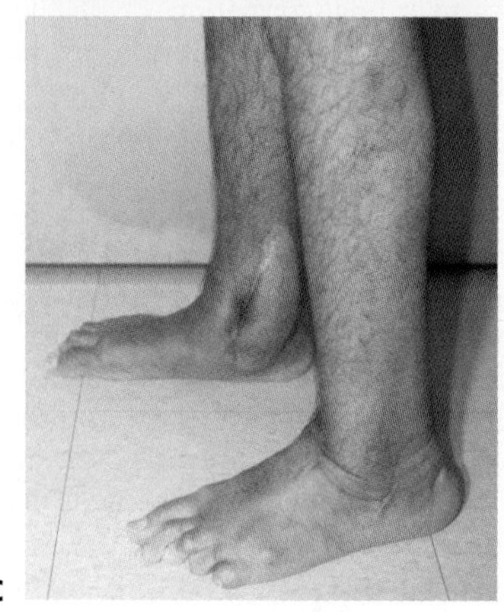

FIG 5 • **A,B.** Bilateral tibial calcaneal arthrodesis nonunion after failed infected ankle arthrodesis and infected total ankle arthroplasty. The patient is on high doses of steroid medication. The infections were eradicated. **C.** Clinical photograph of bilateral tibial calcaneal nonunion with fibrous pseudo-joint. Observe the free flap on the medial ankle. The patient uses a scooter for traveling distances but can walk independently and is independent in activities of daily living.

REFERENCES

1. Blair HC. Comminuted fractures and fracture dislocations of the body of the astragalus: operative treatment. Am J Surg 1943;59: 37–43.
2. Brewster NT, Maffulli N. Reimplantation of the totally extruded talus. J Orthop Trauma 1997;11:42–45.
3. Canale ST, Kelly FB. Fractures of the neck of the talus: long-term evaluation of seventy-one cases. J Bone Joint Surg Am 1978;60A: 143–156.
4. Dennis MD, Tullos HS. Blair tibiotalar arthrodesis for injuries to the talus. J Bone Joint Surg Am 1980;62A:103–107.
5. Dennison MG, Pool RD, Simonis RB, et al. Tibiocalcaneal fusion for avascular necrosis of the talus. J Bone Joint Surg Br 2001;83B: 199–203.
6. Detenbeck LC, Kelly PJ. Total dislocation of the talus. J Bone Joint Surg Am 1969;51A:283–288.
7. Dirschl DR, Duff GP, Dahners LE, et al. High-pressure pulsatile lavage irrigation of intraarticular fractures: effects on fracture healing. J Orthop Trauma 1998;12:460–463.
8. Hiraizumi Y, Hara T, Takahashi M, et al. Open total dislocation of the talus with extrusion (missing talus): report of two cases. Foot Ankle Int 1992;13:473–477.
9. Hutson JJ. Appendix 2: acute shortening to reconstruct fractures and post traumatic deformities with Ilizarov fixators. Technique Orthop 2002;17:110–111.
10. Rochman R, Hutson JJ, Alade O. Tibialcalcaneal arthrodesis using the Ilizarov technique in the presence of bone loss and infection of the talus. Foot Ankle Int 2008;29(10):1001–1008.
11. Johnson EE, Weltmer J, Lian GJ, et al. Ilizarov ankle arthrodesis. Clin Orthop Relat Res 1992;280:160–169.
12. Kile TA, Donnelly RE, Gehrke JC, et al. Tibiotalocalcaneal arthrodesis with an intramedullary device. Foot Ankle Int 1994;15:669–673.
13. Kitaoka HB, Alexander IJ, Adelaar RS, et al. Clinical rating systems for the ankle-hindfoot, midfoot, hallux, and lesser toes. Foot Ankle Int 1994;15:349–353.
14. Lowenberg DW, Van der Reis W. Acute shortening for tibia defects: when and where. Tech Orthop 1996;11:210–215.
15. Mann RA. Chou LB. Tibiocalcaneal arthrodesis. Foot Ankle Int 1995;16:401–405.
16. Marsh JL, Saltzman CL, Iverson M, et al. Major open injuries of the talus. J Orthop Trauma 1995;9:371–376.
17. Ptaszek AJ. Immediate tibiocalcaneal arthrodesis with interposition fibular autograft for salvage after talus fracture: a case report. J Orthop Trauma 1999;13:589–592.
18. Russotti GM, Johnson KA, Cass JR. Tibiotalocalcaneal arthrodesis for arthritis and deformity of the hind part of the foot. J Bone Joint Surg Am 1988;70:1304–1307.
19. Sanders D, Busam M, Hattwick E, et al. Functional outcomes following displaced talar neck fractures. J Orthop Trauma 2004;18: 265–270.
20. Urquhart MW, Mont MA, Michelson JD, et al. Osteonecrosis of the talus: treatment by hindfoot fusion. Foot Ankle Int 1996;17: 275–282.
21. Smith CS, Nork SE, Sangeorzan BJ. The extruded talus: results of reimplantation. J Bone Joint Surg Am 2006;88A:2418–2424.
22. Weber M, Schwer H, Zilkens KW, et al. Tibio-calcaneo-naviculo-cuboidale arthrodesis: 6 patients followed for 1–8 years. Acta Orthop Scand 2002;73:98–103.
23. Whittle AP, Dresher BD, Giel T. Open fractures and dislocations of the talus. Podium presentation, Proceedings of 2004 meeting, Orthopaedic Trauma Association, October 2004.

Chapter **85**

Femoral Head Allograft for Large Talar Defects

Bryan D. Den Hartog

INDICATIONS

- Talar body avascular necrosis with collapse or infection (**FIG 1**) is one indication for femoral head allograft.
- Failed total ankle arthroplasty with insufficient bone remaining for revision (**FIG 2**) also warrants a femoral head allograft.
- Use of a femoral head graft for those patients with severe (> 25 degrees) hindfoot valgus may not be appropriate, because correction of the deformity can cause significant lateral soft tissue tension and lead to tissue necrosis and poor wound healing. In those cases, a tibiocalcaneal fusion with shortening of the medial ankle may be more appropriate.

POSITIONING

- Under a general or spinal anesthetic block, the patient is placed in a supine position on the operating table with the ipsilateral hip bumped to facilitate internal rotation of the leg.
- The lower extremity is prepped and draped in the usual fashion, and a thigh tourniquet inflated to 250 mm Hg is applied after exsanguination of the leg with an Esmarch bandage.

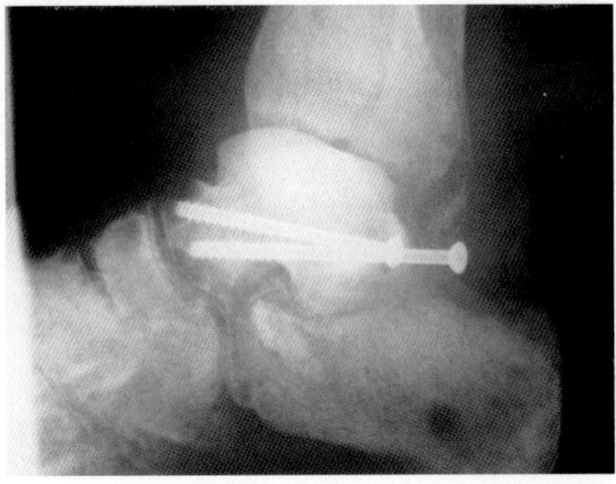

FIG 1 • Lateral radiograph demonstrating avascular necrosis and infection of the talar body after open fracture–dislocation.

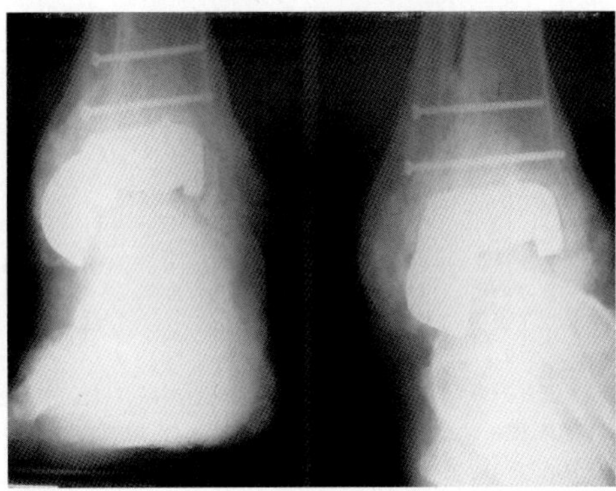

FIG 2 • Radiographs of a failed total ankle arthroplasty with severe loss of talar bone stock.

PREPARATION FOR ALLOGRAFT

- A 12- to 14-cm lateral incision is made along the distal fibula, starting 6 cm above the ankle joint and extending distally along the anterior border of the peroneal tendons to the peroneal tubercle (**TECH FIG 1**).
- The tendons are carefully retracted posteriorly to expose the distal fibula, lateral ankle, and subtalar joints.
- The fibula is osteotomized 6 cm above the joint, then excised and morcelized for later grafting (**TECH FIG 2**).
- Débridement of avascular bone and removal of osteophytes and implant is performed until only viable bone surfaces remain (ie, distal tibial plafond, talar head and neck, and posterior facet of the subtalar joint).
- Determine the size of acetabular reamer from the total hip arthroplasty set that best fits the defect (**TECH FIG 3**).
- Only enough subchondral bone is removed from the tibia, talar neck, and calcaneus to expose viable, softer cancellous bone for fusion to the femoral head graft. If an assistant holds the foot and ankle in the desired position, the

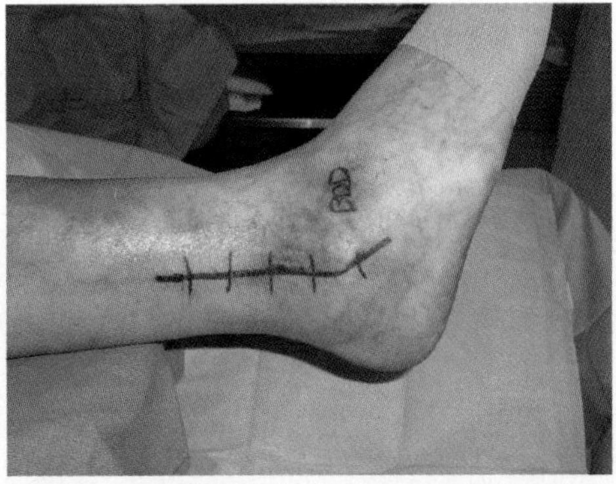

TECH FIG 1 • Patient positioned supine on the operating table. A lateral incision is made over the distal fibula and lateral hindfoot.

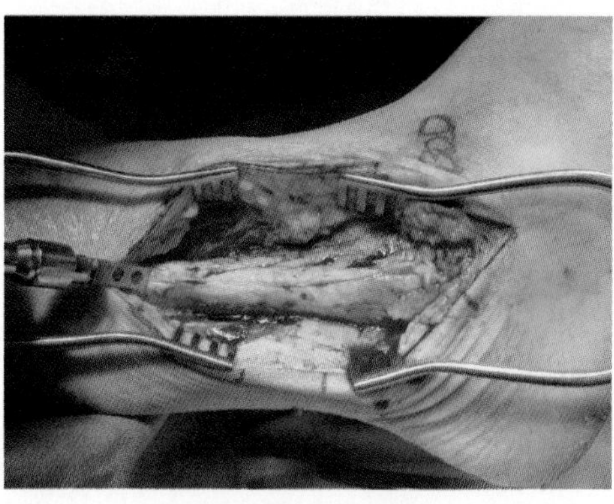

TECH FIG 2 • A fibulectomy is performed to expose the ankle and subtalar joints and lateral calcaneus.

surgeon can ream the defect safely, without the ankle bouncing around. No provisional fixation is necessary: the ankle is still relatively stable even after the ankle implant or necrotic bone is removed.

- With the ankle and hindfoot held in neutral, the defect is reamed (TECH FIG 4). The desired position of fusion is with the ankle in neutral plantar/dorsiflexion flexion and the hindfoot in approximately 5 degrees of valgus in relation to the distal tibia.
- It is critical to protect the soft tissue about the ankle with either Army-Navy or Hohmann retractors while the acetabular reamers are used.
    - Bone shavings are saved and mixed with the morcelized fibular graft.

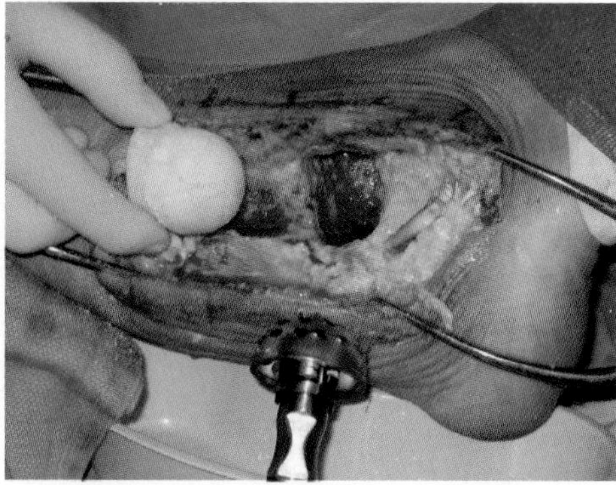

TECH FIG 3 • The defect remaining after talectomy is sized with the male reamers from the hip arthroplasty set.

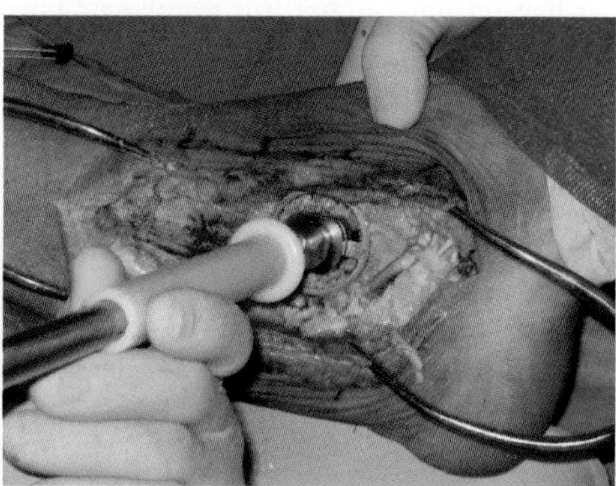

TECH FIG 4 • The bone surrounding the defect is reamed until cancellous bone is exposed on the distal tibia, talar neck, and calcaneus.

PREPARATION AND PLACEMENT OF ALLOGRAFT

- An allograft femoral head is thawed in a warm saline bath at the beginning of the procedure and placed in the bone vice (Allogrip Vice, DePuy), with the three limbs of the vice gripping the femoral neck.
- The female reamer corresponding to the same size male reamer used for reaming the defect is used to decorticate the allograft (TECH FIGS 5 AND 6).
- The head can be drilled multiple times in areas that still contain hard sclerotic bone to facilitate fusion.
- The appropriately sized and decorticated femoral head allograft is then placed in the defect (TECH FIG 7).
    - Ankle and foot position is then checked for neutral position (ie, neutral ankle dorsiflexion–plantarflexion, 5 degrees of hindfoot valgus, and neutral rotation of

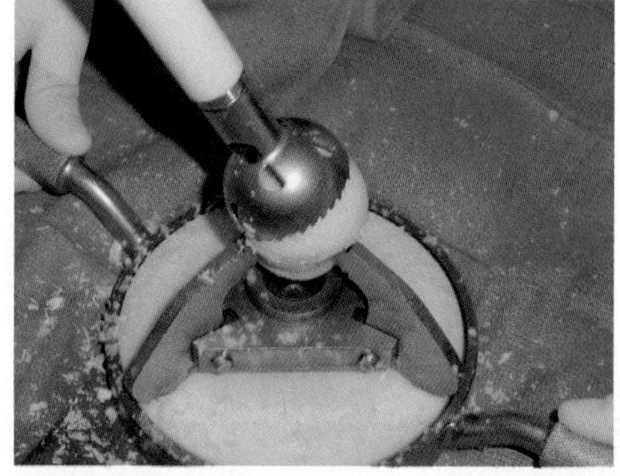

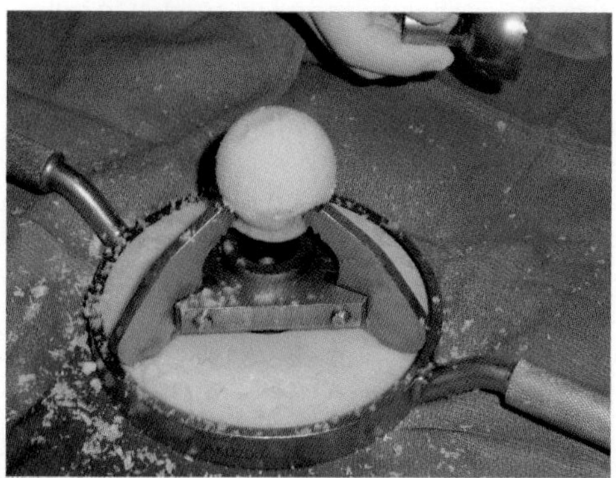

TECH FIG 5 • **A.** A frozen femoral head allograft is thawed and placed in the Allogrip Bone Vice (DePuy). **B.** The female reamer (DePuy) is used to remove the subchondral bone from the allograft to expose cancellous bone and size the graft.

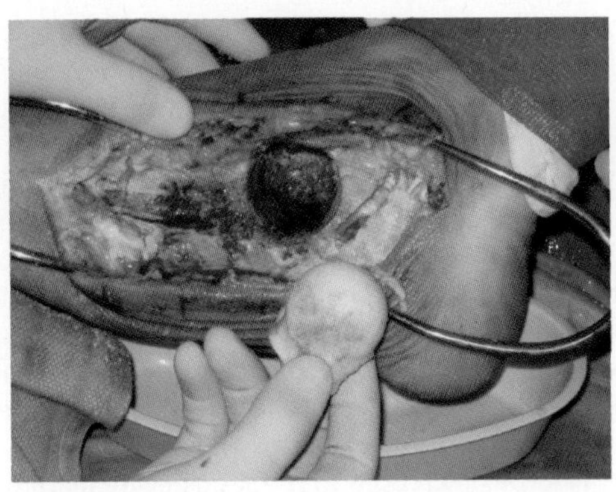

TECH FIG 6 • The femoral head graft is placed in the defect to ensure proper sizing.

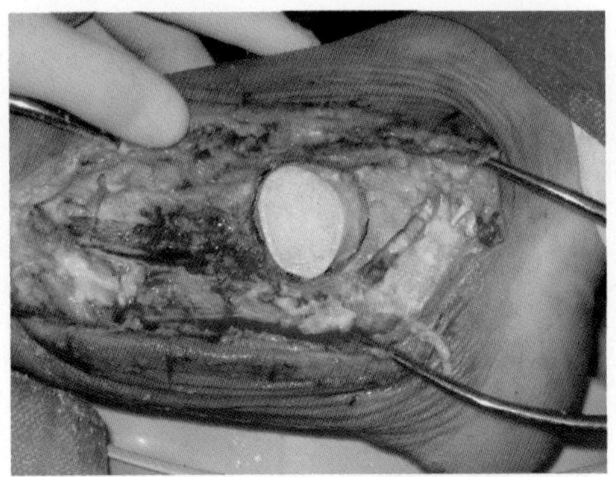

TECH FIG 7 • The femoral head graft is placed in the defect to ensure proper sizing.

the foot on the tibia). Because the femoral head graft is spherical, it is relatively easy to dial in the correct position of the ankle and hindfoot.

- The femoral neck is marked flush with the lateral tibia, the graft is removed, and the femoral neck is cut with a large oscillating saw.
- A bone slurry graft, made up of the autograft from the fibula and male reamers, is then placed in the defect to fill any voids around the fusion site (TECH FIG 8).
- The male reamers can again be placed and used in reverse to evenly spread the graft.
- The femoral head graft is placed back in the defect, and alignment is checked to ensure that it sits flush with the lateral fusion surface. Again, no provisional fixation is needed, as the interference fit between the femoral head and the recipient site is very stable.
  - This will allow unimpeded placement of the lateral blade plate.

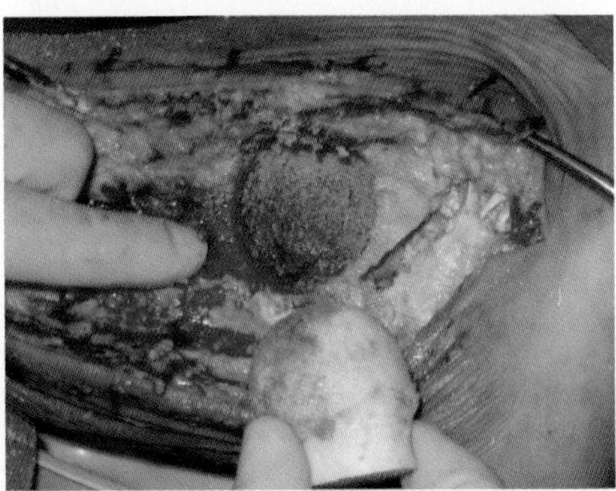

TECH FIG 8 • Once sizing is complete, a slurry of graft reamings is placed in the base of the defect and the reamers placed in reverse to spread the graft.

PLACEMENT OF PLATE AND SCREWS

- The 90-degree blade plate is then sized by placing it along the lateral fusion surface equidistant between the anterior and posterior surfaces of the tibia and femoral head graft.
- In my experience, fixation with six to eight cortical screws in the tibia proximal to the femoral head allograft is desirable; therefore, a blade plate of appropriate length is required. The decision depends on the quality of bone. Typically, for six cortical screws to be positioned in the tibia above the graft, a nine-hole blade plate will be needed.
- The distal end of the plate (the blade end) should line up with the center of the calcaneal body to ensure maximum hold and minimize the chance of fracturing the calcaneus with insertion.
  - Usually a six- to eight-hole plate with the short blade fits well.
- Once the plate size has been selected, place the plate "backward" along the lateral fusion area so the blade is pointing lateral (TECH FIG 9). This technique allows for proper angle of insertion of the guidewire and, therefore, the blade of the plate.

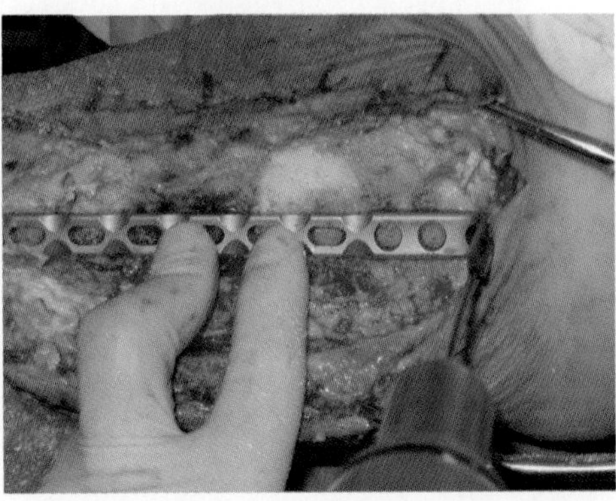

TECH FIG 9 • The blade plate is placed in a "backward" position along the fusion site for sizing. A guidewire is passed through the hole in the blade into the calcaneus.

- Check the hole alignment to ensure that at least one screw hole is over the calcaneus, one in the femoral head allograft, and two or three in the distal tibia.
- Drive the guidewire through the cannulated hole in the blade to the distal cortex of the calcaneus.
  - Pull the plate off the wire.
  - Because the plate could theoretically still rotate on the distal guide pin in the calcaneus, I often place a second wire through the plate. I use one of the screw holes proximally to ensure that when I flip the plate and impact it there is no chance that it will lose its desired proximal position on the tibia and potentially throw off the sagittal alignment or not be seated ideally on the tibia.
- Attach the driving device onto the plate and insert the blade plate over the guidewire (**TECH FIG 10A,B**). The 30-mm blade is most commonly used, because the 40-mm blade can easily penetrate the medial cortex and injure the neurovascular bundle.
  - Be sure to have an assistant apply counterpressure with a padded bolster while driving the plate into the calcaneus.
  - A separate guidewire driven through a proximal hole in the plate may help avoid unwanted twisting or rotation of the plate during insertion.
- Once the plate is seated, the position of the blade is checked to make sure it has not penetrated the medial cortex of the calcaneus. Again, if the 30-mm blade is used, penetration of the medial cortex should not occur.
- The screws (cancellous or cortical, depending on the type and quality of bone) are then inserted (**TECH FIG 10C**). In addition to the blade in the calcaneus, I like to have one additional screw through a distal hole in the plate, immediately above the blade, to enhance fixation in the calcaneus.
- A 7-mm cannulated screw is then placed from the posterolateral side of the distal tibia through the femoral head graft into the talar head and neck.
  - Fluoroscopy is used to check guidewire placement.
  - Avoid penetration into the talonavicular joint.
- A second cannulated screw can be placed from the calcaneal tuberosity into the femoral head graft if the blade-plate fixation to the calcaneus is not stable, as indicated by visible micromotion at the fusion interface or if the patient's bone is osteoporotic. In about half of my patients, this second screw is needed to gain adequate stability of fixation.
- Use the remaining autograft to fill any remaining gaps at the fusion sites anteriorly, posteriorly, and laterally.
- A layered closure over a drain is done, and a bulky Jones dressing applied.

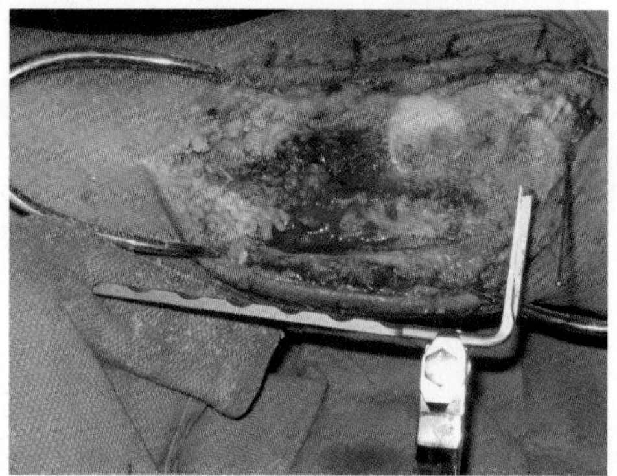

A

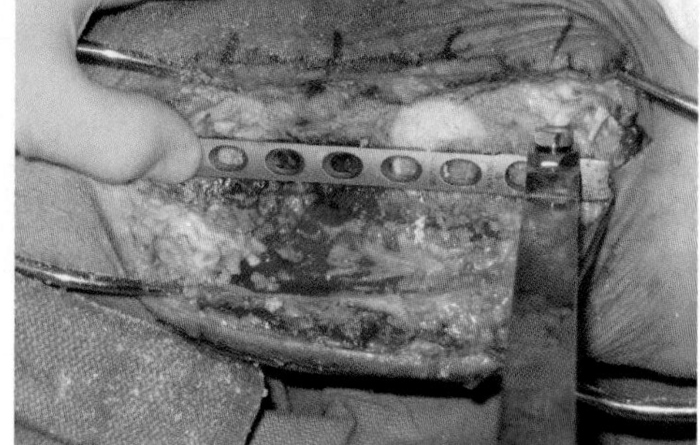

B

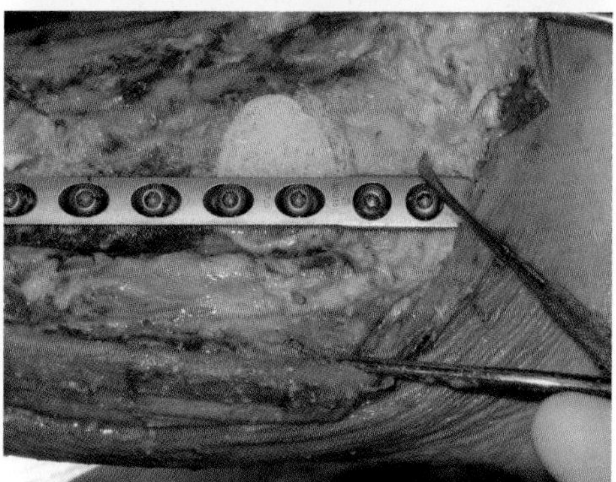

C

TECH FIG 10 • **A.** The blade is pulled off the wire and the driving device attached. **B.** The blade is driven into the calcaneus over the guidewire. **C.** Appropriate length screws are applied.

POSTOPERATIVE CARE

- Remove the bulky dressing 10 to 14 days postsurgery.
- The patient is in a short-leg cast for 6 to 8 weeks, with touch-down weight bearing permitted.
- The patient can begin weight bearing in a cam-soled walker at 2.5 to 3 months postoperatively if radiographs show signs of incorporation of the bone graft placed about the femoral head and fusion between the graft and the surrounding cancellous bone (**FIG 3**).

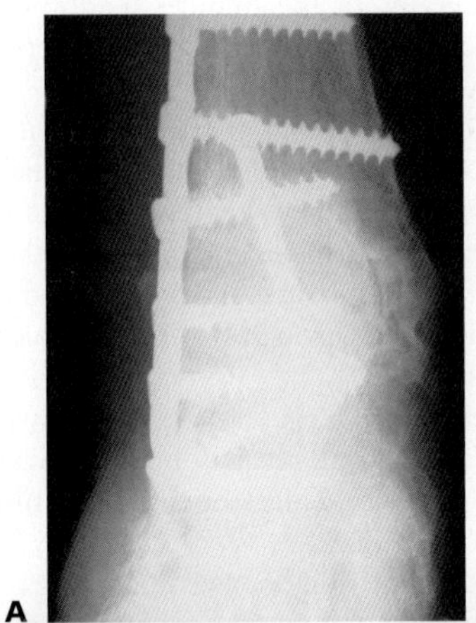

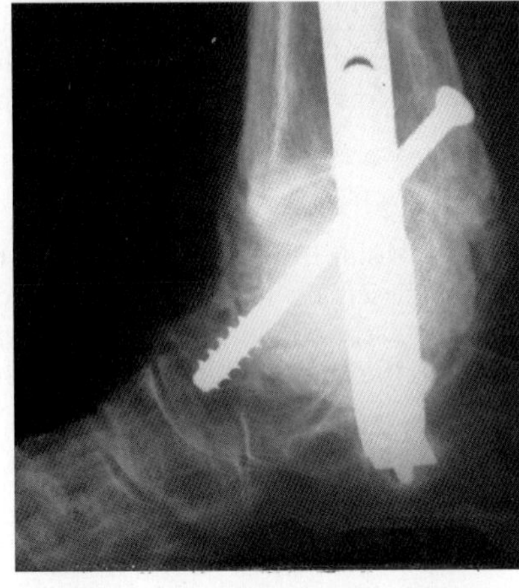

FIG 3 • AP (**A**) and lateral (**B**) radiographs taken 3 months postoperatively demonstrating callus formation about the femoral head allograft.

- We recommend that all of our patients use a non-hinged, light-weight, plastic ankle–foot orthosis (AFO) in a shoe with a soft anatomic cushioned heel indefinitely to protect the remaining joints of the foot.

OUTCOMES

- Our clinical experience with this technique includes five patients who underwent tibiotalocalcaneal fusion over 3 years.[3] Four patients showed radiographic healing by 3 months and began protected weight bearing with a lightweight plastic AFO. One of these four patients subsequently died of a myocardial infarction. The fifth patient was paralytic with severe hindfoot valgus and developed lateral skin breakdown with subsequent methicillin-resistant *Staphylococcus aureus* (MRSA) infection postoperatively over the graft site; that patient eventually underwent below knee amputation.
- Of the four patients who had a good result, the average follow-up was 1.5 years. None of the femoral grafts had collapsed, and all patients had good or excellent relief of their preoperative pain with no loss of leg length. The three surviving patients are community ambulators and use the light-weight AFO for walking outside the home to protect the remaining foot joints from excessive stress.
- The lateral blade–plate–screw construct for stabilizing tibiotalocalcaneal fusions has been previously described as a method to gain exceptional stability in patients with Charcot ankle fracture who had unbraceable deformity and severe instability of the ankle.[1] This fixation construct has been found to be biomechanically superior to an intramedullary rod for this type of fusion.[2]
- Myerson et al[4] have previously described the use of femoral head grafts through an anterior approach to fill large defects of the talar body. They have found them useful for filling large defects and avoiding severe limb shortening.

REFERENCES

1. Alvarez RG, Barbour TM, Perkins TD. Tibiocalcaneal arthrodesis for nonbraceable ankle deformity. Foot Ankle Int 1994;15:354–359.
2. Chiodo CP, Acevedo JI, Sammarco VJ, et al. Intramedullary rod fixation compared with blade-plate-and-screw fixation for tibiocalcaneal arthrodesis: A biomechanical investigation. J Bone Joint Surg Am 2003;85A:2425–2428.
3. Den Hartog BD, Palmer DS. Femoral head allografts for large talar defects. Tech Foot Ankle Surg 2008;7:264–270.
4. Myerson MS, Alvarez RG, Lam PW. Tibiocalcaneal arthrodesis for the management of severe ankle and hindfoot deformities. Foot Ankle Int 2000;21:643–650.

Chapter 86

Posterior Blade Plate for Salvage of Failed Total Ankle Arthroplasty

Mark Ritter, Florian Nickisch, and Christopher W. DiGiovanni

DEFINITION

- The number of total ankle arthroplasties (TAA) both designed and implanted continues to grow rapidly worldwide.
- The success and survivorship of any joint replacement are difficult to determine before a minimum 5-year follow-up. Because the early stage of most new arthroplasties can be marked by a steep learning curve while the later stage is often plagued by some level of polyethylene-induced osteolytic failure, foot and ankle specialists can expect to face increasing numbers of patients requiring revision or salvage surgery—even with the newest-generation TAA designs.
- Failure of a total ankle replacement can broadly be defined as septic or aseptic and usually results from either clinical (recalcitrant pain, instability, or malalignment) or radiographic (progressive loosening, subsidence, or osteolysis) deterioration.
- Implant failure due to septic or aseptic failure typically necessitates removal and leaves the surgeon with extensive areas of bone loss that must be addressed. Other potential problems include wound breakdown, infection, limb length discrepancies, scar formation, instability, malalignment, and, of course, choosing between complex and limited reconstructive options.
- Due to the anatomy and limited bone stock inherent to the ankle and particular to the talus, revision ankle replacement is frequently not possible in these cases, and arthrodesis of the ankle or tibiotalocalcaneal region remains the only viable salvage option.
- Fusion has traditionally been reported and performed through either an anterior or lateral approach. These approaches and the hardware used for them, however, are often limited by wound complications from the thin or previously operated soft tissue envelope, as well as difficulties in assessing rotatory, angular, and longitudinal alignment.
- The posterior approach usually provides the healthiest and deepest soft tissue bed for any postimplant failure reconstruction (through a single incision), permits ready access to the area of greatest potential bone graft harvest (posterior superior iliac spine [PSIS]), uses the fibula to aid in healing and in determining proper alignment, allows use of large fixed-angle devices applied on the tension side to enable safe and early postoperative weight bearing, and facilitates rapid intraoperative assessment of radiographic and clinical position.
- Because the fibula rarely provides enough bone to fill any remaining defect after TAA failure, it is often more useful in its native position as part of the reconstruction as opposed to being partly or completely sacrificed as part of a lateral or combined anterior operative approach.

ANATOMY

- The posterior aspect of the lower leg, ankle, and hindfoot is covered by several layers of well-vascularized soft tissues.
- The superficial posterior compartment contains the gastrocnemius and soleus complex, separated from the deep posterior compartment by a dense investing fascia.
- The sural nerve and the lesser saphenous vein should be carefully avoided as part of the superficial midline dissection in this approach.
- Once the superficial posterior compartment fascia is opened, the gastroc–soleal complex can be mobilized as a unit medially or laterally, or the Achilles tendon can be Z-lengthened to enable immediate access to the deep posterior compartment septum.
- The flexor hallucis longus (FHL) muscle is considered the "lighthouse" to the back of the ankle and hindfoot. It is readily identified by its uniquely low-lying muscle belly within the deep posterior compartment and provides the landmark for the posterior tibial neurovascular bundle, which courses immediately medial to it through the lower aspect of the leg and into the foot (**FIG 1**).
- Once identified, the FHL can be easily swept medially to protect the bundle during retraction and provide maximal exposure of the posterior aspect of the distal tibia, ankle joint, and subtalar joint (**FIG 2**).
- Once the reconstruction has been performed and fixation is indwelling, the deep soft tissue bed present in this region enables the hardware and any bone graft augmentation to thereafter be safely covered by repositioning of the FHL and Achilles complex before untensioned subcutaneous and skin closure.

PATHOGENESIS

- TAA failure can result from many causes, but the predominant mechanism, based on hip and knee replacement data, will likely become aseptic failure. This can occur from polyethylene wear over time, ballooning osteolysis, subsidence of

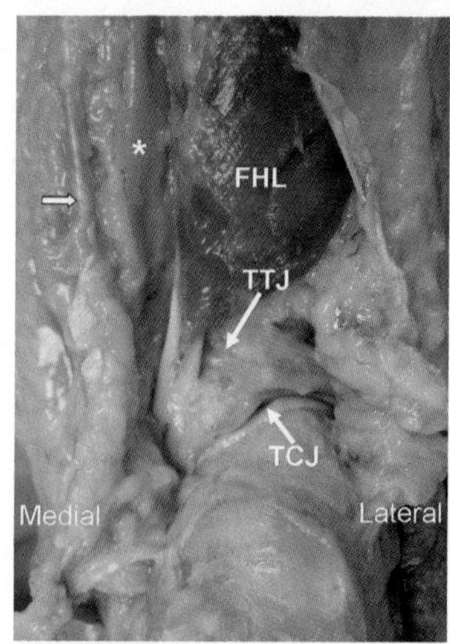

FIG 1 • Anatomy of the posterior ankle. Star, posterior tibial nerve; arrow, posterior tibialis artery. TTJ, tibiotalar joint; TCJ, tibiocalcaneal joint; FHL, flexor hallucis longus.

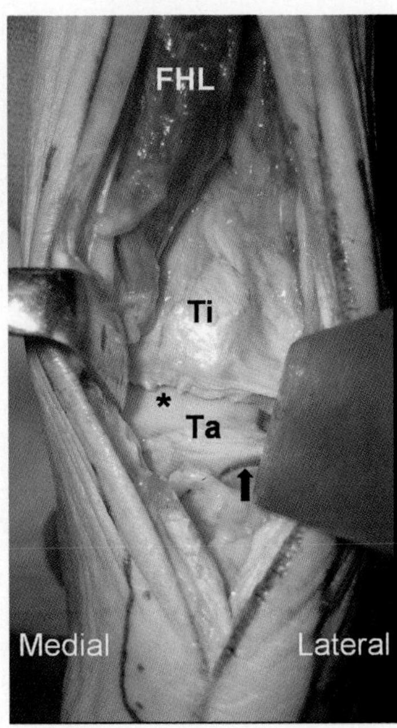

FIG 2 • The flexor hallucis longus is carefully retracted medially, allowing excellent visualization of the ankle (*star*) and subtalar joint (*arrow*).

the implants into surrounding host bone, heterotopic ossification, or frank implant fracture or dislocation. Septic failure can also occur at any point after joint implantation, and if this happens in the nonacute (beyond the first 6 to 12 weeks after surgery) setting, implant removal and some form of exchange or reconstruction as a single or staged procedure is usually required for successful salvage.

NATURAL HISTORY

- Although historically TAA has been in existence since the earliest hip and knee designs of the late 1960s and early 1970s, it has never enjoyed the same clinical success.
- This reason is likely multifactorial but no doubt stems in part from the many unique design aspects of the ankle joint that set it apart from the many other large joints that undergo very successful replacement today. These issues include the ankle's functional dependence upon the alignment and quality of many surrounding nearby joints, its inability to be dislocated during implant insertion, its thin and unforgiving soft tissue envelope, its limited native motion, its size-to-weight bearing ratio, and our present inability to completely resurface it such that the same stress is borne by the same surface area.
- Much of our understanding about ankle joint replacement stems from the adult reconstructive literature regarding hip and knee replacement. Most, if not all, earlier-generation ankle replacement designs have been considered failures by today's standards, and a great number eventuated into fusion or other forms of revision surgery.
- The most recent (third-generation) designs seem to have begun capitalizing on many newer technologies and design concepts ushered in by the successes in the hip, knee, and shoulder, and while early and midterm survivorship data (5 to 10 years) appear to be promising for these modular implants, time of implantation will be the ultimate judge.
- If history is any indication, it is quite possible that the next decade or two of foot and ankle specialists will have to become very familiar with reconstructive salvage of failed TAA in the form of revision replacement or fusion.
- Since the survivorship of the average total hip or knee arthroplasty approaches 90% to 95% at 15 to 20 years and TAA has never approximated this success, the rapidly increasing number of ankle replacement designs being accepted by the FDA and in countries abroad, as well as the seemingly exponential rate of TAA implantation today as an alternative to primary fusion, would suggest that revision ankle replacement surgery will need to be a part of every foot and ankle specialist's armamentarium in upcoming years.

PATIENT HISTORY AND PHYSICAL FINDINGS

- A thorough history and physical examination, as well as an appropriate set of weight-bearing ankle radiographs, are paramount to identifying the patient with a failed TAA.
- Unremitting or new-onset pain is often the chief complaint of a poorly functioning or infected ankle replacement.
- Patients should also be assessed for associated ankle swelling and warmth, which if recent are reasonable indications for a more in-depth evaluation to assess the integrity of the TAA.
- Time from initial implantation as well as any history of prior surgery or implantation in this region should be noted.
- Patients who are diabetic or neuropathic or who have any systemic illness that could predispose them to infection, immunologic compromise, or undetected abnormal wear (Charcot) should also be more carefully assessed.
- Any history of fever, chills, sweats, or recent dental surgery without antibiotic prophylaxis should be noted, as should complaints of ankle or hindfoot instability.
- The examiner should look for obvious ankle or hindfoot deformity, either new or old. Particular attention should be paid to the varus or cavus foot malalignment, which has the highest association with implant failure.
- Restricted range of motion or the presence of pain, crepitance, or grinding on examination should be noted.
- The examiner should look for any surrounding fluctuance, erythema, or draining sinus around the ankle.

IMAGING AND OTHER DIAGNOSTIC STUDIES

- When implant failure is suspected, the initial screening blood work to rule out sepsis should include a complete blood count with differentiation, erythrocyte sedimentation rate, and a C-reactive protein level.
- Weight-bearing, standing plain films of the affected ankle (anteroposterior, lateral, and oblique views) should be obtained. If necessary, particularly when a form of aseptic failure from mechanical malalignment of the foot is suspected, a routine set of plain films of the foot should also be obtained.
- Radiologic signs of loosening include radiolucent lines around the components, as well as malposition and subsidence of any component (**FIG 3**). These are most valuable when they are indentified as acute changes from previous films or shown to be slowly progressive over time.
- Ballooning osteolysis behind an implant is a poor prognosticator for impending implant subsidence and failure. In such

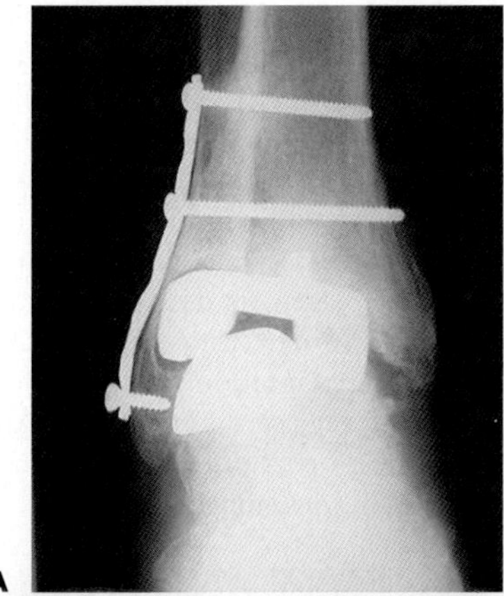

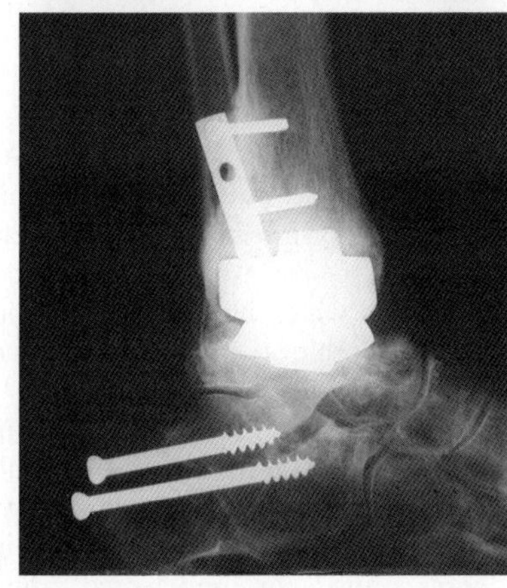

FIG 3 • AP (**A**) and lateral (**B**) radiographs of a failed total ankle arthroplasty. Note lysis around tibial implant and subsidence of the talar component.

patients, polyethylene wear (a narrowed joint space) is often identifiable on plain radiographs.

- An implant should be considered to be infected until proven otherwise when the history, physical examination, and blood work suggest such.
- A bone scan can also be useful as an adjunct for diagnosing septic or aseptic loosening.
- In these patients or in those with an equivocal examination, an office based or radiologically guided aspiration is indicated for routine Gram stain and culture.
- Percutaneous biopsy can also be performed, although intraoperative cultures are considered most sensitive and specific for the etiology of the implant failure. These can be assessed pathologically for polymorphonucleocytes per high-power field, as well as for the presence of bacteria and poly debris.
- In cases of suspected or documented infection, consultation with the infectious disease team is suggested to determine the appropriate microbiologic and chemotherapeutic aspects of the subsequent management.
- Failure can be on one side or both sides of the joint, and hence can involve either the polyethylene spacer (if present), one implant, or all implants in the TAA design. This determination affects whether the TAA can be salvaged.
- CT scanning can be useful to assess the degree of osteolysis and bone destruction, which is often otherwise difficult to discern behind the implants. Such information can also be very useful in planning a revision procedure, as can the integrity of any nearby joints (subtalar, Chopart).

DIFFERENTIAL DIAGNOSIS

- Pain of unknown etiology (implants still well fixed): complex regional pain syndrome, stiffness, fibromyalgia, neuroma, tendon incarceration, neurovascular injury or compromise, heterotopic ossification, occult fracture, syndesmotic nonunion, arthritis or impingement of nearby joints
- Septic failure (infection)
- Aseptic failure (impingement, osteolysis, implant or polyethylene fracture, subsidence, circumferential loosening, malposition, malalignment, dislocation, instability, periprosthetic fracture, syndesmotic nonunion when applicable)

NONOPERATIVE MANAGEMENT

- Nonoperative management is generally not indicated for a septic TAA failure. When these are very acute, these can occasionally respond to serial aspiration and antibiotic therapy, but even in these cases surgical intervention (arthroscopy or single-stage exchange) has proven most effective.
- In cases of aseptic failure, treatment depends on the cause.
  - Gross instability, uncontrollable pain, catastrophic implant failure (fracture), periprosthetic fracture, and aggressive (ballooning) osteolysis are generally best treated surgically.
  - Other causes of aseptic failure can be considered for conservative management, which includes some form of bracing, mechanical offloading with assistive devices, pharmacologic pain control (or osteolytic inhibition), and a RICE protocol.
  - Sometimes simple tolerance is the most appropriate course when the risks of revision surgery might outweigh any of the potential benefits.
  - The risks of such complex surgery, as well as its limitations, must be discussed in detail with any patient in this situation, and this discussion should always include the possibility of below-knee amputation.

SURGICAL MANAGEMENT

- A blade plate or fixed-angle device applied from posteriorly in the prone-positioned patient addresses all the problems associated with arthrodesis of a failed TAA, and it is our preference.
- This procedure can be performed as a single- or two-stage procedure.
- The technique is versatile because it can be used for both tibiotalar or tibiotalocalcaneal arthrodesis, with the only difference being the size of the fixation device.
- Many different implant sizes can be used for this technique, varying from small- to large-fragment fixation, locking or nonlocking constructs, and fixed-angle or straight plates.
- The prone position allows access to a deep and usually healthy, unscarred soft tissue bed capable of accessing or removing the indwelling TAA as well as covering appropriate hardware and bone graft without tension.
- The prone position also allows for the easiest clinical determination of hindfoot position before fusion, and it affords access to the posterior iliac crest for maximal amounts of bone graft procurement. The opposite leg can also be prepared out, if need be, for comparison.
- AP and lateral radiographic images are also easily obtainable, requiring minimal to no manipulation from the surgeon when the operative leg is elevated on two or three folded blankets.

- Lastly, the fixation in this approach is placed on the tension side. This acts to compress the fusion mass under the load of weight bearing, facilitating a more rapid return to ambulation.

Preoperative Planning

- All radiographs and laboratory parameters, as well as the patient's skin envelope, are reviewed before surgery.
- If the patient has an infected TAA, this procedure should be performed in staged fashion and only after the decision has been made not to reimplant an ankle prosthesis at the second stage. A carefully contoured, anatomic polymethylmethacrylate antibiotic spacer impregnated with tobramycin and vancomycin can easily be inserted and removed through the same approach to maintain alignment and soft tissue tension between stages.
- Symptom production from the subtalar joint must be carefully assessed preoperatively (but can also be assessed visually intraoperatively) to determine any potential need for adding subtalar fusion to an isolated tibiotalar arthrodesis. Surrounding bone quality and stock should also be a major factor in making this determination, particularly on the talar side.
- Preoperatively, two-stage office-based or fluoroscopically guided diagnostic differential injections of the talocalcaneal and subtalar joints with local analgesic are well suited for this purpose.
- Precontouring the blade plate (and determining its size) using an ankle sawbones model and a preoperative template saves significant tourniquet time (**FIG 4**).

Positioning

- The patient is positioned prone on an image table with gelpads, using a few folded blankets as a "workbench" under the affected leg to elevate it sufficiently above the contralateral extremity to permit unimpeded imaging of the operated extremity in the cross-table lateral projection (**FIG 5**).
- Gelpads should not be used in the area intended for fluoroscopy, since the material is radiopaque. The image machine should be checked for clearly visible AP and lateral views of the patient's ankle and hindfoot before preparation and draping.

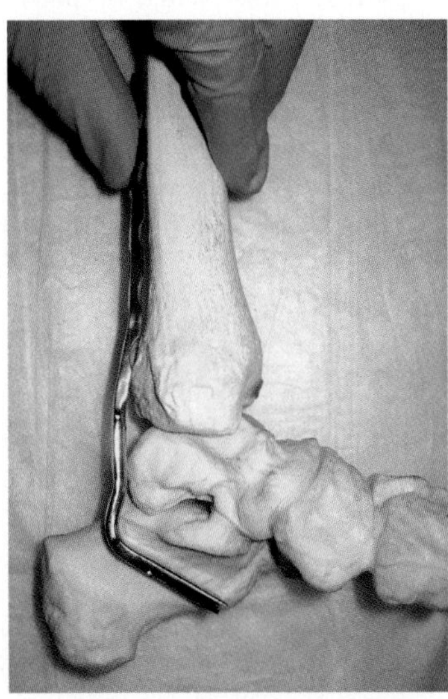

FIG 4 • Precontouring the blade plate with sawbones as template.

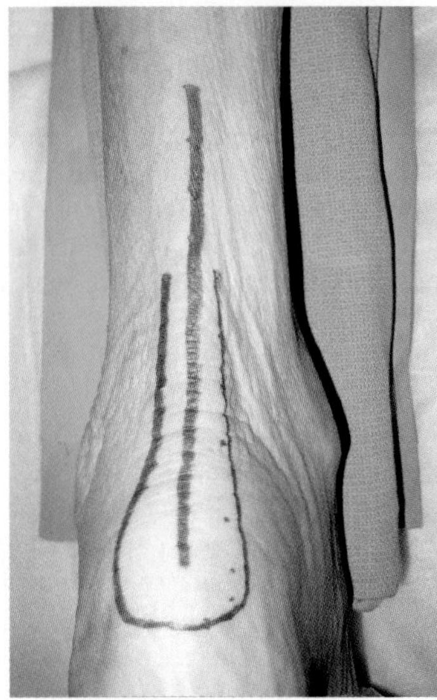

FIG 5 • Posterior midline approach.

- A tourniquet should be placed about the thigh, and the ipsilateral posterior iliac crest should be squared off with preliminary drapes in anticipation of bone graft procurement.

Approach

- The entire ipsilateral leg and PSIS are then prepared and draped in the usual sterile fashion.
- The ankle and hindfoot should be operated on to establish the size of the defect and amount and configuration of bone required before autologous harvest from the PSIS.
- Under tourniquet control, a midline longitudinal incision 12 to 16 cm long is initially made directly posterior to the

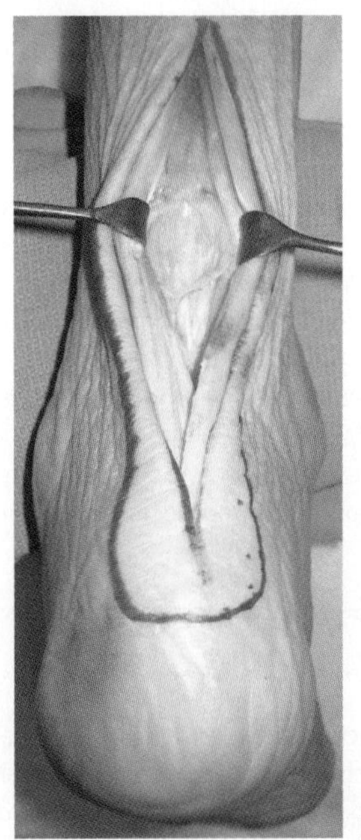

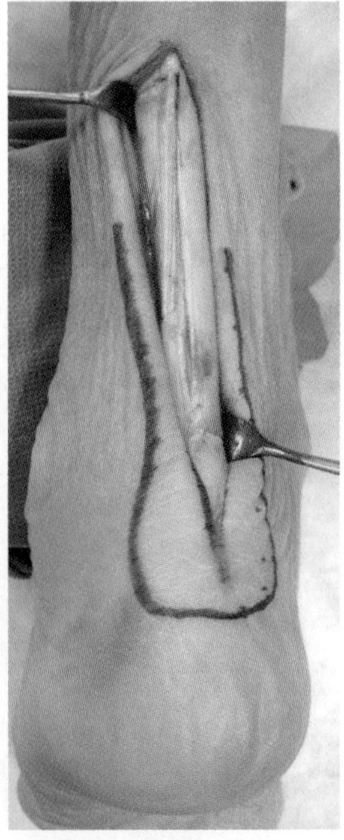

FIG 6 • **A.** Longitudinal split through Achilles tendon. **B.** Z-lengthening of Achilles tendon if additional exposure is required.

ankle and hindfoot (Fig 5). Imaging can be useful at times to establish this position ideally, although we prefer simply centering this over the ankle in the midline. If it is determined intraoperatively that more exposure is required distally to access the subtalar joint, this incision can be easily extended by curving it slightly posteromedially as it courses over the heel.

- No skin retraction is used, and retractors are used only once the deeper tissues are encountered.
- The paratenon of the Achilles and the superficial fascia are first carefully opened with the intention of later closure and separation from overlying skin and subcutaneous tissues in the rare event of wound breakdown.
- A Z-plasty of the Achilles is performed longitudinally to allow access to the deep posterior compartment. Incising the fascia over the superficial posterior compartment can ease tension and improve retractability of the gastrocnemius and soleus during exposure. Care should be taken to maintain full-thickness flaps ("canyon walls") (**FIG 6**).
- The deep posterior compartment fascia is then incised, exposing the FHL and the remaining deep extrinsic musculature.
- The neurovascular bundle is identified but not dissected, and then carefully retracted medially by retracting the lateral side of the FHL.
- This permits unimpaired full access of the posterior tibia, the capsules overlying the ankle and subtalar joints, and the distal fibula immediately beneath a portion of the inferior peroneal musculature (**FIG 7**).

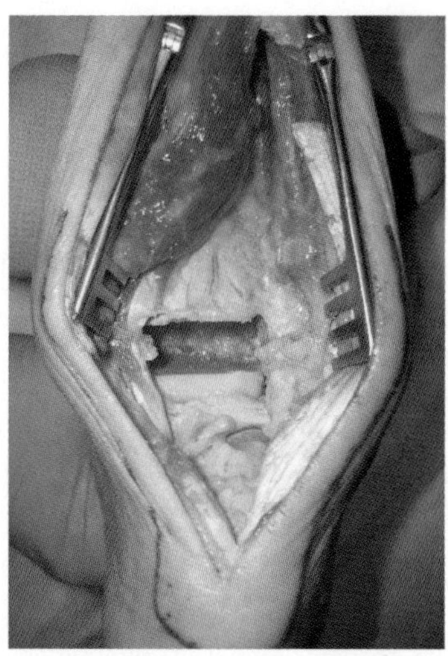

FIG 7 • Deep compartment open, flexor hallucis longus retracted medially. The failed ankle implant has been removed and the defect débrided.

- The inferiormost edge of the peroneals can be removed subperiosteally from the distal fibula as needed to gain access to the ankle joint as well as to expose greater amounts of direct bleeding bone for surface-area healing of the fusion mass. Although not necessary, this permits incorporation of the fibula in the fusion mass when desired.

TECHNIQUES

TAA REMOVAL

- Although most implants are placed through an anterior approach, it is generally not difficult to remove these current designs from a posterior approach.
- Use of a femoral distractor, or, alternatively, an external fixator with medial pins in the tibia and the calcaneus will facilitate distraction of the joint for easy implant removal in the event of soft tissue contracture.
- Once the ankle implants have been removed, any fibrous membrane or other debris within the joint can be excised and the remnant viable bone stock (defect void) and quality can be assessed to plan alignment, bone graft requirements, and implant size for the reconstruction.
- Only healthy, bleeding bone should be left behind amidst a viable soft tissue envelope.
- At this point, the subtalar joint should also be inspected—and fused, if deemed necessary by virtue of its integrity or the remaining available bone stock for fixation. In the case of TAA salvage, this technique is usually recommended.
- Despite any preconceived opinions about the presence or absence of infection, under all circumstances it is advisable to obtain multiple deep tissue samples for pathology and culture. These should be taken ideally before antibiotic prophylaxis is given, and we recommend taking three samples for pathology and three for microbiology, all with separate instruments, from separate sites, labeled with separate identifiers, and placed in separate sterile containers. Under no circumstances should the skin be touched when performing this task, for fear of inadvertent contamination.

INFECTED TAA REMOVAL

- If the joint is infected, or presumed infected, a radical débridement is performed at this time, taking similar cultures and pathology specimens from separate "high-yield" areas.
- In these cases, the ankle joint is then prepared for a second-stage procedure by thorough saline irrigation and interposition of a PMMA antibiotic-laden spacer fashioned to fit the bony defect and maintain alignment, length, and stability (**TECH FIG 1**).
- Since cultures are often not yet indicative of an infecting organism, both vancomycin and tobramycin should be included in the spacer for both gram-negative and gram-positive coverage.

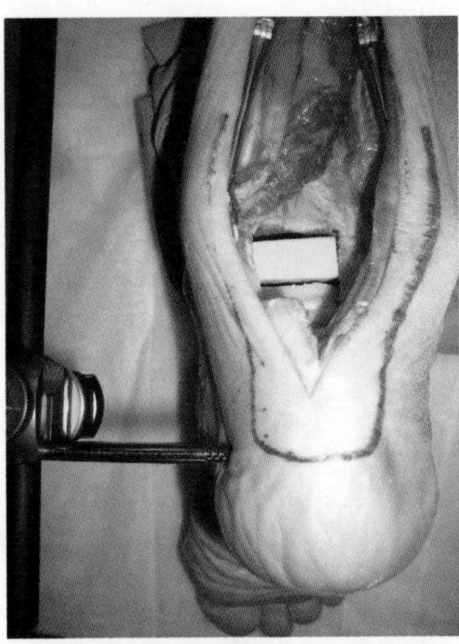

TECH FIG 1 • External fixator medially, antibiotic spacer placed in void after removal of infected implant.

- The soft tissues are copiously reirrigated, and hemostasis is then maintained, and they are completely closed around the spacer.
- The infected patient is treated with adjunctive antibiotics for 6 to 8 weeks, and often an external fixator is added for additional support (in lieu of a splint or cast).
- Before second-stage surgery, the blood work should have returned to normal and the ankle should be reaspirated to verify eradication of infection. All incisions should also have healed uneventfully and be deemed capable of tolerating further surgery.
- At the time of staged reconstruction, the same posterior incision is used, and during exposure a stat Gram stain and frozen sections are taken to quantify white blood cells per high-power field. If these values are within normal limits, the procedure then continues as outlined for primary fusion in the aseptic patient as indicated below.

DECORTICATION AND BONE GRAFTING

- After final takedown and decortication of the ankle (and possibly the subtalar joint) the surgeon can determine how much bone graft to harvest. Occasionally this includes preference of size or shape (eg, tricortical, trapezoidal, cancellous only).
- If the subtalar joint is to be taken down, it is prepared in a similar manner. Bone (laminar) spreaders are very useful for this purpose in both joints.
- Bone graft blocks are taken from the posterior iliac crest with a sagittal saw and osteotomes, and thereafter are fashioned to fit and bridge the resected ankle gap. Generally, tricortical grafts are most amenable to this construct and can be easily contoured into appropriate position to maintain alignment. Once these are taken, the cancellous graft between the remaining inner and outer table of the pelvis can also be harvested for packing the remaining joint space. In all these cases the cancellous bone graft should be mixed with tobramycin and vancomycin powder before being packed into all remaining articular interstices after hardware implantation.

BLADE PLATE APPLICATION

- The foot should be placed in neutral alignment and preliminarily held in reduction with one or two large nonthreaded Steinmann pins. Typically, this alignment includes 0 degrees of ankle flexion with 5 degrees of hindfoot valgus and external rotation appropriate to the opposite side. This step is performed identically for both ankle and tibiotalocalcaneal fusion.
- Hence, once proper length and position are established clinically and radiographically, one or two eighth-inch Steinmann pins are placed through the calcaneus from directly inferiorly, and run into the midtibia to maintain this alignment. Foot and ankle position is then verified in both the lateral and AP planes with imaging. The precontoured 4.5-mm 90-degree fixed-angle blade plate (recommended) is then laid next to this to assess proper contouring and positioning via imaging. Small alterations in this device are best made at this time before it is actually implanted.
- Predrilling a trough for the blade of the plate is usually unnecessary when doing a tibiotalocalcaneal fusion because of the soft cancellous bone found within the calcaneus. In this case, the starting position and angle of insertion are far more important. In the less common circumstance of having enough talar bone to simply fuse only the ankle primarily, a precut trough is advisable before the blade plate is introduced into the denser talus bone. In this latter circumstance, often a smaller blade plate (3.5 mm) is more amenable to this fusion construct.
- In both cases, attention must also be paid to the following:
  - Proper length of the blade to avoid cutout upon implant seating
  - Proper angle of the blade to ensure adequate positioning once seated
  - Number of screw holes traversing the tibia such that adequate fixation is maintained above the fusion mass
  - Proper rotation of the blade such that it sits centrally located along the posterior tibial metadiaphysis once fully seated (**TECH FIG 2**)
- Serial imaging during blade plate insertion can be very helpful in making these determinations before completely bottoming out the implant.
- Once the blade plate is fully seated, the position of the limb clinically and radiographically should be reassessed. After this, the plate can be locked in position by placing

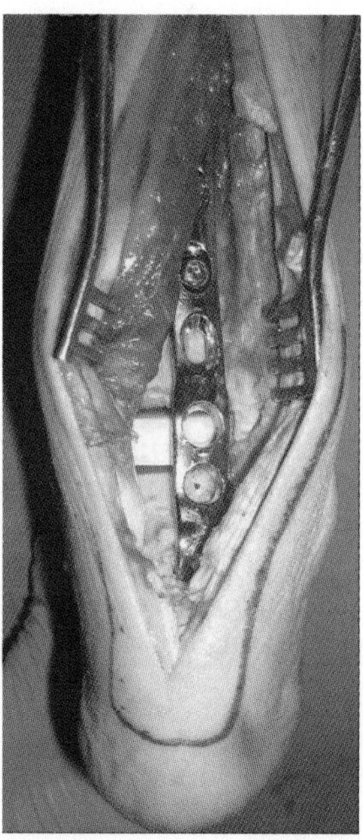

TECH FIG 2 • Blade plate placed posteriorly with foot in neutral position, calcaneus in 5 degrees of valgus, held by Steinmann pin.

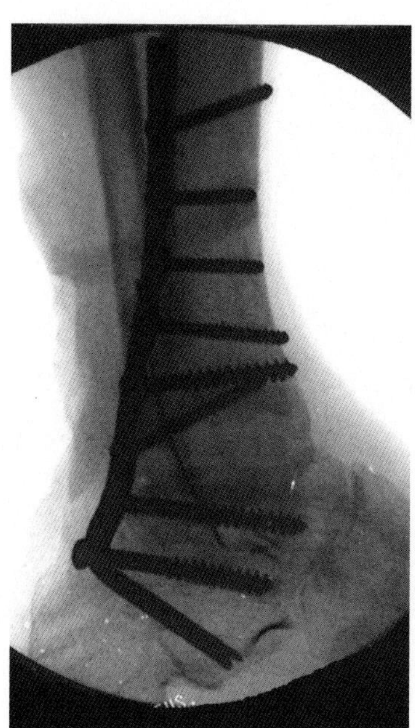

TECH FIG 4 • Lateral fluoroscopic image verifying blade and screw placement and alignment.

a single proximal and distal compressive screw, followed by Steinmann pin removal.

- The remaining compressive screw fixation construct for the plate can then performed in routine fashion, including the use of the articulating tensioning device where applicable.
- Often, several screws can be used to cross several joints not only to enact a neutralization plate construct but also to permit some articular compression across the fusion mass as well.
- After fixation, any residual graft can be packed in and around the plate and joints (**TECH FIG 3**).
- Final films should be taken and saved, and a repeat clinical examination should be performed to ensure satisfactory alignment before final closure (**TECH FIG 4**).
- The deep posterior compartment is then swung back into place to easily cover the plate (**TECH FIG 5**) and the Achilles can be reapproximated in neutral position. A Hemovac drain should be placed at this time before the overlying fascia, subcutaneous tissue, and skin are closed.

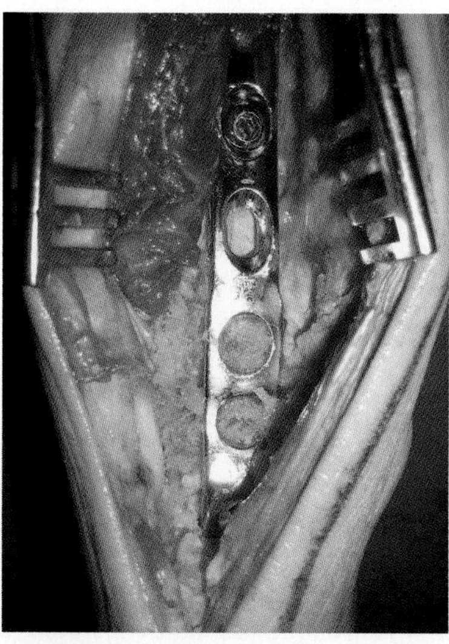

TECH FIG 3 • Additional bone graft is packed around the blade, the ankle, and the subtalar joint.

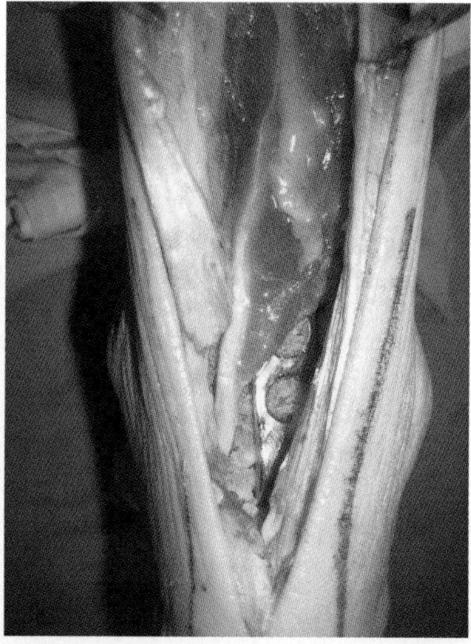

TECH FIG 5 • The flexor hallucis longus is replaced in its anatomic position covering most of the implant.

PEARLS AND PITFALLS

Large bony defect	■ Posterior iliac crest bone graft, corticocancellous
Hard talus bone	■ Predrilling blade trough in talus

POSTOPERATIVE CARE

- An ankle blockade with Marcaine and lidocaine eases pain in the immediate postoperative setting, but it should be placed well above the operative site to avoid wound tension.
- Steri-Strips should be applied across the incision site to distribute stress optimally at this level, and away from the incision itself. To this end, these should be uncut, and benzoin should be avoided to minimize blister formation.
- A meticulously padded Jones dressing, posterior splinting, and taped suction drainage help to avoid edema, hematoma, and pressure sore formation.
- While the patient recovers in bed or rests in a supine position, no pressure should be permitted beneath the lower leg, ankle, and foot. Hence, this area should be "suspended in midair" by placing pillows or blankets underneath the proximal calf, knee, and thigh to avoid pressure on the incision.
- The patient should remain strictly non–weight-bearing for the first 2 weeks postoperatively.
- After the posterior skin wound has healed and sutures have been removed, cast immobilization with partial weight bearing is allowed until week 6. Placing the plate posteriorly across the ankle creates a tension band phenomenon during the gait cycle, helping to compress the fusion site with weight bearing. Physical therapy can also begin during this time interval. At 6 weeks, consideration can be given to transitioning the patient to boot immobilization, depending on the clinical and radiographic progress, and slow progression to full weight bearing can begin.
- All forms of cast or boot immobilization are discontinued after radiographic evidence of healing, usually at about 12 weeks postoperatively (**FIG 8**). The patient can be advanced into a sneaker with a SACH heel or rocker sole.

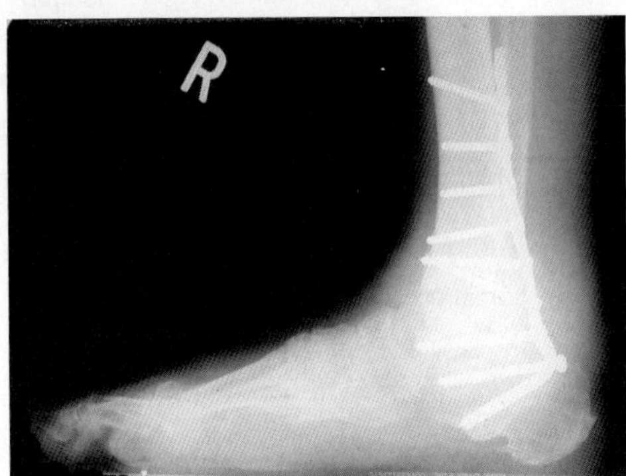

FIG 8 • Weight-bearing lateral radiograph 3 months postoperatively.

OUTCOMES

- In our experience, this operation has been very effective for salvaging difficult revision of failed TAA with reasonable patient satisfaction.
- We have not done enough of these procedures, however, to enable us to reasonably discuss outcome. We do believe, though, that this operation will become more pertinent over time, and that it is a very easy, safe, and versatile technique to address this difficult problem.

COMPLICATIONS

- In our limited experience with this approach, we have encountered no complications, although we believe the potential complication list would certainly be similar to any major revisional fusion operation dealing with intercalary defects.

REFERENCES

1. Bruggeman N, Kitaoka H. Arthrodesis after failed total ankle arthroplasty. Tech Foot Ankle Surg 2002;1:60–68.
2. Hammit MD, Hobgood ER, Tarquinio TA. Midline posterior approach to the ankle and hindfoot. Foot Ankle Int 2006;27:711–715.
3. Hansen T, Cracchiolo A. The use of a 95 degree blasé plate and posterior approach to tibiotalocalcaneal arthrodesis. Foot Ankle Int 2002;23:704–710.
4. Peyvich M, Saltzman C. Total ankle arthroplasty: a unique design. J Bone Joint Surg Am 1998;80A:1410–1420.
5. Quill G. Tibiotalocalcaneal arthrodesis with medullary rod fixation. Tech Foot Ankle Surg 2003;2:135–143.
6. Wapner K. Salvage of failed and infected total ankle replacements with fusion. AAOS Instructional Course Lectures 2002;51:153–157.

Chapter 87 Arthroscopy of the Ankle

Jorge I. Acevedo and Peter Mangone

DEFINITION

- Arthroscopy of the ankle has become an invaluable tool for evaluating and treating pathology in the ankle joint.
- Arthroscopy allows a minimally invasive approach to the structures of the ankle with a magnified view.
- Detailed knowledge of the anatomy surrounding the ankle joint as well as the different structural variations is key to avoiding complications.

ANATOMY

- The anteromedial portal is located medial to the tibialis anterior tendon at the level of the ankle joint (**FIG 1**). Care should be taken to avoid injury to the long saphenous vein and nerve usually located medial to the portal.
- The anterolateral portal lies on the anterior joint line just lateral to the peroneus tertius tendon or alternatively lateral to the extensor digitorum longus tendons (Fig 1). The intermediate cutaneous branch of the superficial peroneal nerve lies in close proximity to this portal.
- Posteromedial and posterolateral coaxial portals lie parallel to the bimalleolar axis (**FIG 2**).
- The posterolateral coaxial portal (**FIG 3**) is located immediately posterior to the peroneus longus tendon, and the posteromedial coaxial portal (**FIG 4**) ideally lies between the posterior colliculus (of the medial malleolus) and the posterior tibial tendon. (Placement between the flexor digitorum longus and the posterior tibial tendon is also acceptable.)

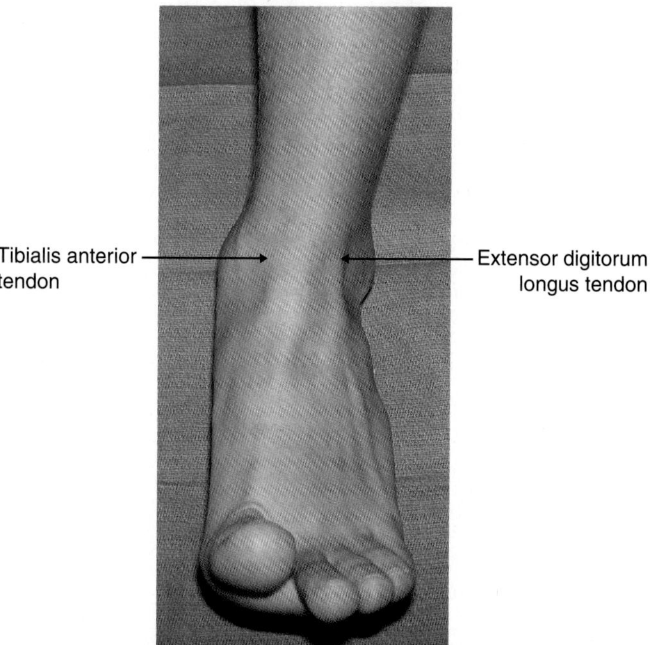

FIG 1 • Anatomic landmarks for anterior ankle arthroscopy. *1*, anteromedial portal site; *2*, anterolateral portal site.

- The sural nerve is located an average of 6.6 mm from this posterolateral portal, while the posterior tibial nerve is found an average of 5.7 mm from the posteromedial portal.

DIFFERENTIAL DIAGNOSIS

- Anterior ankle impingement
- Ankle arthritis or frozen ankle
- Osteochondral tibial or talar defects
- Lateral ankle instability
- Ankle fractures
- Recalcitrant ankle synovitis (often seen in patients with systemic inflammatory disease)

NONOPERATIVE MANAGEMENT

- In general, conservative treatment will include a trial with activity modification, immobilization with a brace, and nonsteroidal anti-inflammatories.

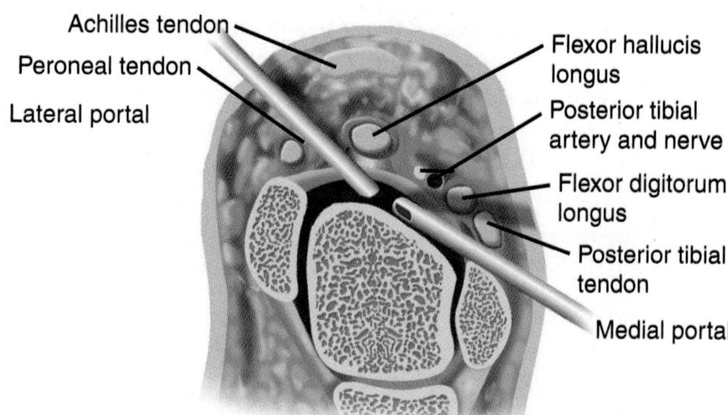

FIG 2 • Coaxial portal cross-sectional anatomy.

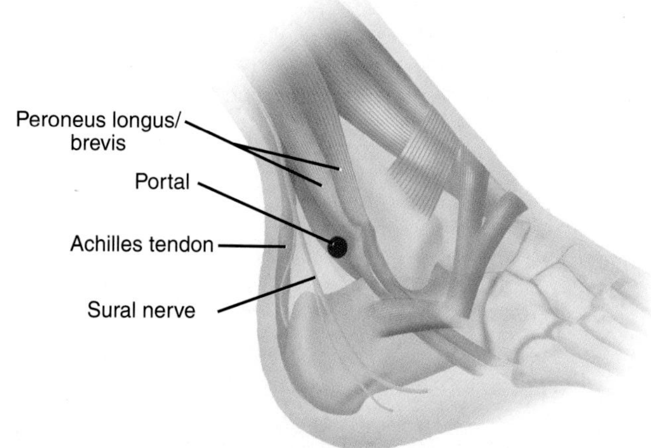

FIG 3 • Coaxial posterolateral portal anatomy.

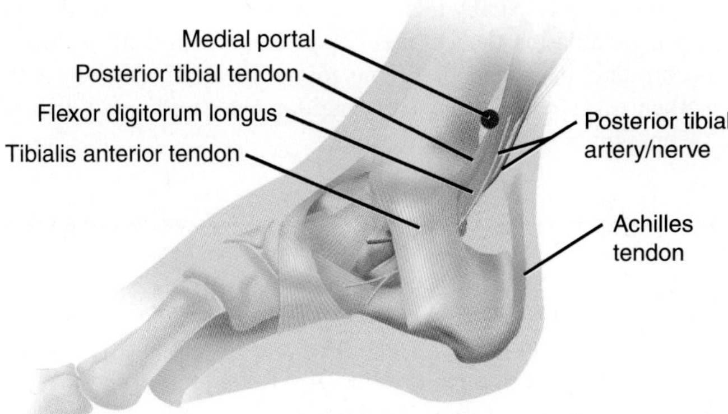

FIG 4 • Coaxial posteromedial portal anatomy.

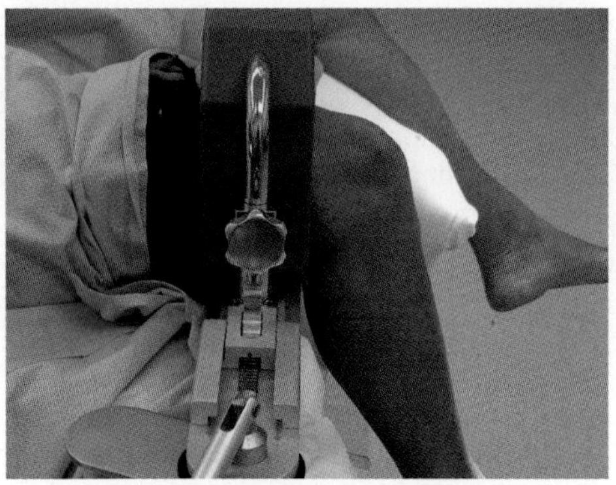

FIG 5 • Leg holder position for posterior portal access.

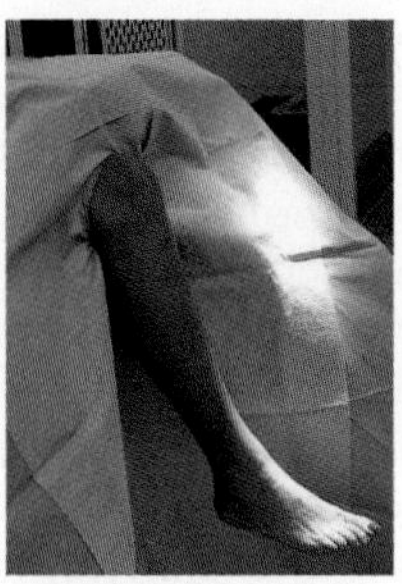

FIG 6 • Bed position for posterior portal access.

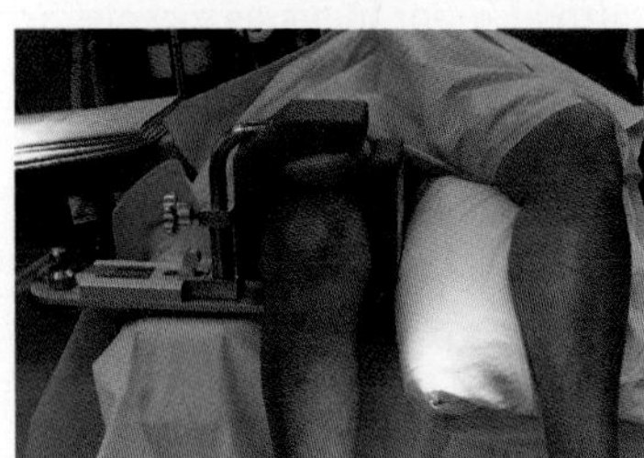

FIG 7 • Position of operative leg and padded contralateral limb.

- Physical therapy using modality treatment, range-of-motion exercises, neuromuscular coordination training (eg, balance board), and strengthening of the secondary or dynamic stabilizing muscles surrounding the ankle is a useful adjunct to most conditions.

SURGICAL MANAGEMENT

Preoperative Planning

- Imaging studies are reviewed to determine ideal portals to be used.
- Standard anteromedial and anterolateral portals are sufficient to access the anterior and central tibiotalar pathology.
- Posterior portals are considered when drilling posterior talar lesions or when it is necessary to address pathology (eg, synovitis, loose bodies) within the posterior capsule.
- A preoperative popliteal block is placed by anesthesia. Over the past 5 years, we have been able to perform 75% of ankle arthroscopies with regional anesthesia and light sedation.
- An examination under anesthesia including anterior drawer as well as a talar tilt test should be performed before positioning.

Positioning

- The patient is placed on a regular operating table with a well-padded tourniquet on the proximal thigh.
- The supine position with a towel roll placed underneath the ankle is used when only anterior portals are necessary. In this situation the tourniquet may be placed on the proximal calf.
- If access to posterior portals is likely, then we lower the leg extension of the bed and use a standard arthroscopy knee holder (**FIG 5**). This restricts thigh motion but allows free leg motion and access to the posterior hindfoot (**FIG 6**). The contralateral leg is placed in a well-padded holder or pillow (**FIG 7**).
- Alternatively a noninvasive ankle distractor is used.

Approach

- Currently the standard working approaches include the anteromedial and anterolateral portals.
- Auxiliary anterior portals (such as the antero-central) should be used with caution because of the high incidence of neurovascular injury.
- The standard posteromedial and posterolateral portals should also be used with extreme caution due to the close proximity of neurovascular structures (**FIG 8**).

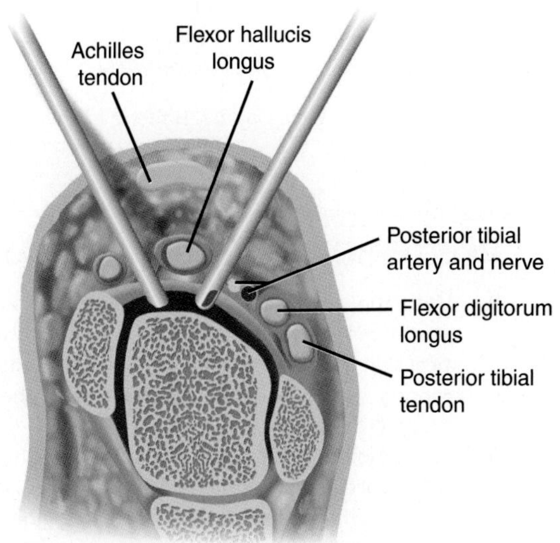

FIG 8 • Conventional posterior portal cross-sectional anatomy.

- We prefer to use posterior coaxial portals parallel to the bimalleolar axis when addressing the posterior ankle joint.
- Although the standard 4-mm arthroscope may be used, we prefer to use the 2.7-mm arthroscopic instruments, which facilitate access and simplify the approach.
- Instruments usually include 2.5-mm shaver, 3.5-mm shaver, thermal ablation device (this is especially helpful for synovectomy and débridement of the joint; however, care must be taken to avoid articular cartilage damage), and small arthroscopic biter and grabber devices.

TECHNIQUES

ANTERIOR PORTAL PLACEMENT

- The operative leg is identified and marked preoperatively.
- The patient is placed supine on the operating table.
- Inject the ankle with 10 cc of sterile saline via the anteromedial ankle. This step also allows identification of the correct orientation and location for the anteromedial arthroscopy portal.
- Make a 5-mm longitudinal skin incision and spread the subcutaneous tissue down to and then through the capsule with a small hemostat. A small gush of fluid confirms the intra-articular location.
- Use the blunt-tip trocar with the arthroscopic cannula to enter the joint. Insert the arthroscope and start the water flow. Place the water pressure about 5 mm Hg above the systolic pressure if possible (no higher than a pressure of 120 mm Hg). This significantly reduces bleeding, which often obscures the view.
- Unless there is severe arthrofibrotic tissue in the anterior ankle, the anterolateral ankle is easily visualized upon introducing the arthroscope (**TECH FIG 1**).
- Introduce an 18-gauge needle from the anterolateral portal location. This serves two purposes: (1) it allows for water flow through the needle, allowing for better visualization and (2) it identifies the correct location of the portal incision in order to access the joint properly.
- Inspect the joint. Distraction allows for much greater joint inspection than otherwise would be possible.
- Make the anterolateral portal in a similar fashion to the anteromedial portal.
- Using both portals, various arthroscopic instruments are used to address the individual patient's pathology.
- The addition of an anteromedial inferior portal is very helpful when dealing with synovitis near the deltoid insertion. This is performed by visualizing the medial gutter with the arthroscope through the anteromedial portal. An 18-gauge needle is introduced under arthroscopic visualization into the inferior medial gutter (usually about 10 mm inferior to the normal anteromedial portal location). Once the needle is confirmed to be in the proper position, a new portal is then made as described earlier. This portal in combination with the conventional anteromedial portal can be used to first inspect and then débride the far inferomedial ankle joint and deltoid insertion.

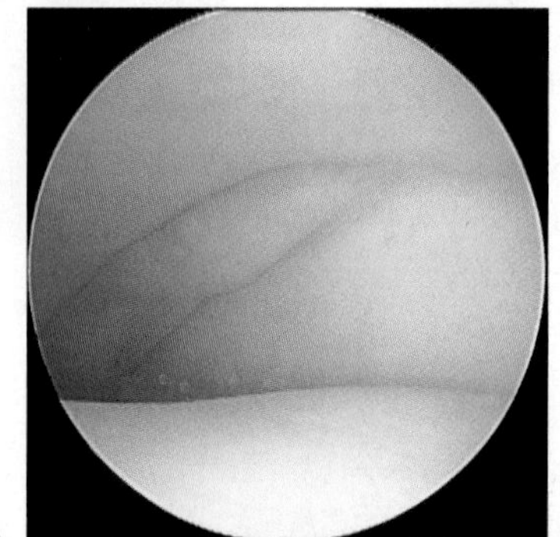

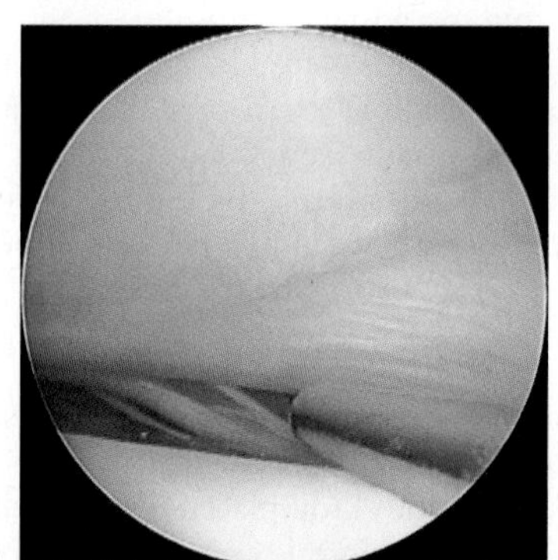

TECH FIG 1 • View of (**A**) anterolateral and (**B**) posterolateral gutter using simple distraction with towel roll underneath ankle.

POSTERIOR COAXIAL PORTALS

- With the arthroscope and inflow in the anterolateral portal, make the posterolateral portal with a small, vertical skin incision immediately posterior to the peroneal tendon sheath and 1.5 cm proximal to the tip of the fibula (**TECH FIG 2**).
- While holding the ankle in neutral dorsiflexion, insert the arthroscopic sheath and blunt trocar anterior and slightly inferior on a plane parallel to the bimalleolar axis. Confirm intracapsular placement by briefly inserting the arthroscope.
- Insert a long switching rod through the cannula and direct it toward the medial malleolus. Use the rod to palpate the posterior colliculus and penetrate just anterior to the posterior tibial tendon (**TECH FIG 3**).
- Tent and incise the skin over the posteromedial ankle. Subsequently, pass a second cannula over the switching stick into the posterior ankle recess.
- Alternatively, the medial portal can be made directly using a small, vertical skin incision posterior to the medial malleolus (posterior colliculus). The arthroscopic

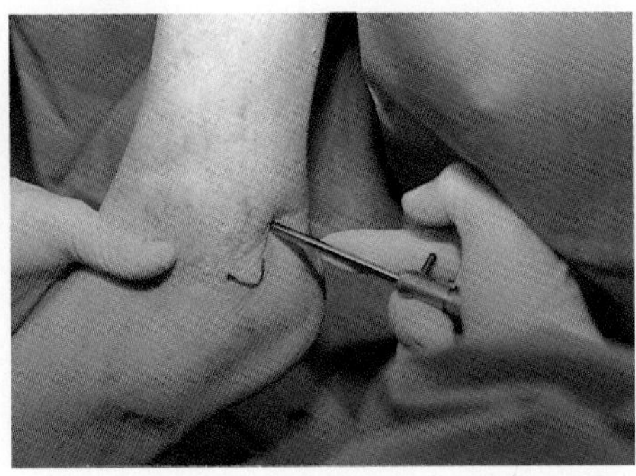

TECH FIG 2 • Lateral coaxial portal: clinical photograph with anatomic correlation.

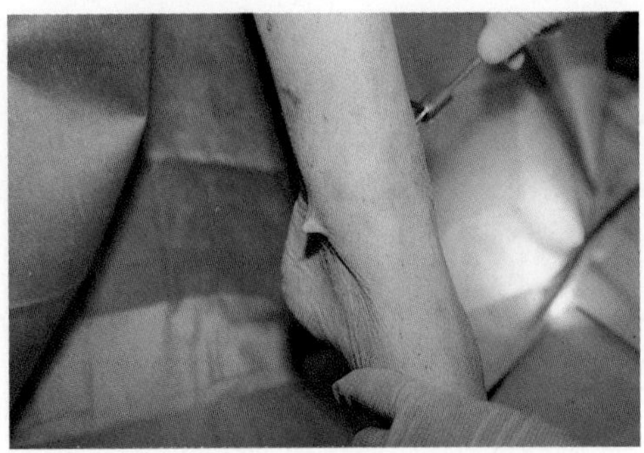

TECH FIG 3 • Medial coaxial portal: clinical photograph with anatomic correlation.

sheath and blunt trocar are inserted anterior and slightly inferior on a plane parallel to the bimalleolar axis. Intracapsular placement is confirmed by briefly inserting the arthroscope (**TECH FIGS 4 AND 5**).

- For synovectomies or posteromedial osteochondral lesions, the arthroscope is placed in the posterolateral cannula while the posteromedial cannula is used as the working portal.

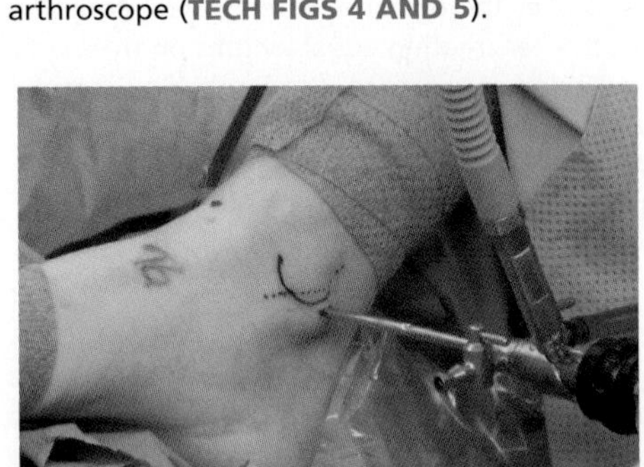

A

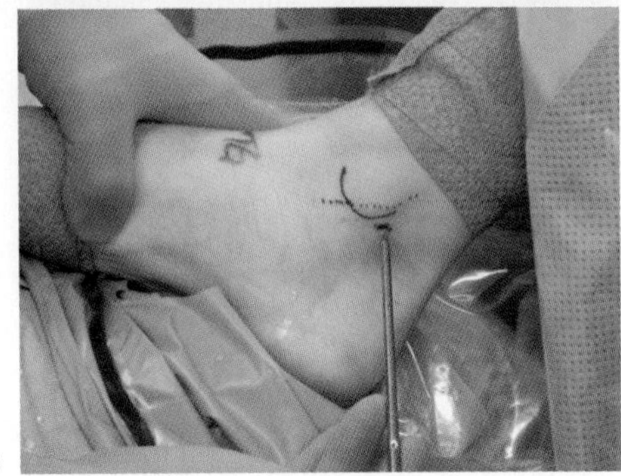

B

TECH FIG 4 • Medial coaxial portal: clinical photograph. (Courtesy of M.T. Busch, MD.)

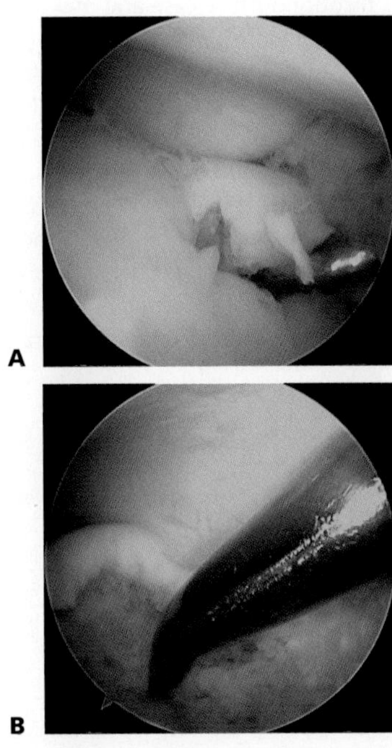

A

B

TECH FIG 5 • Arthroscopic view of instrumentation through medial portal. (Courtesy of M.T. Busch, MD.)

ANKLE DISTRACTOR PLACEMENT

- Inspect all instruments, and confirm that all parts of the noninvasive external distractor are sterile and on the operative field (**TECH FIG 6**).
- The patient is placed supine on the operating table.
- The patient is placed so the foot rests within 10 cm of the end of the bed.
- A bump (made from a rolled blanket) is placed under the hip to rotate the leg so the toes point straight up.
- A tourniquet is placed on the calf below the level of the fibular head to prevent peroneal nerve impingement (**TECH FIG 7**).

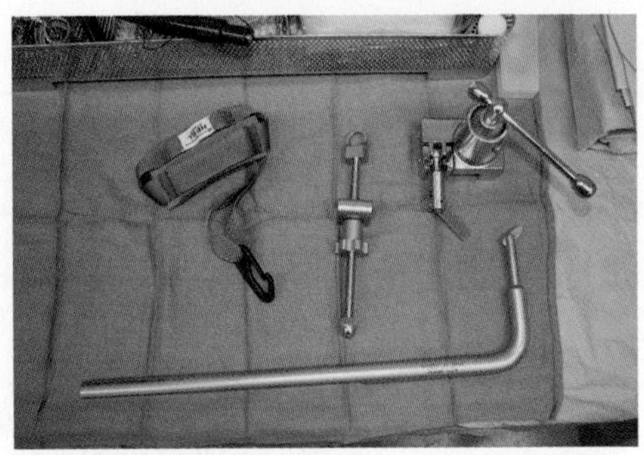

TECH FIG 6 • Distractor set-up: instruments.

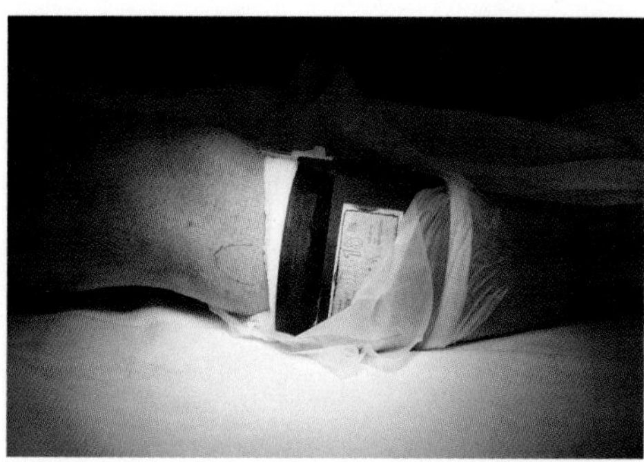

TECH FIG 7 • Distractor set-up: tourniquet placement.

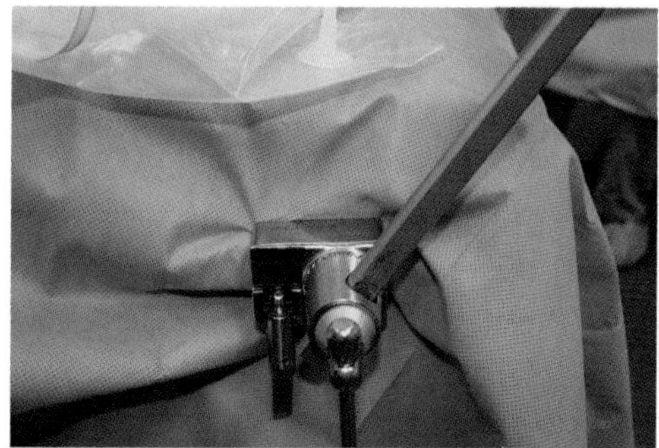

TECH FIG 9 • Distractor set-up: optimal clamp position placed as far distal as possible.

- The hip is flexed 60 degrees and the posterior thigh is placed in a padded thigh holder and secured with straps. It is very important that the thigh holder be placed so that the leg rests in the holder and does not rest in the popliteal fossa. If the thigh holder rests in the popliteal fossa, the pressure on the popliteal vein will increase bleeding throughout the case and make arthroscopic visualization much more difficult. With limited pressure on the popliteal space, the tourniquet is rarely needed during the arthroscopic portion of the case (TECH FIG 8).
- The operative leg and ankle region is prepared and then draped using a standard arthroscopy drape.
- The distal portion of the arthroscopy drape is pulled off the end of the foot to allow for the distractor placement.
- The bed clamp is placed as far distal on the bed as possible. For the clamp to fit properly, the circulating nurse should make sure all of the underlying drapes except the top layer are moved away from the clamp attachment site (TECH FIG 9).
- The external distractor strap is placed with the foam portions over the posterior inferior heel and on the dorsal foot. After creating equal lengths on the medial and lateral sides of the foot, the hook–loop is pulled distally with manual distraction.
- The L-shaped metal post is placed and secured.
- The foot is then pulled manually via the strap and connected to the threaded attachment rod. We recommend the initial placement requires moderate effort to get the hook–loop secured so that initial manual distraction provides the majority of distraction. Once this is connected, use the threaded rod to provide further distraction to the ankle (TECH FIG 10).
- The joint can be flexed or extended while in the distraction device to allow for complete evaluation of the joint.

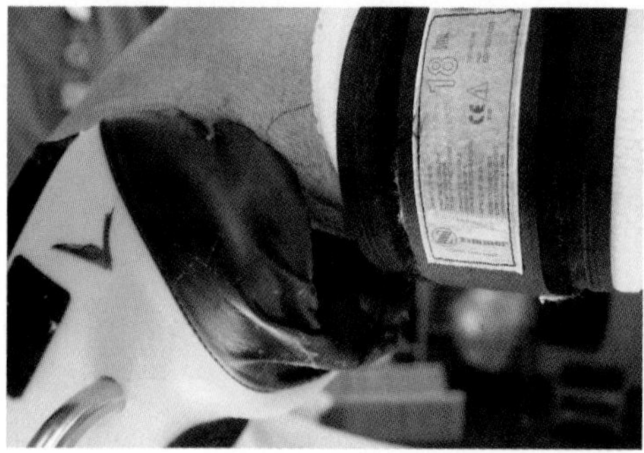

TECH FIG 8 • Distractor set-up: thigh holder placement.

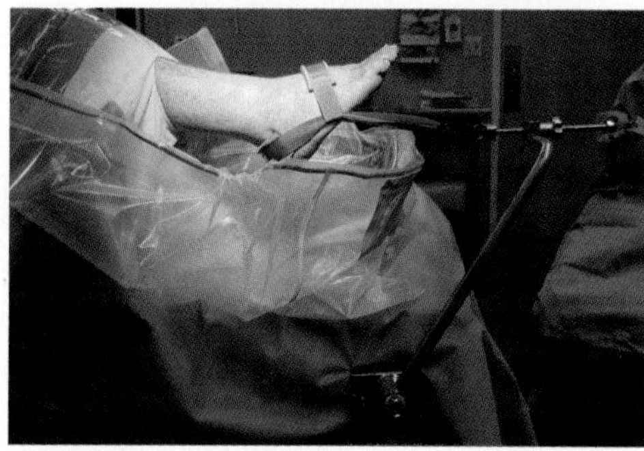

TECH FIG 10 • Distractor set-up: final ankle set-up with manual tensioning.

PEARLS AND PITFALLS

Indications	■ Careful analysis of preoperative films will allow proper planning of necessary portals (anterior only vs. both anterior and posterior).
Coaxial portal placement	■ Spread soft tissues laterally directly behind the peroneals to avoid sural nerve injury. ■ Palpate the posterior colliculus medially with a switching stick before penetrating between the posterior tibial tendon and medial malleolus. ■ Occasionally the medial coaxial portal will occur between the posterior tibial tendon and the flexor digitorum longus. ■ Avoid forceful medial penetration, which can result in tendon splitting. ■ When exposing the medial portal directly, posteromedial skin incision lies along the course of the posterior tibial tendon behind the posterior colliculus. The posterior tibial tendon can be retracted anteriorly or posteriorly to visualize bulging capsule.

Additional equipment needed for posterior portals	■ One additional scope cannula with inflow port (total of two scope cannulas) ■ Small (about 2.5 mm) blunt-tip switching stick
Intra-articular confirmation	■ After joint injection several factors indicate intra-articular placement: (1) inflow of saline without resistance, (2) ballooning of the anterolateral joint capsule, and (3) passive dorsiflexion of the ankle with insufflation of the joint.
Limiting time needed for tourniquet using ankle distraction	■ Care should be taken to avoid thigh holder placement such that direct pressure occurs into the popliteal space when distraction is applied. Direct pressure in the popliteal space decreases outflow through the popliteal vein and will increase venous pressure and intra-articular bleeding.

POSTOPERATIVE CARE

- For most conditions addressed with ankle arthroscopy, patients are placed in a well-padded short-leg splint. Five to seven days postoperatively the splint is removed and patients are allowed weight bearing as tolerated in a brace.
- In cases where drilling, microfracture, or retrograde bone grafting of an osteochondral lesion is performed, a period of non–weight-bearing is emphasized.
- Early range of motion is always encouraged unless a fusion is performed.

OUTCOMES

- Ankle arthroscopy allows the surgeon to address a myriad pathology with a minimally invasive technique. Success of outcomes varies according to underlying pathology but is generally in the range of 85% good to excellent.
- The complication rate ranges from 0.7% to 17%, with neurologic injuries accounting for most of these problems. The superficial peroneal nerve is the most commonly injured nerve, followed by the sural nerve and then the saphenous nerve.[2]
- In one study using the posterior coaxial portals in 29 ankles, no complications were observed at an average 45 months of follow-up.[1]

COMPLICATIONS

- Neurovascular injury
- Cartilage damage
- Reflex sympathetic dystrophy
- Sinus tract formation
- Infection
- Skin necrosis

REFERENCES

1. Acevedo JI, Busch MT, Ganey TM, et al. Coaxial portals for posterior ankle arthroscopy: an anatomic study with clinical correlation on 29 patients. Arthroscopy 2000;16:836–842.
2. Ferkel RD, Guhl JF, Heath DD. Neurological complications of ankle arthroscopy. Arthroscopy 1996;12:200–208.
3. Ferkel RD, Hewitt M. Long-term results of arthroscopic ankle arthrodesis. Foot Ankle Int 2005;26:275–280.
4. Golano P, Vega J, Perez-Carro L, et al. Ankle anatomy for the arthroscopist, part I: the portals. Foot Ankle Clin North Am 2006;11: 253–273.
5. Lui TH, Chan WK, Chan KB. The arthroscopic management of frozen ankle. Arthroscopy 2006;22:283–286.
6. Maiotti M, Massoni C, Tarantino U. The use of arthroscopic thermal shrinkage to treat chronic lateral ankle instability in young athletes. Arthroscopy 2005;21:751–757.
7. Nihal A, Rose DJ, Trepman E. Arthroscopic treatment of anterior ankle impingement syndrome in dancers. Foot Ankle Int 2005;26:908–912.
8. Sim J, Lee B, Kwak J. New posteromedial portal for ankle arthroscopy. Arthroscopy 2006;22:799.e1–799.e2.

Chapter 88

Microfracture for Osteochondral Lesions of the Talus

Hajo Thermann and Christoph Becher

DEFINITION

- The terminology of osteochondral lesions is not uniform: transchondral fractures, osteochondral fractures, flake fractures, and osteochondritis dissecans (OCD) are used to describe the same entity. Most recently, "osteochondral lesions of the talus" (OLT) has emerged as the most common term used to describe these lesions.
- OLTs are characterized by aseptic separation of a fragment of articular cartilage, with or without attached subchondral bone.
- The causes for OLTs remain controversial. The most important distinction to make is if the lesion is acute or chronic.

ANATOMY

- The talar body is trapezoidal. The anterior surface is on average 2.5 mm wider than the posterior surface. The dome is covered by the articular surface, which articulates with the tibial plafond. The medial and lateral facets articulate with the medial and lateral malleoli.
  - About 60% of the talar surface is covered by articular cartilage.
  - Most of the blood supply enters through the neck of the talus via the sinus tarsi.
- Biomechanical studies have shown that the talar cartilage is softest at the posteromedial part, whereas the maximum thickness is found at the posterolateral corner.
  - The tibial cartilage is 18% to 37% stiffer than the corresponding sites on the talus.[2]

PATHOGENESIS

- Lateral lesions are most frequently caused by acute trauma, with a common mechanism being a dorsiflexed ankle forced into inversion. This results in impaction of the talus on the fibula.
  - In our experience, lateral lesions are often located in the anterior part of the talar dome. They tend to be shallower than medial lesions.
- Medial lesions are mostly associated with a single or repetitive supination trauma (microtrauma).
  - Impaction of the medial talus on the tibia with a plantarflexed ankle forced to hindfoot inversion combined with external rotation is regarded as the causative mechanism.
  - Medial lesions are more common (inversion ankle sprains are the most common sports injury) than lateral lesions and occur mostly in the middle or posterior third of the talus. These lesions appear cup-shaped and deeper than lateral lesions.
- Injury to the talar dome associated with supination trauma to the ankle generally exhibits one of two trends in recovery:
  - In most, swelling and pain resolve expediently.
  - Occasionally, swelling and pain persist. In these cases, our investigations using MRI suggest that 20% of these ankles with persistent pain and swelling have an identifiable bone bruise on the medial talar dome.
- The question is the long-term effect of an episode of subchondral effusion (hemorrhage?) on the cartilage layers: Minor trauma on the tide zone with a prolonged separation?
- In our experience, chronic ankle instability creates a medial talar dome lesion with an abrasive character that suggests a repetitive insult. Unlike the classic OCD with a subchondral origin of the pathology, these deteriorations of the cartilage derive from a classic mechanical overload. The long-term damage is a full-thickness cartilage lesion at the medial talus and tibia plafond with varus hindfoot alignment. Medial lesions may be detected bilaterally, mostly with coincidence of bilateral ankle sprains.
- In contrast to chronic osteochondral lesions occurring as a result of repetitive trauma, acute osteochondral injuries result in an acute separation of an osteochondral fragment.
- Other reported causes for OLTs are genetic predisposition and endogenous factors. These causes lack meaningful evidence-based support and represent little more than theories.

NATURAL HISTORY

- Initially, the patient experiences ankle pain with impact activities such as jogging and sports that subsides immediately with rest.
- With time, increasing ankle pain generally forces the patient to stop impact sports activities. The time frame varies from patient to patient based on the patient's pain threshold and age.
- Some cases have an identifiable traumatic incident (ie, ankle sprain) where an initially inapparent lesion is detected and the patient never returns to a pain-free state. (For us this is an interesting phenomenon: does the lesion cause the pain or is there a psychosomatic influence once the lesion is detected on the imaging study?)
- Some OLTs are incidentally discovered with screening imaging studies (radiographs or MRI scans). For instance, an imaging study is obtained for an acute ankle sprain and an obviously nonacute OLT is noted. These patients have an anticipated normal healing course of the ankle injury with complete subsidence of pain and swelling and should never be treated for the asymptomatic OLT.
- Over the past 20 years our clinical experience (H.T.) in treating OLTs suggests that there is no evidence to support that the natural history of untreated OLTs is the development of osteoarthritis of the ankle. We thus view surgical management of OLTs as one of pain relief and not as a salvage procedure to prevent osteoarthritis of the ankle joint.
- McCullough and Venugopal found that in five of six patients treated conservatively for OLTs, radiologic assessment at a mean follow-up of nearly 16 years (range 7 to 28 years) showed that the lesions had failed to heal and that in each instance the ankle joint was relatively asymptomatic, without evidence of diffuse degenerative changes.[15]

PATIENT HISTORY AND PHYSICAL FINDINGS

- Acute OLTs must be ruled out after traumatic events when an OLT or osteochondral fracture is suspected.
- In most cases patients complain of chronic ankle pain with or after sports activities. Swelling and stiffness are accompanied in advanced cases with more constant pain. Occasionally, but not always, mechanical symptoms are present, including catching, locking, and giving way.
- The severity of symptoms may not correlate with the severity of the lesion.
- Physical examination is relatively nonspecific in OLTs.
  - By having the patient plantarflex the foot and ankle, the anterior aspects of the talar dome can be palpated at the anteromedial and anterolateral joint space. Tenderness in the specific area may indicate an osteochondral lesion.
  - Tenderness behind the medial malleolus by having the patient dorsiflex the ankle may indicate a posteromedial lesion.
  - Range of motion of the ankle is tested with the knee flexed to eliminate restriction by shortened gastrocnemius muscles. Range of motion is limited only in case of ankle synovitis and effusion.
- The examination should also include evaluation of associated pathology, taking into account the differential diagnosis.
  - Bony structures, tendons, ligaments, and soft tissue structures should be palpated and tested against resistance to discern tenderness of the specific anatomic part.
  - Ligamentous instability or laxity is assessed with the anterior drawer test and passive varus or valgus stress test.
  - Pushing the ankle against resistance helps identify inflammation or partial tears of tendons of the contracted muscles.
  - Palpation of pulses and neurologic assessment should be part of every examination.

IMAGING AND OTHER DIAGNOSTIC STUDIES

- Standard ankle plain film radiographs should include AP, lateral, and mortise views. However, only 50% to 66% of osteochondral defects can be visualized by plain film radiographs alone.[12] The radiologic signs vary from a small area of compression of subchondral bone to a detached osteochondral fragment.
- The four-stage classification system by Berndt and Harty is still the gold standard based on radiologic appearance:[6]
  - Stage I: Compression lesion, no visible fragment
  - Stage II: Fragment attached
  - Stage III: Nondisplaced fragment without attachment (**FIG 1**)
  - Stage IV: Displaced fragment
- Stress view radiographs are frequently recommended if instability is suspected. However, a thorough clinical examination is more important and in most cases is sufficient for assessment.
- A CT scan offers more accurate staging and characterization of the lesion, with clear definition of the exact dimensions of the osseous portion of the lesion, but subjects the patient to relatively high radiation. We recommend and use limited CT studies with minimal radiation exposure to the patient and sufficient characterization of the OLT.

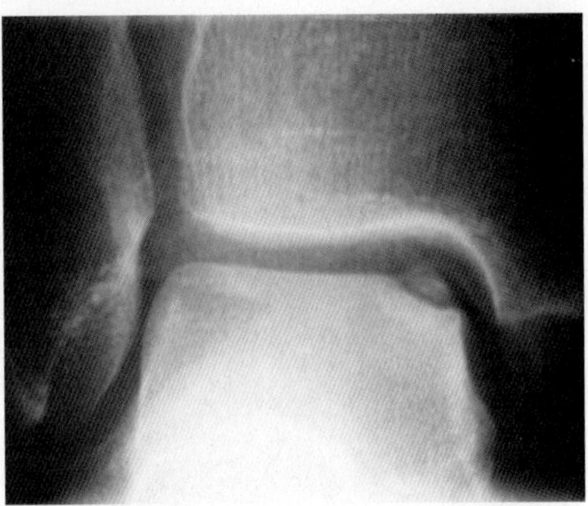

FIG 1 • Osteochondral lesion stage III as per Berndt and Harty's classification.

- MRI is an ideal screening tool and, in our opinion, the method of choice for all patients with suspected OLTs. MRI defines occult injuries of the subchondral bone and cartilage that may not be detected with routine radiographs. Furthermore, the MRI is accurate in diagnosing associated stress fractures and stress reactions—for example, in the medial malleolus. While MRI may demonstrate associated edema in the talar body, in our hands accurate sizing of the OLT is feasible.
- Dipaola et al developed an MRI classification system based on Berndt and Harty's original radiographic system.[7]
  - Stage I: Thickening of articular cartilage and low signal changes
  - Stage II: Articular cartilage breached, low-signal rim behind fragment indicating fibrous attachment
  - Stage III: Articular cartilage breached, high-signal changes behind fragment indicating synovial fluid between fragment and underlying subchondral bone (**FIGS 2 AND 3**).
  - Stage IV: Loose body

DIFFERENTIAL DIAGNOSIS

- Degenerative joint disease (any origin)
- Soft tissue or bony impingement on the ankle joint
- Ankle or subtalar instability

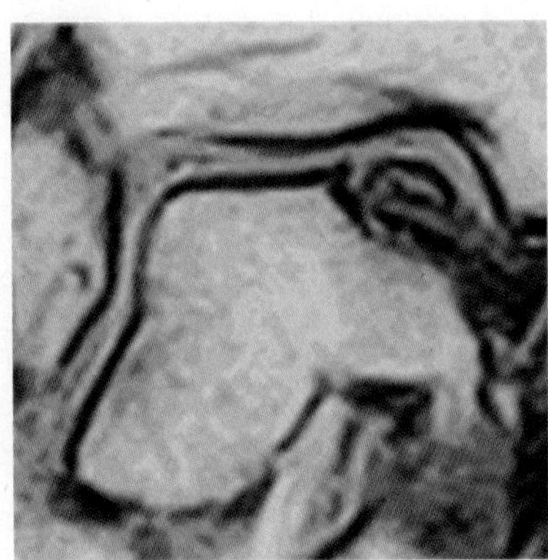

FIG 2 • Coronal MRI (T1-SE-540/20) showing an osteochondral lesion stage III.

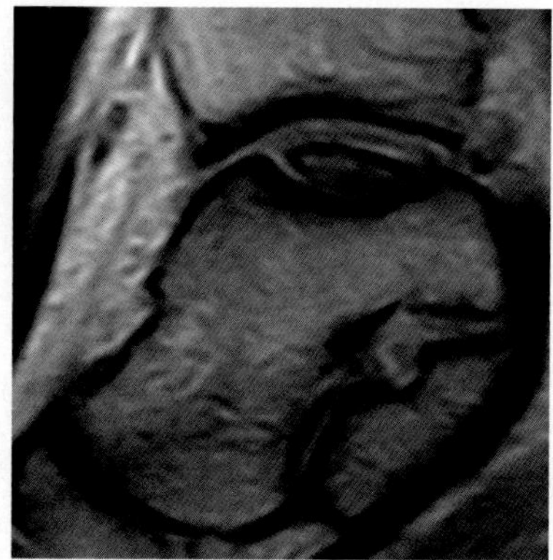

FIG 3 • Sagittal MRI (T2-SE-2000/90) showing an osteochondral lesion stage III.

- Subtalar joint pathologies (ie, chondral lesion, subtalar impingement lesion)
- Tendinitis or partial rupture of the tibialis posterior, tibialis anterior, or peroneal tendons
- Tarsal coalition (talocalcaneal)
- Stress fracture (medial or lateral malleolus; talus)

NONOPERATIVE MANAGEMENT

- The approach and objectives in nonoperative treatment of OLTs vary from those of surgical management.
  - In children and adolescents, the goal is to reverse the cartilage separation and to treat the pain. Partial weight bearing (not unloading) of about 15 kg for 2 to 3 months and nonsteroidal anti-inflammatory agents (NSAIDs) at appropriate doses adjusted for age and weight for 1 to 2 months to relieve the patient's pain are important from physical and psychological standpoints. Given the advantages shown in clinical and experimental trials, we recommend use of the combination of chondroitin and glucosamine sulfate for at least 6 months. We also encourage the daily use of moist heat to enhance vascularity to the ankle and talus. In select cases of extensive talar body edema, we have observed, based on anecdotal experience, that hyperbaric oxygen (HBO) therapy (20 dives, 20 minutes each) results in resolution of edema and pain. We favor low-impact exercise such as biking and swimming for about 1 year. Regardless of MRI findings, the young patient should gradually return to age-appropriate activities once she or he is pain-free. We recommend yearly serial MRI and clinical examinations to monitor talar body status.
  - While osteochondral transfer systems and autologous chondrocyte implantation are accepted salvage procedures, to date we lack an optimal reconstruction of an OLT. Nonoperative treatment for OLTs is the treatment of choice if the adult patient has minor complaints. The goal of nonoperative treatment is not to ameliorate the cartilage lesion but to make the ankle pain-free and resilient. We recommend NSAIDs, physiotherapy, ice or moist heat applications, well-cushioned shoes, biking, swimming, and cross-training for 6 months.
- We allow our adult patients with OLTs activity to tolerance. Immobilization with partial weight bearing has healing potential only for fresh traumatic osteochondral lesions. In an area with little perfusion, some contact pressure is necessary to create a healing response.
  - We rarely use cast or walker boot immobilization because we believe that ankle motion is important. The occasional cast or boot is applied for only brief periods (2 weeks) to reduce pain and patient insecurity. Cast immobilization is associated with inferior results compared with restricting the activity of the patient by partial weight bearing.[20] Flick and Gould concluded that therapy of 4 to 6 weeks with cast immobilization is inadequate immobilization, resulting in poor results for most transchondral fractures.[8]
- In summary, nonoperative treatment is applied for every patient who is opposed to surgical intervention. There is no time frame when a lesion has to be operated on to prevent deterioration. Pain is the benchmark, not the radiographic or MRI findings. In our opinion, an OLT that is primarily cystic and has an intact cartilage surface suggested on MRI (if detectable) should prompt nonoperative rather than operative management.
- If deterioration or no improvement is evident after a period defined by the patient, the optimal means of determining the status of the articular cartilage is arthroscopic probing of the OLT, which is useful in determining the appropriate surgical procedure.

SURGICAL MANAGEMENT

- In our opinion, asymptomatic OLTs should not be treated. Many incidentally discovered OLTs do not become symptomatic and are unrelated to the trauma that prompted the imaging study that led to the detection of the OLT. When, however, the OLT is the most likely source of pain and nonoperative treatment has failed, we recommend arthroscopic surgery for evaluation and treatment of the OLT.
- Retrograde drilling is suggested for a symptomatic subchondral cyst with an overlying intact cartilage surface. High levels of evidence or grades of recommendation for retrograde drilling do not exist. Our theory for the mechanical pain from OLTs is an irreversible separation in the cartilage's tide zone. Drilling may decompress edema but may create heat necrosis and cystic degeneration. Moreover, without 3D CT or navigation, drilling may miss the smaller to intermediate lesions. If the chondral surface is found to be softened and is easily detachable, unstable cartilage and fibrous tissue have to be débrided.
- Our preferred surgical management for stage II to IV OLTs is microfracture to stimulate fibrocartilage formation. After débridement of unstable cartilage in the OLT, microfracture awls designed for small joints are penetrated into the subchondral bone to open the zone of vascularization. Blood from within the talus escapes through the subchondral bone and leads to clot formation in the lesion. This clot contains pluripotent, marrow-derived mesenchymal stem cells that typically produce a fibrocartilage repair with varying amounts of type II collagen content.[11,19]
  - The microfracture technique using dedicated small-joint awls avoids the risk of thermal necrosis associated with other marrow stimulation techniques such as abrasion or drilling.[14] Moreover, all lesions may be accessed without more invasive steps such as transtibial drilling or osteotomy of the medial malleolus.

- If the microfracture technique failed to relieve symptoms, repeat microfracture has been shown to be effective in select cases.[18] However, in our hands, particularly if we performed the index microfracture procedure, we recommend salvage with a matrix-based autologous chondrocyte implantation (MACI).
  - Based on first-generation results after injecting the cultured cells under a periosteal flap, this appeared to be a viable alternative when treating osteochondral or chondral lesions of the talus.[3,13]
  - MACI with cultured cells in scaffolds seems to be more promising and technically less demanding, with good and excellent short-term results.[4]
  - However, costs for the procedure are high, the approach is more invasive, and longer-term results remain to be evaluated to prove superiority over microfracture technique. Moreover, in the United States, MACI lacks FDA approval.
- Osteochondral autograft transfer (OATS) or mosaicplasty is an option in the repair of severe osteochondral lesions with a significant lack of subchondral bone or in cystic lesions.[1,10] The osteochondral plugs can be harvested by either open arthrotomy or arthroscopy of the knee. The option of local osteochondral grafting has also been reported.[17] Major problems with these techniques include the different characteristics of knee (donor) and ankle (recipient) cartilage (different thicknesses and radii of curvature), which may lead to edge loading and graft deterioration. Donor site morbidity can be significant, resulting in a decline of knee function and problems in performing activities of daily living.[16]

Preoperative Planning

- Review of all imaging studies, especially MRIs, is in our opinion most important for preoperative planning. The OLT size, location, topical geography, and depth must be identified to determine the correct approach and technique.
- Ankles must be inspected for severe swelling, warmth, or erythema. We consider elevated blood sample parameters that indicate an acute inflammatory process a contraindication to surgical intervention for OLT management. In our experience, any OLT in any location within the ankle can be treated arthroscopically through standard portals.
  - In some cases, an accessory posterolateral portal facilitates access to posterior OLTs in relatively tight ankles.

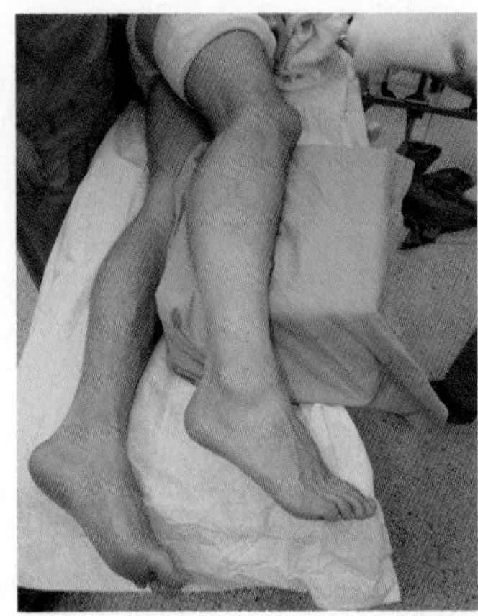

FIG 5 • Positioning of the patient if a posterolateral approach is necessary.

- Examination under anesthesia allows for better assessment of coexisting ankle instability.
  - In case of lateral ligamentous instability, lateral ligament stabilization should be performed along with OLT management. Ankle instability may increase the contact forces and shear stresses on the OLT.

Positioning

- The procedure is performed under general anesthesia with a tourniquet placed at the thigh.
- The patient is preferably positioned with a leg holder that allows the gastrocnemius–soleus complex to be fully relaxed (**FIG 4**).
- We recommend that the patient be positioned in the lateral position if a posterolateral approach may need to be performed (**FIG 5**).
- Noninvasive ankle distraction may be performed using bandages (**FIG 6**).
  - However, in our experience, most OLTs may be safely performed without distraction.

Approach

- We use standard anteromedial and anterolateral arthroscopic portals. The anteromedial portal enters the ankle

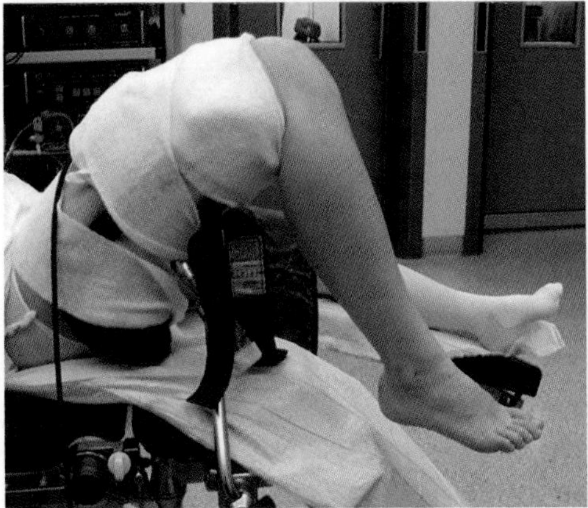

FIG 4 • Positioning of the patient for ankle arthroscopy.

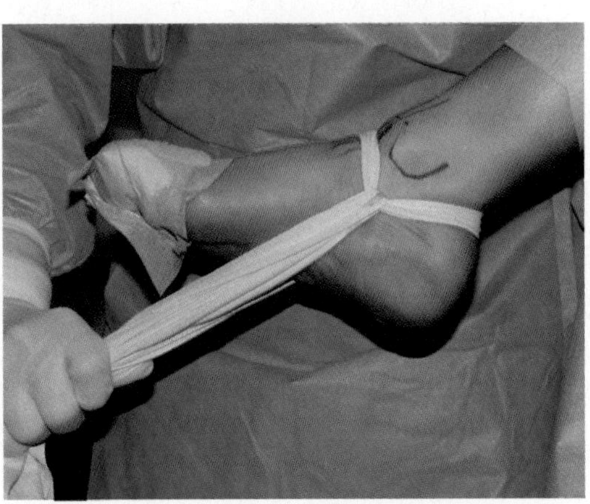

FIG 6 • Atraumatic distraction of the ankle with bandages.

between the medial malleolus and the talar dome 0.5 to 1 cm distal to the joint line and just medial to the anterior tibial tendon. The anterolateral portal enters the joint between the fibula and talus at the same level as the medial portal, lateral to the common extensor tendon.

- If necessary, the posterolateral portal is placed adjacent to the Achilles tendon and behind the peroneal tendon, slightly below the level of the joint line. A Kirschner wire can be directed under vision of the arthroscope from the anteromedial portal posteriorly to find the same location (Wessinger Rod technique). The patient must be fully relaxed and the joint adequately distracted and distended.
- In addition, a superomedial portal located 1 cm above the joint line, medial to the tibialis anterior tendon, might be helpful to achieve more perpendicular angles for microfracturing (**FIG 7**).

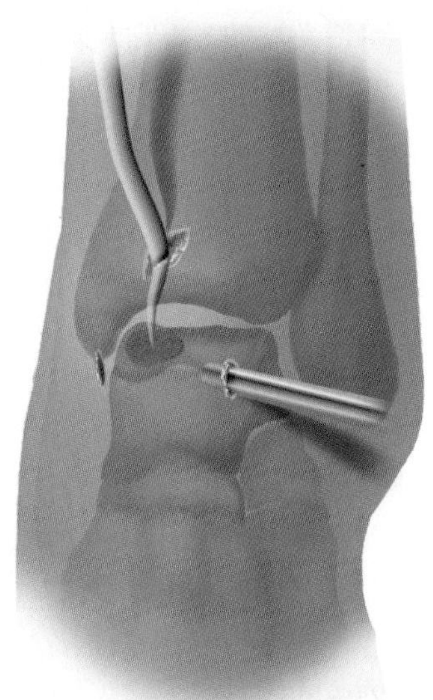

FIG 7 • Superomedial portal for better angles for microfracturing.

TECHNIQUES

ARTHROSCOPY

- Fill the joint with 20 mL saline solution through the anteromedial portal (**TECH FIG 1**).
- We recommend using a 2.5-mm or 2.7-mm arthroscope, with 25- to 30-degree and 70-degree angled lenses, needed to assess and treat defects in all areas of the joint (**TECH FIG 2**).

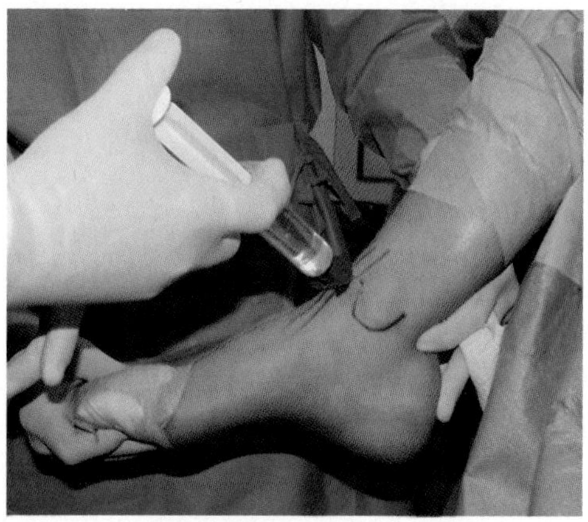

TECH FIG 1 • Filling the joint with 20 mL saline solution.

- Perform a limited synovectomy in all cases. This enhances visibility during the procedure and allows the surgeon to remove inflamed synovium that may contribute to ankle pain and swelling.
- Systematically inspect the ankle and document all pathology.
- Remove loose bodies, if present.
- We assess and probe all articular surfaces of the ankle, including the talar dome, medial and lateral gutters, and the tibial plafond.

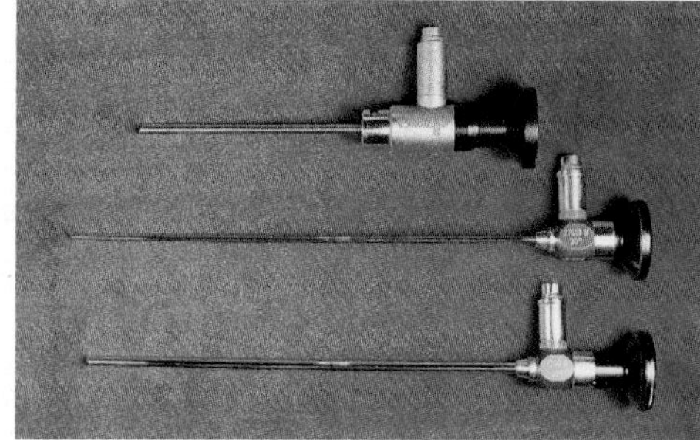

TECH FIG 2 • 2.5-mm and 2.7-mm arthroscopes for ankle arthroscopy.

PREPARATION OF THE LESION

- Identify the lesion with a probe (**TECH FIG 3**).
- Address all unstable cartilage and fibrous tissue of the OLT and the cartilage that lies immediately adjacent to the defect with débridement and curettage (**TECH FIG 4**).
- Create sharp, perpendicular margins to optimize conditions for the attachment of the marrow clot.
- Completely remove the calcified cartilage layer with a burr.

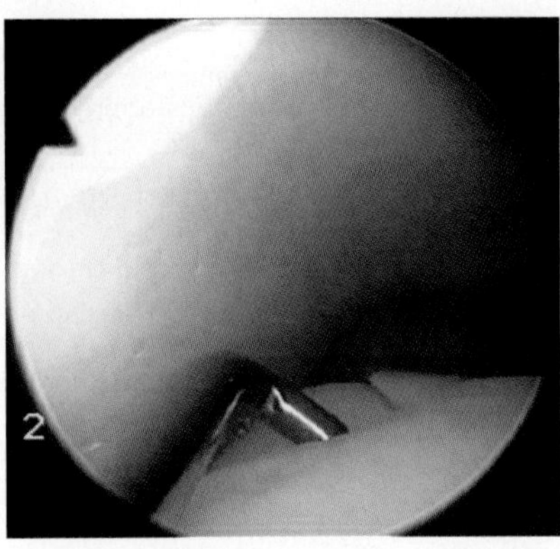

TECH FIG 3 • Probing of the lesion.

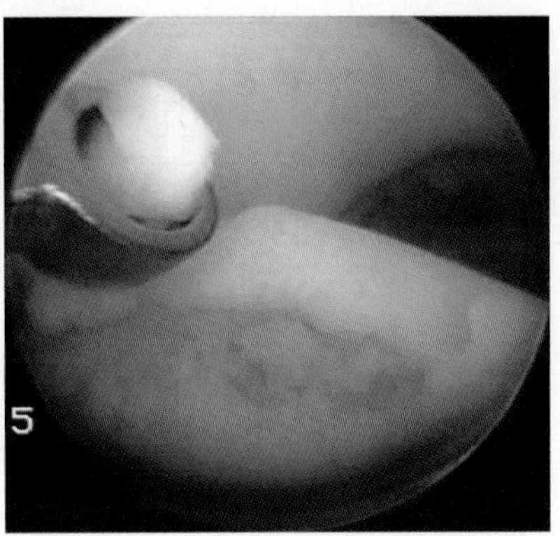

TECH FIG 4 • Débridement and curettage.

MICROFRACTURE

- The microfracture technique is performed if the subchondral bone layer is healthy and intact.
- Arthroscopic awls of different angles permit appropriate perpendicular access to all areas of the prepared OLT. Place the microfractures about 3 to 4 mm apart and 2 to 4 mm deep; fat droplets indicate that the subchondral bone has been adequately penetrated.
- We ensure that the awl is always placed perpendicular to the surface and that penetration of subchondral bone is performed judiciously to maintain the subchondral bone plate integrity and architecture (TECH FIG 5).
- Before removing the arthroscope from the ankle, we release the tourniquet and stop the flow of saline through the ankle to confirm that blood is indeed escaping from the talus into the talar defect (TECH FIG 6).
- We do not routinely use a drain for arthroscopy. Portals are closed in standard fashion.

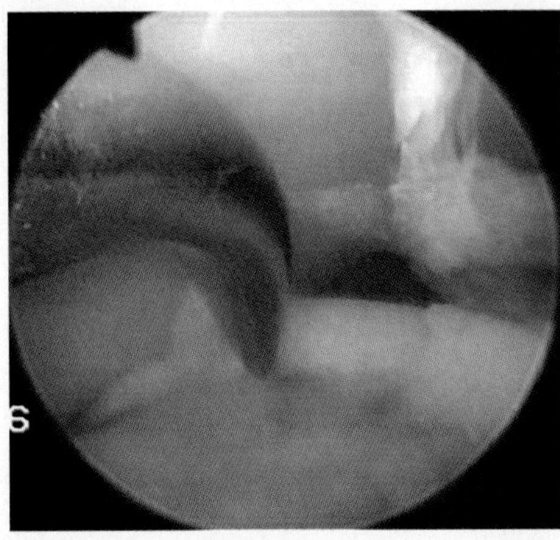

TECH FIG 5 • Microfracture.

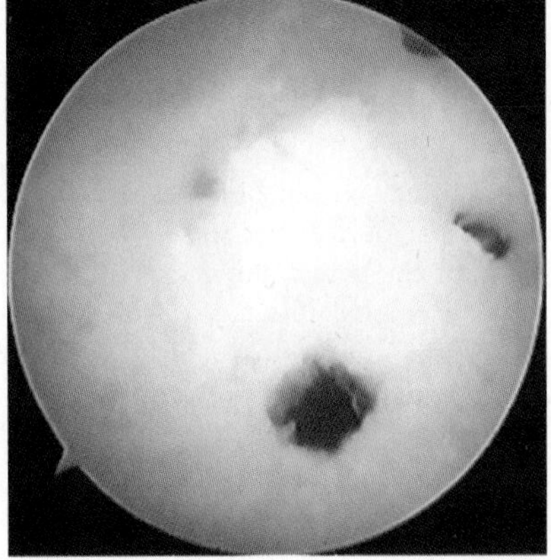

TECH FIG 6 • Release of the tourniquet. Blood enters the joint from the microfractures.

LESIONS ASSOCIATED WITH SUBCHONDRAL CYSTS (CANCELLOUS BONE TRANSLATION TECHNIQUE)

- In OLTs associated with subchondral cysts, we débride the damaged, unhealthy cartilage, perform microfracture, and use the cancellous bone translation technique.
- Fenestrate the cortex at the opposite side, and under fluoroscopic visualization translate the cancellous bone (like a snowplow) with a curved 4-mm AO plunger into the cyst.

PEARLS AND PITFALLS

Indications	▪ Take care to address associated pathology. In case of lateral ligament instability, a stabilizing procedure has to be added to guarantee the success of the microfracture.
Technique	▪ Use a superomedial portal to achieve perpendicular penetration of the awl. Use a swan-neck–shaped awl. ▪ Posterolateral approach with the Wessinger Rod technique: A rod is inserted through the anteromedial portal in a posterolateral direction to identify the optimal entry for the posterolateral portal. ▪ The calcified cartilage layer must be thoroughly removed by a small abrader to provide optimal amount and attachment of repair tissue.[9] ▪ Cancellous bone translation technique

POSTOPERATIVE CARE

- Compressive bandaging is applied up to the thigh. The ankle is elevated and immediate cryotherapy is applied.
- Continuous passive motion (CPM) from the first day, as tolerated by pain and swelling, is used for 6 to 8 hours per day for 4 to 6 weeks.
- Partial weight bearing of 15 kg is allowed for the first 6 weeks, 30 kg for the next 2 weeks. If the ankle is pain-free, then weight bearing can be advanced as tolerated.
- Biking, swimming, and cross-training are permitted after 8 weeks. Impact sports are permitted after 5–6 months if the ankle is pain free with normal activities. Otherwise, we recommend to wait 10–12 months after surgery.
- Dietary supplements (glucosamine and chondroitin sulfate) may have beneficial effects for cartilage regeneration (6 months).

OUTCOMES

- The results of prospective studies have shown significant improvement 2 years after microfracture of the talus.[5]
  - Ninety-five percent of the ankles with osteochondral lesions had excellent or good results.
  - Outcomes did not differ significantly between patients older than 50 years versus younger patients.
  - Location and grade of the defect showed no statistically significant impact on the results.
- MRI studies showed regeneration of tissue in the microfractured area. Subchondral signal changes were observed in almost all postoperative images.[5]
- No distinct correlation between clinical and imaging results was detected.[5]

COMPLICATIONS

- Development of ossifications at the anterior tibia with subsequent restriction in dorsiflexion
- Damage to the deep peroneal nerve with subsequent hyposensitivity in the distribution area
- Infection
- Deep vein thrombosis
- Arthrofibrosis

REFERENCES

1. Assenmacher JA, Kelikian AS, Gottlob C, et al. Arthroscopically assisted autologous osteochondral transplantation for osteochondral lesions of the talar dome: an MRI and clinical follow-up study. Foot Ankle Int 2001;22:544–551.
2. Athanasiou KA, Niederauer GG, Schenck RCJ. Biomechanical topography of human ankle cartilage. Ann Biomed Eng 1995;5:697–704.
3. Baums MH, Heidrich G, Schultz W, et al. Autologous chondrocyte transplantation for treating cartilage defects of the talus. J Bone Joint Surg Am 2006;88A:303–308.
4. Becher C, Thermann H. Autologous chondrocyte transplantation after formerly failed operative treatment for osteochondritis dissecans tali. 12th European Society of Sports Traumatology and Arthroscopy 2000 Congress (ESSKA 2000), 5th World Congress of Sports Trauma, Innsbruck, Austria, 2005, Abstract P-381:417.
5. Becher C, Thermann H. Results of microfracture in the treatment of articular cartilage defects of the talus. Foot Ankle Int 2005;26:583–589.
6. Berndt AL, Harty M. Transchondral fractures (osteochondritis dissecans) of the talus. J Bone Joint Surg Am 1959;41A:97–102.
7. Dipaola JD, Nelson DW, Colville MR. Characterizing osteochondral lesions by magnetic resonance imaging. Arthroscopy 1991;7:101–104.
8. Flick AB, Gould N. Osteochondritis dissecans of the talus (transchondral fractures of the talus): review of the literature and new surgical approach for medial dome lesions. Foot Ankle 1985;5:165–185.
9. Frisbie DD, Morisset S, Ho CP, et al. Effects of calcified cartilage on healing of chondral defects treated with microfracture in horses. Am J Sports Med 2006;34:1824–1831.
10. Hangody L, Kish G, Kárpáti Z, et al. Treatment of osteochondritis dissecans of the talus: use of the mosaicplasty technique—a preliminary report. Foot Ankle Int 1997;18:628–634.
11. Knutsen G, Engebretsen L, Ludvigsen TC, et al. Autologous chondrocyte implantation compared with microfracture in the knee: a randomized trial. J Bone Joint Surg Am 2004;86A:455–464.
12. Loomer R, Fisher C, Lloyd-Smith R, et al. Osteochondral lesions of the talus. Am J Sports Med 1993;21:13–19.
13. Mandelbaum BR, Gerhardt MB, Peterson L. Autologous chondrocyte implantation of the talus. Arthroscopy 2003;19:129–137.
14. Matthews LS, Hirsch C. Temperatures measured in human cortical bone when drilling. J Bone Joint Surg Am 1972;54A:297–308.
15. McCullough CJ, Venugopal V. Osteochondritis dissecans of the talus: the natural history. Clin Orthop Relat Res 1979;144:264–268.
16. Reddy S, Pedowitz DI, Parekh SG, et al. The morbidity associated with osteochondral harvest from asymptomatic knees for the treatment of osteochondral lesions of the talus. Am J Sports Med 2007;35:80–85.
17. Sammarco G, Makwana N. Treatment of talar osteochondral lesions using local osteochondral graft. Foot Ankle Int 2002;23:693–698.
18. Savva N, Jabur M, Davies M, et al. Osteochondral lesions of the talus: results of repeat arthroscopic debridement. Foot Ankle Int 2007;28:669–673.
19. Steadman JR. Microfracture technique for full-thickness chondral defects: technique and clicical results. Operative Tech Orthop 1997;7:300–304.
20. Tol JL, Struijs PA, Bossuyt PM, et al. Treatment strategies in osteochondral defects of the talar dome: a systematic review. Foot Ankle Int 2000;21:119–126.

Chapter 89

Posterior Ankle Impingement Syndrome

Javier Maquirriain

DEFINITION

- Posterior ankle impingement syndrome (PAIS) is a clinical disorder characterized by posterior ankle pain that occurs during forced plantarflexion.[13,14]

ANATOMY

- The posterior ankle region comprises the soft tissues structures situated behind the tibiotalar joint and the dorsal aspect of the calcaneus.
- This region extends superiorly to a horizontal line 4 cm above the tip of the lateral malleolus and inferiorly to a curved line 4 cm below the lateral malleolus.[3]
- The Achilles tendon constitutes the central axis of this region. Neurovascular and musculoskeletal structures in the medial and lateral retromalleolar sulcus surround the calcaneal tendon.
- The posterior talar process protrudes posterior to the articular surface of the ankle joint. The body of the posterior process extends both posteriorly and medially from the talus and has two projections designated as the posteromedial process and posterolateral process. These processes are divided by a groove containing the flexor hallucis longus (FHL) tendon (**FIG 1**).
- The posterolateral process, injuries of which are the most common cause of posterior ankle impingement syndrome, is also called the trigonal process.
- When the posterolateral process remains separated from the talus, it is called os trigonum.

PATHOGENESIS

- The etiology of the posterior ankle pain in forced plantarflexion is varied and may involve any part of the posterior ankle anatomy. PAIS compression pathogenesis has been likened to a "nut in a nutcracker"[9] (**FIG 2**).
- Trigonal process pathology includes fractures, disrupting of a pre-exisitng synchondrosis, or compression/impingement phenomena.
- FHL tendon pathology, including stenosing tenosynovitis and impingement from a prominent posterior talar process, is another cause of PAIS.
- PAIS may be produced by intrinsic tibiotalar pathology resulting from ankle trauma. Articular chondral damage or bony injury may cause pain in extreme plantarflexion.
- Posttraumatic thickened, inflamed, and sometimes calcified soft tissues in the posterior ankle, including the capsule, synovium, and ligaments, may contribute to chronic impingement with ankle plantarflexion.
- A prominence of the posterior calcaneal process also can impinge on the hindfoot.
- In posterior ankle impingement, combined pathologies are common. For example, ballet dancers frequently present with associated trigonal process injury with FHL tenosynovitis.[8]

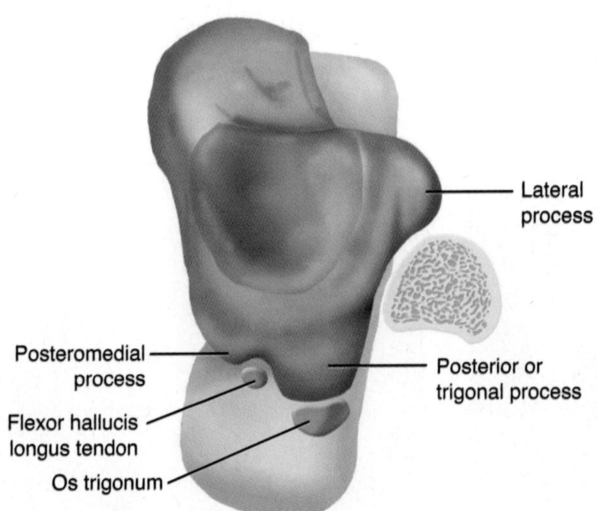

FIG 1 • Posterior talar process anatomy. Superior view of the talus shows the close relationship of the flexor hallucis longus tendon and the trigonal process.

NATURAL HISTORY

- Once injured, patients typically compensate for the loss of plantarflexion by placing the foot in an antalgic position. For example, dancers may begin to assume a more inverted en pointe position to decrease impingement of the posterior structures; doing so, however, may place increased loads on the

Table 1 Etiologic Classification of Posterior Ankle Impingement Syndrome

Trigonal process pathology
Fracture (acute or chronic)
Synchondrosis injury
True compression
Flexor hallucis longus dysfunction
Tenosynovitis
Tibiotalar pathology
Posterior capsuloligamentous injuries
Osteochondritis
Fractures
Synovial cysts
Subtalar pathology
Osteochondritis
Arthritis
Others
Calcified inflammatory tissue
Anomalous muscles
Tumors
Prominent calcaneus posterior process
Combined
Flexor hallucis longus tenosynovitis and os trigonal synchondrosis injury

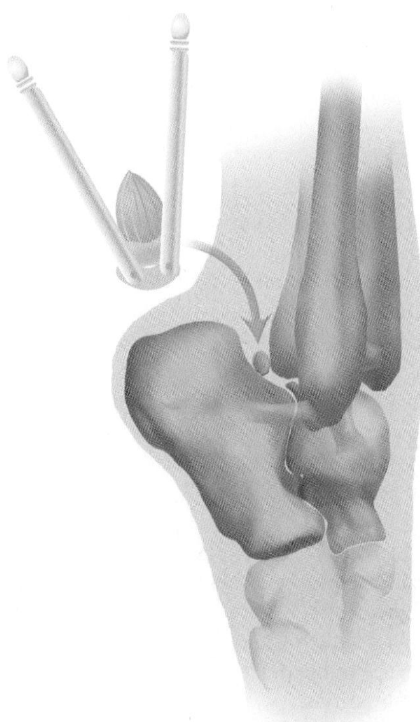

FIG 2 • The "nutcracker" phenomenon involving the os trigonum.

anterior tibiofibular ligament, which thus predisposes the dancers to frequent ankle sprains.

- Calf strain and contractures, plantar foot pain, and toe curling are also typical compensatory problems in dancers that result from efforts to force the foot into a better en pointe position.[7]
- Subtalar joint pathology, especially in posterior articular facets, can produce posterior ankle pain in forced plantarflexion. Furthermore, in chronic PAIS, with limited ankle motion, the subtalar joint may show degenerative changes as a result of higher compensatory loads imposed to maintain ankle range of motion (ROM) during closed kinetic athletic activities.

PATIENT HISTORY AND PHYSICAL FINDINGS

- The patient usually reports chronic or recurrent posterior ankle pain caused or exacerbated by forced plantarflexion or push-off activities, such as dancing, kicking, downhill running, and walking on high heels. Biomechanical analysis showed that ankle plantarflexion is required during the swing limb phase and foot contact with the ball of kicking.[2] Pain is usually deep and mechanical.
- There may be a recent or remote history of ankle trauma, but overuse should be considered.
- Tibiotalar, subtalar, and hallux ROM should be measured and recorded.
- The diagnostic approach should be based on cause-related conditions.
  - The forced plantarflexion test tries to reproduce the typical painful motion of PAIS. It also allows one to estimate the passive ROM limitation.
  - The Maquirriain test tries to reproduce the typical painful motion of PAIS in a closed position. It also allows one to estimate the passive ROM limitation.
  - The one-leg hop test provides valuable functional information to rule out Achilles tendon pathology.

IMAGING AND OTHER DIAGNOSTIC STUDIES

- A complete history and physical examination is often sufficient to diagnose PAIS. However, ancillary imaging studies should be done to establish the cause, thus allowing proper and timely treatment.
- Ankle radiographs should be obtained routinely with lateral view clearly defining trigonal process anatomy. This projection also is used to measure ankle ROM.[14]
- Demonstration of the presence of an os trigonum by conventional radiographs is not necessarily indicative of current clinical relevance.[13] Lateral views may show fracture lines, but they cannot differentiate chronic or acute pathology.
- Bone scintigraphy is a helpful diagnostic tool. Increased activity is present in all patients with an acute fracture of the trigonal process and synchondrosis disruption.[15] A normal bone scan virtually rules out trigonal process pathology.[11]
- MRI is considered the technique of choice to investigate patients with PAIS[5,20] because it enables determination of the nature of the osseous and soft tissue lesions and excludes other causes of posterior ankle pain (**FIG 3A,B**). Bone contusions of the trigonal process are prevalent in individuals with PAIS[5] (**FIG 3C**).

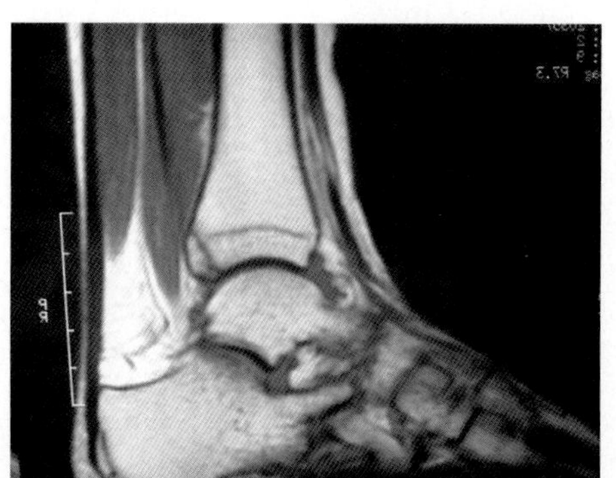

A

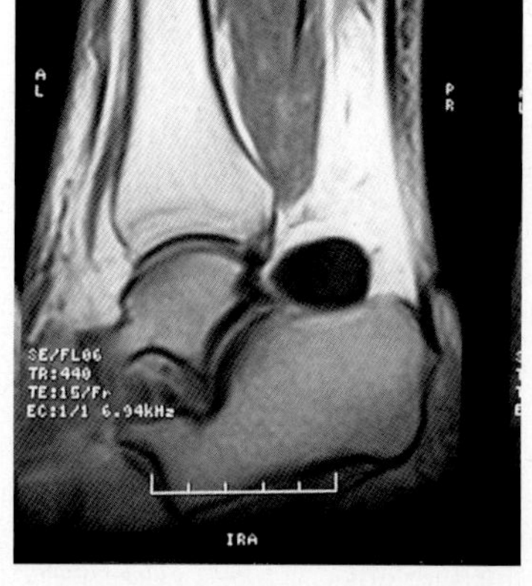

B

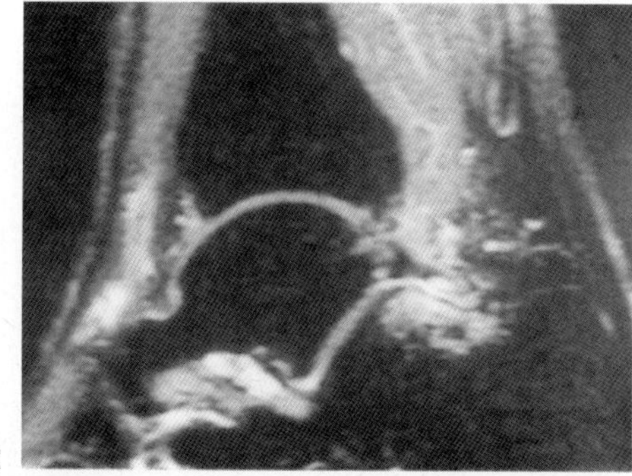

C

FIG 3 • **A.** Parasagittal T1-weighted image showing a posterior tibia fracture, which was occult in the initial radiographs. **B.** Parasagittal T1-weighted image showing a synovial cyst from the tibiotalar joint causing PAIS. **C.** Parasagittal STIR image showing bone marrow edema as a result of contusion in trigonal process injury.

DIFFERENTIAL DIAGNOSIS

- Misdiagnosis is common among patients with posterior ankle pain. Frequently patients had been previously treated for a Achilles tendinopathy.
- When a patient has pain in the posterolateral aspect of the ankle, the differential diagnosis includes Achilles tendinopathy, peroneal tendinopathy or tear, retrocalcaneal bursitis, Sever's disease, and sural neuralgia.
- When the patient has pain in the posteromedial aspect of the ankle, the differential diagnosis includes a posterior deltoid sprain, osteochondral lesion of the talus, soleus syndrome, posterior tibial tendinopathy, tarsal tunnel syndrome, and posteromedial tarsal coalition.

NONOPERATIVE MANAGEMENT

- Initial treatment for PAIS due to overuse includes rest, nonsteroidal anti-inflammatory drugs, cryotherapy, and avoidance of activities that require forced plantarflexion.
- Casting is rarely indicated, but acute articular or bony injuries may benefit from a brief period of immobilization and limited weight bearing.
- Physical therapy is indicated to improve ankle and subtalar ROM, as well as strength and flexibility of regional muscles.
- Successful nonoperative treatment has been reported in about 60% of patients with PAIS.[8]
- Corticosteroid injection for trigonal process pathology and other chronic causes of PAIS can effectively provide pain relief and should be done at least once before surgery is undertaken.[14,15]

SURGICAL MANAGEMENT

- Indications for surgical intervention include failure of nonsurgical treatment and rehabilitation exercises and a positive response to a diagnostic posterior ankle injection.
- Simultaneous bilateral posterior ankle surgery is not recommended.[8] While bilateral mechanical posterior ankle impingement is possible, this presentation should prompt a careful workup for systemic causes of posterior ankle pain.

Preoperative Planning

- All imaging studies are reviewed.
- The ankle–hindfoot score from the American Orthopaedic Foot and Ankle Society (AOFAS) scale is determined.
- Ankle and subtalar ROM are tested under anesthesia.

Positioning

- The patient is placed in a prone position and a tourniquet is applied on the thigh. Both feet are suspended off of the end of the bed, and a small triangular support is placed under the lower leg, making it possible to move the ankle freely and allow fluoroscopic examination. A support is placed at the ipsilateral side of the pelvis to allow slight rotation of the operating table in a safe manner when needed.[19]
- The surgeon must be aware of the potential complications of this position, such as damage to the genitalia, brachial plexus, and ulnar nerves, among other structures.

Approach

- Posterior ankle disorders can be approached by either an open or endoscopic technique.
- Open medial and lateral approaches have been described, with both approaches carrying an inherent risk of damaging neurovascular structures. A posterolateral approach should be used to treat isolated bony impingement.[8] A medial approach should be used when both FHL tendinopathy and bony impingement are being treated.[8]
- In our experience, hindfoot endoscopy is an advanced procedure with a learning curve that needs to be overcome by practicing on cadavers. The difficulty with endoscopic procedure is the initial orientation in the posterior ankle to achieve a safe access to the pathologic structures.[18]

POSTEROMEDIAL APPROACH

- A 4-cm curvilinear incision is made posterior to the medial malleolus at the level of the superior border of the calcaneus, following the underlying course of the neurovascular bundle.
- The bundle and the FHL are retracted posteriorly with a blunt retractor.
- The bony disorder of the posterior talar process (ie, symptomatic os trigonum) is removed.
- The area is rasped smooth, and hypertrophic capsulitis and inflamed tissue are débrided.
- Finally, the FHL excursion is checked and the tunnel is released as needed from proximal to distal to the level of the sustentaculum tali.

POSTEROLATERAL APPROACH

- A curvilinear incision is begun at the posterior ankle mortise in line with the posterior border of the peroneal tendons so that it lies anterior to the sural nerve.[12]
- A capsulotomy is performed with the ankle in slight dorsiflexion, and the lateral talar process or os trigonum is identified lateral to the tunnel. According to Hamilton et al,[8] the fibro-osseous tunnel of the FHL tendon cannot be released safely from the lateral side.
- Adequate osseous decompression is assessed by plantarflexing the foot and palpating for any bone-on-bone impingement.

POSTERIOR ANKLE ENDOSCOPY

- According to van Dijk's technique,[18] the posterolateral portal is made first at the level or slightly above the tip of the lateral malleolus, just lateral to the Achilles tendon; a clamp is directed anteriorly, pointing in the direction of the first interdigital space (**TECH FIG 1A**).
- When the tip of the clamp touches bone, it is exchanged for a 4.5-mm arthroscope shaft with blunt trocar pointing in the same direction. The blunt trocar is situated extra-articularly at the level of the ankle joint, but it is not necessary to enter the joint capsule.
- The posteromedial portal is made just medial to the Achilles tendon at the same level as the posterolateral portal in the horizontal plane.
- A clamp is introduced and directed toward the arthroscope shaft to guide the anterior travel of the clamp.
- The blunt trocar is exchanged for a 30-degree 4.0-mm scope using a lateral view direction to prevent lens damage. The scope in pulled backward until the tip of the clamp comes into view.
- The fatty tissue and adhesions overlying the joint capsule are partially removed using a 3.5-mm full-radius shaver. The posterior compartment of the subtalar joint can be visualized, including the posterior talar process and the FHL tendon. The FHL is an important landmark to prevent damage to the more medially located neurovascular bundle.
- By applying manual distraction to the os calcis, the posterior compartment of the ankle joint opens and allows better visualization. The talar dome can be inspected over almost its entire surface as well as the complete tibial plafond. An osteochondral defect or subchondral cystic lesion can be identified, débrided, and drilled.
- Removal of a symptomatic os trigonum or a nonunion of a fracture of the posterior talar process involves partial detachment of the posterior talofibular ligament and release of the flexor retinaculum, both of which attach to the posterior talar prominence (**TECH FIG 1B,C**).
- Releasing the FHL involves detachment of the flexor retinaculum from the posterior talar process.
- Bleeding is controlled, the new ankle range of motion is checked and recorded, and portals are sutured closed.

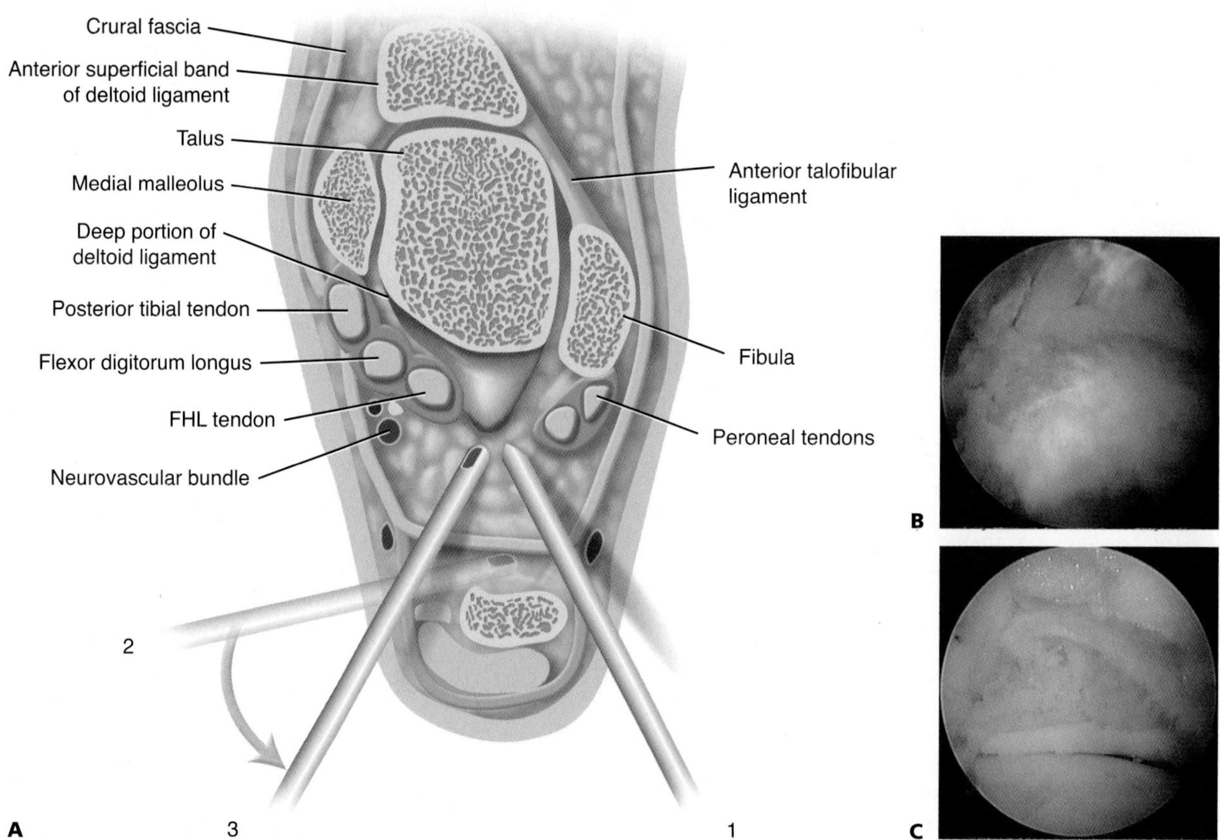

TECH FIG 1 • **A.** Cross-section of the ankle joint at level of the arthroscope. (*1*) The arthroscope is placed through the posterolateral portal, pointing in the direction of the webspace between the first and second toe. (*2*) The full-radius resector is introduced through the posteromedial until it touches the arthroscope shaft. (*3*) It then glides into an anterior direction until it touches bone. **B.** Posterior left ankle endoscopic view. The os trigonum synchondrosis was released, and the ossicle is ready for excision. The FHL tendon is marked. **C.** Posterior ankle endoscopic view after trigonal process resection.

PEARLS AND PITFALLS

- During endoscopy, motion of the hallux intraoperatively is a good marker for identification of the posterior anatomy because of the neurovascular bundle's being medial and the trigonal process's being lateral to the FHL tendon.
- In the hindfoot, the crural fascia can be quite thick. This local thickening is called the Rouvière ligament. During the endoscopic procedure, it needs to be partially excised or sectioned to approach the posterior ankle joint.

POSTOPERATIVE CARE

- An elastic bandage is applied, and the ankle is placed in a walker boot.
- Weight bearing is allowed after 2 or 3 days. Chondral lesion débridement requires longer non–weight-bearing period.
- Early motion (especially plantarflexion) is emphasized.

OUTCOMES

- Most experts agree that results of surgery for PAIS are highly satisfactory.[1,4,6,8–10,14,19,21]
- Outcomes after endoscopic treatment of PAIS reported in the literature compare favorably with results of open surgery.[19] Advantages include decreased morbidity, less scarring, and the potential for faster recovery.[19,21]
  - In a series 55 patients treated endoscopically, van Dijk et al[19] reported an average improvement of the AFOS score from 75 points preoperatively to 90 points after surgery.
- Results may vary according to the cause of symptoms. Patients treated for PAIS caused by overuse have better results than those treated following trauma.[19] Furthermore, patients with osseous impingement do better postoperatively than do patients with soft tissue impingement.
- Involvement in a workers' compensation claim has been shown to influence patient outcome.[1]

COMPLICATIONS

- Sural nerve damage (after posterolateral approach)
- Peroneal tendon fibrosis (after posterolateral approach)
- Tibial nerve injury (after posteromedial approach)
- FHL injury through lateral approach; also during endoscopic technique
- Reflex sympathetic dystrophy
- Infection
- Wound healing problems
- Ankle stiffness
- Deep vein thrombosis

REFERENCES

1. Abramowitz Y, Wollstein R, Barzilay Y, et al. Outcome of resection of a symptomatic os trigonum. J Bone Joint Surg Am 2003; 85:1051–1057.
2. Barfield WR. The biomechanics of kicking in soccer. Clin Sports Med 1998;17:711–728.
3. Bouchet A, Cuilleret J. Región posterior de la garganta del pie. In: Cuilleret BA, ed. Anatomía Descriptiva, Topográfica y Funcional. Buenos Aires: Editorial Médica Panamericana, 1995:223–234.
4. Brodsky AE, Khalil MA. Talar compression syndrome. Am J Sports Med 1986;14:472–476.
5. Bureau NJ, Cardinal E, Hobden R, et al. Posterior ankle impingement syndrome: MR imaging findings in seven patients. Radiology 2000; 215:497–503.
6. Calder JD, Sexton SA, Pearce CJ. Return to training and playing after posterior ankle arthroscopy impingement in elite professional soccer. Am J Sports Med 2010;38:120–124.
7. Frey C. Injuries of the subtalar joint. In Pffeffer GB, ed. Chronic Ankle Pain in the Athlete. Rosemont, IL: American Academy of Orthopedic Surgeons, 2000.
8. Hamilton WG, Geppert MJ, Thompson FM. Pain in the posterior aspect of the ankle in dancers: differential diagnosis and operative treatment. J Bone Joint Surg Am 1996;78A:1491–1500.
9. Hedrick MR, McBryde AM. Posterior ankle impingement. Foot Ankle 1994;15:2–8.
10. Jaivin JS, Ferkel RD. Arthroscopy of the foot and ankle. Clin Sports Med 1994;13.
11. Karasick D, Schweitzer ME. The os trigonum syndrome: imaging features. Am J Radiol 1996;166:125–129.
12. Lawrence SJ, Botte MJ. The sural nerve in the foot and ankle: an anatomic study with clinical and surgical implications. Foot Ankle Int 1994;15:490–494.
13. Lawson JP. Symptomatic radiographic variants in the extremities. Radiology 1985;157:625–631.
14. Maquirriain J. Posterior ankle impingement syndrome. J Am Acad Orthop Surg 2005;13:365–371.
15. Mouhsine E, Crevoisier X, Leyvraz PF, et al. Post-traumatic overload or acute syndrome of the os trigonum: a possible cause of posterior ankle impingement. Knee Surg Sports Traumatol Arthrosc 2004; 12:250–253.
16. Paulos LE, Johnson CL, Noyes FR. Posterior compartment fractures of the ankle. Am J Sports Med 1983;11:439–443.
17. Scholten PE, Sierevelt IN, van Dijk CN. Hindfoot endoscopy for posterior ankle impingement. J Bone Joint Surg Am 2008;90A: 2665–2672.
18. van Dijk CN, Scholten PE, Krips R. A 2-portal endoscopic approach for diagnosis and treatment of posterior ankle pathology. Arthroscopy 2000;16:871–876.
19. van Dijk CN, de Leeuw PA, Scholten PE. Hindfoot endoscopy for posterior ankle impingement. J Bone Joint Surg Am 2009;91A (Suppl 2):287–298.
20. Wakeley CJ, Johnson DP, Watt I. The value of MR imaging in the diagnosis of the os trigonum syndrome. Skel Radiol 1996;25:133–136.
21. Willitis K, Sonneveld H, Amendola A, et al. Outcome of posterior ankle arthroscopy for hindfoot impingement. Arthroscopy 2008; 24:196–202.

Chapter 90 Posterior Ankle Arthroscopy and Hindfoot Endoscopy

C. Niek van Dijk and Tahir Ögüt

DEFINITION

- Because of their nature and deep location, posterior ankle problems pose a diagnostic and therapeutic challenge.
- Arthroscopic evaluation of posterior ankle problems by means of routine ankle arthroscopy using an anteromedial, anterolateral, and posterolateral portal is difficult because of the shape of the ankle joint. In cases in which the ankle ligaments are lax, is it possible to visualize and treat the pathology of the ankle joint itself, but pericapsular or extracapsular posterior pathologic conditions are not accessible through conventional arthroscopic portals.
- A two-portal posterior endoscopic approach with the patient in the prone position affords excellent access to the posterior ankle, the subtalar joint, and the pericapsular and extra-articular structures.[19]

ANATOMY

- Posterior ankle arthroscopy and hindfoot endoscopy enable visualization and accessibility to the posterior half of the tibiotalar joint, the subtalar joint, and extra-articular structures such as the os trigonum, the flexor hallucis longus (FHL) tendon, and the posterior syndesmotic ligaments.
- The posterior intermalleolar ligament, also called the tibial slip or marsupial meniscus, is a structure with consistent location but varying size and width. It is distinct from the posteroinferior tibiofibular ligament and separated from it by a small gap filled with synovial tissue.[2]
- The os trigonum is a secondary center of ossification of the talus. It is present in 1.7% to 7% of normal feet.[4] When this ossification center remains separate from the posterolateral process of the talus (the trigonal process or the Stieda process), it is referred to as the os trigonum. The prevalence of unilateral and bilateral (ununited) os trigona is 10% and 1.402%, respectively.[4,14]
- The FHL tendon originates in the posterior leg then runs within a tendon sheath that begins 1 cm proximal to the subtalar joint and binds the tendon to the posterior talus and calcaneus, forming the fibro-osseous tunnel, which may restrict FHL motion.[6,10]
- The posteromedial neurovascular bundle (tibial nerve and posterior tibial artery) are consistently medial to the FHL tendon throughout its course. Instruments introduced from the posteromedial portal do not risk injuring the neurovascular bundle provided they remain lateral to the FHL.[7] Sitler et al dissected 13 cadavers and found that the tibial nerve was located posterior to the FHL tendon in two specimens.[12]
- A posteromedial portal located 1 cm proximal to the level of the tip of the lateral malleolus is on average 2.9 mm further removed from the medial neurovascular bundle than a portal placed 1 cm more proximally.[7]

PATHOGENESIS

- Posterior ankle pain may be a result of:
  - Posterior ankle impingement or os trigonum syndrome
  - FHL, posterior tibial, or peroneal tendinopathy
  - Posttraumatic calcifications or exostoses
  - Bony avulsions
  - Tibiotalar or subtalar loose bodies
  - Tibiotalar or subtalar osteochondral lesions or arthrosis
  - Any combination of these entities
- Overuse injuries play an important role in the pathogenesis of posterior ankle pain.
- Repetitive minor trauma in the ankle, as seen in athletes, can induce posterior ankle and/or hindfoot osteophyte formation.[15]
- Typically, to produce symptoms, an os trigonum must be disturbed by some traumatic event, such as a supination or forced plantarflexion injuries, dancing on hard surfaces, or pushing beyond physiologic limits.[15]
- The pain is thought to be a result of:
  - Symptomatic motion between the relatively unstable os trigonum and talus
  - Compression of thickened joint capsules (intermalleolar ligament)[1]
  - Impinging scar tissue between the os trigonum and tibia
  - Compression between os trigonum and calcaneus (referred to as "dancers' heel")
  - Irritation of the FHL tendon that courses between the os trigonum and the medial tubercle of the talus[6,15]
- FHL tendinopathy is usually attributable to stenosing tenosynovitis rather than tendinosis or rupture[3]; it has only rarely been reported at sites other than the posteromedial ankle.[3,10] However, immunohistochemical studies have suggested an avascular zone of the tendon in the segment of tendon that passes behind the talus.[11]

NATURAL HISTORY

- Patients present with posterior ankle pain.
- Posterior ankle impingement can be caused by overuse (chronic pain) or trauma (acute pain). It is important to differentiate between these two, because posterior impingement from overuse has a better prognosis.[15]
- Overuse injuries typically occur in ballet dancers, soccer players, and downhill runners.[3,18]
- In chronic conditions, stenosing tenosynovitis of the FHL tendon may coexist with os trigonum syndrome; this leads to poorer outcome if surgical treatment is delayed.[4]
- Nonsurgical treatment for os trigonum syndrome is successful in approximately 60% of patients.[8]

PATIENT HISTORY AND PHYSICAL FINDINGS

- Patients experience deep pain in the posterior aspect of the ankle joint, mainly with forced plantarflexion.

- On examination, there is pain on palpation of the posterior aspect of the talus.
- During the passive forced plantarflexion test, the investigator can apply a rotational movement on the point of maximal plantarflexion, thereby "grinding" the posterior talar process or os trigonum between the tibia and the calcaneus.
- A positive test result, in combination with pain on posterolateral palpation, should be followed by a diagnostic infiltration of an anesthetic (with or without corticosteroid).
- Posteromedial pain on palpation does not necessarily indicate impingement.[15]
- Tenderness on palpation over the musculotendinous junction of the FHL is diagnostic for FHL tendinitis; pain can be elicited by forced simultaneous ankle and first metatarsophalangeal joint dorsiflexion.[3,10]
- "Pseudo hallux rigidus" may coexist with posteromedial ankle pain. Hallux dorsiflexion may be limited with ankle dorsiflexion but restored with ankle plantarflexion. This exam finding/phenomenon has been reported to be secondary to nodular thickening of the proximal FHL that impinges within the fibro-osseous tunnel on the posteromedial ankle.[10]
- Palpation of posterior talar process is a sensitive test for posterior ankle impingement. A positive test should be followed by a hyperplantarflexion test.
- The hyperplantarflexion test is positive when the patient experiences recognizable pain at the moment of impact. It is a highly sensitive test for posterior ankle impingement. A negative test rules out a posterior ankle impingement syndrome.
- If the pain on forced plantarflexion disappears, the diagnosis is confirmed.
- Posteromedial ankle palpation is sensitive for FHL tendinitis.

IMAGING AND OTHER DIAGNOSTIC STUDIES

- In patients with posterior ankle impingement, the AP ankle view typically fails to demonstrate abnormalities (**FIG 1A**).
  - On the lateral view, a prominent posterior talar process or os trigonum can sometimes be recognized.
  - As the posterolaterally located posterior talar process or os trigonum is often superimposed on the medial talar tubercle, detection of an os trigonum on a standard lateral view is often not possible (**FIG 1B**).
  - For the same reason, calcifications can sometimes not be detected by this standard lateral view.
  - We recommend lateral radiographs with the foot in 25 degrees of external rotation in relation to the standard lateral radiographs (**FIG 1C**).
- Bone scintigraphy effectively localizes talar and peritalar injuries.[5]
- Computed tomography defines the exact size and location of calcifications, bony fragments, osteochondral lesions, or intraosseous talar cysts (**FIG 1D**).
- Magnetic resonance imaging (MRI) is useful for detection of bone contusions, edema, posterior capsular or ligament thickening,[1] talar osteochondral lesions, and FHL tenosynovitis.
  - MRI has been reported to accurately identify FHL tendinitis in 82% of patients,[10] represented by intermediate or low signal intensity on T2-weighted images.[4]
  - Fluid in the FHL tendon sheath is frequently seen in MRI without clinical signs of FHL tendinitis. Fluid in the tendon sheath of the FHL must be combined with changes in the tendon itself to be a sign of a tendinitis.
- Bone edema in the os trigonum is an important diagnostic finding.
  - It is a sign of chronic compression of the os trigonum between distal tibia and calcaneus.
  - It can be a sign of degeneration of the cartilage of the undersurface of the os trigonum. In these cases, the bone edema is combined with bone edema of the calcaneus.
  - It can also be a sign of movement between the os trigonum and the talus. In these cases, there is bone edema in the posterior talus as well. These cases represent a pseudoarthrosis type of lesion.

DIFFERENTIAL DIAGNOSIS

- Tarsal tunnel syndrome
- Plantar fasciitis
- Peroneal tenosynovitis
- Posterior tibial tenosynovitis
- Pseudo hallux rigidus (in FHL tenosynovitis)
- Bony avulsions
- Ankle and subtalar arthrosis

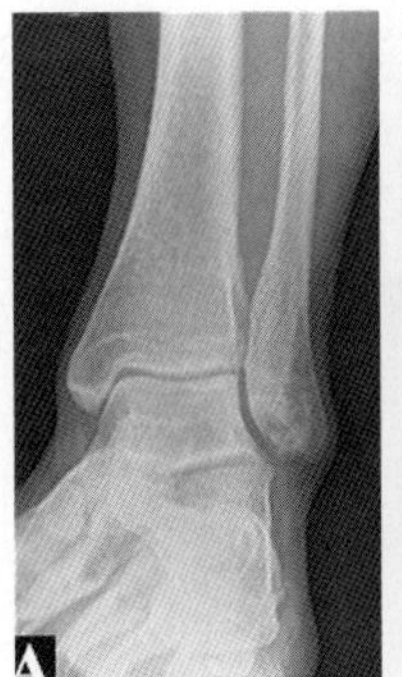

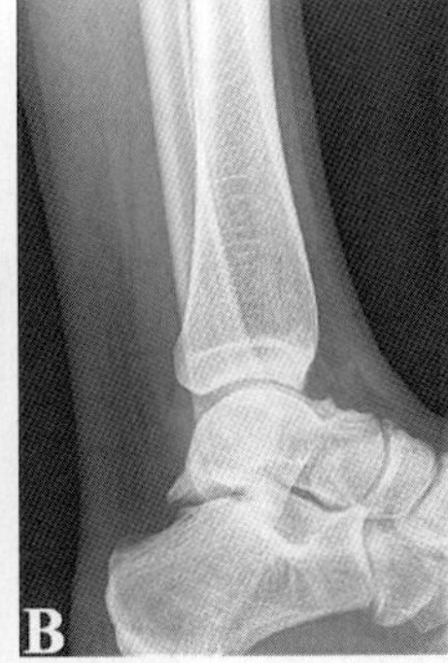

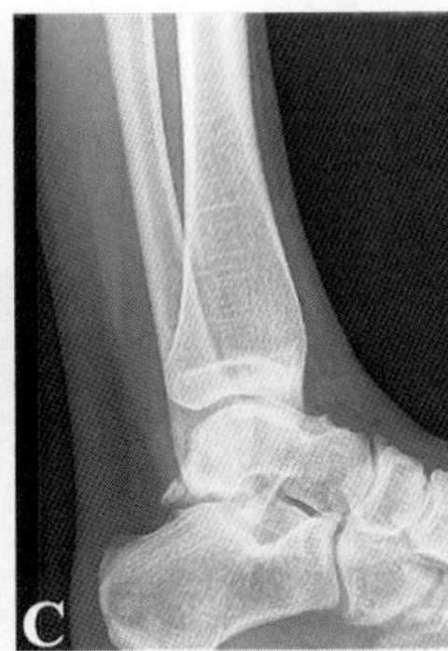

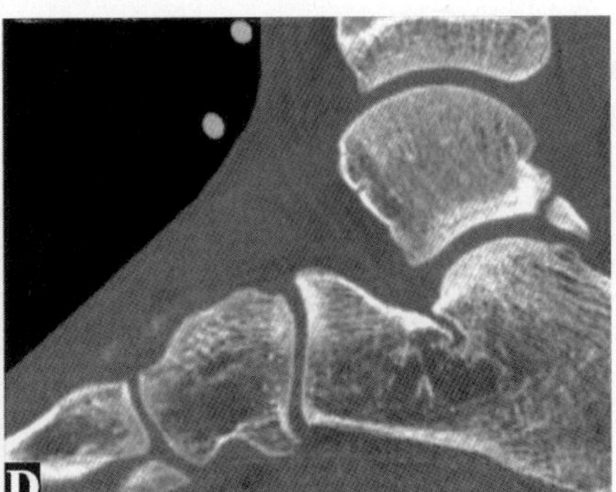

FIG 1 • Imaging posterior ankle impingement. **A.** AP ankle view showing no abnormalities. **B.** Standard lateral view. **C.** Lateral radiograph with the foot in 25 degrees of external rotation. **D.** Sagittal CT scan showing os trigonum.

Table 1 Indications for Posterior Ankle Arthroscopy and Hindfoot Endoscopy

Articular pathology
Posterior compartment ankle joint
Débridement and drilling of osteochondral defects
Removal of loose bodies, ossicles, calcifications, avulsion fragments
Resection of posterior tibial rim osteophytes
Treatment of chondromatosis and chronic synovitis
Posterior compartment subtalar joint
Removal of osteophytes and loose bodies
Subtalar arthrodesis
Treatment of intraosseous talar ganglions by retrograde curetting and drilling
Periarticular pathology
Posterior ankle impingement
Deep portion of deltoid ligament: removal of posttraumatic calcifications or ossicles
Flexor hallucis longus stenosing tenosynovitis: débridement of flexor retinaculum, posterior talofibular ligament, prominent talar process, and opening the sheath of the tendon
Posterior sydesmotic ligaments: hypertrophic ligaments can be excised

NONOPERATIVE MANAGEMENT

- Initial treatment of os trigonum syndrome consists of rest, ice, anti-inflammatory medication, avoidance of forced plantarflexion, and, occasionally, ankle immoblization for 4 to 6 weeks. If there is an established nonunion, immobilization with casting is not recommended.[8]
- Physical therapy, such as progressive resistive exercises and strengthening, may be helpful.[8]
- Corticosteroid injection for os trigonum syndrome can effectively provide temporary pain relief.[4,8]
- Nonsurgical treatment for FHL tenosynovitis includes rest, ice, anti-inflammatories, longitudinal arch supports, standard physical therapy, and stretching exercises.[8,10]

SURGICAL MANAGEMENT

- Indications for posterior ankle arthroscopy and hindfoot endoscopy are listed in Table 1.
- The procedure is performed as outpatient surgery with the patient under general or epidural anesthesia.[17]

Preoperative Planning

- All imaging studies are reviewed to address not only the individual pathology but also the associated bone, cartilage, or ligament injuries, as well as osteophytes, loose bodies, accessory muscles, and calcifications (**FIG 2**).
- Ankle and subtalar joint stability, stability of the peroneal tendons, and Achilles tendon tightness should be determined by examination under anesthesia.
  - Instability is a clinical diagnosis, and these patients are identified by their symptoms. They complain of recurrent giving-way. Laxity can be present without clinical symptoms of giving. If laxity is detected without clinical symptoms of giving-way, it is not an indication for lateral ligament reconstruction.
- For irrigation, a single bag of normal saline with gravity flow can be used.
- A 4.0-mm arthroscope with a 30-degree angle is routinely used for posterior ankle arthroscopy.
- For posterior ankle arthroscopy, a noninvasive distraction device can be used when the ankle joint has to be entered for the diagnosis and treatment of an intra-articular pathology.
- A 4-mm chisel and a periosteal elevator may be needed during posterior arthroscopy for excision of osteophytes and ossicles.

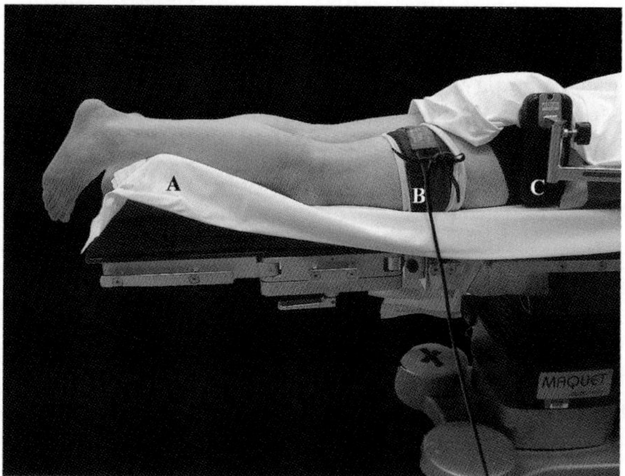

FIG 3 • Positioning for hindfoot endoscopy. Small leg support (*A*), tourniquet (*B*), and leg holder (*C*).

Positioning

- The patient is placed in a prone position. The patient should be placed properly to avoid tension on the brachial plexi, avoid pressure on the ulnar nerve at the elbow, and protect the genitalia.
- A tourniquet is applied around the upper leg, and a small support is placed under the lower leg, making it possible to move the ankle freely (**FIG 3**).

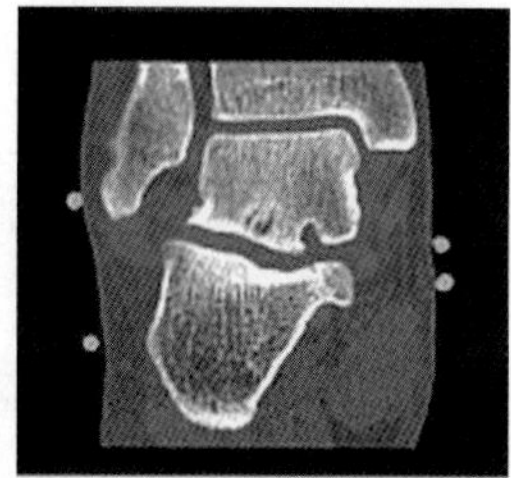
A
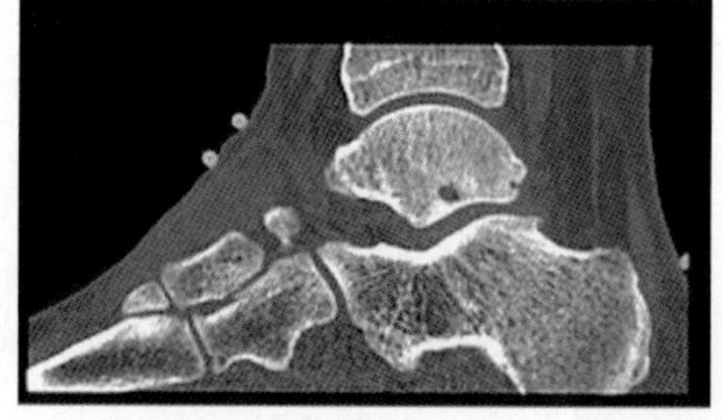
B
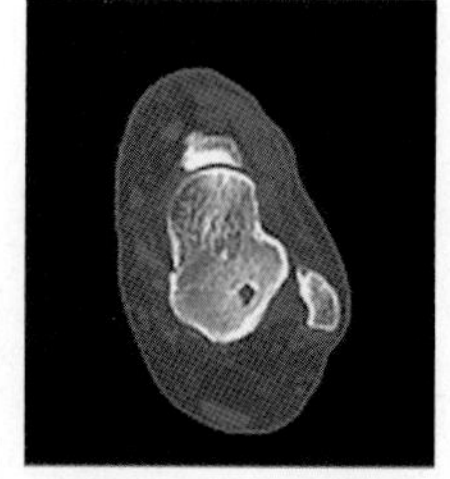
C

FIG 2 • Preoperative planning for débridement and drilling of a subtalar osteochondral cyst lesion in a right ankle. Coronal (**A**), sagittal (**B**), and axial (**C**) CT images showing the subtalar osteochondral defect and secondary cyst lesion.

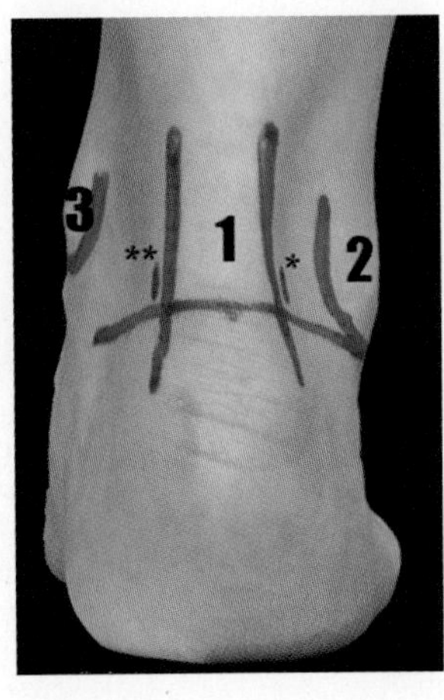

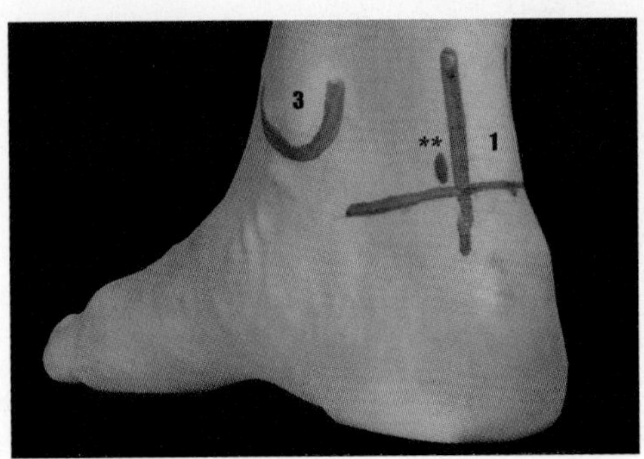

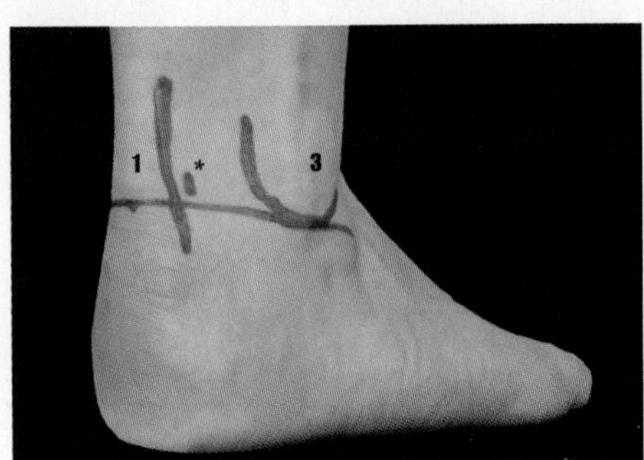

FIG 4 • Posterior (**A**), posteromedial (**B**), and posterolateral (**C**) views of foot and ankle with the cutaneous landmarks for posterior ankle arthroscopy and hindfoot endoscopy. *1,* Achilles tendon; *2,* lateral malleolus; *3,* medial malleolus; *posterolateral portal; **posteromedial portal.

- The foot is placed at the very end of the operating table so that the surgeon can fully dorsiflex the ankle.

Approach

- The landmarks on the ankle are the lateral malleolus, medial and lateral border of the Achilles tendon, and the sole of the foot. With a marking pen, a line is drawn as a reference from the tip of the lateral malleolus to the Achilles tendon, parallel to the sole of the foot.
- Posterolateral and posteromedial portals are made just above this line, at the same level in the horizontal plane, and just lateral and medial to the Achilles tendon (**FIG 4**).

CREATION OF THE POSTEROLATERAL PORTAL

- A vertical stab incision is made for posterolateral portal.
- The subcutaneous layer is split by a mosquito clamp that is directed anteriorly, in the direction of the interdigital web space between the first and second toes (**TECH FIG 1A**).

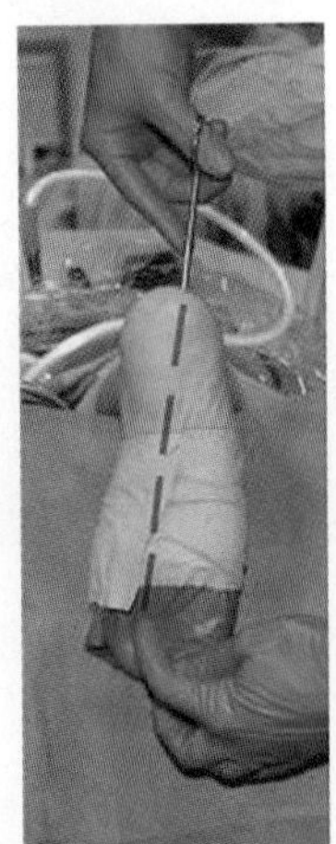

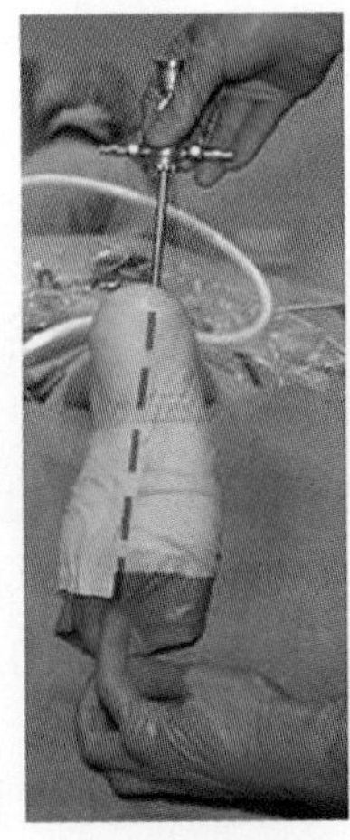

TECH FIG 1 • Creation of the posterolateral portal. **A.** Subcutaneous tissue is dissected by a mosquito clamp in the direction of the first interdigital webs pace. **B.** When the tip of the clamp touches the posterior talar process, it is exchanged for a 4.5-mm arthroscope shaft with the blunt trocar pointing in the same direction.

- When the tip of the clamp touches the bone, it is exchanged for a 4.5-mm arthroscope shaft with the blunt trocar pointing in the same direction (**TECH FIG 1B**).
- The level of the ankle joint and subtalar joint can be distinguished by palpating the bone in the sagittal plane because the prominent posterior talar process or os trigonum can be felt as a posterior prominence between the two joints.
- The trocar is positioned extra-articularly at the level of the ankle joint.
- The trocar is exchanged for the 4-mm arthroscope; the direction of view is 30 degrees to the lateral side.

Creation of the Posteromedial Portal

- A vertical stab incision is made for the posteromedial portal.
- A mosquito clamp is introduced and directed toward the arthroscope shaft at a 90-degree angle (**TECH FIG 2A**).
- When the mosquito clamp touches the shaft of the arthroscope, the shaft is used as a guide for the clamp to move anteriorly in the direction of the ankle joint, touching the arthroscope shaft until it reaches the bone (**TECH FIG 2B**).
- Next, the arthroscope is withdrawn slightly, directly over the mosquito clamp until the tip of the mosquito clamp is visualized (**TECH FIG 2C**).

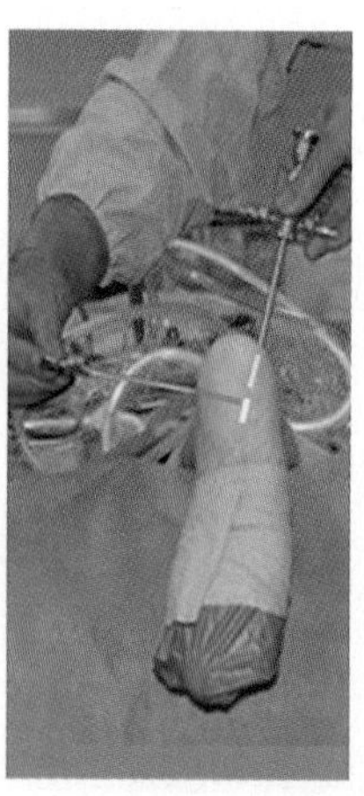
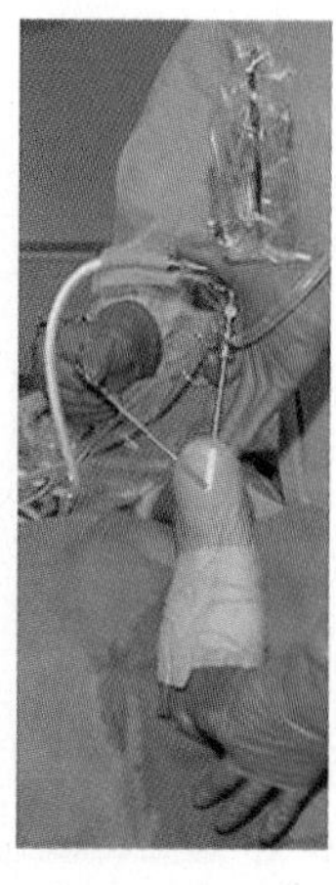
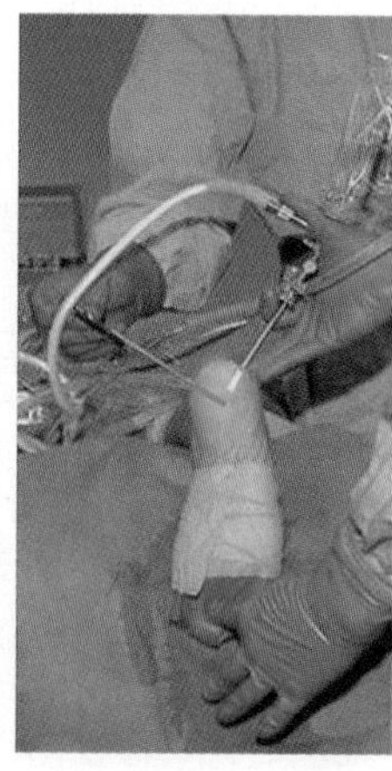

TECH FIG 2 • Creation of the posteromedial portal. **A**. A mosquito clamp is introduced and directed toward the arthroscope shaft at a 90-degree angle. **B.** Touching the arthroscope shaft, the mosquito clamp is slid anteriorly until it reaches the bone. **C.** The arthroscope is now withdrawn slightly and slides over the mosquito clamp until the tip of the mosquito clamp comes into view.

- The clamp is used to spread the extra-articular soft tissue in front of the tip of the lens.
- In situations in which scar tissue or adhesions are present, the mosquito clamp is exchanged for a 5-mm full-radius shaver.
- The tip of the shaver is directed in a lateral and slightly plantar direction toward the posterolateral aspect of the subtalar joint.
- When the tip of the shaver has reached this position, shaving can begin.

Working Posterior to the Ankle

- The joint capsule and adipose tissue can be removed. The adipose tissue is removed first and with it the very thin joint capsule.
- The subtalar joint can now be recognized. The posterior talar fibular ligament that attaches to the talus at this level can be recognized as well.
- After removal of the thin joint capsule, the posterior subtalar joint can be inspected (TECH FIG 3A).
- At the level of the ankle joint, the posterior tibiofibular and talofibular ligaments are identified and the posterior ankle joint can be visualized (TECH FIG 3B).
- The posterior talar process can be freed of scar tissue, and the FHL tendon, an important landmark, is identified. Motion of the hallux helps isolate the fibers of the FHL tendon in the posterior ankle.
- The shaver should never be used medial to the FHL tendon because of the proximity of the posteromedial neurovascular bundle.

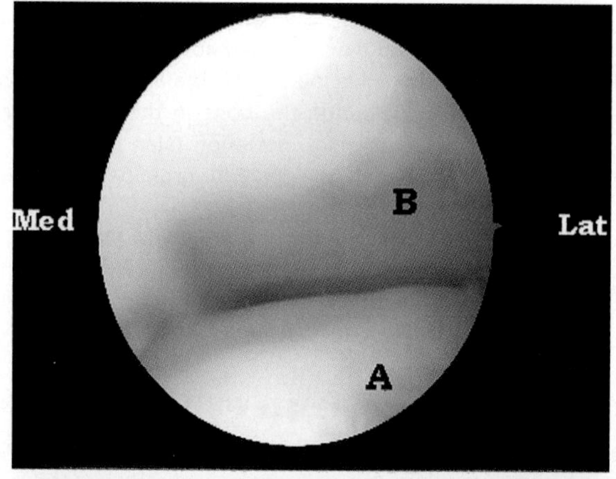

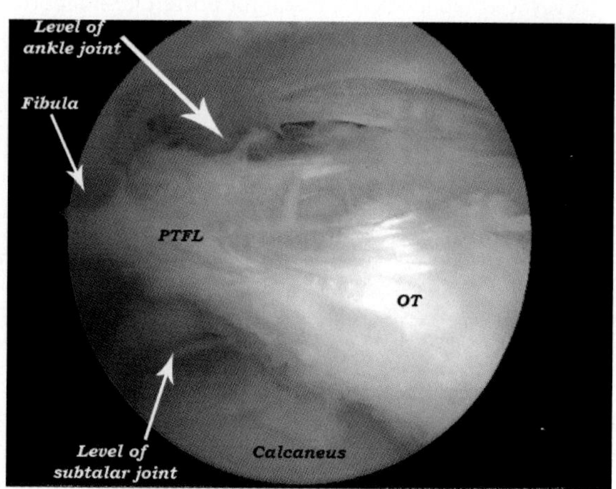

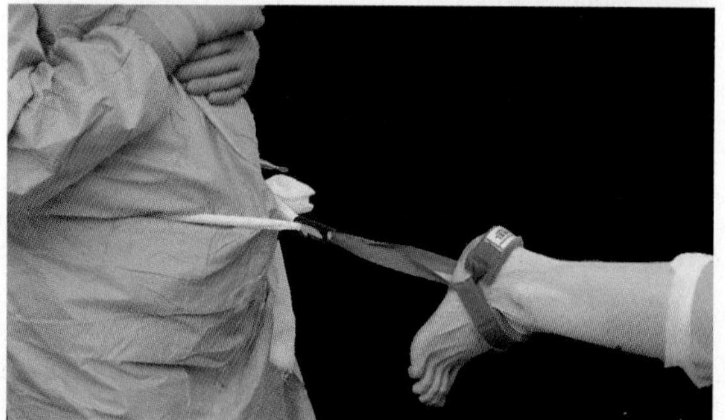

TECH FIG 3 • **A.** Arthroscopic views of the posterior compartment of the subtalar joint showing the calcaneus (*A*) and the talus (*B*). **B.** Endoscopic overview of the posterolateral aspect of the ankle joint. Os trigonum (*OT*) and its connection to the posterior talofibular ligament (*PTFL*). **C.** Application of the soft tissue distractor.

- After removal of the thin posterior ankle joint capsule, the ankle joint is entered with the arthroscope and inspected.
- On the medial side, both the tip of the medial malleolus and the deep portion of the deltoid ligament are visualized.
- By opening the joint capsule from inside out at the level of the medial malleolus, the tendon sheath of the posterior tibial tendon can be opened.
- With manual distraction on the os calcis, the posterior aspect of the ankle joint is opened, and the shaver can be introduced into the tibiotalar joint.
- For greater distraction, a noninvasive ankle distractor can be applied (TECH FIG 3C).
- A total synovectomy or capsulectomy can be performed. In our experience, nearly the entire talar dome tibial plafond can be visualized via this posteior approach.
- An osteochondral defect or subchondral cystic lesion can be identified, débrided, and drilled (TECH FIG 4).

Removal of an Os Trigonum

- The posterior syndesmotic ligaments are inspected and, if hypertrophic, are partially resected.
- Removal of a symptomatic os trigonum (TECH FIG 5), a nonunited fracture of the posterior talar process, or a symptomatic large posterior talar prominence requires partial detachment of the posterior talofibular ligament and release of the flexor retinaculum, both of which attach to the posterior talar prominence.

Release of the Flexor Hallucis Longus Tendon

- Release of the FHL tendon involves detachment of the flexor retinaculum from the posterior talar process by means of a punch (TECH FIG 6).
- A tight, thick crural fascia, if present, can hinder the free movement of instruments. It is helpful to enlarge the hole in the fascia using a punch or shaver.
- Bleeding is controlled by electrocautery at the end of the procedure.

Wound Closure and Dressing

- After removal of the instruments, the stab incisions are closed with 3-0 nylon to prevent sinus formation.
- A sterile compression dressing is applied.
- In patients with combined anterior and posterior symptoms, the posterior pathology is adressed by means of the two-portal hindfoot approach, and the anterior pathology is approached by a two-portal anterior approach.
- This can be done in two ways. The anterior arthroscopy can be performed with the knee flexed and the foot upside down, but we typically prefer a two-stage procedure. First the two-portal hindfoot approach is finished. The patient is then turned and a routine anterior ankle arthroscopy is performed.

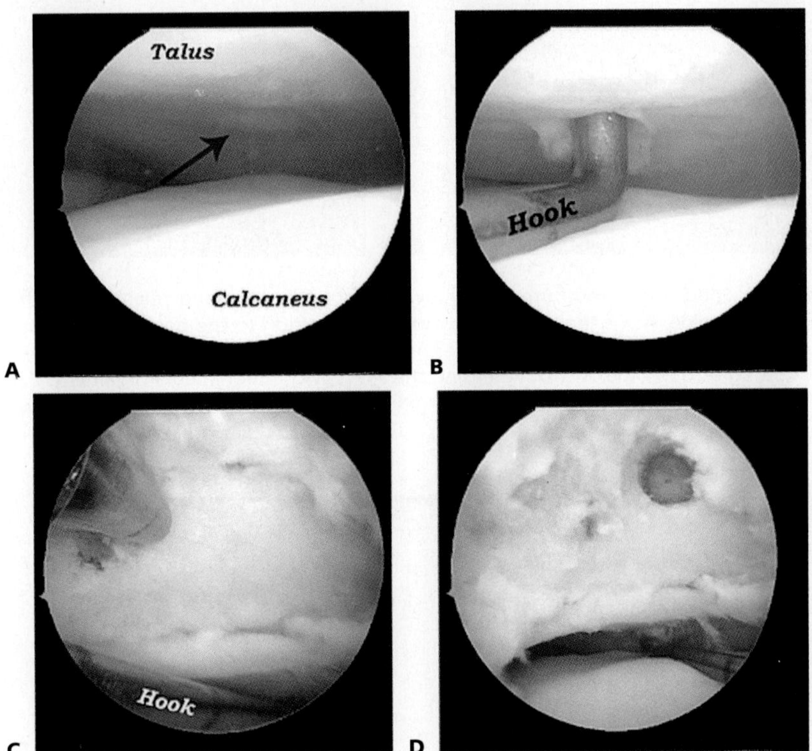

TECH FIG 4 • Endoscopic procedure for débridement and drilling of a subtalar osteochondral cyst lesion in a right ankle (same patient as in Fig 2). **A.** Endoscopic image with an arrow indicating the defect. **B.** A hook is introduced via the posteromedial portal and penetrates the osteochondral defect up to the cyst. **C.** By retrograde drilling, the cyst is reached. The hook is used for guiding the exact direction of the drill. **D.** Postoperative overview.

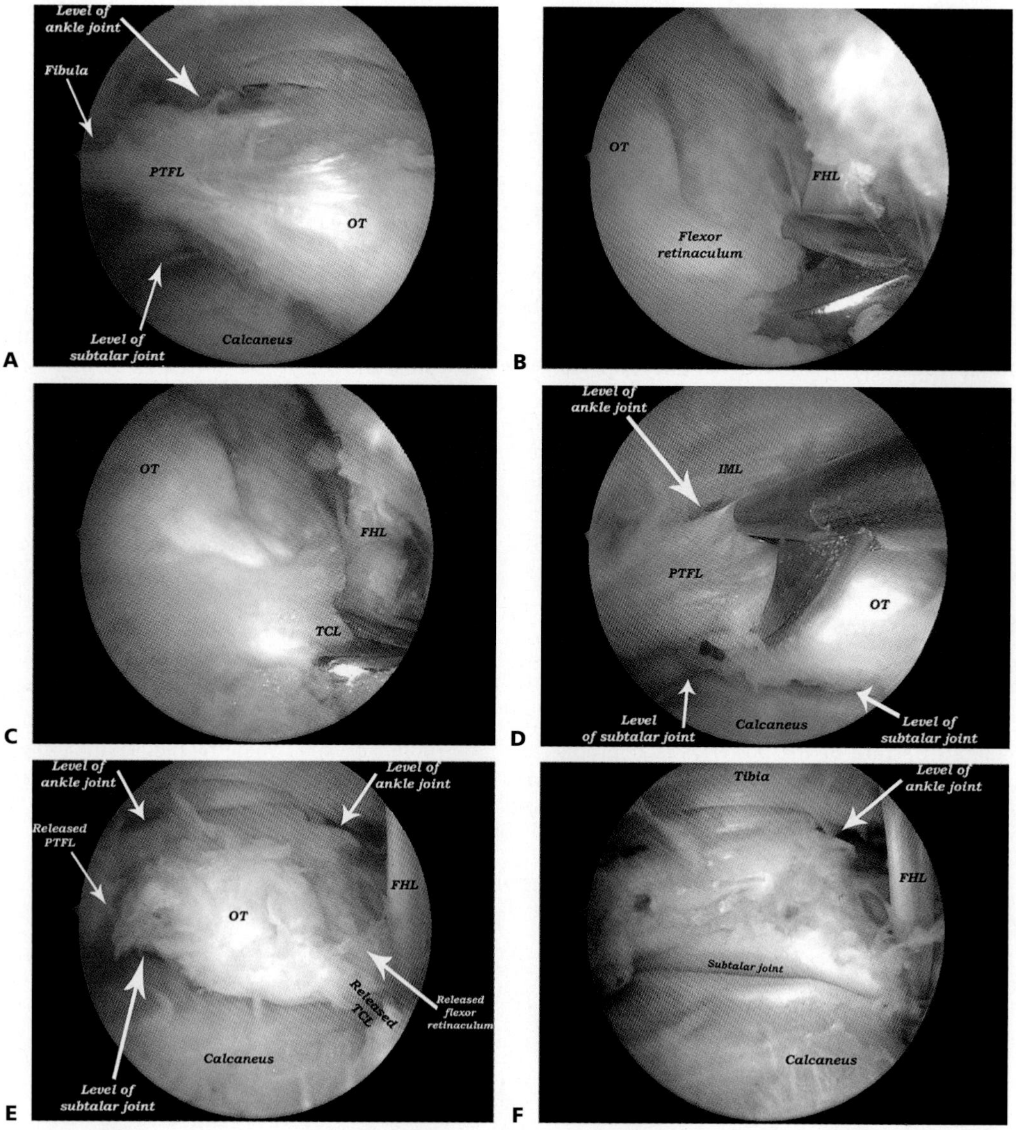

TECH FIG 5 • Endoscopic procedure for removing an os trigonum and releasing the flexor hallucis longus in a left ankle. **A.** Os trigonum (*OT*) with its connection to the posterior talofibular ligament (*PTFL*), flexor retinaculum and talocalcaneal ligament (*TCL*). **B.** Cutting through the flexor retinaculum. **C.** Cutting through the TCL. **D.** Releasing the PTFL. *IML*, intermalleolar ligament. **E.** Overview of the os trigonum released from its related anatomic structures. **F.** Postoperative overview.

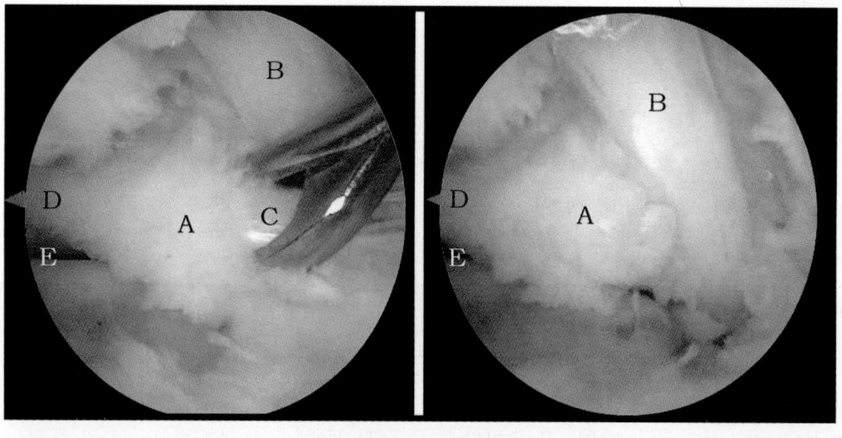

TECH FIG 6 • Endoscopic procedure for releasing of the flexor hallucis longus tendon (*B*) involves detachment of the flexor retinaculum (*C*) from the posterior talar process (*A*) by means of a punch. *D*, talus; *E*, subtalar joint.

PEARLS AND PITFALLS

Position of the arthroscope	▪ The direction of view should always be lateral.
Rouvière ligament	▪ This ligament runs to the FHL retinaculum. ▪ It can be attached to the posterior talar process. ▪ An arthroscopic punch or scissors can be used to enlarge the entry through this ligament. ▪ Usually it has to be detached from the posterior talar process to get to the ankle joint.
Safe areas	▪ The arthroscope should point into the direction of the web space between the first and second toes. ▪ It should be positioned lateral to the FHL tendon. It can be positioned medial to the FHL tendon only when a release of the neurovascular bundle is required (posttraumatic tarsal tunnel syndrome).
Removing the hypertrophic posterior talar process using the chisel	▪ Care should be taken not to place the chisel too far anterior, so as to avoid entering the subtalar joint (**FIG 5**).
How to initially visualize or gain proper orientation in the posterior ankle	▪ The most important trick is to start shaving at the level of the subtalar joint on the lateral side. This is an area in which it is relatively safe to start shaving. The opening of the shaver is directed toward the joint. ▪ Once the subtalar joint has been identified, the posterior talofibular ligament is identified. This ligament attaches to the lateral surface of the talus in this area. ▪ If we move the scope and shaver proximal from the posterior fibular ligament we are at the level of the os trigonum. The soft tissue in this posterolateral area can now be removed. ▪ The ankle joint usually can now be identified by applying some traction to the calcaneus. Dorsiflexing the foot can also help. ▪ Part of the posterior ligaments can be removed to enter the ankle joint when desired. ▪ From the posterolateral corner, the instruments now can be moved over the posterior talar process or os trigonum to the medial side, while staying in contact with the posterior ankle ligaments and the proximal surface of the os trigonum all the way. The flexor hallucis longus then comes into view.

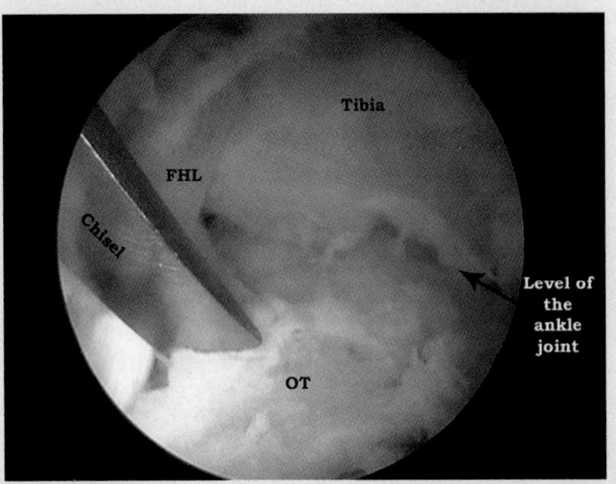

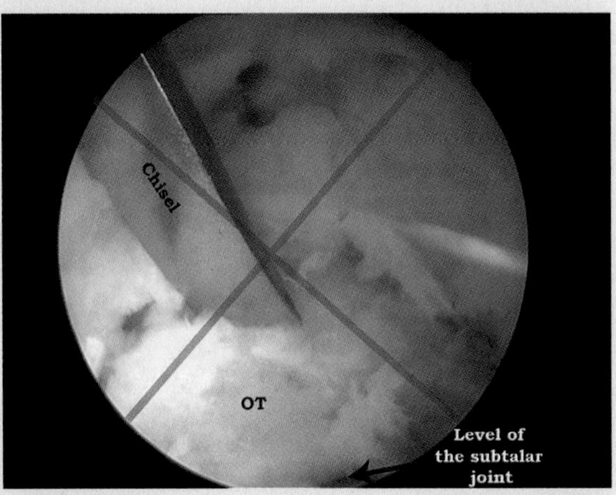

FIG 5 • Removal of the hypertrophic posterior talar process using the chisel. Care should be taken not to place the chisel too far anterior, so as to avoid entering the subtalar joint.

POSTOPERATIVE CARE

- As soon as possible after surgery, the patient is advised to start range-of-motion exercises as tolerated. It is not necessary to immobilize the ankle postoperatively to prevent sinus formation. The posterior ankle joint has a good soft tissue covering. The advantage of the procedure is that patients can start to move the ankle directly postoperatively.
- Postoperatively for 2 or 3 days, the patient is allowed weight bearing on crutches as tolerated.
- The dressing can be removed after 3 days. We remove the sutures 2 weeks postoperatively.
- The patient is reevaluated 1 week postoperatively. If necessary, physical therapy can be prescribed for range of motion, strengthening, and stability.

OUTCOMES

- In a consecutive series of 146 posterior ankle arthroscopies (136 patients) performed at the Academic Medical Center University of Amsterdam between 1994 and 2002, all patients were satisfied postoperatively. There were no complications other than 2 patients who experienced a small area of diminished sensation over the heel pad of the hindfoot.
- The main indication was a posterior ankle impingement syndrome. Procedures, all carried out by the same surgeon, were as follows:
  - Removal of a bony impediment (os trigonum or hypertrophic posterior talar process; n = 52)
  - Additional release of the flexor hallucis longus tendon (n = 37)

- Removal of a soft tissue impediment by a shaver (n = 8)
- Isolated release of the flexor hallucis longus tendon (n = 7)
- Débridement and drilling of an osteochondral defect at the posteromedial talar dome (n = 7), in the tibial plafond (n = 4), or in the posterolateral talar dome (n= 2)
- Removal of calcifications (n=5)
- Total synovectomy (the knee was flexed and an anterior synovectomy was performed by means of the standard anterolateral and anteromedial approach; n= 9)
- Arthroscopic débridement of degenerated subtalar joint (n = 10)
- Removal of a loose body from the subtalar joint (n = 1)
- Curettage, drilling, and grafting of a large intraosseous talar ganglion (n = 3)

- Combined procedures did not cause any technical problems and were successful in most patients. Patients who were treated for a bony impingement did better than patients who were treated for a soft tissue impingement.
- None of these patients had deterioration of the result over time.[16]
- Marumoto and Ferkel treated 11 patients with painful os trigonum by arthroscopic removal of the os trigonum.[9] The average postoperative AOFAS scale was 86.4 points 3 years postoperatively.
  - Jerosch and Fadel applied the same treatment method to 10 patients with symptomatic os trigonum[4]; 9 of them were symptom-free 4 weeks postoperatively, and the average AOFAS scale increased from 43 preoperatively to 87 at a mean follow-up time of 25 months. They observed no complications in these 10 patients.
  - Tey et al endoscopically treated 15 patients with posterior ankle impingement and reported that all but 1 patient (7%) improved at an average 3 years of follow-up.[13]
  - Willits et al performed 24 posterior ankle arthroscopies with an indication of posterior ankle impingement.[20] The average time to return to work was 1 month and to sports was 5.8 months. Mean score on the AOFAS scale was improved to 91 at a mean follow-up time of 32 months postoperatively.

COMPLICATIONS

- Potential complications of this technique include tibial nerve and vascular injury, FHL tendon injury, and sural nerve injury.
- To prevent sural nerve injury it is important to create the posterolateral portal as described previously, close to the Achilles tendon, first making a stab incision and then continuing with blunt dissection by a mosquito clamp.
- Avoiding the potential complications of working through a posteromedial portal, the trick is to angle the instrument (shaver, burr, punch) in the posteromedial portal at 90 degrees to the arthroscope shaft.
- The arthroscope shaft subsequently is used as a guide for the instrument to travel into the direction of the joint. All the way, the mosquito clamp should be felt to touch the arthroscope shaft. In this manner, the neurovascular bundle is passed without problem.
- Precise control of the aspirator and shaver is mandatory to prevent tibialis posterior nerve and vessel injury and to prevent damage to the FHL tendon. In areas close to the neurovascular bundle, the aspirator should be set to a minimum amount of suction.
- We have applied this technique since 1994 without any complications other than two patients who experienced a small area of diminished sensation over the heel pad of the hindfoot.
- When performed in the manner described above, hindfoot endoscopy is a safe and reliable method of diagnosing and treating a variety of posterior ankle problems.
- The decision to treat posterior as well as anterior pathology is made preoperatively. If preoperatively it is decided to treat both anterior and posterior pathology, we start with addressing the posterior pathology by means of the two-portal hindfoot approach. After finishing the posterior procedure, the portals are sutured and the patient is turned and the anterior procedure is performed.

ACKNOWLEDGMENT

The authors would greatly like to thank P.A.J. de Leeuw from the department of orthopaedic surgery in the Academic Medical Center in Amsterdam, The Netherlands, for providing all the images for this chapter.

REFERENCES

1. Fiorella D, Helms CA, Nunley JA. The MR imaging features of the posterior intermalleolar ligament in patients with posterior impingement syndrome of the ankle. Skel Radiol 1999;28:573–576.
2. Golano P, Mariani PP, Rodriguez-Niedenfuhr M, et al. Arthroscopic anatomy of the posterior ankle ligaments. Arthroscopy 2002;18: 353–358.
3. Hamilton WG, Geppert M, Thompson FM. Pain in the posterior aspect of the ankle in dancers. J Bone Joint Surg Am 1996;78A:1491–1500.
4. Jerosch J, Fadel M. Endoscopic resection of a symptomatic os trigonum. Knee Surg Sports Traumatol Arthrosc 2006;14:1188–1193.
5. Johnson RP, Collier D, Carrera GF. The os trigonum syndrome: use of bone scan in the diagosis. J Trauma 1984;24:761–764.
6. Kolettis G, Michell L, Klein JD. Release of the flexor hallucis longus tendon in ballet dancers. J Bone Joint Surg Am 1996;78A:1386–1390.
7. Lijoi F, Marcello L, Baccarani G. Posterior arthroscopic approach to the ankle: an anatomic study. Arthroscopy 2003;19:62–67.
8. Maquirriain J. Posterior ankle impingement syndrome. J Am Acad Orthop Surg 2005;13:365–371.
9. Marumoto JM, Ferkel RD. Arthroscopic excision of the os trigonum: a new technique with preliminary clinical results. Foot Ankle 1997; 18:777–784.
10. Michelson J, Dunn L. Tenosynovitis of the flexor hallucis longus: a clinical study of the spectrum of presentation and treatment. Foot Ankle Int 2005;26:291–303.
11. Petersen W, Pufe T, Zantop T, Paulsen F. Blood supply of the flexor hallucis longus tendon with regard to dancer's tendonitis: injection and immunohistocheical studies of cadaver tendons. Foot Ankle Int 2003;24:591–596.
12. Sitler DF, Amendola A, Bailey CS, et al. Posterior ankle arthroscopy: an anatomic study. J Bone Joint Surg Am 2002;84A:763–769.
13. Tey M, Monllau JC, Centenera JM, Pelfort X. Benefits of arthroscopic tuberculoplasty in posterior ankle impingement syndrome. Knee Surg Sports Traumatol Arthrosc 2007;15:1235–1239.
14. Uzel M, Cetinus E, Bilgic E, et al. Bilateral os trigonum syndrome associated with bilateral tenosynovitis of the flexor hallucis longus muscle. Foot Ankle Int 2005;26:894–898.
15. van Dijk CN. Anterior and posterior ankle impingement. Foot Ankle Clin 2006;11:663–683.
16. van Dijk CN. Hindfoot endoscopy. Foot Ankle Clin 2006;11:391–414.
17. van Dijk CN. Hindfoot endoscopy for posterior ankle pain. Instr Course Lect 2006;55:545–554.
18. van Dijk CN, Lim LS, Poortman A, et al. Degenerative joint disease in female ballet dancers. Am J Sports Med 1995;23:295–300.
19. van Dijk CN, Scholten PE, Krips R. A 2-portal endoscopic approach for diagnosis and treatment of posterior ankle pathology. Arthroscopy 2000;16:871–876.
20. Willits K, Sonneveld H, Amendola A, et al. Outcome of posterior ankle arthroscopy for hindfoot impingement. Arthroscopy 2008;24: 196–202.

Chapter **91**

Endoscopic Treatment of Posterior Ankle Impingement Through a Posterior Approach

Phinit Phisitkul and Annunziato Amendola

DEFINITION

- *Posterior ankle impingement syndrome* is a clinical disorder characterized by posterior ankle pain that occurs in forced plantarflexion. It can be caused by an acute or chronic injury, with the os trigonum or trigonal process of the talus as the most offending structure.[10,19]
- Synonyms used for posterior ankle impingement syndrome include *posterior block of the ankle, posterior triangle pain, talar compression syndrome, os trigonum syndrome, os trigonum impingement, posterior tibiotalar impingement syndrome,* and *nutcracker-type syndrome.*[4,11,20,36]
- The os trigonum is a secondary ossification center of the talus. It mineralizes between the ages of 11 and 13 years in boys and 8 and 11 years in girls. It fuses with the posterior talus within 1 year, forming the posterolateral process, often called the Stieda or trigonal process. The os trigonum remain as a separate ossicle in 1.7% to 7% of normal feet, twice as often unilaterally as bilaterally.[3,8,16,24]

ANATOMY

- The posterior process of the talus is composed of a smaller posteromedial process and a larger posterolateral or trigonal process flanking the sulcus for the flexor hallucis longus (FHL) tendon.
- The os trigonum may be found in connection with the posterolateral tubercle (**FIG 1**). It is completely corticalized and has three surfaces: anterior, inferior, and posterior.
- The anterior surface connects to the posterolateral tubercle via fibrous, fibrocartilaginous, or cartilaginous tissue. The inferior surface forms the posterior part of the talocalcaneal joint.
- The posterior surface is nonarticular and has the attachments of posterior talofibular ligament, posterior talocalcaneal ligament, deep layer of the flexor retinaculum, and the talar component of the fibuloastragalocalcaneal ligament of Rouviere and Canela Lazaro.[28]
- The tibialis posterior tendon, the flexor digitorum longus tendon, and the flexor hallucis longus tendon situate in their own fibrous tunnels in continuity with the fascia of the deep posterior compartment.
- The neurovascular bundles are just medial and posterior to the flexor hallucis longus tendon at the level of the ankle joint, with the tibial nerve as the most lateral structure (**FIG 2**).
- In some variants, the posterior tibial artery can be thin or absent (0–2%), with the dominant peroneal artery traversing across the posterior ankle toward the tarsal tunnel.[2,6]

PATHOGENESIS

- Most cases of posterior ankle impingement syndrome occur in athletes such as ballet dancers or soccer players who have sustained acute or repetitive injuries with the ankle in forced plantarflexion, causing the "nutcracker effect"[12,20](**FIG 3**). Ankle sprain may cause avulsion fracture of the posterior talofibular ligament and secondary impingement.[15,21,25,34]
- Symptoms can be aggravated by any structures localized between the posterior tibial plafond and the calcaneal facet of the posterior subtalar joint, such as the os trigonum, long trigonal process, flexor hallucis longus tendon, posterior inferior tibiofibular ligament, intermalleolar ligament, and any osseous, articular cartilage, capsule, or synovial lesions of the posterior ankle or subtalar joint.
- FHL tenosynovitis is commonly associated with posterior ankle impingement due to the intimate relationship between the tendon and the os trigonum or the trigonal process at the

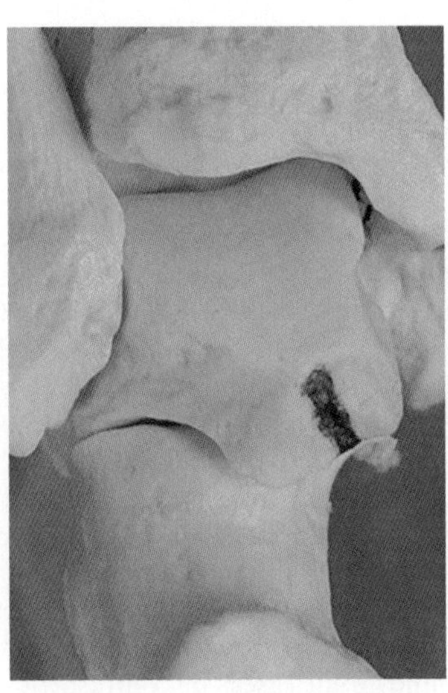

FIG 1 • Os trigonum.

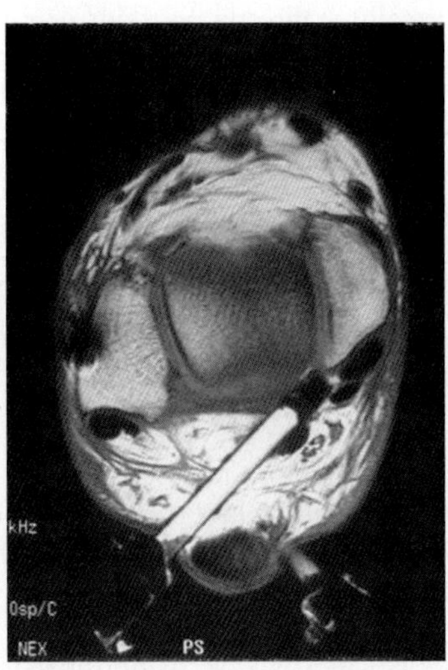

FIG 2 • Neurovascular bundle posteromedial to the FHL tendon.

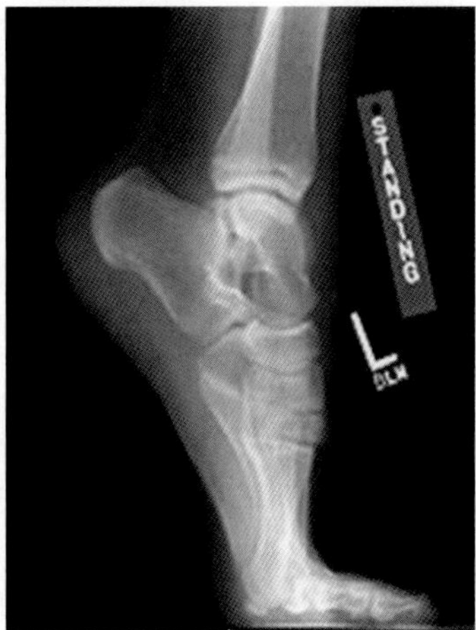

FIG 3 • Forced plantarflexion as a cause of the nutcracker effect in the os trigonum.

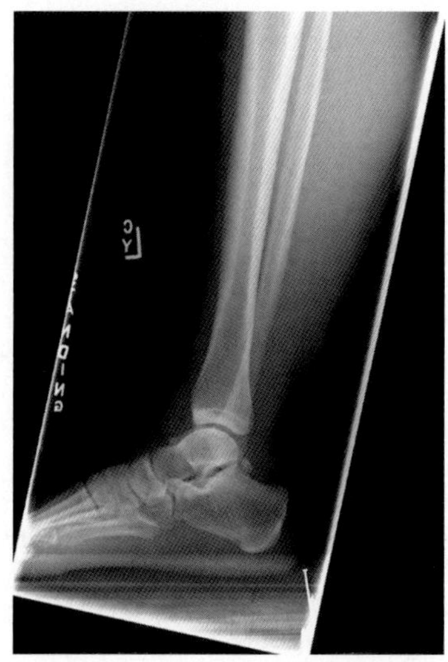

FIG 4 • Lateral radiograph of the ankle.

posterior aspect of the talus. This lesion can be an associated injury or secondary to the inflamed surrounding structures.[17,26,30]

NATURAL HISTORY

- The natural history of posterior ankle impingement is currently unknown. Os trigonum is a benign condition and usually is asymptomatic.
- When symptomatic, nonoperative treatment has been found to be successful in 60% of cases. However, Hedrick and McBryde[10] reported that only 40% of those successfully treated patients could achieve full preinjury activity levels. The prognosis with nonoperative treatment is generally poor in high-activity patients such as ballet dancers.[20]

PATIENT HISTORY AND PHYSICAL FINDINGS

- The routine history should include sex, age, occupation, sports activities, and mechanism of the injury.
- Patients should be asked for the description of pain, its location, and any aggravating positions or activities. Pain from the impingement usually is directly posterior or posterolateral to the ankle joint. Pain in the posteromedial aspect may be associated with tenosynovitis of the FHL tendon, which is usually described as pain along the tendon longitudinally. Aggravation of the symptoms with the ankle in full plantarflexion is essential to the diagnosis.
- Examination must be performed to rule out other pathologies causing posterior ankle and hindfoot pain, such as Achilles tendinopathy, Haglund syndrome, "pump bump" syndrome, tibialis posterior tendinitis, and peroneal tendon injuries. Diligent palpation of the described structures for pain is recommended.
- The physical examination should include:
  - Examination for retromalleolar swelling. Mild swelling occurs in posterior ankle impingement syndrome. Significant swelling should raise the suspicion of peroneal or tibialis posterior tenosynovitis.
  - Passive ankle plantarflexion. In a positive test, sharp pain or crepitus is produced at full plantarflexion.
  - In FHL tenosynovitis, pain is produced with active/passive motion of the hallux while a thumb palpates the tendon for tenderness and crepitus. The presence of FHL tenosynovitis should be documented, and it should be treated accordingly.
  - Tenderness from FHL tenosynovitis is produced with active/passive motion of the hallux while a thumb palpates the tendon for tenderness and crepitus. The presence of FHL tenosynovitis should be documented, and it should be treated accordingly.
  - Tenderness of other posterior ankle structures. Individual palpation of the peroneal tendons, tibialis posterior tendon, Achilles tendon, and posterior aspect of the calcaneal tuberosity is essential to exclude other pathologies. Palpation of the os trigonum itself is difficult due to its depth. Other diagnoses should be considered if there is no pain with passive ankle plantarflexion and the positive test for other possible lesions in spite of the presence of the os trigonum on radiographs.

IMAGING AND OTHER DIAGNOSTIC STUDIES

- A lateral radiograph of the ankle usually demonstrates the osseous lesions sufficiently (**FIG 4**). Lateral radiographs can be taken in full ankle plantarflexion and slight external rotation of the limb to visualize impingement from the os trigonum.[9]
- Bone scanning has been reported to identify the symptomatic os trigonum. It is not routinely obtained, however, and does not replace accurate history taking and physical examination (**FIG 5**). False-positive results in patients with high activity levels make this study less useful.[29]
- CT scan can help clarify osseous or osteochondral lesions, especially when the posteromedial facet fracture is suspected.[7]
- MRI is the most useful imaging examination for posterior ankle impingement syndrome (**FIG 6**). Anatomic variants and a range of osseous and soft tissue abnormalities have been found to be associated with this condition. Posterior tibiotalar synovitis and marrow edema within one or more of the tarsal bones were found in all cases. In contrast, os trigonum was found in only 30% of cases.[5,23,26]
- Diagnostic injection can be helpful when the signs and symptoms are inconclusive.[14,25] The postinjection symptoms have

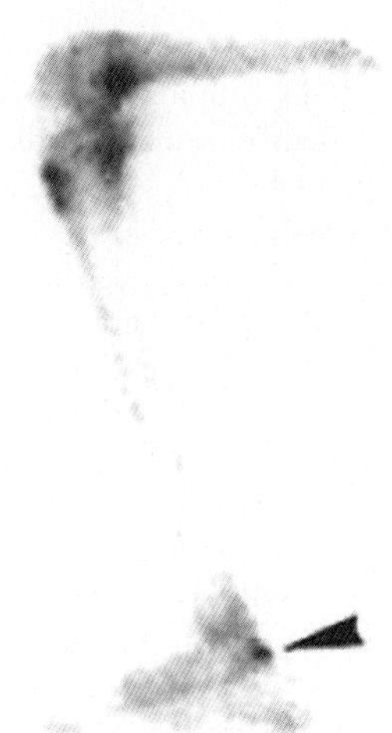

FIG 5 • Positive bone scan.

been shown to be parallel to results after surgical excision of the os trigonum. However, injection directly into the junction between the os trigonum and the talus is difficult and must be done under fluoroscopic guidance in experienced hands.

DIFFERENTIAL DIAGNOSIS

- Haglund syndrome
- Tendinitis (Achilles tendon, peroneal tendons, posterior tibial tendons)
- Loose bodies
- Ankle or subtalar arthritis

NONOPERATIVE MANAGEMENT

- Nonoperative treatment is always the first approach. However, it has shown less than optimal results in the published literature, with, at best, a 60% rate of improvement plus long-term modification of activities.[10]
- Avoidance of aggravating activities such as forced plantarflexion is the most important factor, because it will avoid impingement and aggravation of the inflammatory response. This measure may not be tolerable in athletes who routinely require this position, such as ballet dancers and soccer players.
- Supportive treatments include rest, ice, anti-inflammatory medications, and immobilization in a short-leg walking cast.
- One or two cortisone injections under fluoroscopic guidance have shown more than 80% response rate at 2 years.[25] Its use was not routinely recommended due to the risk of FHL tendon rupture and potential disabilities especially in ballet dancers.
- Physical therapy can be instituted as symptoms improve. It consists of phonophoresis, isometric exercises, heel cord stretching, and selected isometric strengthening.

SURGICAL MANAGEMENT

- Indications
  - Failure of nonoperative treatment after at least 3 months
  - Inability to to return to required activities after nonoperative treatment

Preoperative Planning

- All imaging studies are reviewed. MRI is helpful in the evaluation of associated lesions.
- All the pathologies should be carefully detected. Surgical steps with informed consent can be added accordingly, such as loose body removal, treatment for osteochondritis dissecans lesions, or an open FHL repair.
- When surgery is indicated, the treatment for an os trigonum, an acute or chronic fracture of the trigonal process, or an intact large trigonal process is virtually the same. Further studies, eg, CT scan, to distinguish them may not be necessary.
- If arthroscopic or open surgery is planned, the posterior tibial pulse must be palpable in the soft spot posterior to the medial malleolus, because an absence or a minor artery may be associated with a dominant peroneal artery. This artery traverses across the posterior ankle and is at high risk during arthroscopy.

Positioning

- The patient is placed in the prone position with standard padding (**FIGS 7 AND 8**).
- The patient's ankles are at the level just distal to the end of the bed to leave enough room for possible anterior or lateral arthroscopic portals.
- The surgeon's body can be used to dorsiflex the ankle by leaning forward.

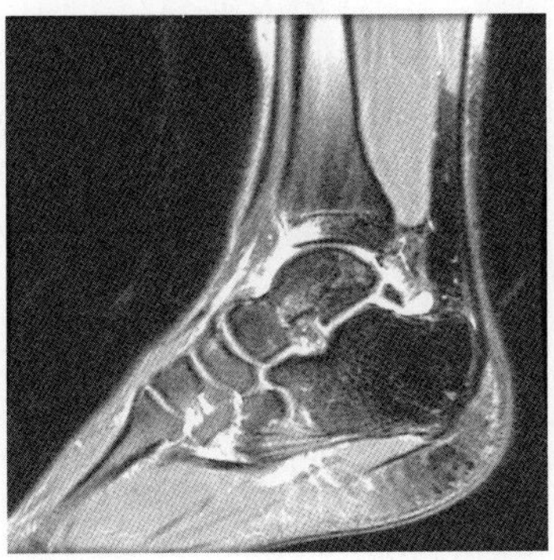

FIG 6 • MRI examination for posterior ankle impingement syndrome.

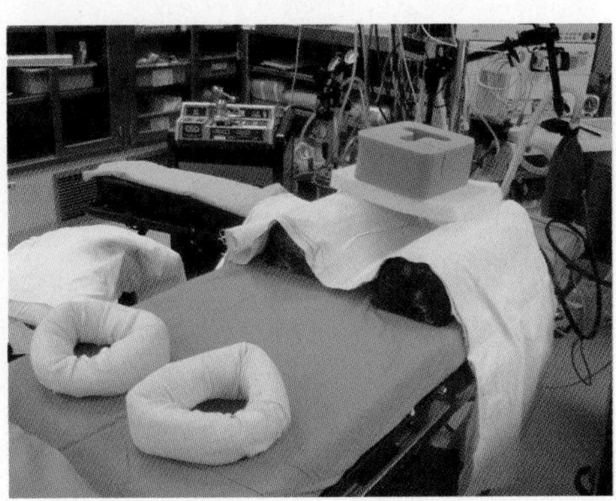

FIG 7 • Prone positioning.

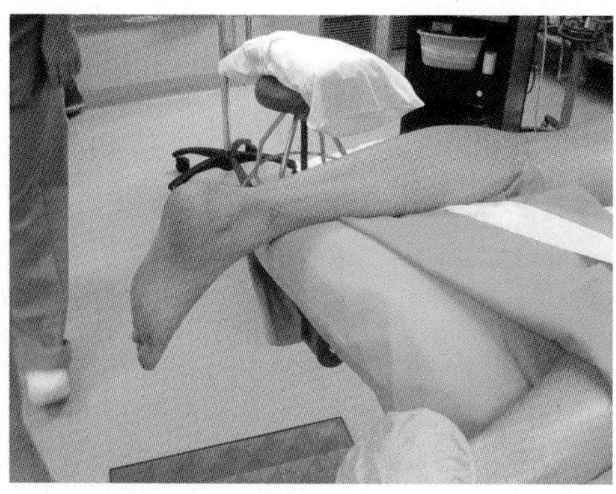

FIG 8 • Ensure adequate padding of all surfaces.

Approach

- The posterior aspect of the ankle and subtalar joints can be accessed open or arthroscopically.
- Open approaches can be posteromedial or posterolateral, on either side of the Achilles tendon.
  - The posteromedial approach is recommended by the author. When the bony impingement is accompanied by pathologies in the neurovascular bundles or lesions in the FHL tendon that may require a repair, a posteromedial approach is advantageous.
  - The posterolateral approach also may be used for cases that require only excision of the os trigonum and trigonal process or release of the FHL tendon.
- The arthroscopic approach has advantages over open surgeries in terms of minimizing surgical injury, postoperative pain, and early return to activities.
  - We prefer the prone over the supine or lateral decubitus position because it provides a more direct approach, minimizing the risk of instrument skiving off toward the neurovascular bundles.
  - Apart from the magnification advantage, we have found that this method also aids in visualization of intra-articular pathologies.[27]
  - This technique requires familiarity with the hindfoot anatomy and arthroscopic skills.

TECHNIQUES

ESTABLISHMENT OF PORTALS

- The anatomic landmarks of the posterior ankle are drawn, including the Achilles tendon, the medial and lateral malleoli, and the superior aspect of the calcaneal tuberosity.
- The posterolateral and the posteromedial portals are located 1.5 cm proximal to the superior aspect of the calcaneal tuberosity on either side of the Achilles tendon (**TECH FIGS 1 AND 2**).
- Ankle joint injection can be performed through the posterolateral portal, but it is not necessary, because the joint will be inspected easily after the os trigonum or the trigonal process has been removed.
- The posterolateral portal is established first with a vertical skin incision, followed by blunt dissection with a straight hemostat. The tip of the hemostat should be kept just next to the Achilles tendon laterally to minimize injury to the sural nerve.
- The dissection proceeds through a fat layer directly anteriorly.
- The os trigonum usually is palpable, and a blunt trocar is inserted toward its superior aspect.
- A 4-mm arthroscope is inserted through the cannula.
- Next, the posteromedial portal is established at the same level just medial to the Achilles tendon.
- A straight hemostat is used to dissect into the same soft tissue tunnel as the arthroscope. The hemostat is advanced while it is kept in contact with the arthroscopic cannula until the tip is seen by the arthroscope.
- The soft tissue is gently dilated. A full-radius 3.5-mm shaver is inserted into the posteromedial portal until the tip is seen (**TECH FIGS 3 AND 4**).

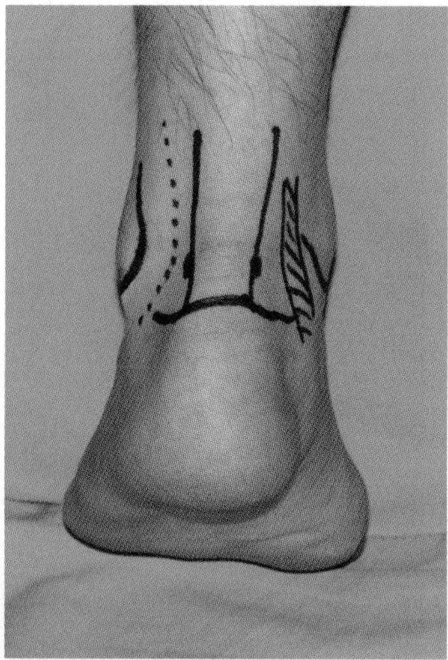

TECH FIG 1 • Placement of posteromedial and posterolateral portals with the patient in the prone position.

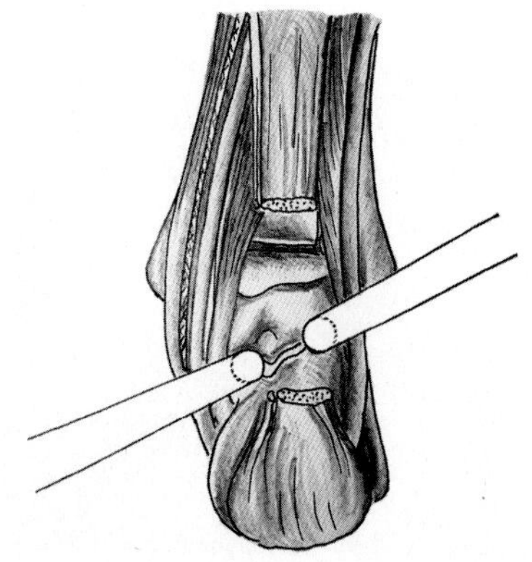

TECH FIG 2 • Topographical landmarks of the pertinent structures.

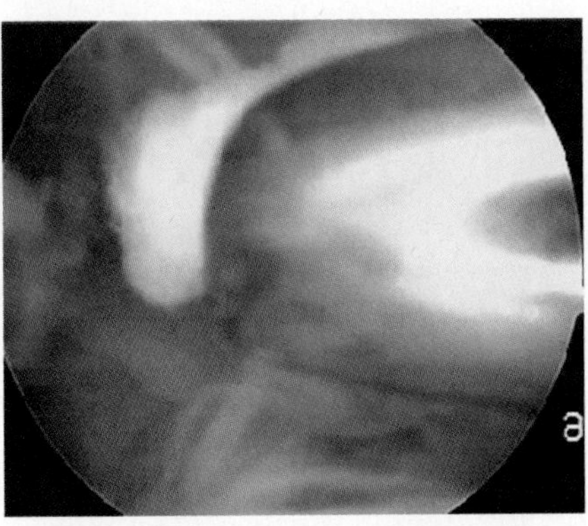

TECH FIG 3 • The hemostat is visualized when creating the second portal.

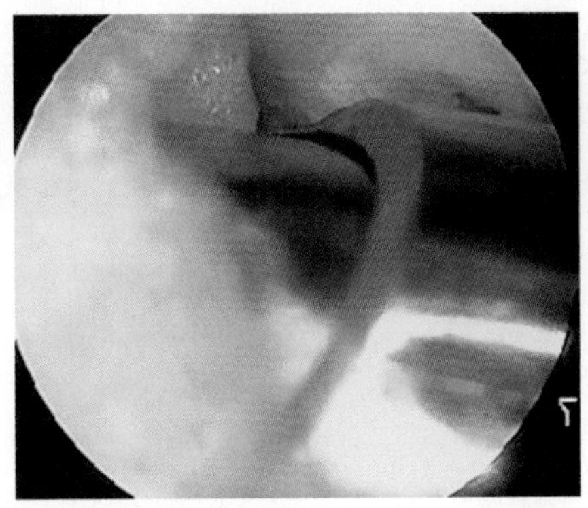

TECH FIG 4 • The 3.5 mm shaver is visualized through the second portal.

DÉBRIDEMENT OF THE SOFT TISSUE

- The initial débridement of the fatty tissue is performed first to make room for the arthroscopic maneuvers. This step will improve visualization tremendously.
- The shaver is kept deep just above or below the os trigonum, with its cutting surface turned laterally.
- The shaver is gradually moved medially until the FHL tendon is seen. The FHL tendon indicates the location of the neurovascular bundles, which lie medial and superficial to it.
- The os trigonum is débrided off all the attached soft tissue circumferentially (**TECH FIG 5**).
- Medially, the retinaculum of the FHL is released off the os trigonum with a shaver or arthroscopic scissors (**TECH FIG 6**).
- Tenosynovitic lesions of the FHL, if seen, may require a release and débridement further distally. Great care is taken to release the fibrous sheath from only the posterior attachment on the calcaneal wall. A partial tear of the FHL can be débrided, but a tear greater than 50% may require an open repair.
- The posterior talofibular ligament attached on the lateral aspect of the os trigonum is released.

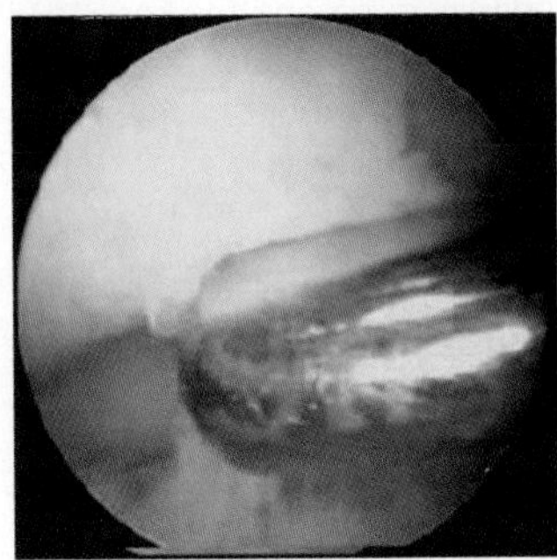

TECH FIG 5 • The os trigonum is débrided of soft tissue attachments with a shaver circumferentially.

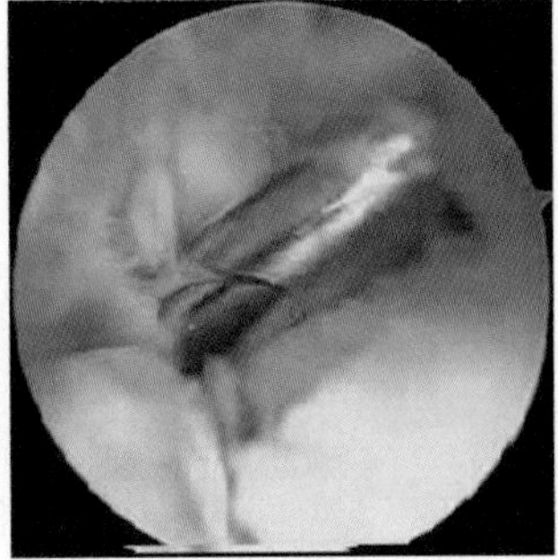

TECH FIG 6 • The FHL is visualized and released from its soft tissue attachments to the os trigonum.

RESECTION OF THE OS TRIGONUM AND TRIGONAL PROCESS

- The synchondrosis is palpated by a Freer elevator coming from the superior aspect.
- Next, the tip of the instrument is pushed into the synchondrosis.
- Cracking of the synchondrosis is performed by levering maneuvers from either the superior or inferior surface (**TECH FIG 7**).

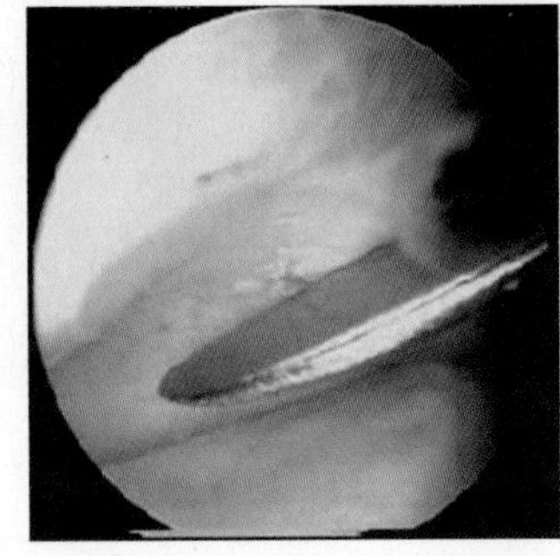

TECH FIG 7 • Lever the os trigonum loose from its talar attachments with a Freer elevator.

- The os trigonum is removed as a whole using a grasper (TECH FIG 8). In the presence of an intact enlarged trigonal process it is removed entirely with a burr.
- The posterior aspect of the talus is evaluated, and any sharp bony edges are rounded off (TECH FIG 9).
- The most posterior aspect of the articular cartilage of the posterior talar facet of the subtalar joint is always removed together with the os trigonum.

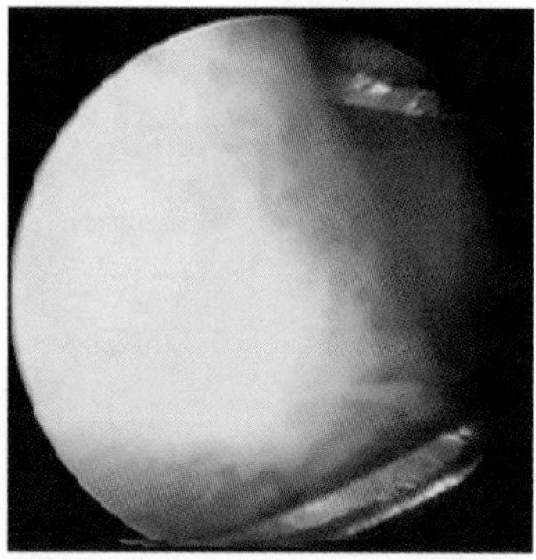

TECH FIG 8 • The os trigonum is removed as a whole using a grasper.

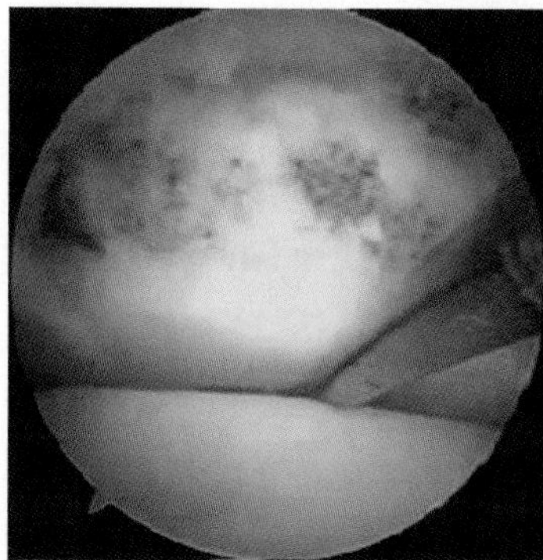

TECH FIG 9 • The posterior aspect of the talus is evaluated and rounded off, particularly around the FHL tendon.

EVALUATION OF ASSOCIATED LESIONS

- The posterior aspect of the ankle joint is evaluated. Synovitis or a thickened intermalleolar ligament is débrided. Stay lateral to the FHL tendon. Loose bodies are removed if present. Intra-articular views of the ankle joint are best achieved with a 2.7-mm arthroscope.
- The subtalar joint is evaluated in the same manner (TECH FIG 10). The dynamic view of the hindfoot is inspected when the ankle is manipulated into full plantarflexion.
- There should be no impingement at the completion of the procedure.
- If arthroscopic evaluation or treatment of the anterior ankle joint is required, it can be performed in two ways.
  - The first way is to reposition the patient into the supine position and redrape the limb.
  - The second way is to bend the knee to 90 degree and perform the anterior ankle arthroscopy in the upside-down manner. This requires experience and familiarity of the ankle anatomy.

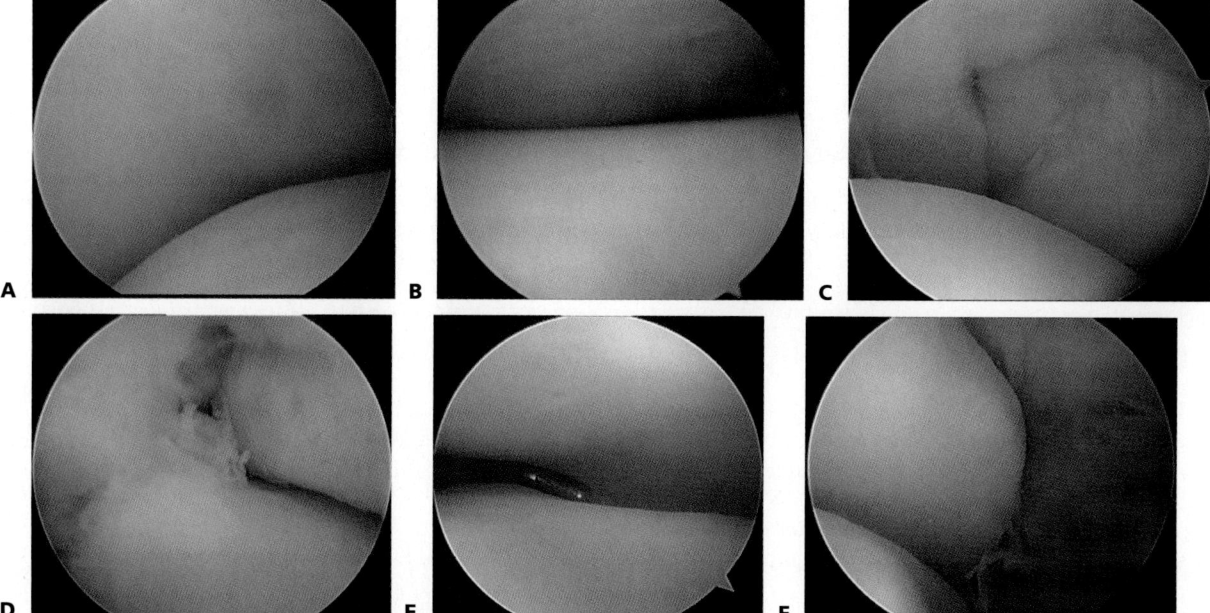

TECH FIG 10 • Multiple views of the ankle and subtalar joint.

PEARLS AND PITFALLS

Diagnosis	▪ Good history taking and physical examination are paramount. ▪ MRI and diagnostic injection can help in questionable cases.
Preoperative planning	▪ Open surgery is preferred when the posterior tibial pulse is not palpable behind the ankle joint. This approach is limited in its access to anterior ankle lesions and may require redraping. However, simple ankle procedures can be performed when the knee is flexed to 90 degrees and the foot held by an assistant. ▪ Patients should be informed of the possibility of conversion to open surgery, especially when a complete rupture of the FHL tendon is anticipated.
Portal placement	▪ The ankle is placed firmly on the bed in true AP or slight external rotated alignment. The incision is made through the skin only. Blunt dissection is used to dissect through the soft tissue planes.
Débridement of soft tissue	▪ The shaver is kept deep on the joint capsule and lateral to the FHL.
Resection of the os trigonum and trigonal process	▪ Palpation with a Freer elevator to identify the synchondrosis. ▪ "Death roll maneuver" is performed before removal of the bony fragment. Adequate portal size is needed.

POSTOPERATIVE CARE

- Portal incisions routinely are left unsutured.
- A compressive soft dressing is applied. The patient is informed about the possibility of some drainage in the first couple of postoperative days. The dressing can be changed if necessary.
- Leg elevation is encouraged.
- No immobilization is required.
- Patients can bear weight as tolerated in a postoperative shoe.
- When acute pain subsides, usually 2 to 3 days postoperatively, patients can begin early range-of-motion and strengthening exercise.
- Full activities are allowed gradually as tolerated.

OUTCOMES

- Nonoperative treatment has not shown promising results, especially in high-demand athletes, but a success rate of more than 80% could be achieved when cortisone injections are routinely given under fluoroscopic guidance.[10,25]
- When nonoperative treatment has failed, excellent outcomes have been reported with either open or arthroscopic resection of the os trigonum.[1,13,18,20,22,32,33]
- Arthroscopic techniques can help minimize morbidities associated with open dissection, such as a painful scar, severe postoperative pain, and wound complications. It requires arthroscopic skills and familiarity with hindfoot anatomy.[31,35]

COMPLICATIONS

- Neurovascular injuries are possible with either arthroscopic or open approaches. Neurapraxia of the tibial, peroneal, and sural nerves has been reported; most patients recovered spontaneously. Permanent sensory deficit and neuroma formation have occurred when the nerves were transected, especially the sural nerve when the open posterolateral approach is used.[1]
- Symptoms can persist after operative treatment. Correct diagnosis and adequate treatment of all associated pathologies are the keys.

REFERENCES

1. Abramowitz Y, Wollstein R, Barzilav Y, et al. Outcome of resection of a symptomatic os trigonum. J Bone Joint Surg Am 2003;85A:1051–1057.
2. Adachi B. Das arteriensystem der Japaner. Kyoto: Maruzen, 1928:215–291.
3. Bizarro A. On sesamoid and supernumerary bones of the limbs. J Anat 1921;55:256–268.
4. Brodsky AE, Khalil MA. Talar compression syndrome. Am J Sports Med 1986;14:472–476.
5. Bureau NJ, Cardinal E, Hobden R, et al. Posterior ankle impingement syndrome: MR imaging findings in seven patients. Radiology 2000;215:497–503.
6. Dubreuil-Chambardel L. Variations des arteres du pelvis et du membre inferieur. Paris: Masson et Cie, 1925:191–271.
7. Giuffrida AY, Lin SS, Abidi N, et al. Pseudo os trigonum sign: Missed posteromedial talar facet fracture. Foot Ankle Int 2003;24:642–649.
8. Grogan DP, Walling AK, Ogden JA. Anatomy of the os trigonum. J Pediatr Orthop 1990;10:618–622.
9. Hamilton WG. Stenosing tenosynovitis of the flexor hallucis longus tendon and posterior impingement upon the os trigonum in ballet dancers. Foot Ankle 1982;3:74–80.
10. Hedrick MR, McBryde AM. Posterior ankle impingement. Foot Ankle Int 1994;15:2–8.
11. Howse AJ. Posterior block of the ankle joint in dancers. Foot Ankle 1982;3:81–84.
12. Iovane A, Midiri M, Finazzo M, et al. Os trigonum tarsi syndrome. Role of magnetic resonance. Radiol Med (Torino) 2000;99:36–40.
13. Jerosch J, Fadel M. Endoscopic resection of a symptomatic os trigonum. Knee Surg Sports Traumatol Arthrosc 2006;14:1188–1193.
14. Jones DM, Saltzman CL, El-Khoury G. The diagnosis of the os trigonum syndrome with a fluoroscopically controlled injection of local anesthetic. Iowa Orthop J 1999;19:122–126.
15. Karasick D, Schweitzer ME. The os trigonum syndrome: Imaging features. AJR Am J Roentgenol 1996;166:125–129.
16. Lawson JP. International Skeletal Society Lecture in honor of Howard D. Dorfman. Clinically significant radiologic anatomic variants of the skeleton. AJR Am J Roentgenol 1994;163:249–255.
17. Lohrer H. Flexor hallucis longus tendon rupture as an impingement lesion induced by os trigonum instability. Sportverletz Sportschaden 2006;20:31–35.
18. Lombardi CM, Silhanek AD, Connolly FG. Modified arthroscopic excision of the symptomatic os trigonum and release of the flexor hallucis longus tendon: Operative technique and case study. J Foot Ankle Surg 1999;38:347–351.
19. Maquirriain J. Posterior ankle impingement syndrome. J Am Acad Orthop Surg 2005;13:365–371.
20. Marotta JJ, Micheli LJ. Os trigonum impingement in dancers. Am J Sports Med 1992;20:533–536.
21. Martin BF. Posterior triangle pain: The os trigonum. J Foot Surg 1989;28:312–318.
22. Marumoto JM, Ferkel RD. Arthroscopic excision of the os trigonum: A new technique with preliminary clinical results. Foot Ankle Int 1997;18:777–784.

23. Masciocchi C, Catalucci A, Barile A. Ankle impingement syndromes. Eur J Radiol 1998;27 Suppl 1:S70–S73.
24. McDougall A. The os trigonum. J Bone Joint Surg Br 1955;37B: 257–265.
25. Mouhsine E, Crevoisier X, Layvraz PF, et al. Post-traumatic overload or acute syndrome of the os trigonum: A possible cause of posterior ankle impingement. Knee Surg Sports Traumatol Arthrosc 2004;12: 250–253.
26. Peace KA, Hillier JC, Hulme JC, et al. MRI features of posterior ankle impingement syndrome in ballet dancers: A review of 25 cases. Clin Radiol 2004;59:1025–1033.
27. Phisitkul P, Tochigi Y, Saltzman CL, et al. Arthroscopic visualization of the posterior subtalar joint in the prone position: a cadaver study. Arthroscopy 2006;22:511–515.
28. Sarrafian S. Anatomy of the Foot and Ankle: Descriptive Topographic Functional, 2nd ed. Philadelphia: JB Lippincott, 1993.
29. Sopov V, Liberson A, Groshar D. Bone scintigraphic findings of os trigonum: A prospective study of 100 soldiers on active duty. Foot Ankle Int 2000;21:822–824.
30. Uzel M, Cetinus E, Bilgic E, et al. Bilateral os trigonum syndrome associated with bilateral tenosynovitis of the flexor hallucis longus muscle. Foot Ankle Int 2005;26:894–898.
31. van Dijk CN, de Leeuw PA, Scholten PE. Hindfoot endoscopy for posterior ankle impingement. Surgical technique. J Bone Joint Surg Am 2009;91A Suppl 2:287–298.
32. van Dijk CN, Scholten PE, Krips R. A 2-portal endoscopic approach for diagnosis and treatment of posterior ankle pathology. Arthroscopy 2000;16:871–876.
33. Veazey BL, Heckman JD, Galindo MJ, et al. Excision of ununited fractures of the posterior process of the talus: A treatment for chronic posterior ankle pain. Foot Ankle 1992;13:453–457.
34. Wenig JA. Os trigonum syndrome. J Am Podiatr Med Assoc 1990;80: 278–282.
35. Willits K, Sonneveld H, Amendola A, et al. Outcome of posterior ankle arthroscopy for hindfoot impingement. Arthroscopy 2008;24: 196–202. Epub 2007 Nov 8.
36. Zeichen J, Schratt E, Bosch U, et al. Os trigonum syndrome. Unfallchirurg 1999;102:320–323.

Chapter 92 Subtalar Arthroscopy

Carol Frey

DEFINITION

- The subtalar joint is a complex and functionally important joint of the lower extremity. It plays a major role in inversion and eversion of the foot.
- Subtalar arthroscopy can be applied as a diagnostic and therapeutic instrument.

ANATOMY

- For arthroscopic purposes, the subtalar joint is divided into anterior (talocalcaneonavicular) and posterior (talocalcaneal) articulations (**FIG 1**).
- The anterior and posterior articulations are separated by the tarsal canal, which has a large lateral opening called the sinus tarsi.
- Within the tarsal canal and sinus tarsi are found the interosseous talocalcaneal ligament, the medial and intermediate roots of the inferior extensor retinaculum, the cervical ligament, fatty tissue, and blood vessels.[5,6,8,12]
  - The lateral ligamentous support of the subtalar joint consists of the lateral talocalcaneal ligament, the posterior talocalcaneal ligament, the lateral root of the inferior extensor retinaculum, and the calcaneofibular ligament (**FIG 2**).
- The anterior subtalar joint is generally thought to be inaccessible to arthroscopic visualization because of the thick interosseous ligament that fills the tarsal canal.[1–4,18] Because of this, the region normally has no connection with the posterior joint complex.
- The posterior subtalar joint has a synovial lining. This joint has a posterior capsular pouch with small lateral, medial, and anterior recesses.

PATHOGENESIS

- One of the most common indications for subtalar arthroscopy is chronic pain in the sinus tarsi, historically referred to as "sinus tarsi syndrome."[2]
- Sinus tarsi syndrome has been described as persistent pain in the tarsal sinus secondary to trauma (80% of the cases reported).[2]
- There are no specific objective findings in this condition.
- The exact etiology is not clearly defined, but scarring and degenerative changes to the soft tissue structure of the sinus tarsi are thought to be the most common cause of pain in this region.
- Therefore, sinus tarsi syndrome is an inaccurate term that should be replaced with a specific diagnosis, as it can include many other pathologies, such as interosseous ligament tears, arthrofibrosis, and joint degeneration.

PATIENT HISTORY AND PHYSICAL FINDINGS

- Patients with subtalar joint pathology often present with lateral ankle pain that is aggravated by standing and walking activities, particularly on uneven terrain.
  - Walking on uneven terrain can result in a feeling of instability.

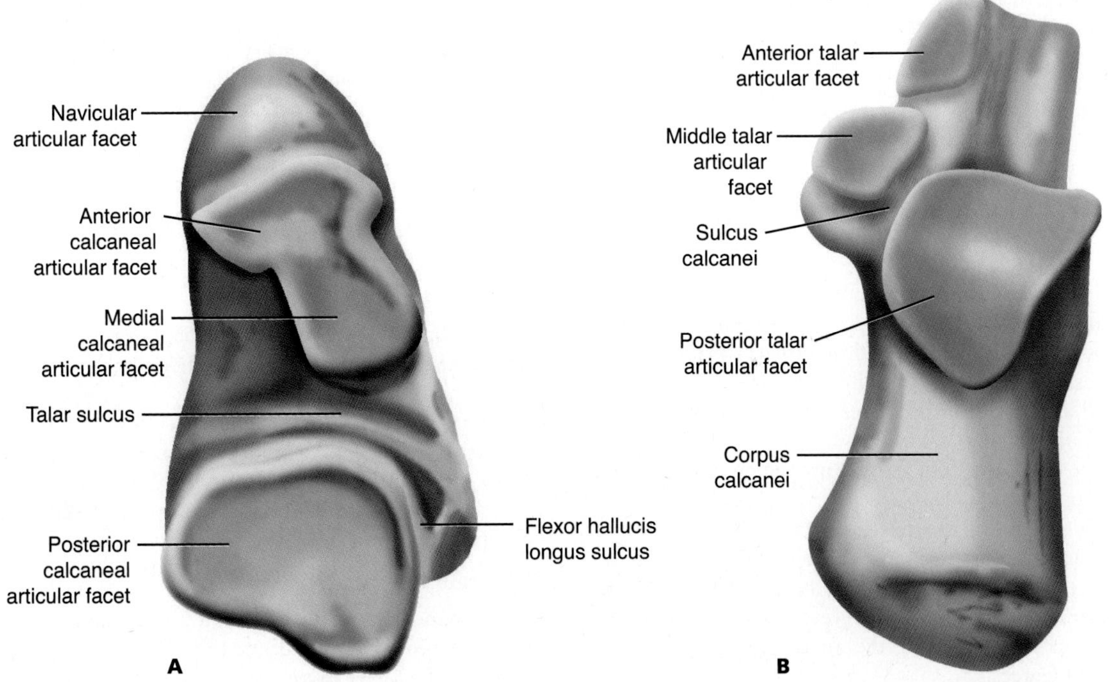

FIG 1 • The subtalar joint is divided into the anterior (talocalcaneonavicular) and posterior joint (talocalcaneal).

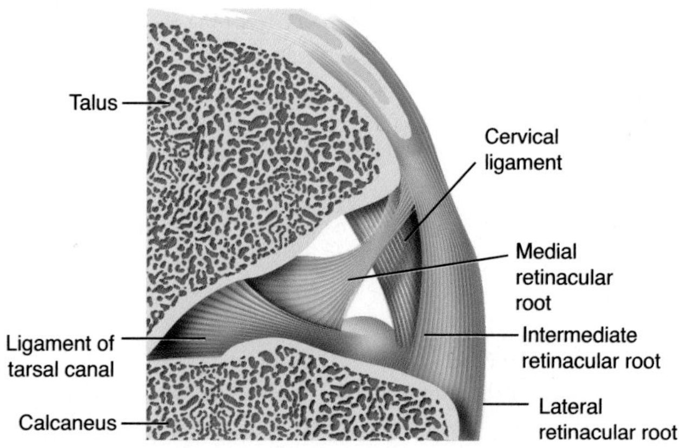

FIG 2 • The ligaments of the subtalar joint.

- Motion of the subtalar joint is not simple inversion and eversion.[8,12] However, motion is best tested by holding the left heel in the right hand and vice versa, then using the opposite hand to hold the forefoot and move the foot from inversion to eversion. This motion should be smooth and painless.
- Inversion and eversion are coming primarily from the talocalcaneal (subtalar) joint. Exact measurements are difficult using standard techniques. Restricted motion may be seen with acute ankle sprain, arthritis, posterior tibial tendon dysfunction, tarsal coalition, fracture, chondral injury, adhesions, synovitis, and inflammatory conditions.
- There may be swelling or stiffness in the joint.
- Subtalar stiffness and pain indicate pathology in and around the subtalar joint but are not specific to one diagnosis.
- Clinical examination reveals pain on the lateral aspect of the hindfoot aggravated by firm pressure over the lateral opening of the sinus tarsi.
- Relief of symptoms with injection of local anesthetic directly into the sinus tarsi confirms the diagnosis of pain or dysfunction in the sinus tarsi.
- Pathology of the interosseous ligaments of the subtalar joint usually is associated with focal pain over the lateral entrance to the sinus tarsi. Patients often have slight restriction and discomfort with passive subtalar motion.

IMAGING AND OTHER DIAGNOSTIC STUDIES

- Differential injections may be required to confirm pathology in the subtalar joint.
- Anteroposterior (AP), lateral, and modified AP views of the foot are necessary to identify the subtalar joint.
- The lateral and posterior processes are better seen on hindfoot oblique views.
- The oblique 45-degree foot films show the anterior portion of the subtalar joint.
- Borden's view shows the posterior facet of the subtalar joint. This view is obtained by rotating the foot medially 45 degrees with dorsiflexion. The x-ray beam is pointed at the lateral malleolus and angled 10 degrees cephalad. Different views are obained by changing the angle of the x-ray beam from 10 to 40 degrees.
- Computed tomographic (CT) scans in the coronal plane are best for visualizing the talar body or posterior and lateral processes of the talus. CT can be used to show intra-articular pathology.
- CT scans in the tranverse or sagittal planes are best to visualize the talar neck and dome.
- Magnetic resonance imaging (MRI) may dectect chronic inflammation or fibrosis within the subtalar joint. Ligament injury, bone contusions, osteochondral lesions, chondral injury, impingement, synovitis, and fibrous or cartilaginous coalitions can be well demonstrated on MRI.
- The preoperative imaging studies predict subtalar cartilage damage less accurately than does arthroscopy.

DIFFERENTIAL DIAGNOSIS

- Chronic lateral ankle pain
- Chronic ankle instability
- Peroneal tendon pathology
- Posterior tibial tendon dysfunction
- Superficial peroneal nerve pathology
- Fracture of the anterior process of the calcaneus
- Fracture of the lateral process of the talus
- Fracture of the posterior proces of the talus
- Navicular fracture
- Calcaneal cuboid arthrosis/subluxation
- Calcaneus fracture
- Coalition

NONOPERATIVE MANAGEMENT

- Injection of anesthetic agent or corticosteroid
- Foot orthosis, including a UCBL
- Anti-inflammatory medication
- Ankle brace with a hindfoot lock
- Peroneal tendon strengthening

SURGICAL MANAGEMENT

- Indications for subtalar arthroscopy include chondromalacia, subtalar impingement lesions, osteophytes, lysis of adhesions with posttraumatic arthrofibrosis, synovectomy, and the removal of loose bodies.[1,2,4,7,11]
- Other therapeutic indications include instability, débridement and treatment of osteochondral lesions, retrograde drilling of cystic lesions, evaluation of coalition, removal of a symptomatic os trigonum, evaluation and excision of fractures of the anterior process of the calcaneus and lateral process of the talus, and subtalar fusion.[9,10,15,16]

Preoperative Planning

- Confirm the diagnosis with diagnositic testing, including differential injections to exclude ankle pathology.
- The absolute contraindications to subtalar arthroscopy must be ruled out. These include localized infection leading to a potential septic joint and advanced degenerative joint disease, particularly with deformity.
- Relative contraindications include severe edema, poor skin quality, and poor vascular status.

Positioning

- The patient is placed in the lateral decubitus position with the operative extremity draped free (**FIG 3**). Padding is placed between the lower extremities, as well as under the contralateral extremity to protect the peroneal nerve.
- A thigh tourniquet is recommended.

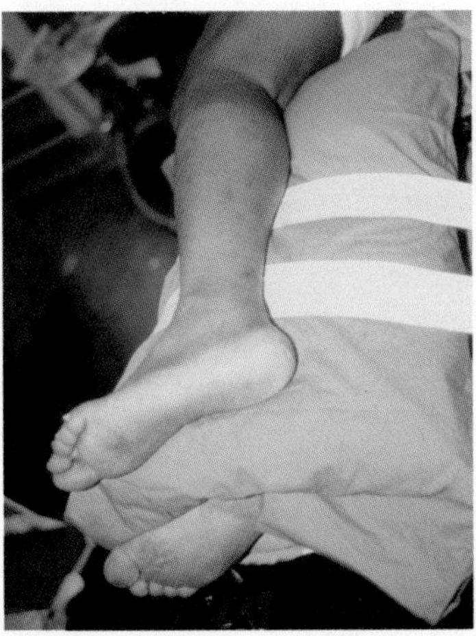

FIG 3 • The patient is placed into the lateral decubitus position with the operative limb draped free.

Approach

Lateral Approach

- Three standard portals are recommended for visualization and instrumentation of the subtalar joint (**FIG 4**). The anatomic landmarks for lateral portal placement are the lateral malleolus, the sinus tarsi, and the Achilles tendon.
- Careful dissection and portal placement help avoid the superficial peroneal nerve branches (anterior portal) and the sural nerve and peroneal tendons (posterior portal).
- The anterior portal is established approximately 1 cm distal to the fibular tip and 2 cm anterior to it (**FIG 5**).

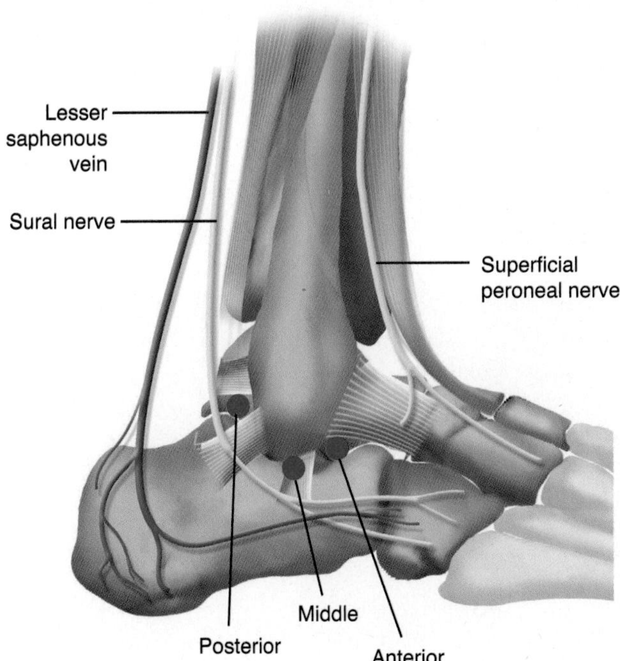

FIG 4 • Standard portals and their positions.

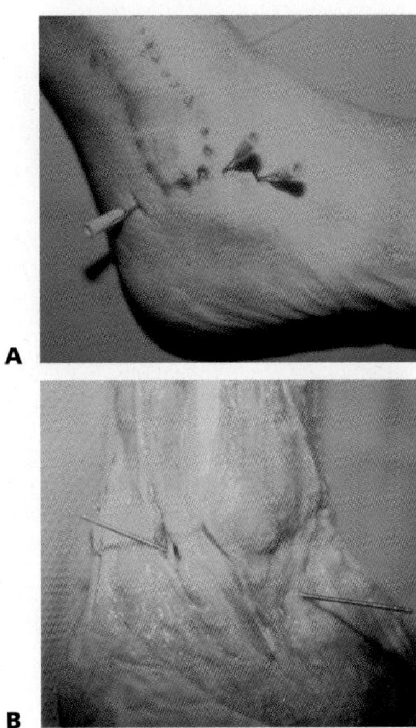

FIG 5 • **A.** Standard subtalar arthroscopic portals demonstrated on a cadaver. **B.** Anterior and posterior portals with the skin stripped away. Note the proximity of the sural nerve to the posterior portal.

- The middle portal is just anterior to the tip of the fibula, directly over the sinus tarsi.
- The posterior portal is at or approximately one finger width proximal to the fibular tip and 2 cm posterior to the lateral malleolus.
- The posterior portal is usually safe when placed behind the saphenous vein and sural nerve and anterior to the Achilles tendon. With placement of the posterior portal, care must be taken to avoid the sural nerve.

Posterior Approach [13,14,17]

- Posterior subtalar arthroscopy can be performed using a posterolateral and a posteromedial portal. This two-portal endoscopic approach to the hindfoot with the patient in the prone position has been credited with offering better access to the medial and anterolateral aspects of the posterior subtalar joint (**FIG 6**).
- The main difference between the two techniques is that the lateral approach for posterior subtalar arthroscopy is a true arthroscopy technique in which the arthroscope and the instruments are placed within the joint, whereas the two-portal posterior technique (using posterolateral and posteromedial portals) starts as an extra-articular approach.
- With the two-portal posterior technique, a working space is first created adjacent to the posterior subtalar joint by removing the fatty tissue overlying the joint capsule and the posterior part of the ankle joint.
- The joint capsule is then partially removed to enable inspection of the joint from the outside in, with the arthroscope positioned at the edge of the joint without actually entering the joint space.
- The maximum size of the intra-articular instruments depends on the available joint space.

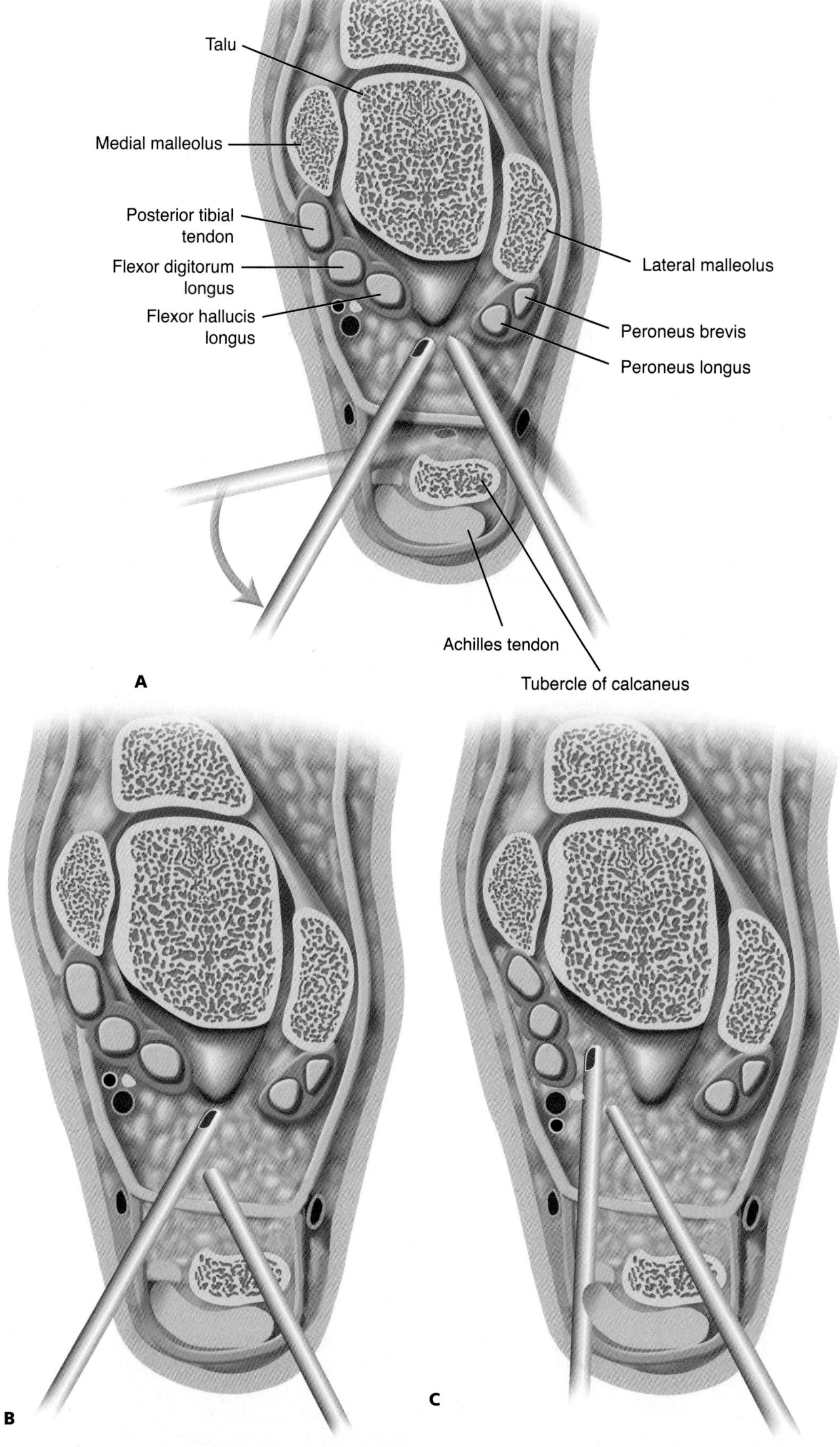

FIG 6 • Posterior endoscopic technique with the use of two portals.

PORTAL PLACEMENT

- Local, general, spinal, or epidural anesthesia can be used for this procedure.
- The anterior portal is identified first with an 18-gauge spinal needle, and the joint is inflated with a 20-mL syringe (TECH FIG 1).
- A small skin incision is made and the subcutaneous tissue is gently spread using a straight mosquito clamp.
- A cannula with a semi-blunt trocar is then placed, followed by a 2.7-mm 30-degree oblique arthroscope.
- The middle portal is placed under direct visualization using an 18-gauge spinal needle and outside-in technique.
- The posterior portal can be placed at this time using the same direct visualization technique. The trocar is placed in an upward and slightly anterior manner.

Inspection From the Anterior Portal

- Diagnostic subtalar arthroscopy examination begins with the arthroscope viewing from the anterior portal (TECH FIG 2A,B). The ligaments that insert on the floor of the sinus tarsi are visualized. It is easy to get disoriented, as the ligaments are closely packed and cross over one another in the sinus tarsi.
- More medially, the deep interosseous ligament (TECH FIG 2C) is observed to fill the tarsal canal.
- The arthroscope should now be slowly withdrawn and the arthroscopic lens rotated to view the anterior process of the calcaneus (TECH FIG 3A,B).
- The arthroscopic lens is then rotated in the opposite direction to view the anterior aspect of the posterior talocalcaneal articulation (TECH FIG 3C).

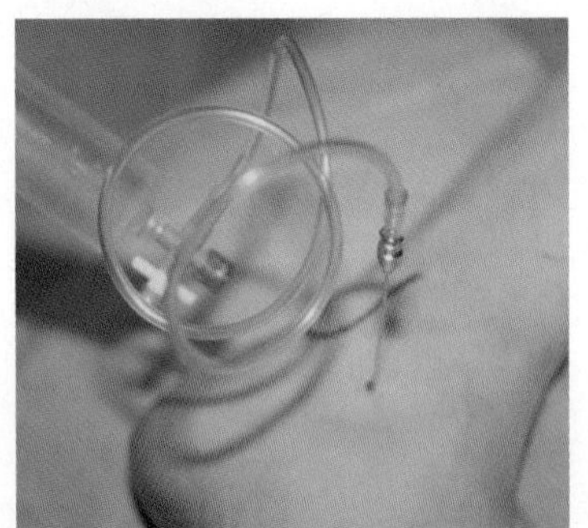
A

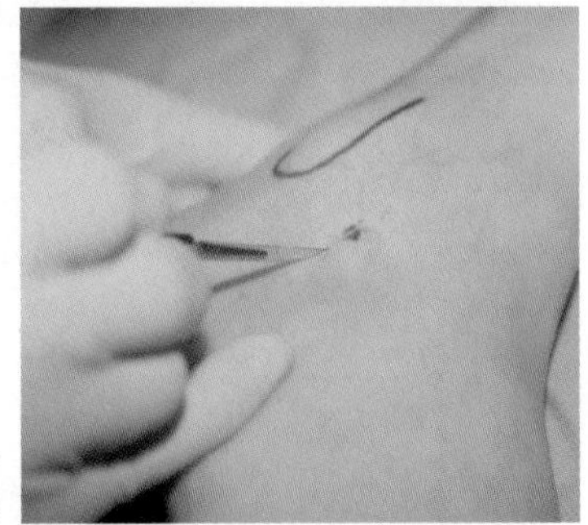
B

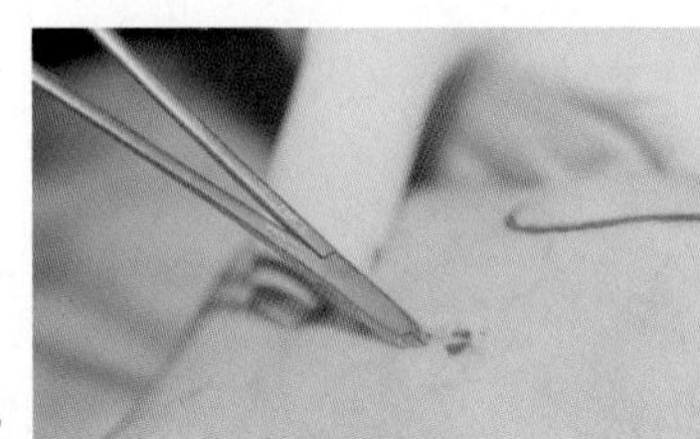
C

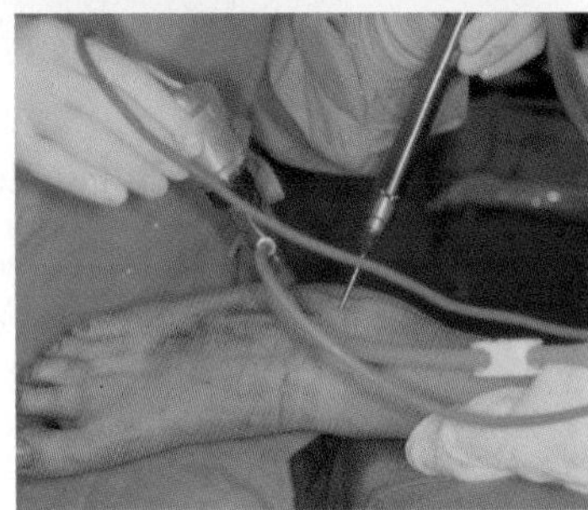
D

TECH FIG 1 • The subtalar joint is entered using an 18-gauge spinal needle. The joint is inflated (**A**) and an incision is made (**B**), followed by blunt dissection (**C**) and entry into the subtalar joint (**D**). The middle portal is made using direct visualization techniques.

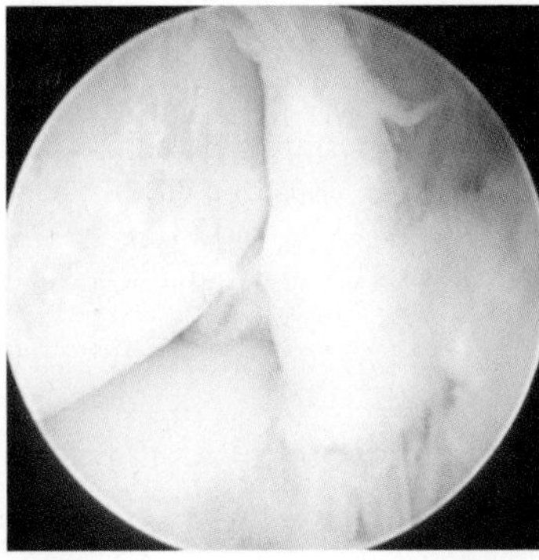
A

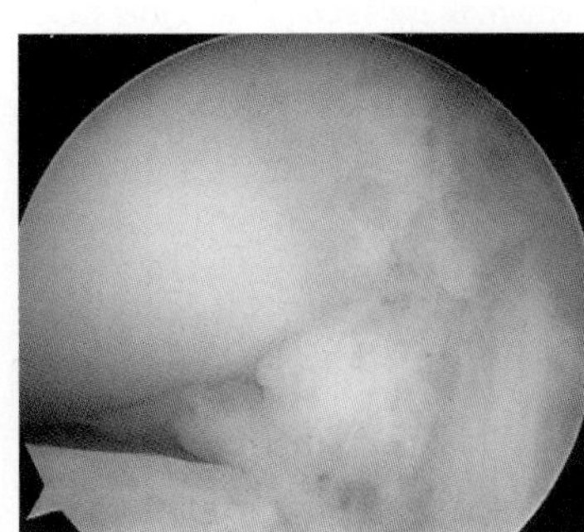
B

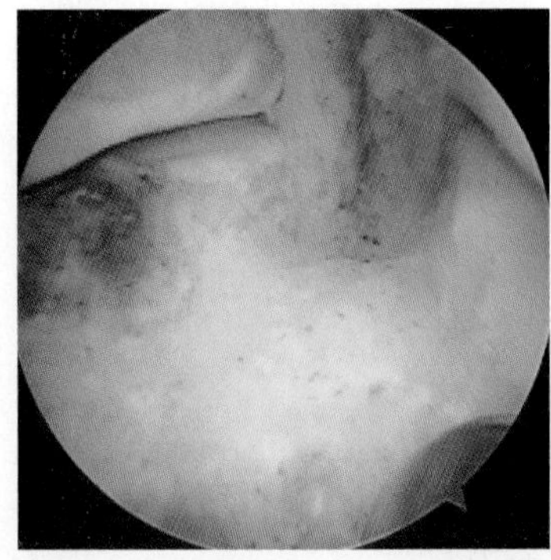
C

TECH FIG 2 • With the arthroscope in the anterior portal, the ligaments that insert on the floor of the sinus tarsi can be visualized. It is often difficult to tell one from the other, especially if they are injured. **A,B.** Examples of a torn interosseous ligament that is impinging into the anterior aspect of the posterior facet of the subtalar joint. This impingement lesion is referred to as the subtalar impingement lesion. **C.** The interosseous ligament of the tarsal canal fills the canal and can be seen with the scope in the anterior portal. The anterior (left) and the posterior (right) facets are well seen.

- Next, the anterolateral corner of the posterior joint is examined, and reflections of the lateral talocalcaneal ligament and the calcaneofibular ligament are observed (**TECH FIG 3D**). The lateral talocalcaneal ligament is noted anterior to the calcaneofibular ligament.
- The arthroscopic lens may then be rotated medially and the central articulation observed between the talus and the calcaneus (**TECH FIG 3E**). The posterolateral gutter may be seen from the anterior portal.
- It is often possible to advance the scope along the lateral and posterolateral gutter and visualize the posterior pouch and Stieda's process (or os trigonum; **TECH FIG 3F**).

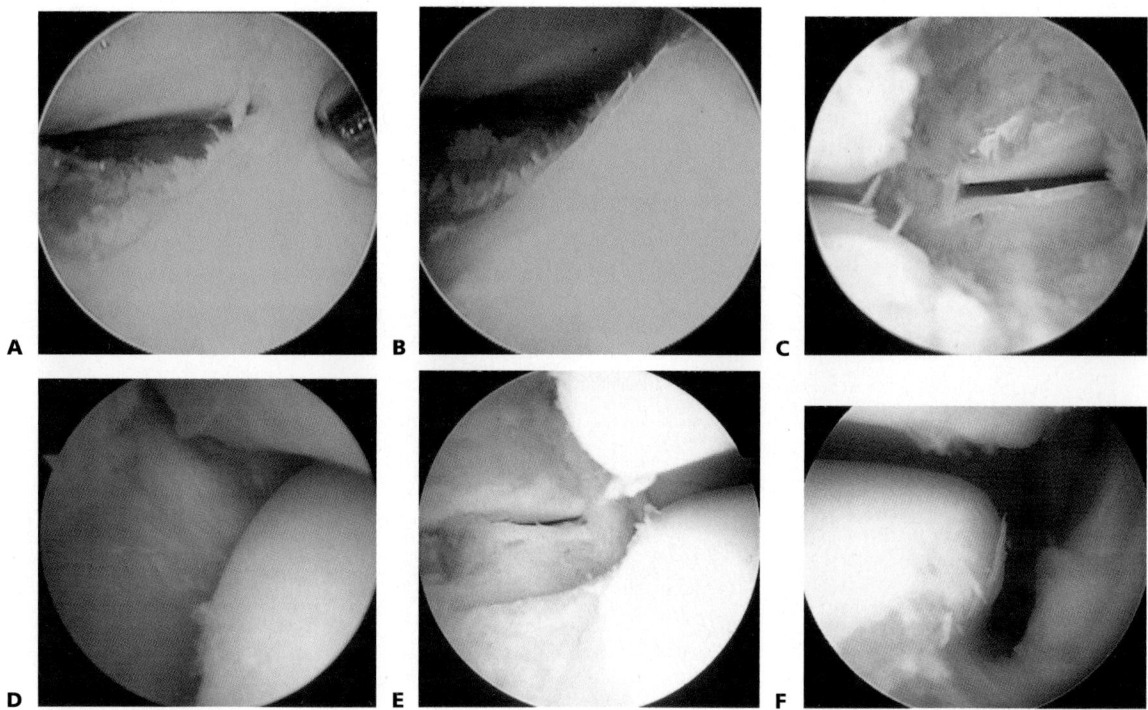

TECH FIG 3 • Views with the arthroscope in the anterior portal. **A.** Anterosuperior process of the calcaneus. This view is useful for inspection and débridement or resection of a fracture in this location. **B.** Closer view of the anterior process. **C.** Anterior aspect of the posterior facet (to the right). **D.** Lateral gutter and lateral talocalcaneal and calcaneofibular ligaments. **E.** Anterior and central aspects of the posterior talocalcaneal articulation (to the right). **F.** It is possible to advance the scope from the anterior portal and visualize the lateral aspect of the posterior capsule and Stieda's process or os trigonum.

INSPECTION FROM THE POSTERIOR PORTAL

- The arthroscope is then switched to the posterior portal. From this view, the interosseous ligament may be seen anteriorly in the joint. As the arthroscopic lens is rotated laterally, the lateral talocalcaneal ligament and calcaneofibular ligament reflections again may be seen.
- The central talocalcaneal joint may then be seen from this posterior view and the posterolateral gutter examined (**TECH FIG 4A**).
- The posterolateral recess, posterior gutter, and posterolateral corner of the talus are visualized (**TECH FIG 4B**). The posteromedial recess and posteromedial corner of the talocalcaneal joint can also be seen from the posterior portal.

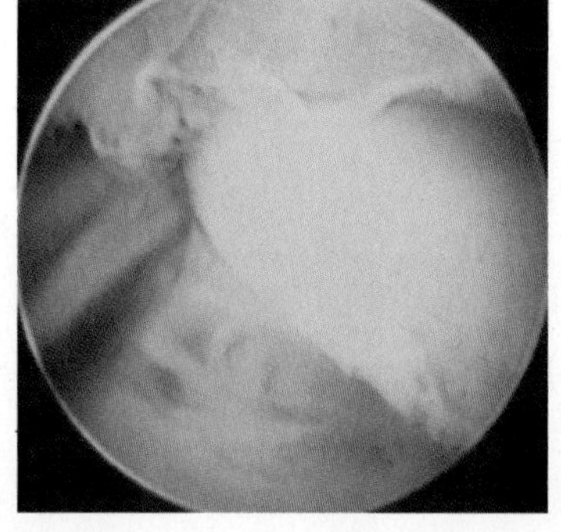

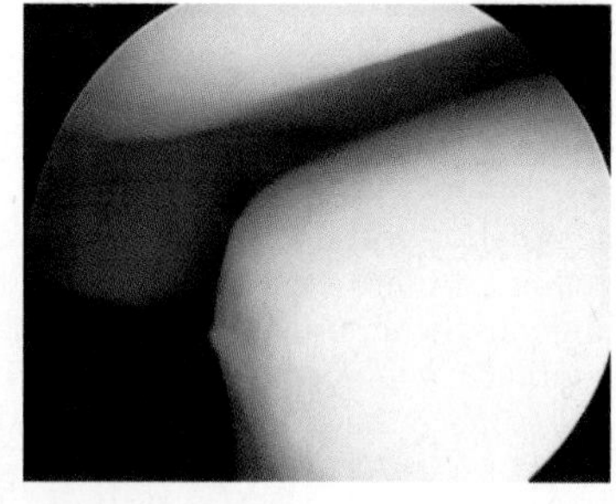

TECH FIG 4 • Views with the arthroscope in the posterior portal. **A.** Posterior and central aspects of the posterior talocalcaneal joint can be seen to the right. The posterior capsule is to the left. **B.** Lateral aspect of the posterior capsule and Stieda's process (*arrow*) or the os trigonum.

SINUS TARSI PATHOLOGY

- The best portal combination for the evaluation and débridement of pathology in the sinus tarsi is the arthroscope in the anterior portal and the instruments in the middle portal.
- One can débride torn interosseous ligaments, remove loose bodies, and perform lysis of adhesions. A radiofrequency wand is a useful tool to access the hard-to-get-to spots in the sinus tarsi and subtalar joint.

OS TRIGONUM PATHOLOGY

- The best portal combination for evaluation and removal of the os trigonum is the arthroscope in the anterior portal and the instrumentation in the posterior portal.
- The os trigonum or a symptomatic Stieda's process can be débrided with a burr or shaver and removed through an arthroscopic portal using a standard arthroscopic grabber (**TECH FIG 5**).
- Rarely, it is necessary to enlarge the portal for delivery of the os trigonum.

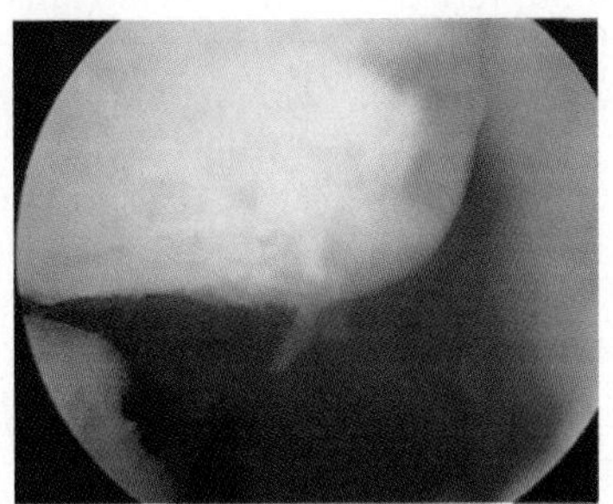

TECH FIG 5 • A fracture of Stieda's process or an injured os trigonum can be removed using standard arthroscopic grabbers. Rarely, the incision must be expanded to deliver the fragment.

ARTHROSCOPIC SUBTALAR ARTHRODESIS

- Both the anterior and posterior portals are used in an alternating fashion during the procedure for viewing and for instrumentation.
- It is important to obtain a fusion of the posterior facet. The anterior facet is generally not fused. A primary synovectomy and débridement are necessary for visualization.
- Débridement and complete removal of the articular surface of the posterior facet of the subtalar joint down to subchondral bone is the next phase of the procedure.
- Once the articular cartilage has been resected, approximately 1 to 2 mm of subchondral bone is removed to expose bleeding cancellous bone.
- Spot-weld holes measuring approximately 2 mm in depth are created on the surfaces of the calcaneus and talus to create vascular channels.
- The posteromedial corner is inspected to insure adequate débridement.
- The guidewire for a large cannulated screw (6.5 to 7 mm) can be visualized as it enters the posterior facet.
- The foot is then put in about 0 to 5 degrees of valgus, the guidewire is advanced, and the screw is placed.
- Screw position and length are confirmed with fluoroscopy.
- Postoperative care is similar to open techniques.
- In general, no autogenous bone graft or bone substitute is needed.

PEARLS AND PITFALLS

The subtalar joint can be difficult to distract, especially the posterior joint.	■ Use of a distraction device is not necessary or very useful for improving visualization of the subtalar joint. A high-flow system and an arthroscopic pump will improve visualization. ■ Rarely, invasive joint distraction, using talocalcaneal distraction with pins inserted from laterally, or tibiocalcaneal distraction can be used in a patient with a tight posterior subtalar joint. The disadvantage of using an invasive distractor is the potential damage to soft tissues (especially the lateral calcaneal branch of the sural nerve) and ligamentous structures and the risk of infection and fracturing the talar neck or body.
Visualization of the anterior joint and sinus tarsi can be difficult. It is easy to get disoriented, as the ligaments are closely packed and cross over one another in the sinus tarsi.	■ The structures in the sinus tarsi, the anterior process of the calcaneus, and occasionally the anterior joint can be visualized best by placing the arthroscope through the anterior portal and instrumentation through the middle portal. This portal combination is recommended for visualization and instrumentation of the sinus tarsi and anterior aspects of the posterior subtalar joint. If the ligaments that insert on the floor of the sinus tarsi are torn or damaged or need débridement, the anterior joint can be visualized and accessed with this portal combination. Furthermore, this portal combination allows excellent visualization and access to the anterior process of the calcaneus.

Visualization of the posterior joint and lateral capsule and access to Stieda's process (os trigonum)	■ The best portal combination for access to the posterior joint is placement of the arthroscope through the anterior portal and instrumentation through the posterior portal. This allows direct visualization and access of nearly the entire surface of the posterior facet, the posterior aspect of the ligaments in the sinus tarsi, the lateral capsule and its small recess, Stieda's process (os trigonum), and the posterior pouch of the posterior joint with its synovial lining.

POSTOPERATIVE CARE

- After completing the procedure, the portals are closed with sutures.
- A compression dressing is applied from the toes to the mid-calf. Ice and elevation are recommended until the inflammatory phase has passed.
- The patient is allowed to ambulate with the use of crutches, and weightbearing is permitted as tolerated.
- The sutures are removed approximately 10 days after the procedure.
- The patient should begin gentle active range-of-motion exercises of the foot and ankle immediately after surgery. Once the sutures are removed, if indicated, the patient is referred to a physical therapist for supervised rehabilitation.
- The patient should be able to return to full activities at 6 to 12 weeks postoperatively.

OUTCOMES

- Compared with open techniques, arthroscopy of the subtalar joint has advantages for the patient, including a faster postoperative recovery period, decreased postoperative pain, and fewer complications.
- Frey et al[2] demonstrated a success rate of 94% good and excellent results in the treatment of various types of subtalar pathology using arthroscopic techniques.
  - All of 14 preoperative diagnoses of sinus tarsi syndrome were changed at the time of arthrosocpy.
  - The most common finding in these cases was a tear of the interosseous ligaments.
- In a more recent study of 126 cases followed for more than 2 years, a significant improvement (61 to 84) was noted using both the AOFAS and Karslon scores. Williams and Ferkelz[19] reported on the 32-month (average) follow-up of 50 patients with hindfoot pain who underwent simultaneous ankle and subtalar arthroscopy.
  - Preoperative diagnoses included degenerative joint disease, sinus tarsi dysfunction, and os trigonum.
  - Good to excellent results were noted in 86% of the patients.
  - Overall, less favorable results were noted with associated ankle pathology, degenerative joint disease, increased age, and activity level of the patient.
  - No operative complications were reported.
- Goldberger and Conti[4] retrospectively reviewed 12 patients who underwent subtalar arthroscopy for symptomatic subtalar pathology with nonspecific radiographic findings.
  - The preoperative diagnoses were subtalar chondrosis in nine patients and subtalar synovitis in three patients.
  - At 17.5 months (average) of follow-up, the postoperative AOFAS hindfoot score was 71 (range 51 to 85) compared with a preoperative score of 66 (range 54 to 79). All patients stated that they would have the surgery again.
- Surgical removal of the contents of the lateral half of the sinus tarsi improves or eradicates symptoms in roughly 90% of cases of patients with sinus tarsi pain or dysfunction.[2]

COMPLICATIONS

- Although rare, the most likely complication to occur after subtalar arthroscopy is injury to any of the neurovascular structures in the proximity of the portals, including the sural nerve and superficial peroneal nerve.
- Other possible complications following subtalar joint arthroscopy include infection, instrument breakage, and damage to the articular cartilage.

REFERENCES

1. Ferkel RD. Subtalar arthroscopy. In: Arthroscopic Surgery: The Foot and Ankle. Philadelphia: Lippincott-Raven, 1996:231–254.
2. Frey C, Feder KS, DiGiovanni C. Arthroscopic evaluation of the subtalar joint: does sinus tarsi syndrome exist? Foot Ankle Int 1999;20: 185–191.
3. Frey C, Gasser S, Feder K. Arthroscopy of the subtalar joint. Foot Ankle Int 1994;15:424–428.
4. Goldberger MI, Conti SF. Clinical outcome after subtalar arthroscopy. Foot Ankle Int 1998;19:462–465.
5. Harper MC. The lateral ligamentous support of the subtalar joint. Foot Ankle 1991;11:354–358.
6. Inman VT. The subtalar joint. In: The Joints of the Ankle. Baltimore: Williams & Wilkins, 1976:35–44.
7. Jaivin JS, Ferkel RD. Arthroscopy of the foot and ankle. Clin Sports Med 1994;13:761–783.
8. Lapidus PW. Subtalar joint, its anatomy and mechanics. Bull Hosp Joint Dis 1955;16:179–195.
9. Lundeen RO. Arthroscopic fusion of the ankle and subtalar joint. Clin Podiatr Med Surg 1994;11:395–406.
10. Mekhail AO, Heck BE, Ebraheim NA, Jackson WT. Arthroscopy of the subtalar joint: establishing a medial portal. Foot Ankle Int 1995; 16:427–432.
11. Parisien JS. Posterior subtalar joint arthroscopy. In: Guhl JF, Parisien JS, Boynton MD. Foot and Ankle Arthroscopy, 3rd ed. New York: Springer-Verlag, 2004:175–182.
12. Perry J. Anatomy and biomechanics of the hindfoot. Clin Orthop 1983;177:9–15.
13. Scholten PE, Altena MC, Krips R, van Dijk CN. Treatment of a large intraosseous talar ganglion by means of hindfoot endoscopy. Arthroscopy 2003;19:96–100.
14. Sitler DF, Amendola A, Bailey CS, et al. Posterior ankle arthroscopy: an anatomic study. J Bone Joint Surg Am 2002;84A:763–769.
15. Tasto JP. Arthroscopic subtalar arthrodesis. Techn Foot Ankle Surg 2003;2:122–128.
16. Tasto JP, Frey C, Laimans P, et al. Arthroscopic ankle arthrodesis. Instr Course Lect 2000;49:259–280.
17. van Dijk CN, Scholten PE, Krips R. A 2-portal endoscopic approach for diagnosis and treatment of posterior ankle pathology. Arthroscopy 2000;16:871–876.
18. Viladot A, Lorenzo JC, Salazar J, Rodriguez A. The subtalar joint: embryology and morphology. Foot Ankle 1984;5:54–66.
19. Williams MM, Ferkel RD. Subtalar arthroscopy: indications, technique, and results. Arthroscopy 1998;14:373–381.

Chapter 93

Osteochondral Transfer for Osteochondral Lesions of the Talus

Mark E. Easley and Justin Orr

DEFINITION

- Medium-sized osteochondral defects of the talar dome
  - May approach the talar shoulder (transition of superior dome cartilage to the medial or lateral talar cartilage)
  - Often associated with subchondral cysts
- Osteochondral defect is reconstructed with a cylindrical osteochondral graft. To provide stability to this graft, the osteochondral defect in the native talus must be *contained* (have circumferential cartilage and subchondral bone).

ANATOMY

- Sixty percent of the talus' surface area is covered by articular cartilage.
- The talus is contained within the ankle mortise.
  - Superior talar dome articulates with the tibial plafond.
  - Medial dome articulates with the medial malleolus.
  - Lateral dome articulates with the lateral malleolus.
- Talar blood supply
  - Posterior tibial artery
    - Artery of the tarsal canal
    - Deltoid ligament branch
  - Peroneal artery
    - Artery of the tarsal sinus
  - Dorsalis pedis artery

PATHOGENESIS

- The pathogenesis for osteochondral lesions of the talus (OLTs) is not fully understood.
- Theories include:
  - Trauma
  - Idiopathic focal avascular necrosis

NATURAL HISTORY

- In general, OLTs do not progress to diffuse ankle arthritis.
- However, large-volume OLTs may lead to subchondral collapse of a substantial portion of the talus and thus create deformity, higher contact stresses, and a greater concern for eventual ankle arthritis if left untreated.

PATIENT HISTORY AND PHYSICAL FINDINGS

- Patients may or may not report a history of trauma.
- Ankle pain, typically on the anterior aspect of the ankle, is a common complaint.
  - Pain is usually experienced on the side of the ankle that corresponds with the OLT, but it may be poorly localized to the site of the OLT. In fact, sometimes medial OLTs produce lateral ankle pain and vice versa.
  - Pain is rarely sharp, unless a fragment of the OLT should act as an impinging loose body in the joint.
  - Typically the pain is a deep ache, with and after activity, and is usually relieved with rest.
- Antalgic gait
- May be associated with malalignment or ankle instability
- Typically tenderness on side of ankle that corresponds with OLT, but not always
- Rarely crepitance or mechanical symptoms
- With chronic OLT, some degree of ankle stiffness is anticipated.

IMAGING AND OTHER DIAGNOSTIC STUDIES

- Plain radiographs
  - Obtain weight-bearing, three views of the ankle
  - Small OLTs may be missed.
  - Large OLTs are usually identified on plain radiographs (**FIG 1**).
  - Often limited in characterizing OLT since the two-dimensional study cannot define the three-dimensional OLT
  - Particularly useful in assessing lower leg, ankle, or foot malalignment that needs to be considered in the management of OLTs
  - May detect incidental OLTs (patient has a radiograph for a different problem and an OLT is incidentally identified on plain radiographs)
- MRI
  - Excellent screening tool when OLT or other foot–ankle pathology is suspected
  - Will identify incidental OLT, but defines other potential soft tissue pathology
  - Demonstrates associated marrow edema that may lead to overestimation of the OLT's size
- CT (**FIG 2**)
  - Ideal for characterizing OLT, particularly large-volume defects
  - Defines OLT size without distraction of associated marrow edema
  - Defines the character of the OLT and extent of its involvement in the talar dome
- Diagnostic injection
  - Intra-articular
  - An anesthetic versus anesthetic plus corticosteroid
  - May have some therapeutic effect, even for several months
  - If the source of pain is the OLT, then intra-articular injection should relieve symptoms from OLT. If the pain is not relieved, then other diagnoses should be considered.

DIFFERENTIAL DIAGNOSIS

- Loose body in ankle joint
- Ankle impingement (anterior or posterior)
- Chronic ankle instability (medial, lateral, or syndesmotic)

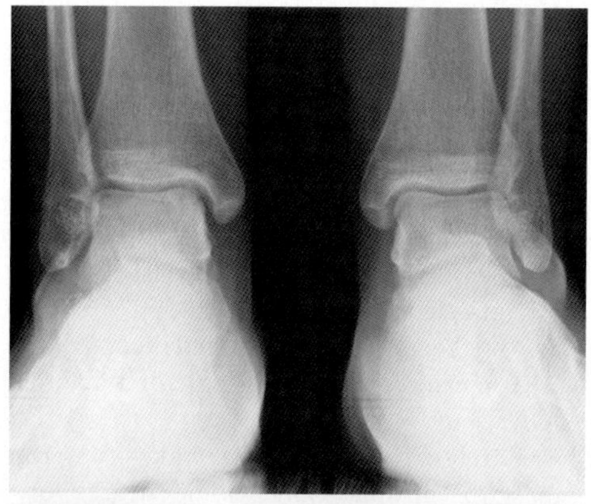

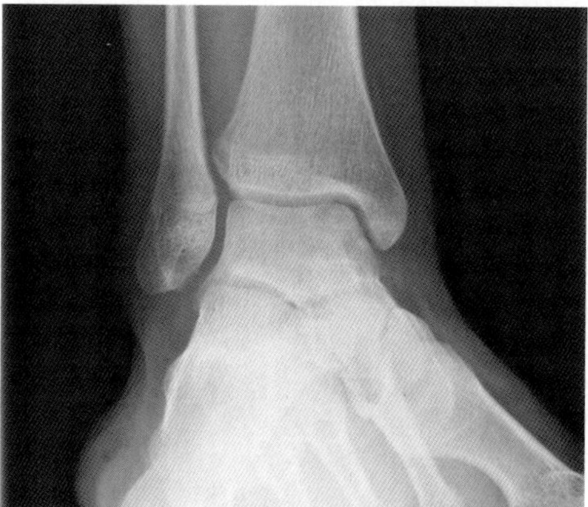

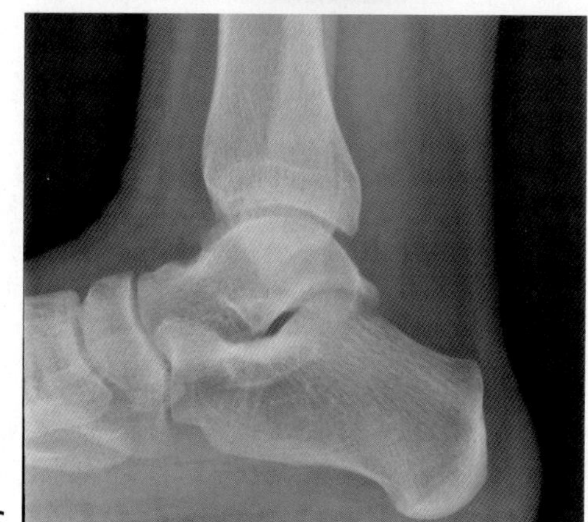

FIG 1 • Radiographs. **A.** AP radiograph of the ankle suggests symmetric alignment and a medial talar dome defect. **B.** Mortise view also suggests medial osteochondral lesion of the talus. **C.** Lateral view shows anatomic alignment, with osteochondral lesion of the talus less obvious.

- Ankle synovitis or adjacent tendinopathy
- Early ankle degenerative change

NONOPERATIVE MANAGEMENT

- Activity modification
- Bracing
- Physical therapy if associated ankle instability
- Nonsteroidal anti-inflammatories or COX-2 inhibitors
- Corticosteroid injection
- Viscosupplementation?

SURGICAL MANAGEMENT

Preoperative Planning

- Indications for this surgery include:
  - Medium-sized OLTs not amenable to other joint-sparing procedures. If associated with a large subchondral cyst, then arthroscopic débridement and microfracture may not be effective, and some surgeons recommend osteochondral transfer as a primary procedure.
  - Failed arthroscopic (débridement and microfracture) management
- Potential sites for graft harvest
  - Patient's ipsilateral knee (superolateral femoral condyle, intracondylar notch)
  - Allograft talus
- Ipsilateral knee versus talar allograft
  - Knee is autograft; however, knee cartilage is thicker than ankle cartilage and may have different biomechanical properties.
  - Allograft talus offers nearly the same cartilage thickness and harvest from the exact location of the native talus' defect; however, it is not the patient's own tissue.
- The surgeon should check for associated pathology that may need to be addressed at the time of allograft talar reconstruction:
  - Osteophyte removal
  - Ligament reconstruction
  - Corrective osteotomies (calcaneal, supramalleolar)

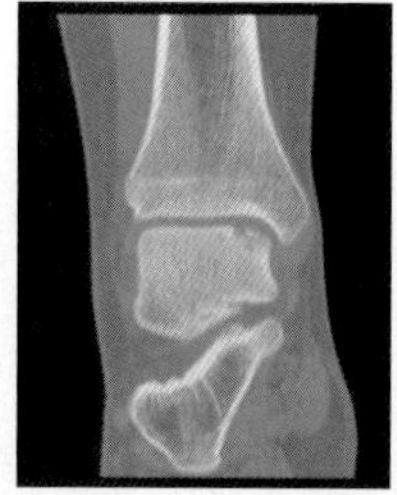

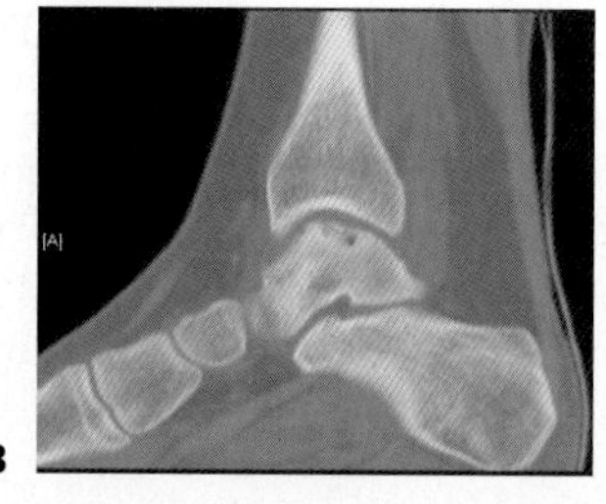

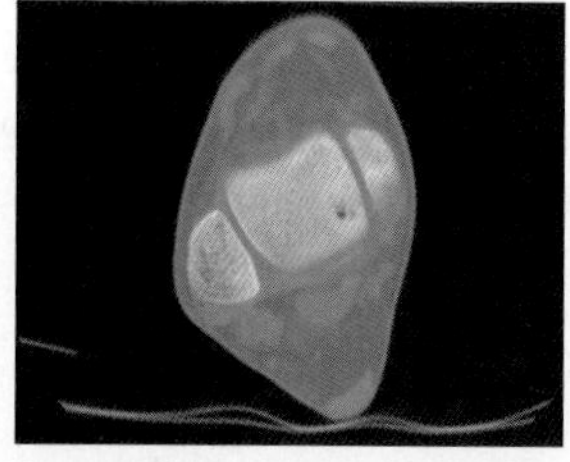

FIG 2 • CT. **A.** Coronal view with medial osteochondral lesion of the talus that approaches talar shoulder but appears contained. **B.** Sagittal view demonstrating rather medial osteochondral lesion of the talus. **C.** Axial view with posteromedial osteochondral lesion of the talus.

- Patient education
  - This is a complex procedure.
  - The patient must understand that the intent is to transfer cartilage and bone from one location to another and expect it to incorporate into the native talus.
  - If allograft is used, there is a negligible but real risk of disease transmission and possible graft rejection by the host.
  - There is no guarantee that the procedure will work, and a revision procedure may be required, such as structural allograft reconstruction or potentially ankle arthrodesis.

Positioning

- The patient is positioned supine (**FIG 3**).
- For a lateral OLT, a bolster under the ipsilateral hip typically affords better access to the lateral talar dome.
- We routinely use a thigh tourniquet.

Approach

- The surgeon must determine the optimal surgical approach:
  - Medial talar dome (usually centromedial or posteromedial) typically warrants a medial malleolar osteotomy.
  - Lateral talar dome (often centrolateral) typically necessitates ligament releases (anterior talofibular and calcaneofibular) with or without lateral malleolar osteotomy.
- The key is that exposure must allow perpendicular access to the OLT; otherwise, the dedicated instrumentation for the osteochondral transfer cannot be used.

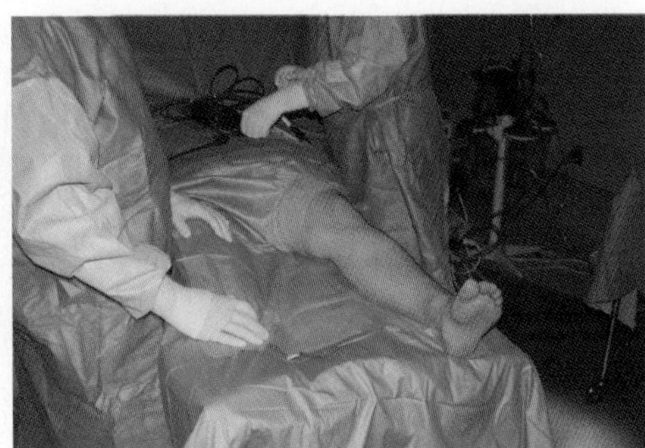

FIG 3 • Positioning is supine, with easy access to the medial ankle but without too much external rotation, which would make access to the lateral knee cumbersome.

MEDIAL APPROACH FOR A MEDIAL OSTEOCHONDRAL LESION OF THE TALUS

- Make a longitudinal incision centered over the medial malleolus (TECH FIG 1A).
- Anterior ankle arthrotomy
  - Identify the joint line (TECH FIG 1B).
  - Visualize the anterior talus and possibly anterior OLT (TECH FIG 1C).
- Open the flexor retinaculum (TECH FIG 1D).
  - Identify and protect the posterior tibial tendon (PTT) (TECH FIG 1E).
- Predrill the intended screw holes for fixation of the osteotomy.
  - Two parallel drill holes in the same orientation are typically used for open reduction and internal fixation (ORIF) of a medial malleolar fracture (TECH FIG 1F).
  - Consider tapping the screw holes as well (traditional malleolar screws are not self-tapping) (TECH FIG 1G).
- Trajectory of the oblique osteotomy
  - Should target tibial plafond at lateral extent of OLT
  - Allows perpendicular access to the OLT with the dedicated instrumentation

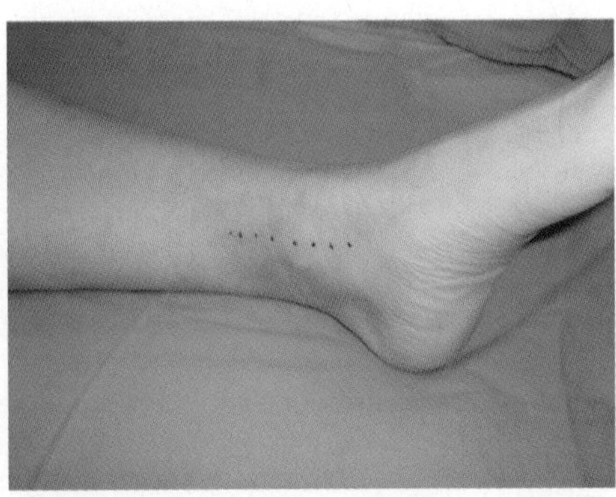

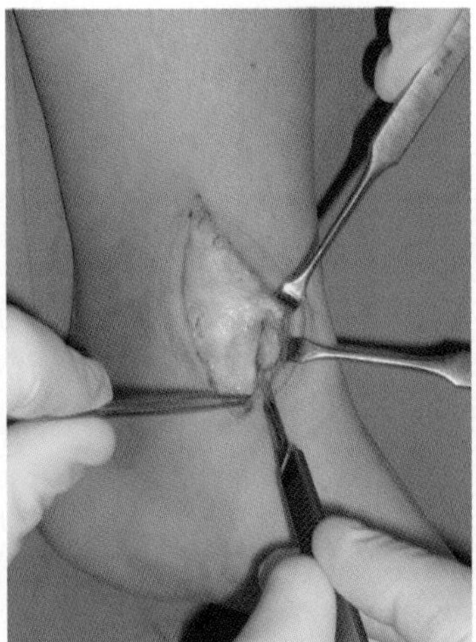

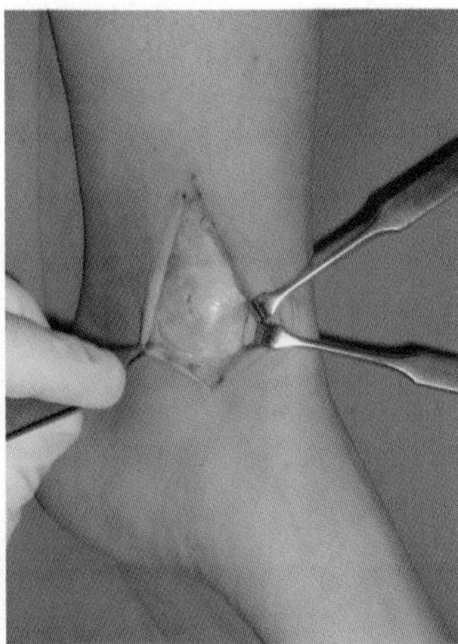

A B C

TECH FIG 1 • **A.** Medial approach is similar to that for open reduction and internal fixation for a medial malleolar fracture. **B, C.** Anterior ankle arthrotomy. **B.** Locating joint and performing the medial capsulotomy. **C.** Medial talar dome visible through the arthrotomy with capsule retracted. This defines the anterior margin for the osteotomy. Rarely, the osteochondral lesion of the talus may be accessed via arthrotomy alone, but this is more common for lateral lesions. *(continued)*

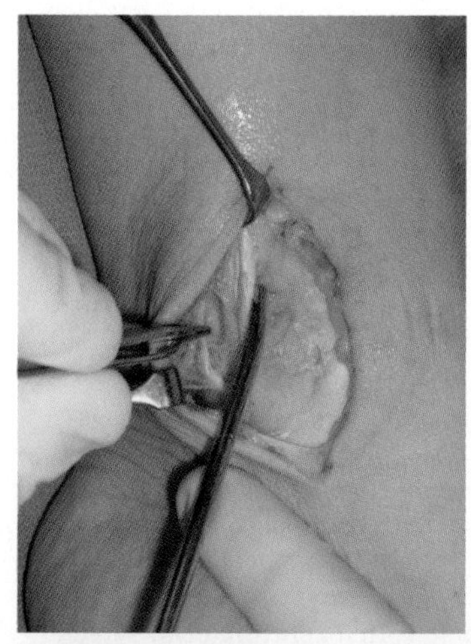
D

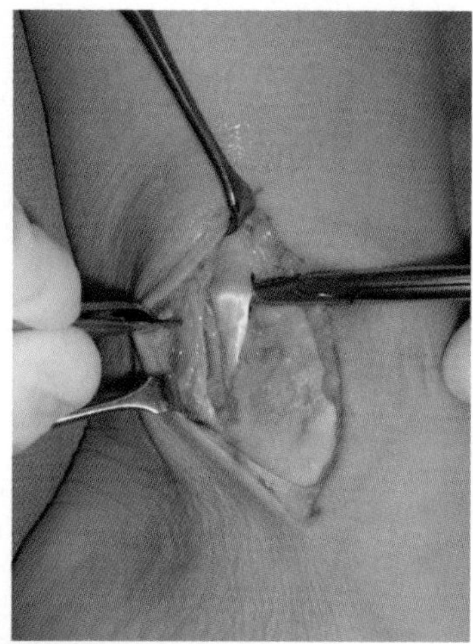
E

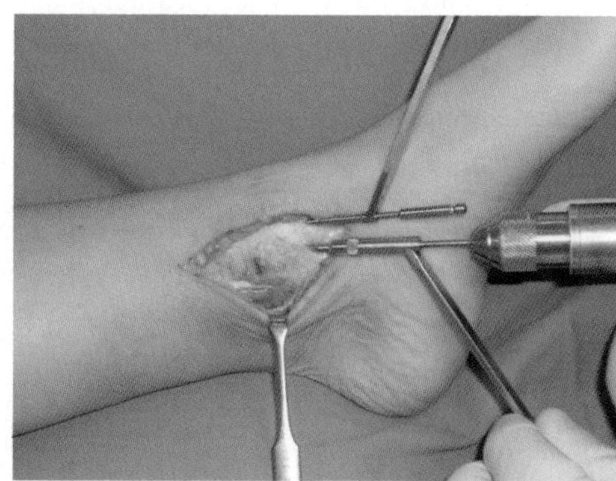
F

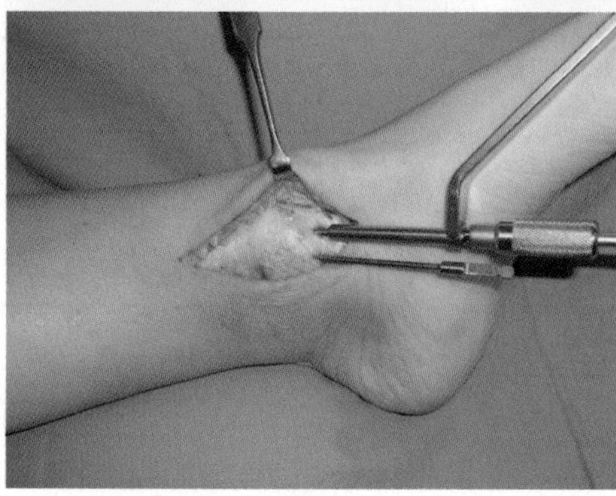
G

TECH FIG 1 • *(continued)* **D, E.** Defining posterior tibia for the osteotomy. **D.** Opening the flexor retinaculum. **E.** Identifying the posterior tibial tendon (to be protected during the osteotomy). **F, G.** Predrilling the medial malleolus. **F.** Drill bit directed as it would be for medial malleolar screws for open reduction and internal fixation of a medial malleolar fracture. **G.** Tap used for screws that are not self-tapping.

- We routinely use a Kirschner wire to determine the trajectory for the osteotomy.
  - Place the wire slightly proximal and lateral to the planned osteotomy so as not to interfere with the saw blade and chisel (**TECH FIG 2A**).
  - Confirm desired Kirschner wire trajectory with fluoroscopy.
- Mark the osteotomy.
  - Across the periosteum and with minimal periosteal stripping (**TECH FIG 2B**)
  - Perpendicular to the tibial shaft axis
- Protect the soft tissues:
  - Tibialis anterior retracted
  - PTT retracted. Do not mistake the flexor digitorum longus for the PTT (PTT rests in a groove directly on the posterior aspect of tibia).
- Performing the osteotomy
  - Microsagittal saw (**TECH FIG 2C**)
    - To the subchondral bone
    - Use cool saline irrigation to limit risk of heat necrosis fo the bone.
  - Chisel (**TECH FIG 2D**)
    - Complete the osteotomy with a chisel.
  - Periodically check the progress of the osteotomy fluoroscopically to confirm trajectory and to avoid injury to the talar dome.
  - Reflect medial malleolus on the deltoid ligament (**TECH FIG 2E**).
    - The PTT sheath must be released from the malleolus to allow full reflection of the malleolus.

Lateral Approach for a Lateral Osteochondral Lesion of the Talus

- Ideal for lateral OLT associated with lateral ankle instability
- Lateral ligaments may be released even without ligament instability.
- Make a longitudinal incision over the distal lateral fibula and curve it slightly anteriorly at the distal margin.
  - Protect the sural nerve and lateral branch of the superficial peroneal nerve.
- Identify the inferior extensor retinaculum and mobilize it to be used as augmentation to lateral ligament repair at the conclusion of the cartilage procedure.
- Identify the peroneal tendons and protect them throughout the procedure.
- Release the joint capsule, with anterior talofibular and calcaneofibular ligaments, from the distal fibula.
- In many patients, plantarflexion and inversion allows sufficient anterior subluxation of the talus to perform osteochondral transfer with the dedicated instruments perpendicular to the osteochondral defect.
- If the exposure is not sufficient with soft tissue release alone, a fibular osteotomy may be performed to gain access to the more posteriorly situated lateral OLT.
- Fibular osteotomy
  - We routinely perform an oblique fibular osteotomy, similar to the pattern of a Weber B ankle fracture.

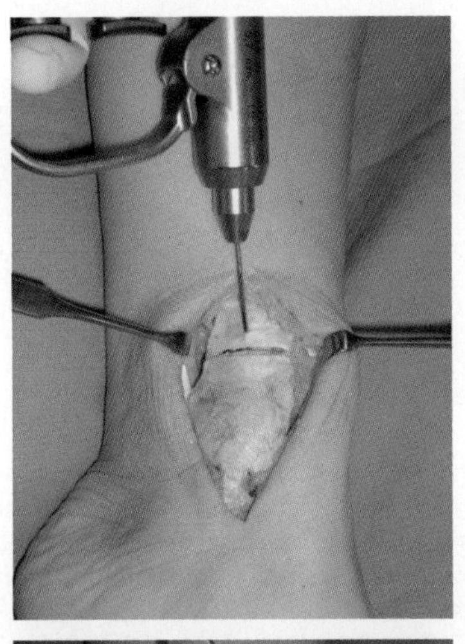
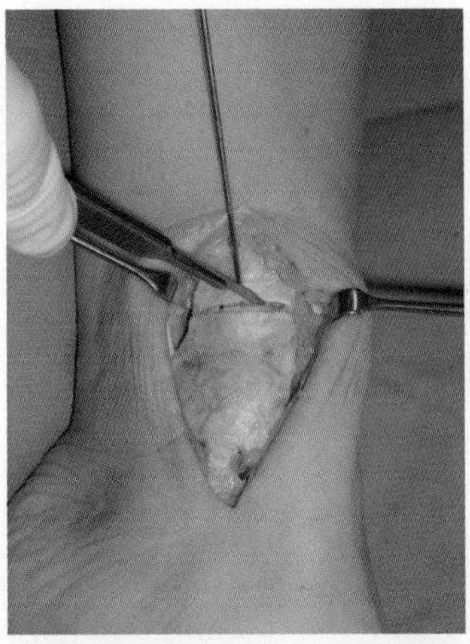
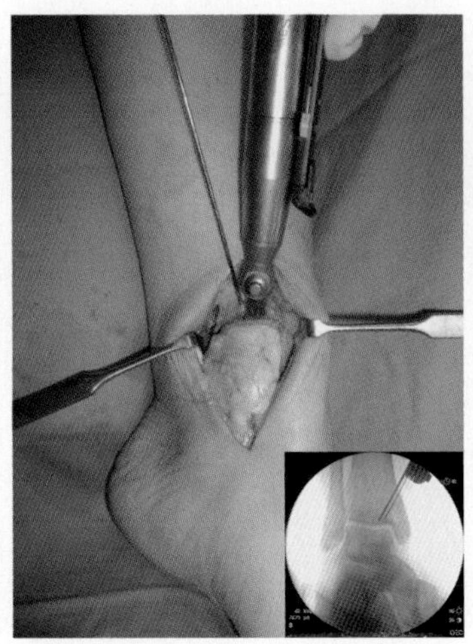
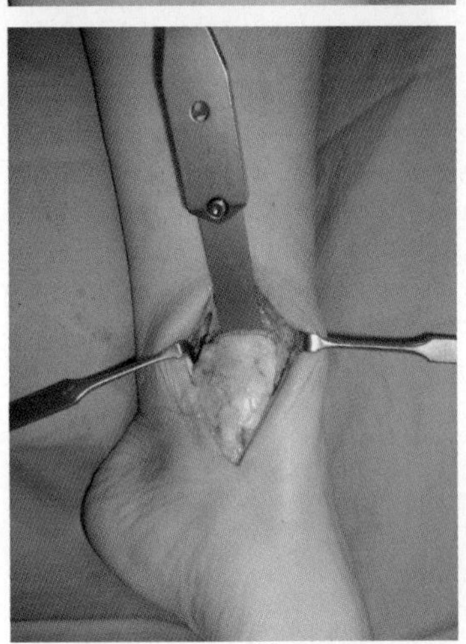
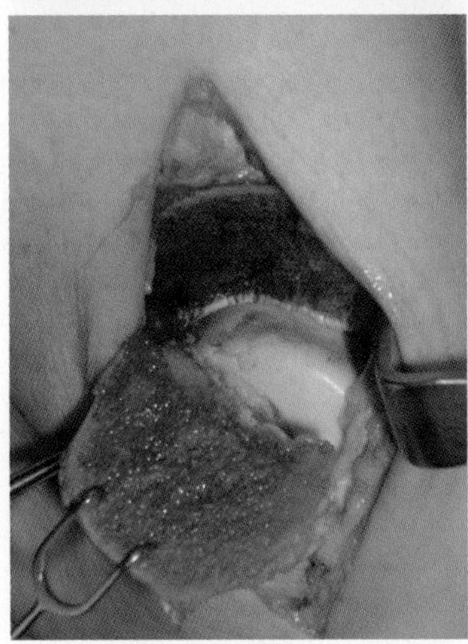

TECH FIG 2 • **A.** Kirschner wire is used to define the trajectory of the osteotomy. So that the wire does not interfere with the saw blade, it is placed slightly more proximal and directly slightly more lateral than the intended osteotomy. **B–D.** Medial malleolar osteotomy. **B.** The periosteum is incised at the starting point, perpendicular to the longitudinal axis of the tibia (virtually no periosteal stripping required). **C.** Microsagittal saw is used to perform the osteotomy. Note the Kirschner wire used to guide the saw. **D.** A chisel is used to carefully complete the osteotomy. **E.** The medial malleolus is reflected, exposing the osteochondral lesion of the talus.

- When performed with the ligament release described above, exposure is markedly enhanced.
- Before performing the osteotomy, we place a small fragment plate on the lateral fibula that spans the proposed osteotomy and predrill the holes.
- With the peroneal tendons and superficial peroneal nerve protected, perform the osteotomy obliquely using a microsagittal saw.
  - Cool saline irrigation to limit bony heat necrosis
  - Avoid injuring intact articular cartilage on talus.
- Syndesmotic ligaments remain intact.

Osteochondral Transfer

- Single-stage operation
- Donor options:
  - Autograft from ipsilateral knee
    - Arthrotomy versus arthroscopic
    - Superolateral femoral condyle versus intracondylar notch
    - Moderate amount of donor graft available
  - Autograft from ipsilateral talus
    - Limited donor graft available
  - Allograft talus
    - Fresh allograft ideal
    - Ideally same side as the native talus to replace the deficient cartilage with cartilage from the exact same location
    - Maximum donor graft available
    - Advantage over knee or talar autograft if the OLT proves not to be contained
- Recipient site preparation
  - Débride the OLT sharply to stable circumferential rim of articular cartilage (TECH FIG 3A).
  - Be sure that the defect is contained.
    - Bony rim circumferentially
    - Interference fit will be compromised if medial talar dome at the defect lacks integrity.
    - If not, then a structural allograft reconstruction should be considered.
  - Assess defect size and orientation with the sizing guide and with reference to preoperative CT scan (TECH FIG 3B). Larger defects may warrant two or even three grafts.
  - Recipient site chisel
    - Assistant will need to position foot in maximal inversion or eversion for medial and lateral OLTs, respectively (TECH FIG 4A).
    - Select appropriate chisel size.
    - Orient chisel perpendicular to defect (TECH FIG 4B).
  - We routinely advance the chisel 11 to 12 mm into the talus (TECH FIG 4C).
    - Maintain proper chisel orientation to the desired depth.

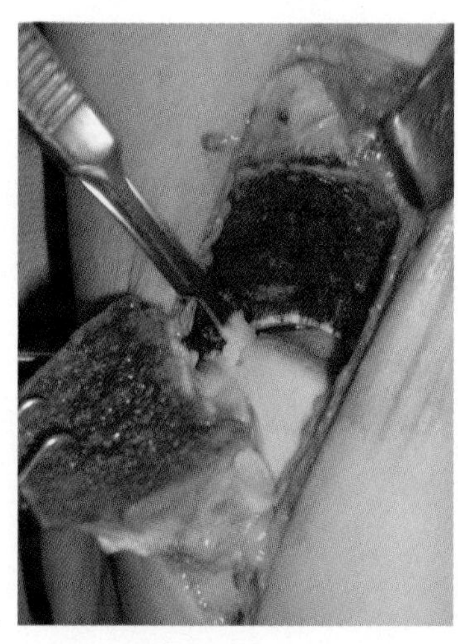

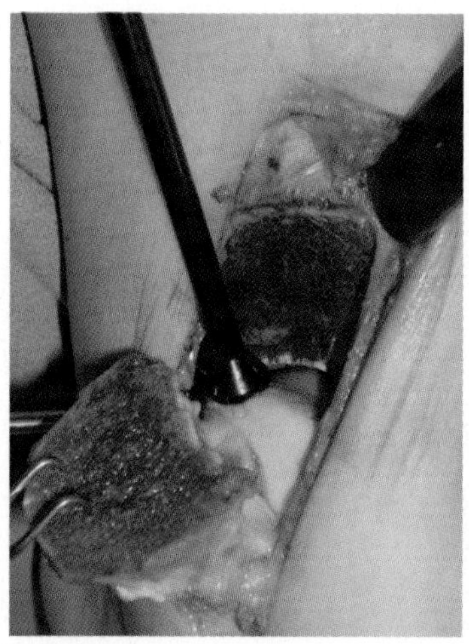

TECH FIG 3 • **A.** The surgeon probes and débrides the osteochondral lesion of the talus to define its superficial dimensions. **B.** The defect is sized to determine optimal recipient chisel size.

  - Do not attempt to change orientation of the chisel once the chisel has been advanced into the subchondral bone.
- Once at the desired depth, twist the chisel forcefully 90 degrees and then 90 degrees again (TECH FIG 4D).
- Gently toggle the chisel to free the diseased cartilage from the surrounding healthy cartilage.
- Extract the diseased osteochondral cylinder (TECH FIG 4E).
- If the subchondral bone is sclerotic, a reamer of corresponding size from an anterior cruciate ligament set may be used to create the recipient site.
  - Use cool saline irrigation to limit the risk of heat necrosis to surrounding native talus.
  - Predrill the guide pin to ensure that the reamer maintains position and proper orientation.
- Donor site preparation and graft harvest (superior lateral femoral condyle)

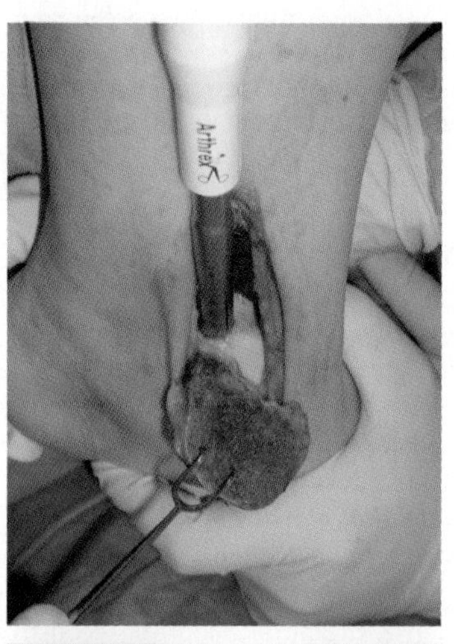

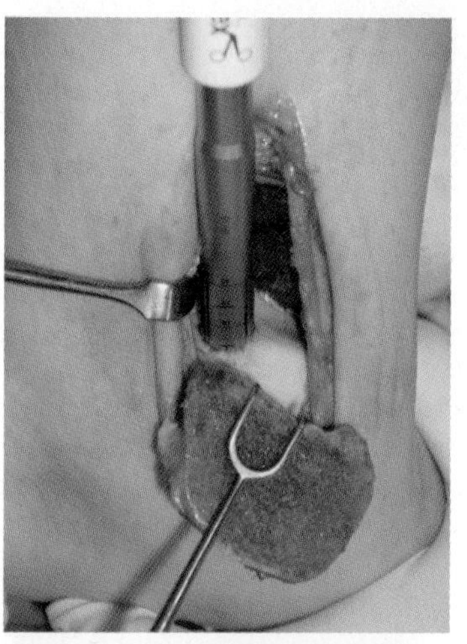

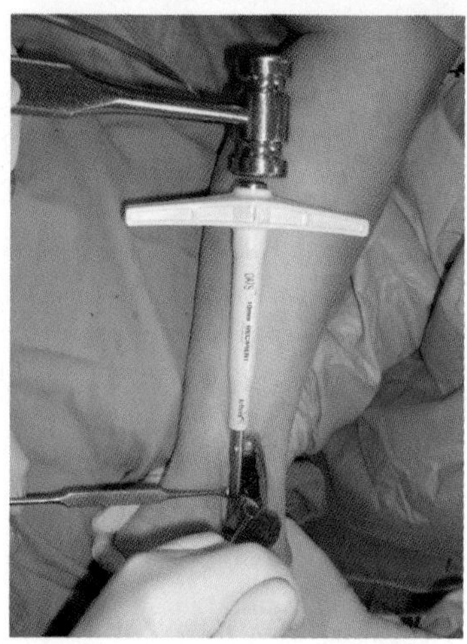

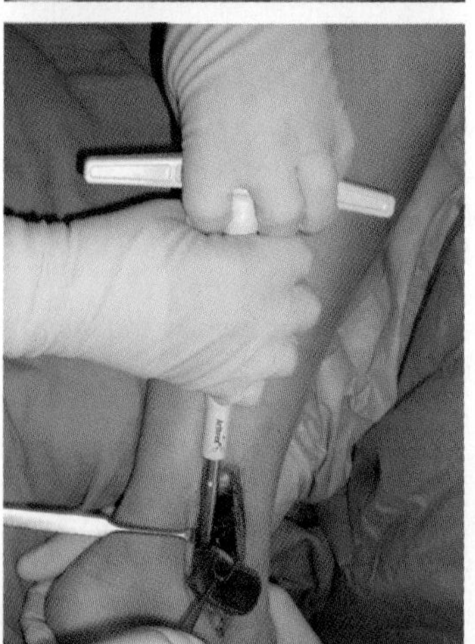

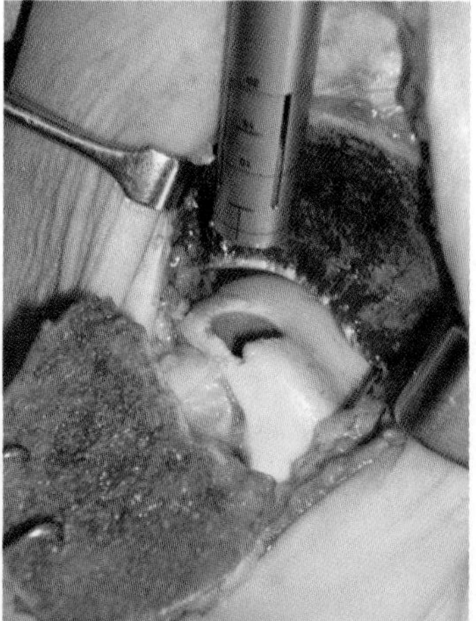

TECH FIG 4 • Preparing the recipient site. **A.** Assistant everts the ankle to permit vertical axis of the recipient chisel. **B.** Recipient chisel is oriented properly on the osteochondral lesion of the talus, approaching without violating the medial talar dome subchondral bone (essential so the defect remains contained). **C.** Mallet to advance the chisel. **D.** Once fully seated, the chisel is aggressively twisted to free the diseased cartilage cylinder. **E.** The recipient site is prepared. Note the slight medial cartilage defect, but the recipient site is still contained.

- Superolateral arthrotomy
  - Knee extended
  - Longitudinal approach immediately lateral to patella (TECH FIG 5A,B), about 5 cm long
  - Avoid injuring cartilage.
- Chose optimal site for graft harvest (TECH FIG 5C).
  - Use the same sizing guide as you did for the recipient site to determine the proper trajectory for the harvesting chisel and to determine the ideal location for graft harvest.
- If multiple grafts are needed, be sure to leave an adequate bridge between harvest sites.
  - Avoid fracturing one harvest site into another, thereby creating a large defect.
- Select the corresponding donor chisel.
  - This chisel is 1 mm larger in diameter than the recipient chisel. This allows for interference fit of the graft into the recipient site.
  - The chisel must be perpendicular to the harvest site (TECH FIG 5D).
  - Be sure not to contact the cartilage surface with the chisel until proper position has been obtained. The chisel is sharp and will cut into the cartilage, even with light pressure.
- Impact the chisel to a depth of 10 mm (TECH FIG 5E).
  - Do not change the orientation of the chisel once it has been advanced into the subchondral bone.
- Once desired depth has been achieved
  - Rotate the chisel 90 degrees and then 90 degrees again (TECH FIG 5F).
  - Toggle the chisel lightly to release the graft.
- Extract the graft from the knee.
  - A fenestration in the chisel allows for visualization of the graft to ensure it is free and advancing from the harvest site with the chisel (TECH FIG 5G,H).

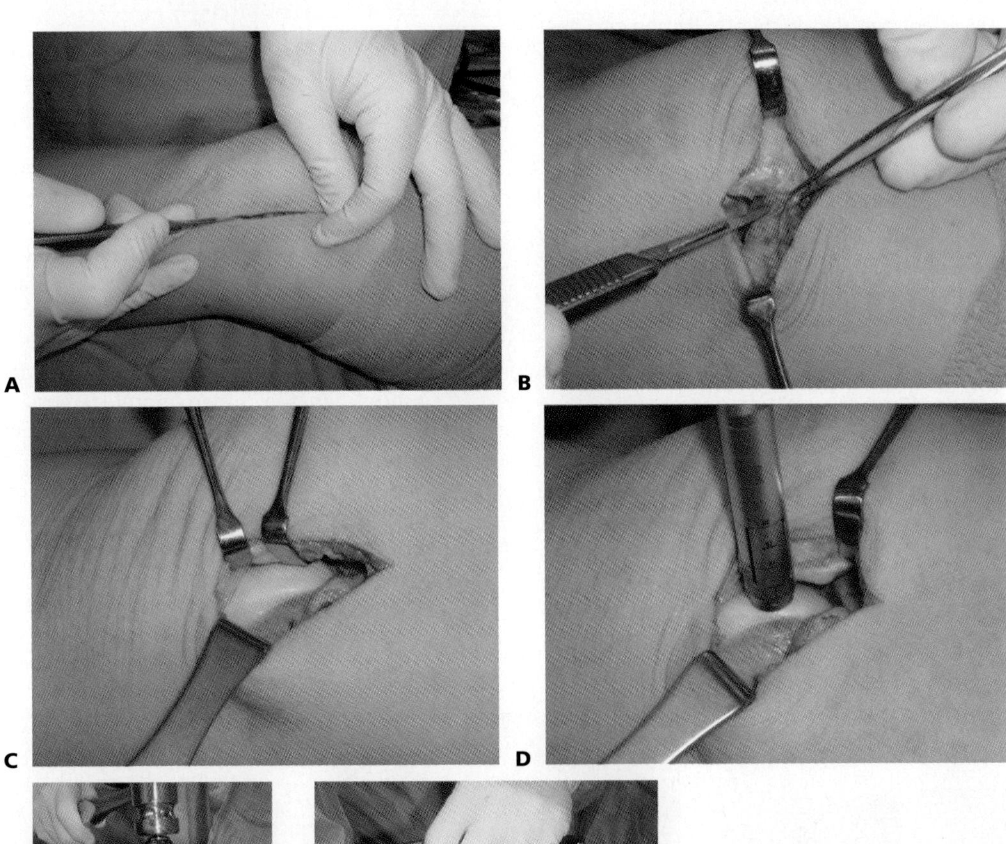

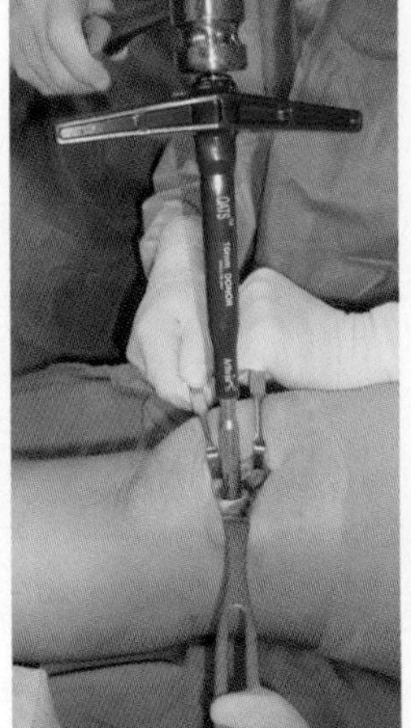

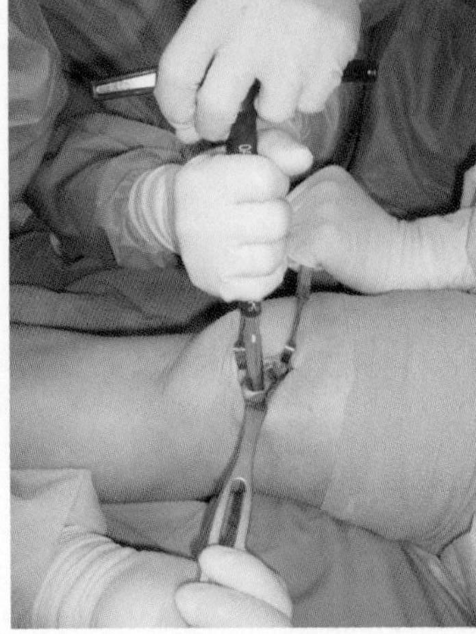

TECH FIG 5 • **A–C.** Exposure of superolateral femoral condyle. **A.** Superolateral approach to knee. **B.** Knee arthrotomy. **C.** Superolateral femoral condyle exposed with patella retracted medially. **D–H.** Harvesting donor graft. **D.** Donor chisel oriented to allow optimal graft harvest. **E.** Harvesting chisel impacted without changing trajectory once chisel introduced. **F.** Once chisel is fully seated, it is aggressively twisted to free the cylindrical graft. *(continued)*

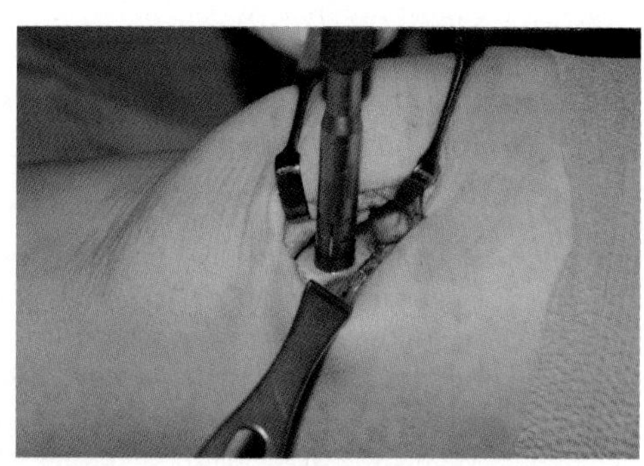

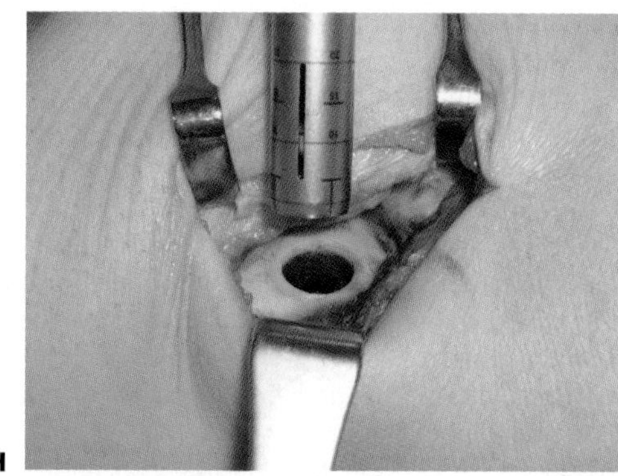

TECH FIG 5 • *(continued)* **G.** Chisel is carefully withdrawn (fenestrations within chisel confirm that the graft is advancing with the chisel). **H.** Graft extracted and harvest site evident.

- The graft does not leave the chisel until it is secured in the recipient site.
- Graft transfer to the recipient site
  - Properly orient the donor chisel over the recipient site, maintaining contact with the chisel directly over the defect (TECH FIG 6A,B).
  - Advance the graft into the recipient site by advancing the tamp in the donor chisel (TECH FIG 6C). Fenestrations in the chisel permit visualization of the graft being advanced.
  - Remove the chisel when the graft is nearly fully seated (TECH FIG 6D,E).
  - The goal is to place the graft flush with the surrounding native articular cartilage.
  - A corresponding tamp or sizing guide may then be used to carefully achieve the final position of the graft (TECH FIG 6F,G).
  - We routinely harvest a 10-mm osteochondral cylinder but prepare an 11- to 12-mm recipient site. While countersinking the graft is a risk, the interference fit typically limits this from occurring. In our opinion it is safer than creating a recipient site that is too shallow, thus potentially leading to forceful tamping of the graft that may lead to shearing of the graft cartilage from its osseous cylinder.

Osteochondral Transfer Incorporating a Small Portion of Medial or Lateral Talar Dome Cartilage

- This technique is used when the OLT involves some of the cartilage on the medial or lateral sides of the talar dome while still being contained.
- Recipient site
  - The recipient site chisel approaches the talar shoulder but is not advanced beyond the subchondral border of the medial or lateral talus.
  - This will extract the dorsal shoulder of the talus, leaving the medial or lateral talar subchondral bone and cartilage intact (still contained).
- Donor site
  - As for the recipient site and chisel, the donor chisel approaches the superolateral femoral condyle's shoulder but is not advanced beyond its border.
  - The dorsal shoulder of the graft will be included in the harvest without violating the lateral femoral condyle's subchondral bone on its lateral margin.
- Transfer
  - Medial OLT
    - The chisel will need to be rotated 180 degrees to fill the articular cartilage defect that extends over the shoulder from the dorsal talar dome.

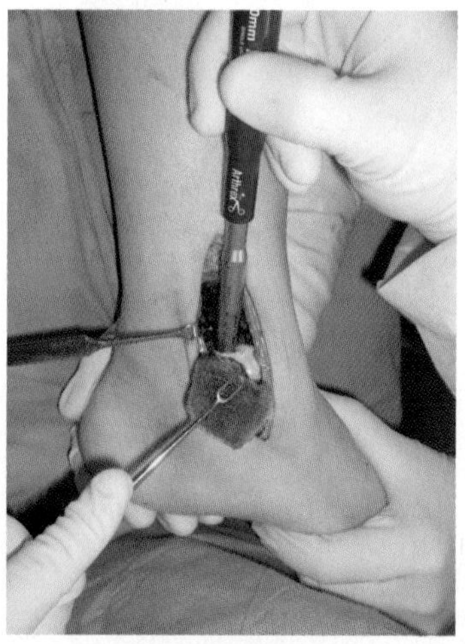

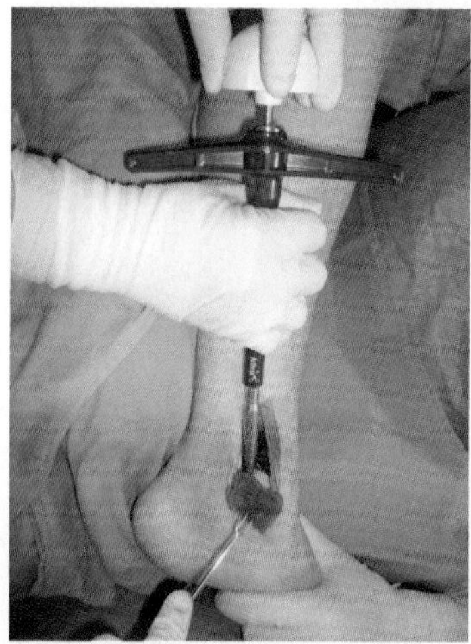

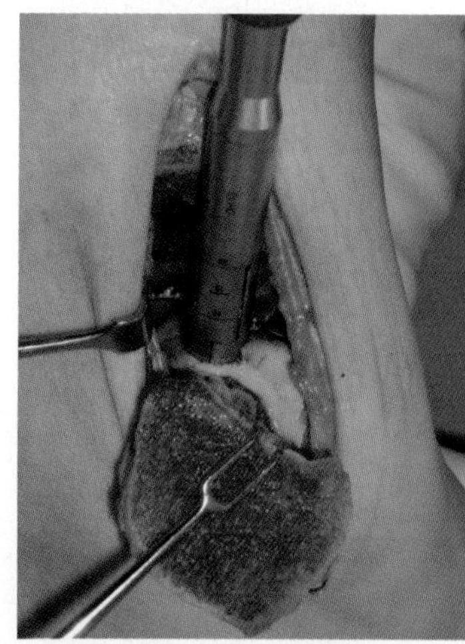

TECH FIG 6 • Transfer of graft to recipient site. **A.** Donor chisel with graft oriented with recipient site. **B.** Tamp within chisel is advanced to transfer the graft into the recipient site. **C.** Fenestrations in chisel confirm that graft is advancing. *(continued)*

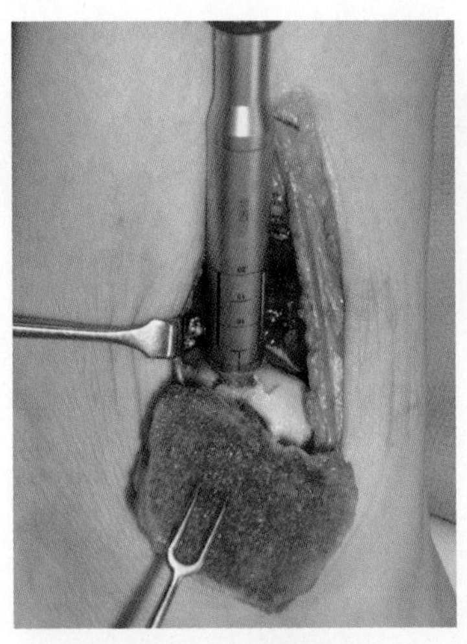
D

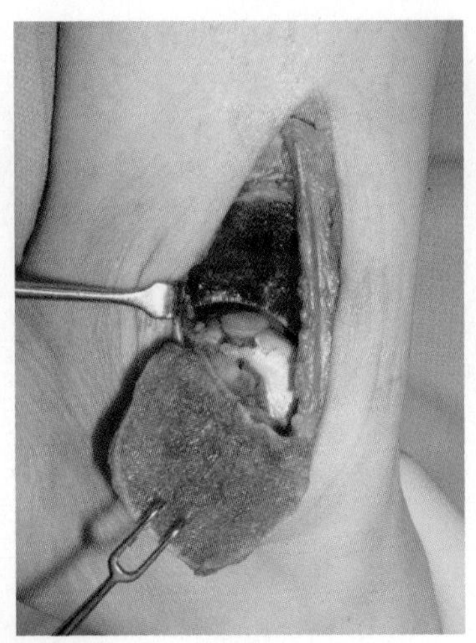
E

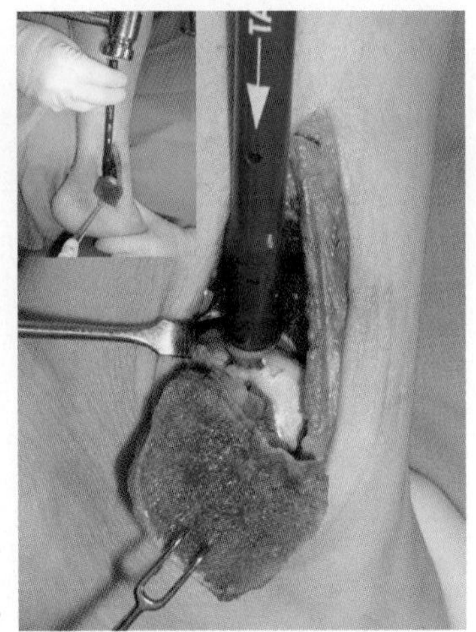
F

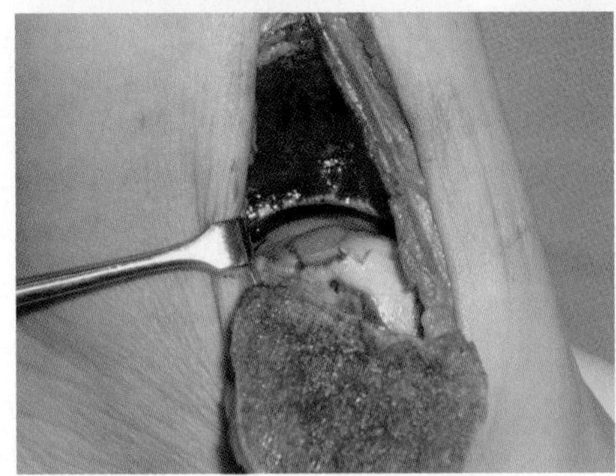
G

TECH FIG 6 • *(continued)* **D.** Chisel typically releases graft before it is fully seated (in our hands, preferred so we can control the final graft position). **E.** Graft sitting slightly proud relative to the adjacent native cartilage. **F.** Dedicated smooth tamp used to perform final seating of graft. Inset shows that the tamp is tapped lightly to advance graft in a graduated manner. **G.** Graft seated flush with surrounding native cartilage. (Note medial articular defect not fully resurfaced, but majority of osteochondral lesion of the talus is resurfaced with stable graft.)

    - Mark the donor chisel during graft harvest to avoid malrotation of the graft in the recipient site.
  - For a lateral OLT this rotation is not necessary when transferring from the ipsilateral knee.

Closure

- Medial closure
  - Reduction of the medial osteotomy after cartilage reconstruction
  - Temporarily place a drill bit in one of the predrilled holes to orient the reduction.
  - Confirm reduction by visualizing the anterior and posterior aspects of the osteotomy at the joint line.
  - We routinely use two partially threaded small fragment cancellous screws to fix the osteotomy under compression (TECH FIG 7A,B).
    - If fixation is suboptimal, two fully threaded cortical screws may be used to engage the opposite cortex.

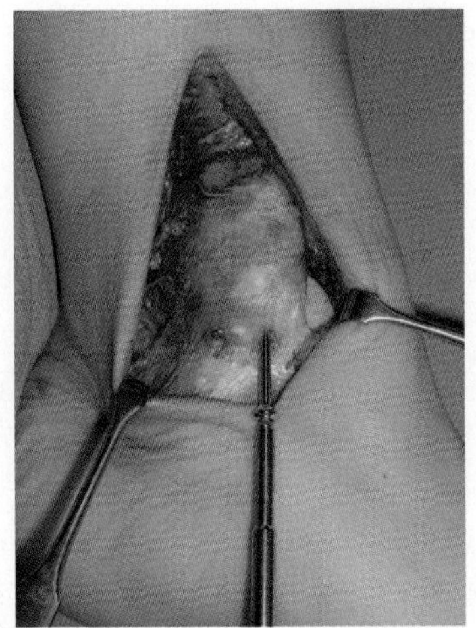
A

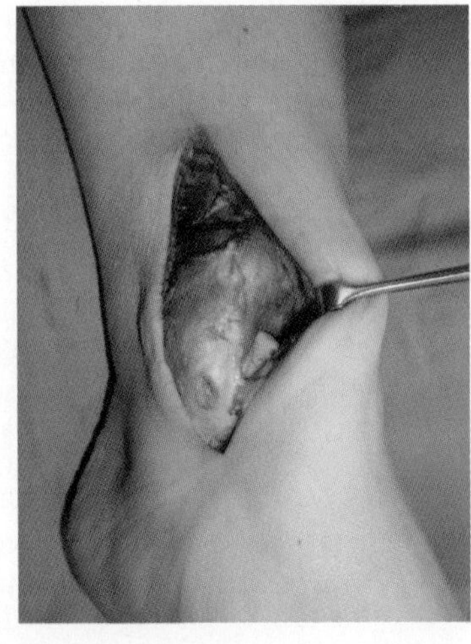
B

TECH FIG 7 • Reducing medial malleolar osteotomy. **A.** Reduced osteotomy is secured with two malleolar screws placed in the predrilled holes. **B.** View through arthrotomy confirms reduction of anterior tibial plafond. *(continued)*

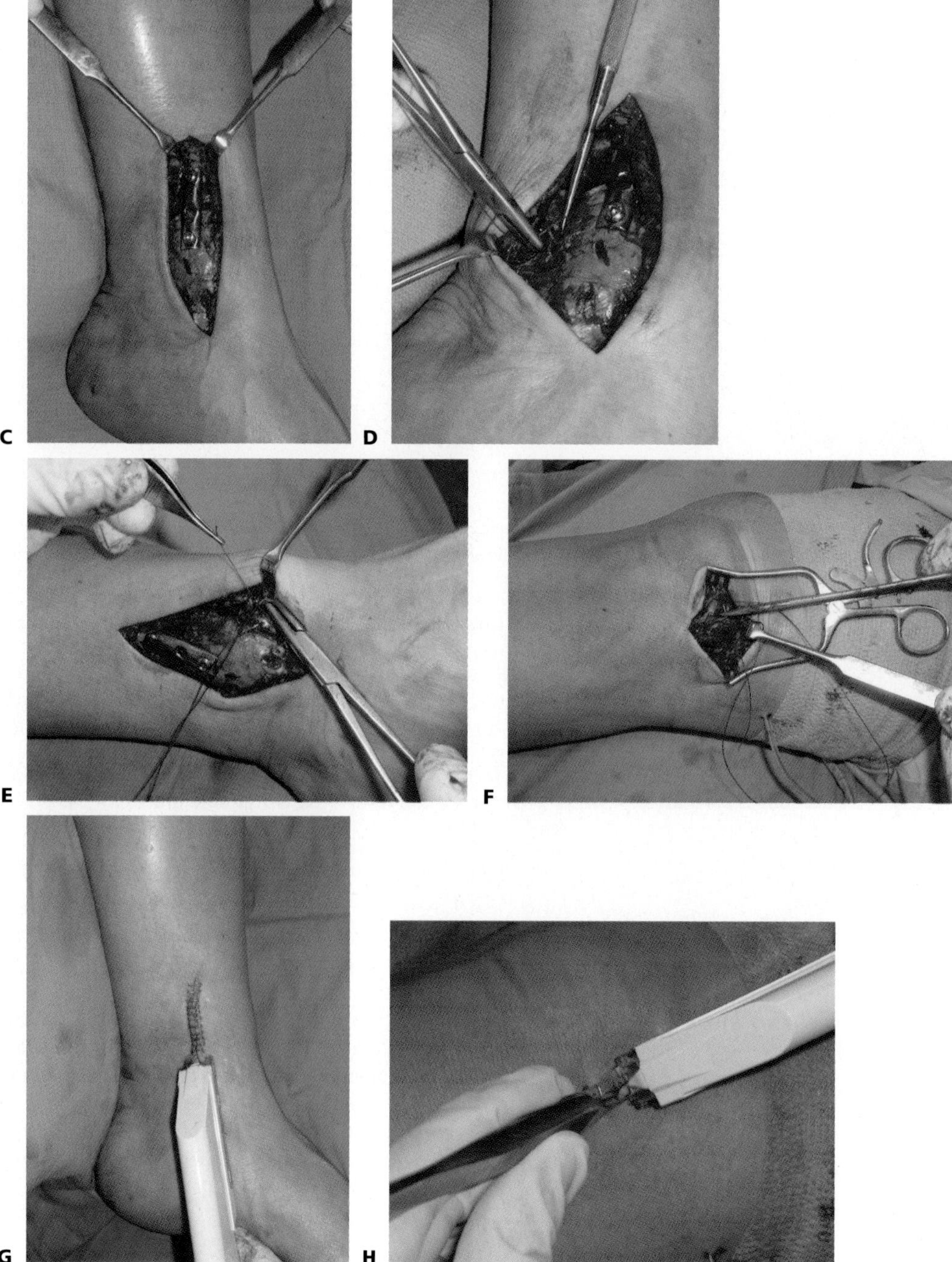

TECH FIG 7 • *(continued)* **C.** Medial buttress plate. **D.** Closing posterior tibial tendon sheath and flexor retinaculum. **E.** Closing anterior capsulotomy. **F.** Closing lateral knee arthrotomy. **G, H.** Skin reapproximation. **G.** Ankle. **H.** Knee.

It may be necessary to use longer cortical screws from a pelvic set to reach the opposite cortex.

- A buttress plate placed at the superior aspect of the osteotomy provides an antiglide effect (**TECH FIG 7C**).
- Confirm fluoroscopically that the osteotomy is anatomically reduced at the plafond.
  - A minimal gap will be present at the osteotomy site despite anatomic reduction, due to the thickness of the saw blade.
  - Reapproximate the flexor retinaculum with the PTT in its anatomic position (**TECH FIG 7D**).
  - Close the anterior arthrotomy (**TECH FIG 7E**).
  - The periosteum over the osteotomy may be reapproximated but must be coordinated with the antiglide plate.
- Lateral closure
- Fibular osteotomy reduction, ligament repair, and closure after cartilage procedure

- Fibular osteotomy is reduced, plate is positioned, and screws are placed in predrilled holes. A small gap at the osteotomy site may be visible on fluoroscopic confirmation despite anatomic clinical reduction; this is secondary to saw blade thickness.
- A modified Brostrom ligament repair serves to reattach the anterior talofibular and calcaneofibular ligaments and augment with the inferior extensor retinaculum. We routinely use suture anchors to reattach the ligaments to the fibula. We use a modified Brostrom ligament reattachment after osteochondral transfer for lateral OLTs.
- Close the superolateral capsule of the knee (**TECH FIG 7F**).
- Close the subcutaneous layer and skin after tourniquet release and meticulous hemostasis for both the knee and ankle (**TECH FIG 7G,H**).
- We use a drain, unless the wounds have minor residual bleeding.

PEARLS AND PITFALLS

Perpendicular access	■ The dedicated chisel must be oriented perpendicular to the articular cartilage. Thus, the exposure (osteotomy) must be adequate to accommodate the perpendicular position of the chisel.
Do not reorient the chisel once it has been advanced into the subchondral bone.	■ Carefully obtain the proper orientation of the chisel before advancing it. If orientation is changed during impaction, you may not be able to extract an intact osteochondral graft.
Graft height and recipient site depth	■ The graft must not be longer than the recipient site. Impaction may lead to shear of the graft's articular cartilage from its osseous cylinder.
Using multiple grafts	■ Do not allow one graft harvest site to fracture into an adjacent harvest site. However, grafts may be overlapped (intersecting circles) to fill the recipient site optimally.
Malleolar osteotomy	■ The medial malleolar osteotomy must have perfect congruency at the tibial plafond when reduced.

POSTOPERATIVE CARE

- We routinely observe these patients overnight for pain control.
- Follow-up is done in about 10 to 14 days.
- Provided the wound and osteotomy (if one was performed) are stable, the patient is transferred into a touch-down weight-bearing cam boot. If not, a touch-down weight-bearing short-leg cast is continued until the wound and osteotomy are stable.
- Intermittent minimal, gentle ankle range of motion (ROM) is encouraged, three or four times a day. If financially feasible, we arrange for an ankle continuous passive motion (CPM) device.
- Touch-down weight bearing is maintained for 8 to 10 weeks, with progressively increasing ankle ROM exercise.
- We routinely obtain simulated weight-bearing radiographs at 6 weeks and 10 weeks, and again at 14 to 16 weeks, depending on the progression of healing. If there was a concern about fixation of the graft or osteotomy, then radiographs are also obtained at the first postoperative visit (**FIG 4**).
- Knee cartilage has a different thickness than ankle cartilage; therefore, an appropriately placed osteochondral graft from the knee may appear recessed on the postoperative radiograph (**FIG 5**).

OUTCOMES

- Good to excellent results with osteochondral autografting at short to intermediate follow-up can be obtained in 90% to 94% of patients.
  - Excellent functional outcomes
  - Improvement in ROM
  - Improved pain scores
- Best results for smaller defects (those that can be managed with a single graft)
- Good to excellent results for OLTs associated with subchondral cysts
- Donor site morbidity was found to be minimal except in a single study, which found poor knee functional scores in 36%.
- No reported complications from malleolar osteotomy
- Results are not worse for osteochondral transfer performed as a secondary procedure after failed arthroscopic treatment compared to osteochondral transfer as a primary procedure. Additionally, there may be no benefit of osteochondral autograft transplantation over chondroplasty or microfracture in the management of primary lesions without subchondral cysts, as demonstrated in a recent randomized prospective trial comparing the three procedures.[9]

COMPLICATIONS

- Infection
- Wound complication
- Failure of graft incorporation
- Graft failure and potential risk of developing degenerative change
- Articular cartilage delamination or fissuring of the graft
- Malleolar osteotomy nonunion
- Persistent pain despite radiographic suggestion of graft incorporation
- Disease transmission with allograft, but with the current screening practices of tissue banks, this risk is negligible
- Donor site morbidity at the knee

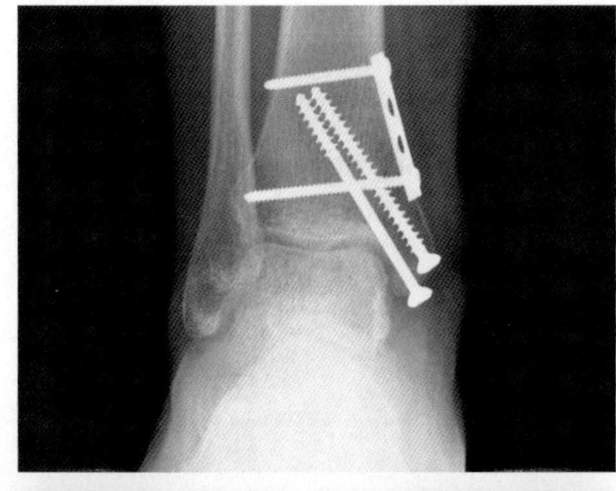

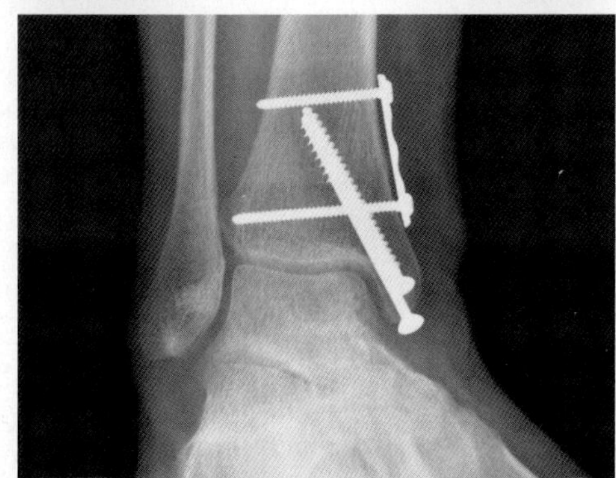

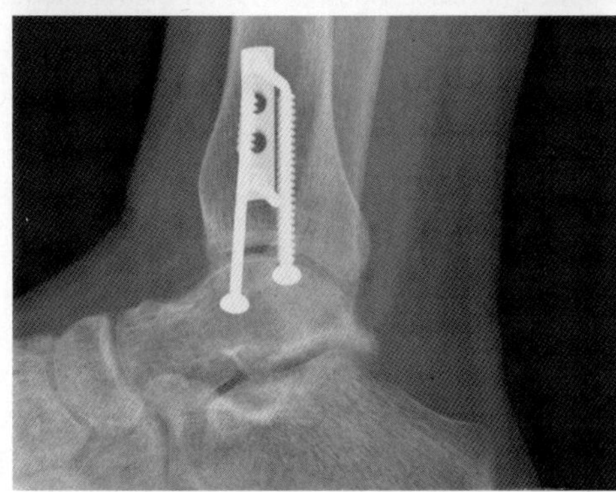

FIG 4 • Postoperative radiographs. **A, B.** AP and mortise views showing anatomic reduction of medial malleolar osteotomy. **C.** Sagittal view.

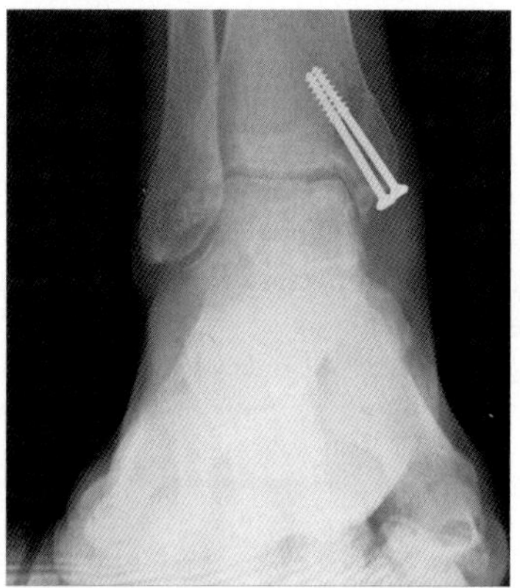

FIG 5 • Different patient undergoing osteochondral transfer. Knee cartilage is thicker than ankle cartilage; thus, despite having anatomic congruency of the graft and adjacent native cartilage, the graft may appear countersunk.

REFERENCES

1. Al-Shaikh RA, Chou LB, Mann JA, et al. Autologous osteochondral grafting for talar cartilage defects. Foot Ankle Int 2002;23:381–389.
2. Baltzer AW, Arnold JP. Bone-cartilage transplantation from the ipsilateral knee for chondral lesions of the talus. Arthroscopy 2005;21: 159–166.
3. Easley ME, Scranton PE, Jr. Osteochondral autologous transfer system. Foot Ankle Clin 2003;8:275–290.
4. Garras DN, Santangelo JA, Wang DW, et al. A quantitative comparison of surgical approaches for posterolateral osteochondral lesions of the talus. Foot Ankle Int 2008;29:415–420.
5. Gobbi A, Francisco RA, Lubowitz JH, et al. Osteochondral lesions of the talus: randomized controlled trial comparing chondroplasty, microfracture, and osteochondral autograft transplantation. [Erratum appears in Arthroscopy 2008 Feb;24(2):A16]. Arthroscopy 2006;22: 1085–1092.
6. Hangody L, Fules P. Autologous osteochondral mosaicplasty for the treatment of full-thickness defects of weight-bearing joints: ten years of experimental and clinical experience. J Bone Joint Surg Am 2003; 85A(Suppl 2):25–32.
7. Hangody L, Kish G, Modis L, et al. Mosaicplasty for the treatment of osteochondritis dissecans of the talus: two to seven year results in 36 patients. Foot Ankle Int 2001;22:552–558.
8. Sammarco GJ, Makwana NK. Treatment of talar osteochondral lesions using local osteochondral graft. Foot Ankle Int 2002;23: 693–698.
9. Scranton PE Jr, Frey CC, Feder KS. Outcome of osteochondral autograft transplantation for type-V cystic osteochondral lesions of the talus. J Bone Joint Surg Br 2006;88:614–619.
10. Tochigi Y, Amendola A, Muir D, et al. Surgical approach for centrolateral talar osteochondral lesions with an anterolateral osteotomy. Foot Ankle Int 2002;23:1038–1039.

Chapter 94 Anterior Tibial Osteotomy for Osteochondral Lesions of the Talus

G. James Sammarco

SURGICAL MANAGEMENT

Patient Positioning

- The patient is positioned supine under appropriate anesthesia, with thigh tourniquet control and a bolster beneath the ipsilateral buttock. The leg, ankle, and foot are prepared and draped from below the knee distally.

Approach

- For a medial lesion a 7-cm anteromedial longitudinal incision is made over the ankle joint parallel to the medial talar facet.
- The soft tissue is dissected to the ankle joint and a capsulotomy performed.
- Enough capsule is stripped from the tibia to expose the medial half of the joint.
- A synovectomy is performed if needed.

TECHNIQUES

TIBIAL OSTEOTOMY USING THE TRAP DOOR

Opening the Tibial Trap Door

- Strip the periosteum proximally along the distal tibial metaphysis to the upper limit of the wound.
  - Make a 1-cm mark on the medial tibial plafond beginning at the angle of Hardy (TECH FIG 1).
  - Make a second mark 3 cm above the joint line.
- Drill two transverse parallel holes across the tibial metaphysis beneath the cortex where the tibial trap door is to be removed. Absorbable pins will be inserted into these predrilled holes when the trap door is replaced after the graft has been inserted in the talar dome.
- Make two vertical parallel saw cuts with a Hall micro-oscillating saw using a no. 64 saw blade (Zimmer, Warsaw, IN) to a depth of 2 cm at the joint surface (TECH FIG 2).
  - Taper these cuts proximally and upward to the anterior tibial metaphysis 3 cm above the joint.
  - To protect the talar surface, insert a Freer elevator between the tibia and talus.
- Make a third horizontal saw cut connecting these cuts at their upper limit.
  - Angle the saw inferiorly and 22 degrees posteriorly from the anterior metaphysis toward the joint surface.
- Use a thin 10-mm osteotome to mobilize the trap door. Remove the trap door and place it aside (TECH FIG 3).

Coring Out the Lesion

- Plantarflex the ankle to deliver the osteochondral lesion into view (TECH FIG 4).
- Probe the lesion to determine its exact location.
- Select the appropriate-size coring instrument (Arthrex, MA): 6, 8, or 10 mm.
- Place the coring instrument at right angles to the talar dome and extract the lesion.
- The removed bone is to be used later.

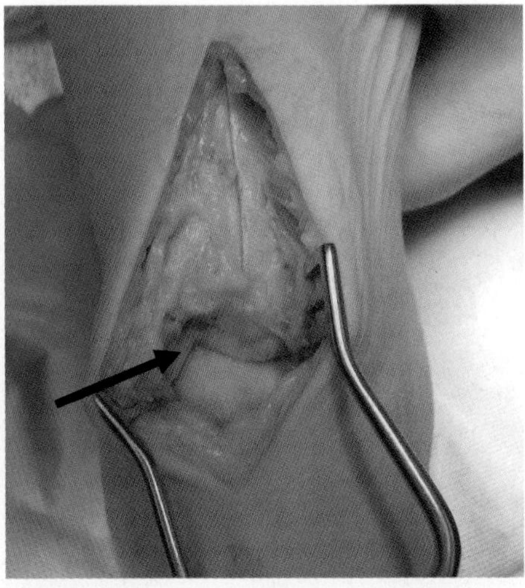

TECH FIG 1 • A 7-cm anteromedial incision exposing the medial half of the ankle joint, showing the angle of Hardy (*arrow*).

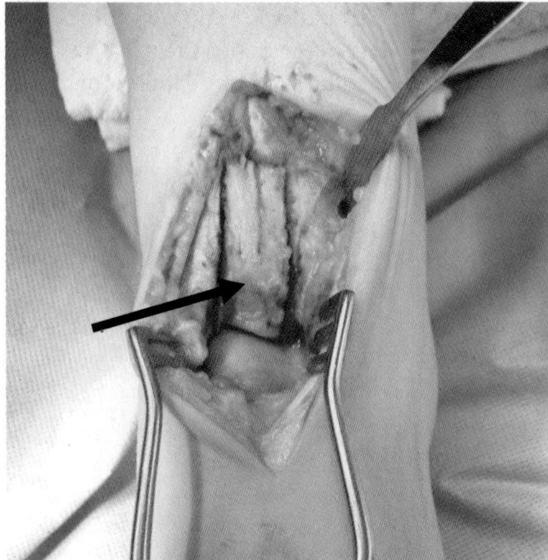

TECH FIG 2 • Saw cuts are made 1 cm wide, 3 cm high, and 2 cm deep (not seen), creating a trap door (*arrow*).

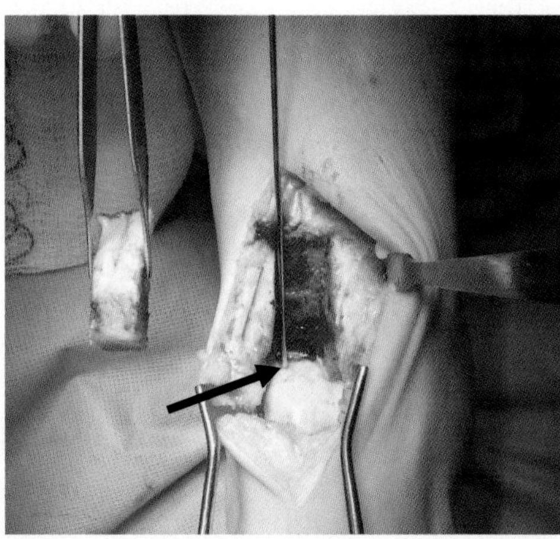

TECH FIG 3 • The trap door is removed and set aside to be replaced after the graft is inserted. A probe has been inserted into the lesion (*arrow*).

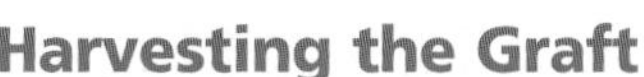

Harvesting the Graft

- Expose the medial facet of the talar body using a mini-Hohmann retractor with the ankle in plantarflexion.
- Position the harvesting instrument on the medial facet 4 mm beneath the talar dome.
- Harvest the graft in such a way that when inserted into the recipient site, the slightly elevated inferior margin of the graft from the medial facet will be oriented toward the medial border of the talar dome, approximating the shape of the normal talar weight-bearing surface (**TECH FIG 5**).

Inserting the Graft

- Débride the talar recipient site and tap the osteochondral graft into place with the inferior medial facet portion oriented toward the medial border of the talus (**TECH FIG 6**).

Filling the Donor Site

- Insert the material that was removed, including the osteochondral lesion, in the donor site.
- This can be augmented with cancellous bone taken from the distal tibia.

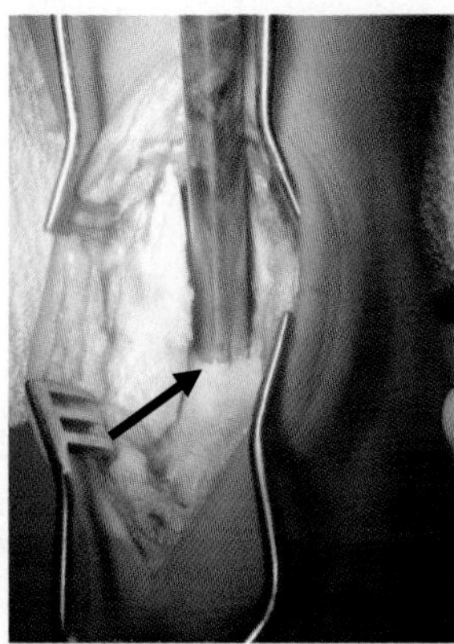

TECH FIG 4 • The ankle is plantarflexed to expose the lesion and a premeasured 8-mm coring device is used to remove the lesion (*arrow*).

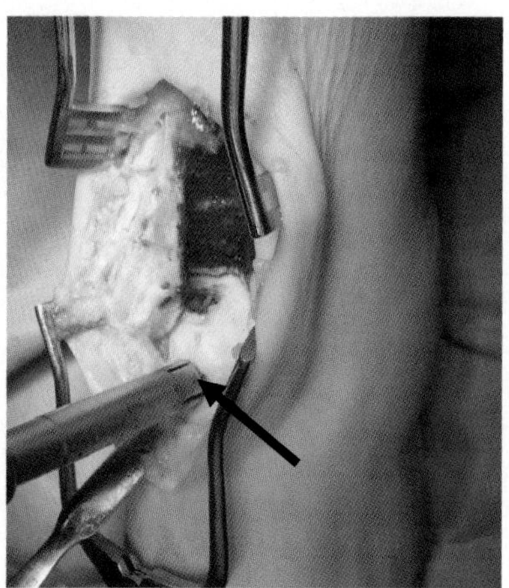

TECH FIG 5 • The osteochondral graft is harvested from the anterior portion of the medial facet 4 mm below the articular surface of the talar dome and at least 10 mm away from the recipient site (*arrow*).

Closing the Trap Door

- Insert the tibial bone block back into its bed and insert bioabsorbable pins (Biosorb, Johnson & Johnson, Princeton, NJ) into the predrilled holes to secure the bone block in place (**TECH FIG 7**).

Wound Closure and Postoperative Care

- Approximate the deep tissues with 3-0 absorbable suture and close the skin with 3-0 monofilament nylon.
- Apply a compression dressing and posterior splint; they are changed at the first follow-up visit.
- Sutures are removed at 2 weeks and a non–weight-bearing short-leg cast is used for 1 month.
- A range-of-motion boot is then prescribed with 50% weight bearing for 3 weeks, after which physical therapy is instituted.

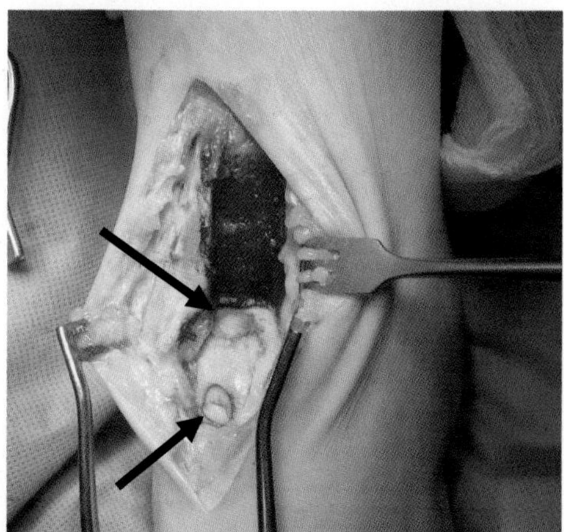

TECH FIG 6 • The osteochondral graft has been inserted into the recipient site (*upper arrow*) and the bony material removed, including attached remaining cartilage from the defect that has been inserted into the donor site (*lower arrow*).

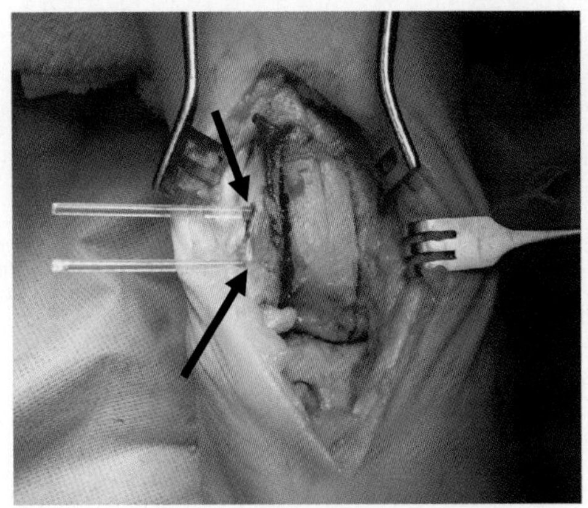

TECH FIG 7 • The trap door is replaced and secured with bioabsorbable pins (*arrows*) placed into predrilled holes.

ADDITIONAL TECHNIQUE

- If the bone at the base of recipient site is excessively sclerotic, it may be drilled using a 0.045 Kirschner wire before inserting the graft in order to encourage vascular ingrowth.
- For lesions on the lateral talar dome, use the same technique but make the most lateral vertical saw cut 2 mm away from the distal tibiofibular syndesmosis to avoid violating the joint.

PEARLS AND PITFALLS

- This technique avoids the need for a medial malleolar osteotomy. It provides excellent visualization of and access to the lesion through a single incision while avoiding a second procedure on an asymptomatic knee to harvest the graft.
- The procedure is best suited for lesions up to 10 mm in diameter and up to 10 mm deep located in the anterior two thirds of the medial or lateral talar dome margins.
- The graft can be placed just beneath the subchondral bone of the medial or lateral facet since these surfaces bear minimal weight, and no complications have been noted in the medial or lateral gutters.
- The surgeon should avoid making the vertical saw cuts more than 3 cm deep at the joint surface or 4 cm in height since this increases the risk of a medial malleolar stress fracture.
- In harvesting the osteochondral graft, the surgeon should avoid taking the graft too near the talar surface or too near the recipient site in order to avoid a stress fracture of the talar dome.
- Patients with arthritis can have progression of the condition even though the graft becomes incorporated and survives.
- The most common minor complaint is occasional aching at the anteromedial joint line with activity.

REFERENCE

1. Sammarco GJ, Makwana NK. Treatment of talar osteochondral lesions using local osteochondral graft. Foot Ankle Int 2002;22:693–698.

Chapter 95 Osteochondral Lesions of the Talus: Structural Allograft

Mark E. Easley, Samuel B. Adams, Jr., and James A. Nunley II

DEFINITION

- Large osteochondral defects of the talar dome, typically involving the talar shoulder (transition of superior dome cartilage to the medial or lateral talar cartilage), and also often associated with large-volume subchondral cysts

ANATOMY

- Sixty percent of the talus' surface area is covered by articular cartilage.
- The talus is contained within the ankle mortise.
  - Superior talar dome articulates with the tibial plafond.
  - Medial dome articulates with the medial malleolus.
  - Lateral dome articulates with the lateral malleolus.
- Talar blood supply
  - Posterior tibial artery
    - Artery of the tarsal canal
    - Deltoid ligament branch
  - Peroneal artery
    - Artery of the tarsal sinus
  - Dorsalis pedis artery

PATHOGENESIS

- The pathogenesis for osteochondral lesions of the talus (OLTs) is not fully understood.
- Theories include:
  - Trauma
  - Idiopathic focal avascular necrosis

NATURAL HISTORY

- In general, OLTs do not progress to diffuse ankle arthritis.
- However, large-volume OLTs may lead to subchondral collapse of a substantial portion of the talus and thus create deformity, higher contact stresses, and a greater concern for eventual ankle arthritis if left untreated.

PATIENT HISTORY AND PHYSICAL FINDINGS

- Patients may or may not report a history of trauma.
- Ankle pain, typically on the anterior aspect of the ankle, is a common complaint.
  - Pain is usually experienced on the side of the ankle that corresponds with the OLT, but it may be poorly localized to the site of the OLT. In fact, sometimes medial OLTs produce lateral ankle pain and vice versa.
  - Pain is rarely sharp, unless a fragment of the OLT should act as an impinging loose body in the joint.
  - It is typically a deep ache, with and after activity, and is usually relieved with rest.
- Antalgic gait
- May be associated with malalignment or ankle instability
- Typically tenderness on side of ankle that corresponds with OLT, but not always
- Rarely crepitance or mechanical symptoms
- With chronic OLT, some degree of ankle stiffness anticipated

IMAGING AND OTHER DIAGNOSTIC STUDIES

- Plain radiographs
  - Small OLTs may be missed.
  - Large OLTs are usually identified on plain radiographs, three views of the ankle, weight-bearing.
  - Radiographs are often limited in characterizing OLTs since the two-dimensional study cannot define the three-dimensional OLT.
  - Particularly useful in assessing lower leg, ankle, or foot malalignment, which needs to be considered in the management of OLTs
  - May detect incidental OLTs (patient has radiograph for a different problem and an OLT is incidentally identified on plain radiographs)
- MRI
  - Excellent screening tool when OLT or other foot–ankle pathology is suspected
  - Will identify incidental OLT, but defines other potential soft tissue pathology
  - Demonstrates associated marrow edema that may lead to overestimation of the OLT's size
- CT
  - Ideal for characterizing OLTs, particularly large-volume defects
  - Defines OLT size without distraction of associated marrow edema
  - Defines the character of the OLT and extent of its involvement in the talar dome
- Diagnostic injection
  - Intra-articular
  - An anesthetic versus anesthetic plus corticosteroid
  - May have some therapeutic effect, even for several months
  - If the source of pain is the OLT, then intra-articular injection should relieve symptoms from OLT (and any intra-articular pathology). If the pain is not relieved, then extra-articular diagnoses should be considered.

DIFFERENTIAL DIAGNOSIS

- Loose body in ankle joint
- Ankle impingement (anterior or posterior)
- Chronic ankle instability (lateral or syndesmosis)
- Ankle synovitis or adjacent tendinopathy
- Early ankle degenerative change

NONOPERATIVE MANAGEMENT

- Activity modification
- Bracing
- Physical therapy if associated ankle instability

- Nonsteroidal anti-inflammatories or COX-2 inhibitors
- Corticosteroid injection
- Viscosupplementation?

SURGICAL MANAGEMENT

Preoperative Planning

- Indications for this surgery include:
  - Large-volume OLTs not amenable to other joint-sparing procedures
  - Failed arthroscopic surgery (débridement and microfracture)
  - Failed open procedures (cylindrical osteochondral transfer)
- Large-volume OLTs typically are not amenable to autologous osteochondral transfer (talus or knee).
- We favor reconstruction of the large talar defect with an allograft talus. While we prefer fresh allograft tissue, we have on occasion used fresh-frozen tissue.
- Scheduling of this procedure with fresh allograft tissue is similar to organ transplantation but with a wider window for implantation after procurement.
  - Multiple tissue banks have the ability to obtain fresh allograft tali.
  - Once a donor talus is identified, the tissue bank performs appropriate screening.
  - If the talus is deemed safe for implantation and represents a match based on radiographic size, on average 14 to 21 days of reasonable chondrocyte viability remains for the talar allograft to be used.
- While fresh structural talar allograft reconstruction for large-volume OLTs has gained a foothold as an accepted treatment among reconstructive foot and ankle surgeons, not all third-party payers cover this procedure. We do not seek an allograft talus for our patients from the tissue banks until our patient has secured insurance coverage for the procedure.
- In seeking an allograft talus that is suited for the patient, the surgeon must:
  - Be sure that the talus is the correct side (right or left)
  - Provide the tissue bank with the optimal size of talar graft. Tissue banks use different methods for talar sizing.
    - Plain radiographic dimensions (if the defect in the diseased talus is particularly large, making measurements difficult, radiographs of the healthy, contralateral talus may be needed)
    - CT scan measurements (may be more accurate, with measurements possible in three dimensions)
- The surgeon should check for associated pathology that may need to be addressed at the time of allograft talar reconstruction:
  - Osteophyte removal
  - Ligament reconstruction
  - Corrective osteotomies
    - Calcaneal
    - Supramalleolar
- The surgeon determines the optimal surgical approach.
  - In our hands, this depends on the amount of talus that will be reconstructed.
  - A portion of the medial talar dome (usually posteromedial) typically warrants a medial malleolar osteotomy.
  - A portion of the lateral talar dome (often centrolateral) typically necessitates ligament releases (anterior talofibular and calcaneofibular) with or without lateral malleolar osteotomy.
  - Involvement of the majority of the medial or lateral talar dome, particularly if involving its respective talar shoulder, usually can be performed through an anterior approach without osteotomy by replacing one third to one half of the talar dome.
- Patient education
  - This is a complex procedure.
  - The patient must understand that the intent is to implant allograft tissue.
  - There is a negligible, but real, risk of disease transmission and possible graft rejection by the host.
  - There is no guarantee that the procedure will work, and a revision procedure may be required, such as arthrodesis, which will eliminate joint motion.

Positioning

- Before anesthesia and moving the patient into the operating room, the surgeon should inspect the allograft to be sure it is the correct side (right or left) and for cartilage defects that may be present directly at the site that the graft is to be harvested.
- The patient is positioned supine.
- For a lateral OLT, a bolster under the ipsilateral hip typically affords better access to the lateral talar dome.
- We routinely use a thigh tourniquet.

Approach

- As noted above, the approach depends on the size and location of the OLT.
- For medial OLTs amenable to reconstruction of only a portion of the medial talar dome: direct medial approach, similar to that for open reduction and internal fixation (ORIF) of a medial malleolar fracture, with a medial malleolar osteotomy
- For lateral OLTs amenable to reconstruction of only a portion of the lateral talar dome: lateral approach, combining typical approaches for ORIF of a fibular fracture and the extensile exposure for a modified Brostrom procedure
- For large medial or lateral OLTs, involving the majority of the medial or lateral talar shoulder: anterior approach, similar to that for ankle arthrodesis or total ankle arthroplasty; typically no malleolar osteotomy is required.

STRUCTURAL ALLOGRAFT RECONSTRUCTION OF CONTAINED MEDIAL OSTEOCHONDRAL LESIONS OF THE TALUS

Approach and Oblique Medial Malleolar Osteotomy

- Make a curvilinear incision over the medial malleolus, similar to that for ORIF of a medial malleolar fracture.
- Protect the saphenous vein and accompanying saphenous nerves.
- Anterior ankle arthrotomy (**TECH FIG 1A**)
  - Defines anterior joint margin for safe performance of medial malleolar osteotomy
  - Allows partial visualization of the OLT and allows confirmation that there is not diffuse articular cartilage degeneration
- Open the posterior tibial tendon sheath–flexor retinaculum, directly on the posterior margin of the tibia and

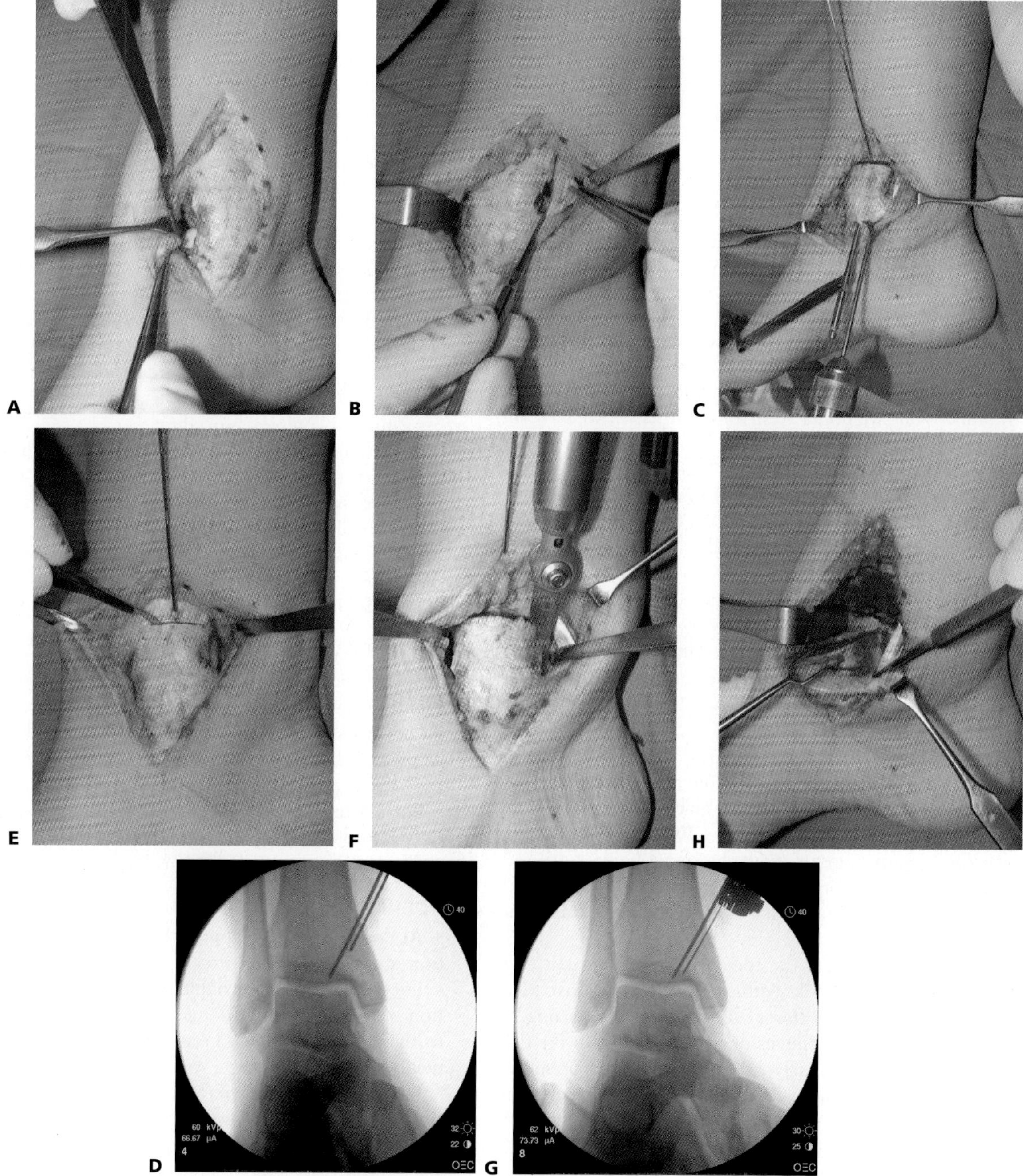

TECH FIG 1 • **A.** Medial incision and anterior ankle arthrotomy. **B.** Opening of the posterior tibial tendon sheath. **C.** Predrilling of medial malleolus. Kirschner wire for trajectory of medial malleolar osteotomy has already been inserted and its position confirmed with fluoroscopy. **D.** Fluoroscopic image demonstrating Kirschner wire being used as a guide to direct the saw. **E.** The periosteum is scored perpendicular to the tibial shaft, at the level of the osteotomy. **F.** Medial malleolar osteotomy. Care must be taken to protect the posterior tibial tendon. **G.** Fluoroscopic image showing near-complete bone cut. **H.** Release of posterior tibial tendon sheath from distal medial malleolus to allow mobilization.

medial malleolus (TECH FIG 1B). Protect the posterior tibial tendon: it rests in a groove immediately posterior to the tibia and is at great risk with a medial malleolar osteotomy.

- Predrill the medial malleolus across the proposed osteotomy site (TECH FIG 1C).
  - We routinely use two small fragment malleolar screws and predrill with the corresponding drill.
  - Obtain fluoroscopic confirmation that the drill bits are in the proper trajectory.
  - Consider passing a tap as well.
- Place a Kirschner wire obliquely to define the trajectory of the medial malleolar osteotomy (TECH FIG 1C).
  - Place it slightly proximal to the desired osteotomy so it can function as a guide but not interfere with the saw (TECH FIG 1D).

- Confirm the optimal Kirschner wire trajectory with intraoperative fluoroscopy.
- Ideally, the Kirschner wire will extend to the lateral margin of the OLT, but with large-volume OLTs that may be too much and unnecessary. However, in our experience, making the osteotomy only to the axilla of the tibial plafond where it meets the medial malleolus will not allow adequate access to perform ideal recipient-site preparation.

- Determine a plane for the osteotomy in the AP plane that is perpendicular to the longitudinal axis of the tibia. We find it helpful to score the osteotomy in the periosteum from anterior to posterior to determine this level (TECH FIG 1E).
- Periosteal stripping is unnecessary; it may be limited to the osteotomy site.
- With a microsagittal saw oriented correctly in both planes, the osteotomy is initiated (TECH FIG 1F).
  - Use cool saline to limit the risk of heat necrosis to the bone.
  - Obtain intraoperative fluoroscopy shortly after initiating the osteotomy; leave the saw blade in place to confirm proper trajectory. If incorrect, a subtle adjustment is still possible (TECH FIG 1G).
- Continue the osteotomy with the saw to the subchondral bone and then complete the osteotomy with a chisel.
  - A fluoroscopic spot view allows the surgeon to confirm that the osteotomy is appropriate and is not violating the talar cartilage.
  - There may be some irregularity to the osteotomy at the posterior margin; this is typical as the osteotomy is mobilized. It may be advantageous as it allows for an interference fit during reduction of the osteotomy and perhaps greater stability.
- Reflect the medial malleolus.
  - The posterior tibial tendon sheath must be released to the distal aspect of the posterior medial malleolus to allow the malleolus to reflect adequately and to gain optimal exposure of the medial talar dome (TECH FIG 1H). Protect the deltoid ligament fibers.

Preparing the Recipient Site

- Define the extent of the OLT (TECH FIG 2A,B).
  - Clinical inspection
  - Review of CT scan
- If the talar defect appears amenable to structural allograft reconstruction, have the donor talus placed on the back table and protected in a saline-soaked sponge.
- Excise the diseased portion of the talus (TECH FIG 2C–F).
  - Reciprocating and microsagittal saw (use cool saline to limit risk of heat necrosis)
  - May need a small curette and rasp as well

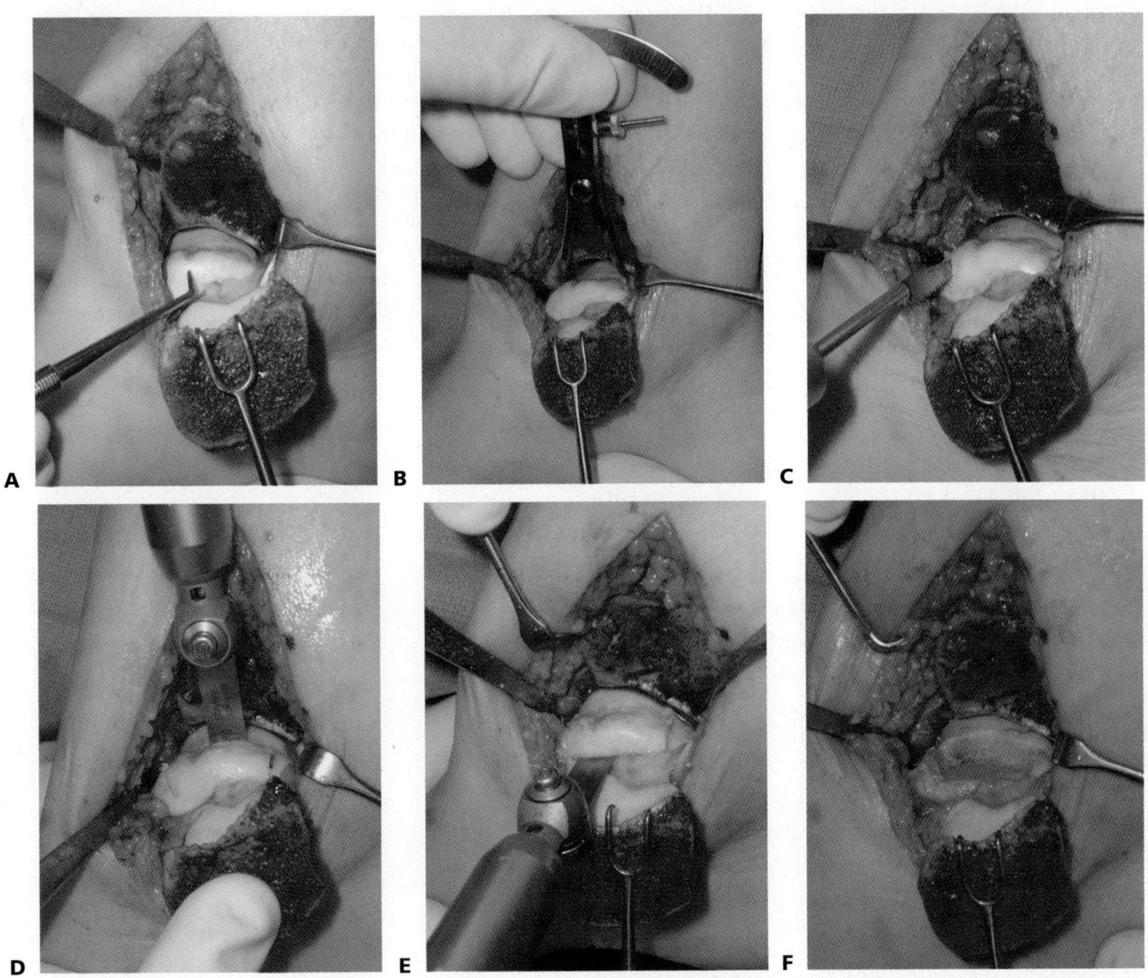

TECH FIG 2 • **A, B.** Identifying the extent of the talar shoulder lesion. **C–E.** Excision of the talar shoulder lesion using the microsagittal and oscillating saws. **F.** Talar shoulder lesion removed.

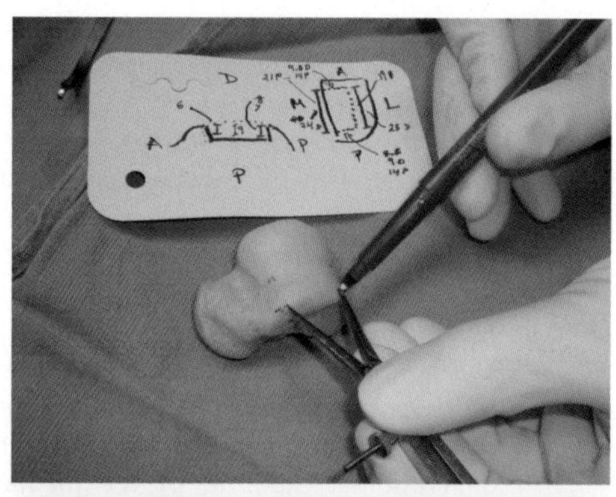

A

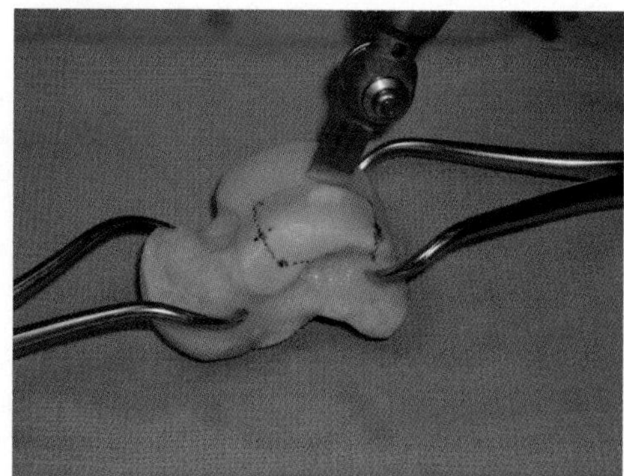

B

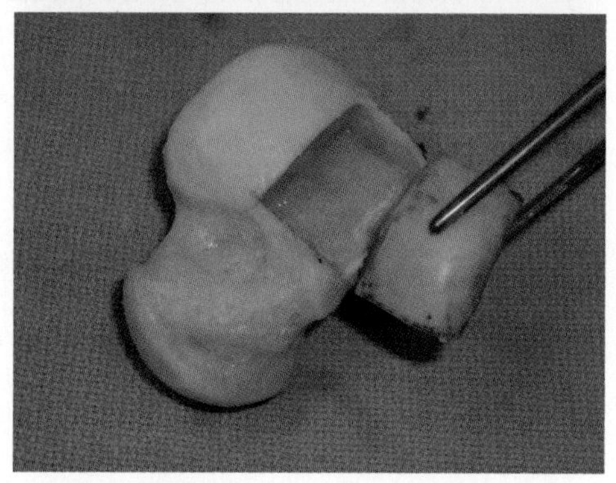

C

TECH FIG 3 • **A.** The dimensions of the recipient site are carefully recorded and transferred to the allograft. **B.** Two pointed reduction clamps are used to stabilize the allograft during preparation. **C.** Donor allograft with newly prepared graft removed.

- Define the dimensions of the recipient site. Use a caliper and a ruler and double-check the measurements.

Harvesting Graft from Donor Talus

- Handle the allograft talus with bone forceps.
- Properly orient the talus (compare to native talus) to ensure that the cuts will be congruent and in the same plane as those for the recipient site.
- Carefully mark the dimensions for graft harvest on the allograft (TECH FIG 3A).
  - Same location on the allograft talus as the recipient site on the native talus
  - If you err, err to have the graft slightly too large. Be sure to account for saw blade thickness.
- "Measure twice and cut once."
  - You have only one opportunity, so be sure the measurements and orientation of the saw blade for each cut are optimal.
  - The allograft can be stabilized with two large pointed reduction clamps (TECH FIG 3B).
- Extract the graft from the donor talus (TECH FIG 3C).
- Reduce the immunogenic load from the graft by washing the graft's cancellous surfaces with saline.

Implanting and Securing the Graft into the Recipient Site

- Only once have we had a graft match perfectly on the first attempt. The graft and recipient site will almost always need to be tailored slightly to allow optimal graft fit.
- It is unlikely that a perfect clinical and fluoroscopic match will be achieved. Attempt to achieve the best clinical match of the graft's articular surface with the surrounding native cartilage (TECH FIG 4A).
- If the clinical match is appropriate, then the fluoroscopic match is not important.
  - There is a lot of variability in cartilage thickness and talar architecture in the human talus.
  - It is difficult to get four surfaces to congruently match.
- Graft fixation
  - Ideally, the graft will have some interference fit.
  - We routinely secure the graft with one or two small-diameter solid screws (1.5 or 2.0 mm in diameter). One is typically placed from dorsal to plantar, the other from medial to lateral (if the depth of the graft will allow) (TECH FIG 4B,C).

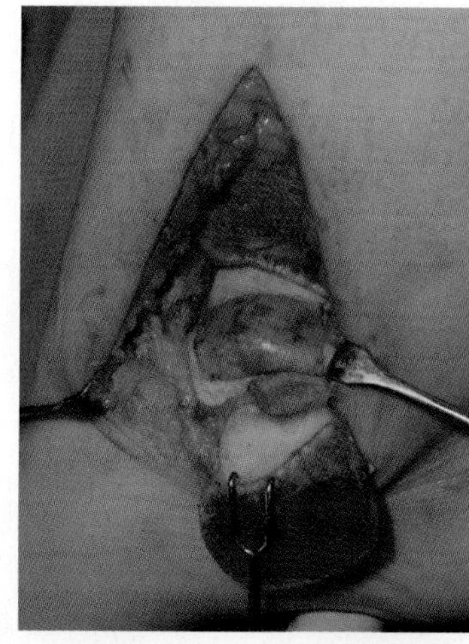

A

TECH FIG 4 • **A–C.** Fitting and securing the graft to the native talus. **A.** After contouring the graft (some minor discoloration from debris while manipulating graft on back table; it is easily washed away). *(continued)*

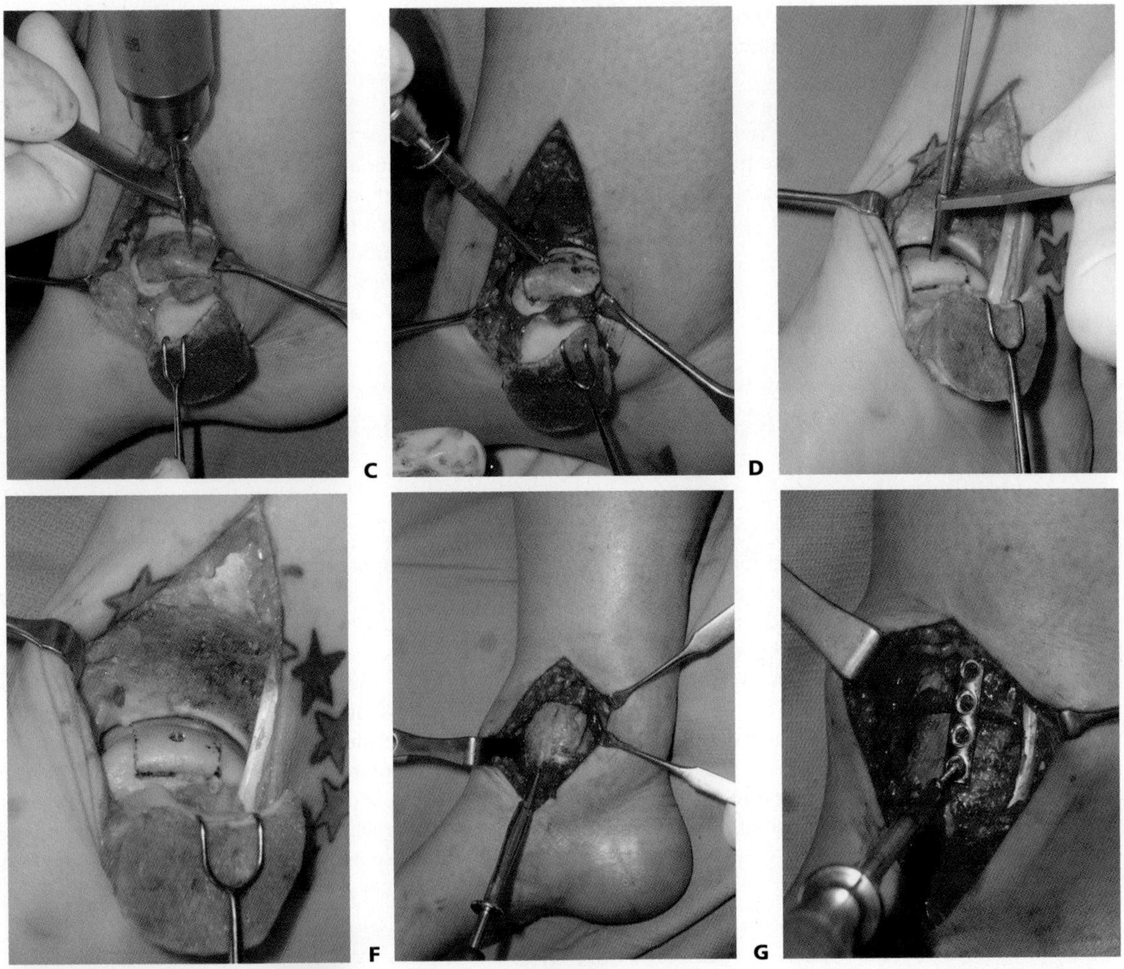

B C D E F G H

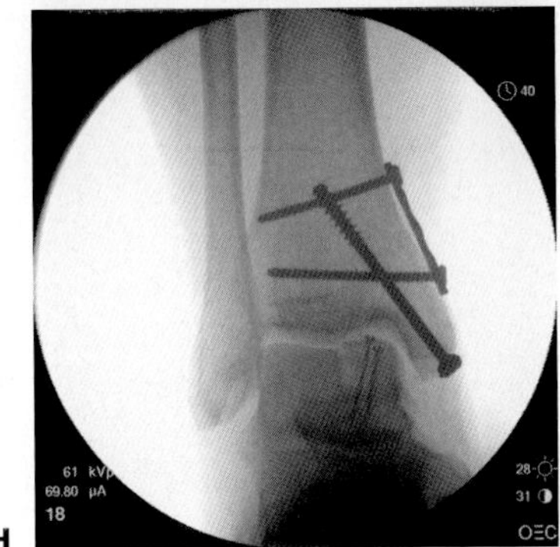

TECH FIG 4 • *(continued)* **B.** Drill hole perpendicular to graft. **C.** Securing graft with two countersunk screws. **D,E.** A different patient with similar graft; excellent interference fit and secured with a single screw. **D.** Screw is inserted in lag fashion. **E.** Screw head is countersunk. **F–H.** Reduction of the medial malleolar osteotomy. **F.** Screw fixation through the predrilled holes. **G.** Antiglide plate. **H.** Final fluoroscopic evaluation of graft and reduction of medial malleolar osteotomy. Despite optimal clinical fit of the graft, rarely does the fluoroscopic appearance suggest anatomic graft match to the native talus, typically due to differing cartilage thicknesses between the donor and the host. While the screws may appear prominent, two-dimensional fluoroscopy is deceiving since the screws are countersunk below the articular surface of the graft and the talar dome is curved.

  - Place the screws in lag fashion.
  - Countersink the screw heads below the articular surface (TECH FIG 4D,E).
- Using fluoroscopy, confirmn that the graft and hardware are in optimal position (TECH FIG 4F–H).
  - The graft will not look perfect fluoroscopically, but as long as the clinical appearance is acceptable, the outcome has a good chance to be favorable.
  - The hardware may appear slightly proud fluoroscopically despite being countersunk. The talar dome is not a flat plane, and therefore the screw may seem to be protruding. Moreover, the articular cartilage is rather thick compared to such a low-profile screw head.

Medial Malleolar Osteotomy Reduction and Closure

- Irrigate the joint.
- Reduce the medial malleolus. Confirm the reduction through the anteromedial arthrotomy and posteriorly behind the posterior tibial tendon.
- Place the two screws in the predrilled holes and tighten the screws.
- While not essential for healing, we favor placing an antiglide plate over the proximal aspect of the osteotomy.
- Using fluoroscopy, confirm reduction of the graft and medial malleolus (see Tech Fig 4).

- Anticipate some incongruencies of the graft–native talus bony interfaces. It is difficult to achieve perfectly congruent apposition.
- There will be a slight gap at the medial malleolar osteotomy site despite anatomic reduction of the medial malleolus. This is due to the thickness of the saw blade. However, it is not acceptable to see a step-off at the osteotomy site where it enters the tibial plafond; this must be anatomic.
- The slight gaps at the graft and medial malleolus do not typically impair healing and should obliterate with eventual remodeling.

- Closure
  - Posterior tibial tendon sheath and flexor retinaculum
  - Anterior arthrotomy
  - Subcutaneous layer
  - Skin to a tensionless closure
  - We routinely use a drain.
  - Dressings, padding, and a posterior–sugar-tong splint with the ankle in neutral position

HEMI-TALUS RECONSTRUCTION OF MEDIAL OSTEOCHONDRAL LESION OF THE TALUS

Preoperative Evaluation

- Patient is a 40-year-old man with chronic ankle pain failing prior arthroscopic débridement and microfracture. Feels he is overloading lateral border of foot.
- Preoperative weight-bearing radiographs suggest large medial OLT and varus malalignment with some varus talar tilt (**TECH FIG 5A,B**).
- CT demonstrates large-volume medial OLT (**TECH FIG 5C–E**).
- Before proceeding to the operating room, confirm that the allograft talus is the one intended for this patient, is available, and has not expired.

Approach

- Anterior approach (**TECH FIG 6**)
  - Similar to anterior approach for ankle arthrodesis and total ankle arthroplasty
  - Protect the superficial peroneal nerve.
  - Divide the extensor retinaculum over the extensor hallucis longus tendon.
  - Protect the deep neurovascular bundle.
  - Anterior capsulotomy. Unlike ankle arthrodesis and total ankle arthroplasty, must protect ankle cartilage.
  - Expose OLT with plantarflexion. Assess mediolateral dimensions and attempt to assess AP dimensions.

A
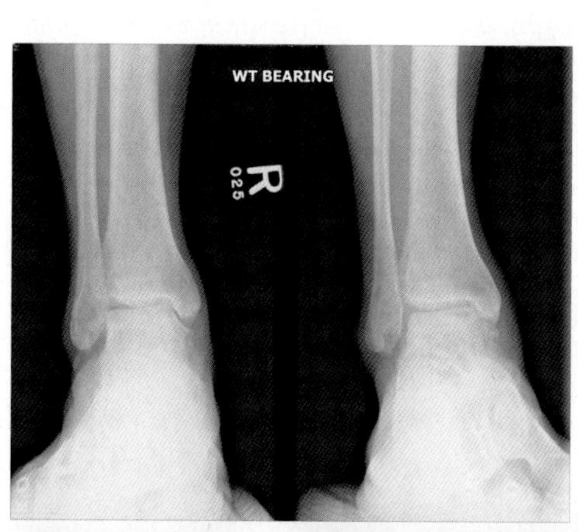

B
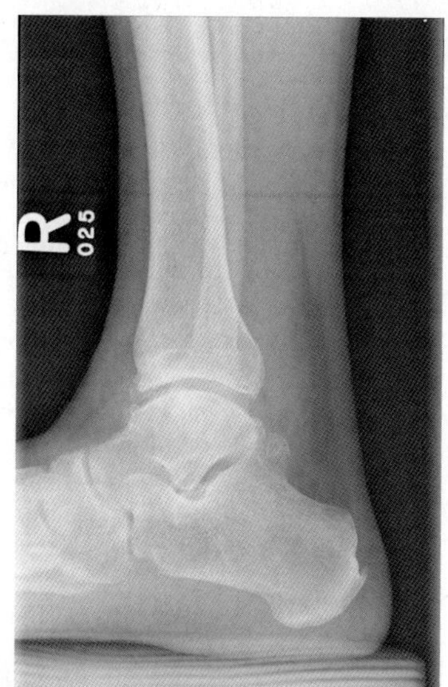

C
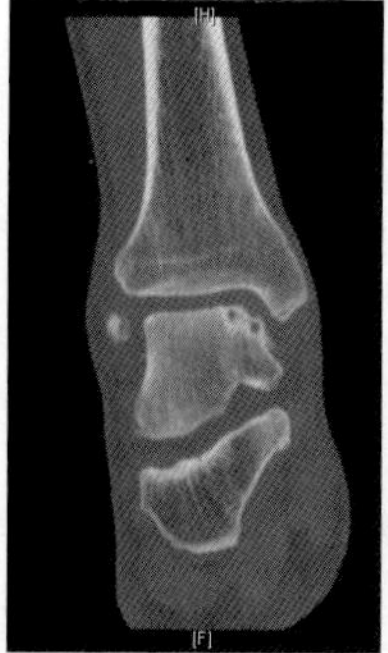

D
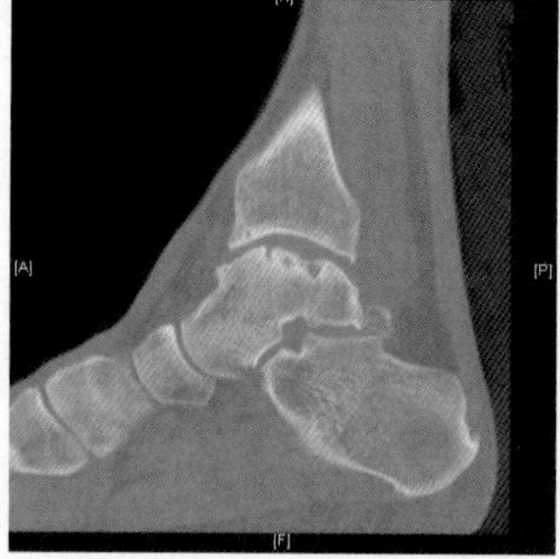

E
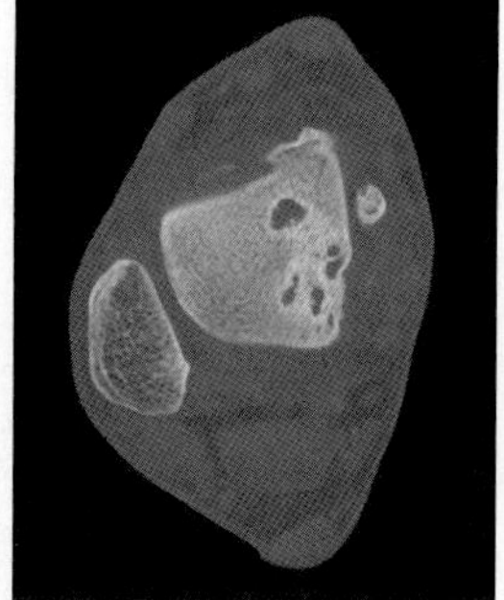

TECH FIG 5 • A, B. Preoperative radiographs. **A.** AP and mortise ankle views suggest large medial talar dome OLT and varus alignment. **B.** Lateral radiograph. **C–E.** Preoperative CT of large-volume OLT. **C.** Coronal view. **D.** Sagittal view. **E.** Axial view.

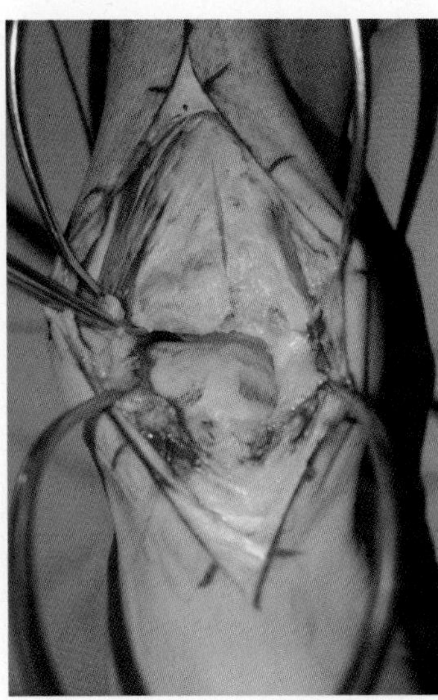

TECH FIG 6 • Anterior approach, similar to that performed for total ankle arthroplasty. Since the entire medial one third to one half of the talar dome will be restructured, a medial malleolar osteotomy is typically not necessary.

- If the talus appears appropriate for an allograft talus, ask to have the donor talus opened and soaking in a warm saline-soaked sponge on the back table. At this point, though, this only expedites the procedure; it is not as though the talus may be returned. . .that patient now owns that talus.

Preparing the Recipient Site

- Joint distraction, preferably with an extra-articular distraction device
- Determine dimensions of diseased talus:
  - Clinical assessment
  - Review and correlate with CT.
- Determine exact lateral sagittal border of OLT.
- Make a vertical (sagittal) cut in the talus 1 mm lateral to the lateral extent of the OLT. The depth of this cut should be conservative until the exact superior-to-inferior dimensions of the OLT can be mapped out on the talus (TECH FIG 7A).
- Horizontal (axial) resection in the talus (TECH FIG 7B)
  - To maintain the proper axis, we routinely use a Kirschner wire placed from anterior to posterior, with its trajectory and depth confirmed on intraoperative fluoroscopy, to avoid misdirection of the axial resection.
  - We use a thin oscillating saw for this cut, also with cold saline irrigation to cool the blade in an attempt to avoid heat necrosis to the bone.
  - Protect the medial malleolar cartilage. Consider using a malleable ribbon retractor in the medial gutter.
- Extract the resected bone (TECH FIG 7C,D).
- Revisit the vertical and horizontal resections with the saw, a rasp, or both. If there is residual OLT in either or both of the prepared surfaces, then consider curetting these and bone grafting, or resecting more native talus (TECH FIG 7E).
- Fluoroscopic evaluation sometimes affords a useful appreciation of the recipient site.
- Determining the exact dimensions of the recipient site:
  - Calipers (TECH FIG 7F)
  - Ruler (TECH FIG 7G)
  - We routinely sketch the dimensions on a drawing of the recipient site on a surgical glove envelope or a sterile label on the back table.

Harvesting Graft from the Donor Talus

- Secure the allograft that has been placed on the back table with a bone-holding forceps.
- Mark the dimensions of the recipient site talus on the donor talus. One challenge is to orient the talus properly

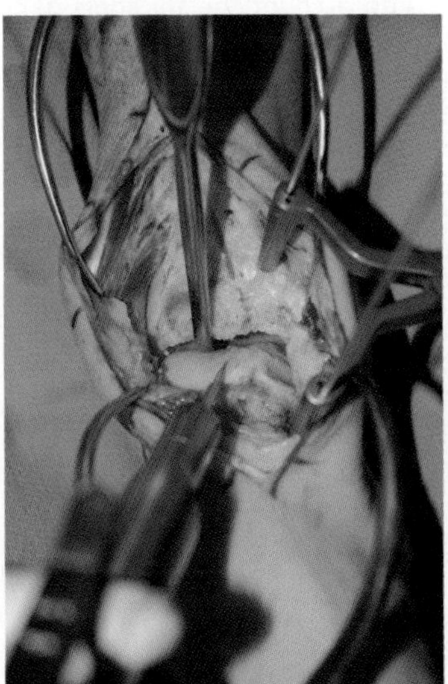

A

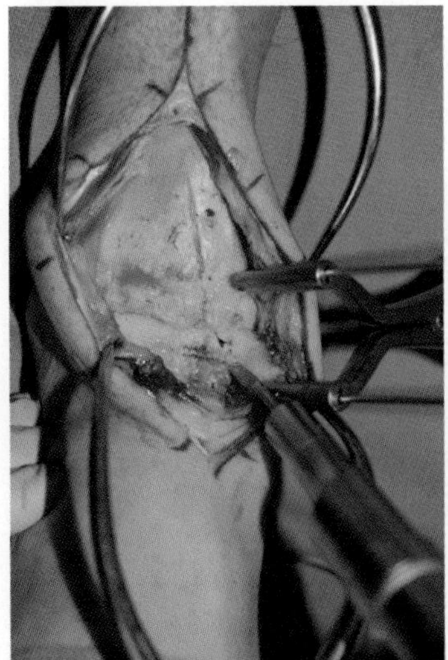

B

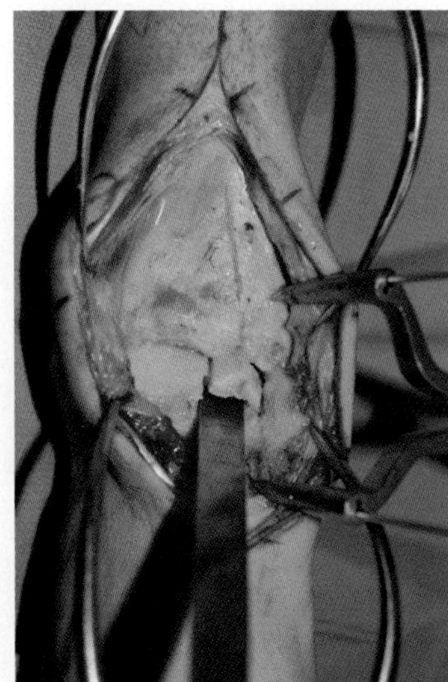

C

TECH FIG 7 • **A–D.** Preparing the recipient site. **A.** Sagittal cut with reciprocating saw. **B.** Axial cut also with reciprocating saw. **C.** Elevating diseased portion of talus with osteotome. *(continued)*

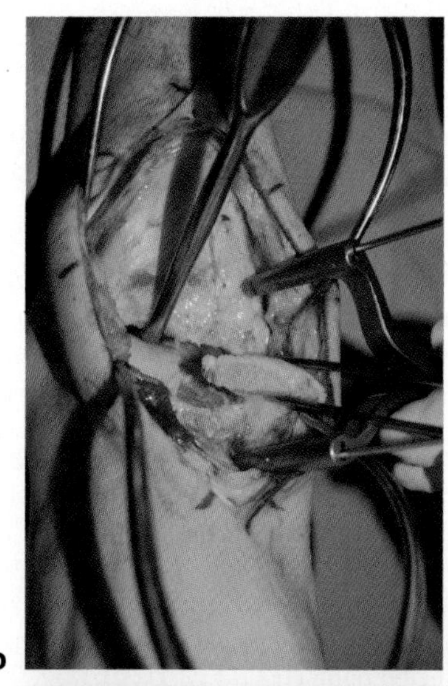

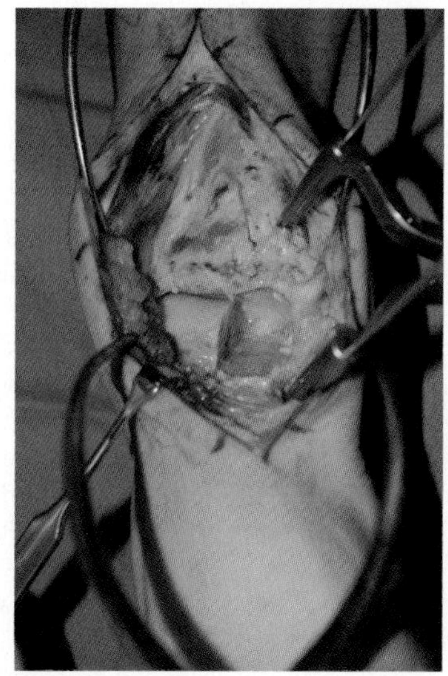

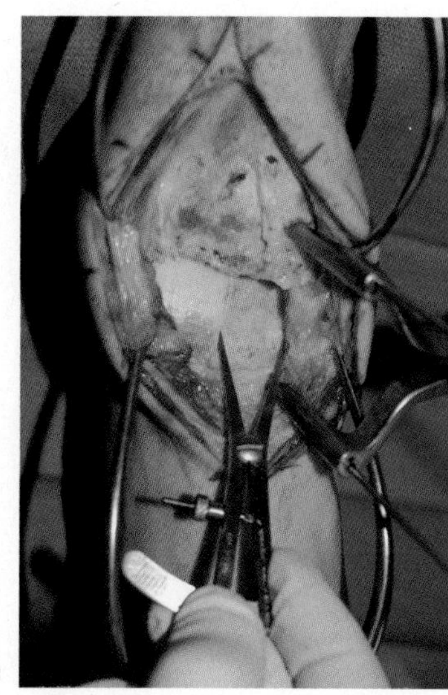

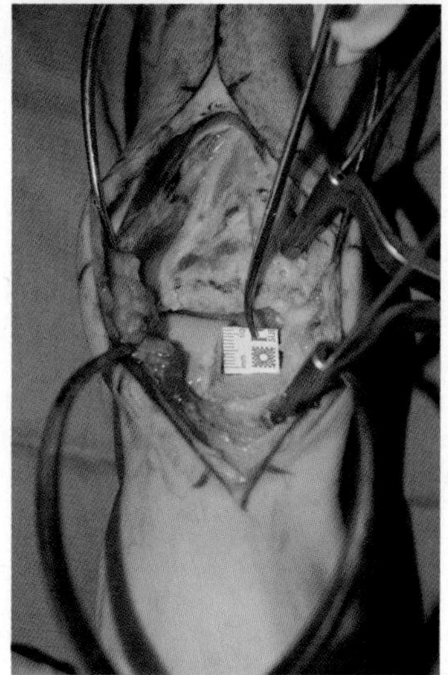

TECH FIG 7 • *(continued)* **D.** Extracting diseased portion. **E.** Further extraction of diseased cartilage until healthy-appearing cancellous surface is apparent. **F,G.** Measuring dimensions of recipient site. **F.** Caliper. **G.** Modified ruler.

to ensure that the two cuts will be in the optimal planes to congruently match the recipient site.

- Double-check the measurements.
  - You have only one chance to harvest this graft.
  - "Measure twice, cut once."
- Make the cuts to harvest the talus (TECH FIG 8).
  - Attempt to match the recipient site dimensions exactly, taking into account the thickness of the saw blade.
  - If you have to err, then err on the side of harvesting a graft that is too large. Fine-tuning the graft is

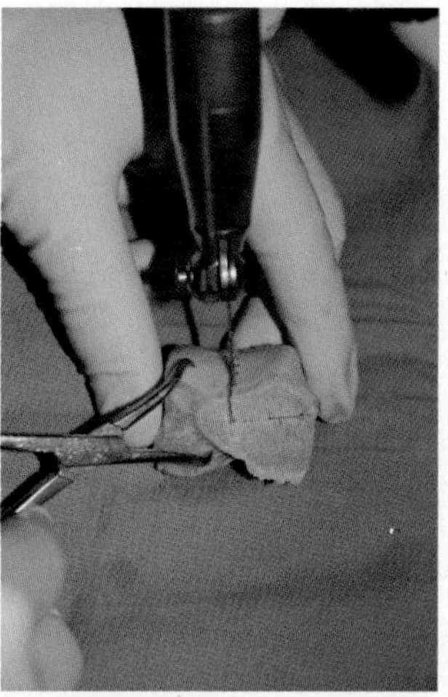

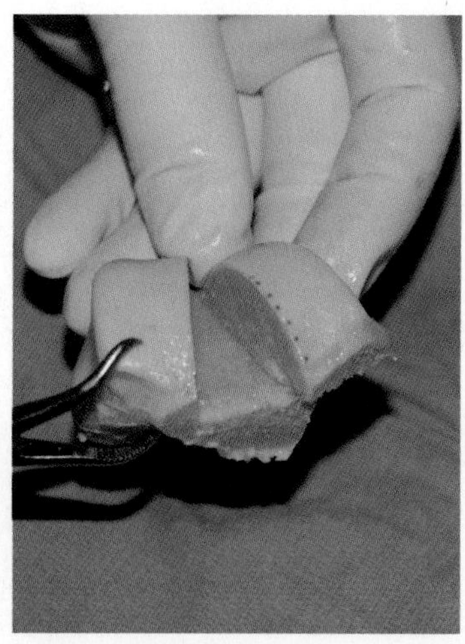

TECH FIG 8 • Harvesting graft from donor talus. **A.** Sagittal cut with oscillating saw. **B.** After completion of axial cut.

sometimes difficult, but it is still possible to downsize it or increase the size of the recipient site; it is not possible to augment the graft or reduce the size of the recipient site once the graft has been harvested.

- We routinely wash the graft's cancellous surfaces with saline in an attempt to decrease the immunogenic load before implantation. However, we have no evidence to support this practice and perform this purely on an empiric basis.

Implanting and Securing Graft into Recipient Site

- Place the graft in the recipient site (TECH FIG 9A,B).
- We have never had a perfect match on the first attempt at seating the graft in the recipient site.
- Tailoring the graft to match the recipient site is often challenging.
  - In our hands this requires a slight deepening of the recipient site and a slight thinning of the graft.
  - Making the corresponding sagittal and axial talar cuts congruently is the most important step in achieving an optimal fit of the graft.
- Only once have we achieved a perfect graft match clinically and fluoroscopically.
  - The human talus is quite variable and regardless of the match, some inconsistencies will be present.
  - While the clinical appearance may suggest a near-perfect match, we routinely see slight incongruencies in the sagittal and axial preparations and what appears to be a slight mismatch to the native subchondral bone.
  - In our experience, however, these are not clinically relevant and some degree of remodeling during graft incorporation is anticipated.
- Fixation of the graft to the native talus (TECH FIG 9C–G)
  - We routinely use two solid small-diameter screws (1.5 or 2.0 mm) placed in lag fashion to secure the graft to the native talus.
  - These are placed anteriorly and countersunk below the articular surface, typically anterior to the tibial plafond with the ankle in neutral position.
  - While we would prefer to avoid violating the cartilage surface, to date we are not aware of any compromised outcome related to the articular defect created by placing the screws.
  - Because the talus is contained within the ankle mortise, in our experience posterior screw fixation is unnecessary.
  - We routinely assess graft position after screw placement fluoroscopically. Since the articular cartilage is not visible and the physiologic talar dome is not in a single plane, the countersunk screws may appear proud fluoroscopically.

Axial Realignment

- Based on the preoperative plan and intraoperative reassessment, consider correction of axial malalignment. This improves the weight-bearing axis of the lower extremity and potentially unloads and protects the graft (eccentric load on the talus may have contributed to development of OLT). The preoperative plan dictates the amount of desired correction. As a rule, 1 mm of medial opening equals 1 degree of correction.
- Through the same incision, perform supramalleolar osteotomy for varus malalignment.
  - Medial opening wedge (TECH FIG 10)
    - Greenstick principle: leave lateral cortical hinge if possible
    - With or without fibular osteotomy, depending on degree of deformity
  - Minimal periosteal stripping
    - Attempt to limit to osteotomy site
  - Protect soft tissues
  - Judicious osteotomy
    - Consider a slightly oblique trajectory to increase surface area.
  - Careful medial opening
    - Protect lateral hinge.
    - If hinge is weak, maintain proper contact; control rotation of two fragments; consider using two plates in two planes for fixation.

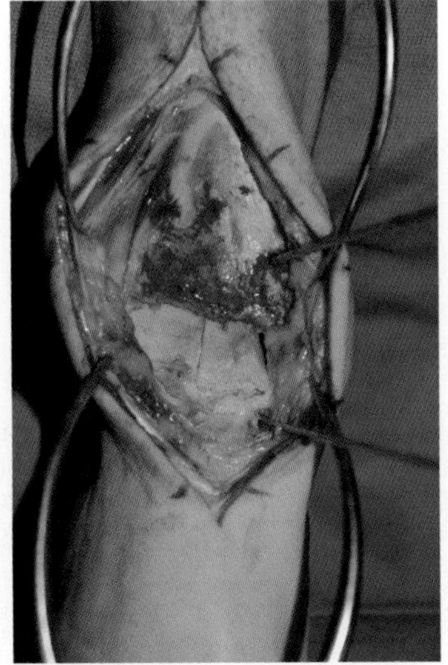

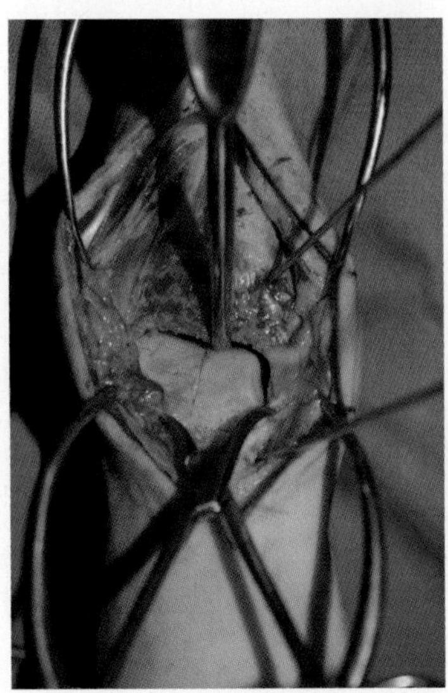

TECH FIG 9 • **A, B.** Optimizing graft position in native talus. **A.** After further "touch-ups" to the graft and recipient site, optimal graft position. **B.** Stabilizing graft to native talus (blunt retractor superiorly and bone reduction clamp for coronal compression). *(continued)*

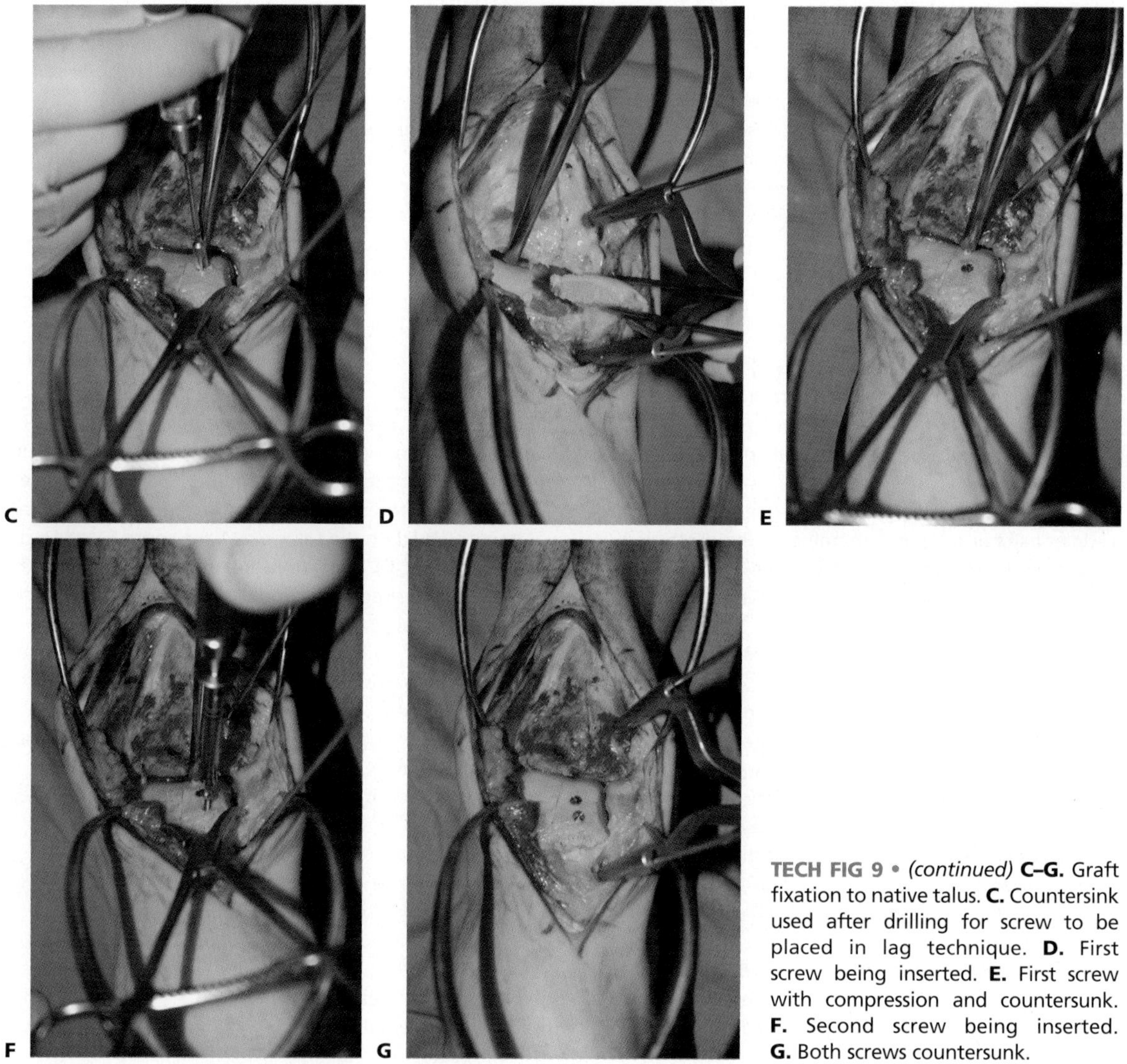

TECH FIG 9 • *(continued)* **C–G.** Graft fixation to native talus. **C.** Countersink used after drilling for screw to be placed in lag technique. **D.** First screw being inserted. **E.** First screw with compression and countersunk. **F.** Second screw being inserted. **G.** Both screws countersunk.

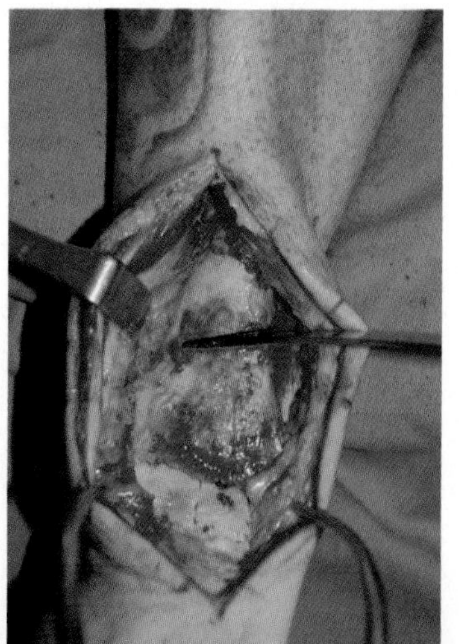

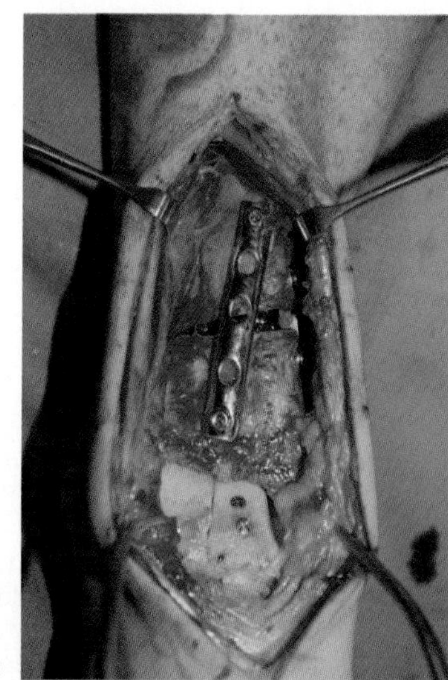

TECH FIG 10 • Realignment medial opening supramalleolar osteotomy. **A.** Osteotomy being carefully opened with an osteotome while preserving the lateral cortical hinge. **B.** Plate fixation.

- We routinely bone graft the opening wedge osteotomy site. However, this is not recommended by all who perform these osteotomies.

Closure

- Perform thorough irrigation.
- Close the capsule.
- Release the tourniquet.
- Reapproximate the extensor retinaculum while protecting the deep neurovascular bundle, extensor tendons, and the superficial peroneal nerve.
- We routinely use a drain for 24 hours.
- Perform subcutaneous closure and tensionless skin reapproximation.
- Dressings, adequate padding, and posterior–sugar-tong splint with the ankle in neutral or even a slightly dorsiflexed position

PEARLS AND PITFALLS

Procuring a talar allograft	■ Be sure it is the correct side (right or left). Be sure the tissue bank leaves the cartilage on the talus (we have had tali delivered from tissue banks that routinely remove the cartilage from the allograft talus!)
Harvesting the graft from the donor talus	■ "Measure twice and cut once." You have only one opportunity to harvest the graft. Use a caliper and a ruler and double-check the measurements.
Orienting the donor talus during graft harvest	■ Take care to orient the donor talus properly, as it should rest in the ankle mortise (compare to the native talus). The sagittal and axial cuts must be congruent for the graft to have an optimal match.
Reducing the immunogenic load of the graft	■ Wash the graft's cancellous surfaces with saline before implantation.
Graft position relative to the native talus	■ Rarely, if ever, is the graft a perfect clinical and fluoroscopic match; there is too much variability in the human talus. Anticipate some remodeling, provided the graft congruency is satisfactory to allow graft incorporation.
Screw fixation	■ Countersink the screws below the articular surface.
Malleolar osteotomy	■ Predrill the position for the screws to fix the malleolus at the conclusion of the surgery. Take into account the thickness of the saw blade; a perfect reduction clinically will demonstrate a slight gap due to bone loss from the saw blade. In our experience, the malleolus heals despite this narrow gap.

POSTOPERATIVE CARE

- We routinely observe these patients overnight for pain control.
- Follow-up is done in about 10 to 14 days.
- Provided the wound and osteotomy (if one was performed) are stable, the patient is transferred into a touch-down weight-bearing cam boot. If not, a touch-down weight-bearing short-leg cast is continued until the wound and osteotomy are stable.
- Intermittent minimal, gentle ankle range of motion (ROM) encouraged, three or four times a day. If financially feasible, we arrange for an ankle continuous passive motion device.

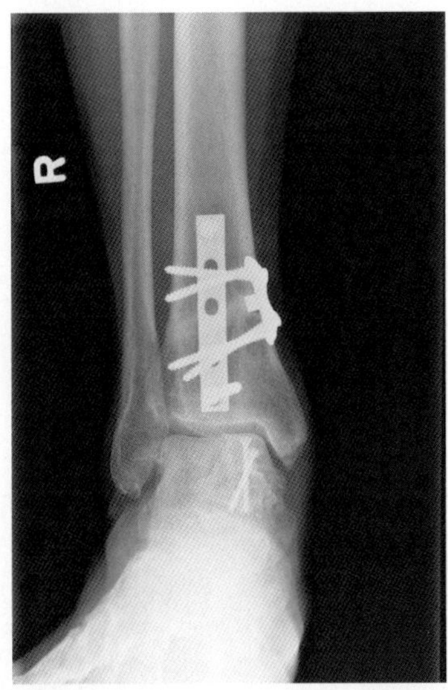

A

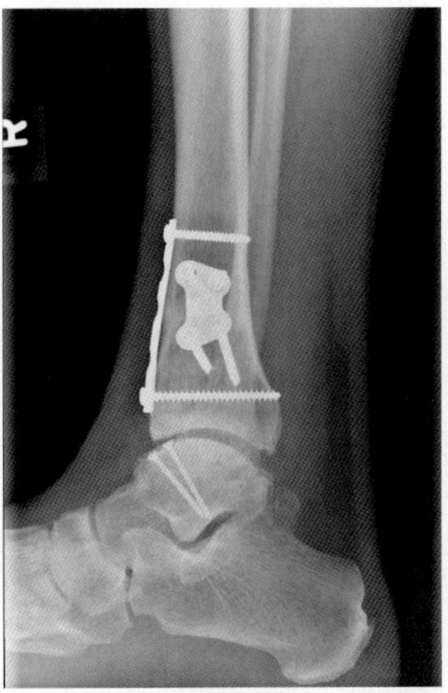

B

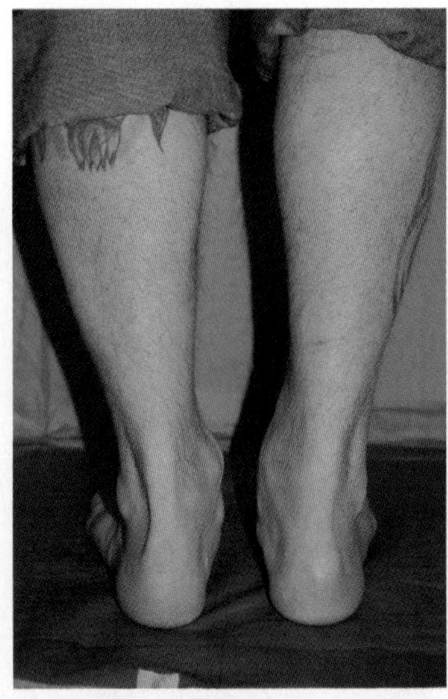
C

FIG 1 • Two-and-a-half-year follow-up. **A.** AP radiograph. **B.** Lateral radiograph. **C.** Clinical correlation.

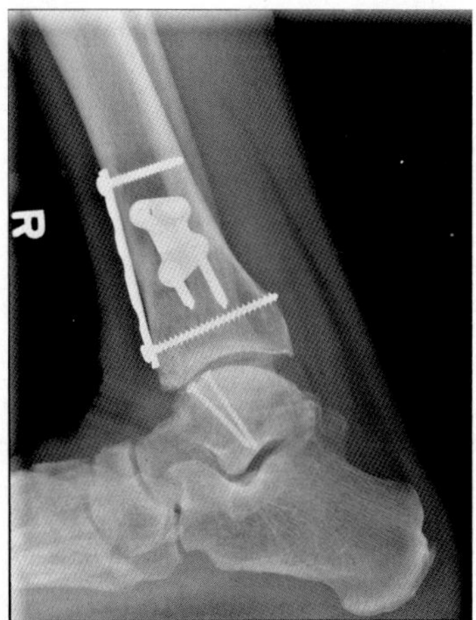

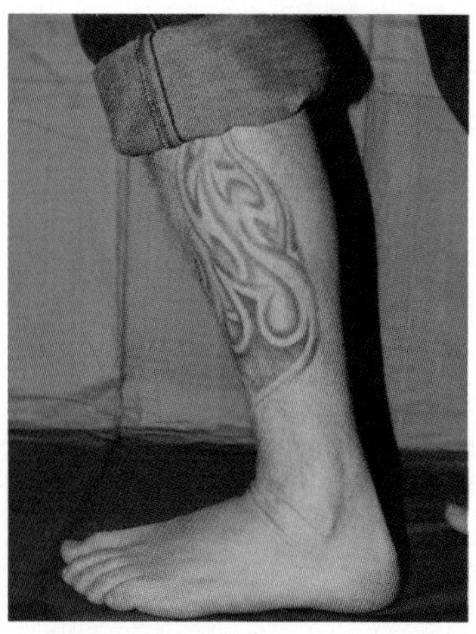

FIG 2 • Dorsiflexion. **A.** Radiograph (although the joint appears to narrow anteriorly, this phenomenon has not changed in 2 years and the patient experiences no pain or impingement). **B.** Clinical appearance.

- Touch-down weight bearing is maintained for 10 to 12 weeks, with progressively increasing ankle ROM exercise.
- We routinely obtain simulated weight-bearing radiographs at 6 weeks and 10 weeks, and again at 14 to 16 weeks, depending on the progression of healing. If there was a concern about fixation of the graft or osteotomy, then radiographs are also obtained at the first postoperative visit (**FIGS 1–3**).

OUTCOMES

- Gross et al[2] reported on nine patients who underwent fresh osteochondral allograft transplantation. At a mean follow-up of 11 years, six grafts remained in situ. The three failed allografts demonstrated radiographic and intraoperative evidence of fragmentation or resorption, and these patients went on to ankle fusion. Standardized outcomes measures for comparison were not used in that study.
- Raikin[3] recently reported on 15 patients who underwent bulk fresh osteochondral allografting for large-volume cystic lesions of the talus. The mean volume of the cystic lesions was 6059 mm^3. At a mean follow-up of 4.5 years, the mean AOFAS ankle–hindfoot score was 83 points. Only two grafts failed and went on to have an ankle arthrodesis. Some form of graft collapse, graft resorption, or joint space narrowing was seen in all patients.
- A retrospective review by Adams et al[1] showed significant improvement in pain and the Lower Extremity Functional Score (LEFS) at a mean follow-up of 48 months in eight patients who underwent osteochondral allograft transplantation of the talus. The mean postoperative AOFAS ankle–hindfoot score was 84 points. Three grafts were found to have graft-host lucencies in one plane on plain radiography. These patients were doing well and no further imaging was obtained. One patient continued to be symptomatic and was thought to have a nonunion of the graft due to circumferential lucency. Second-look arthroscopy demonstrated partial graft cartilage delamination but a stable graft. The patient did not wish to have any further treatment.

COMPLICATIONS

- Infection
- Wound complications
  - Particularly for anterior approach (as is performed for total ankle replacement)
  - Deep retraction only, avoiding direct tension on wound margins, reduces this risk.
- Failure of graft incorporation
- With large structural grafts, graft failure and development of degenerative change
- Articular cartilage delamination or fissuring of the graft
- Malleolar osteotomy nonunion
- Persistent pain despite radiographic suggestion of graft incorporation
- Disease transmission, although with the current screening practices of tissue banks, this risk is negligible

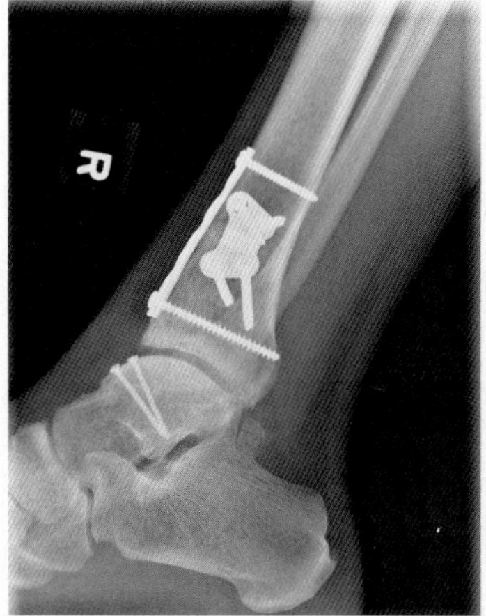

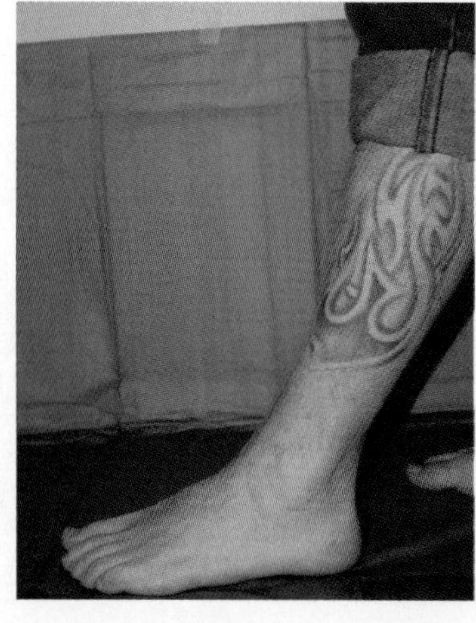

FIG 3 • Plantarflexion. **A.** Radiograph. **B.** Clinical correlation.

REFERENCES

1. Adams SB Jr., Viens NA, Easley ME, et al. Osteochondral lesions of the talar shoulder treated with fresh osteochondral allograft transplantation. American Orthopaedic Foot and Ankle Society (AOFAS) Annual Summer Meeting, July 7–10, 2010.
2. Gross AE, Agnidis Z, Hutchison CR. Osteochondral defects of the talus treated with fresh osteochondral allograft transplantation. Foot Ankle Int 2001;22:385–391.
3. Raikin SM. Fresh osteochondral allografts for large-volume cystic osteochondral defects of the talus. J Bone Joint Surg Am 2009;91A: 2818–2826.

Chapter 96 Autologous Chondrocyte Transplantation

Markus Walther

DEFINITION

- There are several reasons for cartilaginous defects of the ankle:
  - Traumatic injury
  - Osteochondritis dissecans (OCD)
  - Degenerative changes
- The necessity to treat a cartilage defect of the ankle depends on the clinical presentation. Osteochondral lesions of the talus (OLTs) are often found incidentally on screening MRIs obtained for reasons other than suspected intra-articular pathology.
- Autologous chondrocyte transplantation (ACT), also known as autologous chondrocyte implantation (ACI), is one of several surgical treatment options for symptomatic cartilage defects. In my opinion, ACI is best suited for patients between 18 and 50 years of age.
- ACI is indicated for management of symptomatic OTLs failing to respond to débridement, drilling, or microfracture.[1,8,27]
- Primary ACI can be considered in lesions larger than 2 cm^2 or in osteochondral lesions associated with expansive subchondral cysts (stage V lesion).[48]
- Advantages of ACI include:
  - ACI provides a stable cartilage rim that can be maintained at the site of the OLT.
  - Large defects can be readily addressed with this technique.
  - The periosteal flap can be harvested from the adjacent medial tibia.
  - With carefully executed suture technique or with matrix-based chondrocytes, shoulder lesions can be managed.
- Disadvantages of the ACI for the talar dome are:
  - ACI has Food and Drug Administration (FDA) approval only for the knee (as of October 2006).
  - The cost from industry for chondrocyte culture is considerable.
  - The procedure requires two stages to allow time for chondrocyte culture.
- Reports of the traditional technique that requires a periosteal flap under which the transplanted chondrocytes are positioned suggested limitations of the technique for the talus.[47] Many OLTs involve, at least in part, the talar shoulder, an anatomic region poorly suited for anatomic coverage with a periosteal flap. Recently introduced matrix-based autologous chondrocyte transplantation (MACI) may afford advantages since it does not require coverage of the defect with a periosteal flap. Histologic investigations have shown that MACI may offer an improved alternative to traditional treatments for cartilage injury by regenerating hyaline-like cartilage.[48]
- Informed consent and patient education are imperative for ACI. ACI for the ankle lacks FDA approval. However, for larger OLTs, OLTs failing to respond to prior surgical management, or OLT with subchondral cysts, ACI provides patients and their surgeons with a potentially successful treatment avenue that did not exist before ACI. Early favorable outcomes with ACI applied to difficult OLTs justify the extra effort, education, and communication between physician, patients, and third-party payers that may be required to proceed with ACI in the ankle.
- In Europe, harvesting cells for culturing is considered part of a drug-producing process. Therefore, special permission must be sought from the local healthcare administration. Standard operating procedures for harvesting and transportation of the cartilage cells are mandatory for the accreditation process.

ANATOMY

- A slight majority of OLTs are on the medial shoulder of the talus.[42]
  - 62% of lesions are located at the medial talar shoulder; many of these are thought to be a result of OCD rather than posttraumatic.
  - 34% of the lesions are located at the lateral talar shoulder; most are thought to be of traumatic origin.
  - Central OLTs are rare (less than 5%).
  - In the AP direction, the midtalar dome (equator) is much more frequently involved (80%) than the anterior (6%) or posterior (14%) thirds of the talar dome.
- Classification of osteochondral lesions is based on arthroscopic findings[21]
  - Grade I: Intact lesions
  - Grade II: Lesions showing signs of early separation
  - Grade III: Partially detached lesions
  - Grade IV: Craters with loose bodies
- ACI is performed for symptomatic grade II-plus lesions (full-thickness cartilage defects).

PATHOGENESIS

- Traumatic cartilage injuries are caused by short, intensive, greater-than-physiologic strain on the joint resulting in partial detachment of the talar dome cartilage. The depth of these lesions varies from superficial chondral abrasions to full-thickness osteochondral defects.[32,45]
- OCD is a condition most frequently found in adolescents or young adults. While the cause remains poorly defined, theories include:
  - Chronic overload and
  - Local disturbance of blood supply to the subchondral bone associated with the affected cartilage.[25]
- Degenerative cartilage defects (degenerative osteoarthritis) develop from wear and tear of the cartilage surface as part of the aging process. An individual's risk of developing primary osteoarthritis most likely depends on a genetically determined quality of the cartilage. Ankle instability and other conditions that impart eccentric or nonphysiologic loads to the cartilage may accelerate the process of degeneration. In exceptional cases, when such a degenerative process is limited to a focal portion of the talar dome, ACI may be considered for degenerative

cartilage defects, provided the underlying cause leading to focal degeneration (ie, malalignment or chronic instability) is corrected.

NATURAL HISTORY

- The natural history of a focal cartilage injury has not been linked to diffuse ankle arthritis.
  - Posttraumatic arthritis, which differs from an OLT, develops from diffuse injury to the cartilage surface that results in cartilage fibrillation and eventual eburnation. ACI is contraindicated for diffuse ankle arthritis.
  - Injury to a focal portion of the talar dome spans the spectrum from a bone bruise to a detached focal osteochondral fragment. Although an osteochondral fragment may be created at the time of injury, the focal talar dome pathology probably evolves. Many OLTs are probably asymptomatic; we know this from numerous OLTs that are found incidentally on imaging studies of the ankle obtained for reasons other than suspected intra-articular pathology. However, with persistent eccentric stresses, greater-than-physiologic loads, inadequate local blood supply, or inadequate healing time, a stable OLT may progress to an unstable one.
  - The difficulty is also in the symptomatology. While some apparently unstable lesions may be asymptomatic, other OLTs that are clearly stable result in considerable symptoms directly related to the OLT.[28]

PATIENT HISTORY AND PHYSICAL FINDINGS

- While many patients report a specific ankle injury to account for the OLT, many do not present until months after ankle injury. A symptomatic OLT is in the differential diagnosis for an ankle sprain that does not heal. However, many patients with symptomatic OLTs do not recall a specific traumatic event leading to the OLT.[40]
- In my experience, most patients presenting with symptomatic OLTs are between 20 and 40 years of age.
- Men are more commonly affected than women (ratio 1.6:1).[40]
- Patients typically describe an ache in the ankle with activity or with the first steps after a period of rest. Occasionally, sharp ankle pain is noted with weight bearing. In our experience, mechanical symptoms of locking or catching are noted only with a completely detached osteochondral fragment. Paradoxically, OLTs may produce symptoms on the opposite side of the joint from the location of the cartilage defect.
- Our preferred physical examination methods are listed here. Occasionally, symptoms may not be elicited on clinical examination.
  - Locking or catching: found when something interrupts the normal movement of the joint. However, it says nothing about the cause of this condition (eg, scar, joint body, osteochondral fragment and synovitis).
  - Inversion test (calcaneofibular ligament [CFL]): strongly dependent on the cooperation of the patient. If positive, it is highly specific for a ruptured CFL.
  - Medial stability: strongly dependent on the cooperation of the patient. If positive, it is highly specific for a ruptured deltoid ligament.
  - Anterior drawer test (anterior talofibular ligament [ATFL]): strongly dependent on the cooperation of the patient. If positive, it is highly specific for a ruptured ATFL.
  - The medial and lateral corner of the talar dome should be palpated with the ankle maximally flexed to identify anterior or central OLTs; posteromedial palpation immediately posterior to the posterior tibial tendon (PTT) with the ankle maximally dorsiflexed may reproduce symptoms for posteromedial OLTs. While anterolateral OLTs are relatively easy to palpate, posteromedial lesions are difficult to access adequately on physical examination.
- We find it useful to compare the symptomatic ankle to the uninvolved contralateral ankle.
  - The medial and lateral corner of the talar dome should be palpated with the ankle maximally flexed to identify anterior or central OLTs; posteromedial palpation immediately posterior to the PTT with the ankle maximally dorsiflexed may reproduce symptoms for posteromedial OLTs. While anterolateral OLTs are relatively easy to palpate, posteromedial lesions are difficult to access adequately on physical examination.
  - We typically dorsiflex and plantarflex the ankles with axial pressure while simultaneously applying eversion and inversion stresses to reproduce symptoms at the talar defect.
  - Despite appropriate provocative maneuvers, our experience has been that posterior OLTs rarely exhibit obvious clinical findings.
- Associated injuries and other considerations in the differential diagnosis of chronic ankle pain should be evaluated, particularly because OLTs may be incidental findings. These include:
  - Ankle instability: Positive anterior drawer test and inversion testing
  - Chondromatosis of the ankle: Recurrent locking of the joint and persistent effusions are typical physical findings.
  - Intra-articular scaring with load-dependent pain, mostly at the anterior, lateral aspect of the ankle joint
  - Inflammatory arthropathy: While effusion and deep joint pain with weight bearing are commonly present, pain at rest and persistent joint warmth are also common features of inflammatory disease.
  - Pigmented villonodular synovitis (PVNS): Organized nodules of synovitis can mimic loose bodies with locking and effusion. Synovial swelling is not typical for osteochondral defects. MRI with contrast typically confirms the diagnosis of PVNS.

IMAGING AND OTHER DIAGNOSTIC STUDIES

- Plain radiographs of the ankle joint, including AP, mortise, and lateral views, are obtained to rule out late-stage degenerative arthritis.
- MRI with contrast is highly sensitive and specific in diagnosing osteochondral lesions, as well as associated injuries.[23,34]
- Osteochondral lesions were first classified by Berndt and Harty, based on plain radiographs:[7]
  - Stage I: Compression lesion; no visible fragment
  - Stage II: Beginning avulsion of a chip
  - Stage III: Chip, completely detached but in place
  - Stage IV: Displaced chip
- Plain films typically offer limited information on the size and extent of the lesion and may even miss the OLT. MRI, CT, and arthroscopic evaluation provide greater detail of OLTs than plain radiographs.

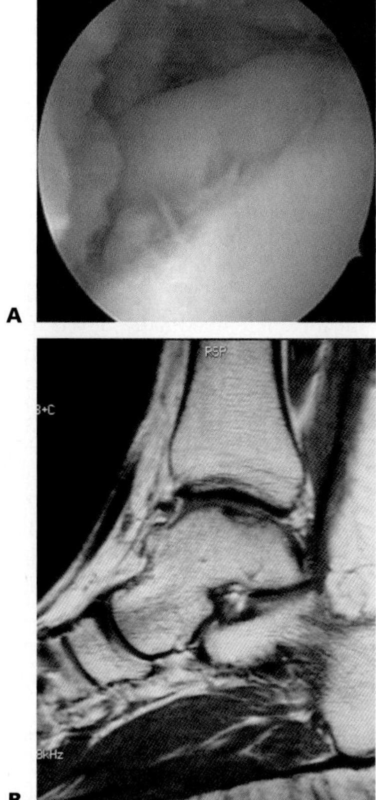

FIG 1 • A. Arthroscopic view of a full-thickness osteochondral defect at the talar dome. B. Corresponding MRI.

- DiPaolo classification of osteochondral lesions based on MRI[11]
  - Stage I: Thickening of articular cartilage and low signal changes
  - Stage II: Articular cartilage breached, low-signal rim behind fragment indicating fibrous attachment
  - Stage III: Articular cartilage breached, high-signal changes behind fragment indicating synovial fluid between fragment and underlying subchondral bone (**FIG 1**)
  - Stage IV: Loose body
- Based on the greater detail of pathologic anatomy, Hepple et al[23] revised the classification and included a type V (subchondral cyst formation)
  - Stage I: Articular cartilage damage only
  - Stage IIa: Cartilage injury with underlying fracture and surrounding bony edema
  - Stage IIb: Stage IIa without surrounding bony edema
  - Stage III: Detached but undisplaced fragment
  - Stage IV: Detached and displaced fragment
  - Stage V: Subchondral cyst formation
- The Ferkel and Sgaglione CT classification is used for preoperative planning purposes and to learn the size of the subchondral defect.[15]
  - Stage I: Cystic lesion of the talar dome with an intact roof
  - Stage IIa: Cystic lesion with communication to the talar dome surface
  - Stage IIb: Open articular surface lesion with an overlying, nondisplaced fragment
  - Stage III: Nondisplaced lesion with lucency
  - Stage IV: Displaced osteochondral fragment

DIFFERENTIAL DIAGNOSIS

- Syndesmosis injury
- Intra-articular scarring
- Subluxation or tear of peroneal tendons
- Fracture or disruption of the os trigonum
- Malleolar avulsion fracture
- Interosseous ligament injury
- Anterior process fracture of the calcaneus
- Lateral shoulder fracture of the calcaneus
- Chondromatosis
- Inflammatory joint disease
- PVNS

NONOPERATIVE MANAGEMENT

- In young patients with open physes, OCD can be managed conservatively with a high rate of complete remission (**FIG 2**).[6,46]
- Acute osteochondral lesions may be treated conservatively. Acute lesions (stage I and II) require 3 weeks of immobilization. Stage III and IV lesions should be treated with a walker and partial weight bearing of 20 kg for 6 weeks.[40] However, unstable osteochondral lesions, particularly those with detached fragments, should be managed operatively.
- Incidentally discovered OLTs and OCD cases in adults are generally treated expectantly with regular follow-up.[13,46]

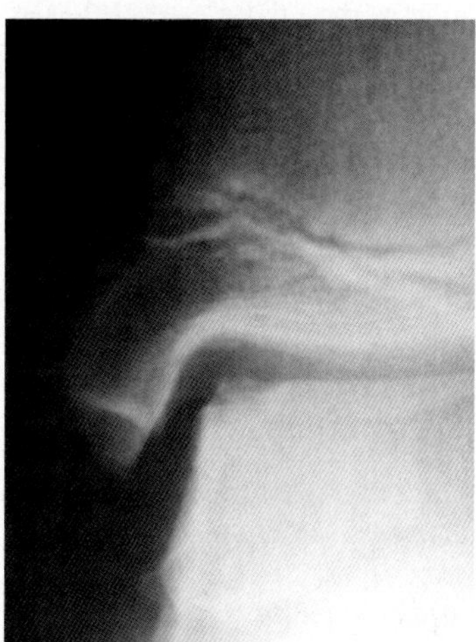

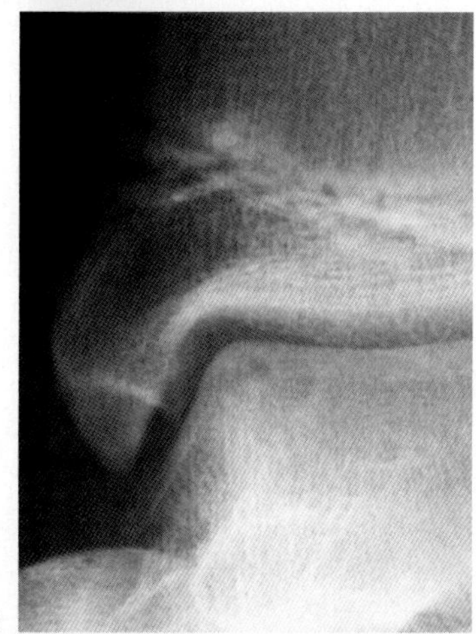

FIG 2 • A. Osteochondritis dissecans in a child with open physis. B. 6 months later, the lesion is healed with conservative treatment.

- The literature suggests that chronic OLTs, even larger lesions, may be treated nonoperatively as well.[43] Nonoperative treatment comprises nonsteroidal anti-inflammatory agents, ankle bracing, physiotherapy, corticosteroid injection, and viscosupplementation. Currently, no conservative treatment of OLTs allows resurfacing or healing of the cartilage defect.

SURGICAL MANAGEMENT

- Microfracture
  - Arthroscopic débridement and microfracture generally represent the initial surgical management for the vast majority of OLTs, with satisfactory results in 65% to 90% of patients.[5,24,39]
  - After arthroscopic débridement of the OLT, the defect's subchondral bone is penetrated with multiple noncontiguous passes of a specialized awl to permit the débrided defect to be populated with undifferentiated stem cells from the deeper tissues.
  - Over the next few months, these cells reorganize into (type II) fibrocartilage.
  - The biomechanical properties of fibrocartilage are different from those of hyaline cartilage; the fibrocartilage does not function in concert with the surrounding physiologic hyaline cartilage. The literature suggests that microfracture is successful in a majority of relatively small OLTs (up to 2 cm^2).[5,19]
- Autologous osteochondral transfer (OATS or mosaicplasty) and ACI are typically secondary surgical procedures when arthroscopic débridement and microfracture and drilling fail.
- Autologous osteochondral cylinder transplantation (OATS or mosaicplasty)[22,41]
  - In the OATS or mosaicplasty technique osteochondral cylinders or plugs are harvested either from a low-load-bearing area of the knee or from the medial or lateral facet of the talus. These plugs are transplanted into the defect area, which has been prepared to the appropriate size.
  - This procedure fills large portions of the defect surface with high-quality hyaline cartilage.[19]
  - The results of this technique are satisfactory, but donor-site morbidity occurs in up to 50% of cases.[37]
  - To limit these harvesting symptoms, OCT can be successfully applied for cartilage defects of up to only about 3 cm^2. Matching defects on the talar shoulder are difficult with this technique, despite technique modifications described by Hangody et al.[22] Moreover, the characteristics of talar cartilage differ from those of cartilage from the knee.[9]
- Allograft osteochondral cylinder transplantation[20]
  - If available, osteochondral cylinders can be taken from a fresh or fresh-frozen cadaver talus.
  - Immunologic reactions have posed little problem to date.[30]

Preoperative Planning

- All imaging studies are reviewed, with MRI providing detail of the cartilage defect and CT providing detail of subchondral bone involvement.[2,12,41]
- Pure cartilage defects or shallow osteochondral defects can be managed with the conventional ACI procedure; deeper osteochondral defects require a "sandwich technique."
- The sandwich technique involves two layers of periosteum. The defect is prepared and bone grafted to recreate the subchondral bone architecture. On this the first layer of periosteum is placed cambium layer up. Then the defect can be treated in the conventional manner: the second layer of periosteum is placed cambium side down. The cultured cartilage cells are injected between these two layers. Alternatively, the cartilage defect may be bone grafted in a first stage, with a conventional ACI procedure being performed in a second stage. This is feasible in the knee but more challenging in the ankle, which may require ligament release or osteotomy for adequate exposure, procedures that should not be performed more than once if not necessary.
- Matrix-based chondrocytes that do not require a periosteal flap can be placed directly on a bone graft, which makes the management of stage V lesions less demanding.
- Ankle malalignment and instability should be identified and corrected in conjunction with ACI if possible.

Positioning

- Harvesting chondrocytes: standard arthroscopy of the ankle or the knee
- Giannini et al. have demonstrated that the detached OLT fragment at the time of index arthroscopy may be an acceptable source of chondrocytes in ACI.[17] Another possible source is the anterior aspect of the talus.[4]
- Transplantation of chondrocytes: Depending on the location of the defect, the patient is positioned supine with a slightly internally or externally rotated leg. If iliac crest graft is to be obtained, the pelvis needs to be prepared and draped as well and the ipsilateral pelvis supported with a bump. Alternatively, bone graft may be harvested from the calcaneus, distal tibia, or proximal tibia, all locations within the surgical field typically prepared for ACI.[14,16,35] A vacuum mattress can be helpful to adjust the patient's position during the procedure (**FIG 3**).

Approach

- Harvesting chondrocytes: Medial and lateral anterior portals and a posterior, lateral portal give an adequate overview of the joint and allow the harvesting of chondrocytes.
- Transplantation: Depending on the location of the OLT, a medial approach between the medial malleolus and the PTT, a medial transmalleolar approach with osteotomy, or a lateral approach (with or without osteotomy) can be considered. ACI demands adequate exposure to properly suture a periosteal patch circumferentially around the OLT.[18,19] Except for OLTs at the anterior or posterior margins of the talar dome, ACI cannot be performed properly without

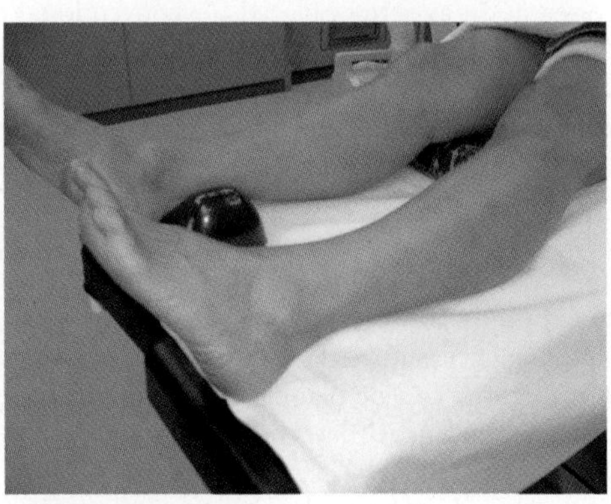

FIG 3 • Standard positioning in a supine position.

medial malleolar osteotomy for extensive medial OLTs and ATFL–CFL release, lateral malleolar osteotomy, or both for extensive lateral OLTs.

- A major advantage compared to mosaicplasty or OATS is that a perpendicular access is not required. Muir et al.[29] demonstrated that the majority of the talar dome can be accessed without osteotomy, but acknowledged that osteotomies are required to adequately expose extensive OLTs.
- Medial OLT: Occasionally, the ACI procedure can be performed for medial OLTs with an anteromedial or posteromedial arthrotomy.[29] In our experience, these are exceptional cases, often requiring extreme intraoperative ankle plantarflexion and dorsiflexion for anteromedial and posteromedial lesions, respectively. An intact deltoid ligament permits little if any translation of the talus relative to the tibia. Access to an anterior defect can be enhanced with a groove created in the anteromedial tibia, but leaves a permanent defect in the anterior weight-bearing surface of the plafond. We appreciate that extreme dorsiflexion allows visualization of some posteromedial OLTs; however, we caution against extreme dorsiflexion that tensions the posteromedial neurovascular bundle in combination with the simultaneous required retraction of the neurovascular bundle to allow proper access to the lesion. One author suggested that a medial malleolar window can be created, obviating the need for osteotomy,[33] but we have no experience with this approach.
- Oblique medial malleolar osteotomy
  - A longitudinal incision is centered over the medial malleolus, similar to that performed for open reduction and internal fixation of medial malleolar fractures.
  - An anterior arthrotomy serves to identify the junction between the medial malleolar and tibial plafond articular surfaces and may allow visualization of the anterior aspect of the OLT.
  - Posteriorly, the flexor retinaculum is opened, and the PTT is identified directly on the posterior tibia. The PTT rests in a groove in the posterior aspect of the medial tibia in its own sheath; the flexor digitorum longus tendon lies directly posterior to the PTT and should not be mistaken for the PTT.
  - With the PTT properly retracted, the posteromedial neurovascular bundle will also be protected.
  - The medial malleolar osteotomy requires minimal periosteal stripping; in fact, we advise leaving as much of the periosteum as possible on the medial malleolar fragment to maintain blood supply for healing.
  - To optimize reduction of the medial malleolar osteotomy after the cartilage repair procedure, we recommend predrilling the medial malleolus. Two parallel drill holes are placed extra-articularly perpendicular across the desired osteotomy, in the same orientation as screws placed for conventional open reduction and internal fixation for medial malleolar fractures. The proper course for these drill holes is confirmed fluoroscopically, both in the AP and lateral planes.
  - Under fluoroscopic guidance a Kirschner wire pin is introduced obliquely to dictate the desired plane of the osteotomy. Typically, we introduce this guide pin slightly more proximal and medial than the intended course of the osteotomy to allow access for the saw blade, chisel, or both without having to remove the pin that guides our osteotomy.
  - The osteotomy can be planned more conservatively as in mosaicplasty, because a perpendicular access to the OLT is not needed. As a rule, we plan to have the osteotomy enter the tibial plafond at the medial extent of the OLT.
  - With the plan for the osteotomy determined, the periosteum is divided transversely, again leaving the majority of the periosteum intact. With cold saline or sterile water irrigation to reduce the risk of osseous heat necrosis, a microsagittal saw is used to perform the oblique osteotomy to the level of the tibial plafond subchondral bone.
  - The joint is penetrated with an osteotome or a chisel. Intermittent fluoroscopic guidance is recommended to confirm proper saw blade or chisel orientation and that the talar dome is not injured during the final stages of the osteotomy.
  - The medial malleolus is then reflected, suspended by the deltoid ligament.
  - Even with careful technique, the osteotomy rarely separates in a uniform plane. Particularly posteriorly, a slight irregularity is observed. This is of little concern, however, as these irregularities will provide greater stability when the osteotomy is reduced.
  - To fully displace the medial malleolar fragment, the PTT sheath must be released from the medial malleolus.
  - At the conclusion of the cartilage resurfacing procedure, the medial malleolus is reduced and secured with two malleolar screws placed in the predrilled tracks with compression.
  - To limit a vertical shear effect, an antiglide screw or plate may be placed at the proximal aspect of the osteotomy. Alternatively, a third screw can be carefully placed from medial to lateral eccentrically across the osteotomy in addition to the two predrilled compression screws.
  - Anatomic reduction is confirmed clinically by visualizing the anterior and posterior aspects of the osteotomy and fluoroscopically in the AP and oblique planes. Fluoroscopy in all three routine views of the ankle confirms proper extra-articular position of the screws.
  - Due to the thickness of the saw blade, a slight, incomplete gap may be visualized at the osteotomy site in select cases; despite this immediate postoperative finding, our anecdotal experience has been that the oblique medial malleolar osteotomy heals in its anatomic position with few complications.
- Lateral OLT
  - ATFL and CFL release: Some lateral OLTs are associated with lateral ankle instability.[26] This combination of pathology is well suited to surgical management, since a modified Brostrom procedure is required to stabilize the ankle. If a lateral OLT is identified without lateral ankle instability, lateral ligament release to allow access to the OLT is readily repaired with a modified Brostrom technique, particularly since the lateral ankle ligaments are not attenuated.[41]
  - The fibula is exposed through a longitudinal incision. If ligament release is inadequate, the extensile longitudinal incision facilitates the addition of a lateral malleolar osteotomy. Moreover, if associated pathology involves the peroneal tendons, the extensile longitudinal approach is necessary.
  - With the sural nerve protected posteriorly and inferiorly and the lateral branch of the superficial peroneal nerve protected anteriorly, the inferior flexor retinaculum is identified and isolated.
  - Deep to the retinaculum and at the distal and posterior margin of the fibula, the peroneal tendons are identified and protected throughout the procedure.

- The ATFL and CFL lie within the lateral ankle capsular complex. Leaving a 1-mm cuff of capsule on the distal fibula, the capsule and the ATFL and CFL are released. The ankle is plantarflexed and inverted; the talus is subluxated anteriorly out of the ankle mortise to expose the OLT.
- After the cartilage resurfacing, the talus is reduced in the ankle mortise and a modified Brostrom procedure is performed. This can be done with suture anchors in the distal fibula, placed to secure the ATFL and CFL components of the lateral ankle capsule in particular or with transosseous sutures.
- During tensioning of the ligament repair, the talus is maintained posteriorly (avoiding anterior translation), with the ankle in a neutral sagittal plane position and the hindfoot in slight eversion. As described by Gould, the inferior extensor retinaculum is advanced to the distal fibula to lend greater stability to the repair.
- Lateral malleolar osteotomy: Several different patterns for lateral malleolar osteotomies exist; surprisingly, few have been described in detail. We typically employ an oblique fibular osteotomy, similar to the pattern created by a simple Weber B ankle fracture. The approach is as described for the ligament release above. As for a medial malleolar osteotomy, periosteal stripping is kept to a minimum, predrilling is preferred, and cold saline or sterile water irrigation is applied to the osteotomy site to limit osseous heat necrosis.
- Before performing the osteotomy, we position a small fragment plate in the desired position and predrill the holes. With the soft tissues protected, in particular the superficial peroneal nerve and the peroneal tendons, the oblique osteotomy is created from anterior to posterior using a microsagittal saw. The syndesmotic ligaments are not disrupted. Release of the ATFL and CFL in combination with the fibular osteotomy can be considered to improve exposure of larger posterolateral OLTs with medial extension.
- At the conclusion of the cartilage repair procedure, the fibula is reduced and secured with the predrilled lateral fibular plate. Reduction is confirmed with intraoperative fluoroscopy. Before placing the plate, a lag screw may be placed across the osteotomy, but we do not routinely do so.
- As for the medial malleolar osteotomy, the thickness of the saw blade may lead to a slight, incomplete gap at the fibular osteotomy site in select cases. Again, despite this immediate postoperative finding, our anecdotal experience has been that the oblique medial malleolar osteotomy heals in its anatomic position with few complications.

- Central defects
  - As observed in the cadaver model of Muir et al.,[29] perpendicular access to the central talar dome is not possible via medial and lateral osteotomies. Tochigi et al.[44] described a Chaput lateral tibial osteotomy, similar to a Tilleaux fracture, to allow greater medial exposure to extensive lateral OLTs; however, Muir et al.[29] noted that this osteotomy still fails to allow access to the central talar dome.
  - The trap door osteotomy described by Sammarco et al.,[38] in which an anterior osteochondral wedge is removed from the distal tibia, may permit access to select anterior central OLTs. Although attractive, the osteotomy must be carefully planned to accommodate the instrumentation at the ideal location for sufficient access, as coronal plane translation of the talus is not possible. Moreover, access to relatively rare posterocentral lesions is still not possible despite this novel approach.

HARVESTING OF CHONDROCYTES

- Complete diagnostic arthroscopy and identify all pathology.
- Using a curette, harvest two or three full-thickness articular grafts that include the superficial layer of subchondral bone (**TECH FIG 1**). The grafts are transferred to a sterile container and transported to the laboratory. Using a patented procedure, the articular cartilage matrix is enzymatically disrupted to isolate the chondrocytes. Culturing of chondrocytes requires about 2 to 6 weeks, depending on the company and the preferred culturing process.
- Ensure that the cells are sent to the company immediately, the "cool chain" is sustained, and the required documents are included in the box.

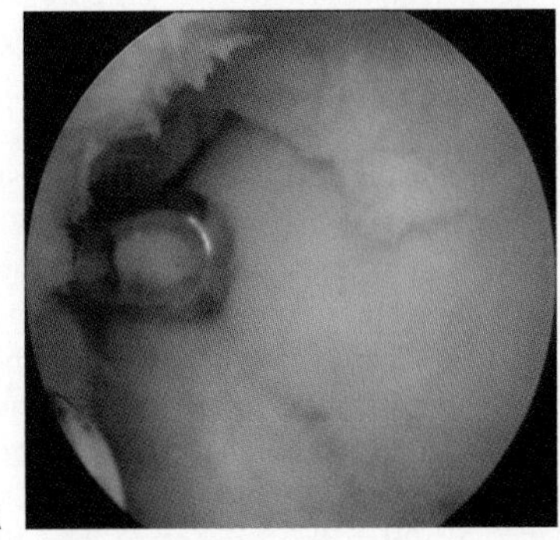
A

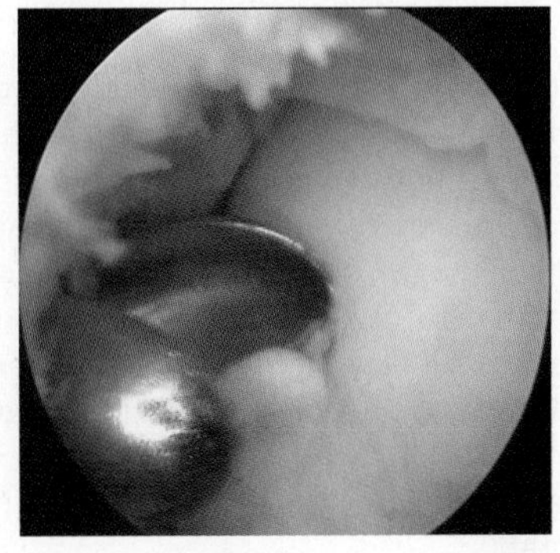
B

TECH FIG 1 • **A.** Harvesting cartilage with a curette from the ventral aspect of the talus. **B.** Grasping the small piece of cartilage for culturing.

TECHNIQUES

AUTOLOGOUS CHONDROCYTE TRANSPLANTATION

- To avoid compromising chondrocyte viability, use a tourniquet to maintain a bloodless field.
- We typically use a thigh tourniquet; although a calf tourniquet is possible, compression of the lower leg musculature may restrict exposure and manipulation of the ankle, thereby compromising exposure.
- Expose the transplantation site. Despite adequate exposure with appropriate osteotomies or ligament releases, performing the second ACI stage for the ankle, in particular suturing the periosteal flap, may prove tedious. Matrix-based transplants, where the chondrocytes for transplantation are already grown in a collagen matrix, provide a significant advantage. These membranes can be fixed with fibrous glue; sutures are optional. For the knee, both techniques have proven to have similar clinical outcomes.[3] At the talus, there is still a lack of scientific evidence, but our extended anecdotal experience has shown similar results in both techniques.
- Débride all unstable cartilage with a curette to create a healthy, stable cartilage rim. The subchondral bone in the defect should be intact.
- If a shallow bony defect exists, remove the sclerotic bone. Despite tourniquet use, some bleeding may be encountered; it should be controlled with an epinephrine sponge or a minimal amount of fibrin glue.
- In the event of a deeper defect, use the "sandwich technique" described above to recreate subchondral support for the transplanted chondrocytes. Any bony cyst has to be filled with autologous bone graft, preferably from the iliac crest or the proximal tibia.[16]
- Impact the graft to provide a smooth surface for the transplantation site.
- Measure the defect and create a template using a small piece of paper (from a sterile glove pack) or aluminum foil (from a suture pack).
- Technique with periosteal flap
  - By exposing the distal tibia just proximal to the ankle, identify an appropriate area for periosteal flap harvest; exposure is to the level of the periosteum without violating it.
  - Place the template on the periosteum and mark an outline 1 to 2 mm greater than the template on the periosteum. The periosteal harvest should be slightly larger than the template as periosteum tends to recoil or shrink slightly after harvest.
  - Perform sharp dissection to bone on the marked periosteum circumferentially. With a sharp periosteal elevator, elevate the periosteum, with its cambium layer, directly off the underlying tibia without creating defects in the periosteal graft. We routinely place a mark on the superficial layer of periosteum before detaching the periosteal flap from the tibia to be certain we can identify the cambium layer at the time of transfer to the talus.
  - Carefully separate overlying fibrous tissue or fat from the periosteal graft.
  - After ensuring that the OLT is bloodless, transfer the periosteal flap to the OLT, with the cambium layer facing the defect.
  - Suture it using interrupted 6-0 Vicryl to the surrounding articular cartilage, with sutures spaced at intervals of about 3 mm. To optimize tensioning, the corners can be anchored first. Place the knots on the articular cartilage rather than the periosteal flap. The final suture is omitted at this point, with the residual defect being at the area of easiest access for chondrocyte transplantation.
  - Apply fibrin glue around the periphery of the periosteal flap's junction with the healthy articular cartilage, particularly between the sutures.
  - Using a flexible angiocatheter, inject sterile saline into the residual opening to confirm a watertight seal; any leakage of saline should emanate only from the residual opening. Add sutures, fibrin glue, or both as needed.
  - The chondrocytes are delivered in a vial that is sterile internally but not externally. The vial can be placed on a separate back table while the surgeon maintains sterile technique while resuspending and extracting the chondrocytes from the vial into a sterile angiocatheter.
  - Through the residual opening under the periosteal flap, introduce the angiocatheter into the defect. The chondrocytes are evenly distributed with the surgeon gently injecting the suspension.
  - Remove the angiocatheter and seal the residual aperture with a final suture and more fibrin glue.
  - After the fibrin glue has cured, ankle range of motion confirms that the periosteal flap is stable.
  - Stabilize the ankle joint with repair of the ligaments or osteotomy, depending on the particular approach.
  - ACI has not been perfected for shoulder lesions of the talus. However, as for the femoral trochlea, a carefully executed suture pattern can allow the periosteum to be draped over a shoulder lesion to recreate, at least to some degree, the physiologic contour of the talus. With the periosteum first tensioned at the shoulder and secondarily on the dorsal and mediolateral aspects of the talus, ACI can be effective for select talar shoulder OLTs.
- Technique with matrix-based chondrocytes (MACI)
  - The technique with matrix-based chondrocytes requires no further preparation after the size of the defect is measured. The matrix is stable and can be fixed directly to the OLT.
  - Take care when removing the transplant from the transport container. In particular, avoid squeezing the transplant (**TECH FIG 2A,B**).
  - Cut the transplant according to the size of the defect. Some companies provide special punches for this step. The size of the transplant should meet exactly the size of the defect. Preparing the transplant 2 mm larger, as recommended for the periosteal flap, can lead to overlaying edges and a lack of stability.
  - Place the transplant into the defect. A first fixation happens due to adhesion forces. The edge can then be stabilized with 6-0 sutures and fibrin glue (**TECH FIG 2C,D**).

- Check the transplant for stability by carefully moving the ankle joint into dorsiflexion and plantarflexion. We recommend that postoperative mobilization be limited so that the transplant is always covered at least partially by the tibial plafond to prevent shear forces. The optimal postoperative rage of motion can be checked in this step.
- Insert one intra-articular tube before closing the wound. Stabilize the ankle joint with repair of the ligaments or osteotomy, depending on the particular approach.

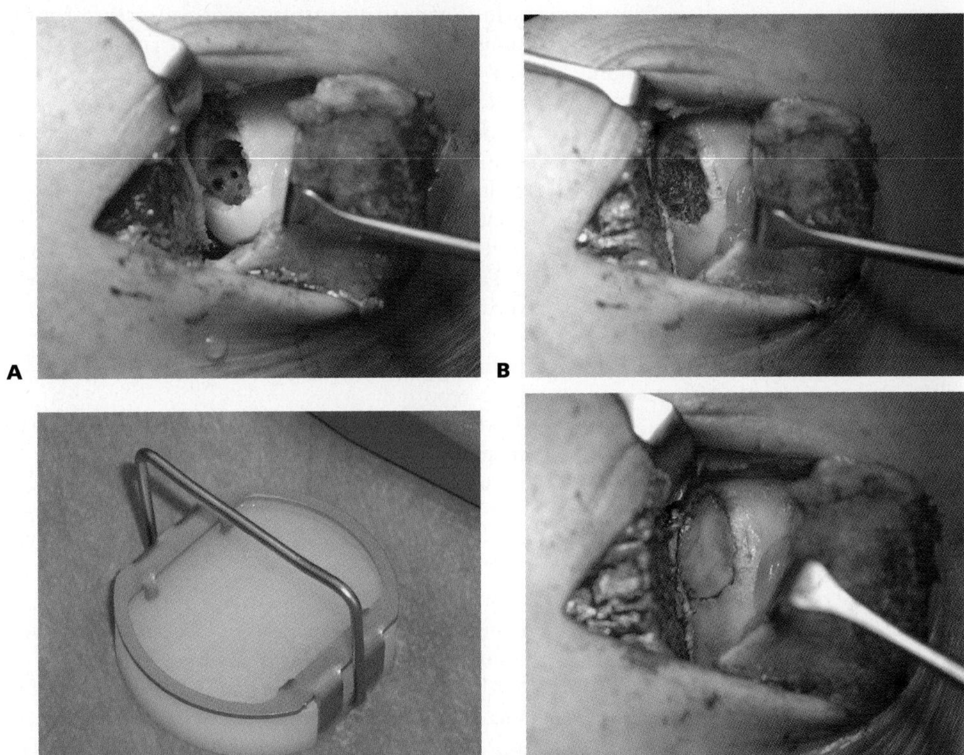

TECH FIG 2 • **A.** Traumatic osteochondral lesion at the lateral talar dome after removing the instable cartilage completely. **B.** Container with the matrix-based chondrocytes, ready for transplantation. **C, D.** Matrix-based chondrocytes transplanted into the defect and fixed with sutures.

PEARLS AND PITFALLS

Indications and planning	■ Address associated pathology. ■ Generalized osteoarthritis is a contraindication. ■ Absence of clinical instability ■ Intact cartilage at the corresponding tibial side ■ The extent of cartilaginous detachment is often underestimated on MR, whereas the bony reaction tends to be overestimated. ■ OLTs with subchondral cysts respond poorly to drilling or microfracturing. In these cases ACI or MACI can be considered as a primary procedure. ■ ACI and MACI are *not* indicated in the face of diffuse ankle arthritis; these procedures are intended for focal defects only.
Harvesting	■ Take extreme care when harvesting the chondrocytes from the ankle or ipsilateral knee joint. ■ If not completely destroyed, the detached cartilage can be harvested. ■ Ensure that the cool chain for transport is appropriate.
Cultivation	■ This service is provided by several companies. They provide the medium for harvesting the chondrocytes and in some cases special tools for harvesting and transplantation.
Transplantation	■ Be careful to prepare the transplant large enough. ■ Adequate exposure is mandatory for ACI or MACI. This often requires a malleolar osteotomy. ■ Intraoperative radiographs should be taken before performing an osteotomy and after the osteosynthesis. The osteotomy should be adequate to gain sufficient access to the OLT. ■ Do not squeeze the transplant (MACI). ■ Be sure that the periosteal flap is watertight before injecting the chondrocytes (ACI).
Rehabilitation	■ Follow the rehabilitation plan; it takes time for the graft to gain its final stability and strength. ■ "Too much, too fast" is the most common reason for failures.

POSTOPERATIVE CARE

- After covering the wounds with sterile dressings, the ankle joint is stabilized with a dorsal splint.
- Immediately postoperatively, the patient should have 48 hours of bed rest. The ankle should not be moved and is fixed with a brace.
- 48 hours postoperatively, drainage tubes are removed and the joint is mobilized with continuous passive motion. Limitations can occur in large defects or extended ligament repair.
- During the first 6 weeks postoperatively, the patients are allowed partial weight bearing (10 kg) and mobilization without weight bearing including accompanying physiotherapy (similar to the postoperative scheme in complex ankle fractures with open reduction and internal fixation).
- After 6 weeks, a gradual increase in joint loading is allowed (20 to 30 kg every 2 weeks) up to full body weight.
- After 12 weeks, full weight bearing in activities of daily life is allowed, including cycling with moderate resistance and swimming.
- After 6 months, increased athletic activities (eg, jogging and skating) can be considered. However, there is little experience in bringing patients with an ACI or MACI back to professional sports. In our anecdotal experience we have seen most patients able to return to recreational sports.
- It is unclear whether patients can return to contact sports and sports that place high physical demands on the ankle joint. So far there are no data available.

OUTCOMES

- There are only limited data on this new treatment concept, and no long-term studies.
- Peterson et al.[8] reported the results of his first 14 consecutive patients managed with ACI for the ankle. At an average follow-up of 45 months, 12 were considered improved, with 11 having good to excellent outcomes.
- Baums et al.[4] found an improvement in the AOFAS ankle score from 43.5 to 88.4 in a prospective study of 12 patients.
- Giannini et al.[18] reported an average AOFAS hindfoot–ankle score improvement from 26 points to 91 points at a mean follow-up of 26 months. Histologic analysis of biopsies obtained at 12 months suggested hyaline cartilage in all eight specimens.
- In another series Giannini et al.[17] demonstrated no statistically significant difference in 16 patients undergoing ACI with chondrocytes cultured from the detached OLT fragment compared to 7 patients undergoing ACI with chondrocytes harvested from the patient's ipsilateral knee. In both groups, the average AOFAS hindfoot–ankle score improved from 54 points to about 89 or 90 points. Histologic appearance, expression of specific cartilage markers, cell viability, cell proliferation in culture, and redifferentiation were favorable, and the morphologic and molecular characters of the cultured chondrocytes from the detached fragment were similar to those of physiologic hyaline cartilage.[17]
- By culturing the chondrocytes from the detached chondral fragment, donor site morbidity can be avoided.[17] However, by taking small chips of cartilage from an unloaded area of the knee, the risk of donor site problems should be significantly lower, as reported for harvesting osteochondral grafts from the ipsilateral knee joint.[37]

COMPLICATIONS

- In rare cases, the harvested chondrocytes are not suitable for culture. Typical causes are avital cells or contamination. In this case, the physician is informed by the laboratory that cultures the cartilage cells. One possibility is to do another arthroscopy to get cartilage cells; however, other treatment options like OATS or allograft can be considered.
- Delayed union in the malleolar osteotomy: Provided progression toward healing, even if very gradual, is observed on serial radiographs, our experience has been that the osteotomies eventually heal without complications. However, prompt revision open reduction and internal fixation with bone grafting is warranted if progression toward healing is not noted, to limit the risk of displacement of the osteotomy.
- Failure of the transplanted tissue includes detachment of the transplant, delamination, or ossification. Especially in the periosteal flap technique, ossification is a common cause of failure.[31] Ossification in the MACI technique has not yet been reported.
- Resorption of the subchondral bone graft in stage V lesions treated using the sandwich technique can lead to a graft failure.
- Hypertrophy: Fibrous tissue may form at the graft–host articular junction or within the ankle, causing impingement, and can be effectively débrided to relieve symptoms. ACI in particular is subject to fibrillation or hypertrophy, and arthroscopic débridement, in select cases, is essential to remove mechanical symptoms and avoid delamination of the graft.[8]
- The source of pain from an OLT remains ill defined, and the success of cartilage resurfacing procedures is certainly not 100%. Therefore, even without any obvious complication, pain may persist.
- If the clinical outcome is not satisfactory and follow-up imaging studies suggest graft compromise, ankle arthroscopy is warranted. While failure of graft incorporation or delamination of the resurfaced articular segment is perhaps irreversible, not all persistent symptoms are necessarily due to such phenomena. Second-look arthroscopy may demonstrate that the cartilage resurfacing procedure was successful but was inadequate to resurface what proved to be a larger area of diseased talus than originally identified.
- In ACI for which the cartilage cells are harvested from the knee, there is a risk of persistent knee symptoms. The reported prevalence of persistent knee symptoms ranges from less than 10%[18,22,41] to 50%.[37] It is important to educate patients about this risk preoperatively. Since Giannini et al[17] has demonstrated no statistically significant difference between chondrocytes cultured from the detached OLT fragment versus chondrocytes harvested from the patient's ipsilateral knee, we always harvest chondrocytes from the ankle joint to minimize the risk of donor site problems.[4] Based on our extended anecdotal experience doing so, we have seen no disadvantage with this concept.
- General surgical complications such as deep venous thrombosis, wound healing problems, or infection are also possible.

REFERENCES

1. Al-Shaikh RA, Chou LB, Mann JA, et al. Autologous osteochondral grafting for talar cartilage defects. Foot Ankle Int 2002;23:381–389.
2. Barnes CJ, Ferkel RD. Arthroscopic debridement and drilling of osteochondral lesions of the talus. Foot Ankle Clin 2003;8:243–257.

3. Bartlett W, Skinner JA, Gooding CR, et al. Autologous chondrocyte implantation versus matrix-induced autologous chondrocyte implantation for osteochondral defects of the knee: a prospective, randomised study. J Bone Joint Surg Br 2005;87B:640–645.
4. Baums MH, Heidrich G, Schultz W, et al. Autologous chondrocyte transplantation for treating cartilage defects of the talus. J Bone Joint Surg Am 2006;88A:303–308.
5. Becher C, Thermann H. Results of microfracture in the treatment of articular cartilage defects of the talus. Foot Ankle Int 2005;26:583–589.
6. Benthien RA, Sullivan RJ, Aronow MS. Adolescent osteochondral lesion of the talus: ankle arthroscopy in pediatric patients. Foot Ankle Clin 2002;7:651–667.
7. Berndt AL, Harty M. Transchondral fractures (osteochondritis dissecans) of the talus. J Bone Joint Surg Am 1959;41A:988–1020.
8. Brittberg M, Peterson L, Sjogren-Jansson E, et al. Articular cartilage engineering with autologous chondrocyte transplantation: a review of recent developments. J Bone Joint Surg Am 2003:85A(Suppl 3):109–115.
9. Cole AA, Margulis A, Kuettner KE. Distinguishing ankle and knee articular cartilage. Foot Ankle Clin 2003;8:305–316.
10. DiGiovanni BF, Fraga CJ, Cohen BE, et al. Associated injuries found in chronic lateral ankle instability. Foot Ankle Int 2000;21:809–815.
11. Dipaola JD, Nelson DW, Colville MR. Characterizing osteochondral lesions by magnetic resonance imaging. Arthroscopy 1991;7:101–104.
12. Easley ME, Scranton PE. Osteochondral autologous transfer system. Foot Ankle Clin 2003;8:275–290.
13. Elias I, Jung JW, Raikin SM, et al. Osteochondral lesions of the talus: change in MRI findings over time in talar lesions without operative intervention and implications for staging systems. Foot Ankle Int 2006;27:157–166.
14. Feeney S, Rees S, Tagoe M. Tricortical calcaneal bone graft and management of the donor site. J Foot Ankle Surg 2007;46:80–85.
15. Ferkel RD, Sgaglione NA. Arthroscopic treatment of osteochondral lesions of the talus: long-term results. Orthop Trans 1993;17:1011.
16. Geideman W, Early JS, Brodsky J. Clinical results of harvesting autogenous cancellous graft from the ipsilateral proximal tibia for use in foot and ankle surgery. Foot Ankle Int 2004;25:451–455.
17. Giannini S, Buda R, Grigolo B, et al. The detached osteochondral fragment as a source of cells for autologous chondrocyte implantation (ACI) in the ankle joint. Osteoarthritis Cartilage 2005:13:601–607.
18. Giannini S, Buda R, Grigolo B, et al. Autologous chondrocyte transplantation in osteochondral lesions of the ankle joint. Foot Ankle Int 2001;22:513–517.
19. Giannini S, Vannini F. Operative treatment of osteochondral lesions of the talar dome: current concepts review. Foot Ankle Int 2004;25: 168–175.
20. Gross AE, Agnidis Z, Hutchison CR. Osteochondral defects of the talus treated with fresh osteochondral allograft transplantation. Foot Ankle Int 2001;22:385–391.
21. Guhl JF. Arthroscopic treatment of osteochondritis dissecans. Clin Orthop Relat Res 1982;167:65–74.
22. Hangody L. The mosaicplasty technique for osteochondral lesions of the talus. Foot Ankle Clin 2003;8:259–273.
23. Hepple S, Winson IG, Glew D. Osteochondral lesions of the talus: a revised classification. Foot Ankle Int 1999;20:789–793.
24. Kelberine F, Frank A. Arthroscopic treatment of osteochondral lesions of the talar dome: a retrospective study of 48 cases. Arthroscopy 1999;15:77–84.
25. Koch S, Kampen WU, Laprell H. Cartilage and bone morphology in osteochondritis dissecans. Knee Surg Sports Traumatol Arthrosc 1997;5:42–45.
26. Komenda GA, Ferkel RD. Arthroscopic findings associated with the unstable ankle. Foot Ankle Int 1999;20:708–713.
27. Mandelbaum BR, Gerhardt MB, Peterson L. Autologous chondrocyte implantation of the talus. Arthroscopy 2003;19(Suppl 1):129–137.
28. McCullough CJ, Venugopal V. Osteochondritis dissecans of the talus: the natural history. Clin Orthop Relat Res 1979;144:264–268.
29. Muir D, Saltzman CL, Tochigi Y, et al. Talar dome access for osteochondral lesions. Am J Sports Med 2006;34:1457–1463.
30. Myerson MS, Neufeld SK, Uribe J. Fresh-frozen structural allografts in the foot and ankle. J Bone Joint Surg Am 2005;87A:113–120.
31. Nehrer S, Spector M, Minas T. Histologic analysis of tissue after failed cartilage repair procedures. Clin Orthop Relat Res 1999;365: 149–162.
32. Outerbridge RE. The etiology of chondromalacia patellae. J Bone Joint Surg Br 1961;43B:752–757.
33. Oznur A. Medial malleolar window approach for osteochondral lesions of the talus. Foot Ankle Int 2001;22:841–842.
34. Radke S, Vispo-Seara J, Walther M, et al. Osteochondral lesions of the talus: indications for MRI with a contrast agent. Z Orthop Ihre Grenzgeb 2004;142:618–624.
35. Raikin SM, Brislin K. Local bone graft harvested from the distal tibia or calcaneus for surgery of the foot and ankle. Foot Ankle Int 2005; 26:449–453.
36. Raikin SM, Elias I, Zoga AC, et al. Osteochondral lesions of the talus: localization and morphologic data from 424 patients using a novel anatomical grid scheme. Foot Ankle Int 2007;28:154–161.
37. Reddy S, Pedowitz DI, Parekh SG, et al. The morbidity associated with osteochondral harvest from asymptomatic knees for the treatment of osteochondral lesions of the talus. Am J Sports Med 2007; 35:80–85.
38. Sammarco GJ, Makwana NK. Treatment of talar osteochondral lesions using local osteochondral graft. Foot Ankle Int 2002;23: 693–698.
39. Schuman L, Struijs PA, van Dijk CN. Arthroscopic treatment for osteochondral defects of the talus: results at follow-up at 2 to 11 years. J Bone Joint Surg Br 2002;84B:364–368.
40. Scranton ES. Osteochondral lesions of the talus. In: Nunley JA, Pfeffer GB, Sanders RW, Trepman E, eds. Advanced reconstruction foot and ankle, 1st ed. Rosemont IL: AAOS, 2004:261–266.
41. Scranton PE, Frey CC, Feder KS. Outcome of osteochondral autograft transplantation for type-V cystic osteochondral lesions of the talus. J Bone Joint Surg Br 2006;88B:614–619.
42. Shea MP, Manoli A. Osteochondral lesions of the talar dome. Foot Ankle 1993;14:48–55.
43. Shearer C, Loomer R, Clement D. Nonoperatively managed stage 5 osteochondral talar lesions. Foot Ankle Int 2002;23:651–654.
44. Tochigi Y, Amendola A, Muir D, et al. Surgical approach for centrolateral talar osteochondral lesions with an anterolateral osteotomy. Foot Ankle Int 2002;23:1038–1039.
45. Toth AP, Easley ME. Ankle chondral injuries and repair. Foot Ankle Clin 2000;5:799–840.
46. Wester JU, Jensen IE, Rasmussen F, et al. Osteochondral lesions of the talar dome in children. A 24 (7-36) year follow-up of 13 cases. Acta Orthop Scand 1994;65:110–112.
47. Whittaker JP, Smith G, Makwana N, et al. Early results of autologous chondrocyte implantation in the talus. J Bone Joint Surg Br 2005;87B:179–183.
48. Zheng MH, Willers C, Kirilak L, et al. Matrix-induced autologous chondrocyte implantation (MACI): biological and histological assessment. Tissue Eng 2007;13:737–746.

Chapter 97

Chevron-Type Medial Malleolar Osteotomy

Bruce Cohen

DEFINITION

- Lesions of the medial talar dome can be very challenging to manage operatively, particularly as they tend to be located in the central or posteromedial aspect of the ankle and are often difficult to access or visualize.
- Various techniques have been described to provide adequate or improved exposure for posteromedial talar dome lesions. Options include arthroscopic techniques, standard arthrotomy, tibial grooving, or medial malleolar osteotomy.
- With the recent interest in new techniques for the treatment of osteochondral lesions of the talar dome, appropriate exposure of both medial and lateral talar dome lesions has become very important.
- Osteochondral allograft insertion and other cartilage replacement techniques are moving to the forefront of orthopaedic foot and ankle care and rely on adequate exposure of the lesion itself. The chevron-type medial malleolar osteotomy is a very stable, reproducible osteotomy that allows excellent exposure to the tibiotalar joint.

ANATOMY

- Pertinent anatomy related to osteotomies of the medial malleolus includes the adjacent structures such as the posterior tibialis tendon and the adjacent neurovascular bundle. The medial malleolus is subcutaneous and convex on its medial border and slightly concave on its lateral surface. The posterior surface includes the malleolar sulcus, which contains the posterior tibialis tendon and the flexor digitorum longus tendon. The distal portion contains the attachment of the deltoid ligament.

PATHOGENESIS

- Lesions of the medial talar dome that require treatment by adjunctive osteotomy include talar body fractures, osteochondral lesions of the talar dome, and other intra-articular lesions.

NATURAL HISTORY

- Advantages proposed for the use of a medial malleolar osteotomy include excellent visualization and wide exposure for débridement or fixation of fragments. Possible disadvantages include the need for prolonged postoperative immobilization and the risk of degenerative ankle arthrosis or nonunion, as well as prominent hardware. No previous study has specifically addressed the results and the morbidity of a medial malleolar osteotomy.

IMAGING AND OTHER DIAGNOSTIC STUDIES

- Standard ankle radiographs are mandatory. Intra-articular lesions, including talar fractures and osteochondral lesions of the talus, can be evaluated with MRI or CT scans.

SURGICAL MANAGEMENT

Preoperative Planning

- Preoperative planning primarily focuses on the planning required for the talar lesion, or fracture, that is being addressed. For comminuted talar body fractures, preoperative CT scans are essential not only for planning the potential fixation but also for evaluating the extent of the articular injury.
- In planning for the treatment of osteochondral lesions, MRI techniques can be helpful in evaluating the size and location of the lesion and the extent of articular involvement and screening for other articular abnormalities.
- CT scans can be helpful in determining the presence of cystic lesions and especially determining whether the lesion is "contained" and appropriate for consideration of osteochondral transplantation.

Positioning

- The patient is positioned supine.

Approach

- A standard medial approach is used, with the incision centered on the medial malleolus and slightly curved distally. Care is taken to avoid injury to the saphenous vein and nerve.

TECHNIQUES

CHEVRON-TYPE MEDIAL MALLEOLAR OSTEOTOMY

- A chevron-type transmalleolar osteotomy is performed in the following manner.
- After standard exposure of the medial malleolus, open the posterior tibialis tendon sheath at the level of the ankle mortise.
- Retract the posterior tibialis tendon itself and protect it posteriorly.
- Predrill and tap the medial malleolus with a 2.5-mm drill.
- Make the chevron-shaped osteotomy with a microsagittal saw. The apex is directed proximally and the limbs of the chevron are extended from the mortise level (**TECH FIG 1A,B**). In the AP plane, the osteotomy is angled toward the junction of the medial malleolus and tibial plafond articular surface (**TECH FIG 1C**).
- Complete the osteotomy with a fine hand osteotome, avoiding a "Kerf" effect within the joint.

- Retract the osteotomized medial malleolus, releasing anterior and posterior soft tissues as necessary for exposure of the talar dome while maintaining the superficial and deep attachments of the deltoid ligament (**TECH FIG 2**).
- At the conclusion of the procedure, stabilize the osteotomy using two 4.0-mm partially threaded cancellous screws (Synthes, USA) (**TECH FIG 3**).

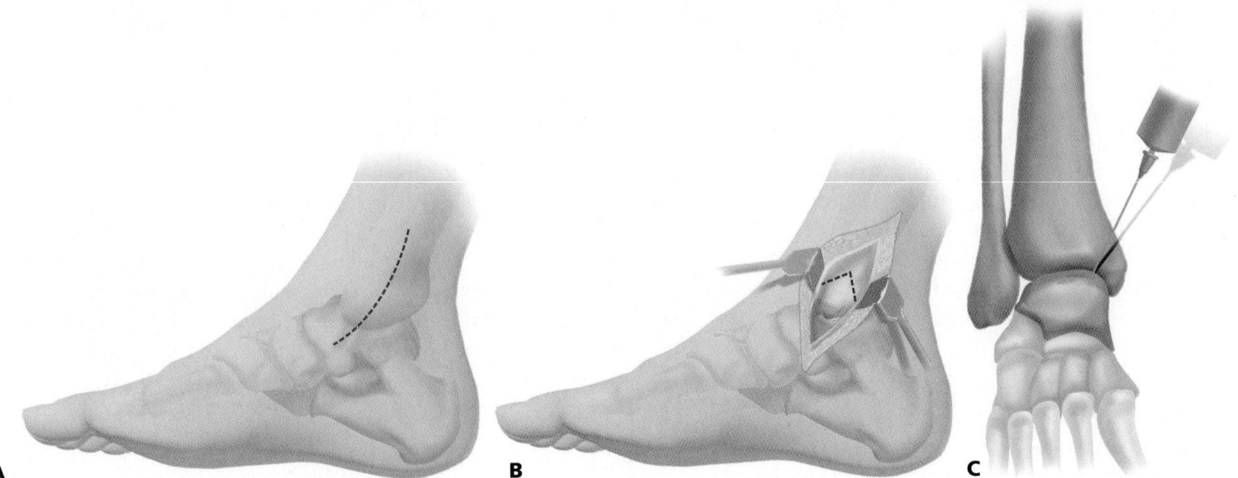

TECH FIG 1 • **A.** Incision for medial malleolar osteotomy. Chevron-type medial malleolar osteotomy in (**B**) lateral plane and (**C**) AP plane.

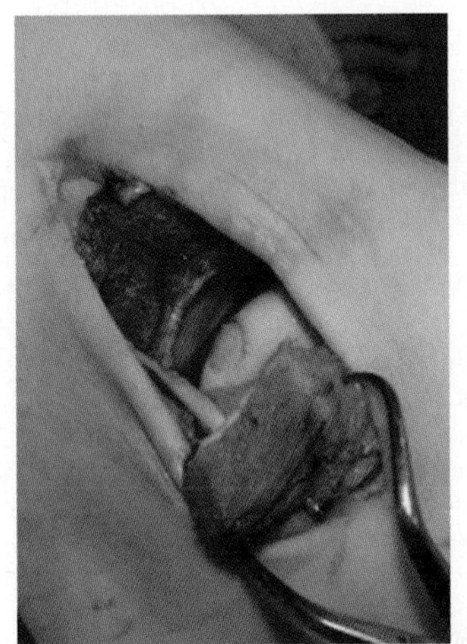

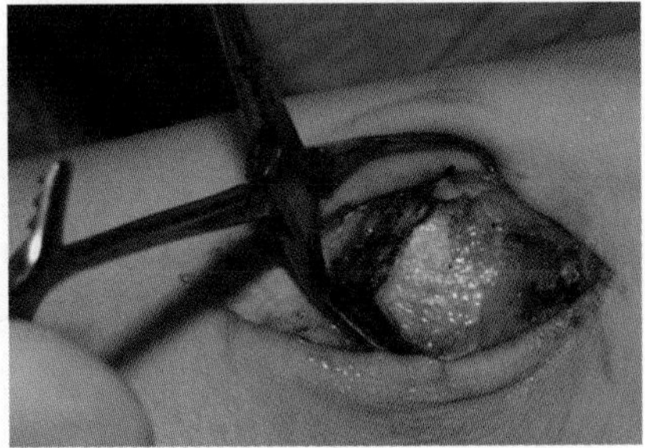

TECH FIG 2 • Intraoperative pictures of osteotomy.

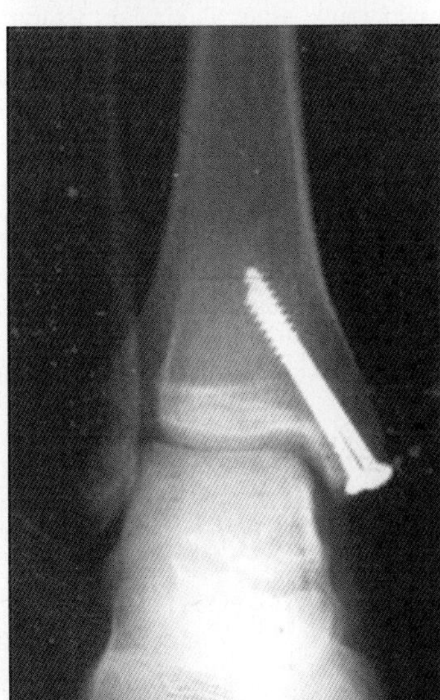

TECH FIG 3 • Postoperative radiographs, AP view.

PEARLS AND PITFALLS

Avoid laceration to posterior tibial tendon.	■ Deep Hohmann retractor is placed after small incision is made in posterior tibial tendon sheath.
Inaccurate reduction	■ Must predrill before osteotomy
Poor visualization	■ Avoid making the exiting areas of the arms of the osteotomy too distal.

POSTOPERATIVE CARE

■ The patient is placed in a plaster splint for 10 to 14 days postoperatively. Active range of motion is begun after 10 to 14 days (or when the wound has sealed) and the patient is placed in a removable short-leg cast brace. Non–weight-bearing ambulation is maintained until radiographs, repeated at about 6 weeks, confirm maintenance of reduction.

OUTCOMES

■ A retrospective review was performed on 19 patients who underwent medial malleolar osteotomy for the treatment of pathology of the talar dome.[6] Chart review, radiographic examination, and clinical examination were performed in all patients. Fifteen patients had osteochondral lesions of the medial talar dome. All patients failed conservative treatment of these lesions, including a period of immobilization and anti-inflammatory medication. The location of the lesion was in the posterior or central portion of the talar dome in all patients.

■ Three patients had medial malleolar osteotomy performed for exposure during internal fixation of displaced talar dome fractures. One additional patient had curettage and bone grafting of a large medial talar cyst.

■ About 50% of the patients had undergone prior surgery on the affected ankle. Six patients had a total of nine prior arthroscopic procedures. The average age of the patients was 32 years (range 14 to 51). The length of follow-up was 12 months (range 6 to 43).

■ All patients achieved union of the osteotomy both clinically and radiographically. The average time to radiographic union was 7 weeks (range 5 to 12). No failures of fixation were noted.

■ Preoperative and postoperative tibiotalar range of motion was measured. At the last follow-up, only 2 of 19 patients had any loss of motion compared to their preoperative evaluation. This decreased range of motion was about 10 degrees of total arc of motion.

■ Four patients had slight (less than 2 mm) displacement at the osteotomy site. This displacement was noted immediately postoperatively and was felt to be due to technical errors during the bone cuts for the osteotomy. No progressive displacement was noted in these patients. All four patients were asymptomatic at the osteotomy site and no progressive ankle arthrosis was noted. Three patients had symptomatic prominent screws that resulted in hardware removal. All the screws were removed as an outpatient procedure under a local anesthetic without complications. No postoperative complications, including infection, nonunion, or delayed wound healing, were noted in the study population.

COMPLICATIONS

■ Nonuion rates for medial malleolar osteotomy are reported as high as 12%. Theoretically the chevron-type provides excellent stability for fixation.

■ Other complications include saphenous nerve injury, with resulting medial ankle numbness or painful subcutaneous neuroma, or posterior tibial tendon laceration, resulting in displacement of the osteotomy and development of progressive arthrosis.

REFERENCES

1. Alexander AH, Lichtman DM. Surgical treatment of transchondral talar-dome fractures (osteochondritis dissecans). J Bone Joint Surg Am 1980;62A:646–652.
2. Alexander IJ, Watson JT. Step-cut osteotomy of the medial malleolus for exposure of the medial ankle joint space. Foot Ankle Int 1991;11:242–243.
3. Berndt AL, Harty M. Transchondral fractures (osteochondritis dissecans) of the talus. J Bone Joint Surg Am 1959;41A:988–1020.
4. Bryant DD, Siegel MG. OCD of the talus: a new technique for arthroscopic drilling. Arthroscopy 1993;9:238–241.
5. Canale ST, Belding RH. Osteochondral lesions of the talus. J Bone Joint Surg Am 1980;62A:97–102.
6. Cohen BE, Anderson RB. Chevron-type transmalleolar osteotomy: an approach to medial talar lesions. Tech Foot Ankle Surg 2002;1: 158–162.
7. Ferkel RD, Fasulo GJ. Arthroscopic treatment of ankle injuries. Orthop Clin North Am 1994;25:17–32.
8. Flick AB, Gould N. Osteochondritis dissecans of the talus (transchondral fractures of the talus): review of the literature and new surgical approach of medial dome lesions. Foot Ankle 1985;5:165–185.
9. Gepstein R, Conforty B, Weiss RE, et al. Closed percutaneous drilling for osteochondritis dissecans of the talus. Clin Orthop Relat Res 1986;213:197–199.
10. Kristensen G, Lind T, Lavard P, et al. Fracture stage 4 of the lateral talar dome treated arthroscopically using Biofix for fixation. Arthroscopy 1990;6:242–244.
11. McCullough CJ, Venegopal V. OCD of the talus: the natural history. Clin Orthop Relat Res 1979;144:264–268.
12. O'Farrell TA, Costello BG. OCD of the talus: the late results of surgical treatment. J Bone Joint Surg Br 1982;64B:494–497.
13. Ove N, Bosse MJ, Reinert CM. Excision of posterolateral talar dome lesions through a medial transmalleolar approach. Foot Ankle 1989; 9:171–175.
14. Parisien JS. Arthroscopic treatment of osteochondral lesions of the talus. Am J Sports Med 1986;14:211–217.
15. Ray RB, Coughlin EJ. Osteochondritis dissecans of the talus. J Bone Joint Surg Am 1947;29A:697–706.
16. Roden S, Tillegard P, Unanderscharin L. Osteochondritis dissecans and similar lesions of the talus. Acta Orthop Scand 1953;23: 51–52.
17. Scharling M. Osteochondritis dissecans of the talus. Acta Orthop Scand 1978;49:89–94.
18. Thompson JP, Looner RL. Osteochondral lesion of the talus in a sports medicine clinic: a new radiographic technique and surgical approach. Am J Sports Med 1984;12:460–463.
19. Yvars MF. Osteochondral fracture of the dome of the talus. Clin Orthop Relat Res 1976;114:185–191.

Chapter 98 Modified Brostrom and Brostrom-Evans Procedures

Paul J. Hecht, Justin S. Cummins, Mark E. Easley, and Dean C. Taylor

DEFINITION

- Lateral ankle injuries are among the most common musculoskeletal injuries in the athletic population.
- Rates as high as 7 per 1000 person-years have been reported in the general population.
- From 10% to 20% of sprains progress to some kind of chronic symptoms.
- Determining whether the patient's instability is functional (ie, subjective giving way) or mechanical (ie, motion beyond the normal physiologic limits) is important for formulating treatment recommendations.

ANATOMY

- The lateral ankle ligament complex consists of the anterior talofibular ligament (ATFL), calcaneofibular ligament (CFL), and posterior talofibular ligament (PTFL).
- The ATFL originates from the anterior aspect of the distal fibula and inserts on the lateral aspect of the talar neck. It is often ill defined and, in the chronically sprained ankle, may be manifest as a capsular expansion.
- The ATFL limits anterior translation of the talus with the ankle in neutral and becomes the primary restraint to inversion when the ankle is plantarflexed.
- The CFL originates from the distal tip of the fibula and inserts on the lateral wall of the calcaneus (**FIG 1AB**).
  - The CFL measures 4 to 6 mm in diameter and 13 mm in length, and is directed posteriorly 10 to 45 degrees from the tip of the fibula.
  - The CFL functions to resist inversion with the ankle in neutral.
- The anterior margin of the talus is wider than the posterior margin, which makes the ankle more susceptible to inversion injuries while in plantarflexion.
- The peroneal tendons provide dynamic stability to the ankle joint.

PATHOGENESIS

- An inversion force with the ankle in plantarflexion is the most common mechanism of injury.
- The ATFL typically is the first ligament injured, followed by the CFL.
- Ligament ruptures are most commonly midsubstance tears or avulsions off of the talus.

NATURAL HISTORY

- Despite a relatively high incidence of lateral ankle injuries, most patients do well with nonoperative management.
- Patients are at increased risk for recurrent lateral ankle sprains after sustaining the initial injury and failing to rehabilitate completely.
- Chronic lateral instability may lead to progressive loss of function and osteoarthritic changes of the ankle.

PATIENT HISTORY AND PHYSICAL FINDINGS

- Patients with chronic ankle instability frequently present with pain as well as complaints of multiple sprains caused by minor provocation.
- Duration of symptoms, the type of incidents that cause sprains, the need for functional bracing, and previous treatments are important for determining treatment recommendations.
- If pain is present between episodes of instability, other lesions about the ankle should also be considered.
- An anterior drawer test with a bony endpoint that is distinctly different from that of the contralateral ankle is considered markedly positive.
- Physical examination techniques include the following:
  - *Palpation.* Palpate the ATFL, CFL, syndesmosis, medial and lateral malleoli, peroneal tendons, base of the fifth metatarsal, and anterior process of the calcaneus.

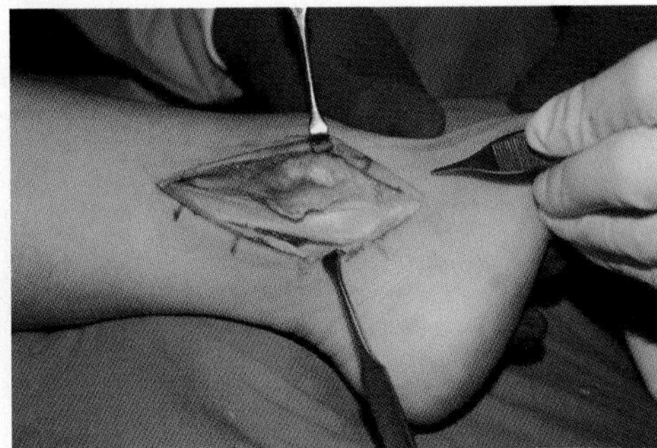

A

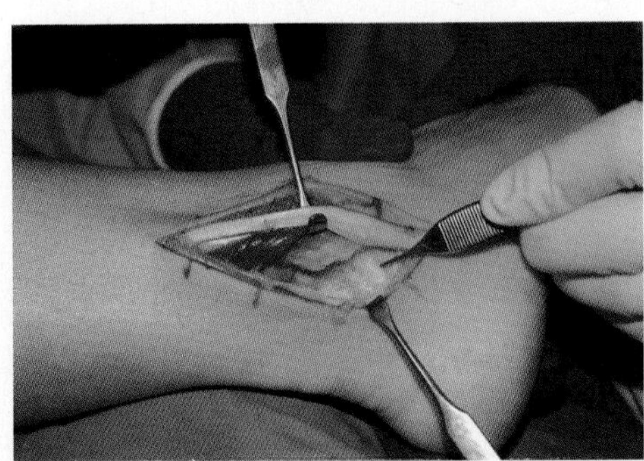

B

FIG 1 • The CFL is directly deep to the peroneal tendons as demonstrated by this surgery to repair peroneal tendon dislocation. **A.** Peroneal tendons in their anatomic location. **B.** CFL identified when peroneal tendons are retracted.

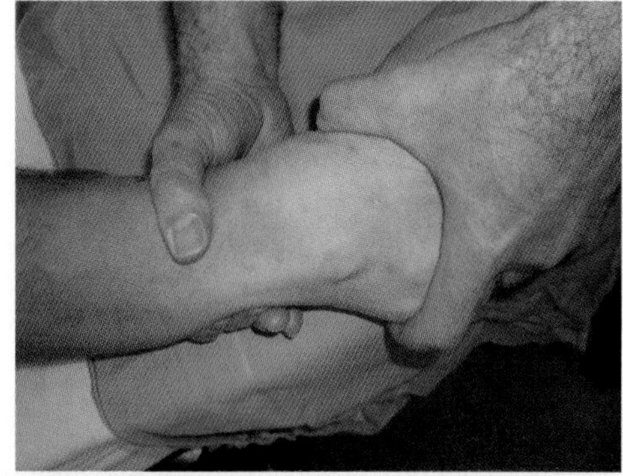

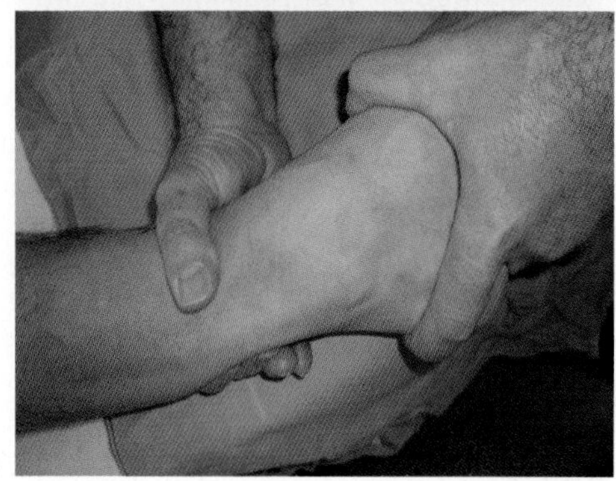

FIG 2 • Anterior drawer test. **A.** Ankle reduced. **B.** Anterior subluxation.

- *Grading ATFL injuries.* I, stretching; II, partial tearing; III, complete rupture. This is most useful in the acute setting to determine which structures are injured.
- *Anterior drawer test* (**FIG 2AB**). The ankle is held in plantarflexion, and the talus is translated forward relative to the tibia. With intact medial structures, the displacement is rotatory. Translation of 5 mm more than the contralateral ankle or absolute translation of 9 to 10 mm is a positive test and suggests an incompetent ATFL. Grading ATFL injuries: I, stretching; II, partial tearing; III, complete rupture; most useful in the acute setting to determine which structures are injured.
- *Talar tilt.* The heel is inverted with the ankle in neutral. Range of motion is compared to the contralateral ankle. Increased inversion is suggestive of a CFL injury.
- *Alignment.* Assess the standing alignment of the hindfoot. Varus hindfoot alignment predisposes the ankle to inversion injury.

IMAGING AND OTHER DIAGNOSTIC STUDIES

- Standard radiographs should include standing anteroposterior (AP), lateral, and mortise views to evaluate for anterior tibial marginal osteophytes, talar exostoses, osteochondral lesions of the talus, or intra-articular loose bodies.
- Talar tilt can be assessed with inversion stress mortise views of the ankle (**FIG 3A**).
  - Comparison views of the contralateral ankle should also be obtained.
  - A talar tilt angle greater than 10 degrees, or 5 degrees greater than the contralateral ankle, is considered pathologic laxity.
- Anterior translation stress radiographs can be obtained by performing the anterior drawer test and shooting a lateral radiograph (**FIG 3B**).
  - Comparison stress views of the contralateral ankle should also be obtained.
  - Anterior translation 5 mm greater than the contralateral ankle, or an absolute value of greater than 9 mm is suggestive of instability.
- Stress radiographs may be helpful, but physical examination remains the gold standard for evaluation of instability.
- MRI can be useful to evaluate the ligamentous injury, as well as peroneal tendon pathology and suspected osteochondral injuries.

DIFFERENTIAL DIAGNOSIS

- Lateral process talar fracture
- Anterior process calcaneus fracture
- Base of the fifth metatarsal fracture
- Tarsal coalition
- Osteochondral lesion of the talus or tibia
- Subtalar instability
- Syndesmosis injury
- Neurapraxia of the superficial peroneal or sural nerve
- Peroneal tendon tear
- Peroneal instability
- Sinus tarsi syndrome
- Anterolateral ankle soft tissue impingement

NONOPERATIVE MANAGEMENT

- Physical therapy should be the initial treatment for patients with chronic instability.
  - Proprioceptive training and peroneal tendon strengthening are the most important features.

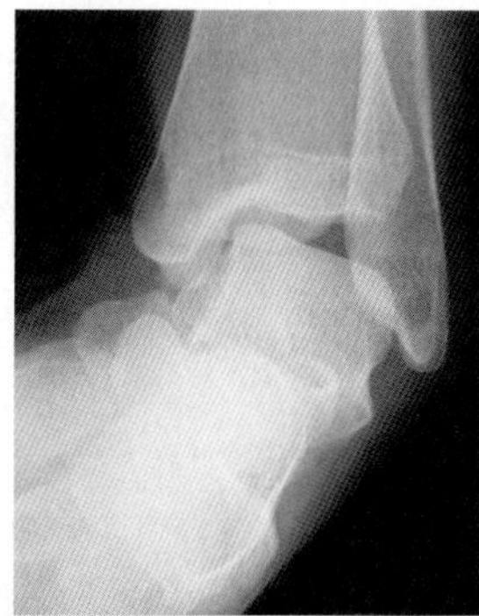

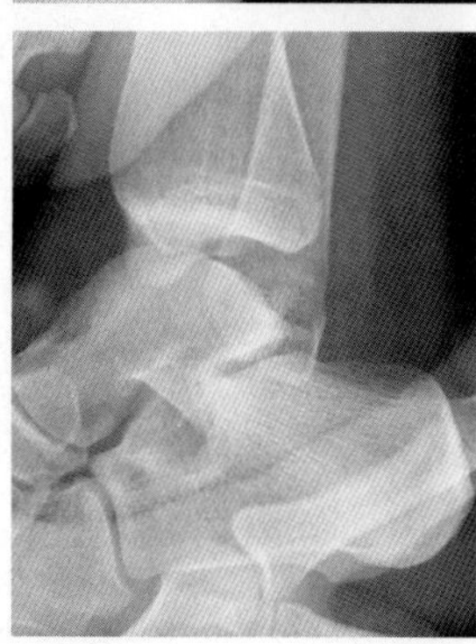

FIG 3 • Radiographic stress tests. **A.** Positive talar tilt test. **B.** Positive anterior drawer test.

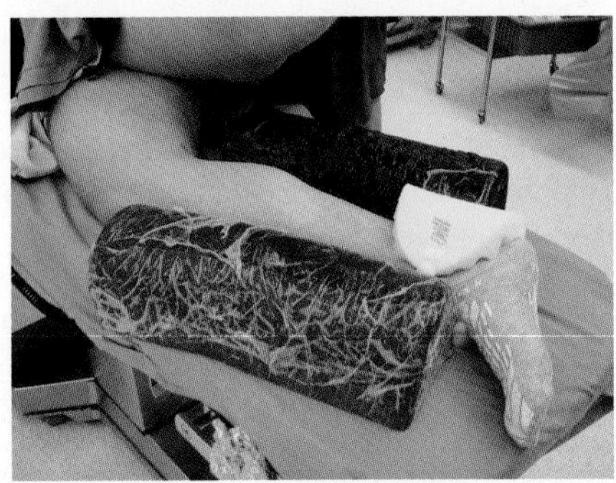

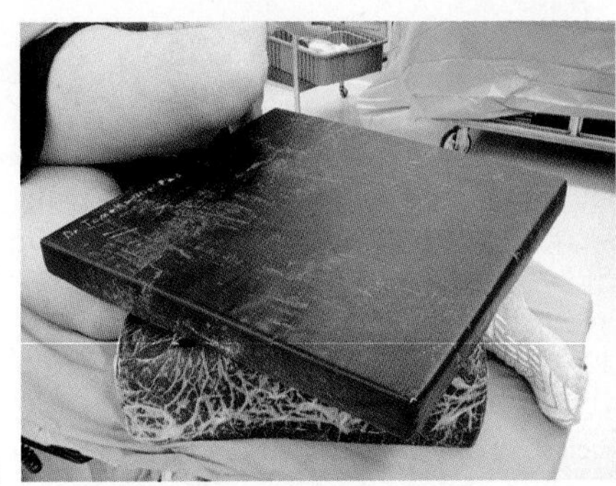

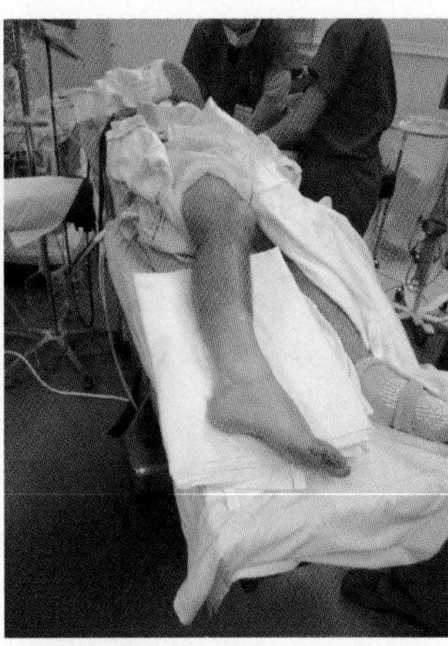

FIG 4 • With the patient in the lateral decubitus position, the nonoperated extremity should be well padded. **A.** Nonoperated leg in a gel pad. **B.** With the nonoperated leg protected, a platform may be used to facilitate positioning of the operated leg. **C.** Alternatively: positioning in the lateral decubitus position, using a stack of folded sheets to serve as a rest for the operated leg.

  - The duration of therapy varies based on strength deficiencies and the intensity of the program.
- External stabilization of the ankle with taping or bracing can be effective.
  - Taping provides tibiotalar stability, but quickly deteriorates with activity.
  - Reusable braces provide similar stability, but do not lose effectiveness with activity.
- Orthotic devices and shoe wear modification can also be used when foot or ankle malalignment contributes to the instability.

SURGICAL MANAGEMENT

- If the patient fails 3 to 6 months of conservative treatment and has persistent signs and symptoms of functional and mechanical instability, he or she becomes a candidate for surgery.

Preoperative Planning

- The history must be considered. A relative contraindication for this anatomic repair is generalized ligamentous laxity as might be encountered in Ehlers-Danlos syndrome.
- Carefully review the physical examination. If a varus heel exists, a Dwyer type calcaneal osteotomy should be considered.
- If an osteochondral lesion is present, the ligamentous reconstruction should be done in conjunction with arthroscopic or open treatment of the osteochondral defect.

Positioning

- The patient is placed in the lateral decubitus position with appropriate padding at bony prominences to avoid damage to subcutaneous structures (**FIG 4AB**).
- An operative platform is created using bolsters or blankets.
- A "bump" made of four or five towels is used either proximal to the ankle to create a varus or inverted position for better exposure or distal to the ankle to create a valgus or everted position to approximate the edges of the repair (**FIG 4C**).

Approach

- Two commonly used approaches
  - J incision (**FIG 5A**)
    - The incision is made from the distal tip of the fibula along its anterior margin proximally to the level of the ankle mortise.
    - Does not afford optimal access to the peroneal tendons
  - Curvilinear extensile exposure (**FIG 5B**)
    - Cuvilinear incision over posterior tip of fibular, extending to sinus tarsi area
    - Affords comprehensive exposure to anterior ankle, ATFL, CFL, and peroneal tendons

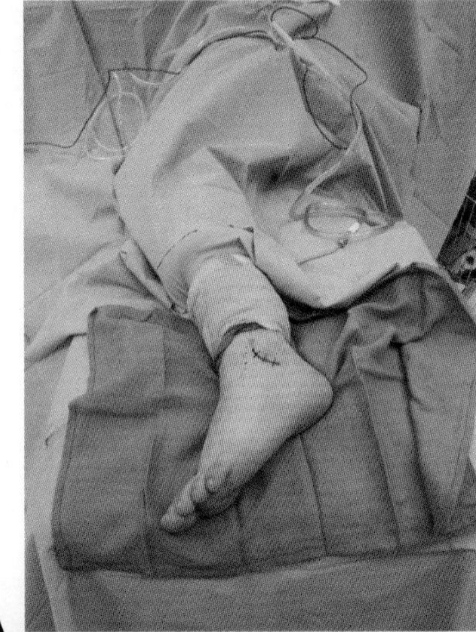

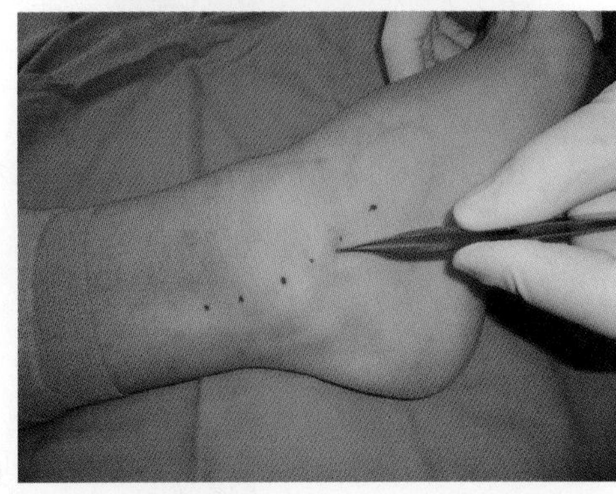

FIG 5 • **A.** A traditional J approach on the anterior distal fibula. **B.** An extensile curvilinear exposure to the lateral ankle. This approach facilitates access to the peroneal tendons should there be associated peroneal tendon pathology.

MODIFIED BROSTROM ANATOMIC LATERAL ANKLE LIGAMENT REPAIR WITH SUTURE ANCHORS

- Perioperative antibiotics are given.
- The patient is positioned as described, a thigh tourniquet is placed, and a standard orthopaedic prep and drape is carried out. The tourniquet is inflated.
- The incision is made as described under Approach in the Surgical Management section (**TECH FIG 1A**).
- With the bump placed proximal to the ankle, a dissection is carried out to isolate the inferior extensor retinaculum.
- The joint capsule is then incised in line with the skin incision and just distal to the leading edge of the fibula. The anterior talofibular (ATF) ligament may or may not be visible as a capsular expansion.
- The CFL is inspected. This inspection, along with the preoperative evaluation, is used to decide whether or not a repair of this ligament is needed.
- The joint is inspected for chondral injury.
- A subperiosteal dissection is carried out at the anterior and lateral aspect of the fibula, raising a flap 3 to 6 mm wide.
- Using curettes and rongeurs, a trough is made in the anterior and lateral aspect of the fibula at its leading edge, about 3 mm deep and 3 mm wide.
- If no CFL repair is needed, a single corkscrew anchor double-armed with no. 2 FiberWire (Arthrex, Inc., Naples, FL) suture is inserted centrally in the trough. If a CFL repair is performed, a second anchor, with no. 2 Fiberwire, is used (**TECH FIG 1B**).
- The joint is thoroughly irrigated, and the actual repair begins. Move the bump so it sits under the lateral border of the foot, placing the subtalar and ankle joints into an everted position before repairing the CFL if necessary.
- The capsular and ATF ligament repair is now performed by bringing the sutures from deep to superficial in a horizontal mattress pattern. The "ligament" is shortened by creating the trough at the fibula. If further shortening is needed, the capsule may be trimmed from the distal cut edge.
- A second reinforcing layer of repair is created by suturing the inferior extensor retinaculum to the periosteal flap with absorbable 2-0 figure 8 sutures.
- The skin is closed in layers with 3-0 absorbable suture in the subcutaneous suture and staples or subcuticular suture used in the skin.
- Dressings are applied, and a short-leg non–weight-bearing splint is applied.

Modified Brostrom Anatomic Lateral Ankle Ligament Repair with Suture Anchor(s) (Courtesy of Mark E. Easley)

- Confirm ankle instability with exam under anesthesia.
- Approach and exposure
  - Curvilinear incision over posterior tip of the fibula and extending to the sinus tarsi (**TECH FIG 2**)
  - Protect sural nerve posteriorly and superficial peroneal nerve anteriorly.
- Prepare the inferior extensor retinaculum.
  - Identify and mobilize the inferior extensor retinaculum (**TECH FIG 3AB**).
  - Relatively thin superficial structure
- Identify, inspect, and protect the peroneal tendons (**TECH FIG 3CD**).
- Anterior arthrotomy
  - Detach the capsule, including the ATFL and CFL (**TECH FIG 4AB**).
  - Protect the peroneal tendons (**TECH FIG 4C**).
  - Excise the anterior inferior tibiofibular ligament (Bassett's ligament) (**TECH FIG 4D**).
    - Usually present in patients after ankle sprain.
    - Potential for anterolateral soft-tissue ankle impingement.
  - Inspect the lateral talar dome for cartilage defect.

A
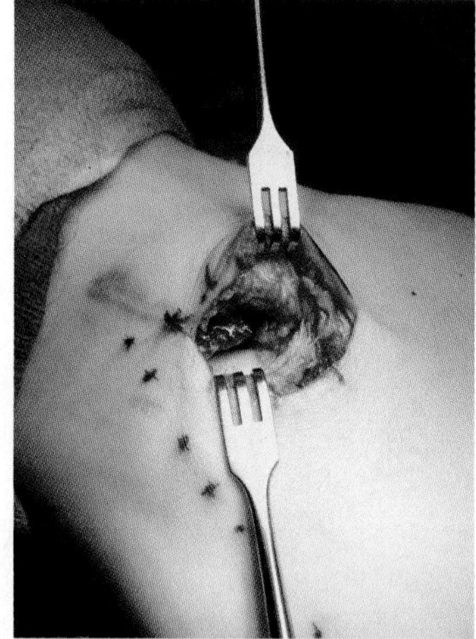

B
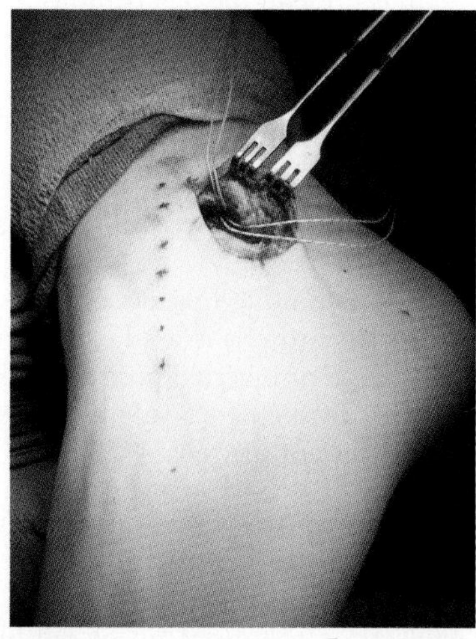

TECH FIG 1 • **A.** Traditional approach to perform the modified Brostrom repair. **B.** Suture anchors placed in the distal fibula.

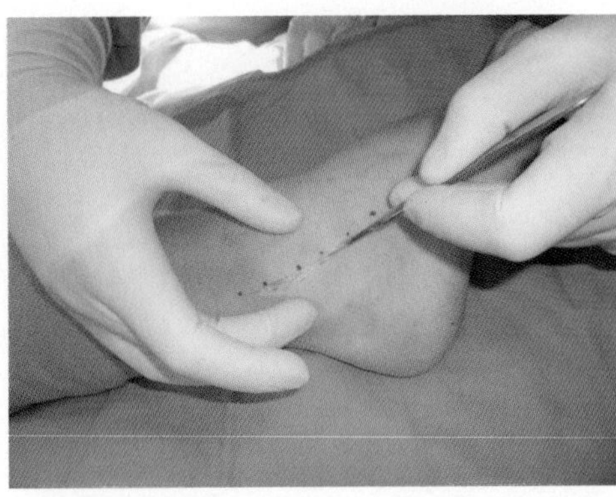

TECH FIG 2 • Curvilinear extensile exposure to the lateral ankle ligaments.

- Identify the ATFL and CFL (TECH FIG 5A–D); these are condensations within the capsular sleeve.
- Develop a distal fibular periosteal flap (TECH FIG 6AB) to use as an additional reinforcement of the repair.
- Prepare anterior distal fibula for reattachment of capsule and ligaments.
  - Create a trough using a rongeur (TECH FIG 6C).
  - Predrill anatomic footprints for ATFL and CFL suture anchor placement (TECH FIG 6DE).
- Place suture anchors (TECH FIG 7AB).
  - Orient them so that they do not:
    - Interfere with one another
    - Violate the joint
    - Violate the posterior cortex of the fibula and irritate the peroneus brevis
  - Test the stability of the suture anchors (TECH FIG 7C).
    - Lift the limb by the anchors; if the anchors are going to fail, we want them to do so now so the problem can be rectified.
- Pass the respective sutures through the CFL, the ajacent capsule, and the ATFL (TECH FIG 7D–F).
- Test the sutures to ensure that they indeed advance the appropriate portion of the capsule to the desired location on the distal fibula (TECH FIG 7G)
- Position the ankle properly for securing the sutures (TECH FIG 8A).
  - Reduce the talus within the ankle mortise
  - Avoid anterior translation of the talus within the mortise
  - Dorsiflex the ankle to neutral
  - Maintain slight hindfoot valgus
- Tie the sutures (TECH FIG 8B–D).
- Check the stability of the repair after the anchor sutures have been tied (TECH FIG 8E).
- Pass the anchor sutures through the distal fibular periosteal flap (TECH FIG 9A–C).
  - This reinforces the repair
  - Place additional sutures from the periosteum to the capsule that has been advanced to the distal fibula (TECH FIG 9D,E)
  - Augment the repair further with the inferior extensor retinaculum

text continues on page 4310

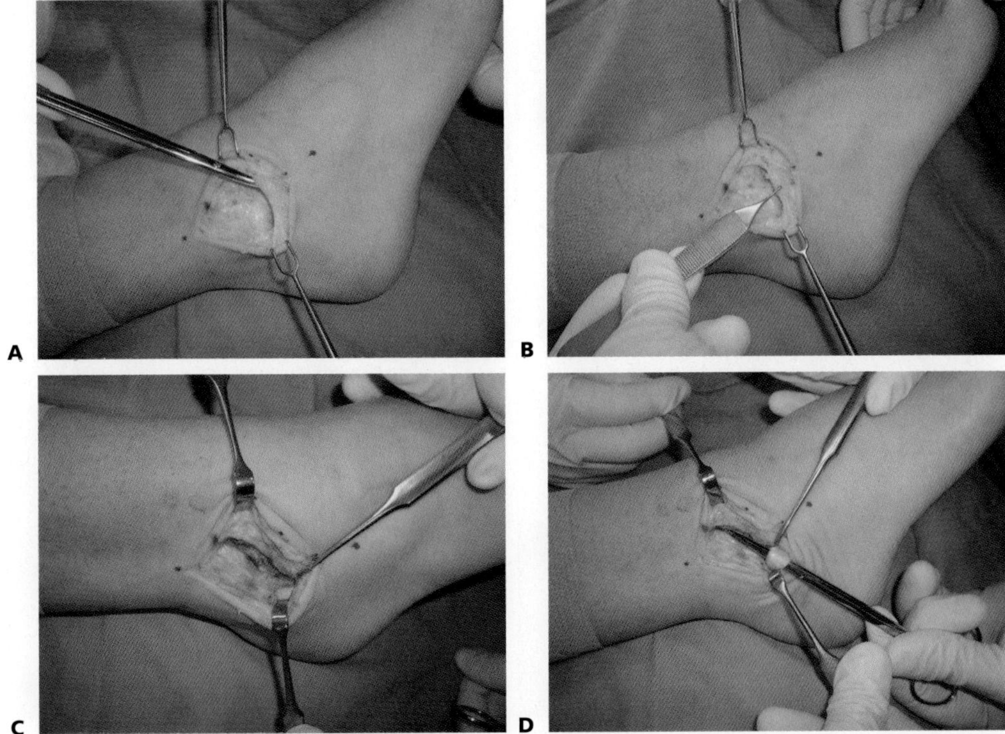

TECH FIG 3 • **A,B.** Mobilize the inferior extensor retinaculum to be used to augment the repair (Gould modification of the Brostrom procedure). **A.** Identify the inferior extensor retinaculum. **B.** Demonstrate that the retinaculum can be advanced. **C,D.** Identify, inspect, and protect the peroneal tendons. **C.** Identify the tendons. **D.** Inspect the tendons.

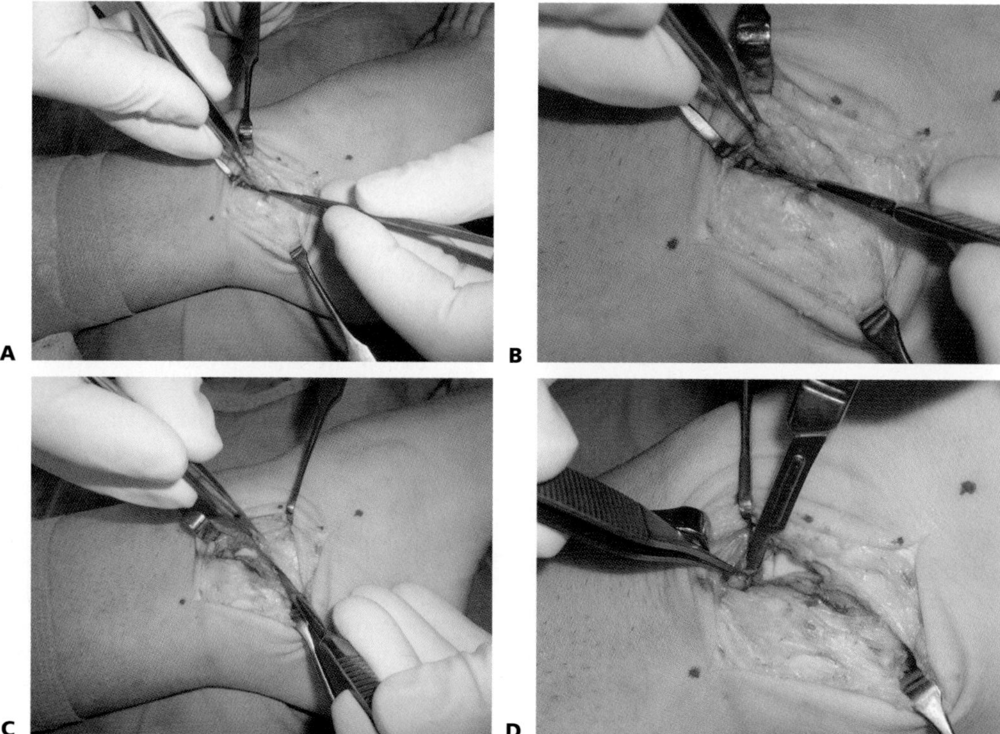

TECH FIG 4 • Anterior arthrotomy. **A–C.** The anterolateral capsule is elevated from the distal fibula. **D.** With the anterolateral tibiotalar joint exposed, the talar articular cartilage may be inspected and the hypertrophied anterior inferior tibiofibular ligament (Basset's ligament) may be excised. (Following multiple ankle sprains, anterolateral soft tissue ankle impingement frequently develops).

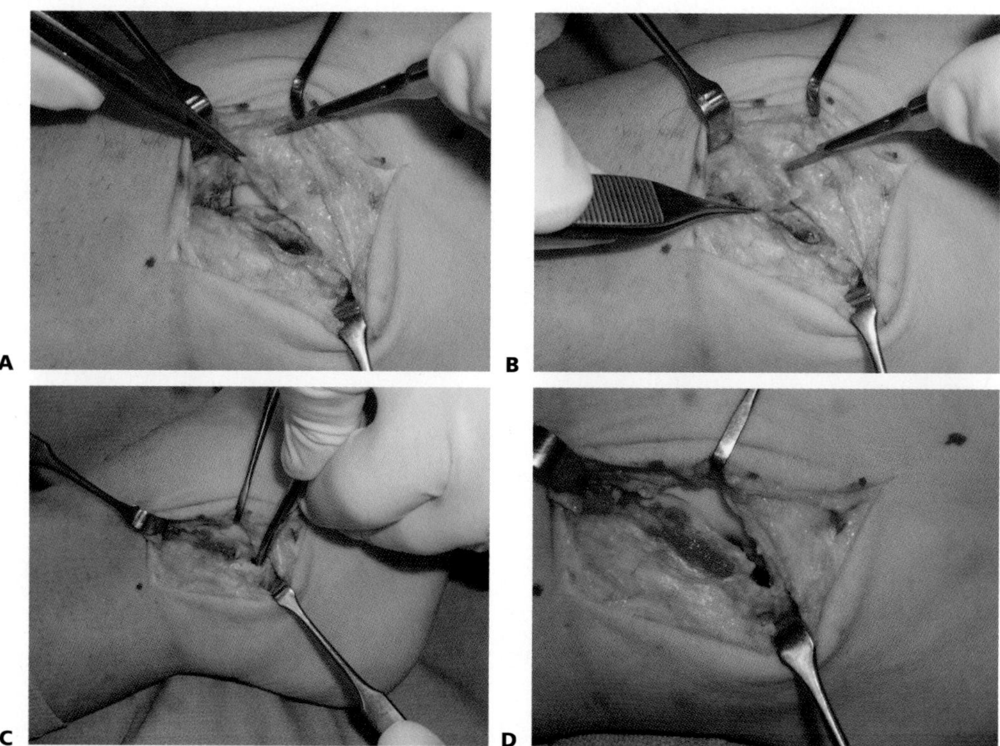

TECH FIG 5 • Identify the ATFL and CFL within the lateral capsule; these structures represent condensations within the lateral capsule. **A,B.** ATFL and its anatomic location on the fibula identified. **C,D.** CFL identified and its competency tested with ankle/hindfoot inversion.

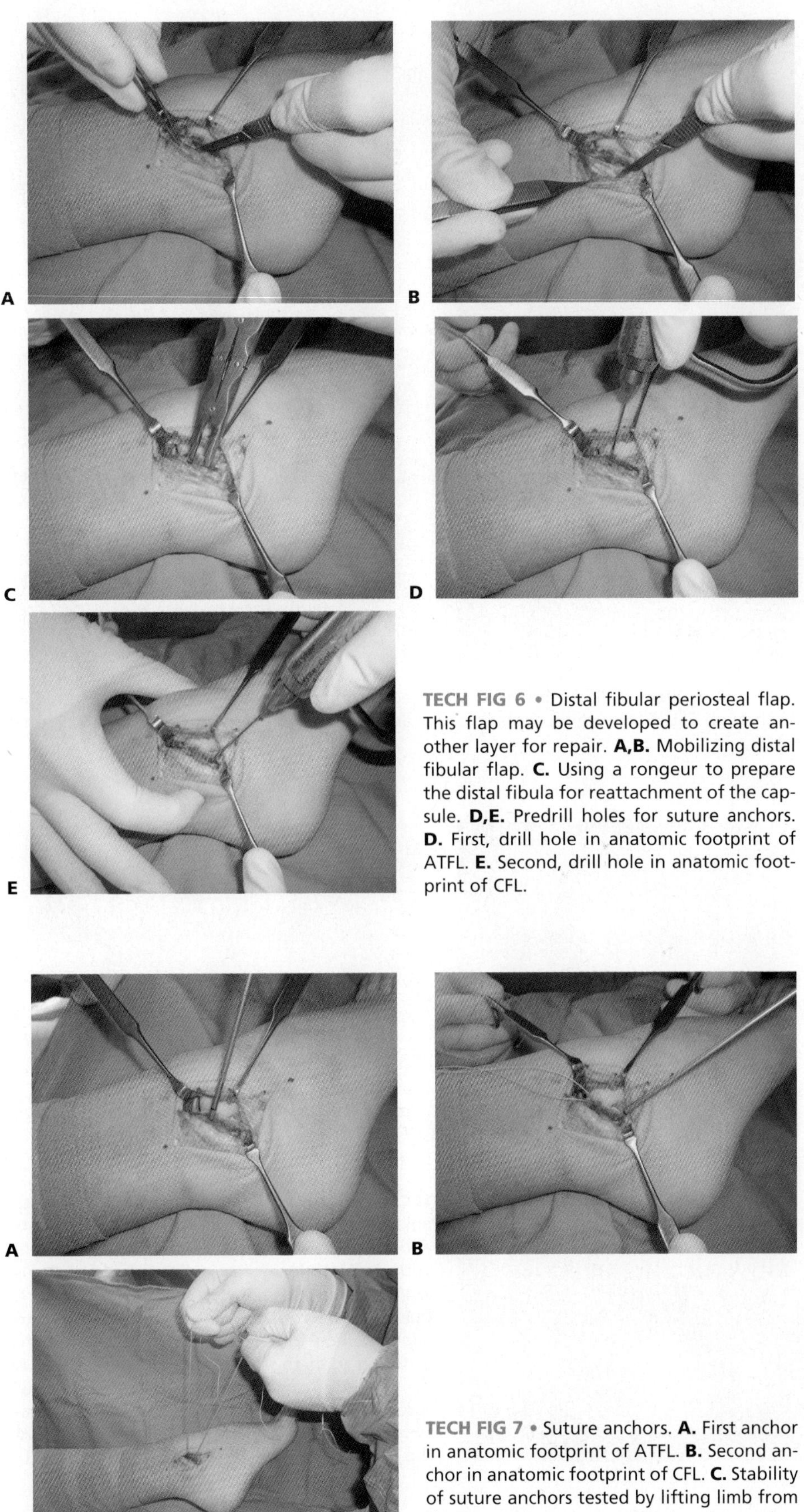

TECH FIG 6 • Distal fibular periosteal flap. This flap may be developed to create another layer for repair. **A,B.** Mobilizing distal fibular flap. **C.** Using a rongeur to prepare the distal fibula for reattachment of the capsule. **D,E.** Predrill holes for suture anchors. **D.** First, drill hole in anatomic footprint of ATFL. **E.** Second, drill hole in anatomic footprint of CFL.

TECH FIG 7 • Suture anchors. **A.** First anchor in anatomic footprint of ATFL. **B.** Second anchor in anatomic footprint of CFL. **C.** Stability of suture anchors tested by lifting limb from the operating room table by the anchor sutures. *(continued)*

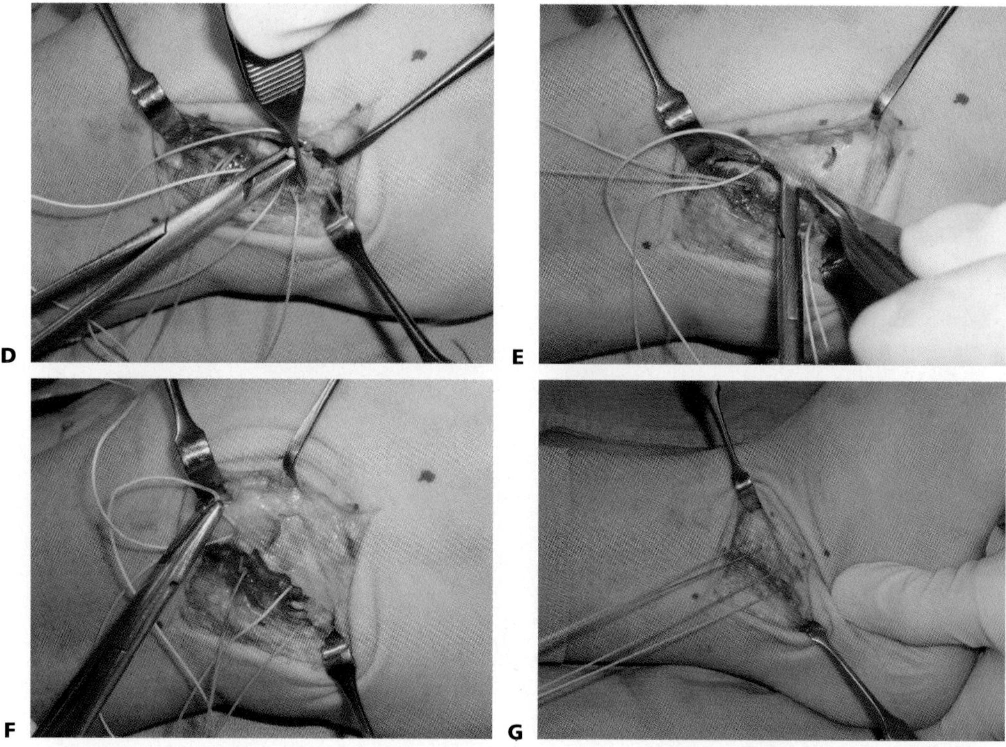

TECH FIG 7 • *(continued)* **D–G.** Anchor sutures passed through respective capsular condensations. **D.** Suture through CFL. **E.** Suture through posterior aspect of capsule adjacent to CFL. **F,G.** Suture through ATFL.

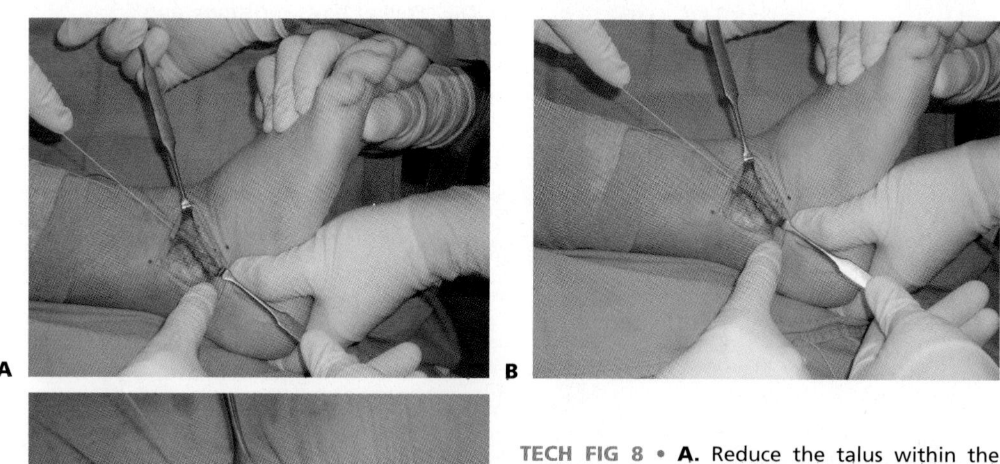

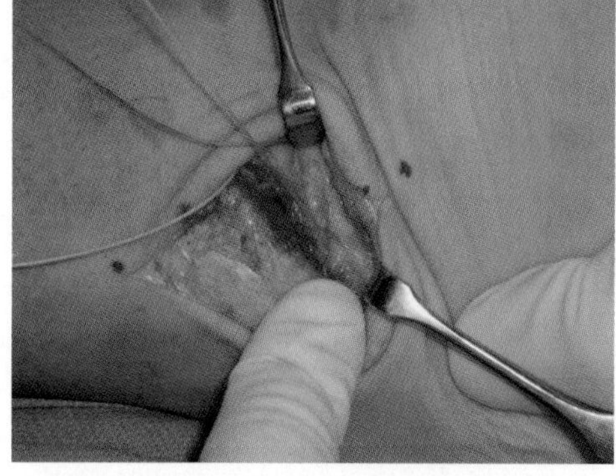

TECH FIG 8 • **A.** Reduce the talus within the ankle mortise before reattaching the ligaments and capsule. The ankle is held in dorsiflexion, with a posterior force maintaining the talus within the ankle mortise. Although covered, a bump has been placed under the distal tibia to allow the heel to translate posteriorly without interfering with the operating table. The heel is maintained in slight valgus. **B–D.** Secure the sutures while ankle is maintained in optimal position. **B.** Protect the peroneal tendons. **C.** Secure the CFL and more posterior capsule. *(continued)*

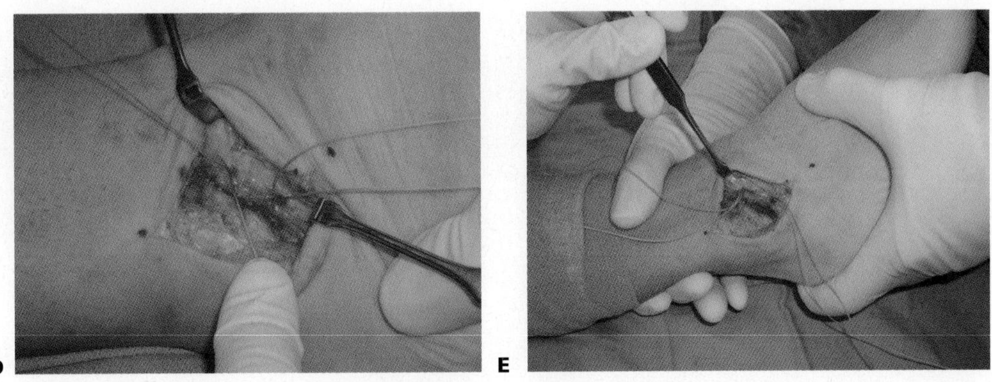

TECH FIG 8 • *(continued)* **D.** Secure the ATFL. **E.** Recheck the anterior drawer test to determine if the primary sutures are securely maintaining ankle stability.

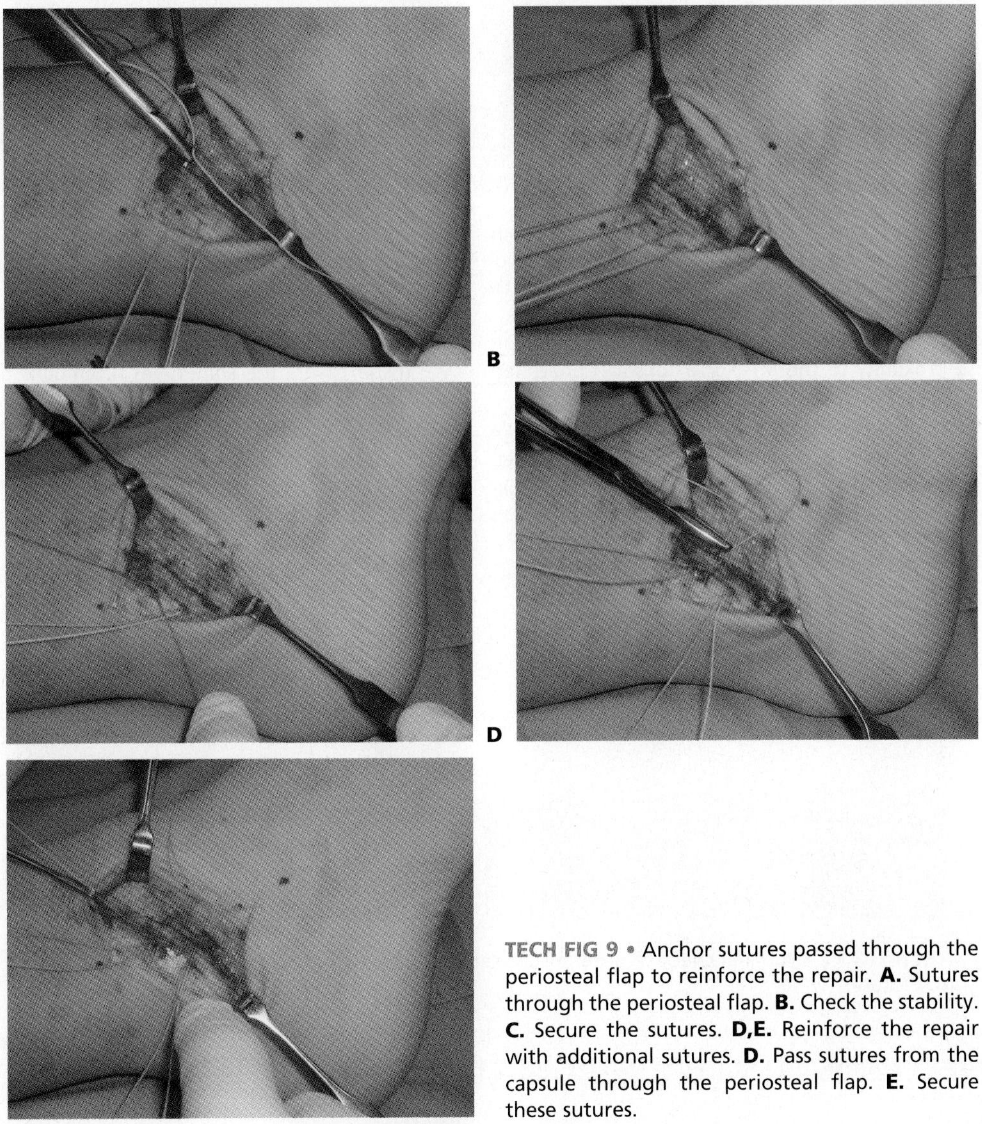

TECH FIG 9 • Anchor sutures passed through the periosteal flap to reinforce the repair. **A.** Sutures through the periosteal flap. **B.** Check the stability. **C.** Secure the sutures. **D,E.** Reinforce the repair with additional sutures. **D.** Pass sutures from the capsule through the periosteal flap. **E.** Secure these sutures.

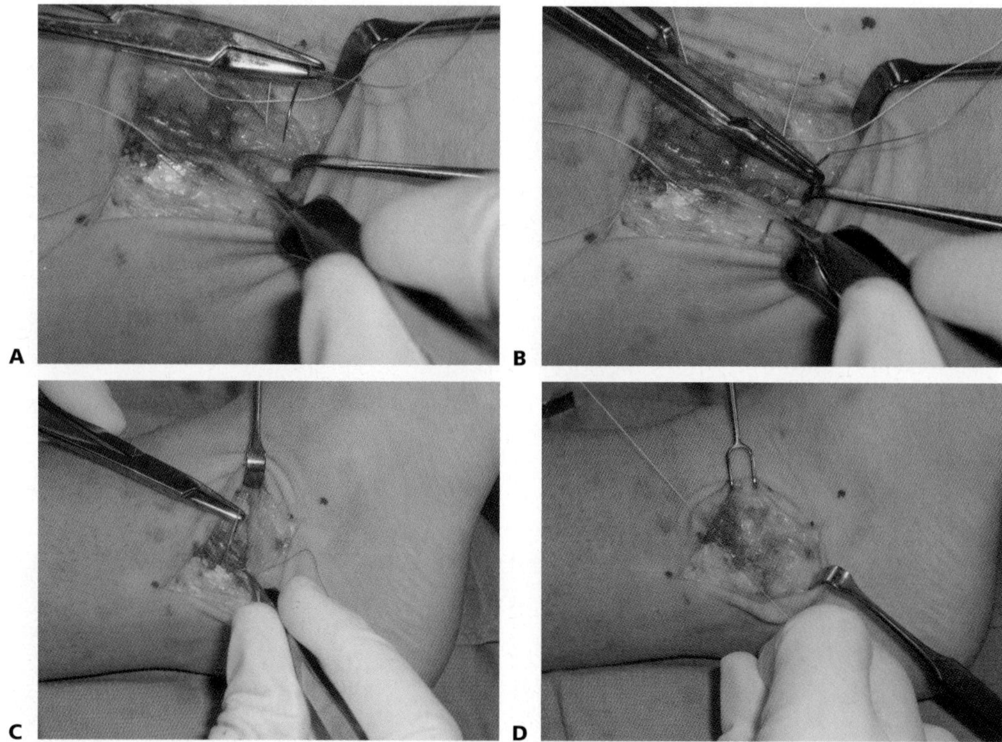

TECH FIG 10 • Gould modification of the Brostrom procedure. **A.** Protect peroneal tendons. **B.** More posterior advancement of the inferior extensor retinaculum. **C.** Anterior advancement. **D.** Attempt to cover the permanent anchor sutures with the retinaculum.

- Protect the peroneal tendons because they are in close proximity to the inferior extensor retinaculum (TECH FIG 10A).
- Advancing the inferior retinaculum to the distal fibula over the capsular advancement is the (Nathaniel) Gould modification of the Brostrom lateral ankle ligament reconstruction (TECH FIG 10B–D).
- If possible. advance the inferior retinaculum so that the tissue covers the sometimes prominent permanent anchors suture knots. Final check of the anterior drawer and talar tilt to ensure that ankle stability has been reestablished (TECH FIG 11A).
- Closure (TECH FIG 11B).

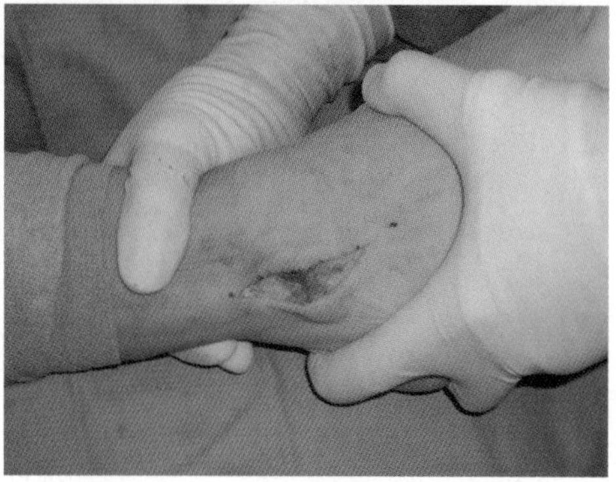

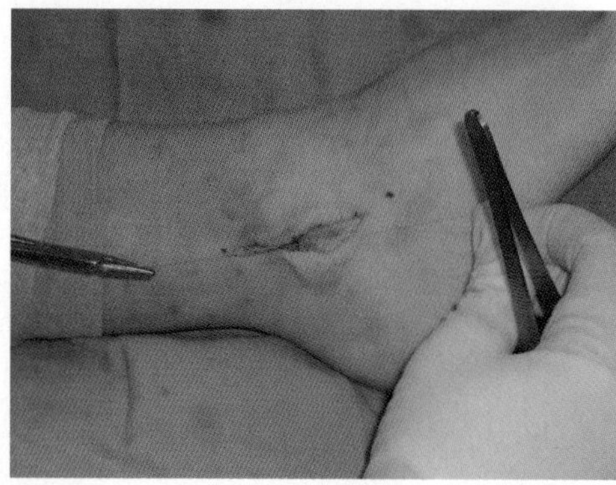

TECH FIG 11 • **A.** Final check of anterior drawer and talar tilt tests to be sure repair is satisfactory. **B.** Closure.

MODIFIED BROSTROM BROSTROM-EVANS PROCEDURE

Definition

- This is a combination of the modified Brostrom procedure described above and the Evans procedure, tenodesing the anterior 50% of the peroneus brevis to the fibula

Indications

- Athlete or patient in whom greater restraint against inversion is desired
  - For example, a football lineman who does not need as much hindfoot flexibility as a running back

- Anatomic repair planned but greater than anticipated instability, particularly with inversion stress, and an intraoperative determination that more restraint to inversion is needed than can be afforded by the modified Brostrom procedure alone.
- Lateral ankle instability in a patient with pre-exisiting longitudinal split tear of the peroneus brevis.

Technique

- Same positioning and approach as for a modified Brostrom procedure
- The ATFL and CFL are released with the capsular sleeve from the fibula the same way as for the modified Brostrom procedure (**TECH FIG 12A**)
- Preparing the peroneus brevis tendon
  - The peroneus brevis (PR) is isolated distal and proximal to the superior peroneal retinaculum (SPR) that is left intact
  - The peroneus brevis is split longitudinally and the anterior 50% is released proximally (**TECH FIG 12B**)
    - While keeping the SPR intact, the PR is split using a suture that is passed beneath the SPR that is used to separate the PR into anterior and posterior limbs, acting as a "saw" to divide the tendon along its longitudinal fibers.
    - Ater being released proximally the anterior limb of the PR is passed beneath the SPR distally
- Passing the anterior limb of the PR through the fibula
  - Drill an oblique tunnel in the distal fibula (**TECH FIG 13A**)
  - Pass the anterior 50% of the PR through the tunnel from distal to proximal (**TECH FIG 13B**)
  - Complete the modified Brostrom procedure (**TECH FIG 13C,D**)
    - The ankle is held in neutral position
    - The talus is maintained in the ankle mortise

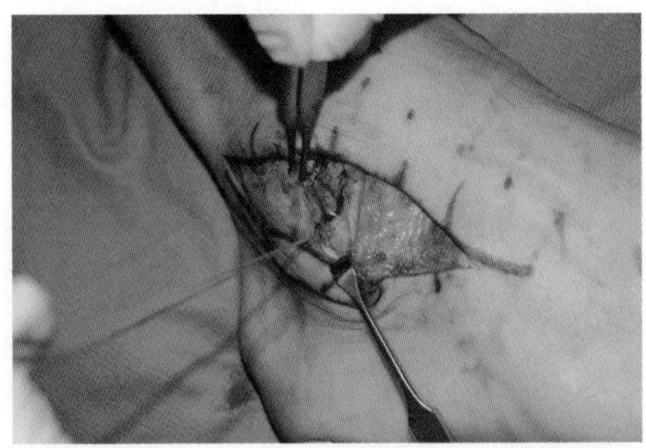
A

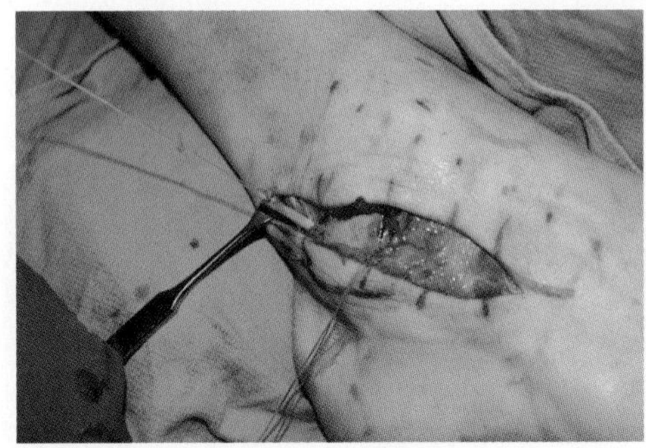
B

TECH FIG 12 • **A.** Prepare the lateral ankle ligament complex as is done for the isolated modified Brostrom procedure. **B.** Isolate the anterior 50% of the peroneus brevis tendon.

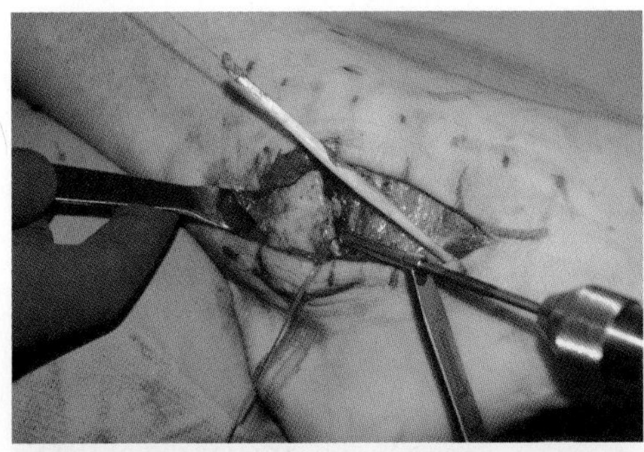
A

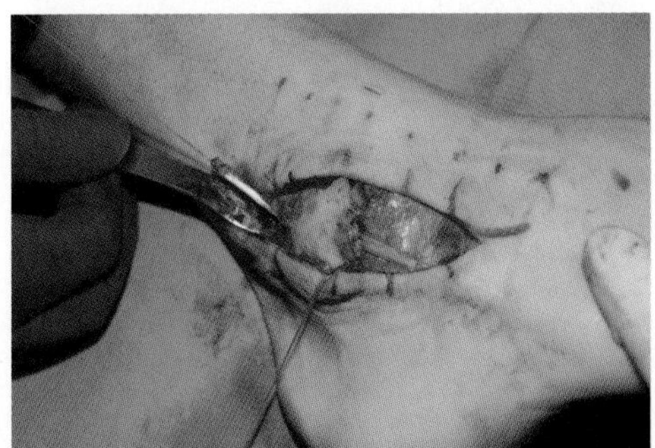
B

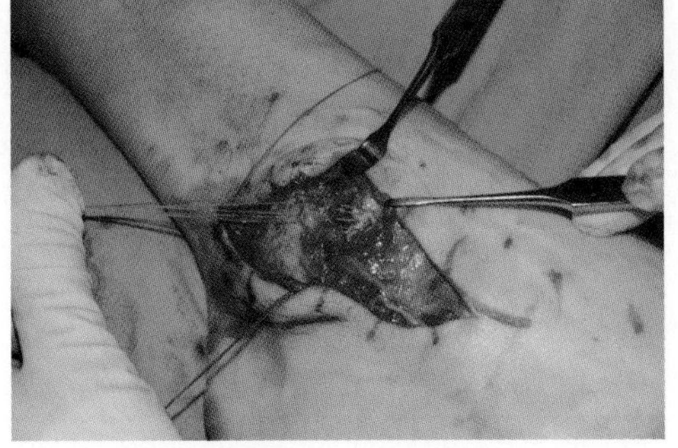
C

TECH FIG 13 • **A.** Transect the anterior 50% of the tendon proximally and pass this half of the peroneus brevis tendon beneath the intact superficial peroneal retinaculum. Drill a fibular tunnel from distal to proximal. **B.** Pass the anterior slip of the peroneus brevis through the tunnel from distal to proximal. **C, D.** Complete the modified Brostrom procedure. *(continued)*

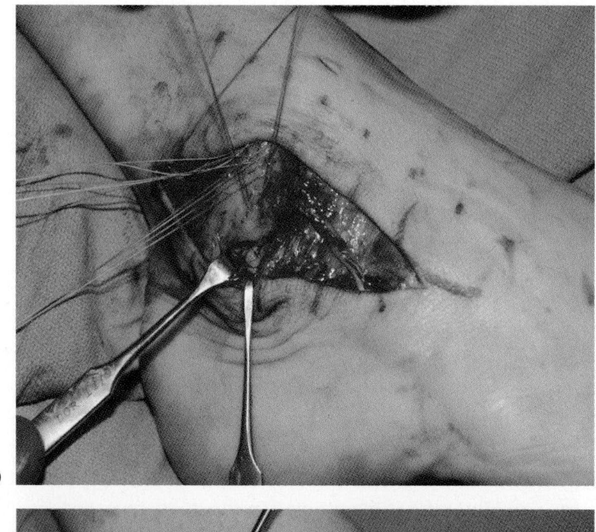
D

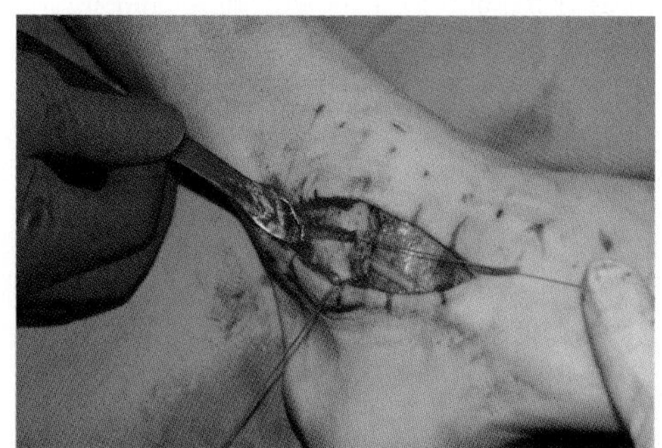
E

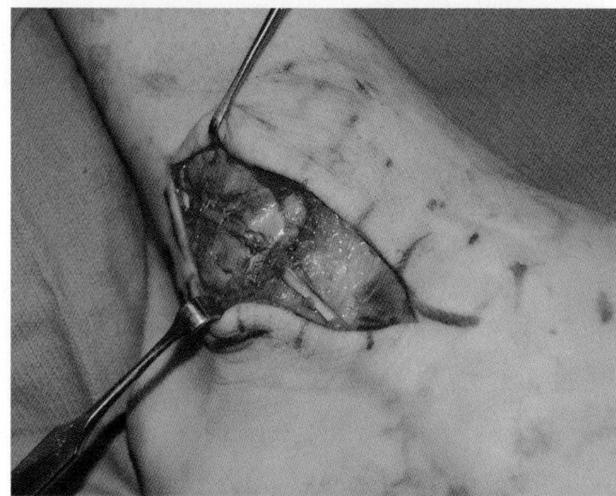
F

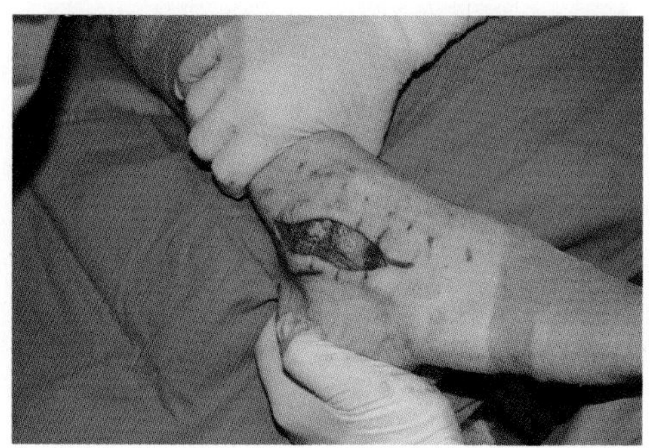
G

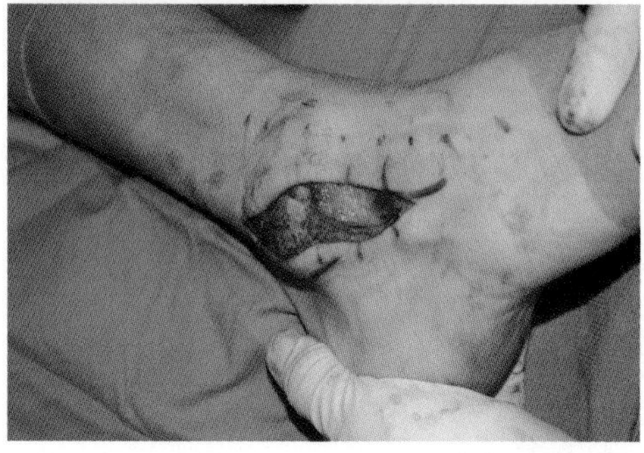
H

TECH FIG 13 • *(continued)* **E, F.** After passing through the fibular tunnel, the anterior slip of the peroneus brevis may be folded distally over the fibula to augment the repair. Check the ankle stability: **(G)** Anterior drawer and **(H)** inversion stress test.

- Slight valgus is maintained in the hindfoot
- Augment the modified Brostrom with the Evans modification
  - The anterior slip of the PR is secured to the fibular periosteum, both at the anterior and posterior aspects of the tunnel
    - Avoid excessive valgus or excessive tensioning as overtightening could occur; the goal is to have a restraint to inversion, not a complete lack of inversion
  - Typically, the anterior slip of the PR can be sewn over the fibula after being passed through the tunnel to further augment the repair (TECH FIG 13E,F)
- Check ankle stability with anterior drawer and particularly inversion stress (TECH FIG 13G,H)

Postoperative Protocol

- Same as for modified Brostrom

PEARLS AND PITFALLS

Incision	■ When making the traditional J incision, be sure it is positioned over the distal fibula and not the lateral process of the talus. Palpate the landmarks carefully.
Use a bump/bolster	■ Position is everything. A bolster under the ipsilateral hip ensures that the leg is maintained in the optimal position, thereby maintaining adequate exposure to the lateral ankle. A bolster under the operated ankle is also useful and improves access to the lateral ankle.
Ankle position when securing the sutures	■ Reduce the talus within the ankle mortise. Dorsiflex the ankle, push the talus posteriorly within the mortise, and maintain slight hindfoot valgus. It is useful to use a bump under the distal tibia so that the foot can be pushed posteriorly.
Protect the superficial peroneal nerve	■ The SPN crosses the anterior aspect of the surgical approach for the classic J incision and potentially for the extensile exposure as well. Be careful not to injure the nerve.

POSTOPERATIVE CARE

- The patient is to remain non–weight-bearing until seen in the clinic for the first cast change in 10 to 14 days.
- At this first postoperative visit, the splint is removed and wound evaluated. If no problems are seen, the skin closure is removed and the patient is placed in a short-leg weight-bearing cast for the subsequent 4 to 5 weeks.
- At the next visit the cast is removed and a physical therapy program is initiated for range of motion, proprioceptive training, and progressive resistive exercise.
- Gradual return to sport is possible at 12 to 16 weeks following surgery.

COMPLICATIONS

- Minimal; avoid injury to the superficial peroneal and sural nerves
- Infection
- Wound dehiscence
- Failure of repair
- Peroneal weakness (postoperative physical therapy program important)
- If the talus was not reduced within the ankle mortise when the sutures were secured, then the repair may prove inadequate.
- With an anatomic repair, overtightening is unlikely.

REFERENCES

1. Black HM, Brand RL, Eichelberger MR. An improved technique for the evaluation of ligamentous injury in severe ankle sprains. Am J Sports Med 1978;6:276–282.
2. Brostrom L. Sprained ankles: VI. Surgical treatment of chronic ligament ruptures. Acta Chir Scand 1966;132:551–565.
3. Burks RT, Morgan J. Anatomy of the lateral ankle ligaments. Am J Sports Med 1994;22:7277.
4. Colville MR. Surgical treatment of the unstable ankle. J Am Acad Orthop Surg 1998; 6:368–377.
5. Colville MR, Marder RA, Boyle JJ, et al. Strain measurement in lateral ankle ligaments. Am J Sports Med 1990;18:196–200.
6. Colville MR, Marder RA, Zarins B. Reconstruction of the lateral ankle ligaments: A biomechanical analysis. Am J Sports Med 1992; 20:594–600.
7. Holmer P, Sondergaard L, Konradsen L, et al. Epidemiology of sprains in the lateral ankle and foot. Foot Ankle Int 1994;15:72–74.
8. Johnson EE, Markolf KL. The contribution of the anterior talofibular ligament to ankle laxity. J Bone Joint Surg Am 1983; 65A:81–88.
9. Peters JW, Trevino SG, Renstrom PA. Chronic lateral ankle instability. Foot Ankle 1991;12:182–191.

Chapter 99

Anatomic Repair of Lateral Ankle Instability

Gregory C. Berlet, Geoffrey S. Landis, Christopher F. Hyer, and Terrence M. Philbin

DEFINITION

- Ankle sprains are the most common athletic-associated injury: they represent up to 40% of all sports-related injuries. The incidence of this inversion type of ankle sprain is around 10,000 people per day.
- Literature has cited that about 50% of patients with ankle sprains have some long-term sequelae of their injury. Many of these people develop ankle instability.
- Ankle instability can be divided into two categories, functional and mechanical.
  - Functional instability refers to the subjective feeling of the ankle giving way during activity.
  - Mechanical instability is the term used when patients show excessive ankle motion, beyond the normal physiologic barriers.

ANATOMY

- The lateral ankle is supported by both dynamic and static structures (**FIG 1**).
- Static structures include the bony architecture of the joints and the ligaments. This bony configuration contributes about 30% of the stability, whereas the remaining 70% of stability comes from the soft tissues.
- The dynamic structures that aid in the stability of the ankle include the peroneus longus and peroneus brevis tendons. These tendons run posterior to the fibula in the peroneal groove. They are kept in this groove by the superior peroneal retinaculum.

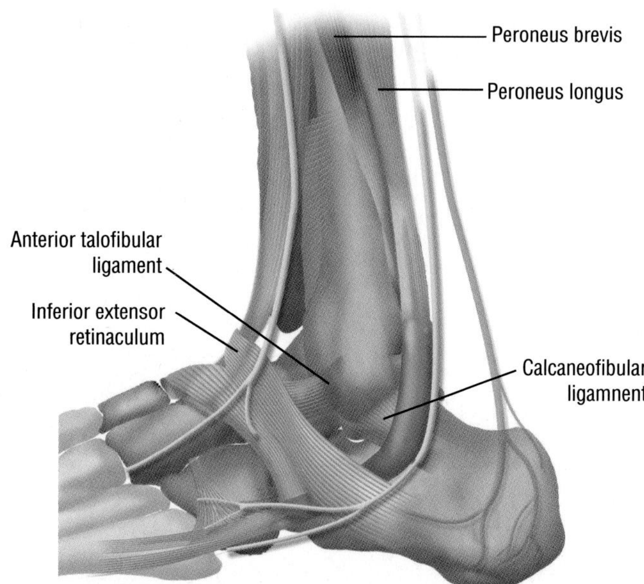

FIG 1 • The relative positions of the sural nerve, the lateral branch of the superficial peroneal nerve, and the inferior extensor retinaculum.

- Once the tendons pass the distal tip of the fibula, they alter their course and run along the lateral border of the calcaneus, under the inferior peroneal retinaculum, with the peroneus brevis inserting on the base of the fifth metatarsal and the peroneus longus making another turn at the cuboid tunnel and inserting on the first metatarsal.
- These two tendons act as the primary evertors of the ankle and also participate in plantarflexion of the ankle. As a result of their course and function, they work in a dynamic fashion to provide stability to the ankle and subtalar joints.
- In addition to the bony configuration of the joint, the static restraints for the lateral aspect of the ankle include the anterior talofibular ligament (ATFL), the calcaneofibular ligament (CFL), and the posterior talofibular ligament (PTFL).
- The ATFL is the most frequently injured ligament and the weakest of the three ligaments. It is flat and broad and originates from the anterior border of the lateral malleolus and continues anteromedially to insert on the talar body, anterior to the articular surface.
- The CFL originates just inferiorly from the ATFL on the anterior border of the lateral malleolus and runs deep to the peroneal tendons, and in a posterior, inferior, and medial direction to insert on the posterior aspect of the lateral calcaneus.
- The PTFL is the strongest of this lateral ankle complex and is rarely injured. It originates from the posterior aspect of the fibula, deep to the peroneals, and inserts on the lateral tubercle of the talus, laterally to the flexor hallucis longus groove.
- With the ankle plantarflexed, the ATFL is taut and becomes vertical, acting as a collateral ligament. In dorsiflexion, the same is true for the CFL.
- The ATFL has been shown to be the primary restraint to inversion in the ankle.

PATHOGENESIS

- Injury to the lateral ligamentous complex of the ankle is common. These inversion ankle injuries often result in attenuation or rupture to one or more of these ligaments.
- With the loss of these static restraints, the ankle becomes mechanically unstable, moving past the normal physiologic restraints for the ankle joint (**FIG 2**).

NATURAL HISTORY

- Once injury to the lateral stabilizers of the ankle has occurred, the patient should undergo immobilization followed by progressive rehabilitation.
- If this approach fails, it is usually related to peroneal weakness, proprioceptive defects, subtalar instability, and mechanical or functional instability.
- Chronic ankle instability can lead to repetitive inversion injuries, with the potential for fracture, osteochondral lesions of the talus, peroneal tendon injury and dislocation, and significant posttraumatic arthritis.

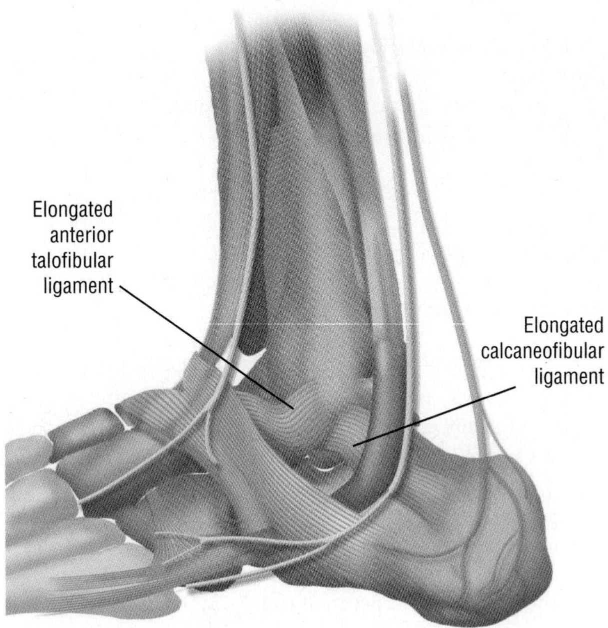

FIG 2 • Position of the elongated anterior talofibular ligament and calcaneofibular ligament.

PATIENT HISTORY AND PHYSICAL FINDINGS

- Patients with chronic lateral ankle instability will describe an inversion injury in the past. As a result, they will report that they have problems with consistent repetitive ankle sprains, a feeling of looseness in the ankle with or without pain.
- The physician should inquire whether the patient is experiencing pain between intervals of repetitive injury. This would point toward the possibility of a secondary problem from instability (ie, osteochondritis dissecans, impingement lesion, synovitis).
- The examination for chronic lateral ankle instability includes evaluation of the joint above (knee) and below (subtalar). Assessment should include overall alignment, range of motion, point of maximal tenderness, anterior drawer testing, evaluation of the peroneal tendons for pathology, ankle proprioception, and evaluation for associated injuries.
- Alignment should be evaluated for both the overall lower limb and the hindfoot. Patients with hindfoot varus alignment are predisposed to ankle inversion injuries and instability. The alignment is assessed in both the seated and standing positions. The flexibility of the hindfoot should be checked.
- Patients whose malalignment cannot be corrected with orthoses should have the alignment addressed at the time of operative ligament repair.
- Tibiotalar as well as subtalar joint motion should be evaluated. Ankle motion has been described as ranging from 13 to 33 degrees of dorsiflexion and 23 to 56 degrees of plantarflexion.
  - The variability is dependent on the operator and the mode of measurement.
  - Accepted values for functional range of motion are 10 degrees of dorsiflexion and 25 degrees of plantarflexion.
  - Range-of-motion testing can always be compared to the uninjured side for comparison.
  - Subtalar motion occurs about an oblique axis running from the medial side of the talar neck to the posterolateral wall of the calcaneus. Total motion for inversion and eversion is an arc of 20 degrees, but this is extremely difficult to assess accurately. The predominance of this motion is inversion.
- The anterior drawer test is designed to test the competency of the ATFL.
  - The test is performed with the patient seated and the knee flexed to 90 degrees. The tibia is stabilized with one hand while the ankle rests in relaxed plantarflexion. The contralateral hand is used to draw the talus anteriorly.
  - If the medial restraints are intact, then the movement has a rotatory component. Increased talar displacement when compared to the contralateral limb indicates a positive test. In addition, excessive motion alone can signify incompetency of the ATFL.
  - Most resources cite an absolute value of 10 mm for a positive test. A firm endpoint should also be noted when testing for ATFL competency.
- Proper examination of the ankle for chronic instability includes the evaluation of the peroneal tendons. These tendons can easily be injured at the time of the varus stress that tears the ATFL as well as with the recurrent instability that follows.
  - Evaluation for swelling in the retrofibular space is performed.
  - Simple palpation of the tendons (for tenderness) and strength testing are mandatory.
  - Peroneal weakness mandates a search for peroneal pathology.
  - The peroneal compression test can be helpful as well. The patient should be examined in a dynamic way to elicit peroneal subluxation or dislocation if it is present.
- Proprioception testing is an essential part of evaluating chronic ankle instability. Defects in proprioception following ankle sprains are well documented in the literature.
  - The modified Romberg test or stabilimetry is the best way to assess proprioception. A modified Romberg test is performed by having the patient stand first on the uninjured limb, with eyes open and then closed; this is then repeated on the injured side.
  - The difference in balance is related to the proprioception pathways of each limb.
  - The limitation of this test is that, to be accurate, there should be a full range of motion of the ankle and the subtalar joint and no pain with full weight bearing.
  - The advantage of the Romberg test is that it requires no special equipment.
  - Stabilimetry measures postural equilibrium and correlates with functional instability, but data generated on total sway in the vertical and horizontal planes require a force plate and computer analysis.
- Finally, the examiner must rule out other possibilities on the differential diagnosis and determine whether there is more than one source of pathology.
  - Point tenderness in the area of the fifth metatarsal base, the anterior calcaneal process, and the lateral talar process could represent fracture.
  - Full evaluation of the ankle joint for loose bodies, osteochondritis dissecans lesions, and impingement lesions should be performed.

IMAGING AND OTHER DIAGNOSTIC STUDIES

- The use of imaging in the patient with the symptoms of ankle instability should begin with three plain radiographic views of the ankle.
  - These films should be evaluated for fractures of the fifth metatarsal, lateral talar process and anterior process of the calcaneus, as well as fractures to the malleoli.
  - In addition, the examiner should be looking for exostoses of the tibia and talus, osteochondral lesions of the talus, and tarsal coalitions.
- Stress radiography can be used to evaluate anterior talar translation and talar tilt. A standardized apparatus would improve reliability and consistency in this measure. The use of the contralateral limb as a control should be included when using this measure for a surgical indication.
- Further studies to evaluate the lateral aspect of the ankle include the use of MRI. MRI can delineate peroneal tendon pathology as well as provide needed information about osteochondral lesions of the talus (**FIG 3**).

DIFFERENTIAL DIAGNOSIS

- Bone
  - Anterior process of calcaneus fracture
  - Lateral–posterior talar process fracture
  - Lateral malleolus fracture
  - Base of fifth metatarsal fracture
  - Tibiotalar bony impingement
  - Tarsal coalition
- Cartilage
  - Osteochondral lesions of talus or tibia
  - Subtalar cartilage flap tear
- Ligamentous
  - Functional lateral ankle instability
  - Mechanical lateral ankle instability
  - Subtalar instability
  - Syndesmosis injury
- Neural
  - Neuropraxia of the superficial peroneal nerve
  - Neuropraxia of the sural nerve, reflex sympathetic dystrophy
- Tendons
  - Peroneus brevis tendon tear
  - Peroneus longus tendon tear
  - Painful os peroneum syndrome
  - Peroneal subluxation or dislocation
- Soft tissue
  - Anterolateral ankle impingement lesion
  - Sinus tarsi syndrome

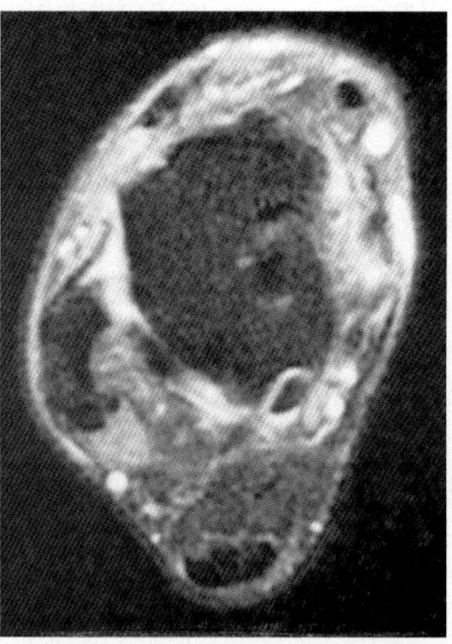

FIG 3 • MRI with torn anterior talofibular ligament.

NONOPERATIVE MANAGEMENT

- Nonsurgical treatment of lateral ankle instability begins with restricted activity and physical therapy.
- Physical therapy should focus on stretching, proprioception, and peroneal tendon strengthening.
- In addition, braces and shoe wear modification can be used. The use of a lateral heel wedge, a flared sole, and a reinforced counter can assist patients with instability.
- External stabilization of the ankle joint with taping or wrap dressings can provide some stabilization. Studies have shown superior initial resistance to inversion with taping, but taping has been shown to lose 50% of this initial effectiveness after 10 minutes of exercise.
- As a result, the use of over-the-counter reusable braces is recommended for nonoperative stabilization of the ankle joint. A University of California Berkeley orthosis, an ankle–foot orthosis (AFO), or a hinged AFO may also be used to help patients avoid surgery.
- In more sedentary patients, these modalities may provide adequate treatment, but for most athletes, they are unacceptable for long-term care.

SURGICAL MANAGEMENT

- Surgery for chronic ankle instability is indicated following a trial of failed nonoperative management.
- Patients with persistent, symptomatic mechanical instability will benefit from ligament reconstruction. This is often the case for athletes as well as patients who cannot tolerate bracing on a long-term basis.
- Relative contraindications for surgery include pain with no instability, peripheral vascular disease, peripheral neuropathy, and inability to comply with postoperative restrictions.
- Many procedures have been described for the management of ankle instability. They can be subdivided into anatomic and nonanatomic reconstruction techniques.
- The authors' choice for lateral ankle ligament reconstruction is influenced and based on the patient's body habitus, activity pattern, and physical demands.
- In patients with the need for full ankle range of motion, such as dancers, an anatomic procedure is recommended.
- In patients who are obese, are at risk for repetitive external varus stresses, have connective tissue disorders (Ehlers-Danlos), or are undergoing revision surgery, a nonanatomic reconstruction such as the Chrisman-Snook is preferred.
- In patients with attenuated tissue, the advent of bioengineered tissue has allowed us to augment the anatomic repair.
- Arthroscopy of the ankle is indicated for patients who have osteochondral lesions of the talus, tibial and talar exostoses, and anterior impingement lesions. We have had excellent results in treating chronic lateral ankle instability with arthroscopic techniques.
- Radiofrequency to provide thermal energy to the ATFL has been used with moderate success to treat patients who require arthroscopy, with the benefits best realized in the functionally unstable ankle.

Preoperative Planning

- Preoperative planning in the case of chronic ankle instability is based on the cause of the instability.
- Patients should be thoroughly evaluated for the possibility of a tarsal coalition.
- Hindfoot alignment should be addressed. Patients with a varus hindfoot are predisposed to suffer inversion injuries, and the possibility of a Dwyer calcaneal osteotomy in addition to the ligament repair should be considered.
- The presence of intra-articular pathology should also be addressed. Patients with clear pathology should have this addressed at the time of surgery.
- Peroneal tendon injuries often accompany ankle instability and should be evaluated and treated at this setting.

Positioning

- Positioning patients for lateral ankle ligament repair and reconstruction should be based on the chosen procedure.
- For anatomic ligament repair, we prefer to place the patient in the lateral decubitus position. This allows direct access to the lateral aspect of the ankle and the ability to address peroneal pathology and perform a calcaneal osteotomy if necessary.
- Patients who are undergoing arthroscopy should be placed in the supine position for arthroscopy. If the surgeon then chooses open ligament repair techniques, a bump can be placed under the ipsilateral hip after the arthroscopic portion of the surgery is complete.

Approach

- The incision for the Brostrom-Gould procedure was originally described as a J-shaped incision, just anterior to the fibula (**FIG 4A**). This allows easy exposure to the anterolateral capsule and ATFL and CFL.
- An alternative to the J incision is a posterior curvilinear incision that allows the surgeon to repair the peroneal tendons and repair the lateral ligament complex (**FIG 4B**). We prefer this curvilinear incision

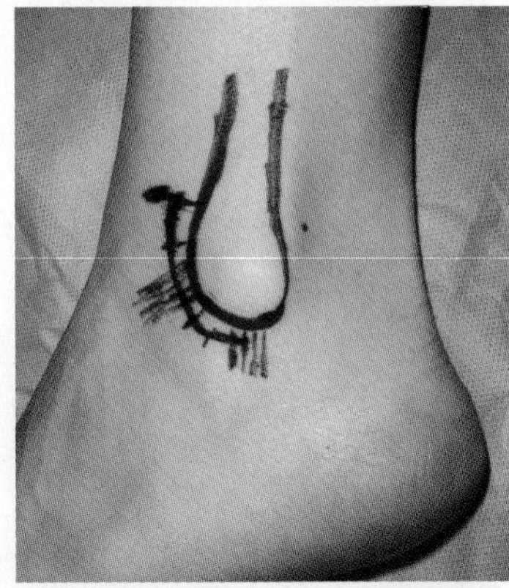

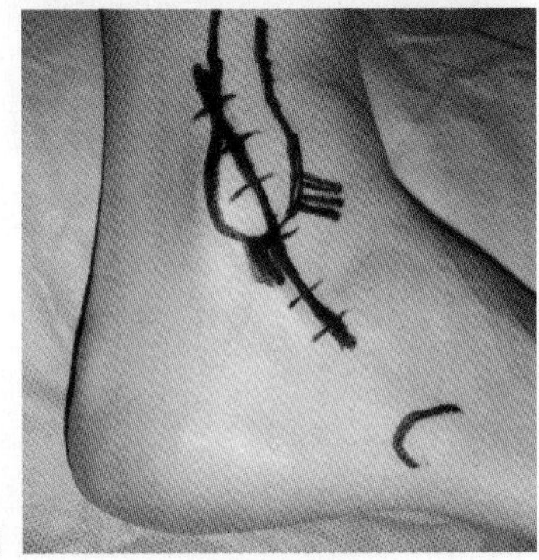

FIG 4 • **A.** Anterior J incision. **B.** Posterior curvilinear incision.

MODIFIED BROSTROM ANATOMIC LATERAL LIGAMENT RECONSTRUCTION

- In 1966, Brostrom reported a series of 60 patients on whom he performed a direct lateral repair of the lateral ligaments of the ankle. The ligaments of the ATFL and the CFL were found to be disrupted but present, and the torn ends were shortened and repaired directly by midsubstance suturing.
- In 1980, Gould modified this procedure by advancing the lateral aspect of the inferior extensor retinaculum to the fibula, reinforcing the repair of the ATFL.
- In addition to reinforcement, the modification limits subtalar instability and provides a checkrein to inversion.
- In this technique the patient is placed in the lateral decubitus position. All bony prominences are padded and an axillary roll is placed to protect the upper extremity. A well-padded thigh tourniquet is placed.
- The choice of an anterior incision or a posterior incision is up to the surgeon.
- The curvilinear incision (**FIG 4B**) extends from 4 to 5 cm proximal to the tip of the fibula and follows the course of the peroneal tendons.
- Distally, carry the incision toward the base of the fifth metatarsal.
- Take care to avoid the superficial peroneal and the sural nerves.
- Take dissection down to the level of the fibular periosteum.
- Mobilize the flaps anteriorly and posteriorly.
- Identify the anterolateral capsule, the peroneal tendons, and the inferior extensor retinaculum.
- The peroneal sheath can be opened proximally and distally, allowing preservation of the superior peroneal retinaculum. Peroneal tendon pathology can then be addressed.
- Make the anterior J-shaped incision along the anterior and distal aspect of the fibula. The incision begins at the level of the ankle joint and stops at the peroneal tendons.
- Carry dissection down to the anterolateral joint capsule, just anterior to the fibula. Take care to avoid any branch of the superficial peroneal nerve.
- In the distal aspect of either incision, identify the inferior extensor retinaculum and mobilize it for later Gould modification. A tag suture can be placed to help retract this tissue during the anatomic repair.
- Identify the lateral gutter of the ankle joint and divide the capsule. Leave a cuff of tissue on the fibula to allow for advancement and imbrication of this tissue.
- Carry the arthrotomy from the level of the tibiotalar joint to the peroneal tendons (**TECH FIG 1A**). Care to protect these tendons during this part of the procedure is paramount.

- This arthrotomy will divide both the ATFL and the CFL in their midsubstance. At this time the surgeon can evaluate the tibiotalar joint.
- Resect scar tissue; up to 5 mm of tissue can be excised.
- Imbricate the ligaments in a pants-over-vest fashion with 0 Vicryl stitches (**TECH FIG 1B–D**).
- Place the sutures but do not tie them until the ankle is held in dorsiflexion and eversion. Be sure to prevent anterior subluxation of the talus at this time.
- After the repair, take the ankle through a range of motion to ensure that the sutures hold.
- Once repair of the arthrotomy has been performed, advance the extensor retinaculum and secure it to the periosteum of the fibula, covering the ligament and capsular repair.
- Perform irrigation and then subcutaneous and skin closure.
- Apply a dressing and splint, placing the ankle is a slightly everted position.

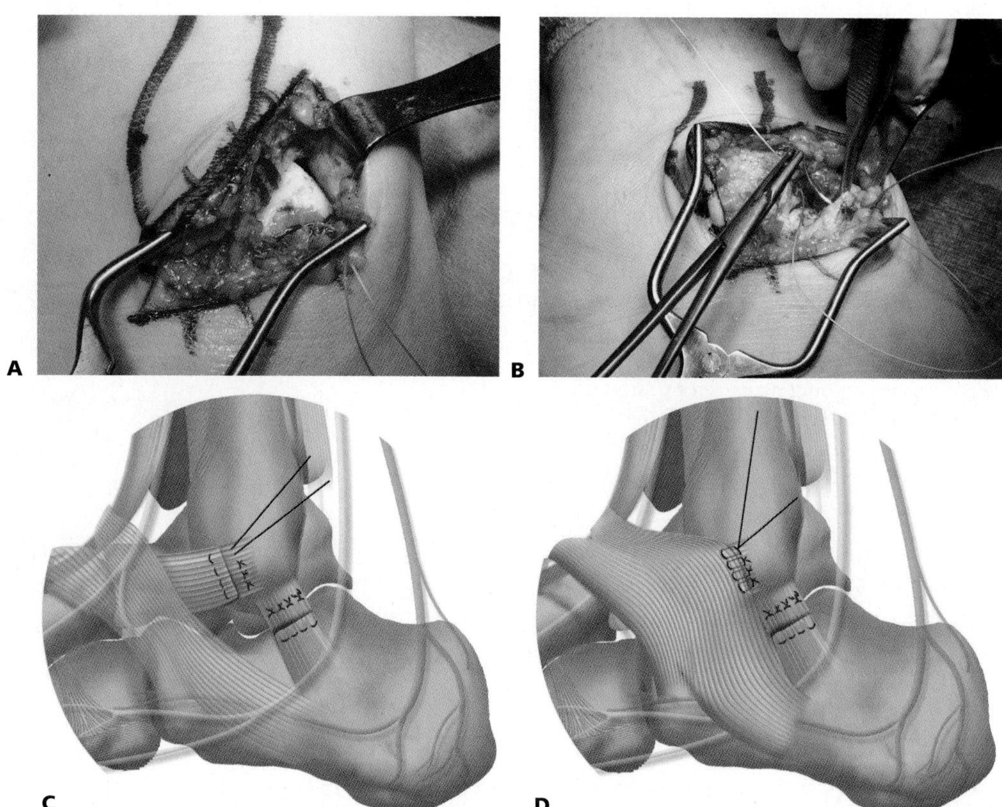

TECH FIG 1 • **A.** Arthrotomy. **B.** Suturing anterior talofibular ligament with pants-over-vest stitch. **C.** After suturing the calcaneofibular and anterior talofibular ligaments, the ankle is ready for inferior extensor retinaculum translocation. **D.** Suturing of the inferior extensor retinaculum to the anterior aspect of the fibula.

MODIFIED BROSTROM ANATOMIC LATERAL LIGAMENT RECONSTRUCTION WITH BIOENGINEERED TISSUE AUGMENTATION

- In patients who have suffered from chronic lateral ankle instability with repeated inversion injuries, often the tissue at the time of surgery is attenuated and of poor quality. In the past, this might have caused failure of the anatomic repair, or caused the surgeon to consider a using an autologous tendon augmentation.
- With the growing orthobiologic market, we have found that these bioengineered tissue augments can provide the surgeon with another option in the case of poor tissue quality, without the morbidity of autogenous tendon harvest.
- The approach is the same as for the standard modified Brostrom repair.
- After performing the arthrotomy, select the preferred tissue graft and prepare it as recommended by the manufacturer.
- Secure the graft distally to the capsule with 0 Vicryl suture.
- After attaching the graft to the distal aspect of the capsule, perform the standard Brostrom repair.
- After tying the sutures through the ATFL and CFL, but before taking the ankle through a range of motion, tension the tissue implant to the fibula through bone tunnels, bone anchors, or suture to the periosteum, with the foot in an everted position.
- Tension the implant to ensure there is no redundancy (**TECH FIG 2**).
- Reef the inferior extensor retinaculum over the implant as well as the anatomic repair and secure it to the fibula.
- Close the subcutaneous tissue and skin and apply a splint in slight eversion.

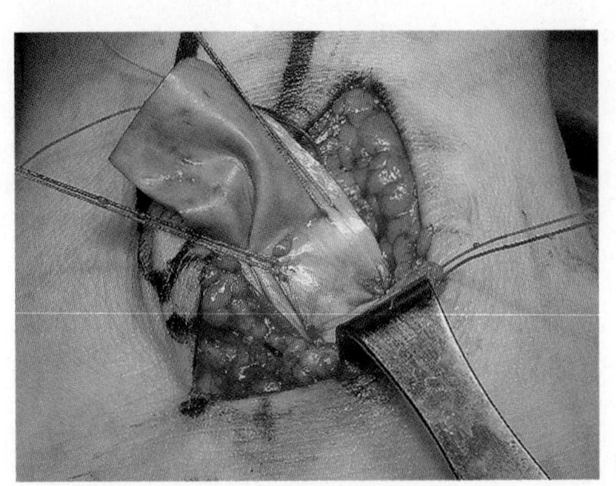

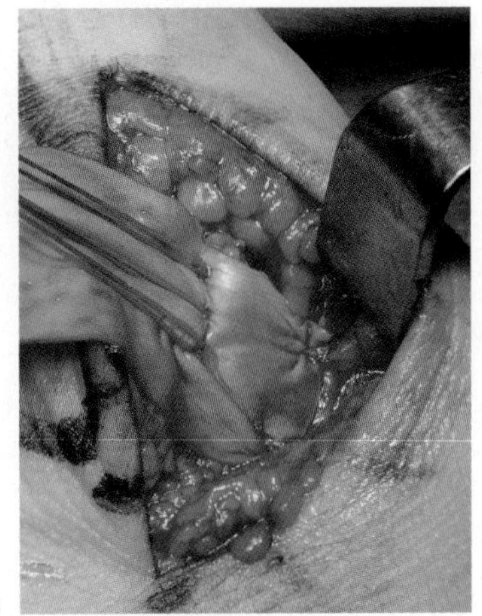

TECH FIG 2 • **A, B.** Tensioning collagen tissue to fibula.

THERMAL CAPSULAR MODIFICATION FOR THE TREATMENT OF CHRONIC LATERAL ANKLE INSTABILITY

- The presence of intra-articular pathology after chronic lateral ankle instability is well documented. The need to address this pathology as well as the lateral ligament instability inspired us to develop an arthroscopic protocol to address both at the same time.
- The patient is placed supine on the operating table.
- A well-padded tourniquet is placed on the upper thigh of the operative leg.
- The operative extremity is then placed into a thigh–knee holder. The holder is padded to ensure there is no pressure on the peroneal nerve and the popliteal space.
- The operative extremity then undergoes sterile preparation and draping.
- A noninvasive ankle distractor strap is applied and the ankle is distracted.
- Introduce a spinal needle into the ankle joint through the area of the standard anteromedial portal and insufflate the joint with 1% lidocaine with epinephrine. This distends the joint and aids in preventing the need for tourniquet use.
- Incise only the skin and carry blunt dissection down to the capsule.
- Use a blunt trocar for a 3.5-mm arthroscope.
- Introduce the arthroscope into the joint and visualize the articular cartilage.
- Once you have confirmed the arthroscope placement, inflow is started to prevent extracapsular extravasation.
- The area of the anterolateral portal is transilluminated, and the surgeon can avoid the dorsal veins of the ankle as well as the branches of the superficial peroneal nerve.
- Use a spinal needle to confirm ankle portal placement and make the skin incision. Again, carry blunt dissection down to the capsule and penetrate the capsule with a blunt trocar.
- Perform a standard 21-point arthroscopic examination. Note any intra-articular pathology (synovitis, osteochondral defects, impingement lesions) and treat it accordingly.
  - In this procedure, we have found that aggressive treatment of the anterolateral impingement lesion is necessary to allow improved visualization of the anterolateral gutter and the ATFL (**TECH FIG 3A**).

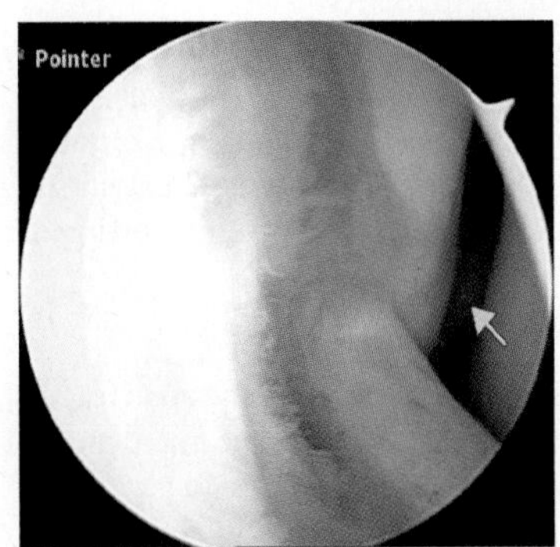

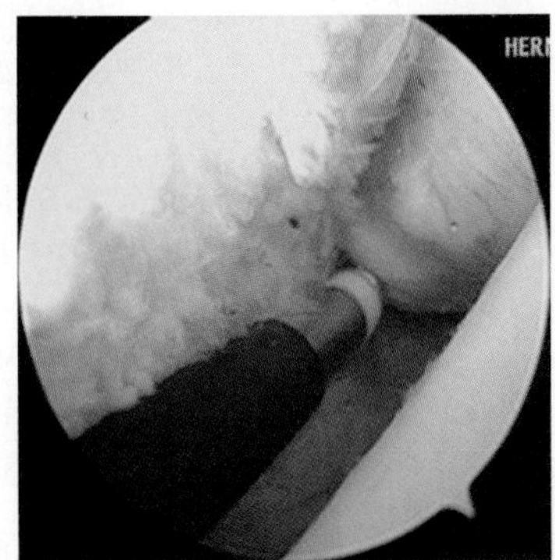

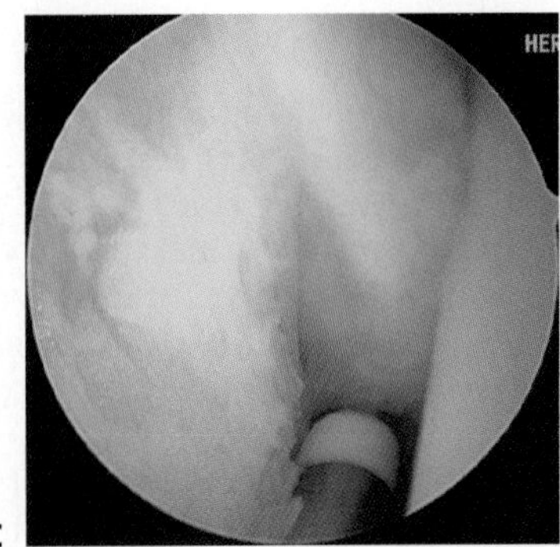

TECH FIG 3 • **A.** Arthroscopic visualization of anterior talofibular ligament. **B.** View after lateral gutter débridement and débridement of impingement lesion and beginning thermal capsulorrhaphy. **C.** View as tissue responds to thermal capsulorrhaphy.

- After treating the intra-articular pathology, introduce the probe for thermal energy delivery.
- Once the wand is in the joint and placed in the posterior recess of the lateral gutter, remove the distraction device from the foot (**TECH FIG 3B**).
  - This is necessary to allow for contraction of the tissues when the thermal energy is delivered.
- Use a painting technique, starting in the area of the CFL and working anteriorly.
- Deliver the treatment only below the "equator" of the lateral ankle portal so as not to cause an impingement lesion (**TECH FIG 3C**).
- Avoid repetitive painting of any one area to prevent injury.
- After adequate exposure to the thermal effects, remove the probe, close the portals, and apply a dressing.
- The patient is placed into a well-padded splint in slight dorsiflexion and eversion.

PEARLS AND PITFALLS

Negative anterior drawer test with history consistent with instability	▪ Beware the restraint of anterior tibial osteophytes. They can cause an abnormally negative drawer test despite a clinical picture of instability.
Failed primary Brostrom procedure	▪ Be sure to evaluate hindfoot anatomy. If the hindfoot is in varus, combine lateral closing-wedge and lateral slide osteotomy with a revision procedure.
Patient activity level	▪ Larger patients (more than 115 kg) and high-demand patients (football players) may require augmentation to the simple Brostrom-Gould procedure.
Anterolateral ankle joint pain, no chronic instability pattern, history of previous ankle sprain	▪ An ankle impingement lesion can act as a primary pain generator.
Global pain in lateral ankle region	▪ Look carefully for secondary pathology. Recurrent instability can result in osteochondritis dissecans of the talus, subluxing or dislocating peroneal tendons, subtalar instability, and other intra-articular lesions of the ankle.

POSTOPERATIVE CARE

- Postoperatively, the patient course is divided into 3-week increments.
  - The first 3 weeks is non–weight-bearing in a cast, the second 3 weeks is weight bearing to tolerance in a cast, and the third 3 weeks is weight bearing in a boot-walker.
- At the 9-week mark, the patient is weaned into an ankle stirrup brace and placed into a physical therapy program to begin range of motion, strengthening, and proprioceptive training.
- Patients are then progressed as tolerated until physical therapy goals are met.
- Patients are allowed to discontinue the brace for daily activities but are asked to brace in situations at risk for 1 year after reconstruction.

OUTCOMES

- The clinical and functional outcome from anatomic repair for chronic lateral ankle instability is good.
- In 1988 Karlsson et al.[6] reported on 152 ankles with a follow-up of 6 years. Good to excellent results were found in 87% of patients. In this study, 86% of athletes reported no deterioration in function. Predictors of poor outcome included more that 10 years of instability, generalized ligamentous laxity, and osteoarthritis of the ankle.
- A prospective outcome comparison study of the Chrisman-Snook and modified Brostrom procedure by Hennrikus et al.[5] demonstrated that both operations provided good or excellent stability in more than 80% of patients, but the Brostrom procedure resulted in higher Sefton scores and a statistically significant decrease in complications when compared to the Chrisman-Snook.
- Recently, a case series on 31 patients by Bell et al.[1] showed 91% good or excellent results 26 years after undergoing the Brostrom procedure.
- Outcome assessment for thermal-assisted capsular modification for ankle instability has shown promise.
  - The senior author has pioneered the use of this technology for the treatment of ankle instability.
  - Initial early-term follow-up studies show clear improvement in patients, with an average increase in AOFAS hindfoot scores of greater than 25 points.
  - We have previously reported on 16 patients with average follow-up of 14.5 months. Good to excellent results were achieved by 80% of the patients.
  - Subsequent publications and presentations have mirrored these results.
- Most recently Maiotti et al[7] reported on 22 patients with 32 months of follow-up. Nineteen of these 22 patients had good to excellent results and 21 of 22 returned to sporting activity.

COMPLICATIONS

- The most common complications after repair of the lateral ligament complex are nerve-related. The incidence of nerve complaints after surgery ranges from 7% to 19%.
- In addition to nerve complications, wound complications and infection, stiffness, and deep venous thrombosis have been reported. These complications are of course present with all surgeries.

- The possibility of recurrent instability is also a possible complication of surgery. This is most often a result of inadequate rehabilitation but can also result if the patient is not appropriately evaluated for hindfoot varus or connective tissue disease.

REFERENCES

1. Bell SJ, Mologne TS, Sitler DF, et al. Twenty-six-year results after Brostrom procedure for chronic lateral ankle instability. Am J Sports Med 2006;34:975–978.
2. Berlet GC, Anderson RB, Davis WH. Chronic lateral ankle instability. Foot Ankle Clin North Am 1999;4:713–728.
3. Berlet GC, Saar WE, Ryan A, et al. Thermal-assisted capsular modification for functional ankle instability. Foot Ankle Clin North Am 2002;7:567–576.
4. Brostrom L. Sprained ankles. VI. Surgical treatment of "chronic" ligament ruptures. Acta Chir Scand 1966;132:551–556.
5. Hennrikus WL, Mapes RC, Lyons PM, et al. Outcomes of the Chrisman-Snook and modified-Brostrom procedures for chronic lateral ankle instability: a prospective, randomized comparison. Am J Sports Med 1996;24:400–404.
6. Karlsson J, Bergsten T, Lansinger O, et al. Reconstruction of the lateral ligaments of the ankle for chronic lateral instability. J Bone Joint Surg Am 1988;70A:585–588.
7. Maiotti M, Massoni C, Tarantino U. The use of arthroscopic thermal shrinkage to treat chronic lateral ankle instability in young athletes. Arthroscopy 2005;21:751–757.

Chapter **100**

Hamstring Autografting/ Augmentation for Lateral Ankle Instability

Alastair Younger and Heather Barske

DEFINITION

- Lateral ligament instability occurs in some patients after an inversion injury.[38] Although an inversion injury is common, only a few patients have ongoing ankle instability severe enough to require surgery. Persistent instability may occur in 15% to 48% of patients.[7,10,15,45]
- Lateral ligament disruption may occur in combination with osteochondral defects, hindfoot varus, peroneal tendon tears, anterior lateral joint impingement, or a tight heel cord.[29,43,48] Any of these concomitant pathologies needs to be sought during the clinical examination and treated if it represents a significant component of the ongoing symptoms.
- Medial ankle instability may occur in combination with lateral ankle instability.[23] In these cases the medial ligament instability may need to be addressed at the same time.

ANATOMY

- The lateral collateral ligaments include the calcaneofibular (CFL) and anterior talofibular ligaments (ATFL).[11] These are condensations within the lateral capsule.
- The CFL runs from the anterior tip of the fibula to the lateral wall of the calcaneus. The ligament passes superficial to the lateral margin of the posterior facet of the subtalar joint and courses deep to the peroneal tendons to insert via a broad base onto the lateral side of the calcaneus.
- The ATFL arises from the anterior portion of the distal fibula and inserts onto the lateral side of the talar neck (**FIG 1**).

PATHOGENESIS

- Lateral ankle instability occurs after an inversion injury to the lateral ligament complex. The injury typically occurs in plantarflexion. Traditionally the ATFL ruptures first and the CFL second. A cavus foot may predispose the ankle to recurrent instability. Osteochondral defects of the talus and peroneal tendon tears are known associated pathologies.[5,23]

NATURAL HISTORY

- Most ankle sprains resolve without the need for surgery. However, a recurrently unstable ankle treated with appropriate physical therapy protocols may benefit from lateral ankle ligament repair or reconstructions. Left untreated, persistent lateral ankle instability may result in fixed varus tilt to the talus within the ankle mortise and eventual ankle arthritis. Most patients present because of the disability associated with the recurrent sprains. Physiotherapy and bracing will improve symptoms in some patients with recurrent instability. There does not appear to be a role for immediate surgery on ruptures of the lateral ligaments.[26]

PATIENT HISTORY AND PHYSICAL FINDINGS

- Patients should remove their socks and shoes before the history is taken so they can directly point to where the symptoms occur. Patients should be asked about pain and its relationship to activity and instability. Pointing to the foot or ankle with one finger will help focus the patient on the area of maximum discomfort and focuses the examination.
- Ankle instability may be difficult for the patient to convey; it may be more subtle than recurrent inversion injuries. Patients should be asked if the ankle gives way; if possible, the position of the foot during the instability episode and circumstances (running, cutting left, cutting right, etc.) should be determined.
- The impact of the instability on sports and work should be determined.
- On physical examination, the patient should be examined standing and walking. He or she should be asked to heel walk and toe walk. The examiner should look for a cavus alignment to the foot. A "peek-a-boo" heel sign may assist in the diagnosis.
- Using the Coleman block: If heel varus corrects, the hindfoot is considered flexible; if heel varus does not correct, the cavus deformity is secondary to a forefoot varus and correction of forefoot will correct the hindfoot through the mobile midfoot. A severe cavus deformity that is rigid may require a calcaneus osteotomy in addition to forefoot correction.

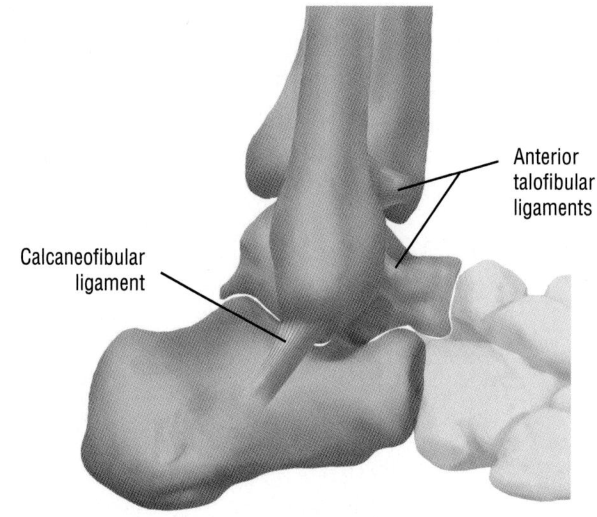

FIG 1 • Anatomy of the calcaneofibular and anterior talofibular ligaments.

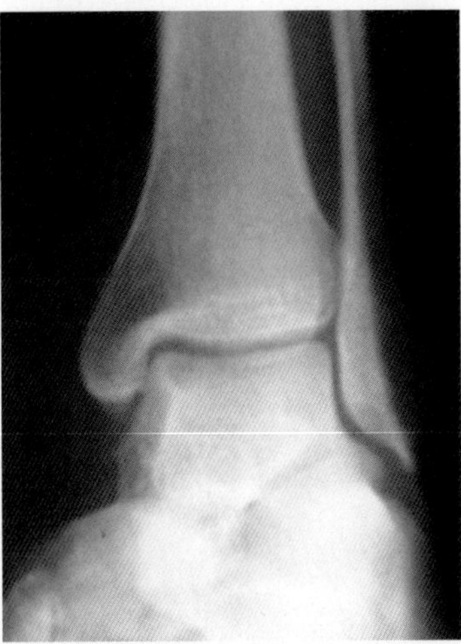

FIG 2 • Radiologic finding of osteochondral lesion of talar dome.

- The area of maximum discomfort and instability should be elicited. We take the ankle and hindfoot through a range of motion independent of one another to determine the joint of maximum discomfort.
- Peroneal tendon pathology may accompany lateral ankle instability. A resisted contraction of ankle eversion should be performed and the tendons palpated for pain and fullness (suggestive of tenosynovitis). The peroneal tendons, which are flexors, are best isolated with the ankle in plantarflexion and testing eversion against resistance. Peroneal tendon weakness accompanies most peroneal pathology due to pain; marked weakness may signify a peroneal tendon tear. In our experience, the combination of chronic ankle instability, varus hindfoot, and marked peroneal tendon weakness should raise the suspicion for a peroneal tendon tear. Occasionally, an equinus contracture may be associated with lateral ankle instability. A Silfverskiold test (ankle dorsiflexion with the knee flexed contrasted with ankle dorsiflexion with the knee extended) allows the examiner to determine whether the contracture is isolated to the gastrocnemius or involves both the gastrocnemius and soleus components of the Achilles complex.
- The ATFL resists anterior translation and medial rotation of the talus on the tibia. A direct anterior draw (pulling the talus anteriorly without plantarflexion and internal rotation) may fail to elicit instability in an unstable ankle as an intact deltoid ligament medially will prevent translation. Instead, the examiner should hold the tibia posteriorly with the left hand while translating the calcaneus anteriorly and internally rotating the foot at the same time. Side-to-side comparison to the contralateral, physiologically stable ankle assists in indentifying ankle instability.
- An inversion stress test determines the integrity of the CFL.
- An injury to the syndesmosis (ie, "high ankle sprain") may be elicited with a squeeze test and by rotating and translating the talus in the ankle mortise in dorsiflexion. A syndesmotic injury must be distinguished from lateral ankle instability since treatment is different.
- We also routinely examine the medial ankle for deltoid instability, since medial and lateral instability may coexist.

IMAGING AND OTHER DIAGNOSTIC STUDIES

- We routinely obtain weight-bearing AP and lateral ankle radiographs; if more information is required, we add a mortise view. Osteochondral defects, anterior osteophytes, and tibiotalar arthritis associated with recurrent instability are generally visualized on standard radiographs of the ankle (**FIG 2**).
- On occasion we add a calcaneal axial view, Saltzman view, or tibial views if we need additional information on limb alignment. Recurrent ankle instability may be secondary to tarsal coalition; if the hindfoot is stiff on clinical examination, then calcaneal axial view and standard foot radiographs may identify the coalition. CT provides greater detail of osteochondral defects, osteophytes, arthritis, and tarsal coalition and should be obtained if these associated findings are suggested on plain radiographs.
- An MRI, particularly an MRI arthrogram, may provide detail of the deficient ligaments. Associated chondral and osteochondral defects as well as soft tissue impingement lesions may also be visualized by an MRI examination (**FIG 3**).
- Selective, diagnostic local anesthetic blocks of the ankle, subtalar, or talonavicular joints may be required to determine localized joint pain.
- When the diagnosis of ankle instability is suspected but remains in question, an inversion stress test done under fluoroscopy, compared to the physiologically stable contralateral ankle, may be useful. Bone scans can assist in determining associated pathology.

DIFFERENTIAL DIAGNOSIS

- Loose body in ankle
- Osteochondral defect
- Syndesmotic instability
- Peroneal tendinopathy or rupture
- Medial ankle instability
- Cavus foot
- Tarsal coalition

NONOPERATIVE MANAGEMENT

- Nonoperative treatment includes bracing and physiotherapy. Patients with recurrent ankle instability may develop peroneal tendon weakness and loss of proprioception.[33,37] Physiotherapy via proprioceptive training and strengthening can resolve the ankle instability. Bracing may help a patient to recover from a sprain and prevent future sprains by strengthening the dynamic, stabilizing peroneal tendons. Nonoperative treatment is less effective if ankle instability is associated with fixed hindfoot varus. Flexible hindfoot varus may be compensated for with a

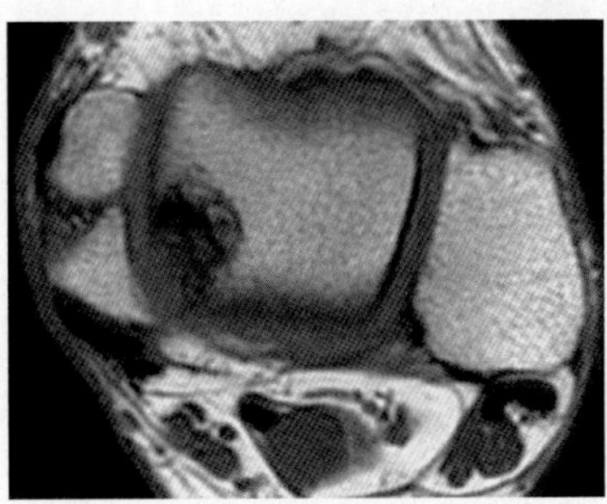

FIG 3 • MRI finding of osteochondral lesion of posteromedial talar dome.

lateral wedge orthotic. If hindfoot varus is driven by a plantarflexed first ray (as determined by the Coleman block test), then the orthotic should be "welled out" under the first metatarsal head, permitting further progression of the hindfoot into physiologic valgus.

SURGICAL MANAGEMENT

- The indication for surgical management of lateral ligament instability is chronic symptoms despite appropriate nonoperative management, including physiotherapy and bracing.
- Surgical management of lateral ankle ligament instability includes repair (anatomic tightening of the lateral ankle ligaments) and reconstruction (reconstitution of the lateral ankle ligaments using more than the local physiologic tissue in the lateral ankle ligamentous complex).
- Lateral ankle ligament reconstruction may be anatomic or nonanatomic.[11] Anatomic reconstruction implies that the ligaments are rebuilt in the physiologically occurring orientation. Nonanatomic reconstruction suggests that lateral ankle support is reconstituted with tissue (typically tendon transfer to substitute for ligament deficiency) that does not follow a physiologic orientation of the ATFL and CFL.
- In our opinion, the literature on this topic favors anatomic over nonanatomic reconstruction; examples of nonanatomic reconstruction include the Evans[2,4,13,17–21,27,28,30–32,34–36,39,40,42] and Watson-Jones procedures.[3,5,13,16,30–32]
- We recommend repairing the lateral ankle ligaments when possible. However, if the ligaments are not repairable or require an augmentation, we perform an anatomic reconstruction. Graft options for reconstruction include autograft (peroneus brevis, plantaris, gracilis) or allograft tendon.

Preoperative Planning

- Plain radiographs, and if further detail is needed other imaging studies of the ankle, must be evaluated for associated conditions, such as malalignment, osteochondral defects, tendon pathology, and arthritis. Adjuvant procedures must be planned so that they may be safely performed in concert with ligament reconstruction.
- We recommend performing stress testing with the patient under anesthesia. In our opinion, the gold standard tests to determine lateral collateral ligament integrity are (a) open anterior drawer and (b) inversion stress test on the table to determine the integrity of the lateral collateral ligaments.

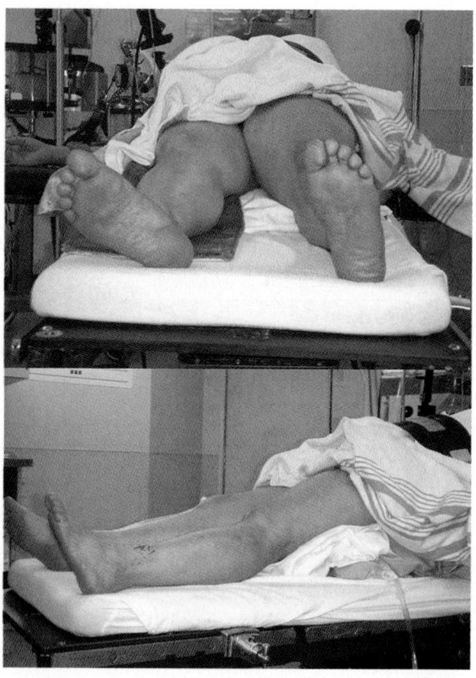

FIG 4 • Patient positioned using bean bag to allow good exposure to the lateral aspect of the ankle.

Positioning

- We routinely use a beanbag or large bump under the ipsilateral hip to rotate the operated extremity and allow full access to the lateral ankle (**FIG 4**).
- A full lateral position is avoided, as it limits access to the proximal medial tibia, making harvest of the gracilis tendon autograft more challenging.

Approach

- We recommend an extensile approach (ie, a longitudinal curvilinear approach) in lieu of the traditional J-shaped incision popularized by Brostrom. The extensile approach affords access to not only the lateral ankle ligaments but also the distal tibia, peroneal tendons, sinus tarsi, and lateral calcaneus for adjuvant procedures that may be warranted.

TECHNIQUES

GRACILIS RECONSTRUCTION THROUGH DRILL HOLES

- We prefer a gracilis autograft tendon, anchored via drill holes, for the anatomic lateral ankle reconstruction and aim to obtain (a) immediate stable fixation, (b) biologic ingrowth to bone in time, and (c) an anatomic reconstruction. The technique is a modification of the plantaris reconstruction described by Anderson (**TECH FIG 1**).[1]
- Place the patient on the operating table with the operative hip as described above. Apply a wide thigh tourniquet. Prepare and drape the leg to just above the knee. Perform anterior drawer and inversion stress tests on the table to confirm the diagnosis.
- Use regional anesthetic blocks if possible to ensure appropriate postoperative pain relief.
- If intra-articular pathology has been preoperatively identified or is suspected, we routinely address this with ankle arthroscopy before lateral ankle reconstruction (**TECH FIG 2**).
- Start the extensile longitudinal lateral incision on the distal fibula, continue it over the lateral malleolus, and curve it anteriorly toward the sinus tarsi (**TECH FIG 3**).
- Expose the superior extensor retinaculum anterior to the fibula while protecting the deep branch of the peroneal nerve, which has variable anatomy. Strip the extensor

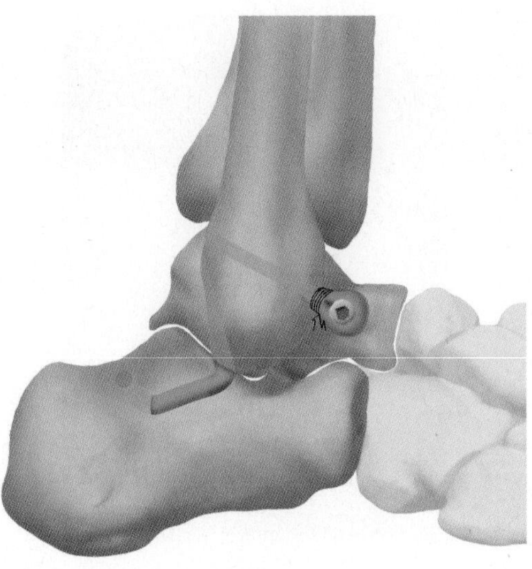

TECH FIG 1 • Free gracilis lateral ligament reconstruction.

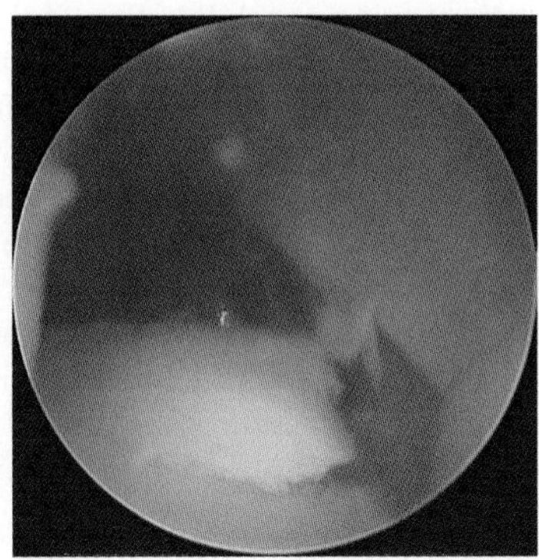

TECH FIG 2 • Osteochondral defect of the talus found on arthroscopy before ligament reconstruction.

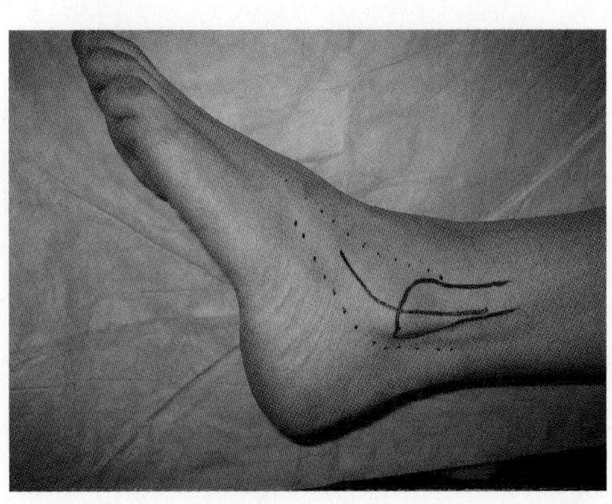

TECH FIG 3 • Lateral incision (*solid line*) with course of sural and superficial peroneal nerves marked (*dotted lines*).

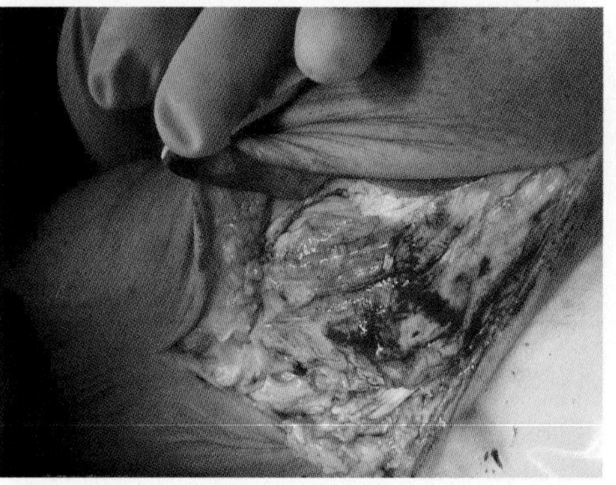

TECH FIG 4 • Lateral dissection anterior to the fibula, sparing the anterior talofibular ligament.

retinaculum off the fibula so that the extensor compartment is exposed. Carry the dissection distally toward the ankle joint to the junction between the tibia, talus, and fibula. Open the joint at this level. This dissection will ensure that no ligaments are damaged during the exposure (**TECH FIG 4**).

- Remove anterior osteophytes using an osteotome.
- Perform an open anterior drawer and inversion stress test (**TECH FIG 5**) to assess the integrity of the lateral collateral ligaments as a final check before proceeding with reconstruction. I will perform a repair if the ligaments are clearly torn off bone, if they are not obviously scarred or thickened, if there is enough length to bridge the gap, or if they have been avulsed with a bone fragment.[9]
- If the ligaments are not considered repairable, then reconstruction is warranted. We favor an autograft gracilis reconstruction, and therefore optimal patient positioning and preparation and draping of the operated extremity are important.
- Perform a standard gracilis tendon harvest with an incision over the medial aspect of the tibial tubercle at the pes anserinus insertion. Carry dissection down through the sartorius fascia and onto the gracilis tendon. Isolate the gracilis with the knee flexed, and use a tendon stripper to release it from its muscle proximally. Reef the tendon using a baseball whipstitch.

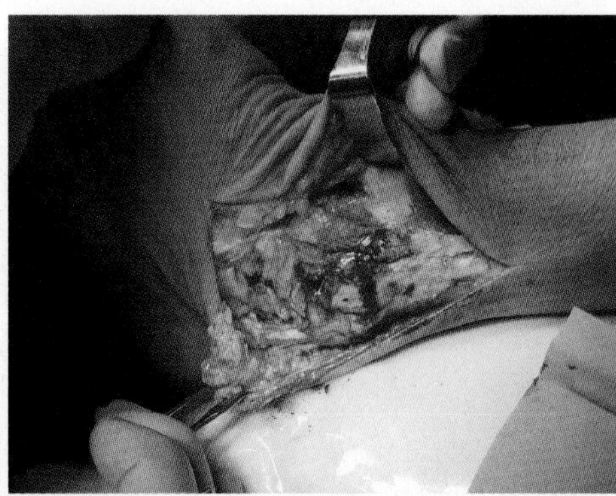

TECH FIG 5 • Open anterior drawer test. Talus is anterior and internally rotated relative to fibula, indicating a positive test and insufficiency of the anterior talofibular ligament.

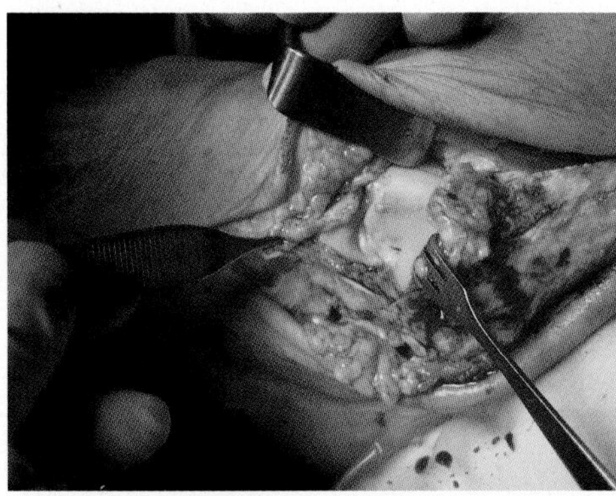

TECH FIG 6 • Dissection of the talus with exposure of the insertion of the anterior talofibular ligament.

- Divide the tendon at its insertion into bone and measure it. Select a drill bit matching the size of the tendon (typically a 3.5-, 4.5-, or 6-mm drill bit). Alternatively, a tendon-anchoring interference screw system may be used, size-matched to the harvested tendon's diameter.
- Expose the fibula first by removing part of the peroneal fascia so that the peroneal tendons and the posterior fibula are exposed (TECH FIG 6). We typically examine the peroneal tendons at this time to rule out or treat associated peroneal tendon pathology. If needed the peroneal retinaculum is incised with a step cut to allow complete exposure of the peroneal tendons for débridement or repair.[29]
- Incise the collateral ligaments and expose the insertions of the CFL and ATFL. Dissect to the origin of both ligaments on the calcaneus and talus. Both areas are dissected clear onto bone (TECH FIG 7). Use a curette to clear the area of the junction of the body and neck of the talus.
- Make a medial incision at the anterior border of the Achilles tendon, and carry dissection down to the bone and tendon at this level (TECH FIG 8).
- Drill through the calcaneus from medial to lateral, adjacent to the Achilles tendon, with the appropriately sized drill bit (depending on harvest tendon diameter), exiting laterally at the origin of the CFL (TECH FIG 9). A cannulated drill or a combined aiming device can be used to target this drill to the calcaneofibular footprint on the calcaneus.
- Make a fibular drill hole starting at the insertion of the CFL and exiting the posterior fibula. Make another fibular drill hole starting at the insertion of the talofibular ligament and exiting in the posterior fibula about 1 cm above the exit point of the previous fibular drill hole (TECH FIG 10).
- Then, make a 2.5-mm drill hole in the center of the junction between the talar body and neck (TECH FIG 11). Measure its depth. A fully threaded cancellous small-fragment screw with a small- and large-fragment washer is readied on the back table.
- With a no. 2 braided nonabsorbable polyester suture, suture the tendon onto the edge of the Achilles medially,

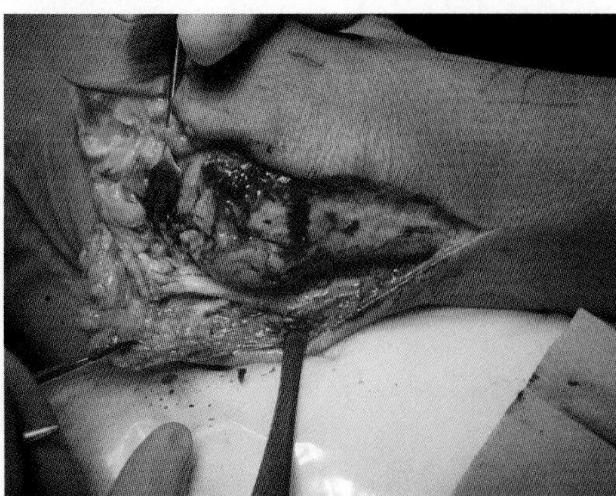

TECH FIG 7 • Dissection posterior to the fibula to expose the peroneal tendons.

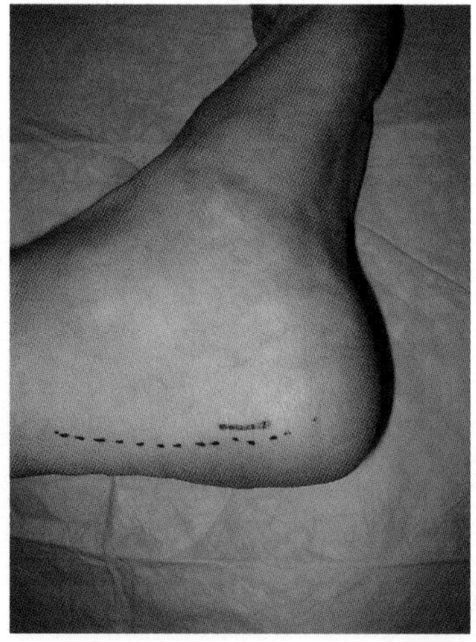

TECH FIG 8 • Location of medial incision.

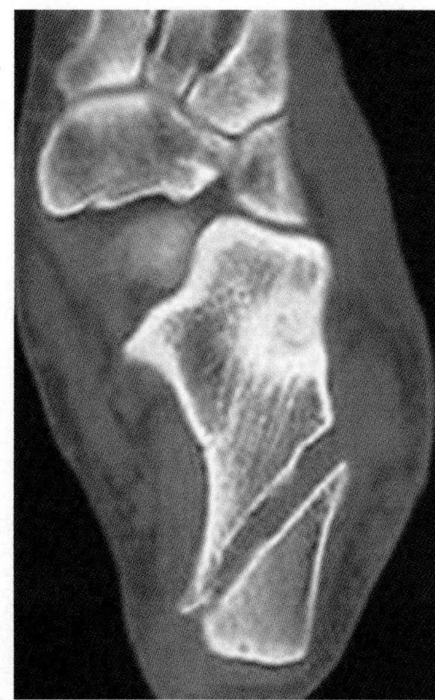

TECH FIG 9 • Postoperative CT demonstrating drill path through calcaneus.

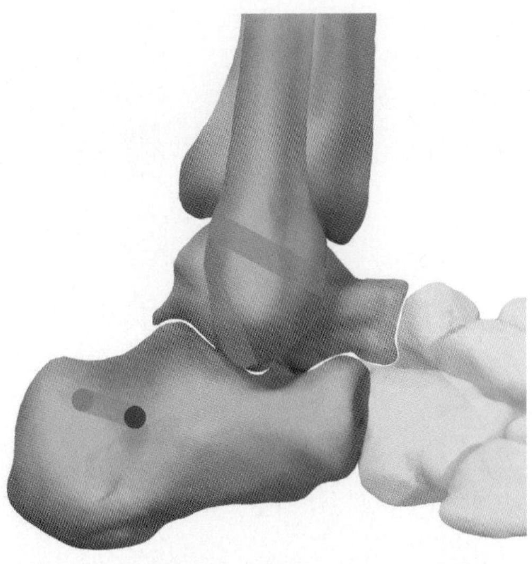

TECH FIG 10 • Drill paths through calcaneus and fibula.

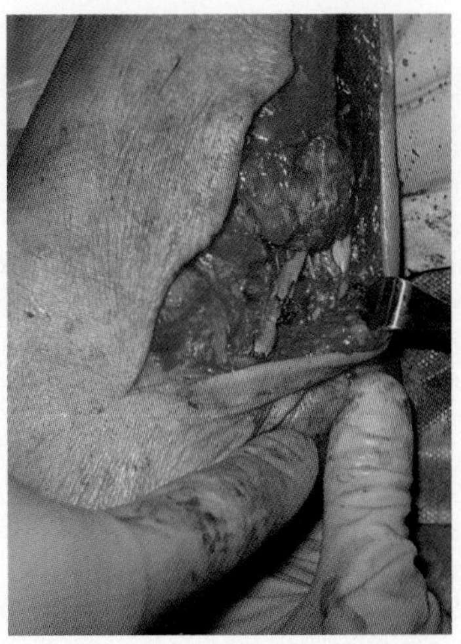

TECH FIG 12 • Gracilis graft passed from calcaneus to fibula.

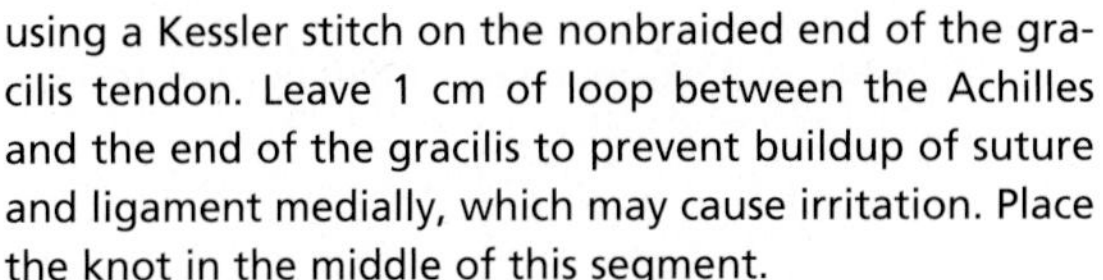

using a Kessler stitch on the nonbraided end of the gracilis tendon. Leave 1 cm of loop between the Achilles and the end of the gracilis to prevent buildup of suture and ligament medially, which may cause irritation. Place the knot in the middle of this segment.

- Use a tendon passer to pass the tendon graft through the calcaneal tunnel to the lateral calcaneus.
- Cycle the tendon a few times to make it tight.
- Pass the tendon through to the posterior aspect of the fibula and pull it tight with the ankle in eversion. Suture the tendon to any remaining tissue on the fibula (**TECH FIG 12**).
- Bring the tendon back through the fibula so that it exits anteriorly at the second drill hole.
- Cycle the tendon in tension and suture it to the cuff of tissue on the fibula at the insertion of the talofibular ligament.
- Start the selected small-fragment screw with the large and small washer into the 2.5-mm hole in the talar neck.

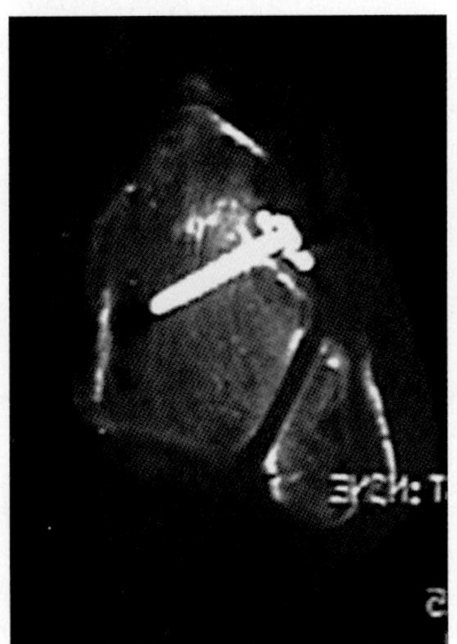

TECH FIG 11 • Postoperative CT scan demonstrating orientation of screw in talus.

- Place the split tendon end over the washer (right side) and under the washer (left side) and secure it around the washer in a clockwise direction. Hold the foot in dorsiflexion and eversion.
- Hold the tendon tight around the washer and screw and tighten the screw home. The tendon will tighten as the screw is placed home (**TECH FIG 13**). Although interference screw systems are effective, our method using standard screws and a simple ligament washer is cost-effective and consistently affords immediate ankle stability.
- Suture the free end of the tendon back onto the tendon segment between the fibula and washer.
- Suture the remainder of the tendon back onto the lateral side of the fibula, and trim the residual tendon end.
- To confirm stability and proper ligament tension of the reconstruction, place the ankle through repeat open anterior drawer and inversion stress tests. Close the wounds using nylon or staples. Use of a drain is at the surgeon's discretion.

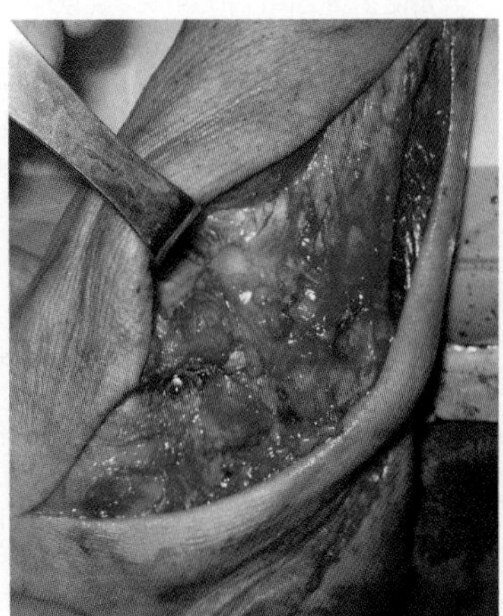

TECH FIG 13 • Gracilis graft tensioned from fibula to talus.

COUGHLIN DRILL HOLES IN BONE

- An alternative technique is to use drill holes through the bone made on the lateral side only.[14] This is a variation of the Emslie technique (TECH FIG 14).
- Use a similar exposure, with no medial incision.
- Make two drill holes on the lateral wall of the calcaneus on each side of the origin of the CFL.
- Pass the tendon through the drill boles and suture it back onto itself.
- Make a single drill hole on the tip of the fibula joining the insertion of both lateral collateral ligaments.
- Make two drill holes on each side of the insertion of the talofibular ligament.
- Pass the tendon through the fibula and through the drill holes on the talus, and tension it and suture it back onto itself.
- We consider this variation more challenging than our described technique, specifically in passing the tendon through bone without fracturing the bone bridges. Moreover, we find it more difficult to ensure anatomic location of the ligaments and optimal tendon tensioning. In our opinion, prolonged postoperative immobilization may be required, depending on the strength of the bone bridges.

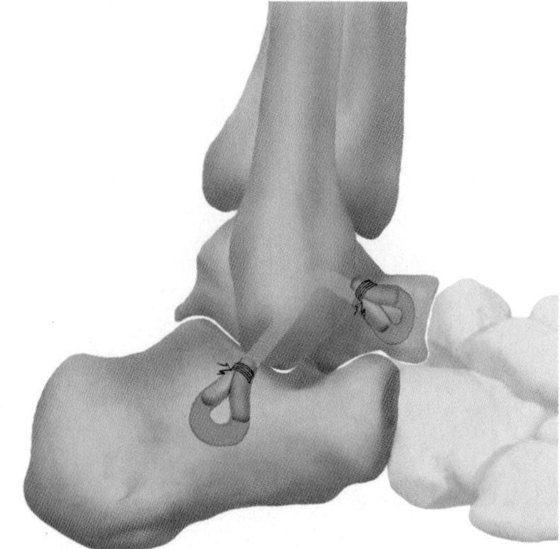

TECH FIG 14 • Coughlin drill holes in bone technique.

BIOTENODESIS SCREW TECHNIQUE

- With this technique a similar exposure and tendon harvest are used (TECH FIG 15). No medial exposure is required.
- Make a drill hole on the lateral side of the calcaneus at the CFL origin. Place the tendon over the tip of a tenodesis screw and secure it to the lateral wall of the calcaneus.
- Pass the tendon through two fibular tunnels at the anatomic locations of the CFL and talofibular ligament, exiting over a posterior fibular bone bridge as described in our technique.
- Make a second drill hole on the lateral side of the talus at the junction of the body and neck to accommodate the tendon and a second biotenodesis screw.
- Our concerns with this alternative are (a) quality of fixation via interference screw in the relatively weak cancellous bone of the calcaneus and (b) the relatively large talar drill hole, which may serve as a stress riser and cause of talar neck fracture.

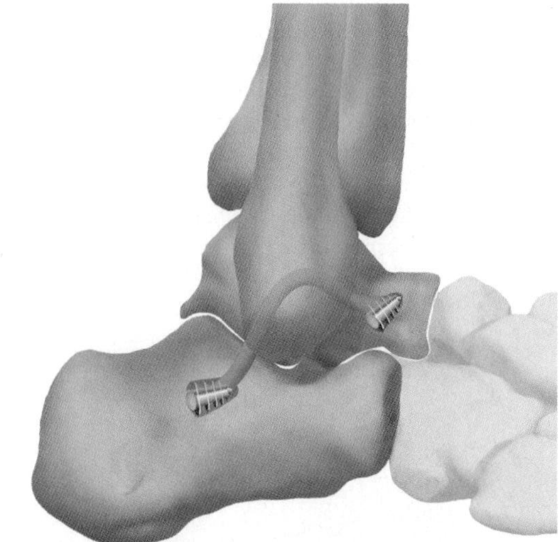

TECH FIG 15 • Biotenodesis screw fixation technique.

MYERSON MINIMAL INCISION TECHNIQUE

- This technique (TECH FIG 16) is similar to the Coughlin technique but is performed through two small incisions.
- Make one incision over the calcaneal drill holes and a second over the region of the talar drill holes. Carry dissection down to bone. Make two connecting drill holes in each location. Tunnel a drill bit and guide subcutaneously to drill the pathway through the fibula.
- Harvest the graft and route it in the same fashion as in the Coughlin technique described earlier.
- While this is a reasonable alternative, as for the Coughlin technique, we have difficulty passing and tensioning the tendon using this technique.

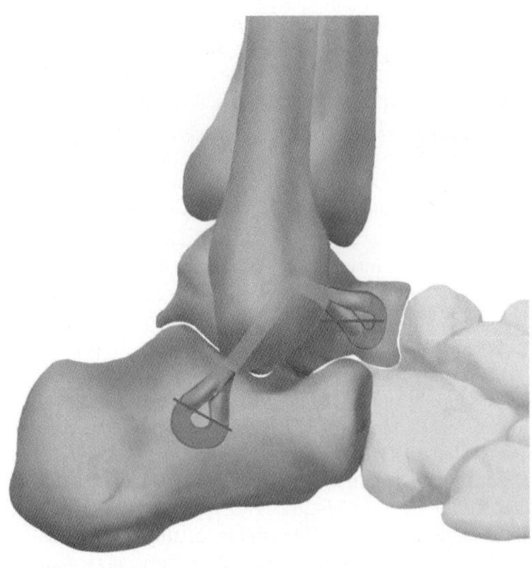

TECH FIG 16 • Myerson minimally invasive technique. Red lines indicate skin incisions.

PEARLS AND PITFALLS

Exposure	▪ Ensure that the exposure goes through the anterior compartment and down into the ankle. This will avoid damage to the ligaments before the open anterior drawer test.
Positioning	▪ Use a bean bag to ensure that the ankle is internally rotated to allow access to the lateral side of the ankle. Different patients have different amounts of internal rotation, and this needs to be accommodated. However, avoid a full lateral position if you plan a gracilis tendon harvest.
Drill holes	▪ Drill the calcaneal hole from medial to lateral. The vector guide can be used to ensure correct positioning of the exit hole and the CFL footprint on the lateral calcaneus.
Drill hole size	▪ The drill hole should closely match the size of the graft to ensure osseous integration. The drills and taps from the anterior cruciate ligament set can be used. The drill hole should be large enough to pass the tendon.
Graft preparation	▪ The graft should be prepared with a whipstitch to ensure that it passes easily through the bone tunnels.
Graft tensioning	▪ Avoid anterior translation of the talus within the ankle mortise when the tendon reconstruction is tensioned. In particular, place a bump under the distal tibia and avoid placing a bump under the heel, which tends to translate the foot and talus anteriorly. Also, after each pass of the tendon through a tunnel, cycle the ankle with the tendon under tension to gain optimal final tension.

POSTOPERATIVE CARE

- With our preferred technique, patients are placed in a walker boot at the time of surgery. At 1 week they are allowed to bear weight as tolerated. The sutures are removed at 2 weeks. Ankle range of motion, supervised by physiotherapy, is initiated at this time. Patients are kept in the walker boot until 10 weeks after surgery during weight bearing. Gait training is started 8 weeks after surgery. Proprioception and single toe raises are started 12 weeks out. Patients may return to sports after 4 months.

OUTCOMES

- There are few retrospective reviews of anatomic reconstructions using various autografts. Despite the paucity of literature all studies have reported good results, with 88% to 100% of patients reporting good outcomes.[1,12,15,46]
- Few studies have specifically looked at the outcome of a gracilis ligament reconstruction. A review of 29 ankles in 28 patients by Coughlin reported a successful outcome in terms of AOFAS and Karlsson scores in all patients. Postoperative follow-up averaged 23 months.[15]
- Sammarco and DiRaimondo used a portion of peroneus brevis through drill holes; 91% good and excellent results were seen in 43 ankles.[44]
- One study looked at the outcome of a semitendinosus graft reconstructing the ATFL; 81% of 23 patients reported an improved outcome.[41]
- There are sufficient studies with poor outcomes in the literature to recommend against nonanatomic reconstruction of the lateral ankle ligaments. Eleven papers in a recent review of lateral ligament reconstructions argued against nonanatomic reconstruction, including the Evans and Watson-Jones procedures.[6,8,22,24,25,28,35,36,39,40,47]

COMPLICATIONS

- Wound healing
- Recurrent instability
- Nerve injury
- Loss of range of motion

REFERENCES

1. Anderson ME. Reconstruction of the lateral ligaments of the ankle using the plantaris tendon. J Bone Joint Surg Am 1985;67A:930.
2. Baltopoulos P, Tzagarakis G, Kaseta M. Midterm results of a modified Evans repair for chronic lateral ankle instability. Clin Orthop Relat Res 2004;422:180.
3. Barbari S, Brevig K, Egge T. Reconstruction of the lateral ligamentous structures of the ankle with a modified Watson-Jones procedure. Foot Ankle 1987;7:362.
4. Baumhauer JF, O'Brien T. Surgical considerations in the treatment of ankle instability. J Athlet Train 2002;37:458.
5. Becker HP, Rosenbaum D. Chronic recurrent ligament instability on the lateral ankle. Orthopade 1999;28:483.
6. Becker HP, Rosenbaum D, Zeithammer G, et al. Gait pattern analysis after ankle ligament reconstruction (modified Evans procedure). Foot Ankle Int 1994;15:477.
7. Bosien WR, Staples OS, Russell SW. Residual disability following acute ankle sprains. J Bone Joint Surg Am 1955;37A:1237.
8. Boszotta H, Sauer G. Chronic fibular ligament insufficiency at the upper ankle joint: late results after modified Watson-Jones plastic surgery. Unfallchirurg 1989;92:11.
9. Boyer DS, Younger AS. Anatomic reconstruction of the lateral ligament complex of the ankle using a gracilis autograft. Foot Ankle Clin 2006;11:585.
10. Brostrom L. Sprained ankles. V. Treatment and prognosis in recent ligament ruptures. Acta Chir Scand 1966;132:537.
11. Colville MR. Surgical treatment of the unstable ankle. J Am Acad Orthop Surg 1998;6:368.
12. Colville MR, Grondel RJ. Anatomic reconstruction of the lateral ankle ligaments using a split peroneus brevis tendon graft. Am J Sports Med 1995;23:210.
13. Colville MR, Marder RA, Zarins B. Reconstruction of the lateral ankle ligaments: a biomechanical analysis. Am J Sports Med 1992;20:594.
14. Coughlin MJ, Matt V, Schenck RC Jr. Augmented lateral ankle reconstruction using a free gracilis graft. Orthopedics 2002;25:31.
15. Coughlin MJ, Schenck RC Jr, Grebing BR, et al. Comprehensive reconstruction of the lateral ankle for chronic instability using a free gracilis graft. Foot Ankle Int 2004;25:231.
16. Eskander M, Macdonald R. Watson-Jones tenodesis for chronic ankle joint instability. J Roy Army Med Corps 1993;139:115.
17. Evans DL. Recurrent instability of the ankle; a method of surgical treatment. Proc Roy Soc Med 1953;46:343.
18. Evans GA, Frenyo SD. The stress-tenogram in the diagnosis of ruptures of the lateral ligament of the ankle. J Bone Joint Surg Br 1979; 61B:347.
19. Evans GA, Hardcastle P, Frenyo AD. Acute rupture of the lateral ligament of the ankle: to suture or not to suture? J Bone Joint Surg Br 1984;66B:209.
20. Fujii T, Kitaoka HB, Watanabe K, et al. Comparison of modified Brostrom and Evans procedures in simulated lateral ankle injury. Med Sci Sports Exerc 2006;38:1025.
21. Girard P, Anderson RB, Davis WH, et al. Clinical evaluation of the modified Brostrom-Evans procedure to restore ankle stability. Foot Ankle Int 1999;20:246.
22. Hedeboe J, Johannsen A. Recurrent instability of the ankle joint: surgical repair by the Watson-Jones method. Acta Orthop Scand 1979; 50:337.
23. Hintermann B, Boss A, Schafer D. Arthroscopic findings in patients with chronic ankle instability. Am J Sports Med 2002;30:402.
24. Horstman JK, Kantor GS, Samuelson KM. Investigation of lateral ankle ligament reconstruction. Foot Ankle 1981;1:338.
25. Juliano PJ, Jordan JD, Lippert FG, et al. Persistent postoperative pain after the Chrisman-Snook ankle reconstruction. Am J Orthop 2000; 29:449.
26. Kaikkonen A, Kannus P, Jarvinen M. Surgery versus functional treatment in ankle ligament tears: a prospective study. Clin Orthop Relat Res 1996;326:194–202.
27. Kaikkonen A, Lehtonen H, Kannus P, et al. Long-term functional outcome after surgery of chronic ankle instability: a 5-year follow-up study of the modified Evans procedure. Scand J Med Sci Sports 1999;9:239.
28. Karlsson J, Bergsten T, Lansinger O, et al. Lateral instability of the ankle treated by the Evans procedure: a long-term clinical and radiological follow-up. J Bone Joint Surg Br 1988;70B:476.
29. Karlsson J, Brandsson S, Kalebo P, et al. Surgical treatment of concomitant chronic ankle instability and longitudinal rupture of the peroneus brevis tendon. Scand J Med Sci Sports 1998;8:42.
30. Karlsson J, Lansinger O. Chronic lateral instability of the ankle in athletes. Sports Med 1993;16:355.
31. Karlsson J, Lansinger O. Lateral instability of the ankle joint. Clin Orthop Relat Res 1992;276:253–261.
32. Karlsson J, Lansinger O: Lateral instability of the ankle joint (1). Non-surgical treatment is the first choice—20 per cent may need ligament surgery. Lakartidningen 1991;88:1399.
33. Karlsson J, Wiger P. Longitudinal split of the peroneus brevis tendon and lateral ankle instability: treatment of concomitant lesions. J Athlet Train 2002;37:463.
34. Kennedy MP, Coughlin MJ. Peroneus longus rupture following a modified Evans lateral ankle ligament reconstruction. Orthopedics 2003;26:1059.
35. Krips R, Brandsson S, Swensson C, et al. Anatomical reconstruction and Evans tenodesis of the lateral ligaments of the ankle: clinical and radiological findings after follow-up for 15 to 30 years. J Bone Joint Surg Br 2002;84B:232.
36. Labs K, Perka C, Lang T. Clinical and gait-analytical results of the modified Evans tenodesis in chronic fibulotalar ligament instability. Knee Surg Sports Traumatol Arthrosc 2001;9:116.
37. Larsen E, Lund PM. Peroneal muscle function in chronically unstable ankles: a prospective preoperative and postoperative electromyographic study. Clin Orthop Relat Res 1991;272:219–226.
38. Mack RP. Ankle injuries in athletics. Clin Sports Med 1982;1:71.
39. Nimon GA, Dobson PJ, Angel KR, et al. A long-term review of a modified Evans procedure. J Bone Joint Surg Br 2001;83B:14.
40. Orava S, Jaroma H, Weitz H, et al. Radiographic instability of the ankle joint after Evans repair. Acta Orthop Scand 1983;54:734.
41. Paterson R, Cohen B, Taylor D, et al. Reconstruction of the lateral ligaments of the ankle using semi-tendinosis graft. Foot Ankle Int 2000; 21:413.
42. Rosenbaum D, Becker H, Sterk J, et al. Functional evaluation of the 10-year outcome after modified Evans repair for chronic ankle instability. Foot Ankle Int 1997;18:765.
43. Rubin A, Sallis R. Evaluation and diagnosis of ankle injuries. Am Fam Physician 1996;54:1609.
44. Sammarco GJ, DiRaimondo CV. Surgical treatment of lateral ankle instability syndrome. Am J Sports Med 1988;16:501.
45. Sammarco VJ. Complications of lateral ankle ligament reconstruction. Clin Orthop Relat Res 2001;391:123–132.
46. Sugimoto K, Takakura Y, Kumai T, et al. Reconstruction of the lateral ankle ligaments with bone-patellar tendon graft in patients with chronic ankle instability: a preliminary report. Am J Sports Med 2002;30:340.
47. van der Rijt AJ, Evans GA. The long-term results of Watson-Jones tenodesis. J Bone Joint Surg Br 1984;66B:371.
48. Vertullo C. Unresolved lateral ankle pain: it's not always "just a sprain." Aust Fam Physician 2002;31:247.

Chapter **101**

Lateral Ankle Ligament Reconstruction Using Allograft and Interference Screw Fixation

William C. McGarvey and Thomas O. Clanton

DEFINITION

- Lateral ankle sprains are the most common injury in sports, accounting for 15% to 20% of all athletic injuries in some parts of the world. These injuries result in compromise or complete disruption of the lateral ankle, and, often subtalar, ligamentous complexes.[12,15]
- Ankle sprains range in severity from mild stretching to complete disruption of the ligamentous structures. Often, the injuries of moderate or medium severity are the most difficult to accurately diagnose and, therefore, manage properly.
- Most acute ankle sprains respond well to a course of nonoperative therapy, including standard rest-ice-compression-elevation (RICE) methods, functional bracing, and even immobilization followed by physical therapy.
- From 30% to 40% of patients will have persistent problems related to pain and swelling for up to 6 months after the injury, and 10% to 20% will have difficulties with recurrent sprains, leading to chronic ankle instability.[10]
  - Chronic ankle instability usually manifests itself in one of two ways: (1) recurring symptoms after an acute episode of ankle sprain, or (2) a pervasive feeling of looseness or "giving way" without warning.

ANATOMY

- The lateral ankle ligamentous complex is made up of three distinct ligaments: the anterior talofibular, the calcaneofibular, and the posterior talofibular ligaments. Other structures contributing to overall lateral ankle stability are the inferior extensor retinaculum and subtalar ligamentous complex.
- The anterior talofibular ligament (ATFL), which blends with the anterolateral joint capsule, is 15 to 20 mm long, 6 to 8 mm wide, and 2 mm thick.
- The ATFL originates from the anterior and distal fibula to insert on the lateral body of the talus, forming an angle of about 75 degrees to the floor.
- The calcaneofibular ligament (CFL) is 20 to 30 mm long, 4 to 8 mm wide, and 3 to 5 mm thick. It originates from the posteromedial portion of the inferior fibula to travel within the peroneal tendon sheath, under the tendons, and attaches to the lateral wall of the calcaneus. The orientation is 10 to 45 degrees posterior to the longitudinal axis of the fibula. The angle formed between the ATFL and CFL is 100 to 105 degrees.
- The posterior talofibular ligament (PTFL) is the largest of the lateral ankle ligaments, at 30 mm in length, 5 mm in width, and 5 to 8 mm in thickness. It has a broad insertion on nearly the entire posterior lip of the talus.
- The ATFL has the lowest load to failure of the three ligaments. Conversely, it has a much higher capacity to withstand strain than the CFL or PTFL, thereby allowing the greatest deformation before failure of all three structures.[16]
- The ATFL is taut with the ankle in plantarflexion, whereas the CFL is relatively loose. The reverse is true for the dorsiflexed ankle. The strength of the CFL and the stability afforded by the bony mortise at the malleoli in a neutral or dorsiflexed ankle make maximal plantarflexion the position of vulnerability for lateral ankle ligament injuries.[1,2]
- The subtalar ligamentous structures include the lateral talocalcaneal ligament, cervical ligament, interosseous talocalcaneal ligament—thought to provide the greatest contribution to stability of the subtalar joint, and the calcaneofibular ligament. These provide some measure of stability to the lateral ankle.

PATHOGENESIS

- Ankle instability is thought to be either acquired, as a result of repetitive trauma, or inherited due to ligamentous laxity, biomechanical abnormality (eg, heel varus, cavus foot position), or a combination of both.
- The ATFL is most commonly injured, accounting for about 75% of injuries to the ligaments of the ankle, followed by the CFL, which accounts for about 20% to 25% of these injuries. Injury to the ligaments occurs when they are either stretched or completely torn, either by avulsion from bone, or, more commonly, from midsubstance tearing.
- Neuromuscular deficits also result from these inversion injuries, leading to slower firing of the peroneal muscles in response to inversion stress, decreased responsiveness in the peronal nerve branches, weakness, and restricted dorsiflexion range of motion due to inadequate muscle forces.
- Repetitive injury can result in accumulated scarring leading to anterolateral mechanical impingement or even sinus tarsi involvement.[6,14]
- Subtalar ligaments also may be injured, although usually to a lesser extent.

NATURAL HISTORY

- Even though most ankle sprains and instability receive some form of treatment, there is little consistency in treatment regimens. The natural history is sketchy as to what would happen in the truly untreated situation.
- In one long-term study, one third of patients treated functionally for ankle sprains had continued complaints of pain, swelling, or instability in the form of recurrent sprains.[10]
- Nearly three fourths had some level of impairment on return to sporting activity, with almost 20% incurring repeated sprains and 4% with pain at rest or severe disability.
- Dysfunction after an acute sprain will persist for 6 months in 40% of injured athletes.[5]
- While it has been suggested that long-term lateral ankle instability and repeated traumatic events to the ankle can lead to advanced stages of degenerative disease, there is no actual proof of this theory.
- Nevertheless, it is presumed that continued ankle injuries as a result of lateral ankle instability can, and often will, lead to osteochondral injuries, abnormal joint mechanics, and neuromuscular dysfunction, predisposing the individual to risk of

more severe injury to the extremity or disabling degenerative arthritis of the ankle and, possibly, the subtalar joints.

PATIENT HISTORY AND PHYSICAL FINDINGS

- Patients experiencing acute ankle sprains often describe a painful tearing or pop after sustaining an inversion type injury. Longer-standing instabilities will cause complaints of lack of confidence in the joint under high demands or frequent giving way; pain and swelling often are less severe and are of secondary concern to the patient.
- Findings on examination in the acute situation are reliably present and include anterolateral ankle pain, swelling, and pain on passive plantarflexion or inversion. In the patient with a chronically unstable ankle, the examination focuses more on the anterior drawer and talar tilt tests and the "suction sign."
- Assessment for structural abnormalities also is important. Heel position should be examined in every patient, by looking at the patient from behind while he or she is standing, to determine the possible presence of varus malalignment.
- Neuromuscular function is another important part of the examination. Peroneal muscle group function, specifically, is critical. Strength and stability of the peroneals should be assessed by resistive muscle grading against plantarflexion and eversion. Provocative maneuvers such as the plantarflexion eversion stress test also should be performed to ensure that the peroneal tendons do not subluxate from the retrofibular groove.
- Sensory nerves should always be inspected to ensure no neurapraxia has taken place as a result of the traction from the injury.
- Syndesmotic integrity should be tested with palpation, the "squeeze" test, and dorsiflexion–external rotation provocative manipulations.

IMAGING AND OTHER DIAGNOSTIC STUDIES

- According to the Ottawa Ankle Rules,[11] nearly 100% sensitivity is approached if the following criteria are used in the acute setting:
  - Tenderness at the posteroanterior edge or tip of the medial or lateral malleolus
  - Inability to bear weight (4 steps) right after the injury or in the emergency room
  - Pain at the base of the fifth metatarsal
- If radiographs are required, anteroposterior, lateral, and mortise views, preferably weight bearing, should be performed, looking for avulsion fractures of the tip of either malleolus, or, less frequently, the lateral calcaneus. One also should inspect for osteochondral fractures, joint malposition, and other fractures that may mimic lateral ankle sprains (see Differential Diagnosis).
- Stress views can be obtained in either the AP (talar tilt) or lateral (anterior drawer) position. Performing the study while stressing the ankle (as described in the section on examination of the patient) can give meaningful information regarding the stability of the joint. Significant controversy exists on what constitutes an abnormal study, but on the basis of the cumulative review of literature on this topic, more than 15 degrees of varus tilt and 5 mm of anterior translation are reasonably considered abnormal.
- MRI is valuable for determining whether the ligamentous structures have been injured and in what time frame. Attenuation, wavy fibers, or disruption in the face of fluid accumulation suggests recent injury, whereas thickening or intrasubstance signal change gives rise to suspicion for a more remote injury. Infrequently, an absence of ligament tissue is noted, reflecting repeated injuries leading to degeneration of the complex.

DIFFERENTIAL DIAGNOSIS

- Acute
  - Lateral malleolar fracture
  - Fifth metatarsal fracture
  - Lateral talar process or "snowboarder's" fracture
  - Peroneal tendon dislocation
  - Osteochondral defect
  - Superficial peroneal neurapraxia
- Chronic
  - Peroneal instability
  - Peroneal split tears
  - Subtalar instability
  - Osteochondral defect
  - Tibiotalar or subtalar arthritis

NONOPERATIVE MANAGEMENT

- Nonoperative management is the mainstay of treatment for both acute and chronic instabilities. Most patients will respond to conservative management; consequently, it is essential that appropriate conservative treatment be tried for all patients before surgery is suggested.
- Acute swelling and pain, whether from a new injury or recent repeat injury, is best managed with RICE. Immobilization in a walking cast or boot should be considered for anyone demonstrating a positive drawer or talar tilt after an acute episode or recurrence.
- Once the acute symptoms have subsided, functional strapping, taping, or bracing should be instituted along with an exercise regimen emphasizing peroneal strengthening, proprioceptive training, and Achilles tendon stretching.
- In the patient with a chronically unstable ankle, shoe wear modifications can be added as the individual returns to sports or activities. Orthoses with lateral heel and sole wedges or flare on the lateral sole of the shoe can promote a valgus moment and help avoid injury in the vulnerable patient. Reducing heel height and stiffening the sole of the shoe also can be helpful.
- Prophylactic brace wear or taping has been shown to have some benefit in prevention of injury. It also has a positive effect on reduction in severity of sprains if reinjury occurs while these measures are in effect.

SURGICAL MANAGEMENT

- Surgery rarely is indicated for an initial acute injury.
  - Acute injuries failing appropriate conservative care, in our opinion, are best treated with an anatomic repair and reinforcement using a modified Brostrom procedure.
- Chronic instability failing appropriate conservative measures is more complex.
  - In a previously unoperated patient with MRI evidence of tissue remnants, an anatomic repair (modified Brostrom procedure) is very effective.

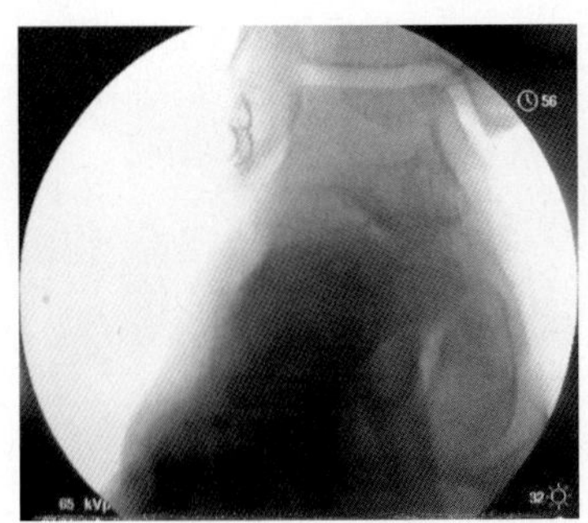

FIG 1 • Plain radiograph of an unstressed, non–weight-bearing ankle after injury and before anatomic repair.

- In patients who have repeated injuries and are left without evidence of ATFL or CFL remnant by MRI, or in patients who have previously undergone an attempt at surgical correction, reconstruction with free tendon graft is our preferred method.[3,4,7,13,17]

Preoperative Planning

- All imaging studies, including MRI, are reviewed, and any adjunctive pathology that may need to be addressed at the time of surgery, such as fragments of bone, OCLs, or peroneal tendon pathology, is noted.
- The joint (and the contralateral joint) is examined under anesthesia to detemine the true nature of instability and also to gauge the effect of the repair (**FIGS 1 AND 2**).
- Graft choice also is an important preoperative consideration. An autogenous hamstring graft can be chosen and harvested in similar fashion to that of ACL graft harvests.[3,4,7,13,17] Alternatively, should the patient be averse to violating his or her own knee, an allograft gracilis tendon has been shown to be a very suitable alternative, with the advantages of reduced pain, no donor site morbidity, and risk and effectiveness virtually the same as using the patient's own tissue.
- The presence of a varus heel may necessitate the addition of a laterally based closing wedge calcaneal osteotomy.

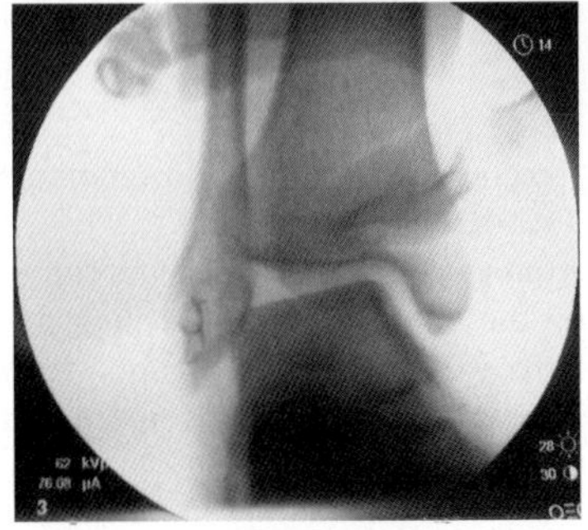

FIG 2 • Preoperative stress radiograph of the same ankle demonstrating talar tilt.

Positioning

- The patient is placed in the supine position, typically with an ipsilateral hip roll to allow access to the posterolateral corner of the ankle.
- Arthroscopic examination is performed to identify any unseen intra-articular pathology.[9] A thigh holder and soft tissue ankle joint distractor often are necessary for the initial portion of the procedure.

Approach

- One of two approaches may be chosen, depending on the degree of pathology that is to be addressed.
  - For ankle ligament reconstruction alone, an anterior curvilinear incision bordering the distal inferior tip of the fibula is preferred.
  - If it is necessary to address peroneal pathology or anterior osteophytes, a more extensile lateral malleolar incision, curving distally after the tip of the fibula, is useful (**FIG 3**).
- An oblique incision over the calcaneus usually can be added to either approach without great concern for increased wound morbidity.

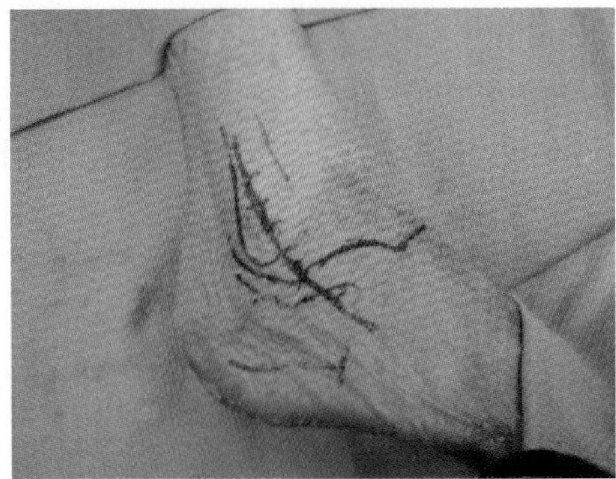

FIG 3 • Surgical approach parallelling the posterior border of the fibula is marked on the skin.

TALAR TUNNEL PLACEMENT

- The lateral ankle is exposed by one of two incisions, as previously described.
- The origin sites of both ATFL and CFL are identified (**TECH FIG 1A**).

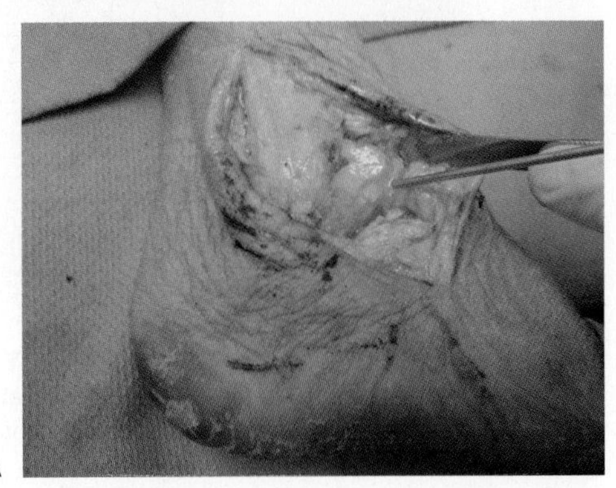

TECH FIG 1 • **A.** The talar tunnel is placed just anterior to the neck–body junction, aiming slightly posterior and lateral. (*continued*)

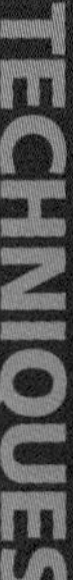

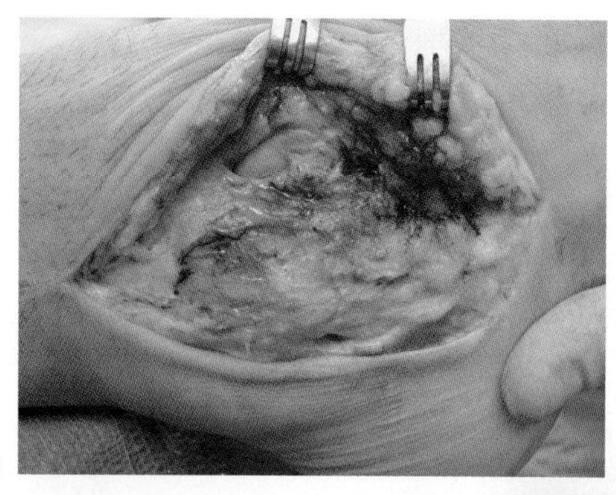

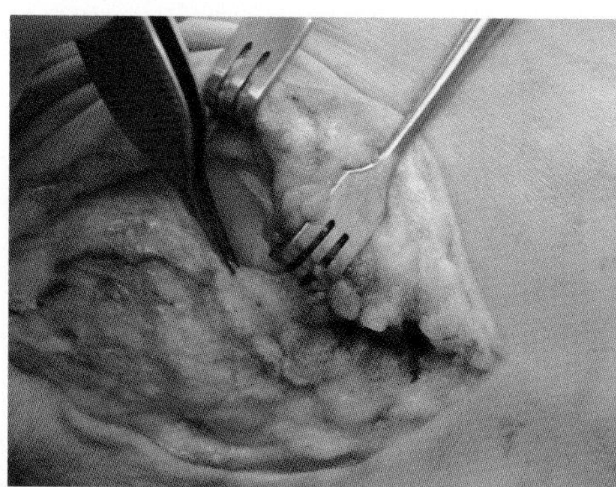

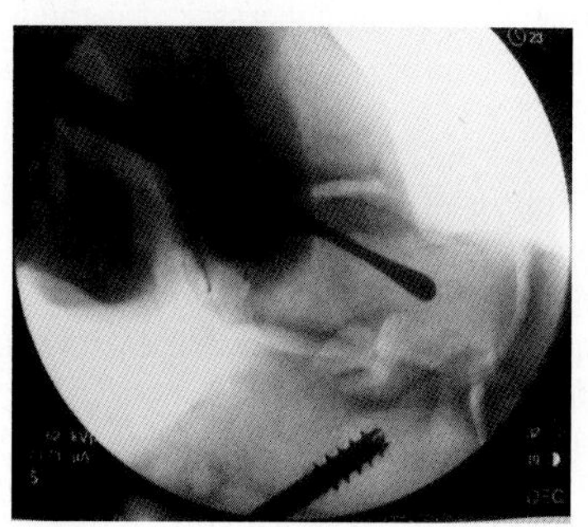

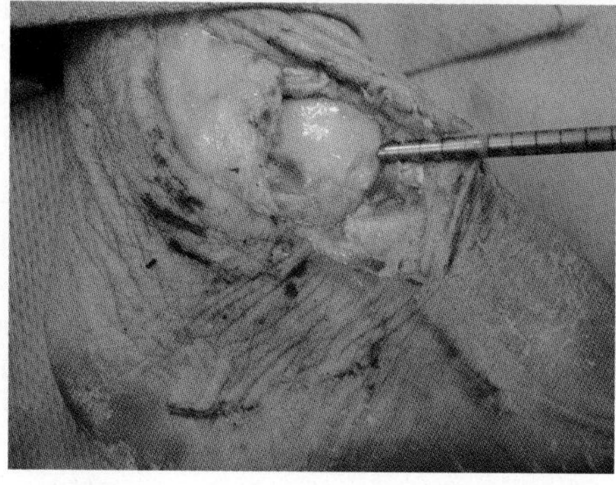

TECH FIG 1 • *(continued)* **B.** A rent in the capsule and previously repaired anterior talofibular ligament (ATFL) is evident. **C.** The area of deficient capsule and ATFL is identified by instrument. **D.** Location of the proposed talar tunnel. **E.** Reaming is performed slightly deeper than the chosen screw length.

- Dissection proceeds to expose the insertion of the ATFL on the lateral talus just at the corner of the lateral process as it blends from the body to the neck (**TECH FIG 1B,C**).
- A 15- to 20-mm tunnel is drilled horizontally at this point with a 4.5- to 6-mm drill to accept the first limb of the tendon graft (**TECH FIG 1D,E**).

FIBULAR TUNNEL PLACEMENT

- The fibula is exposed and a 4.5- to 6-mm tunnel is drilled from the insertion of the ATFL through the posterior fibular cortex (**TECH FIG 2A–C**).
- A second tunnel is made more distally from the CFL insertion to a point about 3 to 4 mm distal to the previous exit point on the posterior fibular cortex. This allows for graft passage over a cortical bridge, and, in addition, the graft can be sutured to periosteum to prevent sliding (**TECH FIGS 2D–F AND 3**).
- An alternative method uses a single tunnel from a point between the ATFL and CFL insertions, not violating the posterior cortex, that would accept a folded or doubled graft fixed with a single interference screw within this single tunnel.

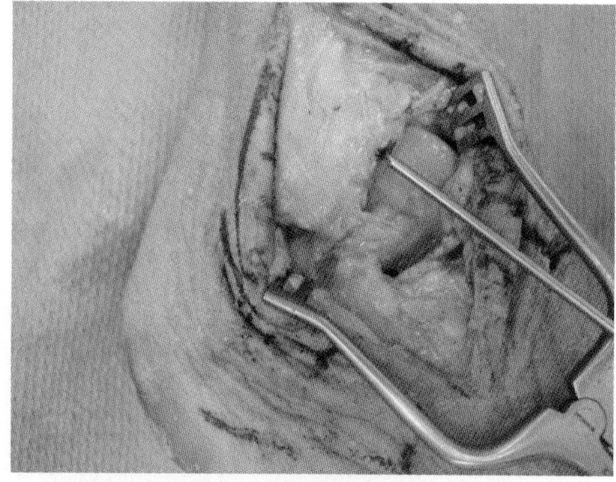

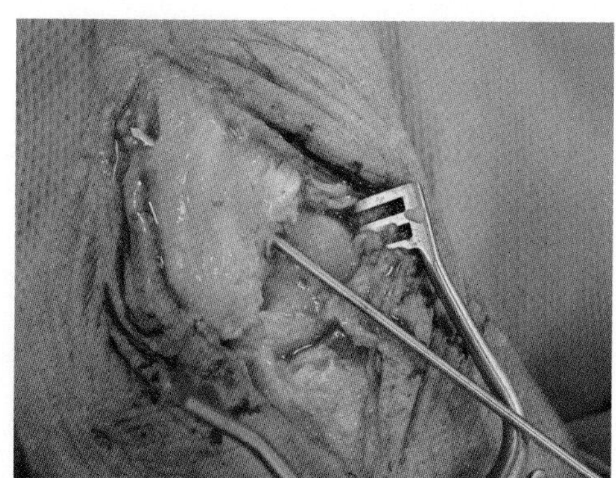

TECH FIG 2 • **A.** The origin of the ATFL is used as the entry point for the first fibular tunnel. **B.** The guide pin is inserted aiming superior and posterior at 45 to 60 degrees to allow for another more inferior tunnel for the calcaneofibular ligament (CFL) limb of the graft. *(continued)*

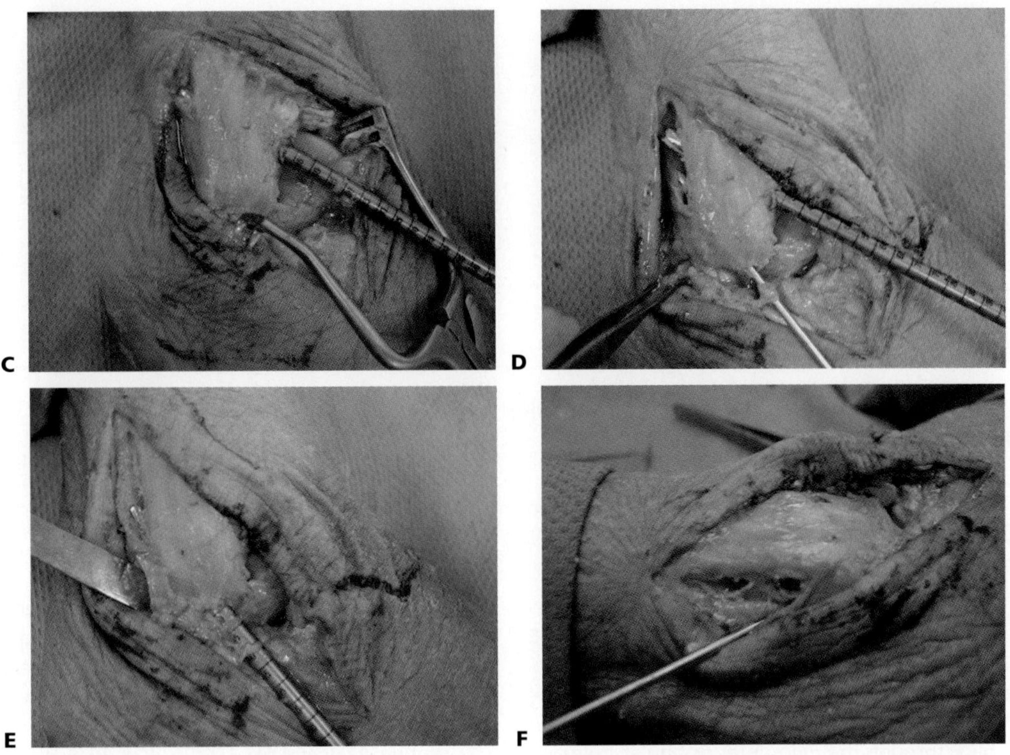

TECH FIG 2 • *(continued)* **C.** Reaming of the first tunnel is done with a size-matched reamer based on screw size and graft diameter. **D.** A second guide pin is inserted from the CFL origin, aiming superior and posterior, but 3 to 4 mm below the previously created tunnel. Care must be taken to avoid tunnel blowout. **E.** Reaming the second fibular tunnel. **F.** A bony bridge is preserved between fibular tunnels.

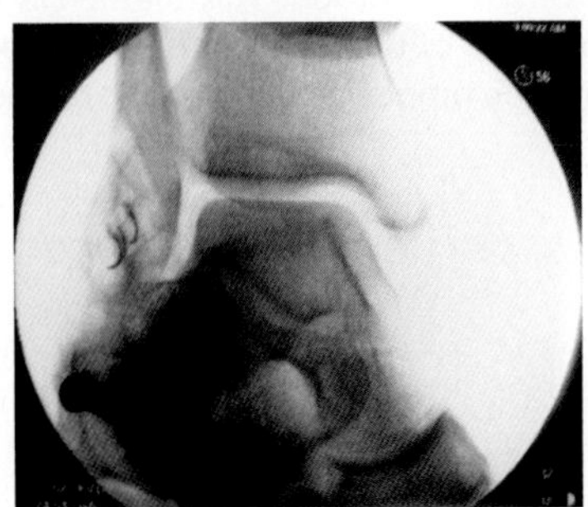

TECH FIG 3 • Postoperative non–weight-bearing radiograph after reconstruction of lateral ligaments with allograft.

CALCANEAL TUNNEL PLACEMENT

- A tunnel of similar size is then drilled bicortically through the lateral calcaneal wall at the level of the CFL insertion (TECH FIG 4).

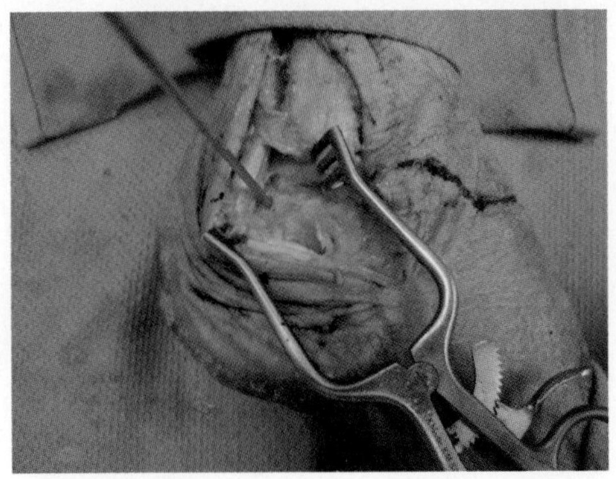

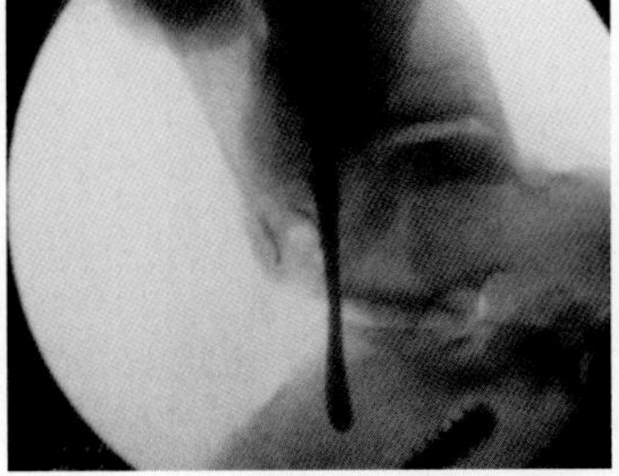

TECH FIG 4 • **A.** The guide pin for the calcaneal tunnel is placed with the peroneal muscle group swept posterior. The tunnel is placed just inferior to the insertion point of the CFL. **B.** Verification of tunnel position. *(continued)*

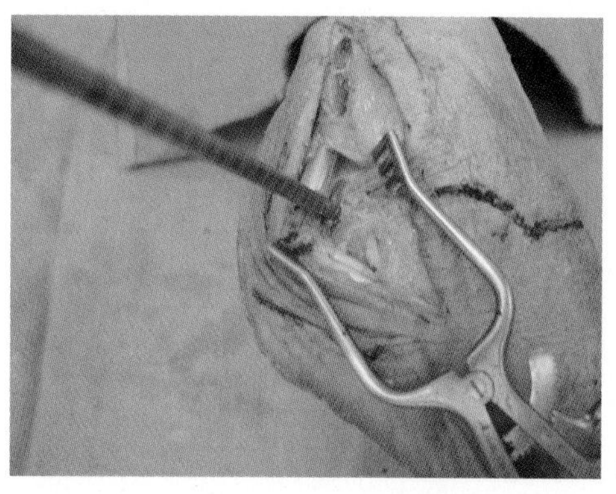

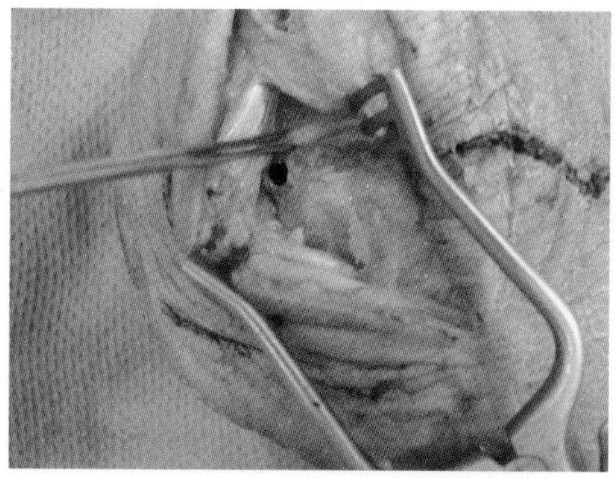

TECH FIG 4 • *(continued)* **C.** Reaming the calcaneal tunnel. **D.** Note the relation between the calcaneal insertion of CFL and the reamed tunnel.

GRAFT PASSAGE

- The sutured tendon is inserted first into the talar tunnel and fixed with an interference screw (**TECH FIGS 5 AND 6**).
- It is then woven through the fibular tunnel from the ATFL insertion, through the more proximal posterior exit tunnel, back through the more inferior fibular hole and out the CFL origin. This gives the most anatomic origin and insertion points (**TECH FIG 7 A–C**).
- Lastly, the graft is passed through the calcaneal tunnel.
- The foot is held neutral to slightly everted, and a roll of towels is placed under the calf to allow a slight posterior drawer effect. The graft is held taut as it is brought through the skin on the medial side (**TECH FIG 8**).
- A second interference screw is placed in the calcaneus (**TECH FIG 9**).
- Range of motion and stability are assessed. If tension does not feel appropriate, the calcaneal screw can be removed, the graft retensioned, and the screw replaced.
- The tendon can receive a few sutures at the fibular tunnels to maintain tension of the individual limbs representing ATFL and CFL (**TECH FIGS 10 A,B AND 11**).
- If the surgeon prefers the single fibular tunnel technique, the interference screw is placed in the fibula with one limb of the graft directed toward the talus (ATFL) and one to the calcaneus (CFL). These are then similarly tensioned and fixed with individual interference screw fixation. This method is more exacting, as the limbs of tendon must be cut to exact length and fit into the proper depths of their respective tunnels.

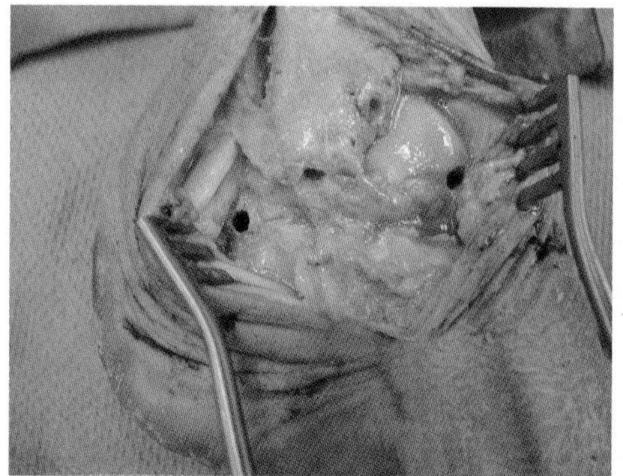

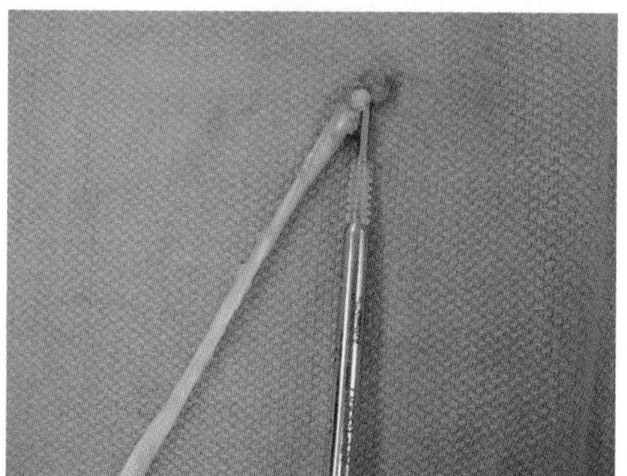

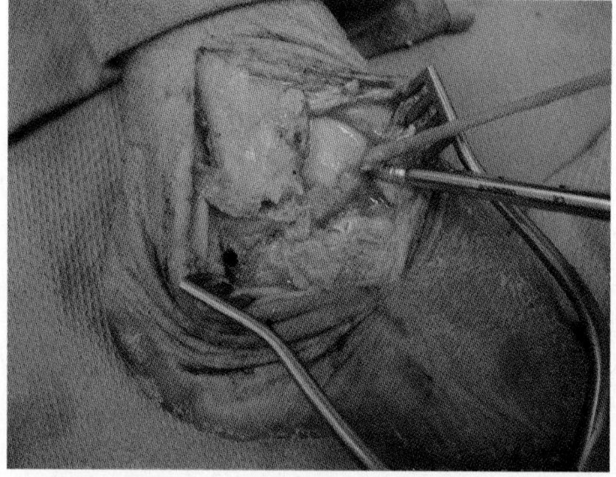

TECH FIG 5 • A. All tunnel holes are reamed in advance of graft passage. **B.** Allograft tendon is mounted for insertion into the tibia tunnel with the first interference screw. **C.** The graft is inserted into the talar tunnel and fixed by interference screw.

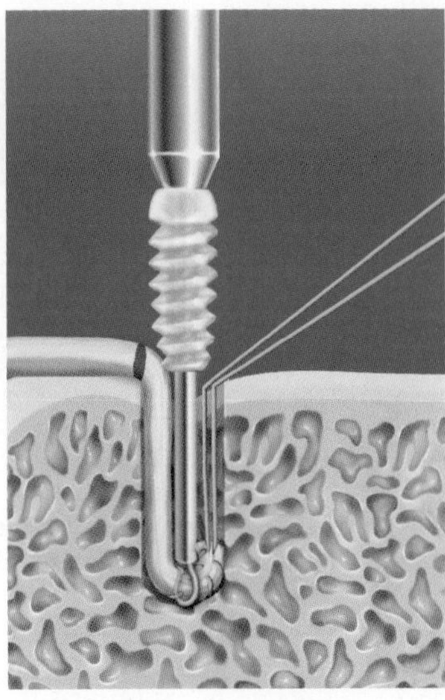

TECH FIG 6 • Schematic of interference fit tenodesis screw.

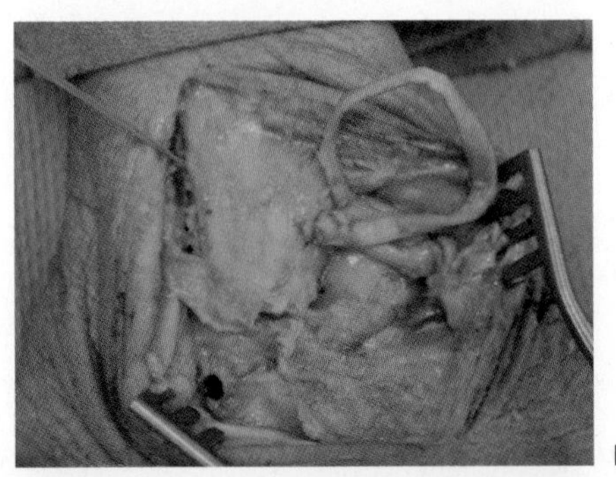

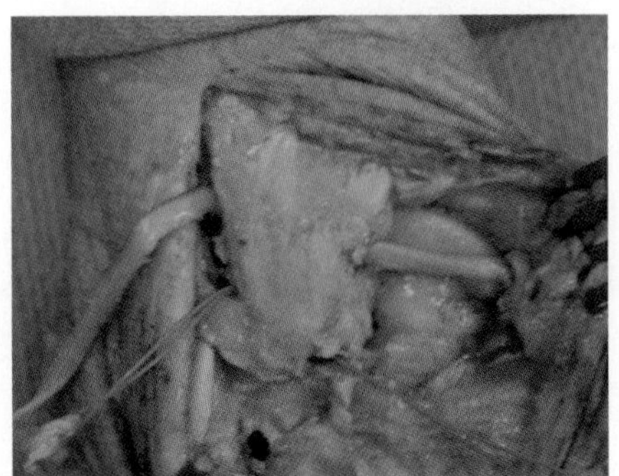

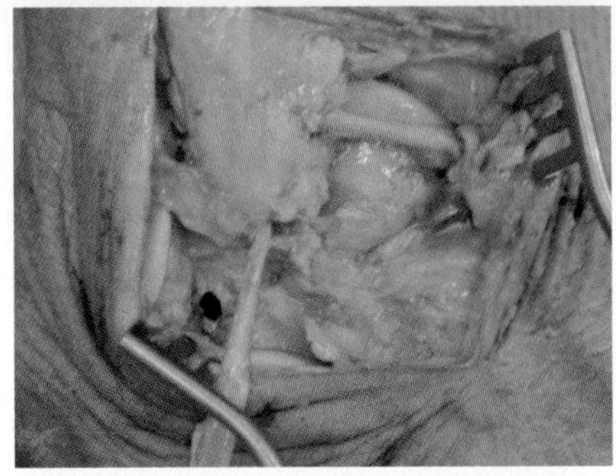

TECH FIG 7 • **A.** The graft is pulled through the first fibular tunnel by a previously placed pull-through suture weave. **B.** The graft is then pulled through the second fibular tunnel and tension maintained. A stay suture can be placed in the graft and the fibular periosteum to maintain the ATFL tension. **C.** Graft pulled through both tunnels.

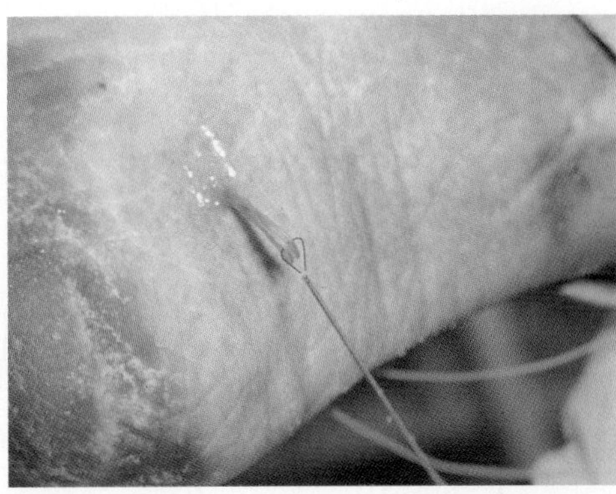

TECH FIG 8 • A Beath pin is used to pull the suture through the medial side of the tunnel and then out through the skin for final tensioning.

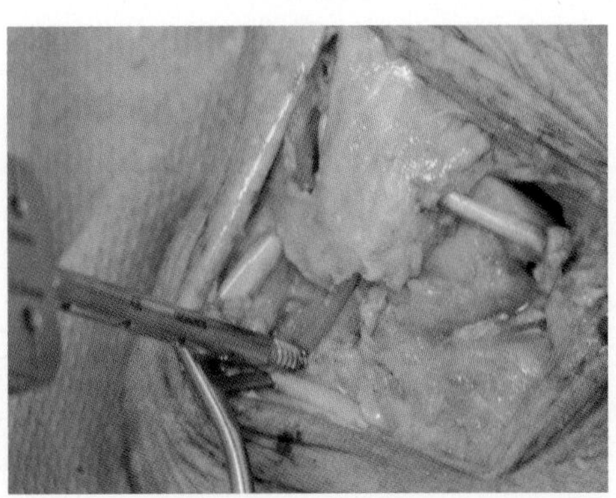

TECH FIG 9 • After appropriate positioning of the ankle and tensioning of the graft, the calcaneal interference screw is inserted.

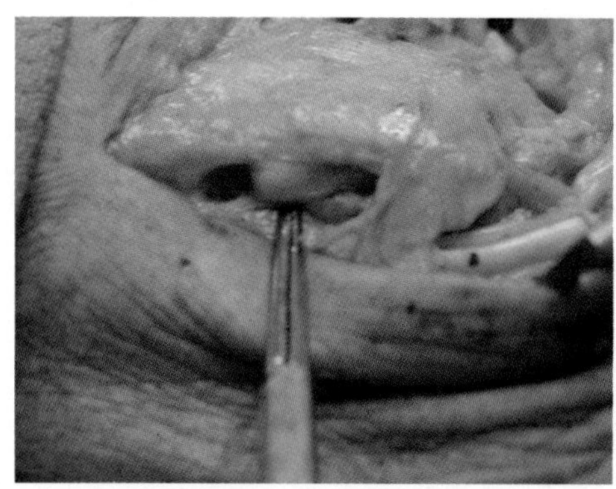

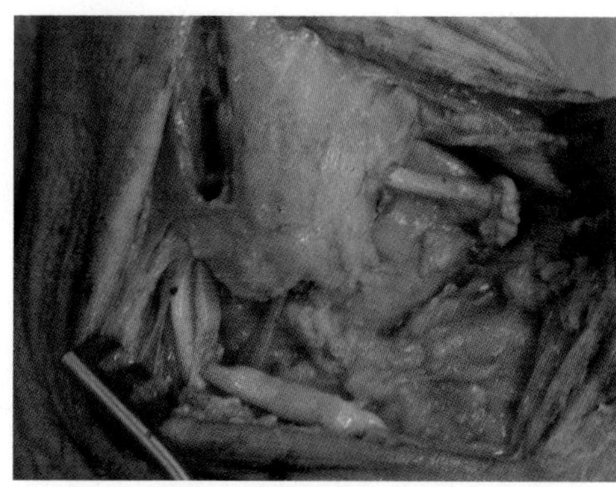

TECH FIG 10 • A. Graft position is supported by a fibular bone bridge. (Without a bony bridge, the graft could subside and thus loosen in the soft cancellous bone trough.) **B.** Finished anatomic ligament weave featuring ATFL and CFL reconstruction.

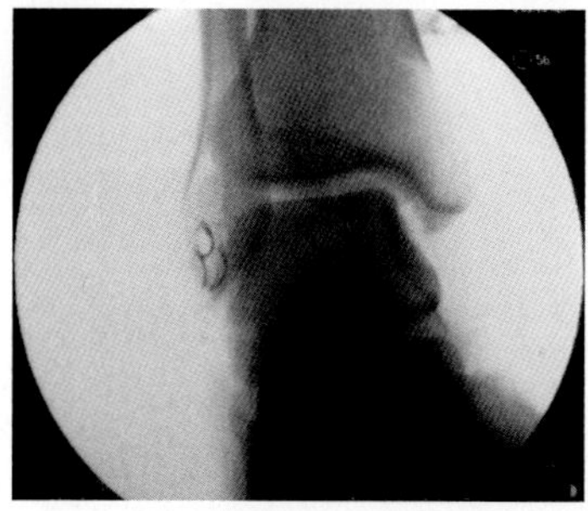

TECH FIG 11 • Postoperative stress radiograph. Note that there is no talar tilt.

WOUND CLOSURE

- Layered closure is performed, usually with a subcutaneous layer of 2-0 Vicryl or monocryl followed by skin sutures with 3-0 nylon.

CALCANEAL OSTEOTOMY

- If heel varus is present, a laterally based closing wedge calcaneal osteotomy may be performed.
- An oblique incision is carried out directly over the area of the planned osteotomy (usually about 2 cm posterior to any other concurrent incision).
- Periosteum is raised in each direction.
- A 1- to 1.5-cm width is marked on the lateral wall of the calcaneal tuberosity verifying that the osteotomy will not breach the bone tunnel.
- Saw cuts are made convergently to meet just before violating medial cortex.
- The wedge is removed and the osteotomy closed.
- Fixation can be achieved through either a large axially directed screw or staples.

PEARLS AND PITFALLS

Graft handling	■ Great care must be taken in harvesting autograft so as to get enough length on the native gracilis. ■ If allograft is used, it must be ordered properly, with enough length to span the distance of the tendon weave (25 cm is plenty). ■ Once the allograft is thawed, it should be bathed in antibiotic solution until ready for use.
Tunnel placement	■ Avoid tunnel breakout. ■ Consider making two separate tunnels on the posterior fibula divided by a cortical bridge between them. This will help resist the chance of graft migration on cancellous bone within the V-shaped tunnel.

Be aware of alignment	■ Persistent heel varus can destroy a perfectly performed ligament reconstruction if not addressed. ■ If necessary, do a calcaneal osteotomy.
Tensioning the graft	■ Hold the foot in the desired neutral position (to about 5 degrees of overeversion), pull the graft taut, and fix it in this position. Ensure mobility and stability at this time. Re-tensioning can be done now with interference screw fixation, but it will not be possible to compensate for this later. ■ Do not overshorten the graft. This will leave the repair too tight or require another harvest.

POSTOPERATIVE CARE

- Bulky, padded splinting in neutral positions are maintained for 10 to 14 days postoperatively.
- Once wounds are healed satisfactorily, the patient may begin protected weight bearing in a cast, as tolerated, for another 4 weeks.
- Gradual transition from cast to boot and introduction of range of motion begin 5 to 6 weeks after surgery.
- Rehabilitation is then instituted focusing on restoration of motion, Achilles stretching, proprioceptive training, and peroneal strengthening.
- Athletic activity usually is withheld for 4 to 6 months.

OUTCOMES

- Anatomic reconstruction for failed acute and chronic instability patterns continues to be our preferred method of lateral ankle ligament reconstruction. This has been shown in the literature to be extremely successful for return to function and reduction or elimination of symptoms in appropriately selected patients.
- When a patient has lost reliable lateral soft tissue structures by virtue of repetitive injury or previous failed procedures, an anatomic free graft lateral ligament reconstruction provides a very good alternative.
- Reconstruction using this method reconstitutes the ATFL and CFL, thus providing restoration of both ankle and subtalar stability.
- Anatomic reconstruction coupled with the preservation of native peroneal tendon function provides an optimum environment for return to function.
- Paterson et al[13] showed 81% complete or substantial symptom resolution in 26 patients at 2-year follow-up by performing reconstruction of the ATFL alone. No significant differences were noted between operated and contralateral ankles with respect to range of motion or uniaxial balancing.
- Coughlin et al[3,4] reported on 2-year follow-up in 28 patients. All patients were rated to have good or excellent outcomes with objective improvement in talar tilt measurements (13 degrees pre- vs 3 degrees postoperatively) and anterior drawer testing (on average, 10 mm pre- vs 5 mm postoperatively).
- Addition of tenodesis or interference screw fixation adds the advantage of being able to promote range of motion earlier with less concern for graft loosening.[8,17]

COMPLICATIONS

- Nerve injury
- Wound problems
- Infection
- Joint stiffness
- Deep venous thrombosis
- Subjective under- or over-tightening

REFERENCES

1. Ardevol J, Bolibar I, Belda V, et al. Treatment of complete rupture of the lateral ligaments of the ankle: A randomized clinical trial comparing cast immobilization with functional treatment. Knee Surg Sports Traumatol Arthrosc 2002;10:371–377.
2. Colville MR, Grondel RJ. Anatomic reconstruction of the lateral ankle ligaments using split peroneus tendon graft. Am J Sports Med 1995;23:210–213.
3. Coughlin MJ, Matt V, Schenck RC. Augmented lateral ankle reconstruction using a free gracilis graft. Orthopedics 2002;25:31–35.
4. Coughlin MJ, Schenck RC, Grebing BR, et al. Comprehensive reconstruction of the lateral ankle for chronic instability using a free gracilis graft. Foot Ankle Intl 2004;25:231–241.
5. Gerber JP. Persistent disability with ankle sprains: A prospective examination of an athletic population. Foot Ankle Intl 1998; 19:653–660.
6. Hertel J. Functional instability following lateral ankle sprain. Sports Med 2000;29:361–371.
7. Jeys LM, Harris NJ. Ankle stabilization with hamstring autograft: A new technique using interference screws. Foot Ankle Intl 2003;24:677–679.
8. Jeys LM, Korrosis S, Stewart T, et al. Bone anchors or interference screws? A biomechanical evaluation for autograft ankle stabilization. Am J Sports Med 2004;32:1651–1659.
9. Komenda GA. Arthroscopic findings associated with the unstable ankle. Foot Ankle Intl 1999;20:708.
10. Konradsen L. Seven years follow-up after ankle inversion trauma. Scand J Med Sci Sports 2002;12:129–135.
11. Lynch S. Assessment of the injured ankle in the athlete. J Athl Train 2002;37:406–412.
12. Maehlum S, Daljord OA. Acute sports injuries in Oslo: A one year study. Br J Sports Med 1984;18:181–185.
13. Paterson R, Cohen B, Taylor D, et al. Reconstruction of the lateral ligaments of the ankle using semitendinosus graft. Foot Ankle Intl 2000;21:413–419.
14. Richie DH. Functional instability of the ankle and the role of neuromuscular control: A comprehensive review. J Foot Ankle Surg 2001;40:240–251.
15. Sandelin J. Acute sports injuries: A clinical and epidemiological study [dissertation]. Helsinki: University of Helsinki; 1988.
16. Siegler S, Block J, Schneck CD. The mechanical characteristics of the collateral ligaments of the human ankle joint. Foot Ankle 1988;8:234–242.
17. Takao M, Oae K, Uchio Y, et al. Anatomical reconstruction of the lateral ligaments of the ankle with a gracilis autograft. A new technique using an interference fit anchoring system. Am J Sports Med 2005;33:814–823.

Chapter 102 Chronic Lateral Ankle Instability

Markus Walther

DEFINITION

- Lateral ligament injuries of the ankle are treated conservatively with good results in most cases. However, several factors may lead to chronic ankle instability with recurring ankle sprains:
  - Inadequate primary treatment
  - Incomplete healing of the ligaments
  - Repetitive trauma with deteriorated tissue quality
- Patients with chronic ankle instability can be divided into two groups:
  - Patients with sufficient tissue quality to perform a local repair
  - Patients with inadequate tissue quality for a local repair
- A Broström procedure for lateral ankle reconstruction is possible, as long as there is sufficient tissue.
- In patients with insufficient local tissue, an augmentation is needed to rebuild or reinforce the lateral ligaments. There are different options of tendon grafts, each with certain advantages and disadvantages:
  - Tenodesis
  - Semitendinosus tendon or gracilis tendon
  - Plantaris longus tendon

ANATOMY

- Laterally, the ankle is stabilized by the anterior (ATFL) and posterior (PTFL) fibulotalar ligament and the calcaneofibular ligament (CFL) (**FIG 1**).[5]
- Additional stability is provided by the bony structures. Especially in dorsal extension, the talus is locked between the medial and lateral malleolus.

PATHOGENESIS

- Torn lateral ligaments are the result of an ankle sprain. Depending on the severity of the sprain, one to three of the lateral ligaments are injured. A rupture of the ATFL is involved in most cases.
- Anatomic classification
  - Grade I: ATFL sprain
  - Grade II: ATFL and CFL sprain
  - Grade III: ATFL, CFL, and PTFL sprain
- AMA (American Medical Association) standard nomenclature system by severity
  - Grade I: Ligament stretched
  - Grade II: Ligament partially torn
  - Grade III: Ligament completely torn
- Grading by clinical presentation symptoms
  - Mild sprain: minimal functional loss, no limp, minimal or no swelling, point tenderness, pain with reproduction of mechanism of injury
  - Moderate sprain: moderate functional loss, unable to toe-rise or hop on injured ankle, limp when walking, localized swelling, point tenderness
  - Severe sprain: diffuse tenderness and swelling, crutches preferred by patient for ambulation
- With each ankle sprain, proprioception of the ankle joint is compromised.
  - The risk for another ankle sprain increases after each injury. In an uninjured person, an ankle sprain will occur in 1:1,000,000 steps. This risk increases to 1:1000 steps after a severe ankle sprain.[11]

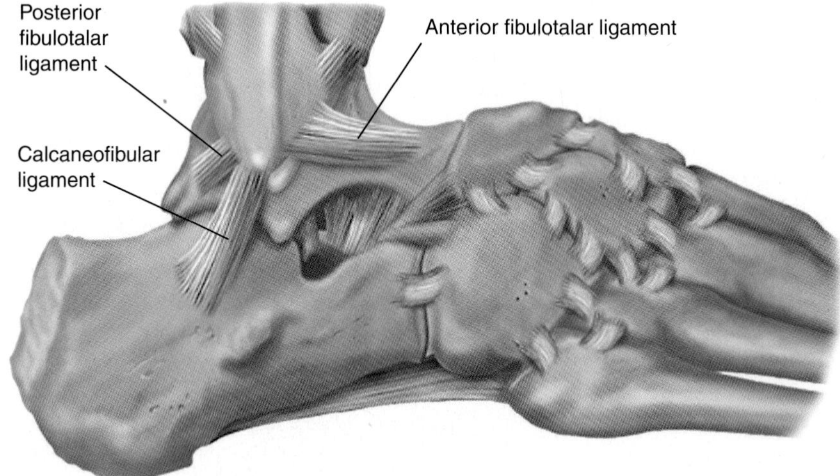

FIG 1 • Anatomy of the lateral ankle showing the three ligaments: anterior and posterior fibulotalar ligament and the calcaneofibular ligament.

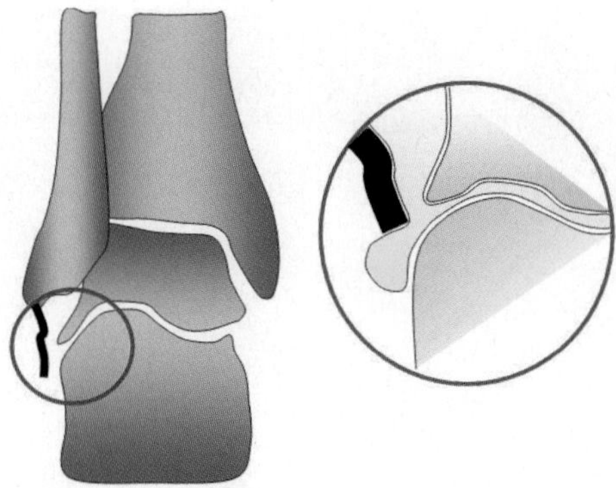

FIG 2 • Synovial fluid between the two ends of torn ligaments can prevent the injury from healing.

- Chronic ankle instability is the combination of insufficient active and ligament stabilization mechanisms.
- There is some evidence that special anatomic variations increase the risk of developing chronic ankle instability after an injury.[13]
- The healing of the ligaments can be compromised by synovial fluid between ligament and bone (**FIG 2**).

NATURAL HISTORY

- Chronic instability is a risk factor for degenerative arthritis of the ankle joint. Valderrabano et al. have shown an increased prevalence of arthritis in patients with chronic ankle instability.[18]
- Recurrent ankle sprains are likely in the future, but this is strongly dependent upon lifestyle and sports activities.

PATIENT HISTORY AND PHYSICAL FINDINGS

- The patient history includes sustained injuries, frequency of ankle sprains, and causes of pain, as well as restrictions in daily living and sports.
- The degree of disability experienced by the patient depends upon the degree of instability and the physical demands.
- Many tests for ankle instability are strongly dependent on patient cooperation. If positive, however, they can be highly specific.
  - The examiner should check the range of motion of the ankle joint with a stretched and a bent knee to rule out a shortening of the gastrocnemius or soleus muscle (or both). Restricted dorsiflexion with a stretched knee joint that is not found with a flexed knee is specific for a shortening of the gastrocnemius muscle (Silfverskiöld test).
  - The inversion test is used to assess for a ruptured CFL.
  - Medial ankle stability is checked in a plantarflexed position of the ankle to avoid a locking of the talus in the joint, which can mimic ligamentous stability. If positive, it is highly specific for a ruptured deltoid ligament.
  - Insufficiency of the fibulocalcaneus ligament often affects the stability of the subtalar joint. The stability is checked in dorsiflexion of the ankle to lock the talus in the upper ankle joint. If positive, it is highly specific for a ruptured CFL in combination with subtalar instability.
  - Effusion can be palpated ventral, but smaller amounts of fluid are difficult to detect.
  - The ankle drawer test strains the ATFL and is highly specific for rupture of this ligament.

IMAGING AND OTHER DIAGNOSTIC STUDIES

- Plain radiographs should be obtained to evaluate potential bony pathology.
- Stress radiographs: The AP view shows the lateral opening of the joint. An anterior talar shift can be seen on the lateral stress view (**FIG 3**).
- MRI gives valuable information on the lateral ligaments and other pathology. In chronic instability scarring is often found. However, it is impossible to judge functional stability in an MRI. Frequent additional pathologies visible on MRI are tears of the peroneal tendons, osteochondral lesions, and bone edema.

DIFFERENTIAL DIAGNOSIS

- Articular injury (chondral or osteochondral fractures)
- Nerve injuries (sural, superficial peroneal, posterior tibial)
- Tendon injury (peroneal tendon tear or dislocation, tibialis posterior)
- Other ligamentous injuries (syndesmosis, subtalar, bifurcate, calcaneocuboid)
- Impingement (anterior osteophyte, anteroinferior tibiofibular ligament, scars)
- Unrelated pathology, masked by routine sprain (undetected rheumatoid condition, diabetic neuroarthropathy, tumor)

NONOPERATIVE MANAGEMENT

- The goals of nonoperative treatment are improving proprioception and strength. This can be achieved by physiotherapy and exercises.
- Shoe modifications include a lateral wedge or a flare.
- Means of external fixation are orthoses, braces, or taping. However, those methods are limited.
  - Tape loses 30% of its stability after 200 steps. Skin problems are reported in up to 28%.
  - Within the group of orthoses, semirigid, warped types provide the highest degree of stability.[2]
- For many patients with symptomatic instability or pain, nonsurgical measures are not acceptable as a long-term solution. Usually these patients require a lateral ligament repair.

SURGICAL MANAGEMENT

- In patients with no previous surgery and good tissue quality, the Broström procedure is a good option, reinserting the original ligaments in place.[3] Especially with modern anchor techniques, this procedure has regained a great deal of popularity.

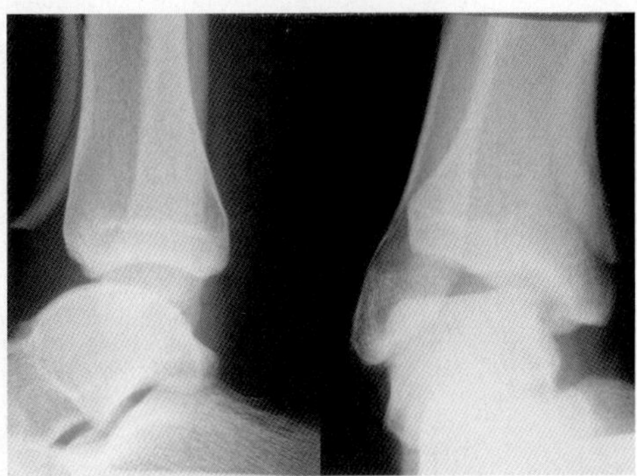

FIG 3 • Stress radiographs of a patient with a chronic high-grade instability of the ankle joint.

Broström showed in his work that even after a longer period of chronic instability, a reconstruction of the original ligaments is possible, providing sufficient stability and function of the ankle joint.[4]

- However, most patients with a history of recurrent inversion trauma do not have adequate tissue quality to perform a Broström procedure.[6,10,16]
- Insufficient local tissue can be augmented or replaced by a tendon graft.
- There are different options of tendon grafts, each with certain advantages and disadvantages.
  - Tenodesis: The major disadvantage of tenodesis procedures (eg, Evans or Watson-Jones) is that they often end up in persistent pain[14,15] in combination with an increasing lack of stability over time.[12,17]
  - Autologous or homologous semitendinosus tendon or gracilis tendon can be used as graft. Although in general tolerated well, there is some risk of donor site morbidity after harvesting those tendons.[1] If a homologous graft is used, there is a small risk of infection.
  - A local tendon that can easily be harvested with a minimum of donor site morbidity is the plantaris longus tendon.[7]

Preoperative Planning

- In about 3% of the patients, no plantaris longus tendon can be found or it is not long enough for transplantation. A strategy has to be discussed with the patient as to how to proceed in this case. An option is to change to a technique using another transplant (eg, the gracilis or semitendinosus tendon).

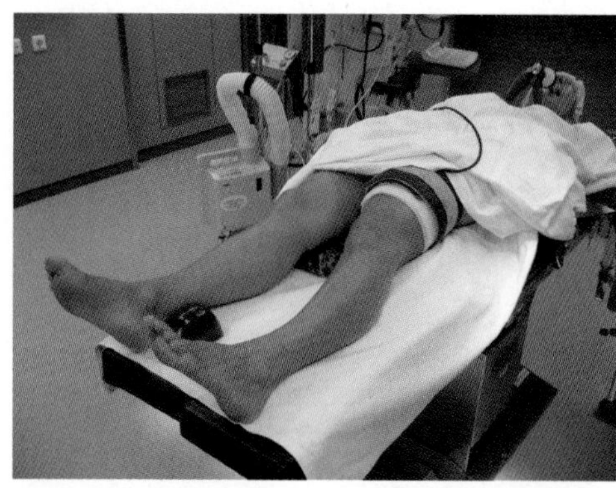

FIG 4 • The patient is positioned supine with a sand sack under the injured side.

- Examinations performed under anesthesia include range of motion of the ankle joint and the ankle stress tests to confirm the previous results, without an active stabilization of the ankle joint by the patient.
- Additional intra-articular pathology is a common finding. In most cases, it is advisable to do an arthroscopy of the ankle joint before the final reconstruction.[9]

Positioning

- The patient is positioned supine with a sand sack under the injured side.
- The procedure is performed with a tourniquet (**FIG 4**).

Approach

- The plantaris longus tendon is harvested using a medial cut between the soleus and gastrocnemius muscle (**FIG 5A**).
- The procedure is performed with a standard lateral approach, straight, from the fibula directed to the base of the fifth metatarsal (**FIG 5B**).

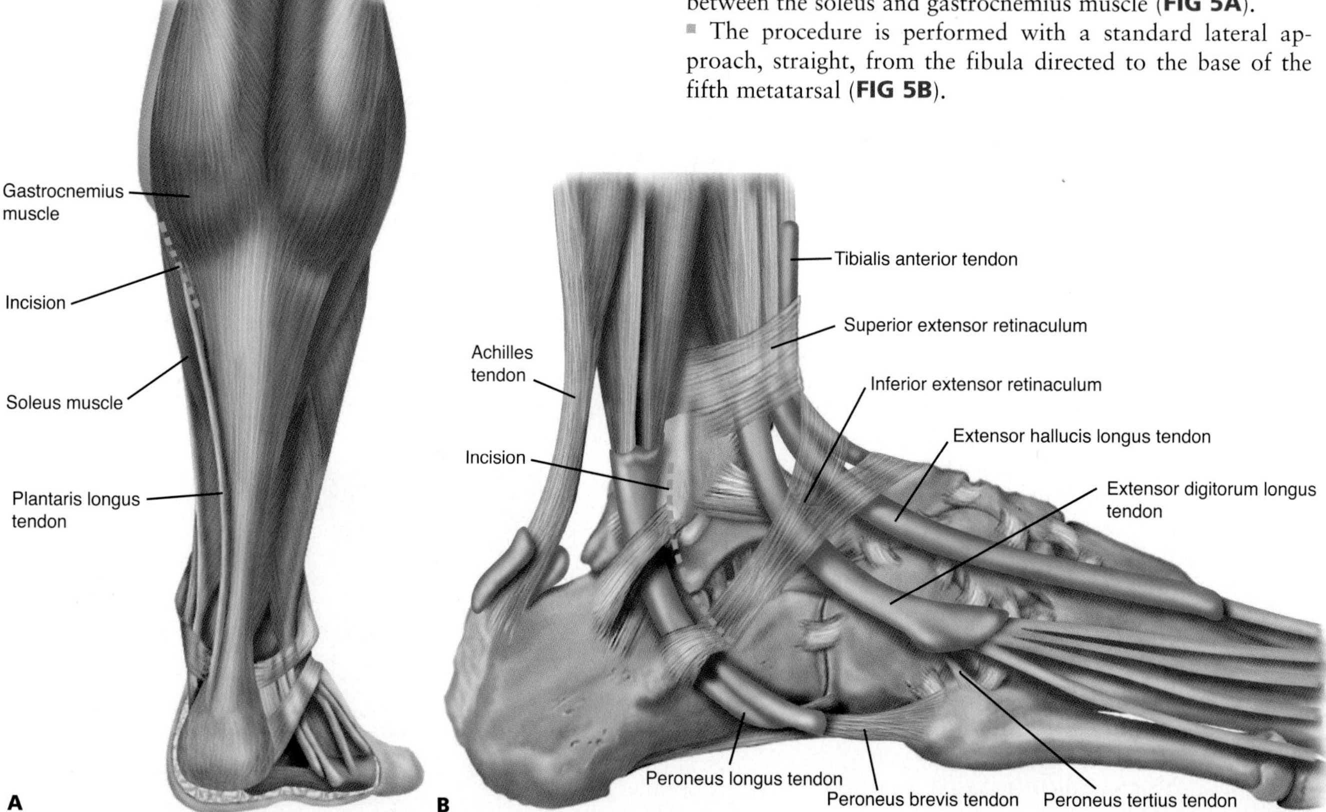

FIG 5 • **A.** Medial approach to harvest the plantaris longus tendon. **B.** Lateral approach with a 6- to 8-cm cut from the fibula toward the base of the fifth metatarsal.

HARVESTING OF PLANTARIS LONGUS

- Make a 3-cm cut at the medial aspect of the calf where the muscle has its highest volume (TECH FIG 1).
- When the muscular fascia is split, the soleus and the gastrocnemius can be bluntly separated.
- The tendon structure found medially between the two muscles is the plantaris longus tendon, which can easily be harvested with a tendon stripper. The plantaris longus tendon often is much easier to identify at this location than at the medial aspect of the calcaneus.
- If it is not possible to mobilize the plantaris longus tendon distally with the tendon stripper, the tendon can be cut through a small longitudinal incision (about 1 cm).
- Free the tendon from any muscular or fatty tissue.
- Reinforce one end of the tendon with a 0 nonabsorbable suture.
- Store the tendon in a moist compress.

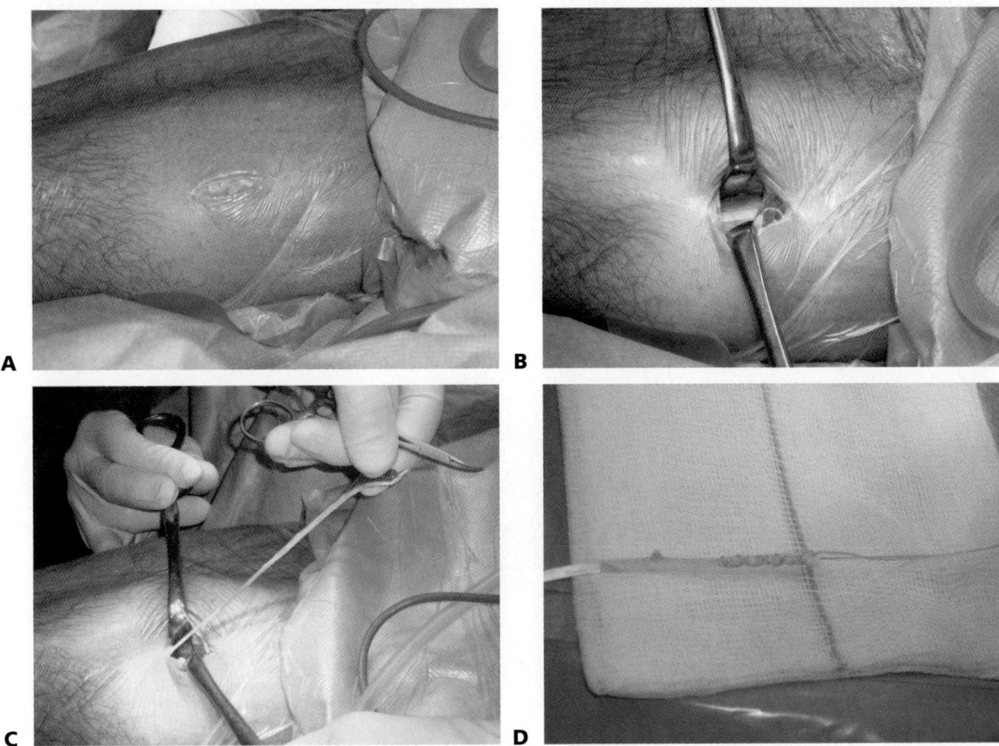

TECH FIG 1 • Harvesting of the plantaris longus tendon. **A.** Medial incision between the soleus and gastrocnemius muscle. The fascia is directly under the fatty tissue. **B.** After a longitudinal incision of the fascia, the plantaris longus tendon is found right between the soleus and gastrocnemius muscle. **C.** The tendon is mobilized with a tendon stripper. **D.** The end of the plantaris longus is reinforced with a 0 nonabsorbable suture and stored in a moist compress.

ANATOMIC RECONSTRUCTION OF THE LATERAL LIGAMENTS WITH THE PLANTARIS LONGUS TENDON

- Expose the lateral ligaments and the distal fibula via a lateral approach.
- The tissue of the sinus tarsi can be reamed, especially if there is any evidence of inflammation.
- Inspect the quality of ligaments and local tissue.
- Drill two holes at the ventral aspect of the fibula with a diameter of 3.2 mm and a distance of 7 and 13 mm from the tip of the fibula (TECH FIG 2).
- Drill a third hole on the lateral side.
- With a small Weber forceps, connect the ventral holes and flatten the sharp edges surrounding them.
- Drill another two holes at the lateral aspect of the neck of the talus with a diameter of 3.2 mm and a distance of about 8 mm. The holes are located just at the border of the cartilage. In quite a few cases, remnants of the original ligaments can be found at this location.
- Again, create a canal with the Weber forceps.
- Retract the peroneal tendons, and have the assistant position the hindfoot in maximum pronation. Drill two holes and connect them, 13 mm from the joint line of the subtalar joint, similar to the technique mentioned before.

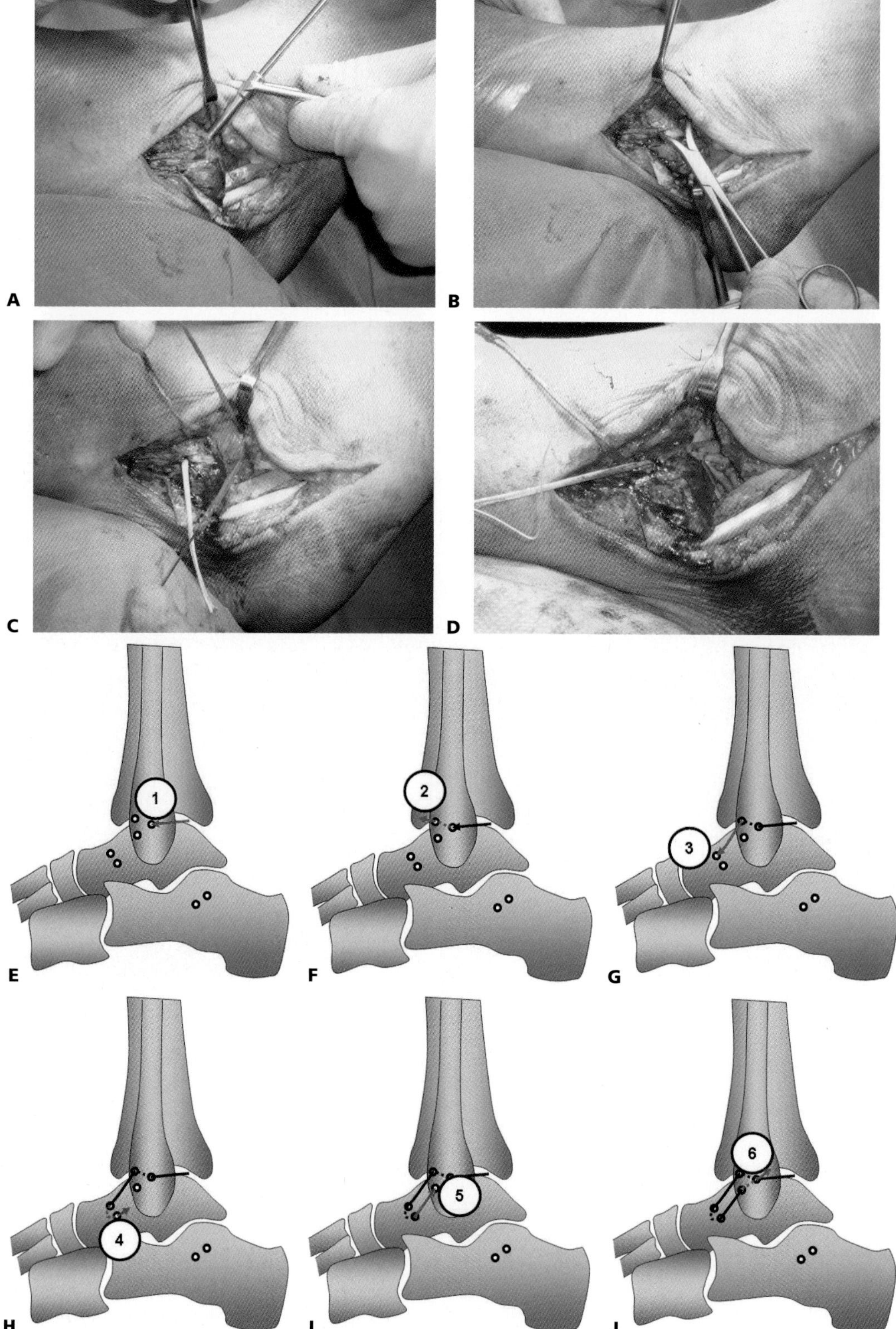

TECH FIG 2 • Anatomic reconstruction with the plantaris longus tendon. **A.** Drilling a hole at the anatomic insertion of the anterior talofibular ligament. **B.** Creating a canal between the drill holes with a Weber forceps. **C.** Routing the tendon through the drill holes. **D.** Any spare tissue of the tendon can be used for a further reinforcement. **E–O.** Routing the tendon through the drill holes.*(continued)*

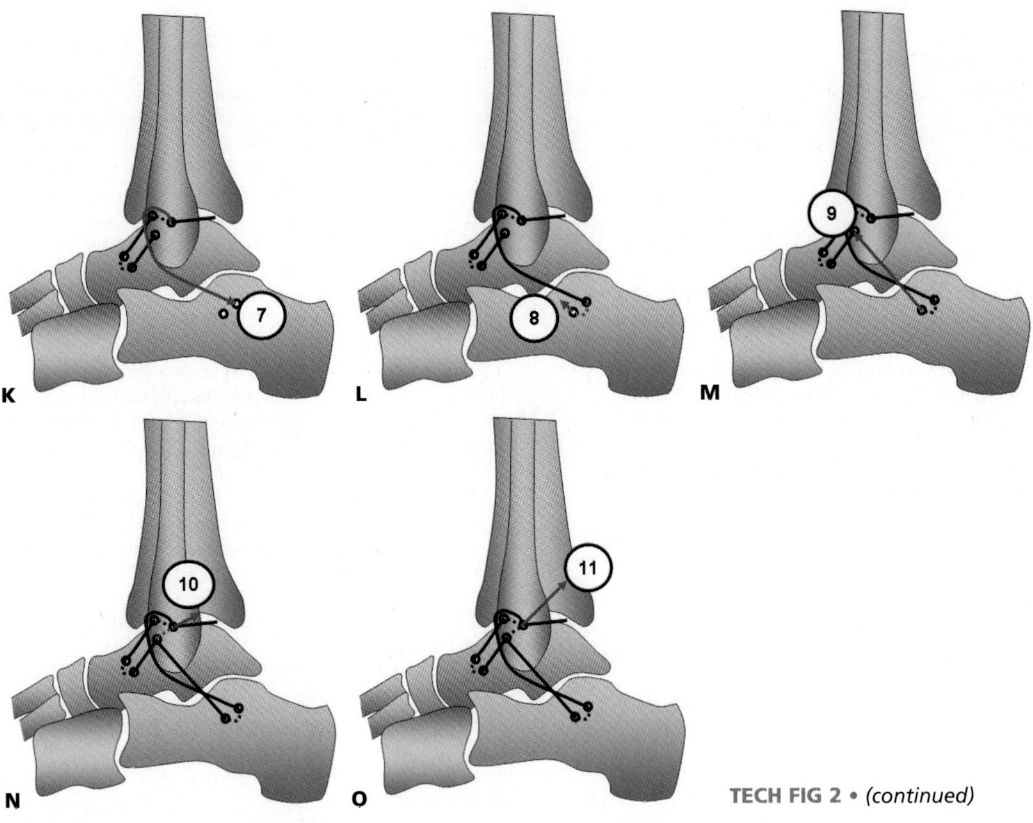

TECH FIG 2 • *(continued)*

- The plantaris longus transplant (which is armed with 0 nonabsorbable sutures) can be pulled through the holes with a sharp needle.
- When bringing the transplant under tension, the foot should be in a neutral position.
- Connect both ends of the transplant with 0 nonabsorbable sutures.
- If there are parts of the transplant left, they can be used to augment the reconstructed ligaments and held in place with side-to-side sutures.

PEARLS AND PITFALLS

Indications	▪ A complete history and physical examination should be performed. ▪ Care must be taken to address associated pathology. ▪ Graft augmentation is always indicated when the local tissue is insufficient.
Graft management	▪ A strategy has to be discussed with the patient if the plantaris longus tendon cannot be identified or is not suitable for transplantation. ▪ Extreme care should be taken when harvesting and preparing grafts. ▪ Graft should be secured at all times and handled carefully.
Fixation problems	▪ If the tendon does not go through the holes, try again to smooth the edges with a Weber forceps. ▪ If the plantaris longus tendon is too short for the whole routing, use a single layer, where the local tissue is best. ▪ Fracture of the bony bridges between the drill holes can be managed with anchors or with a transosseous suture of the graft.

POSTOPERATIVE CARE

▪ All patients are kept in a walking boot or walking cast for 2 weeks, and weight bearing is limited to 10 kg. After 2 weeks they get an ankle brace for another 4 weeks with full weight bearing in normal shoes. The ankle brace should be used day and night. In addition, physiotherapy with active stabilization is started in the third week. Cycling is normally possible after 4 to 6 weeks, running after 8 to 10 weeks. The patient should avoid contact sports, including soccer, for 3 to 5 months.

OUTCOMES

▪ Hintermann and Renggli[8] published a series on this technique and found 78% excellent, 18% good, and 4% satisfying results in the AOFAS hindfoot score. Those good results match our experience.

▪ Especially athletic patients benefit from anatomic repair of the ligaments, which seems to produce more reliable and much better results than tenodesis.

COMPLICATIONS

- Intraoperative graft mishandling
- Graft failure or rupture
- Fracture of the fibula
- Deep venous thrombosis
- Infection
- Loss of motion

REFERENCES

1. Adachi N, Ochi M, Uchio Y, et al. Harvesting hamstring tendons for ACL reconstruction influences postoperative hamstring muscle performance. Arch Orthop Trauma Surg 2003;123:460–465.
2. Beynnon B. The use of taping and bracing in treatment of ankle injury. In: Chan KM, Karlson J. World consensus conference on ankle instability. Stockholm, International Federation of Sports Medicine, 2005:38–39.
3. Broström L. Sprained ankles. VI. Surgical treatment of "chronic" ligament ruptures. Acta Chir Scand 1966;132:551–565.
4. Broström L. Sprained ankles. V. Treatment and prognosis in recent ligament ruptures. Acta Chir Scand 1966;132:537–550.
5. Burks RT, Morgan J. Anatomy of the lateral ankle ligaments. Am J Sports Med 1994;22:72–77.
6. Colville MR, Marder RA, Zarins B. Reconstruction of the lateral ankle ligaments. A biomechanical analysis. Am J Sports Med 1992; 20:594–600.
7. Hintermann B. Anatomische Rekonstruktion des Außenbandapparates mit der Plantarissehne. Oper Orthop Traumatol 1998;10:210–218.
8. Hintermann B, Renggli P. Anatomic reconstruction of the lateral ligaments of the ankle using a plantaris tendon graft in the treatment of chronic ankle joint instability. Orthopade 1999;28:778–784.
9. Hintermann B, Boss A, Schafer D. Arthroscopic findings in patients with chronic ankle instability. Am J Sports Med 2002;30: 402–409.
10. Karlsson J, Bergsten T, Lansinger O, et al. Surgical treatment of chronic lateral instability of the ankle joint: a new procedure. Am J Sports Med 1989;17:268–273.
11. Konradsen L, Olesen S, Hansen HM. Ankle sensorimotor control and eversion strength after acute ankle inversion injuries. Am J Sports Med 1998;26:72–77.
12. Krips R, van Dijk CN, Halasi PT, et al. Long-term outcome of anatomical reconstruction versus tenodesis for the treatment of chronic anterolateral instability of the ankle joint: a multicenter study. Foot Ankle Int 2001;22:415–421.
13. Mei-Dan O, Kahn G, Zeev A, et al. The medial longitudinal arch as a possible risk factor for ankle sprains: a prospective study in 83 female infantry recruits. Foot Ankle Int 2005;26:180–183.
14. Rosenbaum D, Becker HP, Sterk J, et al. Long-term results of the modified Evans repair for chronic ankle instability. Orthopedics 1996;19:451–455.
15. Rosenbaum D, Becker HP, Wilke HJ, et al. Tenodeses destroy the kinematic coupling of the ankle joint complex: a three-dimensional in vitro analysis of joint movement. J Bone Joint Surg Br 1998; 80B:162–168.
16. Rudert M, Wulker N, Wirth CJ. Reconstruction of the lateral ligaments of the ankle using a regional periosteal flap. J Bone Joint Surg Br 1997;79B:446–451.
17. Snook GA, Chrisman OD, Wilson TC. Long-term results of the Chrisman-Snook operation for reconstruction of the lateral ligaments of the ankle. J Bone Joint Surg Am 1985:67A:1–7.
18. Valderrabano V, Hintermann B, Horisberger M, et al. Ligamentous posttraumatic ankle osteoarthritis. Am J Sports Med 2006; 34:612–620.

Chapter **103**

Deltoid Ligament Reconstruction

Eric M. Bluman and Richard J. deAsla

DEFINITION

- Deltoid ligament deficiency is present when both the deep and superficial components of the medial collateral ligament complex of the ankle are ruptured or are insufficient.
- Deltoid ligament deficiency may result from degenerative (eg, late-stage adult acquired flatfoot deformity), postoperative,[6–8] or traumatic or athletic[4] causes.

ANATOMY

- The deltoid ligament complex is a multiunit structure that provides support and restraint for the tibiotalar joint, subtalar joint, spring ligament, and talonavicular joint.
- There is wide agreement that the deltoid ligament complex is made up of both deep and superficial components.
- The deep portion of the complex originates from the intercollicular groove and posterior colliculus of the medial malleolus and inserts on the medial face of the talar body near the center of rotation of the tibiotalar joint. These short and stout fibers are intra-articular but extrasynovial. It is made up of anterior and posterior fascicles.
- There has not been agreement over the superficial components of the complex. In one of the more detailed anatomic studies Pankovich and Shivaram[5] described the superficial layer as being made up of the tibionavicular, tibiocalcaneal, and tibiotalar ligaments. These fibers represent a triangular array originating on the distal medial malleolus and extending in a fan shape to their respective insertions. The relative contribution of these components to both ankle and foot biomechanics is still a topic of investigation.

PATHOGENESIS

- The most common cause of deltoid ligament disruption is supination–external rotation ankle (SER) fractures. The most severe form of these fractures has either a medial malleolus fracture or a deltoid ligament rupture, in conjunction with a lateral malleolus fracture. The variant with an intact medial malleolus and disrupted medial collateral ligaments is termed SER IV-deltoid. This latter form is the most common form of deltoid ligament disruption.
- It has been very well established that deltoid reconstruction is not indicated for disruptions that occur in conjunction with ankle fractures. Reduction and fixation of the fracture component with re-establishment of the mortise morphology leads to healing of the deltoid ligament in the vast majority of those with these combined injuries.[9]
- A smaller proportion of patients with deltoid ligament insufficiency will have developed this as a component of stage IV adult acquired flatfoot disorder (AAFD).[2]
- Deltoid ligament insufficiency without concomitant ankle fractures resulting from the acute injury has been described but will not be discussed here. This chapter will concentrate on deltoid ligament insufficiency arising from degenerative causes.

NATURAL HISTORY

- As the posterior tibial tendon becomes deficient, the ability to bring the hindfoot into varus actively is lost.
- As the mechanical axis of the leg is shifted medially (relative to the foot) and the hindfoot deformity becomes more severe and eventually stiff, tension is progressively increased on the soft tissues of the medial ankle. The medial collateral ligament complex becomes unable to resist the loads placed upon it, with eventual insufficiency and lengthening.[7,8]
- Progression to stage IV AAFD occurs when the deltoid ligament becomes incompetent and the valgus force from the preexisting hindfoot deformity causes the talus to tilt within the mortise.

PATIENT HISTORY AND PHYSICAL FINDINGS

- Aspects of the history and physical examination of stage IV AAFD will be similar to those found in the earlier stages of this AAFD.
- There will be hindfoot valgus.
- Because of the chronic nature of posterior tibial tendon involvement, strength will be greatly diminished and likely absent because of rupture. The patient will neither be able to resist hindfoot eversion nor actively bring the forefoot across midline.
- Because of the decreased working length of the triceps surae resulting from chronic hindfoot valgus, there will be contracture of these muscles. A fixed hindfoot deformity may give a falsely optimistic impression of tibiotalar dorsiflexion. Reestablishment of ankle and hindfoot alignment without an appropriate lengthening of the heel cord will create or exacerbate an equinus deformity.
- There may be significant forefoot supination.
- Lateral pain may represent sinus tarsi or subfibular impingement, lateral ankle joint arthritis, or in severe cases distal fibular stress fracture.
- Pain in the sinus tarsi is frequently unrecognized or underappreciated before palpation by the clinician.
- Callosity and pain below the talar head may be present if substantial dorsolateral peritalar subluxation has caused a prominence in the medial plantar midfoot.
- It is essential to determine whether the tibiotalar valgus deformity that is a hallmark of stage IV AAFD is rigid or reducible. This is further explained under surgical management.
- Clinical determination of the presence of valgus tibiotalar deformity is greatly enhanced with radiologic examination.
- The integrity of the lateral collateral ligament complex needs to be determined. A severe valgus deformity may lead to erosion and incompetence of these structures.
- The surgeon must also evaluate for the presence of ipsilateral knee valgus. If this is significant, consideration should be given to correcting the proximal deformity before the foot and

ankle surgery. Correction of the leg–ankle–foot axis without attention to knee deformity may not adequately relieve valgus stress through the reconstructed lower limb and result in recurrence of deformity.

- Methods for examining the deltoid ligament include:
  - Palpating the area inferior to the medial malleolus. Tenderness may represent incipient or recent deltoid rupture and may only be present early in stage IV disease.
  - Joint line palpation. The presence of valgus tilt indicates insufficiency of the deltoid ligament.
  - Weight-bearing AP ankle radiographs. Valgus tilt greater than 4 degrees indicates deltoid ligament insufficiency.

IMAGING AND OTHER DIAGNOSTIC STUDIES

- The preferred radiologic views include the three-view weight-bearing series. The AP standing view will provide the most information. Patients with deltoid ligament insufficiency will demonstrate tibiotalar valgus tilting (**FIG 1**).
- Cross-sectional imaging is required only when plans are made for performing reconstruction using native peroneus longus tendon (discussed later). In this case MRI is used to confirm the integrity of the peroneus brevis before the longus is harvested.
- Selective intra-articualar blocks often help the clinician localize the exact source of pain.

DIFFERENTIAL DIAGNOSIS

- Stage II or III AAFD
- Medial malleolus fracture nonunion
- Tibiotalar arthritis (with eccentric lateral joint erosion)
- Osteonecrosis of the talus with lateral collapse
- Distal tibial supramalleolar valgus malalignment (resulting from distal tibiofibular fracture or pilon fracture)
- Valgus malunion of pronation abduction-type ankle fracture with lateral plafond impaction or comminution

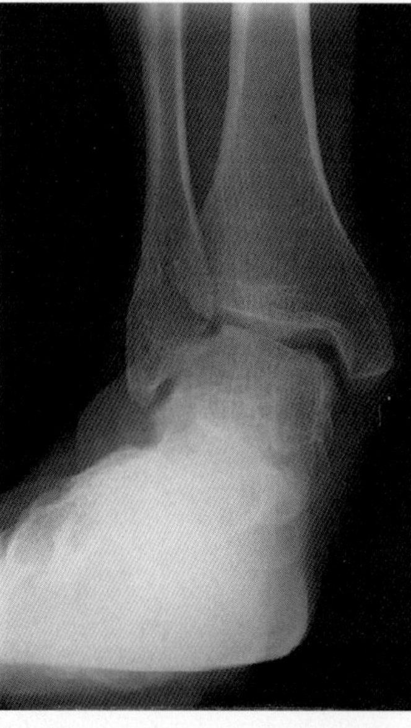

FIG 1 • Standing AP weight-bearing radiograph of the ankle demonstrating valgus tibiotalar tilt resulting from insufficiency of the deltoid complex.

NONOPERATIVE MANAGEMENT

- In contrast to acute deltoid deficiency presenting in conjunction with an ankle fracture, we believe that nonoperative care has a very limited place in patients with chronic deltoid ligament insufficiency resulting from degenerative causes (eg, stage IV AAFD). All but patients with medical comorbidities contraindicating surgery should undergo surgical reconstruction.
- Conservative therapy may also be needed to relieve pain and temporize deformity while related orthopaedic conditions are corrected.
- Should conservative therapy be chosen, custom-molded rigid orthotics that extend to the calf, such as the Arizona brace, provide the best chances of preventing progression of the disease.
- Although halting the progression of the disease may be possible with conservative therapy, the deformities of stage IV cannot be corrected with bracing alone.

SURGICAL MANAGEMENT

- Healing of a chronically insufficient deltoid ligament to a functional structure does not occur in AAFD. Reefing and other surgical techniques attempting to incorporate this diseased tissue into the repair do not produce reliable results. Allograft or autograft reconstructions of the deltoid ligament give the best chances for success.
- Once a diagnosis of stage IV AAFD is made, an operative plan to correct all components of the deformity is needed.
- Evaluation of the ability to passively correct the tibiotalar deformity is central to whether the deltoid ligament may be reconstructed for salvage of the ankle joint.
- Tibiotalar valgus deformity that can be corrected passively may benefit from deltoid reconstruction in conjunction with bony and tendon work. Rigid tibiotalar deformity of stage IV AAFD should be reconstructed with tibiotalocalcaneal or pantalar fusion.
- It is essential to correct all components of the foot deformity along with deltoid reconstruction so that the forces that resulted in the native deltoid ligament insufficiency are neutralized and do not cause failure of the reconstructed ligament.
- If lateral collateral ligament insufficiency is found on examination, the surgical plan should include reconstruction of these structures.

Preoperative Planning

- Imaging studies are reviewed.
- Examination under anesthesia (EUA) should be accomplished before positioning the patient. Intraoperative fluoroscopy may be very useful during the EUA.
- It is also important to re-evaluate the lateral collateral ligaments during the EUA.
- All foot reconstructive procedures needed to restore plantigrade alignment should be done at the same surgical sitting if possible. These procedures should be done immediately before deltoid ligament reconstruction.

Positioning

- The patient should be positioned supine on the operating table.
- Retrograde application of an Esmarch bandage followed by inflation of an upper thigh tourniquet may be used to create a relatively bloodless field.
- Access to the medial ankle may be improved by placing a soft support under the contralateral hip.

- The surgeon should ensure that the lower extremity is prepared and draped to a level above the knee so that limb–foot alignment may be evaluated intraoperatively.

Approach

- The approach for the minimally invasive deltoid ligament reconstruction (MIDLR) requires a longitudinal incision from the tip of the medial malleolus to just inferior to the prominence of the sustentaculum tali. This incision may need to be carried through incompetent fibers of the superficial deltoid ligament (**FIG 2**).
- The approach for the peroneal grafting method uses a straight longitudinal incision over the peroneal tendons to harvest the peroneus longus tendon and then a medial incision through which the tendon is brought before threading it through and securing it to the tibia. The patient should be initially positioned with a bump under the ipsilateral hip, which may be removed when increased access to the medial ankle is required.

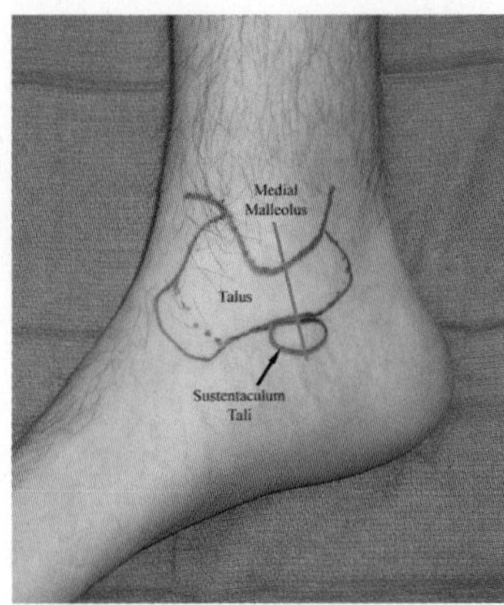

FIG 2 • Approach for the minimally invasive deltoid ligament reconstruction technique marked out on the medial ankle. The locations of the medial malleolus, talus, and sustentaculum tali are indicated.

MINIMALLY INVASIVE DELTOID LIGAMENT RECONSTRUCTION

- This technique[1,2] reconstructs components of both the superficial and deep layers of the deltoid ligament without sacrificing any host tissue for graft.

Forked Allograft Preparation

- Cadaveric allograft from the posterior tibial tendon or the peroneal tendon provides a graft of good size. Larger grafts (eg, Achilles tendon) may be used but should be cut to appropriate thickness. Do not use grafts smaller than the posterior tibial tendon or peroneals.
- The graft should be about 20 cm in length and 6 to 7 mm in diameter. Split one end longitudinally, leaving about 5 cm of the opposite end unsplit.
- Place Krackow stitches of no. 00 nonabsorbable woven suture in all three limbs of the tendon (**TECH FIG 1**).
- After preparation, wrap the graft in moistened gauze and set it aside.

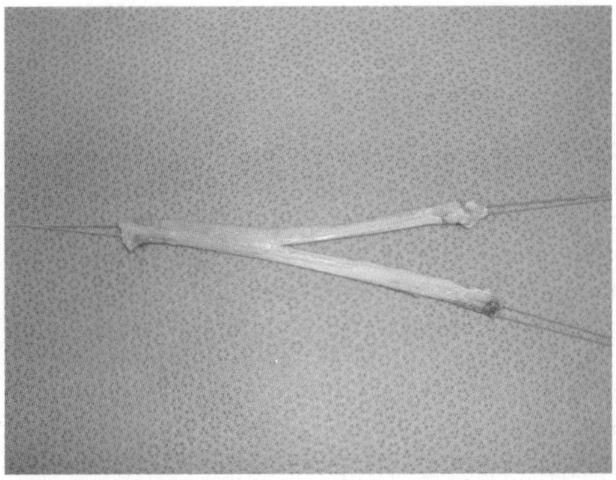

TECH FIG 1 • Preparation of forked graft. A allograft tendon about 20 cm long and 7 mm in diameter is chosen and split longitudinally for about two thirds of its length. Final appearance of the forked graft, showing Krackow sutures placed in all three ends of its limbs.

Tibial Limb Placement

- Above the medial malleolus, in the midcoronal plane, choose a level about 1 cm above the plafond at which the tibial limb of the graft will be anchored. This is approximated well by the level of the distal tibial physeal scar. Intraoperative fluoroscopy is very helpful in locating a proper site. The saphenous vein and nerve should be anterior to the entry site chosen.
- At the level for insertion, make a 1-cm longitudinal incision down to medial tibial cortex. Advance a guidewire from medial to lateral parallel to the plafond (**TECH FIG 2**). Make a 6.0-mm blind tunnel over the guidewire for a distance of 25 mm. Remove the guidewire.
- Secure the tibial limb (unsplit end) of the forked graft in the blind tibial tunnel using a 6.25-mm soft tissue interference screw (**TECH FIG 3**). Use manual testing to ensure that the graft is adequately anchored in the tunnel.

Talar Limb Placement

- The path of the tunnel through the talus starts at the medial center of tibiotalar rotation. This is most easily approximated by drilling the insertion point for the native deep deltoid ligament. The lateral exit of the tunnel is located at the lateral junction of the talar dome and neck. This lateral exit point is located by palpation. If this junction cannot be palpated, a small incision may need to be made to locate the lateral neck body junction. Advance a guidewire for a cannulated 5.0-mm drill along this axis. Confirm the position of the guidewire with AP and lateral fluoroscopic views.
- Drill a 5.0-mm tunnel over the guidewire. Pass one end of the sutured tendon through the tunnel from medial to lateral using a suture passer. Place appropriate tension on the graft and place a 5.0-mm soft tissue interference screw in the medial aspect of the tunnel to secure the graft. Advance the interference screw so that it is countersunk 1 to 2 mm into the tunnel.

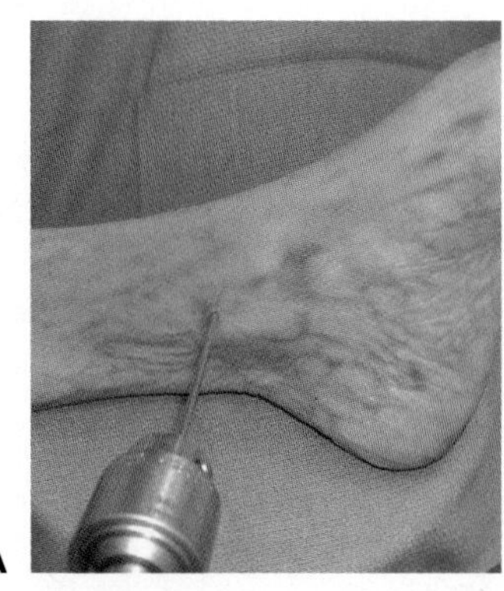

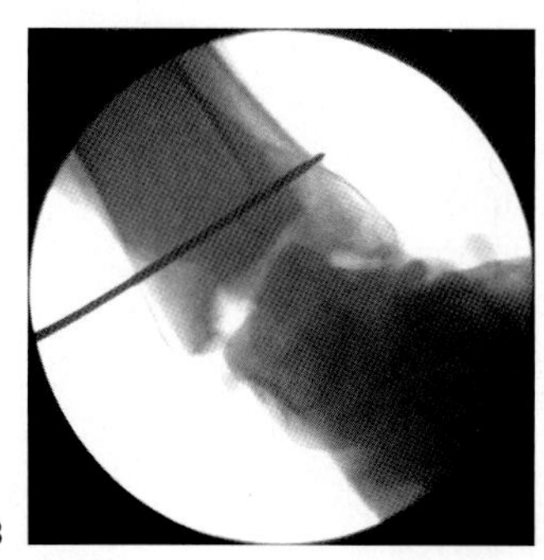

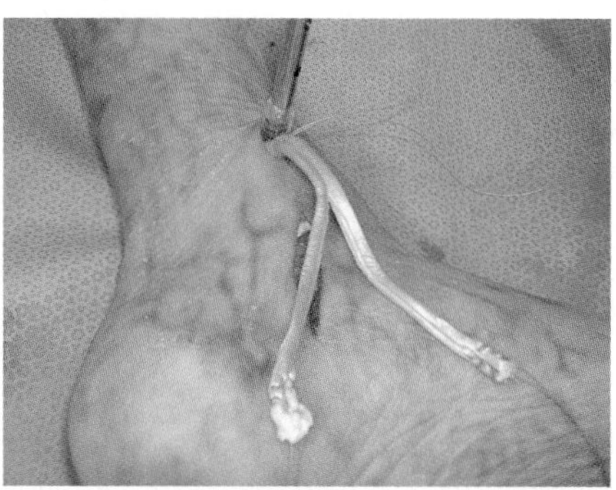

TECH FIG 2 • Insertion of tibial limb. **A.** Starting point for tibial guidewire placement should be at the level of the distal tibial physeal scar. **B.**Tibial guidewire placement as shown by AP view with fluoroscopy. **C.** Securing the tibial limb of the graft with a soft tissue interference screw.

Calcaneal Limb Placement

- Using palpation, locate the medial border of the sustentaculum tali. Once it is found, carefully dissect the posterior tibial tendon sheath away from the bone and retract it inferiorly. Insert the guidewire for the cannulated drill along an axis from the midportion of the sustentaculum tali to a point about 1 cm superior to the peroneal tubercle on the lateral side of the calcaneus (**TECH FIG 4A**). Placing the guidewire in this location allows for centralization in the sustentaculum and - minimizes the chances of breaching the subtalar joint. Check the position of the guidewire using fluoroscopy.
- Create a 5.0-mm tunnel over this guidewire.
- Pass the free end of the remaining limb of the tendon graft through the sustentacular tunnel and out the skin overlying the lateral calcaneus. A small slit may need to be made to allow the graft to be pulled fully through. Perform tensioning and tibiotalar joint position manually and check it under fluoroscopy.
- When appropriate tension is achieved, insert a 5.0-mm interference screw from medial to lateral into the sustentacular tunnel.
- The appearance of the final construct in situ is illustrated in **TECH FIG 4B**. An illustration of the position of the graft after insertion and fixation is shown in **TECH FIG 4C**.
- Close the wounds in a layered fashion.

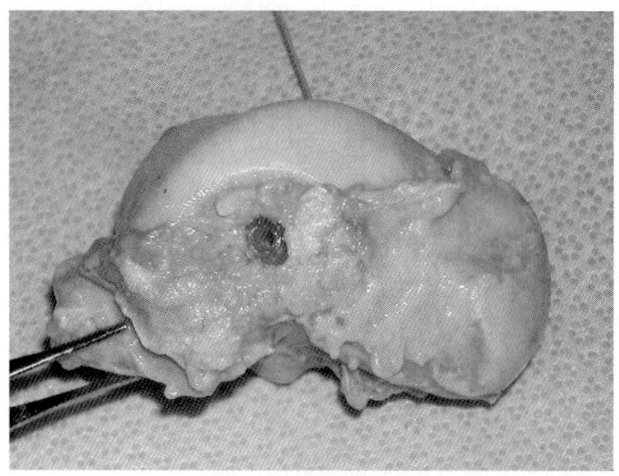

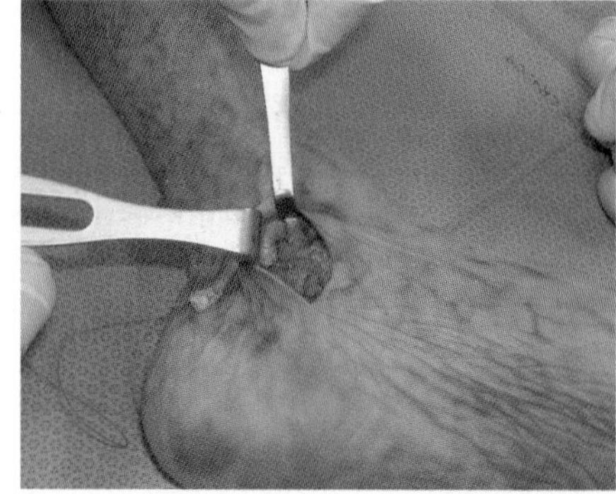

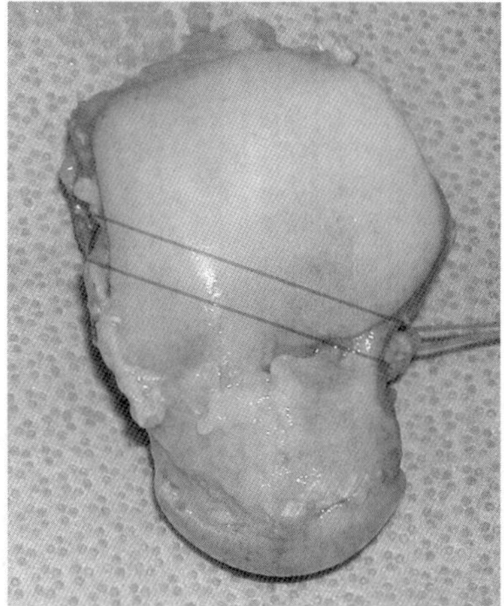

TECH FIG 3 • Talar limb placement. **A.** Starting point for the talar tunnel is approximated by the footprint of the deep deltoid ligament insertion on the medial face of the talus. Shown is the medial talar surface of a cadaveric dissection specimen. A soft tissue interference screw has been placed in the medial portion of the talar tunnel. The talar head is oriented to the right in this image. **B.** Path of the talar tunnel as seen from a dorsoplantar view of a cadaveric talus. The talar head is toward the bottom and the medial talus is at the left side of the image. The lines represent the path of the tunnel through the talus. **C.** Medial aspect of ankle after talar limb has been inserted, tensioned, and secured.

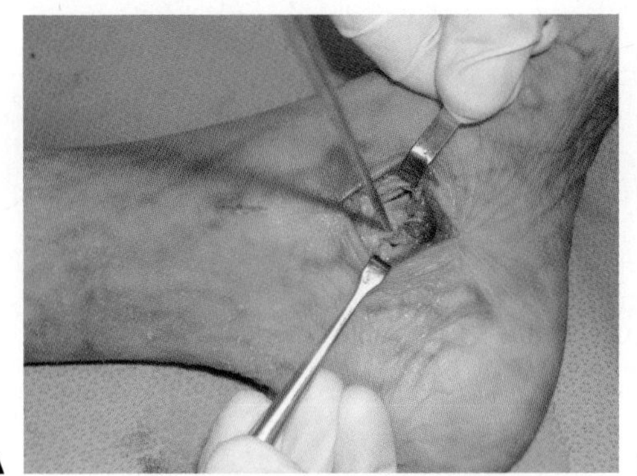

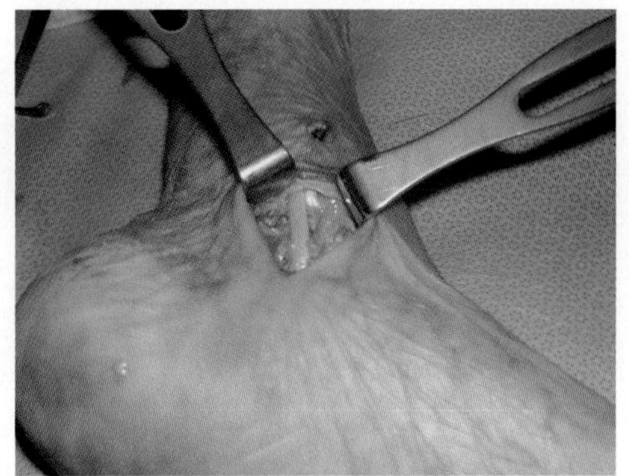

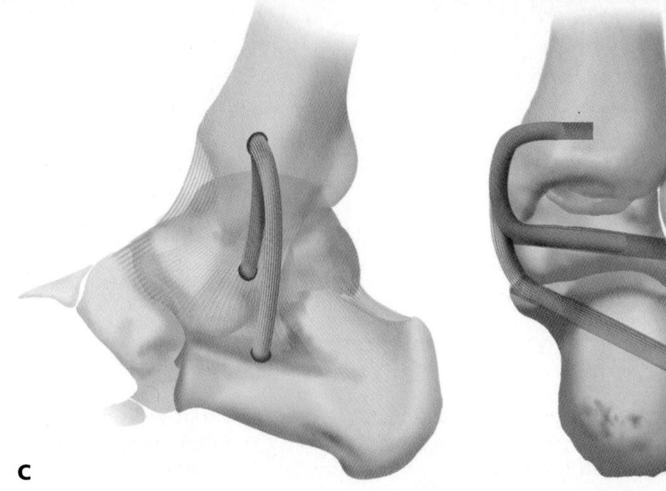

TECH FIG 4 • Calcaneal limb placement. **A.** Starting point for the calcaneal limb with guidewire advanced so as to avoid the subtalar joint and exit out the lateral calcaneal cortex. **B.** Completed minimally invasive deltoid ligament reconstruction in situ from the medial aspect. **C.** Completed minimally invasive deltoid ligament reconstruction from the medial aspect and from a posteroanterior view.

PERONEUS LONGUS GRAFT TENDON HARVESTING

- Harvest the peroneus longus tendon through a lateral incision that extends from the fourth metatarsal base to about midway up the calf.[3]
- Tenodese the proximal stump of the transected peroneus longus tendon to the peroneus brevis.
- After securing a Krackow locking suture to the free end of the peroneus longus tendon, wrap it in a piece of moist gauze.

Talar Tunnel Construction

- Make a medial incision centered over the medial malleolus, extending distally over the fibers of the superficial deltoid.
- Divide the fibers of the attenuated deltoid ligament, exposing the medial aspect of the talus.
- Pass an intraosseous guidewire from the lateral talar neck–body junction to the estimated center of rotation on the medial aspect of the talus inferior to the tip of the medial malleolus.
- Verify guidewire position fluoroscopically and clinically by dorsiflexing and plantarflexing the ankle to determine if the center of rotation has been localized.
- Create a tunnel using a cannulated reamer about 4 to 5 mm in diameter.

Tibial Tunnel Construction

- Create a second bony tunnel from the tip of the medial malleolus to a point in the lateral distal tibia. The exit point is about 5 to 6 cm proximal to the tibial plafond and anterior to the fibula. We recommend saving the shavings from the reamer to be used later as bone graft.

Graft Passage and Fixation

- Pass the tendon through the tibial tunnel from distal-medial to proximal-lateral.
- Tension the tendon first at the medial talar tunnel and then at the lateral tibial exit site, with correction of valgus talar tilt.
- Secure the tendon to the lateral tibia under maximal tension with a soft tissue washer or staple. Pack bone graft obtained from reaming in the bony tunnels. A schematic of the final construct is depicted in TECH FIG 5.
- Close the wounds.

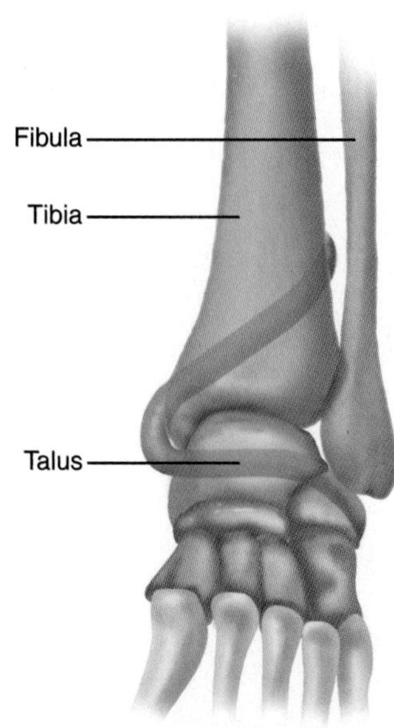

TECH FIG 5 • Peroneus longus autograft construct. Completed peroneus longus autograft has been passed through the talar tunnel, into the medial malleolus, and out the lateral tibia, where it is fixed to the lateral cortex.

PEARLS AND PITFALLS

Need for concomitant procedures	▪ Deltoid reconstruction as described here is intended to reconstitute a functional restraint to valgus tibiotalar tilting. ▪ Be sure to correct any malalignment or deformity that will tend to produce valgus angulation at the tibiotalar joint at the same time that the deltoid reconstruction is done. ▪ Failure to do this may result in the correction being inadequate or may even lead to outright failure of the graft.
Fixation problems: graft pullout	▪ Ensure that the tendon ends are reinforced with Krackow sutures to allow for secure passage of the tendons and to prevent interference screw laceration of the graft.
Tunnel placement	▪ Make sure the talar tunnel starts medially at the insertion of the deep deltoid ligament. Substantial deviation of the starting point of the talar tunnel from this location will result in increased shearing forces across the tendon. ▪ The superficial (calcaneal) limb of the graft must be centered within the sustentaculum. Eccentric placement may result in the medial facet of the subtalar joint or the inferior cortex of the sustentaculum being breached. Breaching the medial facet could lead to subtalar arthritis. Breaching the inferior sustentacular cortex could result in flexor hallucis longus paratenonitis or abrasion.
Nerve injury	▪ Make small incisions over the exit of the talar and calcaneal limbs to prevent damage to branches of the superficial peroneal and sural nerves.
Indications	▪ These techniques are designed to aid in the surgical correction of stage IV AAFD. Other treatment methods may need to be used for either acute deltoid injuries or deltoid insufficiency associated with disease processes other than AAFD.

POSTOPERATIVE CARE

▪ In the immediate period after tibiotalar joint-sparing reconstruction of stage IV posterior tibial tendon rupture, a plaster splint is applied in neutral position. Physiotherapy starts after the incisions have healed, usually about 2 weeks postoperatively. Therapy consists of passive and active mobilization of the ankle joint as well as intrinsic muscle exercises. Weight bearing is started progressively but is not full until 12 weeks postoperatively. Gait training is instituted as needed after weight bearing is commenced.

OUTCOMES

▪ There are no long-term results for these methods because both were recently developed. Studies on outcomes are made difficult by the small number of patients who present with stage IV AAFD. Ongoing studies are evaluating the ability to maintain the correction and stability obtained with these methods.

▪ Two-year clinical results for the forked graft method are just becoming available at the time of the writing of this chapter. Initial short-term results are promising, with maintenance of tibiotalar joint motion and stability in those who have undergone the procedure.

▪ Short-term follow-up data are available for the peroneus longus graft method. In the five patients evaluated after undergoing this procedure, four had tibiotalar valgus correction to 4 degrees or less that was maintained 2 years after the procedure.

COMPLICATIONS

- Breaching tibiotalar joint with misplaced tibial or talar tunnel
- Breaching subtalar joint with misplaced calcaneal tunnel (forked graft method)
- Damage to superficial peroneal nerve
- Damage to deep peroneal nerve (peroneal graft method)
- Damage to the sural nerve on calcaneal limb pull-through (forked graft method)
- Infection
- Graft failure or rupture

REFERENCES

1. Bluman EM, Khazen G, Haraguchi N, et al. Minimally invasive deltoid ligament reconstruction: a biomechanical and anatomic analysis. Presented at American Orthopaedic Foot and Ankle Society 21st Annual Summer Meeting, Boston, MA, 2005.
2. Bluman E, Myerson M. Stage IV posterior tibial tendon rupture. Foot Ankle Clin 2007;12:341–362.
3. Deland JT, de Asla RJ, Segal A. Reconstruction of the chronically failed deltoid ligament: a new technique. Foot Ankle Int 2004;25:795–799.
4. Hintermann B, Valderrabano V, Boss A, et al. Medial ankle instability: an exploratory, prospective study of fifty-two cases. Am J Sports Med 2004;32:183–190.
5. Pankovich AM, Shivaram MS. Anatomical basis of variability in injuries of the medial malleolus and the deltoid ligament. I. Anatomical studies. Acta Orthop Scand 1979;50:217–223.
6. Pell RF, Myerson MS, Schon LC. Clinical outcome after primary triple arthrodesis. J Bone Joint Surg Am 2000;82A:47–57.
7. Resnick RB, Jahss MH, Choueka J, et al. Deltoid ligament forces after tibialis posterior tendon rupture: effects of triple arthrodesis and calcaneal displacement osteotomies. Foot Ankle Int 1995;16:14–20.
8. Song SJ, Lee S, O'Malley MJ, et al. Deltoid ligament strain after correction of acquired flatfoot deformity by triple arthrodesis. Foot Ankle Int 2000;21:573–577.
9. Zeegers AV, van der Werken C. Rupture of the deltoid ligament in ankle fractures: should it be repaired? Injury 1989;20:39–41.

Chapter 104

Medial Ankle/Deltoid Ligament Reconstruction

Beat Hintermann and Victor Valderrabano

DEFINITION

- Pronation injuries of the ankle joint complex may result in a partial or complete disruption of the superficial anterior bundles of the deltoid ligament.
- Chronic medial ankle instability may cause a secondary posterior tibial dysfunction over time, as the tendon may become elongated, ruptured, or both.
- Medial ankle instability may also be the result of a posterior tibial dysfunction with chronic overload of the deltoid ligaments and consecutive step-by-step disruption.
- Medial ankle instability must be suspected if the patient complains of "giving way," especially medially, when walking on even ground, downhill, or downstairs, pain at the anteromedial aspect of the ankle, and sometimes pain on the lateral ankle, especially during dorsiflexion of the foot.

ANATOMY

- The deltoid ligament is a multibanded complex with superficial and deep components.
- It may be wise to differentiate the superficial and deep portions of the deltoid complex with respect to the joints they are spanning. The superficial ligaments cross two (the ankle and the subtalar joints) and the deep ligaments cross one joint (only the ankle joint), although differentiation is not always absolutely clear.[10]
- The three superficial and more anterior bands are the tibionavicular, tibiospring, and tibiocalcaneal ligaments; the three deep bands are the anterior, intermediate, and posterior tibiotalar ligaments (**FIG 1**).[1]
- As the tibioligamentous portion of the superficial deltoid has a broad insertion on the "spring ligament," this ligament complex may interplay with the deltoid ligament in the stabilization of the medial ankle joint, and thus functionally not be separated from it (Fig 1).[3]

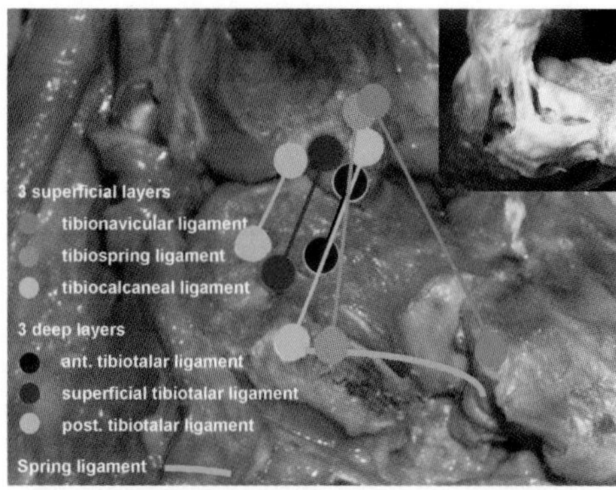

FIG 1 • Anatomic situs of medial ankle. The superficial and deep deltoid consists of three distinct bundles each.

PATHOGENESIS

- Acute injuries to the medial ankle ligaments can occur during running downstairs, landing on an uneven surface, and dancing while the body is simultaneously rotated in the opposite direction. A key feature of the history is whether the patient has sustained a pronation (eversion) trauma—for instance, an outward rotation of the foot during simultaneous inward rotation of the tibia.
- Complete deltoid ligament ruptures are sometimes seen in association with lateral malleolar fractures, or in specific bimalleolar fractures.
- Chronic deltoid ligament insufficiency can be seen in a number of conditions, including posterior tibial tendon disorder, traumatic and sports-related deltoid disruptions, as well as valgus talar tilting in patients with previous triple arthrodesis or total ankle arthroplasty.

NATURAL HISTORY

- There is evidence that the medial ankle ligaments are more often injured than generally believed.[4,5,7,8]
- Several structures contribute to the stabilization of the medial ankle, and in the case of injury they are not involved in a uniform way. Medial ankle instability is thus not a single entity, and this has most important consequences for treatment.
- The findings of an exploratory, prospective study on 51 patients (53 ankles) have supported our belief that medial ankle instability without posterior tibial tendon dysfunction does exist as an entity.[7] It is, however, not clear yet whether, or to what extent, such a medial ankle instability may cause a secondary posterior tibial dysfunction over time, as the tendon may become elongated, ruptured, or both.
- What is clear from the literature is that a coexisting pronation deformity of the foot will lead to further deterioration over time, as the medial ankle ligaments are chronically overstretched.

PATIENT HISTORY AND PHYSICAL FINDINGS

- The diagnosis of medial ankle instability is made on the basis of the history and the results of physical examination, including special maneuvers, and plain roentgenography.
- Medial instability is suspected if the patient complains of "giving way," especially medially, when walking on even ground, downhill, or downstairs, pain at the anteromedial aspect of the ankle, and sometimes pain on the lateral ankle, especially during dorsiflexion of the foot.
- A history of chronic instability, manifested by recurrent injuries with pain, tenderness, and sometimes bruising over the medial and lateral ligaments, is considered to indicate combined medial and lateral instability that is thought to result in rotational instability of the talus in the ankle mortise.
- Acute injuries may present with tenderness and hematoma at the side of the deltoid ligament.

- Physical examination methods for chronic medial ankle instability should include:
  - Standing test. Inspect for malalignment, deformity, asymmetry, and swelling. Asymmetric planus and pronation deformity of the affected foot may indicate medial ankle instability: distinct, moderate, important.
  - Palpation of anteromedial ankle. Pain in the medial gutter is typically provoked by palpation of the anterior border of the medial malleolus. It is the result of underlying synovitis due to chronic shifting of the talus within the ankle mortise.
  - Anterior drawer test is a highly sensitive test for medial ankle instability.
- A complete examination of the hindfoot should also include evaluating associated injuries and ruling out other possible causes. These include, among others:
  - Fracture of medial malleolus: After an acute injury, radiographic analysis must be performed routinely to exclude a fracture of the medial malleolus (eg, bony avulsion of the deltoid ligament) or fibula fracture with or without syndesmotic disruption.
  - Loss of posterior tibial function after partial or complete rupture: The patient cannot correct the deformity while standing or create supination power to the foot.
  - Talonavicular coalition: The subtalar joint is not mobile; so there is no varusization of the heel while going into the tiptoe position.
  - Neurologic disorder: There is partial or complete palsy of one or more muscles due to deficient neurologic control.

IMAGING AND OTHER DIAGNOSTIC STUDIES

- Acute injury: Plain radiographs, including AP and lateral views, should be obtained to rule out bony avulsion fractures or associated injuries.
- Chronic injury: Plain weight-bearing radiographs, including AP views of the foot and ankle and a lateral view of the foot, should be obtained to rule out old bony avulsion fractures, secondary deformity of the foot (eg, valgus malalignment of the heel, dislocation at the talonavicular joint), and tibiotalar alignment (eg, medial gapping of the joint due to incompetence of the deltoid ligament) (**FIG 2**).

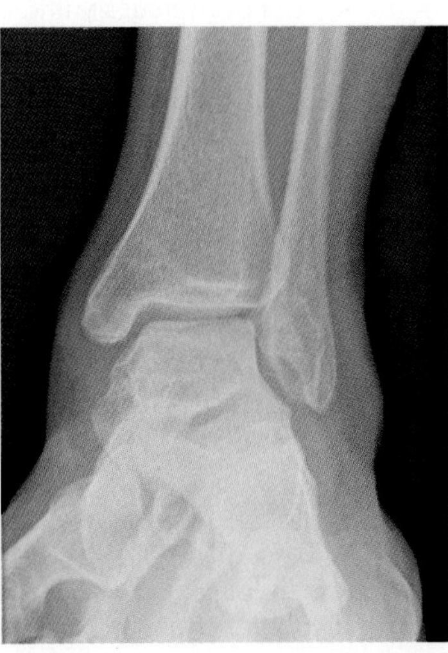

FIG 2 • Incompetence of deltoid ligament. AP weight-bearing radiograph shows a gapping of the medial tibiotalar joint.

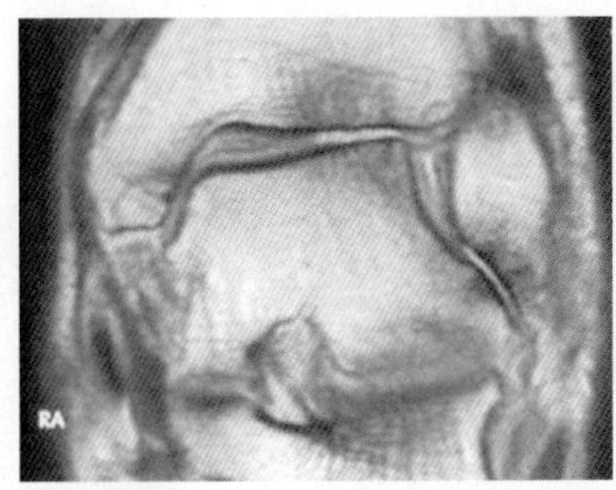

FIG 3 • Proximal avulsion of deltoid ligament. AP MR imaging reveals a complete avulsion of the deltoid ligament to the medial malleolus, resulting in a medial gapping of the tibiotalar joint.

- Stress radiographs may be helpful to identify incompetence of the deltoid ligament in the treatment of acute ankle fractures,[13] but they are not helpful in chronic conditions.[10]
- A CT scan may be obtained to detect a talocalcaneal coalition or bony fragmentation that involves the articular surfaces.
- MR imaging may show an injury to the deltoid ligament (**FIG 3**), particularly in acute conditions, and it may also reveal pathologic conditions of the posterior tibial tendon.

DIFFERENTIAL DIAGNOSIS

- Bony avulsion fracture of the medial malleolus (with or without fracture of the fibula or syndesmotic disruption)
- Fixed flatfoot deformity (eg, acquired flatfoot deformity in adults after posterior tibial dysfunction)
- Osteochondral injury
- Talocalcaneal coalition

NONOPERATIVE MANAGEMENT

- Although nonoperative management is controversial, patients with less instability, particularly whose who have less of a "giving-way" feeling, and those who are less involved with high-level pronation sports activities, may be treated nonoperatively.
- Nonoperative treatment consists of three components:
  - Medial foot arch supports
  - Physiotherapy for strengthening the invertor muscles
  - A neuromuscular rehabilitation program

SURGICAL MANAGEMENT

Preoperative Planning

- All imaging studies are reviewed.
- Plain films should be reviewed for fractures, cartilage lesions, hindfoot and midfoot malalignment, and the presence of any hardware (from previous procedures) or foreign bodies.
- Associated fractures, cartilage lesions, foot malalignment, and tendon disruption should be addressed concurrently.
- Examination under anesthesia should be performed to compare with the contralateral ankle.

Positioning

- The patient is in the supine position with the feet at the edge of the table.
- A commercially available knee holder is used to support the distal femur and to place the foot into a hanging position (**FIG 4**).
- This allows the surgeon to move the foot freely while arthroscopy is done before open reconstruction.
- After the arthroscopy, the knee holder is removed, leaving the foot on the table.

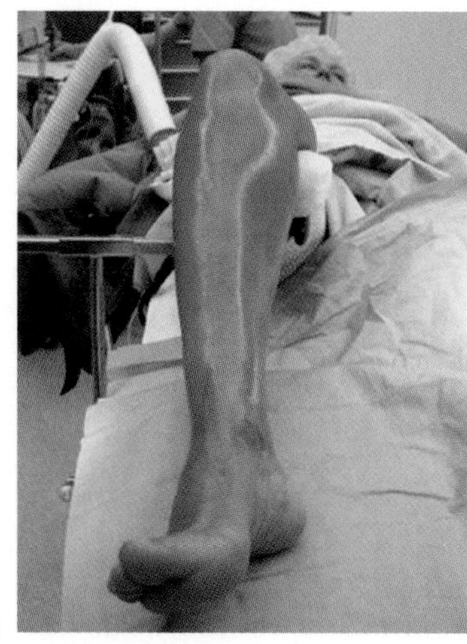

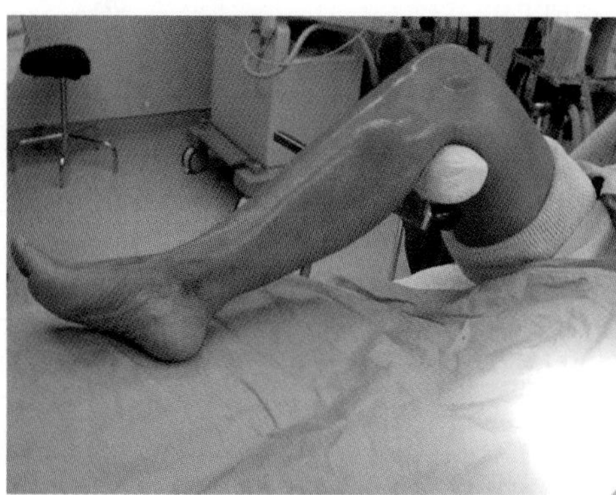

FIG 4 • Positioning for arthroscopy and medial ligament reconstruction. A knee holder is used to support the distal femur so that the foot is hanging on the table. **A.** View from the bottom of the table. **B.** Medial view.

Approach

- An anteromedial approach is used for ankle arthroscopy.[4]
- A gently curved incision of 3 to 5 cm is made, starting 1 cm cranially of the tip of the medial malleolus and running toward the medial aspect of the navicular bone.
- If there is additional instability of the lateral ankle ligaments, as found on the clinical examination and confirmed by arthroscopy, a lateral approach to the ankle is also performed to explore the anterior talofibular and calcaneofibular ligaments.

TECHNIQUES

ANKLE ARTHROSCOPY

- Arthroscopy is done to visualize the internal structures and to assess medial and lateral ankle stability.[4]
- After visual evaluation of the ligaments, test lateral and medial ligament stability by applying gentle varus, valgus, and anterior pull stress to the ankle joint under arthroscopic control.
- Ligament lesions are graded as distended if the ligament is thinned or elongated, and as ruptured if continuity is lost.[7] Because most ligament tears are located on the proximal insertion, this is usually best seen by a completely free insertion area of the ligament on the malleoli (**TECH FIG 1**).
- As the foot is everted and pronated, the deltoid ligament is considered incompetent when it is tensioned, but obviously no strong medial buttress is created with this maneuver (**TECH FIG 2**). An excessive lifting away of the talus from the medial malleolus by pulling the foot anteriorly is also considered an indicator of stretching of this ligament.
- Lateral instability is considered to be present when talar tilting occurs by supination stress of the foot.
- As evaluated for both the medial and lateral side, the ankle joint is graded as stable when there is some translocation of the talus, but not enough to open the tibiotalar joint by more than 2 mm (as measured by the 2-mm hook) and not enough to introduce the 5-mm arthroscope into the tibiotalar space; as moderately unstable when the talus moves to some extent out of the ankle mortise, allowing introduction of the 5-mm arthroscope into the tibiotalar space, but not enough to open the tibiotalar joint by more than 5 mm; and as severely unstable when the talus moves easily out of the ankle mortise, typically allowing free insight into the posterior aspect of the ankle joint without significant pulling stress on the heel.[7]

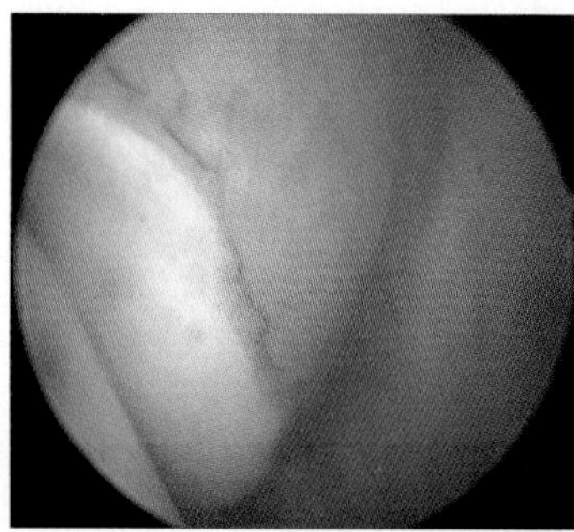

TECH FIG 1 • Avulsion of anterior superficial layers from medial malleolus. Arthroscopy typically reveals a completely free insertion area of the ligament on the medial malleolus.

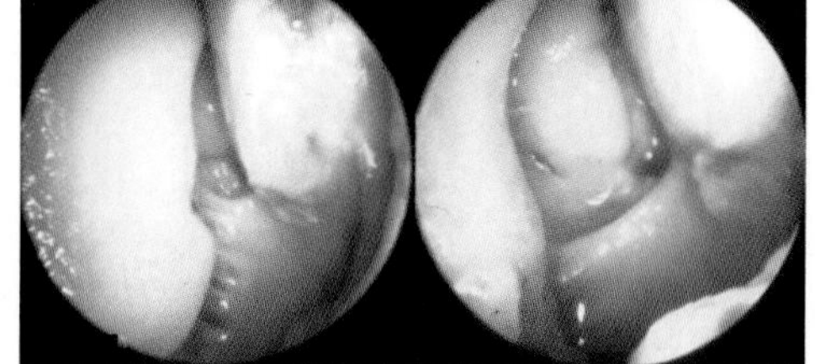

TECH FIG 2 • Incompetent deltoid ligament. **A.** As the foot is everted and pronated, the deltoid ligament is considered incompetent when it is tensioned, but obviously no strong medial buttress is created with this maneuver. **B.** An excessive lifting away of the talus from the medial malleolus by pulling the foot anteriorly is also considered an indicator of stretching of this ligament.

MEDIAL ANKLE LIGAMENT RECONSTRUCTION

- Complete acute rupture: Because the rupture is mostly situated proximally of the deltoid ligament (**TECH FIG 3**), reattachment to the medial malleolus is achieved by interosseous sutures; a bony anchor can also be used for refixation to the bone.[8]
- Chronic ruptures of the superficial deltoid ligament are classified as shown in Table 1.[7,8]
- Chronic rupture of the superficial deltoid ligament (type I lesion): Expose the anterior border of the medial malleolus by making a short longitudinal incision between the tibionavicular and tibiospring ligaments, where there is usually a small fibrous septum without adherent connective fibers between the two ligaments (**TECH FIG 4A**). After roughening the medial aspect of the medial malleolus, place an anchor (Panalock®) 6 mm above the tip of the malleolus (**TECH FIG 4B**); this serves for refixation of

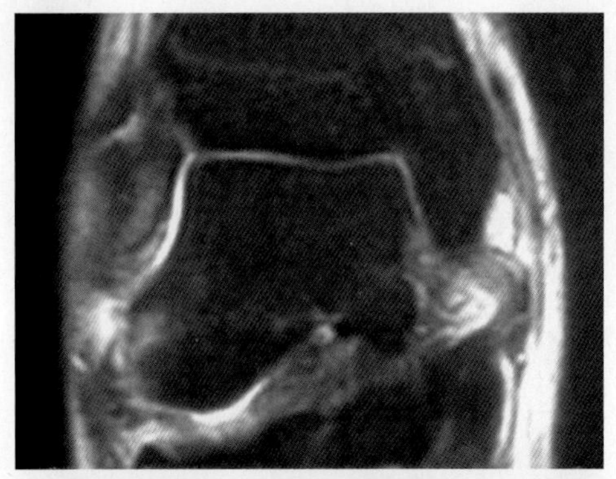

A

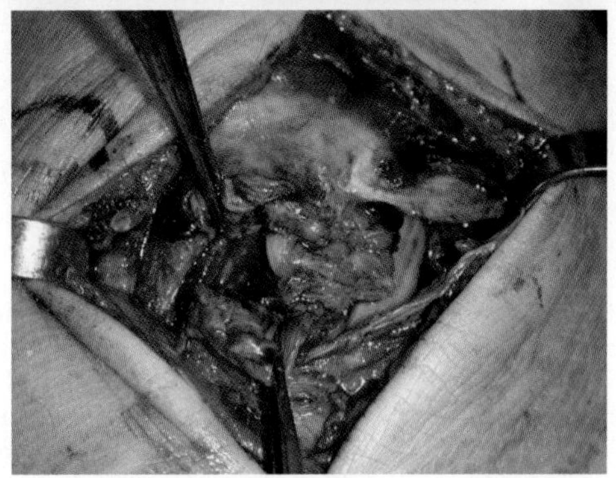

B

TECH FIG 3 • Acute deltoid rupture. This 28-year-old soccer player sustained a valgus trauma, causing an acute "giving way" of the foot. **A.** MR imaging reveals complete disruption of the ligament close to its proximal insertion to the medial malleolus. **B.** Surgical exploration confirms complete disruption of the deltoid ligament, although the posterior tibial tendon remained intact.

Table 1 **Classification of Chronic Superficial Lesions of Deltoid Ligament**

Lesion	Location of Tear
Type I lesion	Proximal tear/avulsion of deltoid ligament
Type II lesion	Intermediate tear of deltoid ligament
Type III lesion	Distal tear/avulsion of deltoid and spring ligaments

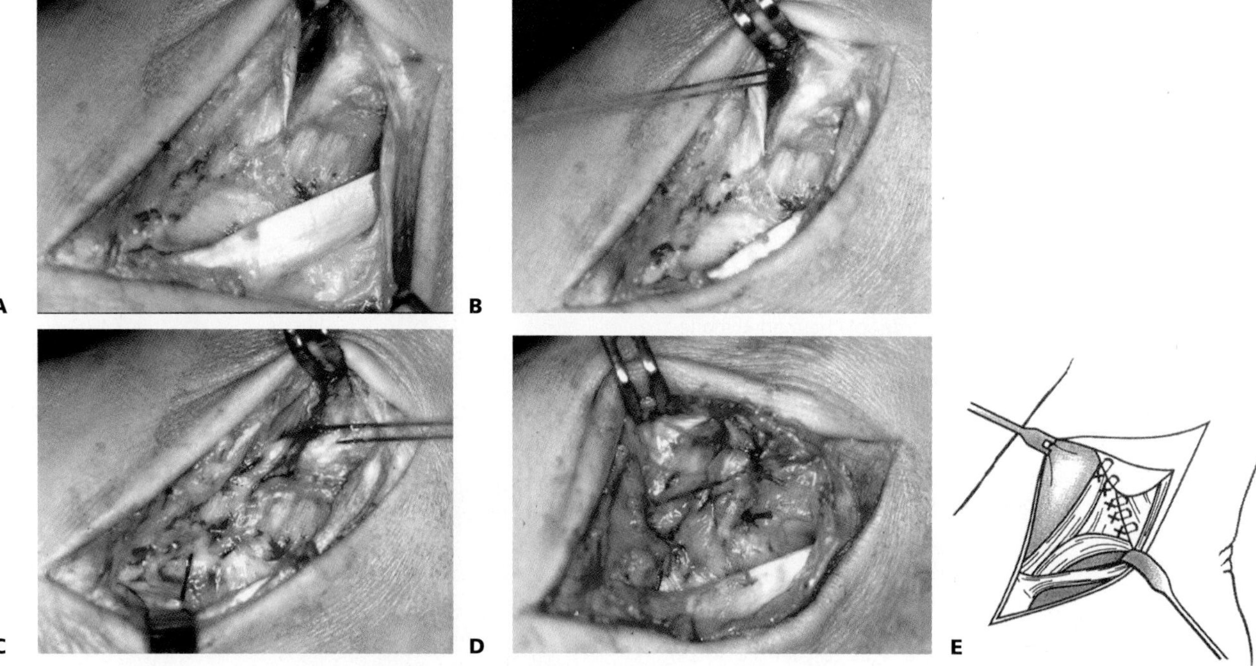

TECH FIG 4 • Chronic rupture of the superficial deltoid ligament (type I lesion). **A.** The rupture is located between the tibionavicular and tibiospring ligaments, where a small fibrous septum without adherent connective fibers between the two ligaments is usually present. **B.** After roughening the medial aspect of the medial malleolus, an anchor (Panalock®) is placed 6 mm above the tip of the malleolus. **C.** It serves for refixation of the tibionavicular and tibiospring ligaments to the medial malleolus, and to shorten both ligaments. **D.** Final reconstruction after some additional no. 0 resorbable sutures. **E.** Principle of reconstruction.

the tibionavicular and tibiospring ligaments to the medial malleolus, and to shorten both the tibionavicular and tibiospring ligaments (TECH FIG 4C–E). Use additional no. 0 resorbable sutures to refix the tibionavicular and tibiospring ligaments.

- Chronic rupture of the superficial deltoid ligament (type II lesion): Divide the scarred insufficient ligament (TECH FIG 5A) into two flaps: the deep flap remains reattached distally; the superficial flap remains reattached to the medial malleolus. Place two anchors (Panalock®) 6 mm above the tip of the malleolus (TECH FIG 5B), and place one anchor (Panalock®) at the superior edge of the navicular tuberosity (TECH FIG 5C). Two anchors serve for refixation of the deep flap to the medial malleolus (TECH FIG 5D), and the superficial flap to the navicular tuberosity (TECH FIG 5E), thereby creating a strong and well-tightened ligament reconstruction (TECH FIG 5F). The second superior anchor on the medial malleolus serves for reattachment of the tibionavicular ligament (TECH FIG 5G). Use additional no. 0 resorbable sutures to further stabilize the reconstructed tibionavicular and tibiospring ligaments (TECH FIG 5H,I).
- Chronic rupture of the superficial deltoid ligament (type III lesion): If necessary, débride the tear (TECH FIG 6A). Then place two nonresorbable sutures in the spring ligament (TECH FIG 6B). If the tibionavicular ligament is completely detached from its insertion, place an anchor (Panalock®) at the superior edge of the navicular tuberosity. After tightening the sutures (TECH FIG 6C,D), use additional no. 0 resorbable sutures to further stabilize the reconstructed tibionavicular and spring ligaments.
- Chronic rupture of the deep deltoid ligament: Because this condition usually includes an extended tear of the superficial anterior bundles of the deltoid ligament, any

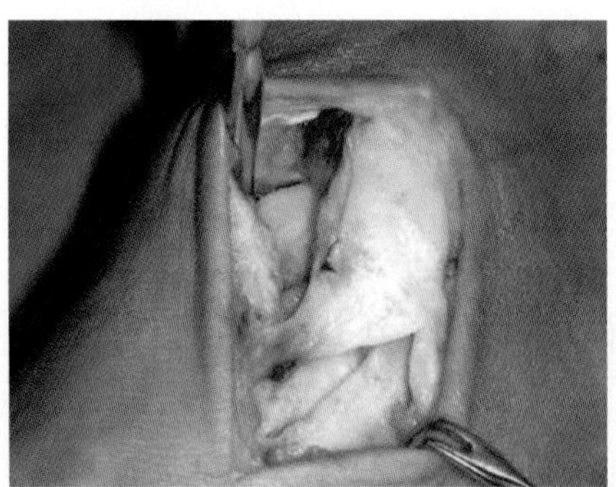

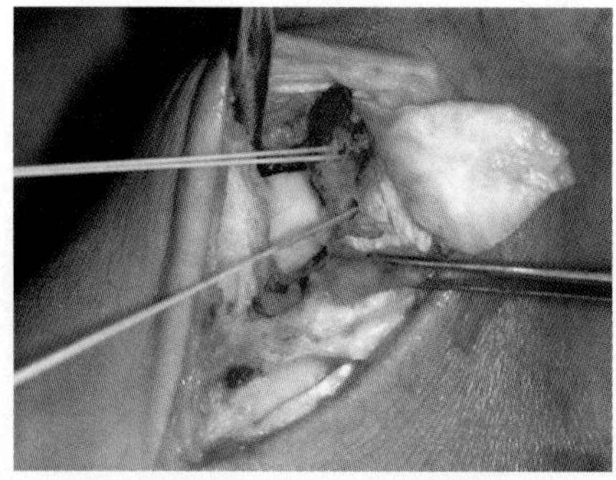

TECH FIG 5 • Chronic rupture of the superficial deltoid ligament (type II lesion). **A.** The superficial deltoid ligament is scarred and incompetent. **B.** Two anchors (Panalock®) are placed 6 and 9 mm above the tip of the medial malleolus. *(continued)*

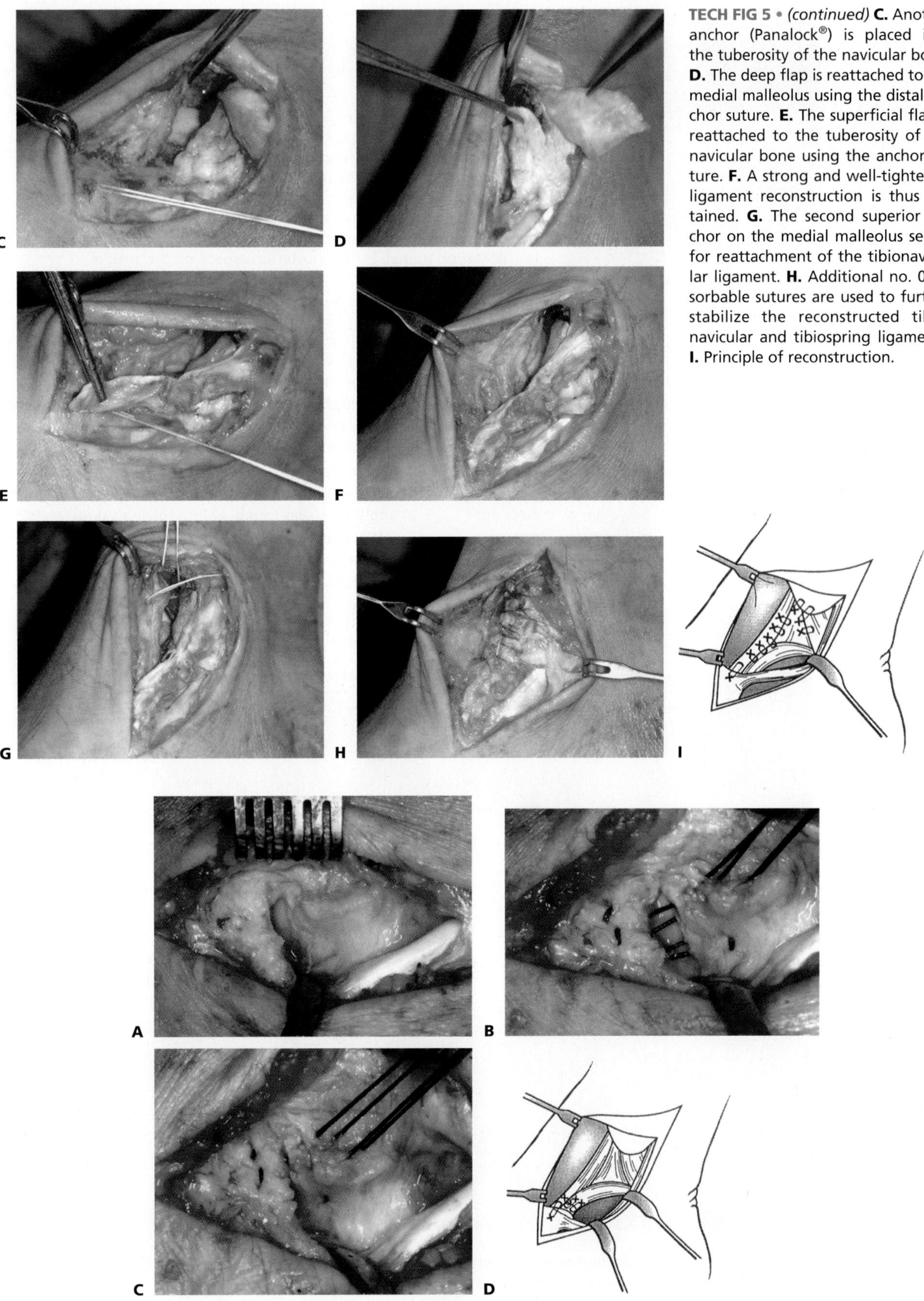

TECH FIG 5 • *(continued)* **C.** Another anchor (Panalock®) is placed into the tuberosity of the navicular bone. **D.** The deep flap is reattached to the medial malleolus using the distal anchor suture. **E.** The superficial flap is reattached to the tuberosity of the navicular bone using the anchor suture. **F.** A strong and well-tightened ligament reconstruction is thus obtained. **G.** The second superior anchor on the medial malleolus serves for reattachment of the tibionavicular ligament. **H.** Additional no. 0 resorbable sutures are used to further stabilize the reconstructed tibionavicular and tibiospring ligaments. **I.** Principle of reconstruction.

TECH FIG 6 • Chronic rupture of the superficial deltoid ligament (type III lesion). **A.** The distal tear in the spring ligament is exposed and débrided. **B.** Two nonresorbable sutures are placed in the spring ligament. **C.** The sutures are tightened. **D.** Principles of reconstruction.

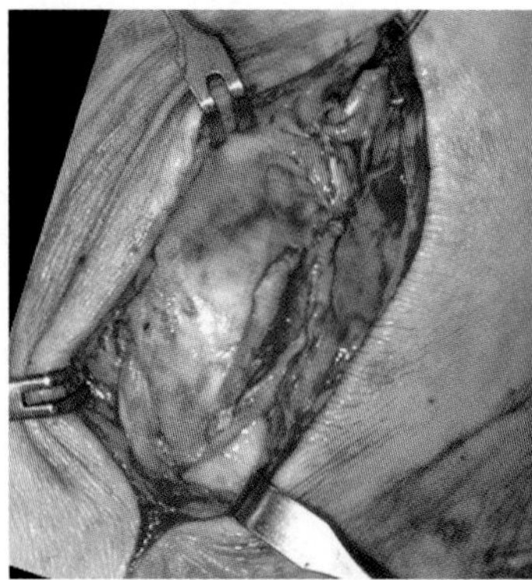

TECH FIG 7 • Chronic rupture of the deep deltoid ligament. After the posterior tibial tendon has been split into two bundles, both bundles are inserted into a drill hole at the tip of the medial malleolus (*arrow*). One bundle is conducted through the anterior tunnel at the anterior aspect of the medial malleolus, and the posterior bundle is conducted through the posterior tunnel at the posterior aspect of the medial malleolus.

reconstructive surgery should attempt to address the whole deltoid ligament. The posterior tibial tendon can be used as a graft for augmentation of the reconstructed deltoid ligament by passing it through a drill hole from the tip of the medial malleolus to the medial aspect of the distal tibia (**TECH FIG 7**). This technique was found to be disappointing, however, as it does not sufficiently reinforce the deep tibiotalar ligaments (Hintermann, unpublished data). Most recently, the use of a bone–tendon–bone transplant has been proposed for reconstruction of the deltoid ligament (**TECH FIG 8**).[2] In this in vitro study, two limbs were created on a distal transplant; one was fixed to the medial aspect of the talus and the other to the sustentaculum tali. The proximal end was fixed to the distal tibia, the medial malleolus, or the lateral tibia. Less than 2.0 degrees of angulation was found while applying valgus stress of 5 daN for all fixation methods. However, the authors advised against fixation of the proximal limb in the medial malleolus.

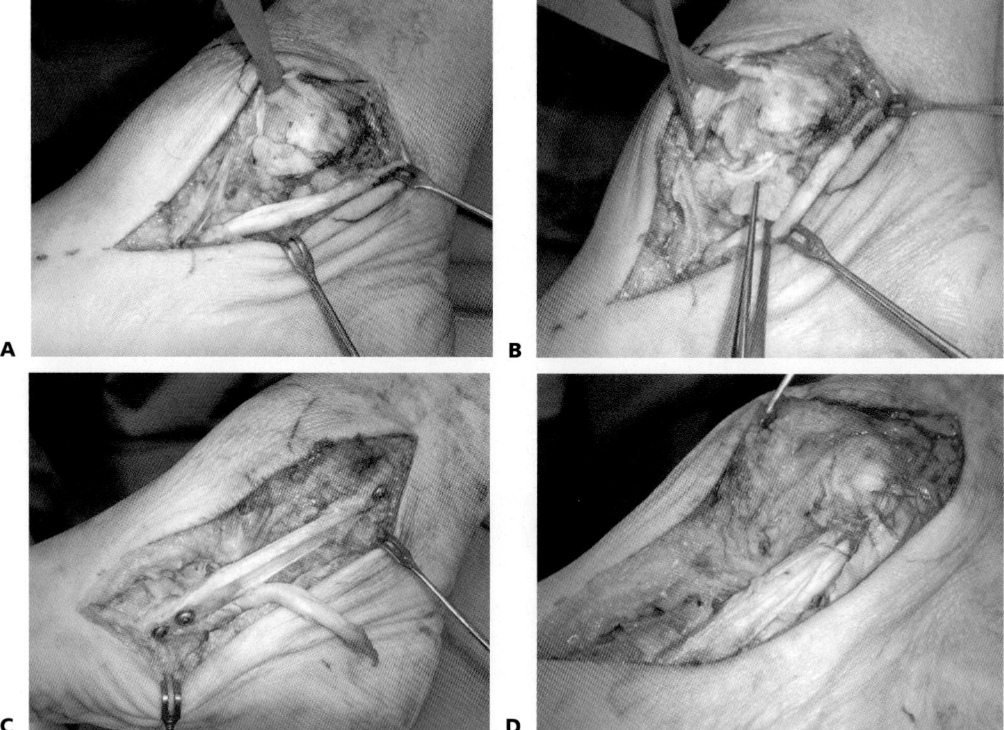

TECH FIG 8 • Chronic rupture of the deep deltoid ligament. **A.** Exposure of the posterior tibial tendon reveals a tear. **B.** Exposure of the deltoid ligament reveals an extended disruption and incompetence of the superficial and deep layers. **C.** A bone–tendon–bone transplant is fixed by screws distally into the navicular bone and, after tightening, proximally to the posterior aspect of the medial malleolus. **D.** Multiple nonabsorbable and absorbable sutures are used for further reconstruction of the ligament.

LATERAL ANKLE LIGAMENT RECONSTRUCTION

- About 75% of patients with chronic medial ankle instability were found to have an associated avulsion of the anterior talofibular ligament that resulted in a complex rotational instability of the talus within the ankle mortise.[7]
- If the condition of the anterior talofibular ligament and the calcaneofibular ligament allows an adequate primary repair, these ligaments can be reconstructed by shortening and reinsertion (**TECH FIG 9**).
- When no substantial ligamentous material is present, augmentation with a free plantaris tendon graft is performed (**TECH FIG 10**).[12]

Posterior Tibial Débridement and Reconstruction

- Inspect the posterior tibial tendon meticulously during surgery, especially in the case of a type II or type III lesion of the anterior deltoid ligament.
- If there is degeneration of the tendon, débride the tendon.
- If there is elongation of the tendon, consider shortening the tendon.
- If there is an accessory bone (os tibiale externum), consider reattaching the bone with the tendon insertion; the posterior tibial tendon can also be tightened if the bone is reattached more distally to the navicular bone (**TECH FIG 11**).[9]
- A transfer of the flexor digitorum tendon might be considered in the case of a diseased or ruptured tendon, but this is seldom the case.

Lateral Lengthening Calcaneal Osteotomy

- This procedure is considered in the case of a pre-existing valgus and pronation deformity of the foot (eg, when a valgus and pronation deformity is also present on the contralateral, asymptomatic foot) or in the case of a severe attenuation or defect of the tibionavicular, tibiospring, or spring ligaments.
- A calcaneal osteotomy is performed along and parallel to the posterior facet of the subtalar joint, from lateral to medial, preserving the medial cortex intact (**TECH FIG 12A–D**).[6]
- As the osteotomy is widened, the pronation deformity of the foot is seen to disappear (**TECH FIG 12E**).
- Fashion a tricortical graft from the iliac crest to the length required and place it into the osteotomy site (**TECH FIG F–H**).

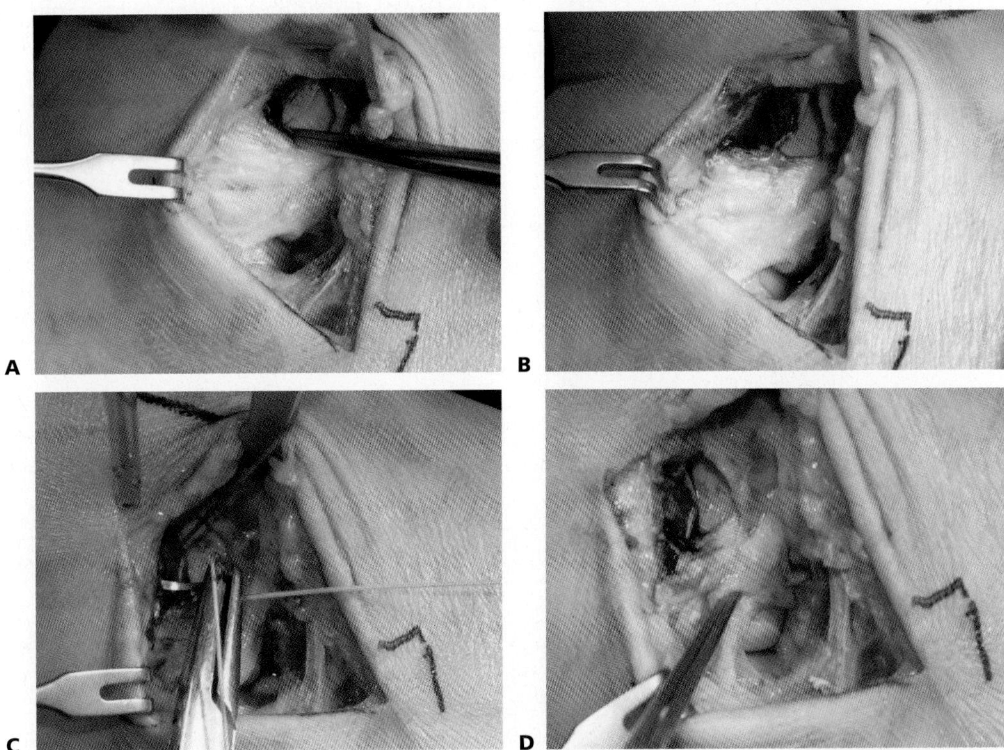

TECH FIG 9 • Primary anatomic repair of lateral ankle ligaments. **A.** Exposure of lateral ligaments and arthrotomy of ankle and subtalar joints that are débrided. The scarred anterior portion of the lateral ligaments is widely disconnected from the anterior border of the fibula. **B.** The anterior border of the fibula is roughened. **C.** An anchor or transosseous sutures are used to reattach the avulsed lateral ligaments (eg, the anterior tibiofibular and calcaneofibular ligaments at their common insertion 8 to 10 mm above the tip of lateral malleolus). **D.** A strong and well-tightened ligament reconstruction is thus obtained.

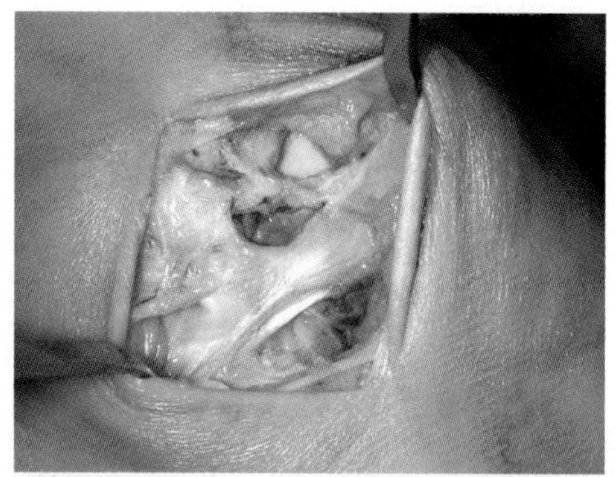

A

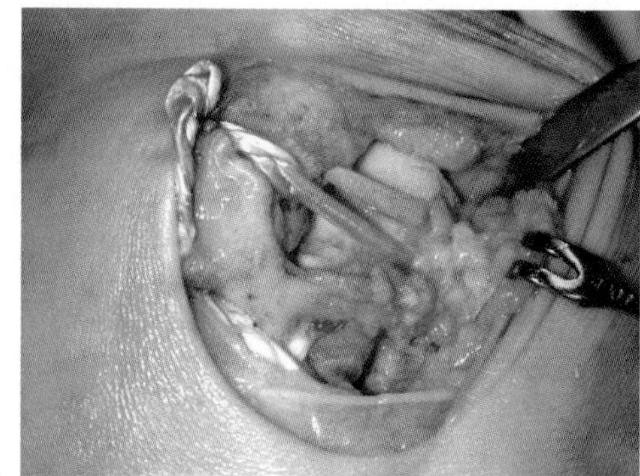

B

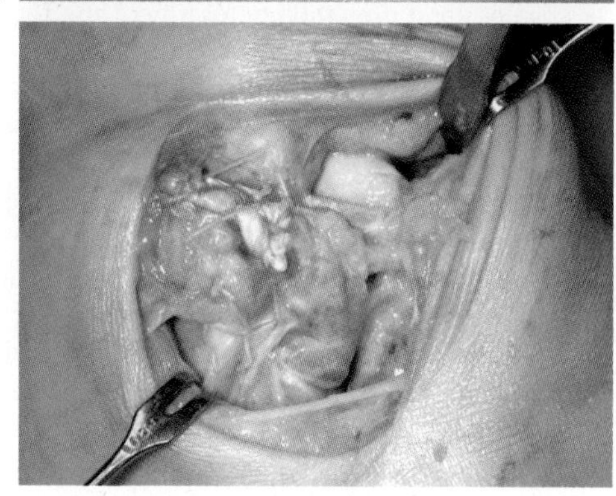

C

TECH FIG 10 • Reconstruction of lateral ankle ligaments with a free plantaris tendon graft. **A.** The remaining scarred ligaments do not allow primary repair of lateral ankle ligaments. **B.** A free plantaris tendon graft is used for reconstruction of the anterior talofibular and the calcaneofibular ligaments. **C.** A strong and well-tightened ligament reconstruction is thus obtained.

Double Arthrodesis

- This procedure is considered when the medial ankle instability is so excessive that a valgus tilt of the talus within the mortise is seen on a standard AP view of the ankle while the foot is loaded (Fig 2).[11]
- Be sure to fully correct the whole deformity (eg, valgus malalignment of the heel, and the peritalar dislocation of talus).
- Expose the talonavicular joint from medially through the same incision (**TECH FIG 13A,B**).
- Use a distraction spreader (Hintermann spreader) to open the joint; this allows for cartilage removal and débridement (**TECH FIG 13C,D**).
- Expose the subtalar joint from medially through the same incision.

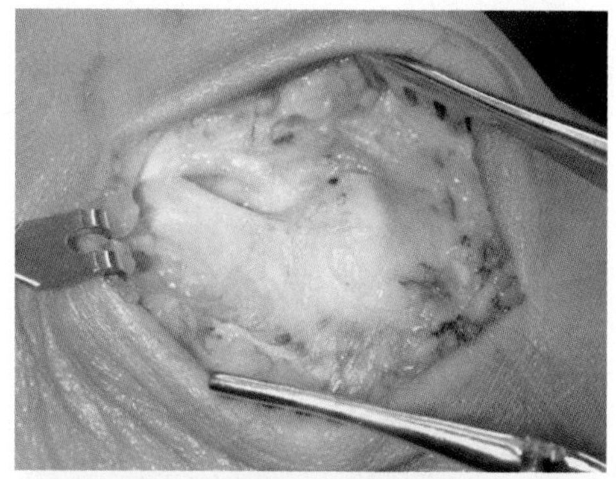

A

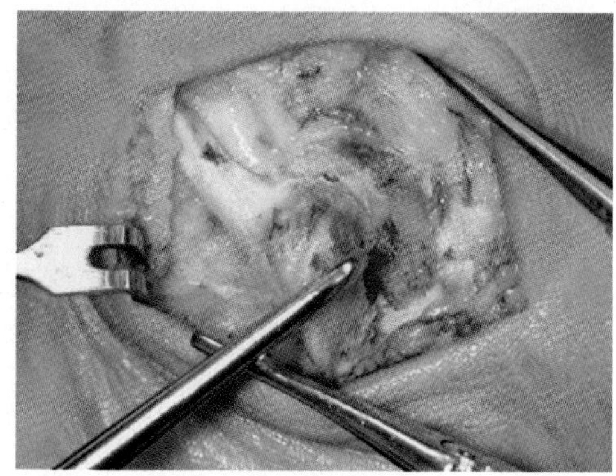

B

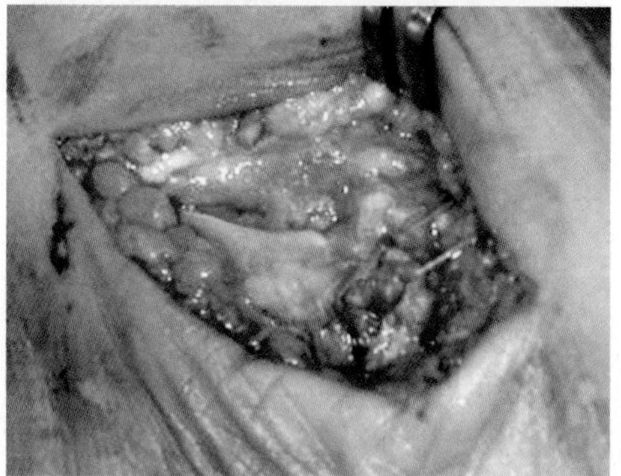

C

TECH FIG 11 • Unstable os tibiale externum. **A.** An unstable accessory bone (os tibiale externum) is found to weaken the pull of posterior tibial tendon. **B.** The accessory bone is mobilized and 3 to 5 mm of bone is removed on both sides of the pseudarthrosis. **C.** This allows for reattachment of the accessory bone more distally to the navicular bone, using screws and nonabsorbable sutures.

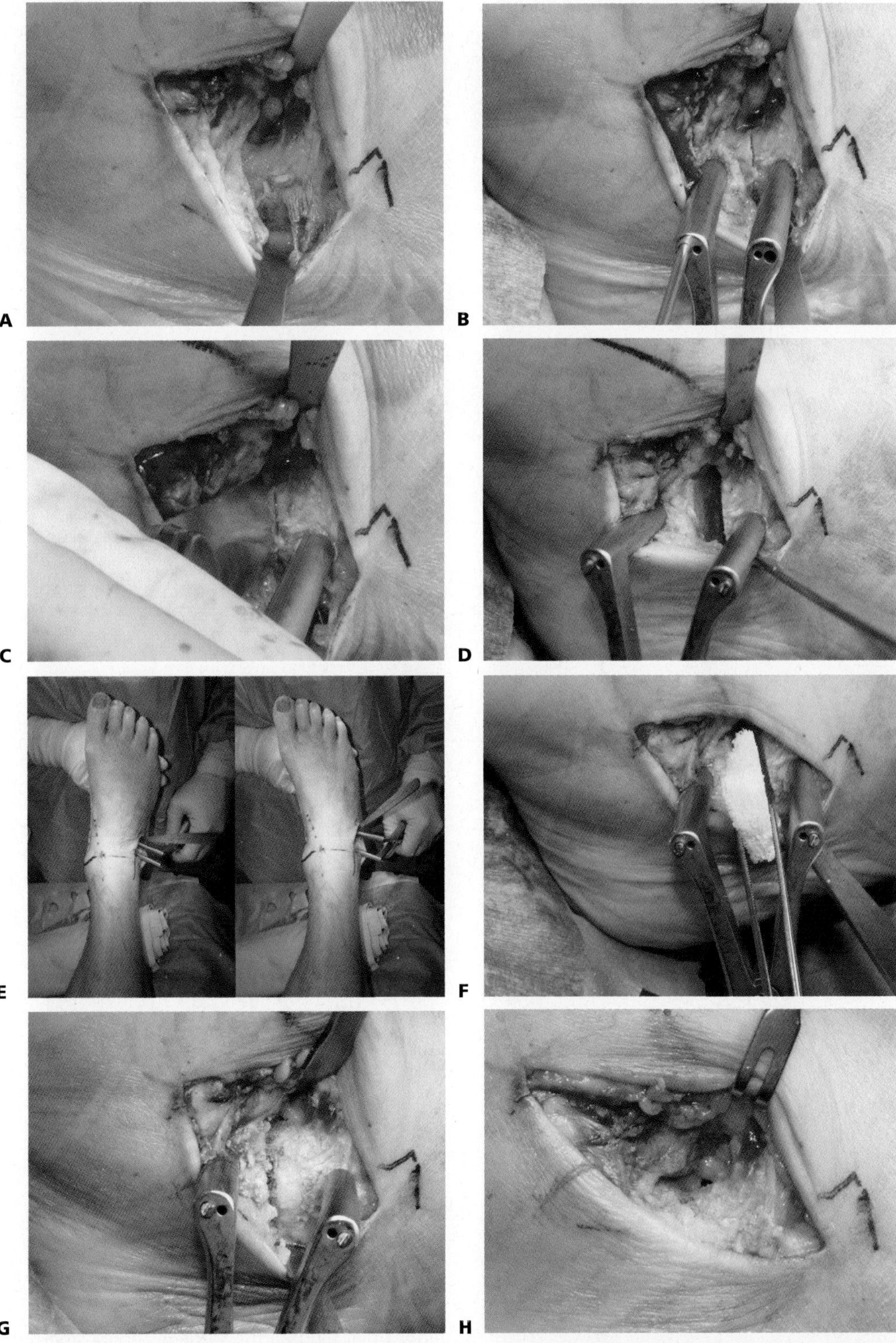

TECH FIG 12 • Calcaneal lengthening osteotomy. **A.** The neck of the calcaneus is exposed using a lateral incision. **B.** The osteotomy is marked by a cisel to be directed through the sinus tarsi along the anterior border of the posterior facet of the subtalar joint. Two Kirschner wires for the Hintermann retractor are inserted. **C.** Osteotomy is performed using a saw. **D.** The osteotomy is opened using the retractor. **E.** As the osteotomy is widened, the pronation deformity of the foot is seen to disappear. **F.** A tricortical graft from the iliac crest or an allograft is fashioned to the length required and placed into the osteotomy site. **G.** The border of the inserted graft is smoothed. **H.** A regular bony contour on the bottom of the sinus tarsi is thus obtained.

- Use the distraction spreader to open the joint; this allows for cartilage removal and débridement (**TECH FIG E–G**).
- Correct the deformity first by reducing the former talonavicular joint, making sure to correct the frontal plane position of the navicular (eg, to achieve full correction of any forefoot supination deformity) (**TECH FIG 13H–L**).
- Stable fixation is achieved by triple screw fixation at the talonavicular and double screw fixation at the subtalar joint (**TECH FIG 13M–O**).

Wound Closure

- Close the wounds in layers.
- Close the subcutaneous tissue and skin in standard fashion.

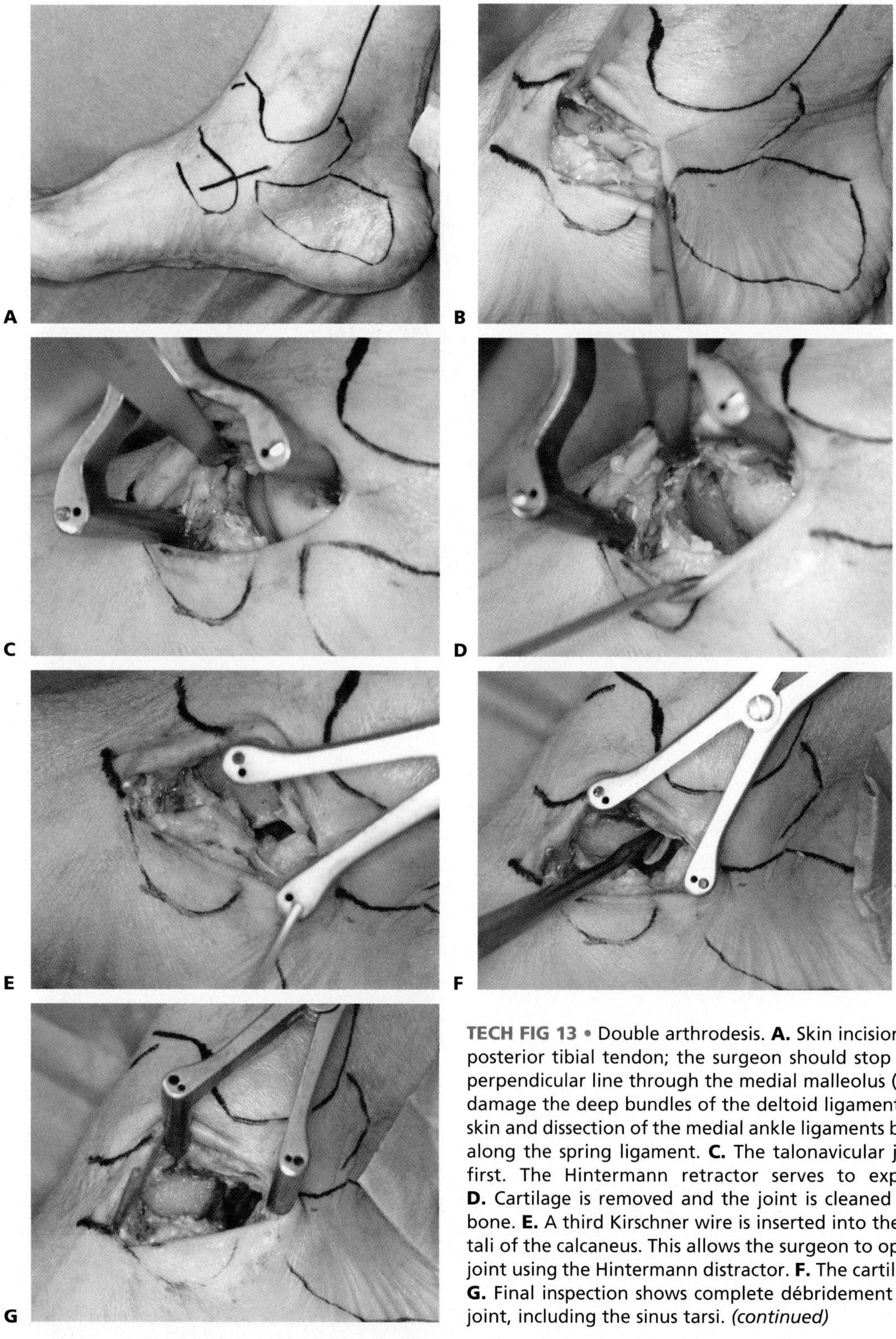

A B

C D

E F

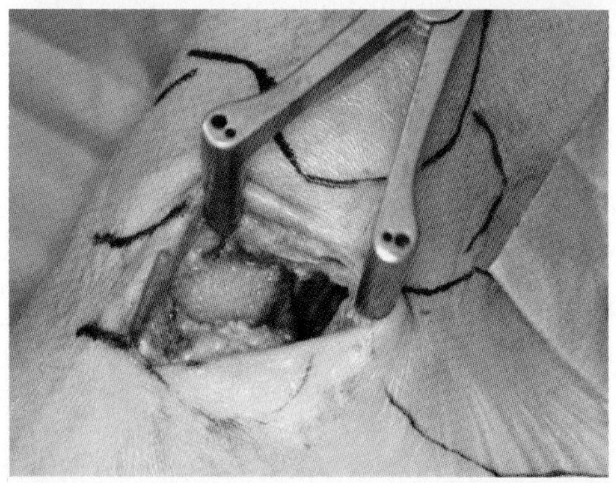

G

TECH FIG 13 • Double arthrodesis. **A.** Skin incision just above the posterior tibial tendon; the surgeon should stop proximally at a perpendicular line through the medial malleolus (eg, so as not to damage the deep bundles of the deltoid ligament). **B.** Incision of skin and dissection of the medial ankle ligaments by sharp incision along the spring ligament. **C.** The talonavicular joint is exposed first. The Hintermann retractor serves to expose the joint. **D.** Cartilage is removed and the joint is cleaned to subchondral bone. **E.** A third Kirschner wire is inserted into the sustentaculum tali of the calcaneus. This allows the surgeon to open the subtalar joint using the Hintermann distractor. **F.** The cartilage is removed. **G.** Final inspection shows complete débridement of the subtalar joint, including the sinus tarsi. *(continued)*

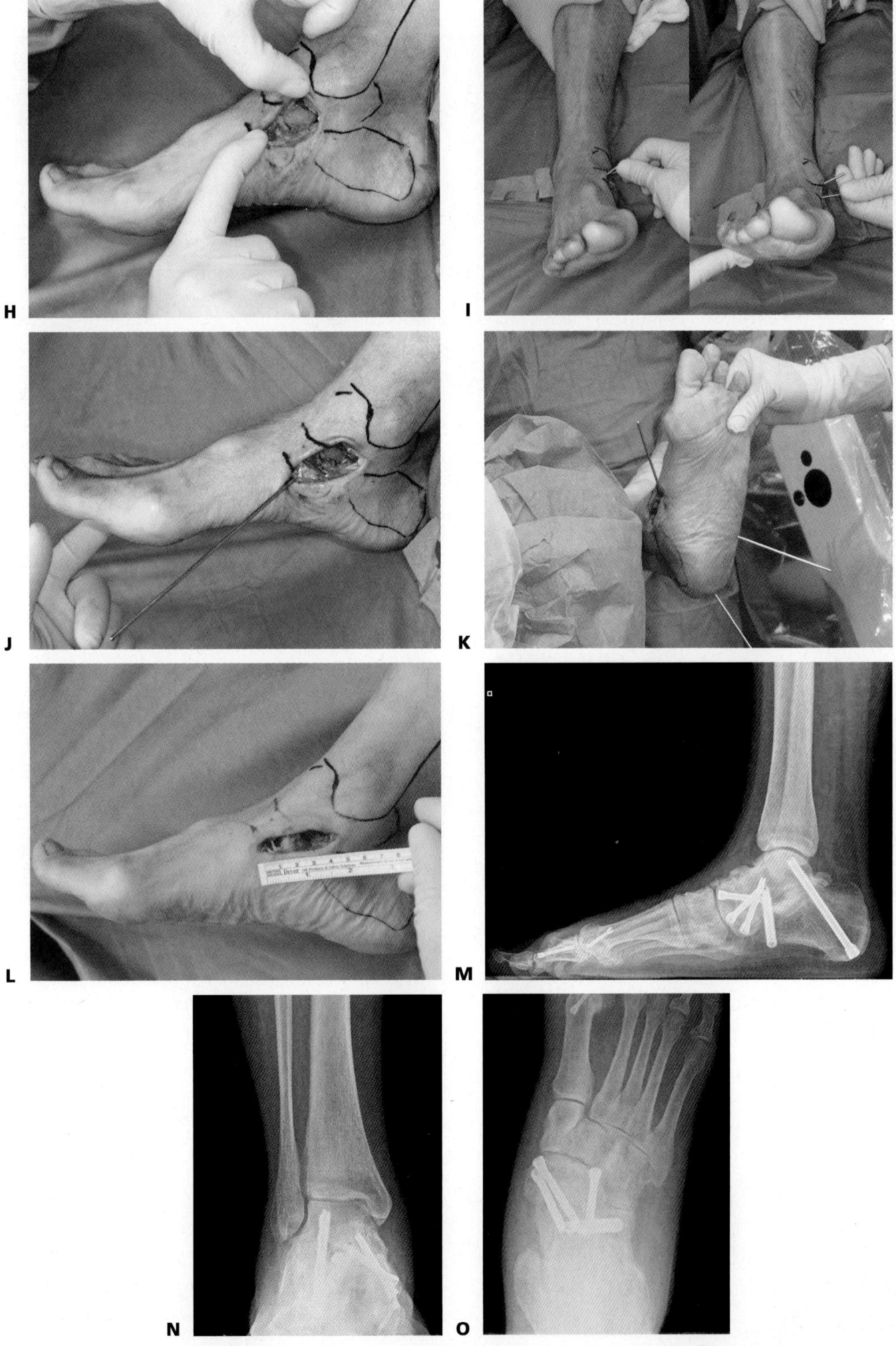

TECH FIG 13 • *(continued)* **H.** The Kirschner wires in the navicular and talar bones are kept in place and serve to reduce the talonavicular joint properly. **I.** Frontal view showing the frontal realignment at the talonavicular joint using both Kirschner wires as joysticks. **J.** A first guiding Kirschner wire is inserted through the tuberosity of the navicular into the talus. Afterwards, two other guidewires will be used to properly stabilize the talonavicular joint in the frontal plane. **K.** After inserting two additional guidewires from the bottom through the subtalar joint, fluoroscopy is used to insert the cannulated screws (QUIX, Newdeal/Integra). **L.** The deltoid ligament is reattached to the spring ligament using nonabsorbable sutures. The foot looks properly positioned at the end of surgery. Note the short incision that is used for this procedure. At 2 months, weight-bearing radiographs are obtained. **M.** Lateral view. **N.** AP view of the ankle. **O.** AP view of the foot.

PEARLS AND PITFALLS

Diagnosis	■ Medial ankle instability is a clinical diagnosis; therefore, a complete and careful history and physical examination should be performed.
Indication	■ Care must be taken to address associated pathologies.
Suture techniques	■ Transosseous sutures or anchor sutures should be used for proper fixation of the ligaments to the bone. ■ Slowly resorbable or nonresorbable suture material should be used for fixation to bone.
Ligament reconstruction	■ Nonanatomic reconstruction of ligaments is responsible for most failures. ■ Careful exploration of the injured or incompetent ligament should be done routinely.
Additional procedures	■ Careful assessment of the foot while weight bearing is mandatory to identify associated malalignment and deformity problems. ■ Reconstruction of the medial ankle ligaments will fail if such associated problems are neglected or inappropriately addressed.

POSTOPERATIVE CARE

- The foot is protected by a plaster cast for 6 weeks, and full weight bearing is allowed as soon as pain-free loading is possible. In the case of double arthrodesis, initial plaster immobilization for 8 weeks is recommended.
- The rehabilitation program starts after cast removal. It includes passive and active mobilization of the ankle joint, training of the muscular strength, and protection with a walker or stabilizing shoe when walking.
- A walker or stabilizing shoe can be used for 4 to 6 weeks after cast removal, depending on regained muscular balance of the hindfoot.
- We recommend continued use for walks on uneven ground, for high-risk sports activities, and for professional work outside.

OUTCOMES

- With appropriate surgical technique, success rates for ligament reconstruction of the medial ankle are on the order of 85% to 90% in terms of return to former sports and professional activities.[7]
- As associated malalignment has been addressed more aggressively in the last years, the success rate has further increased.
- The most troubling problem remains a chronic incompetence of the deep deltoid ligament, which results in valgus tilt of the talus while loading the foot. Despite the use of tendon augmentation, most attempts at isolated ligament reconstruction have failed; the main step is probably a double arthrodesis in getting a stable and well-aligned hindfoot. An alternative may be a tibiocalcaneal arthrodesis.

COMPLICATIONS

- Deficient stability because of inappropriate ligament reconstruction
- Recurrent instability because valgus deformity was not addressed
- Suture granuloma at the anterior margin of the medial malleolus when using nonresorbable sutures and placing the suture knot onto a bony surface
- Deep venous thrombosis
- Infection
- Scarring in the anteromedial ankle causing soft tissue impingement

REFERENCES

1. Boss AP, Hintermann B. Anatomical study of the medial ankle ligament complex. Foot Ankle Int 2002;23:547–553.
2. Buman EM, Khazen G, Haraguchi N, et al. Minimally invasive deltoid ligament reconstruction: a comparison of three techniques. Proceedings of the 36th Annual Winter Meeting, Specialty Day, AOFAS, Chicago, March 25, 2006, p. 25.
3. Harper MC. Deltoid ligament: an anatomical evaluation of function. Foot Ankle 1987;8:19–22.
4. Hintermann B, Boss A, Schäfer D. Arthroscopic findings in patients with chronic ankle instability. Am J Sports Med 2002;30:402–409.
5. Hintermann B. Medial ankle instability. Foot Ankle Clin 2003;8: 723–738.
6. Hintermann B, Valderrabano V. Lateral column lengthening by calcaneal osteotomy. Techn Foot Ankle Surg 2003;2:84–90.
7. Hintermann B, Valderrabano V, Boss AP, et al. Medial ankle instability: an exploratory, prospective study of 52 cases. Am J Sports Med 2004;32:183–190.
8. Hintermann B, Knupp M, Pagenstert GI. Deltoid ligament injuries: diagnosis and management. Foot Ankle Clin 2006;11:625–637.
9. Knupp M, Hintermann B. Reconstruction in posttraumatic combined avulsion of an accessory navicular and the posterior tibial tendon. Techn Foot Ankle Surg 2005;4:113–118.
10. Milner CE, Soames RW. The medial collateral ligaments of the human ankle joint: anatomical variations. Foot Ankle Int 1998; 19:289–292.
11. Nelson DR, Younger A. Acute posttraumatic planovalgus foot deformity involving hindfoot ligamentous pathology. Foot Ankle Clin 2003;8:521–537.
12. Pagenstert GI, Hintermann B, Knupp M. Operative management of chronic ankle instability; plantaris graft. Foot Ankle Clin 2006;11: 567–583.
13. Tornetta P, III. Competence of the deltoid ligament in bimalleolar ankle fractures after medial malleolar fixation. J Bone Joint Surg Am 2000;82A:843–848.

Chapter 105 Open Achilles Tendon Repair

Sameh A. Labib

DEFINITION

- The Achilles tendon is the strongest tendon in the body and is the primary plantarflexor of the ankle joint.[15]
- Sudden stretch of the tendon tissue can result in complete or partial rupture, with an estimated incidence of 18 per 100,000 persons.[3]
- With complete rupture, the ruptured ends of the tendon may pull apart, leading to a significant plantarflexion weakness and to the creation of a gap that is palpated clinically.
- A common source of confusion is that patients may continue to have active ankle plantarflexion due to the action of other flexors of the ankle.
- As a result, the diagnosis is initially missed in an estimated 20% to 25% of cases.[5]

ANATOMY

- Three calf muscles—the medial, lateral gastrocnemius, and soleus—converge together to form the "triceps surae" or the Achilles tendon (**FIG 1**).
- The plantaris muscle originates from the lateral femoral condyle and passes obliquely between the gastrocnemius and soleus to reside medial to the Achilles tendon and inserts into it or the calcaneus. In an anatomic study, the plantaris muscle was absent in 7.3% of specimens.[15]
- The Achilles tendon courses distally, rotates 90 degrees internally, the soleus contribution being medial to that of the gastrocnemius, and inserts into the middle third of the flat surface of the posterior calcaneal tuberosity.[10]
- The middle section of the tendon, 2 to 6 cm proximal to its insertion site, is a hypovascular zone.
  - This zone is the narrowest in cross-section and corresponds to the most common site of tendon pathology, including paratenonitis, tendinosis, and tendon rupture.[10]
- The tendon is surrounded by a paratenon that has a single layer of cells with variable structure, not a true tenosynovium.
- Webb et al[16] documented the highly variable position of the sural nerve in relation to the Achilles tendon.
  - As measured from the calcaneal insertion, the sural nerve crossed the tendon from medial to lateral at a mean distance of 9.8 cm, then coursed distally to lie a mean of 18.8 mm lateral (**FIG 2**).

PATHOGENESIS

- Achilles ruptures are usually caused by noncontact injuries. Common injury mechanisms leading to Achilles rupture are forceful push-off with an extended knee, sudden unexpected ankle dorsiflexion, or violent dorsiflexion of a plantarflexed foot.[13]

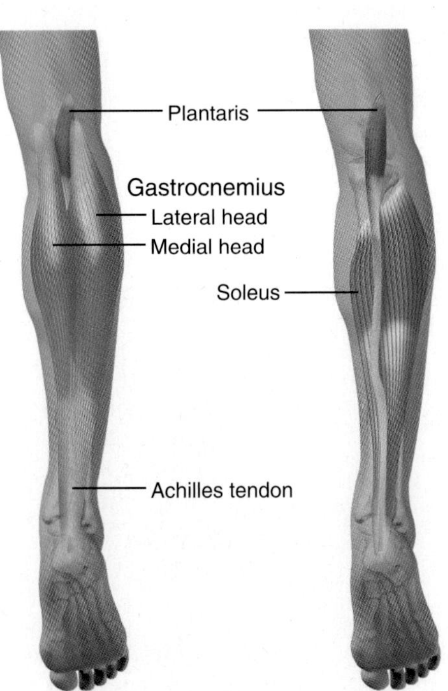

FIG 1 • The "triceps surae" (Achilles tendon) is formed by the convergence of the medial, lateral gastrocnemius, and soleus muscles.

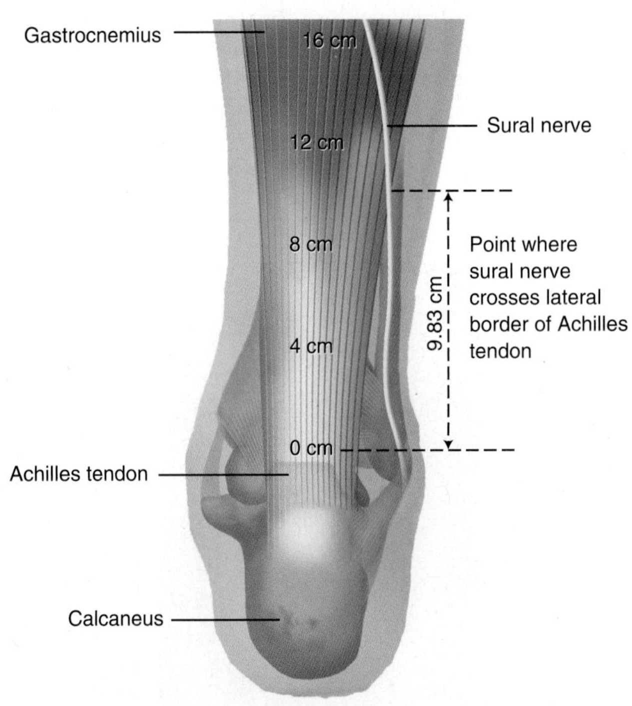

FIG 2 • Position of the sural nerve in relation to the Achilles tendon. (Adapted from Webb J, Moorjani N, Radford M. Anatomy of the sural nerve and its relation to the Achilles tendon. Foot Ankle Int 2000;21:475–477.)

- Achilles rupture can occur high, near the muscle–tendon juncture (9%), at the tendon midportion (72%), or at the calcaneal insertion (19%).[5]
- Concomitant injuries such as ankle ligament sprains or ankle or tarsal fractures should be ruled out.

NATURAL HISTORY

- Most Achilles ruptures do not have any antecedent symptoms.
  - A study of histologic scores comparing ruptured tendons with unruptured tendons, however, showed that there were significant histopathologic changes in the ruptured group that were not present in the older, asymptomatic, unruptured group. Therefore, tendinosis may play a role, but the extent of this role remains unknown.[14]
- Achilles rupture is more common in men. Studies have shown a male/female ratio of up to 12:1.
- From an epidemiologic standpoint, middle-aged men with white-collar professions and recreational athletic activity constitute most of the patients.
  - Other predisposing factors are leg muscle imbalance, training errors, foot pronation, and use of corticosteroids and fluoroquinolones.[13]
- The contralateral risk of rupture was estimated at 26% on return to the same level of sports activities.[15]

PATIENT HISTORY AND PHYSICAL FINDINGS

- Most ruptures occur during athletic activity. Patients usually describe a sudden painful snap or shooting pain followed by sudden weakness to foot push-off.
- Athletes will be unable to bear weight and will report distal leg swelling and stiffness.
- Examination for ruptured Achilles tendon can include:
  - Palpable gap test. A gap present indicates complete Achilles rupture with separation of the ruptured ends. It is more reliable when done early after rupture. It is 73% sensitive.[13]
  - Calf squeeze test (Thompson test). With patient prone, squeeze the calf and observe foot movement. Compare with the contralateral side.

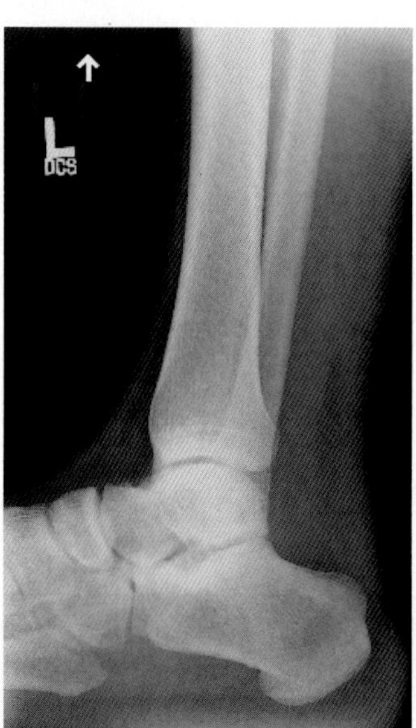

FIG 3 • Ankle radiograph showing a disrupted Kager triangle.

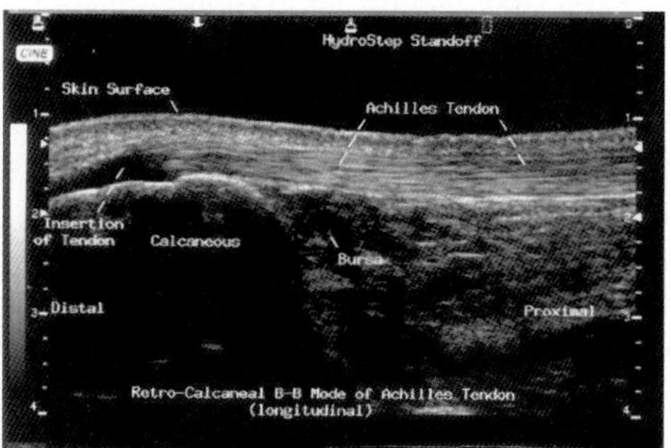

FIG 4 • Normal Achilles ultrasound image.

  - Knee flexion test. With patient prone, patient actively flexes knee. Observe foot position and compare with other.
  - Active plantarflexion. This is poorly sensitive and unreliable because powerful plantarflexion may still be possible due to the action of other ankle plantarflexors.

IMAGING AND OTHER DIAGNOSTIC STUDIES

- AP, lateral, and mortise view plain radiographs of the ankle should be obtained to rule out concomitant fractures or calcific changes of the Achilles tendon.
  - On a lateral view, the examiner should look for a disruption of the normal triangular fat pad seen anterior to the Achilles tendon (Kager triangle; **FIG 3**).
- Ultrasonography can provide a dynamic study of the tendon structure and accurately measure gapping of the ruptured tendon ends.
  - The quality of images is highly dependent on the equipment and operator (**FIG 4**).
- MRI is highly sensitive and specific in diagnosing Achilles tendon rupture.
  - It provides valuable information about tendon degeneration or other associated injuries (**FIG 5**).
  - MRI was found to be superior to ultrasound in diagnostic specificity of chronic Achilles tendinopathy.[2]

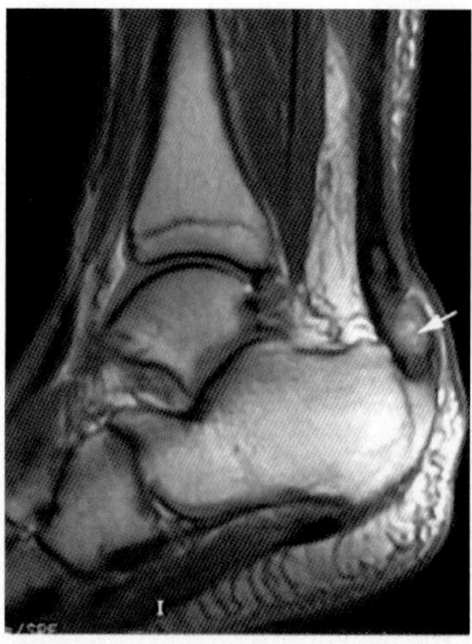

FIG 5 • Ankle MRI (T1-weighted image) showing a distal Achilles tendon rupture.

DIFFERENTIAL DIAGNOSIS

- Rupture of the medial gastrocnemius
- Plantaris tendon rupture
- Baker cyst rupture
- Acute deep venous thrombosis
- Leg or calf contusion
- Tibia distal shaft fracture
- Posterior ankle impingement or symptomatic os trigonum

NONOPERATIVE MANAGEMENT

- Nonoperative treatment usually entails casting the foot in plantarflexion to allow apposition of the tendon ends, followed by casting the foot in neutral. Treatment continues for 12 weeks.
  - In a recent retrospective review, early recognition and initiation of nonoperative management within 48 hours of injury resulted in a successful functional outcome that was comparable to surgical repairs.[17]
  - Nonetheless, nonoperative treatment carries up to threefold increase in the rerupture rate and may result in weakness of push-off secondary to healing of the tendon in a lengthened position.
- Nonoperative treatment is often reserved for elderly, sedentary patients and also for patients with diabetes, tobacco use, and steroid use who are at high risk for surgical wound healing.[4]

SURGICAL MANAGEMENT

- Operative repair and early mobilization is considered the treatment of choice for younger patients with active lifestyles. In most patients, it is established that operative repair results in a favorable functional outcome with a significantly lower rerupture rate.
- Numerous surgical techniques have been described, including open repair, percutaneous repair, limited open repair, and open repair with augmentation.[1]
  - In a comprehensive review of the recent literature, Wong et al[18] concluded that in terms of outcome and the complication rate, the best results could be achieved with open repair and early mobilization.

Preoperative Planning

- Plain radiographs are reviewed and any displaced fractures are treated at the same surgical sitting.
- MRIs are reviewed to evaluate the quality of tendon tissue and the level of rupture and to measure the tendon gap if present.
- Severe tendon degeneration or a large gap may require a larger incision or tendon lengthening or augmentation; the surgeon should take this into account during preoperative patient counseling.

Positioning

- Achilles tendon repair is performed with the patient prone (**FIG 6**). We prefer to use a Wilson frame and commercially available foam head rest.
- A thigh tourniquet is used for intraoperative hemostasis. A leg tourniquet is not recommended because it may tether the calf muscles and prevent intraoperative tendon apposition.
- Some surgeons prefer to drape both legs for intraoperative comparison and accurate restoration of the resting tendon length. The operated leg should be clearly marked.

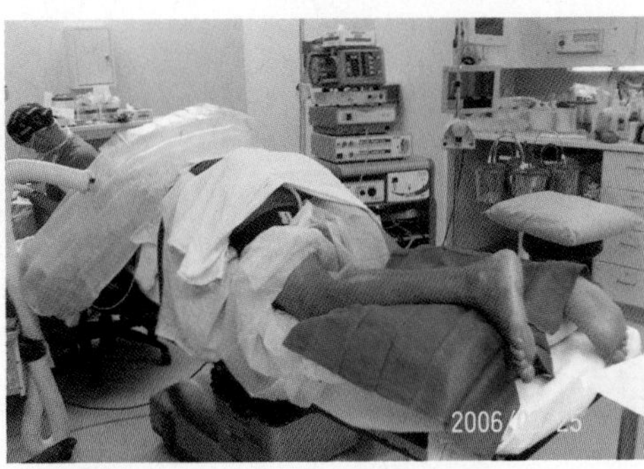

FIG 6 • Patient is in prone position with both legs prepared and draped for surgery.

Approach

- Open Achilles repair is usually performed through a longitudinal medial, midline, or lateral incision.
- Primary end-to-end repair is done with heavy nonabsorbable suture.
- Modified Bunnell, Kessler, Krackow, and triple-bundle techniques have been described.[5]
  - In a biomechanical study, Jaakkola et al[6] showed that the triple-bundle technique (**FIG 7**) provided the strongest suture repair. They credited its superior strength to the use of multiple strands and to tying the knots away from the repair site. However, the authors expressed concern over the large amount of suture material used and its possible negative effect on the vascularity of the tendon.
- At our institution, we have designed a modification of the Krackow technique in which the free ends of one suture are

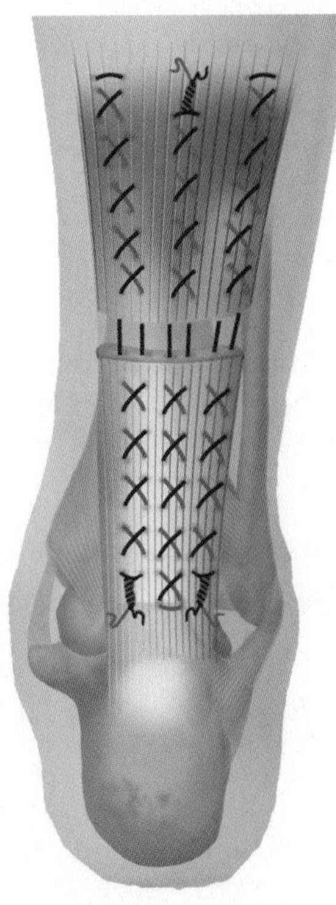

FIG 7 • Triple-bundle technique of Achilles repair.

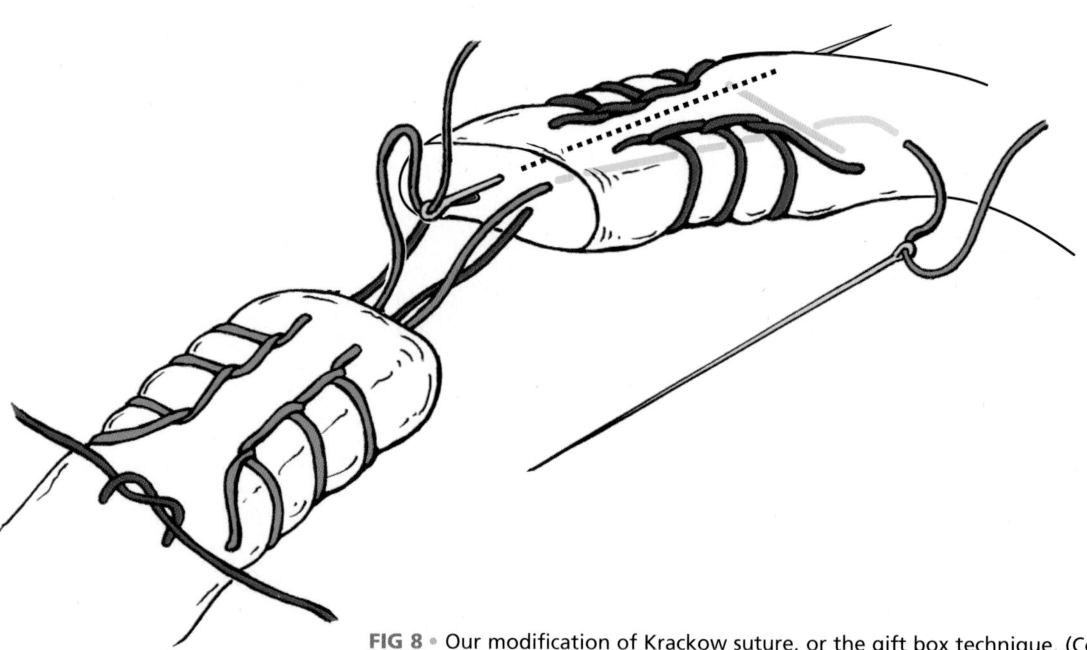

FIG 8 • Our modification of Krackow suture, or the gift box technique. (Copyright Sam Labib.)

passed peripherally to encircle the transverse limb of the opposite suture (**FIG 8**).

- We likened this scheme to wrapping a gift box and named it the gift box technique.
- We have performed biomechanical pull-out studies on 13 Achilles cadaveric pairs comparing the gift box technique to the standard Krackow suture and documented more than a twofold increase in suture pull-out strength.[12]
- We believe that the modification is simple to perform, minimizes suture material use, and preserves the vasculature of the healing tendon.

TECHNIQUES

INCISION

- A longitudinal incision over the medial border of the tendon provides excellent exposure and access to the plantaris tendon and avoids the sural nerve (**TECH FIG 1**).
  - Mobilize the thick skin and subcutaneous layer laterally, and take great care to preserve the paratenon.
  - Protect the sural nerve and lesser saphenous vein as they course lateral to the paratenon.
  - Enter the paratenon through a midline incision (away from the skin incision).
  - Limit dissection at the tendon–paratenon plane, especially anterior to the tendon, to preserve the vascular supply of the tendon.

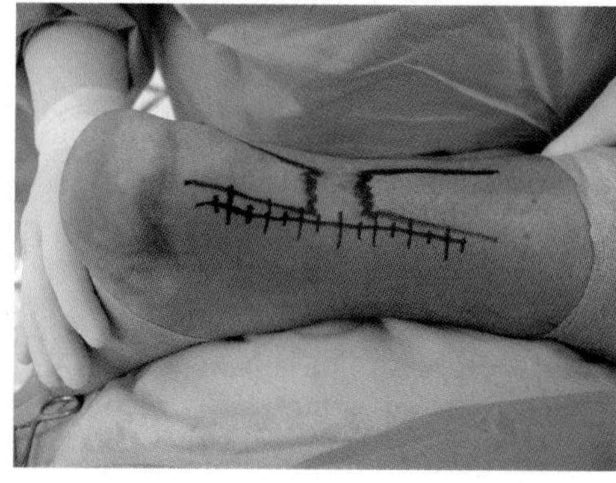

TECH FIG 1 • Medial longitudinal incision centered over the rupture site.

MODIFIED KRACKOW SUTURE (GIFT BOX) TECHNIQUE

- Débride the ends of the ruptured tendon in a limited manner.
- Two no. 2 fortified polyester sutures (Herculine, Linvatec) are used.
  - Four loop Krackow locking sutures[9] are passed on the medial side and four on the lateral side, avoiding the middle third of the tendon width.
  - Unlike the classic Krackow suture, we pass our transverse limb in the middle of the tendon as we transition from one side to the other (**TECH FIG 2**).
- Use straight Keith needles to pass the free suture ends across the rupture site into the opposite end of the tendon.

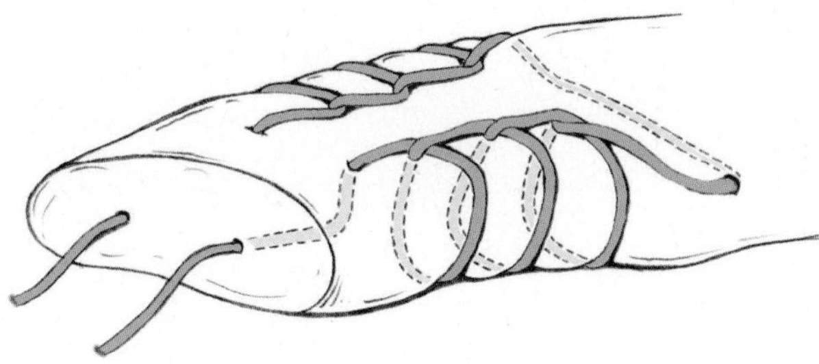

TECH FIG 2 • The transverse limb of the gift box suture is passed through tendon midsubstance. (Copyright Sam Labib.)

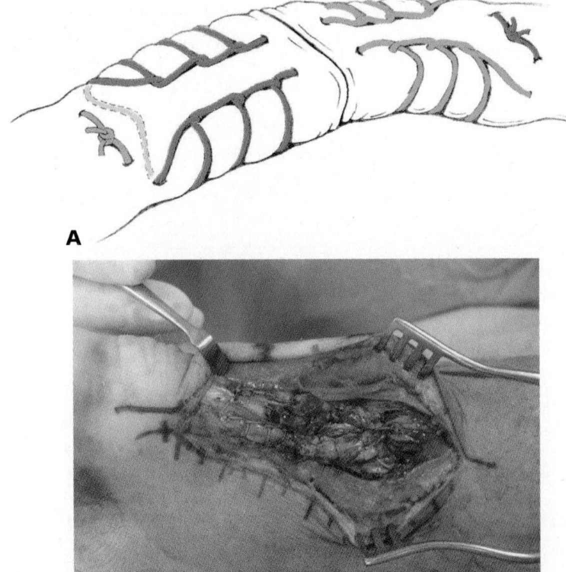

TECH FIG 3 • **A.** The gift box suture completed and tied. Note the tension created on the transverse limb of the suture, which helps tendon apposition. **B.** Intraoperative photograph of the completed gift box suture. (**A**, Copyright Sam Labib.)

  - Sutures should emerge one superficial and one deep to the transverse limb of the opposite Krackow suture (Fig 8).
  - Thus, four suture strands are passed across the rupture site.
- Tie the surgical knots away from the rupture site—in other words, proximal and distal to the Krackow suture.
  - Excellent apposition is usually achieved as the knots push on the transverse limbs of opposing sutures and the desired tendon length is recreated (TECH FIG 3).
- Use epitendinous running Prolene no. 3-0 suture to oversew the tendon ends together.
- Meticulously repair the paratenon with no. 3-0 braided polyglycolic absorbable suture (Vicryl, Ethicon) (TECH FIG 4).
  - This can be facilitated by placing the ankle in maximum plantarflexion to relax the tendon tissue.
  - We believe that midline placement of the paratenon incision facilitates its repair and minimizes the chance of skin tethering to the repaired tendon.
- Perform subcuticular skin closure with no. 4-0 monofilament absorbable suture (Monocryl, Ethicon).

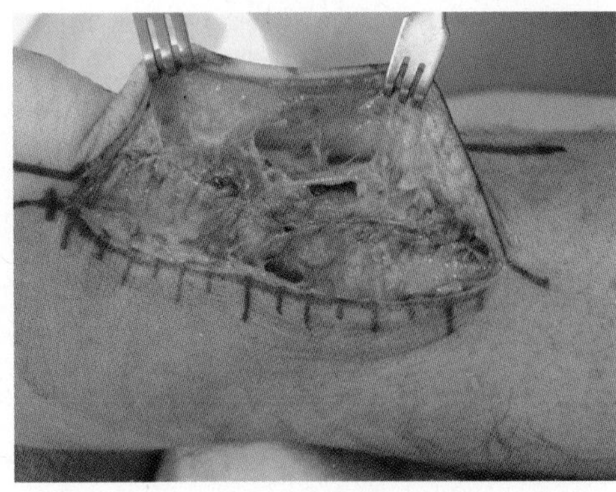

TECH FIG 4 • Intraoperative photo after closure of the Achilles paratenon.

TRIPLE-BUNDLE SUTURE TECHNIQUE

- Beskin et al popularized an open repair of the Achilles tendon using no. 1 nonabsorbable polyester suture (Ethibond, Ethicon).
- Three rows of sutures are placed, creating six strands of suture that are tied away from the rupture site (Fig 7).
- The technique provides the strongest suture repair available to date but is technically difficult to perform, requires a large amount of suture material, and may lead to vascular compromise of the tendon during healing.[6]

PRIMARY REPAIR WITH AUGMENTATION

- Multiple authors have advocated primary augmentation of Achilles repair, with some preferring plantaris tendon, flexor tendon (TECH FIG 5), or artificial tendon implants.[13]
- A study by Jessing and Hansen,[7] however, found no evidence that such augmentation was superior to a nonaugmented end-to-end repair.

TECHNIQUES

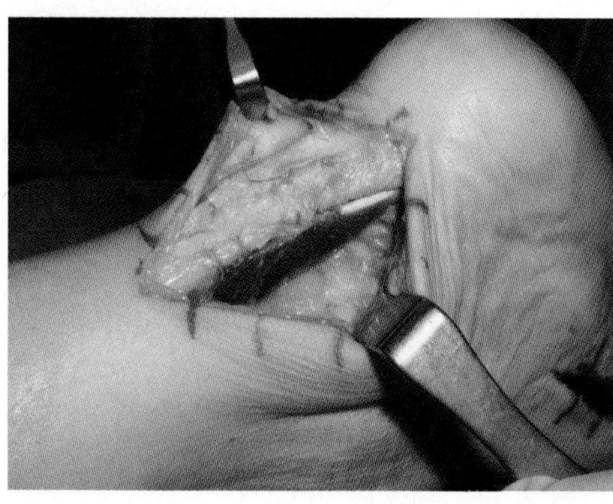

TECH FIG 5 • Flexor hallucis longus tendon used to augment Achilles tendon repair.

PEARLS AND PITFALLS

Clinical evaluation	■ Diagnosis of complete rupture can be missed due to other active ankle flexors. ■ Ultrasonography or MRI may be needed to verify the diagnosis. ■ Care is taken to evaluate concomitant bony or tendon injury.
Nonoperative treatment	■ Should be initiated early, with cast application in plantarflexion preferably within 48 hours of injury. ■ Tendon gapping should be looked for and corrected. ■ Strongly considered for patients with poor skin or vascular compromise. Poorly controlled diabetes and tobacco or steroid use are relative contraindications for surgical treatment.
Approach	■ Midline incisions may result in a painful scar. ■ A lateral incision places the sural nerve at an added risk of injury. ■ Poor tissue handling may result in wound slough or dehiscence.
Tendon tension	■ Aggressive trimming of tendon ends may result in significant shortening and undue tension on the repair. ■ Use the contralateral limb as your guide to appropriate restoration of resting tendon length.
Suture technique	■ Avoid strangulating locking suture techniques, which may compromise tendon healing and promote scar formation. ■ Paratenon preservation and repair is mandatory for tendon repair and healing.

POSTOPERATIVE CARE

- Early functional mobilization was shown to yield improved tendon healing.[8]
- A posterior splint holding the site in mild plantarflexion is used for 14 days. Labib et al showed no significant difference in tension when the repaired tendon was positioned in 30, 20, and 10 degrees of plantarflexion.[11]
- Wound inspection is done, a non–weight-bearing cast boot is applied with heel lifts, and daily active range of motion is started.
- The patient is kept non–weight-bearing for a total of 6 weeks, but recent evidence suggest that weight bearing can be started before 6 weeks with no added risk of rerupture or gap formation.[8]
- The patient is allowed gradual return to full weight bearing over an additional 6 weeks.
- At 3 months, full weight bearing is permitted, with low-impact activities.
- At 6 months, full activities are permitted as tolerated.

OUTCOMES

- Based on a literature review, there is overwhelming support for open operative repair and early functional mobilization of Achilles tendon rupture in healthy active individuals. On average, a success rate of 85% to 95% is often quoted.[5]
- Wong et al[1] conducted an extensive literature review and concluded that the best results with regard to outcome and complication rate could be achieved with open repair and early mobilization.
- Most authors agree that surgical repair provides a significantly lower rerupture rate and better functional outcome, but these advantages should be weighed against the possible risks of wound dehiscence or infection.
- Recent studies showed a significant temporal improvement in surgical outcome coupled with a net decrease in surgical complications.[5]

COMPLICATIONS

- Delayed or missed diagnosis
- Intraoperative devitalization of tendon, leading to wound infection
- Failure to preserve and repair the paratenon, leading to scarring and skin tethering
- Sural nerve injury and neuroma formation
- Wound dehiscence
- Tendon rerupture
- Loss of ankle motion
- Calf weakness

REFERENCES

1. Assal M, Jung M, Stern R, et al. Limited open repair of Achilles tendon ruptures: a technique with a new instrument and findings of a prospective multicenter study. J Bone Joint Surg Am 2002;84A:161–170.
2. Aström M, Gentz CF, Nilsson P, et al. Imaging in chronic Achilles tendinopathy: a comparison of ultrasonography, magnetic resonance imaging and surgical findings in 27 histologically verified cases. Skel Radiol 1996;25:615–620.
3. Bhandari M, Guyatt GH, Siddiqui F, et al. Treatment of acute Achilles tendon ruptures; a systemic overview and meta-analysis. Clin Orthop Relat Res 2002;400:190–200.
4. Bruggeman NB, Turner NS, Dahm DL, et al. Wound complications after open Achilles tendon repair: an analysis of risk factors. Clin Orthop Relat Res 2004;427:63–66.
5. Coughlin MJ. Surgery of the Foot and Ankle, 7th ed. Mosby, 1999: 835–850.
6. Jaakkola JI, Hutton WC, Beskin JL, et al. Achilles tendon rupture repair: biomechanical comparison of the triple bundle technique versus the Krackow locking loop technique. Foot Ankle Int 2000; 21:14–17.
7. Jessing P, Hansen E. Surgical treatment of 102 tendo Achilles ruptures: suture or tenontoplasty? Acta Chir Scand 1975;141: 370–377.
8. Kangas J, Pajala A, Ohtonen P, et al. Achilles tendon elongation after tendon repair; a randomized comparison of 2 postoperative regimens. Am J Sports Med 2007;35:59–64.
9. Krackow KA, Thomas SC, Jones LC. A new stitch for ligament-tendon fixation. J Bone Joint Surg Am 1986;68A:764–766.
10. Labib SA, Gould JS. Achilles tendonitis. Orthopedic Board Review Hyperguide, 2000. www.ortho.hyperguide.com/Sports Medicine.
11. Labib SA, Hage WD, Sutton K, et al. The effect of ankle position on the tension in the Achilles tendon before and after operative repair: a biomechanical cadaver study. Foot Ankle Int 2007;28:478–481.
12. Labib SA, Rolf RH, Dacus R, et al. The "giftbox" open repair of the Achilles tendon: a modification of the traditional Krackow technique that increases the strength of the repair. Foot Ankle Int 2009;30: 410–414.
13. Maffulli N. Rupture of the Achilles tendon, current concept review. J Bone Joint Surg Am 1999;81A:1019–1036.
14. Maffulli N, Barrass V, Ewen SWB. Light microscopic histology of Achilles tendon ruptures: a comparison with unruptured tendons. Am J Sports Med 2000;28:857–863.
15. Sarrafian SK. Anatomy of the Foot and Ankle, 2nd ed. Philadelphia Lippincott, 1993.
16. Webb J, Moorjani N, Radford M. Anatomy of the sural nerve and its relation to the Achilles tendon. Foot Ankle Int 2000;21:475–477.
17. Weber M, Niemann M, Lanz R, et al. Nonoperative treatment of acute rupture of the Achilles tendon: results of a new protocol and comparison with operative treatment. Am J Sports Med 2003;31: 685–691.
18. Wong J, Barrass V, Maffulli N. Quantitative review of operative and nonoperative management of Achilles tendon ruptures. Am J Sports Med 2002;30:565–575.

Chapter 106

Limited Open Repair of Achilles Tendon Ruptures: Perspective 1

Mathieu Assal

DEFINITION

- Achilles tendon ruptures usually occur 3 to 4 cm above the calcaneal tuberosity.
- Although most injuries are "complete" ruptures, "partial" injuries have been described.

ANATOMY

- The Achilles tendon is about 9 cm long and 0.9 cm in diameter.
- The proximal part is composed of the gastrocnemius and soleus tendons.
- The distal portion inserts onto the posterior aspect of the tuberosity of the calcaneus.
- The Achilles tendon is surrounded by the paratenon, a delicate envelope that contributes to tendon vascularization.
- There is an area of poor vascularity located between 2.5 cm and 5 cm above the calcaneal tuberosity.

PATHOGENESIS

- Rupture of the Achilles tendon is a common injury among high-level athletes, recreational sports enthusiasts, or even sedentary individuals.
- Rupture of the Achilles tendon usually occurs during forceful dorsiflexion of the ankle.
- Patients often describe hearing or feeling a "pop" in the back of their ankle.
- Intratendinous degeneration can be found histologically.
- Association with cortisone and fluoroquinolone use has been demonstrated.
- This is typically a lesion of middle age, with peak incidence during the third and fourth decades.

NATURAL HISTORY

- There is a great deal of controversy concerning the treatment of an acute rupture of the Achilles tendon.
- Conservative treatment is found to have a higher rate of tendon rerupture and loss of strength because the tendon heals in an elongated position.
- The major factor motivating surgeons to use a nonoperative approach appears to be avoiding the wound complications that occur with an operative repair.
- An increasing number of reports in the literature have tended to favor operative treatment of an acute rupture of the Achilles tendon.
- The exact type of operative procedure and the postoperative regimen remain controversial.[1–9] Mini-invasive techniques are associated with a lower complication rate.[10–13]
- If soft tissue complications are avoided, excellent functional results and full return to previous activity can be expected.

PHYSICAL FINDINGS

- Physical examination reveals moderate swelling about the posterior aspect of the ankle.
- Patients are usually able to walk, although with moderate pain.
- With the patient prone, spontaneous excess dorsiflexion of the involved ankle is noted.
- In most cases a tender defect ("soft spot") can be palpated in the Achilles tendon between 2.5 and 5 cm proximal to its insertion into the calcaneal tuberosity.
- The Thompson squeeze test is positive.
- Patients have difficulty walking on their toes or rising up on their heels.

IMAGING AND DIAGNOSTIC STUDIES

- History and physical examination are sufficient to confirm the diagnosis.
- Since these injuries occur in a traumatic setting, plain radiographs of the ankle are strongly advised.
- There have been many reports of associated ankle fractures (medial malleolus).[14]
- Calcaneal (tuberosity) avulsion will appear on the lateral view.
- Ultrasound and MRI are not required for the diagnosis of Achilles tendon rupture but may be of value when the diagnosis is questionable.

DIFFERENTIAL DIAGNOSIS

- Ankle sprain
- Ankle fracture
- Tennis leg (gastrocnemius tear)
- Acute paratenonitis
- Calcaneal (tuberosity) avulsion
- Plantaris tendon rupture

NONOPERATIVE MANAGEMENT

- Nonoperative treatment of acute Achilles tendon ruptures involves prolonged immobilization.
- Prolonged immobilization is associated with musculoskeletal changes (atrophy), increased time necessary for rehabilitation, and delayed return to work and preinjury activities.
- In randomized studies the rerupture rate has been found to be much higher in the nonoperative group.
- However, nonoperative treatment avoids surgical complications.
- Nonoperative treatment should be considered in elderly patients with limited functional expectations, patients with significant tobacco or alcohol addictions, patients receiving chronic cortisone treatment, patients with vascular disease, and patients with severe comorbidities such as renal failure.

Indications and Contraindications

- The indication for this technique is an acute (less than 3 weeks) Achilles tendon rupture occurring between 2.0 and 7.0 cm above the tuberosity of the calcaneus.
- Greater than 90 percent of ruptures of the Achilles tendon occur in the area between 2 and 8 cm above the calcaneal tuberosity.[15]
  - We believe that ruptures occurring more than 8 cm above the tuberosity (muscular ruptures) can be treated nonoperatively, while ruptures occurring less than 2 cm from the tuberosity necessitate fixation directly to bone.
- Contraindications include chronic rupture greater than 3 weeks in duration, previous local surgery, steroid use, open ruptures and lacerations greater than 6 hours in duration, complex open ruptures with soft tissue defects, and ruptures not occurring between 2 and 8 cm above the tuberosity of the calcaneus.

SURGICAL MANAGEMENT

Preoperative Planning

- Plain films should be reviewed for fracture, avulsion, and calcific tendinopathy.
- All imaging studies are reviewed.
- An examination under anesthesia should be performed before positioning the patient to reconfirm the side of injury.

Positioning

- The patient is placed prone on the operating table.
- A tourniquet is applied around the upper thigh.
- Both legs are included in preparation and draping to compare Achilles tendon tension and spontaneous plantarflexion intraoperatively.
- Plastic draping is not used (the technique involves percutaneous steps).
- Patients receive antibiotic prophylaxis.

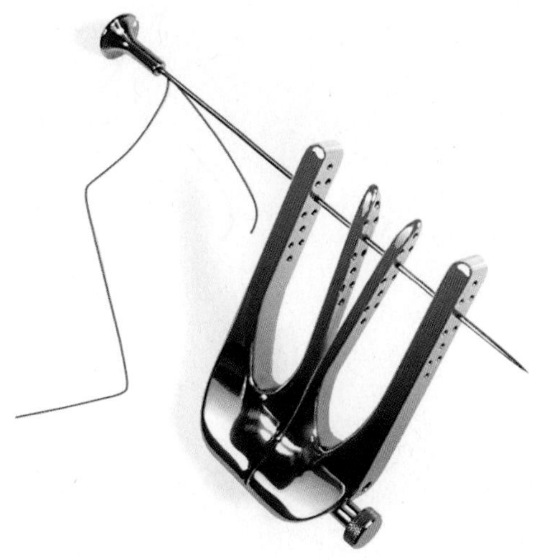

FIG 1 • The Achillon® instrument, with a straight needle and suture passed through one of the levels of holes.

Instrumentation

- The Achillon (Newdeal, Integra Life Science) was designed by this author and is made of either a rigid polymer or stainless steel (**FIG 1**).
- It is designed to guide the passage of the sutures.
- It is composed of a pair of internal branches connected to a pair of external branches, with each branch having a line of apertures at the same level to allow easy and accurate passage of the sutures through all four branches.
- The two internal branches are at an 8-degree angle to each other, following the V-shaped anatomic form of the tendon.
- A micrometric screw allows for varying the opening of the branches according to tendon morphology.
- A straight needle with its attached suture is used with a needle driver, designed to provide a larger support surface to push the needle through the soft tissues and at the same time protect the surgeon by preventing perforation of the glove from the end of the needle.

TECHNIQUES

- Palpate the site of injury, represented by the gap or soft spot (**TECH FIG 1A**).
- The incision is paratendinous and medial (**TECH FIG 1B**), beginning at the soft spot and extending about 2.0 cm proximally.
- Gently retract the skin and subcutaneous tissue with hooks and identify the paratenon (**TECH FIG 2A**).
- Carefully open the sheath and tag each edge with a stay suture (**TECH FIG 2B**).
- Identify both stumps of the ruptured tendon (**TECH FIG 3A**) and carefully note the exact site of rupture.
- Introduce the Achillon in the closed position under the paratenon in a proximal direction, holding the tendon stump with a small clamp under the instrument (**TECH FIG 3B**).
- The tendon stump is located between the two internal branches (**TECH FIG 3C**).
- As the instrument is introduced, progressively widen it, holding the tendon stump firmly with the clamp.
- Confirm the position of the guide by external palpation; you should feel the tendon between the central (internal) branches of the instrument.
- Pass three sutures from lateral to medial, usually beginning with the most proximal hole of the instrument (**TECH FIG 4A,B**).
- Hold the end of each suture with a small clamp to keep them separate from each other.
- Slowly withdraw the instrument while progressively closing the branches (**TECH FIG 5A**).
- This maneuver results in the sutures sliding from an extracutaneous position to a peritendinous position, and thus the tendon itself is the only tissue held by the sutures (**TECH FIG 5B**).
- Apply traction to the three suture pairs to ensure they are firmly anchored in the tendon, and individually clamp them to prevent any confusion.
- Perform the same sequence on the distal stump: introduce the instrument under the tendon sheath and push it until it touches the calcaneus (**TECH FIG 6A**).

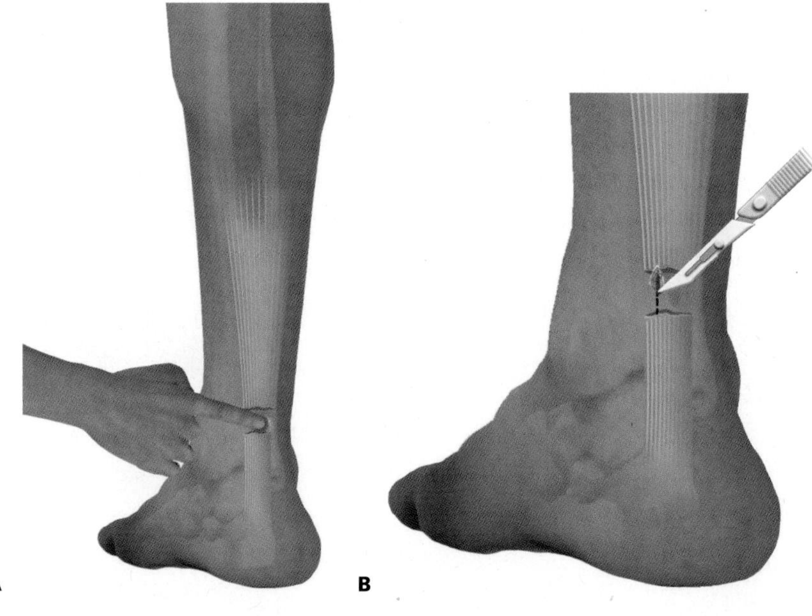

TECH FIG 1 • Illustration showing the skin incision, begun at the gap or soft spot (**A**), paratendinous and medial, and extended one and one-half to two centimeters proximally (**B**).

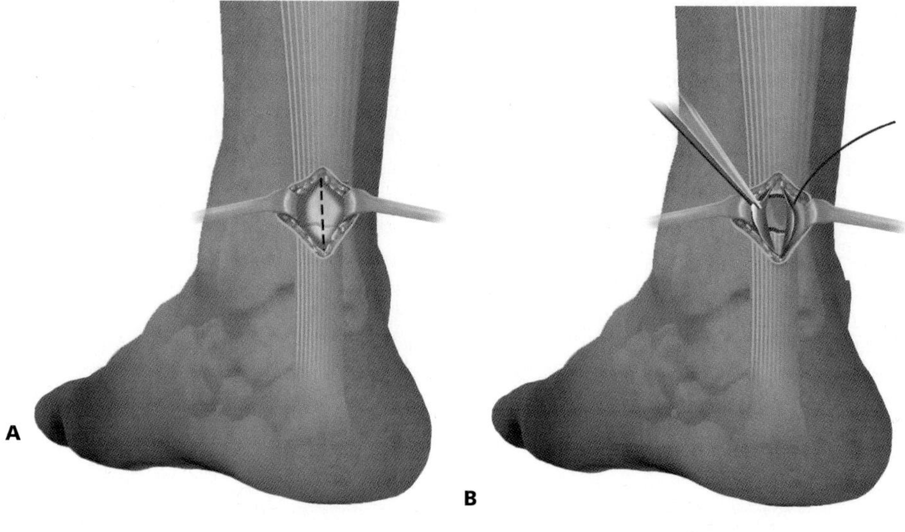

TECH FIG 2 • Illustration showing the sheath opened longitudinally in the midline (**A**) and a stay suture in place (**B**).

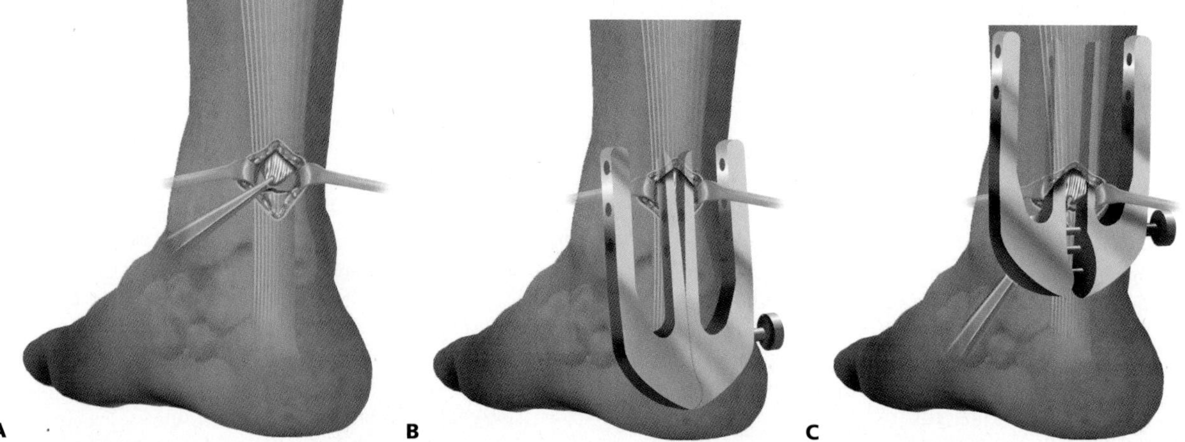

TECH FIG 3 • Illustration showing the forceps grasping the proximal tendon stump (**A**), and introduction of the instrument proximally under the paratenon (**B,C**).

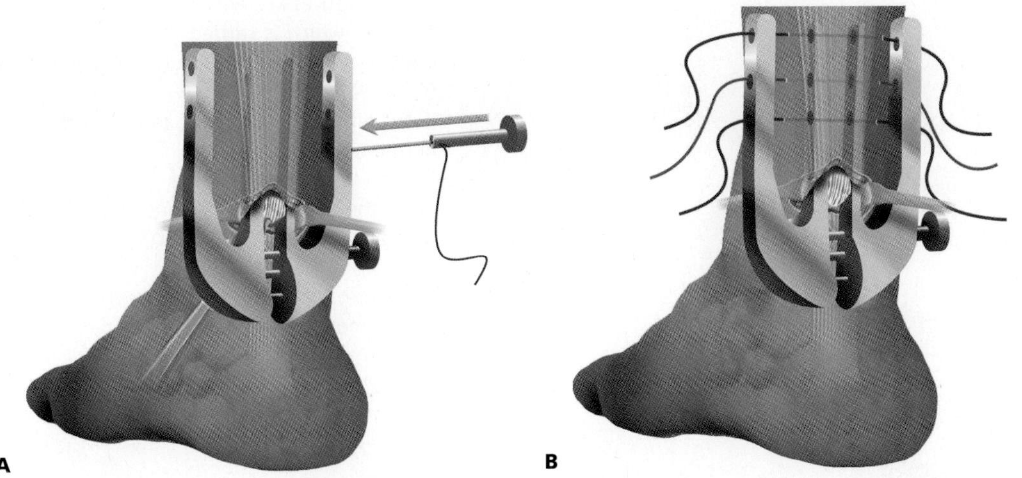

TECH FIG 4 • Illustration showing introduction of the first needle (**A**), and illustration showing all three sutures in the proximal tendon (**B**).

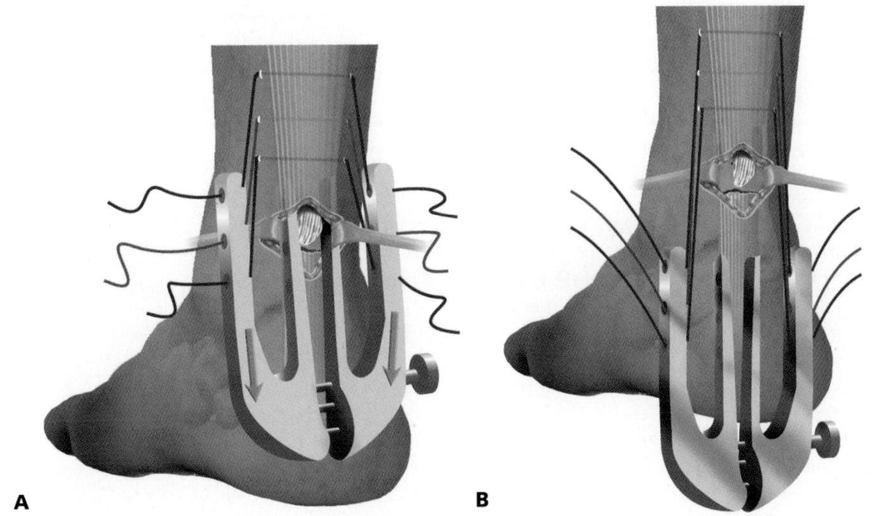

TECH FIG 5 • Illustration showing the instrument being withdrawn (**A**) bringing the sutures from an extra-cutaneous to a peritendinous position (**B**).

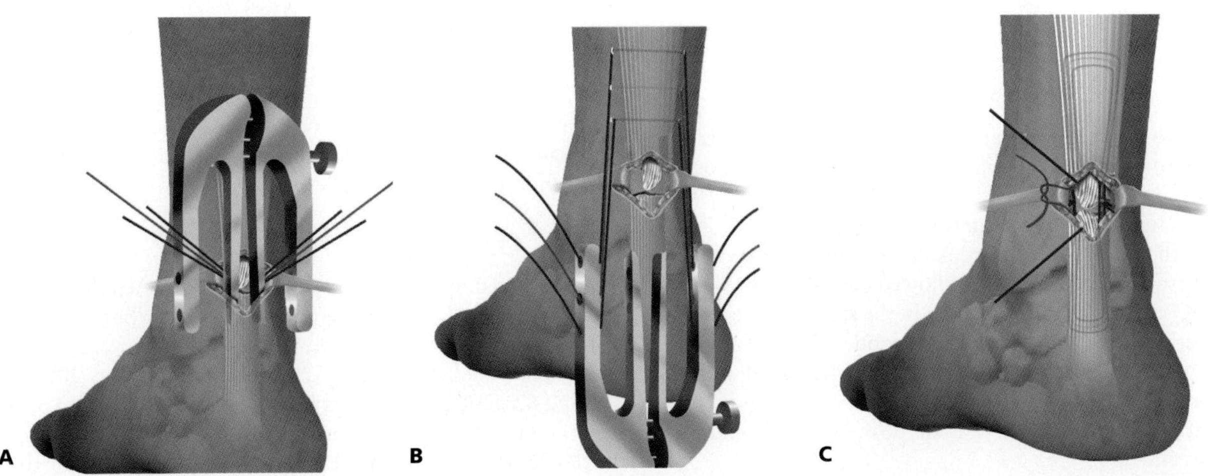

TECH FIG 6 • Illustration showing the exact same sequence performed on the distal stump. (**A**) Introduce the instrument under the tendon sheath and push it until it touches the calcaneus. (**B**) Illustration showing the sutures organized for tightening. (**C**) Illustration showing the tendon reduction performed under direct vision, confirming apposition of the tendon ends. *(continued)*

TECHNIQUES

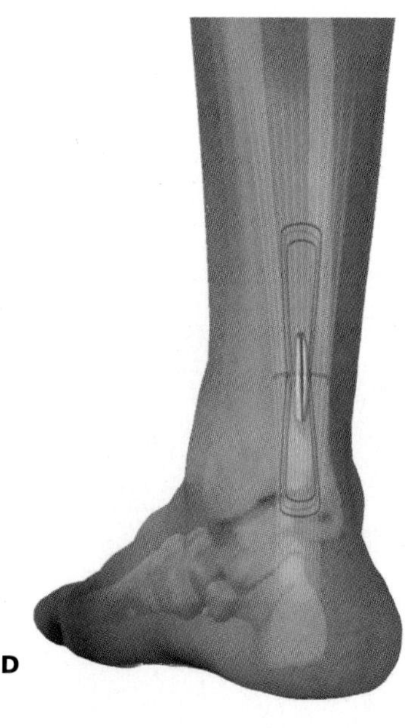

TECH FIG 6 • *(continued)* (**D**) Illustration showing closure of the skin with intradermal sutures.

- All the sutures are now organized for tightening (**TECH FIG 6B**), which is carried out with corresponding pairs, and the tendon reduction is under direct visual control (**TECH FIG 6C**).
- If it is difficult to ascertain tendon length and reduction because the ends are too frayed, compare the tendon tension to the opposite leg.
- Close the tendon sheath, and then the skin with intradermal sutures (**TECH FIG 6D**).
- No drain is used.
- Apply a splint holding the ankle in 30 degrees of flexion before moving or waking up the patient.

PEARLS AND PITFALLS

- Be sure to note the soft spot or gap in the tendon to accurately plan the site of incision.
- Carefully open the paratenon and tag with stay sutures.
- Note exact site of rupture.
- Hold tendon stump with clamp while introducing Achillon instrument under the paratenon.
- Progressively open the instrument as it is introduced.
- After suture insertion carefully withdraw instrument while branches are progressively closed.
- Carefully organize all sutures for tying with ankle placed in equinus.
- Tendon reduction must be carefully controlled under direct vision.
- Orthosis is applied prior to moving or waking the patient.
- Failure to accurately locate the exact site of rupture prior to making incision.
- Failure to tag the paratenon with stay sutures.
- Failure to hold tendon stump with clamp while introducing Achillon instrument.
- Failure to progressively open the Achillon instrument as it is being inserted.
- Failure to keep each of the three sutures separate from each other.
- Failure to apply traction to the three suture pairs to ensure that they are firmly anchored in the tendon.
- Failure to individually clamp each of the three suture pairs to avoid confusion.
- Failure to control tendon reduction under direct visual control.
- Failure to apply orthosis prior to moving or waking the patient.

POSTOPERATIVE CARE

- Low-molecular-weight heparin (subcutaneous administration) is used to prevent deep vein thrombosis for 3 weeks postoperatively.
- Our early functional rehabilitation program, carefully supervised by the physical therapist, is divided into four stages.
- For the first 2 weeks patients are allowed partial weight bearing (30 to 45 pounds) and maintained in the splint full time.
- Then gentle ankle range of motion (flexion and extension) is begun, as well as thigh muscle exercises and the use of a stationary bicycle.
- The goal is to reach a neutral ankle position by the end of the third week.
- After 3 weeks, full weight bearing is allowed with continuous use of the protective splint.
- At the end of 8 weeks the splint is discontinued and weight bearing is allowed without any external support.
- A more intensive program of ankle range of motion, stretching, and isometric and proprioceptive exercises is instituted.
- Jogging is allowed at 3 months, and more demanding sports at 5 months.

OUTCOMES

- This limited open procedure with use of the Achillon instrument provides the advantage of an open repair but avoids the soft tissue problems associated with open repair.
- We published a prospective multicenter study in 2002 including 82 patients.[12] Results showed no wound healing problems and no infections. No patient noted a sensory disturbance in the sural nerve distribution. All patients returned to their previous professional or sporting activities. The mean AOFAS score was 96 points (range 85 to 100 points).
- Complications occurred in three patients. Two of them were noncompliant and removed the orthosis within the first

Table 1 Concentric Peak Torque Measured with Isokinetic Dynamometry in Fifty Patients

Angular Velocity *(deg/sec)*	Mean Torque (and Standard Deviation) *(Nm)*	
	Injured Side	Unaffected Side
30	111.4 ± 19	118.9 ± 30
60	95.4 ± 19	101.3 ± 25

3 weeks postoperatively, thus disrupting the repair by a new injury. One patient fell 12 weeks after the surgery and sustained a rerupture. All three new injuries were repaired with an open surgical procedure.

- Isokinetic results: The concentric peak torque was performed with the ankle in plantarflexion at 30°/s and 60°/s of angular velocity, after correction for dominance. There was no significant difference between the injured and uninvolved sides (Table 1). Endurance testing at 120°/s also revealed no difference between sides.
- Three recent reports describe similar excellent results using the exact surgical technique and Achillon instrument, thus providing further confirmation of its important role in the repair of acute Achilles tendon ruptures.

COMPLICATIONS

- Disruption of the repair related to the patient's noncompliance with the rehabilitation protocol (before the third month postoperatively)
- Rerupture of the healed Achilles tendon (after the third month postoperatively)
- Sural nerve injury
- Infection
- Deep venous thrombosis

REFERENCES

1. Cetti R, Christensen SE, Ejsted R, et al. Operative versus nonoperative treatment of Achilles tendon rupture. A prospective randomized study and review of the literature. Am J Sports Med 1993;21: 791–799.
2. Leppilahti J, Orava S. Total Achilles tendon rupture. A review. Sports Med 1998;25:79–100.
3. Maffulli N. Rupture of the Achilles tendon. J Bone Joint Surg Am 1999;81:1019–1036.
4. Soldatis JJ, Goodfellow DB, Wilber JH. End-to-end operative repair of Achilles tendon rupture. Am J Sports Med 1997;25:90–95.
5. Bradley JP, Tibone JE. Percutaneous and open surgical repairs of Achilles tendon ruptures. A comparative study. Am J Sports Med 1990;18:188–195.
6. Mandelbaum BR, Myerson MS, Forster R. Achilles tendon ruptures. A new method of repair, early range of motion, and functional rehabilitation. Am J Sports Med 1995;23:392–395.
7. Haji A, Sahai A, Symes A, et al. Percutaneous versus open tendo Achillis repair. Foot Ankle Int 2004;25:215–218.
8. Cretnik A, Kosanovic M, Smrkolj V. Percutaneous versus open repair of the ruptured Achilles tendon: a comparative study. Am J Sports Med 2005;33:1369–1379.
9. Calder JD, Saxby TS. Independent evaluation of a recently described Achilles tendon repair technique. Foot Ankle Int 2006;27:93–96.
10. Ma GW, Griffith TG. Percutaneous repair of acute closed ruptured Achilles tendon: a new technique. Clin Orthop 1977;(128):247–255.
11. Kakiuchi M. A combined open and percutaneous technique for repair of tendo Achillis. Comparison with open repair. J Bone Joint Surg Br 1995;77:60–63.
12. Assal M, Jung M, Stern R, et al. Limited open repair of Achilles tendon ruptures: a technique with a new instrument and findings of a prospective multicenter study. J Bone Joint Surg Am 2002;84-A: 161–170.
13. Rippstein P, Easley M. "Mini-open" repair for acute Achilles tendon ruptures. Tech Foot Ankle Surg 2006;5:3–8.
14. Assal M, Stern R, Peter R. Fracture of the ankle associated with rupture of the Achilles tendon. Case report and review of the literature. J Ortho Trauma 2002;16:358–61.
15. DiStefano VJ, Nixon JE. Achilles tendon rupture: pathogenesis, diagnosis, and treatment by a modified pullout wire technique. J Trauma 1972;12:671–677.

Chapter 107 Mini-Open Achilles Tendon Repair: Perspective 2

Mark E. Easley, Marc Merian-Genast, and Mathieu Assal

DEFINITION

- Achilles tendon ruptures usually occur 3 to 4 cm above the calcaneal tuberosity.
- Although most injuries are "complete" ruptures, "partial" injuries have been described.
- An increasing number of reports in the recent literature favor operative treatment of a fresh rupture of the Achilles tendon; mini-invasive techniques are associated with a lower complication rate.

ANATOMY

- The Achilles tendon is about 9 cm long and 0.9 cm in diameter.
- The proximal part is composed of the gastrocnemius and soleus tendons.
- The distal portion inserts onto the posterior aspect of the tuberosity of the calcaneus.
- The Achilles tendon is surrounded by the paratenon, a delicate envelope that contributes to tendon vascularization.
- There is an area of poor vascularity located between 2.5 cm and 5 cm above the calcaneal tuberosity.

PATHOGENESIS

- Rupture of the Achilles tendon is a common injury among high-level athletes, recreational sports enthusiasts, or even sedentary individuals.
- Rupture of the Achilles tendon usually occurs during forceful dorsiflexion of the ankle.
- Patients often describe hearing or feeling a "pop" in the back of their ankle.
- Intratendinous degeneration can be found histologically.
- Association with cortisone and fluoroquinolone use has been demonstrated.
- This is typically a middle-age lesion, with peak incidence during the third and fourth decades.

NATURAL HISTORY

- There is a great amount of controversy concerning the treatment of an acute rupture of the Achilles tendon.
- Conservative treatment is found to have a higher rate of tendon rerupture and loss of strength due to the tendon healing in an elongated position.
- The major factor motivating surgeons to use a nonoperative approach appears to be avoiding the wound complications that occur with an operative repair.
- An increasing number of reports in the literature have tended to favor operative treatment of an acute rupture of the Achilles tendon.
- The exact type of operative procedure and the postoperative regimen remain controversial.
- If soft tissue complications are avoided, excellent functional results and full return to previous activity can be expected.

PATIENT HISTORY AND PHYSICAL FINDINGS

- Physical examination reveals moderate swelling about the posterior aspect of the ankle.
- Patients are usually able to walk, although with moderate pain.
- With the patient prone, spontaneous excess dorsiflexion of the involved ankle is noted.
- In most cases a tender defect ("soft spot") can be palpated in the Achilles tendon between 2.5 and 5 cm proximal to its insertion into the calcaneal tuberosity.
- The Thompson squeeze test is positive.
- Patients have difficulty walking on their toes or rising up on their heels.

IMAGING AND OTHER DIAGNOSTIC STUDIES

- History and physical examination are sufficient to confirm the diagnosis.
- Since these injuries occur in a traumatic setting, plain radiographs of the ankle are strongly advised.
- There have been many reports of associated ankle fractures (medial malleolus).
- Calcaneal (tuberosity) avulsion will appear on the lateral view.
- Ultrasound and MRI are not required for the diagnosis of Achilles tendon rupture but may be of value when the diagnosis is questionable.

DIFFERENTIAL DIAGNOSIS

- Ankle sprain
- Ankle fracture
- Tennis leg (gastrocnemius tear)
- Acute paratenonitis
- Calcaneal (tuberosity) avulsion
- Plantaris tendon rupture

NONOPERATIVE MANAGEMENT

- Nonoperative treatment of acute Achilles tendon ruptures involves prolonged immobilization.
- Prolonged immobilization is associated with musculoskeletal changes (atrophy), increased time necessary for rehabilitation, and delayed return to work and preinjury activities.
- In randomized studies the rerupture rate has been found to be much higher in the nonoperative group.
- However, nonoperative treatment avoids surgical complications.
- Nonoperative treatment should be considered in elderly patients with limited functional expectations, patients with significant tobacco/alcohol addictions, patients under chronic cortisone treatment, patients with vascular disease, and patients with severe comorbidities (eg, renal failure).

SURGICAL MANAGEMENT

Preoperative Planning

- Plain films should be reviewed for fracture, avulsion, and calcific tendinopathy.
- All imaging studies are reviewed.
- Examination under anesthesia should be performed before positioning the patient to reconfirm the side of injury.

Preoperative Planning

- The surgeon should have available the Achillon® (Integra Life Sciences, Plainsboro, NJ) Achilles tendon repair system and two sets each of no. 2 nonabsorbable suture.
- The surgeon should be prepared to convert to an open procedure should the mini-open procedure not be feasible (severe shear injury pattern to the tendon).

Positioning

- The patient is placed in the prone position.
- The patient's brachial plexi and ulnar nerves at the elbow are well protected from tension and untoward pressure, respectively.
- The patient's genitalia must be protected.
- We routinely use a thigh tourniquet applied with the patient still supine on the stretcher before placing the patient in the prone position on the operating table.
  - This facilitates effective tourniquet placement and avoids hyperextension of the back during tourniquet placement with the patient already prone.
- The feet are suspended over the end of the bed, with firm padding under the ankles.
- Both lower extremities are prepared into the operative field to determine the appropriate tension of the repair.

TECHNIQUES

APPROACH AND IDENTIFICATION OF RUPTURED TENDON ENDS

- Mini-open incision (TECH FIG 1A)
  - Make a longitudinal skin incision about 2 cm long at the level of the rupture.
    - The incision is longitudinal in the event the procedure has to be converted to a full open procedure.
- Divide the paratenon to gain control of the ruptured tendon ends (TECH FIG 1B).
  - The plantaris tendon may occasionally be intact despite complete Achilles tendon rupture (TECH FIG 1C).
  - Tag the two tendon ends with suture (TECH FIG 1D,E).

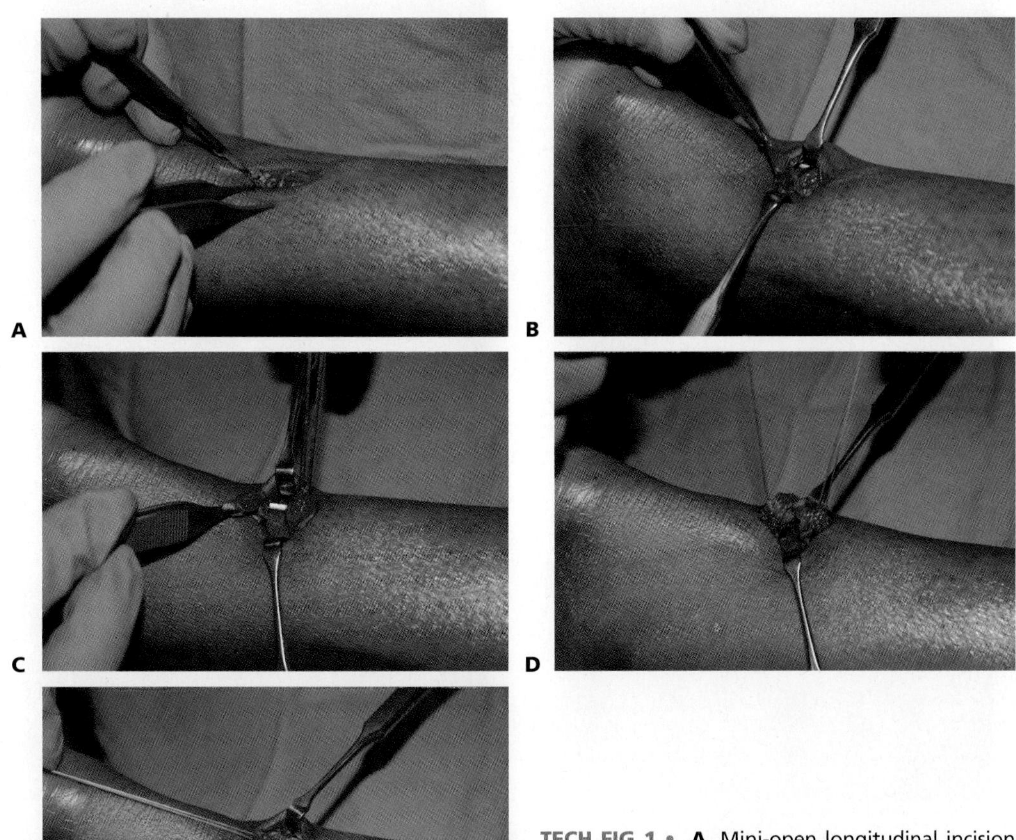

TECH FIG 1 • **A.** Mini-open longitudinal incision directly over tendon rupture. **B.** Paratenon is divided to gain access to tendon ends. **C.** The plantaris tendon may remain intact despite complete Achilles tendon rupture. **D.** Tag sutures are placed on the mobilized tendon ends. **E.** Tension is applied to tag sutures, approximating the tendon ends.

PLACING PERMANENT SUTURES IN PROXIMAL ASPECT OF THE RUPTURED TENDON

- Using the proximal tag sutures, apply tension to the proximal tendon stump.
- Place retractors within the paratenon to define the interval between the tendon and the paratenon.
- Advance the Achillon device within the paratenon on the medial and lateral aspects of the tensioned proximal tendon (**TECH FIG 2A,B**).
- Typically, the tendon is palpable between the arms of the Achillon device.
- In succession from closest to farthest from the rupture, pass three sutures through the tensioned proximal tendon (**TECH FIG 2C–F**).
- By retracting the Achillon device distally back into the wound, secure the sutures in the tendon, within the paratenon, and exiting within the wound (**TECH FIG 3A,B**).
  - Tension must be placed on the sutures before proceeding to the next step to ensure the sutures are properly anchored in the proximal tendon (**TECH FIG 3C**).
  - If the sutures pull out, repeat the three aforementioned steps, with careful palpation to be sure that the tendon is indeed between the arms of the Achillon device.

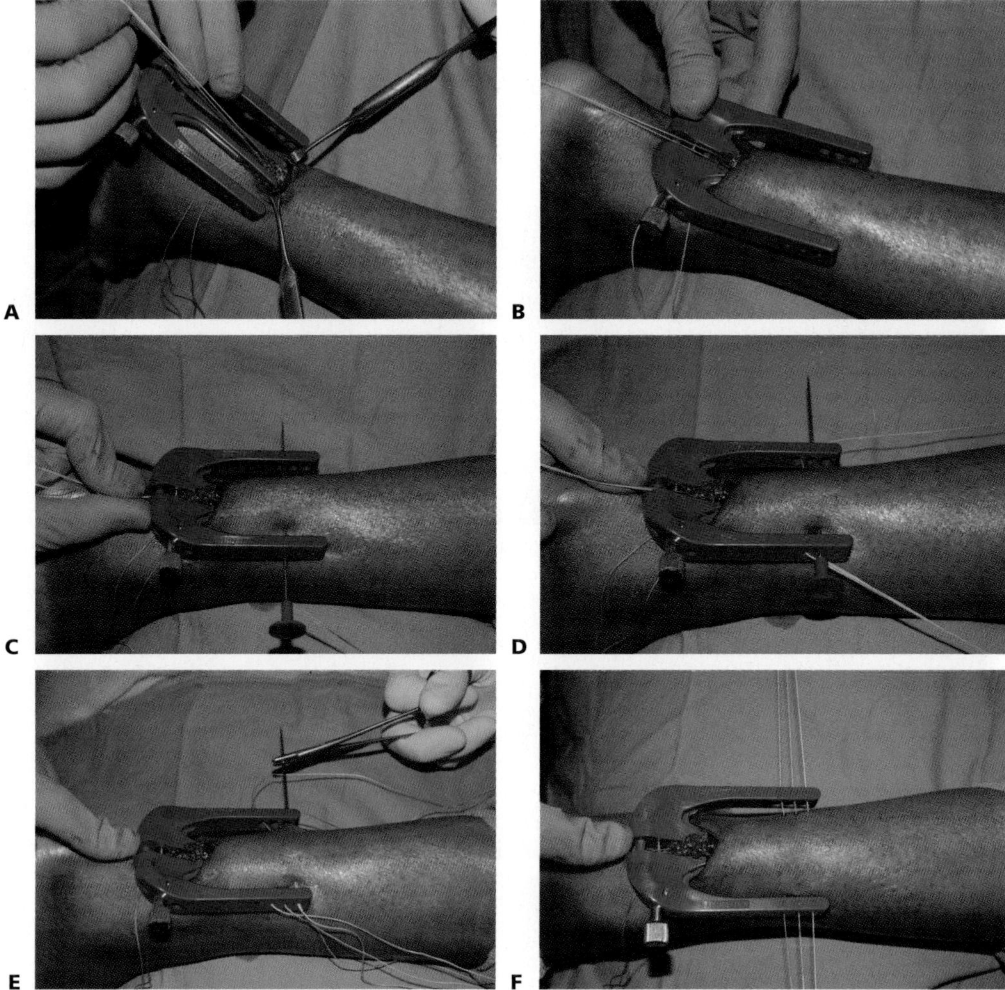

TECH FIG 2 • **A.** The Achillon device is advanced within the paratenon. **B.** Longitudinal tension placed on the tag suture while advancing the Achillon device facilitates optimal positioning of the tendon between the two arms of the Achillon device. **C.** The suture closest to the rupture is inserted first. Tension is maintained on the tag suture. **D.** The second suture is passed through the tendon. **E.** The third suture is passed. Tension is still maintained on the tag suture, and the tendon is centered between the two arms of the Achillon device that are within the paratenon. **F.** All three sutures are passed through the proximal tendon and organized.

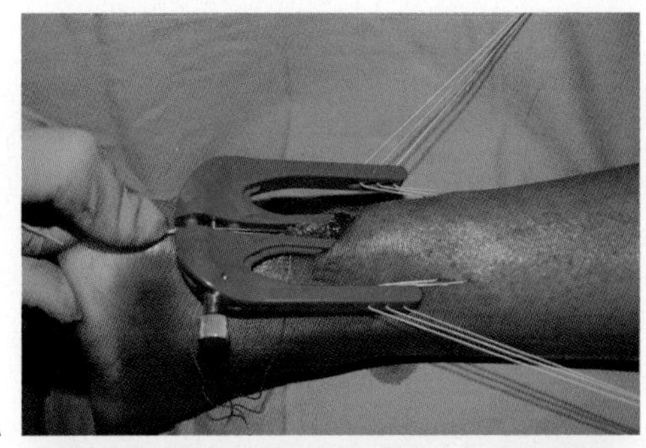

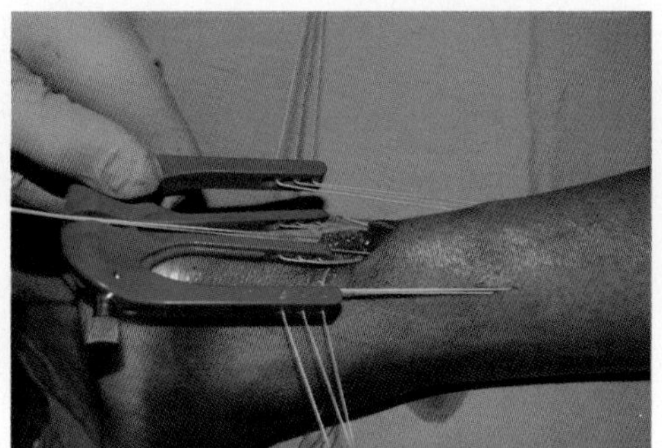

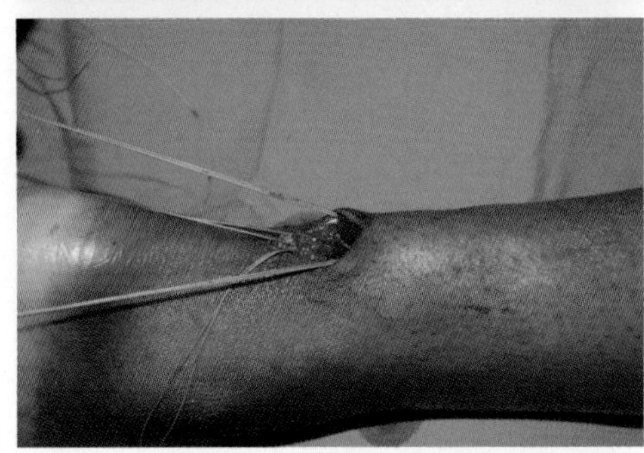

TECH FIG 3 • A, B. By retracting the device from the wound, the three sets of sutures remain in the tendon, are within the paratenon, and exit at the wound. **C.** Longitudinal traction is placed on the sutures to ensure that they are secure within the proximal tendon.

PLACING PERMANENT SUTURES IN DISTAL ASPECT OF THE RUPTURED TENDON

- This is essentially the mirror image of placing sutures in the proximal tendon.
- With distal ruptures, the Achillon device must be advanced as close to the Achilles insertion on the calcaneus as possible to optimize the sutures' purchase in tendon.
- Advance the Achillon device's inner arms on either side of the Achilles tendon, within the paratenon (**TECH FIG 4A**).
  - Palpate to be sure that the tendon is indeed between the two arms of the Achillon device.
- Place the three sutures (similar to those in the proximal tendon), from closest to farthest from the rupture, into the distal tendon, with tension applied to the tag sutures (**TECH FIG 4B–E**).
- Retract the Achillon device from the wound, thereby bringing the three sutures within the paratenon and into the wound, ready for repairing the rupture (**TECH FIG 4F**).
- To ensure that the purchase of the sutures in the distal tendon is satisfactory, apply forceful tension to the sutures.
  - Tension should plantarflex the ankle (**TECH FIG 4G**).
  - Should the sutures pull out, repeat the steps described above so that acceptable purchase of the sutures in the distal tendon is achieved. In our opinion, palpation of the tendon between the arms of the Achillon device is helpful.

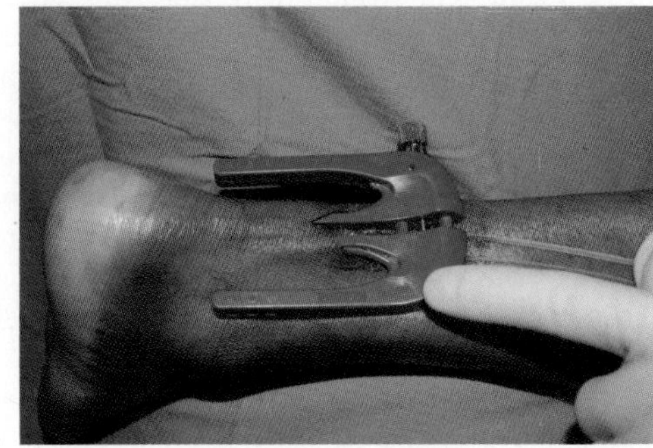

TECH FIG 4 • A. The Achillon device is advanced within the paratenon on the medial and lateral aspects of the distal tendon. *(continued)*

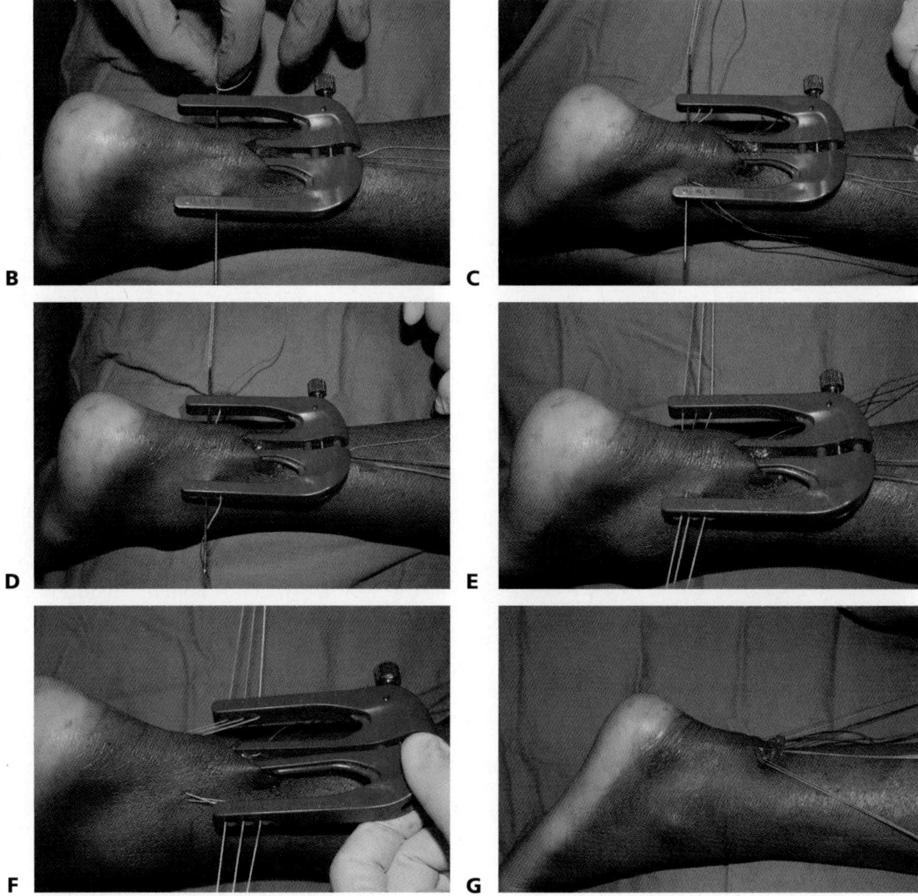

TECH FIG 4 • *(continued)* **B–E.** The three sutures are placed in the distal tendon and organized. **F.** The Achillon device is retracted from the wound so that the three sutures remain within the tendon, are within the paratenon, and exit at the wound. **G.** Longitudinal traction ensures that the sutures are secure within the distal tendon. Note the plantarflexion of the ankle with tension on the sutures.

TENDON REPAIR

- Approximate the two tendon ends by tensioning the sutures (**TECH FIG 5A**).
- The sutures must be carefully organized so that corresponding sutures are secured to one another.
- Passive plantarflexion of the ankle with a bump placed under the dorsum of the foot or maintained by an assistant takes tension off the tendon during repair.
- Secure the two sets of sutures closest to the rupture to one another first.
  - With tenson maintained on one side, secure the other side with a surgeon's knot (**TECH FIG 5B**).
  - Then secure the other side, applying tension first to remove residual slack in the suture (**TECH FIG 5C**).
- Repeat the suture technique described for the initial set of sutures for the other sets (**TECH FIG 5D**).
  - Secure the intermediate set of sutures to one another, followed by the sets farthest from the rupture.
  - If the sutures more distant from the rupture are overtensioned during the repair, then the tension gained with the previously secured sutures is forfeited. Therefore, overtensioning of each successive set of sutures is unnecessary.
- With the opposite, uninjured extremity prepared into the operative field, the resting tension of the repair may be compared to what is deemed physiologic (**TECH FIG 5E**).
  - Setting the resting tension of the repair slightly greater than that of the contralateral extremity is acceptable and, in our opinion, preferred.
  - Avoid undertensioning of the repair.
- As for flexor tendon repairs for the hand, we recommend reinforcing the repair with additional sutures directly at the rupture (**TECH FIG 5F**).
  - In our opinion, this is important because the mini-open technique described above only serves the function of an internal splint. When the repair site is directly palpated after repair with only the three sets of sutures, invariably there is mostly suture at the repair site and relatively little collagen.
  - We routinely perform this reinforcement with a running, absorbable suture.
  - This not only reinforces the tendon repair but tends to bring more tendon collagen directly to the repair site.
  - Place the running or alternatively multiple interrupted sutures circumferentially at the repair site.

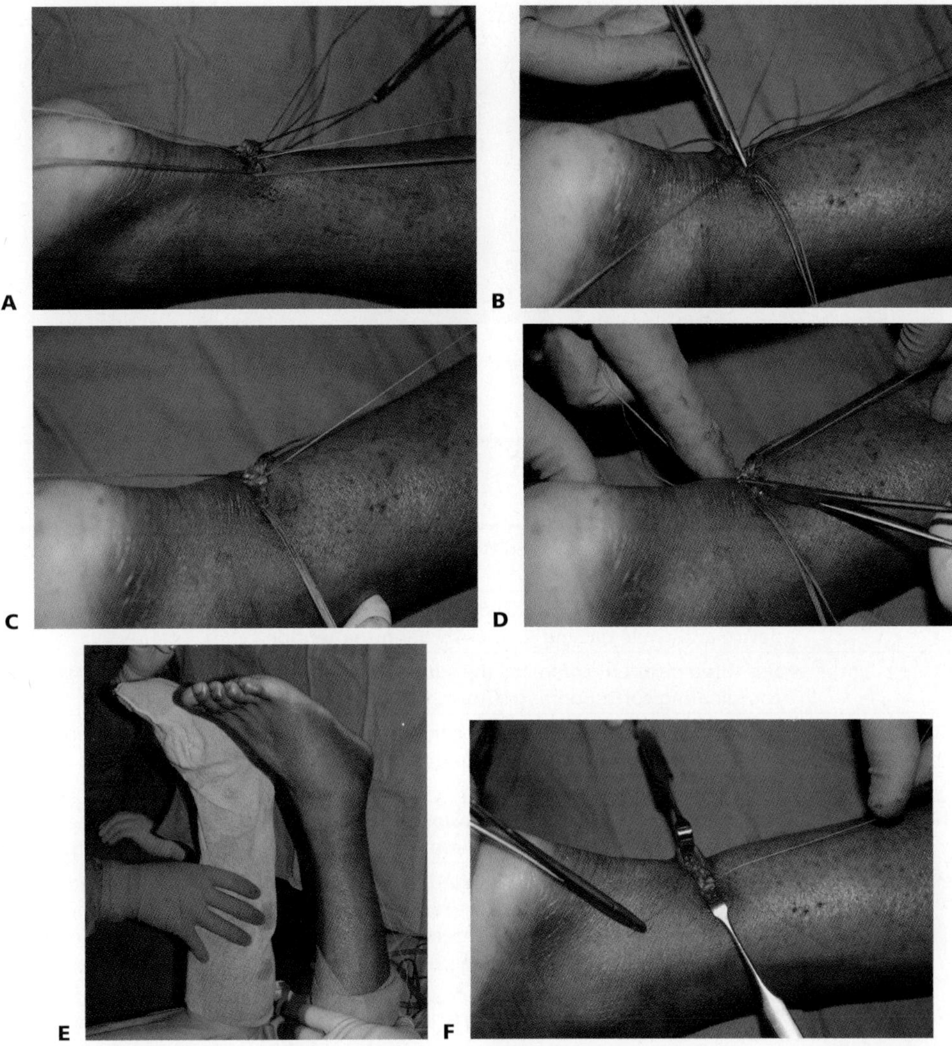

TECH FIG 5 • A. The ruptured tendon ends are approximated by tensioning both sets of sutures. **B.** One side of the corresponding sutures closest to the rupture is tied. Tension should be maintained on the other side of this set of sutures. **C.** After removing slack in the suture, the other side of this first set of sutures is tied. **D.** The second and third set of sutures are secured. Overtensioning of each successive set of sutures should be avoided since this will cause the previous set to lose its tension. **E.** The resting tension of the repair should match that of the other uninjured extremity. Preferably, the tension should be slightly greater in the repair. **F.** The repair is reinforced with a single running or multiple interrupted sutures directly at the rupture.

CLOSURE

- Repair the paratenon and fascial layer over the tendon to a "water-tight" closure (**TECH FIG 6A**).
- Reapproximate the subcutaneous layer and skin to a tensionless closure (**TECH FIG 6B,C**).

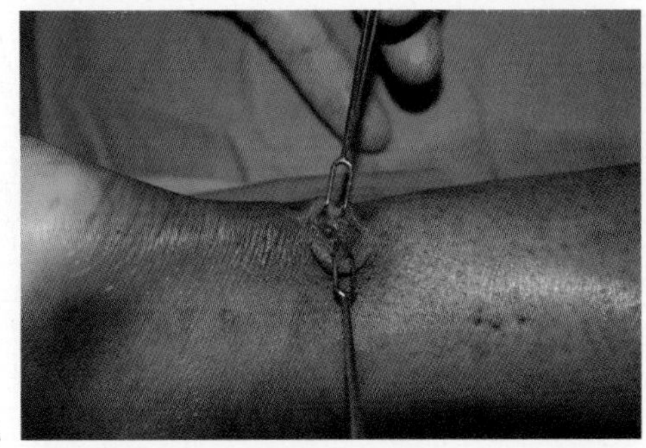

TECH FIG 6 • A. The paratenon and fascial layer are reapproximated. *(continued)*

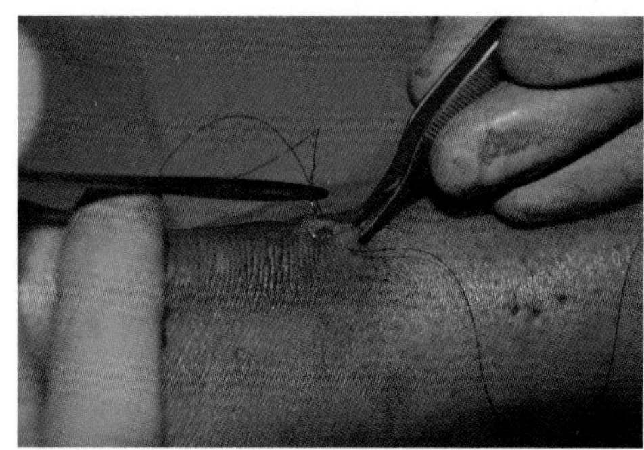
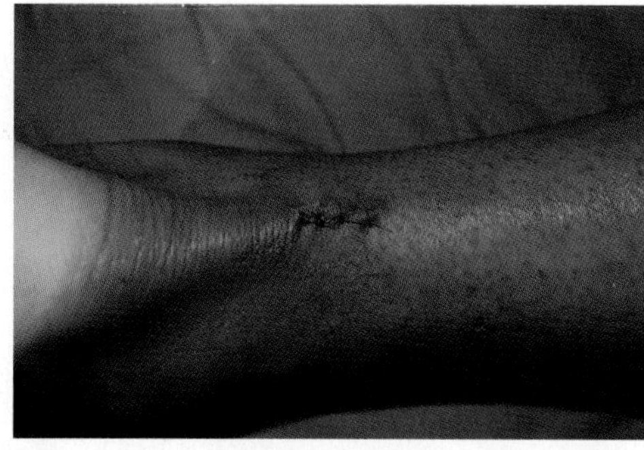

B C

TECH FIG 6 • *(continued)* **B, C.** The subcutaneous layer and skin are reapproximated to a tensionless closure.

PEARLS AND PITFALLS

Ensure that the tendon is between the arms of the Achillon device.	■ Palpate the tendon between the Achillon device arms during suture insertion.
Gain maximum purchase of the sutures in the tendon.	■ Use tag sutures in the ruptured tendon ends to apply tension while advancing the Achillon device and while passing sutures through the tendon.
Organize the sutures.	■ Use three different colors for the sutures on either side of the repair to facilitate coordinating corresponding sutures for the repair.
Ensure that the sutures are indeed secured in the tendon ends before repair.	■ Apply tension to the sutures after they have been passed through the tendon and have been organized within the paratenon; if they should pull out, then they will need to be passed again.
Optimal tensioning of the repair	■ In our experience, setting the tension slightly greater than the opposite extremity's physiologic resting tension is appropriate and leads to an optimal outcome.
Assess the rupture pattern.	■ Although mini-open, the tendon ends may be assessed through the limited approach. Occasionally, shear patterns of the rupture are not amenable to this technique and a more traditional open technique is warranted. We therefore recommend that the mini-open technique be performed through a short longitudinal incision that can easily be extended if necessary.

POSTOPERATIVE CARE

- Low-molecular-weight heparin (subcutaneous administration) is used for prophylactic anticoagulation for 3 weeks postoperatively.
- We institute an early functional rehabilitation program, carefully supervised by the physical therapist, which is divided into four distinct stages.
- For the first 2 weeks patients are allowed partial weight bearing (30 to 45 pounds) and maintained in the splint full time.
- Then gentle ankle range of motion (flexion and extension) is begun, as well as thigh muscle exercises and the use of a stationary bicycle.
- The goal is to reach a neutral ankle position by the end of the third week.
- After 3 weeks, full weight bearing is allowed with continuous use of the protective splint.
- At the end of 8 weeks the splint is discontinued and weight bearing is allowed without any external support.
- A more intensive program of ankle range of motion, stretching, and isometric and proprioceptive exercises is instituted.
- Jogging is allowed at 3 months, and more demanding sports at 5 months.

OUTCOMES

- This limited open procedure with use of the Achillon instrument provides the advantage of an open repair but avoids the soft tissue problems associated with open repair.
- Assal et al published a prospective multicenter study[1] including 82 patients. Results showed no wound healing problems and no infections. No patient noted a sensory disturbance in the sural nerve distribution. All patients returned to their previous professional or sporting activities. The mean AOFAS score was 96 points (range 85 to 100 points).
- Complications occurred in three patients. Two of them were noncompliant and removed the orthosis within the first 3 weeks postoperatively, thus disrupting the repair by a new injury. One patient fell 12 weeks after the surgery and sustained a rerupture. All three new injuries were repaired with an open surgical procedure.
- Isokinetic results: The concentric peak torque was performed with the ankle in plantarflexion at 30°/sec and 60°/sec of angular velocity, after correction for dominance. There was no significant difference between the injured and uninvolved sides. The endurance testing at 120°/sec also revealed no difference between sides.
- Three recent reports describe similar excellent results using the exact surgical technique and Achillon instrument, thus providing further confirmation of its important role in the repair of acute Achilles tendon ruptures.

REFERENCE

1. Assal M, Jung M, Stern R, et al. Limited open repair of Achilles tendon ruptures: a technique with a new instrument and findings of a prospective multicenter study. J Bone Joint Surg Am 2002;84A:161–170.

Chapter **108**

Percutaneous Achilles Tendon Repair: Perspective 1

Karen M. Sutton, Sandra L. Tomak, and Lamar L. Fleming

DEFINITION

- Achilles tendon ruptures typically occur about 2 to 6 cm proximal to the tendon's insertion site on the calcaneus.
- This injury is relatively common among both high-performance athletes and the recreational athlete, particularly the "weekend warrior."
- Ruptures occur most often in men between 30 and 50 years of age.

ANATOMY

- Tendinous portions of the gastrocnemius and soleus muscles coalesce to form the Achilles tendon (**FIG 1**).
- The plantaris muscle is a distinct entity medial to the Achilles tendon.
- The soleus tendon originates as a band proximally on the posterior surface of its muscle, and the gastrocnemius tendon emerges from the distal margin of the muscle bellies.
- The length of the tendon formed from the gastrocnemius and soleus range from 11 to 26 cm and 3 to 11 cm, respectively.

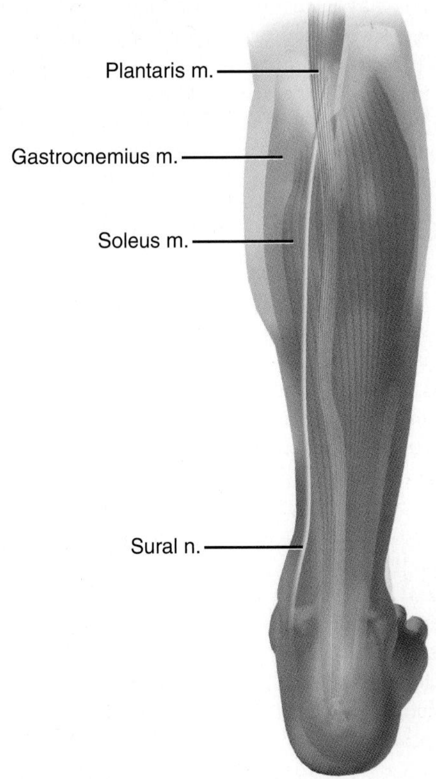

FIG 1 • Merging of the gastrocnemius and soleus muscles to form the Achilles tendon.

- Viewed from proximal to distal, the Achilles tendon progressively becomes thinner in its anteroposterior dimensions, particularly from 4 cm proximal to the calcaneus to its insertion on the calcaneus.[4]
- Ninety-five percent of the tendon collagen is type I collagen; a small percentage is elastic. Seventy percent of the dry weight of the tendon is collagen.[17]
- The blood supply to the Achilles tendon arises from the musculotendinous junction, the osseous insertion, and multiple mesotenal vessels.
- The tendon is most poorly vascularized at its midportion, receiving its blood supply from the paratenon.[20] The mesotenal vessels decrease in number 2 to 6 cm proximal to the osseous insertion.[21]
- The Achilles tendon receives much of its nutrition from the tenosynovial fluid that bathes the tendon and is contained within the paratenon.

PATHOGENESIS

- Ruptures occur most commonly during athletic activities.
- Both hyperpronation and cavus foot alignment are associated with Achilles tendon injuries. The cavus foot is thought to place more stress on the lateral side of the Achilles tendon and to absorb shock poorly.[19]
- Inconsistent training, including sudden increases in training intensity; excessive training; training on hard surfaces; and running on sloping, hard, or slippery roads have been implicated in Achilles tendon problems.[19]
- Mechanisms of injury, leading to eccentric loads on the Achilles tendon, include pushing off with the weight-bearing forefoot while extending the knee, unexpected dorsiflexion of the ankle, or violent dorsiflexion of a plantarflexed foot.[1]
- With normal aging, the Achilles tendon decreases in cell density, collagen fibril diameter and density, and fiber waviness. These changes may make the aging athlete more susceptible to injury.[21]
- Spontaneous rupture of the Achilles tendon has been associated with corticosteroid use,[11] inflammatory or autoimmune conditions,[6,15] collagen abnormalities,[5] infectious diseases,[2] neurologic conditions,[15] and fluoroquinolone use.[18]

NATURAL HISTORY

- Chronic Achilles tendon injuries typically result in the patients's inability to complete everyday tasks such as climbing stairs.[8]

PATIENT HISTORY AND PHYSICAL FINDINGS

- The patient reports sudden pain in the affected leg.
- Some patients recall an audible pop or snap.

- With Achilles tendon ruptures, patients occasionally experience a sensation as though they were "kicked" or "hit" in the injured calf.
- Patients report an inability to bear weight and have weakness of the affected lower extremity.
- Physical examination should include the following:
  - Palpation of gap: Palpate along the posterior aspect of the lower leg, and a gap may be felt along the course of the tendon.
    - Positive: appreciable gap
  - Thompson test: With the patient prone, squeeze the proximal portion of the calf.
    - Positive: no plantarflexion of the ankle
    - False-positive results may be obtained with an intact plantaris tendon.
  - Knee flexion test: With the patient prone, have him or her actively flex both knees to 90 degrees.
    - Positive: asymmetric resting tension of both ankles; the affected foot may even fall into neutral or dorsiflexion.
  - Needle test: Insert a hypodermic needle into the calf medial to the midline and 10 cm proximal to the insertion of the tendon. The ankle is put through passive range of motion.
    - Positive: the needle points proximally on dorsiflexion.
    - This test is usually only performed if there remains a high index of suspicion with the other tests being equivocal.

IMAGING AND OTHER DIAGNOSTIC STUDIES

- Plain radiographs (rarely required in evaluation of Achilles tendon ruptures)
  - In a lateral radiograph, the fat-filled triangular space (ie, Kager's triangle) anterior to the Achilles tendon and between the posterior aspect of the tibia and the superior aspect of the calcaneus loses its regular configuration.
- MRI (**FIG 2**) (rarely required in evaluation of Achilles tendon ruptures)
  - T1- and T2-weighted images in the axial and sagittal planes should be used to evaluate Achilles tendon ruptures.

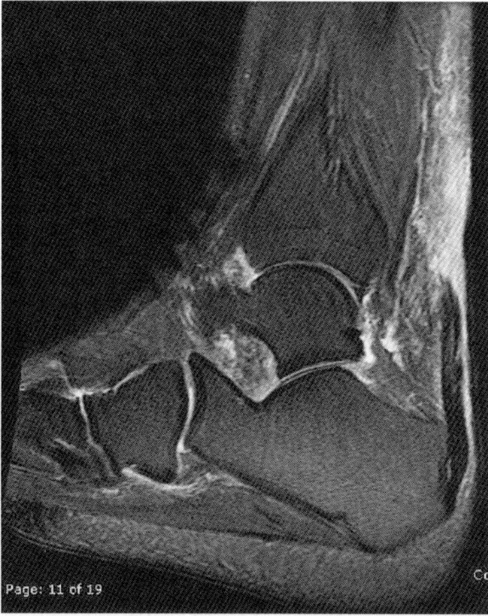

FIG 2 • T2-weighted MRI scan displaying a complete rupture of the Achilles tendon about 5 cm proximal to the insertion site on the calcaneus.

  - T1-weighted: a complete rupture of the Achilles tendon is identified as a disruption of the signal within the tendon.
  - T2-weighted: a complete rupture is demonstrated as a generalized increase in signal intensity, and the edema and hemorrhage at the site of the rupture are seen as an area of high signal intensity.[10]
- Ultrasound (useful because it can be performed in the office setting)
  - Rupture seen as an acoustic vacuum with thick irregular edges
  - May also be used for postoperative evaluation to assess the structure of the tendon and integrity of repair[14]

DIFFERENTIAL DIAGNOSIS

- Typically, rupture of the Achilles tendon does not conjure up a differential diagnosis.
- Because four other muscles plantarflex the ankle, Achilles tendon ruptures may be initially mistaken for ankle sprains; although increasingly less common, it has been reported that up to 20% of Achilles tendon ruptures may be missed by the first doctor to examine the patient.[9]

NONOPERATIVE MANAGEMENT

- Equinus short-leg cast or plantarflexed cam boot for 6 to 8 weeks
- At 6 to 8 weeks, start gentle range-of-motion exercises.
- A heel lift is used in the transition to wearing normal shoes.
- The patient may return to running in 4 to 6 months.
- Considered for elderly or sedentary patients, poor surgical candidates (vascular compromise and/or poor skin quality), or patients favoring nonoperative treatment
- The rerupture rate after nonoperative management is about 12.1%, compared with the rerupture rate for surgical repair, which is only 2.2%.[12]

SURGICAL MANAGEMENT

- In our hands, percutaneous repair is reserved for acute tears, a minimal tendon gap, and compliant patients.
- Advantages of percutaneous repair are as follows:
  - Low risk of wound complications
  - Preservation of blood supply for tendon healing
  - Performed as outpatient procedure
  - Requires only local anesthetic
  - Maintenance of tendon length
  - Earlier return to function when compared to closed treatment
- Disadvantages include:
  - Potential sural nerve injury
  - Higher rerupture rate versus open repair
  - Limited patient population
  - Need for compliance postoperatively
- Percutaneous repair is contraindicated in chronic tears, tendon gap, noncompliant patients, and high-level athletes (relative).

Positioning

- Prone position
- No tourniquet
- Injured foot in about 25 degrees of plantarflexion

Approach

- Percutaneous

PERCUTANEOUS ACHILLES TENDON REPAIR

- The repair is performed under local anesthesia (TECH FIG 1.)
- A size 0 monofilament polydioxanone suture with two Keith needles, one on either end, is used.
- Medial and lateral stab incisions are made on either side of the Achilles tendon using a no. 15 blade in the following locations: at the level of the rupture; 2.5 cm and 5 cm above the rupture; and 2.5 cm below the rupture. A total of eight stab incisions are made (TECH FIG 2).
- The subcutaneous tissues at each incision site are spread using a hemostat.
- Beginning at the most proximal lateral wound, the needle is passed transversely, and the suture is then manipulated until equal lengths are established on either side (TECH FIG 3).
- The suture is then advanced distally from both sides through the ipsilateral proximal incisions in a crisscross fashion through the tendon at 45-degree angles (TECH FIG 4).
- The previous step is repeated at both 5 cm and 2.5 cm proximal to the rupture (TECH FIG 5).
- The suture, now emerging at the level of the rupture, is then tensioned to ensure that ist is secured in the proximal Achilles tendon stump.
- The suture is then advanced distally across the rupture site, in a fashion similar to the previous step (TECH FIG 6).
- The lateral suture is passed through the ipsilateral incision transversely, from lateral to medial, where the ends of the sutures are pulled simultaneously, and then tied; closing the tendon gap.
- A hemostat is used to bury the knot and to be sure there is no skin puckering at any of the incision sites.
- Staples are placed to approximate the skin.

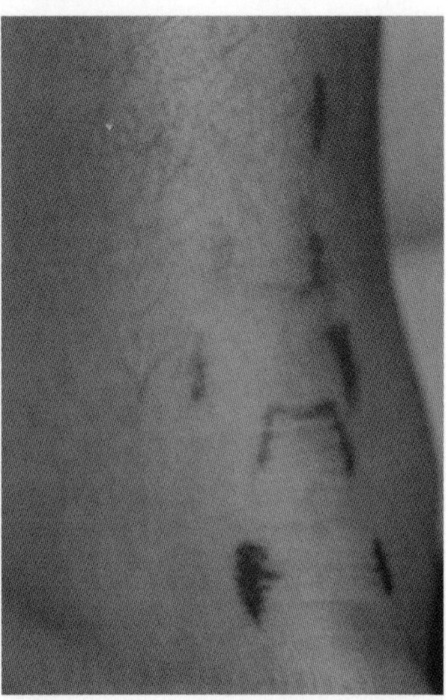

TECH FIG 2 • Incision locations: at the level of the tear, 2.5 cm and 5 cm above the tear, and 2.5 cm below the tear.

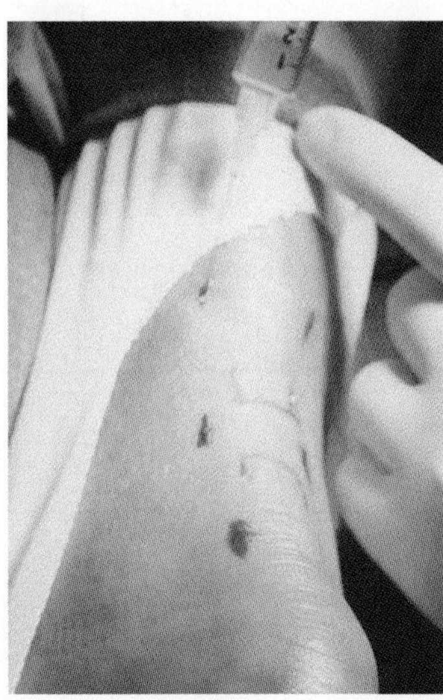

TECH FIG 1 • Local anesthetic used for the procedure.

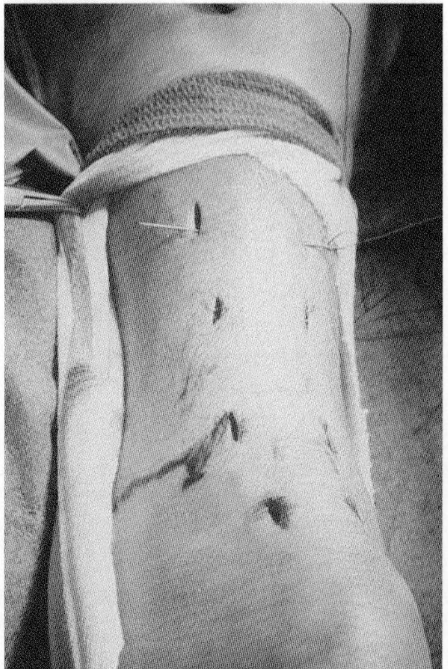

TECH FIG 3 • The needle is passed transversely, and the suture is manipulated until equal lengths are obtained.

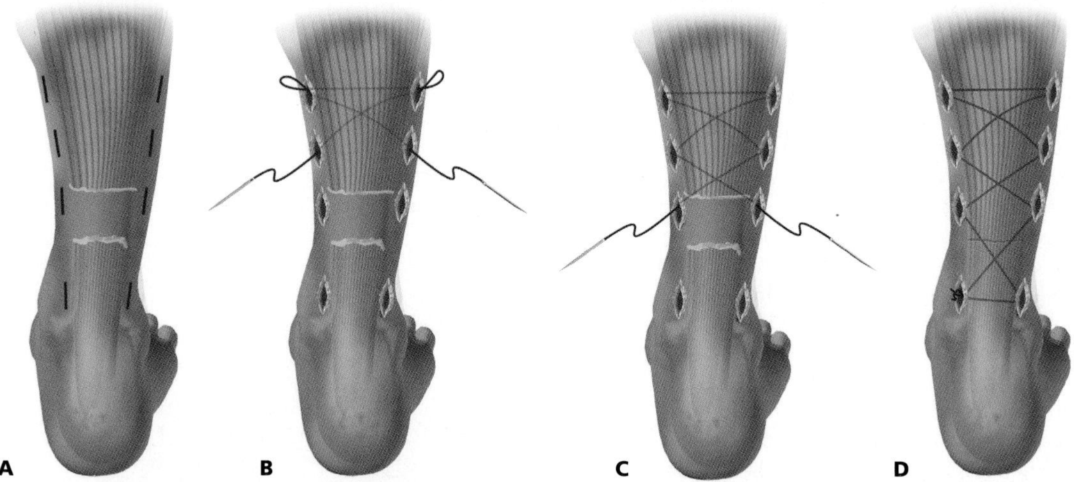

TECH FIG 4 • Diagram outlining the technique used for percutaneous repair of an acute Achilles tendon rupture. **D.** The finished repair. (Adapted with permission from Tomak SL, Fleming LL. Achilles tendon rupture: An alternative treatment. Am J Orthop 2004;33:9–12.)

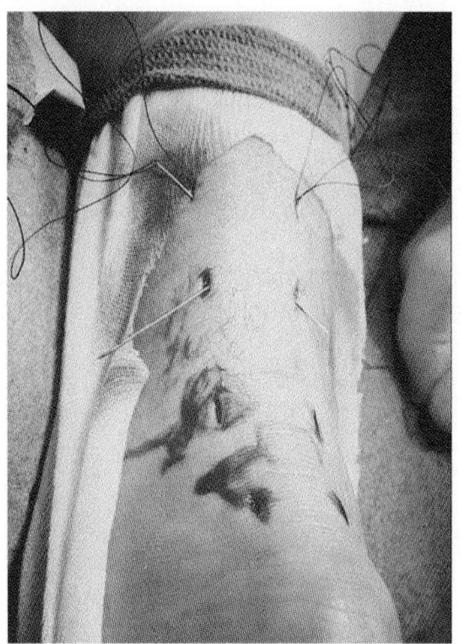

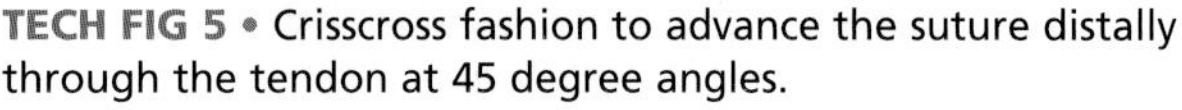

TECH FIG 5 • Crisscross fashion to advance the suture distally through the tendon at 45 degree angles.

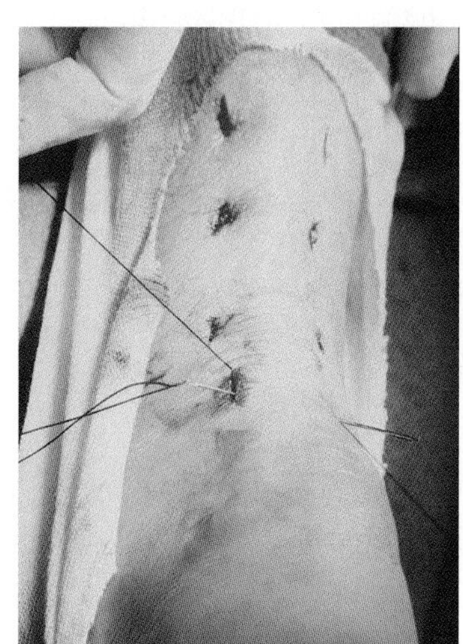

TECH FIG 6 • Suture is advanced distally across the rupture site.

PEARLS AND PITFALLS

- No need for antibiotic prophylaxis
- Perform technique with two Keith needles.
- To avoid sural nerve injury, use the "nick and spread" technique or lengthen the lateral incisions at the level of the rupture and at the musculotendinous junction to 1.0 to 1.5 cm. Use two small Langenbeck retractors to further visualize the location of the sural nerve lying superficial to the fascia.[16]

POSTOPERATIVE CARE

- Throughout the rehabilitation period: light active dorsiflexion, muscle strengthening, proprioception exercises, stationary cycling with heel push, soft tissue treatments
- For the first 2 weeks: immobilization and non–weight-bearing of the foot and ankle in an adjustable boot locked in 20 degrees of plantarflexion (**FIG 3**). Gentle plantigrade movement of the foot, straight leg raises, and knee range of motion are begun.
- Week 2: the boot is adjusted to 10 degrees of plantarflexion.
- Week 4: Orthosis is adjusted to neutral; partial weight bearing is initiated.

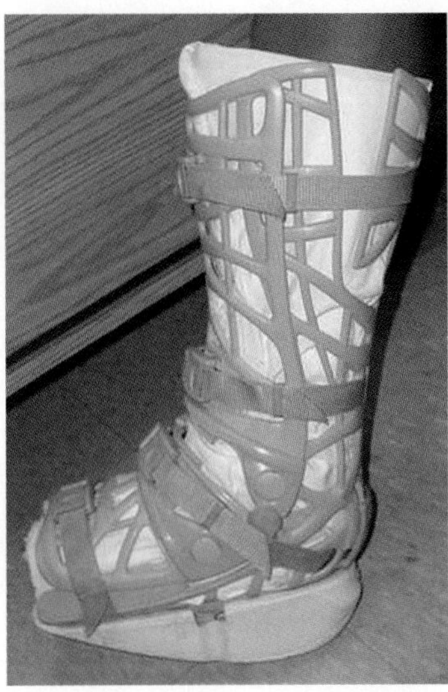

FIG 3 • Orthosis used for rehabilitation.

- Week 6: Full weight bearing is permitted.
- Week 8: The foot is placed in a shoe with a heel lift.
- Month 3: The patient starts closed-chain exercises, cycling, and elliptical trainer.
- Month 6: Running, jumping, and sports activities may be resumed.

OUTCOMES

- Retrospective review of 10 consecutive patients with acute Achilles tendon ruptures[22]:
  - No reruptures
  - No major complications
  - One sural nerve injury
  - Mean return to full activity at 6.1 months
  - American Orthopaedic Foot and Ankle Society (AOFAS) ankle hindfoot rating: average score 94
  - Mean difference of 1.58 cm in calf circumference, with the involved leg having the smaller circumference
  - Mean plantarflexion peak torque of the uninvolved leg and the involved leg of 67.8 and 52.8 foot-pounds, respectively (at a speed of 30 degrees per second)
- Comparative studies of percutaneous versus open Achilles tendon repair
  - Lim et al[13] reported significantly fewer wound complications/infections with percutaneous Achilles repair when compared to open repair. There was no significant difference between the two groups with respect to the duration of the immobilization, return to functional activity, and other complications.
  - Haji et al[7] reported: Mean operative times of 28.5 minutes and 25.9 minutes (statistically significant) and rerupture rates of 2.6% versus 5.7% (not statistically significant), respectively for percutaneous versus open repair.
  - Cretnik et al[3] noted significant increased tendon thickness and increased loss of dorsiflexion in the openly treated patients.
    - Out of 133 percutaneously repaired tendons, 1 patient (0.7%) sustained a complete rerupture, and 4 patients (3%) sustained a partial rupture, compared with 3 (2.8%) and 0 patients, respectively, in the open repair group.
    - Sural nerve injury occurred in 6 patients (4.5%) in the percutaneous repair group and 3 patients (2.8%) in the open repair group.
  - Wagnon and Akayi[23] compared the Webb-Bannister percutaneous technique to open repair.
    - The open repair group had an 8.6% incidence of wound complications (no wound dehiscence occurred in the percutaneous repair group).
    - Two patients out of 35 experienced rerupture after open repair; 1 patient (out of 22) experienced a rerupture after percutaneous repair.
    - Patients returned to work a mean of 4 months after open repair and 3.75 months after the Webb-Banister percutaneous repair.
    - No sural nerve complications occurred.

COMPLICATIONS

- Sural nerve injury
- Palpable suture knot which may necessitate excision
- Rerupture
- Deep venous thrombosis[3]

REFERENCES

1. Arner O, Lindholm A. Subcutaneous rupture of the Achilles tendon. A study of 92 cases. Acta Chir Scand 1959(suppl):239.
2. Arner O, Lindholm A, Orell S. Histologic changes in subcutaneous rupture of the Achilles tendon. A study of 74 cases. Acta Chir Scandinavica 1958–1959;116:484–490.
3. Cretnik A, Kosanovic M, Smrkolj V. Percutaneous versus open repair of the ruptured Achilles tendon: A comparative study. Am J Sports Med 2005;33:1369–1379.
4. Cummins E, Anson B, Carr B, et al. The structure of the calcaneal tendon (of Achilles) in relation to orthopaedic surgery. With additional observations on the plantaris muscle. Surg Gynecol Obstet 1946;83:107–116.
5. Dent CM, Graham GP. Osteogenesis imperfecta and Achilles tendon rupture. Injury 1991;22:239–240.
6. Dodds WN, Burry HC. The relationship between Achilles tendon rupture and serum uric acid level. Injury 1984;16:94–95.
7. Haji A, Sahai A, Symes A, et al. Percutaneous versus open tendo achillis repair. Foot Ankle Int 2004;25:215–218.
8. Hattrup SJ, Johnson KA. A review of ruptures of the Achilles tendon. Foot Ankle 1985;6:34–38.
9. Inglis AE, Scott WN, Sculco TP, et al. Ruptures of the tendo achillis. An objective assessment of surgical and non-surgical treatment. J Bone Joint Surg Am 1976;58:990–993.
10. Kabbani YM, Mayer DP. Magnetic resonance imaging of tendon pathology about the foot and ankle. Part I. Achilles tendon. J Am Podiatr Med Assoc 1993;83:418–420.
11. Kennedy JC, Willis RB. The effects of local steroid injections on tendons: A biomechanical and microscopic correlative study. Am J Sports Med 1976;4:11–21.
12. Kocher MS, Bishop J, Marshall R, et al. Operative versus nonoperative management of acute Achilles tendon rupture: Expected-value decision analysis. Am J Sports Med 2002;30:783–790.
13. Lim J, Dalal R, Waseem M. Percutaneous vs. open repair of the ruptured Achilles tendon—a prospective randomized controlled study. Foot Ankle Int 2001;22:559–568.
14. Maffulli N. Rupture of the Achilles tendon. J Bone Joint Surg Am 1999;81:1019–1036.
15. Maffulli N, Irwin AS, Kenward MG, et al. Achilles tendon rupture and sciatica: A possible correlation. Br J Sports Med 1998;32:174–177.
16. Majewski M, Rohrbach M, Czaja S, et al. Avoiding sural nerve injuries during percutaneous Achilles tendon repair. Am J Sports Med 2006;34:793–798.

17. O'Brien M. Functional anatomy and physiology of tendons. Clin Sports Med 1992;11:505–520.
18. Royer RJ, Pierfitte C, Netter P. Features of tendon disorders with fluoroquinolones. Therapie 1994;49:75–76.
19. Saltzman CL, Tearse DS. Achilles tendon injuries. J Am Acad Orthop Surg 1998;6:316–325.
20. Schmidt-Rohlfing B, Graf J, Schneider U, et al. The blood supply of the Achilles tendon. Internat Orthop 1992;16:29–31.
21. Strocchi R, De Pasquale V, Guizzardi S, et al. Human Achilles tendon: Morphological and morphometric variations as a function of age. Foot Ankle 1991;12:100–104.
22. Tomak SL, Fleming LL. Achilles tendon rupture: An alternative treatment. Am J Orthop 2004;33:9–12.
23. Wagnon R, Akayi M. The Webb-Bannister percutaneous technique for acute Achilles' tendon ruptures: A functional and MRI assessment. J Foot Ankle Surg 2005;44:437–444.

Chapter 109 Percutaneous Achilles Tendon Repair: Perspective 2

Nicholas A. Ferran, Ansar Mahmood, and Nicola Maffulli

DEFINITION

- Rupture of the Achilles tendon is common.
- More than 20% of acute injuries are misdiagnosed, leading to chronic or neglected ruptures.[4]

ANATOMY

- The two heads of the gastrocnemius arise from the condyles of the femur, the fleshy part of the muscle extending to about the midcalf. As the muscle fibers descend they insert into a broad aponeurosis that contracts and receives the tendon of the soleus on its deep surface to form the Achilles tendon.[9]
- The Achilles tendon is the thickest and strongest tendon in the body. About 15 cm long, it originates in the midcalf and extends distally to insert into the posterior surface of the calcaneus. It receives muscle fibers from the soleus on its anterior surface throughout its length.[9]

PATHOGENESIS

- The most common mechanism of injury is pushing off with the weight-bearing forefoot while extending the knee. Sudden unexpected dorsiflexion of the ankle or violent dorsiflexion of a plantarflexed foot may also result in ruptures.[5]
- Corticosteroids, fluoroquinolone use, tendon pathology, and poor vascularity of the Achilles tendon have been associated with rupture.[5]

NATURAL HISTORY

- A delay in treatment of Achilles tendon rupture results in the formation of a discrete gap. The gap between ruptured tendon ends may fill with fibrous nonfunctional scar. Patients find walking and ascending stairs difficult, and standing on tiptoes on the affected limb impossible.

PATIENT HISTORY AND PHYSICAL FINDINGS

- Patients often give a history of feeling a blow to the posterior aspect of the leg and may describe an audible snap followed by pain and inability to bear weight.
- In acute tendon ruptures, a gap in the Achilles tendon is usually palpable. In delayed presentation, edema may fill this gap, making palpation unreliable.
- Active plantarflexion of the foot is usually preserved due to the action of the tibialis posterior and the long toe flexors.
- The calf squeeze test, first described by Simmonds in 1957[7] but often credited to Thompson, is performed with the patient prone and the ankles clear of the table. The examiner squeezes the fleshy part of the calf, causing deformation of the soleus, and resulting in plantarflexion of the foot if the Achilles tendon is intact. The affected leg should be compared to the contralateral leg.
- The knee flexion test is performed with the patient prone and the ankles clear of the table. The patient is asked to actively flex the knee to 90 degrees. During this movement the foot on the affected side falls into neutral or dorsiflexion and a rupture of the Achilles tendon can be diagnosed.[6]

IMAGING AND OTHER DIAGNOSTIC STUDIES

- The diagnosis of acute ruptures is usually a clinical one.
- Plain lateral radiographs may reveal an irregular configuration of the fat-filled triangular space anterior to the Achilles tendon and between the posterior aspect of the tibia and the superior aspect of the calcaneus.

DIFFERENTIAL DIAGNOSIS

- Ankle sprain

NONOPERATIVE MANAGEMENT

- Acute ruptures may be managed conservatively in an equinus cast for 6 to 8 weeks before being converted to a functional brace.
- Conservative management may result in tendon lengthening, thus altering function.[1]

SURGICAL MANAGEMENT

- Percutaneous repair[3] was originally described as a compromise between open surgery and conservative management. A percutaneous repair aims to provide the optimal functional outcome of open repair while decreasing the problems associated with it in terms of wound healing and skin breakdown.

Preoperative Planning

- Once the diagnosis is made, an assessment of general health and comorbidities should be performed.
- The preoperative functional status should be noted.
- The skin quality and neurovascular status of the affected limb should be examined.
- The status of the sural nerve should be documented.
- We recommend that the patient be maintained on deep venous thrombosis prophylaxis.
- The procedure can be performed under general anesthesia or a local anesthetic, with a 50:50 mixture of 10 mL of 2% lignocaine hydrochloride (Antigen Pharmaceuticals Ltd, Roscrea, Ireland) and 10 mL of 0.25% bupivacaine hydrochloride (Astra Pharmaceuticals Ltd, Kings Langley, England) instilled into an area of between 8 and 10 cm around the ruptured Achilles tendon.

Positioning

- The patient is placed prone, and a pillow is placed beneath the anterior aspect of the ankles to allow the feet to hang free.
- The operating table is angled down 20 degrees cranially to reduce venous pooling in the feet and ankles.
- A tourniquet is not necessary for this procedure.

Approach

- Previous approaches such as those described by Ma and Griffith[3] using three medial and three lateral stab incisions have been abandoned in light of the relatively increased incidence of sural nerve entrapment.
- We will present two techniques that we employ. The first is an approach similar to that described by Webb and Bannister.[8] Three 3-cm transverse skin incisions are made. The middle one is made over the palpable gap, and the proximal and distal incisions are placed 4 cm proximal and distal to the middle incision respectively (**FIG 1**). The second is currently our favored technique: the results for acute ruptures are as good as the first technique, but it is even less invasive.
- In the first technique the proximal incision is made more medial to the others to avoid the sural nerve. The stab incisions used in the five-incision latter procedure do not usually give rise to sural nerve problems.

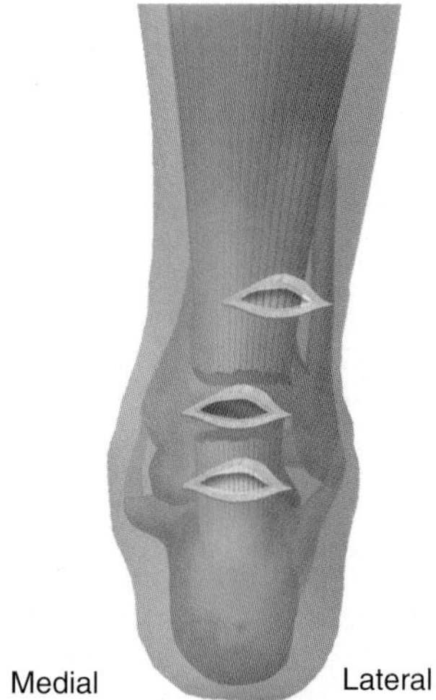

FIG 1 • Incisions. The proximal incision is placed medially.

TECHNIQUES

MINIMALLY INVASIVE REPAIR OF ACUTE ACHILLES TENDON RUPTURE WITH MODIFIED KESSLER SUTURE PATTERN

- Use a small hemostat to free the tendon sheath from the overlying subcutaneous tissue.
- Pass a 1 PDS II (Ethicon, Johnson & Johnson Intl, Brussels, Belgium) double-strand suture on a long curved needle transversely through the distal incision, passing through the substance of the tendon and out through the same incision (**TECH FIG 1A**).
- Reintroduce the needle medially into the distal incision through a different entry point in the tendon, and pass it longitudinally through the tendon to lock the tendon. Direct the needle toward the middle incision and out through the ruptured tendon end (**TECH FIG 1B**).
- Rethread the suture still protruding from the distal incision onto the needle and reintroduce it laterally into the distal

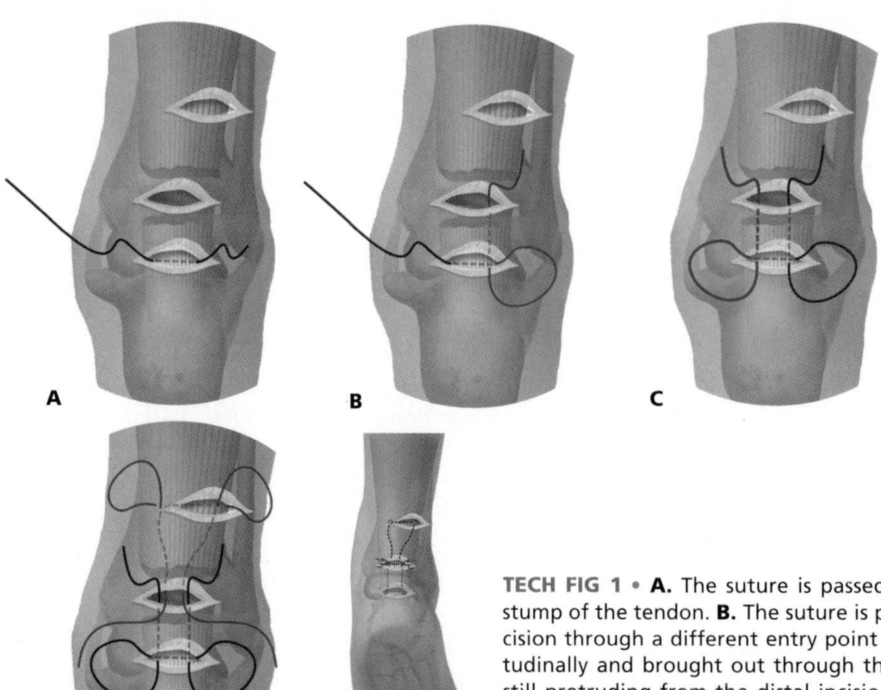

TECH FIG 1 • **A.** The suture is passed transversely through the distal stump of the tendon. **B.** The suture is passed medially into the distal incision through a different entry point in the tendon and passed longitudinally and brought out through the middle incision. **C.** The suture still protruding from the distal incision is rethreaded onto the needle and reintroduced laterally into the tendon and brought out through the medial incision. **D.** The procedure is repeated in the proximal stump. **E.** The suture ends are then tied with the ankle in physiologic plantarflexion.

incision and into the tendon. Pass it proximally through the tendon to exit from the middle incision (**TECH FIG 1C**).

- Apply traction to the suture to ensure satisfactory grip of the tendon.
- Carry out the same procedure for the proximal stump of the ruptured tendon (**TECH FIG 1D**).
- A further 1 PDS II (Ethicon) double-stranded suture can be placed in the tendon ends as described above to produce an eight-strand repair.
- Tie the sutures with the ankle in physiologic plantarflexion (**TECH FIG 1E**).
- Assess the tension by observing the contralateral limb as the sutures are tied.
- Close the skin wounds with undyed subcuticular 3-0 Vicryl (Ethicon, Edinburgh, UK) suture and apply nonadherent dressings.
- Apply a full plaster-of-Paris cast in the operating room with the ankle in physiologic equinus.

PERCUTANEOUS REPAIR OF ACUTE ACHILLES TENDON RUPTURE USING FIVE STAB INCISIONS

- Local anesthetic infiltration is used. Instill a 50:50 mixture of 10 mL of 2% lignocaine hydrochloride (Antigen Pharmaceuticals) and 10 mL of 0.25% bupivacaine hydrochloride (Astra Pharmaceuticals) into an area 8 to 10 cm around the ruptured Achilles tendon.
- The patient is placed prone, and a pillow is placed beneath the anterior aspect of the ankles to allow the feet to hang free.
- Angle the operating table down about 20 degrees cranially to reduce venous pooling in the feet and ankles.
- The affected leg is prepared with antiseptic and sterile draped. We do not use a tourniquet.
- Make five stab incisions over the Achilles tendon (**TECH FIG 2A**). The first is directly over the palpable defect and measures about 2 cm in a transverse direction.
- The other incisions are about 4 cm proximal and 4 cm distal to the first incision and are vertical 1-cm stab incisions on the medial and lateral aspect of the Achilles tendon.
- We advocate blunt dissection with a small hemostat directly onto the Achilles tendon. This avoids damaging the sural nerve, which crosses the lateral border of the Achilles tendon about 10 cm proximal to its insertion into the calcaneus.
- Use a small hemostat to free the tendon sheath from the overlying subcutaneous tissue (Tech Fig 2A).
- Pass a 1 PDS II (Ethicon) double-stranded suture on a long curved needle transversely through the lateral proximal stab incision, passing it through the substance of the tendon and out through the medial proximal stab incision (**TECH FIG 2B**).
- Reintroduce the needle into the medial proximal stab incision through a different entry point in the tendon and pass it longitudinally and distally through the tendon to lock into the tendon. Direct the needle toward the middle incision and out through the ruptured tendon end (**TECH FIG 2C**).
- Rethread the suture that is still protruding from the lateral proximal stab incision onto the needle and reintroduce it via the lateral proximal stab incision into the tendon substance. Also pass it longitudinally and distally through the tendon to exit from the middle incision. Apply traction to the suture to ensure a satisfactory grip within the tendon. If the suture pulls through, repeat the procedure. We sometimes use an eight-stranded method by doubling the sutures used for the Kessler-type technique we are describing.
- Carry out the same procedure for the distal half of the ruptured tendon.
- Tie the sutures with the ankle in physiologic plantarflexion and bury them into the tissues using a hemostat (**TECH FIG 2E**).
- Close the skin wounds with undyed subcuticular 3-0 Vicryl (Ethicon) suture and apply nonadherent dressings.
- Apply a full plaster-of-Paris cast in the operating room with the ankle in physiologic equinus. Split the cast on both medial and lateral sides to allow for swelling (**TECH FIG 2F**).

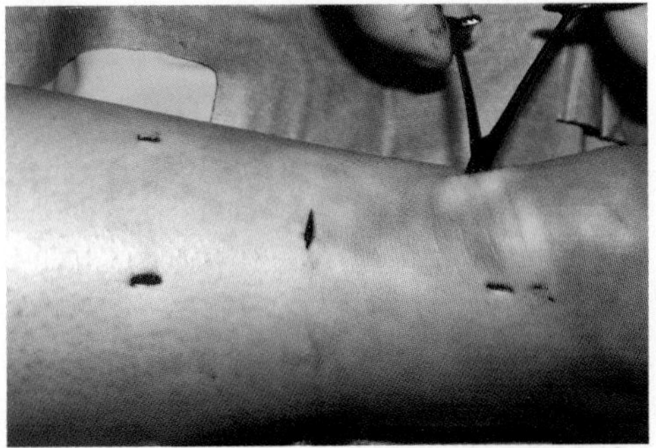
A

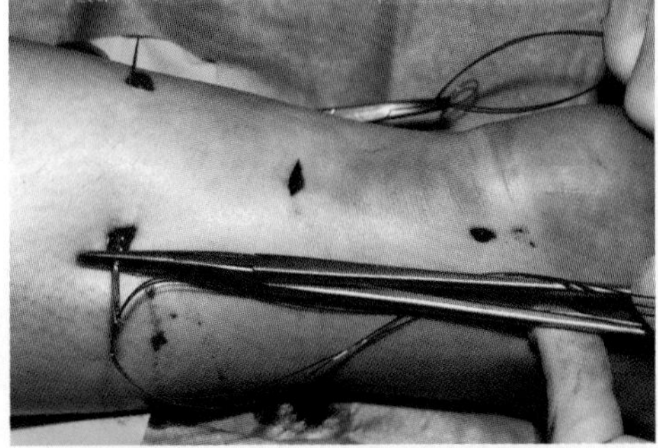
B

TECH FIG 2 • **A.** The five stab incisions around the Achilles tendon rupture. A hemostat is used to free the Achilles from any subcutaneous and peritendinous adhesions. **B.** The needle is introduced into the lateral proximal stab incision through the substance of the tendon. *(continued)*

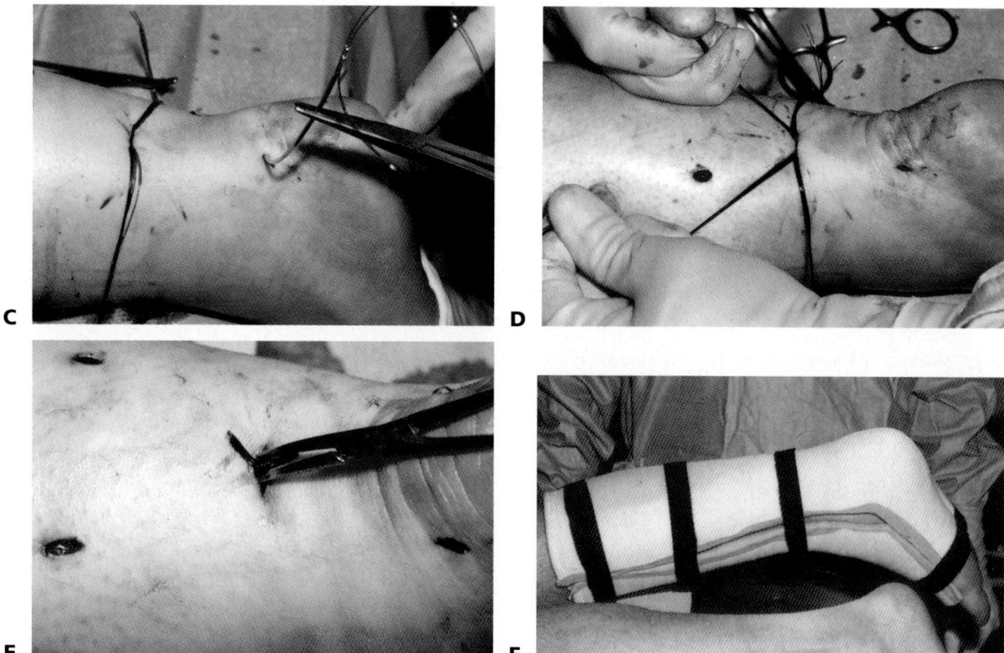

TECH FIG 2 • *(continued)* **C.** The needle is reintroduced into the medial proximal stab incision through a different entry point in the tendon and passed longitudinally and proximally through the tendon, directed toward the middle incision and out through the ruptured tendon end. The same is done with the suture protruding from the lateral proximal stab incision once it is rethreaded onto a needle. Traction is applied to the suture to ensure a satisfactory grip within the tendon. The same procedure is then repeated for the distal segment. **D.** The sutures are then tied with the ankle in physiologic plantarflexion. **E.** A hemostat is used to bury the suture into the tissues. **F.** A full plaster-of-Paris cast is applied in the operating room with the ankle in physiologic equinus. The cast is split on both medial and lateral sides to allow for swelling.

PEARLS AND PITFALLS

Tourniquet	■ Avoiding the use of the tourniquet allows identification and hemostasis of bleeding points, reducing the incidence of postoperative hematoma.
Incision	■ A medially placed proximal incision reduces the risk of sural nerve injury.

POSTOPERATIVE CARE

- The postoperative care regimen and rehabilitation are similar for both techniques.
- Patients are discharged on the same day of the operation.
- The neurovascular status of the limb is assessed.
- After assessment by a physiotherapist, making sure that the patient is safe and comfortable in the cast, the patient can be discharged.
- The full cast is retained for 2 weeks, and patients are allowed to bear weight as comfort allows. During the period in the cast, patients are advised to perform gentle isometric contractions of the gastroc–soleus complex.
- At 2 weeks, patients are reviewed as outpatients, the cast is split, and the wounds are inspected. An anterior splint is worn with the foot in plantarflexion for a further 4 weeks.
- Patients are advised to mobilize with partial weight bearing initially, increasing to weight bearing as able by 4 weeks.
- The splint is then removed, and physiotherapy follow-up for gentle mobilization is arranged. Light weight-bearing exercise can be started 2 weeks after cast removal, and the patient should be fully weight bearing by 10 weeks.

OUTCOMES

- Lim et al,[2] in a randomized controlled trial, advocated percutaneous repair over open surgical techniques after finding no significant differences in functional results, a lower infection rate with the percutaneous repair, and a subjectively more acceptable cosmetic appearance of the percutaneous operative site.
- We reviewed 31 patients who underwent percutaneous repair in our tertiary referral center between 2001 and 2003.[10] Eleven patients (35.5%) received general anesthesia and 20 (64.5%) had local anesthesia. The average length of cast time was 5.97 weeks. One (3.2%) patient sustained a

major complication, a small pulmonary embolism, which was managed successfully with warfarin. There were no reruptures, and six (19.4%) patients had minor wound complications.

COMPLICATIONS

- Early complications include sural nerve damage and hematoma.
- Intermediate superficial and deep wound infections may occur.
- The most important late complication is rerupture.

REFERENCES

1. Bohnsack M, Ruhmann O, Kirsch L, et al. Surgical shortening of the Achilles tendon for correction of elongation following healed conservatively treated Achilles tendon rupture. Z Orthop Ihre Grenzgeb 2000;138:501–505.
2. Lim J, Dalal R, Waseem M. Percutaneous vs. open repair of the ruptured Achilles tendon: a prospective randomized controlled study. Foot Ankle Int 2001;22:559–568.
3. Ma GWC, Griffith TG. Percutaneous repair of acute closed ruptured Achilles tendon: a new technique. Clin Orthop Relat Res 1977;128:247–255.
4. Maffulli N. Clinical tests in sports medicine: more on Achilles tendon. Br J Sports Med 1996;30:250.
5. Maffulli N. Rupture of the Achilles tendon. J Bone Joint Surg Am 1999;81A:1019–1036.
6. Matles AL. Rupture of the tendo Achilles: another diagnostic sign. Bull Hosp Joint Dis 1975;36:48–51.
7. Simmonds FA. The diagnosis of the ruptured Achilles tendon. Practitioner 1957;179:56–58.
8. Webb JM, Bannister GC. Percutaneous repair of the ruptured tendo Achillis. J Bone Joint Surg Br 1999;81B:877–880.
9. Williams PL. Gray's Anatomy, 38th ed. Edinburgh: Churchill Livingstone, 1995.
10. Young J, Sayana MK, McClelland D, et al. Percutaneous repair of acute rupture of Achilles tendon. Tech Foot Ankle Surg 2006;5:9–14.

Chapter **110**

Chronic Achilles Tendon Ruptures Using V-Y Advancement and FHL Transfer

Steven M. Raikin

DEFINITION

- Achilles tendon rupture results in loss of plantarflexion function of the ankle through disruption of the gastroc–soleus–Achilles (GSA) mechanism.
- Chronic rupture is usually defined as a rupture not appropriately treated within 8 weeks of injury.
- Chronic or neglected ruptures result in retraction of the proximal myotendinous portion and diastasis between the ruptured tendon ends.
- Functional deficits result from loss of plantarflexion strength and dorsiflexion; check reign of the GSA mechanism.
- This chapter presents a combined reconstruction and augmentation technique for repairing chronic or neglected Achilles tendon ruptures.

ANATOMY

- The triceps surae complex is composed of the two heads of the gastrocnemius and the soleus muscle combining to form a single tendon—the Achilles tendon, making up the GSA complex.
- The GSA complex originates from the distal femoral condyles and inserts into the posterior calcaneal tuberosity, making it one of the few muscle–tendon complexes to cross three joints (knee, ankle, and subtalar joints) in the human body.
- The tendon is loosely surrounded by a paratenon, which allows the tendon to slide about 1.5 cm.
- The blood supply to the tendon emanates from the muscle proximally and the calcaneal insertion distally, leaving a watershed area of relatively avascular tendon 4 to 5 cm from the calcaneal insertion.[3]

PATHOGENESIS

- Seventy-five percent of Achilles tendon ruptures occur during sporting activities.
- A history of prior Achilles tendinitis is present in about 15% of ruptures.
- Ruptures occur most commonly in the 30- to 40-year age group, with a male predominance.
- Eighty percent of Achilles tendon ruptures occur in the watershed area 2 to 6 cm above the insertion.
- Mechanism of injury resulting in rupture can be forceful plantarflexion or hyperdorsiflexion of the ankle.
- Achilles tendon ruptures are frequently missed or misdiagnosed as ankle sprains on initial assessment.
- Failure of immobilization or repair will allow continued contracture of the gastrocsoleus muscle, resulting in retraction of the proximal myotendinous portion of the GSA complex and subsequently in the development of a gap between the tendon ends.

NATURAL HISTORY

- Missed or neglected ruptures of the Achilles tendon result in plantarflexion weakness and loss of the dorsiflexion; check reign of the GSA complex.
- Without treatment patients develop gait dysfunction, particularly walking up stairs, inclines, or ladders, as well as balance difficulties, with a tendency to fall forward.

PATIENT HISTORY AND PHYSICAL FINDINGS

- Patients frequently recall the primary event, and often describe feeling like they had been "shot" or "hit" on the back of the heel when the rupture occurred.
- Silent or spontaneous ruptures may occur in the presence of systemic inflammatory diseases, steroid use, or chronic underlying Achilles tendinosis.
- Patients are usually able to walk on the limb and plantarflex the ankle without significant pain despite the chronic rupture.
- Primary complaints are:
  - Weakness of plantarflexion (walking up inclines, stairs, ladders)
  - Gait and balance difficulties
- Clinical examination
  - Inability to walk on tiptoes
  - Inability to perform a single-leg toe raise (difficulty with double-leg raise)
  - Direct evaluation should be performed with the patient lying prone with both knees flexed to 90 degrees (both sides are examined and compared):
    - Decreased resting tension of the Achilles tendon (normal resting tension of the unaffected side holds the ankle at 20 to 30 degrees of plantarflexion, while the ruptured side will usually be neutral [zero degrees plantarflexion]).
    - Hyperdorsiflexibility of the ankle compared to the unaffected side
    - Plantarflexion may be present (due to the effect of the posterior tibial tendon, flexor hallucis longus [FHL], and digitorum longus, and the peroneal tendons) but is weaker than the unaffected side.
    - A palpable gap may be present between the ruptured tendon ends (**FIG 1**) when the tendon is followed from the insertion proximally. Careful palpation can usually detect the proximal end, and the gap can be estimated, although it is difficult to measure clinically.
    - The Thompson test (squeezing the calf) will not result in symmetrical ankle plantarflexion (compared to the unaffected side), although some degree of plantarflexion is usually present in chronic rupture cases.

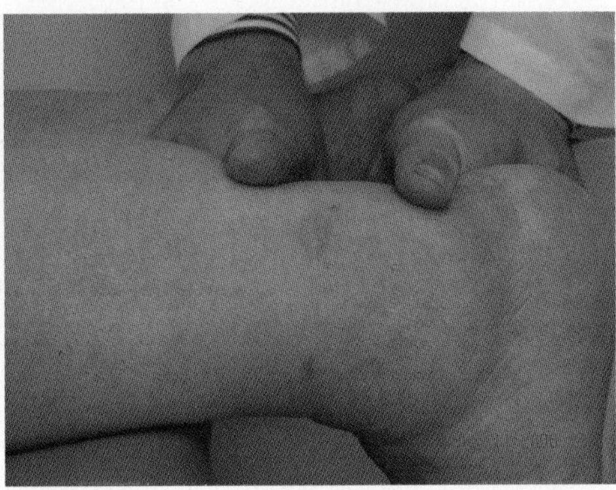

FIG 1 • A large palpable gap can usually be felt between the ruptured ends.

IMAGING AND OTHER DIAGNOSTIC STUDIES

- The diagnosis of an Achilles tendon rupture (acute or chronic or neglected) can usually be made on careful clinical evaluation alone.
- If one is uncertain or wishes to better quantify the rupture gap, ultrasound or MRI can be performed.
  - Both tests are highly reliable in confirming the diagnosis and in obtaining an accurate measurement of the gap.
  - No difference in diagnostic accuracy has been shown, although the MRI may yield more information about the degree of atrophy and fibrosis within the gastrocsoleus muscle.
  - This will not affect the treatment options but may help prognosticate the outcome of reconstruction.
- MRI evaluation is useful in neglected ruptures to quantify the gap between the tendon ends.

NONOPERATIVE MANAGEMENT

- Brace management can be used for patients who are not candidates for surgical reconstruction.
  - These include patients with medical risk factors, poor distal circulation, and impaired wound healing potential (including patients on steroids or immunosuppressive medications, and those with diabetes mellitus).
  - Patients with more moderate functional deficits, with low physical demands, may choose nonsurgical management.
- Management consists of a custom-molded ankle–foot orthosis (MAFO) made of polypropylene.
- An ankle hinge spring-loaded MAFO can be fashioned to add plantarflexion torque and further aid push-off.
- Long-term braces tend to be poorly tolerated in many patients with more active lifestyles.

SURGICAL MANAGEMENT

- The choice of surgical reconstruction depends on the size of the rupture gap. The ability to mobilize the retracted muscle tends to be the major limiting factor.
- Defects less than 1 cm can usually be mobilized and repaired with end-to-end anastomosis.
- For defects of 1 to 3 cm, direct end-to-end anastomosis can usually be obtained. Stretching of the retracted muscle is usually required via longitudinal traction over about a 10-minute time period to close the gap.
- Defects of 3 to 7 cm require an advancement procedure of the Achilles tendon, performed as a V-to-Y lengthening. Further augmentation with a FHL tendon transfer results in additional strength and function of the repair. This technique will be outlined in more detail below.
- For defects of more than 7 cm, reconstruction involves either an Achilles turndown procedure (if enough tendinous tissue is available proximally) or an allograft replacement of the Achilles tendon.

Preoperative Planning

- MRI or ultrasound should be reviewed to determine the gap size and to aid in the location of the ruptured ends (**FIG 2**).
- Examination under anesthesia should be performed as described above.
- General endotracheal or spinal anesthesia can be used for this procedure.
- Surgery is usually performed on an outpatient basis.

Positioning

- Once the patient is anesthetized, a well-padded thigh tourniquet should be applied.
  - It is technically easier to apply the tourniquet while the patient is still in a supine position.
  - The surgeon must ensure that the connection for the tubing is placed posteriorly or laterally to allow attachment after positioning, and to prevent pressure problems from the patient lying on the connection or tubing.
  - A calf tourniquet should not be used because it may limit the surgeon's exposure and puts squeeze on the gastrocsoleus muscle, preventing muscle mobilization.
- The patient is turned into a prone position.
- Chest rolls should be used if the patient is asleep for the procedure (this is usually not needed if the procedure is performed under spinal anesthesia).
- Both lower extremities should be prepared and draped. This allows the unaffected side to be used as a template against which the resting tension of the repair can be assessed.
  - The legs should be prepared and draped to above the level of the knee joints.

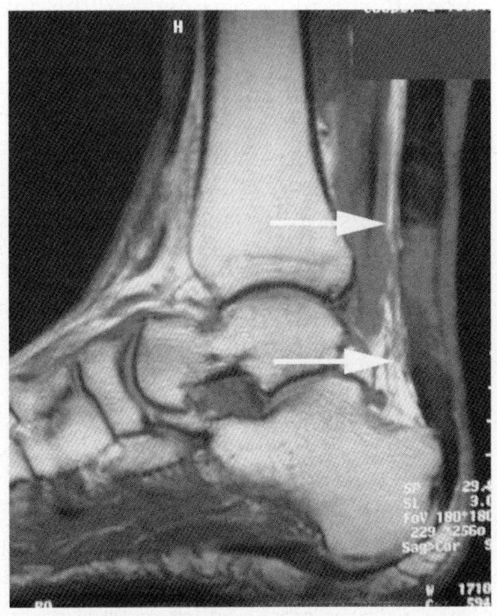

FIG 2 • MRI shows a neglected Achilles tendon rupture. The *white arrows* indicate the proximal and distal stump ends, with a 5-cm gap.

INCISION

- After Esmarch exsanguination of the limb, the tourniquet is inflated and left inflated until a compressive dressing has been applied at the end of the procedure.
- The approach to the repair involves an extensile incision over the posterior calf (**TECH FIG 1A**).
- Place the distal incision, over the region of the rupture and gap, medial to the Achilles tendon.
  - This prevents injury to the sural nerve, which runs 5 mm lateral to the Achilles tendon, and keeps the incision away from the posterior aspect of the heel, where it could rub against a shoe counter, causing irritation.
  - This usually involves the most distal 10 cm of the incision.
- Continue the incision sharply full thickness down to and through the paratenon. Reflect the paratenon off the tendon and preserve it for later repair.
- Proximally, curve the incision centrally and continue it up the posterior midline of the calf up to the proximal extent of the myotendinous junction.
- The sural nerve in the calf crosses from lateral to central over the myotendinous junction region and then passes under the medial head of the gastrocnemius muscle proximally.
  - The nerve must be identified (**TECH FIG 1B**) within the subcutaneous tissue, retracted, and protected throughout the rest of the procedure.
  - The nerve runs with the lesser saphenous vein, which aids in identifying its location, and the vein too should be preserved if possible.
- Expose the entire tendon up to a level proximal to the myotendinous junction.
- Carefully reflect the paratenon off the proximal tendon and preserve it for later repair.

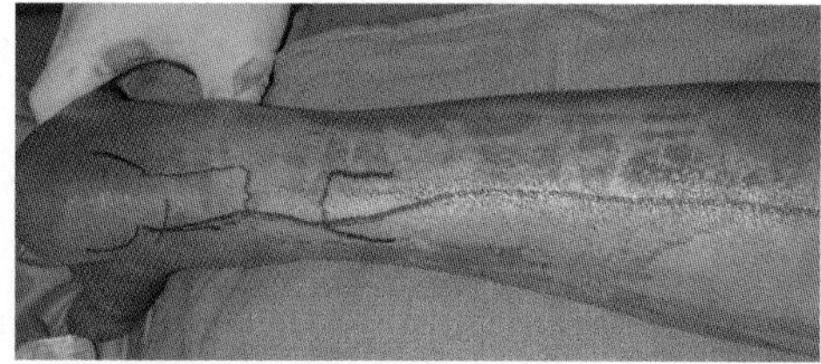

A

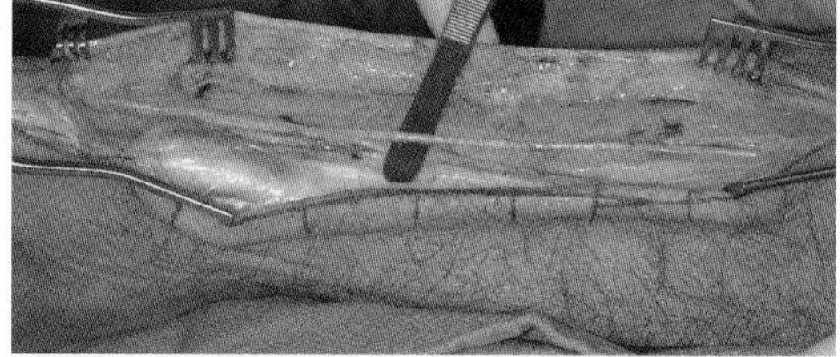

B

TECH FIG 1 • **A.** The incision required to address a neglected Achilles rupture with a large gap between tendon ends. **B.** The sural nerve should be isolated as it traverses from the lateral aspect of the tendon distally to the posterior midline within the calf.

MEASUREMENT OF THE GAP

- Once the ruptured region is identified, measure the gap. A scar pseudo-tendon is frequently identified within the rupture gap, and this should be resected together with the nonviable ends of the tendon.
- Measure the true tendon gap (**TECH FIG 2**) with the knee flexed to 30 degrees and the ankle plantarflexed to 20 degrees to match the resting tension of the unaffected side.

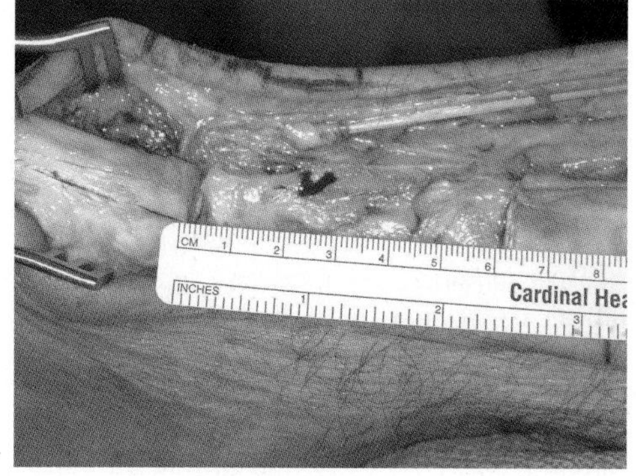

TECH FIG 2 • The true tendon gap is measured with the ankle in neutral resting tension (compared to the unaffected side).

V-TO-Y LENGTHENING

- Make an inverted-V incision through the tendinous portion only of the myotendinous junction of the GSA complex.
- Leave the underlying muscle fibers intact and attached to the proximal muscle body.
- Place the apex of the V in the midline at the most proximal portion of the myotendinous junction.
- The limbs of the V then diverge to exit at the medial and lateral borders of the tendon, respectively. The V limbs should be at least one-and-a-half times longer than the length of the measured gap (**TECH FIG 3A**). In our experience with these more extensive gaps (greater than 5 cm), we recommend that the limbs of the V are at least twice the length of the rupture gap to allow adequate lengthening to be obtained.
- Use a heavy braided nonabsorbable suture (we use no. 2 Fiberwire [Arthrex Inc., Naples, FL], but no. 5 Ethibond [Ethicon-J&J, Piscataway, NJ] can also be used) for the end-to-end tendon anastomosis after the lengthening.

- Use a locking Krackow technique, placing at least five locking loops in a running style along the medial and lateral aspect of the tendon, on each end of the rupture (TECH FIG 3B).
- Insert the suture into the free end of the tendon and then loop it in a locking pattern up the side of the tendon. Attempt to capture about one third to one half of the tendon width with each loop of the suture. Once five loops have been thrown, pass the suture through the substance of the tendon, exiting at the same level on the opposite side of the tendon. Throw another five locking loops toward the end of the tendon, with the suture exiting again at the free end of the tendon.
- We have found that a single continuous suture is adequate for the repair.
- Apply traction to the suture material within the proximal tendon stump in a distally directed longitudinal direction (TECH FIG 3C). This is a firm continuous traction, allowing the muscle fibers to gently stretch out and slide. A weight can be hung over the end of the table to facilitate traction. While some force is required to create this advancement slide, take patience and great care not to detach the tendon from the muscle, which would devascularize the tendon.
- While this is being applied, gently tease the muscle fibers of the myotendinous junction longitudinally, allowing the myotendinous junction to slide distally.
- Continue traction until the tendon ends can be approximated with the ankle resting tension matching the unaffected side.
- Repair the V incision in the tendon, creating an inverted-Y configuration (TECH FIG 3D). The long arm of the inverted Y is the length that the tendon has been elongated—equal to the length of the measured gap.

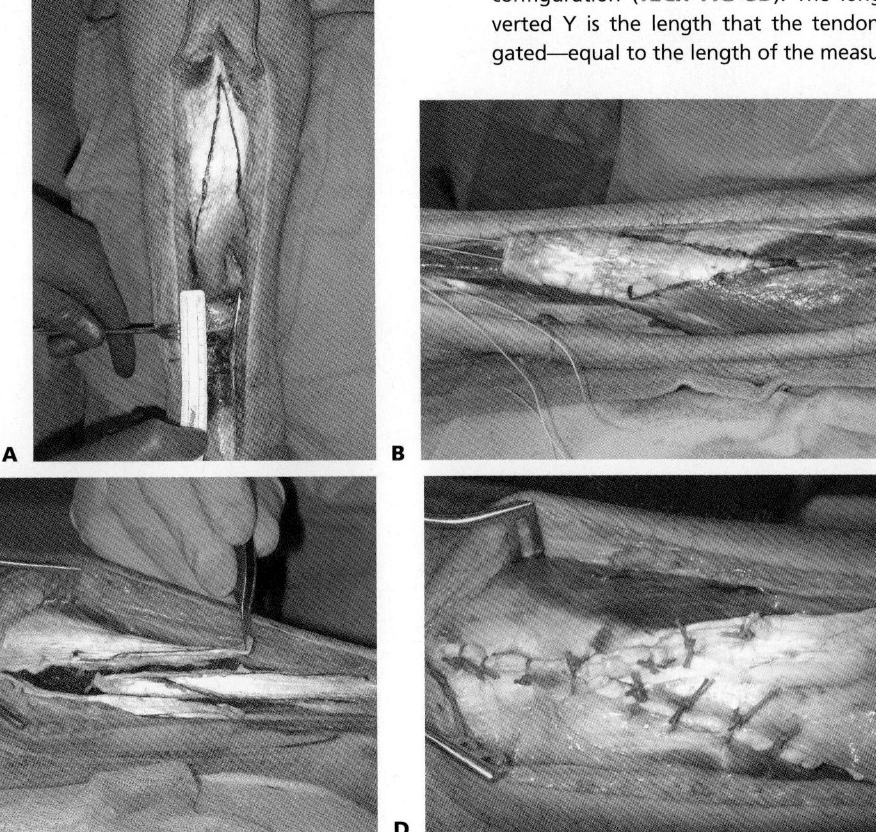

TECH FIG 3 • **A.** The inverted V is made within the myotendinous zone. The limbs of the V are twice the length of the rupture gap. **B.** A locking Krackow-type stitch is placed in each end of the ruptured tendon, using at least five locking loops of braided no. 2 nonabsorbable suture. **C.** The inverted V is cut through the tendinous portion only, leaving the underlying muscle fibers intact. The underlying muscle fibers are allowed to slide after the V release is made in the tendinous portion. **D.** Once lengthened the V cut is repaired into a Y configuration.

FLEXOR HALLUCIS LONGUS AUGMENTATION

- Before repairing the ends of the tendon together, harvest the FHL tendon and transfer it to augment the repair.
- The FHL muscle lies in the deep posterior compartment of the leg immediately posterior to the Achilles tendon in this region. With the Achilles tendon and muscle belly reflected, the deep posterior compartment fascia can be incised and released, exposing the FHL muscle and tendon. The muscle of the FHL usually extends distally down to the level of the tibiotalar joint, making it easy to identify (it is frequently referred to as "beef at the heel") (TECH FIG 4A). Identify the tendon at the distal end of the muscle and digitally retract it.

- The hallux should be seen to flex on traction of the tendon, confirming that the correct tendon has been identified.
- Immediately medial to the FHL muscle and tendon is the medial neurovascular bundle (including the tibial nerve and posterior tibial artery); take care to avoid injury to these structures.
- Follow the FHL tendon around the medial malleolus (dissection should be performed along the lateral aspect of the tendon as the sheath is released behind the ankle to avoid inadvertent injury to the bundle) (**TECH FIG 4B**).
- With the ankle and hallux held fully flexed and maximum traction placed on the FHL tendon, transect the tendon as distally as possible. In almost all cases, adequate length of tendon can be obtained using this technique (**TECH FIG 4C**).
- Measure the tendon diameter (**TECH FIG 4D**); a corresponding-sized bone tunnel will be drilled into the posterior tubercle of the calcaneus directly anterior to the attachment of the distal stump of the Achilles tendon.

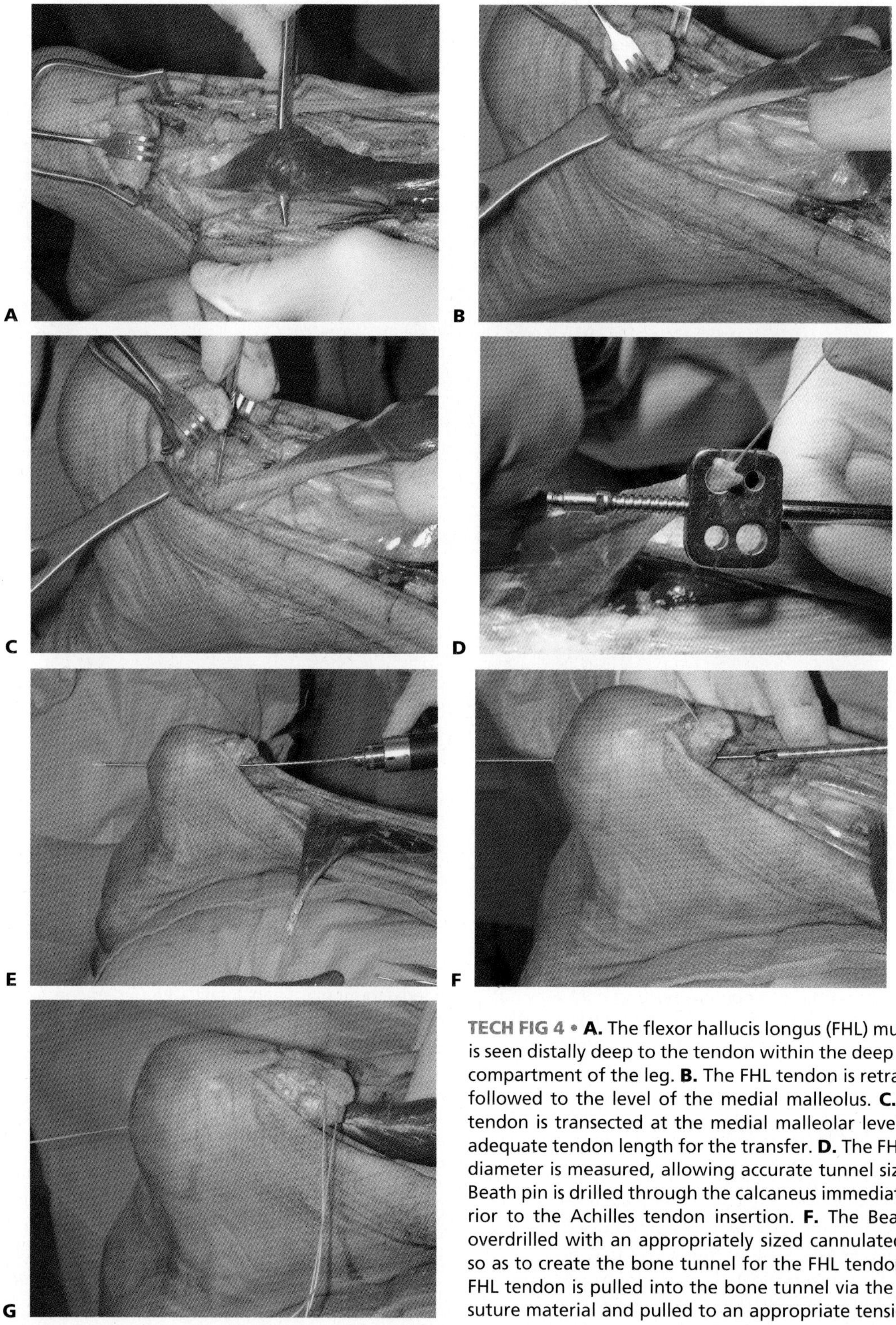

A

B

C

D

E

F

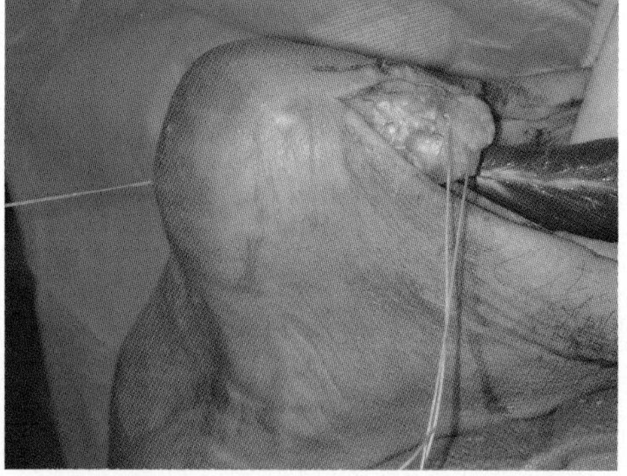
G

TECH FIG 4 • **A.** The flexor hallucis longus (FHL) muscle belly is seen distally deep to the tendon within the deep posterior compartment of the leg. **B.** The FHL tendon is retracted and followed to the level of the medial malleolus. **C.** The FHL tendon is transected at the medial malleolar level, leaving adequate tendon length for the transfer. **D.** The FHL tendon diameter is measured, allowing accurate tunnel sizing. **E.** A Beath pin is drilled through the calcaneus immediately anterior to the Achilles tendon insertion. **F.** The Beath pin is overdrilled with an appropriately sized cannulated drill bit so as to create the bone tunnel for the FHL tendon. **G.** The FHL tendon is pulled into the bone tunnel via the attached suture material and pulled to an appropriate tension.

- Place a Krackow locking suture in the distal portion of the FHL tendon and pull the tendon into the bone tunnel. This is done using a Beath pin (long pin with a suture eyelet), pulling the suture ends out of the plantar aspect of the foot (**TECH FIG 4E**). Create the bone tunnel with a size-specific cannulated drill bit over the Beath pin (**TECH FIG 4F**). Traction can be applied to the suture to hold the tendon within the bone tunnel at the appropriate tension.
- Pull the tendon to the required tension before fixation. The ideal tension holds the ankle at a resting tension of the ankle equal to that of the contralateral side (**TECH FIG 4G**).
- Fix the tendon into the bone tunnel using an interference screw of the same size as the bone tunnel. We use an absorbable biotenodesis screw (Arthrex) (**TECH FIG 5**).

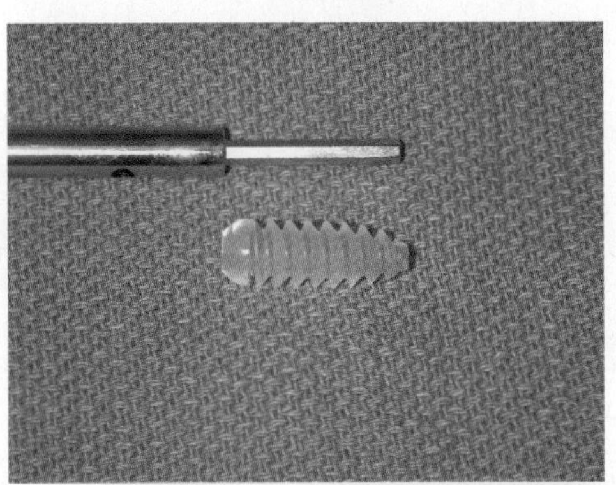

A

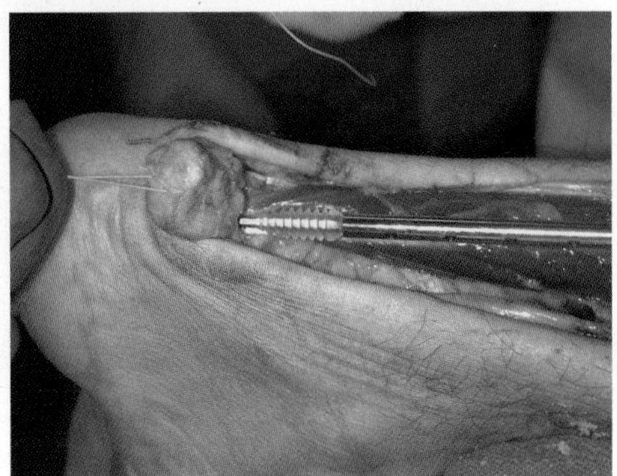

B

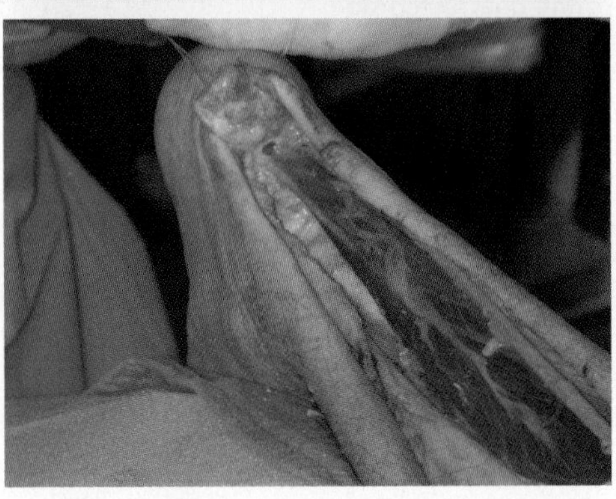

C

TECH FIG 5 • A bioabsorbable interference screw (noncutting threads) is inserted into the bone tunnel holding the flexor hallucis longus tendon, obtaining interference fit between the tendon and the bone and completing the tendon transfer.

ALTERNATE TECHNIQUE FOR FLEXOR HALLUCIS LONGUS HARVEST

- If additional length of the FHL tendon is required, the tendon can be harvested from the midfoot.
- This requires a separate incision to be made over the medial side of the foot from the plantar aspect of the talonavicular joint extending to the midshaft of the first metatarsal.
- Reflect the abductor hallucis and flexor hallucis brevis dorsally, exposing the long flexor tendons.
- Identify the FHL and flexor digitorum longus (FDL) tendons at the master knot of Henry (beware of the medial plantar nerve!) and cut the FHL tendon.
- The FHL stump can be tenodesed to the FDL tendon, but multiple communications exist between these two tendons and this is usually not necessary.
- Retract the FHL through the posterior calf incision.
- This technique allows the FHL tendon to be passed through a transverse bone tunnel in the posterior tuberosity of the calcaneus and looped back onto itself.
- The double strands of tendon are theoretically stronger than a single strand, but no advantage has been shown clinically with this technique.
- I prefer to use the first single-incision technique, limiting the risks of an additional incision and the risks to the structures dissected in the approach, including the medial plantar nerve and its branches.

ACHILLES TENDON REPAIR

- After the FHL transfer is completed, attention is moved back to the Achilles tendon.
- Oppose the proximal and distal ends of the tendon appropriately (via the V-Y slide) and tie them together with intratendinous knots, using the aforementioned nonabsorbable braided suture (**TECH FIG 6A**).
- Once again, confirm that the ankle resting tension remains equal to the contralateral side to avoid overtightening of the repair (**TECH FIG 6B**).
- Gently dorsiflex the ankle to ensure that no diastasis occurs between the tendon ends, confirming adequate integrity of the repair strength.

TECHNIQUES

- Suture the muscle belly of the FHL to the back of the Achilles tendon at the level of the repair with absorbable suture. This provides a vascular bed to the relatively disvascular level of the ruptured Achilles tendon, theoretically increasing the healing potential of the repair.
- Repair the paratenon over the repaired Achilles tendon as a separate layer, using absorbable suture.
- Close the skin in layers via routine closure.
- Apply a well-padded posterior plaster splint with the ankle maintained at its resting level of plantarflexion (equal to the contralateral side), and release the tourniquet.

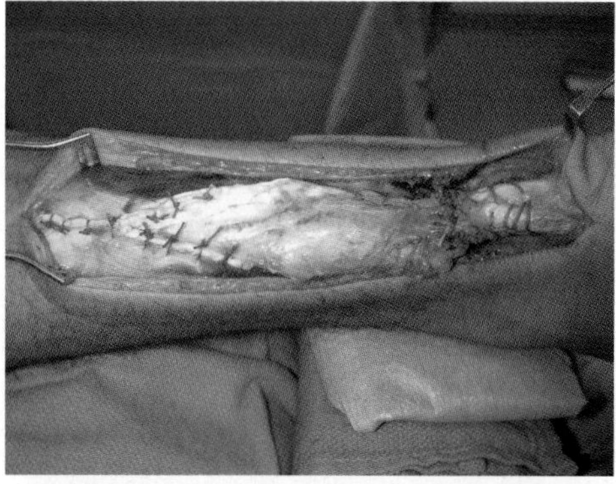

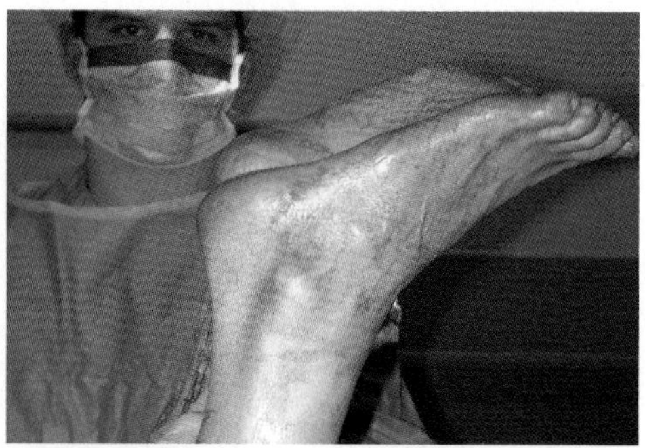

TECH FIG 6 • A. The ruptured Achilles tendon ends are approximated after the V-Y lengthening, allowing direct end-to-end repair of the tendon. **B.** The final resting tension of the repaired Achilles tendon is compared to and matched with that of the unaffected side.

PEARLS AND PITFALLS

Indications	■ As with any Achilles tendon surgery, wound edge necrosis remains a major risk factor. Patients need to be adequately assessed for vascularity, skin quality, and healing potential.
Surgical approach	■ The sural nerve may be trapped in scar tissue after the rupture and should be carefully dissected and protected.
V-Y lengthening	■ Ensure that adequate length is used for the limbs of the V. Twice the rupture gap length is recommended. ■ Avoid excess traction of the proximal tendon, which may result in complete disruption of the myotendinous portion of the GSA complex.
FHL harvest	■ Beware of the deep neurovascular bundle immediately medial and adjacent to the FHL muscle and tendon at the distal tibial level. ■ Dissect the FHL tendon to at least the level of the medial malleolus to ensure enough tendon length is available. ■ When drilling the Beath pin, ensure that the ankle is dorsiflexed so that the bone tunnel direction is colinear with that of the Achilles tendon and the proposed tendon transfer. ■ Ensure that adequate interference fit has been obtained with the screw in the bone tunnel by pulling on the tendon after insertion. ■ Ensure that the FHL tendon is placed at adequate tension to match the unaffected side.
Closure	■ Care should be taken in repairing the paratenon. This has a rich vascular supply, which is important to the tendon repair, and aids in preventing adhesions to the tendon to the skin and subcutaneous tissue.

POSTOPERATIVE CARE

- Postoperatively patients are splinted for 2 weeks in slight equinus (equal to the resting tension of the unaffected side).
- They are kept strictly non–weight-bearing for the first 6 postoperative weeks.
- At 2 weeks after surgery incisions are checked and sutures removed.
- Patients are placed into Achilles-type fracture boots (Bledsoe Inc., Grand Prairie, TX) with three heel wedges, and instructed to remove one wedge after 2 weeks.
- After 6 weeks patients are allowed to start bearing weight on the affected extremity as comfort allows in their protective Achilles boot braces (with two wedges in place at this point).
- Patients are then instructed to remove one wedge every 2 weeks thereafter.
- Physical therapy is performed two or three times a week for the subsequent 10 weeks and includes passive Achilles stretching, an Achilles strengthening program, and gait training. This is performed with the boot brace removed.
- Twelve weeks after surgery, if the ankle is in a neutral alignment, the boot brace is discontinued for ambulation, with the patient continuing the therapy program.
- Patients are instructed to slowly resume their activity as comfort allows, but to avoid sudden acceleration and cutting or jumping activities until at least 6 months after surgery.

OUTCOMES

- Outcomes of chronic or neglected Achilles tendon rupture repair are uniformly inferior to those of acute rupture repair.
- Using a V-Y advancement alone, Us et al[5] reported up to 22% deficiency in peak torque compared to the unaffected side in 6 patients.
- Wapner et al[6] reported on using the FHL tendon without V-Y advancement through a two-incision approach (with the second incision made in the medial longitudinal arch, where the FHL was harvested at the level of the master knot of Henry).
  - On Cybex testing they reported 29.5% average decrease in strength at 30°/s and decreases in torque and work generated by plantarflexion of the ankle as being 41.8% and 51% respectively compared to the nonoperated side.
- In a recent study by Raikin et al[4] using the combined V-Y lengthening and FHL augmentation described above on 15 patients with a minimum gap of 5 cm, a 7.7 N-m (−22.3%) loss of plantarflexion torque at 60°/s and a 3.5 N-m (−13.5%) loss of plantarflexion torque at 120°/s was seen on Cybex testing compared to the unaffected side.
  - Patients had an average 5-degree loss of active motion arc of the ankle joint in the sagittal plane. AOFAS ankle hindfoot scores improved from an average 58.4 out of 100 preoperatively to an average 94.1 out of 100 postoperatively.
  - Eight of 15 patients were able to perform more than 10 repetitions of a single-leg heel raise at 2-year follow-up.
  - All patients were satisfied with their outcome (rated good or very good).

COMPLICATIONS

- Wound edge necrosis
- Rerupture
- Plantarflexion weakness
- Sural neuritis or nerve injury
- Deep vein thrombosis

REFERENCES

1. Jozsa L, Kvist M, Balint BJ. The role of recreational sport activity in Achilles tendon rupture: a clinical, pathoanatomical and sociological study of 292 cases. Am J Sports Med 1989;17:338–343.
2. Lagergren C, Lindholm A. Vascular distribution in the Achilles tendon; an angiographic and microangiographic study. Acta Chir Scand 1959;116:491–495.
3. Mandelbaum BR, Myerson MS, Forster R. Achilles tendon ruptures: a new technique of repair, early range of motion and functional rehabilitation. Am J Sports Med 1995;23:392–395.
4. Raikin SM, Elias I, Bessler MP, et al. Reconstruction of retracted Achilles tendon rupture with V-Y lengthening and FHL tendon. Foot Ankle Int 2007;28:1238–1248.
5. Us AK, Bilgin SS, Aydin T, et al. Repair of neglected Achilles tendon ruptures: procedures and functional results. Arch Orthop Trauma Surg 1997;116:408–411.
6. Wapner KL, Pavlock GS, Hecht PJ, et al. Repair of chronic Achilles tendon rupture with flexor hallucis longus tendon transfer. Foot Ankle Int 1993;14:443–449.

Chapter 111

Chronic Achilles Tendon Ruptures Using Hamstring/Peroneal Tendons

Nicholas A. Ferran and Nicola Maffulli

DEFINITION

- Rupture of the Achilles tendon is common.
- More than 20% of acute injuries are misdiagnosed, leading to chronic or neglected ruptures.[3]
- Most authors define chronic rupture as a rupture with a delay in diagnosis or treatment for more than 4 weeks.[2,8,9]

ANATOMY

- The two heads of the gastrocnemius (medial and lateral) arise from the condyles of the femur, the fleshy part of the muscle extending to about the middle of the calf. As the muscle fibers descend they insert into a broad aponeurosis, which contracts and receives the tendon of the soleus on its deep surface to form the Achilles tendon.[14]
- The Achilles tendon is the thickest and strongest tendon in the body. About 15 cm long, it originates in the middle of the calf and extends distally to insert into the posterior surface of the calcaneum. Throughout its length, it receives muscle fibers from the soleus on its anterior surface.[14]

PATHOGENESIS

- The most common mechanism of injury is pushing off with the weight-bearing forefoot while extending the knee. However, sudden unexpected dorsiflexion of the ankle or violent dorsiflexion of a plantarflexed foot may also result in ruptures.[4]
- Corticosteroids, fluoroquinolones, previous tendon pathology, and poor vascularity of the Achilles tendon have been associated with rupture.[4]
- Patients with chronic ruptures of the Achilles tendon recall either minimal trauma or an injury misdiagnosed as an ankle sprain. They commonly complain of a limp and difficulties with activities of daily living, particularly ascending stairs.[5]

PATIENT HISTORY AND PHYSICAL FINDINGS

- Methods for examination include the following:
  - *Palpable gap*. Gap is not always palpable in chronic ruptures.
  - *Calf squeeze test (Simmonds test* or *Thompson test)*[12]: positive or negative. False positive may be possible if plantaris is present and intact.
  - *Knee flexion test (Matles test)*[6]: A false positive may occur when there is neurologic weakness of the Achilles tendon.
- Patients may present with a limp.
- In acute tendon ruptures, a gap in the Achilles tendon is usually palpable. This gap may be absent in chronic ruptures, as the gap is usually bridged by scar tissue.
- Active plantarflexion of the foot is usually preserved due to the action of tibialis posterior, the peroneal tendons, and the long toe flexors.
- The calf squeeze test, first described by Simmonds in 1957,[12] but often credited to Thompson, who redescribed it in 1962, is performed with the patient prone and ankles clear of the couch. The examiner squeezes the fleshy part of the calf, causing the deformation of the soleus and resulting in plantarflexion of the foot if the Achilles tendon is intact. The affected leg should be compared to the contralateral leg.
- The knee flexion test is performed with the patient prone and ankles clear of the table. The patient is asked to actively flex the knee to 90 degrees. During this movement the foot on the affected side falls into neutral or dorsiflexion and a rupture of the Achilles tendon can be diagnosed.[6]

IMAGING AND OTHER DIAGNOSTIC STUDIES

- As clinical diagnosis of chronic ruptures can be problematic, imaging can be useful.
- Plain lateral radiographs may reveal an irregular configuration of the fat-filled triangular space anterior to the Achilles tendon and between the posterior aspect of the tibia and superior aspect of the calcaneus (this space is known as the triangle of Kager).
- Ultrasonography of a chronic rupture usually demonstrates an acoustic vacuum with thick irregular edges (**FIG 1**).
- T1-weighted MR images will show disruption of signal within the tendon substance, while T2-weighted images show generalized high signal intensity.

DIFFERENTIAL DIAGNOSIS

- Acute rupture of the Achilles tendon, rerupture of the Achilles tendon, tear of the musculotendinous junction of the gastrocnemius-soleus and the Achilles tendon.

NONOPERATIVE MANAGEMENT

- Consensus is that the most appropriate treatment for chronic Achilles tendon ruptures is surgical.[8]

SURGICAL MANAGEMENT

- A delay in presentation of Achilles tendon rupture results in filling of the gap between the ruptured tendon ends with fibrous nonfunctional scar, which needs excision. To re-establish tendon continuity, surgeons may consider the use of

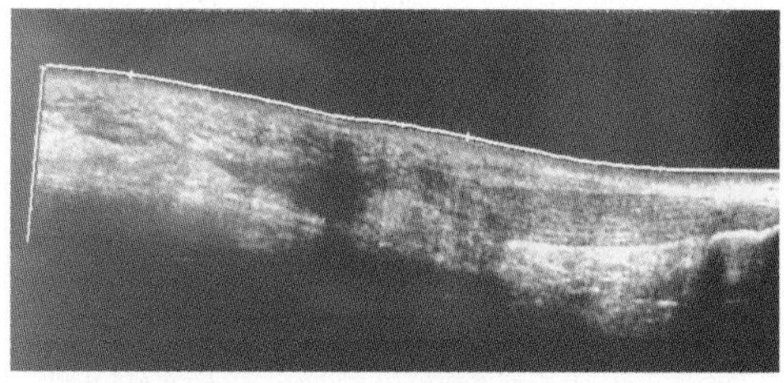

FIG 1 • Ultrasound of ruptured Achilles tendon. Acoustic vacuum demonstrated with irregular edges.

the following: (1) the residual Achilles tendon, (2) adjacent tendons, (3) autologous free tendon grafts, (4) allografts.[15]

Preoperative Planning

- All imaging should be reviewed to estimate the tendon gap.
- If the gap in maximum plantarflexion is 5 to 9 cm, peroneus brevis transfer can be used.[7,10,13,16]
- If the gap is 9 to 12 cm, we recommend a free autologous gracilis tendon graft.[5]
- If these tendons have already been used for other reconstructive procedures, alternative surgical options will have to be considered.

Positioning

- Under general anesthesia, the patient is placed prone with the ankles clear of the operating table.
- A tourniquet is applied to the limb to be operated on. The limb is exsanguinated, and the tourniquet is inflated to 250 mm Hg.

Approach

- The traditional midline longitudinal approach over the Achilles tendon has been associated with wound healing problems and a risk of sural nerve injury when extended proximally.
- We do not use the lateral approach, given the high risk of sural nerve injury.
- We employ a 10- to 12-cm curvilinear approach medial to the medial border of the tendon with sharp dissection through the subcutaneous fat to the paratenon. This incision avoids the sural nerve.[13]
- Maintaining thick skin flaps is vital to reduce the incidence of wound breakdown.

PERONEUS BREVIS TENDON TRANSFER FOR CHRONIC ACHILLES TENDON RUPTURE

- The Achilles tendon is exposed by longitudinal incision of the paratenon in the midline for the length of the skin incision.
- The ends of the Achilles tendon are freshened by sharp dissection, producing a defect between the freshened ends. The proximal stump is gently dissected out and mobilized distally (**TECH FIG 1**).
- Through the base of the wound, the deep fascia overlying the deep flexor compartment and the compartment containing the peronei muscles can be seen.
- The internervous plane lies between the peroneus brevis (supplied by the superficial peroneal nerve) and the flexor hallucis longus (supplied by the tibial nerve).
- The peroneus brevis tendon can be identified toward the medial side.
- The tendons of the peroneus longus and brevis can be distinguished from each other at this level by the fact that although both are tendinous in the distal third of the lower leg, the peroneus brevis is muscular more distally than the peroneus longus. The deep fascia overlying the peroneal tendons is incised and the peroneal tendons are mobilized.
- Make a 2.5-cm longitudinal incision over the base of the fifth metatarsal. Identify the peroneus brevis tendon, place a stay suture in the distal end of the peroneus brevis tendon, and detach the tendon from its insertion and mobilize it proximally.
- Deliver the tendon through the posteromedial wound using gentle continuous traction as it is pulled through the inferior peroneal retinaculum. In this fashion, the tendon of the peroneus brevis retains its blood supply from the intermuscular septum.
- Weave the peroneus brevis tendon through the Achilles tendon ends.

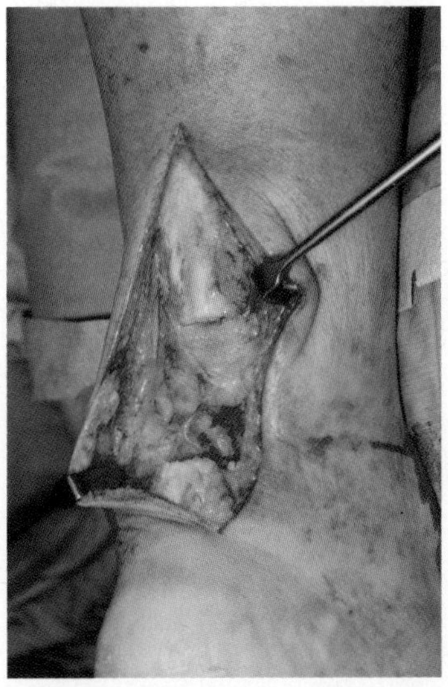
A

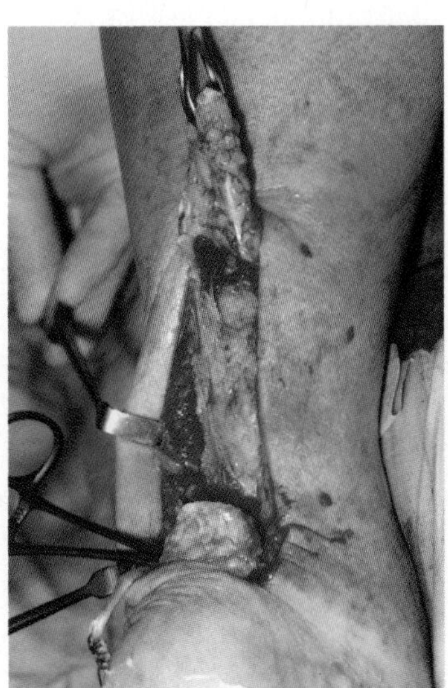
B

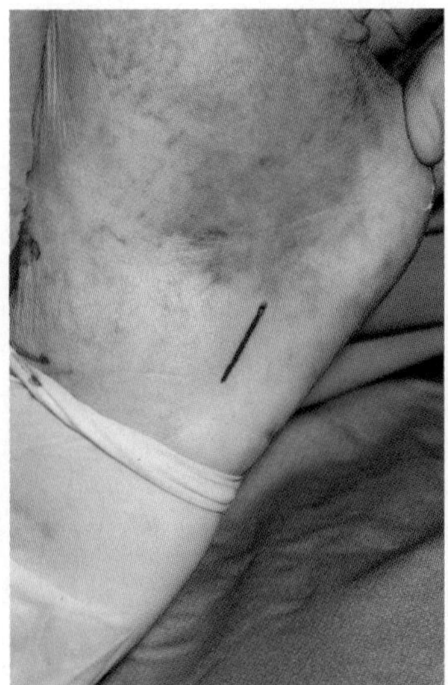
C

TECH FIG 1 • Repair of chronic Achilles tendon rupture with peroneus brevis. **A.** Tendon ends are débrided to demonstrate true defect. **B.** Proximal stump mobilized into wound. **C.** Incision made over insertion of peroneus brevis on the base of the fifth metatarsal. *(continued)*

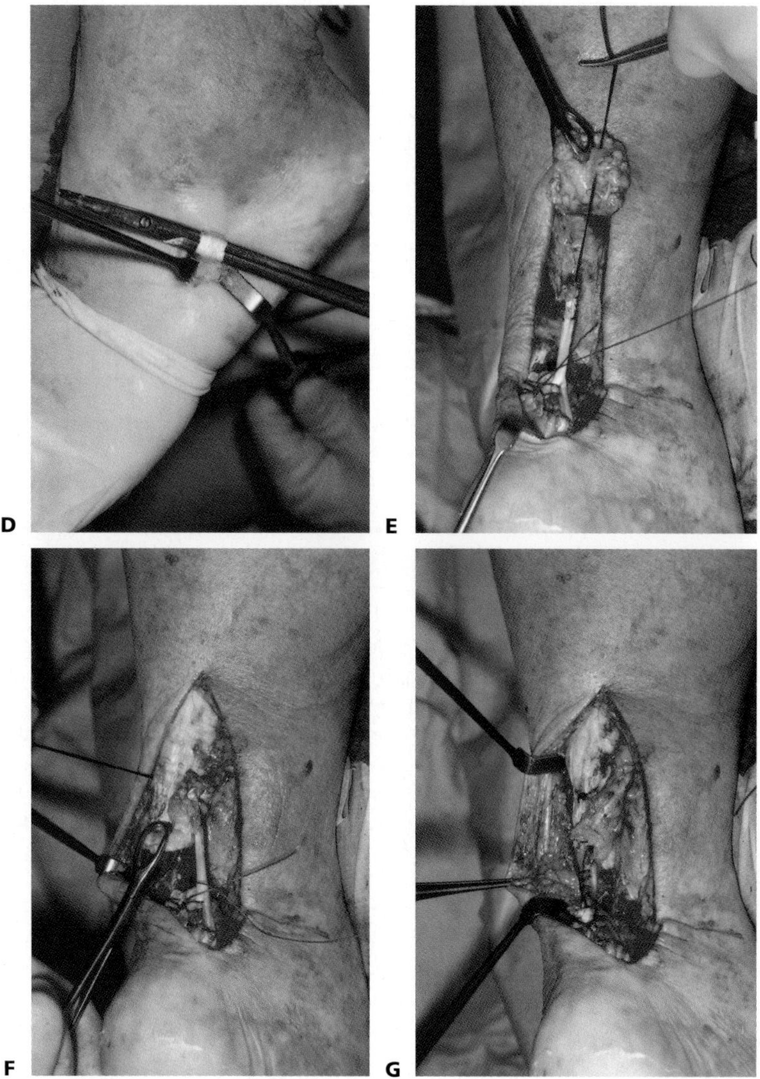

TECH FIG 1 • *(continued)* **D.** Peroneus brevis insertion dissected. **E.** Tendon passed from lateral to medial in distal stump. **F.** Tendon passed from medial to lateral in proximal stump. **G.** Completed repair.

- First pass it from lateral to medial through the distal stump via coronal incisions medially and laterally in the Achilles tendon.
- Suture the edges of the coronal incisions in the Achilles tendon to the peroneus brevis tendon to prevent progression of the incision that would lead to the peroneal tendon cutting out through the Achilles tendon.
- Pass the tendon through the proximal stump from medial to lateral, with the foot maximally plantarflexed.
- Suture the peroneal tendon to the Achilles tendon stumps using 3-0 Vicryl. This is usually sufficient, but, if there is a very large defect, the tendon of the plantaris can be harvested, if present. This is then used to reinforce the reconstruction.
- In most cases of neglected ruptures of the Achilles tendon, the paratenon is either not present or not viable. If present, one can generally manage to close it over the proximal stump using 2-0 Vicryl.
- Close the skin with a continuous 2-0 subcuticular Vicryl suture. Steri-Strips are applied and the wound is dressed.
- The tourniquet is deflated and the time recorded.

FREE GRACILIS TENDON GRAFT FOR CHRONIC RUPTURES OF THE ACHILLES TENDON

- Make a 12- to 15-cm longitudinal, slightly curvilinear skin incision medial and anterior to the medial border of the Achilles tendon.
- The paratenon, if not disrupted, is incised longitudinally in the midline for the length of the skin incision.
- The Achilles tendon is thus exposed, and gentle continuous traction is applied to the proximal stump of the ruptured tendon to further deliver it into the wound (TECH FIG 2).
- Excise scar tissue in both the proximal and distal stumps to reach viable tendon.

A 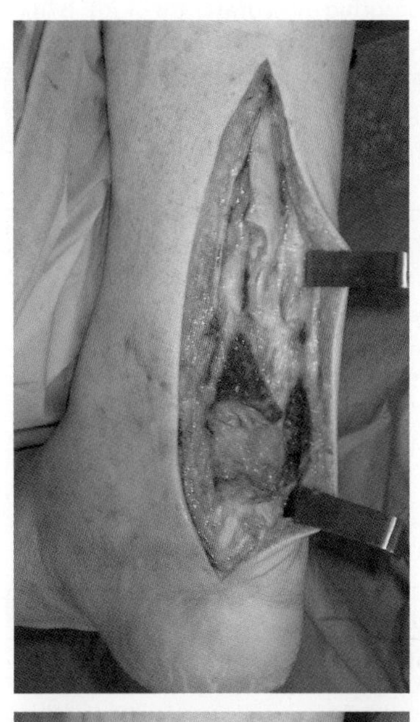

B 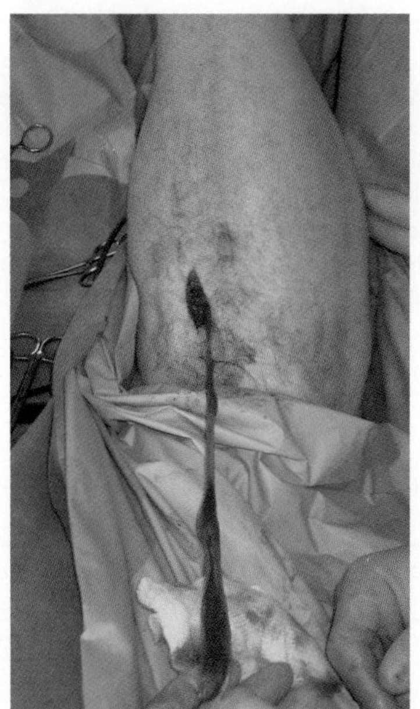

C 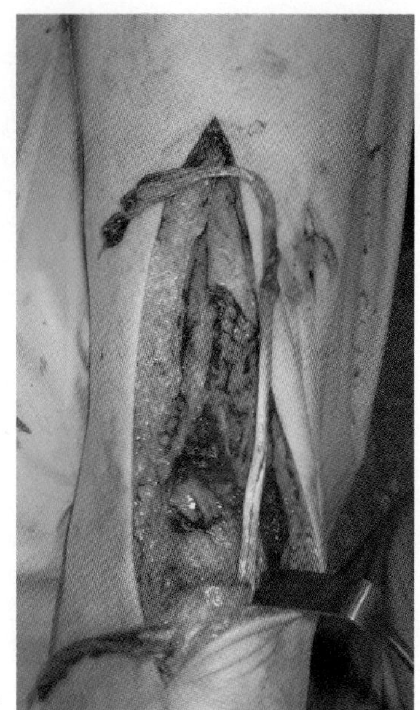

D 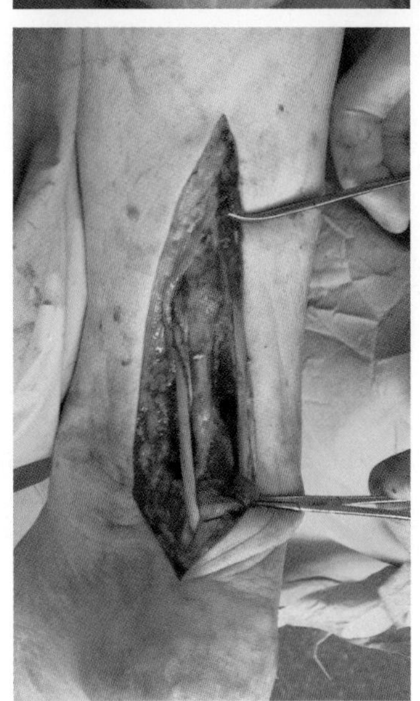

E 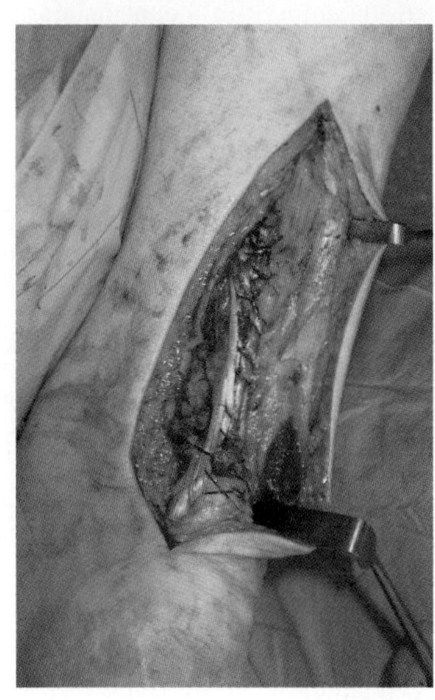

TECH FIG 2 • Repair of chronic Achilles tendon rupture with gracilis tendon graft. **A.** Tendon ends débrided to reveal true defect. **B.** Gracilis harvested. **C.** Tendon passed from medial to lateral in distal stump. **D.** Tendon passed from lateral to medial in proximal stump. **E.** Completed repair.

- If the remaining gap in the Achilles tendon is greater than 9 cm, we proceed to harvest the gracilis tendon.
- Make a vertical 2- to 3-cm longitudinal incision on the medial aspect of the tibial tuberosity, centered over the distal insertion of the pes anserinus.
- A venous plexus is often encountered at the distal end of the wound, and care should be taken to diathermy this.
- Carry out dissection deep to the fat both medially and superiorly with a small swab on an artery forceps to expose the sartorius fascia.
- Insert a curved retractor and make a curved incision, 1 cm long, along the superior margin of the pes anserinus into the sartorius fascia, taking care to avoid the saphenous nerve.
- Use blunt dissection with Mackenrodt scissors to produce a window within the superior border of the sartorius allowing access to the tendon of gracilis.
- The gracilis tendon lies more superiorly than the neighboring tendon of the semitendinosus and can be retrieved with a curved Moynihan clip.
- As the tendon is brought into the wound, use of an arthroscopic probe helps to identify the possible tendon's proximal vincular attachments. The vincula are sectioned to achieve distal traction on the tendon.
- Before using a tendon stripper to harvest the tendon, all attachments to the tendon must be completely released. An assistant places his or her hand over the calf, and, by applying firm traction longitudinally, excludes the presence of remaining tendinous attachments by the absence of calf tethering.
- Harvest the gracilis tendon with the tendon stripper by directing the instrument in line with the tendon fibers, parallel to the thigh.

TECHNIQUES

- Once the gracilis tendon is freed of fat and muscle fibers on the back table, pass it from medial to lateral through a small transverse incision in the distal stump of the Achilles tendon made with a no. 11 scalpel blade.
- Pull the gracilis tendon proximally and through a small incision in the substance of the proximal stump of the Achilles tendon in a lateral-to-medial direction.
- Suture the gracilis tendon to the Achilles tendon at each entry and exit point using 3-0 Vicryl (Polyglactin 910 braided absorbable suture).
- Before fully securing the graft, the foot is maximally plantarflexed.
- In most patients with neglected ruptures of the Achilles tendon, the paratenon is either not present or not viable. If present, one can generally manage to close it over the proximal stump using 2-0 Vicryl.
- Close the skin with a continuous 2/0 subcuticular Vicryl suture. Steri-Strips are applied and the wound is dressed.
- The tourniquet is deflated and the time recorded.

PEARLS AND PITFALLS

Diagnosis	▪ Diagnosis is usually made on a clinical basis, but this can be difficult in cases of chronic rupture. ▪ Imaging can be useful in clinching the diagnosis and in preoperative planning.
Indications	▪ We recommend peroneus brevis transfer for Achilles tendon defects less than 9 cm.
	▪ For defects greater than 9 cm we recommend free gracilis graft.
Positioning	▪ Prone position, with thigh tourniquet
Incision	▪ An incision placed medial and anterior to the medial border of the Achilles tendon reduces the likelihood of sural nerve injury.
Gracilis harvesting	▪ The tendon must be completely freed of its attachments before harvesting.

POSTOPERATIVE CARE

- Before the patient is taken off the operating table, a below-knee plaster-of-Paris cast is applied to the operated leg, with the patient prone and the ankle in maximal equinus.
- The operated leg is elevated until discharge.
- Patients are usually discharged on the day after surgery after having been taught to use crutches by an orthopaedic physiotherapist.
- Thromboprophylaxis is provided with Fragmin 2500 units (dalteparin sodium) subcutaneously once daily, or with 150 mg acetylsalicylic acid orally daily until removal of the cast.
- Patients are told to bear weight on the operated leg as able, but to keep it elevated as much as possible at home for the first 2 postoperative weeks.
- The cast is removed at the second postoperative week, and a synthetic anterior below-knee slab is applied with the foot in maximal equinus.
- The synthetic slab is secured to the leg with three or four removable Velcro straps for 4 weeks.
- Patients can graduate to full weight bearing as soon as comfort allows.
- A trained physiotherapist supervises the introduction of gentle mobilization exercises of the ankle, isometric contraction of the gastrocsoleus complex, and gentle concentric contraction of the calf muscles. Inversion and eversion of the ankle is also encouraged.
- At 6 weeks postoperatively, the patient is followed up and the anterior slab removed.
- Physiotherapists supervise gradual stretching and strengthening exercises.
- Cycling and swimming are started at 8 weeks postoperatively. Patients are encouraged to increase the frequency of their exercise.
- Patients are allowed to return to their sport at the fifth postoperative month.

OUTCOMES

- We have reported on 22 patients with chronic Achilles tendon ruptures using peroneus brevis tendon transfer. All were satisfied with the procedure. Despite subjective patient satisfaction, however, objective evaluation demonstrated greater loss of isokinetic strength variables at high speeds, and greater loss of calf circumference when compared with patients undergoing open repair of fresh Achilles tendon ruptures.[11]
- Gallant et al[1] assessed eversion and plantarflexion strength after repair of Achilles tendon rupture using peroneus brevis tendon transfer and found mild objective eversion and plantar flexion weakness. However, subjective assessment revealed no functional compromise.
- In a study by Pintore et al,[11] of 21 patients treated with a free gracilis graft, 2 had excellent results, 15 had good results, and 4 had fair results. All returned to their preinjury occupation. Fifteen returned to leisure activities, including sports such as tennis, squash, and bowling.
  - Maximum calf circumference was significantly decreased in the operated leg at both presentation and follow-up.
  - The operated limb showed a lower peak torque than the nonoperated one, but patients did not perceive this as hampering their daily or leisure activities.[5]

COMPLICATIONS

- Wound healing problems
- Infection
- Sural nerve injury
- Rerupture of Achilles tendon
- Deep vein thrombosis

REFERENCES

1. Gallant GG, Massie C, Turco VJ. Assessment of eversion and plantar flexion strength after repair of Achilles tendon rupture using peroneus brevis tendon transfer. Am J Orthop 1995;24:257–261.
2. Jennings AG, Sefton GK. Chronic rupture of tendo Achilles: long-term results of operative management using polyester tape. J Bone Joint Surg Br 2002;84B:361–363.
3. Maffulli N. Clinical tests in sports medicine: more on Achilles tendon. Br J Sports Med 1996;30:250.
4. Maffulli N. Rupture of the Achilles tendon. J Bone Joint Surg Am 1999;81A:1019–1036.
5. Maffulli N, Leadbetter WB. Free gracilis tendon graft in neglected tears of the Achilles tendon. Clin J Sport Med 2005;15:56–61.
6. Matles AL. Rupture of the tendo Achilles: another diagnostic sign. Bull Hosp Joint Dis 1975;36:48–51.
7. McClelland D, Maffulli N. Neglected rupture of the Achilles tendon: reconstruction with peroneus brevis tendon transfer. Surgeon 2004;2: 209–213.
8. Miskulin M, Miskulin A, Klobucar H, et al. Neglected rupture of the Achilles tendon treated with peroneus brevis transfer: a functional assessment of 5 cases. J Foot Ankle Surg 2005;44:49–56.
9. Nellas ZJ, Loder BG, Wertheimer SJ. Reconstruction of an Achilles tendon defect utilizing an Achilles tendon allograft. J Foot Ankle Surg 1996;35:144–148.
10. Perez-Teuffer A. Traumatic rupture of the Achilles tendon: reconstruction by transplant and graft using the lateral peroneus brevis. Orthop Clin North Am 1974;5:89–93.
11. Pintore E, Barra V, Pintore R, et al. Peroneus brevis tendon transfer in neglected tears of the Achilles tendon. J Trauma 2001;50: 71–78.
12. Simmonds FA. The diagnosis of the ruptured Achilles tendon. Practitioner 1957;179:56–58.
13. Turco V, Spinella AJ. Achilles tendon ruptures: peroneus brevis transfer. Foot Ankle 1987;7:253–259.
14. Williams PL. Gray's Anatomy, 38th ed. Edinburgh: Churchill Livingstone, 1995.
15. Young J, Sayana MK, Maffulli N, et al. Technique of free gracilis tendon transfer for delayed rupture of the Achilles tendon. Tech Foot Ankle Surg 2005;4:148–153.
16. Young JS, Sayana MK, McClelland D, et al. Peroneus brevis tendon transfer for delayed Achilles tendon ruptures. Tech Foot Ankle Surg 2005;4:143–147.

Chapter 112

Chronic Achilles Tendon Ruptures Using Allograft Reconstruction

Andrew P. Molloy and Mark S. Myerson

DEFINITION

- Chronic Achilles tendon ruptures are defined as those of greater than 3 months' duration.
- There are three indications for this technique:
  - A defect between healthy ends of tendon of at least 5 cm. Procedures using local tissue or autograft tendon augmentation generally suffice for lesser defects.
  - An expectation of recovery of function that would not be provided by Achilles tendon direct repair or advancement or flexor hallucis longus transfer
  - Failed reconstruction using autologous tendon advancement or augmentation
- This technique may also be considered for patients with severe chronic Achilles tendinopathy that warrants resection of an extensive degenerated section of the tendon, leaving a gap similar to that observed in chronic Achilles tendon rupture.

ANATOMY

- The Achilles tendon is the condensation of the two heads of the gastrocnemius and soleus muscles. The musculotendinous junction is about 6 to 8 cm from its insertion into the central third of the posterior calcaneus.
- The enthesis is composed of cartilage and fibrocartilage, typically over an area of 6 cm^2. The posterior calcaneal tuberosity and retrocalcaneal bursa lie anterosuperiorly.
- The tendon is surrounded by paratenon consisting of both parietal and visceral layers. These relatively pliable layers provide tendon blood supply, nutrition, and lubrication. The approximate physiologic excursion of the Achilles tendon is 1.5 cm.
- Blood supply, from vessels running the entire length of the paratenon, approach the tendon from its anterior surface via the mesotenon. The concentration and diameter of these vessels vary along the course of the paratenon, with the fewest being at the relatively hypovascular area 4 cm proximal to the insertion. The blood supply at the Achilles insertion on the calcaneus is also relatively avascular.[4]

PATHOGENESIS

- Rupture occurs when the tendon is stressed beyond its yield point. The magnitude of this depends on the force and speed of loading, cross-sectional area of the tendon, and diminution of tendon quality by any pathologic process.
- Predisposing factors
  - Achilles tendinopathy
  - Corticosteroids (oral or locally infiltrated), anabolic steroids
  - Low normal level of exercise, aging
  - Gout, hyperthyroidism, renal insufficiency, arteriosclerosis
  - Fluoroquinolones
- Pathogenesis of tendinopathy and chronic tears
  - Chronic Achilles tendon tears most commonly occur with preexisting tendinopathy, tendinopathy that frequently was asymptomatic. Eighty percent of tears occur in the relatively hypovascular area 2 to 6 cm above the insertion; the second most common location for tendinopathy or chronic tears to develop is at the insertion on the calcaneus.
  - Tendinopathy is a result of microtrauma, hypovascularity, degeneration, and failure of healing. With progression, fibrovascular proliferation from the paratenon, accompanied by a marked lymphocytic and histiocytic response, develops in the degenerative tendon, leading to fibrinous and myxanthomatous degeneration of the Achilles tendon. These changes decrease the threshold for tendon rupture.
- Pathologic changes in untreated ruptures
  - There is initial retraction of the tendon ends due to inherent muscle tension.
  - Within 2 weeks, fibrous organization of the tendon ends and hematoma occur.
  - There is a gradual transformation in shape of the tendon ends, with the distal and proximal portions respectively becoming more bulbous and conical. Moreover, the tendon ends tend to adhere to the investing fascia of the deep posterior compartment.
  - The hematoma in the gap between the tendon ends gradually organizes into fibrous scar tissue, which appears to reestablish tendon continuity but lacks contractile strength.
  - The fibroblasts remain disorganized rather than aligning in a physiologically correct longitudinal formation.
  - The resultant fibrous mass is rarely capable of withstanding the physiologic tensile forces of the gastrocnemius–soleus complex and thus develops further elongation and weakness.
- Rupture of the Achilles tendon may lead to (1) loss of plantarflexion power, (2) lack of control of the second rocker during the stance phase of gait, and (3) subjective and objective decrease in ankle stability.[12,13]

NATURAL HISTORY

- Most chronic ruptures present in older patients.
  - Occasionally a prodrome of Achilles tendon symptoms is reported; however, there may have been only the typical palpable and visual changes that occur with tendinopathy.
  - The patient will describe a sudden onset of pain of varying intensity either on stumbling (eccentric loading) or on push-off (concentric loading).
  - The pain is usually associated with swelling and weakness, although if the tendon was previously dysfunctional due to tendinopathy, the difference may be small.
  - Medical attention is often not sought because plantarflexion function, albeit weak, remains due to the contribution of the other ankle plantarflexors (flexor hallucis longus, flexor digitorum longus, peroneal tendons, and the posterior tibial tendon).
- The amount of disability with an untreated rupture is often determined by the patient's premorbid status.

- A marked limp, inability to run, acquired pes planus, and difficulty climbing stairs are often noted.
- Inability to repetitively perform a single leg raise and subjective weakness and instability are generally present.[1,12,13]

PATIENT HISTORY AND PHYSICAL FINDINGS

- Physical examination methods include the following:
  - Thompson–Simmond test: Abnormal result signifies a functional tear of Achilles tendon.
  - Plantarflexion power: A score less than 4 indicates that a tear is likely; a score of 4 or 5 indicates that a tear is unlikely.
  - Palpation of gap in Achilles tendon: Mild = end-to-end repair; Moderate = V–Y advancement; severe = Achilles tendon allograft
- A complete history and physical examination should be done to determine associated injuries and predisposing factors.
- Inspection
  - Gap in tendon
  - Calf atrophy
  - Resting tension of the foot with the patient prone and knee flexed, relative to the uninjured contralateral extremity
- Gait
  - Antalgic
  - Vertical oscillation of pelvis with increased hip and knee flexion[13]
  - Ankle instability[13]
- Palpation of gap between tendon ends gives some indication of repair technique, should surgical reconstruction be considered.
  - 1 to 2 cm: usually end-to-end repair with or without tenodesis augmentation
  - 2 to 5 cm: usually V–Y advancement with or without tenodesis augmentation
  - More than 5 cm: autograft or allograft tendon transfer or reconstruction
- Range of motion: excessive dorsiflexion (**FIG 1**)
- Plantarflexion
  - May still be present due to recruitment of tibialis posterior, flexor hallucis longus, flexor digitorum longus, and peroneal tendons
  - Decreased power
- Thompson–Simmond test[11,14]

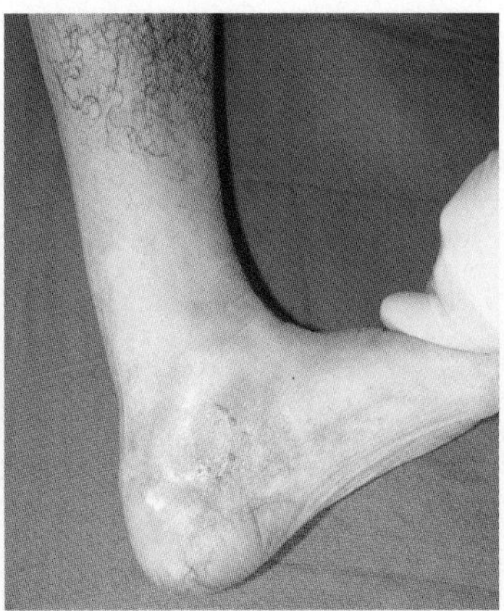

FIG 1 • Excessive dorsiflexion due to chronic rupture of Achilles tendon.

- Premorbid conditions: skin quality, smoking, neurovascular status, diabetes mellitus

IMAGING AND OTHER DIAGNOSTIC STUDIES

- Imaging studies for chronic Achilles tendon ruptures are typically not indicated.
- Plain radiographs may reveal calcification within the tendon, suggestive of a degenerative process leading to rupture.
- Plain radiographs may also demonstrate a bony avulsion from the calcaneus.
- Ultrasound and magnetic resonance imaging (MRI) are unnecessary but confirm clinical findings and provide some understanding of the extent of diseased tendon or gap in contrast to healthy tendon. This additional information may be useful in surgical planning for an Achilles tendon allograft since clinical examination may not accurately define the extent of diseased tendon that will need to be resected.

NONOPERATIVE MANAGEMENT

- The extent of nonoperative treatment depends on level of symptoms and required level of functional improvement. Despite the seemingly devastating functional consequences of chronic Achilles tendon rupture, not all patients require a reconstructive procedure.
- Bracing
  - The level of hindfoot and ankle stabilization required is determined by the power of plantarflexion power afforded by secondary muscles and to a lesser extent by the patient's weight.
  - A relatively lightweight carbon-fiber ankle–foot orthosis (AFO) may enhance gait during push-off by transferring elastic recoil gained during dorsiflexion to plantarflexion to compensate for lack of Achilles tendon function. In our experience, this treatment is less suitable for heavier patients.
  - A clamshell AFO that encompasses the foot and ankle may be of greater benefit than a traditional AFO for patients with a combination of severe loss of plantarflexion function and poor ankle stability. The addition of an anterior component to the conventional AFO provides the advantage of resisting excessive ankle dorsiflexion.
  - In select patients, a double-upright brace attached to a stiffer-soled shoe and locked at the ankle may be as effective as a conventional or clamshell AFO.
- Physical therapy
  - Physical therapy should focus on strengthening the secondary ankle plantarflexors (flexor hallucis longus, flexor digitorum longus, posterior tibial tendon, and peroneals)
  - Gait training, stabilization, and proprioception exercises

SURGICAL MANAGEMENT

- Advantages of allograft versus autograft
  - No morbidity or loss of function and pain from donor site
  - Quality and amount of autogenous tendon may be insufficient
  - Shorter operative time as no harvesting is required
  - Satisfactory mechanical properties of allograft are proven[8–10]
- Disadvantages
  - Cost
  - Theoretical risk of transmission of host infectious diseases[2,3]

Preoperative Planning

- Vascular status is assessed.
- The surgeon should ensure that the posterior lower leg skin is amenable to surgical intervention; if concern exists, the threshold for plastic surgery consultation should be low.
- The contralateral limb is assessed for natural resting tension of the gastrocnemius–soleus complex.
- Imaging studies, if obtained, may provide some understanding of the extent of degenerated Achilles tendon.

Positioning

- Before positioning, a well-padded tourniquet is applied. This should be on the thigh as to prevent tethering of the gastrocnemius–soleus complex and potential inaccuracies in allograft tensioning.
- We prefer a popliteal block for postoperative pain management in conjunction with general anesthesia to permit the patient to tolerate the thigh tourniquet. Depending on surgeon preference, a more proximal regional anesthetic, spinal, or epidural may be considered. The advantage to a popliteal block is improved leg function and potentially safer mobilization in the immediate postoperative period, since the proximal limb girdle muscle function is not forfeited.
- Prone positioning with adequate padding, maintenance of airway, avoidance of brachial plexus tension, and safe positioning of the patient's genitalia are all important.
- The lower limb is prepared and draped in the standard sterile fashion to above the knee.
- The limb is exsanguinated and the tourniquet is inflated. (Care must be taken to avoid excessive hip and lower back extension.)

Approach

- A posterior approach to the distal lower leg is used with a midline incision of about 20 cm centered over the Achilles tendon and central posterior calcaneus. While this is our preferred technique, the surgical approach must respect prior surgical approaches to the Achilles tendon (**FIG 2**).

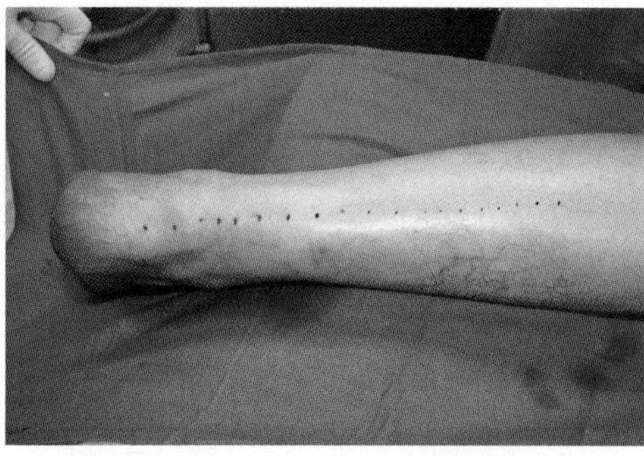

FIG 2 • Marked skin incision for allograft reconstruction.

TECHNIQUES

ALLOGRAFT RECONSTRUCTION OF CHRONIC ACHILLES TENDON RUPTURE

- The Achilles tendon allograft tissue, comprising the distal Achilles tendon with its insertion into a block of allograft calcaneus, is carefully inspected to ensure it has been properly screened, has not expired, and is appropriate for the proposed procedure.
- Make a longitudinal incision in the midline. If preexisting incisions are present, maintain a midline approach as best as possible while respecting the previous approach or approaches.
- Create full-thickness flaps and retract only the deeper tissues to minimize wound complications.
- Incise the tendon sheath longitudinally and reflect it.
- Define and mobilize the tendon ends.
- Débride the proximal tendon end, leaving only healthy tendon. With allograft Achilles tendon reconstruction, the distal Achilles tendon stump is resected completely (**TECH FIG 1**).
- Contour the block of allograft calcaneus attached to the Achilles allograft with a saw, rongeur, or both for insertion and fixation into the patient's calcaneus.
- Use an oscillating saw to create a matching corticocancellous trough in the posterior aspect of the patient's calcaneus. We prefer to use a flexible chisel to fine-tune this trough, which will accommodate the allograft bone (**TECH FIG 2**).
- After fully inserting the allograft's bony portion into the patient's calcaneal trough, secure the bony block using two fully threaded cancellous 4.0-mm titanium screws (DePuy ACE Screw System, Warsaw, IN) (**TECH FIGS 3–5**).

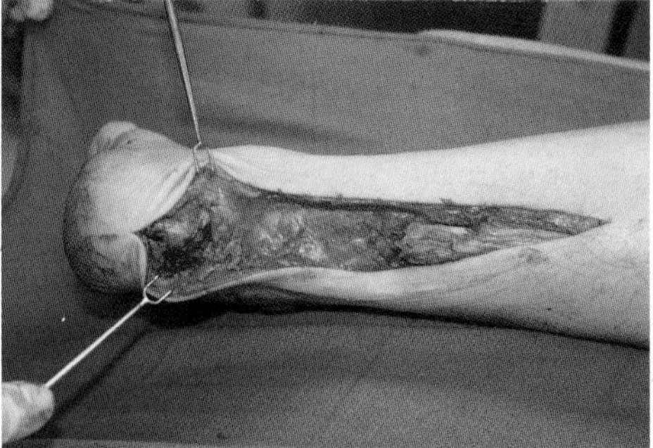

TECH FIG 1 • Intraoperative view after resection of diseased Achilles tendon.

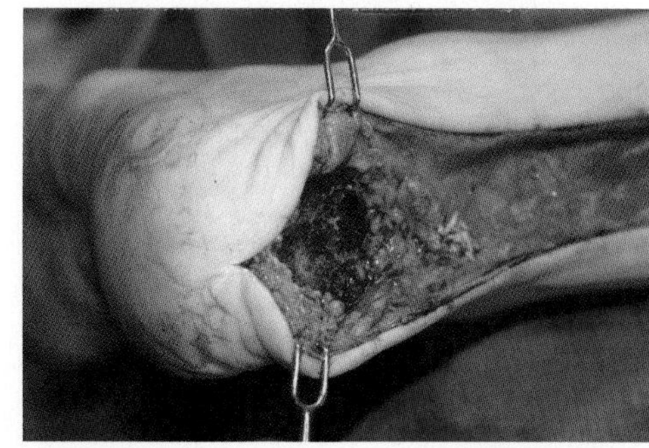

TECH FIG 2 • Preparation of posterior calcaneus for allograft.

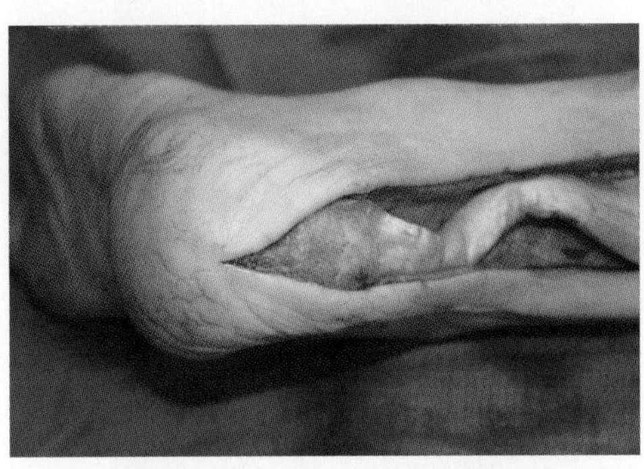

TECH FIG 3 • Determining proper allograft fit.

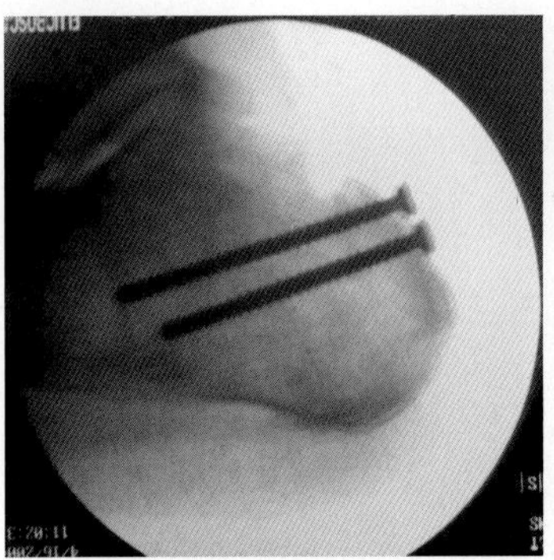

TECH FIG 5 • Intraoperative fluoroscopy of fixation of bony segment of allograft.

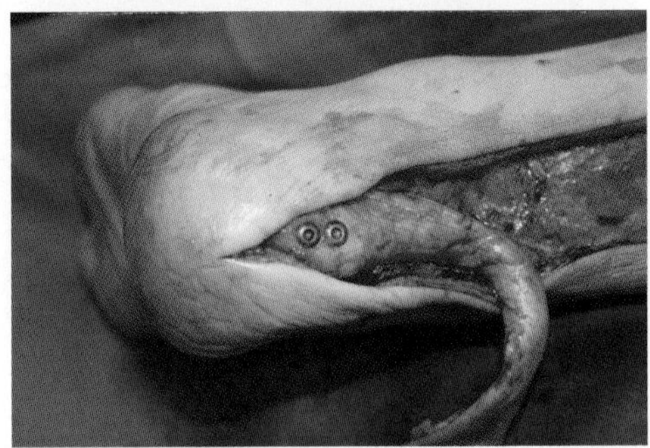

TECH FIG 4 • Fixation of distal bone segment of allograft.

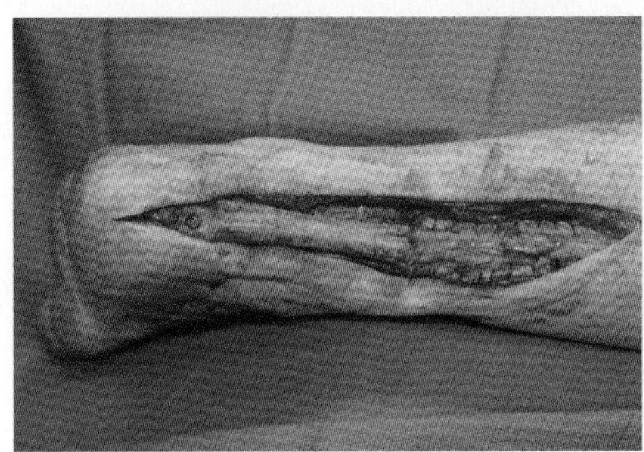

TECH FIG 6 • Intraoperative view of properly tensioned allograft reconstruction.

- Insert a running nonabsorbable no. 2 whip suture (Ethibond, Ethicon, Somerville, NJ) on either side of the allograft tendon (TECH FIG 6).
- By proximally tensioning the sutures, the ankle assumes a position of maximum equinus as the graft spans the defect. This tension is maintained until the allograft is adequately secured to the patient's residual native Achilles tendon, with the no. 2 nonabsorbable suture being woven into the host tissue or secured to a symmetric no. 2 whip suture placed into the host tissue.
- With healthy residual proximal host Achilles tendon, we recommend performing an end-to-end repair between allograft and host tendon. When the patient's residual tendon is adequate but with suspect quality at the most distal portion of the host tissue, we routinely perform an overlapping, imbricated reconstruction.
- Augment the repair or reconstruction with a running 2–0 Vicryl suture (Ethicon).
- Close the paratenon with 4-0 Vicryl.
- Reapproximate the subcutaneous layer with 4-0 Vicryl and close the skin with 4-0 nylon, while maintaining careful handling of the skin margins.

PEARLS AND PITFALLS

Indications	▪ Careful assessment of soft tissues and cause of the chronic Achilles rupture
Approach	▪ Delaminating of skin flaps must be avoided; full-thickness flaps must be created. Retractors are not to be placed on the skin margins; only deep retraction of full-thickness flaps should be performed.
Achilles tendon débridement	▪ Débridement of diseased tendon must be adequate to leave only healthy host Achilles tendon.
Graft tensioning	▪ Maximum equinus positioning during graft tensioning to optimize graft resting tension at follow-up
Skin coverage	▪ Careful respect of soft tissue, meticulous closure, and appropriate immobilization typically lessen soft tissue complications.

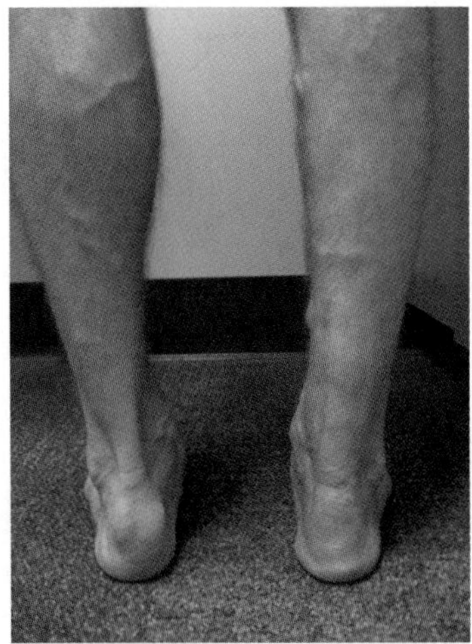

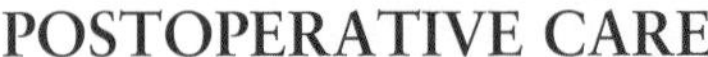

FIG 3 • Six-month follow-up after allograft reconstruction.

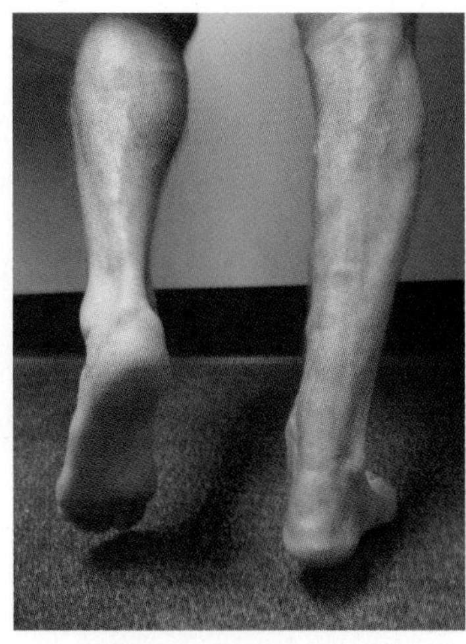

FIG 4 • Single-leg toe-raise on affected side at 6-month postoperative stage.

POSTOPERATIVE CARE

- Immobilization in equinus in a bulky splint for 2 weeks
- Suture removal at 2 weeks
- Immobilization in a hinged cam walker (Bledsoe Platform Boot, Medical Technology Inc., Grand Prairie, TX) set to neutral dorsiflexion block and block at 20 degrees of plantarflexion. The foot is kept in equinus by inserting heel pads into the boot.
- Partial weight bearing (25 kg) is commenced at 2 weeks. This is increased by increments of 25 kg per week until full weight bearing is achieved.
- At 8 to 10 weeks the boot is swapped for a 1- to 2-cm heel raise inside a shoe.
- Gentle passive and active range-of-motion exercises and isometric exercises are commenced at 4 weeks.
- Gentle passive stretching is started at 4 weeks and effort is gradually increased until at 10 weeks, standing calf-stretching exercises are commenced.
- Elastic band exercises are started upon removal of the boot. Stationary bike riding is started at 10 to 12 weeks, with gradual progression of exercise up to 18 weeks, when active push-off exercises are initiated.

OUTCOMES

- In our hands, outcomes with this technique have been satisfactory and without wound complications (**FIG 3**).
- Typically, at 20 weeks the patient can perform single-leg toe-raises and begin jogging and light sporting activities, if previously able (**FIG 4**).
- In our experience, most patients return to their preoperative exercise level and return to their prior occupation.

COMPLICATIONS

- Infection
- Wound dehiscence
- Rupture of repair
- Incorrect tensioning
- Aseptic necrosis of graft

REFERENCES

1. Barnes MJ, Hardy AE. Delayed reconstruction of the calcaneal tendon. J Bone Joint Surg Br 1986;68B:121–124.
2. Buck BE, Resnick L, Shah SM, et al. Human immunodeficiency virus cultured from bone: implications for transplantation. Clin Orthop Relat Res 1990;251:249–253.
3. Buck BE, Malinin TI, Brown MD. Bone transplantation and human immunodeficiency virus: an estimate of risk of acquired immunodeficiency syndrome (AIDS). Clin Orthop Relat Res 1989;240:129–136.
4. Carr AJ, Norris SH. The blood supply of the calcaneal tendon. J Bone Joint Surg Br 1989;71B:100–101.
5. Falconiero R, Pallis M. Chronic rupture of a patellar tendon: a technique for reconstruction with Achilles allograft. Arthroscopy 1996;12:623–626.
6. Haraguchi N, Bluman EM, Myerson MS. Reconstruction of chronic Achilles tendon disorders with Achilles tendon allografts. Tech Foot Ankle Surg 2005;4:154–159.
7. Lepow GM, Green JB. Reconstruction of a neglected Achilles tendon rupture with an Achilles tendon allograft: a case report. J Foot Ankle Surg 2006;45:351–355.
8. Levitt R, Malinin T, Posada A, et al. Reconstruction of anterior cruciate ligaments with bone-patella-tendon-bone and Achilles tendon allografts. Clin Orthop Relat Res 1994;303:67–78.
9. Linn RM, Fischer DA, Smith JP, et al. Achilles tendon allograft reconstruction of the anterior cruciate ligament-deficient knee. Am J Sports Med 1993;21:825–831.
10. McNally PD, Marcelli EA. Achilles allograft reconstruction of chronic patellar tendon rupture. Arthroscopy 1998;14:340–344.
11. Simmond FA. The diagnosis of the ruptured Achilles tendon. Practitioner 1957;179:56–58.
12. Simon SR, Mann RA, Hagy JL et al. Role of posterior calf muscles in normal gait. J Bone Jont Surg Am 1978;60A:465–472.
13. Sutherland DH, Cooper L, Daniel D. The role of the ankle plantar flexors in normal walking. J Bone Joint Surg Am 1980;62A:354–363.
14. Thompson TC, Doherty JH. Spontaneous rupture of tendon Achilles: a new diagnostic test. J Trauma 1962;2:126.
15. Yuen JC, Nicholas R. Reconstruction of a total Achilles tendon and soft-tissue defect using an Achilles allograft combined with a rectus muscle free flap. Plast Reconstr Surg 2001;107:1807–1811.

Chapter 113 Soft Tissue Expansion in Revision/Complex Achilles Tendon Reconstruction

Jorge I. Acevedo

SURGICAL MANAGEMENT

- Indications include neglected ruptures requiring secondary repair or revision surgery.
- Soft tissue expansion over the Achilles tendon and subsequent repair of the tendon are performed as a staged, two-part procedure about 3 to 4 weeks apart.
- This can be particularly effective when performing augmented procedures that increase the girth at the distal tendon or when the local skin is contracted.

Preoperative Planning

- MRI studies are reviewed to determine the ideal placement of the expander and to plan second-stage repair.
- The patient is instructed on the rationale for the staged procedure and the importance of weekly follow-up visits between each stage.

Positioning

- The prone position allows the best access when approaching the Achilles tendon.
- A well-padded pillow is placed underneath the knees and anterior tibia–ankle.
  - This allows for free plantarflexion and dorsiflexion of the ankle.

Approach

- The preferred approach is a posteromedial incision adjacent to the Achilles tendon. This allows the surgeon to avoid injury to the short saphenous vein and sural nerve.
- Simple extension of the incision is performed for the second-stage definitive repair.
- The posteromedial incision may be extended into a lazy-S, L shape, or a direct medial approach.

TECHNIQUES

IMPLANTATION OF EXPANDER

- The initial stage of treatment involves subcutaneous placement of a 70-mL, rectangular soft tissue expander (McGhan, Santa Barbara, CA) between the Achilles tendon and the skin (**TECH FIG 1**).
- After sterile preparation, make a longitudinal incision along the medial aspect of the ankle, adjacent to the course of the Achilles tendon.
- Perform superficial subcutaneous elevation until a pocket about 6 × 4 cm is created.
- Insert a McGhan tissue expander into this cavity and place the injection catheter away from the implant.
- Subcuticular closure is followed by reapproximation of the skin.
- 10 mL of normal saline is initially injected into the implant via the injection port.
- The patient is seen 1 week postoperatively for further inflation of the implant.
  - Ten mL of normal saline is added to the expander weekly.

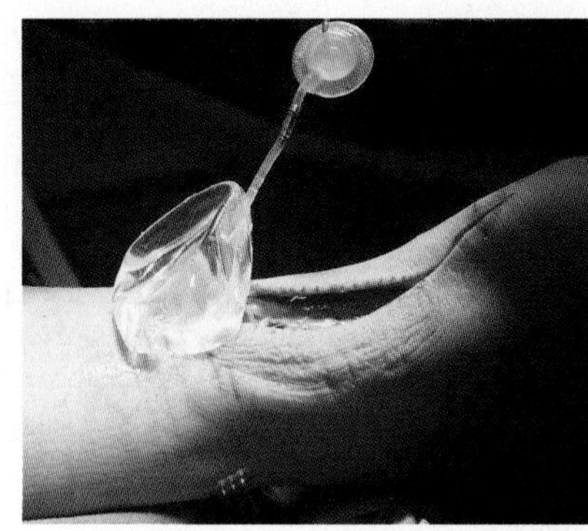

TECH FIG 1 • McGhan 70-mL soft tissue expander.

REMOVAL OF EXPANDER AND TENDON REPAIR

- The expander is removed 3 to 4 weeks postoperatively (**TECH FIG 2**). At that time, removal of the tissue expander and Achilles repair are performed.
- The previously created incision is accessed and extended as necessary. The expansion balloon is then easily removed from its subcutaneous pocket.
- Surgical repair of the injured tendon is carried out in the surgeon's preferred fashion.

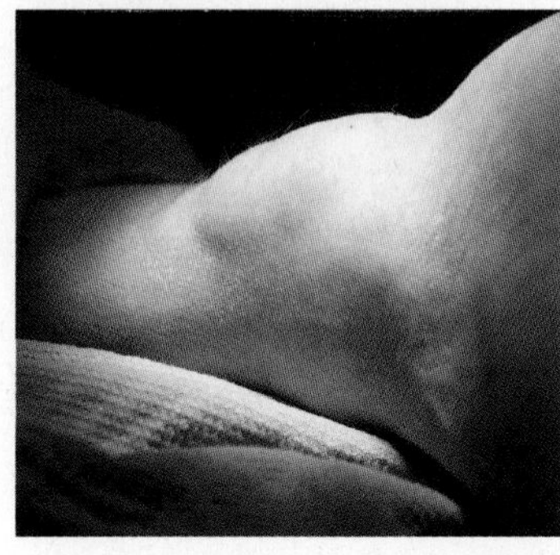

TECH FIG 2 • Inflated soft tissue expander in place subcutaneously.

- Careful repair of the paratenon overlying the Achilles tendon is essential at this stage to re-establish the fragile blood supply to this area.
- Upon completion of the repair, subcutaneous closure is achieved and reapproximation of the wound is then afforded by the lack of tension at the expanded skin margins (**TECH FIG 3**).

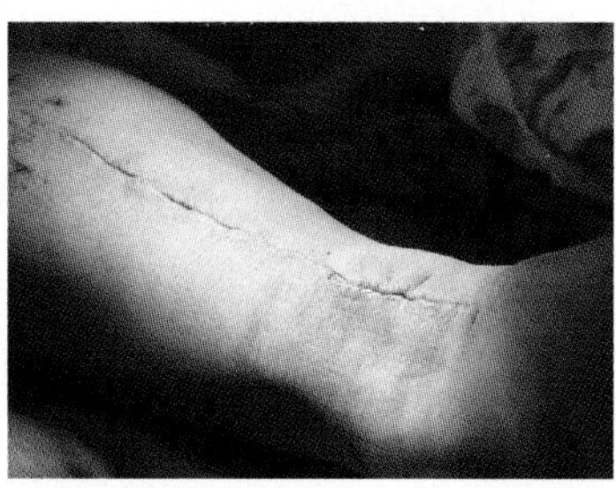

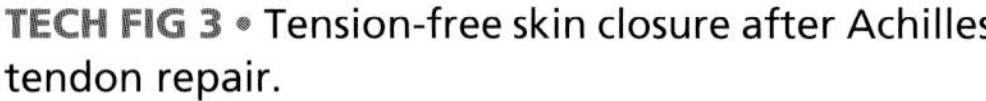

TECH FIG 3 • Tension-free skin closure after Achilles tendon repair.

PEARLS AND PITFALLS

Indications	■ This technique should be avoided in patients with diabetes, peripheral vascular disease, immunocompromise, or a history of tobacco use.
Soft tissue expander inflation	■ Patients rarely tolerate more than 30 to 40 cc of total volume within the implant. The expansion rate may need adjustment (from 10 mL/week) depending on individual skin pliability.

POSTOPERATIVE CARE

- After the initial stage of insertion, the patient is followed weekly for subsequent expander inflation. The inflation rate is 10 mL per week for 3 to 4 weeks.
- After expander removal and second-stage reconstruction the operative limb is placed into a short-leg splint in 10 to 15 degrees of plantarflexion.
- Non–weight-bearing with immobilization in a short-leg cast is maintained for 3 weeks. Range-of-motion exercises are initiated at 3 to 4 weeks postoperatively. Finally, weight bearing is allowed at 6 weeks after surgical repair (**FIG 1**).

OUTCOMES

- This technique has been used successfully in our practice with no complications related directly to soft tissue expansion.

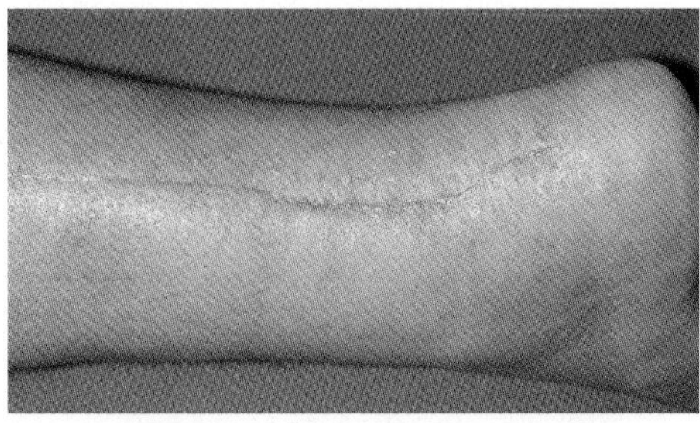

FIG 1 • Outcome 8 weeks after second-stage surgery.

COMPLICATIONS

- Infection
- Seroma
- Sural nerve injury
- Fibrotic reaction

REFERENCES

1. Abraham E, Pankovich AM. Neglected rupture of the Achilles tendon. J Bone Joint Surg Am 1975;57:253–255.
2. Acevedo JI, Weber KS, Eidelman DI. Avoiding wound complications after neglected Achilles tendon repair: tissue expansion technique. Foot Ankle Int 2007;28:393–395.
3. Ademoglu Y, Ozerkan F, Ada S, et al. Reconstruction of skin and tendon defects from wound complications after Achilles tendon rupture. J Foot Ankle Surg 2001;40:158–165.
4. Dalton G, Wapner K, Hecht P. Complications of Achilles and posterior tibial tendon surgeries. Clin Orthop Relat Res 2001;391: 133–139.
5. Kumta SM, Maffulli N. Local flap coverage for soft tissue defects following open repair of Achilles tendon rupture. Acta Orthop Belg 2003;69:59–66.
6. Leppilahti J, Kaarela O, Teerikangas H, et al. Free tissue coverage of wound complications following Achilles tendon rupture surgery. Clin Orthop Relat Res 1996;328:171–176.
7. Ozaki J, Fujiki J, Sugimoto K, et al. Reconstruction of neglected Achilles tendon rupture with Marlex mesh. Clin Orthop Relat Res 1989;238:204–208.
8. Paavola M, Orava S, Leppilahti J, et al. Chronic Achilles tendon overuse injury: complications after surgical treatment. Am J Sports Med 2000;28:77–82.
9. Parker R, Repinecz M. Neglected rupture of the Achilles tendon: treatment by modified Strayer gastrocnemius recession. J Am Podiatry Assoc 1979;69:548–555.

Chapter 114 Retrocalcaneal Bursoscopy

Angus M. McBryde and Fred W. Ortmann

DEFINITION

- Patrick Haglund in 1928 described an enlarged posterior border of the os calcis.[3]
- This anatomy, Haglund deformity, becomes very important when external shoeing and repeated hyperdorsiflexion causes contact between the Achilles tendon, the retrocalcaneal bursa, and the posterior proximal border of the calcaneus.
  - As a result, Haglund syndrome is commonly characterized by inflammation within the retrocalcaneal or Achilles tendon bursa and often secondarily presents as insertional Achilles tendinopathy.
- The posterior heel pain and swelling associated with Haglund syndrome is the result of mechanical irritation by the calcaneal prominence on the surrounding soft tissues and the Achilles tendon.
- After conservative measures have failed, Haglund deformity and retrocalcaneal bursitis can be treated surgically using either an open or an endoscopic technique.
  - The endoscopic technique is an outpatient treatment that is associated with low morbidity and high outpatient satisfaction. There is a short recovery time and a short time to gain preprocedure activity level.
  - Appropriate visualization of the Achilles tendon and removal of the calcaneal prominence and retrocalcaneal bursa can be effectively accomplished using an endoscopic technique.

PATHOGENESIS

- The retrocalcaneal space has been described as a disc space bursa covering the posterior superior angle of the calcaneus.[2] The bursa walls may become diseased and hypertrophied with repeat hindfoot movement.
- Achilles tendinopathy is a degenerative process within the tendon substance causing microtears, edema, and reactive fibrosis with scar formation. These changes cause secondary mechanical irritation of the surrounding tissues and can even stimulate an inflammatory process.

PATIENT HISTORY AND PHYSICAL FINDINGS

- Clinical evaluation may help differentiate between retrocalcaneal bursitis and Achilles tendinopathy, although the two often coexist.
- Pathology within the retrocalcaneal space is detected on clinical examination with point tenderness along the anteromedial and anterolateral aspects of the Achilles tendon and an associated prominence of the calcaneus.
- Palpation of the affected hindfoot often reveals tenderness at the distal portion of the Achilles tendon proximal to its insertion on the calcaneus. The pain can be reproduced with passive or active dorsiflexion.

IMAGING AND OTHER DIAGNOSTIC STUDIES

- Imaging can assist with documenting the presence or absence of tendinopathy (**FIG 1A**).
- It can be difficult to distinguish whether symptoms are caused by retrocalcaneal bursitis or insertional Achilles tendinosis or tendinitis, and the two conditions often coexist.
- MRI can be used preoperatively to better demonstrate the coexistence of the two diagnoses (**FIG 1B**).
- Normal-appearing and diseased tendons can be distinguished endoscopically.

NONOPERATIVE MANAGEMENT

- Nonoperative measures for the treatment of posterior heel pain include the use of nonsteroidal anti-inflammatory medication, shoe wear modification (such as avoiding backless shoes), physical therapy for icing, other modalities, stretching exercises, pressure-release inserts, and hands-on friction massage.
- Local injections can be given in the retrocalcaneal space, but the concomitant use of local anesthesia and corticosteroids may further weaken the substance of the Achilles tendon and risk weakness and further micro- or macro-rupture of the tendon.[4]

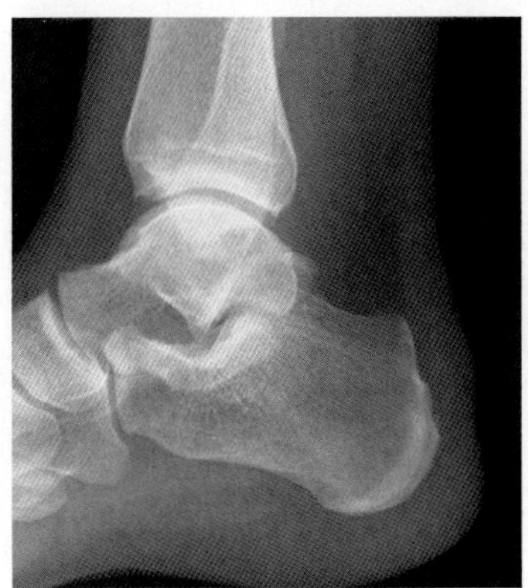

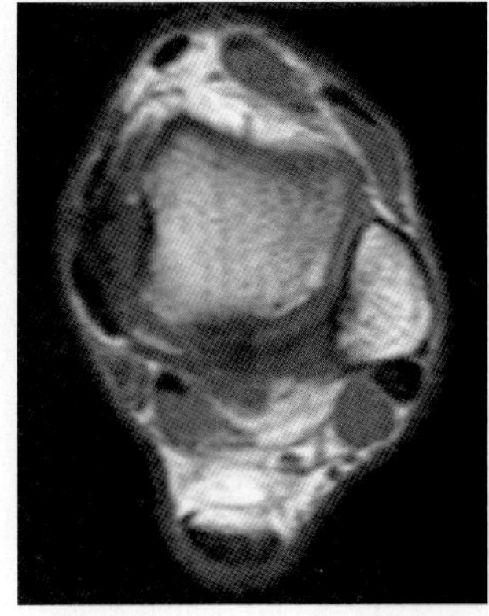

FIG 1 • **A.** Preoperative lateral foot film showing Haglund exostosis. **B.** MRI showing retrocalcaneal bursa involvement and insertional tendinopathy. (From Ortmann FW, McBryde AM. Endoscopic bony and soft-tissue decompression of the retrocalcaneal space for the treatment of Haglund deformity and retrocalcaneal bursitis. Foot Ankle Int 2007;28:149–153.)

SURGICAL MANAGEMENT

- The goal of treatment of Haglund deformity and syndrome is to remove the calcaneal prominence and to decompress the inflamed surrounding soft tissues.
- Open surgical correction is an alternative for patients who have failed to respond to nonoperative measures, especially if augmentation is advisable.
  - Open procedures include resection of the calcaneal prominence proximal to the Achilles tendon insertion with retrocalcaneal bursa removal.
  - A dorsal closing wedge osteotomy can rotate the posterior calcaneus to less prominence.
  - Achilles tenolysis and partial resection of the diseased portion of the tendon may be necessary, often with augmentation by the flexor hallucis longus or flexor digitorum.
  - Complete Achilles removal at its insertion is occasionally necessary.
  - Complications associated with these procedures include hematomas, tendon or skin breakdown, nonunion, Achilles tendon avulsion, tenderness around the operative scar, cosmetic problems, altered sensation around the heel, and stiffness.[1,6,8,10,11] Rehabilitation can be prolonged.
- The endoscopic technique of decompressing the retrocalcaneal space was developed to reduce morbidity and decrease the functional time to recovery for patients with retrocalcaneal bursitis.[12]
  - The endoscopic technique has been shown to have fewer complications and a better cosmetic appearance than an open procedure.[7]
- Here, we describe retrocalcaneal bursoscopy using our method of endoscopic bony and soft tissue decompression of the retrocalcaneal space and the results from our patient series.[9] Hindfoot endoscopy is being increasingly used for numerous problems.

Positioning

- The operation is performed with the patient in the supine position and under either general or regional anesthesia.
  - A high thigh tourniquet is inflated to 300 mm Hg after Esmarch ischemia.
  - The foot is positioned at the edge of the operating table. This enables the surgeon to place the foot against his or her body while using both hands to operate the arthroscopic instruments.
  - The leg rests on a firm padded 12-inch-long and 4-inch-diameter cylindrical bump that allows the surgeon ample room to work and to control ankle dorsiflexion and plantarflexion.
- Alternatively, the prone position can be used.
- Both positions allow the patient's foot to be controlled against the chest of the surgeon, who can then have both hands free for the instruments.

TECHNIQUES

PORTAL PLACEMENT AND EXPOSURE

- Make a lateral portal through a vertical incision at the level of the superior aspect of the calcaneus (**TECH FIG 1A**).
- The incision is slightly anterior to the Achilles tendon and posterior to the sural nerve. It is important to bluntly dissect and spread the soft tissues when making the lateral portal to minimize the risk of injury to the sural nerve.
- Enter the retrocalcaneal space with a blunt trocar to develop working space.
- Place a 4.0-mm arthroscope into the retrocalcaneal space.
- Establish the medial portal similarly just anterior to the Achilles tendon, using the light of the arthroscope as a guide (**TECH FIG 1B**).

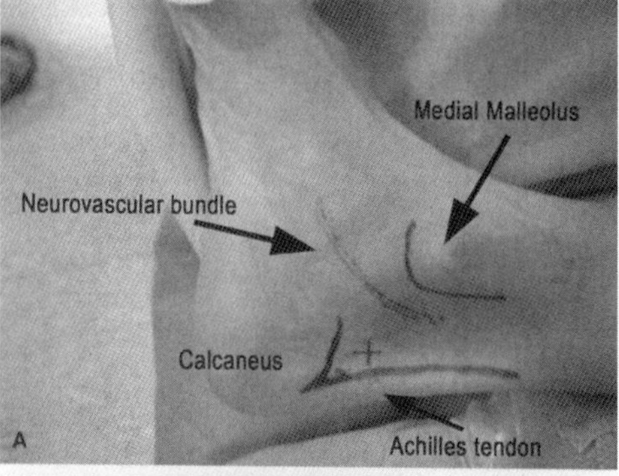

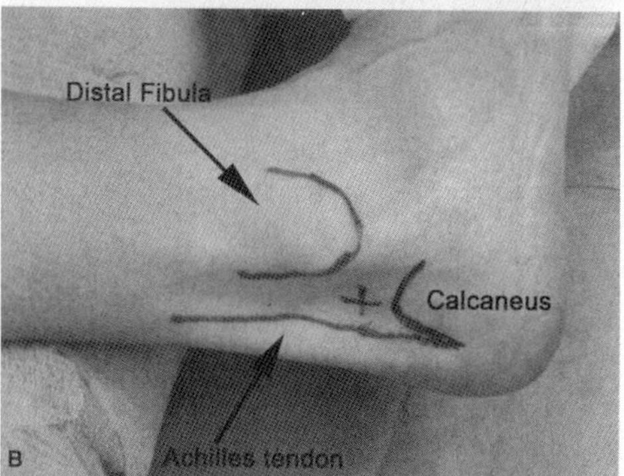

TECH FIG 1 • Establishing landmarks and planning portal placement medially (**A**) and laterally (**B**).

RESECTION AND DECOMPRESSION

- Introduce a 3.5-mm arthroscopic shaver (for larger hindfeet, a 4.5-mm arthroscope can be used) into the medial portal and remove the bursal tissue. This expanded working space creates visualization and access to the posterior calcaneus and the Achilles tendon attachment.

- Depending on the quality of the bone, use either the arthroscopic shaver or a 4-mm arthroscopic burr to resect the posterior superior calcaneal prominence (**TECH FIG 2**).
- Keep the hooded portions of the instruments toward the anterior direction.
- Take special care to stop the rotating or oscillating shaver or burr usage when the instrumentation enters or exits the portal.
- Carry out the resection both medially and laterally into the sulcus of the calcaneal tendon (retrocalcaneal bursa) and distally to the attachment of the Achilles tendon.
- Visually confirm adequate exposure and resection of the osseous prominence until there are no areas of Achilles tendon impingement.
  - In a few cases, the use of the mini C-arm (Mini 6600 series; GE OEC Medical Systems, Salt Lake City, UT) is needed to determine, document, and confirm adequate resection.
- Damaged or diseased Achilles tendon can be selectively exposed and with a nerve hook or probe identified.
- Limited bone or tendinopathy can be removed with the arthroscopic shaver.
- An 18-gauge needle can be inserted several times into the tendon to promote blood ingress and collagen scar where there is myxoid or degenerative change.
  - The rationale for this is to initiate a vascular response within the tendons for healing; it is performed with or without débridement.
- Insert an arthroscopic probe into the retrocalcaneal space to confirm continuing effective attachment of the Achilles tendon.

A 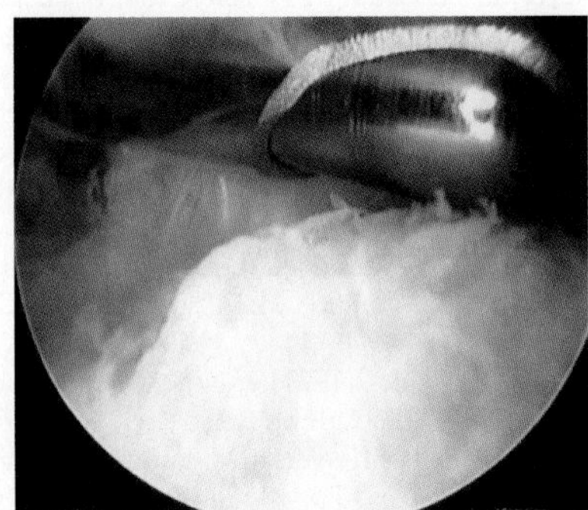

B 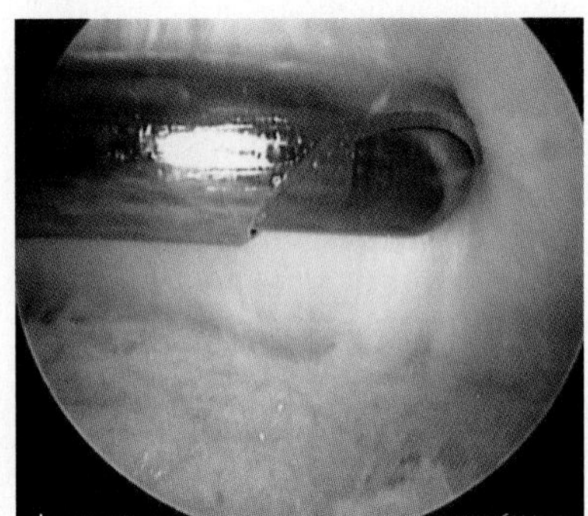

TECH FIG 2 • An arthroscopic shaver is used to resect the posterior superior calcaneal prominence. A 4-mm arthroscopic burr can also be used. (From Ortmann FW, McBryde AM. Endoscopic bony and soft-tissue decompression of the retrocalcaneal space for the treatment of Haglund deformity and retrocalcaneal bursitis. Foot Ankle Int 2007;28:149–153.)

COMPLETION AND WOUND CLOSURE

- Hyper-plantarflex and dorsiflex the foot with the anterior chest and abdomen to verify any last areas of impingement.
- Irrigate and suction the retrocalcaneal space to remove any loose tissue.
- Close the portal sites with two 4-0 nylon skin horizontal mattress sutures.
- Inject local anesthetic (0.25% Marcaine without epinephrine) into the portal sites.
- Apply a compression dressing and splint the foot into slight equinus with the posterior splint and sugar-tong "trilaminar splint."

PEARLS AND PITFALLS

- Set up with heels directly at the end of operating room table so can manage position of ankle/foot in dorsiflexion and plantarflexion with chest/abdomen.
- Develop entire operative field from posteromedial to posterolateral corner so panoramic view of Achilles tuberosity attachment.
- MRI is necessary preoperatively to document insertional tendinopathy. If more than 25% of the cross-sectional area of the tendon is involved, open repair may be necessary (author's opinion).
- Experience enables removal of paratenon and further removal of small ruptures and/or ossification in selected cases and situations.
- Postoperative routine is (a) non–weight-bearing for 2 to 3 weeks, (b) partial weight-bearing for 2 to 3 weeks, and (c) to maximize strength of posterior tibial and peroneals as soon as mobilization permits.

POSTOPERATIVE CARE

- The average time until full weight bearing is 4 weeks.
- Patients wear shoes with a heel counter and return to normal daily function in 8 weeks.
- All athletes returned to their previous level of activity in an average of 12 weeks.
- Patients may need a longer period of cast immobilization after débridement of the Achilles tendon or significant Achilles tendinopathy.

OUTCOMES

- In our study of endoscopic bony and soft tissue decompression of the retrocalcaneal space for the treatment of Haglund deformity and retrocalcaneal bursitis,[9] 32 heels in 30 consecutive patients underwent endoscopic decompression. The time of surgery after diagnosis of retrocalcaneal bursitis averaged 20 months. All patients had failed to respond to nonoperative measures, and none had undergone previous surgery.
- Indications for operative intervention included failed nonoperative measures, history and physical examinations consistent with retrocalcaneal bursitis, and Haglund deformity causing mechanical impingement or Achilles tendinopathy.
- Patients were prospectively followed from 1997 to 2003, with a mean follow-up of 35 months (range 3 to 62 months).
- Thirty heels completed subjective and objective measures using the American Orthopaedic Foot and Ankle Society (AOFAS) ankle–hindfoot scale.[5]
  - Twenty-eight patients had an average preoperative AOFAS score of 62 points. Postoperative AOFAS scores averaged 97 points.
- Twenty-six patients had excellent results and three had good results. There was one poor outcome and one major complication. An excellent result was defined as pain-free activity with complete return to activity, and a poor result was defined as having persistent symptoms and inability to return to activity.
- The cohort was stratified into "daily athletic activity" and "athletic" groups and the groups were compared. No statistical differences in outcome between the two groups existed.
- All patients reported satisfaction with the cosmetic appearance of their portal sites.
- These results compared with those published by van Dijk et al[13]: their 20 patients resumed participating in sports at an average of 12 weeks.

COMPLICATIONS

- One major complication occurred among the 30 heels: a patient sustained a proximal Achilles tendon rupture (of an unprotected tendon) 19 days after having undergone endoscopic decompression while ambulating without a prescribed protected walker boot.[9]
- There were no intraoperative or skin or soft tissue complications (ie, wound dehiscence and postoperative infection).
- No patients reported a painful scar or neuroma-type symptoms.

REFERENCES

1. Angermann P. Chronic retrocalcaneal bursitis treated by resection of the calcaneus. Foot Ankle Int 1990;10:285–287.
2. Frey C, Rosenburg Z, Shereff MJ, et al. The retrocalcaneal bursa: anatomy and bursography. Foot Ankle Int 1992;13:203–207.
3. Haglund P. Beitrag zur Klinik der Achillessehne. Zeitschr Orthop Chir 1928;49:49–58.
4. Kennedy JC, Willis RB. The effects of local steroid injections on tendons: a biomechanical and microscopic correlative study. Am J Sports Med 1976;4:11–21.
5. Kitaoka HB, Alexander IJ, Adelaar RS, et al. Clinical rating systems for the ankle–hindfoot, midfoot, hallux, and lesser toes. Foot Ankle Int 1994;15:349–353.
6. Leach RE, Dilorio E, Harney RA. Pathologic hindfoot conditions in the athlete. Clin Orthop Relat Res 1983;177:116–121.
7. Leitze Z, Sella EJ, Aversa JM. Endoscopic decompression of the retrocalcaneal space. J Bone Joint Surg Am 2003;85A:1488–1496.
8. Miller AE, Vogel TA. Haglund's deformity and the Keck and Kelly osteotomy; a retrospective analysis. J Foot Surg 1989;28:23–29.
9. Ortmann FW, McBryde AM. Endoscopic bony and soft-tissue decompression of the retrocalcaneal space for the treatment of Haglund deformity and retrocalcaneal bursitis. Foot Ankle Int 2007;28:149–153.
10. Pauker M, Katz K, Yosipovitch Z. Calcaneal ostectomy for Haglund disease. J Foot Surg 1992;31:588–589.
11. Scheider W, Niehus W, Knahr K. Haglund's syndrome: disappointing results following surgery—a clinical and radiographic analysis. Foot Ankle Int 2000;21:26–30.
12. van Dijk CN, Scholten PE, Krips R. A 2-portal endoscopic approach for diagnosis and treatment of posterior ankle pathology. Arthroscopy 2000;16:871–876.
13. van Dijk CN, van Dyk GE, Scholten PE, et al. Endoscopic calcaneoplasty. Am J Sports Med 2001;29:185–189.

Chapter 115 Insertional Achilles Tendinopathy

Mark E. Easley and Matthew J. DeOrio

DEFINITION

- Insertional Achilles tendinopathy is posterior heel pain at the insertion of the Achilles tendon.
- The clinical diagnosis is acute and chronic pathology of the Achilles tendon insertion and its surrounding tissues.

ANATOMY

- The Achilles tendon, the condensation of the gastrocnemius and soleus tendons, inserts on the posterior calcaneal tuberosity.
- The insertion is not only posterior but also on the medial and lateral aspects of the calcaneus.
- A dorsal-posterior calcaneal prominence is most obvious on a lateral radiograph. The Achilles tendon inserts distal to this, directly posterior on the calcaneus.
- Between the distal Achilles tendon and the dorsal-posterior calcaneal prominence, immediately proximal to the Achilles insertion, is the retrocalcaneal bursa.
- A pre-Achilles bursa is superficial to the distal Achilles tendon.

PATHOGENESIS

- While not fully understood, repetitive microtrauma to the Achilles tendon insertion is thought to be the cause.
- Most likely some initial injury occurs, followed by multiple minor reinjuries that lead to chronic symptoms.
- In the acute phase, the process may have some inflammatory characteristics; however, the chronic process is degenerative, with a relative paucity of inflammatory tissue.
- Without histologic confirmation, the diagnosis of Achilles tendinitis or tendinosis cannot be made; therefore, the pathologic process at the Achilles tendon insertion is viewed as "tendinopathy" without tissue confirmation.

PATIENT HISTORY AND PHYSICAL FINDINGS

- The patient may recall an inciting event but typically reports chronic acitivity-related aching or even sharp pain at the posterior heel.
- In addition, the patient notes a progressively enlarging prominence on the posterior heel.
- This ache is usually accompanied by exquisite tenderness directly posteriorly on the calcaneus, at the Achilles tendon insertion, with manual pressure, on contact from the shoe's heel counter, or when the posterior heel is rested on a hard surface.
- Putting the Achilles tendon on stretch aggravates the symptoms, such as when the patient walks uphill.
- Physical examination reveals the following:
  - A prominence is evident on the posterior heel, at the Achilles tendon insertion (**FIG 1**).
  - Tenderness is felt directly on the posterior calcaneal prominence.
  - No tenderness is found in the Achilles tendon proximal to its insertion on the calcaneus.
  - Thompson's test is negative.

IMAGING AND OTHER DIAGNOSTIC STUDIES

- A lateral weight-bearing radiograph of the foot often demonstrates irregularities and calcifications at the Achilles tendon insertion on the posterior calcaneus (**FIG 2A**).
- While unnecessary to make the diagnosis, magnetic resonance imaging (MRI) defines the extent of tendon involvement at the insertion and the presence of retrocalcaneal and perhaps even pre-Achilles bursitis (**FIG 2B**).

DIFFERENTIAL DIAGNOSIS

- Pre-Achilles bursitis
- Retrocalcaneal bursitis
- Calcaneal stress fracture
- Haglund's deformity (prominent dorsal-posterior calcaneal tuberosity impinging on the Achilles tendon)
- Calcaneal stress fracture
- Posterior ankle impingement
- Plantar fasciitis
- Noninsertional Achilles tendinopathy

NONOPERATIVE MANAGEMENT

- Activity modification (avoidance of activities that place the Achilles tendon on stretch)
- Nonsteroidal anti-inflammatory agents
- Heel lift or a shoe with a heel to unload the Achilles tendon
- Open-backed shoe or a shoe with a soft heel counter

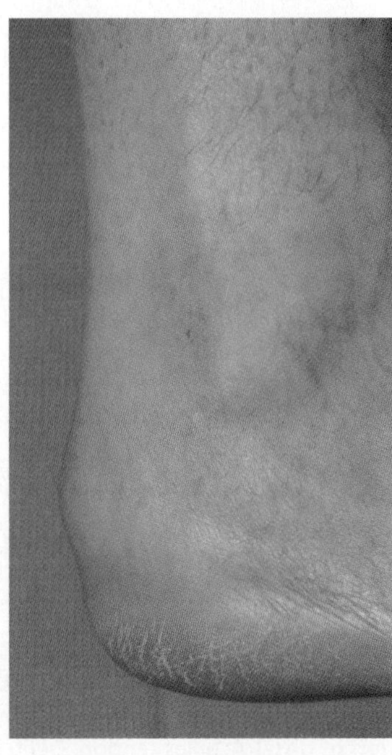

FIG 1 • Example of posterior calcaneal prominence characteristic of insertional Achilles tendinopathy.

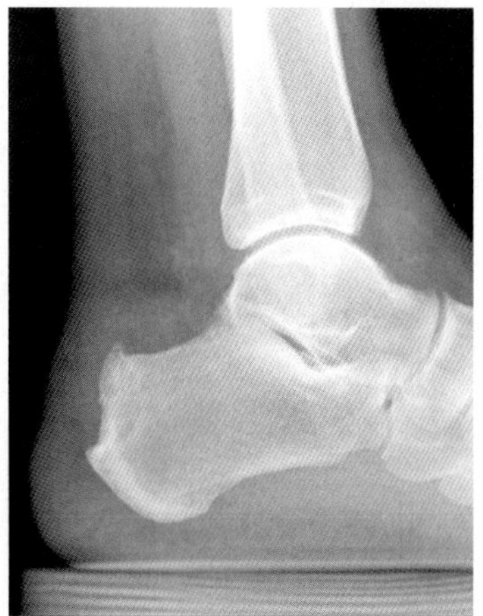

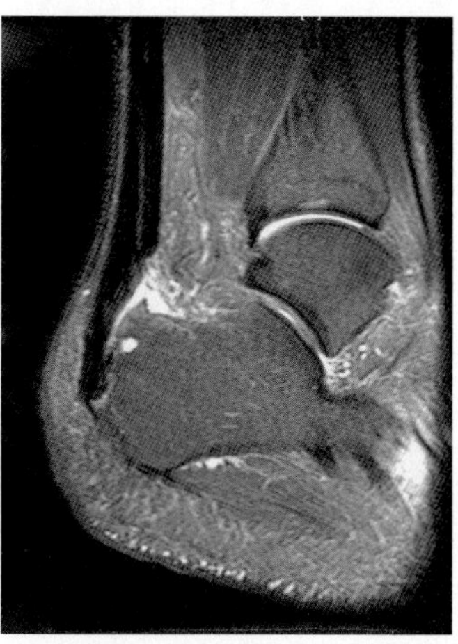

FIG 2 • **A.** Lateral foot radiograph demonstrating the posterior calcaneal prominence and calcification within the Achilles tendon insertion. **B.** T2-weighted sagittal MRI of patient with insertional Achilles tendinopathy. Signal change in the distal tendon and retrocalcaneal bursitis can be seen.

- Physical therapy
  - Focus on eccentric strengthening exercises
  - In our experience the common practice of aggressive Achilles stretching must be avoided as it will aggravate the symptoms.
  - Modalities: ultrasound, iontophoresis
- Extracorporal shockwave therapy may have some benefit but is largely unproven.
- Corticosteroid injection may lead to Achilles rupture and is contraindicated unless the process is isolated to retrocalcaneal bursitis, in which case a judicious injection of only the retrocalcaneal bursa can be performed.

SURGICAL MANAGEMENT

- The primary surgical indication is nonoperative management.
- Up to 50% of insertional Achilles tendinopathy can be successfully managed without surgery, even when there is a large posterior calcaneal prominence.
- Insertional Achilles teninopathy with central calcific tendinosis may be less amenable to nonoperative management.

Preoperative Planning

- Preoperative medical clearance
- Even in healthy patients, the thin skin on the posterior heel is at risk. Carefully inspect skin to be sure that the patient is a reasonable candidate for a posterior approach to the Achilles tendon insertion.
- With extensive Achilles tendon degeneration (confirmed with preoperative MRI), an augmentation of the insertion may be warranted. Therefore, preoperative planning should include the anticipation that the flexor hallucis longus (FHL) tendon may need to be harvested and transferred to the posterior calcaneus. The FHL tendon lies immediately deep to the deep compartment fascia that is anterior to the Achilles tendon and can readily be harvested through the same approach.
  - As a rough estimate, we perform an FHL augmentation in less than 10% of cases but routinely have our preferred anchoring system available should the transfer be warranted.
  - We educate all of our patients undergoing surgical management for insertional Achilles tendinopathy that, based on our intraoperative findings, an FHL tendon transfer may be necessary.
- The recovery following surgical management for insertional Achilles tendinopathy is prolonged and may take a full year before the patient returns to full activity. We educate our patients that the recovery is not rapid.

Positioning

- The patient is placed prone on the operating table.
- We routinely inflate the thigh tourniquet with the patient supine on the stretcher, then flip the patient to the prone position on the operating room table. This facilitates proper tourniquet position and avoids stressing the patient's lumbar spine, which may be stressed when placing the tourniquet with the patient in the prone position.
- The chest and pelvis are well padded.
- The brachial plexi and ulnar nerves at the elbows are protected and relaxed.
- The genitalia are protected.

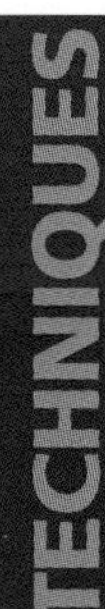

TECHNIQUES

APPROACH AND REFLECTION OF THE ACHILLES TENDON INSERTION

- A central approach is undertaken, directly over Achilles tendon and posterior calcaneus (TECH FIG 1A).
- The scalpel is moved through skin and into central portion of distal Achilles tendon. Deep incision is continued distally, directly to bone.
  - The goal is to avoid unnecessary delamination of the soft tissues and to elevate full-thickness flaps.
- We then elevate medial and lateral slips of Achilles tendon from the calcaneus (TECH FIG 1B,C).
  - More than half of the Achilles tendon insertion can be elevated without compromising the integrity of the insertion. One study suggests that up to 75% can be released.
  - We elevate the Achilles tendon until all the diseased portion of tendon can be excised.

- Another study suggests that the entire insertion of the Achilles tendon should be routinely elevated and excised to ensure that all diseased tissue is removed. Reattachment is facilitated by a proximal Achilles tendon lengthening that also serves to unload the Achilles tendon.
- We do not routinely elevate the entire Achilles tendon, but should one or both of the Achilles tendon slips become detached, we have uniformly been able to reattach the tendon to the calcaneus with a successful outcome.

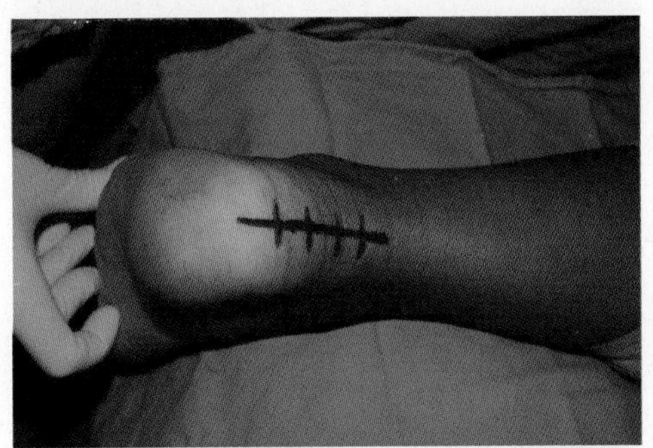

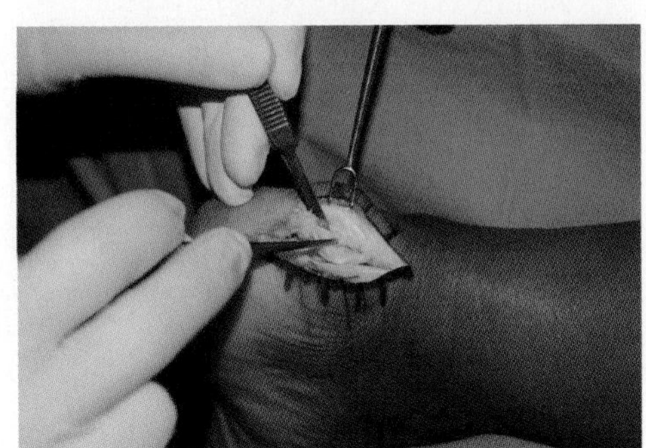

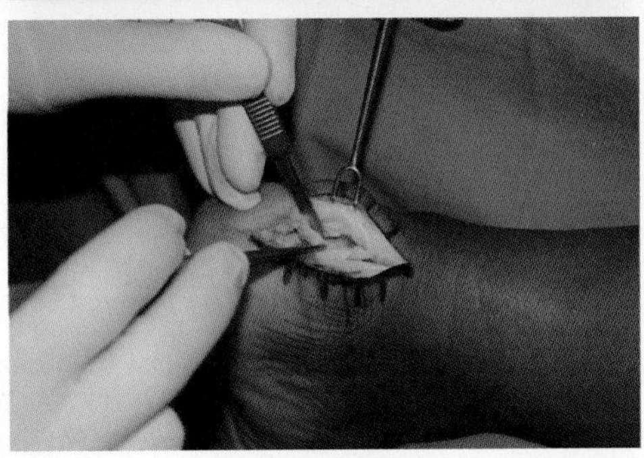

TECH FIG 1 • **A.** Central posterior approach. The foot is hanging from the end of the bed. After a full-thickness incision is made through the diseased portion of the tendon, lateral (**B**) and medial (**C**) tendon slips are developed.

DÈBRIDEMENT OF THE DISEASED PORTION OF ACHILLES TENDON

- The diseased portion of tendon is gradually pared from the Achilles insertion, until only healthy fibers remain (**TECH FIG 2A–C**).
  - Healthy Achilles fibers have an organized, longitudinal pattern.
  - Degenerated Achilles tendon substance is unorganzied and may be likened to crab meat (**TECH FIG 2D,E**).
- Calcific tendinosis may be present, and all calcifications within the residual Achilles tendon must be excised (**TECH FIG 2F**).

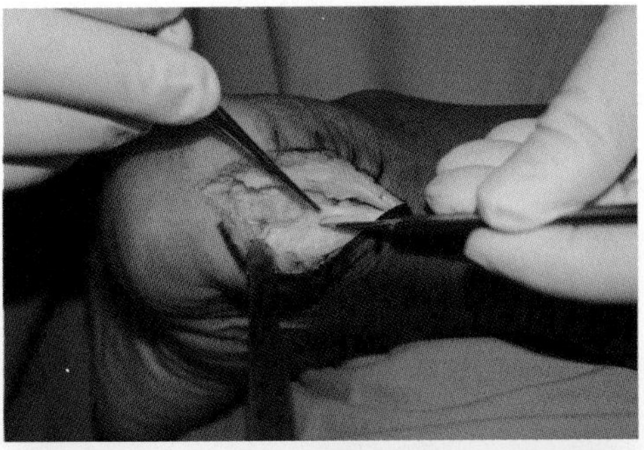

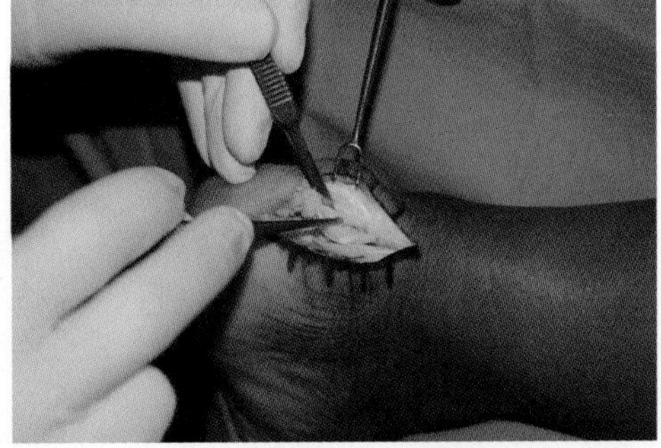

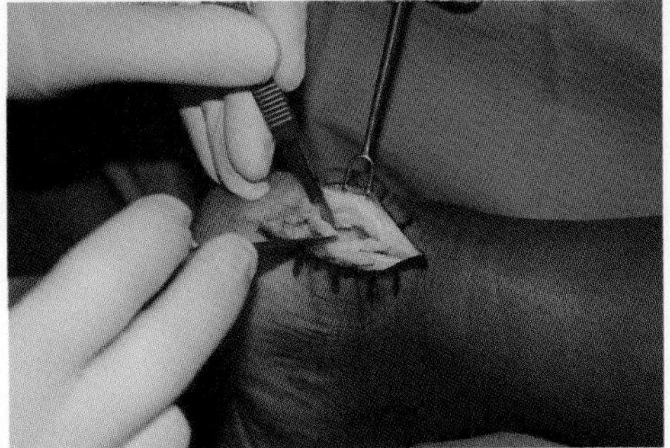

TECH FIG 2 • Débriding the diseased portion of the tendon. **A.** Medial tendon slip débridements. **B,C.** Lateral tendon slip débridement. (*continued*)

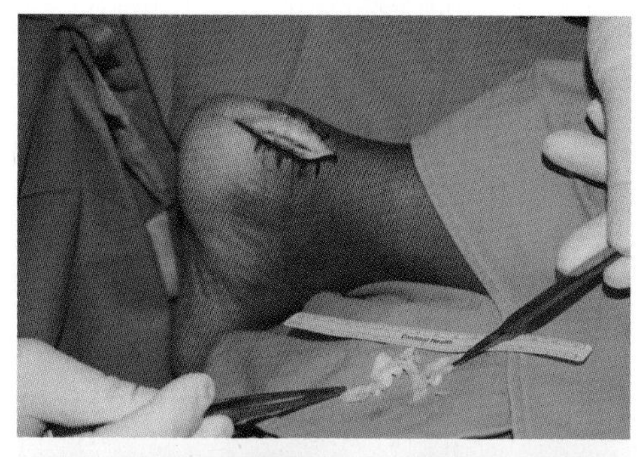
D

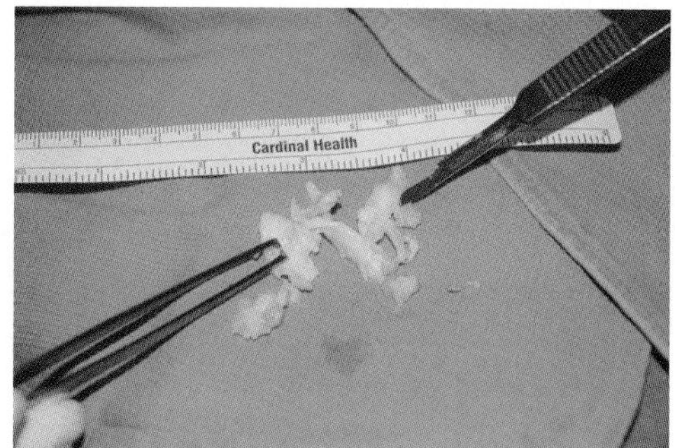

E

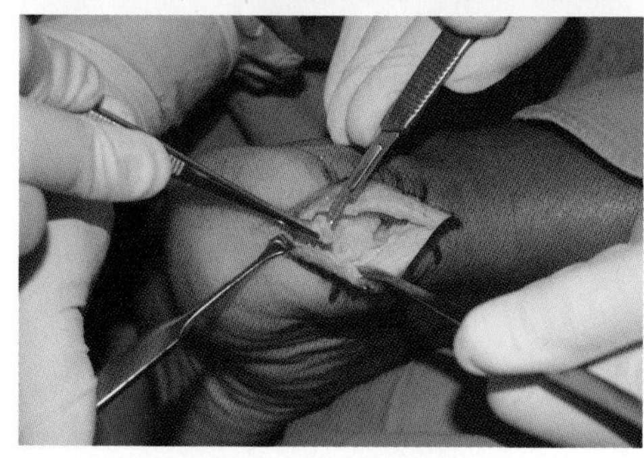
F

TECH FIG 2 • (*continued*) **D, E.** Collection of the excised diseased portion of tendon. **F.** Calcific tendinosis. It is important to débride the calcifications within the residual tendon.

CALCANEAL EXOSTECTOMY

- Retractors are used to protect the medial and lateral Achilles tendon slips.
- We routinely use a microsagittal saw to perform the exostectomy.
- We first define the exit point on the dorsal calcaneus in order to avoid the tendency to take unnecessary calcaneal bone (**TECH FIG 3A**).
  - If necessary, a single fluoroscopy spot image may be used to define the trajectory of the saw blade.
  - As a general rule, it is steeper (more vertical) than anticipated (**TECH FIG 3B**).
- The bony prominence is mobilized with a chisel and removed with a rongeur (**TECH FIG 3C,D**).
- Commonly, the exostectomy must be "touched up" to remove all of the prominence (**TECH FIG 3E**).
- With the Achilles tendon slips still protected, the medial and lateral chamfers are removed (**TECH FIG 3F,G**).
  - This helps narrow the heel and reduce the bulk of the residual calcaneus, medial, and lateral prominences that may lead to persistent pressure and impingement experienced by the patient.
  - While these chamfers are near the medial and lateral insertion points of the Achilles tendon, typically they can be excised without compromising the residual tendon attachment.

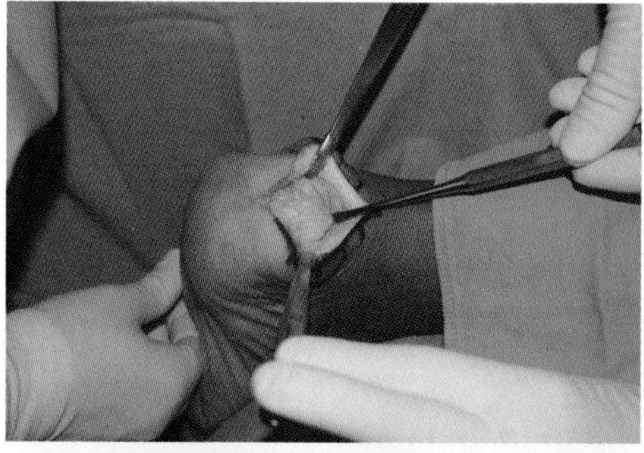
A

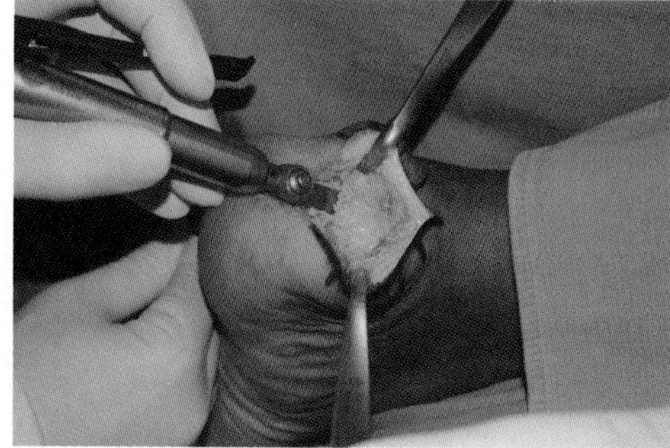
B

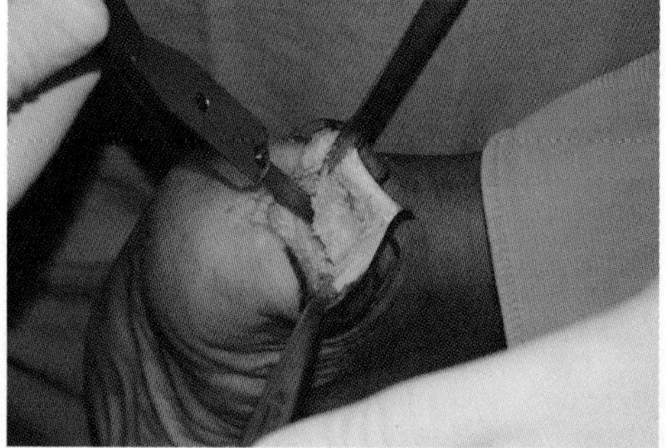
C

TECH FIG 3 • Calcaneal exostectomy. **A.** Planning the trajectory for the saw blade. **B.** A microsagittal saw is used to perform the exostectomy. **C.** A chisel is used to mobilize the excised fragment. (*continued*)

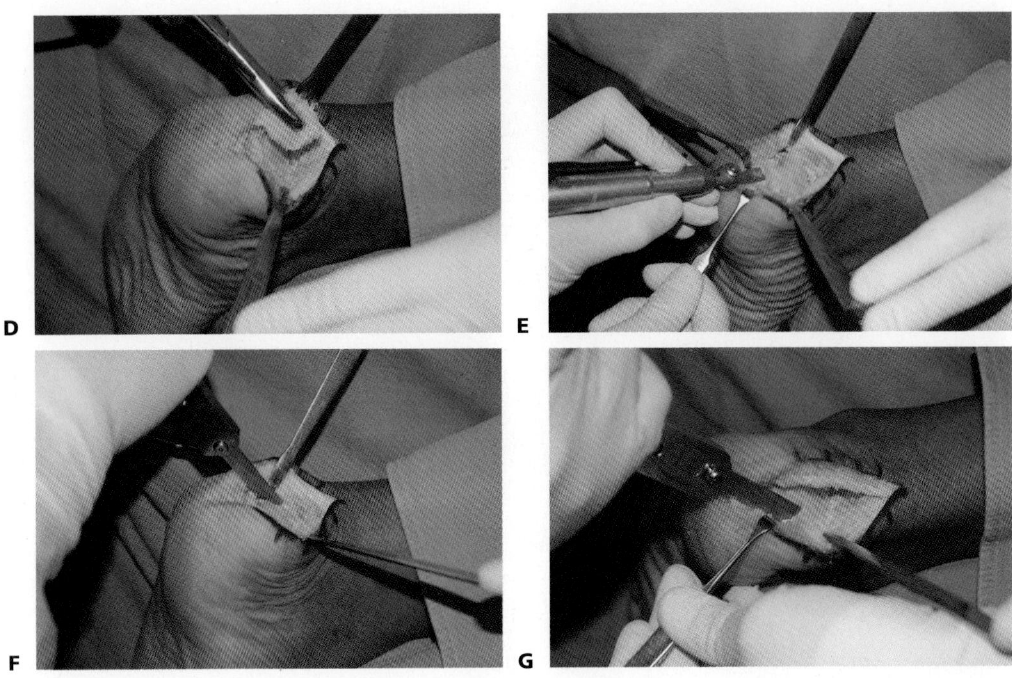

TECH FIG 3 • (*continued*) **D.** A rongeur is used to remove the resected bone. **E.** Touch-up to ensure an appropriate amount of bone was removed and an adequate "healing" cancellous surface is exposed. Chamfer preparation to decompress the lateral (**F**) and medial (**G**) dimensions of the prominent calcaneus.

REATTACHMENT OF RESIDUAL HEALTHY ACHILLES TENDON

Primary Sutures

- With only healthy Achilles tendon fibers remaining and the calcaneus decompressed posteriorly, medially, and laterally, the Achilles tendon should be reattached to the calcaneus.
- While one study suggested that up to 75% of the tendon attachment can be released without compromising the integrity of the insertion, we routinely reattach the elevated portion of tendon to the exposed cancellous calcaneal surface.
- In our opinion, reattachment not only strengthens the repair but also facilitates direct tendon healing to the calcaneus.
- We routinely use two or three suture anchors:
  - One anchor for each tendon slip
  - Occasionally, an additional anchor to augment the reattachment of both tendon slips
- The anchors are positioned relatively symmetrically on the exposed cancellous surface, in a position that will allow for each respective tendon slip to be reapproximated to the calcaneus in a balanced fashion (**TECH FIG 4A,B**).
- The anchors must be strong enough to lift the foot from the bed (**TECH FIG 4C–E**). If they should fail, we would prefer for them to fail now so we can rectify the problem.

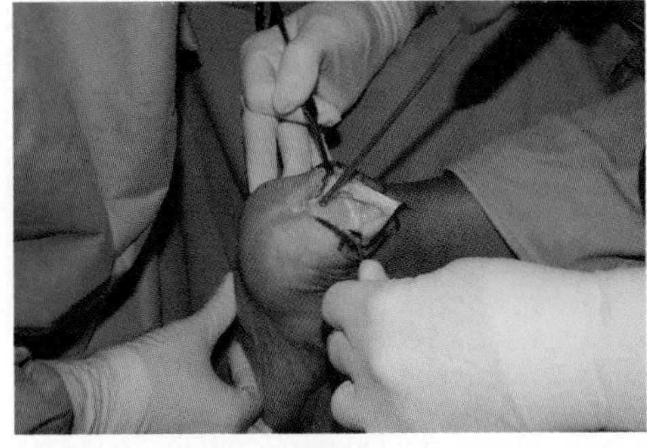

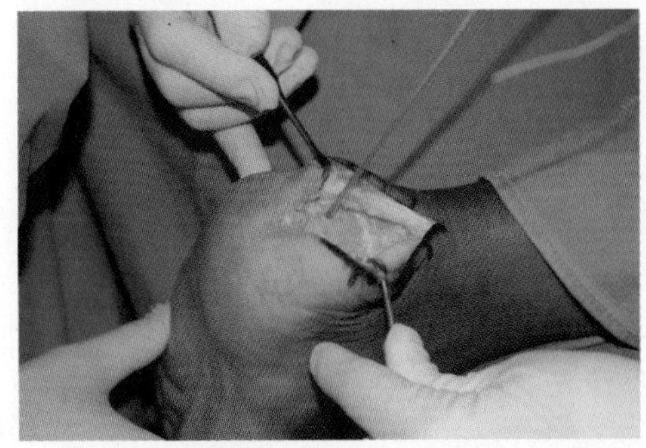

TECH FIG 4 • **A.** Anchor being started into bone. **B.** Anchor secured to bone. (*continued*)

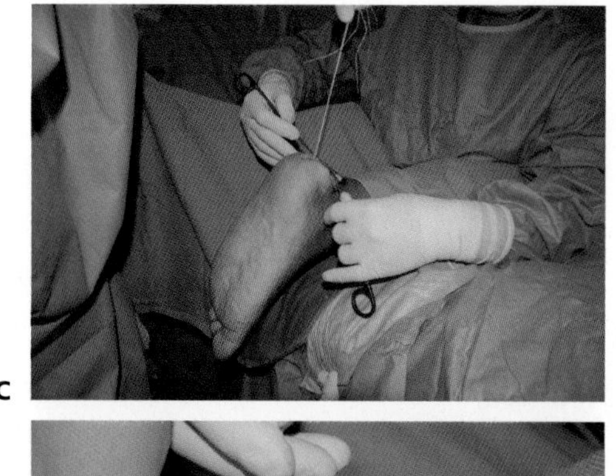

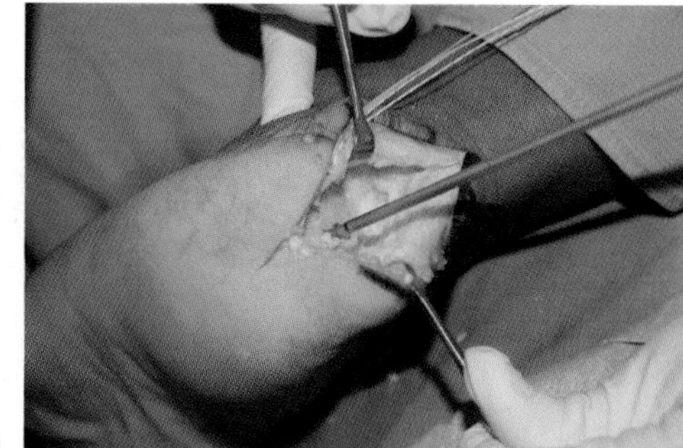

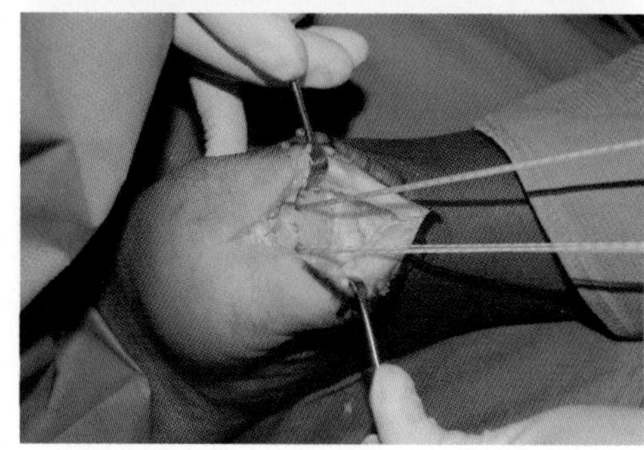

TECH FIG 4 • (*continued*) **C.** Testing the stability of the anchor by lifting the limb off the table. The medial suture anchor (**D**) is placed symmetrically relative to the lateral anchor and secured to bone (**E**).

Balancing and Securing the Sutures

- The anchor sutures are then passed in through their respective tendon slip, also in a balanced manner to ensure that the tendon slips have near equal tension once the sutures are secured (**TECH FIG 5A–C**).
- We routinely check the anticipated tension by pushing the tendon slip to bone while tensioning the sutures after they have been passed through the tendon.
- If the tension does not appear to be equal in the two slips, we readjust the position of the sutures.
- The sutures must not only be tensioned appropriately in the longitudinal plane but must also be balanced well in the medial-to-lateral plane, so that the two tendon slips may also be reapproximated side to side and reconfigure the physiologic Achilles attachment.
- The sutures are then secured (**TECH FIG 5D,E**). Have the assistant hold the ankle in plantarflexion so that the tendon slips fully contact the calcaneus.

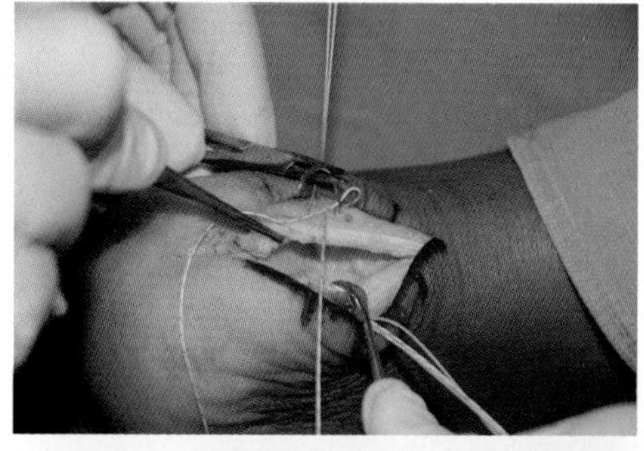

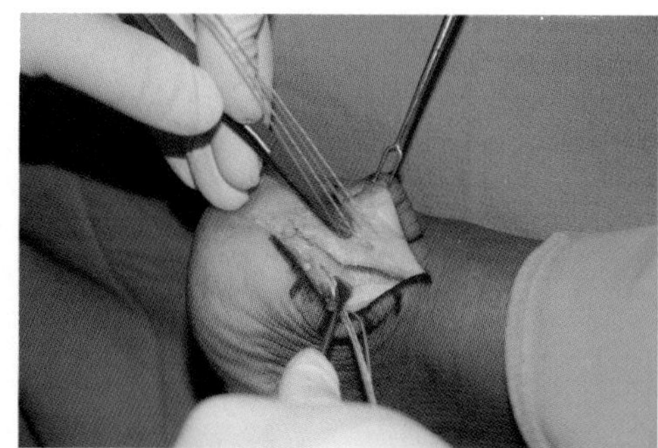

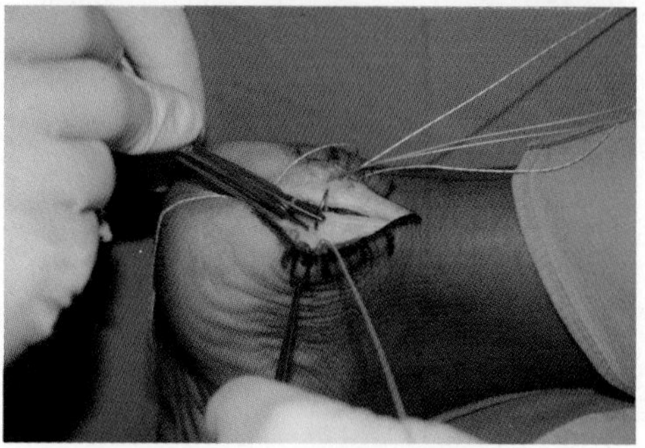

TECH FIG 5 • **A.** the suture is passed through the tendon. **B.** Confirming the optimal balance of the tendon slip on the anchor. **C.** Passing the sutures through the second tendon slip. (*continued*)

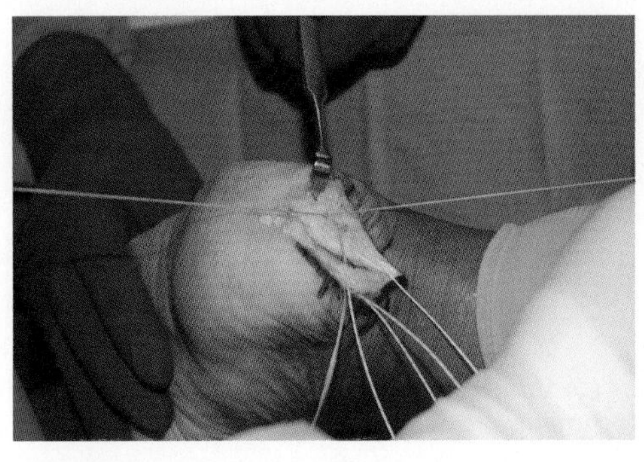

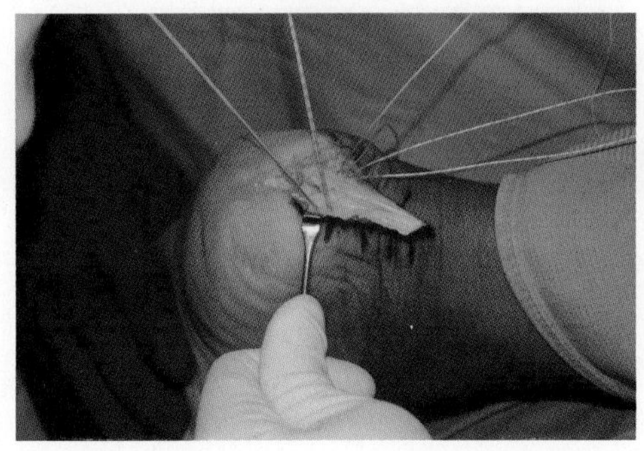

TECH FIG 5 • (*continued*) **D.** Lateral tendon slip fully approximated to bone. Note that the ankle is held in plantarflexion to facilitate tendon approximation. **E.** Medial tendon slip being attached.

Additional Sutures

- We have a low threshold to place a third suture anchor to further stabilize both Achilles slips distally on the calcaneus (TECH FIG 6A–C).
- Finally, the most distal Achilles fibers are reapproximated to the fascial tissue immediately distal to the calcaneus (TECH FIG 6D,E).
  - Avoid trapping fat in this portion of the repair as it may lead to fat necrosis.
- The two Achilles slips are then reapproximated to one another with an absorbable suture (TECH FIG 6F).
- Gently test dorsiflexion. The ankle should typically still reach neutral without compromising the repair. If it does not, however, it is not a problem.
  - Patients rarely if ever develop equinus contracture.
  - Once the Achilles tendon insertion is again healthy and asymptomatic, it has been our experience that the gastrocnemius and soleus muscles accommodate.

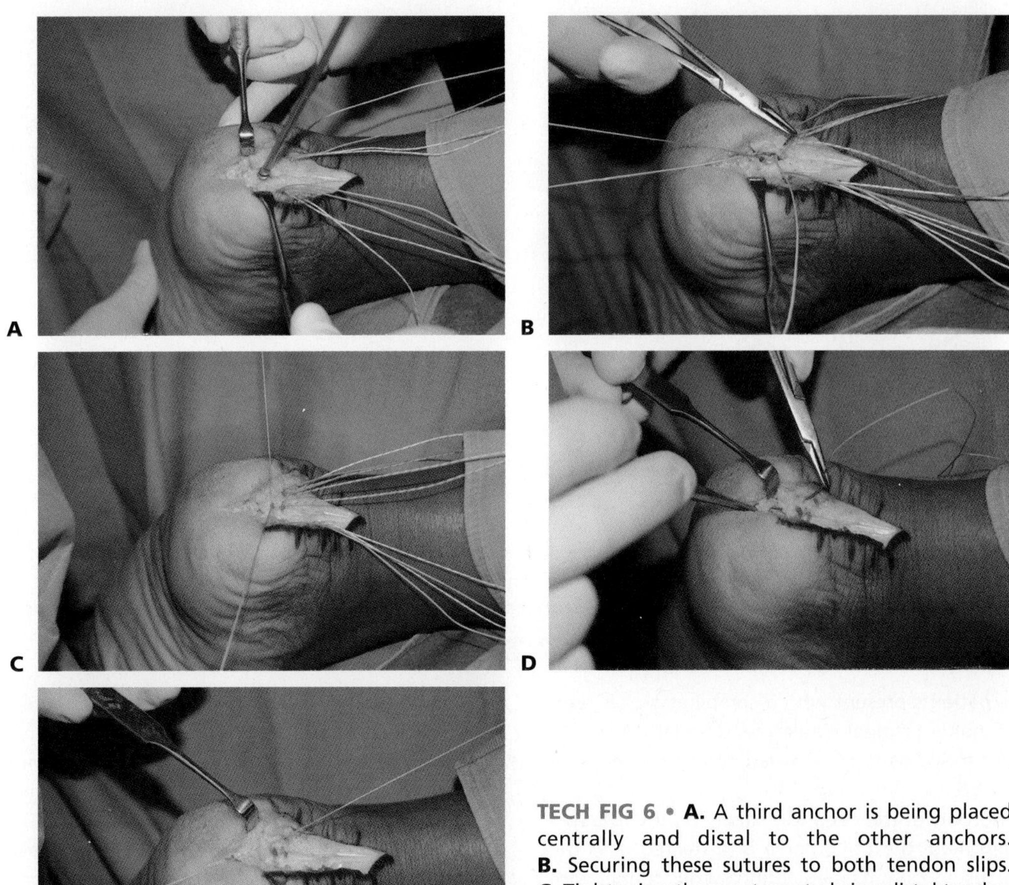

TECH FIG 6 • **A.** A third anchor is being placed centrally and distal to the other anchors. **B.** Securing these sutures to both tendon slips. **C.** Tightening these sutures to bring distal tendon slips to bone. **D–F.** Reapproximating the tendon slips to the distal fascia. **D.** Passing suture. **E.** Fully closing the gap between the distal tendon and the fascia. (*continued*)

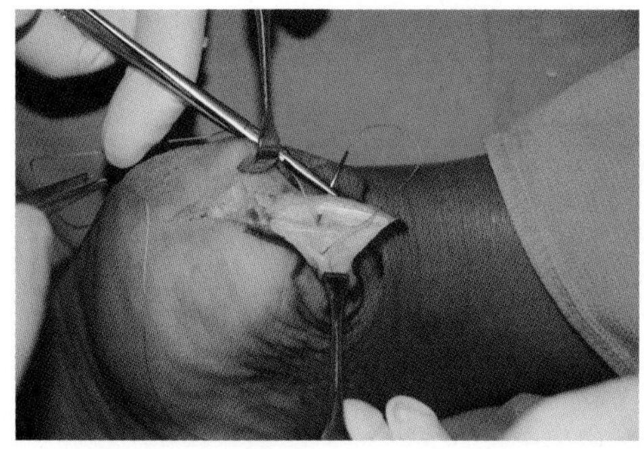

TECH FIG 6 • (*continued*) **F.** Reapproximating two tendon slips proximal to the reattachment.

CLOSURE

- Close the paratenon (TECH FIG 7A).
- Reapproximate the subcutaneous tissues (TECH FIG 7B).
- Perform a tensionless closure. We routinely use staples in the proximal wound but favor suture in the distal wound, where the skin does not evert as readily (TECH FIG 7C).
- Sterile dressings, abundant padding, and a posterior splint with the ankle in its resting tension complete the closure.

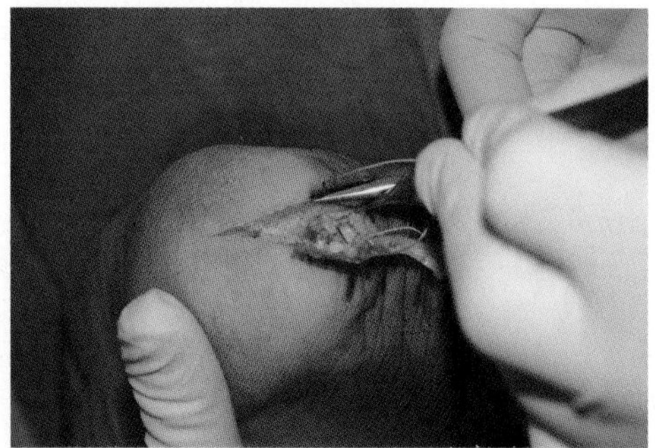

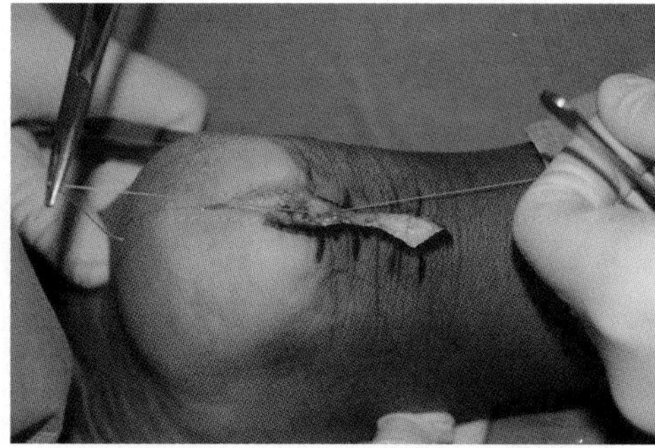

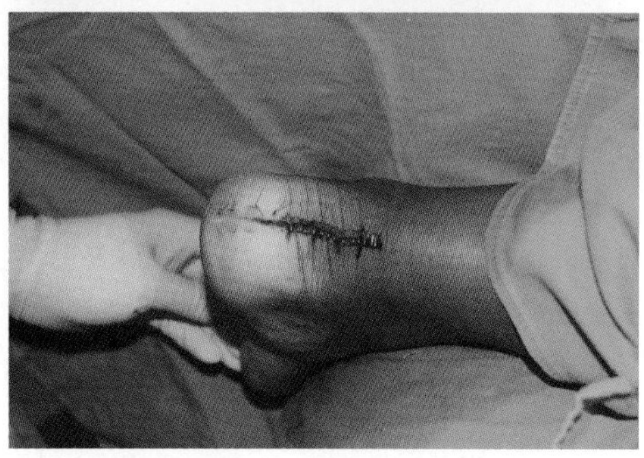

TECH FIG 7 • Closure. **A.** Paratenon. **B.** Subcutaneous tissue. **C.** Skin (sutures are used distally to ensure that skin margins did not invert).

FLEXOR HALLUCIS TENDON AUGMENTATION

- Only rare patients present with a combination of insertional and noninsertional Achilles tendinopathy.
- Extensive dèbridement of diseased tendon is required (TECH FIG 8A,B).
- After fasciotomy of the deep compartment, the FHL tendon is identified, the tibial nerve is protected, and the FHL is harvested from its medial fibrosseous tunnel with the ankle and hallux interphalangeal joint in maximum plantarflexion (TECH FIG 8C).
- With this local (short) harvest of the FHL, in contrast to a long harvest from the plantar foot via a separate incision, the tendon length is ample for augmentation of the Achilles reattachment (TECH FIG 8D).
- The FHL tendon is anchored via an interference screw in the central calcaneus, within the exposed cancellous surface created after exostectomy (TECH FIG 8E).
  - A suture goes through the plantar calcaneus to allow optimal tensioning of the FHL tendon (TECH FIG 8F).
- Suture anchors for reattachment of the the Achilles slips are balanced on either side of the FHL anchor point (TECH FIG 8G).

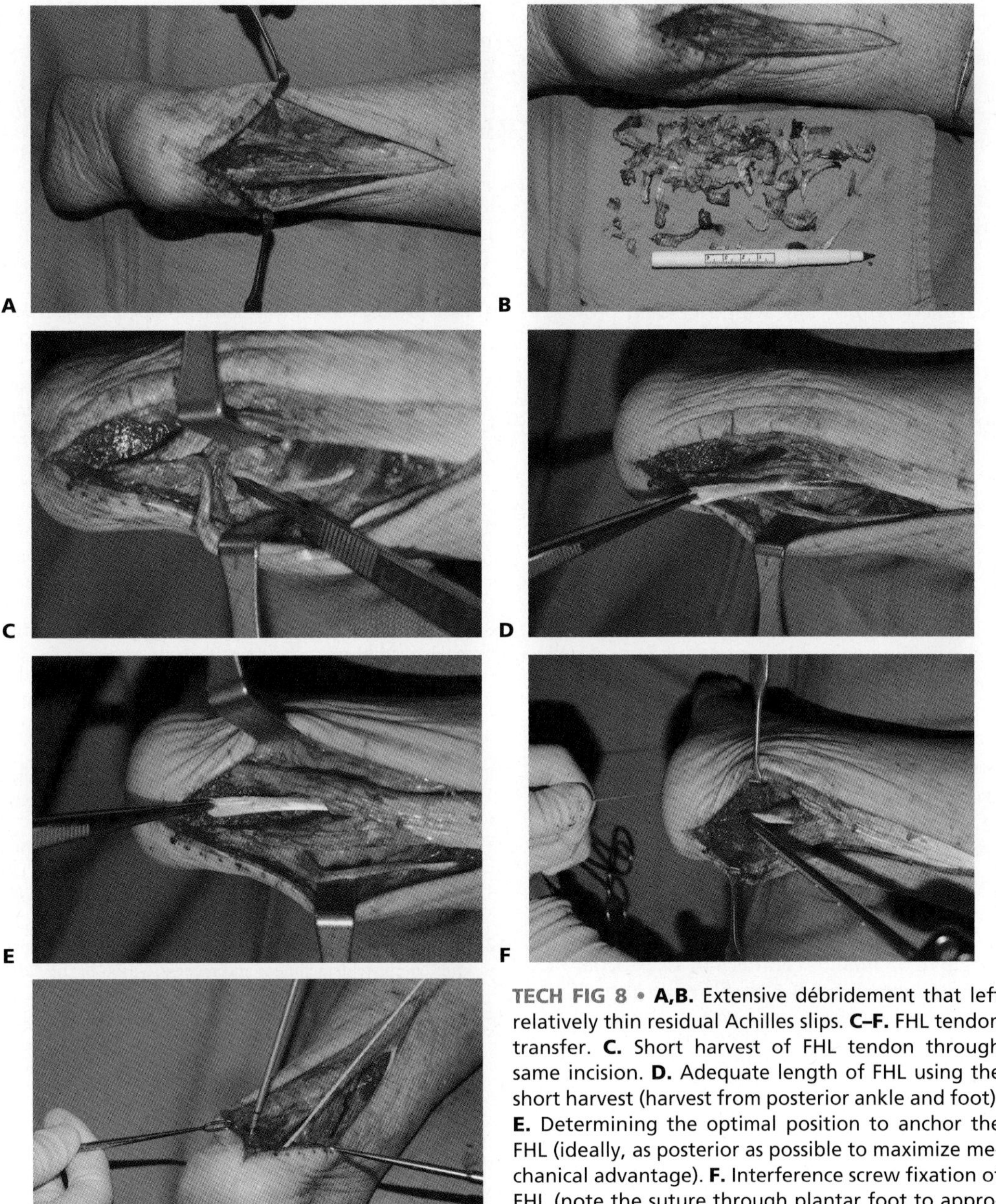

TECH FIG 8 • **A,B.** Extensive débridement that left relatively thin residual Achilles slips. **C–F.** FHL tendon transfer. **C.** Short harvest of FHL tendon through same incision. **D.** Adequate length of FHL using the short harvest (harvest from posterior ankle and foot). **E.** Determining the optimal position to anchor the FHL (ideally, as posterior as possible to maximize mechanical advantage). **F.** Interference screw fixation of FHL (note the suture through plantar foot to appropriately tension the FHL). **G.** Suture anchors are placed symmetrically for reattachment of Achilles slips, without interfering with the FHL anchor point.

PEARLS AND PITFALLS

Calcific tendinosis	■ Be sure not only to dèbride the unhealthy tendon fibers but also to remove all calcifications within the tendon.
Reattachment of the healthy Achilles tendon to the calcaneus	■ The two Achilles tendon slips should be reattached in a balanced manner on the exposed cancellous surface of the calcaneus. ■ Before tying the sutures of the suture anchors, check that the tension appears nearly equal for the two tendon slips.
Paratenon	■ As for repair of acute Achilles tendon ruptures, be sure to close the paratenon over the tendon.
FHL tendon augmentation	■ This is an intraoperative decision and, in our experience, rarely necessary. If augmentation is needed, perform an FHL harvest through the same incision via a deep compartment fasciotomy. Be sure to identify and protect the tibial nerve that will be immediately adjacent to the FHL tendon. Transfer the tendon as far posteriorly on the exposed cancellous surface of the calcaneus as possible for the greatest mechanical advantage.

POSTOPERATIVE CARE

- Weeks 0 to 2: Posterior splint with the ankle in resting tension of plantarflexion
- At 2 weeks: Return to clinic for suture removal and casting
- Weeks 2 to 5: Short leg, plantarflexed (5 to 10 degrees) weight-bearing cast, with weight bearing permitted but use of an assistive device encouraged
- At 5 weeks: Return to clinic for cast removal and transfer to a cam boot
- Weeks 5 to 8: Cam walker boot with a 5- to 10-degree heel lift; initiate a physical therapy program, with a gradual progression to careful resistance exercises
- Weeks 8 to 12: Progression to a regular shoe with a heel lift or an open-back shoe with a slight heel; physical therapy with a progressive eccentric strengthening exercises
- Between 3 and 6 months: return to full activities; home program for physical therapy
- It may take a full year before patients "can forget about this Achilles tendon."
- Maintain independent basic physical therapy exercises for a lifetime.

OUTCOMES

- Most patients undergoing surgical management of insertional Achilles tendinopathy have good to excellent results, albeit without returning to full activity for 6 to 12 months.
- However, most studies note that there are patients that do not return to full activity and while they are improved, they are not pain-free.
- Johnson et al[5] reported a mean improvement in the AOFAS ankle outcomes score from 53 to 89 points for 22 patients at 34 months' average follow-up.
- McGarvey et al[9] noted an 82% satisfaction rate in 22 patients at mean follow-up of 33 months. Thirteen of 22 patients were pain-free and and an equal number could return to full acitivities.

COMPLICATIONS

- Wound dehiscence
- Infection
- Avulsion of Achilles tendon from anchors on calcaneus
- Persitent pain despite apparent successful procedure
- Suture reaction or irriation

REFERENCES

1. Calder JD, Saxby TS. Surgical treatment of insertional Achilles tendinosis. Foot Ankle Int 2003;24:119–121.
2. Den Hartog BD. Insertional Achilles tendinosis: pathogenesis and treatment. Foot Ankle Clin 2009;14:639–650.
3. DeOrio MJ, Easley ME. Surgical strategies: insertional Achilles tendinopathy. Foot Ankle Int 2008;29:542–550.
4. Furia JP. High-energy extracorporeal shock wave therapy as a treatment for insertional Achilles tendinopathy. Am J Sports Med 2006; 34:733–740.
5. Johnson KW, Zalavras C, Thordarson DB. Surgical management of insertional calcific Achilles tendinosis with a central tendon splitting approach. Foot Ankle Int 2006;27:245–250.
6. Knobloch K, Kraemer R, Lichtenberg A, et al. Achilles tendon and paratendon microcirculation in midportion and insertional tendinopathy in athletes. Am J Sports Med 2006;34:92–97
7. Kolodziej P, Glisson RR, Nunley JA. Risk of avulsion of the Achilles tendon after partial excision for treatment of insertional tendonitis and Haglund's deformity: a biomechanical study. Foot Ankle Int 1999;20:433–437.
8. Maffulli N, Testa V, Capasso G, Sullo A. Calcific insertional Achilles tendinopathy: reattachment with bone anchors. Am J Sports Med 2004;32:174–182.
9. McGarvey WC, Palumbo RC, Baxter DE, Leibman BD. Insertional Achilles tendinosis: surgical treatment through a central tendon splitting approach. Foot Ankle Int 2002;23:19–25.
10. Nicholson CW, Berlet GC, Lee TH. Prediction of the success of nonoperative treatment of insertional Achilles tendinosis based on MRI. Foot Ankle Int 2007;28:472–477.
11. Rompe JD, Furia J, Maffulli N. Eccentric loading compared with shock wave treatment for chronic insertional Achilles tendinopathy: a randomized, controlled trial. J Bone Joint Surg Am 2008;90A: 52–61.
12. Wagner E, Gould J, Bilen E, et al. Change in plantarflexion strength after complete detachment and reconstruction of the Achilles tendon. Foot Ankle Int 2004;25:800–804.
13. Wagner E, Gould JS, Kneidel M, et al. Technique and results of Achilles tendon detachment and reconstruction for insertional Achilles tendinosis. Foot Ankle Int 2006;27:677–684.

Chapter **116**

Surgical Management of Calcific Insertional Achilles Tendinopathy Using a Lateral Approach

Anthony Watson

DEFINITION

- Calcific Achilles tendinopathy is the most common cause of posterior heel pain.
- Intratendinous degeneration results in ectopic calcification and ossification at the Achilles tendon insertion to the calcaneus.

ANATOMY

- The Achilles tendon inserts over the inferior half of the posterior calcaneal tuberosity (**FIG 1**).
- The insertion expands over the tuberosity to become the calcaneal periosteum.
- The inferior half of the posterior calcaneal tuberosity has a rough surface with an extensive Sharpey fiber network.
- The superior half of the posterior calcaneal tuberosity has a smooth, almost articular surface.
- The retrocalcaneal bursa occupies the interval between the Achilles tendon and the superior half of the posterior calcaneal tuberosity. The bursa also extends superiorly over the posterosuperior process of the calcaneus.
- The ossification–calcification typically develops at the insertion, extends proximally into the tendon, and may comprise several segments within the more proximal tendon.

PATHOGENESIS

- The pathogenesis is not well understood.
- Two patient groups are typically affected: athletically active individuals in their 30s and 40s and overweight women in their 50s and 60s.
- Biochemical and histologic findings include:
  - Degenerative changes[2]
  - An anaerobic environment[1]
  - Longitudinal tears of the Achilles tendon[2,5]
  - Chondral metaplasia and endochondral ossification without insertional fibers from the tendon[3,5]

NATURAL HISTORY

- Symptoms compromise the patient's ability to wear shoes with a heel counter and participate in activity ranging from walking to intense athletic activity.
- Symptoms may improve in at least 50% of cases with activity modification, physical therapy, or shoe modifications.[6]
- Disabling symptoms that do not improve with nonoperative treatment may benefit from surgery.
- Achilles tendon rupture in the presence of insertional calcification is extremely rare, even without any form of treatment.

PATIENT HISTORY AND PHYSICAL FINDINGS

- The typical patient complaint is posterior heel pain aggravated by activity or shoe wear.
- Symptoms develop insidiously over time.
- Inflammatory enthesopathies such as psoriasis, Reiter syndrome, and inflammatory bowel disease may be present.
- Tenderness localized to the Achilles insertion on palpation (the examiner should press directly posteriorly on the heel where the Achilles tendon inserts) confirms the diagnosis.
- Tenderness may also be present in the Achilles tendon itself or over the retrocalcaneal bursa. The examiner should lightly squeeze the tendon between the index finger and thumb; squeezing hard on the tendon can result in a false-positive result. A thickened or painful tendon will require MRI to determine whether tendon transfer reconstruction is necessary.
- Peritendinous swelling is rare, but increased caliber of the Achilles tendon may be present.
- Weakness is rare, but Achilles tendon contracture is common.
- Achilles tightness should be addressed with stretching before considering nonoperative treatment a failure.
- Pain with resisted plantarflexion suggests more extensive tendinosis.

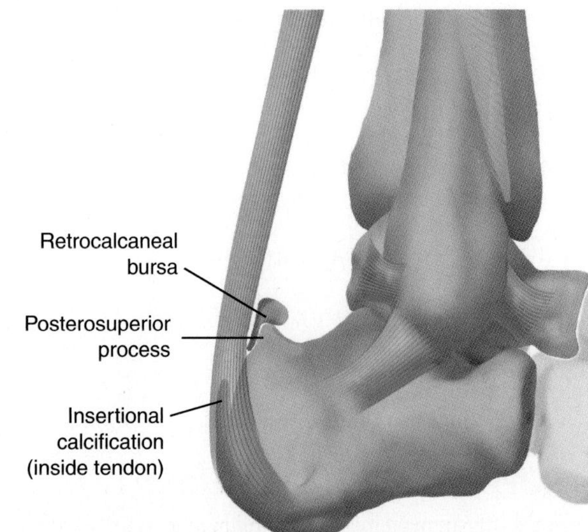

FIG 1 • Anatomy of insertional calcification of the Achilles tendon. Note expansion of Achilles tendon fibers over posterior calcaneal tuberosity and intratendinous location of calcification.

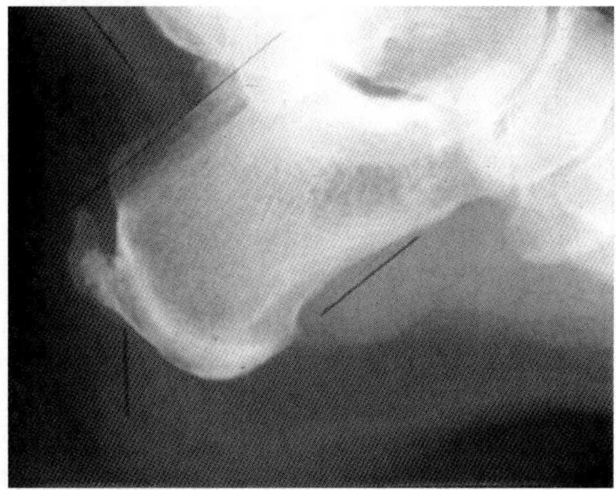

FIG 2 • Lateral radiograph of heel with insertional calcification of the Achilles tendon.

- Pain with maximum passive plantarflexion suggests inflammation of the paratenon.
- Palpation of the retrocalcaneal bursa will differentiate retrocalcaneal bursitis from insertional tendinosis because a tender retrocalcaneal bursa may benefit from bursectomy.
- Pain with toe walking supports the diagnosis. Inability to do either suggests the need for rehabilitation before considering surgery.
- The surgeon must accurately assess the neurovascular status of the foot and the presence and appearance of any previous incisional scars.

IMAGING AND OTHER DIAGNOSTIC STUDIES

- Lateral radiograph of heel (**FIG 2**)
  - The examiner should identify insertional ossification, characterize the size of the posterosuperior process of the calcaneus, and identify intratendinous calcification more proximally.
- Parallel pitch lines and the Fowler angle provide no diagnostic, therapeutic, or prognostic information.
- MRI is indicated when the tendon is thickened, tender, or calcified to determine whether greater than 50% of the cross-sectional area of the tendon is involved (**FIG 3**).

DIFFERENTIAL DIAGNOSIS

- Retrocalcaneal bursitis
- Calcaneal stress fracture
- Plantar fasciitis
- Calcaneal periostitis
- Achilles tendinosis without insertional calcification

NONOPERATIVE MANAGEMENT

- Nonoperative management is helpful in at least 50% of cases.
- Initial treatment is with a removable walker boot with removable wedges.
- Two or three wedges are used for 2 weeks, and then a wedge is removed every 2 weeks.
- Use of the boot is continued for 2 weeks after removal of the last wedge.
- Weight bearing as tolerated is permitted in the boot.
- Physical therapy is started upon completion of removable walker boot immobilization and should include eccentric closed-chain strengthening exercises.[6]
- Corticosteroid injection is contraindicated.

SURGICAL MANAGEMENT

- Surgical treatment is indicated for disabling symptoms that do not improve with thorough nonoperative treatment.
- Patients should be counseled that recovery can be a lengthy and sometimes frustrating process, as it is often 12 to 18 months before maximum improvement occurs, especially in nonathletic patients.[4,7]
- Recurrent prominence occurs in 50% of cases but is rarely symptomatic.[7]

Preoperative Planning

- It may be helpful to have patients undergo crutch training preoperatively.
- A flexor hallucis longus tendon transfer reconstruction of the Achilles tendon will be necessary if an MRI demonstrates that greater than 50% of the cross-sectional area of the Achilles tendon is involved with degenerative tendinosis.

Positioning

- The lateral or prone position is necessary. The heel is more accessible in older or heavier patients when positioned prone. Anesthesia concerns may require lateral positioning.

Approach

- Lateral, medial, posterior, and combined approaches have all been described. The lateral approach will be described here.
- Advantages of the lateral approach are:
  - Direct exposure of the insertional calcification
  - Less compromise of the Achilles insertion expansion than other approaches because the strongest insertion is medial
  - The scar is less likely to be irritated by shoes, as with the posterior approach.

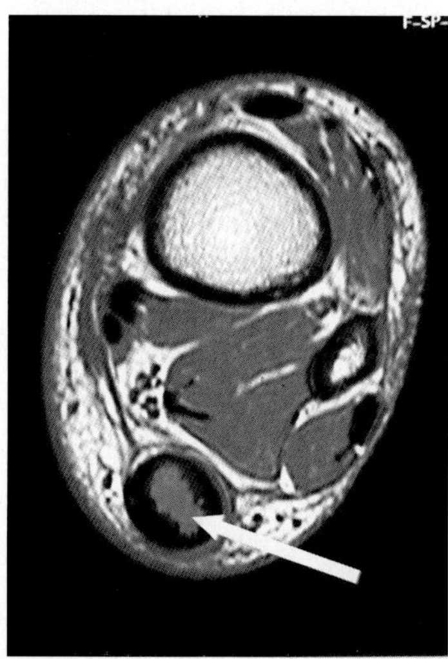

FIG 3 • Axial T1-weighted MRI showing intratendinous degeneration comprising greater than 50% of the cross-sectional area of the Achilles tendon (*white arrow*).

RETROCALCANEAL DECOMPRESSION BY LATERAL APPROACH

- After administration of anesthesia, position the patient lateral decubitus or prone.
- Apply a thigh tourniquet.
- Prepare and drape the leg, exsanguinate the leg, and inflate the tourniquet.
- Make a longitudinal incision along the lateral heel anterior to the anterior margin of the Achilles tendon. The incision should extend distally to nearly the plantar surface and proximally superior to the retrocalcaneal bursa (**TECH FIG 1**).
- Carefully perform sharp dissection to create full-thickness flaps, taking care to identify and protect any branches of the sural nerve.

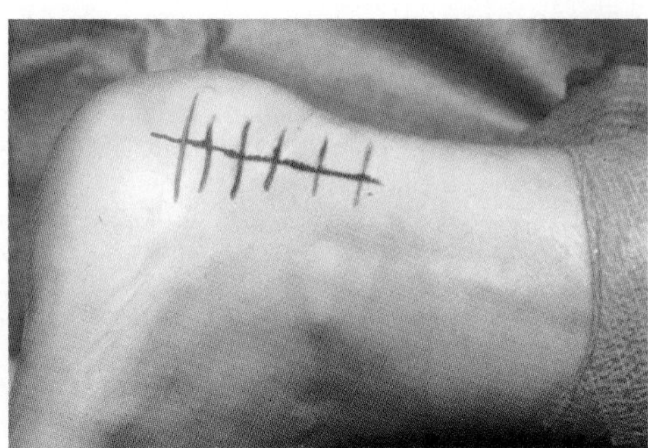

TECH FIG 1 • Location of incision.

- Make a longitudinal periosteal incision and extend it proximally through the retrocalcaneal bursa, and excise the retrocalcaneal bursa.
- Elevate the periosteum anteriorly, then elevate it posteriorly.
- Continue sharp elevation of the calcaneal periosteum and Achilles tendon insertion expansion medially along the posterior calcaneal tuberosity all the way to the medial aspect of the tuberosity.
- Subperiosteal exposure of the insertional ossification requires careful dissection to preserve the Achilles sleeve.
- Resect any degenerative tendinosis of the Achilles tendon. If preoperative MRI showed tendinosis affecting greater than 50% of the cross-sectional area of the Achilles tendon, a flexor hallucis longus tendon transfer, described elsewhere, will be necessary.
- Resect the posterior calcaneus along a line from inferior to the insertional ossification to anterior to the posterosuperior process of the calcaneus using a saw or osteotome (**TECH FIG 2**).
- Round over the sharp edges medially and laterally with a rasp or rongeur.
- Place two suture anchors in the cancellous bone left after ostectomy and repair the Achilles tendon to the calcaneus (**TECH FIG 3**).
- Repair the periosteum laterally.
- Close the incision.
- Apply a sterile dressing and plaster posterior mold splint with the ankle in resting plantarflexion.

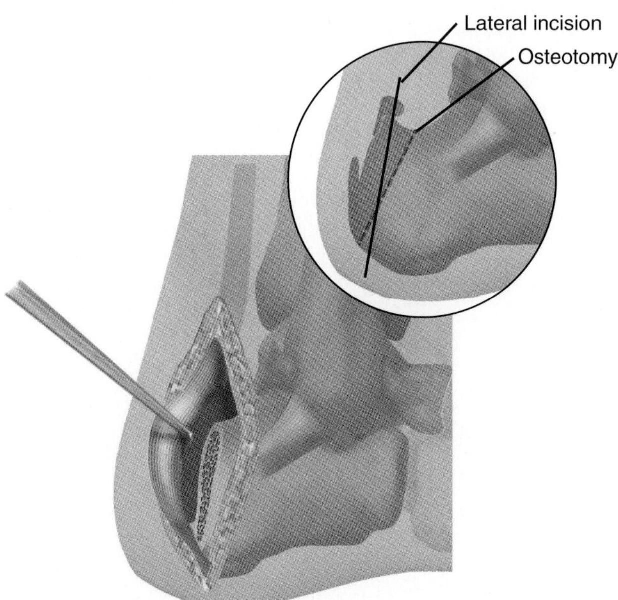

TECH FIG 2 • Location of ostectomy to include the posterosuperior process of the calcaneus and the insertional calcification.

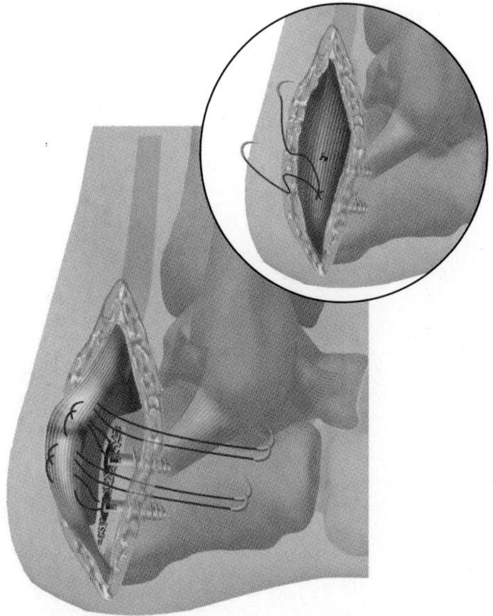

TECH FIG 3 • Location of suture anchors and repair of Achilles tendon to ostectomy surface of calcaneus.

PEARLS AND PITFALLS

Exposure	■ Do not be afraid to lengthen the incision to avoid tension from retraction. ■ The incision is posterior to the sural nerve, but there may be a branch to the calcaneus in the field, which should be protected. ■ Creating full-thickness tissue flaps and avoiding blunt dissection minimize the risk of wound dehiscence.
Decompression	■ Elevating the periosteum anterior to the ostectomy will facilitate later repair of the Achilles to the calcaneus. ■ Be sure to perform ostectomy anterior to the posterosuperior process of the calcaneus, but be careful to avoid the posterior facet of the subtalar joint. ■ A secure repair of the Achilles to the calcaneus permits early motion with minimal risk of early avulsion.

POSTOPERATIVE CARE

- Non–weight-bearing is continued for 4 weeks postoperatively.
- Two weeks after surgery, the postoperative splint is changed to a removable walker boot with an Achilles wedge like that used for nonoperative care.
- The removable walker boot is continued for 6 weeks, for a total of 8 weeks of immobilization.
- Active, nonresistive ankle and hindfoot range-of-motion exercises are begun once the incision has healed.
- Physical therapy begins 8 weeks after surgery.

OUTCOMES

- Fifty to 85% of patients report good or excellent results 2 years after surgery.[4,7]
- The percentage of good or excellent results is higher in athletic than nonathletic patients.[4]
- Radiographically recurrent insertional calcification occurs in 50% of patients, but symptoms do not always recur with radiographic recurrence.[7]
- Some patients have recurrent symptoms without radiographic recurrence.[7]
- Maximum symptomatic relief may not occur until 12 to 18 months after surgery.
- A 1- to 2-month period of temporary symptomatic recurrence often occurs 7 to 10 months after the surgery.[7]

COMPLICATIONS

- Superficial or deep infection is especially common in diabetic and overweight patients.
- Delayed wound healing is also especially common in diabetic and overweight patients.
- Paresthesias and hypoesthesias can be avoided by identifying and protecting the sural nerve and its calcaneal branch.
- Achilles avulsion
- Deep venous thrombosis
- Recurrence

REFERENCES

1. Alfredson H, Bjur D, Thorsen K, et al. High intratendinous lactate levels in painful chronic Achilles tendinosis: an investigation using microdialysis technique. J Orthop Res 2002;20:934–938.
2. Astrom M, Rausing A. Chronic Achilles tendinopathy: a survey of surgical and histopathologic findings. Clin Orthop Relat Res 1995;316:151–164.
3. Maffulli N, Reaper J, Ewen SW, et al. Chondral metaplasia in calcific insertional tendinopathy of the Achilles tendon. Clin J Sports Med 2006;16:329–334.
4. Maffulli N, Testa V, Capasso G, et al. Surgery for chronic Achilles tendinopathy yields worse results in nonathletic patients. Clin J Sports Med 2006;16:123–128.
5. Rufai A, Ralphs JR, Benjamin M. Structure and histopathology of the insertional region of the human Achilles tendon. J Orthop Res 1995;13:585–593.
6. Shalabi A, Kristoffersen-Wilberg M, Svensson L, et al. Eccentric training of the gastrocnemius-soleus complex in chronic Achilles tendinopathy results in decreased tendon volume and intratendinous signal as evaluated by MRI. Am J Sports Med 2004;32:1286–1296.
7. Watson AD, Anderson RB, Davis WH. Comparison of results of retrocalcaneal decompression for retrocalcaneal bursitis and insertional Achilles tendinosis with calcific spur. Foot Ankle Int 2000;21:638–642.

Chapter 117

Flexor Hallucis Longus Tendon Augmentation for the Treatment of Insertional Achilles Tendinosis

William C. McGarvey and Thomas O. Clanton

DEFINITION

- The term *insertional Achilles tendinitis* (IAT) is actually a misnomer. The condition is more typically a degenerative process, and the nomenclature should reflect this condition, more appropriately, as a tendinosis or tendinopathy.[5,7,8,9,14]
- As the name suggests, insertional Achilles tendinopathy is identified by a painful condition at the musculotendinous insertion of the tendo Achilles on the posterior calcaneus.
  - It represents about 10% to 20% of all Achilles pathology.[2]
  - It is most commonly seen as an overuse injury in athletes, eg., runners and "push-off" athletes such as basketball or volleyball players, or in more sedentary patients as a degenerative process.

ANATOMY

- The Achilles tendon (TA) is the largest tendon in the body. Its chief function is plantarflexion of the foot and ankle.
- It is viscoelastic and strong, elongating up to 15% under loads and bearing up to 10 times body weight in single-legged stance during running.[5,9]
- The Achilles insertion is a broad expanse that envelops the entire tuberosity of the os calcis and sends Sharpey's fibers to the medial, lateral, and plantar borders of the bone.[1]
- Immediately anterior to the Achilles tendon lie the retrocalcaneal bursa and a variably sized posterolateral prominence of calcaneus, often known as *Haglund's deformity.*
- More anteriorly lies the deep posterior compartment musculature, which includes the flexor hallucis longus (FHL), the neurovascular bundle, including the tibial nerve, and vessels.
- The FHL originates from the fibula and interosseous membrane, travelling obliquely and distally to pass under the sustentaculum tali, through a fibro-osseous tunnel, and on to the master knot of Henry to attach to the hallux.

PATHOGENESIS

- Repetitive stress can lead to a combination of inflammatory and degenerative changes.
- Degeneration or tendinosis occurs as the already compromised vascularity of the tendon is further reduced by age and injury.[8,9]
  - Microscopic and macroscopic changes occur, leading to scarring and slow regeneration or repair.
  - Tenocytes are reduced in number and quality, contributing to poor repair potential.
- Inflammatory changes are manifested as paratenonitis involving the investing layer surrounding the TA, but not the tendon itself. This leads to thickening and adherence of the paratenon to the TA.
- Additionally, the continuum of injury and inadequate repair capacity create a cycle of collagen and calcium deposition in an effort to stabilize the musculotendinous enthesis, leading to enlargement of the insertion site; generation of abundant, poor quality tissue; and irritation of the surrounding tisssues, causing a painful thickening of the insertion of the TA.

NATURAL HISTORY

- Untreated IAT has not been studied extensively. However, surgical findings and histologic analyses have provided some information.
- Persistent IAT leads to continued pain and swelling of the retrocalcaneal heel.
- A vicious cycle occurs in which further injury induces more attempts at repair and scar formation, leading to more irritation of surrounding tissues, decreased vascularity, and further microscopic injury.
- The posterior heel is more difficult to accommodate in a shoe.
- Range of motion is reduced, leading to increased susceptibilty to injury with any activity that places the TA under strain.
- Calcific debris is generated, both as reactive tissue reponse to injury and intratendinous hematoma formation as a result of injury. This compromises the viscoelasticity and, therefore, the integrity of the tendon, making it more apt to tear, either partially or completely.[4,14]
- A less pliable, less resilient TA is the end product. Insertional avulsion or rupture may occur, presenting a difficult treatment dilemma.

PATIENT HISTORY AND PHYSICAL FINDINGS

- Patients provide fairly accurate descriptions and complain of pain at the bone–tendon interface on the retrocalcaneal heel.
- Pain may be worse after activity, but gradually becomes more pervasive.
- Athletes may note an increase in symptoms with increases in training intensity or duration or changes in surface or shoes.
- Examination demonstrates tenderness directly posteriorly on the heel or, often, posterolaterally.
- In advanced cases, thickening, nodularity, or hardening may be palpated.
- Dorsiflexion of the ankle may be reduced compared with the contralateral leg.
- Methods for examining the Achilles tendon and its insertion include:
  - Direct palpation
    - The posterior heel and TA are inspected for visual or palpable swelling, tenderness, nodularity, or gapping, all of which are suggestive of diseased tendon.
  - Thompson test
    - With the patient prone, squeeze the calf at the gastrocnemius–soleus junction to elicit plantarflexion of the foot.

Compare with the contralateral side. A positive test is identified when the excursion of the injured side is far less than its uninjured counterpart. This is evidence for complete rupture.

IMAGING AND OTHER DIAGNOSTIC STUDIES

Radiographs

- Radiographs often are not necessary for diagnosis, but they are helpful in determining the presence of calcific debris, which is a poor prognostic sign[14] (**FIG 1**).
- Plain lateral and axial radiographic views usually are sufficient.

Ultrasonography

- Ultrasonography is a relatively inexpensive and accurate way to determine tendon quality, integrity, and function.
  - It has the advantage of being used dynamically to watch active tendon excursion, if so desired. It also may be used to follow the course of healing.
  - It is a highly user-dependent tool.

MRI

- MRI probably is the most comprehensive study available for investigation and evaluation of a damaged Achilles tendon (**FIG 2 A,B**).
- This study gives the most accurate information regarding degree of TA involvement, quality of surrounding tissue, presence or absence of rupture, and other concomitant pathology.

DIFFERENTIAL DIAGNOSIS

- Retrocalcaneal bursitis
- Haglund syndrome
- Inflammatory arthritides
- Seronegative spondyloarthropathies
- Gout
- Familial hyperlipidemia
- Sarcoidosis
- Diffuse idiopathic skeletal hyperostosis
- Pharmacologically induced pathology
  - Fluoroquinolone use
  - Chronic corticosteroid use

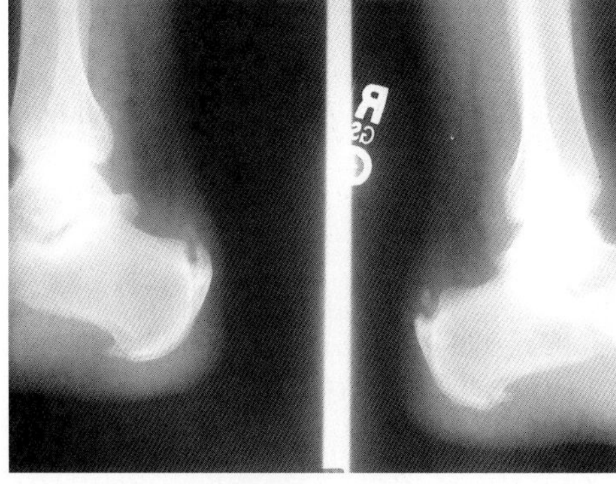

FIG 1 • Plain radiographs demonstrate intratendinous calcification at the Achilles insertion.

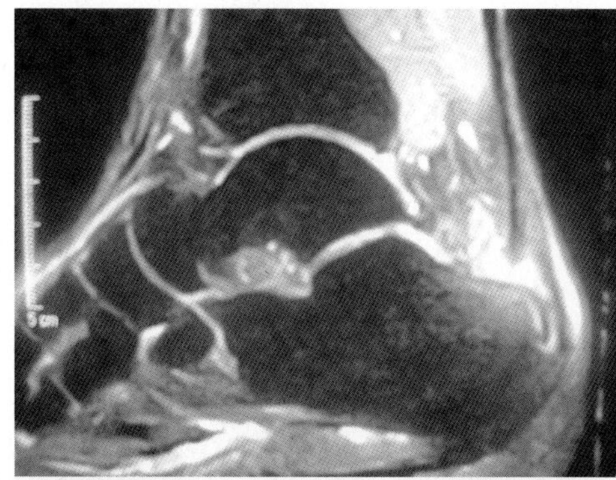

A

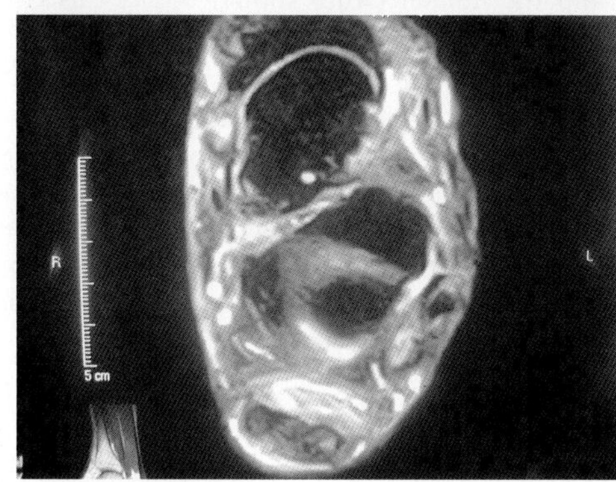

B

FIG 2 • MRI scan of insertional Achilles tendinosis. In this T2 sequence, the degenerative areas of tendon are demonstrated by increased uptake within the substance of the tendon in the sagittal (**A**) and axial (**B**) planes.

NONOPERATIVE MANAGEMENT

- Nonoperative treatment is successful in over 90% of patients with this process.[5,8]
- Success rates decline in the face of greater age at time of presentation, longstanding symptoms, and evidence of calcific tendinosis.[8]
- Initial phases of treatment include NSAID use, heel lifts, eccentric stretching, and shoe modifications to widen and soften the heel counter.
- More advanced situations may call for formal orthsoses to correct any biomechanical abnormallity, night splinting to apply continual stretch to the TA, and therapy modalities such as ice, contrast baths, and iontophoresis.
- Severe cases may require immobilzation in a cast or boot, followed by gradual reintroduction to cross-training before return to regular sports or activities.

SURGICAL MANAGEMENT

- Surgical decision making should reflect failed conservative efforts and continued symptoms and functional impairments.
- Younger, more athletic patients often respond to a simple débridement of damaged TA, which usually accounts for less than 50% of the total tendon. A midline tendon-splitting approach to this débridement is our preferred procedure for these patients.

Preoperative Planning

- Tendon integrity becomes more questionable with involvement of more than 50%, so augmentation is entertained at this point. This extensive involvement may become evident on preoperative testing or, alternatively, on intraoperative evaluation.

- Ideally, the surgeon will already have a good idea before beginning the procedure as to whether an augmentation is necessary.
  - This is readily apparent on imaging.
  - One must be ready to add this procedure if it is found to be necessary intraoperatively.

Positioning

- The patient is placed in the prone position (**FIG 3**).
- Both feet are prepped into the surgical field, up to the level of the knees.

Approach

- A midline incision currently is preferred (**FIG 4**), beginning about 2 to 3 cm proximal to the insertion and extending distally to expose the entire insertion of the TA.

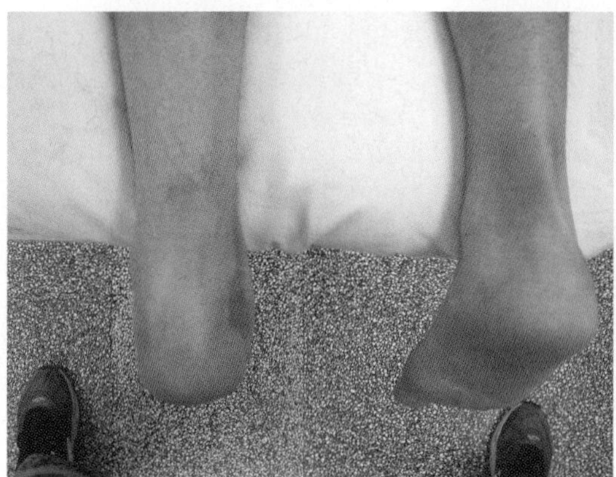

FIG 3 • Positioning for flexor hallucis longus (FHL) transfer. The patient is in the prone position with both feet prepped into the surgical field. Note the evidence of acute Achilles avulsion as resting tension on the foot is lost.

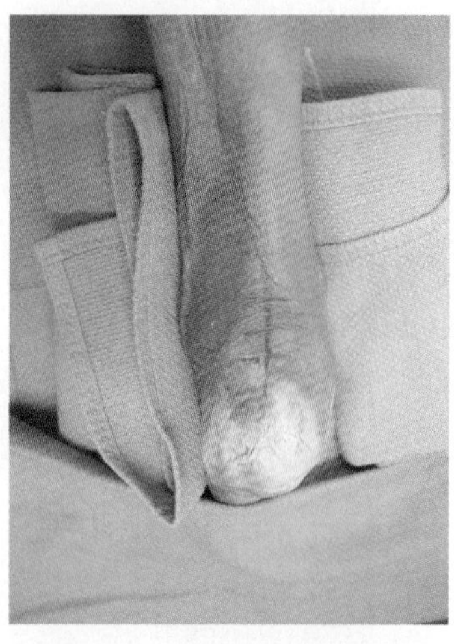

FIG 4 • Surgical approach. The planned incision for Achilles insertional débridement and FHL transfer is marked on the skin.

TECHNIQUES

RETROCALCANEAL DÉBRIDEMENT

- Full-thickness flaps should be developed medially and laterally, including the substance of the Achilles tendon (**TECH FIG 1A**).
- All nonviable or suspect-appearing tissue should be removed (**TECH FIG 1B**).
- Once adequate débridement takes place, the retrocalcaneal bursa also can be excised.
- Any enlarged or impinging posterolateral prominence of calcaneus should be aggressively removed with a rongeur, oscillating saw, or osteotome.

A

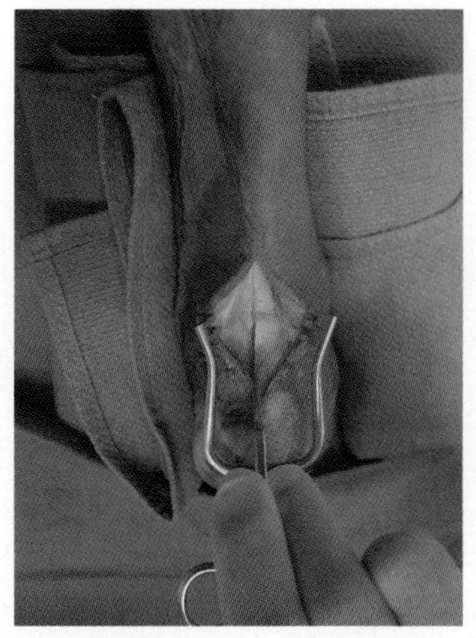

B

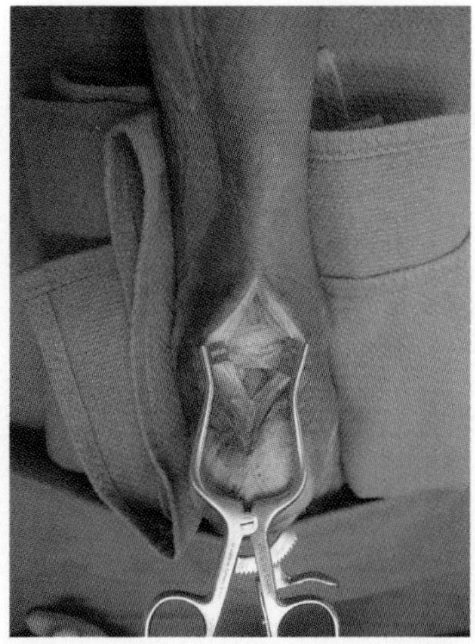

TECH FIG 1 • **A.** A midline tendon-splitting incision is made with full-thickness flaps through the TA. **B.** The retrocalcaneal bursa is visualized through the tendon.

FLEXOR HALLUCIS LONGUS HARVEST

- The FHL muscle belly usually is easily visible after the débridement is complete (TECH FIG 2A).
- Trace the FHL into its fibro-osseous tunnel (TECH FIG 2B,C).
- Plantarflex the ankle and hallux maximally.
- With a no. 15 blade, transect the tendon as distally as possible while an assistant pulls posteriorly on the proximal portion of the tendon (TECH FIG 2D).
- An interlocking suture of 2-0 braided nonabsorbable material is sewn into the tendon stump.

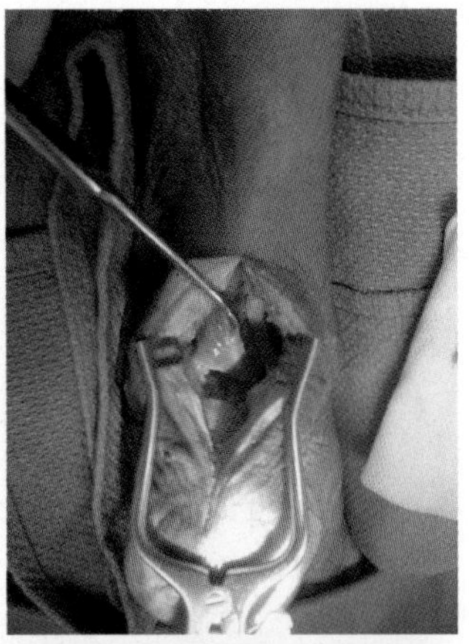

A

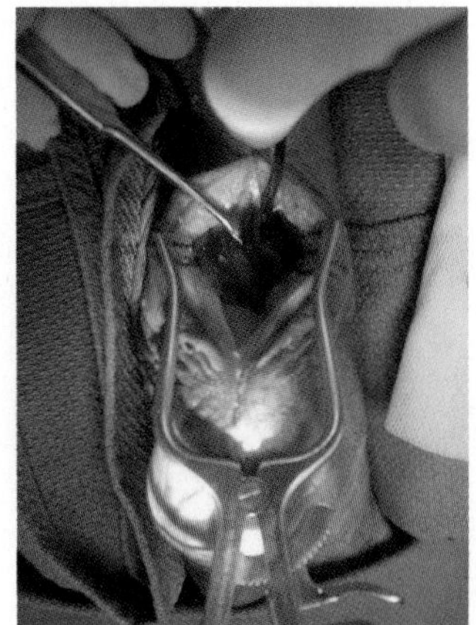

B

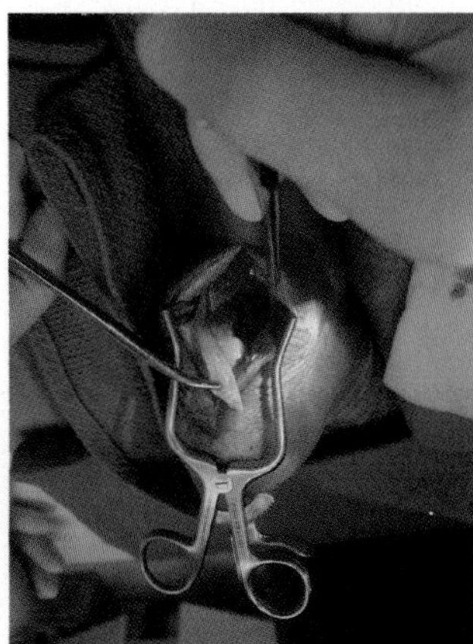

C

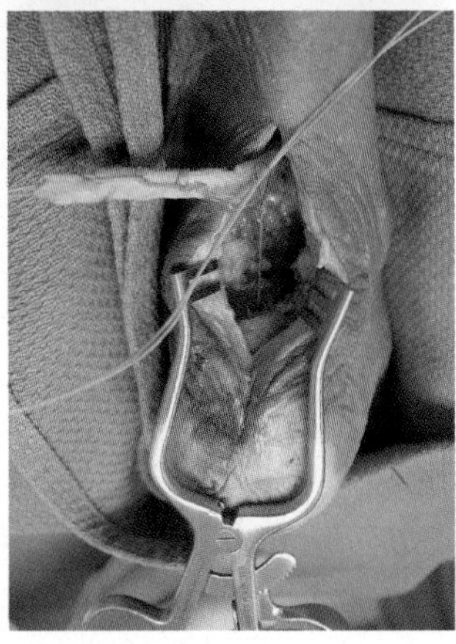

D

TECH FIG 2 • **A, B.** The flexor hallucis longus (FHL) tendon and the tibial nerve (medial or to the right) lie parallel and in close proximity to one another separated by a fibro-osseous sheath. **C.** The FHL is harvested throught the posterior incision, with care taken to avoid injuring the nerve, which lies just outside or medial to the fibro-osseous tunnel. **D.** A Krackow interlocking suture technique is used to secure the FHL to be brought into the tunnel.

ATTACHING THE GRAFT

- A 6.5-mm vertical tunnel is created in the posterior calcaneus about 1 cm anterior to the previous Achilles insertion (TECH FIG 3A).
- The FHL suture is passed through the tunnel and through the plantar skin with a Beath pin, bringing the FHL tendon into the tunnel (TECH FIG 3B).
- Tensioning is ensured by using the other foot as a reference at about 15 to 20 degrees of resting equinus. If the most medial and lateral remnants of native Achilles are maintained, they will also serve as reference for proper tensioning.
- An absorbable interference screw is introduced for graft fixation (TECH FIG 3C).
- Tension and range of motion are assessed and should be roughly equal to that of the unijnjured limb (TECH FIG 3D).
- The FHL muscle belly is then sewn in a side-to-side tenodesis fashion to the remaining TA to promote vascularity and help restore power to push-off (TECH FIG 3E).

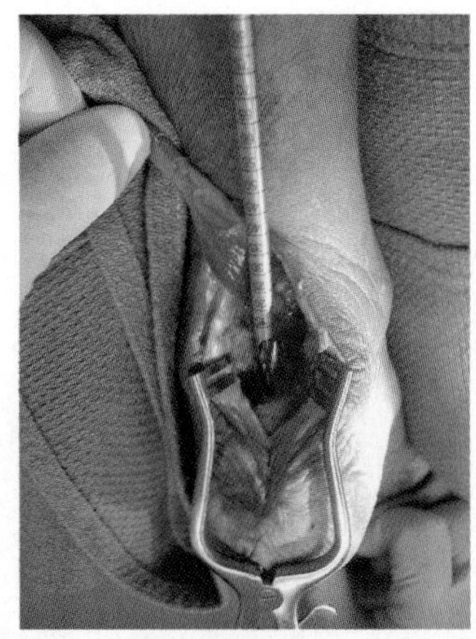

A

TECH FIG 3 • **A.** A bony tunnel is reamed to match the size of the interference screw to be used. *(continued)*

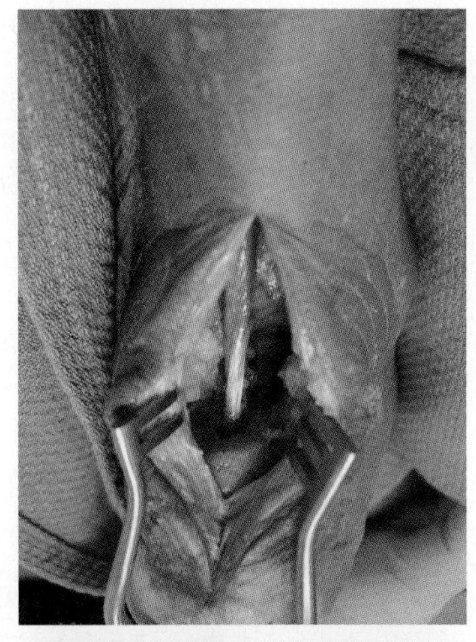
B

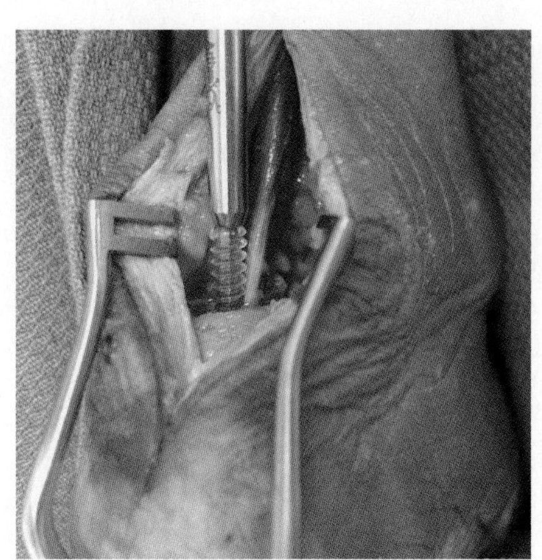
C

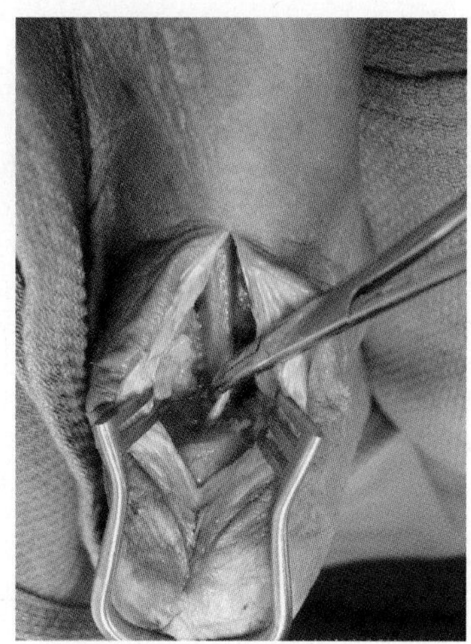
D

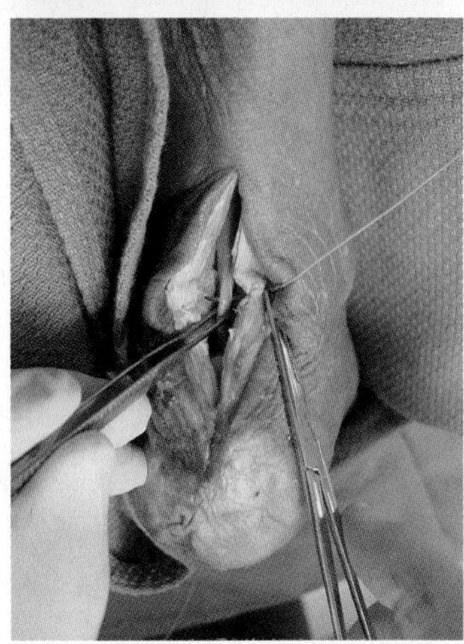
E

TECH FIG 3 • *(continued)* **B.** FHL pulled through the bony tunnel with tension equal to that of the other leg. **C.** Interference screw placement. **D.** Completed FHL transfer. **E.** A side-to-side tenodesis connecting the FHL muscle belly to the Achilles remnant is performed.

WOUND CLOSURE

- Layered closure is performed with a 2-0 absorbable monofilament in the paratenon, if any is left.
- 2-0 monocryl suture is used for subcutaneous fat.
- Skin is closed with 3-0 nylon suture.

PEARLS AND PITFALLS

Decision to augment	■ All studies must be evaluated thoroughly and the tendon inspected carefully at the time of surgery to ensure TA insertional integrity. Any question regarding stability of insertion should prompt consideration for augmentation. ■ Prep both feet into the field to permit evaluation of the uninjured side during the procedure.
Incision	■ Full-thickness flaps are essential for reliable healing. Avoid undermining the skin. Perform the débridement through the tendon. ■ A midline incision appears to have better angiosomal blood supply than either medial or lateral incisions.
FHL harvest	■ The muscle belly is easy to identify, but the tendon and tibial nerve are similar in appearance, consistency, and location as they course into the foot. ■ Follow the FHL from muscle to tendon and stay within the fibro-osseous tunnel under the sustentaculum. ■ Transect the tendon from medial to lateral up against the medial calcaneal wall.
Insertional débridement	■ Be aggressive in removal of injured TA tissue and inflamed bursa. ■ Be generous in resecting the calcaneal prominence.
Bone tunnel	■ Do not wallow out the tunnel while drilling. The calcaneus is predominantly cancellous, and this is easy to do.
Tensioning	■ Leaving a few TA fibers attached medially and laterally can demonstrate the patient's natural resting tension to help with this step.

POSTOPERATIVE CARE

- Immediately postoperatively, the foot is splinted in 15 to 20 degrees of equinus for 2 weeks.
- The patient is then placed in a walking boot with a 2-inch heel lift for another 2 weeks and allowed to gently touch down to the floor. (Noncompliant patients receive a walking cast.)
- At 1 month, patients are instructed on gentle active-assisted range of motion and permitted to progress to full weight bearing as tolerated.
- Over the next 2 months, the heel lift is gradually reduced in height until a painless plantigrade foot is achieved.
- Physical therapy is begun at 6 to 8 weeeks after surgery.

OUTCOMES

- Treatment of IAT by simple débridement is useful in younger patients, but more unpredictable as the extent of disease or patient age increases.[8]
- Several studies have shown substantial healing times after débridement alone, and even further compromise and poor predictability with evidence of intratendinous calcific debris.[14]
- The success of the procedure depends on how thoroughly débridement of involved tissue is performed; however, beyond 50% tendon compromise, the stability of the insertion comes into question.
- Augmentation with the FHL tendon has been shown to be technically reproducible and statistically successful.[6,12,13,15]
  - In one series, 20 patients undergoing this procedure for chronic Achilles tendon insufficiency revealed no postoperative reruptures, tendinopathy recurrences, or wound complications.[15]
  - Despite presumed and reported differences in calf circumference and push-off strength, these differences seem well tolerated and acceptable to patients when compared to the substantial amount of pain relief and restoration of function they receive.[15]
- The technique, as described, modifies classic descriptions in several ways:
  - Deviation from the classic two-incision technique,[6,12,13] thus reducing morbidity of another surgical site
  - Maintaining more native FHL bulk and function by preserving distal vincular tendon[11] attachments at the master knot of Henry. Theoretically, this will reduce the push-off strength morbidity associated with this procedure.
  - Decision regarding augmentation can be made after Achilles débridement determines insertional integrity, because the FHL harvest may be performed through the same incision as the débridement of the TA.
- Less tendon is needed because tendon transfer fixation is equal to or better than the side-to-side single-looped method because of interference screw fixation of the tendon directly to bone.[3,10]

COMPLICATIONS

- Wound complications
- Inadequate tendon débridement
- Inadequate bone resection
- Tibial nerve injury
- Fracture through bone tunnel
- Over- or under-tensioning the tendon transfer

REFERENCES

1. Chao W, Deland JT, Bates JE, Kenneally SM: Achilles tendon insertion: An anatomic in vitro study. Foot Ankle Intl 1997;18:81–84.
2. Clain MR, Baxter DE. Achilles tendonitis. Foot Ankle Intl 1992; 13:482–487.
3. Cohn JM, Sabonghy EP, Godlewski CA, et al. Tendon fixation in flexor hallucis longus transfer: A biomechanical study comparing a traditional technique versus bioabsorbable interference screw fixation. Tech Foot Ankle Surg 2005;4:4214–4221.
4. Fiamengo SA, Warren RF, Marshall JL, et al. Posterior heel pain associated with a calcaneal step and Achilles tendon calcification. Clin Orthop Relat Res 1982;167:203–211.
5. Gerken AP, McGarvey WC, Baxter DE. Insertional Achilles tendinitis. Foot Ankle Clin 1996;1:237–248.
6. Kann JN, Myerson MS. Surgical management of chronic ruptures of the Achilles tendon. Foot Ankle Clin 1997;2:535–545.
7. Marks RM. Achilles tendinopathy, peritendinitis, pantendinitis, and insertional disorders. Foot Ankle Clin 1999;4:789–810.
8. McGarvey WC, Palumbo RC, Baxter DE, et al. Insertional Achilles tendinosis: Surgical treatment through a central tendon splitting approach. Foot Ankle Intl 2002;23:19–25.
9. Myerson MS, McGarvey WC. Disorders of the Achilles tendon insertion and Achilles tendinitis. Instr Course Lect 1999;48:211–218.
10. Sabonghy EP, Wood RM, Ambrose, et al. Tendon transfer fixation: Comparing a tendon to tendon technique versus bioabsorbable interference-fit screw fixation. Foot Ankle Intl 2003;24:260–262.
11. Wapner KL, Hecht PJ, Shea JR, et al. Anatomy of second muscular layer of the foot: Consideration for tendon selection in transfer for Achilles and posterior tibial tendon reconstruction. Foot Ankle Intl 1994;15:420–423.
12. Wapner KL, Hecht PJ. Repair of chronic Achilles tendon rupture with flexor hallucis longus tendon transfer. Oper Tech Orthop 1994;4:132–137.
13. Wapner KL, Pavlock GS, Hecht PJ, et al. Repair of chronic Achilles tendon rupture with flexor hallucis longus tendon transfer. Foot Ankle 1993;14:443–449.
14. Watson AD, Anderson RB, Davis WH. Comparison of retrocalcaneal decompression for retrocalcaneal bursitis and insertional Achilles tendinosis with calcific spur. Foot Ankle Intl 2000; 21:638–642.
15. Wilcox DK, Bohay DR, Anderson JG. Treatment of chronic Achilles tendon disorders with FHL tendon transfer augmentation. Foot Ankle Intl 2000;21:1004–1010.

Chapter 118 Open Management of Achilles Tendinopathy

Nicola Maffulli and Umile Giuseppe Longo

DEFINITION

- Tendinopathy of the Achilles tendon involves clinical conditions in and around the tendon arising from overuse.[1]
- Tendinopathy of the Achilles tendon is common both in athletic and nonathletic individuals. It can affect several regions of the tendon.
- One particularly common site is the main body of the tendon, 2 to 4 cm from its insertion on the calcaneus.[2]

ANATOMY

- The two heads of gastrocnemius (medial and lateral) arise from the condyles of the femur, the fleshy part of the muscle extending to about the midcalf. As the muscle fibers descend they insert into a broad aponeurosis that contracts and receives the tendon of the soleus on its deep surface to form the Achilles tendon.[3]
- The Achilles tendon is the thickest and strongest tendon in the body. About 15 cm long, it originates in the midcalf and extends distally to insert into the posterior surface of the calcaneum. Throughout its length, it receives muscle fibers from the soleus on its anterior surface.[4]

PATHOGENESIS

- To date, the etiopathogenesis of Achilles tendinopathy remains unclear.
- Tendinopathy has been attributed to a variety of intrinsic and extrinsic factors.[6]
- It has been linked to overuse vascularity, dysfunction of the gastrocnemius-soleus, age, gender, body weight and height, endocrine or metabolic factors, deformity of the pes cavus, lateral instability of the ankle, the use of quinolone antibiotics, excessive movement of the hindfoot in the frontal plane, marked forefoot varus, changes in training pattern, poor technique, previous injuries, footwear, and environmental factors such as training on hard, slippery, or slanting surfaces.[1–6]
- Most of the above factors should be considered associative, not causative, evidence, and their role in the cause of the condition is therefore still debatable.[7]

NATURAL HISTORY

- Although Achilles tendinopathy has been extensively studied, there is a clear lack of properly conducted scientific research to clarify its cause, pathology, natural history, and optimal management.[8]
- The management of Achilles tendinopathy lacks evidence-based support, and tendinopathy sufferers are at risk of long-term morbidity with unpredictable clinical outcome.[9]
- Most patients respond to conservative measures, and the symptoms can be controlled, especially if the patients accept that a decreased level of activities may be necessary.[9]
- In 24% to 45.5% of patients with Achilles tendinopathy, conservative management is unsuccessful, and surgery is recommended after exhausting conservative methods of management, often tried for 3 to 6 months. However, longstanding Achilles tendinopathy is associated with poor postoperative results, with a greater rate of reoperation before reaching an acceptable outcome.[10,11]
- As the biology of tendinopathy is being clarified, more effective management regimens may come to light, improving the success rate of both conservative and operative management.[12]

PATIENT HISTORY AND PHYSICAL FINDINGS

- Patients typically present with pain located 2 to 6 cm proximal to the insertion of the tendon and felt after exercise.
- As the pathologic process progresses, pain may occur during exercise, and, when severe, may interfere with activities of daily living.
- Runners experience pain at the beginning and at the end of a training session, with a period of diminished discomfort in between.
- The foot and the heel should be inspected for malalignment, deformity, obvious asymmetry in the size of the tendon, localized thickening, a Haglund heel, and any previous scars.[11–13]
- The tendon should be palpated to detect tenderness, heat, thickening, nodularity, and crepitation.
- The "painful arc" sign helps to distinguish between lesions of the tendon and paratenon. In paratendinopathy, the area of maximum thickening and tenderness remains fixed in relation to the malleoli from full dorsiflexion to plantarflexion, whereas lesions within the tendon move with movement of the ankle.[14]

IMAGING AND OTHER DIAGNOSTIC STUDIES

- Plain soft tissue radiography is useful in diagnosing associated or incidental bony abnormalities.[9]
- Ultrasound is the primary imaging method, since it correlates well with the histopathologic findings despite being operator-dependent.[12]
- Ultrasound promptly identifies hypoechoic areas, which have been shown at surgery to consist of degenerated tissue, and increased thickness of the tendon.
- MRI studies should be performed only if the ultrasound scan remains unclear.
- MRI provides extensive information on the internal morphology of the tendon and the surrounding structures and is useful in evaluating the various stages of chronic degeneration and in differentiating between peritendinitis and tendinosis. Areas of mucoid degeneration are shown on MRI as a zone of high signal intensity on T1- and T2-weighted images.[13]

DIFFERENTIAL DIAGNOSIS

- Paratendinopathy of the Achilles tendon, acute or chronic rupture of the Achilles tendon, rerupture of the Achilles tendon, tear of the musculotendinous junction of the gastrocnemius-soleus and the Achilles tendon[12]

NONOPERATIVE MANAGEMENT

- There is weak evidence of a modest benefit of nonsteroidal anti-inflammatory drugs (NSAIDs) for the alleviation of acute symptoms.[5]
- Low-dose heparin, heel pads, topical laser therapy, and peritendinous steroid injection produced no difference in outcome when compared with no treatment.[8]
- Medications shown to be effective in randomized controlled trials include peritendinous injection of aprotinin, topical application of glyceryl trinitrate, and the use of ultrasound-guided sclerosing injections in the area of neovascularization.[9]
- Painful eccentric calf-muscle training can be an effective treatment for noninsertional Achilles tendinopathy.[13]
- Eccentric loading and low-energy shock-wave therapy show comparable results.[14]

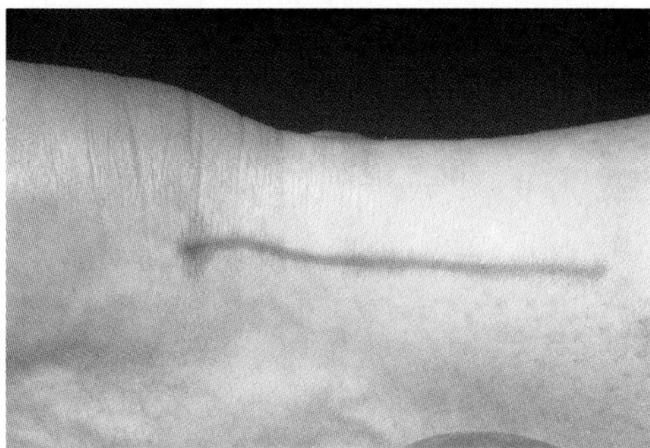

FIG 1 • Incision used for open surgery: it lies just posterior to the medial border of the Achilles tendon. It avoids the sural nerve and the short saphenous vein, and the scar is away from the shoe counter.

SURGICAL MANAGEMENT

- Conservative management is unsuccessful in 24% to 45.5% of patients with tendinopathy of tendo Achilles.[14]
- Surgery is recommended after at least 6 months of conservative management.[11]
- The objective is to excise fibrotic adhesions, remove degenerated nodules, and make multiple longitudinal incisions in the tendon to detect intratendinous lesions and to restore vascularity, possibly stimulating the remaining viable cells to initiate a response in the cell matrix and healing.[14]
- The defect can be sutured in a side-to-side fashion or left open.
- Reconstruction procedures may be required if large lesions are excised.

Preoperative Planning

- Preoperative imaging studies can guide the surgeon in the placement of the incision and in incising the tendon sharply in line with the tendon fiber bundles.

Positioning

- Under locoregional anesthesia, the patient is placed prone with the ankles clear of the operating table.
- The prone position allows excellent access to the affected area.
- Alternatively, the patient can be positioned supine with a sandbag under the opposite hip and the affected leg positioned in a figure 4 position.
- A tourniquet is applied to the limb to be operated on. The limb is exsanguinated, and the tourniquet is inflated to 250 mm Hg.[4]

Approach

- The incision is made on the medial side of the tendon to avoid injury to the sural nerve and short saphenous vein (**FIG 1**).
- A straight posterior incision may also be more bothersome with the edge of the heel counter pressing directly on the incision.
- Maintaining thick skin flaps is vital to reduce the incidence of wound breakdown.[10]

TECHNIQUES

- Expose the paratenon and the Achilles tendon (TECH FIG 1).
- Identify and incise the paratenon (TECH FIG 2).
- In patients with evidence of coexisting paratendinopathy, the scarred and thickened tissue is generally excised.
- Based on preoperative imaging studies, the tendon is incised sharply in line with the tendon fiber bundles (TECH FIG 3).
- The tendinopathic tissue can be identified as it generally has lost its shiny appearance and it frequently contains disorganized fiber bundles that have more of a "crabmeat" appearance (TECH FIG 4).
- Sharply excise this tissue (TECH FIG 5).
- The remaining gap can be repaired using a side-to-side repair, but we leave it unsutured (TECH FIG 6).

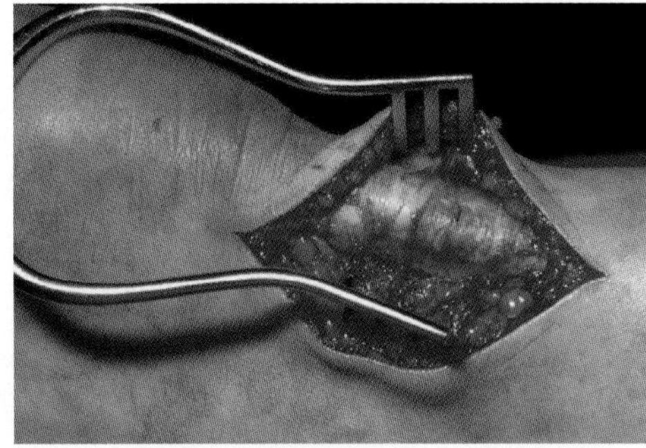

TECH FIG 1 • Paratenon and the Achilles tendon exposed.

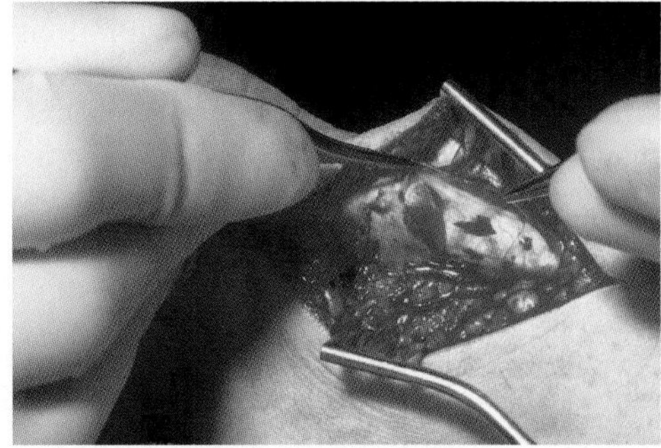

TECH FIG 2 • The paratenon is excised.

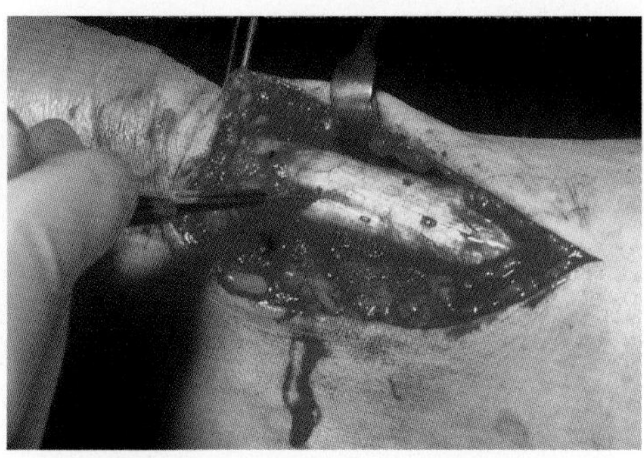

TECH FIG 3 • Longitudinal tenotomy along the tendon fibers. Note that as the tendon fibers rotate 90 degrees, the longitudinal tenotomy has to follow them.

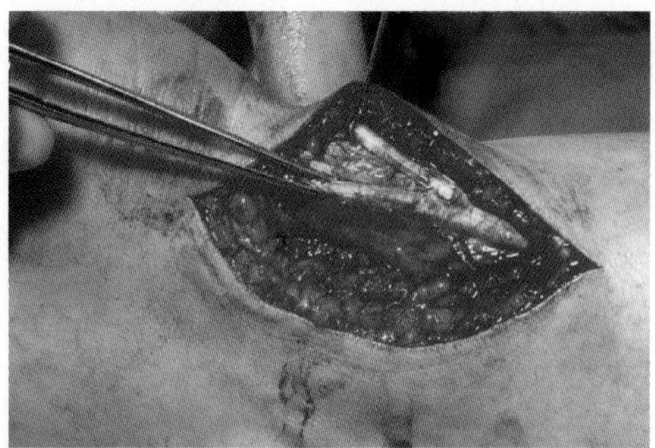

TECH FIG 4 • The macroscopic appearance of the tendinopathic area is visualized.

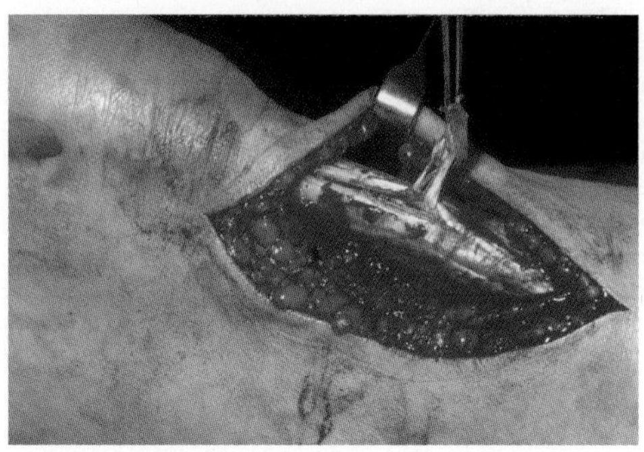

TECH FIG 5 • The tendinopathic tissue is excised.

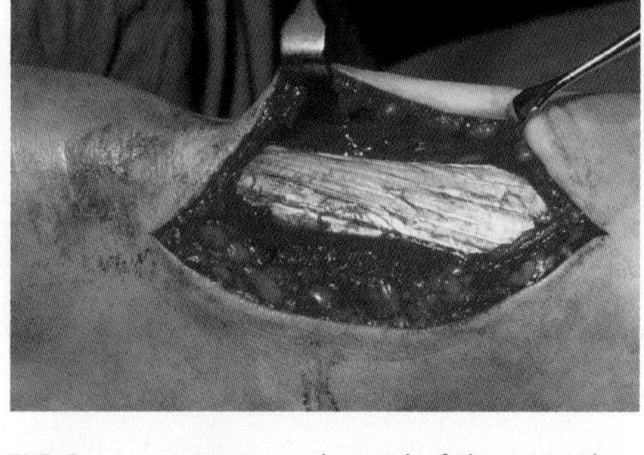

TECH FIG 6 • Appearance at the end of the procedure.

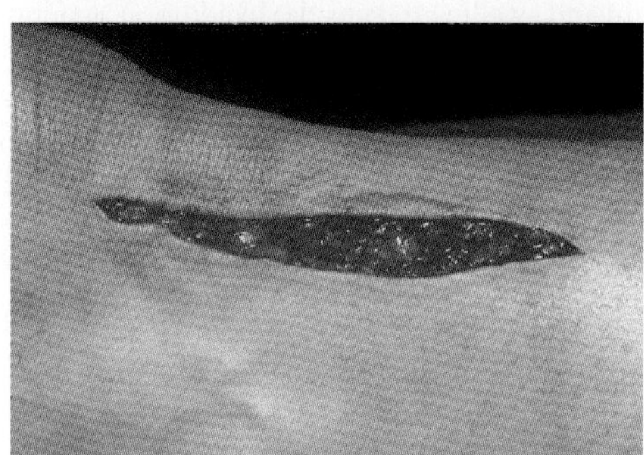

TECH FIG 7 • The skin wound after suture of the deep tissues.

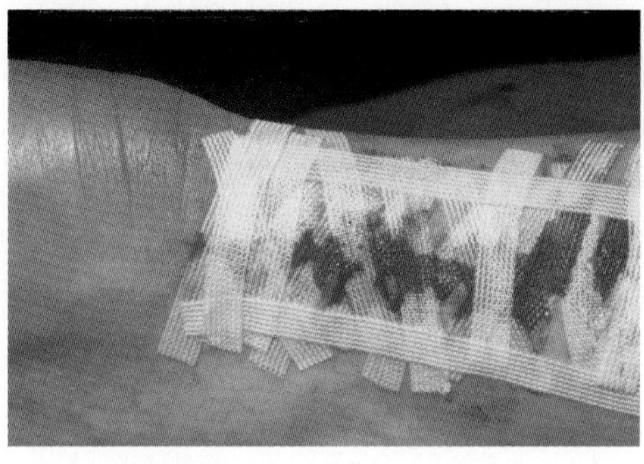

TECH FIG 8 • Steri-Strips are applied to the surgical wound before a routine compressive bandage. The limb is then immobilized in a below-knee synthetic weight-bearing cast with the foot plantigrade.

- Suture the subcutaneous tissues with absorbable material (**TECH FIG 7**).
- The skin edges are juxtaposed with Steri-Strips (**TECH FIG 8**) and then a routine compressive bandage. The limb is immobilized in a below-knee synthetic weight-bearing cast with the foot plantigrade.
- If significant loss of tendon tissue occurs during the débridement, consider a tendon augmentation or transfer.
- A tendon turndown flap has been described for this purpose. With a turndown procedure, one or two strips of tendon tissue from the gastrocnemius tendon are dissected out proximally while leaving the strip attached to the main tendon distally. It is then flipped 180 degrees and sewn in to cover and bridge the weakened defect in the distal tendon.
- A plantaris weave has also been reported for this purpose. The plantaris tendon can be found on the medial edge of the Achilles tendon. It can be traced proximally as far as possible and detached as close as possible to the muscle tendon junction to gain as much length as possible.
- It can be left attached distally to the calcaneus, looped and woven through the proximal Achilles tendon, and sewn back onto the distal part to the tendon.
- Alternatively, the plantaris can be detached distally as well and used as a free graft.
- The tourniquet is deflated and the time recorded.[7]

PEARLS AND PITFALLS

Diagnosis	▪ Diagnosis is usually made on a clinical basis, including a careful history and physical examination. ▪ Ultrasound can identify hypoechoic areas, which have been shown at surgery to consist of degenerated tissue, and increased thickness of the tendon. ▪ MRI studies should be performed only if the ultrasound scan remains unclear.
Positioning	▪ Prone position, with thigh tourniquet
Incision	▪ An incision placed medial and anterior to the medial border of the Achilles tendon reduces the likelihood of injury to the sural nerve and short saphenous vein.

POSTOPERATIVE CARE

▪ A period of initial splinting and crutch walking is generally used to allow pain and swelling to subside. In addition, wound healing complications are difficult to manage and an initial period of immobilization may promote skin healing.

▪ After 14 days, the wound is inspected and motion exercises are initiated. The patient is encouraged to start daily active and passive ankle range-of-motion exercises. The use of a removable walker boot can be helpful during this phase. Weight bearing is not limited according to the degree of débridement needed at surgery, and early weight bearing is encouraged. However, extensive débridements and tendon transfers may require protected weight bearing for 4 to 6 weeks postoperatively.

▪ After 6 to 8 weeks of mostly range-of-motion and light resistive exercises, initial tendon healing will have been completed. More intensive strengthening exercises are started, gradually progressing to plyometrics and eventually running and jumping.[13,14]

OUTCOMES

▪ The surgical procedure is commonly successful, but patients should be informed of the potential failure of the procedure, risk of wound complications, and at times prolonged recovery time.[6]

▪ Rehabilitation is focused on early motion and avoidance of overloading the tendon in the initial healing phase.

COMPLICATIONS

- Wound healing problems
- Infection
- Sural nerve injury
- Rupture of Achilles tendon
- Deep vein thrombosis

REFERENCES

1. Maffulli N. Re: Etiologic factors associated with symptomatic Achilles tendinopathy. Foot Ankle Int 2007;28:660–661.
2. Maffulli N, Kader D. Tendinopathy of tendo achilles. J Bone Joint Surg Br 2002;84B:1–8.
3. Maffulli N, Kenward MG, Testa V, et al. Clinical diagnosis of Achilles tendinopathy with tendinosis. Clin J Sport Med 2003;13: 11–15.
4. Maffulli N, Khan KM, Puddu G. Overuse tendon conditions: time to change a confusing terminology. Arthroscopy 1998;14:840–843.
5. Maffulli N, Reaper J, Ewen SW, et al. Chondral metaplasia in calcific insertional tendinopathy of the Achilles tendon. Clin J Sport Med 2006;16:329–334.
6. Maffulli N, Sharma P, Luscombe KL. Achilles tendinopathy: aetiology and management. J R Soc Med 2004;97:472–476.
7. Maffulli N, Testa V, Capasso G, et al. Results of percutaneous longitudinal tenotomy for Achilles tendinopathy in middle- and long-distance runners. Am J Sports Med 1997;25:835–840.
8. Maffulli N, Testa V, Capasso G, et al. Similar histopathological picture in males with Achilles and patellar tendinopathy. Med Sci Sports Exerc 2004;36:1470–1475.
9. Maffulli N, Testa V, Capasso G, et al. Surgery for chronic Achilles tendinopathy yields worse results in nonathletic patients. Clin J Sport Med 2006;16:123–128.
10. Maffulli N, Testa V, Capasso G, et al. Calcific insertional Achilles tendinopathy: reattachment with bone anchors. Am J Sports Med 2004;32:174–182.
11. Maffulli N, Wong J. Rupture of the Achilles and patellar tendons. Clin Sports Med 2003;22:761–776.
12. Maffulli N, Wong J, Almekinders LC. Types and epidemiology of tendinopathy. Clin Sports Med 2003;22:675–692.
13. Rompe JD, Nafe B, Furia JP, et al. Eccentric loading, shock-wave treatment, or a wait-and-see policy for tendinopathy of the main body of tendo Achilles: a randomized controlled trial. Am J Sports Med 2007;35:374–383.
14. Sayana MK, Maffulli N. Eccentric calf muscle training in non-athletic patients with Achilles tendinopathy. J Sci Med Sport 2007;10:52–58.

Chapter 119

Flexor Hallucis Longus Transfer for Achilles Tendinosis

Bryan D. Den Hartog

DEFINITION

- Insertional and midsubstance Achilles tendinosis is a painful degenerative process that arises due to mechanical and vascular factors and affects the paratenon and collagen fibers.
- It is most commonly seen in patients in their mid-40s and older.

ANATOMY

- The Achilles tendon, the largest tendon in the body, connects the gastroc–soleus complex to the calcaneus (**FIG 1**).
- It is covered by a paratenon without a definite tendon sheath.
- The blood supply of the tendon arises distally from calcaneal arterioles and proximally from intramuscular branches. There is a relatively hypovascular, or watershed, area 2 to 4 cm proximal to the tendon insertion.

PATHOGENESIS

- Mechanical and vascular factors contribute to the development of tendinosis. The process begins with mechanical pressure on the insertion of the Achilles tendon from internal factors, a Haglund's deformity, or external factors, such as a firm heel counter. Retrocalcaneal bursitis develops initially without Achilles tendon involvement. Increasing prominence of the posterolateral calcaneal tuberosity or hindfoot malalignment (ie, varus heel), can cause tendon collagen fiber injury and further inflammation of the retrocalcaneal bursa.
- Progressive thickening of the retrocalcaneal bursa and peritendinous tissue increases mechanical pressure on the tendon, impeding blood flow and hampering the normal repair process, leading to a thickened, degenerative tendon.

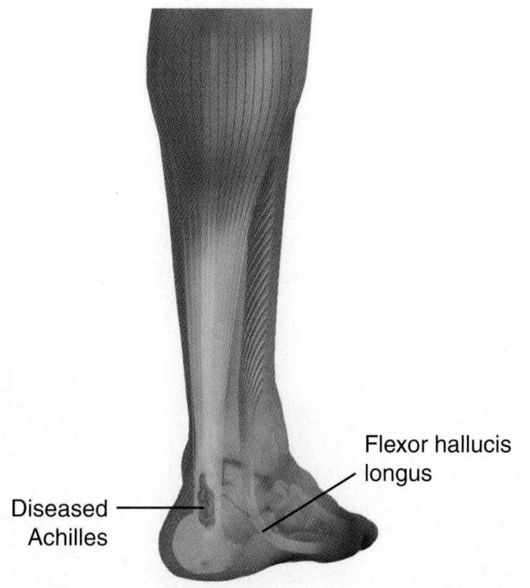

FIG 1 • The Achilles tendon and its relationship to the flexor hallucis longus tendon.

- With dysvascular changes associated with aging, the tendon becomes increasingly thick and painful. Radiographs at this point may show a spur or calcification at the Achilles insertion.

NATURAL HISTORY

- The natural history of the pathologic process most likely is a continuum that begins with retrocalcaneal bursitis and ends in chronic Achilles tendinosis.
- Patient activity becomes more restricted due to increased pain and weakness.
- Age-dependent changes in collagen quality and decreased vascularity contribute to the development of tendinosis.
- As the degenerative process becomes chronic, the tendon becomes mechanically deficient and more susceptible to rupture.
- Symptoms become unremitting as the disease progresses.

PATIENT HISTORY AND PHYSICAL FINDINGS

- Achilles tendinosis causes pain and swelling of the diseased segment of tendon.
- Pain increases with physical activity and with direct pressure on the affected tendon.
- Patients with seronegative arthropathies, spondyloarthropathies, hypercholesterolemia, sarcoidosis, and renal transplant have an increased incidence of Achilles tendinopathy.
- The patient should be assessed for hyperpronation or heel varus deformities, which can cause eccentric Achilles tendon loading. If either is present, an orthosis to keep the hindfoot in neutral may be necessary.
- Ankle dorsiflexion is measured with the knee flexed and extended to assess for gastrocnemius or Achilles tendon tightness. If excessive tightness is present, a gastrocnemius recession should be considered along with the flexor hallucis longus (FHL) transfer.
- With the patient prone on the examining table, the Achilles tendon is palpated to localize the area of thickening and tenderness (either insertional or noninsertional). Assess the size of the calcaneal tuberosity; if it is enlarged, excision of this prominence should be considered to reduce mechanical pressure on the diseased Achilles tendon.

IMAGING AND OTHER DIAGNOSTIC STUDIES

- Radiographs are useful in evaluating the extent of tendon calcification and presence of a Haglund's deformity (**FIG 2**).
- Although MRI scanning is not essential for preoperative planning, it can be beneficial in estimating the amount of degenerative tendon to be excised (**FIG 3**).

DIFFERENTIAL DIAGNOSIS

- Haglund's deformity
- Os trigonum

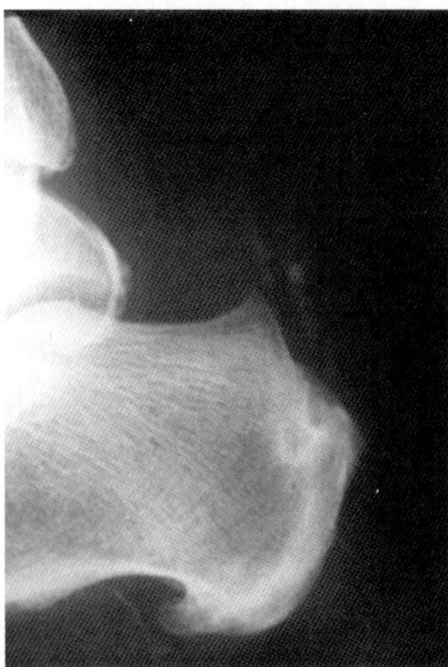

FIG 2 • Lateral radiograph of the heel revealing a prominent calcaneal tuberosity and calcification of the Achilles insertion.

- Retrocalcaneal bursitis
- Peritendinitis
- Seronegative spondyloarthropathy
- Insertional tendinopathy
- Achilles tendinosis

NONOPERATIVE MANAGEMENT

- Nonsurgical treatment of insertional or noninsertional Achilles tendinosis includes rest, immobilization, and rehabilitation.
- Immobilization can include casting, a cast brace, and a custom molded ankle foot orthosis (AFO).
- Structural abnormalities such as heel varus are addressed with wedges or orthotics, or both.
- Training regimens are modified to reduce stress on the affected tendon.
- Physical therapy for heavy-load eccentric strengthening exercises has been found to be effective for Achilles tendinopathy and may be superior to conventional treatment regimens and comparable to open débridement of the tendon.

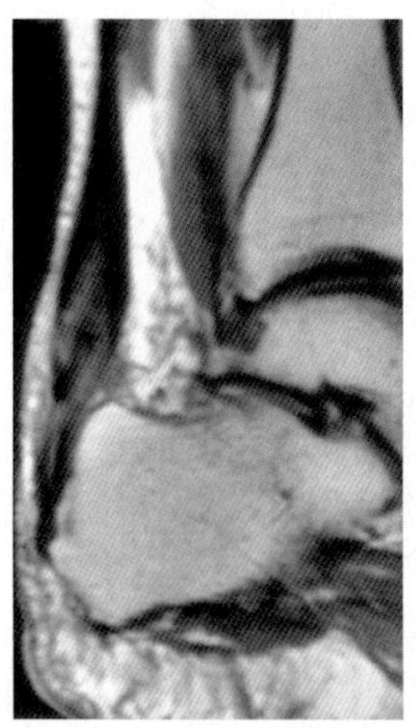

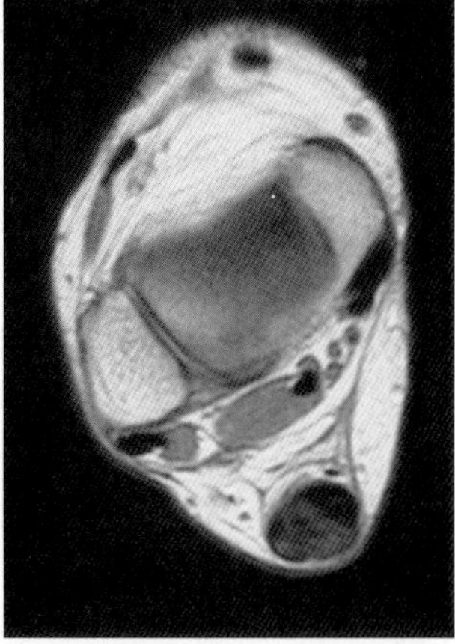

FIG 3 • **A.** This sagittal MRI scan demonstrates increased signal in the Achilles insertion. **B.** This axial MRI scan of the Achilles insertion reveals diseased fibers.

SURGICAL MANAGEMENT

- Surgery is performed only on those patients who have intractable pain and impaired function or those who have failed previous tendon débridement or Haglund's resection alone. Most people in this patient group have a chronic Achilles tendon deficiency, and are sedentary, overweight, and have radiographic or MRI evidence of a thickened, calcific Achilles insertion.
- Most treatments that have been described focus on removing mechanical pressure from the diseased tendon (eg, excising the posterosuperior calcaneal tuberosity), débridement of the diseased tendon, or augmentation of the remaining, débrided tendon (ie, FHL, peroneus brevis, plantaris).
- The bulk of surgical treatment is discussed in the following sections and in the Techniques section.

Preoperative Planning

- The extent and location of diseased tendon must be identified. The area of tendon degeneration most often is the distal 2 to 4 cm. The degeneration also may be isolated at the midsubstance.
- The patient must understand preoperatively that the time to maximum improvement could be prolonged (average 8.2 months).
- If the surgeon wants to loop the transferred FHL through the calcaneus at the time of the transfer and more tendon length consequently will be needed, the FHL should be harvested from the midmost at Henry's knot and pulled out the posterior incision.

Positioning

- The patient is placed prone on the operating table with a soft bump anterior to the ankle (**FIG 4**).

Approach

- Various incisions have been used to approach the diseased tendon.
  - Incisions that have been recommended include central splitting, medial and/or lateral longitudinal pretentious, or medial with a transverse L-shaped extension distally.
  - All of these incisions can be used successfully to expose and débride diseased tissue, but if augmentation of the Achilles tendon is anticipated, a medial incision will give the best access to the FHL.
- Whatever incision is selected, it should be done sharply through the subcutaneous tissue to the paratenon, taking care not to dissect horizontally, thus reducing the risk of vascular compromise of the soft tissues overlying the tendon.

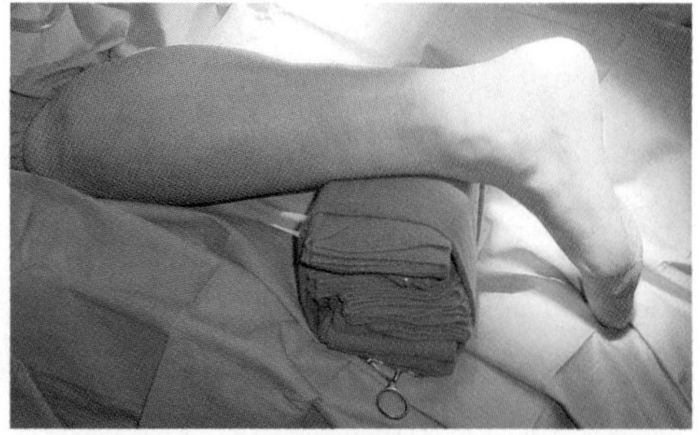

FIG 4 • The patient is positioned prone on the operating table.

FLEXOR HALLUCIS LONGUS TRANSFER OR AUGMENTATION FOR ACHILLES TENDINOSIS

- A 10-cm posteromedial incision is made starting near the junction of the proximal and middle thirds of the Achilles tendon and stopping distally at the tendinous insertion into the calcaneal tuberosity. The incision is made sharply through the subcutaneous tissue to the paratenon, taking care not to dissect horizontally, thereby reducing the risk of vascular compromise of the soft tissue overlying the Achilles tendon. An L-shaped extension of the incision distally is performed if extensive débridement of the Achilles tendon is anticipated and better exposure of the lateral tendon insertion is needed (**TECH FIG 1**).
- The substance of the tendon is carefully inspected. Any amorphous (codfish-flesh appearing), calcified, or ossified tissue of the tendon is excised, leaving only relatively healthy, normally striated tissue. Usually, more than 50% of the cross-section is removed. The degenerative, calcified area of tendon is best excised by removing a wedge-shaped piece of tissue from the insertion of the Achilles tendon (**TECH FIG 2**).
- In all cases, a partial calcaneal ostectomy is performed at the superoposterior aspect to decompress the Achilles tendon insertion (**TECH FIG 3**). This also improves exposure to the anterior aspect of the tendon, aiding in tendon inspection and débridement.
- With the degenerative tissue removed, the triangular fat pad anterior to the Achilles tendon is excised, exposing the deep posterior fascia (**TECH FIG 4**).
- The fascia overlying the posterior compartment of the leg is incised longitudinally to the proximal extent of the FHL muscle body. The FHL tendon is identified (**TECH FIG 5**). The flexor retinaculum is released along the medial aspect of the hindfoot to further expose the FHL.
- Gentle retraction of the neurovascular bundle with a blunt retractor allows safe visualization of the tendon distally (**TECH FIG 6**). The FHL is transected as far distal as possible with the ankle and hallux in maximum plantarflexion. Transection of the tendon is done medial to lateral to avoid accidental injury to the neurovascular structures.
- The tendon is brought posteriorly and positioned at the calcaneus between the two limbs of the remaining débrided Achilles insertion (**TECH FIG 7**). If more length of the FHL is needed, the origin of the more distal muscle fibers of the FHL can be detached bluntly from the fibula and interosseous ligament to increase the excursion of the FHL. Proper tensioning of the FHL transfer is determined by dorsiflexing the ankle to place the Achilles tendon at maximal stretch. With the FHL appropriately tensioned, any excess length of the tendon is removed to allow optimal pull of the transferred tendon to the calcaneus.

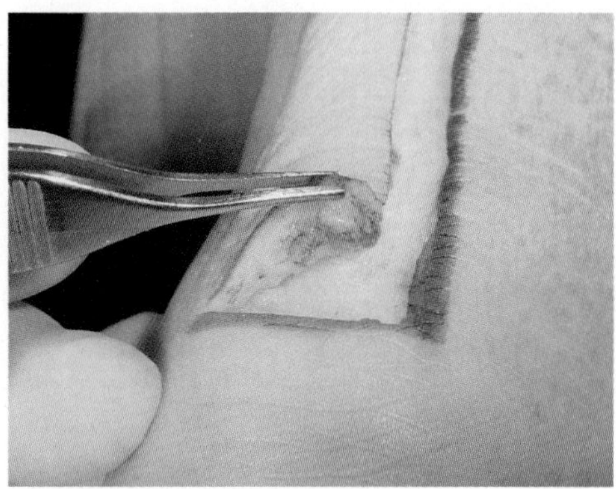

TECH FIG 1 • Full-thickness, L-shaped incision to increase exposure of the diseased Achilles tendon.

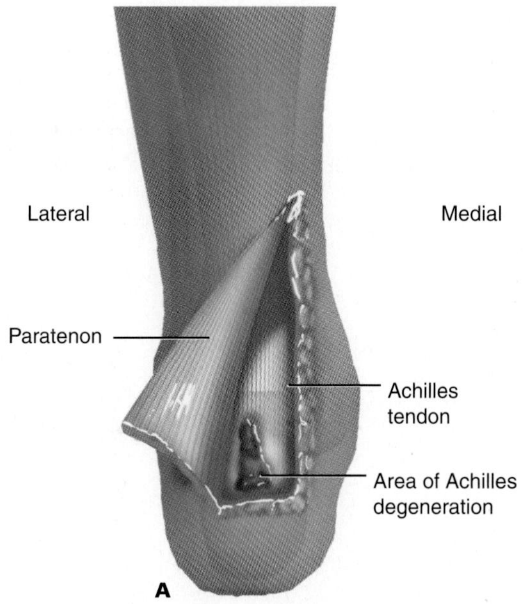

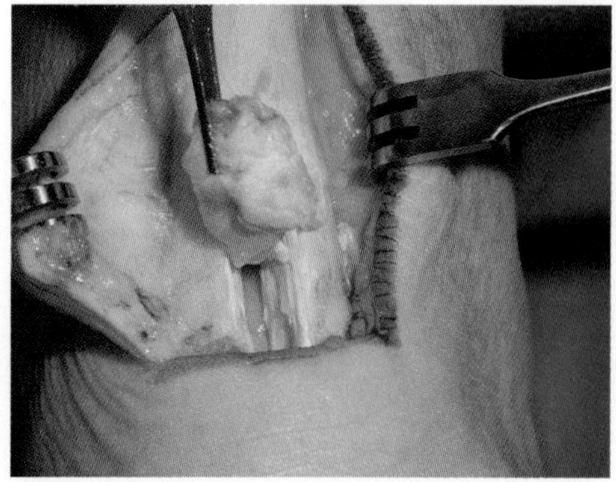

TECH FIG 2 • **A.** Drawing of typical location of diseased Achilles. **B.** Area of wedge resection of the Achilles insertion in preparation for repair.

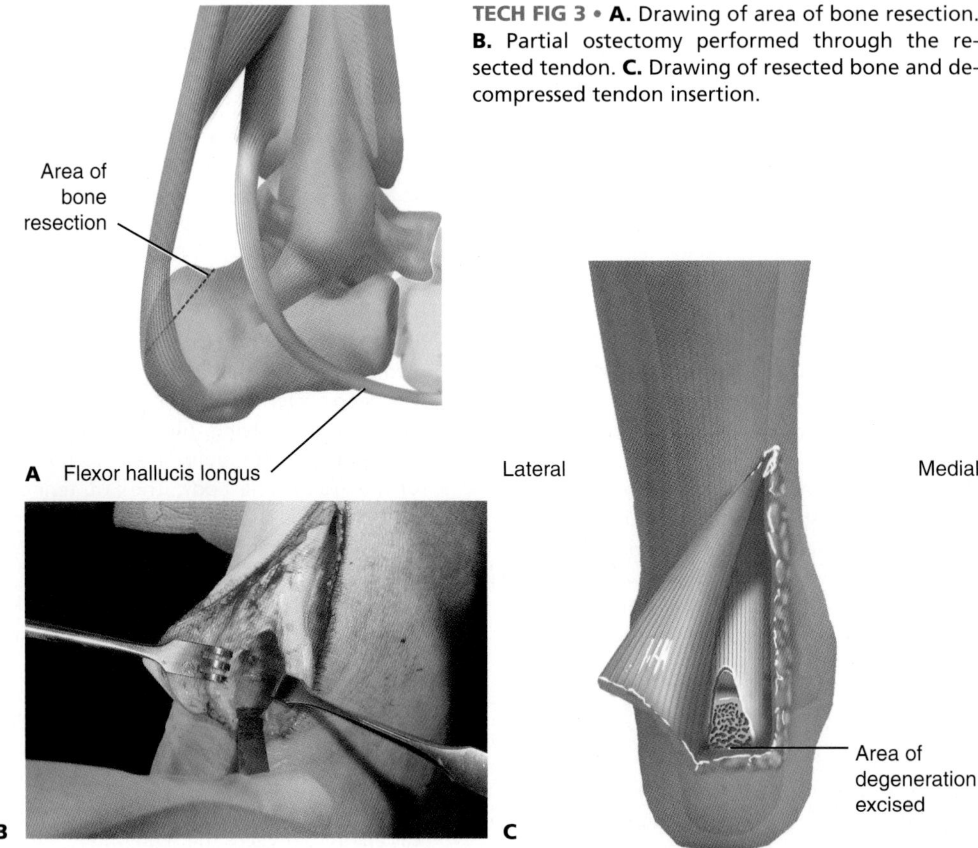

TECH FIG 3 • A. Drawing of area of bone resection. **B.** Partial ostectomy performed through the resected tendon. **C.** Drawing of resected bone and decompressed tendon insertion.

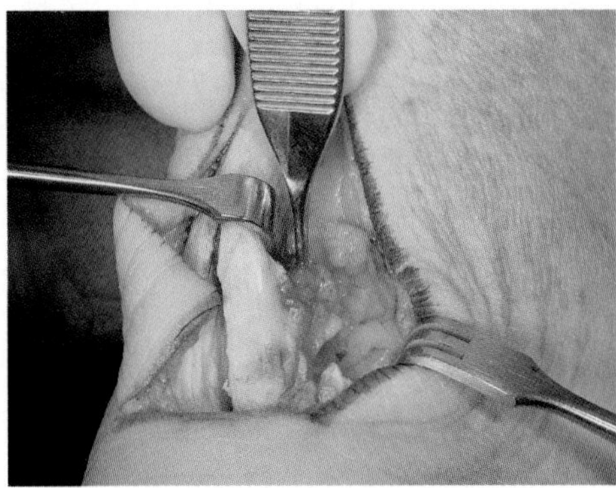

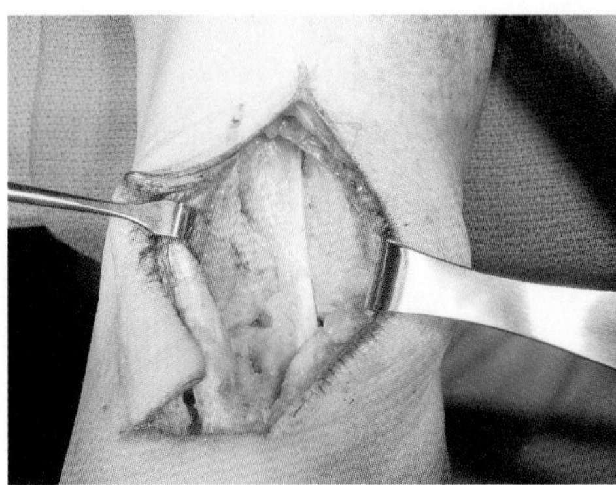

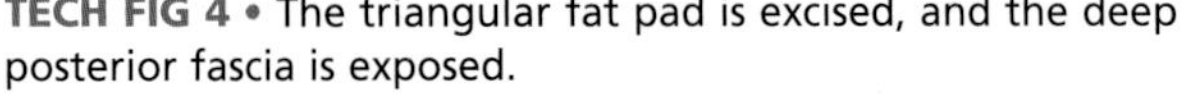

TECH FIG 4 • The triangular fat pad is excised, and the deep posterior fascia is exposed.

TECH FIG 5 • The flexor hallucis longus (FHL) tendon is exposed after the deep fascia is split.

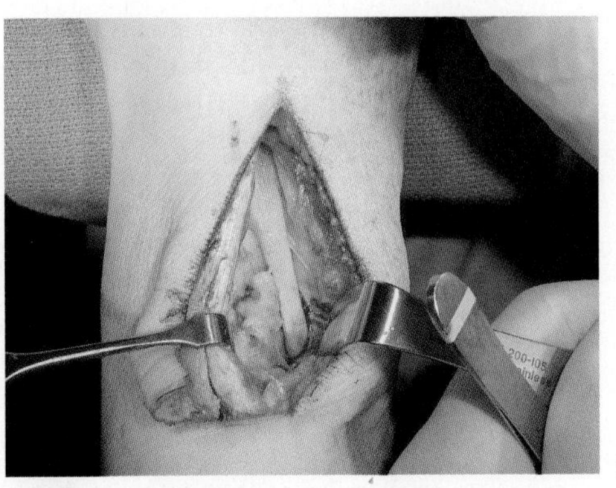

A

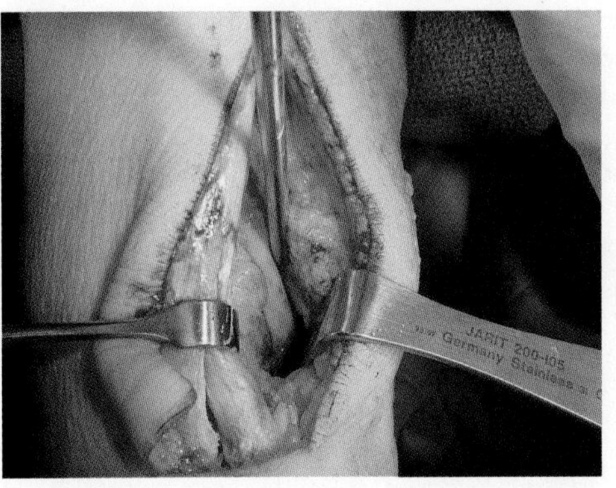

B

TECH FIG 6 • A. The flexor retinaculum is split to expose the FHL distally. **B.** The neurovascular bundle is protected with a deep retractor.

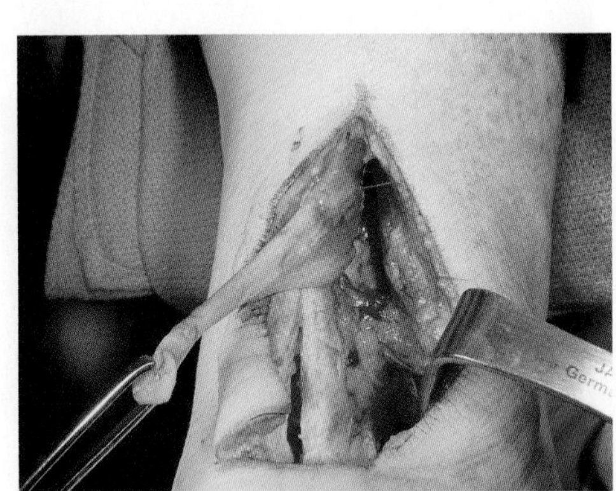

A

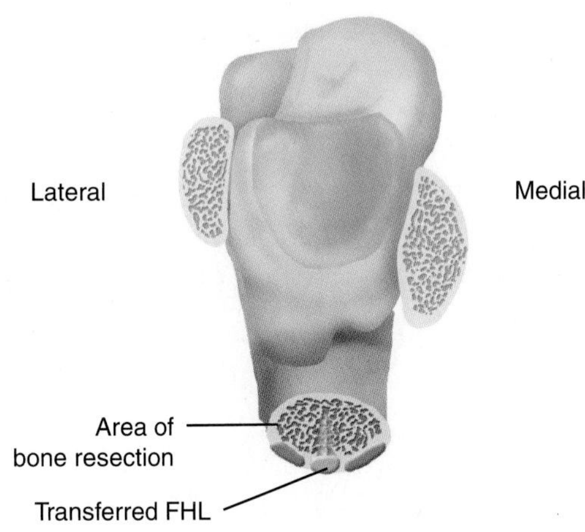

B

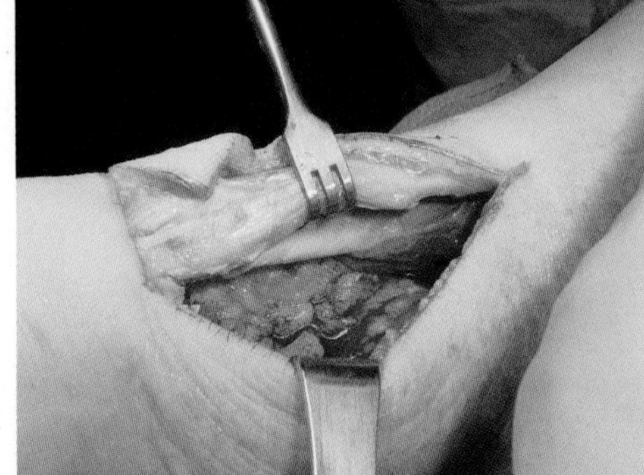

C

TECH FIG 7 • A. The FHL is pulled posteriorly and checked for length. **B.** Drawing of FHL placement between the limbs of the remaining Achilles tendon. **C.** The FHL is tightly positioned against the Achilles tendon.

- The transferred tendon is held with a two-strand suture anchor (**TECH FIG 8**). The first strand of suture is used in modified Kessler fashion to secure the FHL to the calcaneus at the proper tension (**TECH FIG 9**). The second strand is used as a whipstitch to add pullout strength (**TECH FIG 10**). The FHL tendon is sutured to the Achilles tendon in side-to-side fashion with nonabsorbable braided suture (**TECH FIG 11**).
- A careful, layered closure of the paratenon, subcutaneous tissue, and skin is performed.

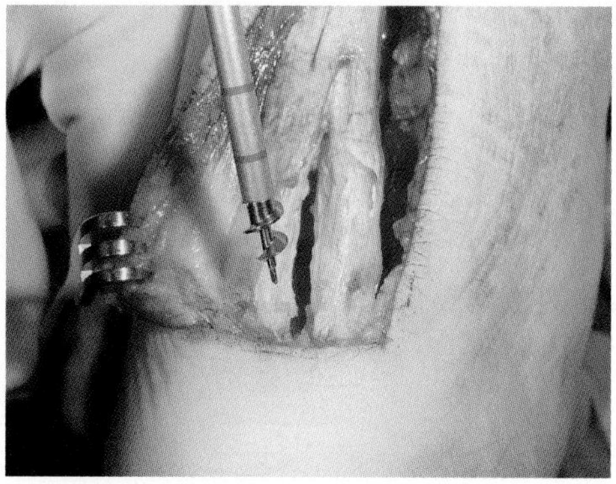

TECH FIG 8 • Two-strand suture anchor.

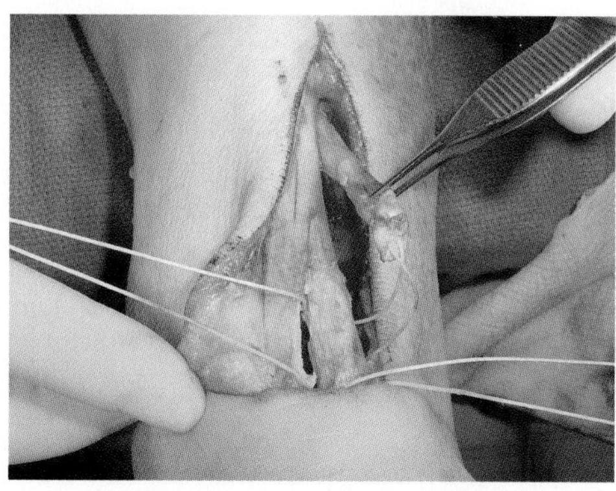

TECH FIG 9 • A positioning stitch is applied to the tendon, and appropriate FHL tension is determined.

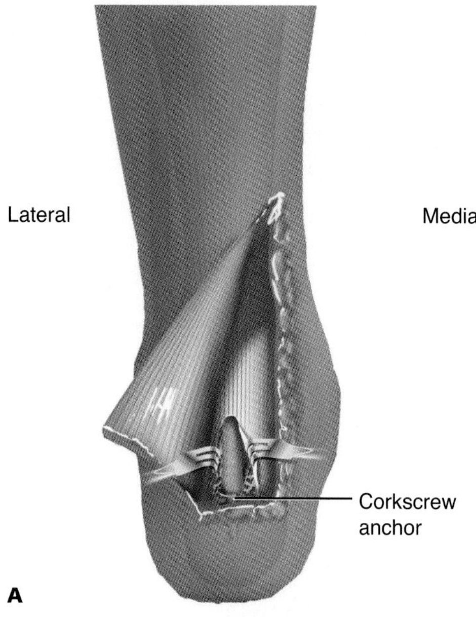

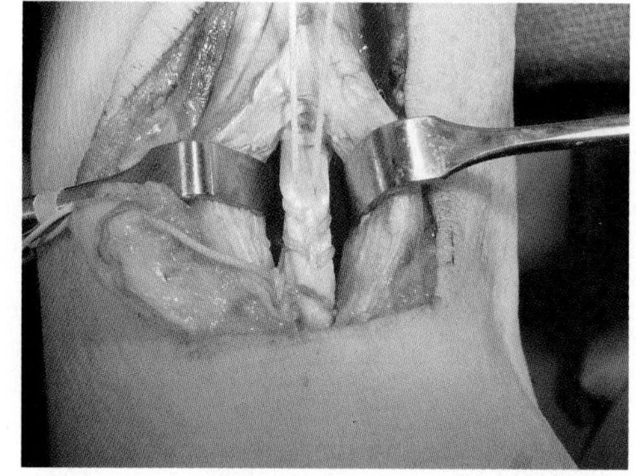

TECH FIG 10 • **A.** Drawing of the anchored tendon. **B.** The FHL is secured with whipstitch.

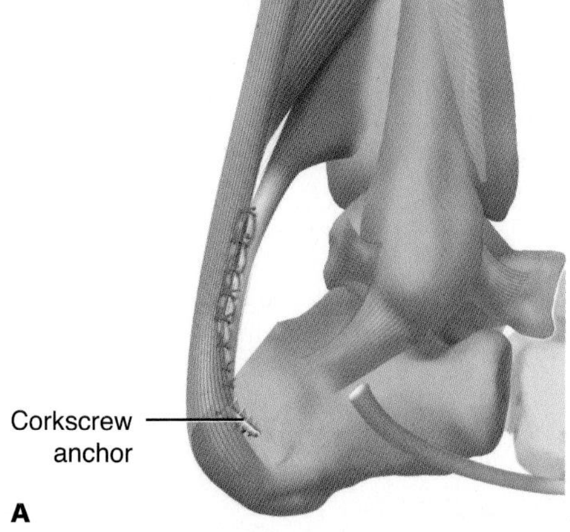

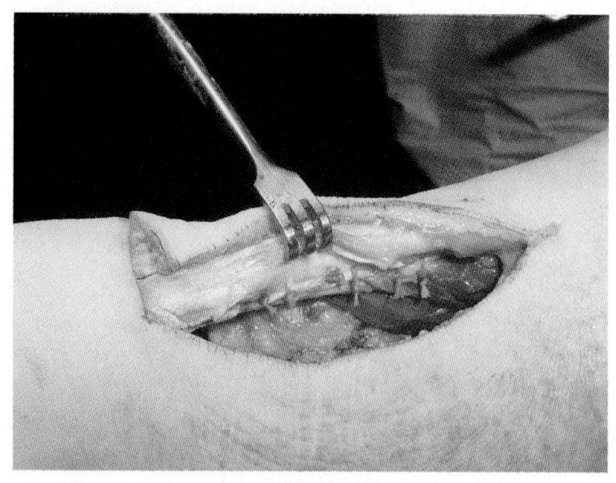

TECH FIG 11 • **A.** The FHL is sutured to the Achilles tendon in side-to-side fashion. **B.** Photograph of the FHL sutured to the Achilles tendon.

PEARLS AND PITFALLS

Skin incision	▪ Care must be taken to make a full-thickness incision from the skin to the paratenon without undermining the soft tissue layer, to avoid skin slough.
Achilles tendon débridement	▪ Make sure to excise all diseased Achilles tendon to reduce the risk of persistent pain postoperatively.
FHL harvest	▪ Protect the neurovascular bundle with a deep retractor through the medial incision while exposing the FHL for transfer to avoid injuring adjacent vital structures. ▪ Cut the tendon with a no.15 blade medial to lateral to avoid injury to the neurovascular bundle. ▪ Maximally plantarflex the ankle and great toe, and pull on the FHL before cutting the tendon to obtain adequate length of the transferred tendon.
FHL transfer	▪ Dorsiflex the foot while placing the FHL transfer at maximal stretch to determine the proper insertion point and tensioning of the transferred tendon. ▪ Make sure there is good apposition between the FHL and remaining Achilles tendon by excising all interposed fat and using nonabsorbable sutures to hold the repair.
Skin closure	▪ Perform careful, separate layer closure, starting with the paratenon, to avoid excessive scarring.

POSTOPERATIVE CARE

- A compressive dressing with splints is applied in the operating room with the ankle in neutral position. The initial dressing is kept in place for 10 to 14 days. At that time, if the incision is well healed and the reconstruction was deemed stable at the time of operation, the patient is placed in a controlled ankle motion (CAM)-soled walker, and weight bearing as tolerated is allowed.
- If more than 75% of the Achilles tendon has been débrided, a weight-bearing cast is applied for 4 weeks to provide extra support for the healing tendon.
- Range-of-motion and strengthening exercises are begun 6 to 8 weeks postoperatively if clinical improvement (decreased pain and swelling) is evident.
- The patient is weaned from the CAM-soled walker at 10 to 12 weeks as symptoms of pain and swelling allow.

OUTCOMES

- Hansen[5] reported a proximal FHL transfer technique with good or excellent results. Emphasis was placed on thoroughly excising the diseased tendon.
- Wapner[11] reported good to excellent pain relief and improved function in seven patients with Achilles débridement and FHL transfer harvested from the midfoot for tendinosis.
- Wilcox et al,[13] using the American Orthopaedic Foot and Ankle Society (AOFAS) hindfoot score and the SF-36 Health Survey, reported overall good results with FHL transfer in 20 patients with recalcitrant Achilles tendinosis but found that patient function may not improve.
- Den Hartog[3] reported significant improvement in the postoperative AOFAS hindfoot scores in 29 patients who underwent FHL transfer for severe Achilles tendinosis.

COMPLICATIONS

- Rerupture of the augmented Achilles
- Wound necrosis secondary to undermining of soft tissues
- Infection
- Scarring secondary to inadequate repair of the paratenon
- Persistent pain and swelling

REFERENCES

1. Carr AJ, Norris SH. The blood supply of the calcaneal tendon. J Bone Joint Surg Br 1989;71B:100–110.
2. Coull R, Flavin R, Stephens MM. Flexor hallucis longus tendon transfer: Evaluation of postoperative morbidity. Foot Ankle Int 2003;24:931–934.
3. Den Hartog BD. Use of proximal flexor hallucis longus transfer in severe calcific Achilles‘ tendinosis. Tech Foot Ankle Surg 2002;1:145–150.
4. Den Hartog BD. Flexor hallucis longus transfer for chronic Achilles tendinosis. Foot Ankle Int 2003;24:233–237.
5. Hansen ST Trauma to the heel cord. In Jahss MH, ed. Disorders of the Foot and Ankle, ed 2. Philadelphia: WB Saunders, 1991:2357.
6. Mann RA, Holmes GB, Seale KS, et al. Chronic rupture of the Achilles: A new technique of repair. J Bone Joint Surg Am 1991;73A:214–219.
7. McGarvey WC, Palumbo RC, Baxter DE, et al. Insertional Achilles tendinosis: Surgical treatment through a central tendon splitting approach. Foot Ankle Int 2002;23:19–25.
8. Pudda G, Ippolito E, Postacchini F. A classification of Achilles tendon disease. Am J Sports Med 1976;4:145.
9. Schepsis AA, Leach RE. Surgical management of Achilles tendonitis. Am J Sports Med 1987;15:308–315.
10. Turco VJ, Spinella AJ. Achilles tendon rupture—peroneus brevis transfer. Foot Ankle 1987;7:253–259.
11. Wapner KL, Pavlock GS, Hecht PJ, et al. Repair of chronic Achilles tendon rupture with flexor hallucis longus tendon transfer. Foot Ankle 1993;14:443–449.
12. Watson AD, Anderson RB, Davis HW. Comparison of results of retrocalcaneal decompression for retrocalcaneal bursitis and insertional Achilles tendinosis with calcific spur. Foot Ankle Int 2000;21:638–642.
13. Wilcox DK, Bohay DR, Anderson JG. Treatment of chronic Achilles tendon disorders with flexor hallucis longus transfer/augmentation. Foot Ankle Int 2000;21:1004–1010.

Chapter 120

Proximal Mini-Invasive Grafting of Plantaris Tendon

Geert I. Pagenstert and Beat Hintermann

DEFINITION

- The plantaris tendon is an ideal source for soft tissue augmentation for ligament reconstructions or tendon repair.[1,14]
- The plantaris tendon has high tensile strength with the structured collagen characteristic of physiologic tendons.
- Harvest of the plantaris tendon rarely creates appreciable donor site morbidity.
- The goal of this chapter is to provide the foot and ankle surgeon with a simple and reliable method to harvest readily available local tissue for plantaris tendon grafting even if its harvest was not originally planned.

ANATOMY

- The plantaris muscle originates from the lateral femoral condyle, courses along the lower leg's superficial posterior compartment, and has its musculotendinous junction just distal to the level of the knee joint.
- The proximal plantaris tendon is situated between the gastrocnemius and the soleus muscle. Distally, it lies immediately adjacent to the Achilles tendon in the distal third of the lower leg and typically inserts in the calcaneal tuberosity (**FIG 1A**).
- The length of the plantaris tendon ranges from 30 to 45 cm.[11]
- The plantaris tendon insertion is variable.[3,4,11]
  - In addition to inserting on the calcaneal tuberosity, it may insert at the bursa calcanei, retinaculum flexorum, ankle capsule, plantar aponeurosis, or blend with the Achilles tendon or intermuscular septum (**FIG 1B**).
  - Because of this variability, distal harvesting procedures are unsuccessful in about 12% to 20% of cases.[4,9,12]
- In about 6% to 7% of individuals, the plantaris tendon is absent. In humans, the plantaris muscle and tendon serve little function; however, early in evolution, it was far more developed in monkeys.[3,8,10,11] Therefore, harvesting the plantaris tendon in humans causes no appreciable donor site morbidity.[2,7–9]
- Bohnsack et al[1] compared highest tensile strength per cubic millimeter (N/mm^3) of commonly used autografts:
  - Peroneus longus, 61 N/mm^3
  - Peroneus brevis, 41 N/mm^3
  - Plantaris, 94 N/mm^3
  - Achilles split, 36 N/mm^3
  - Fascia lata, 27 N/mm^3
  - Periosteal flap, 2 N/mm^3
  - Corium, 12 N/mm^3
  - Anterior talofibular ligament, 8 N/mm^3
- They found the plantaris tendon to have the highest N/mm^3.

PATHOGENESIS

- Chronic joint instability and chronic tendon ruptures develop over months to years.
  - In joint instability, acutely torn ligaments eventually scar in an elongated state.

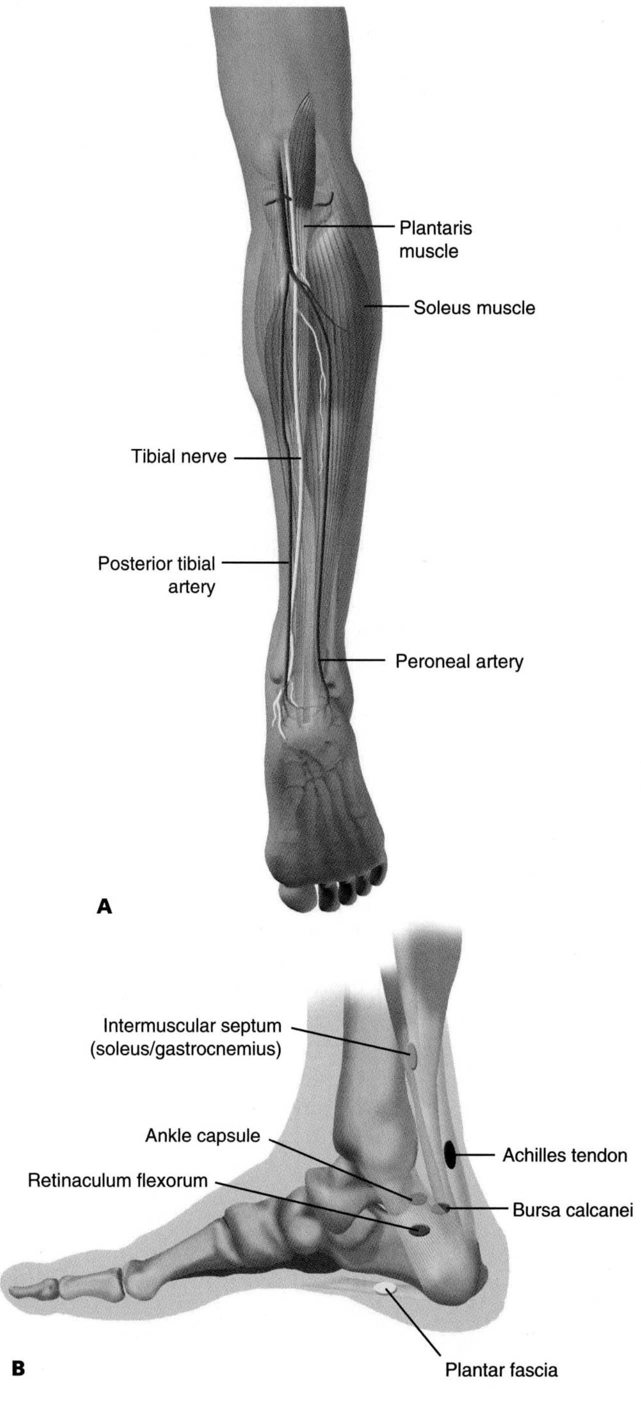

FIG 1 • Anatomy of the plantaris tendon. **A.** The only tubular structure between the soleus and the gastrocnemius muscles is the plantaris tendon. Therefore, blind dissection between these muscles does not risk nerves and vessels. Major vessels run underneath the soleus muscle. **B.** Insertions of the plantaris tendon are variable and may complicate the successful harvesting procedure.

- Acute untreated tendon ruptures, similarly, eventually demonstrate degeneration and elongation.

- Both chronic ligament and tendon injuries eventually may become so degenerated that surgical reconstruction is not possible with residual local tissue, especially in the case of chronically attenuated ligaments or tendons that have been subjected to repeated trauma or microtrauma. These situations lend themselves well to plantaris autografting.

PATIENT HISTORY AND PHYSICAL FINDINGS

- Although isolated plantaris tendon ruptures have been reported, no specific physical examination technique has been developed that can isolate the plantaris tendon to confirm in advance that it is present when plantaris tendon harvest is being considered.

IMAGING AND OTHER DIAGNOSTIC STUDIES

- Ultrasound is useful in identifying the presence of a plantaris tendon and has a high specificity.[10]
- When MRI is used to evaluate an injury to the ankle ligament or tendon, the imaging study also may prove useful in identifying the presence of an ispsilateral plantaris tendon that may be used for tissue augmentation.[7,8,13]

SURGICAL MANAGEMENT

- The plantaris tendon is ideal tissue for most ligament or tendon augmentations in the foot and ankle, especially because it typically is in the sterile field for virtually every foot and ankle procedure.

Preoperative Planning

- If an MRI scan was obtained to determine the initial pathology, it can be used to identify the existence of the plantaris tendon before surgery.[8,13]
- If not, a preoperative ultrasound examination is helpful.[10,13]

Positioning

- Harvest of the plantaris tendon is relatively simple, regardless of which patient position is dictated by the particular foot and ankle procedure.
- No tourniquet is needed for plantaris tendon harvesting.

Approach

- The proximal approach is a 2-cm longitudinal incision about 30 cm proximal to the medial malleolus (**FIG 2**).
- The distal approach is a 2-cm longitudinal incision at the medial Achilles insertion on the medial calcaneal tuberosity (**FIG 3**).

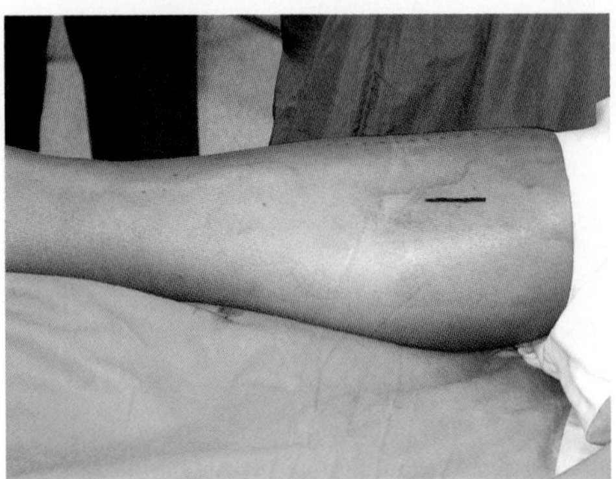

FIG 2 • The authors' preferred technique of proximal plantaris harvesting. A 2-cm incision is made at the proximal quarter of the medial calf.

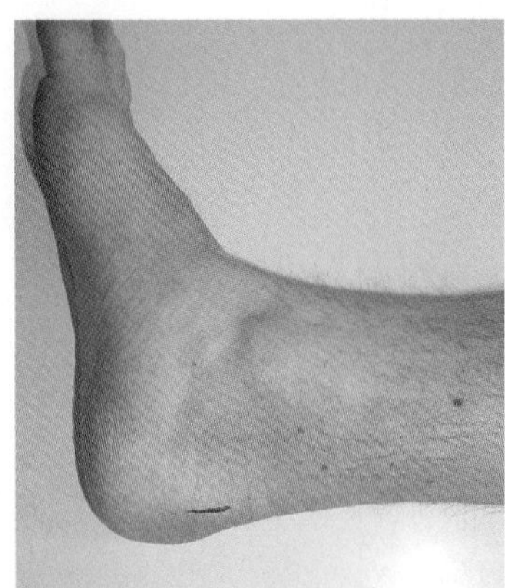

FIG 3 • Distal plantaris harvesting using a 2-cm skin incision at the medial border of the Achilles tendon insertion at the medial calcaneal tuberosity.

TECHNIQUES

- The plantaris may be harvested from a proximal or distal approach; for both approaches, only a minimally invasive, 2-cm incision is required.

AUTHORS' PREFERRED TECHNIQUE FOR PROXIMAL PLANTARIS HARVESTING[6,7]

- Subcutaneous blunt dissection to the fascia is performed with care taken to protect the saphenous nerve and vein (**TECH FIG 1A**). A 2-cm longitudinal incision is made in the fascia to enable the surgeon's finger to enter the intermuscular space (**TECH FIG 1B**). The only tubular structure that runs between the gastrocnemius and the soleus muscle bellies is the plantaris tendon. No nerves or vessels are at risk.[13]
- The tendon is mobilized with the finger or a nerve retractor (**TECH FIG 1C**).
- The plantaris tendon is isolated in a distal direction using a blunt tendon stripper. The tendon stripper is ad-

vanced while maintaining the tendon under tension (**TECH FIG 1D**).

- At the level of the calcaneus, the inner cylinder of the stripper is rotated to transect the tendon. The tendon is stored in a wet sponge for later use (**TECH FIG 1E**).
- The fascia is reapproximated with absorbable suture, and wound closure is performed with a subcuticular running stitch (**TECH FIG 1F**). We routinely use adhesive strips to promote an optimal cosmetic appearance to the healed wound.

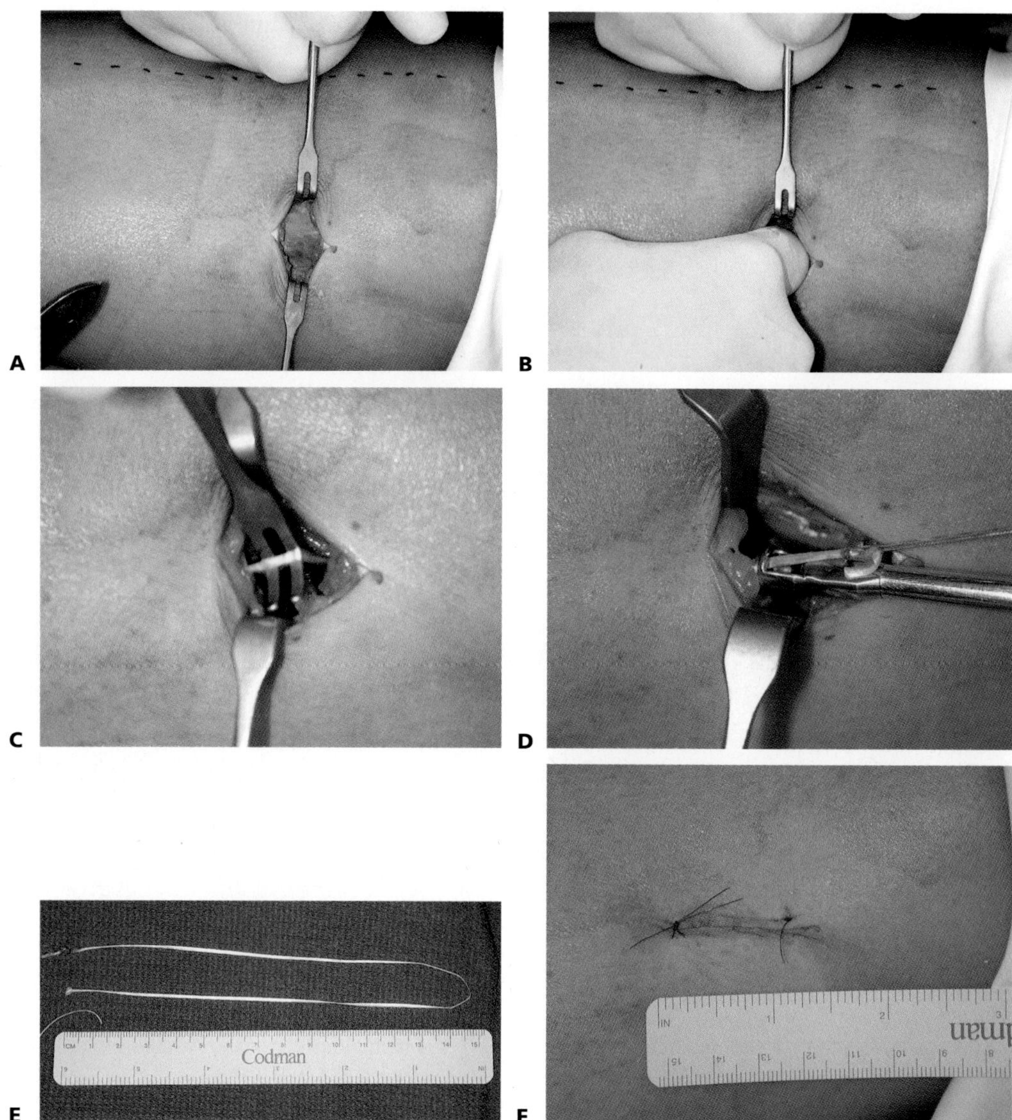

TECH FIG 1 • **A**. Blunt spreading of the subcutaneous fat down to the fascia without damage to the saphenous nerve or vein. **B.** A 2-cm fascial incision is made, and blunt dissection is carried out further down between the gastrocnemius and soleus muscles with the surgeon's finger. **C.** The plantaris tendon is developed with a nerve retractor. **D.** Introduction of the tendon stripper. **E.** The harvested autograft usually is about 30 cm long.

DISTAL PLANTARIS HARVEST

- A 2-cm skin incision is made at the medial border of the Achilles tendon insertion at the calcaneal tuberosity (see Fig 3).
- Blunt dissection is carried down to the Achilles tendon and the plantaris tendon. The variability of the plantaris insertions may necessitate a slightly more involved dissection to identify the distal extent of the plantaris tendon (see Fig 1B).
- The tendon is mobilized and harvested with a blunt tendon stripper from distal to proximal (**TECH FIG 2A**).
- At the level of the popliteal fossa, the inner cylinder of the stripper is rotated to transect the tendon (**TECH FIG 2B**). The tendon is stored in a wet sponge until it is needed for ligament or tendon augmentation.
- The skin is closed with interrupted sutures and adhesive strips.

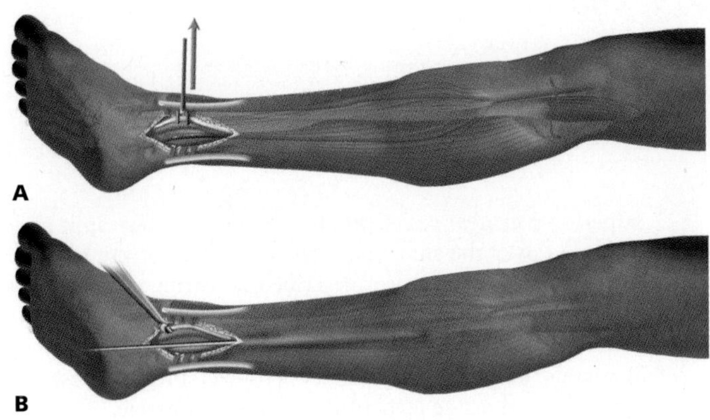

TECH FIG 2 • **A.** The plantaris tendon is located by blunt dissection. **B.** The tendon stripper is advanced from distal to proximal up to the popliteal fossa. Then the inner cylinder of the stripper is rotated to cut the tendon.

PEARLS AND PITFALLS

Indication	■ We prefer the plantaris tendon over the peroneal tendons when grafting for chronic lateral ankle reconstruction. Use of this tendon will not further decrease dynamic control of lateral ankle instability.[2,5,6]
Technique	■ A proximal approach to a plantaris autograft will increase the success of the grafting procedure, because the distal tendon course is variable and may be difficult to find.[6,7] ■ A proximal approach to the plantaris tendon will reduce complications—making the incision at the calcaneal tuberosity could cause hypertrophic scarring and resultant shoe wear irritation.[6,7] ■ If the plantaris tendon cannot be located with distal harvesting technique, a small, medial, split Achilles tendon graft can be harvested with the tendon stripper advanced from distally to proximally.

POSTOPERATIVE CARE

- Adhesive wound strips can reduce skin tension and broadening of the scar.
- After wound healing the patient may use scar massage to reduce subcutaneous adhesions.

OUTCOMES

- The proximal harvesting procedure of the plantaris tendon was reported in a clinical study of plantaris tendon autograft for lateral ligament reconstruction of chronic ankle instability.[7] In 52 cases (93%), a strong 25- to 35-cm tendon graft was harvested. In one case (2%) the plantaris tendon was deemed too weak to serve as appropriate donor material. In three (5%) of 56 ankle reconstructions the plantaris tendon could not be located during surgery without preoperative imaging or ultrasound. This observation was consistent with incidence studies of the plantaris tendon in cadavers (absence ranged between 6% and 7%).[8,10,13]
- Use of the distal approach to harvest the plantaris tendon also has been reported. Investigators failed to locate the plantaris tendon distally in 12% to 20% of cases in these studies.[4,9,12,13]

COMPLICATIONS

- We have performed proximal plantaris harvesting in 102 cases with only one case of mild dysesthesia at a broadened scar. This did not create any functional deficits for the patient.
- Despite the close proximity of the saphenous nerve and vein, we have not observed any saphenous nerve or vein injuries.
- In 36 patients we have performed a distal approach plantaris harvest. Four of these patients (11% of cases) developed a hypertrophic or hypersensitive scar that created shoe irritation.

REFERENCES

1. Bohnsack M, Surie B, Kirsch IL, et al. Biomechanical properties of commonly used autogenous transplants in the surgical treatment of chronic lateral ankle instability. Foot Ankle Int 2002;23:661–664.
2. Brunner R, Gaechter A. Repair of fibular ligaments: Comparison of reconstructive techniques using plantaris and peroneal tendons. Foot Ankle 1991;11:359–367.
3. Daseler EH, Anson BH. The plantaris muscle. An anatomical study of 750 specimens. J Bone Joint Surg 1943;25:822–827.
4. Harvey FJ, Chu G, Harvey PM. Surgical availability of the plantaris tendon. J Hand Surg Am 1983;8:243–247.
5. Hintermann B. Biomechanics of the unstable ankle joint and clinical implications. Med Sci Sports Exerc 1999;31:459–469.
6. Pagenstert GI, Hintermann B, Knupp M. Operative management of chronic ankle instability: Plantaris graft. Foot Ankle Clin 2006; 11:567–583.
7. Pagenstert GI, Valderrabano V, Hintermann B. Lateral ankle ligament reconstruction with free plantaris tendon graft. Tech Foot Ankle Surg 2005;4:104–112.
8. Saxena A, Bareither D. Magnetic resonance and cadaveric findings of the incidence of plantaris tendon. Foot Ankle Int 2000;21:570–572.
9. Segesser B, Goesele A. [Weber fibular ligament-plasty with plantar tendon with Segesser modification]. Sportverletz Sportschaden 1996;10:88–93.
10. Simpson SL, Hertzog MS, Barja RH. The plantaris tendon graft: An ultrasound study. J Hand Surg Am 1991;16:708–711.
11. Tillmann B, Toendury G. Flexorengruppe der unteren Extremität. In: Leonhardt H, Tillmann B, Toendury G, et al., eds. Bewegungsapparat, 3rd ed. Stuttgart-New York: Thieme, 1987:584–793.
12. Weber BG, Hupfauer W. Zur Behandlung der frischen fibularen Bandruptur und der chronischen fibularen Bandinsuffizienz. Arch Orthop Trauma Surg 1969;65:251–257.
13. Wening JV, Katzer A, Phillips F, et al. [Detection of the tendon of the musculus plantaris longus—diagnostic imaging and anatomic correlate]. Unfallchir 1996;22:30–35.
14. White WL. The unique, accessible and useful plantaris tendon. Plast Reconstr Surg 1960;25:133–141.

Chapter 121

Repair of Peroneal Tendon Tears

Brad Dresher and Brian Donley

DEFINITION

- Peroneal tendon tears are a disruption of the fibers, most commonly of the peroneal brevis tendon.
- Acute tears rarely may be the result of an ankle fracture or severe sprain.
- The most common type of tear, an attrition tear, is the result of multiple subluxations or peroneal tendinitis.

ANATOMY

- The peroneus longus and peroneus brevis tendons both originate in the lateral compartment of the leg.
- The peroneus brevis inserts into the base of the fifth metatarsal and the longus into the proximal plantar first metatarsal and the first cuneiform.
- Both muscles are innervated by the superficial peroneal nerve.
- The peroneus longus courses posterior to the peroneus brevis tendon as they pass through the common peroneal synovial sheath proximal to the lateral malleolus.
- The superior peroneal retinaculum prevents subluxation of the peroneal tendons, forming a 1- to 2-cm fibrous sling from the posterolateral aspect of the distal fibula to the anterior Achilles sheath and lateral wall of the calcaneus.
- The inferior peroneal retinaculum covers the tendons 2 to 3 cm distal to the lateral malleolus.
- The peroneal tubercle of the calcaneus separates the peroneus longus and brevis into separate sheaths.

PATHOGENESIS

- Traumatic rupture may occur with ankle fractures or severe sprains[3] but is rare.
- Partial longitudinal tears are commonly associated with peroneal tenosynovitis.
- Peroneus longus tears often are seen with a painful os peroneum, an enlarged peroneal tubercle, or pathology at the cuboid or calcaneus.
- Instability of peroneal tendons at the level of the superior peroneal retinaculum may be a cause of tendinitis leading to tears.
- Brevis tendon tears can be caused by compression between the lateral ridge of the malleolus and the peroneus longus tendon.[3]
- Brevis tears are commonly at the level of the distal lateral malleolus.

NATURAL HISTORY

- Injury to the peroneal tendons is a frequently overlooked cause of persistent lateral ankle pain.
- There have been two mechanisms described by Munk and Davis[6] leading to a tear of the peroneus brevis tendon.
  - Subluxation of the peroneus brevis tendon may occur as a result of chronic ankle instability, and the tearing of the superior peroneal retinaculum. The tendon may split as it subluxes over the sharp posterolateral edge of the fibula.[6]
  - The second mechanism described is tearing of the brevis tendon caused by compression between the posterior fibula and the peroneus longus tendon.[1]
- Peroneus longus tears, unlike peroneus brevis tears, are commonly seen at the level of the peroneal tubercle.

PATIENT HISTORY AND PHYSICAL FINDINGS

- The evaluation of a patient with suspected peroneal pathology should start with a thorough history from the patient. Pain, swelling, and warmth may be caused by an acute injury or prolonged repetitive activity.
- The patient should be asked to pinpoint the area of pain to the examiner.
  - Peroneus brevis tendon tears cause pain and persistent swelling along the peroneal tendon sheath and commonly behind the fibula.[4]
  - Peroneus longus tendon tears present with pain in the cuboid groove, in the plantar aspect of the foot, or at the level of the peroneal tubercle.[8]
- Patients should be asked about other existing conditions. Rheumatoid arthritis, psoriasis, hyperparathyroidism, diabetic neuropathy, calcaneal fractures, and local injections have been associated with an increased risk of peroneal tendon tears.[8]
- A history of subluxation or dislocation (**FIG 1**) can also give rise to peroneal tendon pathology.
- Physical examination of the peroneal tendons should include:
  - Assessment for posterolateral hindfoot swelling. Swelling indicates pathology; swelling about the lateral or posterolateral side of the ankle could represent tendinitis, tenosynovitis, repetitive subluxation, or tear.
  - Inspection for hindfoot alignment. Any varus position from neutral is a positive finding. Varus position is associated with an increased rate of peroneal tendon disorders.[5]

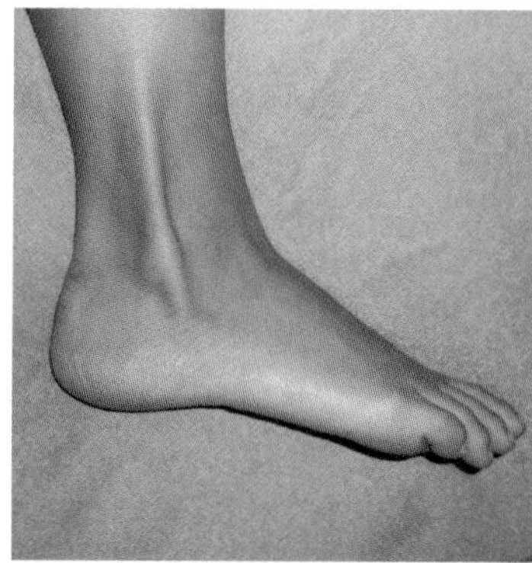

FIG 1 • Dislocation of peroneal tendons.

- Palpation along the course of the peroneal tendons should be performed to identify areas of tenderness. Any tenderness along tendons is a positive finding. Tenderness along the peroneal tendons may represent tendinitis, tenosynovitis, or tear.
- Strength: ankle and foot eversion strength against resistance. Weakness in eversion is probably pathology, but near-normal eversion strength may not rule out peroneal pathology due to recruitment of other muscle groups. Strength may be decreased due to pain or tendon rupture.
- Neurovascular assessment: sensory examination along the sural nerve distribution. Pain along the sural nerve distribution is assessed to rule out sural nerve neuritis.
- Peroneal tunnel compression test. The foot is dorsiflexed and everted while manual pressure is applied along the retrofibular region. A positive finding (pain) indicates possible tendinitis, tenosynovitis, or tear.
- Plantarflexion of the first ray. With the foot in neutral, active plantarflexion of the first ray is tested. Loss of plantarflexion of the first ray compared to the unaffected side is a positive sign. Loss or limitation of plantarflexion of the first ray is consistent with dysfunction of the peroneus longus tendon.
- Testing for peroneal tendon dislocation or subluxation involves active rotation of the ankle, with subluxation or dislocation on palpation and visualization noted. Dislocation or subluxation gives rise to tendinitis or tears.

IMAGING AND OTHER DIAGNOSTIC STUDIES

- Plain radiographs and weight-bearing views of the ankle and foot are obtained. An axillary heel view will allow evaluation of the peroneal tubercle and the retromalleolar groove. Radiographs are important in ruling out fractures, arthrosis, tumors, and impingement.
- MRI is the study of choice when evaluating the peroneal tendons. Heterogeneity or discontinuity of the tendon, a fluid-filled tendon sheath, marrow edema along the lateral calcaneal wall, and a hypertrophied peroneal tubercle are all indications of peroneal tendon tears (**FIG 2**).
- Often the MRI underestimates the extent of pathology with regard to tears of the peroneus longus tendon.[8]
- Peroneal tenography allows indirect visualization of the tendons by injecting contrast into the sheaths. Tenography may be useful to test for external compression, dislocation, and complete rupture.

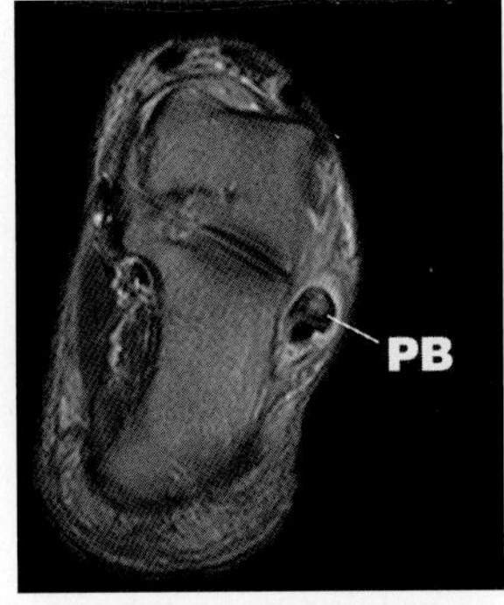

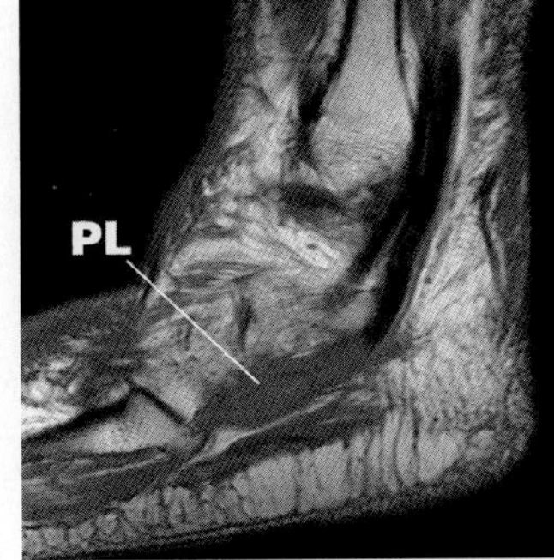

FIG 2 • MRI findings.

- Ultrasound is noninvasive and does not expose the patient to radiation. Complete ruptures are seen as discontinuities in the tendon and partial tears are represented by focal lucencies. However, ultrasound has limited usefulness in imaging disorders of the peroneal tendons and is very dependent on the quality of the ultrasonographer.
- CT scanning may be a useful tool in the assessment of peroneal tendons. Soft tissue imaging allows tendons to be differentiated from adjacent structures. Rupture, impingement, dislocation, and tenosynovitis may demonstrated.[3]

DIFFERENTIAL DIAGNOSIS

- Sural nerve neuritis
- Calcaneus fractures
- Os peroneum fracture
- Lateral malleolar avulsion fractures
- Lateral ankle impingement
- Hypertrophic peroneal tubercle
- Bony spurring at the posterior lateral fibular groove of the calcaneus
- Prominent exostoses
- Hindfoot arthrosis
- Tumor

NONOPERATIVE MANAGEMENT

- Nonoperative management consists of nonsteroidal anti-inflammatory medication, rest, activity modification, a lateral heel wedge, rarely use of an ankle–foot orthosis, and in difficult cases immobilization in a short-leg cast or walking boot for 6 weeks.
- Use of corticosteroid injections have been reported, but tendon splitting and rupture should be considered as possible complications of injection.[3]

SURGICAL MANAGEMENT

- Redfern and Myerson[7] describe an algorithm for surgical treatment, evaluating functional tendons, mobility of the remaining peroneal musculature, ankle stability, and position of the heel.
- After an MRI and clinical examination indicate a tear or rupture and the patient has failed to respond to conservative treatment, surgery is indicated.
- The procedure is finalized when intraoperative examination is performed.
- Upon gross examination three types of tears or ruptures are evaluated:
  - Type I: Both tendons are grossly intact.
  - Type II: One tendon is torn, the other usable.
  - Type III: Both tendons are torn and unusable.

Preoperative Planning

- All imaging studies are reviewed.
- MRI has been reported to both underestimate and overestimate the degree of tendon pathology.[7]
- Operative planning should rest on the clinical evaluation, failure of conservative treatment, and occasionally injection of local anesthetic into the tendon sheath.[7]
- Deformity of the hindfoot or laxity of the ankle ligaments that could cause recurrent tendon tears should be noted preoperatively and addressed in a single procedure with any peroneal tendon pathology.

Positioning

- The patient is positioned supine with a bump under the ipsilateral hip.
- A well-padded tourniquet is placed on the ipsilateral thigh.
- Blankets are used under the operative ankle to elevate the operative extremity.
- The contralateral leg is secured to the table with tape.

Approach

- Following the course of the peroneal tendons, a slightly curved 10-cm incision is made posterior to the lateral malleolus and carried distally along the course of the tendons.
- Blunt dissection is taken to the peroneal sheath, while protecting the sural nerve (**FIG 3**).

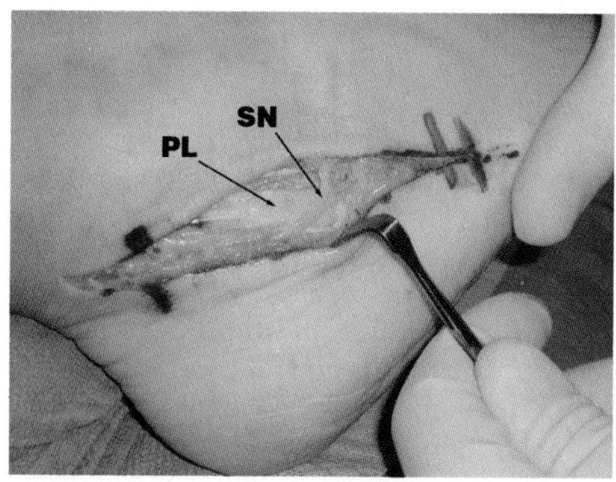

FIG 3 • Sural nerve position during approach.

TECHNIQUES

TYPE I: BOTH TENDONS GROSSLY INTACT

- Perform the standard approach.
- Open the peroneal sheath in line with the tendons.
- Perform an intraoperative examination of the peroneal tendons to evaluate the amount of degeneration or tears (**TECH FIG 1A**).
- Perform a synovectomy, followed by removal of any degenerated tendon (**TECH FIG 1B**).
- If the remaining usable tendon is 50% or more of the original diameter, then a repair is indicated.
- Use a running 3-0 absorbable Vicryl suture to tubularize the tendon and return it to a smooth surface (**TECH FIG 1C**).
- Obtain hemostasis.
- Repair the sheath using 2-0 suture, followed by subcutaneous closure, and use nonabsorbable suture for the skin.

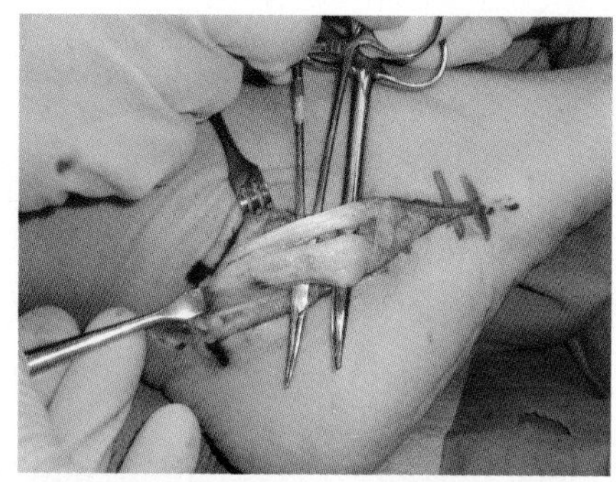

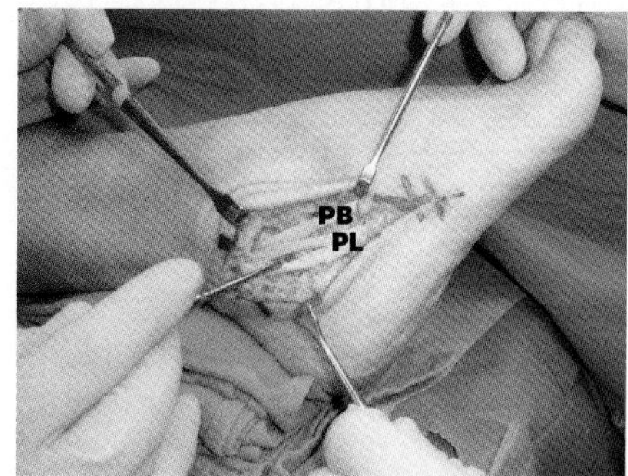

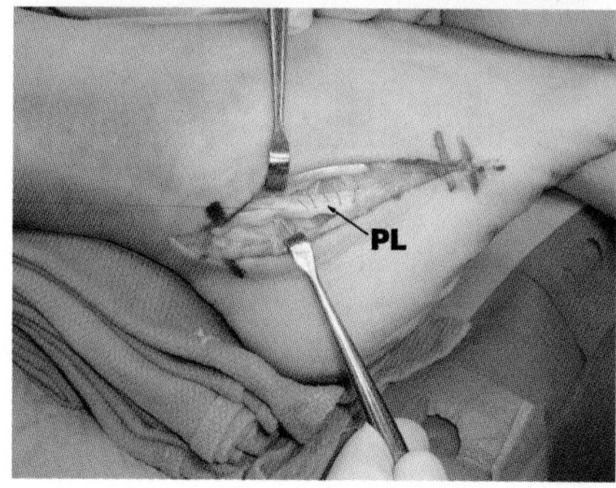

TECH FIG 1 • **A.** Thickened peroneus longus, normal-appearing brevis. **B.** Débridement of peroneus longus. **C.** Repair of tendon.

TYPE II: ONE TENDON TORN AND THE OTHER USABLE

- Perform the standard approach.
- Open the peroneal sheath in line with the tendons.
- Perform an intraoperative examination of the peroneal tendons to evaluate the amount of degeneration or tears.
- If one tendon is found to be more than 50% unusable, then a tenodesis is indicated.
- Perform the tenodesis side to side to the usable tendon proximal.[7]
- The sheath should remain open.
- Obtain hemostasis.
- Subcutaneous closure and use nonabsorbable suture for the skin.

TYPE III: BOTH TENDONS TORN OR UNUSABLE

- Perform the standard approach.
- Open the peroneal sheath in line with the tendons.
- Perform an intraoperative examination of the peroneal tendons to evaluate the amount of degeneration or tears.
- In type III, both peroneal tendons are more than 50% degenerated or torn.
- Examine for excursion of the proximal muscle.
- If no excursion is present due to scarring and fibrosis, a tendon transfer is indicated.
- If excursion is present and the tissue bed is scarred, then a staged allograft with silicone rod is considered.
- If excursion is present and the tissue bed is free from scarring, then an onstage allograft or tendon transfer is considered.[7]

PEARLS AND PITFALLS

MRI	■ MRI has been shown to underestimate and overestimate the degree of peroneal tendon pathology compared with the intraoperative findings.[7] It must be correlated with the clinical examination findings.
Intraoperative	■ The surgeon should be ready to evaluate the peroneal tendons during the procedure and proceed with the proper repair or reconstruction, as physical examination and current imaging findings have been described to both overestimate and underestimate the degree of pathology.
Intraoperative	■ The surgeon may need to resect a portion of the distal muscle belly of the peroneus brevis to make room in the peroneal sheath behind the fibula.
Intraoperative	■ The surgeon must evaluate the posterior fibula for an exostosis, which may be the cause of a peroneus brevis tear.

POSTOPERATIVE CARE

- A posterior splint is applied in the operating room.
- At 1 week the splint is changed to a partial weight-bearing cast.
- At 3 weeks a wound check with suture removal is done, followed by a walking boot for 3 more weeks.
- At 6 weeks a prefabricated ankle brace is applied and active range-of-motion exercises are started.
- Physical therapy for calf strength is initiated at 6 weeks.
- Return to activities is considered at 3 months, with an orthotic containing lateral posting.

OUTCOMES

- A study by Redfern and Myerson[7] assessed 29 feet with peroneus longus and brevis tears.
  - 31% had normal peroneal strength postoperatively, and 59% had moderate peroneal strength.
  - 9% had postoperative complications.
  - 50% continued to experience some painful symptoms postoperatively; in all but three patients, pain was mild.

COMPLICATIONS

- Wound infection
- Sural nerve neuritis
- Complex regional pain syndrome
- Adhesive tendinitis
- Failed repair

REFERENCES

1. Bassett FH III, Speer KP. Longitudinal rupture of the peroneal tendons. Am J Sports Med 1993;21:354–357.
2. Bonnin M, Tavernier T, Bouysset M. Split lesions of the peroneus brevis tendon in chronic ankle laxity. Am J Sports Med 1997;25: 699–703.
3. Clarke H, Kitaoka HB, Ehman RL. Peroneal tendon injuries. Foot Ankle Int 1998;19:280–288.
4. Krause J, Brodsky J. Peroneus brevis tendon tears: pathophysiology, surgical reconstruction and clinical results. Foot Ankle Int 1998; 19:271–279.
5. Manoli A II. The subtle cavus foot, "the underpronator," a review. Foot Ankle Int 2005;26:256–263.
6. Munk R, Davis P. Longitudinal rupture of the peroneus brevis tendon. J Trauma 1976;16:803–806.
7. Redfern D, Myerson M. The management of concomitant tears of the peroneus longus and brevis tendons. Foot Ankle Int 2004; 25:695–707.
8. Selmani E, Gjata V, Gjika E. Current concepts review: peroneal tendon disorders. Foot Ankle International 2006;27:221–228.

Chapter **122**

Reconstruction of Chronic Peroneal Tendon Tears

Keith L. Wapner, Selene G. Parekh, and Wen Chao

DEFINITION

- Pathology of the peroneal tendons may cause chronic lateral ankle pain.[1,3]
- Chronic lateral ankle pain can have many causes.
- Isolated tears of the peroneus brevis and longus are rare, but fissuring and longitudinal splitting of the brevis and longus tendons have been reported as a cause of chronic ankle pain and functional instability.
- Histologic evaluation of these splits has shown chronic wear with cystic and myxoid degeneration of the tendon.
- When recognized early, direct repair is possible with good results.[4,5]

ANATOMY

- The peroneus brevis tendon can be identified at the level of the lateral malleolus since it is closest to the malleolus.
- The peroneus longus tendon is directly posterior to the brevis tendon.
- Both the longus and brevis tendons are tethered at the level of the lateral malleolus by the superior peroneal retinaculum, which is a band of deep fascia that extends from the tip of the lateral malleolus to the calcaneus (**FIG 1**).
- The tendons lie within the fibular groove; the most common location for longitudinal peroneus brevis tendon tears is at the fibular groove[10] (**FIG 2**).
- The flexor hallucis longus tendon (FHL) has a strength percentage of 3.6 and can substitute for the peroneus brevis muscle–tendon unit, which has a strength percentage of 2.6.
- The FHL is an in-phase muscle with an axis of contracture similar to the peroneal muscle–tendon unit as it arises off the posterior fibula.
- This technique inserts the FHL into the residual stump of the peroneus brevis tendon.
- Our technique does not restore function of both peroneal tendons, since the distal portion of the peroneus longus tendon is too enmeshed in scar to serve as a viable insertion point for the FHL tendon.

PATHOGENESIS

- The pathogenesis of chronic peroneal tendon ruptures is unclear. Many theories have been suggested, including a zone of critical hypovascularity,[11] mechanical impingement from the fibular groove,[6,9,12] incompetence of the peroneal retinaculum,[2,8] the presence of a sharp posterior fibular ridge,[6,9,12] dynamic compression between the peroneus longus and brevis tendons,[7] or the presence of a peroneus quartus muscle.[13,14]

NATURAL HISTORY

- Patients typically present with advanced pathology of both tendons, such that neither can be salvaged in their entirety.
- These patients tend to be middle-aged individuals who were active, working adults before their injuries. They will not wear bracing full-time or accept a surgical fusion of their hindfoot.
- Most patients have a history of at least one failed surgical procedure to attempt a primary repair or anastomosis of the peroneus brevis and longus tendons.
- The goal of this procedure is to provide dynamic stabilization of the ankle and restore the function of the peroneal tendons.

PATIENT HISTORY AND PHYSICAL FINDINGS

- These patients present with chronic lateral ankle pain and tenderness, swelling, and lateral ankle instability.
- Patients have considerable weakness and painful inversion and eversion compared with the contralateral limb.
- A fully functional FHL tendon must be demonstrated.
- Alignment of the affected lower extremity, including the hip, knee, tibia, ankle, hindfoot, and forefoot, must be assessed. A fixed hindfoot varus deformity may need to be corrected at the time of surgery.
- If mechanical instability of the ankle is present, a ligament reconstruction at the time of the first stage can be included.
- Muscle strength and balance should be evaluated, particularly inversion and eversion.
- The single heel rise is helpful to evaluate the normal inversion–varus alignment of the hindfoot.
- Manual muscle testing for FHL is helpful to evaluate the functionality and strength of the FHL motor unit.
- The anterior drawer test is used in evaluating the integrity of the anterior talofibular ligament and the calcaneofibular ligament.

IMAGING AND OTHER DIAGNOSTIC STUDIES

- Weight-bearing ankle and foot radiographs must be obtained.
- MRI of the involved ankle demonstrates chronic thickening, fissuring, scarring, and stenosis of the remaining peroneal structures (**FIG 3A**). Tears in the substance of the tendon and fluid in the sheaths may also be visualized (**FIG 3B**). Associated pathology of the ankle can be identified as well.

DIFFERENTIAL DIAGNOSIS

- Fibular fracture, stress fracture
- Peroneal tendon tear
- Ankle instability, involving the anterior talofibular ligament or calcaneofibular ligament
- Lateral process fracture of the talus
- Syndesmosis or subtalar sprains
- Impingement lesions
- Osteochondral lesions of the talus
- Tarsal coalition

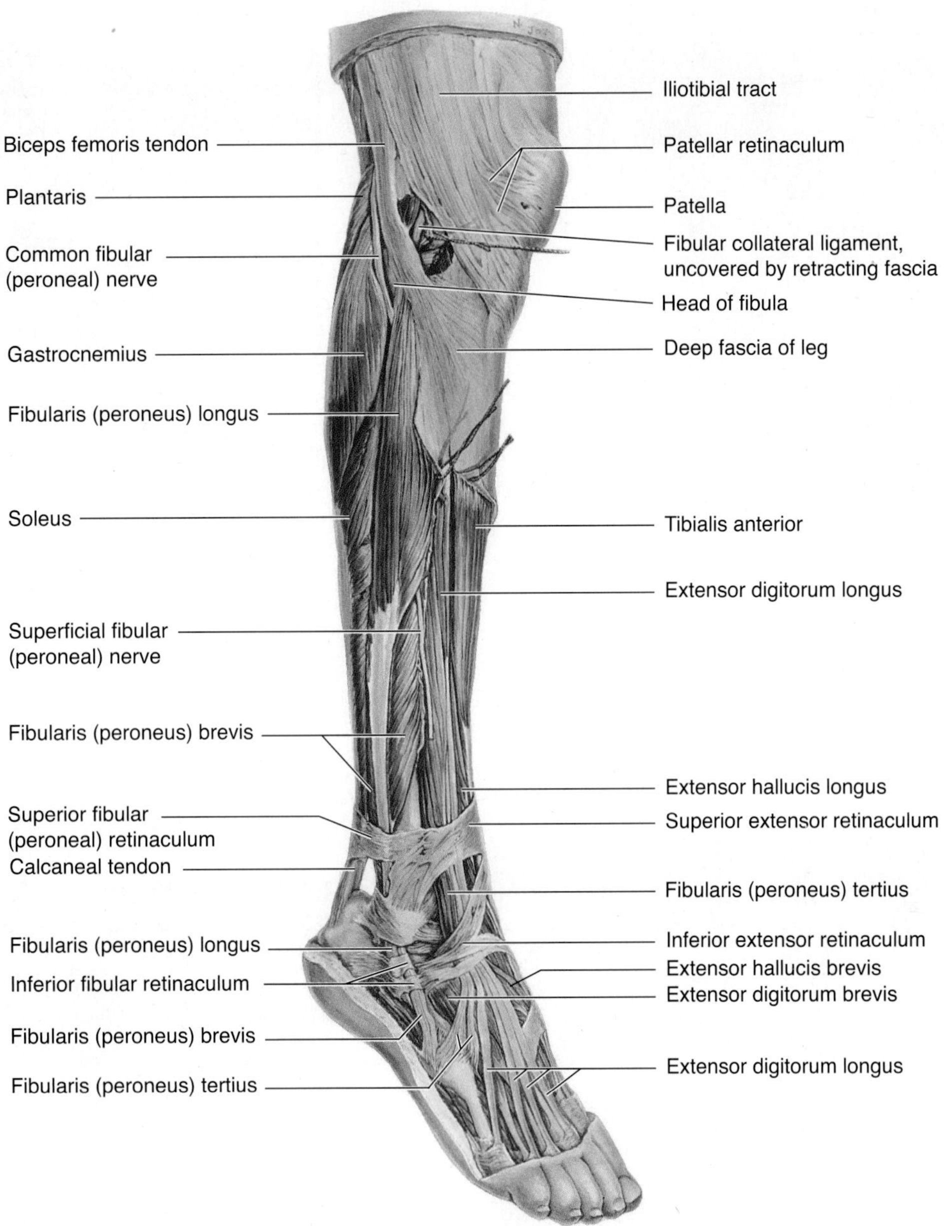

FIG 1 • The peroneus longus and brevis tendons are tethered at the level of the lateral malleolus by the superior peroneal retinaculum, which extends from the tip of the lateral malleolus to the calcaneus. (Source: Moore KL, Dalley AF. Clinically Oriented Anatomy, 4th ed. Philadelphia: Lippincott Williams & Wilkins, 1999.)

NONOPERATIVE MANAGEMENT

- Functional rehabilitation includes range of motion for the ankle and hindfoot, concentric and eccentric muscle strengthening, endurance training with particular attention to the peroneal musculature, and proprioceptive training.
- Proprioceptive exercises improve dynamic stability and are an essential part of the rehabilitation program.
- Functional bracing or taping may be useful to help prevent recurrent injury during "at-risk" activities.

SURGICAL MANAGEMENT

- The technique is staged in two parts. During each stage, the patient is positioned in the same manner. Perioperative antibiotics are given. A pneumatic thigh tourniquet is applied as needed.

Preoperative Planning

- All imaging studies must be reviewed.
- Plain films must be reviewed for degenerative changes, malalignment, fractures, and the presence of hardware from previous surgeries.

Positioning

- The patient is placed supine on the operating table. Some prefer to place the patient on a beanbag and approach the lateral aspect of the ankle in a lazy lateral or lateral decubitus

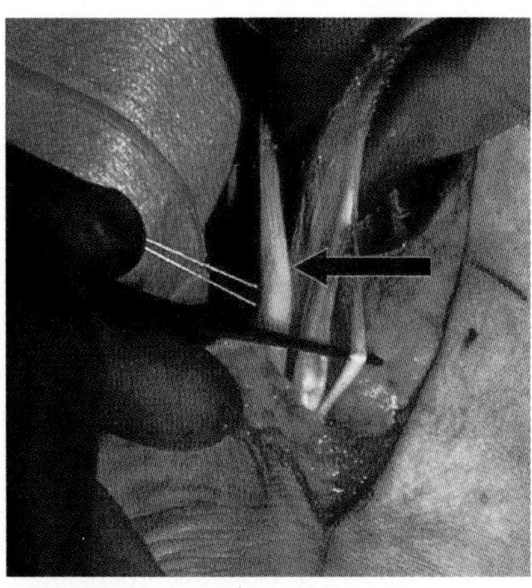

FIG 2 • Intraoperative photograph of a longitudinal peroneus brevis tear located in the fibular groove.

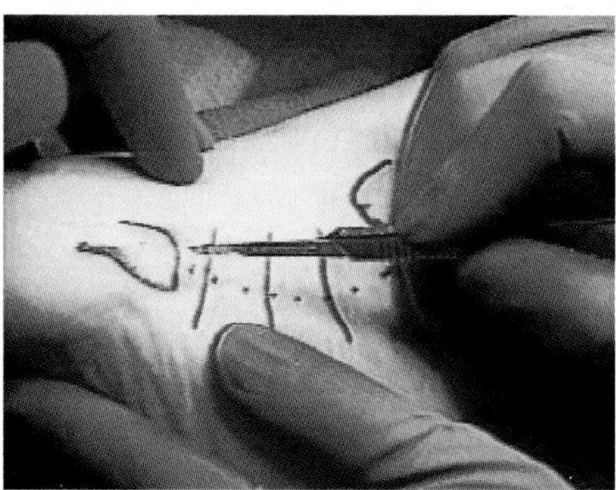

FIG 4 • Intraoperative photograph demonstrating the peroneal incision, from over the peroneals to the base of the fifth metatarsal.

position. We place saline bags under the ipsilateral hip to achieve this lazy lateral position.

Approach

- A longitudinal incision is centered over the course of the peroneal tendons, beginning 1 cm posterior and proximal to the tip of the fibula.
- The incision is extended to the base of the fifth metatarsal (**FIG 4**).
- Care must be taken to protect the sural nerve in the distal aspect of the incision, which is subcutaneous and just posterior to the incision.
- The surgeon carefully dissects through the extensive scar tissue (**FIG 5**).

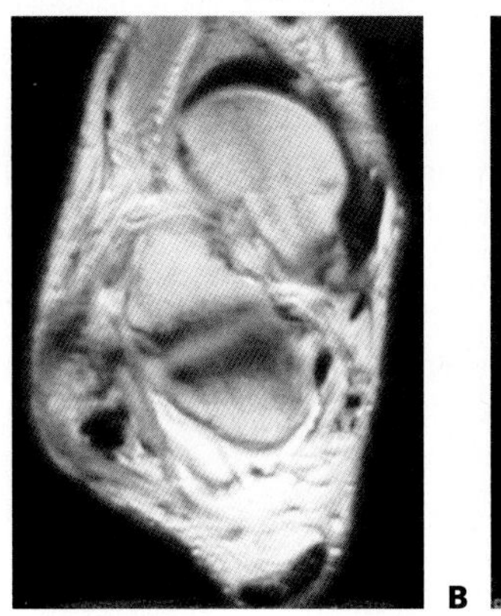

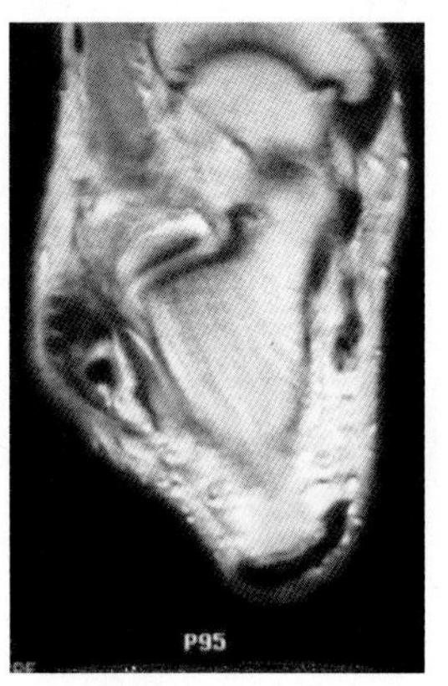

FIG 3 • Axial T2 MRI image demonstrating (**A**) a tear in the peroneal tendon and (**B**) fluid around the sheath of the tendon.

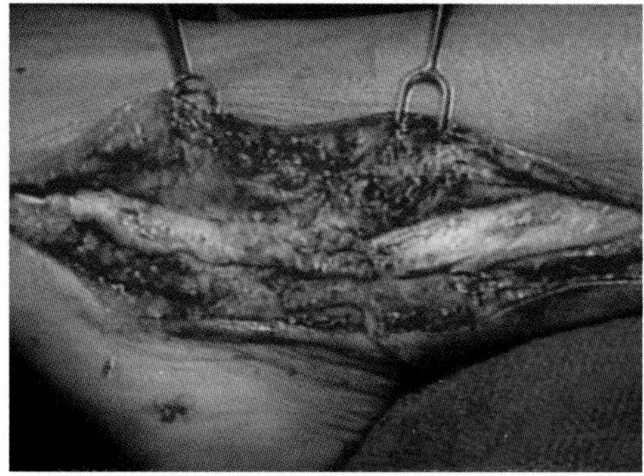

FIG 5 • Extensive scar tissue is evident overlying the peroneal tendons in this multiply operated patient.

TECHNIQUES

STAGE 1: DÉBRIDING THE PERONEAL TENDON AND SHEATH REMNANTS

- If present, identify the peroneal sheath. Incise the sheath proximally through the superior peroneal retinaculum to the musculotendinous junction. Distally, open the sheath as far as needed.
- The first stage of reconstruction consists of débriding the remaining peroneal tendon tissue and the tendon sheath (**TECH FIG 1**).

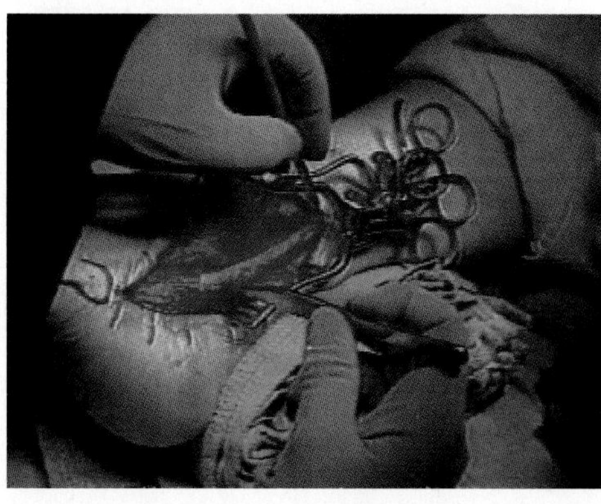

TECH FIG 1 • The peroneal tendon sheath and tendon are débrided.

STAGE 1: INSERTING THE HUNTER ROD

- Insert a 6–mm Hunter rod into the bed of the peroneal sheath. Suture the Hunter rod to the remaining stump of the peroneus brevis tendon distally with nonabsorbable suture. Proximally, the rod remains free in the sheath (**TECH FIG 2**).
- Trim the sheath of any redundancy and close it over the Hunter rod (**TECH FIG 3**).

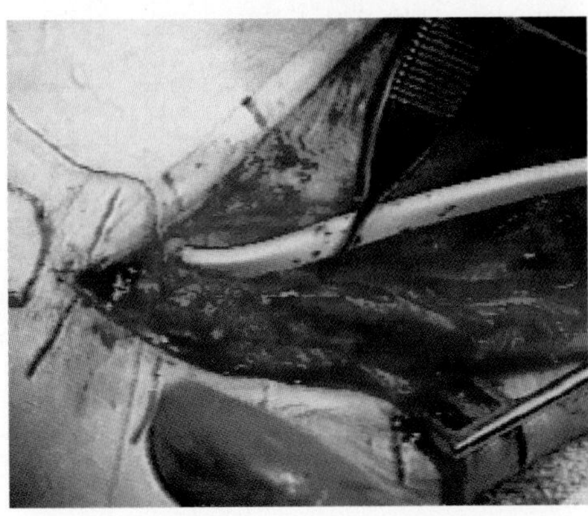

TECH FIG 2 • A 6-mm Hunter rod is placed into the bed of the peroneal sheath. The Hunter rod is sutured into the remaining stump of the peroneus brevis tendon distally with nonabsorbable suture. Proximally, the rod remains free in the sheath.

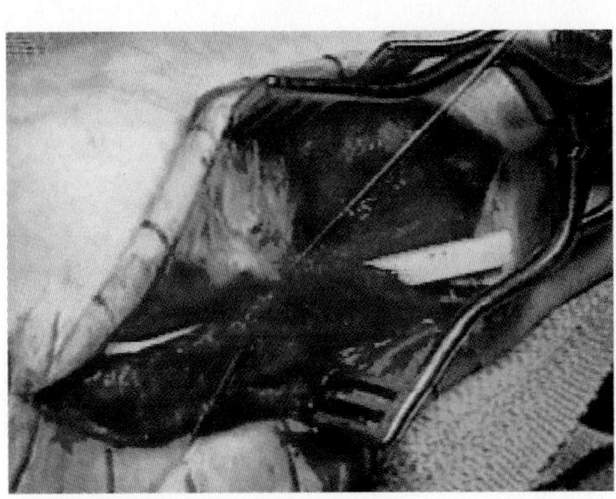

TECH FIG 3 • The sheath is trimmed of any redundancy and closed over the Hunter rod.

STAGE 2: HARVESTING THE FHL

- Make an incision along the medial border of the midfoot, just above the level of the abductor muscle, from the navicular to the head of the first metatarsal.
- Identify the abductor hallucis fascia and reflect the abductor muscle plantarly.
- Place a small Weitlaner retractor in the wound and reflect the flexor hallucis brevis plantarward as well. Release the origin of this muscle.
- Identify the FHL and flexor digitorum longus (FDL) tendons within the midfoot. This is facilitated by placing a finger over the lateral aspect of the short flexors and plantarflexing and dorsiflexing the hallux interphalangeal joint.
- Release the FHL as far distally as possible, generally at the level of the midshaft of the first metatarsal. An adequate distal stump of the FHL must be maintained to suture the distal stump to the FDL tendon with all five toes in a neutral posture. It is important to stay within the second muscle layer of the foot deep to the fat pad that overlies the neurovascular structures that sit just plantar to the long tendons.
- Tag the proximal stump of the FHL with a suture.

STAGE 2: EXCHANGING THE HUNTER ROD FOR THE FHL TENDON

- With the FHL harvested, make a small incision at the proximal aspect of the previously made lateral incision overlying the proximal aspect of the Hunter rod, staying proximal to the lateral malleolus.
- Identify the FHL in the deep posterior compartment at its origin on the posterior fibula. Pull it into the lateral incision (**TECH FIG 4**).

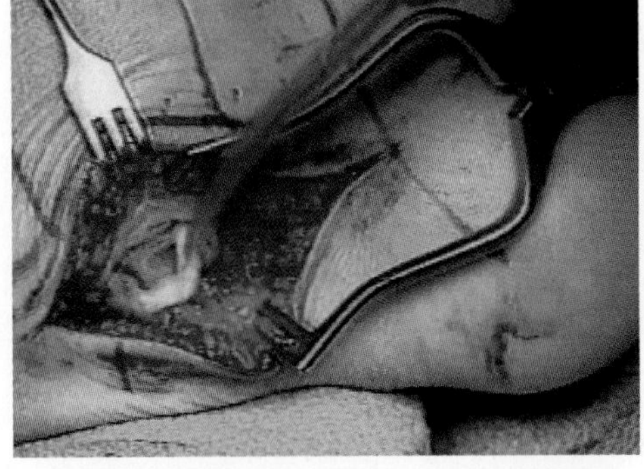

TECH FIG 4 • After the flexor hallucis longus is released from the plantar surface of the foot, it is identified in the deep posterior compartment at its origin on the posterior fibula. It is then pulled into the lateral incision.

- Identify the proximal portion of the Hunter rod and attach the FHL to the proximal aspect of the Hunter rod.
- Make a small distal incision over the distal suture site of the Hunter rod and the remaining portion of the peroneus brevis (**TECH FIG 5**).
- Release the Hunter rod from this suture site and pull it distally, allowing the FHL tendon to slide into the newly formed tendon sheath.
- Attach the FHL to the remaining stump of the peroneus brevis tendon using a Pulvertaft weave (**TECH FIG 6**).

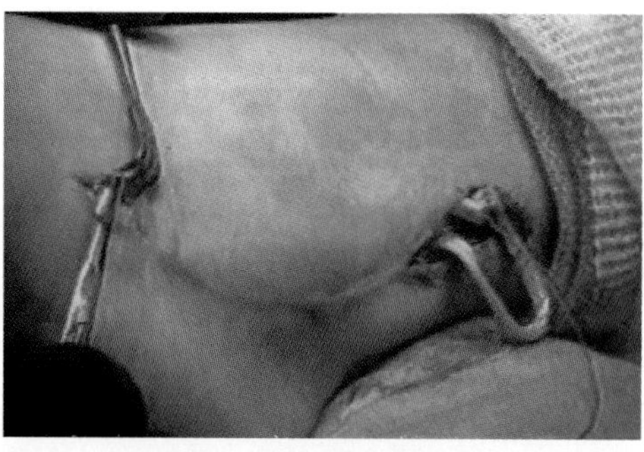

TECH FIG 5 • A small distal incision is made over the distal suture site of the Hunter rod and the remaining portion of the peroneus brevis.

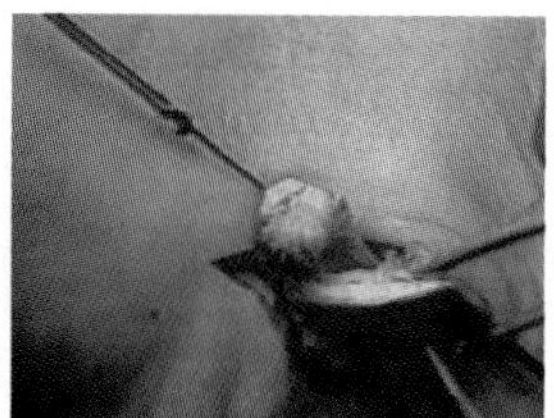

TECH FIG 6 • The flexor hallucis longus is attached to the remaining stump of the peroneus brevis tendon using a Pulvertaft weave.

PEARLS AND PITFALLS

Indication	■ Complete history and physical examination ■ Address associated malalignment and pathology. ■ For patients with chronic tendinosis of both peroneal tendons that have failed previous surgical repair ■ Address additional pathology such as ligament instability or heel varus at the first stage of reconstruction.
Incision	■ Avoid injury to the sural nerve. Preoperative testing is necessary to assess whether there is preexisting damage from the patient's previous surgeries. By staying over the course of the peroneal tendons the surgeon can generally avoid the sural nerve as it sits about 1 cm posterior.
Hunter rod placement	■ Use a nonabsorbable suture to attach the Hunter rod distally to avoid displacing the rod from the distal peroneus brevis stump. ■ Perform adequate débridement on the peroneal tendons and surrounding scar.
FHL harvest	■ Do not harvest the FDL. ■ During exposure, be careful of the neurovascular structures. ■ Tenodese the distal stump of the FHL to the FDL tendon with all five toes held in a neutral position.

POSTOPERATIVE CARE

- Postoperatively, after the insertion of the Hunter rod, patients are initially placed in a bulky Jones dressing for the first 2 weeks. Thereafter, they are allowed to bear weight as tolerated in a removable short-leg walking boot. They are instructed to remove the boot four times a day and perform active and passive range-of-motion exercises of the ankle and hindfoot in all planes of motion.
- Three months after the Hunter rod placement, the patient is brought back to the operating room for a transfer of the FHL tendon. Postoperatively, again, he or she is placed in a bulky Jones-type dressing for 2 weeks. Thereafter, the patient is advanced to a removable short-leg cast walker and maintained non–weight-bearing until 4 weeks. From week 4 to week 8, the patient is advanced to partial weight bearing in a removable cast walker. The patient is instructed to begin active and passive range-of-motion exercises of the ankle and hindfoot in all planes of motion. Home strengthening exercises are begun at 8 weeks, and the patient is advanced to an ankle stirrup at 12 to 14 weeks based on his or her strength. All patients are enrolled in formal physical therapy for functional rehabilitation of the ankle starting at 8 weeks.

OUTCOMES

- Data on the 8-year follow-up of seven patients has been published by the senior author (KLW). All wounds healed without complications. One workers' compensation patient had continued pain and ambulates with a molded ankle–foot orthosis. The remaining six patients report complete relief of preoperative symptoms and a return to preinjury levels of activity. There were five excellent results, one good result, and one fair result.[15,16]

COMPLICATIONS

- Wound complications
- Sural nerve injury
- Chronic pain

REFERENCES

1. Bassett FH III, Speer KP. Longitudinal rupture of the peroneal tendons. Am J Sports Med 1993;21:354–357.
2. Beck E. Operative treatment of recurrent dislocation of the peroneal tendons. Arch Orthop Trauma Surg 1981;98:247–250.
3. Brage ME, Hansen ST Jr. Traumatic subluxation/dislocation of the peroneal tendons. Foot Ankle 1992;13:423–431.
4. Burman M. Stenosing tendovaginitis of the foot and ankle; studies with special reference to the stenosing tendovaginitis of the peroneal tendons of the peroneal tubercle. AMA Arch Surg 1953;67:686–698.
5. Cox D, Paterson FW. Acute calcific tendinitis of peroneus longus. J Bone Joint Surg Br 1991;73B:342.
6. Edwards ME. The relations of the peroneal tendons to the fibula, calcaneus and cuboideum. Am J Anat 1928;42:213–253.
7. Gray JM, Alpar EK. Peroneal tenosynovitis following ankle sprains. Injury 2001;32:487–489.
8. Kojima Y, Kataoka Y, Suzuki S, et al. Dislocation of the peroneal tendons in neonates and infants. Clin Orthop Relat Res 1991;266:180–184.
9. Lamm BM, Myers DT, Dombek M, et al. Magnetic resonance imaging and surgical correlation of peroneus brevis tears. J Foot Ankle Surg 2004;43:30–36.
10. Sammarco GJ, DiRaimondo CV. Chronic peroneus brevis tendon lesions. Foot Ankle 1989;9:163–170.
11. Sobel M, Geppert MJ, Hannafin JA, et al. Microvascular anatomy of the peroneal tendons. Foot Ankle 1992;13:469–472.
12. Sobel M, Geppert MJ, Olson EJ, et al. The dynamics of peroneus brevis tendon splits: a proposed mechanism, technique of diagnosis, and classification of injury. Foot Ankle 1992;13:413–422.
13. Sobel M, Levy ME, Bohne WH. Congenital variations of the peroneus quartus muscle: an anatomic study. Foot Ankle 1990;11:81–89.
14. Zammit J, Singh D. The peroneus quartus muscle: anatomy and clinical relevance. J Bone Joint Surg Br 2003;85B:1134–1137.
15. Wapner KL, Parekh SG, Pedowitz DI, et al. Reconstruction of chronic peroneal tendon ruptures with staged Hunter rods and a flexor hallucis longus transfer. Tech Foot Ankle Surg 2005;4:202–206.
16. Wapner KL, Taras J, Lin SS, et al. Staged reconstruction for chronic rupture of both peroneal tendons using Hunter rod and flexor hallucis longus tendon transfer: a long-term follow-up study. Foot Ankle Int 2006;27:591–597.

Chapter 123 Repair of Dislocating Peroneal Tendons: Perspective 1

Sheldon Lin, Karl Bergmann, Vikrant Azad, Virak Tan, Enyi Okereke, and Siddhant Mehta*

DEFINITION

- Subluxation or dislocation of the peroneal tendon is a relatively uncommon injury, with the majority of the cases attributed to a traumatic event. Chronic subluxation has also been reported without any history of a specific event. Numerous surgical procedures have been described for the treatment of peroneal tendon subluxation, which may be classified into three categories: primary repair, soft tissue augmentation, and bony reconstruction. Primary repair of the superior peroneal retinaculum (SPR) is a commonly used surgical procedure. However, the effectiveness of primary repair depends upon the quality of the retinaculum and its ability to contain the peroneal tendons. When the SPR tissue is deficient or insufficient, then other procedures are necessary.
- Soft tissue procedures other than primary repair involve the augmentation of tissue already present or the rerouting of tissue from other structures to recreate the SPR.
- Bony procedures attempt to recreate a more stable fibular sulcus by deepening the fibular groove or extending the fibular rim. In this chapter we present a soft tissue augmentation procedure using a periosteal-based flap of the retrofibular sulcus.

ANATOMY

- Along the lateral aspect of the lower leg there are two muscles in the lateral compartment, the peroneus longus (PL) and peroneus brevis (PB). These two muscles arise at the proximal fibula and become tendinous before crossing the ankle.
- The peroneal tendons are contained in a single sheath located posterior and immediately distal to the fibula. Roughly at the level of the peroneal tubercle on the lateral calcaneus, the tendons separate into separate sheaths. The PB muscle belly extends more distal than the PL, and it becomes tendinous about 1.5 cm before the tip of the fibula. The PB tendon lies directly posterior to the fibula and anteromedial to the PL tendon as the two tendons course behind the fibula.
- The peroneal tendon sheath comprises the SPR, the calcaneofibular ligament (CFL), and the fibular sulcus. Respectively, the fibular sulcus represents the anterior border, the SPR the lateral border, portions of the SPR and CFL the posterior border, and portions of the CFL and posterior talofibular ligament the medial border of the peroneal tendon sheath.[12]
- The PB inserts on the dorsal base of the fifth metatarsal, while the PL courses lateral to medial on the plantar aspect of the foot and inserts on the lateral sides of the base of the first metatarsal and medial cuneiform bones.
- The SPR is the primary restraint against subluxation of the peroneal tendons within the fibular groove. The SPR can have an extremely varied anatomy, with differences in width, thickness, and insertional patterns. Most commonly, the SPR inserts into both the Achilles tendon and the calcaneus.[3] There is no distinct insertion point of the SPR; instead, it blends into the periosteum of the fibula.
- The anatomy of the fibula is varied as well. About 50% of fibulae have a bony ridge about 2 to 4 mm that augments the fibular sulcus.[2] A cadaveric study by Edwards[5] found that 82% of the time a sulcus was present at the posterior edge of the distal fibula. The average sulcus dimension was 3 mm deep and 6 mm wide. He found that 11% of the cadavers had no groove and that 7% of the cadavers had a convex fibula. A fibrocartilaginous rim was deficient in 48% of all cadavers and was absent in 30%.

PATHOGENESIS

- According to Zoellner and Clancy,[16] in acute injury, the peroneal tendons tend to dislocate anteriorly over the lateral malleolus in people who have an anatomic predisposition. The fibular groove that serves as the pulley for the tendons can be shallow or convex, and the SPR may be absent or lax. A low-lying PB muscle belly can also cause subluxation (**FIG 1**). In a study of the effect of a low-lying PB muscle belly, Geller et al[7] measured the location of the musculotendinous junction (MTJ) in 30 cadaveric specimens with respect to the fibula tip and peroneal tubercle, and also the width of the PB tendon.

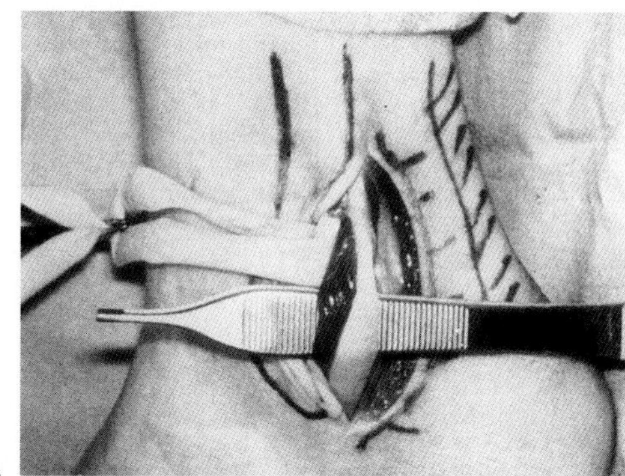

A

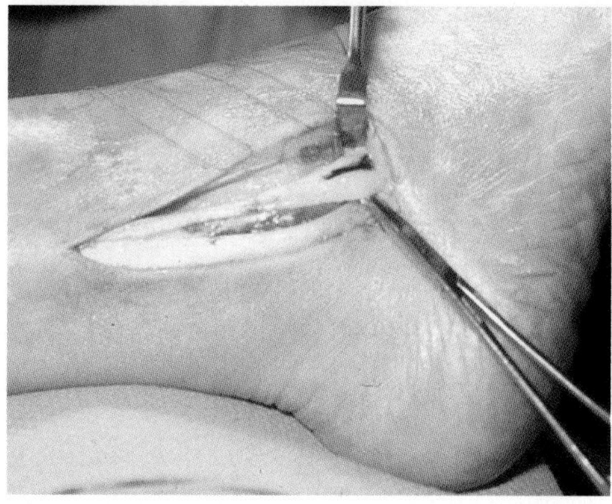

B

FIG 1 • **A, B.** Anatomic dissection of a peroneus muscle belly that is too distal. Note the distance to the fibular tip.

*Deceased

Table 1 **Low-lying Muscle Belly of PB and its Relationship to PB Tears**

Specimen Data	Average Distance To Fibula Tip (cm)	Average Distance Peroneal Tuberosity	Average Width (cm)
No tear (n = 26)	1.62 ± 1.38	3.39 ± 1.3	1.19 ± 0.37
Tear (n = 4)	0.04 ± 1.51	2.13 ± 0.83	1.44 ± 0.39

The PB MTJ was significantly more distal and the tendons had a significantly greater diameter in torn (4/30) versus untorn (26/30) specimens (Table 1). The authors suggested that the location of the peroneus brevis MTJ may have an influence on the development of degenerative tears.

- Recurrent dislocations are the result of an inciting acute traumatic episode of forceful ankle dorsiflexion with a simultaneous powerful contraction of the peroneal muscles that causes failure of the SPR. The dorsiflexion causes the SPR to tighten, thereby decreasing its diameter. This force is theorized to cause the retinaculum to be avulsed from its periosteal attachment. Eckert and Davis[4] stated that the SPR's attachment on the edge of the fibula does not adhere to a strong band of collagen, but instead blends into the periosteum of the lateral malleolus. They proposed that this weak insertion point is responsible for tendon dislocation secondary to avulsion of the fibular fibrocartilaginous lip and stripping of the SPR from the fibula.
- The prototypical mechanism is in skiers as they forcefully contract the peroneal muscles to grab the ski edge into the snow.
- Eckert and Davis[4] classified SPR injury into three different grades according to severity:
  - Normally, the peroneal tendons are contained within the fibular sulcus by the SPR.
  - Grade 1 injury: Separation of the retinaculum from the cartilaginous lip and the lateral malleolus
  - Grade 2 injury: The distal 1- to 2-cm dense fibrous lip is elevated along with the SPR.
  - Grade 3 injury: Avulsion of a thin fragment of bone along with the collagenous lip attached to the deep surface of the SPR and deep fascia. (Radiographically, this may be represented by a "fleck sign.")
  - In grade 1 injuries the peroneal tendons are easily reducible and are unstable under tension only.
  - In grade 2 and 3 injuries the peroneal tendons fail to remain reduced even without tension.

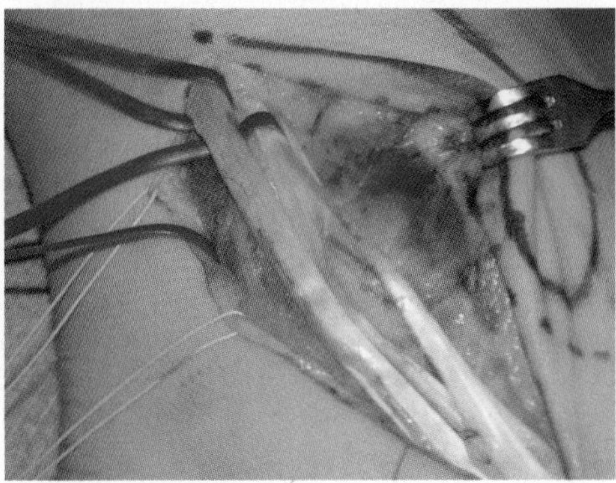

FIG 2 • The split peroneus brevis tendon, with the peroneus longus running more posterior.

NATURAL HISTORY

- Based on our experience, symptomatic recurrent subluxation does not resolve spontaneously.
- Often, peroneal tendon dislocation continues to be misdiagnosed as a chronic ankle sprain. As the tendons dislocate and relocate, direct tendon injury occurs due to repetitive trauma.
- Zone 1 tendon injuries occur at the fibular groove and usually involve the PB tendon. The action of the PB tendon snapping over the sharp ridge of the fibula leads to a longitudinal tear within the tendon substance (**FIG 2**).
- Zone 2 injuries occur distal to the fibular tip, usually affecting the PL tendon. These injuries are caused by the PL coursing over the lateral wall of the calcaneus and turning 45 degrees at the cuboid facet. As the tears propagate, an inflammatory response may lead to tenosynovitis, tendinopathy, and potential tendon rupture. Peroneal tendon subluxation and dislocation is thought to accentuate the symptoms.

PATIENT HISTORY AND PHYSICAL FINDINGS

- The patient may not be able to recall a traumatic event preceding the usual complaints of lateral ankle swelling and pain posterior to the lateral malleolus. Most patients report that the pain radiates proximally. Patients complain of persistent lateral ankle pain and swelling with a sensation of snapping or popping and may note a "pop" laterally before the tendon gives way.
- On physical examination, the lateral ankle will be swollen and tender and may be ecchymotic in the acute setting. This can easily be confused with a lateral ankle sprain (Table 2), but the location of the pain may be used to differentiate between the two. Tenderness posterior to the fibula is indicative of peroneal tendinopathy; in contrast, tenderness at the anterior distal fibula suggests an anterior talofibular ligament injury (ankle sprain). However, since the CFL is the floor of the

Table 2 **Clinical Differentiation of Ankle Subluxation from Ankle Sprain**

Signs and Symptoms	Subluxation	Sprain
Tenderness	Proximal to tip of fibula	Distal to tip of fibula
Swelling	Posterolateral	Anteroinferior
History	Snapping	Giving way
Worse on uneven ground?	Possible	Probable
Worse on circumduction?	Yes	No
Worse on flexion–inversion?	No	Yes

peroneal tendon sheath, there may still be some confusion with more severe ankle sprains. A negative anterior drawer test and pain experienced when the foot is stressed against resisted eversion are more indicative of an injury to the SPR.

- Peroneal tendon subluxation test: In the prone position, with the knee flexed to 90 degrees, ankle dorsiflexion and forced hindfoot eversion against resistance is performed. Apprehension and peroneal tendon subluxation or dislocation with this provocative maneuver typically confirms the diagnosis.[8]
- Acutely dislocated peroneal tendons are occasionally seen on physical examination, but more commonly the tendons are reduced upon presentation and are dislocated only with the peroneal tendon subluxation test.
- Likewise, chronic peroneal tendon subluxation or dislocation may not present with the tendons frankly dislocated. Chronic subluxation and dislocation are generally best diagnosed by testing the ankle through a range of motion of inversion and plantarflexion to maximum eversion and dorsiflexion with resistance.
- Peroneal compression test: Direct compression of the peroneal tendon sheath to identify peroneal tendon injury

IMAGING AND OTHER DIAGNOSTIC STUDIES

- Standard weight-bearing ankle radiographs (AP, lateral, and mortise) define the bony ankle anatomy alignment. In cases of peroneal tendon subluxation, radiographs are usually negative. In a grade 3 injury a "fleck" of bone can be seen off the posterior distal fibula and is considered pathognomonic of an SPR injury (**FIG 3**).
- MRI affords detail of the soft tissues. Injury to the SPR, the peroneal tendons, or other supporting tissues may be identified: anomalous structures such as the peroneus quartus or a low-lying PB muscle belly may be suggested (**FIG 4**). A MRI is useful for preoperative planning, as other pathology (PB tear, low-lying MJT, fibular sulcus) may also need to be surgically addressed concomitant with repair of the subluxation or dislocating peroneal tendons. We also use MRI to define the morphology of the fibular sulcus. While MRI may identify dislocated or subluxated peroneal tendons, the tendons are often reduced while the patient is relaxed in the MRI scanner; however, occasionally dislocated tendons may be identified on axial MRI views.

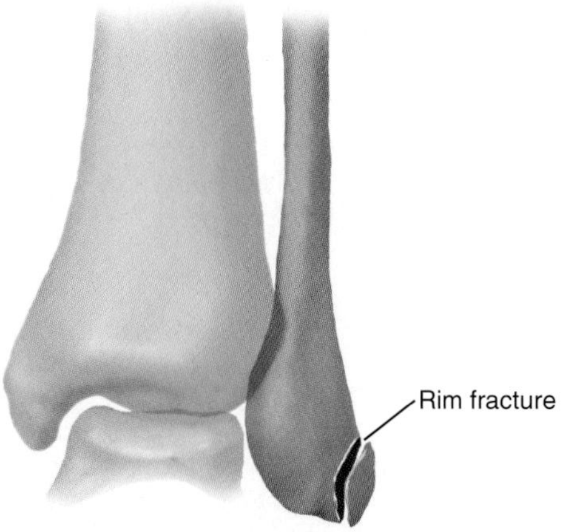

FIG 3 • "Fleck" sign on a radiograph. The best view to see this on is the mortise view.

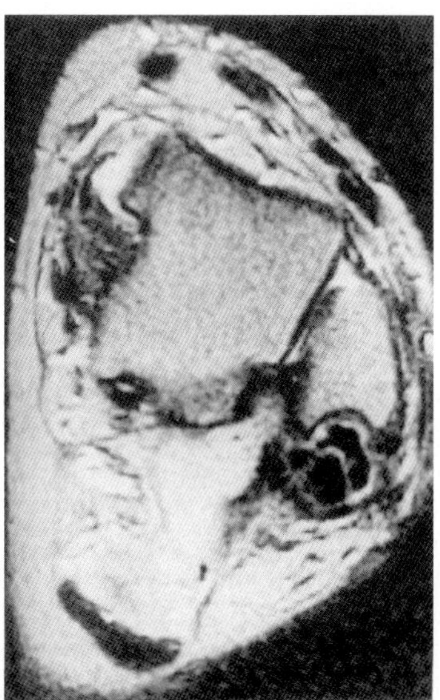

FIG 4 • An MRI in the axial plane demonstrating the peroneus brevis tendon splitting over the cartilage lip of the fibula.

- CT scan is rarely indicated in preoperative planning of dislocated peroneal tendons.

DIFFERENTIAL DIAGNOSIS

- Injury to the lateral ligament complex
- Fracture of lateral malleolus, lateral process of the talus, anterior process of the calcaneus, or fracture at the base of the fifth metatarsal
- Osteochondral defect on the talar dome
- Peroneal tendon pathology

NONOPERATIVE MANAGEMENT

- Initial treatment of an acute injury consists of a well-molded, short-leg cast for 6 weeks. Successful outcomes of nonoperative management range from 14% in a study by Eckert and Davis[4] to up to 56% as reported by McClennan,[9] while other investigators have also reported variable outcomes in small case series.[6,10,11,14] At best, only half of all patients become better. Therefore, as part of initial injury counseling, it is necessary to inform the patient that an operation will still be necessary, in most instances, despite conservative treatment. For patients with chronic subluxation, nonoperative treatment has not been shown to help; usually pain and symptoms recur once the short-leg cast is removed. In addition, more athletic, higher-demand patients tend to demand more reliable treatment and wish to proceed with operative repair.

SURGICAL MANAGEMENT

- Illustrated here is a modified surgical technique for soft tissue augmentation representing an alternative procedure for the treatment of peroneal tendon subluxation. No absolute contraindications exist for the procedure, but relative contraindications include:
  - The presence of a previous fracture or surgery that alters the local morphology and tissue quality
  - An Eckert and Davis grade 3 fracture, with a thin fragment of bone along the cartilaginous lip attached to the deep surface of the peroneal retinaculum; the anterior portion of

the SPR is already compromised and would not make a good surgical candidate.

- Patients with collagen disorders (Marfan, Ehlers-Danlos), where the strength and integrity of the periosteal flap could be suspect

Preoperative Planning

- Routine ankle radiographs are essential to identify or rule out a rim fracture of the distal fibula, which occurs in 15% to 50% of all cases of peroneal subluxation.[1]
- Typically, the ankle radiographs appear normal. We routinely obtain an MRI to identify potential peroneal tendon tears, other soft tissue anomalies such as a peroneus quartus, or other causes of lateral ankle pain and instability that need to be addressed concomitant to SPR augmentation.[13]
- MRI axial cuts define the morphology of the fibular sulcus and are helpful in staging a bony procedure if necessary during the superior retinaculoplasty.

Positioning

- Either general or regional anesthesia is acceptable for this procedure, and the surgeon's preference determines which anesthetic method to use.
- The patient is placed in an oblique lateral position using a beanbag or large support under the ipsilateral hip. Adequate rotation of the limb facilitates access to the posterior fibula.
- We routinely use a thigh tourniquet and carefully pad all bony prominences.
- An examination under anesthesia with provocative maneuvers such as the anterior drawer and rotary subluxation test may identify associated instability and locking or popping of the unstable peroneal tendons.

Approach

- The standard lateral approach is used.
- Care should be taken not to injure the sural nerve.

TECHNIQUES

SUPERIOR PERONEAL RETINACULOPLASTY

- We use a standard lateral incision along the course of the peroneal tendons, taking care not to injure the sural nerve.
- Carry the incision down to the level of the peroneal tendon sheath (**TECH FIG 1A**).
- Inspect the SPR. Usually, it is attenuated and deficient, especially along its anterior border. The retinaculum often is lifted off its fibular attachment, thus allowing the peroneal tendons to subluxate.
- Make an incision in the peroneal sheath along the posterior border of the fibula.

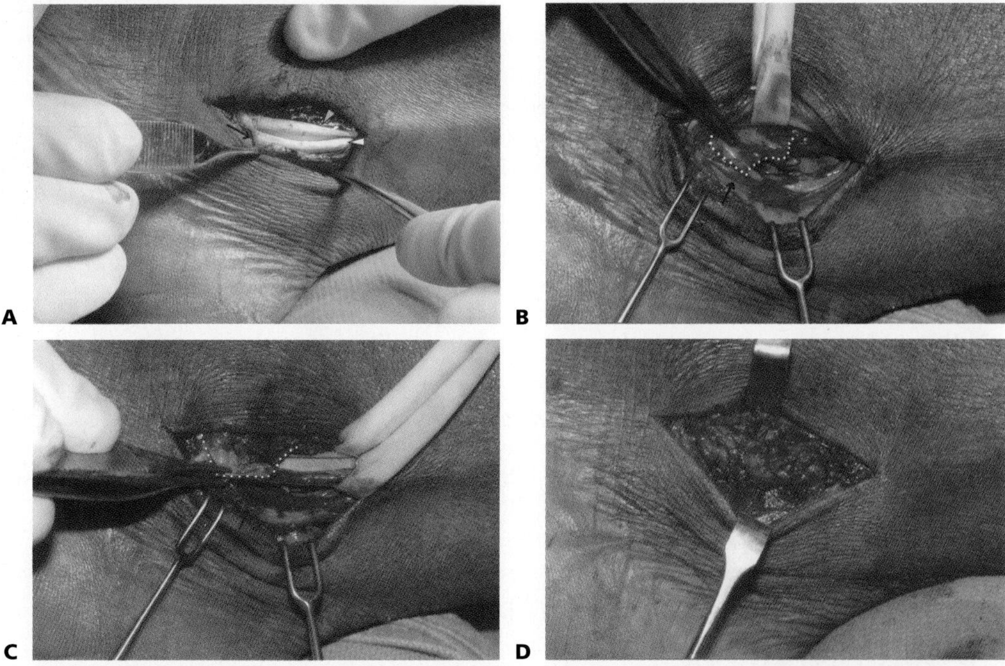

TECH FIG 1 • A. Intraoperative photograph of a left ankle (lateral approach) shows the peroneal tendons subluxing anteriorly (brevis is the *gray arrow*, longus is the *white arrow*, superior peroneal retinaculum [SPR] is the *black arrow*). **B.** The peroneal tendons have been retracted anteriorly by the Penrose drain. Elevation of an anterior-based periosteal flap (outlined by *dots*) from the fibular groove has been completed. The *black arrow* shows the remnant of the SPR posteriorly. **C.** The tendons are relocated, after a groove-deepening procedure, into the recreated groove. The *white dots* outline the anteriorly based periosteal flap. It is then brought over to the posterior remnant of the SPR (*black arrow*). **D.** The flap is sutured to the remnant SPR with nonabsorbable sutures, completing the superior peroneal retinaculoplasty.

- Retract the peroneal tendons anteriorly (**TECH FIG 1B**).
- Occasionally, a small tear may be noticed in the PB tendon, warranting débridement or repair.
- If a shallow or convex fibular groove is present, we typically perform a groove-deepening procedure.
- We routinely reinforce the SPR with a soft tissue periosteal flap elevated from the fibular groove from a posterior to anterior direction.
- Raise the periosteal flap, measuring about 1.0 × 3.0 cm, sharply, from posterior to anterior. After the flap is raised, a groove-deepening procedure may be performed when indicated.
- Use a burr to deepen the groove 6 to 9 mm with all raw bony edges. The groove should extend from the fibular tip to 5 cm proximal. We use bone wax to smooth the groove.
- Reduce the peroneal tendons and use the periosteal flap to contain the tendons, with the visceral side of the periosteum facing the tendons (**TECH FIG 1C**).
- Suture the flap to the posterior remnant of the SPR with a series of 3-0 polybraided nonabsorbable sutures (**TECH FIG 1D**).
- Range the ankle to evaluate the soft tissue repair, being sure that the tendons are free to move within the reconstructed peroneal tendon sheath.
- Close the skin in usual fashion, and place the leg into appropriate dressings and splints with compressive bandages.

DETAILED SURGICAL TECHNIQUE (COURTESY OF MARK E. EASLEY, MD, AND JAMES K. DEORIO, MD)

Positioning and Approach

- Patient positioned in lateral decubitus position
- Regional anesthesia
- Thigh tourniquet
- Posterolateral approach
  - Immediately posterior to posterior margin of the distal fibula
  - Expose SPR.
  - Protect sural nerve.
  - Release SPR 1 to 2 mm posterior from posterior fibular margin.
    - Peroneal tendons will be dislocated, so determining exactly where to release SPR will be distorted.
  - Chronically dislocated tendon may be located in a "pocket" lateral to the distal fibula (**TECH FIG 2**).
  - Inspect the tendons, particularly the more anterior peroneus brevis, for a tear.
    - Peroneal tendon dislocations predispose the tendons to longitudinal split tears as the tendon repeatedly subluxates around the posterolateral fibula.

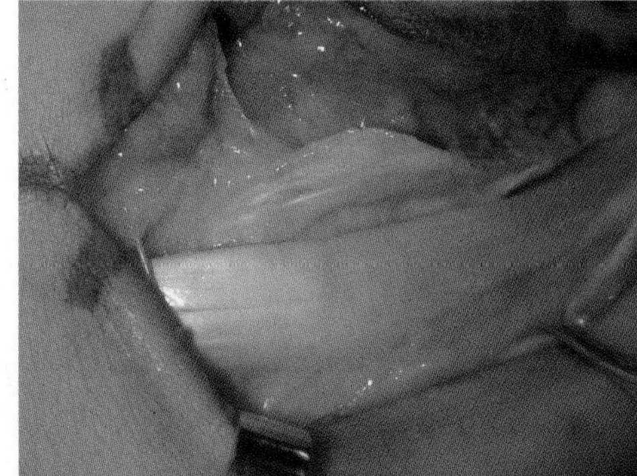

A

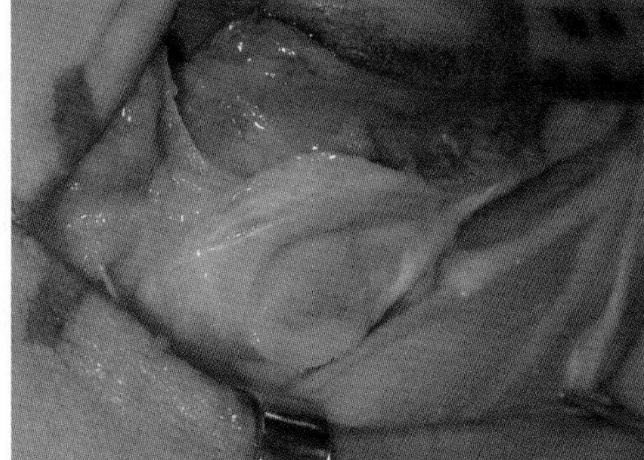

B

TECH FIG 2 • Chronically dislocated peroneal tendons. **A.** Tendons in a pseudogroove on the lateral fibula. **B.** With peroneal tendons reduced, a "new gliding surface" and pocket of displaced superior peroneal retinaculum is evident.

TRADITIONAL GROOVE-DEEPENING PROCEDURE ("TRAP DOOR TECHNIQUE")

- Creating the "trap door" in the posterior distal fibula
  - Maintain the peroneal tendons dislocated anteriorly to protect them during the fibular groove deepening.
  - Using a microsagittal saw, weaken the posterior cortex within the fibular groove (**TECH FIG 3A**).
  - While the fibula may be weakened only on the posterolateral margin, it is often necessary to weaken the "hinge" on the posteromedial margin as well (**TECH FIG 3B**).
  - The fibular groove also needs to be weakened transversely, at the proximal margin of the trap door (**TECH FIG 3C**).
  - Next, the trap door is completed at its distal margin, where the fibular groove rounds the distal fibula (**TECH FIG 3D**).

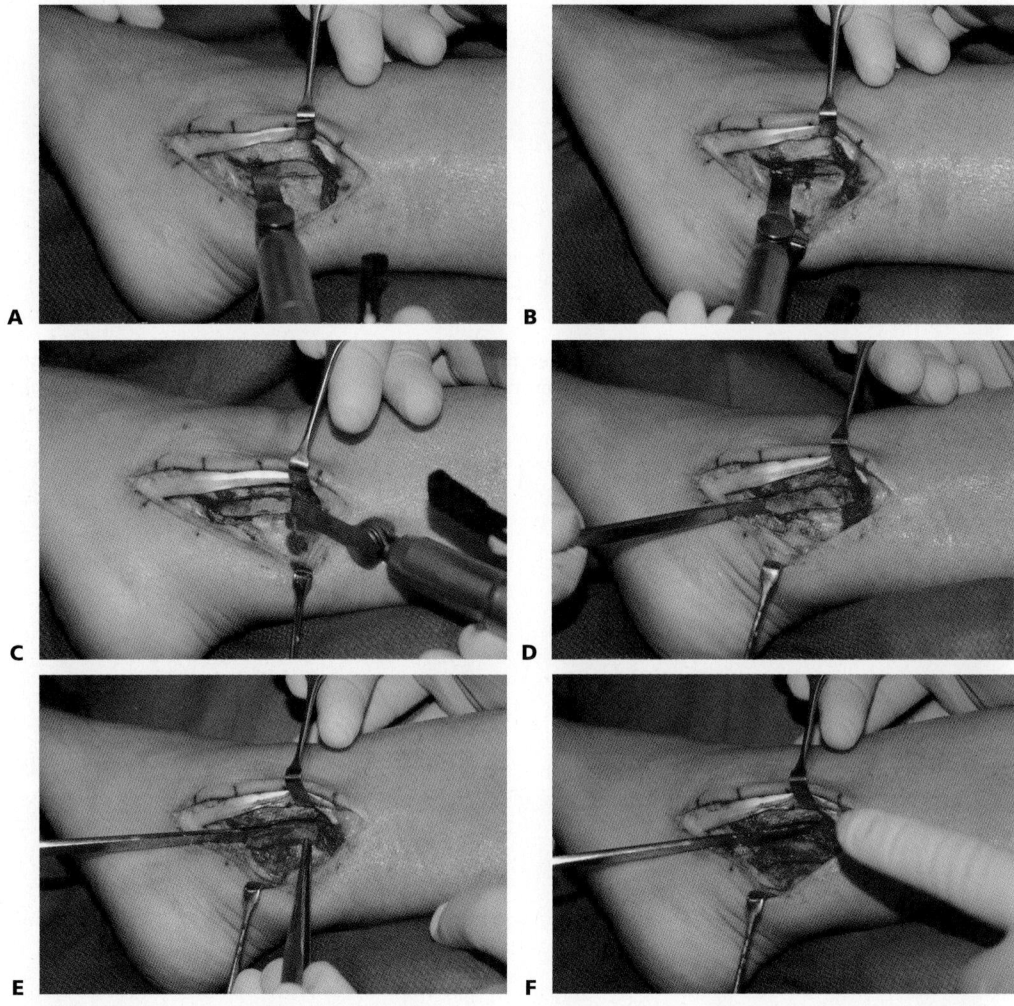

TECH FIG 3 • **A.** Weakening the posterolateral aspect of the fibula to create the "trap door." **B.** Weakening the hinge of the trap door. **C.** Transverse osteotomy to ensure that the trap door can open. **D–F.** Elevating the trap door. **D.** Osteotome introduced into distal posterior fibula. **E.** Posterior fibula elevated at its posteromedial hinge. **F.** Trap door completely open.

  - Elevate the trap door and reflect it posteriorly on its hinge (**TECH FIG 3E,F**). If the hinge should be separated completely, it is not a problem.
- Decancellate the distal fibula. We typically use a high-speed burr to evacuate the cancellous bone from the distal fibula (**TECH FIG 4**), but a curette may also be used.
- Replace the "trap door" into the deepened fibular groove.

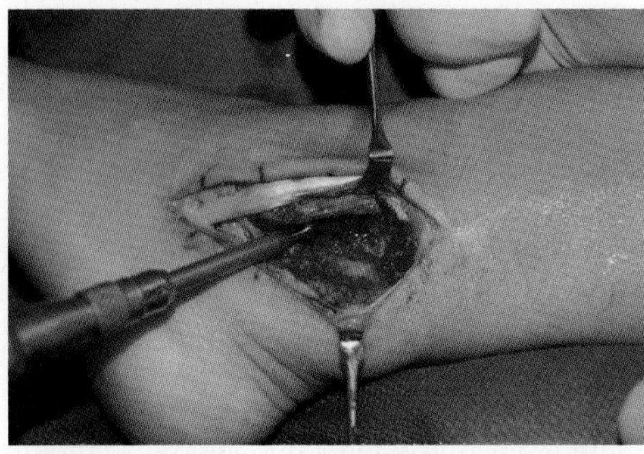

TECH FIG 4 • High-speed burr is used to remove cancellous bone from distal fibula.

  - Impact the posterior fibular bone that was elevated, but try to preserve the smooth surface so that the peroneal tendons have a smooth gliding surface with little risk of impingement or creation of adhesions (**TECH FIG 5A**).
  - The groove should be deep enough to keep the peroneal tendons reduced without manually restricting them (**TECH FIG 5B**). If it is not, then further decancellation may be necessary.
- Repair the SPR.
  - With the tendons reduced, repair the SPR by advancing the intact leading edge of the SPR from its posterior position to the posterolateral rim of the distal fibula from which the SPR was displaced by the tendon dislocation and elevated for the surgical exposure (**TECH FIG 6A**).
  - We routinely create drill holes in the distal posterolateral fibula to anchor the SPR (**TECH FIG 6B**).
- Be sure that the tendons glide well within the new fibular groove and are not stenosed by the repair (**TECH FIG 6C,D**).
- Standard closure

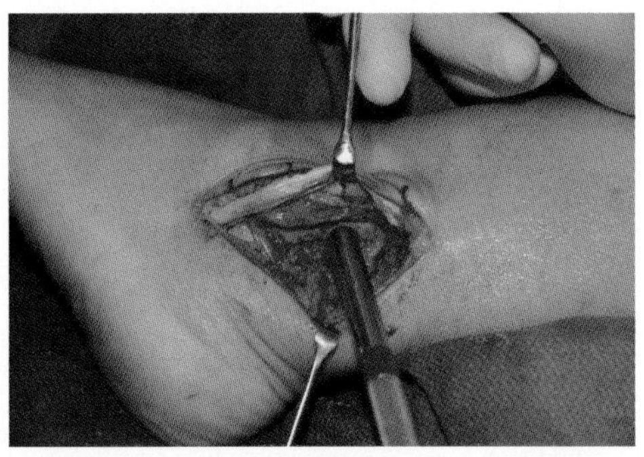

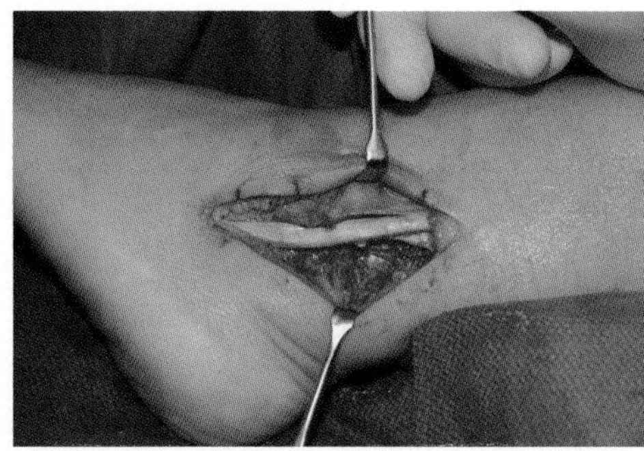

TECH FIG 5 • A. Trap door reduced in deepened fibular groove, with impactor being used to recess the bone and deepen the groove maximally. **B.** Peroneal tendons remaining reduced, even without repair of the superior peroneal retinaculum.

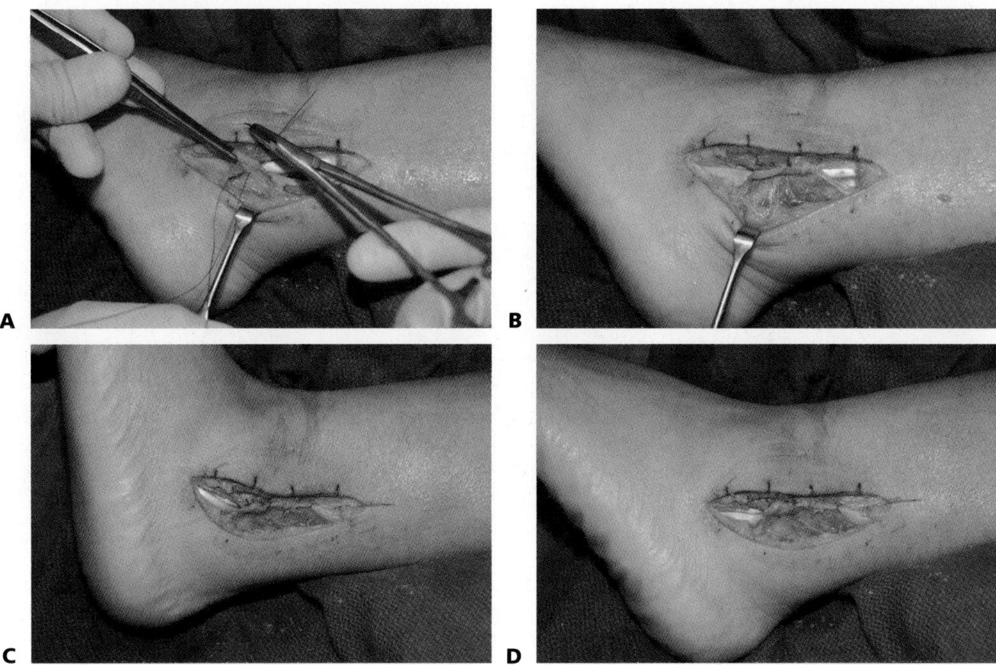

TECH FIG 6 • A, B. Superior peroneal retinaculum (SPR) repair to posterior fibula. **A.** Sutures to the posterolateral fibula to advance the SPR. **B.** Drill holes used to anchor SPR to posterolateral fibula. **C, D.** Peroneal tendons gliding without being stenosed within new fibular groove. **C.** Dorsiflexion. **D.** Plantarflexion.

MODIFIED TECHNIQUE USING A LARGE-DIAMETER DRILL BIT (AS DESCRIBED BY ROBERT B. ANDERSON, MD)

- Chronically dislocated peroneal tendons may create a new pocket and even gliding surface on the lateral fibula (**TECH FIG 7**).
- Protect the dislocated tendons and adjacent soft tissues from the drill bit.
- From the distal fibular tip, introduce progressively larger-diameter drill bits to weaken the distal fibula and ream away the distal fibular cancellous bone (**TECH FIG 8**).
- While simple impaction of the posterior fibula to deepen the groove is possible at this point, we prefer to first weaken the cortex with a microsagittal saw as described for the traditional fibular groove-deepening procedure (**TECH FIG 9A**).
- To protect the smooth surface on the posterior fibula, a tamp can be placed longitudinally in the groove and impacted so as to avoid disruption of the smooth gliding surface for the peroneal tendons (**TECH FIG 9B**).
- The peroneal tendons should remain reduced without manually restraining them (**TECH FIG 10A**). If not, then deepen the groove further with a larger-diameter drill bit and perform further impaction of the posterior fibular surface.
- Reattach the SPR to the posterolateral fibular margin via drill holes.
- Be sure the peroneal tendons glide well without restriction in the deeper fibular groove (**TECH FIG 10B**).
- Standard closure

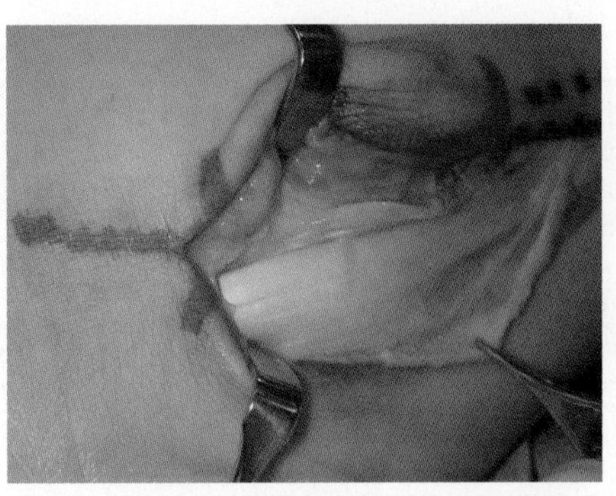

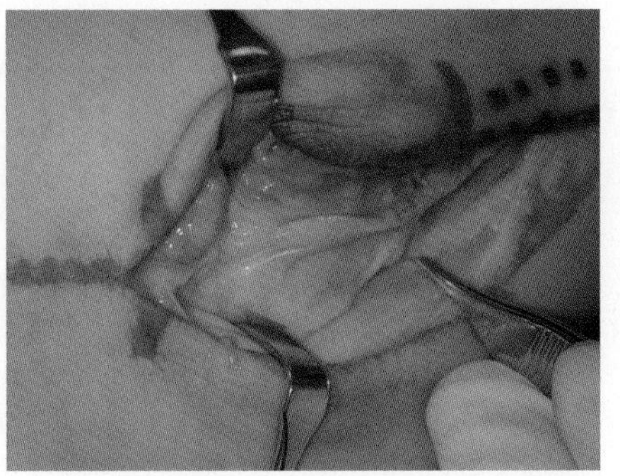

TECH FIG 7 • Pseudogroove created on lateral fibula. **A.** Peroneal tendons lateral to fibula. **B.** With tendons reduced, the pseudogroove is visible, with the displaced and attenuated superior peroneal retinaculum.

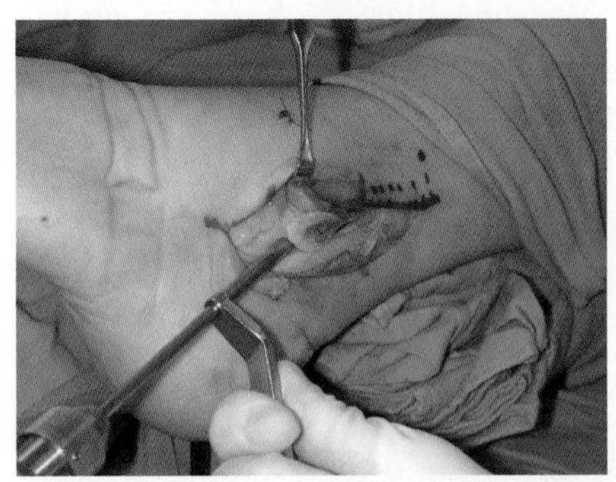

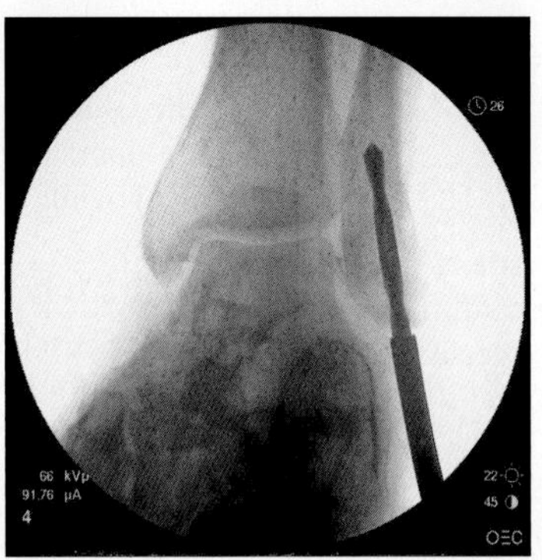

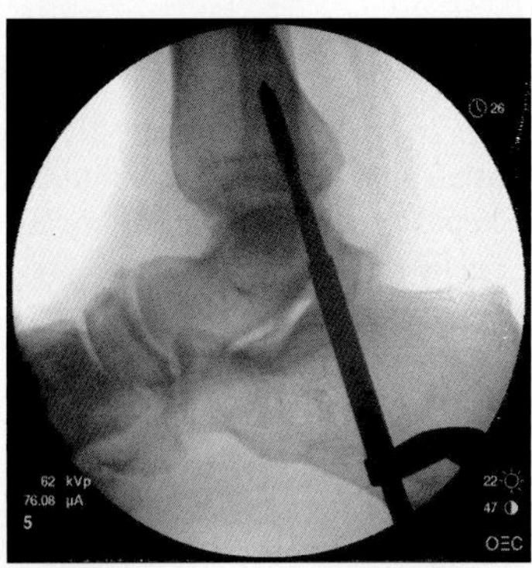

TECH FIG 8 • A. Drill bit introduced to decancellate the distal fibula. **B, C.** Fluoroscopic confirmation of proper drill bit position in distal fibula. **B.** AP view. **C.** Lateral view.

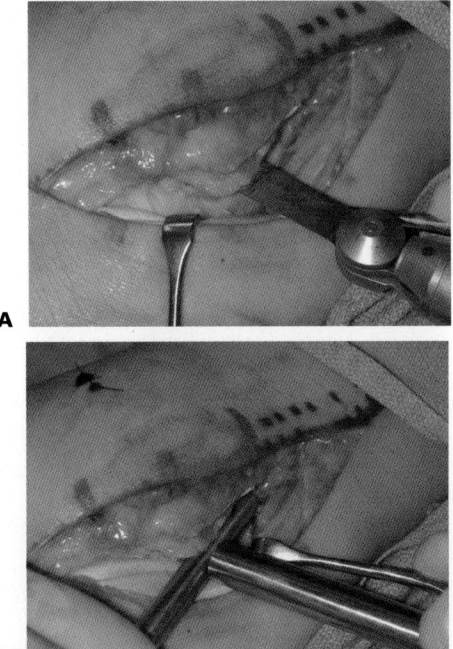

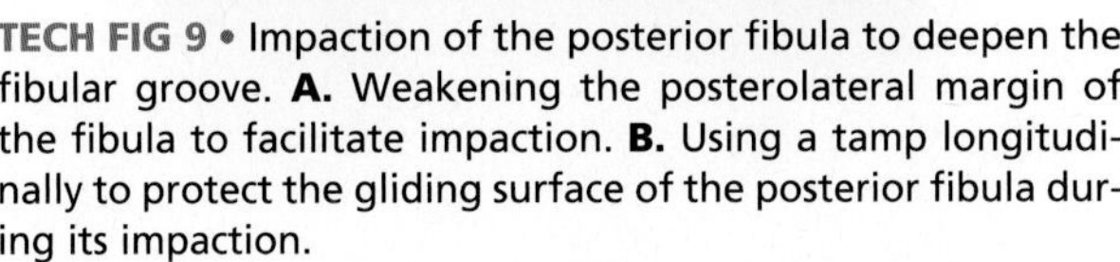

TECH FIG 9 • Impaction of the posterior fibula to deepen the fibular groove. **A.** Weakening the posterolateral margin of the fibula to facilitate impaction. **B.** Using a tamp longitudinally to protect the gliding surface of the posterior fibula during its impaction.

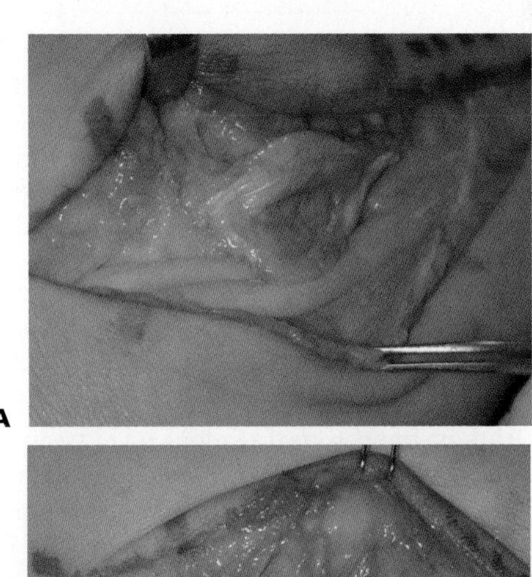

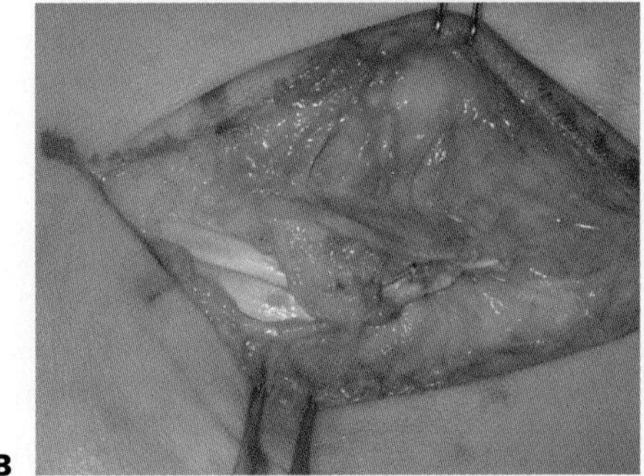

TECH FIG 10 • A. Peroneal tendons remaining reduced in the deepened fibular groove, even without superior peroneal retinaculum (SPR) repair. **B.** SPR repaired without stenosis of the peroneal tendons.

PEARLS AND PITFALLS

Harvest of periosteal flap	■ The peroneal tendons must be retracted anteriorly to allow visualization of the flap donor site to ensure sufficient harvest and to avoid damage to the peroneal tendons. ■ The flap should maintain its continuity, anteriorly, with the fibrocartilage ridge. Use of a no. 69 Beaver blade is critical for flap elevation. ■ The flap should be elevated before any groove-deepening procedure. If the groove is deepened before this, the periosteum will be destroyed.
Flap-to-tendon adhesions	■ No issues with tendon-to-flap adhesions have been reported; nonetheless, early range of motion starting at 4 weeks minimizes any chance of adhesions developing.
Peroneal tendon tears	■ Tears in the tendons need to be débrided and repaired or reconstructed. Successful peroneal tendon reduction with persistent symptoms secondary to peroneal tendon tears may lead to a poor outcome.
Avoid overtightening the peroneal tendon sheath reconstruction.	■ This will lead to stenosing flexor tenosynovitis. Overtightening is unnecessary; the tendons simply need to remain reduced.

POSTOPERATIVE CARE

- Postoperatively, the patient is immobilized in a short-leg cast and is kept non–weight-bearing for a total of 6 weeks.
- After 4 weeks the cast is removed and the patient is given a removable stiff-ankle rocker-bottom boot and remains non–weight-bearing for an additional 2 weeks while beginning physical therapy with ankle range-of-motion exercises.
- At the end of 6 weeks the patient is progressed to weight bearing as tolerated in the brace, after which the patient is weaned from the stiff-ankle boot and is started with ankle strengthening with inversion and eversion exercises.

OUTCOMES

- A favorable outcome of the procedure depends not only on how well the surgical procedure is performed but also on the appropriate treatment of other associated conditions. Often tendon injuries coexist with subluxation and dislocation and must be treated simultaneously. If tendon pathology such as a tear or degeneration is present and left untreated, pain may persist after surgery no matter how well the surgery was performed.
- In a preliminary study by Tan et al.[15] conducted at two centers (University of Pennsylvania and University of Medicine and Dentistry of New Jersey), 10 patients with subluxation or dislocation of the peroneal tendons were treated with this technique. Nine of 10 patients had good to excellent results. One patient required a groove-deepening procedure.

COMPLICATIONS

- Peroneal tendon adhesions: Early range-of-motion exercises starting at 4 weeks can minimize this complication.
- Stenosing flexor tenosynovitis: Overtightening of the peroneal tendon sheath is unnecessary; the tendons simply need to remain reduced posterior to the fibula.
- Sural and superficial peroneal nerve injury

The editor and coauthors of this chapter wish to acknowledge the contribution of Dr. Enyi Okereke. Dr. Okereke passed away while on a medical mission to Enugu, Nigeria.

REFERENCES

1. Church CC. Radiographic diagnosis of acute peroneal tendon dislocation. AJR Am J Roentgenol 1977;129:1065–1068.
2. Clanton TO, Porter DA. Primary care of foot and ankle injuries in the athlete. Clin Sports Med 1997;16:435–466.
3. Davis WH, Sobel M, Deland J, et al. The superior peroneal retinaculum: an anatomic study. Foot Ankle Int 1994;15:271–275.
4. Eckert WR, Davis EA Jr. Acute rupture of the peroneal retinaculum. J Bone Joint Surg Am 1976;58A:670–672.
5. Edwards ME. The relations of the peroneal tendons to the fibula, calcaneus, and cuboideum. Am J Anat 1928;42:213–253.
6. Escalas F, Figueras JM, Merino JA. Dislocation of the peroneal tendons: long-term results of surgical treatment. J Bone Joint Surg Am 1980;62A:451–453.
7. Geller J, Lin S, Cordas D, et al. Relationship of a low-lying muscle belly to tears of the peroneus brevis tendon. Am J Orthop (Belle Mead NJ) 2003;32:541–544.
8. Magee DJ. Lower leg, ankle, and foot. In: Orthopedic Physical Assessment, enhanced edition. St. Louis: Saunders Elsevier, 2006:765–845.
9. McLennan JG. Treatment of acute and chronic luxations of the peroneal tendons. Am J Sports Med 1980;8:432–436.
10. Oden RR. Tendon injuries about the ankle resulting from skiing. Clin Orthop Relat Res 1987;216:63–69.
11. Sarmiento A, Wolf M. Subluxation of peroneal tendons: case treated by rerouting tendons under calcaneofibular ligament. J Bone Joint Surg Am 1975;57A:115–116.
12. Sarrafian SK. Biomechanics of the subtalar joint complex. Clin Orthop Relat Res 1993;290:17–26.
13. Sobel M, Bohne WH, Markisz JA. Cadaver correlation of peroneal tendon changes with magnetic resonance imaging. Foot Ankle 1991;11:384–388.
14. Stover CN, Bryan DR. Traumatic dislocation of the peroneal tendons. Am J Surg 1962;103:180–186.
15. Tan V, Lin SS, Okereke E. Superior peroneal retinaculoplasty: a surgical technique for peroneal subluxation. Clin Orthop Relat Res 2003;410:320–325.
16. Zoellner G, Clancy W Jr. Recurrent dislocation of the peroneal tendon. J Bone Joint Surg Am 1979;61A:292–294.

Chapter 124 Repair of Dislocating Peroneal Tendons: Perspective 2

Florian Nickisch, Scott B. Shawen, and Robert B. Anderson

DEFINITION

- Peroneal tendon subluxation or dislocation from the retrofibular groove is a rare cause of ankle pain and disability. The acute injury often remains unrecognized or is misdiagnosed as an ankle sprain.
- Untreated or misdiagnosed acute injury predisposes a patient to recurrent peroneal dislocation, potential peroneal tendon tear, or chronic dislocation.

ANATOMY

- The peroneus longus and brevis muscles are the two major structures within the lateral compartment of the leg, both arising from the proximal fibula (**FIG 1**).
- Both structures become tendinous before crossing the ankle joint and remain in a common sheath. As they course distally the tendon of the peroneus brevis lies against the posterior surface of the distal fibula, anterior and medial to the tendon of the peroneus longus.
- Distal to the fibula each tendon enters a distinct tendon sheath, separated by the peroneal tubercle.
- Posterior to the distal fibula both tendons are stabilized in the retrofibular groove by the superior peroneal retinaculum (SPR) (**FIG 2**).
- The posterior surface of the distal fibula is covered by a layer of fibrocartilage to allow smooth gliding of the peroneal tendons. The depth and width of the retrofibular (peroneal) groove is highly variable. A definite groove is present in about 80%. In the remaining cases the posterior surface of the fibula is flat or convex.[5] A fibrocartilage rim on the lateral border of the fibula that adds an additional 2 to 4 mm to the depth of the sulcus is often present.
- The SPR, the primary restraint to peroneal instability, is composed of a band of the deep fascia that is continuous with the periosteum of the distal fibula but does not attach to the fibrocartilage rim or the posterolateral edge of the bone.[11] It is extremely variable in width and thickness, and five distinct insertional patterns have been described, the most common being a band to both the Achilles tendon and the calcaneus.[3]
- The fiber orientation of the SPR is parallel to those of the calcaneofibular ligament, and therefore inversion injuries of the calcaneofibular ligament may also cause injury to the SPR.[6,10]

PATHOGENESIS

- Acute subluxation or dislocation of the peroneal tendons usually occurs while the foot is forcefully dorsiflexed with the peroneal muscles strongly contracted; it commonly occurs during a forward fall in Alpine skiing or in springboard diving.[8]
- Resisted plantarflexion and inversion while the peroneals contract may also cause subluxation or dislocation of the peroneal tendons, and in this case it is commonly associated with lateral instability of the ankle.

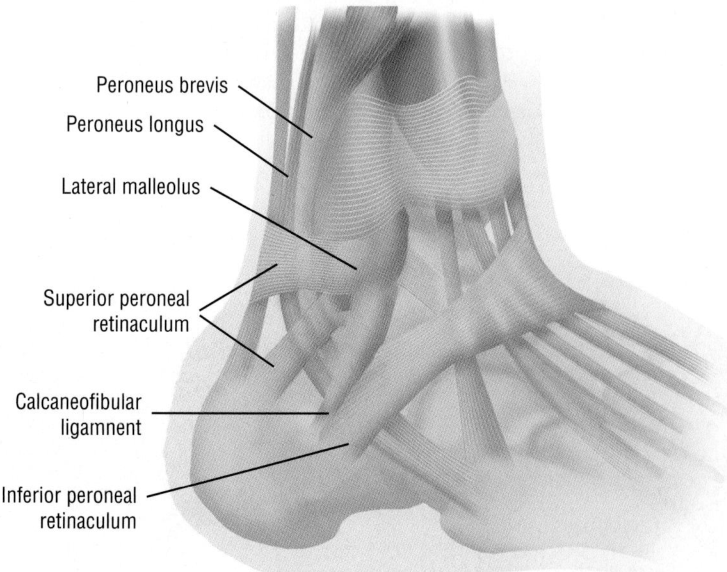

FIG 1 • Lateral view of the ankle showing the peroneal tendons as well as the superior and inferior peroneal retinacula. Note the vertical orientation of a portion of the superior peroneal retinaculum that corresponds to the orientation of the calcaneofibular ligament. (From Davis WH, Sobel M, Deland J, et al. The superior peroneal retinaculum: an anatomic study. Foot Ankle Int 1994;15:273.)

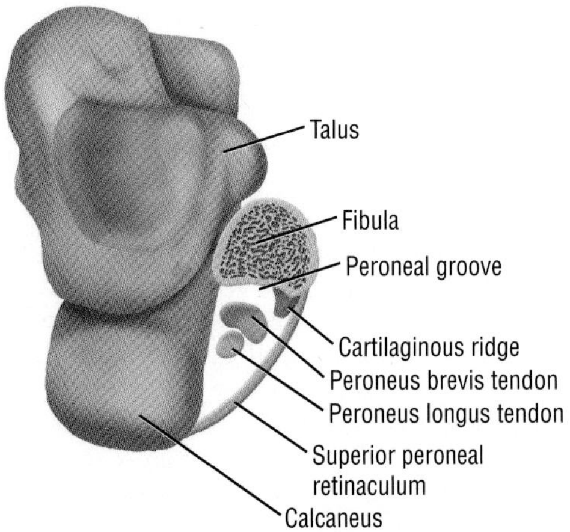

FIG 2 • Superior view of the ankle region shows the relationship of the fibular groove, superior peroneal retinaculum, peroneal tendons, and cartilaginous ridge. (From Coughlin MJ, Mann RA, eds. Surgery of the Foot and Ankle, 7th ed. St. Louis, MO: Mosby, 1999, p. 819.)

- Peroneal dislocation may also occur as a sequela to severe calcaneal fractures with lateral displacement of the calcaneus.[5,7]
- Peroneal dislocations can be classified into three grades depending on the pathoanatomy of the injury[4] (**FIG 3**).
- As a result of subluxation or dislocation, inherent injuries to the tendons can occur. Depending on the location of the tendon injury they are divided into zone I, II, and III.
  - Zone I injuries are defined as those involving the fibular groove and most often affect the peroneus brevis tendon. As the tendons sublux in the groove, the brevis is forced onto the sharp posterolateral bony ridge of the distal fibula, causing a longitudinal split in the tendon from the strain of a 45-degree course change as well as compression by the overlying longus tendon.
  - Zone II injuries are located between the tip of the fibula and the cuboid tunnel.
  - Zone III injuries are located in the cuboid tunnel and primarily involve the peroneus longus tendon and possibly a painful os peroneum.

NATURAL HISTORY

- If diagnosed early, in acute peroneal dislocation the tendons can be manually reduced and held in a reduced position for a 4- to 6-week period of immobilization. In this situation, functional rehabilitation leads to maintenance of tendon reduction and complete recovery in about 50% of cases.[1]
- With delayed diagnosis and treatment, recurrent subluxation and chronic dislocation is common and may lead to degeneration and tearing of the peroneal tendons.[9]

PATIENT HISTORY AND PHYSICAL FINDINGS

- Most patients present well beyond the acute phase complaining of vague posterolateral ankle pain that radiates proximally with or without a popping sensation during activity.[12]
- There may be a history of forced dorsiflexion trauma associated with a pop on the lateral aspect of the ankle.
- Often a history of an inversion–supination sprain and possible lateral ankle instability is reported.[10]
- On physical examination peroneal tendinopathy is characterized as fullness along the tendons with diffuse tenderness. Localized tenderness over the posterior ridge of the fibula should raise suspicion for progression of the injury to a peroneal tendon split tear.
- Pain may be elicited with inversion stretch or active resisted eversion.
- Tendon subluxation typically presents as snapping or popping and pain with eversion against resistance. The peroneal tunnel compression test consists of having the patient perform this motion while palpating the posterior border of the fibula. Circumduction of the ankle may demonstrate dislocation of the tendons with eversion and dorsiflexion and spontaneous relocation with plantarflexion and inversion (**FIG 4**).
- Chronic dislocation of the tendons is characterized by a palpable ridge over the lateral distal fibula often associated with chronic swelling.
- Eversion strength may be limited by pain. Significant weakness of active eversion without much pain should raise suspicion for a complete tear of the peroneal tendons.

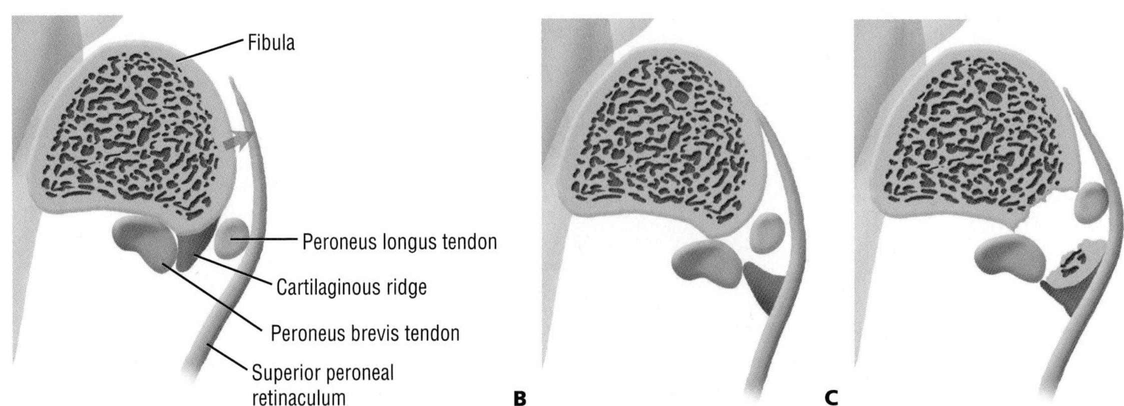

FIG 3 • Classification by Eckert and Davis of peroneal tendon subluxation/dislocation. **A.** Grade I: superior peroneal retinaculum (SPR) stripped off fibula; peroneus longus dislocated anteriorly. **B.** Grade II: fibrous rim avulsed from posterolateral aspect of fibula along with SPR; peroneus longus dislocated anteriorly. **C.** Grade III: bony rim avulsion fracture attached to SPR with anterior dislocation of peroneus longus. (From Coughlin MJ, Mann RA, eds. Surgery of the Foot and Ankle, 7th ed. St. Louis, MO: Mosby, 1999, p. 821, modified from Eckert WR, Davis EAJ. Acute rupture of the peroneal retinaculum. J Bone Joint Surg Am 1976;58A:670–672.)

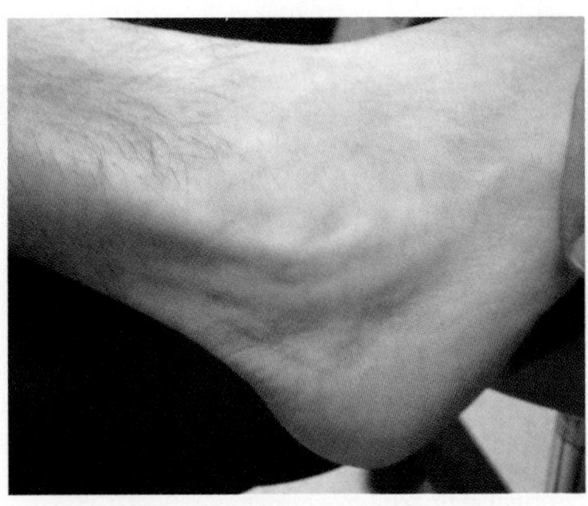

FIG 4 • Dislocated peroneal tendons during resisted eversion.

- A complete examination of the ankle should also include evaluation of associated injuries ruling out differential diagnoses. This includes (but is not limited to) the following:
  - Lateral ankle instability: history of frequent sprains, cavovarus foot, increased laxity with anterior drawer or inversion stress test compared to the contralateral side
  - High ankle sprain (syndesmotic sprain): pain over anterior ankle syndesmosis, pain with provocative maneuvers (calf squeeze test, external rotation stress test)
  - Painful os trigonum or posterior talar process fracture: pain with forced plantarflexion, pain with resisted plantarflexion of the great toe

IMAGING AND OTHER DIAGNOSTIC STUDIES

- Plain radiographs including AP, mortise, and lateral views of the ankle should be obtained to rule out fracture or large osteochondral defects of the talus.
- Occasionally a "fleck" sign, an avulsion fracture off the posterior distal fibula, can be seen on AP or mortise views. If present this is considered pathognomonic for a grade III injury to the SPR with peroneal dislocation.[4] As shown in **FIGURE 5A**, this may be difficult to see without the use of a "hot lamp."
- Stress views may be helpful to rule out lateral ankle instability.
- CT may be helpful in uncertain diagnosis to evaluate the anatomy of the fibular groove and detect small avulsion fractures, which may be difficult to see on plain films[2] (**FIG 5B**). Axial CT scan images may also confirm peroneal tendon dislocation.
- MRI can identify injury to the SPR, subluxated or dislocated tendons, and intrasubstance degeneration and split tears of the tendons (**FIG 6**).
- Ultrasound, while operator-dependent, allows a dynamic, real-time examination to evaluate subluxation during provocative maneuvers.

DIFFERENTIAL DIAGNOSIS

- Peroneal tendinopathy or tears
- Lateral ankle instability
- High ankle sprain
- Osteochondral defect of the talus
- Painful os trigonum or posterior talar process fracture
- Retrocalcaneal bursitis

NONOPERATIVE MANAGEMENT

- Acute peroneal subluxation or dislocation can be treated nonoperatively if the peroneal tendons can be reduced and held in a reduced position.
- In this case treatment consists of short-leg cast immobilization in slight plantarflexion and inversion for 4 to 6 weeks, followed by functional rehabilitation. U- or J-shaped foam or felt pads can be placed in the cast to apply pressure around the distal fibula and maintain the position of the peroneal tendons.
- In our opinion, there is no role for nonoperative treatment for symptomatic chronic peroneal dislocation or recurrent subluxation.

SURGICAL MANAGEMENT

- All irreducible peroneal tendon dislocations and those associated with a rim avulsion fibular fracture should be considered for acute surgical reduction and repair.
- Operative treatment is also indicated for all chronic injuries in patients with pain or functional limitations.
- Five basic categories of repair have been described: (1) anatomic reattachment of the retinaculum, (2) bone block procedures, (3) reinforcement of the superior peroneal retinaculum with local tissue transfers, (4) rerouting of the tendons behind the calcaneofibular ligament, and (5) groove-deepening procedures.[8]
- The goal of groove-deepening procedures is to increase the height of the posterolateral fibular rim to prevent the peroneal tendons from subluxating.

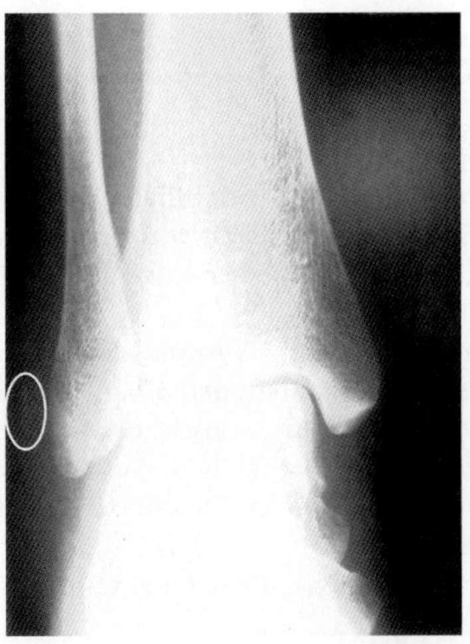

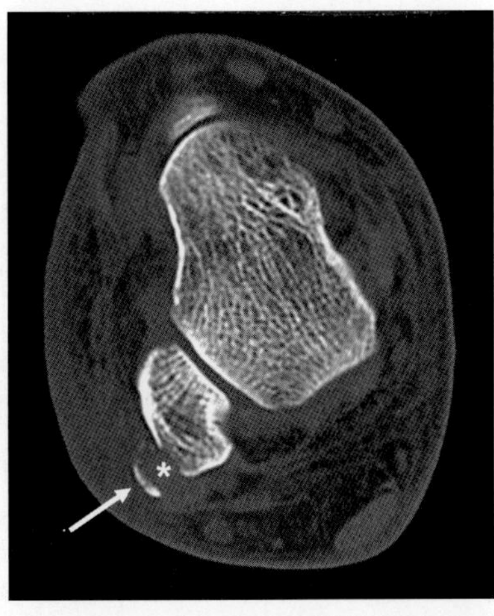

FIG 5 • **A.** AP radiograph of the ankle under a "hot lamp" showing a lateral rim fracture off the distal fibula (fleck sign, *circle*). **B.** Axial CT scan showing a grade III injury with an avulsion fracture of the lateral edge of the distal fibula (fleck sign, *arrow*) and dislocated peroneal tendon (*asterisk*).

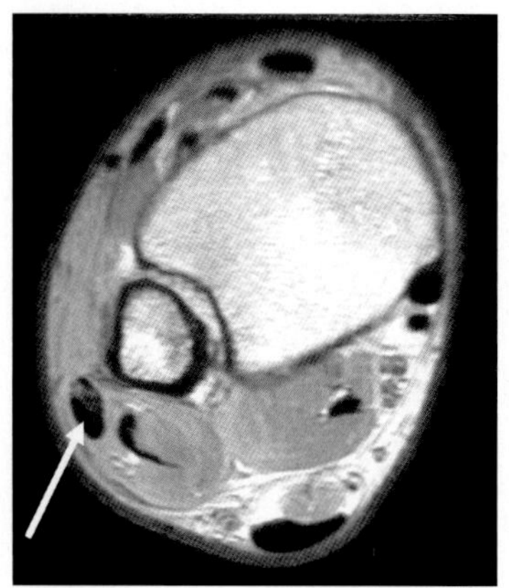

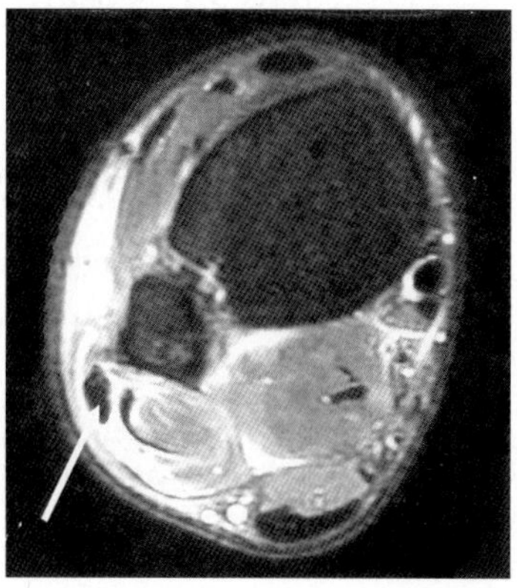

FIG 6 • T1-weighted (**A**) and T2-weighted (**B**) axial MRI images showing dislocated peroneal tendons (*arrow*) with abundant tenosynovitis. Note the shallow retrofibular groove and the torn superior peroneal retinaculum.

- General contraindications to surgical intervention include peripheral vascular disease, skin breakdown or vasculitis, and patients who are "voluntary" subluxators. These are usually patients with generalized ligamentous laxity. Physical examination usually shows the peroneal tendons to subluxate to the lateral rim of the fibular on both ankles, but not over it.

Preoperative Planning

- We recommend reviewing all imaging studies preoperatively to plan for not only fibular groove deepening but also any procedures to address associated pathology. Plain films should be reviewed for fractures, loose bodies, ankle and foot alignment, and the presence of any hardware (from previous procedures).
- Associated fractures, osteochondral lesions, and lateral ankle instability should be addressed concurrently.
- We routinely perform an examination under anesthesia on the operating table before making an incision to assess the ankle and subtalar joint. The peroneal tendons may also be assessed under anesthesia, but without the patient being able to evert against resistance, this is of limited value.

Positioning

- The procedure is performed with the patient in the semilateral position (**FIG 7**). A bean bag is used to maintain the position of the body with a 10-lb sandbag underneath the ipsilateral hip. This allows the physician to readily access the posterior fibula and obtain fluoroscopic AP and lateral ankle views of the ankle without moving the C-arm from the standard AP position. Regional or general anesthesia may be used and a thigh tourniquet is applied.

Approach

- The standard surgical approach is through a longitudinal, curvilinear incision on the posterior aspect of the fibular following the course of the peroneal tendons to roughly the level of the peroneal tubercle (Fig 7).
- This allows excellent visualization of the SPR, the peroneal tendons, and the posterior aspect of the distal fibula and also provides sufficient access to the lateral tibiotalar joint in cases where concomitant lateral ligament reconstruction is indicated.
- If lateral ankle instability and injury to the peroneal tendons distally have been ruled out preoperatively or with the examination under anesthesia, the approach can be limited to a longitudinal incision just posterior to the fibula.

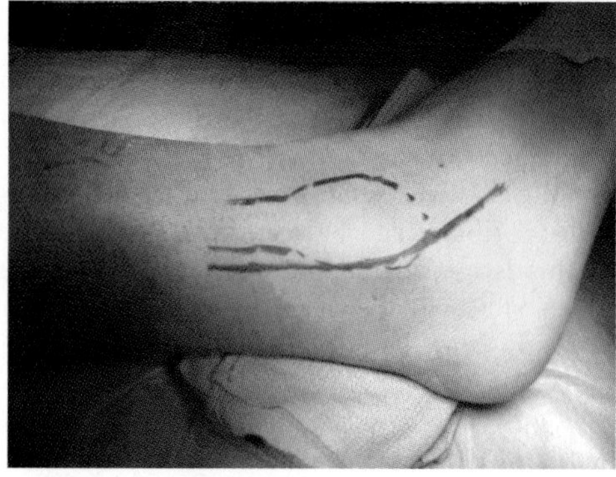

FIG 7 • Utilitarian posterolateral approach for peroneal repair and indirect fibular groove deepening.

TECHNIQUES

INDIRECT FIBULAR GROOVE DEEPENING

- Make a curvilinear incision along the posterior aspect of the distal fibula. It extends toward the base of the fifth metatarsal but usually ends at the level of the peroneal tubercle.
- Develop full-thickness skin flaps to avoid skin necrosis.
- Protect the sural nerve and branches of the superficial peroneal nerve.
- Incise the peroneal sheath distal to the fibula. If the SPR is still intact, incise it over the bone and then sharply elevate it off the fibula, leaving a cuff of tissue on the distal fibula. Retract the edges of the SPR posteriorly with two small hemostats to facilitate later repair.
- Inspect the peroneal tendons, excise inflamed tenosynovium, and débride and repair split tears in the tendons with buried nonabsorbable suture (**TECH FIG 1A,B**).
- Excise any low-lying peroneus brevis muscle from the tendon. Also excise a normal anatomic variant, the peroneus quartus, a supernumerary muscle of the lateral compartment of the leg, if present. These additional procedures tend to make room in the groove for the peroneal tendons (**TECH FIG 1C**).
- Expose the distal fibular tip, avoiding injury to the calcaneofibular ligament.

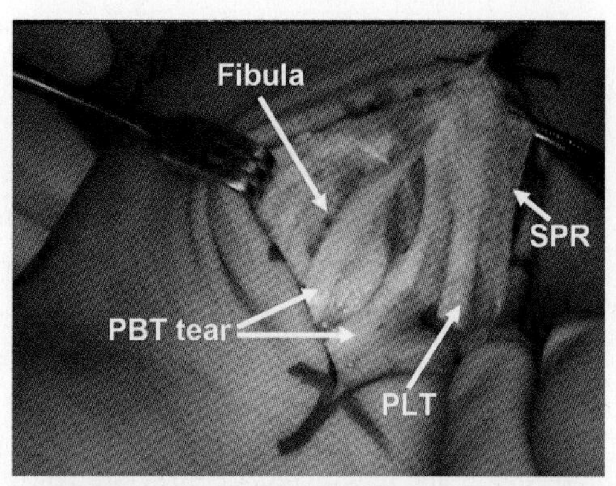

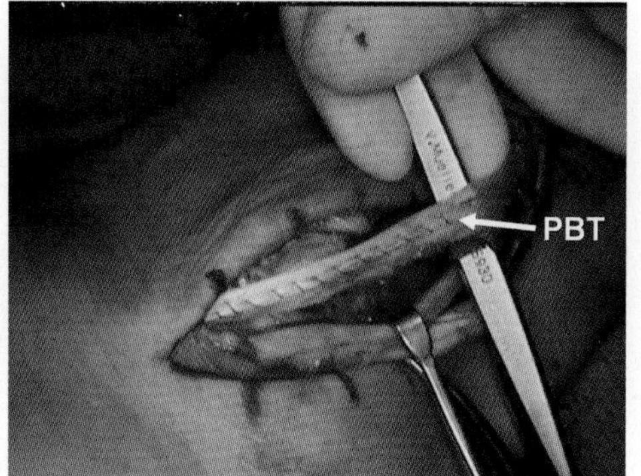

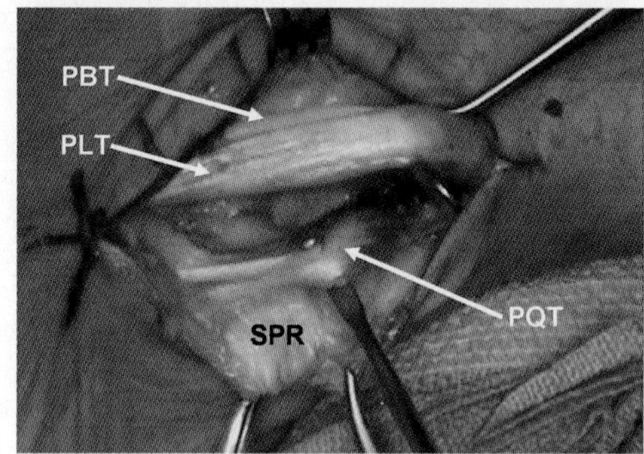

TECH FIG 1 • A. The superior peroneal retinaculum is incised longitudinally and retracted with two hemostats. A longitudinal split tear of the peroneus brevis tendon (PBT) is often identified in chronic dislocations. *PLT*, peroneus longus tendon. **B.** Split tears of the PBT are débrided or repaired. **C.** The low-lying peroneus brevis muscle and if present the peroneus quartus (PQT) are excised to create room for the peroneal tendons.

- Place an intramedullary guide pin from distal to proximal inside the fibula, in line with the posterior cortex (**TECH FIG 2A**). Thin the posterior cortex by sequential reaming over the guidewire (usually 7 to 8 mm) (**TECH FIGS 2B AND 3**). We routinely use suitably sized reamers from the biotenodesis screw system (Arthrex, Naples, FL) or any anterior cruciate ligament instrument set. Alternatively, consider using progressively larger drill bits from a standard trauma set or cannulated drills from a dedicated fifth metatarsal (Jones fracture) set (Wright Medical, Memphis, TN).

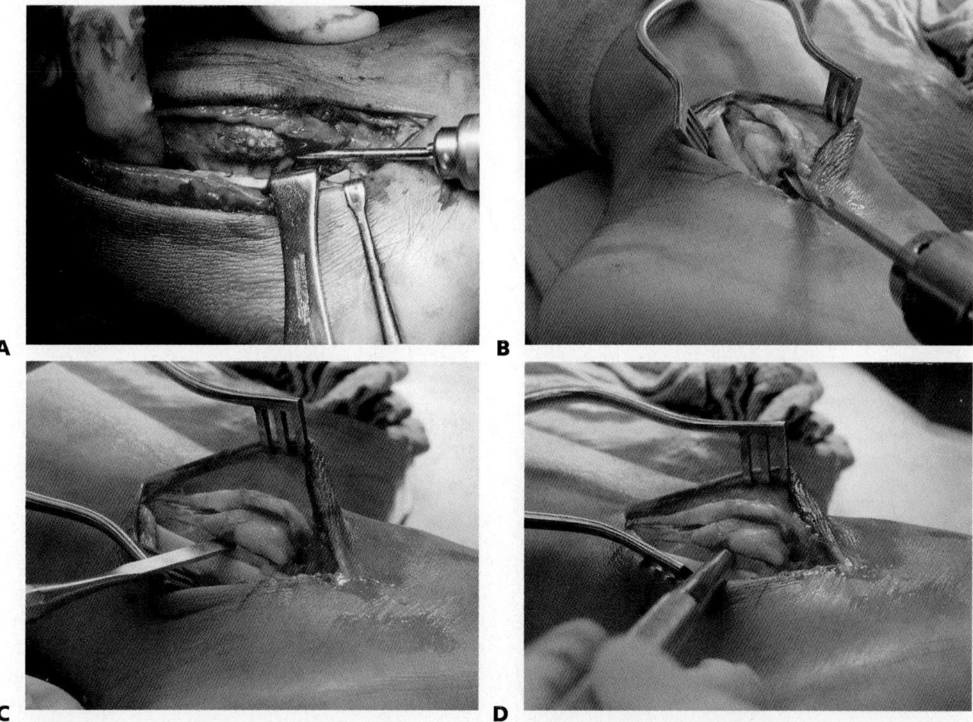

TECH FIG 2 • A. An intramedullary guide pin is placed into the distal fibula parallel to the posterior cortex. **B.** The posterior cortex of the fibula is thinned by intramedullary reaming with cannulated reamers over the guide pin. **C.** To avoid fracture of the edge of the fibula during impaction the posterolateral cortex is perforated with an osteotome (this is necessary only in very hard bone). **D.** The posterior cortex of the fibula is impacted into the void created by the reamers with an appropriate-size tamp.

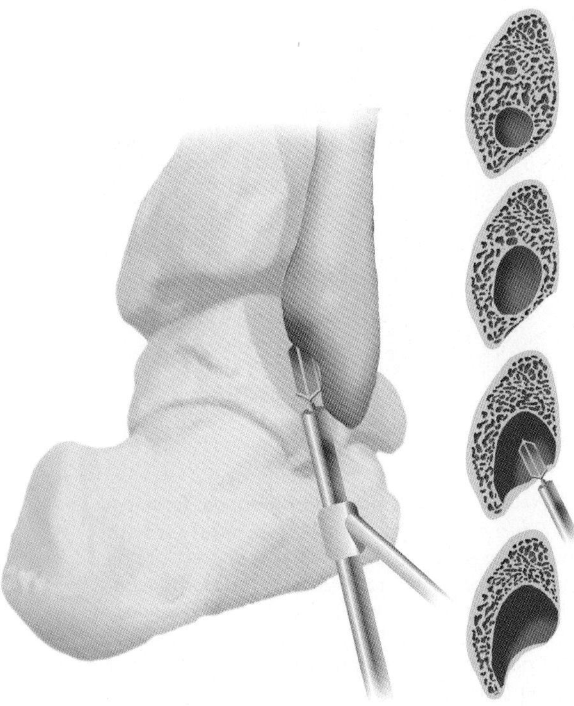

TECH FIG 3 • Schematic drawing of technique for indirect fibular groove deepening (original drawing by Robert B. Anderson).

- Once the posterior cortex is sufficiently thinned, impact it into the void created by the reamers using an appropriately sized bone tamp (TECH FIGS 2D AND 3). This preserves the physiologic gliding surface covering the groove, making it a smooth bed for tendon excursion. If the bone is very hard and impaction cannot be performed easily, the posterolateral cortex of the fibula can be perforated with an osteotome or microsagittal saw to facilitate impaction of the posterior cortex (TECH FIG 2C).
- Also tamp the very distal tip of the fibula inward to avoid a sharp edge that would otherwise impinge on the peroneal tendon as it courses into the foot.
- When done correctly the entire peroneus brevis and at least 50% of the peroneus longus tendon should be covered by the fibular rim with the tendons in a resting position.
- After completing groove deepening, tendon débridement, and tendon repair, repair the SPR.
- Sharply elevate the remainder of the cuff on the fibula off bone, exposing the lateral cortex, which is then roughened to bleeding bone with a rasp or rongeur.
- Excise any redundant SPR tissue and advance the remaining SPR to the previously prepared cortical bed; secure it through either drill holes or suture anchors.
- Place three or four drill holes or suture anchors about 1 cm apart proximally from the tip of the fibula (TECH FIG 4A). Reattach the posterior flap of the SPR to the prepared bone with 2-0 suture in a "pants-over-vest" technique, making sure that the space between the bony surface of the lateral malleolus and the SPR is obliterated. Suture the anterior portion of the retinaculum over the repair with interrupted 2-0 suture (TECH FIG 4B,C).
- Test the stability of the repair by ranging the ankle through a full range of motion. Verify free excursion of reduced tendons; the tendons should not be trapped by the repair. Overtightening of the SPR repair is not necessary; the goal is to keep the peroneal tendons reduced posterior to the fibula.

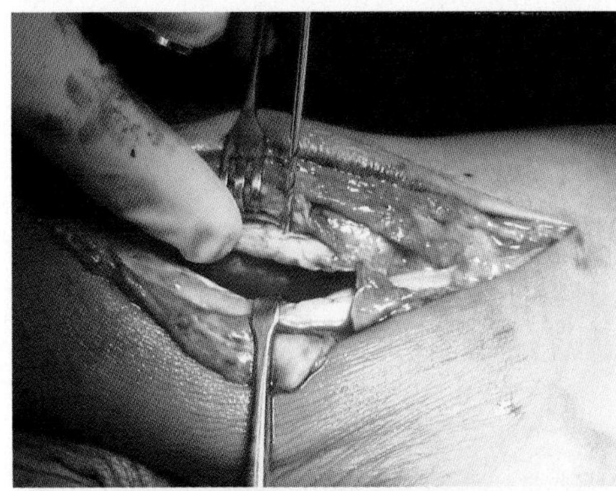

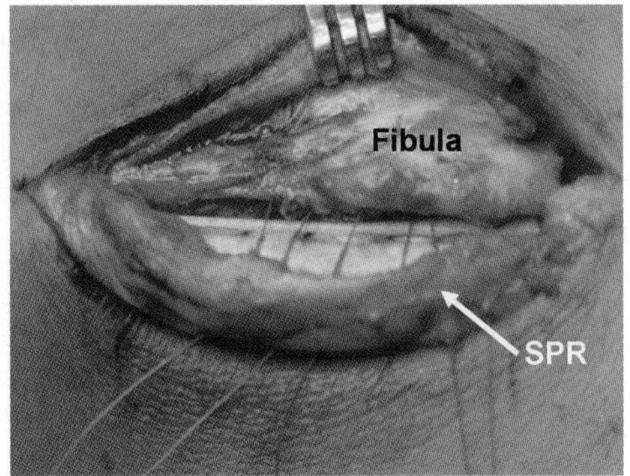

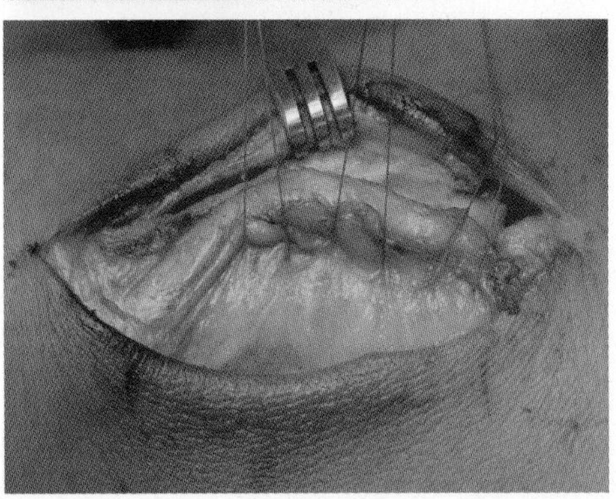

TECH FIG 4 • After deepening of the retrofibular groove the lateral cortex of the fibula is roughened with a rongeur or rasp and the superior peroneal retinaculum is repaired. **A.** Six drill holes are created in the posterolateral edge of the fibula (alternatively two or three suture anchors can be used). **B,C.** The superior peroneal retinaculum is then repaired to the distal fibula with 2-0 suture in a "pants-over-vest" fashion.

PEARLS AND PITFALLS

Avoid surgery on voluntary dislocators.	■ High risk of recurrence
Maintain the operated limb in a semilateral position (use a large bump under the ipsilateral hip or a bean bag).	■ It is difficult to gain access to the posterior aspect of the fibula with the patient in a supine position.
Incise the SPR on the posterior margin of the fibula, not too far posteriorly.	■ This allows excision of redundant tissue and a secure SPR repair to bone.
Create adequate room for the peroneal tendons.	■ Excise all low-lying peroneus brevis muscle and the entire peroneus quartus if present.
Inspect both peroneal tendons for tears.	■ Débride and repair as necessary.
Avoid fibular stress fracture.	■ Reaming the fibula may not weaken the posterior fibula adequately, particularly in young, healthy patients with good bone quality. Weaken the posterior fibular cortex with an osteotome or microsagittal saw before impaction to control the fibular groove deepening.
Avoid creating stenosis of the peroneal tendons when repairing the SPR.	■ Observe satisfactory tendon excursion with ankle and hindfoot range of motion after SPR repair.

POSTOPERATIVE CARE

- Immediately postoperatively the leg and ankle are placed into a posterior and U-splint in neutral position and the patient is kept non–weight-bearing for 2 weeks.
- Sutures are removed at 2 weeks. A short-leg walking cast is applied and the patient is allowed to bear weight as tolerated.
- At 6 weeks the cast is removed and a cam walker boot is applied to avoid ankle inversion, while allowing plantarflexion and dorsiflexion. Active range-of-motion exercises are initiated at that time.
- Peroneal strengthening is started at about 8 to 10 weeks after surgery.
- Full return to activities is expected between 4 and 6 months postoperatively.
- In elite athletes, given a stable reconstruction, we have been more aggressive with the rehabilitation, to include biking and pool activities by 4 weeks.

OUTCOMES

- As many variations of fibular groove-deepening techniques have been described, all reported results in the literature are derived from small retrospective series. There are no published prospective randomized studies comparing different surgical techniques.
- In general, results of fibular groove-deepening techniques have been good, as long as the underlying pathology is correctly addressed.[8]
- In our hands, indirect grooving has provided excellent overall results while minimizing the surgical dissection and morbidity. We have not had recurrent dislocations using this technique.
- We recommend that fibular groove deepening should be performed with every SPR reconstruction for chronic peroneal dislocation.

COMPLICATIONS

- Infection
- Delayed wound healing
- Sural nerve injury
- Recurrent dislocation
- Loss of motion

REFERENCES

1. Brage ME, Hansen ST Jr. Traumatic subluxation/dislocation of the peroneal tendons. Foot Ankle 1992;13:423–431.
2. Clanton TO, Porter DA. Primary care of foot and ankle injuries in the athlete. Clin Sports Med 1997;16:435–466.
3. Davis WH, Sobel M, Deland J, et al. The superior peroneal retinaculum: an anatomic study. Foot Ankle Int 1994;15:271–275.
4. Eckert WR, Davis EAJ. Acute rupture of the peroneal retinaculum. J Bone Joint Surg Am 1976;58A:670–672.
5. Edwards M. The relations of the peroneal tendons to the fibula, calcaneus, and cuboideum. Am J Anat 1927;42:213–252.
6. Geppert MJ, Sobel M, Bohne WH. Lateral ankle instability as a cause of superior peroneal retinacular laxity: an anatomic and biomechanical study of cadaveric feet. Foot Ankle 1993;14:330–334.
7. Karlsson J, Eriksson BI, Sward L. Recurrent dislocation of the peroneal tendons. Scand J Med Sci Sports 1996;6:242–246.
8. Maffulli N, Ferran NA, Oliva F, et al. Recurrent subluxation of the peroneal tendons. Am J Sports Med 2006;34:986–992.
9. McLennan JG. Treatment of acute and chronic luxations of the peroneal tendons. Am J Sports Med 1980;8:432–436.
10. McGarvey W, Clanton T. Peroneal tendon dislocations. Foot Ankle Clin 1996;1:325–342.
11. Niemi WJ, Savidakis J Jr, DeJesus JM. Peroneal subluxation: a comprehensive review of the literature with case presentations. J Foot Ankle Surg 1997;36:141–145.
12. Sammarco GJ. Peroneal tendon injuries. Orthop Clin North Am 1994;25:135–145.
13. Shawen SB, Anderson RB. Indirect groove deepening in the management of chronic peroneal tendon dislocation. Tech Foot Ankle Surg 2004;3(2):118–125.

Chapter 125 Reconstruction of Tibialis Anterior Tendon Ruptures

James Santangelo and Mark E. Easley

DEFINITION

- Tibialis anterior rupture may present as an acute injury or as a chronic painless foot drop.
- The diagnosis is often delayed.
- Recommended treatment is surgical for active patients and nonsurgical for low-demand patients. Surgical options include direct repair and reconstruction.

ANATOMY

- The tibialis anterior muscle originates from the lateral tibial condyle and interosseous membrane.
- Its insertion is the medial side of the medial cuneiform and the inferomedial base of the first metatarsal.
- The musculotendinous junction is at the junction of the middle and distal thirds of the tibia.
- The tendon courses within a synovial sheath from the musculotendinous junction to its insertion,[2] deep to the extensor retinaculum of the ankle and foot.
- Innervation is the deep peroneal nerve.
- The tibialis anterior muscle controls deceleration of the foot after heel strike and dorsiflexes the ankle.

PATHOGENESIS

- Younger individuals with healthy tibialis anterior tendons rarely suffer spontaneous rupture; instead, their mechanism of injury is laceration from penetrating trauma or distal tibia fracture.
- Spontaneous ruptures typically occur in older individuals with degenerative tendinopathy of the tibialis anterior tendon. Minor trauma may be associated with these ruptures, with a mechanism of plantarflexion–eversion. Ruptures typically occur within 3 cm of the tendon's insertion on the medial cuneiform.[1]

NATURAL HISTORY

- The natural history of tibialis anterior rupture is inferred from studies documenting the results of nonoperatively treated patients. These patients will ambulate with a slap-foot gait and sometimes have difficulty negotiating uneven terrain. Most patients are functional; however, they may require a brace.
- Nonoperatively treated patients tend to be older and lower-demand. The natural history for younger, more active patients may indicate less desirable results.
- Definite conclusions regarding the natural history of tibialis anterior ruptures are limited due to the low number of reported cases in the literature and lack of natural history studies.

PATIENT HISTORY AND PHYSICAL FINDINGS

- Physical examination methods include:
  - Examining for swelling. The examiner should palpate along the course of the tibialis anterior muscle–tendon. Swelling with discontinuity of the tendon indicates a tendon rupture. An anterior ankle mass may be the presenting complaint.
  - Gait disturbance. The examiner should observe the patient ambulating, looking for slap-foot gait or foot drop. Chronic ruptures may present with minimal gait disturbance; the patient may have difficulty ambulating only when on uneven surfaces. Inability to heel-walk indicates tibialis anterior dysfunction. The patient may need to hyperflex the hip and knee to clear the foot during the swing phase of gait, since the ankle does not dorsiflex adequately.
  - Muscle strength is evaluated with manual motor testing. No contraction or weak ankle dorsiflexion suggests tibialis anterior dysfunction. Patients will substitute the toe extensors for the tibialis anterior during ankle dorsiflexion, exhibiting toe hyperextension when asked to dorsiflex the ankle.
- The examiner should note any heel cord tightness. Subacute and chronic injuries often present with heel cord contractures, since the major antagonist to ankle plantarflexion is forfeited with tibialis anterior tendon rupture. As a rule, at least 10 degrees of ankle dorsiflexion must be present for a tibialis anterior repair or reconstruction, and thus surgical management may require adding Achilles tendon or gastrocnemius lengthening.
- The examiner should completely assess the involved extremity to rule out other diagnoses. The most common errors in diagnosis are:
  - Lumbar radiculopathy: presents with diminished sensation, positive straight-leg raise test
  - Peroneal nerve palsy: affects the toe extensors and peroneal musculature in addition to the tibialis anterior. Preservation of extensor hallucis longus and toe extensor function will distinguish tibialis anterior rupture from peroneal nerve palsy.[1]

IMAGING AND OTHER DIAGNOSTIC STUDIES

- Imaging studies are generally not required in the evaluation of tibialis anterior tendon ruptures, since the diagnosis is usually simple to make on clinical examination alone.
- Radiographs are nondiagnostic and rarely required in the evaluation of tibialis anterior tendon ruptures. Radiographs are, however, useful to assess associated injures (tibia fractures).
- MRI may be useful in chronic cases where patients do not recall a history of trauma.[1] MRI demonstrates lack of continuity in the tibialis anterior and signal change in the tendon, particularly with pre-existing tendinopathy. Because the tibialis anterior tendon courses from lateral to medial across the anterior ankle and retracts with rupture, occasionally it is difficult to assess.
- If there is uncertainty in the diagnosis, electrodiagnostic studies may identify common peroneal palsy or lumbar radiculopathy.

DIFFERENTIAL DIAGNOSIS

- Peroneal nerve palsy
- Lumbar radiculopathy
- Rarely, a peripheral neuropathy may present as isolated tibialis anterior tendon dysfunction.

NONOPERATIVE MANAGEMENT

- Low-demand patients may be treated with an ankle–foot orthosis (AFO).

SURGICAL MANAGEMENT

- Direct repair of the tendon is occasionally possible, but delay in diagnosis may preclude direct repair due to muscle contracture.
- A sliding tibialis anterior tendon grafting technique has been described to gain tendon length to allow repair, and allograft tendon transfers have been proposed in the absence of tibialis anterior myofibrosis.
- Our preferred reconstruction for tendons that cannot be directly repaired is to augment the repair with the adjacent, native extensor hallucis longus (EHL) tendon (**FIG 1**).

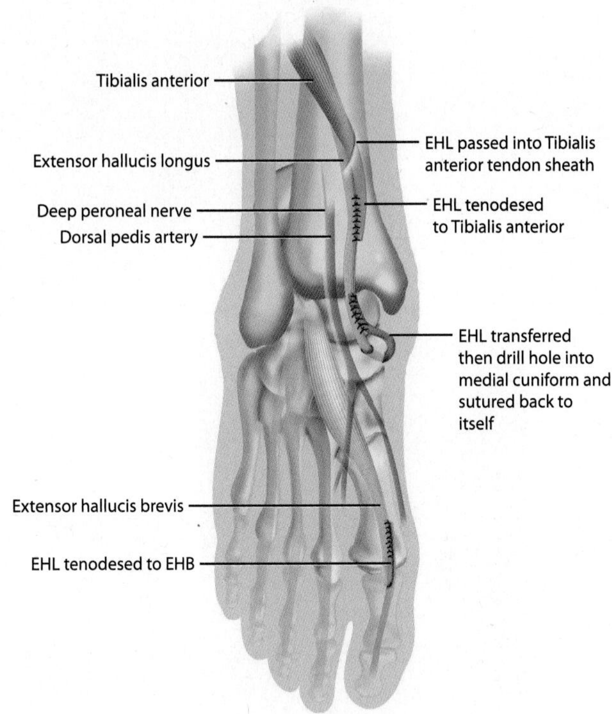

FIG 1 • Extensor hallucis longus transfer to medial cuneiform. The proximal end of the tibialis anterior tendon is tenodesed to the extensor hallucis longus. Distally, the extensor hallucis brevis is tenodesed to the extensor hallucis longus distal end to preserve hallux interphalangeal joint extension.

Preoperative Planning

- Imaging studies are reviewed when available to appreciate the extent of pre-existing tendinopathy and to potentially identify the approximate site of the rupture.
- The surgeon should prepare for Achilles tendon lengthening or gastrocnemius–soleus recession to achieve adequate (at least 10 degrees) dorsiflexion.

Positioning

- The patient is positioned supine. A bump may be placed under the ipsilateral hip, but this is typically not necessary since access is required only to the anteromedial ankle.

Approach

- An anterior approach is made directly over the course of the tibialis anterior tendon.
- As has been learned from total ankle arthroplasty and open reduction and internal fixation of tibial pilon fractures, careful soft tissue handling is essential.

EXTENSOR HALLUCIS LONGUS TRANSFER TO MEDIAL CUNEIFORM

- Perform gastrocnemius recession or Achilles tendon lengthening if indicated.
- Use an anterior approach with an incision over the course of the tibialis anterior tendon (**TECH FIG 1A,B**).
- Divide the superior and inferior extensor retinaculum and tibialis anterior sheath.
- Isolate the remnant of the tibialis anterior tendon. Occasionally direct repair is possible, rarely by advancing the residual tendon to bone, but instead to the residual tendon stump on the medial cuneiform. If inadequate tendon is available or muscle excursion is poor, then proceed with EHL transfer.
- Expose the EHL tendon. Proximally the EHL is in a separate sheath adjacent to the tibialis anterior.
- Through a separate 3- to 5-cm incision over the distal EHL immediately proximal to the first metatarsophalangeal joint, divide the EHL tendon distally. Leave enough distal stump to suture to the adjacent tendon of the extensor hallucis brevis. Place a whipstitch consisting of no. 2 nonabsorbable suture in the free end of the EHL.
- Pass the EHL under the skin bridge and through the tibialis anterior sheath proximally. The EHL will now occupy the previous sheath for the tibialis anterior (**TECH FIG 1C,D**).
- Drill a vertical hole in the medial cuneiform for attachment of the EHL. Sequentially drill using 2.5-mm, 3.5-mm, and 4.5-mm drill bits. Enlarge the hole with a

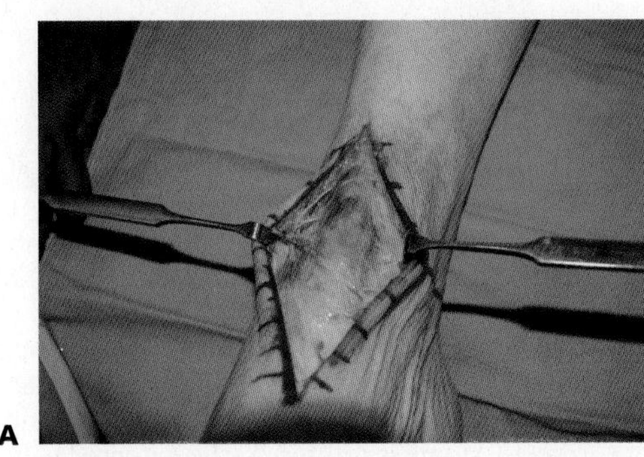

TECH FIG 1 • **A.** Anterior approach over tibialis anterior. *(continued)*

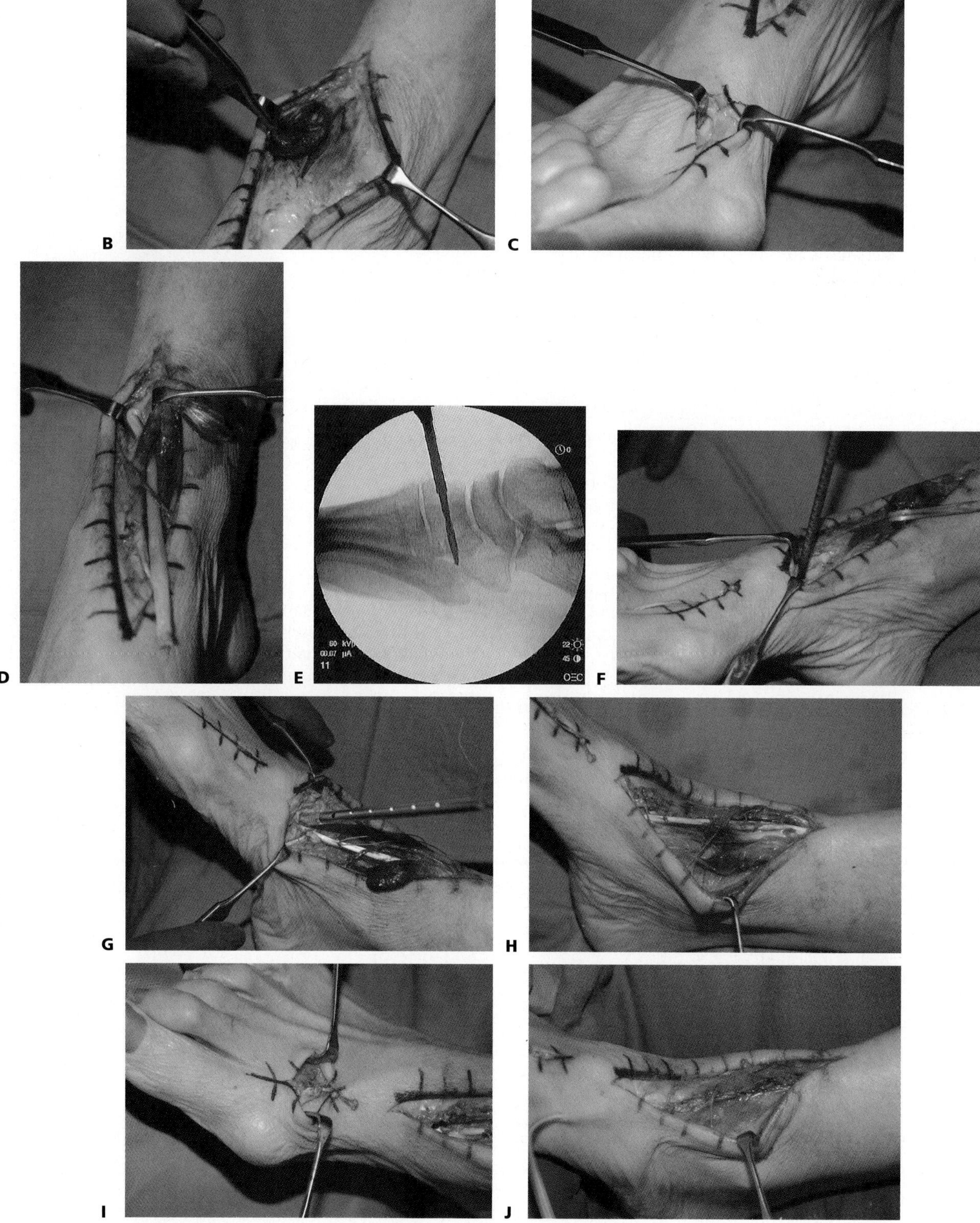

TECH FIG 1 • *(continued)* **B.** The tendon sheath is opened, exposing the torn retracted end of the tibialis anterior. The sheath is carefully preserved for later repair. **C.** The extensor hallucis longus (EHL) tendon is harvested by dividing it at the level of the metatarsophalangeal joint. **D.** The EHL tendon sheath is entered proximally. The EHL tendon is passed into the tibialis anterior sheath and pulled distally. **E.** A drill hole is placed from dorsal to plantar at the midpoint of the medial cuneiform. **F.** The drill hole is sequentially enlarged. **G.** Fixation using a biotenodesis screw (Arthrex, Naples, FL). The graft is also looped around the medial cuneiform and sutured to itself and surrounding soft tissue. **H.** Proximally, the EHL is tenodesed to the tibialis anterior stump. **I.** The EHL stump is sutured to the extensor hallucis brevis. **J.** The tibialis anterior sheath is closed.

curette as needed to allow graft passage. Leave enough periosteum to provide additional points of attachment for suturing the graft in place.

- Secure the graft with the ankle in 10 degrees of dorsiflexion (**TECH FIG 1E–H**).
- Pass the EHL graft from dorsal to plantar. Fixation may be accomplished with an interference screw or by looping the graft around the medial cuneiform and suturing it to surrounding periosteum and back on itself. The EHL tendon may be further anchored to the residual distal fibers of the torn tibialis anterior tendon.
- The transferred EHL tendon serves to bridge the gap created by the tibialis tendon rupture. However, the relative strength of the EHL muscle is far less than that of the tibialis anterior muscle. Therefore, in the absence of myofibrosis of the tibialis anterior, we recommend sewing the residual tibialis anterior tendon stump to the transferred EHL tendon under some tension.
- Attach the distal EHL stump to the extensor hallucis brevis, and we recommend dorsiflexing the hallux about 10 to 15 degrees to compensate for anticipated stretching of this tendon transfer postoperatively (**TECH FIG 1I**).
- Close the tibialis anterior tendon sheath, superior extensor retinaculum, and wound in layers (**TECH FIG 1J**).
- Place a splint or bivalved cast with the ankle in 10 degrees of dorsiflexion. Avoid plantarflexion as this places tension on the wound edges and tendon transfer.

PEARLS AND PITFALLS

Misdiagnosis	■ Perform a complete history and physical examination to rule out conditions that may mimic tibialis anterior rupture.
Failure to address heel cord tightness	■ Note ankle dorsiflexion as part of the preoperative evaluation and perform Achilles tendon lengthening or gastrocnemius recession as indicated.
Inadequate EHL graft length	■ Expose and divide the distal end of the EHL at the metatarsophalangeal joint level.
Wound breakdown	■ Carefully close the tibialis anterior sheath, superior extensor retinaculum, and subcutaneous tissue before skin closure. Immobilization in at least 5 degrees of dorsiflexion is important to avoid tension on the wound edges.
Graft failure	■ Secure fixation with proper use of an interference screw and adequate graft length to suture back on itself and surrounding tissues ■ Postoperative immobilization ■ Avoidance of early aggressive rehabilitation

POSTOPERATIVE CARE

- A short-leg cast is worn for 6 weeks, followed by an ankle–foot orthosis (AFO) for an additional 6 weeks.

OUTCOMES

- Sammarco et al[5] presented a series of 18 patients with acute and chronic tibialis anterior tendon ruptures managed with direct repair or interpositional graft. There was significant improvement in the average hindfoot score. The authors concluded that surgical repair of a ruptured tibialis anterior tendon can be beneficial regardless of age, sex, medical comorbidities, or delay in diagnosis.
- Ouzounian et al[4] reported on seven patients with tibialis anterior rupture treated with a variety of surgical reconstructive techniques. All patients had an increase in strength and function.
- Markarian et al[3] failed to show a significant difference between operative and nonoperatively treated groups. The lack of statistical significance was possibly due to the bimodal age distribution in the study, with older, more sedentary patients receiving nonoperative treatment.
- The literature is scarce regarding the results and complications of surgical reconstruction of the tibialis anterior tendon due to the rarity of this injury.

COMPLICATIONS

- Intraoperative graft complications
- Neuroma
- Wound dehiscence
- Infection
- Graft failure

REFERENCES

1. Coughlin MJ. Disorders of tendons. In: Coughlin MJ, Mann RA, eds. Surgery of the Foot and Ankle, 7th ed. St Louis: Mosby, 1999:790–795.
2. Cracchiolo A. Anterior tibial tendon disorders. In: Nunley JA, Pfeffer GB, Sanders RW, et al, eds. Advanced Reconstruction Foot and Ankle. Rosemont, IL: American Academy of Orthopaedic Surgery, 2003:173–177.
3. Markarian GG, Kelikian AS, Brage M, et al. Anterior tibialis tendon ruptures: an outcome analysis of operative vs. nonoperative treatment. Foot Ankle Intl 1998;19:792–801.
4. Ouzounian TJ, Anderson R. Anterior tibial tendon rupture. Foot Ankle Intl 1995;16:406–410.
5. Sammarco V, Sammarco G, Henning C, et al. Surgical repair of acute and chronic tibialis anterior tendon ruptures. J Bone Joint Surg Am 2009;91A:325–332.

Chapter 126 Tendon Transfer for Foot Drop

Mark E. Easley and Aaron T. Scott

DEFINITION

- Pathology leading to a spectrum of motor function loss that includes loss of ankle dorsiflexion
  - Common peroneal nerve palsy, L5 radiculopathy, cerebrovascular accident
    - Loss of ankle dorsiflexion and hindfoot eversion
    - Retained posterior tibial tendon (PTT) function
  - Hereditary sensory motor neuropathy
    - A constellation of motor function deficits and associated deformity
    - Includes loss of dorsiflexion and hindfoot eversion
    - Retained PTT function
  - Flaccid paralysis
    - Global loss of motor function to the ankle and foot

ANATOMY

- Posterior tibialis
  - Muscle originates on the posterior tibia, interosseous membrane, and fibula.
  - Muscle and then tendon course in the deep posterior compartment.
  - Tendon travels directly posterior to the medial malleolus.
  - Tendon has numerous insertions on bones of plantar midfoot, spring ligament, and medial aspect of navicular.
- Interosseous membrane (IOM) and distal tibia–fibula syndesmosis
  - Thick fibrous bands between tibia and fibula
  - Distal tibia–fibula syndesmosis is narrow, with little space for tendon transfer even when a generous window is created in the distal IOM.
- Inferior extensor retinaculum
  - On the dorsum of the foot to prevent bowstringing of the extensor tendons as they transition across the anterior ankle to the dorsal foot
- Sciatic nerve
  - Comprises tibial and common peroneal nerves that separate immediately proximal to the popliteal fossa
  - Common peroneal nerve often affected in these neuropathies
  - Superficial peroneal nerve
    - Motor function to anterior and lateral compartment muscles
      - Dorsiflexion and eversion, respectively
    - Sensory distribution to dorsum of the foot
  - Deep peroneal nerve
    - Courses between tibialis anterior and extensor hallucis longus tendons proximal to the ankle
    - Located directly on the dorsum of midfoot
      - Immediately deep to extensor hallucis brevis muscle belly
    - Motor function to intrinsic muscles of foot
    - Sensory distribution to first web space
- Tibial nerve function typically spared
- Tibial nerve must be intact to create a dynamic tendon transfer
- If tibial nerve is not intact, then transfer can only be a tenodesis
- Anterior ankle and dorsal midfoot neurovascular structures at risk
  - Superficial peroneal nerve (may be insensate as part of the neuropathy)
  - Deep neurovascular bundle
    - Anterior tibial artery
    - Deep peroneal nerve (may also be insensate as part of the neuropathy)
  - Peroneal artery branch
    - Situated directly on anterior distal IOM

PATHOGENESIS

- Loss of common peroneal nerve function
- Loss of ankle dorsiflexion and hindfoot eversion
- Loss of major antagonists
  - Eventual equinus contracture
    - Imbalance of hindfoot inverter (PTT) and everters (peroneus brevis) and usually, but not always, peroneus longus)
  - Eventual hindfoot varus deformity
    - Imbalance of hindfoot inverters (PTT) and everter (peroneus longus)
- Flaccid paralysis
  - Tibial and common peroneal nerve palsies
  - No motor function distal to knee
  - Since both sets of major antagonists lost, typically no contractures

NATURAL HISTORY

- Foot drop may eventually recover.
  - Tendon transfers should not be considered until a chance for recovery has been ruled out.
- Common peroneal nerve palsy may lead to progressively worsening equinocavovarus foot deformity due to overpull of plantarflexors and inverters powered by intact tibial nerve and loss of dorsiflexors and everters powered by compromised common peroneal nerve.
- Flaccid paralysis remains relatively stable since both sets of antagonists are compromised.

PATIENT HISTORY AND PHYSICAL FINDINGS

- Gait abnormality
  - "Slap foot gait"
    - Inability to dorsiflex ankle and control tibialis anterior from heel strike to stance phase
  - Exaggerated hip and knee flexion
    - Inability to dorsiflex ankle or great toe from push-off through swing phase
    - Compensation to allow toes to clear during swing phase

- Hindfoot inversion
  - Patient walks on lateral border of foot.
- Inability to dorsiflex ankle
  - May check by asking patient to walk on heels
  - Manual muscle testing with patient seated on examining table with knee flexed
- Lack of eversion
  - Varus hindfoot
  - Over time, may become a fixed inversion contracture
- In some disease processes (eg, Charcot-Marie-Tooth disease) toe dorsiflexion is spared, creating claw toe deformities.
  - Patient attempts to compensate for lack of ankle dorsiflexion with toe extensors, worsening claw toe deformities.
- Even when toe extensors are involved in the palsy, flexor tendons may become contracted.
  - Passive dorsiflexion of the ankle will reveal this.
- With equinocavovarus foot contracture, calluses may form under metatarsal heads, particularly the fifth.
- Sensation may be diminished on the dorsal and lateral aspects of the foot.

IMAGING AND OTHER DIAGNOSTIC STUDIES

- Imaging is typically unnecessary for patients with foot drop except in the following situations:
  - Consideration should be given to MRI:
    - If there is concern for mass effect creating a compressive neuropathy: lumbar spine, common peroneal nerve at fibular head
    - To rule out tibialis anterior tendon rupture (should be evident on clinical examination alone)
  - Consideration should be given to radiographs of foot or ankle:
    - To rule out stress fracture
    - To better define bony deformity (fixed deformity, associated ankle or foot arthritis; important because arthrodesis may need to be considered in lieu of or in combination with tendon transfer)
- Electrodiagnostic studies
  - Absence of recovery at 1 year and particularly at 18 months is highly suggestive that recovery of nerve function will not occur.
  - Nerve conduction studies and electromyography
  - Baseline and follow-up studies to determine if any recovery evident
  - Important to determine if tendon transfer is warranted
  - Tendon transfer should not be performed if nerve function may recover!
  - Absence of recovery at 1 year and particularly at 18 months is highly suggestive of no recovery.
  - We recommend consultation with a neurologist to confirm interpretation of electrodiagnostic studies.
  - Studies may also define function of PTT.
    - Important when considering dynamic PTT transfer versus PTT tenodesis
    - A tendon transfer of a healthy tendon immediately reduces its strength on manual muscle testing from 5/5 to 4/5, so if it is already compromised, then the tendon transfer will do little more than create a tenodesis.
  - Useful in determining if a more proximal compressive neuropathy exists

DIFFERENTIAL DIAGNOSIS

- Tibialis anterior tendon rupture
- Cerebrovascular accident
- Lumbar spine radiculopathy
- Hereditary sensorimotor neuropathy
- Leprosy
- Poliomyelitis
- Cerebral palsy (spastic)

NONOPERATIVE MANAGEMENT

- Bracing with an ankle–foot orthosis (AFO)
  - Requires a fixed AFO in flaccid paralysis
  - May be a flexible AFO with common peroneal palsy
    - Requires plantarflexion stop
  - Equinus contracture may need to be corrected to facilitate bracewear.
    - Achilles stretching
    - Botulinum toxin injection
    - Tendo Achilles lengthening (TAL)
  - Varus deformity
    - If flexible may be corrected with bracing
    - If fixed, bracing is difficult.

SURGICAL MANAGEMENT

Preoperative Planning

- The surgeon must confirm that motor function will not recover before proceeding with tendon transfer.
  - Serial clinical examination
  - Serial electrodiagnostic studies (at least one compared to baseline)
- The surgeon must determine what motor function persists:
  - Tibial nerve
    - PTT (inversion)
    - Gastrocnemius–soleus (plantarflexion)
  - None (flaccid paralysis)
- The surgeon must evaluate for equinus contracture.
  - The surgeon should be prepared to perform TAL if necessary (see Tech Fig 1A–D).
- Flexible versus fixed deformities
  - Flexible deformity typically corrects with tendon transfer alone.
  - Fixed deformity
    - May require capsular release or even arthrodesis
- Toe contractures
  - Although claw toe deformity may not be evident with the ankle plantarflexed, once the deformity is corrected, toe contractures may become obvious.
    - Dorsiflexing the ankle will put the contracted flexor hallucis and digitorum on stretch, thereby revealing the toe contractures.
    - The surgeon should be prepared to address toe contractures as part of the procedure.
- Tendon transfer anchoring
  - We routinely use interference screws to anchor tendon transfers to bone.
  - Need to have an anchoring system available
  - Alternatively, anchoring to existing distal tendon or existing soft tissues in the foot may be possible.
- In our experience, anesthesia should maintain complete muscle relaxation and paralysis during the procedure; otherwise, the success of the tendon transfer may be compromised.

- At the conclusion of the procedure we often perform botulinum toxin injections into the gastrocnemius–soleus complex to further protect the tendon transfer postoperatively.

Positioning

- Supine
- If the PTT will be transferred through the IOM or if a peroneal tendon will be used for correction of flaccid paralysis, we routinely place a bolster under the ipsilateral hip to afford optimal lateral exposure. Once the lateral tendon is harvested or the PTT transferred through the IOM, the bolster may be removed.
- We routinely use a thigh tourniquet.

Approach

- Multiple relatively small incisions are needed; extensile exposures are unnecessary.
- PTT harvest
  - Medial harvest over navicular
  - Posteromedial tibia at musculotendinous junction of PTT
- PTT transfer through the IOM
  - Incision over distal IOM
  - Incision over dorsolateral foot
- PTT transfer anterior to tibia
  - Incision over central midfoot
- Bridle procedure
  - Same PTT harvest
  - PTT transfer through IOM with incision directly anterior over distal tibia; may be extended to dorsal foot. Alternatively, separate small incision over centrodorsal midfoot.
  - Lateral incisions: incision over musculotendinous junction of peroneus longus and another incision over lateral cuboid where peroneus longus courses around cuboid

TECHNIQUES

ACHILLES LENGTHENING

- Indications
  - Not always necessary, but typically required when foot drop occurs
    - Without active dorsiflexion the gastrocnemius–soleus' antagonist is lost, often leading to an Achilles contracture.
    - Occasionally patients maintain an active stretching program, thereby avoiding an Achilles contracture.
  - Weakening of the gastrocnemius–soleus complex may be beneficial since a transfer of a healthy muscle–tendon unit is subject to an automatic one-grade loss of power (5/5 manual muscle testing drops to 4/5 with transfer).
    - Occasionally we use botulinum toxin in the gastrocnemius–soleus complex when performing a PTT transfer for foot drop.
- Technique
  - Determined by the Silfverskiold test
    - Equinus contracture with the knee in extension and flexion (**TECH FIG 1A**)

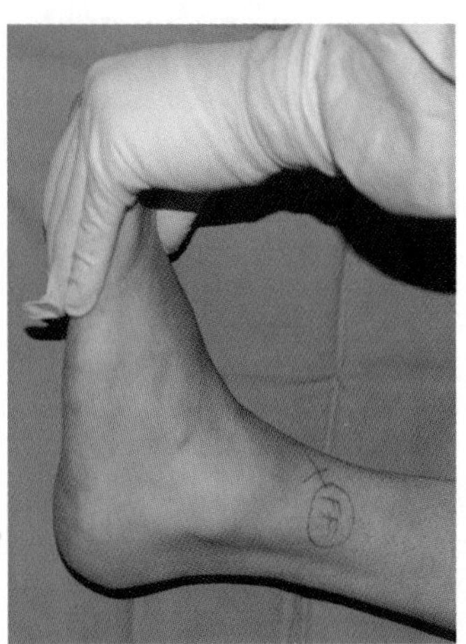
A

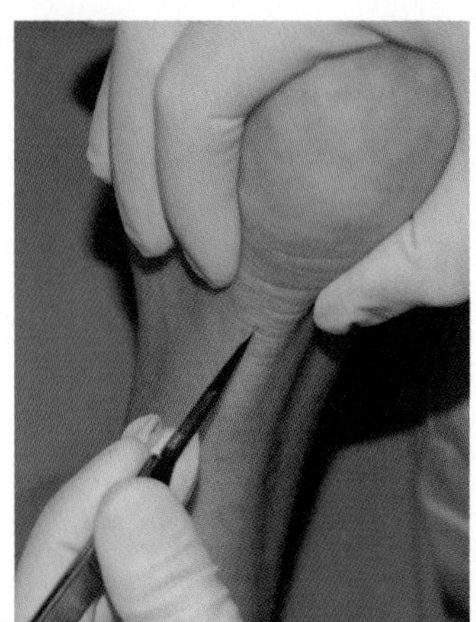
B

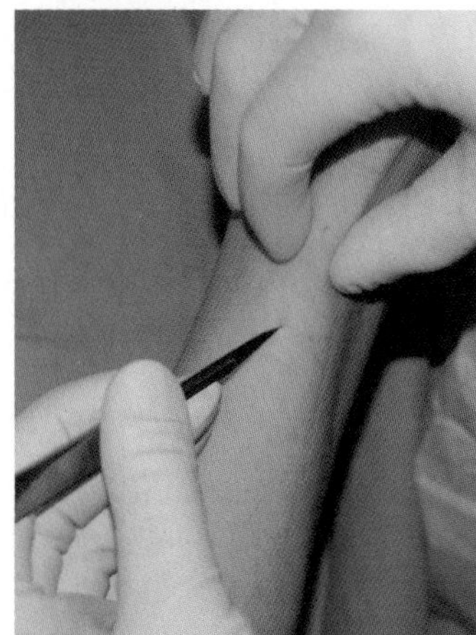
C

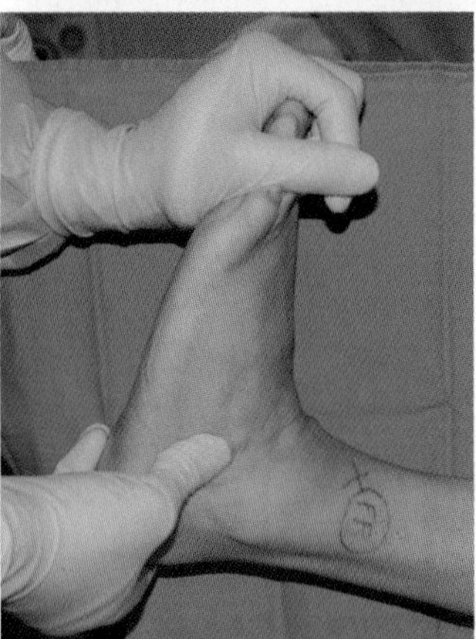
D

TECH FIG 1 • Tendo Achilles lengthening. **A.** Equinus with knee in flexion and extension suggests tight gastrocnemius and soleus. **B.** Initial Achilles hemisection. **C.** Second Achilles hemisection (opposite direction from first), to be followed by third and final hemisection in same direction as first. **D.** Dorsiflexion re-established after Achilles lengthening.

- Triple hemisection (Hoke procedure) because both the gastrocnemius and soleus are contracted (**TECH FIG 1B–D**)
- Equinus contracture only with the knee in extension: gastrocnemius–soleus recession (Strayer procedure) because only the gastrocnemius is contracted

Posterior Tibial Tendon Transfer Through the Interosseous Membrane

- Advantages
  - PTT in direct line from its muscle through the IOM to the lateral cuneiform (our preferred site for tendon anchoring)
  - Anchor point slightly lateral of midline to promote dorsiflexion and eversion
- Disadvantage
  - PTT may be constricted and stenosed within narrow window created in distal IOM.

Posterior Tibial Tendon Harvest

- Make a 4-cm longitudinal incision over the medial navicular and PTT on the medial foot.
- Open the PTT sheath to expose the tendon.
- Release the PTT insertion on the medial navicular.
- Alternatively, use a chisel to elevate some medial navicular bone with the PTT release from the medial navicular (may allow for another centimeter of tendon for transfer) (**TECH FIG 2A**).
- Isolate the PTT attachment on the medial navicular and the tendon fibers that begin to course to the plantar midfoot (**TECH FIG 2B**).
- With the PTT fibers isolated, transect them to release the PTT distally.
  - Be sure to fully isolate the PTT fibers; the medial plantar nerve and the plantar medial complex of veins is in close proximity.
    - Accidentally transecting the nerve leads to loss of sensation in the plantar medial forefoot.
    - Violating the veins may make it difficult to achieve satisfactory hemostasis as these veins may then retract under the foot.
- Thin the distal stump of the PTT to be transferred to facilitate its transfer into an osseous tunnel that will be created in the foot (**TECH FIG 2C**).

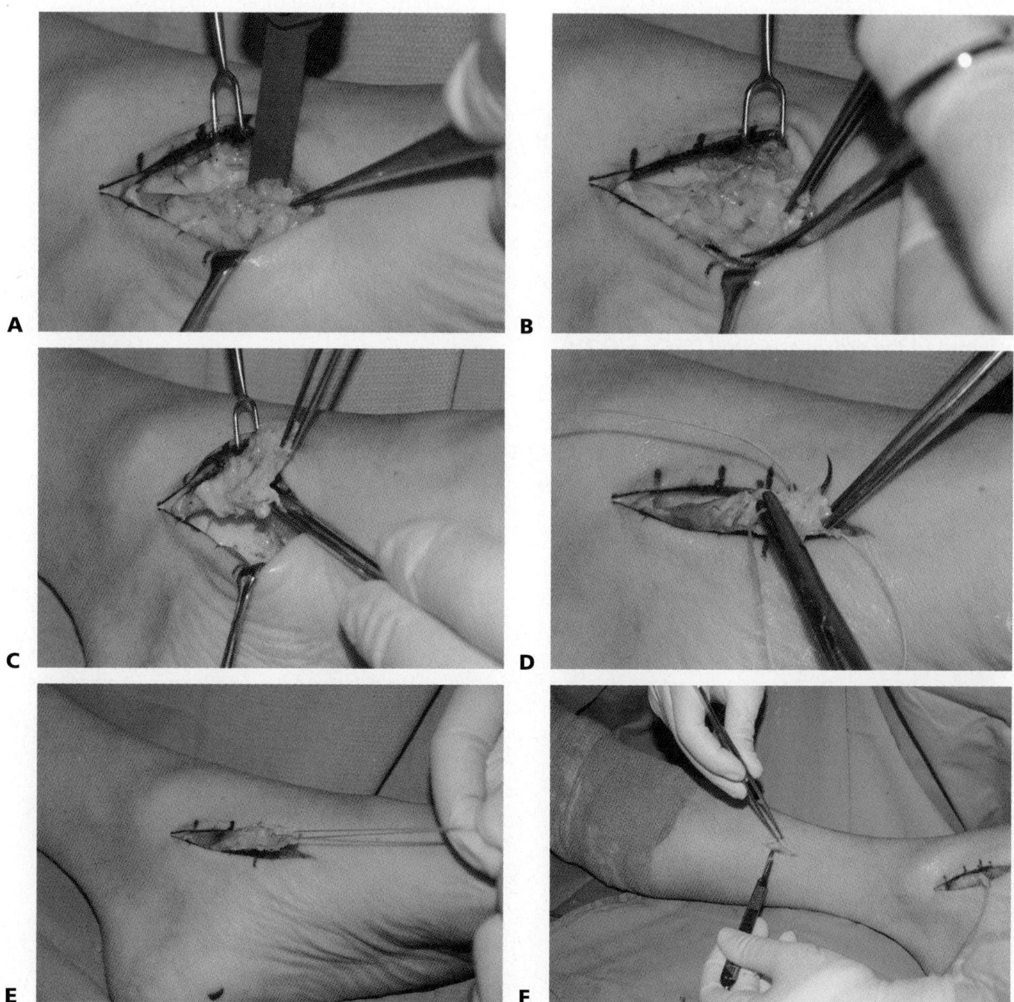

TECH FIG 2 • Posterior tibial tendon (PTT) harvest **A.** Elevating PTT with a sliver of medial navicular may allow longer tendon harvest. **B.** Isolating PTT. **C.** Distal PTT needs to be trimmed to allow it to pass into dorsal foot osseous tunnel. **D, E.** Tag suture in distal PTT. **F.** Transfer of PTT to proximal medial wound. A 3-cm incision is made over PTT musculotendinous junction. *(continued)*

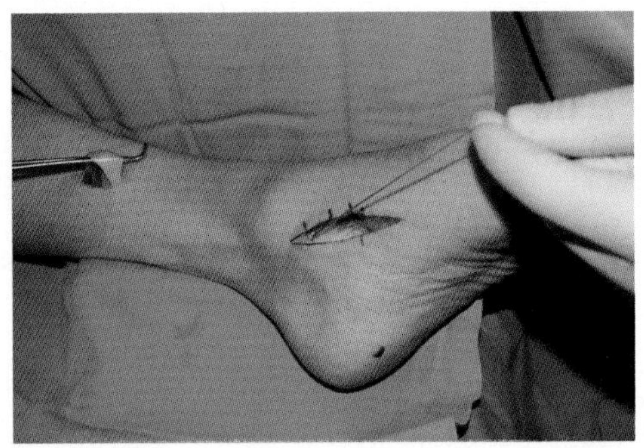

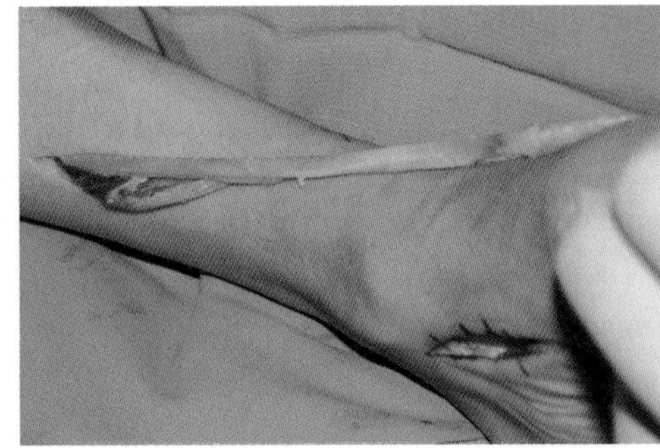

TECH FIG 2 • *(continued)* **G.** Tendon transfer is mobilized. **H.** PTT is transferred to proximal wound.

- Place tag sutures in the distal PTT (**TECH FIG 2D,E**).
- Make a more proximal medial incision at the PTT musculotendinous junction on the posterior tibia.
  - 3-cm incision (**TECH FIG 2F**)
    - Flexor digitorum tendon is usually encountered first.
    - Deep to the FDL, directly on the posteromedial tibia, the PTT is identified.
    - Place a blunt retractor around the PTT through this more proximal wound to isolate it.
- Mobilize the distal PTT.
  - Alternate tension on the proximal tendon through the proximal wound and the distal tag sutures (**TECH FIG 2G**), then apply tension proximally only.
  - This may not work.
  - The medial incision may need to be extended proximally to allow access to the posterior medial malleolus, a common location where the tendon may bind.
  - Once mobilized, the distal aspect of the PTT may be transferred to the proximal wound (**TECH FIG 2H**).
    - Tendon will desiccate rapidly, so we keep it tucked in the proximal medial wound.

Posterior Tibial Tendon Transfer Through the Interosseous Membrane

- Lateral incision on anterior aspect of distal fibula, at distal tibiofibular syndesmosis
- Careful exposure of anterior IOM
  - Elevate the anterior compartment soft tissues.
- A branch of the peroneal artery courses on the anterior IOM and is at risk.
- Create a generous window in the distal IOM (**TECH FIG 3A**).
  - From tibia to fibula
  - About 3 to 4 cm long
- Pass a tonsil clamp through the IOM directly on the posterior aspect of the tibia to exit in the proximal medial wound (**TECH FIG 3B**).
  - The posterior neurovascular structures (tibial nerve and posterior tibial artery) are at risk, so be sure the clamp is *directly* on the posterior tibia.

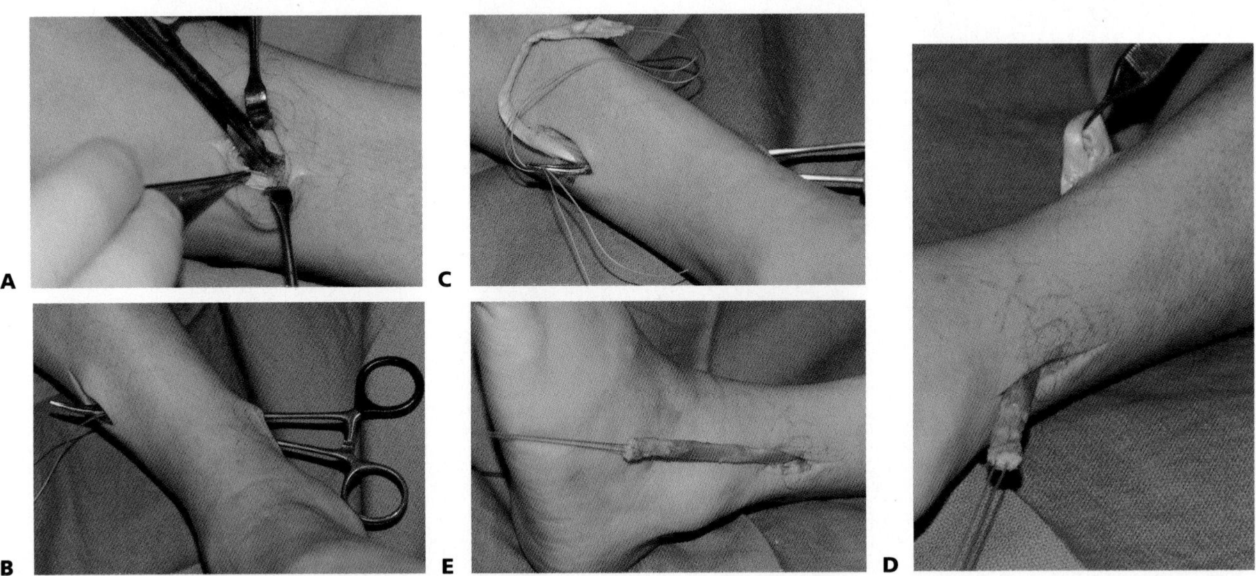

TECH FIG 3 • PTT transfer through the interrosseous membrane (IOM). **A.** A window is carefully created in the interosseous membrane (IOM) (perspective with view of lateral distal leg [foot to the left and knee to the right]). **B.** A blunt clamp is passed through IOM, *directly* on posterior tibia. **C.** Posterior tibial tendon (PTT) tag sutures are grasped. **D.** PTT is transferred to anterolateral wound, with tendon immediately on posterior tibia. **E.** The surgeon must be sure tendon does not bind in IOM window.

- Use the tonsil clamp to grasp the tag sutures of the PTT (TECH FIG 3C).
- Pull the tag sutures and PTT from the medial wound to the lateral wound, keeping the tendon directly on the posterior aspect of the tibia (TECH FIG 3D,E).
- Be sure that the window in the IOM does not impinge on the transferred tendon.
  - If there is stenosis, then further enlarge the window so that the tendon easily glides between the tibia and fibula.
- Keep the tendon end in the wound to limit desiccation.

Preparation of the Dorsal Foot Anchor Site

- Fluoroscopically identify the center of the lateral cuneiform.
  - Oblique foot views usually best define the lateral cuneiform (TECH FIG 4A).
- Center a 3- to 4-cm longitudinal skin incision directly over the lateral cuneiform.
- Dissect to the lateral cuneiform.
  - Protect the superficial peroneal nerve and extensor tendons.
  - Deep neurovascular bundle is usually medial to this approach.
- Expose and define the cuneiform.
  - We routinely use small-gauge hypodermic needles or Kirschner wires to mark the joints surrounding the lateral cuneiform and fluoroscopically confirm that the lateral cuneiform is defined by these markers (TECH FIG 4B).
  - Periosteum and capsular tissue are left intact.
- Create an osseous tunnel in the center of the lateral cuneiform.
  - We routinely predrill the center with a Kirschner wire and confirm the starting point and trajectory of the wire fluoroscopically.
  - Remove the wire and introduce sequentially larger drill bits to enlarge the tunnel (TECH FIG 4C).

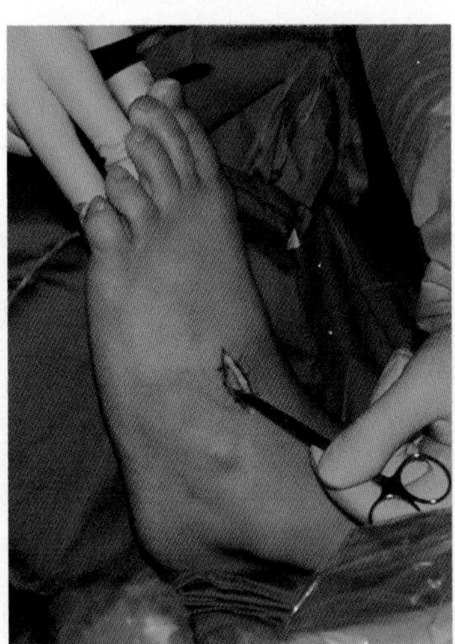
A

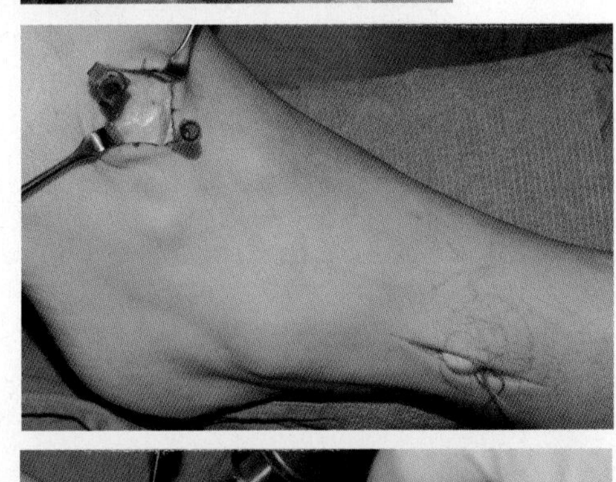
B

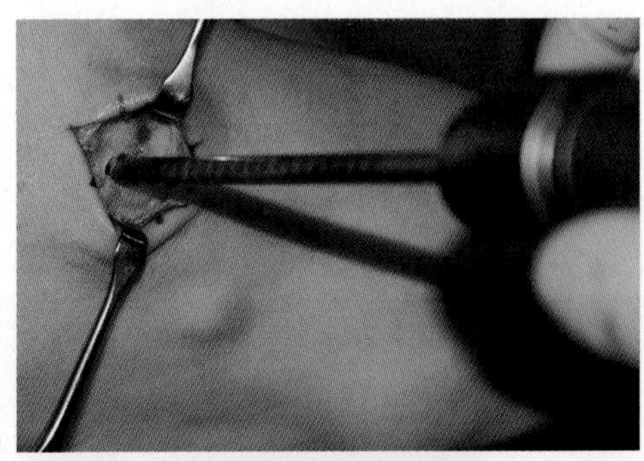
D

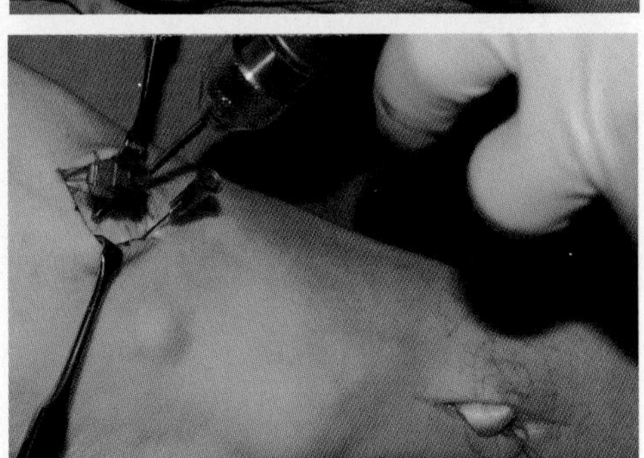
C

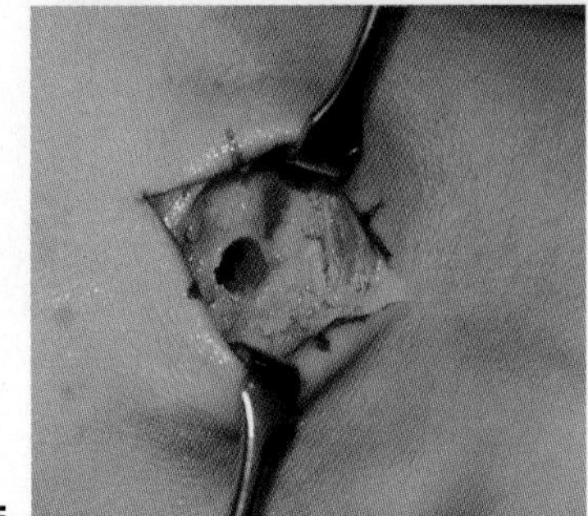
E

TECH FIG 4 • Preparing dorsal foot osseous tunnel. **A.** Lateral cuneiform is identified fluoroscopically. **B.** Borders of lateral cuneiform are exposed and marked. **C.** Drill hole is created in lateral cuneiform and proper position is confirmed fluoroscopically. **D.** Osseous tunnel is gradually enlarged, first with drill bits, then dedicated reamer system for interference screw. **E.** Prepared osseous tunnel in lateral cuneiform.

- We use drill bits to a diameter of 4.5 mm.
- With fluoroscopic confirmation, slight adjustments may be made with each successive drill bit to center the tunnel optimally in the cuneiform.
- Introduce the reamer system for the interference screw system to enlarge the tunnel to the desired diameter (**TECH FIG 4D**).
  - Typically, we enlarge the tunnel to 6.5 to 7.0 mm in the lateral cuneiform (**TECH FIG 4E**).

Posterior Tibial Tendon Transfer to Dorsum of Foot

- Transferring the PTT deep to the extensor retinaculum with the extensor tendons diminishes the power of the transfer (which is by definition already weakened by one grade with transfer).
- Create a subcutaneous soft tissue tunnel from the dorsal foot incision to the more proximal and lateral lower leg incision using a curved Kelly or tonsil clamp (**TECH FIG 5A**).
- Use the clamp to grasp the tag sutures and pull the tendon through the subcutaneous tunnel to the dorsal foot incision (**TECH FIG 5B**).
- Before anchoring the tendon in the osseous tunnel, pull the tendon via the tag sutures into the tunnel to be sure that the tunnel diameter is appropriate.
  - Pass a Beath pin or drill bit (has an eye to place suture) through the tunnel and the plantar skin (**TECH FIG 5C**).
    - Because of the midfoot arch and the drill hole centered in the lateral cuneiform foot this pin or the drill bit will exit in the medial arch (**TECH FIG 5D**).
  - Dorsiflex the ankle.
  - With the tag sutures secured, pull the pin or drill bit through the plantar skin, thereby pulling the distal tendon end into the tunnel (**TECH FIG 5E**).
    - If the tunnel does not accommodate the tendon, then the tendon and tag sutures must be withdrawn and the tunnel enlarged.
    - Because of the angle at which the tendon enters the tunnel, we often need to guide the tendon into the tunnel with a forceps.
  - Anchoring the tendon to bone
    - Some degree of stretching or accommodation is anticipated, so we routinely anchor the tendon with the ankle maintained in 10 degrees of dorsi-

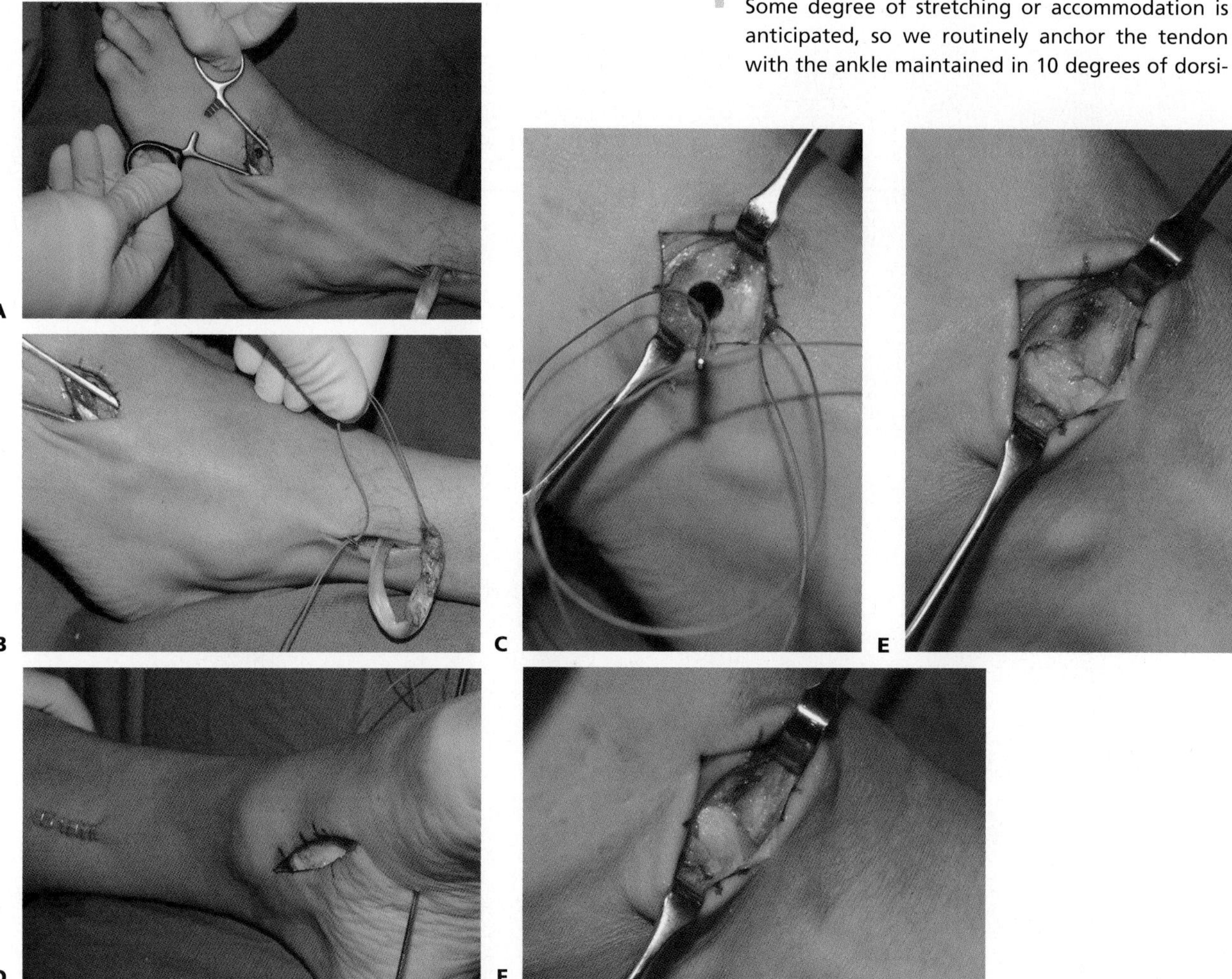

TECH FIG 5 • Posterior tibial tendon (PTT) transfer from lateral lower leg wound to dorsum of foot. **A.** Subcutaneous tunnel created with a blunt clamp. **B.** Grasping tag sutures. **C.** Passing Beath drill with tag sutures through osseous tunnel. **D.** Pulling Beath drill through plantar foot. **E.** The surgeon must be sure the tendon fits appropriately into the osseous tunnel. **F.** Tendon tensioning. Tendon advances appropriately into osseous tunnel (note ankle is held in dorsiflexion). *(continued)*

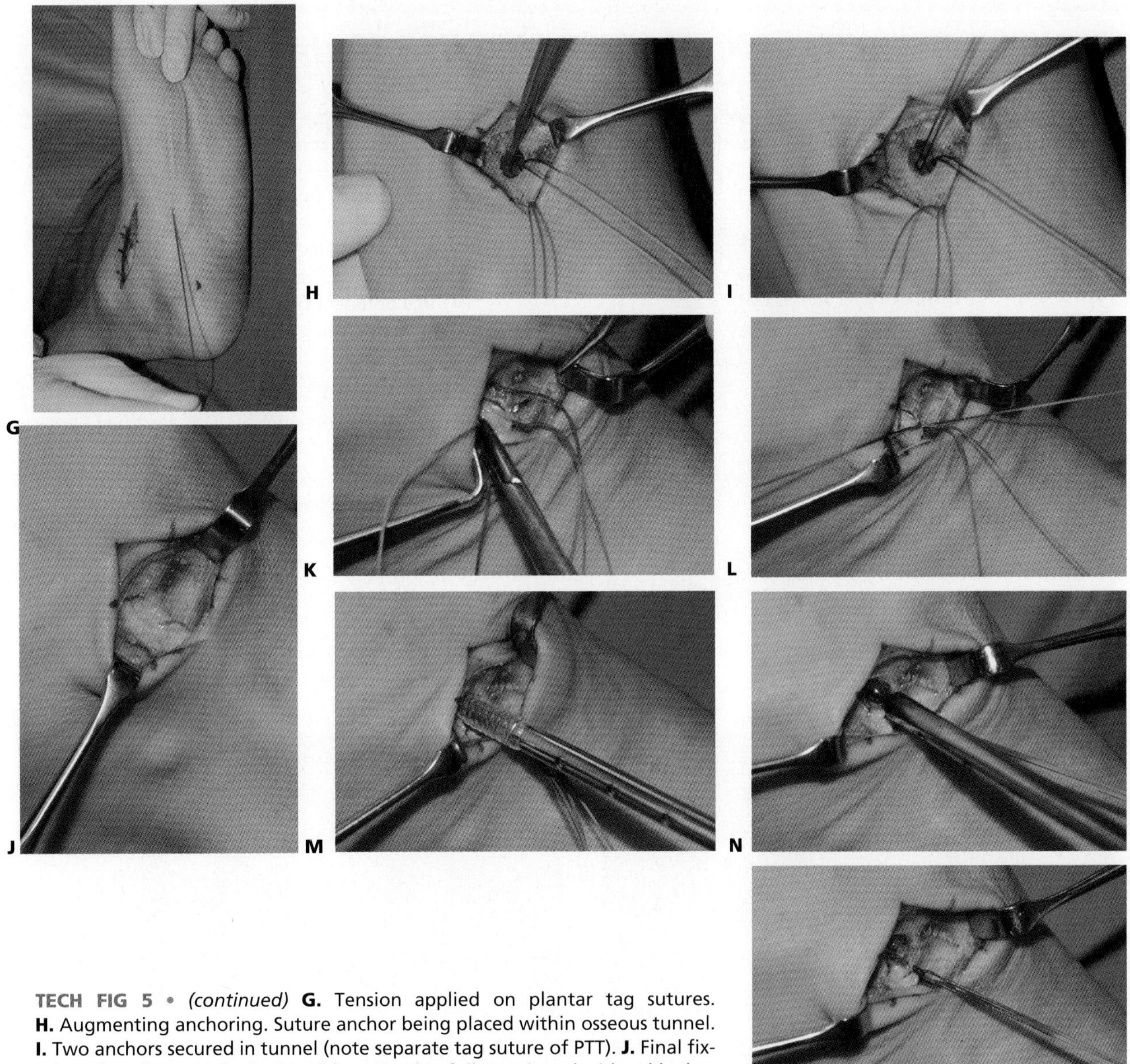

TECH FIG 5 • *(continued)* **G.** Tension applied on plantar tag sutures. **H.** Augmenting anchoring. Suture anchor being placed within osseous tunnel. **I.** Two anchors secured in tunnel (note separate tag suture of PTT). **J.** Final fixation of tendon transfer in dorsal foot. Tendon fully tensioned with ankle dorsiflexed. **K, L.** Securing tendon to anchors and adjacent periosteum. **M.** Interference screw positioned. **N.** Screw advanced. **O.** Screw fully seated.

flexion and pull firmly on the plantar suture (**TECH FIG 5F,G**).

- A properly sized isolated interference screw is probably adequate.
- However, we typically augment the anchor point with several nonabsorbable sutures from the periosteum surrounding the tunnel to the tendon directly at the entrance to the tunnel.
- To further augment the anchor point: before advancing the tendon and tag suture into the tunnel, place one or two suture anchors within the tunnel (**TECH FIG 5H,I**). Then advance the tendon into the tunnel and secure the tendon with the anchors (**TECH FIG 5J,K**). By tightening these sutures, the tendon may be pulled even further into the tunnel (**TECH FIG 5L**). An interference screw and periosteal sutures may still be used (**TECH FIG 5M–O**).
- Have the assistant maintain full ankle dorsiflexion and tension on the tag sutures on the plantar foot.
- We usually cut the tag sutures so they retract beneath the skin.
- Rarely, we have used a well-padded button on the plantar foot to further augment the tendon's anchor point. We do not routinely do so because of the risk for plantar skin necrosis from the button despite adequate padding.
- In select patients, the dorsiflexed ankle will unmask claw toes due to flexor hallucis longus and flexor digitorum longus contractures. Consider flexor hallucis longus and flexor digitorum longus lengthenings, posterior to the ankle and tibia via the more proximal medial approach, or percutaneous tenotomies at the plantar toes.

POSTERIOR TIBIAL TENDON TRANSFER ANTERIOR TO THE TIBIA

- Advantages
  - PTT has no opportunity to stenose in the IOM.
  - Glides smoothly around anteromedial tibia
  - Anchor point slightly lateral of midline to promote dorsiflexion and eversion

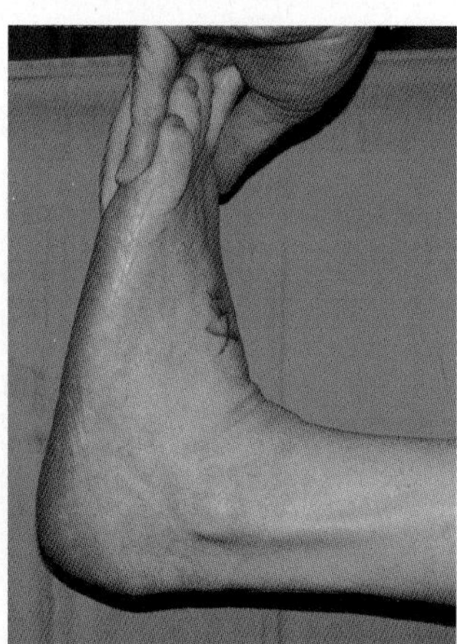

TECH FIG 6 • Adequate dorsiflexion (essential for successful tendon transfer to re-establish dorsiflexion).

- Disadvantage
  - PTT is not in direct line from its origin to anchor point in the foot; it must travel around medial tibia.
  - Anchor point is in the middle (second) cuneiform.
    - Central location so it cannot provide an eversion moment
    - However, typically unimportant since with PTT transfer the agonist–antagonist balance between PTT and peroneus brevis is again re-established by being neutralized.

Achilles Lengthening

- Same as for PTT transfer through IOM described earlier (**TECH FIG 6**)

Posterior Tibial Tendon Harvest

- Same as for PTT transfer through IOM described earlier (**TECH FIG 7**)

Preparation of the Dorsal Foot Anchor Site

- Similar to preparation of dorsal foot anchor site described earlier for PTT transfer through IOM

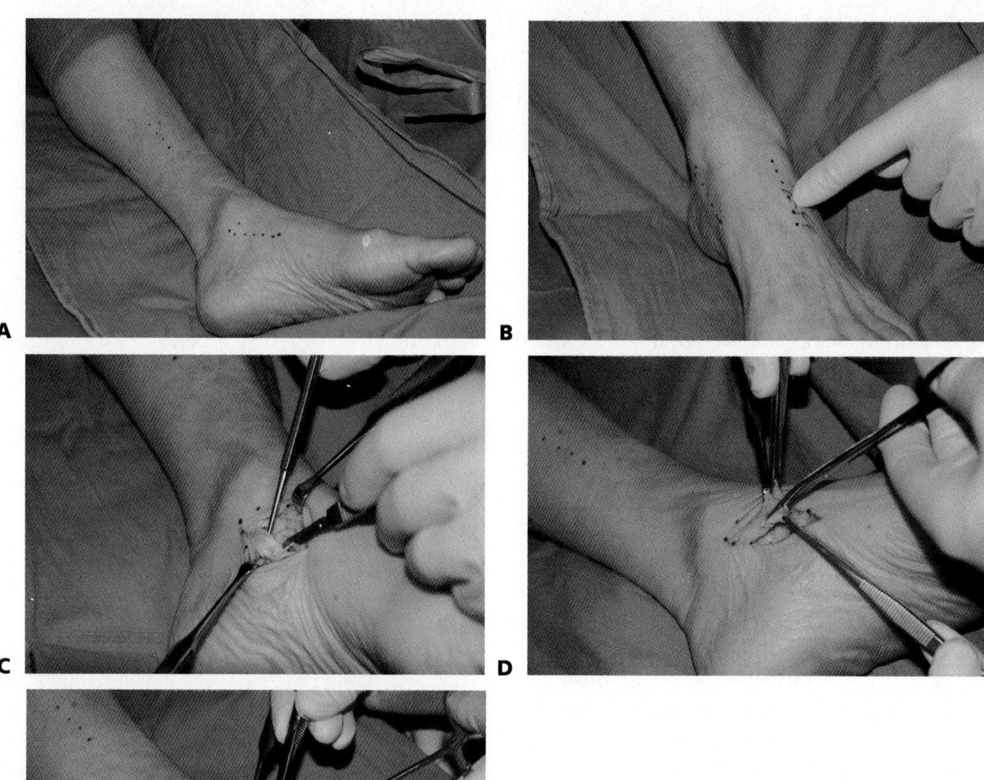

TECH FIG 7 • Approach to posterior tibial tendon (PTT) harvest. **A.** The two planned medial incisions. **B.** Planned dorsal foot incision. **C–E.** Harvesting PTT. **C.** PTT is isolated. **D.** Distal tendon is trimmed (contoured). **E.** Tag suture in distal end of tendon. *(continued)*

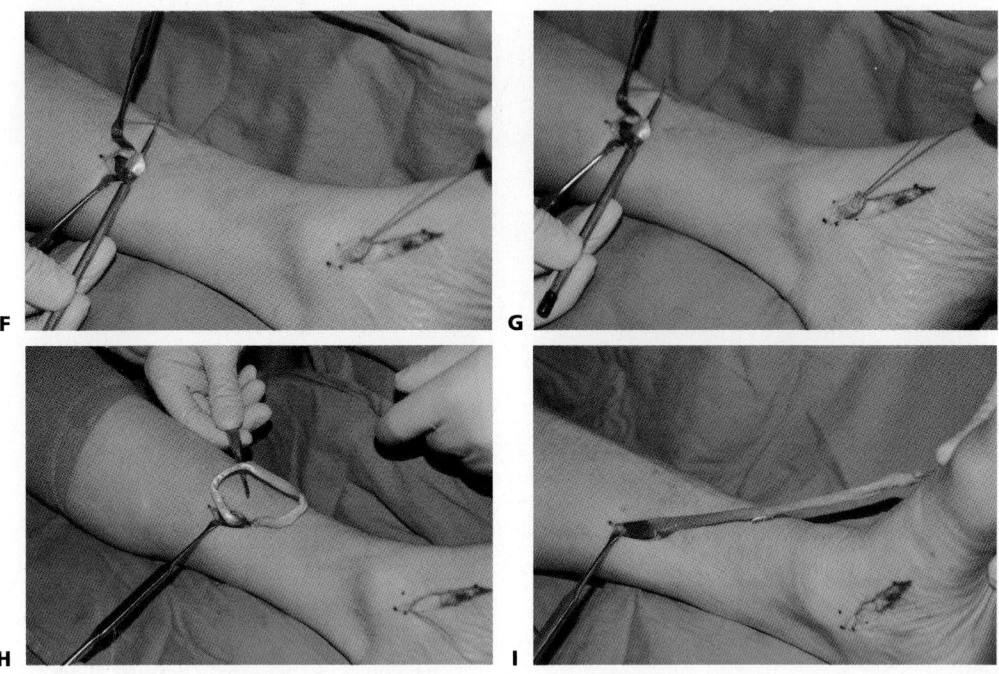

TECH FIG 7 • *(continued)* PTT is mobilized. **F.** PTT is identified at its musculotendinous junction. **G.** PTT is mobilized to allow transfer to proximal wound. **H, I.** Transferring PTT to proximal medial wound. **H.** Tendon is pulled into proximal wound. **I.** Proposed course for transfer to dorsum of foot.

- However, when transferring the PTT through the IOM we typically anchor the tendon to the lateral (third) cuneiform.
- In contrast, when we transfer the PTT anterior to the medial tibia, we typically anchor the tendon in the middle (second) cuneiform.
- Middle cuneiform is smaller than the lateral cuneiform.
  - In our experience, greater risk of fracture with drill hole, tendon transfer, and interference screw
- Fluoroscopically identify the center of the middle cuneiform.
  - AP and sometimes oblique foot views best define the middle cuneiform.
- Center a 3- to 4-cm longitudinal skin incision directly over the middle cuneiform.
- Dissect to the middle cuneiform.
  - Protect the superficial peroneal nerve and extensor tendons (TECH FIG 8A).
  - Protect the deep neurovascular bundle, usually encountered in this approach; it is directly deep to the muscle of the extensor hallucis brevis.
- Expose and define the cuneiform.
  - We routinely use small-gauge hypodermic needles or Kirschner wires to mark the joints surrounding the medial cuneiform and fluoroscopically confirm that the medial cuneiform is defined by these markers (TECH FIG 8B).
  - Leave the periosteum and capsular tissue intact.
- Create an osseous tunnel in the center of the medial cuneiform.
  - We routinely predrill the center with a Kirschner wire and confirm the starting point and trajectory of the wire fluoroscopically.
  - Remove the wire and introduce sequentially larger drill bits to enlarge the tunnel (TECH FIG 8C).
    - We use drill bits to a diameter of 4.5 mm.
    - With fluoroscopic confirmation, slight adjustments may be made with each successive drill bit to center the tunnel optimally in the cuneiform.

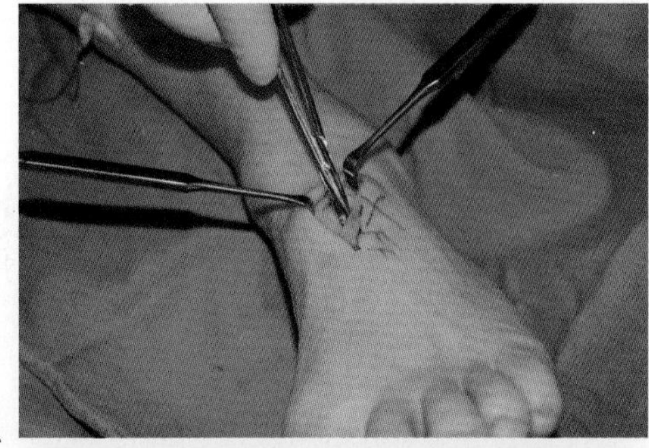

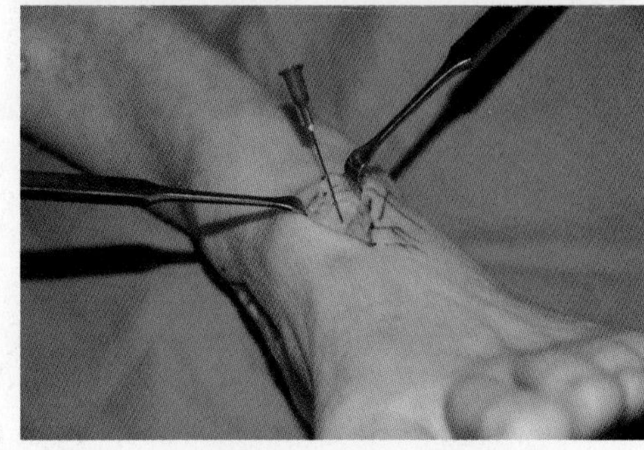

TECH FIG 8 • Preparation of dorsal foot osseous tunnel. **A.** Dorsal incision over middle cuneiform. **B.** Middle cuneiform is identified and marked. *(continued)*

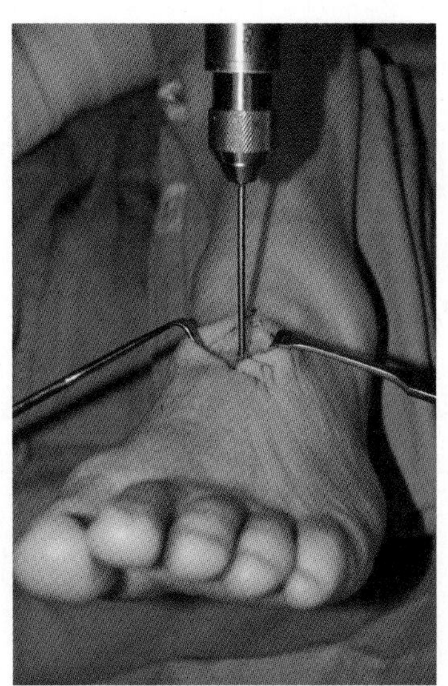

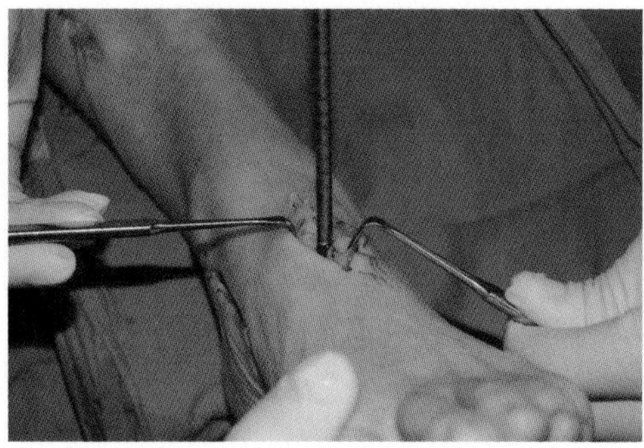

TECH FIG 8 • *(continued)* **C.** Increasingly larger-diameter drill bits. **D.** Increasingly larger reamers (judiciously, since the middle cuneiform is not particularly large).

- Use the reamer from the interference screw system to enlarge the tunnel to the desired diameter (**TECH FIG 8D**).
- Typically, we enlarge the tunnel to 5.5 to 6.0 mm in the medial cuneiform.

Posterior Tibial Tendon Transfer to Dorsum of Foot

- Transferring the PTT deep to the extensor retinaculum with the extensor tendons diminishes the power of the transfer (which is by definition already weakened by one grade with transfer).
- Create a subcutaneous soft tissue tunnel from the dorsal foot incision to the more proximal and medial lower leg incision using a curved Kelly or tonsil clamp (**TECH FIG 9A,B**).
- Use the clamp to grasp the tag sutures and pull the tendon through the subcutaneous tunnel to the dorsal foot incision.
- Before anchoring the tendon in the osseous tunnel, pull the tendon via the tag sutures into the tunnel to be sure that the tunnel diameter is appropriate.
  - Pass a Beath pin or drill bit (has an eye to place suture) through the tunnel and the plantar skin (**TECH FIG 9C,D**). Because of the midfoot arch, this pin or drill bit will exit in the medial arch (**TECH FIG 9E**).
  - Dorsiflex the ankle.
  - With the tag sutures secured, pull the pin or drill bit through the plantar skin, thereby pulling the distal tendon end into the tunnel (**TECH FIG 9F**).
    - If the tunnel does not accommodate the tendon, then the tendon and tag sutures must be withdrawn and the tunnel enlarged.

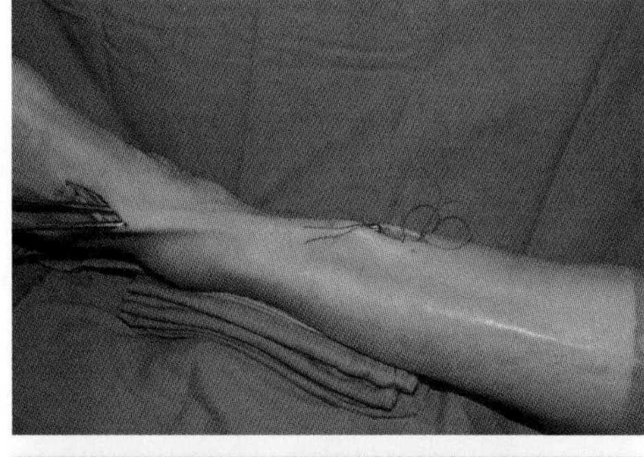

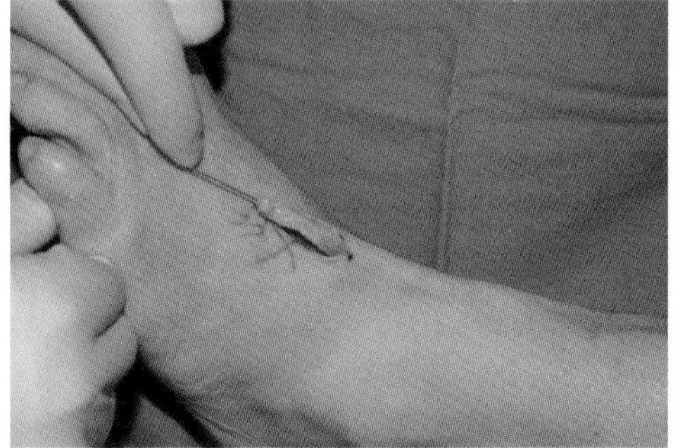

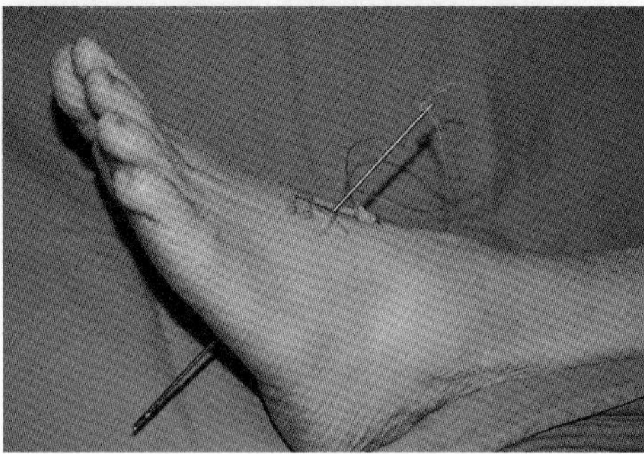

TECH FIG 9 • Transfer of posterior tibial tendon (PTT) to dorsum of foot. **A.** Subcutaneous tunnel for blunt clamp to grasp tag suture in PTT. **B.** PTT is transferred subcutaneously to dorsum of foot. **C–F.** Ensuring that PTT will pass through osseous tunnel in middle cuneiform. **C.** Beath drill through tunnel with tag suture from PTT secured. *(continued)*

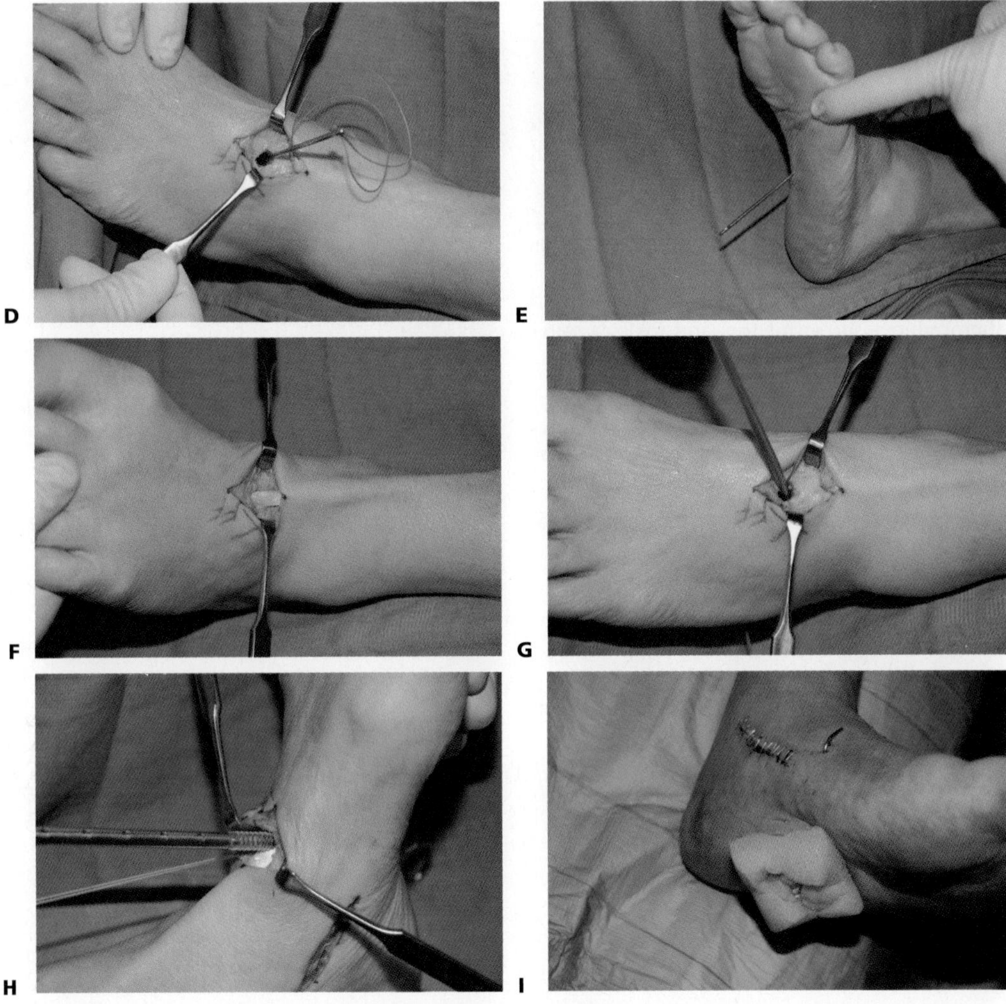

TECH FIG 9 • *(continued)* **D.** Entry point of Beath drill in dorsal tunnel. **E.** Exit of Beath drill in plantar foot. **F.** Tendon advancing appropriately with ankle in dorsiflexion and tension on tag sutures passed through plantar foot. **G, H.** Tendon fixation. **G.** Augmentation possible with suture anchors placed directly in tunnel before advancing tendon into tunnel. **H.** Interference screw with ankle dorsiflexed and tension maintained on plantar tag suture. **I.** Suture button. In this case middle cuneiform fractured with insertion of interference screw and therefore a suture button was used. Note also the use of two Kirschner wires in the medial foot to further stabilize fracture in cuneiform.

  - Because of the angle at which the tendon enters the tunnel, we often need to guide the tendon into the tunnel with a forceps.
- Anchoring the tendon to bone
  - Some degree of stretching or accommodation is anticipated in the posterior tibial muscle and tendon, so we routinely anchor the tendon with the ankle maintained in 10 degrees of dorsiflexion.
  - A properly sized isolated interference screw is probably adequate.
  - However, we typically augment the anchor point with several nonabsorbable sutures from the periosteum surrounding the tunnel to the tendon directly at the entrance to the tunnel.
  - To further augment the anchor point
    - Before advancing the tendon and tag suture into the tunnel, place one or two suture anchors within the tunnel (TECH FIG 9G).
    - Then advance the tendon into the tunnel and secure the tendon with the anchors. By tightening these sutures, the tendon may be pulled even further into the tunnel. An interference screw and periosteal sutures may still be used (TECH FIG 9H).
  - Have the assistant maintain full ankle dorsiflexion and tension on the tag sutures on the plantar foot.
  - We usually cut the tag sutures so they retract beneath the skin.
  - Rarely, we have used a well-padded button on the plantar foot to further augment the tendon's anchor point (TECH FIG 9I). We do not routinely do so because of the risk for plantar skin necrosis from the button despite adequate padding.

BRIDLE PROCEDURE

- Advantages
  - The "bridle" creates a balance to the foot and ankle.
  - Potentially can make the patient with flaccid paralysis brace-free
- Disadvantage
  - With flaccid paralysis, the tendon transfer is static, not dynamic.
  - Functions as a tenodesis
    - If procedure is successful, foot and ankle remain in neutral position at all times.

Achilles Lengthening

- Same as for PTT transfer through IOM described earlier

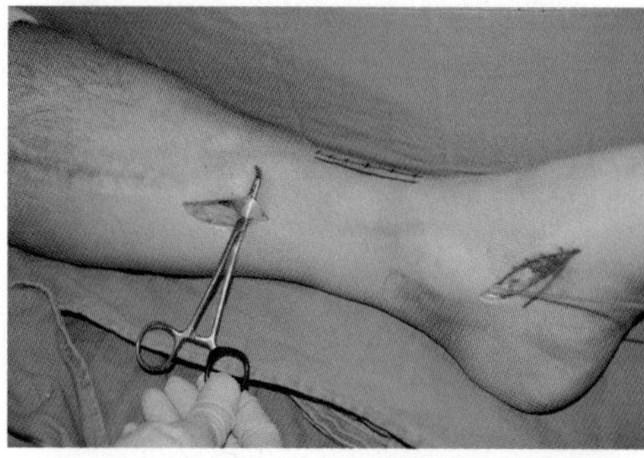

TECH FIG 10 • Harvest of posterior tibial tendon for bridle procedure.

Posterior Tibial Tendon Harvest

- Same as for PTT transfer through IOM described earlier (**TECH FIG 10**)

Harvest of the Peroneus Longus

- With an adequate skin bridge from the anterior ankle distal tibial incision, make a 2- to 3-cm incision immediately posterior to the fibula, about 8 cm proximal to the tip of the fibula at the level of the peroneus longus' musculotendinous junction (**TECH FIG 11A**).
- Protect the superficial peroneal nerve. However, with common peroneal nerve palsy, an injury to this terminal sensory branch will probably be inconsequential.
- Sharply divide the peroneal retinaculum 2 to 3 cm longitudinally over the musculotendinous junction of the peroneus longus.
- Divide the peroneus longus tendon at its musculotendinous junction (**TECH FIG 11B**).
- Place a tag suture in the transected distal end of the tendon.
- Make another 2- to 3-cm incision over the lateral cuboid (**TECH FIG 11A**).
  - Protect the sural nerve.
  - Isolate the peroneus longus tendon and pull its released proximal portion through this lateral foot wound (**TECH FIG 11C,D**).
- Tuck the peroneus longus tendon in the distal lateral foot wound to keep it from desiccating.
- The peroneus longus tendon will be passed to the anterior ankle wound (see below).

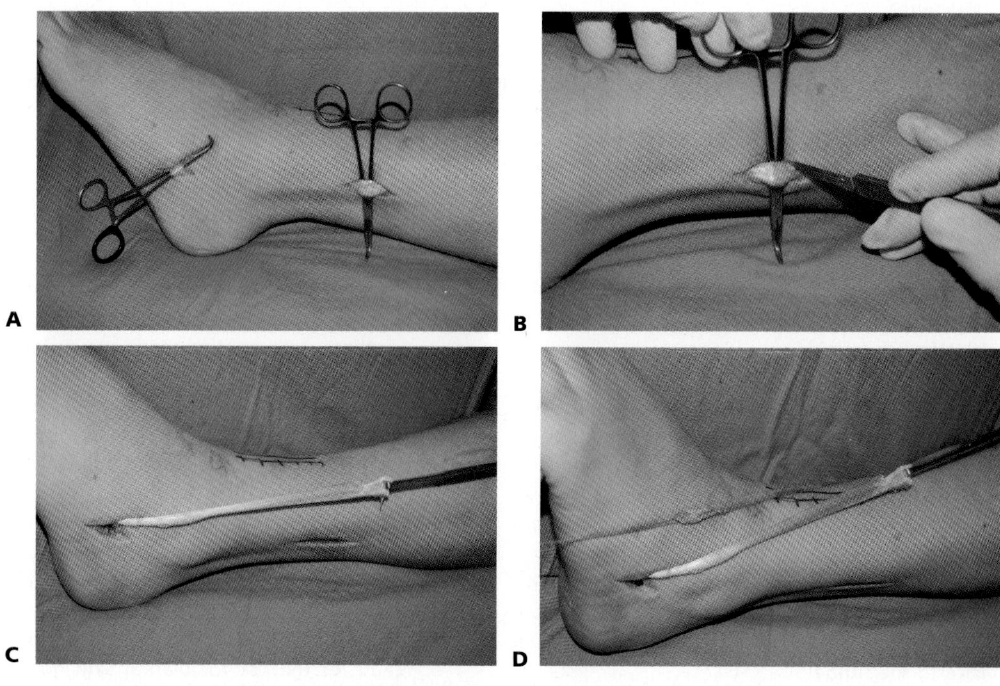

TECH FIG 11 • **A–C.** Harvest of peroneus longus for bridle procedure. **A, B.** Two small incisions, the first at the musculotendinous junction of peroneus longus and the second where the tendon courses around the cuboid. **C.** Peroneus longus transferred to distal lateral incision. **D.** Anticipated course for peroneus longus in bridle procedure (note also approximate course of posterior tibial tendon transfer).

Posterior Tibial Tendon Transfer Through the Interosseous Membrane

- Make an incision over the lateral aspect of the distal anterior tibia.
- Carefully expose the anterior IOM (TECH FIG 12A).
- Protect the superficial peroneal nerve.
  - Divide the extensor retinaculum over the tibialis anterior and extensor hallucis longus tendons.
  - Protect the deep neurovascular bundle (TECH FIG 12B).
- Protect the peroneal artery branch that courses on the anterior IOM.
- Create a generous window in the distal IOM (TECH FIG 12C).
  - From tibia to fibula
  - About 4 cm long
- Pass a curved Kelly or tonsil clamp through the IOM directly on the posterior aspect of the tibia to exit in the proximal medial wound (TECH FIG 12D).
  - The posterior neurovascular structures (tibial nerve and posterior tibial artery) are at risk, so be sure the clamp is *directly* on the posterior tibia.
- Use the tonsil clamp to grasp the tag sutures of the PTT.
- Pull the tag sutures and PTT from the medial wound to the lateral wound, keeping the tendon directly on the posterior aspect of the tibia (TECH FIG 12E).
- Be sure that the window in the IOM does not impinge on the transferred tendon. If there is stenosis, then further enlarge the window so that the tendon easily glides between the tibia and fibula.
- Keep the tendon end in the wound to limit desiccation.

Transfer of the Peroneus Longus

- Using a Kelly clamp, create a subcutaneous tunnel from the anterior distal tibial wound to the lateral foot wound (TECH FIG 13A).
  - Spread this tissue carefully with the clamp to avoid any soft tissue impingement within the tunnel.
  - Grasp the tag suture in the peroneus longus and pull the tendon from the lateral foot wound to the anterior distal tibial wound (TECH FIG 13B).

Transfer of Posterior Tibial Tendon Through the Tibialis Anterior Tendon

- Make a stab incision in the tibialis anterior tendon with proximal tension placed on the tibialis anterior tendon while the ankle is held in dorsiflexion.
  - This will tension the distal extent of the tibialis anterior tendon before it is secured to the PTT.
  - Avoid simply creating an incision in the tibialis anterior tendon in situ; this will render the tension in the medial aspect of the "bridle" ineffective.

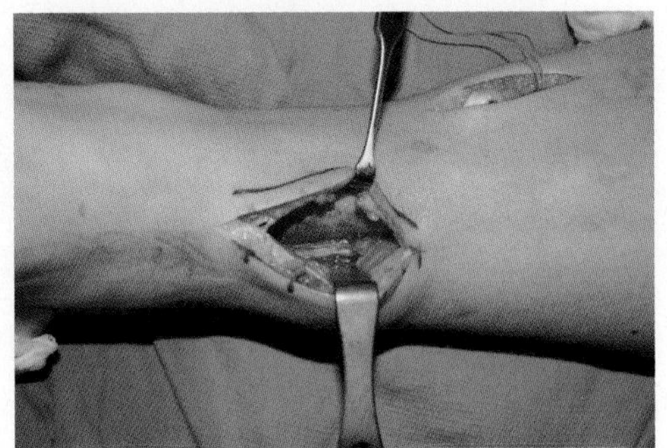
A

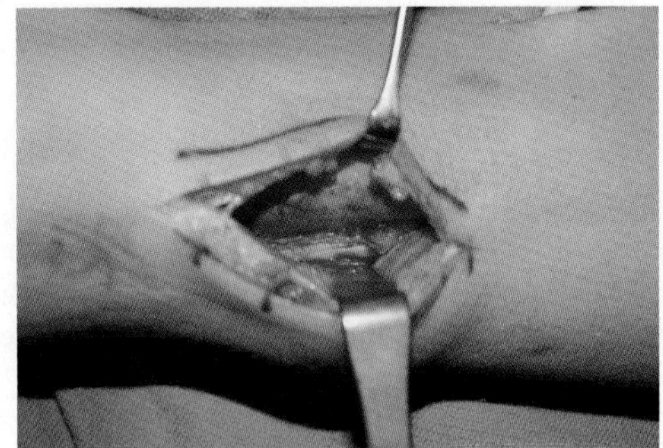
B

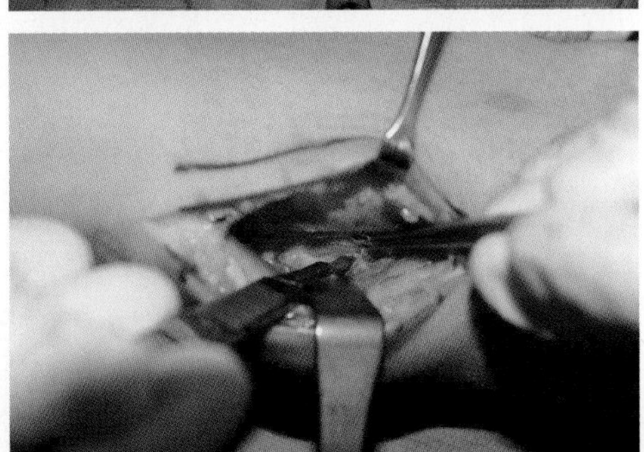
C

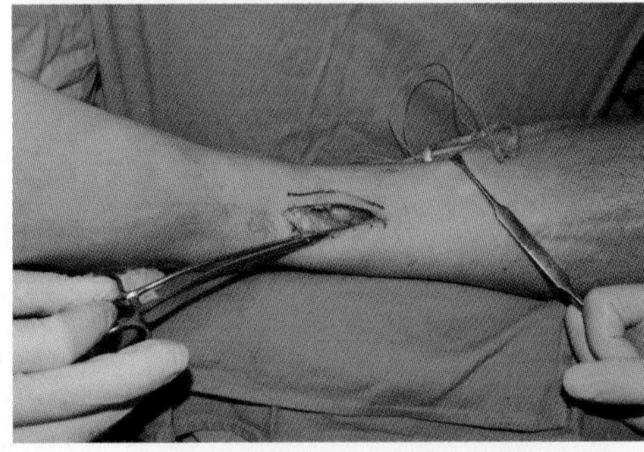
D

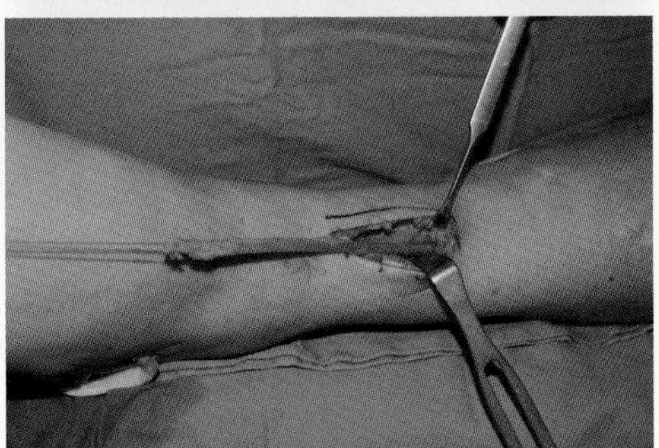
E

TECH FIG 12 • Creating an interosseous membrane (IOM) window to transfer the posterior tibial tendon to the anterior lower leg. **A.** Approach. **B.** Protecting deep neurovascular bundle and peroneal artery. **C.** Creating the window in the IOM. **D, E.** Transfer of the posterior tibial tendon (PTT) to the anterior lower leg. **D.** Blunt clamp is passed *directly* on the posterior tibia from anterior to proximal medial wound to grasp tag suture in PTT. **E.** Ensuring that the tendon does not bind in the IOM window.

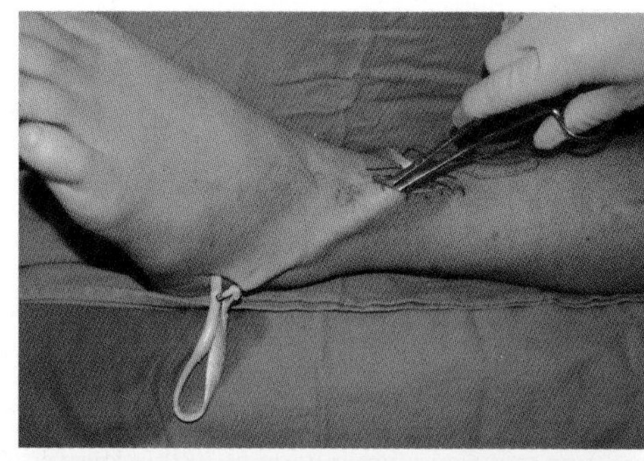

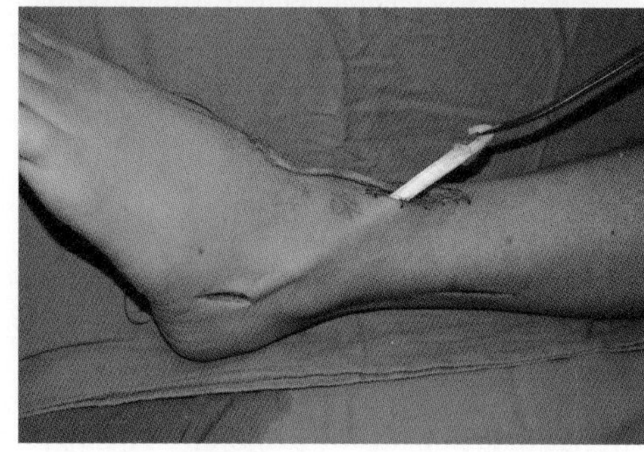

TECH FIG 13 • Transferring peroneus longus tendon from distal lateral foot wound to anterior lower leg wound. **A.** Subcutaneous tunnel to grasp free end of peroneus longus. **B.** Tendon transferred.

- Pass the PTT through this stab incision in the tibialis anterior (**TECH FIG 14**).
- If a more secure fixation between the tibialis anterior and PTT is desired, then consider a Pulvertaft weave.
  - While more weaving of the PTT through the tibialis anterior may afford greater fixation, it may in turn diminish the excursion of the PTT, thereby limiting the amount of distal PTT that will rest within the middle cuneiform's osseous tunnel.

Preparation of the Dorsum of the Foot and Anchoring the Posterior Tibial Tendon

- Similar to that described for PTT transfer anterior to the tibia (see earlier)
  - Transfer to the middle cuneiform
- A separate incision may be made (two limited incisions anteriorly) or the anterior distal tibial approach may be extended to the dorsum of the foot (single extensile anterior incision).
- Create an osseous tunnel in the middle cuneiform (**TECH FIG 15A**).
- Create a subcutaneous soft tissue tunnel from the dorsal foot incision to the more proximal and anterior lower leg incision using a curved Kelly clamp.
- Use the clamp to grasp the tag sutures and pull the tendon through the subcutaneous tunnel to the dorsal foot incision (**TECH FIG 15B**).
- Before anchoring the tendon in the osseous tunnel, pull the tendon via the tag sutures into the tunnel to be sure that the tunnel diameter is appropriate.
  - Pass a Beath pin or drill bit (has an eye to place suture) through the tunnel and the plantar skin (**TECH FIG 15C**). Because of the midfoot arch, this pin or drill bit will exit in the medial arch (**TECH FIG 15D**).
  - Dorsiflex the ankle.
  - With the tag sutures secured, pull the pin or drill bit through the plantar skin, thereby pulling the distal tendon end into the tunnel (**TECH FIG 15E**).

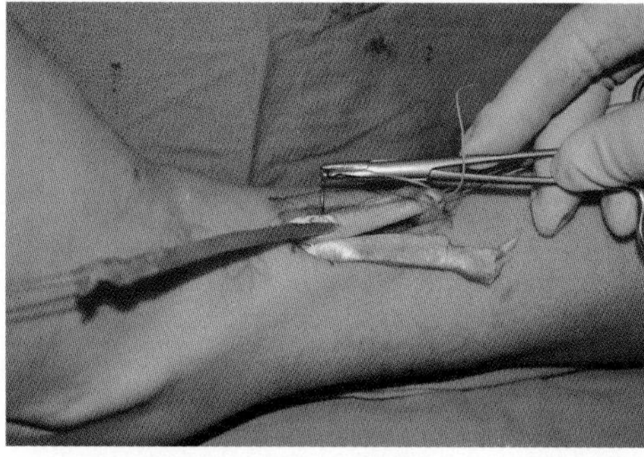

TECH FIG 14 • Posterior tibial tendon is transferred through the tibialis anterior. Note the pretensioning of the tibialis anterior to optimize tension in the bridle.

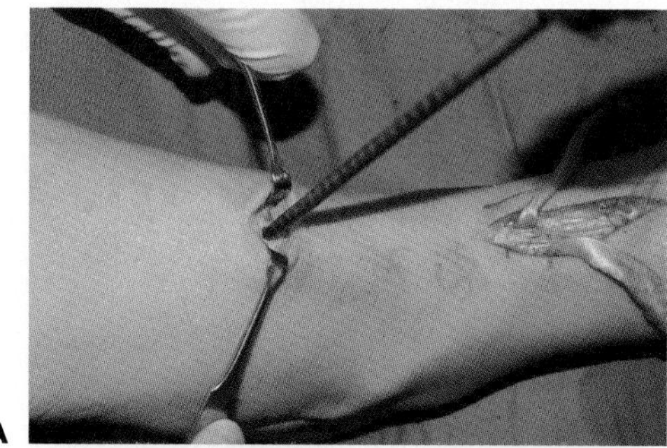

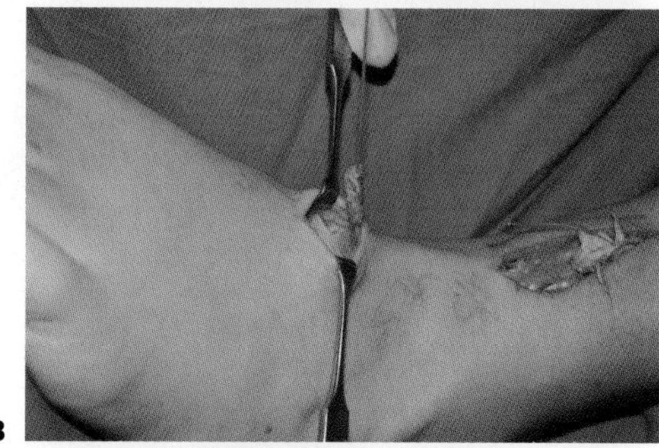

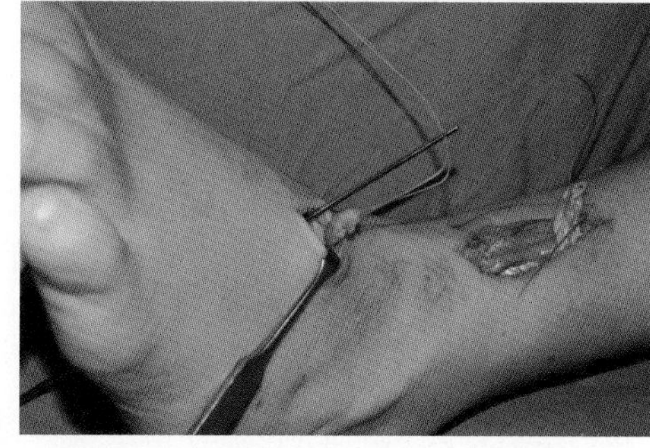

TECH FIG 15 • **A.** Creating the osseous tunnel in middle cuneiform. **B–G.** Transferring posterior tibial tendon (PTT) from anterior lower leg wound to dorsum of foot. **B.** Tendon passed through subcutaneous tunnel to dorsum of foot. **C.** Beath needle with tag sutures from PTT passed through osseous tunnel. *(continued)*

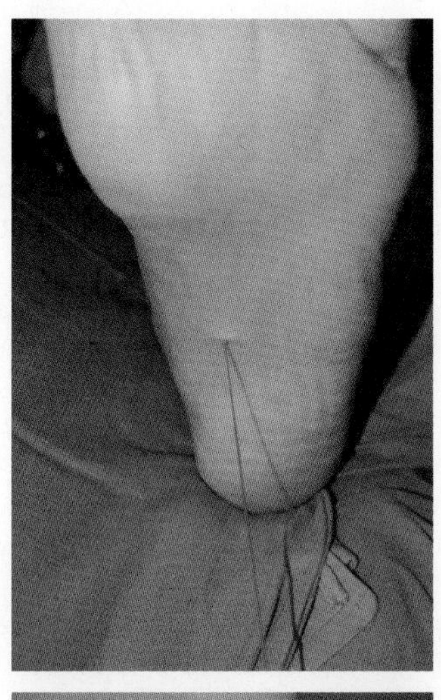

D

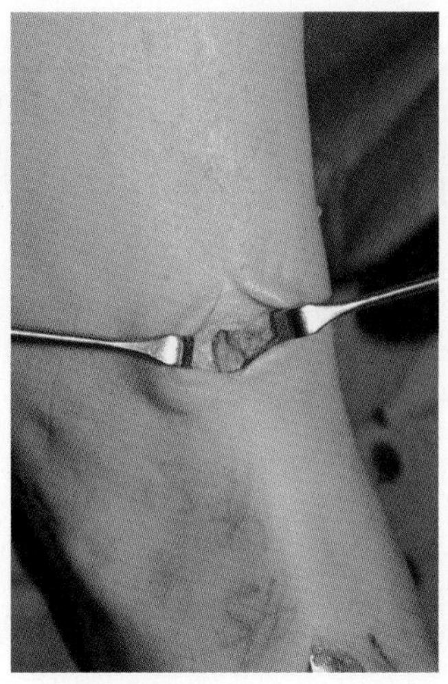

E

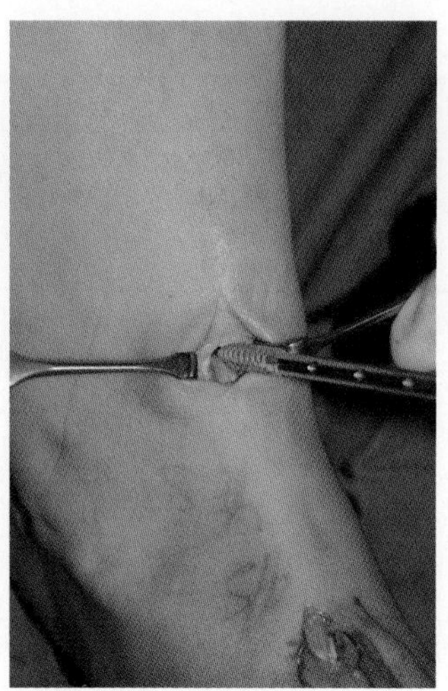

F

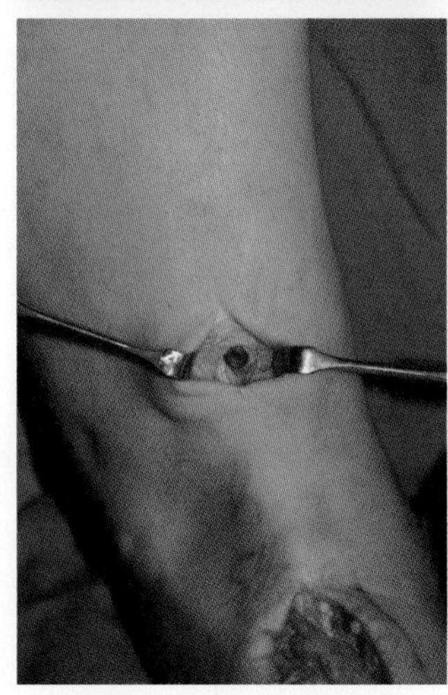

G

TECH FIG 15 • *(continued)* **D.** Tension on tag sutures on plantar foot. **E.** Tendon passed into middle cuneiform osseous tunnel. **F.** Positioning interference screw. **G.** Interference screw fully seated with appropriate PTT tension achieved.

- With the PTT properly tensioned in the second cuneiform's osseous tunnel, the PTT is anchored in a manner similar to that described earlier for the other techniques (interference screw with or without suture anchor in tunnel) (TECH FIG 15F,G).

Securing and Tensioning Tibialis Anterior and Peroneus Longus to the Posterior Tibial Tendon

- Maintain the ankle in 10 degrees of dorsiflexion.
- Balance the foot with respect to varus or valgus; it should have a neutral to slight valgus heel.
- Tibialis anterior
  - Tension the tibialis anterior proximally and suture the tibialis anterior and PTT to one another at the point where the PTT passes through the tibialis anterior.
  - Reinforce this connection with several more side-to-side sutures between the two tendons, both proximal and distal to where the PTT passes through the tibialis anterior.
- Peroneus longus
  - Approximate the peroneus longus to the PTT where it passes anterior to the distal tibia and ankle, with maximum tension applied (TECH FIG 16).
- Without support, the ankle should maintain dorsiflexed ankle and neutral hindfoot positions.

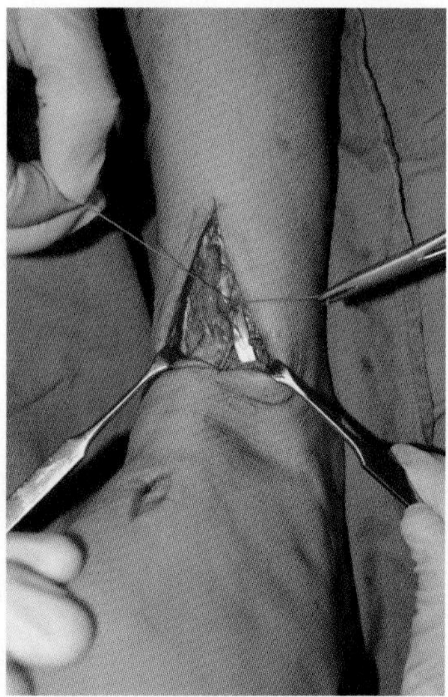

TECH FIG 16 • With the foot balanced, tibialis anterior and peroneus longus are secured to posterior tibial tendon transfer to create the bridle.

PEARLS AND PITFALLS

Tension of tendon transfer	■ Overtension rather than undertension, as some "stretching out" of the transfer is anticipated.
Achilles lengthening	■ The threshold to lengthen the gastrocnemius–soleus complex should be low. Obviously, with an Achilles contracture, lengthening is warranted. Transferring the PTT immediately reduces its power by one grade, so weakening the transfer's antagonist may be prudent. Overlengthening must be avoided.
Residual muscle function	■ Be sure the PTT is fully functional; if not, the transfer will not be dynamic but instead simply a tenodesis. This is the objective in flaccid paralysis, but not for a foot drop secondary to a common peroneal nerve palsy.
Route of PTT transfer	■ PTT transfer through the IOM may lead to stenosis. Provided there is no residual peroneal (eversion) function, then transferring the PTT anterior to the tibia may lead to an effective transfer without the risk of stenosis.
Bridle procedure	■ Balance the foot with proper tensioning of the tibialis anterior and peroneus longus components of the transfer.
Anchoring the transfer	■ With newer anchoring techniques, placing a suture button on the plantar foot secured to the tag suture is typically unnecessary.

POSTOPERATIVE CARE

- We routinely place a well-padded short-leg cast in the operating room to protect the transfer, with the ankle in maximum dorsiflexion.
- At first follow-up (2 to 3 weeks), we remove the cast while maintaining ankle dorsiflexion.
  - To protect the transfer, the ankle should not be allowed to plantarflex.
  - A new short-leg cast is applied, one that allows touch-down weight bearing.
- Follow up at 5 to 6 weeks from surgery.
  - The short-leg cast is removed, again protecting dorsiflexion.
  - Wound inspection
    - Without allowing the ankle to plantarflex, the cast is removed.
  - Consideration may be given to creating a temporary AFO.
  - We typically place the patient in a short-leg walking cast at this point, with the ankle in near-maximum dorsiflexion. The patient is encouraged to walk.
- At 8 to 10 weeks
  - The patient can typically discontinue use of the cast.
  - AFO for ambulation is typically worn until 4 to 5 months after surgery. During the final month of brace wear, the surgeon can consider hinging the AFO and placing a plantarflexion stop at neutral.
  - A cam boot is used for sleeping; it is typically worn until 4 to 5 months after surgery.
  - A physical therapy program is initiated to train the PTT to function as an ankle dorsiflexor.
- Return to brace-free full function is not recommended before 6 months.

OUTCOMES

- Select case series of PTT transfers for foot drop and bridle procedures suggest a satisfactory outcome in a majority of cases.

COMPLICATIONS

- Infection
- Wound dehiscence. The wound must be healed before initiating active dorsiflexion (usually not a problem because cast is maintained for at least 8 weeks).
- Failure of the tendon transfer anchoring point; less common with newer anchoring system
- Imbalance of bridle procedure: tibialis anterior and peroneus longus must be properly tensioned intraoperatively

REFERENCES

1. Elsner A, Barg A, Stufkens SA, et al. Lambrinudi arthrodesis with posterior tibialis transfer in adult drop-foot. Foot Ankle Int 2010;31:30–37.
2. Hove LM, Nilsen PT. Posterior tibial tendon transfer for drop-foot: 20 cases followed for 1–5 years. Acta Orthop Scand 1998;69:608–610.
3. Mizel MS, Temple HT, Scranton PE Jr, et al. Role of the peroneal tendons in the production of the deformed foot with posterior tibial tendon deficiency. Foot Ankle Int 1999;20:285–289.
4. Morita S, Muneta T, Yamamoto H, et al. Tendon transfer for equinovarus deformed foot caused by cerebrovascular disease. Clin Orthop Relat Res 1998;350:166–173.
5. Rodriguez RP. The Bridle procedure in the treatment of paralysis of the foot. Foot Ankle 1992;13:63–69.
6. Soares D. Tibialis posterior transfer for the correction of foot drop in leprosy: long-term outcome. J Bone Joint Surg Br 1996 Jan;78(1):61–2.
7. Sundararaj GD. Tibialis posterior transfer (circumtibial route) for foot-drop deformity. Indian J Lepr 1984;56:555–562.

Exam Table for Foot and Ankle

Examination	Technique	Illustration	Grading & Significance
Achilles tendon rupture: Active plantarflexion test	With the patient supine, active plantarflexion power is tested.		Positive: Weak plantarflexion power graded 1 to 5 Poorly sensitive and unreliable, as powerful plantarflexion may still be possible due to the action of other ankle plantarflexors.
Achilles tendon rupture: Knee flexion test	While prone, the patient actively flexes the knee. The examiner observes foot position and compares it with the other side.		Positive: Foot falls into neutral or dorsiflexion. Negative: Foot maintains plantarflexion posture. Less reliable test; may be difficult to perform due to acute pain. 88% sensitive.
Achilles tendon rupture: Palpable gap test	Gentle palpation of the tendon reveals a defect at the rupture site.		Gap present or absent. Gap present indicates complete Achilles rupture with separation of the ruptured ends. More reliable when done early after rupture; 73% sensitive.
Achilles tendon rupture: Thompson or Simmonds test	With the patient in prone position, the examiner squeezed the calf at the gastrocsoleus muscle level. Limited ankle plantarflexion occurs (as compared to the unaffected side).		Positive test if ruptured, demonstrating limited ankle plantarflexion. Not as reliable in chronic ruptures as it is in acute ruptures due to formation of "pseudo tendon" scar between ruptured ends.
Ankle instability: Anterior drawer test	The patient sits on the edge of the examination table with the legs dangling and the feet in a few degrees of plantarflexion. The examiner places one hand on the anterior aspect of the tibia and grasps the calcaneus with the palm of the other hand. The examiner then pulls the calcaneus anteriorly while pushing the tibia posteriorly. This tests the anterior talofibular ligament. To test the calcaneofibular ligament, the same maneuver is performed with the ankle in a dorsiflexed position.		Typically, anterior drawer is increased when the foot is externally rotated (vs. internally rotated); this is a highly sensitive test for medial ankle instability. The examiner should look for a difference of 3 to 5mm in the relationship between the lateral talus and the anterior aspect of the fibula. On side-to-side comparison the unstable side will have a greater degree of translation. Indicates an insufficient anterior talofibular ligament.

(continued)

Examination	Technique	Illustration	Grading & Significance
Ankle instability: Suction sign test	Anterior drawer test as described above.	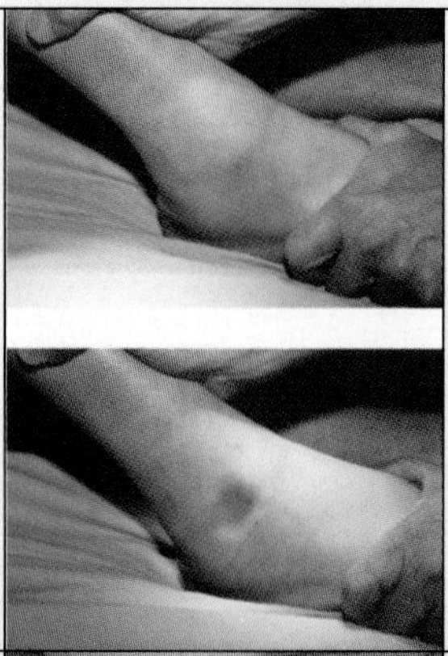	As the heel is delivered from the back of the ankle in an unstable ankle, a dimpling will occur in the region just anterior and inferior to the tip of the fibula as a vacuum is created by the talus sliding out from the mortise.
Distal tarsal tunnel test	The examiner palpates for medial hindfoot tenderness (plus or minus swelling) at the "soft spot"—the distal edge of the abductor hallucis muscle about 5 cm anterior to the posterior of the heel at the intersection of the plantar and medial skin.	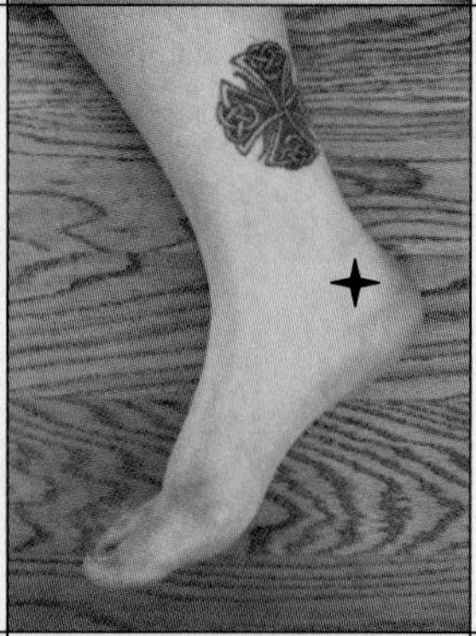	Tenderness corresponds with the course of the lateral plantar nerve and its first branch and is associated with nerve entrapment or neuritis.
Equinus contracture	The hindfoot is held in neutral position and the midfoot is aligned by internal rotation of the navicular. Then the forefoot is placed into pronation and the medial ray is held firm. Then the examiner manipulates the foot into dorsiflexion with the knee extended as well as with the knee flexed.	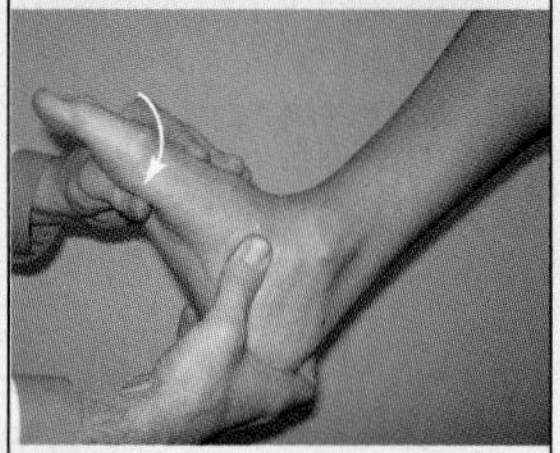	With knee extended: isolated gastrocnemius contracture when unable to achieve neutral dorsiflexion. Gastrocsoleus contracture is present when the examiner cannot get the ankle to neutral with the knee flexed. May need to perform a gastrocnemius recession or Achilles lengthening procedure concomitantly when there is 5 degrees of equinus in the ankle.
Equinus contracture: Silfverskiold test	With the patient sitting, the ankle is maximally dorsiflexed with the knee extended and the foot held in a neutral position. The knee is then flexed and the ankle dorsiflexed again.	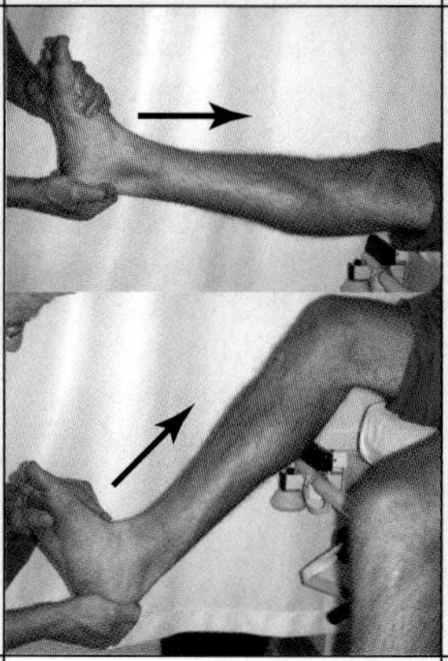	Positive: When the foot is held in equinus correcting to above neutral with the knee flexed; indicates a tight Achilles tendon within the gastrocnemius muscle. The deformity may aggravate an unstable ankle.
First MTP joint grind test	The examiner grinds the MTP joint with an axially directed force.	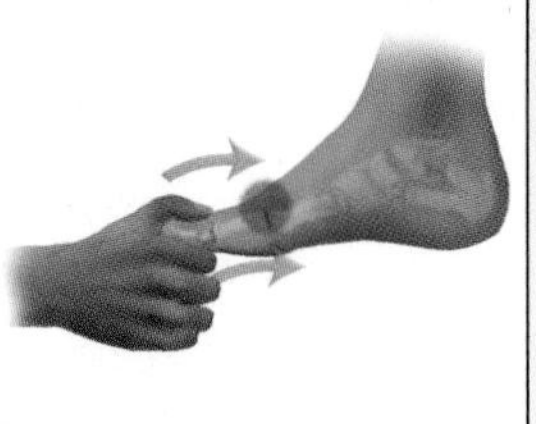	Pain at MTP joint associated with osteochondral lesion or severe degeneration. Usually not symptomatic in mild cases. If this test causes severe pain, one may consider imaging studies. Not normally painful unless an osteochondral defect is present or degeneration is advanced. If painful, then arthrodesis is indicated.

Examination	Technique	Illustration	Grading & Significance
First MTP joint hypertension test to distinguish hallux rigidus from sesamoid pathology	The big toe is hyperextended.	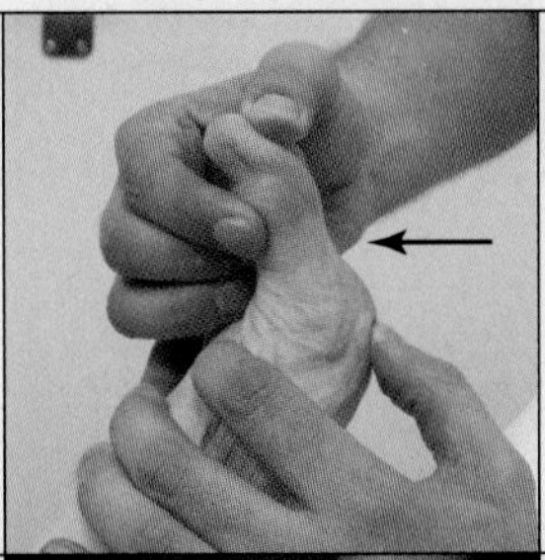	The examiner must discern between rising pain at the plantar (sesamoid) or dorsal (hallux rigidus) aspect of the MTP joint. High specificity with appropriate history, but otherwise not specific.
First tarsometatarsal hypermobility test (perspective 1)	The examiner grasps the lesser metatarsal heads with one hand and passively plantarflexes and dorsiflexes the first metatarsal with the other hand.	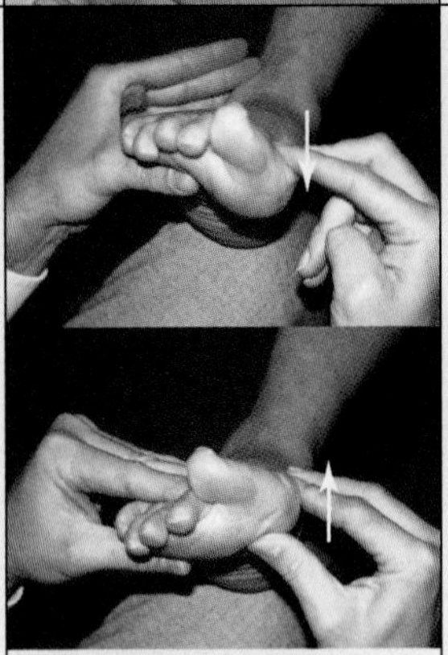	Hypermobility has been defined as an elevation of 5 to 8 mm above the level of the second metatarsal, but the diagnosis of hypermobility is often more subjective. Hypermobility at the tarsometatarsal joint creates a valgus moment at the MTP joint that may contribute to failure of distal hallux valgus correction.
First tarsometatarsal joint excursion (perspective 2)	One hand is placed with the thumb and index finger located plantar and dorsal to the first metatarsal head and the opposite thumb and index finger placed plantar and dorsal to the second metatarsal hand. The first ray is then dorsiflexed and plantarflexed to end range of motion and the intervals between the thumb and index finger of both hands are noted and measured.	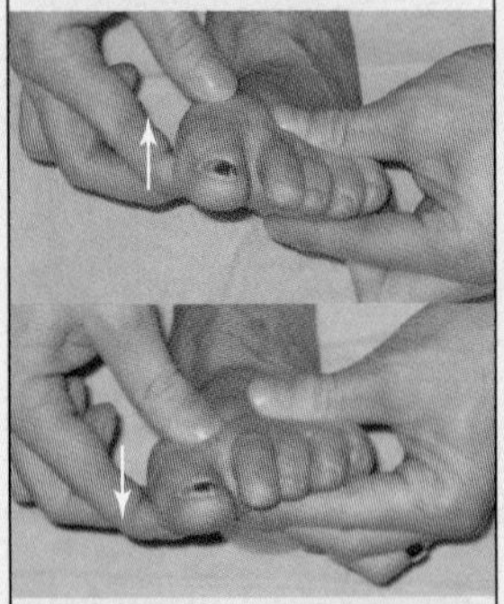	The normal first ray excursion is 10 mm (5 mm of dorsiflexion and 5 mm of plantarflexion). Hypermobility can be defined as total excursion >15 mm. Hypermobility of the first ray is significant when contemplating a surgical procedure for the hallux valgus deformity. If hypermobility is present, a first tarsometatarsal joint fusion may be more appropriate.
Fixed forefoot varus	The calcaneus is held in a neutral position (out of valgus) and any fixed elevation of the first ray relative to the fifth is noted.	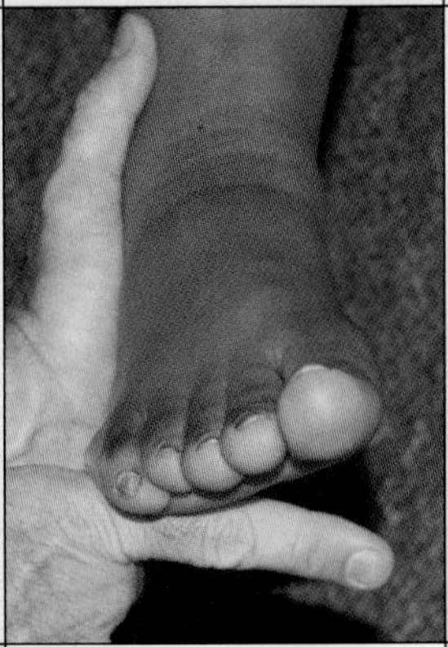	The severity of deformity is noted in degrees. Fixed forefoot varus must be accounted for in any treatment algorithm and is usually the first component of the deformity to become rigid.
Flexor hallucis longus tenosynovitis	The pain is produced with active–passive motion of the hallux while a thumb palpates the tendon for tenderness and crepitus.	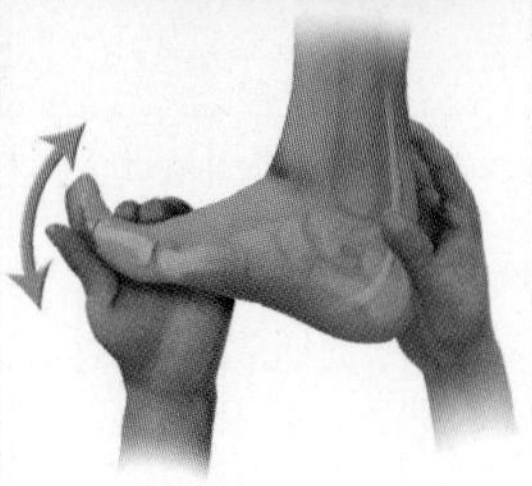	The presence of flexor hallucis longus tenosynovitis should be documented and treated accordingly.

(continued)

Examination	Technique	Illustration	Grading & Significance
Forced dorsiflexion of the first MTP joint	The examiner gradually increases dorsiflexion of the first MTP joint.		Pain is associated with impingement of the base of the proximal phalanx and metatarsal head. The amount of dorsiflexion obtained is measured as well. Maximum extension is characteristically limited and pain is sometimes present. Also, the osteophytic ridge can be best palpated in the dorsolateral portion of the joint. Pain associated with stretching of the extensor hallucis longus, capsule, and inflamed synovium; often occurs earlier in the disease process. Maximal flexion is sometimes limited, but pain is best brought out. Tenderness is commonly identified in the dorsolateral aspect of the joint.
Lesser MTP joint pushup test	With the patient seated and knee flexed, the examiner dorsiflexes the ankle to neutral by applying pressure under the metatarsal heads. The correction of the toe deformity with this manuver is noted.		If the deformity is flexible, with the pushup test the MTP joint will flex to its normal position. If not, it will remain extended defining a fixed deformity. Semiflexible deformities are those that correct partially with the pushup test. A flexible deformity is amenable to soft tissue procedures, including tendon transfers. Fixed deformities will need extensive procedures, including osteotomies. This test is also useful in the operating room to assess residual MTP joint contracture after the hammertoe has been corrected at the proximal interphalangeal joint. Residual MTP joint contracture necessitates additional surgical correction at the MTP joint, such as extensor tendon lengthening, capsular release, or collateral ligament release.
Lesser MTP joint stability test	The metatarsal bone and the proximal phalanx are stabilized and stress is placed in a dorsoplantar direction, attempting to subluxate the joint.		Stage 0: no laxity to dorsal translation; stage 1: the base of the proximal phalanx can be subluxated with the dorsal stress; stage 2: the proximal phalangeal base can be dislocated and relocated; stage 3: the base of the proximal phalanx is fixed in a dislocated position. For the initial stages (0, 1, 2) a tendon transfer associated with a dorsal MTP soft tissue release will stabilize the deformity. For fixed MTP dislocations a bone-shortening procedure should be added to the soft tissue procedures.
Lesser toe manipulation test	Gentle manual straightening of the toe to assess the ability of the toe to correct to neutral.		If the toe completely corrects to neutral it is considered a flexible deformity. If the toe does not completely correct, it is considered a fixed deformity. A flexible deformity can be addressed with a soft tissue procedure such as a flexor-to-extensor tendon transfer. A fixed deformity will require bone resection for surgical correction.

Examination	Technique	Illustration	Grading & Significance
MTP joint vertical Lachman test	The examiner stabilizes the hallux metatarsal with the thumb and index finger of one hand while attempting to translate the proximal phalanx in a dorsal–plantar direction with the thumb and index finger of the other hand.	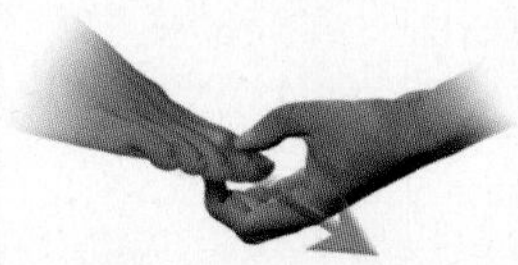	A positive test is any laxity greater than the contralateral side.
Mulder test for Morton's neuroma	With the patient prone and the knee flexed 90 degrees, the examiner deeply palpates the plantar aspect web space with the index finger. Maintaining this pressure, the examiner gently squeezes the forefoot.	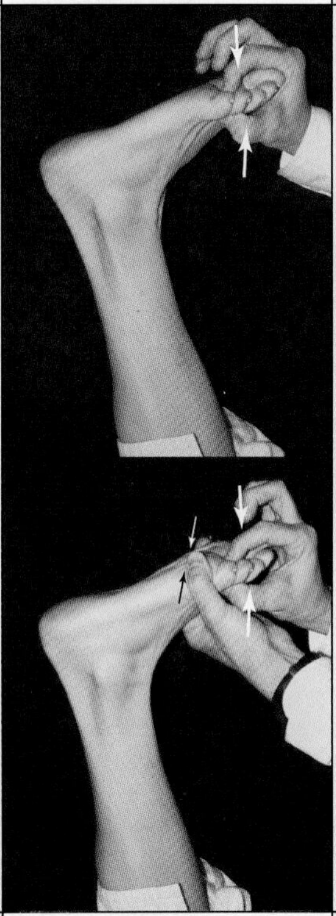	Palpable "click" and reproduction of symptoms help confirm the diagnosis.
Percussion test for neuralgia	Percussion over the dorsomedial hallucal nerve or terminal hallucal branch of the deep peroneal nerve in the first web space.	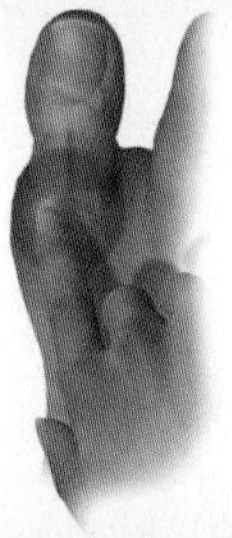	Hypesthesias or radiating symptoms can occur in the terminal nerve branches because of compression from synovitis or dorsal osteophytes. Most clinicians simply note a positive or negative percussion test. Large dorsal osteophytes may compress the dorsal medial or lateral digital nerve.
Posterior ankle impingement: Maquirriain	In the seated position (90 degrees hip flexion, 90 degrees knee flexion, neutral ankle position), the subject is asked to slide both feet forward while maintaining full contact on the floor. Limited ankle plantarflexion or posterior ankle pain will be evidenced by the inability to maintain forefoot contact.	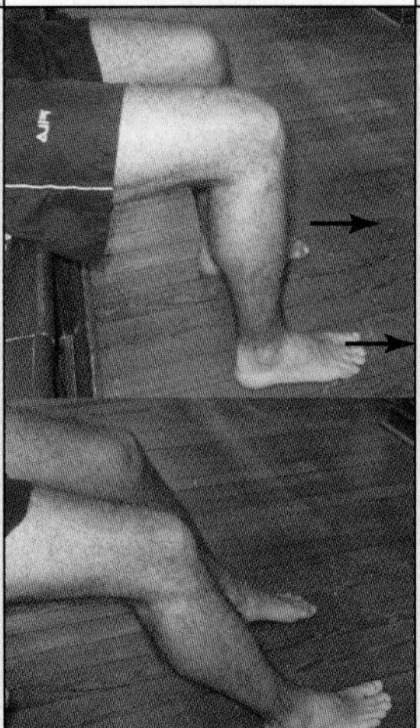	Negative: symmetric motion; positive: asymmetric motion due to posterior ankle pain or limited ankle plantarflexion. In this office test the examiner should try to reproduce typical painful motion of posterior ankle impingement syndrome in closed position. It also allows the examiner to estimate the passive ROM limitation.

(continued)

Examination	Technique	Illustration	Grading & Significance
Posterior ankle impingement: Passive forced plantarflexion test (perspective 1)	With the patient in prone position with both feet out of the table, the physician performs a forced plantarflexion maneouver. Limitation of range of motion can also be estimated.		Discomfort; posterior ankle pain. Normal ankle ROM is 18 degrees dorsiflexion and 48 degrees plantarflexion. In this office test the examiner should try to reproduce typical painful motion of posterior ankle impingement syndrome. It also allows the examiner to estimate the passive ROM limitation.
Posterior ankle impingement: Passive forced plantarflexion test (perspective 2)	The ankle is passively flexed while the subtalar joint is held in neutral position. The opposite thumb and index finger are used to palpate the retromalleolar regions for any crepitus.		Sharp pain or crepitus is produced at full plantarflexion with a positive test.
Tibiotalar joint line palpation	Digital palpation of medial joint line with simultaneous application of valgus force.		Valgus tilt present or absent. Presence of valgus tilt indicates insufficiency of deltoid ligament.
Toe palpation	The examiner palpates the distal and proximal interphalangeal joints and the MTP joint for points of maximal tenderness.		The proximal interphalagneal joint should be the area of maximal tenderness, but the tip of the toe may be painful as well.
Windlass mechanism test	The examiner palpates the affected versus unaffected plantar fascia while recreating the windlass mechanism (by combining passive ankle dorsiflexion and 1–5 MTP joint dorsiflexion).		Less firm or tense plantar fascia compared to the opposite side indicates chronic attenuation or incompetence of the plantar fascia.

INDEX

Page numbers followed by *f* and *t* indicated figures and tables, respectively.

B

CCS0311